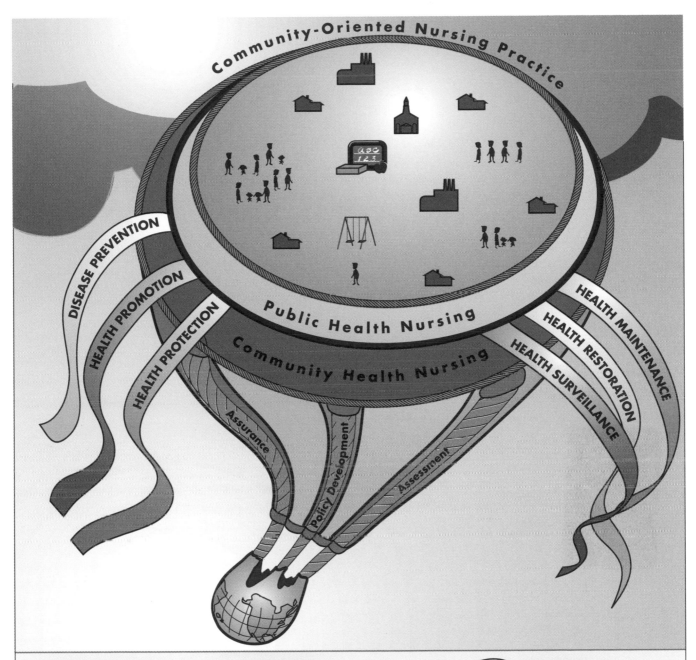

Overarching Concept
- Community-oriented nursing practice

Subconcepts
- Community health nursing
- Public health nursing

Foundational Pillars
- Assurance
- Assessment
- Policy development

Settings
- Community
- Environment
- School
- Industry
- Church
- Prisons
- Playground
- Home

Clients
- Individuals
- Families
- Groups
- Populations
- Communities

Interventions
- Disease Prevention
- Health Promotion
- Health Protection
- Health Maintenance
- Health Restoration
- Health Surveillance

Services
- Personal Health Services
- Populations/Aggregate Services
- Community Services

CONGRATULATIONS

You now have access to Mosby's "Get Smart" Bonus Package!

Here's what's included to help you "Get Smart"

sign on at:

http://www.mosby.com/MERLIN/community_stanhope

A Web site just for you as you learn pediatric nursing with the new 5th edition of
Community and Public Health Nursing

what you will receive:

Whether you're a student, an instructor, or a clinician, you'll find
information just for you. Things like:
- Content Updates ● Links to Related Products
- Author Information . . . and more

plus:

WebLinks

An exciting new program that allows you to directly access
hundreds of active web sites keyed specifically to the content
of this book. The WebLinks are continually updated, with new
ones added as they develop. **Simply peel off the sticker on this page
and register with the listed passcode.**

If passcode sticker is removed, this
textbook cannot be returned to Mosby, Inc.

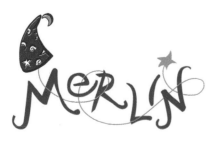

Mosby's **E**lectronic **R**esource **L**inks & **I**nformation **N**etwork

Mosby

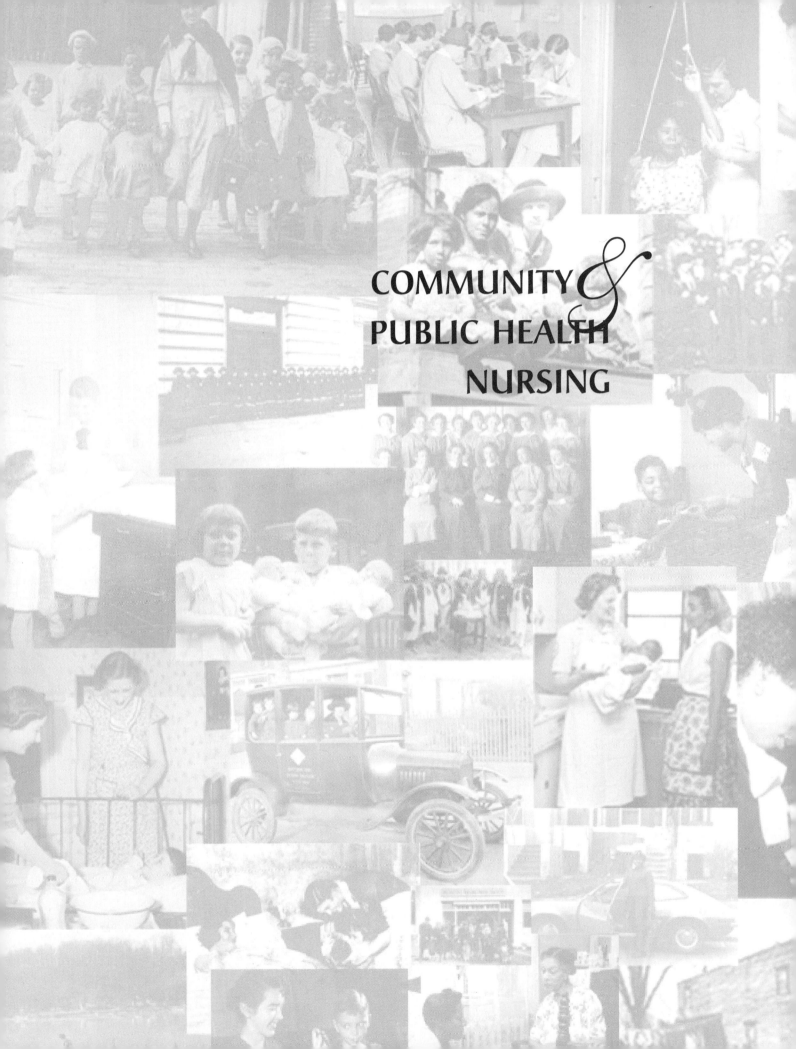

COMMUNITY& PUBLIC HEALTH NURSING

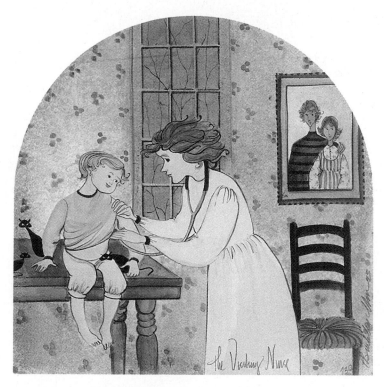

Visiting Nurse, by P. Buckley Moss
Copyright 1993, P. Buckley Moss
From the archives of the P. Buckley Moss Museum
Waynesboro, Virginia

COMMUNITY&
PUBLIC HEALTH
NURSING **FIFTH EDITION**

Marcia Stanhope, RN, DSN, FAAN, c
Professor and Associate Dean
College of Nursing
University of Kentucky
Lexington, Kentucky

Jeanette Lancaster, RN, PhD, FAAN
Dean and Sadie Heath Cabaniss Professor
School of Nursing
University of Virginia
Charlottesville, Virginia

Illustrated

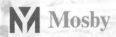 Mosby

St. Louis Baltimore Boston Carlsbad Chicago Minneapolis New York Philadelphia Portland
London Milan Sydney Tokyo Toronto

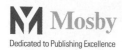
Mosby
Dedicated to Publishing Excellence

Editor-in-Chief Sally Schrefer
Executive Editor June D. Thompson
Senior Developmental Editor Linda Caldwell
Project Manager Dana Peick
Senior Production Editor Jeffrey Patterson
Designer Amy Buxton

*Front Cover and Part Opener photos provided courtesy of
the Visiting Nurses Association of Washington, DC*

FIFTH EDITION

Copyright © 2000 by Mosby, Inc.

Previous editions copyrighted 1984, 1988, 1992, 1996

NOTICE

Pharmacology is an ever-changing field. Standard safety precautions must be followed, but as new research and clinical experience broaden our knowledge, changes in treatment and drug therapy may become necessary or appropriate. Readers are advised to check the most current product information provided by the manufacturer of each drug to be administered to verify the recommended dose, the method and duration of administration, and contraindications. It is the responsibility of the licensed health care provider, relying on experience and knowledge of the patient, to determine dosages and the best treatment for each individual patient. Neither the publisher nor the editor assumes any liability for any injury and/or damage to persons or property arising from this publication.

Mosby, Inc.
A Harcourt Health Sciences Company
11830 Westline Industrial Drive
St. Louis, Missouri 63146

Printed in the United States of America

International Standard Book Number   0-323-00749-X

99 00 01 02 03 GW/KPT 9 8 7 6 5 4 3 2 1

About the Authors

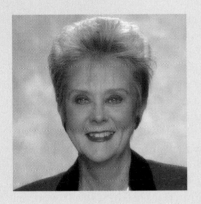

Marcia Stanhope, RN, DSN, FAAN, c

Marcia Stanhope is currently Associate Dean and Professor at the University of Kentucky College of Nursing in Lexington, Kentucky. She has practiced community and home health nursing and has served as an administrator and consultant in home health, and she has been involved in the development of two nurse-managed centers. She has taught community health, public health, epidemiology, primary care nursing, and administration courses. Dr. Stanhope formerly directed the Division of Community Health Nursing and Administration at the University of Kentucky. She has been responsible for both undergraduate and graduate courses in community health nursing. She has also taught at the University of Virginia and the University of Alabama, Birmingham. Her presentations and publications have been in the areas of home health, community health and community-based nursing practice, and primary care nursing. Dr. Stanhope holds a diploma in nursing from the Good Samaritan Hospital in Lexington, Kentucky, and a bachelor of science in nursing from the University of Kentucky. She has a master's degree in public health nursing from Emory University in Atlanta and a doctorate of science in nursing from the University of Alabama, Birmingham. Dr. Stanhope is the co-author of three other Mosby publications: *Handbook of Community-Based and Home Health Nursing Practice, Public and Community Health Nurse's Consultant,* and *Case Studies in Community Health Nursing Practice: A Problem-Based Learning Approach.*

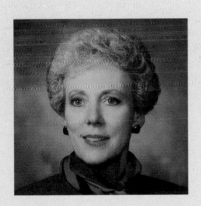

Jeanette Lancaster, RN, PhD, FAAN

Jeanette Lancaster is currently the Sadie Heath Cabaniss Professor of Nursing and Dean at the University of Virginia School of Nursing in Charlottesville, Virginia. She has practiced psychiatric nursing and taught both psychiatric and community health nursing. She formerly directed the master's program in community health nursing at the University of Alabama, Birmingham, and served as dean of the School of Nursing at Wright State University in Dayton, Ohio. Her publications and presentations have been largely in the areas of community and public health nursing, leadership and change, and the significance of nurses to effective primary health care. Dr. Lancaster is a graduate of the University of Tennessee, Memphis, College of Nursing. She holds a master's degree in psychiatric nursing from Case Western Reserve University and a doctorate in public health from the University of Oklahoma. Dr. Lancaster is the author of another Mosby publication, *Nursing Issues in Leading and Managing Change.*

Dedication

This text, now in its fifth edition, has spanned 2 decades and with this edition crosses into a second century of existence. The expertise and energy of the contributors and their quest to make a difference in the health of our clients, in the future of nursing professionals, and to excellence in practice is reflected in all of the editions, past and present. This edition of the text is dedicated to all contributors who have been involved in this project in its 18-year history, with special thanks to you as an aggregate of scholars and as individual experts. Thanks also to Peg Teachey for assisting me in completing this edition of the text and to Jeanette for her endurance over time.

A special dedication to my friend Dottie Carter and to the memory of Jim Carter. The Carters were instrumental in making my first community-oriented project a success. You were very important to the launching of my career.

Marcia Stanhope

None of us succeeds in meeting our career goals without the support, encouragement, and friendship of many caring people. As I reflect back over my many years in nursing, I realize that there have been many family members, friends, and colleagues who have inspired, urged, and prodded me to achieve as much as was humanly possible. Special thanks to my parents, Howard and Glada Miller, who simply thought nothing was impossible and who were always so pleased by my accomplishments no matter how large or small. Over the years, my husband, Wade, and my daughters, Melinda and Jennifer, have been tremendous sources of inspiration and colleagueship. While I am indebted to many, three people stand out as caring, giving, and supportive over time: Virginia Jarratt, my first dean; Marcia Stanhope, friend and colleague through five editions of this text; and Brenda Carsley, my assistant and "right-hand woman." Thanks to each of you for being such a wonderful friend and supporter. I also pay special thanks to Teresa Carroll and Leslie Sadler, who served as administrative interns and provided immense help with the fifth edition.

Jeanette Lancaster

Contributors

Dyan Aretakis, MSN, FNP
Project Director
Teen Health Center
University of Virginia Health Sciences Center
Charlottesville, Virginia

Ruth D. Berry, RN, MSN
Assistant Professor, Community Health Nursing
  Administration
University of Kentucky
Coordinator, Parish Nurse Services
Coordinator, Nurse-Managed Clinic for Homeless
Lexington, Kentucky

Christine DiMartile Bolla, RN, DNSc
Adjunct Professor
Department of Nursing
Western University of Health Sciences
Chico, California

Joyce Bonick, RN, JD
Nursing Regulation Consultant
Kentucky Board of Nursing
Louisville, Kentucky

Marjorie Buchanan, RN, MS
Senior Program Officer
Independence Foundation
Philadelphia, Pennsylvania

Angeline Bushy, PhD, RN, CS
Professor - Bert Fish Endowed Chair
Community Health Nursing
University of Central Florida
Daytona Beach, Florida

Jacquelyn C. Campbell, PhD, RN, FAAN
Anna D. Wolf Endowed Professor
Associate Dean for Doctoral Education Programs and
  Research
School of Nursing
Johns Hopkins University
Baltimore, Maryland

Ann H. Cary, PhD, MPH, RN, A-CCC
Professor and Coordinator of Doctoral Nursing Program
George Mason University
College of Nursing
Fairfax, Virginia

Marcia K. Cowan, MSN, CPNP
Pediatric Nurse Practitioner
St. Thomas Pediatric Center
Tullahoma, Tennessee

Cynthia E. Degazon, PhD, RN
Associate Professor
Hunter Bellevue School of Nursing
Hunter College of the City University
New York, New York

Janna Dieckmann, PhD, RN
Visiting Assistant Professor
School of Nursing
University of North Carolina at Chapel Hill
Chapel Hill, North Carolina

Mary Eure Fisher, RN, MSN
Public Health Nurse Manager
Thomas Jefferson Health District
Clinical Instructor
University of Virginia School of Nursing
Charlottesville, Virginia

Kathleen Fletcher, RN, MSN, CS, GNP
Director, Geriatric Services
University of Virginia Health Systems
Charlottesville, Virginia

Beverly C. Flynn, PhD, RN, FAAN
Professor, Department of Environments for Health
Director, Institute of Action Research for Community
  Health
Head, World Health Organization Collaborating Center in
  Healthy Cities
Indiana University School of Nursing
Indianapolis, Indiana

Sara T. Fry, PhD, RN, FAAN
Henry R. Luce Professor of Nursing Ethics
School of Nursing
Boston College
Boston, Massachusetts

Jean Goeppinger, PhD, RN, FAAN
Professor and Chair
Department of Community and Mental Health
School of Nursing
University of North Carolina
Chapel Hill, North Carolina

Patty J. Hale, RN, PhD, FNP
Associate Professor
Department of Nursing
Lynchburg College
Lynchburg, Virginia

Shirley May Harmon Hanson, RN, PMHNP, PhD, FAAN, LMFT, CFLE
Professor
School of Nursing
Oregon Health Sciences University
Portland, Oregon

Susan B. Hassmiller, PhD, RN
Senior Program Officer
The Robert Wood Johnson Foundation
Princeton, New Jersey

Patricia B. Howard, PhD, RN, CNAA
Associate Professor and Coordinator
Advanced Practice Psychiatric/Mental Health Nursing
College of Nursing
University of Kentucky
Lexington, Kentucky

Kathleen Huttlinger, PhD, RN
Director, Grants and Sponsored Programs
Samuel Merritt College
Oakland, California

L. Louise Ivanov, DNS, RN
Associate Professor
School of Nursing
University of Virginia
Charlottesville, Virginia

Cheryl B. Jones, RN, PhD, CNAA
Expert, Center for Primary Care Research
Agency for Health Care Policy and Research
Center for Primary Care Research
Rockville, Maryland

Kim Dupree Jones, RNC, MN, FNP
Doctoral Student
Oregon Health Sciences University
Portland, Oregon

Joanna Rowe Kaakinen, RN, PhD
Associate Professor
School of Nursing
University of Portland
Portland, Oregon

Katherine K. Kinsey, PhD, RN, FAAN
Associate Professor and Independence Foundation Chair
Director: Neighborhood Nursing Center
LaSalle University School of Nursing
Philadelphia, Pennsylvania

Thomas Kippenbrock, MSN, EdD
Chair
Department of Nursing
Arkansas State University
State University, Arkansas

Joyce Splann Krothe, DNS, MSN, BSN, RN
Associate Professor
Indiana University School of Nursing
Bloomington, Indiana

Pamela A. Kulbok, RN, DNSc
Associate Professor
School of Nursing
University of Virginia
Charlottesville, Virginia

Shirley Cloutier Laffrey, PhD, MPH, RN, CS
Associate Professor, Community Health Nursing
School of Nursing
The University of Texas, Austin
Austin, Texas

Kären M. Landenburger, RN, PhD
Associate Professor
Nursing Program
University of Washington–Tacoma
Tacoma, Washington

Peggye Guess Lassiter, BSN, MSN
Assistant Professor
Howard University
College of Pharmacy, Nursing and Allied Health Sciences
Division of Nursing
Washington, DC

Shirleen Lewis-Trabeaux, MN, RN
Assistant Professor
Course Coordinator of Community Health
Baccalaureate Nursing Program
Nicholls State University
Thibodaux, Louisiana

Susan C. Long-Marin, DVM, MPH
Manager, Epidemiology
Mecklenburg County Health Department
Charlotte, North Carolina

Carol J. Loveland-Cherry, PhD, RN, FAAN
Associate Professor and Director
Division of Health Promotion and Risk Reduction
School of Nursing
University of Michigan
Ann Arbor, Michigan

Lois W. Lowry, DNSc, RN
Professor
College of Nursing
East Tennessee State University
Johnson City, Tennessee

Karen S. Martin, RN, MSN, FAAN
Health Care Consultant
Martin Associates
Omaha, Nebraska

Mary Lynn Mathre, RN, MSN, CARN
Nurse Consultant
Addictions Consult Services
University of Virginia Health System
Charlottesville, Virginia

Mary Ann McClellan, MN, CPNP, ARNP
Assistant Professor
College of Nursing
University of Oklahoma
Oklahoma City, Oklahoma

Robert E. McKeown, PhD
Associate Professor
Department of Epidemiology and Biostatistics
School of Public Health
University of South Carolina
Columbia, South Carolina

Lillian H. Mood, RN, BSN, MPH, FAAN
Director of Risk Communication and Community Liaison
Environmental Quality Control
South Carolina Department of Health and Environmental
  Control
Columbia, South Carolina

Marie Napolitano, RN, PhD, FNP
Assistant Professor
Primary Care Nurse Practitioner Program
Oregon Health Sciences University
Portland, Oregon

Julie C. Novak, DNSc, RN, CPNP
Theresa A. Thomas Professor of Primary Care
Family Health Care Division Chair
Primary Care Nurse Practitioner Program Chair
School of Nursing
University of Virginia
Charlottesville, Virginia

Lisa C. Onega, PhD, RN, CS, FNP, GNP
Assistant Professor of Gerontological Nursing
Oregon Health Sciences University
Portland, Oregon

Demetrius J. Porche, DNS, RN, CS, CCRN
Director and Associate Professor
Nicholls State University
Adjunct Assistant Professor, Community Health Sciences
Tulane University School of Public Health and Tropical
  Medicine
Thibodaux, Louisiana

Bonnie Rogers, DrPH, COHN-S, FAAN
Associate Professor, Director
Public Health Nursing and the Occupational Health
  Nursing Program
School of Public Health
University of North Carolina
Chapel Hill, North Carolina

Molly A. Rose, RN, PhD
Associate Professor
Coordinator, Community Systems Administration
Thomas Jefferson University
College of Health Professions, Department of Nursing
Philadelphia, Pennsylvania

Linda M. Sawyer, PhD, RN, CS
Assistant Clinical Professor
Department of Community Health Systems
School of Nursing
University of California
San Francisco, California

Cheryl Pandolf Schenk, RN, MN, CS
Nurse Practitioner
Division of Endocrinology
Veterans Administration
Medical Center
Decatur, Georgia

Juliann G. Sebastian, PhD, RN, CS
Assistant Dean for Advanced Practice Nursing
College of Nursing
University of Kentucky
Lexington, Kentucky

George F. Shuster, III, RN, DNSc
Associate Professor
College of Nursing
University of New Mexico
Albuquerque, New Mexico

Marcia Stanhope, RN, DSN, FAAN, c
Associate Dean and Professor
College of Nursing
University of Kentucky
Lexington, Kentucky

Francisco S. Sy, MD, DrPH
Associate Professor of Epidemiology and Biostatistics
School of Public Health
University of South Carolina
Columbia, South Carolina

Karen MacDonald Thompson, RN, MSN
Doctoral Candidate
University of Virginia
Consultant, The Epsilon Group
Charlottesville, Virginia

Sally P. Weinrich, PhD
Professor
College of Nursing
University of South Carolina
Columbia, South Carolina

Cynthia J. Westley, RN, MSN, ANP-C
Community C&E Manager
University of Virginia Health System
Charlottesville, Virginia

Carolyn A. Williams, PhD, RN, FAAN
Dean and Professor
College of Nursing
University of Kentucky
Lexington, Kentucky

Judith Lupo Wold, PhD, RN
Associate Professor and Director
School of Nursing
Georgia State University
College of Health and Human Sciences
Atlanta, Georgia

■ Contributors to Canadian Boxes

Jo-Ann Ackery, RN, BScN
Manager, Communicable Disease, STD, HIV/AIDS
  Program
Toronto Public Health
Toronto, Ontario, Canada

Maureen Cava, BScN, MS
Clinical Nurse Specialist
Toronto Public Health
Assistant Professor, Faculty of Nursing
University of Toronto
Toronto, Ontario, Canada

Catherine Clarke, RN, BScN, MN
Program Manager
Toronto Public Health
Toronto, Ontario, Canada

Karen Janine Foster, RN, BScN, MEd
Public Health Nurse
Toronto Public Health
Nursing Instructor, School of Nursing
Ryerson Polytechnical University
Toronto, Ontario, Canada

Jann Houston
Manager, Vaccine Preventable Diseases
Toronto Public Health
Toronto, Ontario, Canada

Lianne Patricia Jeffs, RN, BScN, MSc
Policy Analyst/Coordinator
Center for Professional Development
Registered Nurses Association of Toronto
Clinical Instructor, Faculty of Nursing
University of Toronto
Toronto, Ontario, Canada

Barbara Mildon, RN, MN
President-Elect
Community Health Nurses Association of Canada
Toronto, Ontario, Canada

Pat Sanagan, RN, BScN, MEd
Substance Abuse Prevention Coordinator
Toronto Public Health, North York Office
Toronto, Ontario, Canada

Karen E. Wade, RN, BN, MScN
Clinical Nursing Specialist
Toronto Public Health
Assistant Professor, Faculty of Nursing
University of Toronto
Toronto, Ontario, Canada

■ Reviewers

Paula Mastrilli, RN, BScN, MScN
Faculty of Nursing
University of Toronto
Ryerson Polytechnic
Toronto, Ontario, Canada

Lorraine Noll, MSN, RNC
Associate Professor
Professional Nursing Program
University of Wisconsin—Green Bay
Green Bay, Wisconsin

Jane Baker Nunnelee, RN, MS, GNP
Assistant Clinical Professor
Texas Woman's University
Private Practice/Consultant
Dallas, Texas

Alwilda Scholler-Jaquish, RN, MN, MS, PhD, CS
Assistant Professor
School of Nursing
Texas Tech University Health Sciences Center
Lubbock, Texas

Foreword

The challenge of today's nursing educator is the preparation of the practitioners and leaders of the future. Rather than focus on giving lectures and providing "content," the model of the effective educator is increasingly being conceptualized as that of a "coach" whose expertise is directed to assessing the needs of students and identifying resources and opportunities that they can use in addressing their learning needs. Although a wide range of materials and experiences may be useful in assisting students to meet their goals, the need for a progressive, authoritative, and readable textbook persists. Stanhope and Lancaster's fifth edition of *Community and Public Health Nursing* remains a compelling choice.

This latest edition of what has become a classic resource in the field of community and public health nursing maintains the strengths of the four previous editions and incorporates new material to deal with current health problems and management strategies. In one single volume the user has access to guidance from acknowledged experts and leaders in community and public health nursing, who consider a wide range of topics from the history of the field and conceptual foundations to models for program planning and evaluation. Contemporary epidemics and concerns such as AIDS, adolescent pregnancy, substance abuse, and homelessness are addressed, as are the latest approaches to advocacy, nursing diagnosis, and case management in community-oriented services. Additionally,

the text highlights the renewal of the public health system in the United States and a return to the core functions of public health and nursing with emphasis on assessment, policy and program development, and assurance of personal health services for vulnerable populations.

The provision of high-quality, direct care nursing service to individuals is the heart of nursing, but for a profession that aspires to make a difference, a focus that is limited to direct care clinical concerns at the individual level is not a sufficient response to the present and future health care needs of the nation. If nursing is to have a positive and significant impact, its practitioners must become seriously involved in structuring the political agenda and adopting strategies to deal with promoting health and providing health care services at the community level. With the aging of the population, the growing recognition that the ever increasing cost of medical care must be slowed, and the emphasis on capitated managed care, it has never been more important to focus attention on community-oriented, population-focused approaches to health promotion and disease prevention. For those who seek to understand the elements and strategies inherent in practice and the essence of community and public health nursing, and for those who seek to prepare for the challenges and rewards that go with it, Stanhope and Lancaster's text continues to be the resource of choice.

Carolyn A. Williams, RN, PhD, FAAN

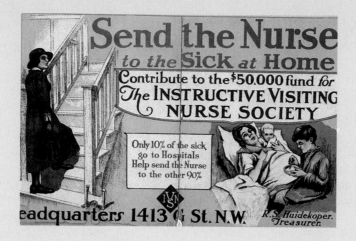

Congratulations *to* Public Health Nursing
for over 100 Years of Service *1893 to 2000*

Public health nursing in the United States traces its origins to those first graduate nurses who provided nursing services to poor people in their homes across the nation. These nurses provided care to those in need with little or no financial compensation, and they were frequently the only providers of care to these underprivileged people. The beginning of public health nursing in the United States was the founding of the first organized public health nursing agency or settlement house in New York City in 1893. This agency went beyond the individual efforts of community nurses of previous times and began a large-scale national movement to ensure that "public health nurses" would be available to those in need. The vision of this movement came from Ms. Lillian Wald, a nurse and the founder of the Henry Street Settlement in 1893–the first district nursing agency in the United States. Homes, workplaces, schools, street corners, clinics . . . anywhere people in need could be found, so one could find public health nurses.*

Congratulations *to* Visiting Nurses Association, Washington, DC
for 100 Years of Service *1900 to 2000*

The rich history of the Visiting Nurses Association (VNA) of Washington, D.C. is depicted on the cover of this text and at the beginning of each section of this text.† The year was 1900, and Washington was a city in transition. Swamps were still being cleared, cattle no longer roamed the Mall, and the streets were being cleared for residential and industrial development. A social order had risen after the Civil War, and many beautiful mansions graced the downtown area, but still Washington was a city of congested slums, dirt, poverty, and disease. Tuberculosis was a common and usually fatal illness. The infant mortality rate was astronomically high. New discoveries in medicine were taking their time reaching the city's poor. Many had not heard of "germs" and were unaware of sanitary measures to guard against infections. The city's poor and low-income residents could not afford physicians and could not access the very few government or social welfare programs.

It was during these conditions, in April 1900, that four individuals founded the Instructive Visiting Nurse Society (renamed the Visiting Nurses Association of Washington, D.C. in 1953). Before the end of their first year of service, a total of four nurses, who were put in the field to give care to 1851 patients, made 7864 home visits.

Since their early humble beginnings, the VNA of Washington, D.C. has remained a strong and proactive organization, creating a community health care network. It pioneered early programs in home visiting; child welfare, including the first prenatal home care program; TB prevention programs; school nursing; and more recently the region-wide Fight the Flu immunization program, HIV/AIDS care, mental health care, and hospice services. Through wartime, social advancement, and dramatic changes in health care, the VNA of Washington, D.C. has been a trendsetter of improvements in home health services. Although the organization is now 100 years old, its goal remains the promotion of health and well-being in the individuals and families they serve through preventive, educational, and therapeutic services, just as they did 100 years ago.

---

*From *A century of caring: a celebration of public health nursing in the United States 1893-1993*, Introduction by Audrey Davis, Moira Shannon, Janet Horan.

†Front Cover, Part Opener photos, and above photo provided courtesy of the Visiting Nurses Association of Washington, DC.

Preface

For a long time, the health care system in the United States, especially the public health system, has been in trouble. It has been widely accepted that a good health care system should address the structure of the system, the cost, quality of care, and access to health care. In recent years, considerable time and attention have been devoted to what is called "health care reform." In truth, what is actually being reformed is the way in which medical care is organized, financed, and delivered. To be able to properly address health care reform, a changed public health system is thought to be critical. Because of the recent move toward managed care as a means of reorganizing care delivery, the public health system has begun to reorganize itself to be a partner in the changing health care environment. In many states, public health reform is occurring, with a renewed focus on the core functions of public health: the assessment of a community's health status and resources, policy development aimed at proposals that encourage better health, and assurance that personal health services are available for those in need.

Despite the fact that more money is spent per capita in the United States for illness care than in any other country, Americans are not the healthiest of all people. Lifestyle continues to play an enormous role in morbidity and mortality. For example, half of all deaths are still attributed to tobacco, alcohol, and illicit drug use; diet and activity patterns; microbial agents; toxic agents; firearms; sexual behavior; and motor vehicle accidents. Over the years the most significant improvements in the health of the population have come from advances in public health such as improved sanitation, food pasteurization, refrigeration, immunizations, and the emphasis on personal lifestyle and environmental factors that affect health. Changes in the public health system are essential if the health of the people in the United States is to improve.

The need to focus attention on health promotion, lifestyle factors, and disease prevention led to the development of a healthy public policy for the nation. This policy was designed by a large number of people representing a wide range of groups interested in health. The policy is reflected in the document *Healthy People 2000* and the updated document *Healthy People 2010*, which identify a comprehensive set of national health promotion and disease prevention objectives.

The most effective disease prevention and health promotion strategies designed to change personal lifestyles are developed by the establishment of partnerships between government, business, voluntary organizations, consumers, communities, and health care providers. According to *Healthy People 2000*, these partnerships aim to reduce health disparities among Americans by targeting care to children, minorities, elderly, and the uninsured; to increase the healthy life span of Americans; and to achieve access to preventive services. The overall goals are to protect and promote health of populations, to prevent disease and injury, and to develop healthy communities. To develop healthy communities, individuals, families, and the communities must commit to those goals. Also society, through the development of health policy, must support better health care, the design of improved health education, and the financing of strategies to alter health status.

What does this mean for the public health or community health nurse? Because people do not always know how to improve their health status, the challenge of nursing is to initiate change. Public health nursing is a practice that is focused on the health of the population as a whole, while community health nurses often focus on the delivery of personal health services directed toward all age groups. Community health and public health nursing takes place in a variety of public and private settings and includes disease prevention, health promotion, health protection, education, maintenance, restoration, coordination, management, and evaluation of care of individuals, families, and populations, including communities.

To meet the demands of a constantly changing health care system, nurses must be visionary in designing their roles and identifying their practice areas. To do so effectively, the nurse must understand concepts and theories of public health, the changing health care system, the actual and potential roles and responsibilities of nurses and other health care providers, the importance of a health promotion and disease prevention orientation, and the necessity to involve consumers in the planning, implementation, and evaluation of health care efforts.

Since its initial publication 18 years ago, this text has achieved wide acceptance and popularity among public health and community health nursing students and nursing faculty in baccalaureate, BSN-completion, and graduate programs. The text was written to provide nursing students and practicing nurses with a comprehensive source book that provides a foundation for designing community and public health nursing strategies for individuals, families, and populations, including communities. The unifying theme for the book is the integration of health promotion and disease prevention concepts into the multifaceted role of community-oriented practice. The prevention focus emphasizes traditional public health practice with increased attention to the effects of the internal and external environment on health. The focus on interventions for the individual and family emphasizes community health practice with attention to the effects of all of the determinants of health, including lifestyle, on personal health.

The title of this edition has been changed to *Community and Public Health Nursing*. Also, the term *community-oriented* is now used to reflect the orientation of community and public health nursing. In 1998, the Quad Council of Public Health Nursing, comprised of members from the American Nurses Association Council on Community, Primary, and Long-Term Care; the American Public Health Association Public Health Nursing section; the Association of Community Health Nursing Educators; and the Association of State and Territorial Directors of Public Health Nursing developed a statement on the *Scope of Public Health Practice*. Through this statement, the leaders in community-oriented nursing attempted to clarify the differences between *public health nursing* and the newest term introduced into nursing's vocabulary during health care reform of the 1990s, *community-based nursing*. The Quad Council recognized that the terms *public health nursing* and *community health nursing* have been used interchangeably since the 1980s to describe population-focused, community-oriented nursing practice and community-based practice. However, they decided to make a clearer distinction between community-oriented and community-based nursing practice.

In this textbook, we suggest these same two levels of care in the community: community-oriented care and community-based care. We also suggest three role functions for nursing practice in the community: public health nursing, community health nursing, and community-based nursing.

ORGANIZATION

The text is divided into seven sections:
- **Part One, Perspectives in Health Care Delivery and Community and Public Health Nursing,** describes the historical and current status of the health care delivery system, public and community health nursing practice both domestically and internationally.
- **Part Two, Influences on Health Care Delivery and Community-Oriented Nursing,** addresses specific issues and societal concerns that affect public and community health nursing practice.
- **Part Three, Conceptual Frameworks Applied to Community-Oriented Nursing Practice,** provides conceptual models for public and community health nursing practice, and selected models from nursing and related sciences are also discussed.

- **Part Four, Issues and Approaches in Community-Oriented Health Care,** examines the management of health care and select community environments, as well as issues related to managing cases, programs, disasters, and groups.
- **Part Five, Issues and Approaches in Family and Individual Health Care,** discusses risk factors and health problems for families and individuals throughout the lifespan.
- **Part Six, Vulnerability: Community-Oriented Nursing Issues for the Twenty-First Century,** covers specific health care needs and issues of populations at risk.
- **Part Seven, Community and Public Health Nurses: Roles and Functions,** examines diversity in the role of community and public health nurses and describes the rapidly changing roles, functions, and practice settings.

NEW TO THIS EDITION

Additional new chapters have been included in the fifth edition of *Community and Public Health Nursing* to ensure that the text remains a complete and comprehensive resource:
- **Chapter 45, Community Health Nurse as Parish Nurse and Block Nurse,** describes the services provided by the emerging new role of parish nurse while revisiting the role of the block nurse, a role that dates back to the early history of public health nursing.
- **Chapter 46, Public Health Nursing in the Local Health Department,** is included. There is a renewed interest in public health nurses' contributions to the health of populations and their role in governmental health activities.

Additional new content includes the following:
- Focused information on forensic nursing is added to Chapter 37, Violence and Human Abuse
- *Healthy People 2000* and *Healthy People 2010* objectives and public and community health nursing interventions designed to obtain them are incorporated in appropriate chapters throughout the text.
- More emphasis is placed on the aspects of the home visit in Chapter 25, Family Health Risks, and Chapter 40, Community Health Nurse in Home Health and Hospice.

PEDAGOGY

Full color has been added throughout for better accessibility of content and for visual enhancement. Other key features of this edition are detailed below.

Each chapter is organized for easy use by students and faculty. Chapters begin with an outline to alert students to the structure and content of the chapter. Also at the beginning of the chapter are objectives, which guide student learning and assist faculty in knowing what students should gain from the content. Key terms are identified at the beginning of the chapter and defined either in the chapter or in the glossary to assist the student in understanding unfamiliar terminology.

Students say:

"... *helpful in identifying what the chapter is about and what ideas are important*"

DID YOU KNOW? boxes provide students with a fact of interest and lend insight into the topic of the chapter.

Students say:

"... *interesting and thought provoking. Related well to topics being covered*"
"... *effective and very informative*"

WHAT DO YOU THINK? boxes are designed to stimulate debate and discussion.

Students say:

"... *effective study questions that help to engage the reader in critical thinking* ..."
"... *had me thinking about what is the right thing to do.*"
"*Good discussion questions!*"

NEW! **HOW TO** boxes provide specific, application-oriented information.

Students say:

"*Good and useful information in boxes!*"
"*Great information!*"

NEW! **NURSING TIPS** emphasize special clinical considerations for nursing practice.

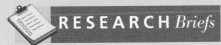 **RESEARCH** *Briefs* in each chapter illustrate the use and application of the latest research findings in public health, community health, and nursing.

Students say:

"*Enjoyed reading!*"
"... *interesting* ... *added to my body of knowledge regarding research.*"

NEW! Canadian boxes, written by practicing Canadian public health nurses, offer the Canadian perspective on community and public health nursing issues and practice for Canadian readers and promote an international view of nursing care.

Students say:

"... *a very interesting insight into other systems of health care.*"

clinical applications at the end of each chapter provide the reader with an understanding of how to apply chapter content in the clinical setting through the presentation of a case situation with questions that students will want to think about as they analyze the case.

Students say:

"... *gives the reader real life scenarios and engages him or her in problem solving* ..."

Key Points provide a summary in list form of the most important points made in the chapter.

Students say:

"... *help to reiterate the essentials.*"
"*Helps to reinforce the content just read.*"

critical thinking activities stimulate student learning by suggesting a variety of activities that encourage both independent and collaborative effort.

Students say:

"... *get the reader thinking about ways in which he or she can apply what they have learned in their community.*"
"*Great! Good activities to engage people in getting involved in their community.*"

The **Bibliography** offers both references used to develop chapter materials and additional readings to expand the student's knowledge of the chapter topics.

In the back of the book are additional important sources of information in the Appendixes, the Answers to Clinical Applications, and the Glossary:

The **Appendixes** provide additional resources and key information.

The **Glossary** offers complete definitions of all key terms and other important concepts.

NEW! **Answers to Clinical Applications.** In this edition answers to each Clinical Application are provided.

Students say:

"*I found this text to be reader friendly and easy to follow* ..."
"*The content throughout the chapter was clear and comprehensible* ..."
"*Interior design is very attractive and reader friendly.*"
"... *the boxes and tables highlight vital information, which assists the reader to integrate previous knowledge.*"
"*Great color illustrations!*"

TEACHING AND LEARNING PACKAGE

Several ancillaries have been developed to assist instructors and students in the teaching and learning process:
- Instructor's Resource Kit with five text sections:
  - Lecture Outlines and Chapter Summaries
  - Critical Thinking
  - Multimedia Resources
  - Printed test bank, with 900 questions
  - 69 transparency masters
- Computerized test bank, with same 900 questions
- *Mosby's Community Health Nursing Video Series* (eight-part series)
- A CD-ROM workbook: *Real World Community Health Nursing: An Interactive CD-ROM*
- A website: MERLIN www.mosby.com/MERLIN/ community_stanhope

ACKNOWLEDGMENTS

We would like to thank our families, friends, and colleagues who supported us in the completion of this edition. Special thanks go to our coworkers at the University of Kentucky College of Nursing and the University of Virginia School of Nursing who provided generous support and assistance. We especially thank June Thompson and Linda Caldwell at Mosby and the peer reviewers for their time and thoughtfulness in completing the revisions.

We would like to extend special thanks to the contributors of edition four of the book. Their expertise and commitment to community health nursing continue to be reflected in this edition: Teresa Acquaviva (Poverty and Homelessness), Sara Barger (Nursing Centers), Patricia Birchfield (Elder Health), Jeanne Bucsela (Environmental Health), Douglas Forness (Educational Theories), Carol Garrison (Epidemiology), Beth Hibbs (Environmental Health), Judith Igoe (School Health), Max Lum (Environmental Health), Diana Narkunas (Environmental Health), Charlene Ossler (Occupational Health), Lynelle Phillips (Environmental Health), and Sudie Speer (School Health).

Marcia Stanhope   *Jeanette Lancaster*

Contents

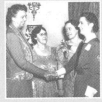

PART *One*

Perspectives in Health Care Delivery and Community and Public Health Nursing

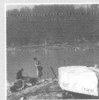

PART *Two*

Influences on Health Care Delivery and Community-Oriented Nursing

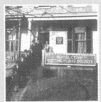

PART *Three*

Conceptual Frameworks Applied to Community-Oriented Nursing Practice

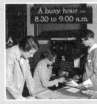

PART *Four*

Issues and Approaches in Community-Oriented Health Care

PART *Five*

Issues and Approaches in Family and Individual Health Care

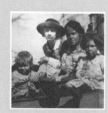

PART *Six*

Vulnerability: Community-Oriented Nursing Issues for the Twenty-First Century

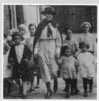

PART *Seven*

Community and Public Health Nurses: Roles and Functions

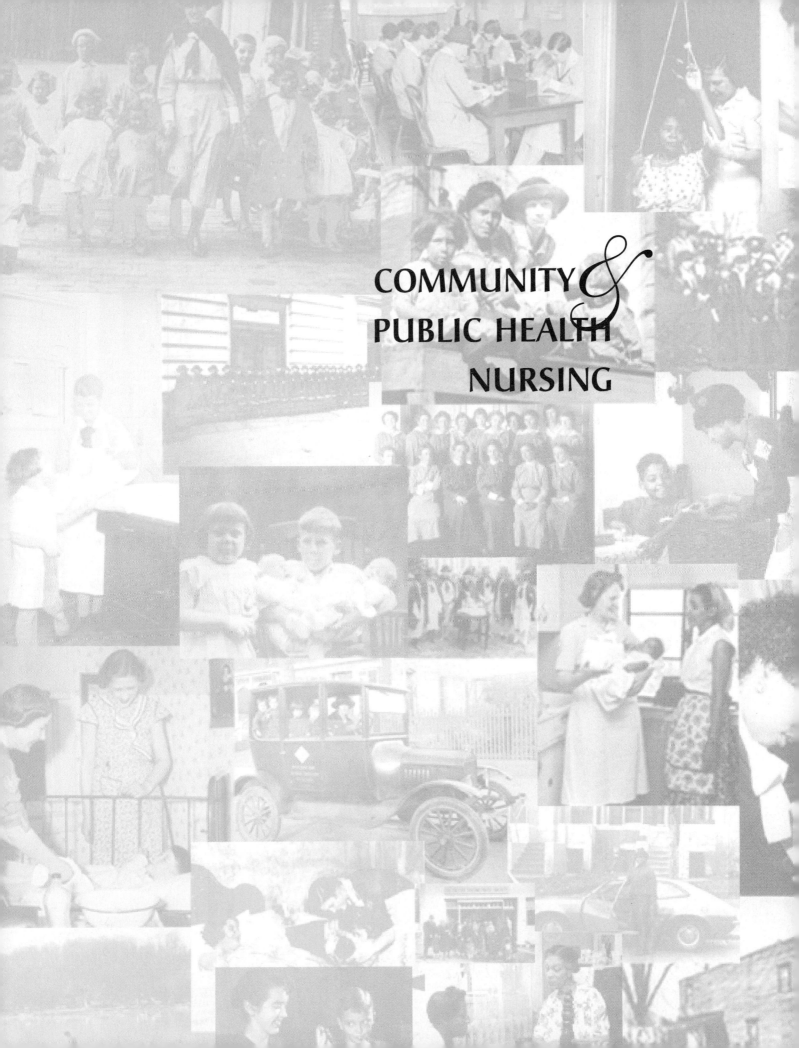

COMMUNITY & PUBLIC HEALTH NURSING

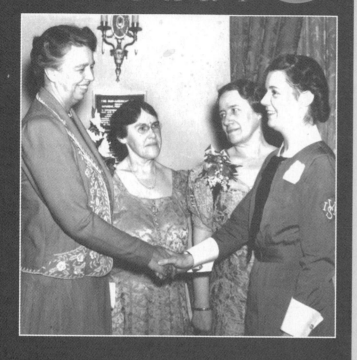

PART *One*

Perspectives in Health Care Delivery and Community and Public Health Nursing

Since the late 1800s, public health nurses have led many of the improvements in the quality of health care for individuals, families, and communities. Also, as nurses around the world meet and learn about one another, it is clear that community and public health nursing, from one country to another, has more similarities than differences.

Significant changes in health care occurred during the 1990s. The federal initiative to reform health care and initiate a national plan failed. This led to a shift of health care from the control of hospitals and health care professionals to control by insurers, investors, and venture capitalists. The positive aspects of the proposed health care reform plan were largely lost in the scramble for groups to carve out market share and develop profitable systems of health care delivery.

The public health system, as a subset of the overall health care system, has been affected by the changes in health care organization, ownership, and financing. Specifically, public health is realigning with the traditional core functions and moving away from the provision of primary health care. If community and public health nurses are to be effective in promoting the health of people, they must understand the history of public health nursing and the current status of the public health system.

Part One presents information about significant factors affecting health in the United States. Some contrasts and comparisons in health care are made to health care in Canada. Playing an instrumental role in changing the level and quality of services and the priorities for funding requires informed, courageous, and committed nurses. The chapters in Part One are designed to provide essential information so that community health nurses can make a difference in health care by understanding the roles of community and public health health nurses and nurses in community-based practice as well as understanding how the public health system differs from the primary care system.

Chapter 1 explains exactly what makes community and public health nursing unique. Often people confuse community and public health nursing with community-based nursing practice. There is a core of knowledge known as "public health" that forms the foundation for community and public health nursing. Working with people in the community may not necessarily be community health or public health nursing. Such nursing practice involves more than the care of a person or family whose care has been moved from the hospital to the community.

1 Community-Oriented Population-Focused Practice: The Foundation of Specialization in Public Health Nursing

CAROLYN A. WILLIAMS

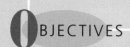BJECTIVES

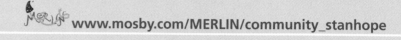 www.mosby.com/MERLIN/community_stanhope

After reading this chapter, the student should be able to do the following:

- State the mission and core functions of public health and the essential public health services.
- Describe specialization in public health nursing and community health nursing and the practice goals of each.
- Contrast clinical community health nursing practice with population-focused practice.

- Describe what is meant by population-focused practice.
- Name barriers to acceptance of population-focused practice.
- State key opportunities for population-focused practice.

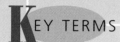EY TERMS

aggregate
capitation
community-based nursing
community-based nursing
  care

community health nurse
cottage industry
integrated system
managed care
population

population-focused
population-focused
  pratice
public health
public health nursing

public health core
  functions
subpopulations

See Glossary for definitions

CHAPTER OUTLINE

As the twenty-first century begins the United States continues to grapple with ways to improve the health of the American people. The goal is to improve the functioning of the complicated array of public and private organizations involved in health care or health-related activities. Despite the failure of the Clinton administration's efforts to make fundamental changes in health care, private market forces and federal and state initiatives are bringing about changes in the health care system. With the changes have come new concerns about the growth of managed care, access to care, the ability to maintain affordable insurance coverage, quality of services, and new warnings about possible increases in costs. Because of these factors the goals of protecting health, promoting health, and preventing disease and disability, and the role of public health in achieving these goals, have gained new prominence. In short, there has been a revival of interest in public health and in population-focused thinking about health and health care in the United States.

Although populations have historically been the focus of public health practice, populations are also the focus of the "business" of **managed care.** Thus public health practitioners and managed care executives share a population orientation. Increasingly managed care executives and program managers are using the basic sciences and analytic tools of the field of public health, particularly epidemiology and statistics, to develop databases and approaches to making decisions at the level of a defined population or subpopulation. Thus a **population-focused** approach to planning, delivering, and evaluating nursing care has never been more important.

This is a crucial time for public health nursing, a time of opportunity and challenge. The issue of growing costs together with the changing demography of the United States population, such as the aging of the population, is expected to put increased demands on resources available for health care. Most important to the public health community is the emergence of modern-day epidemics and causes of mortality, many of which affect the young, such as infants and teenagers. Most of the causes are preventable. What has all of this to do with nursing? Understanding the importance of community-oriented, population-focused nursing practice and developing the knowledge and skills to practice it will be critical to attaining a leadership role in health care regardless of the practice setting. Those who practice population-focused nursing in the context of community-based populations will be in a strong position to affect the health of populations and how scarce resources will be used.

PUBLIC HEALTH PRACTICE: THE FOUNDATION FOR HEALTHY POPULATIONS AND COMMUNITIES

Within the last decade, attention has focused on proposals to reform the American health care system. These proposals have focused primarily on cost containment in medical care financing. They have also focused on strategies for providing health insurance coverage to a higher portion of the population. Since medical treatment is estimated to account for up to 99% of all health expenses (U.S. Public Health Service, 1993), it is understandable that health insurance would be the emphasis. However, many times the most benefit from the least expenditure is sought for in the wrong place. As stated in the U.S. Public Health Services Report on the *Core Functions of Public Health,* reform of the medical insurance system is necessary, but it is not adequate to improve the health of Americans. Historically, gains in the health of populations have come largely from public health changes. Safety and adequacy of food supplies, the provision of safe water, sewage disposal, and personal behavioral changes including reproductive behavior are a few examples of public health's influence. The dramatic increase in life expectancy for Americans during the 1900s, from less than 50 years in 1900 to more than 75 years in 1990, is credited primarily to improvements in sanitation, the control of infectious diseases through immunizations, and other public health activities (U.S. Public Health Service, 1993). "Population-based preventative programs launched in the 1970s are also largely responsible for the more recent changes in tobacco use, blood pressure control, dietary patterns (except obesity), automobile safety restraint, and injury control measures that have fostered declines of more than 50% in stroke deaths, 40% in coronary heart disease deaths, and 25% in overall death rates for children" (U.S. Public Health Service, 1993, p. 2).

DID YOU KNOW? *The concept of using a population/aggregate approach in the practice of public health nursing began to be seriously discussed in the 1970s.*

Another way of looking at the benefits of public health practice is to look at how early deaths can be prevented. The U.S. Public Health Service estimates that medical treatment can prevent only about 10% of all early deaths in the United States. However, "population-wide public health approaches have the potential to help prevent some 70 percent of early deaths in America through measures targeted to the factors that contribute to those deaths. Many of these contributing factors are behavioral such as tobacco use and diet and sedentary lifestyles; others are environmental in nature"(U.S. Public Health Service, 1994/1995, p. 2).

Public health practice is of great value. The U.S. Public Health Service estimated in 1993 that only 0.9% of all national health expenditures support population-focused public health functions, yet the impact is enormous. Unfortunately, the public is largely unaware of the contributions of public health practice. The proportion of expenditures for public health activities has actually declined by about 25% over the last 10 years. Some of this decline in the 1980s and 1990s has been related to public health agencies providing personal care services as the provider of last resort to persons who could not receive care elsewhere.

The result has been a shift of resources and energy away from public health's traditional and unique population-focused perspective (U.S. Public Health Service, 1994/1995). Because of the importance of influencing a population's health and in providing a strong foundation for the health care system, the U.S. Public Health Service and other groups are strongly advocating a renewed emphasis on the population-focused essential public health functions and services that have had the most effect on improving the health of the entire population. As part of this effort, the statement on public health in America presented in Figure 1-1 was developed by a working group made up of representatives of federal agencies and organizations concerned about public health. The list of essential services presented in Figure 1-1 represents the fundamental obligations of public health for the core functions of assessment, assurance, and policy development discussed later. Box 1-1 further explains these essential services. More complete discussions can be found in the reference section (U.S. Public Health Service, 1993, 1994/1995).

Definitions in Public Health

In 1988 the Institute of Medicine published a report on the future of public health. In the report, **public health** was defined as "what we, as a society, do collectively to assure the conditions in which people can be healthy" (Institute of Medicine, 1988, p. 1). The committee stated that the mission of public health was "to generate organized community effort to address the public interest in health by applying scientific and technical knowledge to prevent disease and promote health" (Institute of Medicine, 1988, p. 1; Williams, 1995). It was clearly noted that the mission could be accomplished by many groups, public and private, and by individuals. However, the government has a special function "to see to it that vital elements are in place and that the mission is adequately addressed" (Institute of Medicine, 1988, p. 7). To clarify the governmental role in fulfilling the mission, the report stated that assessment, policy development, and assurance are the **public health core functions** at all levels of government.

- *Assessment* refers to systematic data collection on the population, monitoring of the population's health status, and making information available on the health of the community.
- *Policy development* refers to the need to provide leadership in developing policies that support the health of the population, including the use of the scientific knowledge base in making decisions about policy.
- *Assurance* refers to the role of public health in making sure that essential community-oriented health services are available, which may include providing essential personal health services for those who would otherwise not receive them. Assurance also refers to making sure that a competent public health and personal health care workforce is available.

Public Health Core Functions

The Core Functions Project, a working group within the U.S. Public Health Service, developed a useful illustration, the Health Services Pyramid (Fig. 1-2), that shows that population-focused public health programs with the goals of disease prevention, health protection, and health promotion provide a foundation for primary, secondary, and tertiary health care services. All levels of services shown in the pyramid are important to the health of the population and thus must be part of a health care system with health as a goal. It has been said that "the greater the effectiveness of services in the lower tiers, the greater is the capability of higher tiers to contribute efficiently to health improvement"(U.S. Public Health Service, 1994/1995, p. 3). Because of the importance of the basic public health programs, members of the Core Functions Project argued that "financing any tier of the overall health care system at the expense of those below it undermines the system's integrity" (U.S. Public Health Service, 1994/1995, p. 3). Thus the goal of health of populations may never be reached.

Several new efforts to enable public health practitioners to be more effective in implementing the core functions of assessment, policy development, and assurance have been undertaken at the national level. In 1997 the Institute of Medicine published *Improving Health in the Community: A Role for Performance Monitoring* (Institute of Medicine, 1997). This monograph was the product of an interdisciplinary committee, co-chaired by a public health nursing specialist and a physician, whose purpose was to determine how a performance monitoring system could be developed and used to improve community health. The major outcome of the committee's work was the Community Health Improvement Process (CHIP), a method for improving the health of the population on a community-wide basis. The method brings together key elements of the public health and personal health care systems in one framework. A second outcome of the project was the development of a set of 25 indicators that could be used in developing a community health profile (e.g., measures of health status, functional status, quality of life, health risk factors, and health resource use). A third product of the committee's work was a set of indicators for specific public health problems that could be used by public health specialists as they carry out their assurance function and monitor the performance of public health and other agencies.

The Centers for Disease Control and Prevention (CDC) established a Task Force on Community Preventive Services. The Task Force is working to collect evidence on the effectiveness of a variety of community interventions to prevent morbidity and mortality. It was anticipated that late in 1999 the efforts of the Task Force would be published as a document. This document will be a population-focused guide to providing services much like the *Guide to Clinical Preventive Services* for personal care, the report of the

PUBLIC HEALTH IN AMERICA

Vision:

Healthy people in healthy communities

Mission:

*Promote physical and mental health and
prevent disease, injury, and disability*

Public health

- Prevents epidemics and the spread of disease
- Protects against environmental hazards
- Prevents injuries
- Promotes and encourages healthy behaviors
- Responds to disasters and assists communities in recovery
- Ensures the quality and accessibility of health services

Essential public health services

- Monitors health status to identify community health problems
- Diagnoses and investigates health problems and health hazards in the community
- Informs, educates, and empowers people about health issues
- Mobilizes community partnerships to identify and solve health problems
- Develops policies and plans that support individual and community health efforts
- Enforces laws and regulations that protect health and ensure safety
- Links people to needed personal health services and ensures the provision of health care when otherwise unavailable
- Ensures a competent public health and personal health care workforce
- Evaluates effectiveness, accessibility, and quality of personal and population-based health services
- Researches for new insights and innovative solutions to health problems

Source: Essential Public Health Services Work Group of the Core Public Health Functions Steering Committee
Membership: American Public Health Association
        Association of State and Territorial Health Officials
        National Association of County and City Health Officials
        Institute of Medicine, National Academy of Sciences
        Association of Schools of Public Health
        Public Health Foundation
        National Association of State Alcohol and Drug Abuse Directors
        National Association of State Mental Health Program Directors
        U.S. Public Health Service
           Centers for Disease Control and Prevention
           Health Resources and Services Administration
           Office of the Assistant Secretary for Health
           Substance Abuse and Mental Health Services Administration
           Agency for Health Care Policy and Research
           Indian Health Service
           Food and Drug Administration

FIG. 1-1 Public health in America.

BOX 1-1 How to Participate in the Essential Services of Public Health

PUBLIC HEALTH NURSES

1. Monitor health status to identify community health problems.

Activities:
- Participate in community assessment.
- Identify subpopulations at risk for disease or disability.
- Collect information on interventions to special populations.
- Define and evaluate effective strategies and programs.
- Identify potential environmental hazards.

2. Diagnose and investigate health problems and hazards in the community.

Activities:
- Understand and identify determinants of health and disease.
- Apply knowledge about environmental influences of health.
- Recognize multiple causes or factors of health and illness.
- Participate in case identification and treatment of persons with communicable disease.

3. Inform, educate, and empower people about health issues.

Activities:
- Develop health and educational plans for individuals and families in multiple settings.
- Develop and implement community-based health education.
- Provide regular reports on health status of special populations within clinic settings, community settings, and groups.
- Advocate for and with underserved and disadvantaged populations.
- Ensure health planning, which includes primary prevention and early intervention strategies.
- Identify healthy population behaviors and maintain successful intervention strategies through reinforcement and continued funding.

4. Mobilize community partnerships to identify and solve health problems.

Activities:
- Interact regularly with many providers and services within each community.
- Convene groups and providers who share common concerns and interests in special populations.
- Provide leadership to prioritize community problems and development of interventions.
- Explain the significance of health issues to the public and participate in developing plans of action.

5. Develop policies and plans that support individual and community health efforts.

Activities:
- Participate in community and family decision-making processes.
- Provide information and advocacy for consideration of the interests of special groups in program development.

- Develop programs and services to meet the needs of high-risk populations as well as broader community members.
- Participate in disaster planning and mobilization of community resources in emergencies.
- Advocate for appropriate funding for services.

6. Enforce laws and regulations that protect health and ensure safety.

Activities:
- Regulate and support safe care and treatment for dependent populations such as children and the frail elderly.
- Implement ordinances and laws that protect the environment.
- Establish procedures and processes that ensure competent implementation of treatment schedules for diseases of public health importance.
- Participate in development of local regulation that protects communities and the environment from potential hazards and pollution.

7. Link people to needed personal health services and ensure the provision of health care that is otherwise unavailable.

Activities:
- Provide clinical preventive services to certain high-risk populations.
- Establish programs and services to meet special needs.
- Recommend clinical care and other services to clients and their families in clinics, homes, and the community.
- Provide referrals through community links to needed care.
- Participate in community provider coalitions and meetings to educate others and to identify service centers for community populations.
- Provide clinical surveillance and identification of communicable disease.

8. Ensure a competent public health and personal health care workforce.

Activities:
- Participate in continuing education and preparation to ensure competence.
- Define and support proper delegation to unlicensed assistive personnel in community settings.
- Establish standards for performance.
- Maintain client record systems and community documents.
- Establish and maintain procedures and protocols for client care.
- Participate in quality assurance activities such as record audits, agency evaluation, and clinical guidelines.

9. Evaluate effectiveness, accessibility, and quality of personal and population-based health services.

Activities:
- Collect data and information related to community interventions.

From Association of State and Territorial Directors of Nursing: *Public health nursing: a partner for progress*, Washington, DC, 1998, the Association.

BOX 1-1 How to Participate in the Essential Services of Public Health—cont'd

- Identify unserved and underserved populations within the community.
- Review and analyze data on health status of the community.
- Participate with the community in assessment of services and outcomes of care.
- Identify and define enhanced services required to manage health status of complex populations and special risk groups.
10. **Research for new insights and innovative solutions to health problems.**
Activities:
- Implement nontraditional interventions and approaches to effect change in special populations.

- Participate in the collecting of information and data to improve the surveillance and understanding of special problems.
- Develop collegial relationships with academic institutions to explore new interventions.
- Participate in early identification of factors that are detrimental to the community's health.
- Formulate and use investigative tools to identify and impact care delivery and program planning.

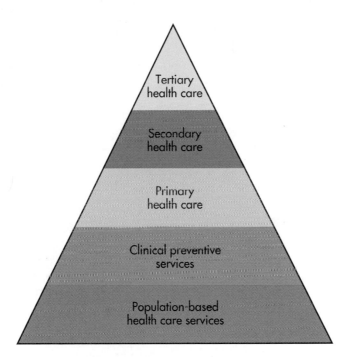

FIG. 1-2 Health services pyramid.

U.S. Preventive Services Task Force (1996). These efforts are important because they provide conceptual and methodologic tools for public health practitioners, many of whom are public health nursing specialists, to enable them to be more effective in dealing with core functions.

PUBLIC HEALTH NURSING AS A FIELD OF PRACTICE: AN AREA OF SPECIALIZATION

What is public health nursing? Is it really a specialty, and if so, why? Public health nursing is a specialty because it has a distinct focus and scope of practice, and it requires a special knowledge base. The following factors distinguish public health nursing as a specialty:

- *Population focused.* Primary emphasis is on *populations* that are free-living in the *community,* as opposed to those that are institutionalized.
- *Community oriented.* 1) Concern for the connection between health status of the population and the environment in which the population lives (physical, biologic, sociocultural). 2) An imperative to work *with* members of the community to carry out core public health functions.
- *Health and preventive focus.* Predominant emphasis on strategies for health promotion, health maintenance, and disease prevention, particularly primary and secondary prevention.

- *Interventions at the community and/or population level.* The use of political processes to affect public policy as a major intervention strategy for achieving goals.
- *Concern for the health of all members of the population/ community, particularly vulnerable subpopulations*

⋮ NURSING TIP

The primary features of the public health specialty are population focus, community orientation, emphasis on health promotion and disease prevention, and concern for and interventions on a population basis.

In 1981 the public health nursing section of the American Public Health Association developed the *Definition and Role of Public Health Nursing in the Delivery of Health Care* to describe the field of specialization. This statement was reaffirmed in 1996 (APHA, 1996). Central elements of their definition are as follows:

Public health nursing synthesizes the body of knowledge from the public health sciences and professional nursing theories. The implicit over-riding goal is to improve the health of the community. Public health nursing practice is a systematic process by which:

1. The health and health care needs of a population are assessed in collaboration with other disciplines in order to identify subpopulations (aggregates), families, and individuals at increased risk of illness, disability, or premature death.
2. A plan for intervention is developed to meet these needs, which includes resources available and those activities that contribute to health and its recovery, the prevention of illness, disability, and premature death.
3. A health care plan is implemented effectively, efficiently, and equitably.
4. An evaluation is made to determine the extent to which these activities have an impact on the health status of the population (APHA, 1981, pp. 3, 4; 1996, pp. 1, 2).
5. The results of the process are used to influence and direct the current delivery of care, use of health resources, and the development of local, regional, state, and national health policy and research to promote health and prevent diseases (APHA, 1996, p. 2).

The American Nurses Association, with input from several other nursing organizations—the Public Health Nursing Section of the American Public Health Association, the Association of State and Territorial Directors of Public Health Nursing, and the Association of Community Health Nurse Educators—has worked on the development of a statement on the *Scope and Standards of Public Health Nursing Practice.* Public health nursing is described as population-focused, community-oriented nursing practice that emphasizes the prevention of disease and disability. Public health nursing practice takes place through assessment, policy development, and assurance activities of nurses working in partnerships with nations, states, communities, organizations, groups, and individuals. Nurses would be expected to have organizational and political skills along with nursing and public health knowledge to assess the needs and strengths of the population, design interventions to mobilize resources for action, and promote equity of opportunity for health.

Educational Preparation for Public Health Nursing

Targeted and specialized education for public health nursing practice has a long history. In the late 1950s and early 1960s, before the integration of public health concepts into the curriculum of baccalaureate nursing programs, special baccalaureate curricula were established in several schools of public health to prepare nurses to become public health nurses. Now it is generally assumed that a graduate of a baccalaureate nursing program has the necessary basic preparation to function as a beginning staff public health nurse.

Since the late 1960s there has been agreement among public health nursing leaders that master's preparation is necessary to specialize in public health nursing. This agreement occurred several years before the current expectation that a master's degree in nursing is necessary to be eligible to sit for the nurse practitioner certification examination. Perhaps because of the absence of a certification examination specifically for public health nursing, the expectation of a master's degree for the specialty has not been widely recognized nor required. The general educational expectations for public health nursing were reaffirmed at a 1984 Consensus Conference on the Essentials of Public Health Nursing Practice and Education sponsored by the U. S. Department of Health and Human Services (USDHHS) Division of Nursing. The participants agreed "that the term 'public health nurse' should be used to describe a person who has received specific educational preparation and supervised clinical practice in public health nursing" (Consensus Conference, 1985, p. 4). At the basic or entry level, a public health nurse is one who "holds a baccalaureate degree in nursing that includes this educational preparation; this nurse may or may not practice in an official health agency but has the initial qualifications to do so" (Consensus Conference, 1985, p. 4). Specialists in public health nursing are defined as those who are prepared at the graduate level, either master's or doctoral, "with a focus in the public health sciences" (Consensus Conference, 1985, p. 4).

The consensus statement specifically pointed out that the public health nursing specialist "should be able to work with population groups and to assess and intervene successfully at the aggregate level" (Consensus Conference, 1985, p. 11). Areas considered essential for the preparation of such specialists were "Epidemiology, Biostatistics, Nursing theory, Management theory, Change theory, Economics, Politics, Public health administration, Community assessment, Program planning and evaluation, Interventions at the aggregate level, Research, History of public health, and Issues in public health" (Consensus Conference, 1985, p. 11).

Population-Focused Practice Versus Practice Focused on Individuals

As mentioned previously, one key factor that distinguishes specialization in public health nursing from other areas of nursing practice is the focus on populations that are free living in the community. A population focus is historically consistent with public health philosophy, and while such practice is built on basic clinical nursing practice, it is different from clinical nursing practice. It may be helpful to define what is meant by the term *population* and to comment on what is meant by population-focused practice.

A **population** or **aggregate** is a collection of individuals who have one or more personal or environmental characteristic in common. Those who are members of a community are defined either in terms of geography (e.g., a county, group of counties, or a state) or a special interest (e.g., children attending a particular school) and can be seen as constituting a population. Often there are **subpopulations** within the larger population. Examples of a subpopulation within a population of a county are high-risk infants under the age of 1 year, unmarried pregnant adolescents, or individuals exposed to a particular event such as a chemical spill. In **population-focused practice,**

problems are defined (assessments/diagnoses), and solutions (interventions) such as policy development or providing a given preventive service are implemented for or with a defined population or subpopulation as opposed to diagnoses, interventions, and treatment carried out at the individual client level.

Basic professional education in nursing, medicine, and other clinical disciplines focuses primarily on developing competence in decision making at the individual client level by assessing health status, making management decisions (ideally with the client), and evaluating the effects of care. Figure 1-3 illustrates three levels at which problems can be identified. For example, community-based nurse clinicians, nurse practitioners, and sometimes community health nurses focus on individuals they see either in a home or clinic setting. This individual focus is depicted by an individual person or the individual family in any subpopulation (see the "c" arrows). In such a situation the provider's emphasis is on defining and resolving a problem for individuals, with each individual seen one at a time. In Figure 1-3 the individual clients are also grouped into three separate subpopulations, each of which has a characteristic in common (see the shaded areas and the "b"

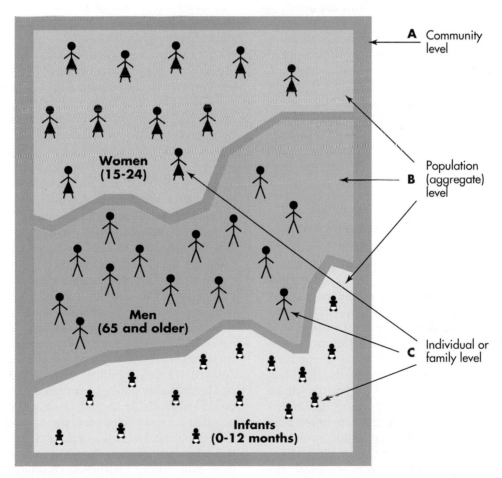

FIG. 1-3 Levels of health care practice. (Courtesy C.A. Williams, College of Nursing, University of Kentucky, Lexington, Ky.)

arrows). Subpopulations or aggregates are often the focus of attention of public health nursing specialists who define problems at the subpopulation or aggregate level as opposed to an individual level. Population-level decision making is different from decision making in clinical care and demands the specialty preparation described previously. For example, in a clinical direct-care situation the community health nurse may determine that a client is hypertensive and explore options for intervening. At the population level the public health nursing specialist would explore the answer to a set of questions:

1. What is the prevalence of hypertension among various age, race, and sex groups?
2. Which subpopulations have the highest rates of untreated hypertension?
3. What programs could reduce the problem of untreated hypertension and thereby lower the risk of further cardiovascular morbidity and mortality?

Usually public health nursing specialists are concerned with more than one subpopulation. Frequently, they are concerned with the health of the entire community, shown in Figure 1-3 as the entire box containing all of the subgroups within the community (see arrow "a"). In the real world there are many more subgroups than those reflected in this figure. Those concerned with the health of a given community must consider the total population, which is made up of multiple and sometimes overlapping subpopulations. Such an example could be adolescents at risk for unplanned pregnancies, which would overlap with the female population 15 to 24 years of age. A subpopulation that would overlap with infants under 1 year of age would be children from 0 to 6 years of age. In addition, a population focus requires considering those who may need particular services but have not entered the health care system (e.g., children without immunizations or clients with untreated hypertension).

Public Health Nursing Specialists and Core Public Health Functions: Selected Examples

The core public health function of *assessment* includes activities that involve the collection, analysis, and dissemination of information on both the health and health-relevant aspects of a community or a specific population. Questions such as whether the health services of the community are available to the population and are adequate to address needs are considered. Assessment also includes an ongoing effort to monitor the health status of the community or population and the services provided. Excellent examples of assessment at the national level are the efforts of the USDHHS to organize the goal setting, data collection and analysis, and monitoring necessary to develop the series of publications describing the health status and health-related aspects of the U.S. population. These efforts began with *Healthy People* in 1980 and continued with *Promoting Health, Preventing Disease: 1990 Health Objectives for the Nation* and *Healthy People 2000*. They are now moving into the future with *Healthy People 2010* objectives (USDHHS, 1998). Many states and other jurisdictions have developed publications describing the health status of a defined community, set of communities, or populations. Unfortunately, it is difficult to find descriptions of health assessments on particular communities unless they demonstrate new methods or reveal unusual findings about a community. Such working documents and data sets should be available and used by public health practitioners to develop services in specific settings like a county or state health department.

A recent survey was conducted to determine the extent to which local health departments were performing the core public health functions. The questions asked about assessment included 1) whether there was a needs assessment process in place that describes the health status of the community and community needs, 2) whether there has been a survey of behavioral risk factors within the last 3 years, and 3) whether an analysis has been done of "the determinants and contributing factors of priority health needs, adequacy of existing health resources, and the population groups most affected" (Turnock, Handler, and Miller, 1998, p. 28). It should be part of the public health nurse specialist's role within a local health department to participate in and provide leadership for assessing community needs, health status of populations within the community, environmental and behavioral risks, looking at trends in the health determinants, identifying priority health needs, and determining the adequacy of existing resources within the community (see Research Brief by Moore and colleagues).

Policy development is both a core function of public health and a core intervention strategy used by public health nursing specialists. Policy development in the public arena seeks to build constituencies that can help bring about change in public policy. In an interesting case study of her experience as director of public health for the state of Oregon, Gebbie (1999) describes her experiences in developing a constituency for public health. This enabled her to mobilize efforts to develop statewide goals for *Healthy People 2000* and also to update Oregon's disease reporting laws. Gebbie's experiences as a state director of public health illustrate how a public health nursing specialist can provide leadership at a very broad level. Gebbie left Oregon to go to Washington, D.C. to serve in the federal government as President Clinton's key official in the national effort to control AIDS. Clearly, Gebbie is an example of an individual who has provided leadership in policy development both at the state and national levels.

The third core public health function, *assurance*, focuses on the responsibility of public health agencies to make certain that activities have been appropriately carried out to meet public health goals and plans. This may result in public health agencies requiring others to engage in activities to meet goals, encouraging private groups to undertake certain activities, or in some instances actually offering services directly. Assurance also includes the development of partnerships between public and private agencies to make sure that needed services are available and that assessing the quality of the activities is carried out (see Research Brief by Barnes-Boyd and colleagues).

PUBLIC HEALTH NURSING AND COMMUNITY HEALTH NURSING VERSUS COMMUNITY-BASED NURSING

A broad understanding of public health should include concern for all populations within the community, both free living and institutionalized. Further, it should consider the match between the health needs of the popula-

tion and the health care resources in the community, including those services offered in institutional settings. Although all direct care providers may contribute to the community's health in the broadest sense, not all are primarily concerned with the population focus, or the "big picture." All nurses in a given community, including those working in hospitals, physicians' offices, and health clinics, contribute positively to the health of the community. However, the special contributions of public health nursing specialists include looking at the community or population as a whole; raising questions about its overall health status and factors associated with that status, including environmental factors (physical, biologic and social-cultural); and working *with the community* to improve the population's health status.

Figure 1-4 is a useful illustration of all possible arenas of practice. Since most community health nurses and many staff public health nurses, historically and at present, focus on providing direct personal care services, including health education, to persons or family units outside of in-

RESEARCH *Brief*

The following illustrates an assessment effort led by two public health nursing specialists. The assessment focused on a target population of 1-year-old Mexican-American and Caucasian non-Hispanic infants who were enrolled in a Medicaid-managed care demonstration project. This systematic effort generated findings that should provide direction for future programming. It was found that, despite the fact that the infants had access to care, differences remained between the immunization levels of the Mexican-Americans as compared with the Caucasian non-Hispanic infants. The Mexican-Americans completed fewer doses of both DPT (diphtheria-pertussis-tetanus) and polio vaccine. They were less likely to complete the recommended immunization series by 1 year of age than the Caucasian non-Hispanic infants. In fact, the Mexican-American infants received less than 60% of the three DPTs.

This shows that continuous enrollment in a Medicaid-managed care system does not ensure that there will be a high rate of immunization coverage. The strongest predictor of the number of immunizations received was the number of siblings. Those infants with fewer siblings received more immunizations, which was true for both ethnic groups. After controlling for a set of potential explanations the multiregression analysis showed that the ethnic group was not a predictor of immunization levels. Significant predictors of a higher number of immunization levels included fewer siblings for both the Hispanic and non-Hispanic groups and higher maternal education for the Caucasian non-Hispanic, but not for the Hispanic group. This assessment clearly showed that factors other than enrollment in Medicaid influence immunization rates. This assessment process provided considerable information for the public health nursing specialists about which subgroup of infants in this target population was at risk for incomplete immunization coverage.

Moore P et al: Indicators of differences in immunization rates of Mexican Americans and white non-Hispanic infants in a Medicaid managed care system, *Public Health Nurs* 13:21, 1996.

RESEARCH *Brief*

An example of leadership by public health nurses in the area of assurance is provided by an account of a home visiting program (REACH-Resources, Education and Care in the Home) designed to reduce preventable causes of morbidity among socially disadvantaged infants in selected high-risk, high-need Chicago communities. The target population was normal infants born into socially deprived homes and thus living in a high-risk environment. The intervention was designed to put in place a monitoring effort, as well as to provide clinical services and instruction. Information was provided to the mothers to help them reduce the development of preventable causes of morbidity and mortality. The results indicated that repeated home visits with ongoing infant monitoring and culturally sensitive teaching helped mothers maintain good health practices and early identification of infant problems.

This project is an example of ensuring that a target group of infants in a high-risk environment received careful attention during an important and vulnerable period of their lives. It was designed and put in place by public health nursing specialists, but the actual clinical encounters were provided by teams consisting of community-based nurses working for a hospital and community lay workers. It is a clear example of a partnership between a public health agency and a hospital organization to meet the specific needs of a target population.

Barnes-Boyd C, Norr KF, Macion KW: Evaluation of an interagency home visiting program to reduce post-neonatal mortality in disadvantaged communities, *Public Health Nurs* 13:201, 1996.

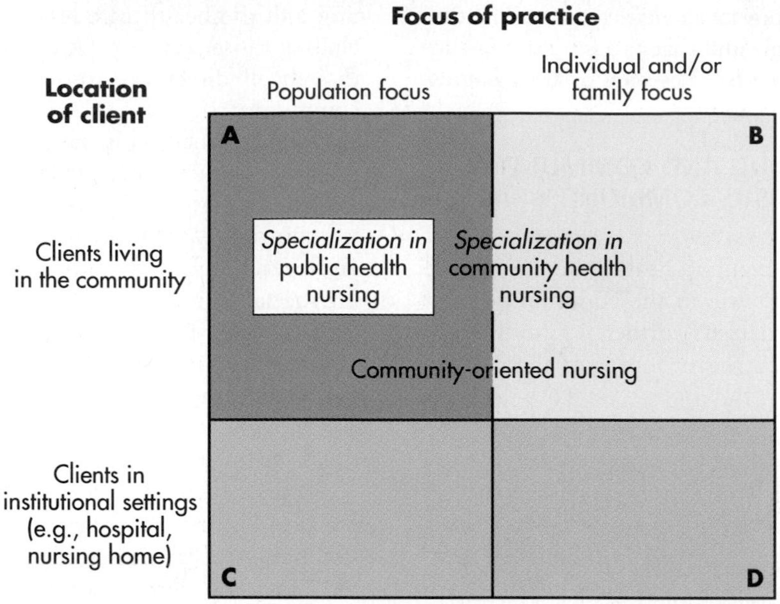

Focus of practice

| Location of client | Population focus | Individual and/or family focus |

FIG. 1-4 Arenas for health care practice. (Courtesy C.A. Williams, College of Nursing, University of Kentucky, Lexington, Ky.)

stitutional settings (either in the client's home or in a clinic environment), such practice falls into the upper right quadrant (section B) of Figure 1-4. However, specialization in public health nursing is community oriented and population focused and is represented by the box in the upper left quadrant (section A) (see the Nursing Tip earlier in this chapter).

In addition to the population focus, there are three additional reasons that the most important practice arena for public heath nursing is represented by section A, the population of noninstitutionalized clients:

1. Preventive strategies can have the greatest impact on noninstitutionalized populations, which represent the majority of a community most of the time.
2. The major interface between health status and the environment (physical, biologic, sociocultural) occurs in the noninstitutional population.
3. For philosophical, historical, and economic reasons, population-focused practice is most likely to flourish in organizational structures that serve noninstitutionalized populations (health departments, health maintenance organizations [HMOs], health centers, etc.).

What roles in the health care system do public health nursing specialists (those in section A) have? Options include director of nursing for a health department, director of the health department, state commissioner for health, or director of maternal and child health services for a state or local health department. Although nurses have in the past occupied and currently do occupy all of these roles, with the exception of the director of nursing for a health department, they are in the minority. Frequently, nurses who occupy these roles are seen as administrators and not as public health *nursing* specialists, which is a tragedy.

Where does the staff public health nurse or community health nurse fit on the diagram? Their fit depends on the focus of that nurse's practice. In many settings most of the staff nurse's time is spent in community-based direct care activities where the focus is on dealing with individual clients and individual families, which falls into section B. However, although a staff public health nurse or a community health nurse may not be a public health nurse specialist, this nurse may spend some of his or her time carrying out core public health functions with a population focus, and thus that part of the role would be represented in section A of the diagram. The field of public health nursing can be seen as primarily encompassing two groups of nurses:

- Public health nursing specialists whose practice is community-oriented *and* is focused on using population-focused strategies for carrying out the core public health functions (section A).
- Staff public health nurses or community health nurses who are community-based and may be clinically oriented to the individual client and combine some population-focused, community-oriented strategies and direct care clinical strategies in programs serving specified populations (section B).

Figure 1-4 also shows that specialization in public health nursing, as it has been defined in this chapter, can be viewed as a specialized field of practice with certain attributes within the broad arena of community health nursing and community-based nursing. This view is consistent with recommendations developed at the Consensus Conference on the Essentials of Public Health Nursing Practice and Education mentioned previously. One of the outcomes of the conference was consensus on the use of the terms *community health nurse* and *public health nurse*. It was agreed that the term **community health nurse** could apply to all nurses who practice in the community, whether or not they have had preparation in public health nursing. Thus nurses providing secondary or tertiary care in a home setting, school nurses, and nurses in clinic settings (in fact, any nurse who does not practice in an institutional setting) may fall into the category of "community health nurse." Nurses with a master's degree or a doctoral degree who are practicing in community settings could be referred to as "community health nurse specialists" regardless of the area of nursing in which the degree was earned. According to the conference statement, "the degree may be in any area of nursing, such as maternal-child health, psychiatric-mental health, or medical-surgical nursing or some subspecialty of any clinical area" (Consensus Conference, 1985, p. 4). However, the definitions of the three areas of practice have changed as clearer thinking has occurred about the three areas of practice: public health nursing, community health nursing, and community-based nursing.

In 1998, the Quad Council of Public Health Nursing developed a statement on the *Scope of Public Health Practice*. They attempted to clarify the differences between public health nursing and the newest term introduced into nursing's vocabulary during health care reform of the 1990s, **community-based nursing.** The authors recognized that the terms *public health* and *community health nursing* have been used interchangeably since the 1980s to describe population-focused, community-oriented nursing practice and community-based practice. However, they decided to make a clearer distinction between community-oriented and community-based nursing practice. The definition of public health nursing is the same as the one found on p. 8. In contrast, **community-based nursing care** is referred to as the provision or ensurance of personal care to individuals and families in the community. The editors of this text suggest two levels of care in the community: community-oriented care and community-based care. They also suggest three role functions for nursing practice: public health nursing, community health nursing, and community-based nursing.

In the middle of Figure 1-4 is a box labeled "Specialization in community health nursing," which is partly in section A and partly in section B. This suggests that there is a need and a place for specialization in community health nursing that is more focused than simply being a master's-prepared clinical specialist who practices in a community-based setting, as was suggested by the Consensus Conference 15 years ago. Although in 1985 these nurses were referred to as *community health nurses,* today they are referred to as *nurses in community-based practice.* Those who provide community-oriented service to specified subpopulations in the community and who provide some clinical services to those populations may be seen as specialists in community health nursing. Although such practitioners may be community-based, they are also com-munity-oriented as public health specialists but are usually focused on only one or two special subpopulations. Preparation for this specialization includes a master's degree in community health with emphasis in a direct-care clinical area, such as school health or occupational health, and ideally some education in the public health sciences. Examples of roles such specialists might have in direct clinical care areas include case manager, supervisor in a home health agency, school nurse, occupational health nurse, parish nurse, and a nurse practitioner who also manages a nursing clinic.

Sections C and D of Figure 1-4 represent nurses who focus on institutionalized populations. Nurses who provide direct care in hospital settings fall into section D, and those who have administrative responsibility for nursing services in institutional settings fall into section C. Box 1-2 presents detailed definitions of the four key nursing areas in the community that are depicted in Figure 1-4.

⫶ WHAT DO YOU THINK? *Are public health nursing, community health nursing, and community-based nursing practice all the same?*

ROLES IN PUBLIC HEALTH NURSING

Within public health and community health nursing circles, there has been a tendency to talk about public health nursing and community health nursing from the point of view of a role rather than the functions related to the role. This is limiting. In discussing such nursing roles there is a preoccupation with the direct care provider orientation. Even in discussions about how a practice can become more population-focused, it is interesting that the focus frequently is on how an individual practitioner, such as an agency staff nurse, can adopt a population-focused practice philosophy. Rarely is attention given to how nurse administrators in public health, one role for public health nursing specialists, might reorient their practice toward a population focus, which is particularly important and more feasible for an administrator than for the staff nurse. This is because in many agencies nursing administrators, supervisors, or others (sometimes program directors who are not nurses) make the key decisions about how staff nurses will spend their time and what types of clients will be seen and under what circumstances. Public health nursing administrators who are prepared to practice in a population-focused manner will be more effective than those who are not prepared to do so.

Staff nurses would benefit from having a clear understanding of population-focused practice for three reasons. First, it would give them professional satisfaction to see how their individual client care contributes to health at the population level. Second, it would help them understand and appreciate the practice of associates who are population-focused specialists. Third, it would give them a better basis for providing clinical input into decision making at the program or agency level, a necessary contribu-

Population-Based Practice in Community and Public Health Nursing in Canada

Lianne Jeffs, Registered Nurses Association of Ontario and University of Toronto

THE HEALTH CARE MOVEMENT

The medical model, focusing on treatment, cure, institutional care, and medical interventions, dominated the Canadian health care arena until the mid 1970s. A national Medicare program was established in 1968. The Provincial Committee on the Costs of Health Services (Canada, 1969), the Hastings Report (Canada, 1973), and the Mustard Report (Ontario, 1974) all emphasise the need for less expensive community care, organizational and structural changes, and a focus on health promotion and disease prevention. Out of this emerged the lifestyle, or behavioural approach, decade (1974-1984). In 1974, Lalonde's *A New Perspective on the Health of Canadians* was released and emphasised that the health care system was not the most important factor in determining health. In 1978, the World Health Organization's Alma Ata Declaration became the basis for primary health care (see Appendix A-4). In the 1980s, in response to the acknowledgement of the broader determinants of health, *Achieving Health for All: A Framework for Health Promotion* and the *Ottawa Charter of Rights for Health Promotion* were released. These documents have served as blueprints for more recent efforts in the health care movement that emphasise a focus on population-based health promotion and disease prevention strategies (e.g., the *Jakarta Declaration of Health Promotion in the 21st Century* and the *Population Health Promotion Model*).

EVOLUTION OF COMMUNITY HEALTH NURSING AND PUBLIC HEALTH NURSING

In Canada, the terms *community health nursing* and *public health nursing* have been used interchangeably and debated in terms of nature of practice and nature of client. Definitions of the public health nurse and community health nurse vary throughout the provinces and territories. The current discussion focuses on whether community health nursing refers only to registered nurses in traditional public health practice in health units, nurses in public health and home health services, or all nurses in community-based practice. Both public health nursing and community health nursing have evolved over the years as a result of the shift within the health care system from a medical model to a population-based health promotion focus. The role of public health nursing practice has diversified into the areas of health education, health promotion, illness and injury prevention, and primary health care for populations. Public health nurses have been defined as community health nurses who have sound knowledge of public health science, nursing science, and the social sciences, and practice to promote, protect, and preserve the health of the population (Community Health Nurses Inter-

est Group, 1998). Public health nurses provide services in the home, schools, workplaces, community centres, and other community agencies and institutions. Community health nursing emerged in the 1970s out of the growing industry of home care nursing in Canada.

The increased emphasis of home health care to individuals and families together with the downloading of public health services to municipalities may jeopardise critically important population-based health promotion and illness and injury prevention programs. Municipalities and regions finding themselves unable to afford certain services may opt to eliminate these services. In this context, a distinction between public health nursing and community health nursing is essential. It is recommended that *community health nursing* be used as the inclusive or umbrella term for community-based nursing practice, including public health nursing, home care nursing, community mental health nursing, and occupational health nursing (King et al, 1996). *Public health nursing* is defined as community-based nursing practice including population-focused health promotion and illness and injury prevention strategies working with individuals, families, groups, and communities (King et al, 1996).

EDUCATIONAL PREPARATION

The educational preparation for community health nursing and public health nursing is at the baccalaureate level and in some cases a post-RN diploma in public health. In some provinces, legislation exists that provides educational requirements for entry into public health nursing practice (e.g., in Ontario, the Health Promotion and Protection Act of 1984 restricts the use of the title of Public Health Nurse to those working in official programs who possess a baccalaureate or post-RN diploma in public health). Despite the need for baccalaureate-level education for public health nursing, a discrepancy between educational preparation and the actual practice requirements emerging from the primary health care movement has been reported (Working Group, 1991). Epidemiological surveillance, partnerships with groups and communities, population-based approaches, and community development have been identified as areas that need more emphasis within nursing curricula. Relatively few community health and public health nursing graduate programs are currently available in Canada (Dalhousie University, University of Ottawa, University of Toronto, University of Calgary, and Memorial University). The discrepancy of educational preparation in community health nursing practice and the limited availability of graduate programs are barriers to recognising and maximising the unique scope of practice of both public health nursing and community health nursing.

Continued efforts are needed to ensure that more graduate programs in community health nursing and public health nursing are developed in Canada and that nursing

Population-Based Practice in Community and Public Health Nursing in Canada–cont'd

curricula reflect the emerging primary health care principles and emphasis on epidemiology, population-based health promotion, and illness and injury prevention. In the current health care reform context, it is imperative to clearly describe both the roles of the community health nurse and the public health nurse in order to ensure that primary health care, including population-based health promotion and illness and injury prevention strategies, and programs are at the core of public health and community health services.

Bibliography

Community Health Nurses Interest Group of the Registered Nurses Association of Ontario: *Public health nursing position statement*, Toronto, 1998, the Association.

King M, Harrison MJ, Reutter LI: Public health nursing or community health nursing: what's in a
name? In Stewart MJ, editor: *Community nursing: promoting canadians' health*, Toronto, 1995, W.B. Saunders Canada.
Pinder L: The federal role in health promotion: art of the possible. In Pederson A, O'Neill M,
Rootman I, editors: *Health promotion in Canada provincial, national and international perspectives*, Toronto, 1994, W.B. Saunders Canada.
Working Group: *Report of the Working Group on the Educational Requirements of Community
Health Nurses* (Cat.No. H39-235/1991E), Ottawa, 1991, Minister of Supply and Services.

Canadian spelling is used.

---

tion to effective and efficient population-focused practice. Clearly it is desirable that staff nurses have a population perspective, although their opportunities to make decisions at that level are more limited than those of the nurse who has administrative responsibility.

Recently, a curriculum plan was proposed by representatives of key public health nursing organizations and other individuals that would prepare the staff public health nurse, or generalist, to function as a community-oriented practitioner. Content areas such as nursing and public health processes; core public health functions; history; legal, ethical, political, and economic issues; communication skills, partnership development, leadership, group process, epidemiology, quality and outcomes evaluation, community assessment, program management, community mobilization, environmental health, conflict resolution, negotiation, and change theory are essential to the development of community-oriented practice (ASTDN, 1998). The above content required for the preparation of the public health nurse generalist at the baccalaureate level can be found in this text.

It is important not to think too narrowly about nursing roles because present role functions are frequently too limited to allow for population-focused practice. Also, roles that might include the suggested population-focused decision making may not be defined as nursing roles. Examples include directorships of health departments, state or regional programs, units of health planning and evaluation, and directorships of programs such as preventive services within a managed care organization. If population-focused public health nursing is to be taken seriously and strategies for implementing the role functions of assessment, policy development, intervention, and evaluation are to be applied at the population level, more consideration must be given to organized systems for assessing population needs and managing care. Such a view of public health nursing

BOX 1-2 Definitions of the Four Key Nursing Areas in the Community

Community-Oriented Nursing Practice is a philosophy of nursing service delivery that involves the generalist or specialist public health and community health nurse. The nurse provides "health care" through community diagnosis and investigation of major health and environmental problems, health surveillance, and monitoring and evaluation of community and population health status for the purposes of preventing disease and disability and promoting, protecting, and maintaining "health" in order to create conditions in which people can be healthy.

Public Health Nursing Practice is the synthesis of nursing theory and public health theory applied to promoting and preserving the health of populations. The focus of public health nursing practice is the community as a whole and the effect of the community's health status (resources) on the health of individuals, families, and groups. Care is provided within the context of preventing disease and disability and promoting and protecting the health of the community as a whole.

Community Health Nursing Practice is the synthesis of nursing theory and public health theory applied to promoting, preserving, and maintaining the health of populations through the delivery of personal health care services to individuals, families, and groups. The focus of community health nursing practice is the health of individuals, families, and groups and the effect of their health status on the health of the community as a whole.

Community-Based Nursing Practice is a setting-specific practice whereby care is provided for "sick" individuals and families where they live, work, and attend school. The emphasis of community-based nursing practice is acute and chronic care and the provision of comprehensive, coordinated, and continuous services. Nurses who deliver community-based care are generalists or specialists in maternal-infant, pediatric, adult, or psychiatric-mental health nursing.

clearly places those who specialize in this area in the position of dealing with health care policy. In other words, public health nurse specialists must move into situations in which policy formation is a recognized component. To do this, however, some nurses may have to assume positions that are not traditionally considered nursing positions or nursing roles. This is true because, at present, much of the policy making that directly affects provision of nursing services to certain populations occurs outside the range of what are normally referred to as nursing roles.

Defining nursing roles so that they fit into the present structure of nursing services may have unfortunate limitations. For the immediate future it may be more useful to concentrate on identifying the skills and knowledge needed to make decisions in population-focused practice. It is also more important to define where in the broader community and health care system such decisions are made and to develop nurses with the knowledge, skills, and political understanding necessary for success in such positions. Some of these positions are within nursing settings, particularly roles such as administrator of the nursing service and top level staff nurse supervisors. However, as suggested earlier, other such positions may be outside of what are traditionally viewed as nursing roles, such as the commissioner of a health department.

CHALLENGES FOR THE FUTURE
Barriers to Specialization in Public Health Nursing

There are several barriers to the development of specialization in public health nursing. One of the most serious is the mind-set of many nurses that the only role for a nurse is at the bedside or at the client's side (i.e., the direct care role). Clearly, the heart of nursing is the direct care provided in personal contacts with clients. On the other hand, two things should be clear. First, whether a nurse is able to provide direct care services to a given client depends on many decisions made by individuals within and without of the care system. Second, nurses need to be involved in those fundamental decisions. Perhaps the one-to-one focus of nursing and past cultural expectations of the "proper role" of women have influenced nurses to view less positively other ways of contributing, such as administration, consultation, and research.

However, two things have changed. First, in all fields, in and out of nursing, women have taken on every role imaginable. The second change is that the number of male nurses is consistently growing. The cultural view of nursing as a female occupation is changing, and this is opening doors to new roles that may not have been considered appropriate for nurses in the past.

A second barrier to the type of practice implied in population-focused public health nursing is the structures within which nurses work and the process of role socialization within those structures. The fact that a particular role might not exist within the nursing unit may suggest that it is undesirable or impossible for nurses. For example, nurses interested in using political strategies to make changes in health-related policy, an activity clearly within the practice domain of public health nursing, may run into a number of barriers if their goals are different from the agenda of other health care groups. Such groups may use subtle but effective maneuvers to lead nurses to conclude that involvement takes them from the client and is not in their own or the client's best interests.

A third barrier is that few nurses receive graduate level preparation in the concepts and strategies of disciplines basic to public health (e.g., epidemiology, biostatistics, community development, service administration, and policy formation). One of the problems mentioned previously, which continues to be a problem in master's level preparation for public health nursing, is that in many programs the skills necessary for population assessment and management are not given the in-depth attention that other parts of the curriculum receive, particularly the direct care aspects. In short, with few exceptions, within the graduate programs in public health nursing and community health nursing, there is no aggressive effort to develop the population-focused skills that are needed (Josten et al, 1995). Many nurses see these skills as less important than clinical skills. However, for individuals specializing in public health nursing, these skills are as essential as direct care skills; they are just as difficult to develop, and they should be given more attention in graduate programs that prepare nurses for specialization in public health nursing. With the current revival in public health, there is a growing awareness among key decision makers that graduate preparation for nurses in community health and public health need to have a solid core of public health science.

Establishing Population-Focused Nurse Leaders

The massive organizational changes occurring in the delivery system present a unique opportunity to establish new roles for nurse leaders who are prepared to think in population terms. In the 1980s, Starr (1982) described the trend toward the use of private capital in financing health care, particularly institutional-based care and other health-related businesses. The movement can be thought of as the "industrialization" of health care, which until recently has operated very much like a **cottage industry.**

The implications and consequences of this movement are enormous, with a goal of providing investors a return on their investment. Today major developments in health care delivery include more attention to primary care and community-based care delivery in a variety of settings; less emphasis on specialty care; the development of partnerships, alliances, and other linkages across settings in an effort to build **integrated systems,** which would provide a broad range of services for the population it serves; and a growing adoption of **capitation,** a payment arrangement in which insurers agree to pay providers a fixed sum for each person per month or per year, independent of the costs actually incurred. With the spread of capitation has come serious interest throughout the health care system in the concept of populations, sometimes referred to by financial officers and others as *covered lives* (e.g., individuals with insurance that pays on a capitated basis). For public health specialists it is a new experience to see individuals involved in the business aspects of health care and frequently employed by hospitals thinking in population terms and taking a population approach to decision making.

This new focus on populations coupled with the integration that is occurring in some health care systems will likely create new roles for individuals, hopefully nurses, who will span inpatient and community-based settings and will focus on providing a wide range of services to the population served by the system. Such a role might be director of patient care services for a health care system. In addition to those who will have the administrative responsibility for a large programmatic area, there will be a demand for individuals who can design programs of preventive and clinical services to be offered to targeted subpopulations. Who will decide what services will be given to which subpopulation and by which providers? Large systems and consultant firms are currently offering courses designed to prepare physicians for such roles (Advisory Board Company, 1994). How will nurses be prepared for leadership in the emerging and future structures for health care delivery and health maintenance?

Just as physician leaders are recognizing that other physicians need to be prepared to use population-focused methods, such as epidemiology and biostatistics, to make evidence-based decisions in the development of programs and protocols, the attention being given to preparing nurses for administrative decision making seems to be declining. This may be a result of the recent lack of federal support for preparing nurse administrators and of the growing popularity of nurse practitioner programs. However, it is time that nurse leaders give more attention to preparing nurses for leadership in the area of population-focused practice. Perhaps it is time to combine specialization in public health nursing and nursing administration as suggested some time ago (Williams, 1985). Regardless of how the population is defined, there will be a growing need for nurses with population-level assessment, management, and evaluation skills. The primary focus of the health care system of the future will be on community-oriented strategies for health promotion and disease prevention and community-based strategies for primary care and much of secondary care. Directing more attention to developing the specialty of public health nursing as a way to provide nursing leadership may be a good response to the health care system changes. To prepare for such population-focused decision making will require more attention to developing master's- and doctoral-level programs that have a stronger basis in the public health sciences, while providing for better preparation of baccalaureate-prepared nurses in community health and community-based practice.

Some observers of public health have anticipated that if universal health insurance coverage for all Americans becomes a reality, public health practitioners can turn over the delivery of personal primary care services to other providers, such as HMOs and integrated health plans, and return to the core public health functions. However, as described previously, assurance, making sure that basic services are available to all, is a core function of public health. Thus, even under the condition of universal coverage, there will still be a need to monitor subpopulations in the community to ensure that necessary care is available and that quality is at an acceptable level and, when it is not, to see that it is provided. Universal coverage, however, has not become a reality. Because of pressures in the health care system to cut costs, there is now a growing concern that the problem of access to basic primary care will get worse before it gets better, particularly for special, vulnerable populations (e.g., the homeless, the frail, the elderly, and persons with HIV).

The history of public health nursing shows that a common feature of leaders is to move forward to deal with unresolved problems in a positive, proactive way. This is the legacy of Lillian Wald at the Henry Street Settlement and many others who have met a need with innovation. Within the context of the core public health function of assurance, there clearly is an opportunity for public health nursing to develop population-focused outreach programs directed to "the matching of the needs of vulnerable groups in the community with the services that hold promise for helping them"(Aiken and Salmon, 1994, p. 328). As a specialty, public health nursing can have a positive impact on the health status of populations, but to do so "it will be necessary to have broad vision; to prepare nurses for leadership roles in policy making and in the design, development, management, monitoring, and evaluation of population-focused health care systems and to develop strategies to support nurses in these roles" (Williams, 1992, p. 268).

clinical application

The basic thesis of this chapter is that population-focused nursing practice is different from clinical nursing care delivered in the community. If one accepts the thesis of this chapter that specialization in public health nursing is population-focused and encompasses a unique body of knowledge, then it is useful to debate where and how public health nursing specialists practice and how their practice compares with what has been defined as specialization in community health nursing and community-based nursing.

In your public/community health class, debate with classmates which of the nurses in the following categories are practicing population-focused nursing:

A. School nursing
B. Staff nurses in home care
C. Director of nursing for a home care agency
D. Nurse practitioners in a health maintenance organization

E. Vice-president of nursing in a hospital
F. Staff nurses in a public health clinic or community health center
G. Director of nursing in a health department

Choose three categories in the list, and interview at least one nurse in each category. Determine what their scope of practice is. Are they carrying out population-focused practice? Could they? How?

Answers are in the back of the book.

KEY POINTS

- Public health is what we, as a society, do collectively to ensure the conditions in which people can be healthy.
- Assessment, policy development, and assurance are the core public health functions at all levels of government.
- *Assessment* refers to systematic data collection on the population, monitoring of the population's health status, and making information available on the health of the community.
- *Policy development* refers to the need to provide leadership in developing policies that support the health of the population, including the use of the scientific knowledge base in making decisions about policy.
- *Assurance* refers to the role of public health in making sure that essential community-wide health services are available, which may include providing essential personal health services for those who would otherwise not receive them. *Assurance* also refers to making sure that a competent public health and personal health care workforce is available.
- *Setting* is frequently viewed as the feature that distinguishes public health nursing from other specialties. A more useful approach is to use characteristics such as the following: a focus on populations that are free-living in the community; the emphasis on prevention; the concern for the interface between health status of the population and the living environment (physical, biologic, sociocultural); and the use of political processes to affect public policy as a major intervention strategy for achieving goals.

- According to the 1984 Consensus Conference sponsored by the Nursing Division for the U. S. Department of Health and Human Services, specialists in public health nursing are defined as those who are prepared at the graduate level, either master's or doctoral, "with a focus in the public health sciences" (Consensus Conference, 1985).
- Specialization in public health nursing is seen as a subset of community health nursing.
- Population-focused practice is the focus of specialization in public health nursing. This focus on populations and the emphasis on health protection, health promotion, and disease prevention are the fundamental factors that distinguish public health nursing from other nursing specialties.
- *Population* is defined as a collection of individuals who share one or more personal or environmental characteristics. The term *population* may be used interchangeably with the term *aggregate*.

critical thinking activities

1. Define for your personal understanding
   a. Essential functions of public health
   b. Specialist in public health nursing
   c. Specialist in community health nursing
2. State your opinion of the similarities and/or differences between a clinical nursing role and the population-focused role of the public health nursing specialist.
3. Review the models of public health nursing practice of the ANA and APHA as described in this chapter.
4. With three or four of your classmates, develop a plan for identifying two or three nurses in your community who are in an administrative role and discuss with them the following:
   a. How they define the populations they are serving
   b. Strategies they use to monitor the population's health status
   c. Strategies they use to ensure that the populations are receiving basic needed services
   d. What initiatives they are taking to address problems

Bibliography

Advisory Board Company: *Capitation 1:the new American medicine*, Washington, DC, 1994, Advisory Board Company.

Aiken LH, Salmon ME: Health care workforce priorities: what nursing should do now, *Inquiry* 31:318, 1994.

American Nurses Association, Division of Community Health Nursing: *Conceptual model of community health nursing*, Pub No CH-10, Kansas City, Mo, 1980, the Association.

American Nurses Association: *Scope and standards of public health nursing*, Washington, DC, in press, the Association.

American Public Health Association: *The definition and role of public health nursing: a statement of the APHA public health nursing section, March 1996 Update*, Washington, DC, 1996, the Association.

American Public Health Association: *The definition and role of public health nursing in the delivery of health care: a statement of the public health nursing section*, Washington, DC, 1981, the Association.

Association of State and Territorial Directors of Nursing: *Public health nursing: a partner for Progress*, Washington, DC, 1998, the Association.

Barnes-Boyd C, Norr KF, Nacion KW: Evaluation of an interagency home visiting program to reduce postneonatal mortality in disadvantaged communities, *Public Health Nursing* 13:201, 1996.

Consensus Conference on the Essentials of Public Health Nursing Practice and Education, Rockville, MD, 1985, US Department of Health and Human Services, Bureau of Health Professions, Division of Nursing.

Gebbie K: Building a constituency for public health, *J Public Health Manage Pract* 3:1, 1999.

Institute of Medicine: *Improving health in the community: a role for performance monitoring*, Washington, DC, 1997, National Academy Press.

Institute of Medicine: *The future of public health*, Washington, DC, 1988, National Academy Press.

Josten L et al: Public health nursing education: back to the future for public health sciences, *Fam Community Health* 18:36, 1995.

Moore P et al: Indicators of differences in immunization rates of Mexican-American and White non-Hispanic infants in a Medicaid managed care system, *Public Health Nursing* 13:21, 1996.

Starr P: *The social transformation of American medicine,* New York, 1982, Basic Books.

Turnock B, Handler AS, Miller CA: Core function–related local public health practice effectiveness, *J Public Health Manage Pract* 4:26, 1998.

US Department of Health and Human Services: *Healthy people 2010 objectives,* 1998 (Draft for public comment).

US Preventive Services Task Force: *Guide to clinical preventive services,* ed 2, Baltimore, 1996, Williams & Wilkins.

US Public Health Service: *A time for partnership,* Prevention Report, Washington, DC, Dec 1994/Jan 1995, Office of Disease Prevention and Health Promotion.

US Public Health Service: *The core functions project,* Washington, DC, 1993, Office of Disease Prevention and Health Promotion.

Williams CA: Beyond the Institute of Medicine Report: a critical analysis and public health forecast. *Family Community Health* 18:12, 1995.

Williams CA: Population-focused community health nursing and nursing administration: a new synthesis. In McCloskey JC, Grace HK, editors: *Current issues in nursing,* ed 2, Boston, 1985, Blackwell Scientific Publications.

Williams CA: Public health nursing: does it have a future? In Aiken LH, Fagin CM, editors: *Charting nursing's future: agenda for the 1990s,* Philadelphia, 1992, JB Lippincott.

CHAPTER

2

History of Public Health and Public and Community Health Nursing

JANNA DIECKMANN

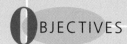 **www.mosby.com/MERLIN/community_stanhope**

OBJECTIVES

After reading this chapter, the student should be able to do the following:

- Interpret the focus and roles of community and public health nurses through an historical approach.
- Trace the ongoing interaction between the practices of public health and nursing.
- Identify the dynamic relationship between changes in social, political, and economic contexts and community-oriented nursing practice.
- Outline the professional and practice impact of individual leadership on community and public health nursing, especially the leadership of Florence Nightingale and Lillian Wald.

- Identify structures for delivery of community-oriented nursing care such as settlement houses, visiting nurse associations, official health organizations, and schools.
- Recognize major organizations that contributed to the growth and development of community-oriented nursing.
- Relate the impact of legislative initiatives to changing opportunities for community-oriented nursing practice.

KEY TERMS

American Nurses Association
American Public Health Association
American Red Cross
Mary Breckinridge
district nursing

district nursing association
Frontier Nursing Service
instructive district nursing
Metropolitan Life Insurance Company
National League for Nursing

National Organization for Public Health Nursing
Florence Nightingale
official health agencies
William Rathbone
settlement houses
Sheppard-Towner Act

Social Security Act of 1935
Town and Country Nursing Service
visiting nurse associations
visiting nurses
Lillian Wald
See Glossary for definitions

CHAPTER OUTLINE

Change and Continuity
Historical Measures to Provide for the Public's Health
America's Colonial Period and the New Republic
Nightingale and the Origins of Trained Nursing
America Needs Trained Nurses
School Nursing in America
The Profession Comes of Age
Public Health Nursing in Official Health Agencies
World War I and the Importance of Public Health Nursing

Paying the Bill for Community and Public Health Nurses
Efforts to Shape Public Policy
Between the Two World Wars: Economic Depression and the Rise of Hospitals
Increasing Federal Action for the Public's Health
World War II: Extension and Retrenchment in Community and Public Health Nursing
The Rise of Chronic Illnesses
Failure of Financing for Community-Oriented Nursing

Consolidation of National Nursing Organizations
New Forms of Payment for Community-Oriented Nursing
Community Organization and Professional Change
Community and Public Health Nursing from the 1970s to the Present
Community and Public Health Nursing Today

The author acknowledges the important foundational work for this chapter developed by Dr. Jeanette Lancaster in previous editions of this book.

Nurses use an historical approach to illuminate both the profession's present and future. Several different questions might be asked:

- Who are community and public health nurses?
- How does the past contribute to who they are today?
- What are the places and times in which community and public health nurses have worked and continue to work?
- When is a conscious process of critique and insight employed to look into past actions of the specialty, and what can be discovered from the process?
- Can agreement with and endorsement of these past actions be achieved?
- How might knowledge of community and public health nursing history serve not only as a source of inspiration, but also as a stimulus to solve creatively the emerging problems of this contemporary period?

This chapter serves as an introduction to consideration of these questions.

CHANGE AND CONTINUITY

For over 100 years, public health nurses in the United States have created intervention strategies to respond effectively to prevailing public health problems. The history of community and public health nursing reflects changes in the specific focus of the profession while emphasizing continuity in approach and style. Community and public health nurses have sought to improve the health status of individuals, families, and populations, especially those who belong to vulnerable groups. Part of the appeal of community and public health nursing has been its autonomy of practice and independence in problem solving and decision making, done in the context of a multi-disciplinary practice. Many of the varied and challenging roles of public health nurses can be traced to the late 1800s when public health efforts focused on environmental conditions such as sanitation, control of communicable diseases, education for health, prevention of disease and disability, and care of sick persons in their homes.

Although threats to health from communicable diseases, the environment, chronic illness, and the aging process have changed over time, the foundational principles and goals of public health nursing have remained the same. While many communicable diseases, such as diphtheria, cholera, and typhoid fever, have been largely controlled in the United States, other communicable diseases continue to affect many lives, including illnesses such as human immunodeficiency virus (HIV) and acquired immunodeficiency syndrome (AIDS), measles, tuberculosis, and hepatitis. Even though environmental pollution in residential areas has been reduced, communities are now threatened by overcrowded garbage dumps and pollutants affecting the air, water, and soil. Finally, with growth in the elderly population of the United States and their preference to remain at home, additional nursing services are required to sustain frail elders and the chronically ill in the community.

The roles of the community and public health nurse in the United States developed from several sources and are a product of various social, economic, and political forces. This chapter describes the societal circumstances that influenced nurses to establish community based and community-oriented practices. As community-oriented nurses rely heavily on public health science, in addition to their focus on nursing science and practice, major events in public health are also noted. The nation's need for community and public health nurses, the practice of community-oriented nursing, and the organizations influencing community and public health nursing in the United States during the nineteenth and twentieth centuries are outlined in this chapter.

HISTORICAL MEASURES TO PROVIDE FOR THE PUBLIC'S HEALTH

Concern for the health and care of individuals in the community has characterized human existence. All people and all cultures have been concerned with the events surrounding birth, death, and illness. They have sought to prevent, understand, and control disease. Their ability to preserve health and treat illness has depended on the contemporary level of science, use and availability of technologies, and degree of social organization. For example, ancient Babylonians emphasized hygiene and possessed some medical skills, such as the use of medications to treat sick persons. Using principles of observation and empirical knowledge, the Egyptians of about 1000 BC developed a variety of pharmaceutical preparations and constructed earth privies and public drainage systems. The Mosaic health code of the Old Testament Jews directed practices to maintain and prolong life for individuals, families, and communities (Rosen, 1958).

The ancient Greeks sought a harmonious relationship with nature by linking individual health to the environment. The privileged classes valued personal cleanliness, exercise, diet, and sanitation, although the lives of the majority might have been different. The classical Roman civilization viewed medicine from a community health and social medicine perspective, emphasizing regulation of medical practice and punishment for negligence; provision of pure water through a complex system of settling basins, aqueducts, and reservoirs; establishment of sewage systems and drainage of swamps; and supervision of street cleaning and public food preparation. During the rule of the Roman Empire, women visited and cared for sick persons (Pellegrino, 1963).

The decline of the Greco-Roman civilization led to both a decay of urban culture and a disintegration of community health organization and practice (Rosen, 1958). During the Middle Ages (between 500 and 1500 AD), health risks in European cities were characterized by high population density, lack of clean water, and poor handling of refuse and body waste. Poor sanitary conditions and residential crowding led to increased prevalence and periodic pandemics of communicable diseases such as cholera, smallpox, and bubonic plague. Although most people were responsible for securing their own health care services, religious convents and monasteries established hospitals to care for the sick, poor, and neglected, including the aged, disabled, and orphaned (Rosen, 1958). Health education and personal hygiene knowledge also increased during the latter portion of the Middle Ages, as demonstrated in surviving manuscripts that encouraged healthful living and moderate eating.

During the Renaissance (from the fourteenth through the sixteenth centuries AD), recognition of human dignity and worth increasingly influenced health practices (Kalisch and Kalisch, 1995). Although the growth of science and technology during this period supported the advance of medicine and public health, public health measures continued to be rudimentary. For example, although increased social organization led to improved management of cities, many areas continued to depend upon private enterprise for water supply and completely lacked systems of sewage disposal. In England, the Elizabethan Poor Law of 1601 guaranteed medical care for poor, blind, and "lame" individuals. This minimal care was most often provided in almshouses supported by the local government, which sought as much to regulate the poor as to provide care during illness. Table 2-1 presents milestones of public health efforts that occurred during the seventeenth, eighteenth, and nineteenth centuries.

The Industrial Revolution in nineteenth century Europe, with its tremendous advances in transportation, communication, and other forms of technology, led to deep social upheaval. Previous caregiving structures, which had depended on assistance of family, neighbors, and friends, became inadequate because of migration, urbanization, and changing demand. During this period, Roman Catholic and Protestant women continued to provide

nursing care in institutions and sometimes in the home, but their numbers were small. For example, Mary Aikenhead, also known by her religious name, Sister Mary Augustine, started the Irish Sisters of Charity in 1812 in Dublin, where the nuns visited the poor population (Kalisch and Kalisch, 1995).

Many women who performed nursing functions in almshouses and early hospitals in Great Britain were poorly educated and untrained, sometimes referred to as the "dregs of the community, dirty, drunken, and dishonest" (Swinson, 1965). With the increasingly complex practice of medicine in the mid-1800s, hospital work required a more skilled caregiver. Physicians and hospital administrators sought to advance the practice of nursing. Early experiments yielded some improvement in care, but the efforts of Florence Nightingale would be credited with beginning a revolution.

AMERICA'S COLONIAL PERIOD AND THE NEW REPUBLIC

In the early years of America's settlement, as in Europe, the care of the sick was usually informal and was provided by household members, almost always women. The female head of the household was responsible for caring for all household members, which meant more than only nursing them in sickness and during childbirth. She was also responsible for growing or gathering healing herbs in season for use throughout the year. For the increasing numbers of urban residents in the early 1800s, this traditional system became insufficient.

American ideas of social welfare and the care of the sick were strongly influenced by the traditions of British settlers in the New World. Just as American jurisprudence is based on English common law, colonial Americans established systems of care for the sick, poor, aged, mentally ill, and dependent based on the model of the Elizabethan

TABLE 2-1 Milestones in History of Public Health and Community Health Nursing: 1600 to 1865

Year	Milestone
1601	Elizabethan Poor Law written
1617	Sisterhood of the Dames de Charite organized in France by St. Vincent de Paul
1789	Baltimore Health Department established
1798	Marine Hospital Service established; later became Public Health Service
1812	Sisters of Mercy established in Dublin where nuns visited the poor
1813	Ladies' Benevolent Society of Charleston, South Carolina founded
1836	Lutheran deaconesses provide home visits in Kaiserwerth, Germany
1851	Florence Nightingale visits Kaiserwerth for 3 months of nurse training
1855	Quarantine Board established in New Orleans; beginning of tuberculosis campaign in the United States
1859	District nursing established in Liverpool by William Rathbone
1860	Florence Nightingale Training School for Nurses established at St. Thomas Hospital in London
1864	Red Cross established

Poor Law. Early county or township government was responsible for the care of all dependent residents but provided almshouse charity carefully, economically, and only for their own. Those who were residents elsewhere were returned to their home counties for care. Few hospitals existed, and they were only in the larger cities. In 1751, Pennsylvania Hospital was founded in Philadelphia, the first hospital in what would become the United States.

Early colonial public health efforts included the collection of vital statistics, improved sanitation, and control of communicable diseases that were introduced through seaports. The colonists lacked a continuing and organized mechanism for ensuring that public health efforts would be supported and enforced. Epidemics intermittently taxed the limited local organization for health during the seventeenth, eighteenth, and nineteenth centuries (Rosen, 1958).

After the American Revolution, the threat of disease, especially yellow fever, brought public support for establishing government-sponsored, or official, boards of health. By 1800, with a population of 75,000, New York City had established a public health committee for monitoring water quality, sewer construction, drainage of marshes, planting of trees and vegetables, construction of a masonry wall along the waterfront, and burial of the dead (Rosen, 1958).

Increased urbanization and beginning industrialization contributed to increased incidence of disease, including epidemics of smallpox, yellow fever, cholera, typhoid, and typhus. Tuberculosis and malaria remained endemic with a high incidence rate, and infant mortality was about 200 per 1000 live births (Pickett and Hanlon, 1990). American hospitals in the early 1800s were generally unsanitary and staffed by poorly trained workers. Physicians received a limited education through proprietary schools or simple apprenticeship. Medical care was difficult to secure, although public dispensaries (similar to outpatient clinics) and private charitable efforts attempted to address gaps in the availability of sickness services, especially for the urban working class and poor. Environmental conditions in urban neighborhoods, including inadequate housing and sanitation, were additional risks to health.

The federal government's early efforts for public health were targeted toward securing its maritime trade and seacoast cities by providing health care for merchant seamen and by protecting seacoast cities from epidemics. The Public Health Service, which remains the most important federal public health agency today, was established in 1798 as the Marine Hospital Service. The first Marine Hospital was opened in Norfolk, Virginia in 1800. Additional legislation to establish quarantine legislation for seamen and immigrants was passed in 1878.

During the early 1800s, experiments in providing nursing care at home usually focused on moral elevation and illness intervention. The Ladies' Benevolent Society of Charleston, South Carolina provided charitable assistance to the poor and sick beginning in 1813. In Philadelphia, lay nurses oriented in a brief training program cared for postpartum women and their newborns in their homes. In Cincinnati, Ohio, the Sisters of Charity began a visiting nurse service in 1854 (Rodabaugh and Rodabaugh, 1951). Although these early programs were significant in providing services at the local level, they were not adopted elsewhere, and their influence on later community health nursing is unclear.

During the middle of the nineteenth century, national interest grew to address public health problems and improve urban living conditions. The roles of urban boards of health reflected changing ideas of public health. Rather than solely addressing environmental hazards as they had in the past, communicable disease became an interest. Soon after it was founded in 1847, the American Medical Association (AMA) formed a hygiene committee to carry out sanitary surveys and to develop a system for collecting vital statistics. The Shattuck Report, published in 1850 by the Massachusetts Sanitary Commission, called for major innovations: the establishment of a state health department and local health boards in every town; sanitary surveys and collection of vital statistics; environmental sanitation; food, drug, and communicable disease control; well-child care health education; tobacco and alcohol control; town planning; and the teaching of preventive medicine in medical schools (Kalisch and Kalisch, 1995). However, these actions were not implemented in Massachusetts until 19 years later.

NIGHTINGALE AND THE ORIGINS OF TRAINED NURSING

Florence Nightingale's vision of trained nurses and her model of nursing education influenced the development of professional nursing and, indirectly, public health nursing in the United States. In 1850 and 1851, Nightingale had carefully studied nursing "system and method" by visiting Pastor Theodor Fliedner at his School for Deaconesses in Kaiserwerth, Germany. Pastor Fliedner had visited Mennonite deaconesses in Holland engaged in parish work for the poor and the sick, as well as Elizabeth Fry, the English prison reformer. Thus mid-nineteenth century efforts to reform the practice of nursing drew upon a variety of mutually interacting innovations across Europe.

The Kaiserwerth Lutheran deaconesses incorporated care of the sick at home with care in their hospital, and their system of **district nursing** (community health nursing) had spread to other cities in Germany. American requests for assistance from the deaconesses to respond to epidemics of typhus and cholera in Pittsburgh proved temporary because of a lack of local women interested in the work. Their early efforts in the United States were focused on institutional care (Nutting and Dock, 1935).

During the Crimean War (1854 to 1856), the British military established hospitals for sick and wounded soldiers in Scutari in Asia Minor. The care of soldiers was severely deficient, with cramped quarters, poor sanitation, lice and rats, insufficient food, and inadequate medical supplies (Kalisch and Kalisch, 1986; Palmer, 1983). When the British public demanded improved conditions, Florence Nightingale sought appointment to address the chaos. Because of her wealth, social and political connections, and knowledge of hospitals, the British government sent her to Asia Minor with 40 ladies, 117 hired nurses, and 15 paid servants.

In Scutari, Nightingale progressively improved the soldiers' health using a population-based approach that yielded improvements in environmental conditions and nursing care. Using simple epidemiology measures, she documented a decreased mortality rate from 415 per 1000 at the beginning of the war to 11.5 per 1000 at the end (Cohen, 1984; Palmer, 1983). Like Nightingale's efforts in Scutari, public health nurses typically identify health care needs that affect the entire population, mobilize resources, and organize themselves and the community to meet these needs.

After the Crimean War and her return to England in 1856, with her fame established, Nightingale organized hospital nursing practice and nursing education in hospitals to replace untrained lay nurses with Nightingale nurses. Nightingale not only focused on the role of hospital nursing but also emphasized public health nursing: "The health of the unity is the health of the community. Unless you have the health of the unity, there is no community health" (Nightingale, 1894, p. 455). She differentiated "sick nursing" from "health nursing," which emphasized that nursing should strive to promote health and prevent illness. Nightingale (1946, p. v) found the task of nursing to be to "put the constitution in such a state as that it will have no disease, or that it can recover from disease." Proper nutrition, rest, sanitation, and hygiene were necessary for health. Community and public health nurses continue to focus on the role of health promotion, disease prevention, and environment in their practice with individuals, families, and communities, respectively.

Nightingale's contemporary, British philanthropist **William Rathbone,** founded the first **district nursing association** in Liverpool, England. Rathbone's wife had received outstanding nursing care from a Nightingale-trained nurse during her terminal illness at home. Rathbone became inspired to offer similar care to relieve the suffering poor unable to afford private nurses. With Rathbone's verbal and economic support between 1859 and 1862, the Liverpool Relief Society divided the city into nursing districts and assigned a committee of "friendly visitors" to each district to provide health care to needy people (Kalisch and Kalisch, 1995). Based on the Liverpool experience, Rathbone and Nightingale recommended steps to provide nursing in the home, and district nursing was organized throughout England. Florence Sarah Lees Craven shaped the profession through her *Guide to District Nurses* that recommended, for example,

that the district nurse gain influence to improve the status of the whole family through the illness of one member of the family (Craven, 1889).

AMERICA NEEDS TRAINED NURSES

With increased urbanization during the Industrial Revolution, the number of jobs for women rapidly increased. Educated women could become elementary school teachers, secretaries, or saleswomen, whereas less educated women worked in factories of all kinds. The idea of becoming a trained nurse increased in popularity. During the 1870s, the first nursing schools based on the Nightingale model opened in the United States.

Trained nurse graduates of the first Nightingale-style schools in the United States usually worked in private duty nursing or held the few positions of hospital administrators or instructors. These private duty nurses might live with families of patients receiving care. Although the trained nurse's effect on improving American hospitals was clear, the cost of private duty nursing care for the sick at home was prohibitive for all but the wealthy. Community health nursing in the United States was beginning to organize to meet urban health care needs, especially for the disadvantaged. Nurses became active as **visiting nurses** and in establishing community **settlement houses.**

The care of the sick poor at home was made economical by having home-visiting nurses attend several families in 1 day rather than attend only one as the private duty nurse did. In 1877 the Women's Board of the New York City Mission hired Frances Root, a graduate of Bellevue Hospital's first nursing class, to visit sick poor persons to provide nursing care and religious instruction (Bullough and Bullough, 1964). In 1878 the Ethical Culture Society of New York hired four nurses to work in dispensaries. In the next few years, **visiting nurse associations** were established in Buffalo, NY (1885), Philadelphia (1886), and Boston (1886). Wealthy people interested in charitable activities funded both settlement houses and visiting nurse associations. Upper class women, freed of some of the social restrictions that had previously limited their public life, became interested in the charitable work of creating, supporting, and supervising the new visiting nurses.

The public was interested in limiting disease among all classes of people, partly for religious reasons, partly as a form of charity, but also because the middle and upper classes feared the impact of diseases believed to originate in the large communities of new immigrants from Europe. In New York City in the 1890s, about 2.3 million people were packed into 90,000 tenement houses. The environmental conditions of immigrants in tenement houses and sweatshops were familiar features of urban life across the northeastern United States and into the upper Midwest. "Slum dwellers were ravaged by epidemics of typhus, scarlet fever, smallpox, and typhoid fever, and many of them died or developed tuberculosis" (Kalisch and Kalisch, 1995, p. 172). From the beginning, community

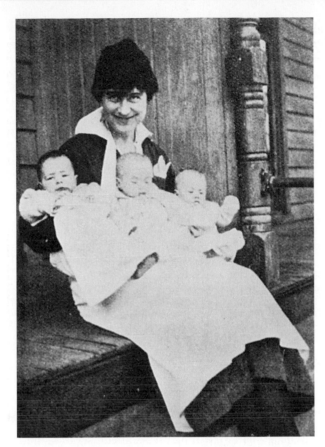

FIG. 2-1 Teaching well-child care was a significant public health nursing role. (Courtesy Instructional Visiting Nurse Association of Richmond, Va.)

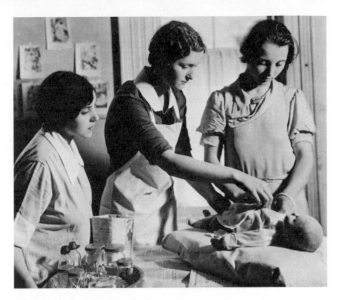

FIG. 2-2 Public health nurse demonstrating well-child care during a home visit. (Courtesy the Visiting Nurse Service of New York.)

health nursing practice included teaching and prevention (Fig. 2-1). Community and public health nursing interventions, improved sanitation, economic improvements, and better nutrition were credited with reducing the incidence of acute communicable disease by 1910.

New scientific explanations of communicable disease suggested that preventive education would reduce illness. The visiting nurse became key to communicating the prevention campaign through the home visit and well baby clinics. These community health visiting nurses worked with physicians, gave selected treatments, and kept temperature and pulse records. The nurses emphasized education of family members in the care of the sick and in personal and environmental prevention measures, such as hygiene and good nutrition (Fig. 2-2). Many early visiting nurse agencies employed only one nurse, who was supervised by members of the agency board, usually composed of wealthy or socially prominent ladies. These ladies were critically important to the success of visiting nursing through their efforts to open new agencies, financially support existing agencies, and make the services socially acceptable.

For example, in 1886, two Boston women approached the Women's Education Association to seek support for

district nursing. To increase the likelihood of financial support, they used the term **instructive district nursing** to emphasize the relationship of nursing to health education. Support was also secured from the Boston Dispensary, which provided free medical care on an outpatient basis. In February of 1886 the first district nurse was hired, and in 1888 the Instructive District Nursing Association became incorporated as an independent voluntary agency. Sick poor persons, who paid no fees, were cared for under the direction of a trained physician (Brainard, 1922).

Other nurses established settlement houses, neighborhood centers that became hubs for health care and social welfare programs. For example, in 1893 **Lillian Wald** and Mary Brewster, both trained nurses, began visiting the poor on New York's lower east side. The nurses' settlement they established became the Henry Street Settlement and later the Visiting Nurse Service of New York City. By 1905, the public health nurses had provided almost 48,000 visits to over 5000 patients (Kalisch and Kalisch, 1995). Lillian Wald emerged as the established leader of public health nursing during its early decades (Box 2-1, Fig. 2-3).

In 1909, Yssabella Waters published her survey, *Visiting Nursing in the United States*. Visiting nurse services were concentrated in the northeastern quadrant of the country. Emphasizing the rapid and divergent development of visiting nursing, in 1909, New York City had 58 different organizations with 372 trained nurses providing care in the community. However, nationally, 68% of visiting nurses were employed in single-nurse agencies. In addition to visiting nurse associations and settlement houses, many different types of organizations sponsored visiting nurses, such as boards of education, boards of health, mission boards, clubs, churches, social service agencies, and tuber-

BOX 2-1 Lillian Wald: First Public Health Nurse in the United States

Public health nursing evolved in the United States in the late nineteenth and early twentieth centuries largely because of the pioneering work of Lillian Wald. Born on March 10, 1867, Lillian Wald decided to become a nurse after Vassar College refused to admit her at 16 years of age. She graduated in 1891 from the New York Hospital Training School for Nurses and spent the next year working at the New York Juvenile Asylum. To supplement what she thought had been inadequate training in the sciences, she enrolled in the Woman's Medical College in New York (Frachel, 1988).

Having grown up in a warm, nurturing family in Rochester, New York, her work in New York City introduced her to an entirely different side of life. In 1883, while conducting a class in home nursing for immigrant families on the lower east side of New York City, Wald was asked by a small child to visit her sick mother. Wald found the mother in bed, having hemorrhaged for 2 days. This home visit confirmed for Wald all of the injustices in society and the differences in health care for poor persons versus those persons able to pay (Frachel, 1988).

She simply could not tolerate seeing poor people with no access to health care. With her friend Mary Brewster and the financial support of two wealthy laypeople, Mrs. Solomon Loeb and Joseph H. Schiff, she moved to the east side and occupied the top floor of a tenement house on Jefferson Street. This move eventually led to the establishment of Henry Street Settlement. In the beginning, Wald and Brewster helped individual families. Wald believed that the nurse's visit "should be like that of a very interested friend rather than that of an impersonal, paid visitor" (Dolan, 1978).

Ever discontent to deal only with the present and convinced that environmental conditions as well as social conditions were the causes of ill health and poverty, Wald became actively involved in using epidemiological methods to campaign for health-promoting social policies. Not only did she write *The House on Henry Street* to describe her own public health nursing work, but also she led in the development of payment by insurance companies for nursing services (Frachel, 1988).

In 1909, with Lee Frankel, Lillian Wald established the first community health nursing program for workers at the Metropolitan Life Insurance Company. Believing that keeping workers healthier would increase their productivity, she urged that nurses at agencies such as Henry Street Settlement provide skilled nursing care. Wald convinced the company that it would be more economical to use the services of community health nurses than to employ their own nurses. She also convinced them that services could be available to anyone desiring them, with fees graduated according to the ability to pay. This nursing service designed by Wald continued for 44 years and contributed several significant accomplishments to community health nursing, including the following (Frachel, 1988):
1. Providing home nursing care on a fee-for-service basis
2. Establishing an effective cost-accounting system for visiting nurses
3. Using advertisements in both newspapers and the radio to recruit nurses
4. Reducing mortality from infectious diseases

Lillian Wald also believed that the nursing efforts at the Henry Street Settlement should be aligned with an official health agency. Therefore she arranged for nurses to wear an insignia that signified that they served under the auspices of the Board of Health. Also, she established rural health nursing services through the Red Cross. Her other accomplishments included helping to establish the Children's Bureau and fighting in New York City for better tenement living conditions, city recreation centers, parks, pure food laws, graded classes for mentally handicapped children, and assistance to immigrants (Backer, 1993; Dock, 1922; Frachel, 1988; Zerwekh, 1992).

culosis associations. With tuberculosis responsible for at least 10% of all mortality during this time, visiting nurses contributed to its control through gaining "the personal cooperation of patients and their families" to modify the environment and personal behavior (Buhler-Wilkerson, 1987, p. 45). Most visiting nurse agencies depended on the philanthropy and social networks of metropolitan areas. As today, service delivery in less densely populated (rural) areas presented additional challenges.

NURSING TIP

Securing information about the organizational history of a practice agency, such as a visiting nurse association, may provide important perspectives on current agency values, decision-making structures, service areas, and clinical priorities.

The **American Red Cross,** through its Rural Nursing Service (later the **Town and Country Nursing Service**), initiated home nursing care in areas outside larger cities. Lillian Wald secured initial donations to support this agency, which provided care of the sick, provided instruction in sanitation and hygiene in rural homes, and improved living conditions in villages and isolated farms. The Town and Country nurse addressed diseases such as tuberculosis, pneumonia, and typhoid fever with a resourcefulness born of necessity. The rural nurse might use hot bricks, salt, or sandbags to substitute for hot water bottles; chairs as back rests for the bedbound; and boards padded with quilts as stretchers (Kalisch and Kalisch, 1995). Immediately after World War I, the 100 existing Red Cross Town and Country Nursing Services expanded to 1800 in less than 2 years, eventually growing to almost 3000 programs in small towns and rural areas. This service demonstrated the importance and feasibility of public

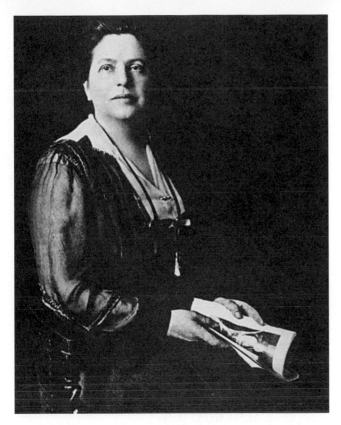

FIG. 2-3 Lillian Wald. (Courtesy the Visiting Nurse Service of New York.)

health nursing across the country at local and county levels. Once established, these agencies were passed on to be maintained by local voluntary agencies or local government.

Occupational health nursing began as industrial nursing and was a true outgrowth of early home visiting efforts. In 1895, Ada Mayo Stewart began work with employees and families of the Vermont Marble Company. As a free service for the employees, Stewart provided obstetric care, sickness care, and some postsurgical care but very few services for work-related injuries (Kalisch and Kalisch, 1995).

SCHOOL NURSING IN AMERICA

In New York City in 1902, more than 20% of children could be absent from school on a single day, suffering from such common conditions as pediculosis, ringworm, scabies, inflamed eyes, discharging ears, and infected wounds. School medical inspection began in 1897 but was focused on excluding infectious children from school rather than on providing or obtaining medical treatment so that children might return to school. Familiar with this community-wide problem from her work with the Henry Street Nurses' Settlement, Lillian Wald sought to emulate English innovations by providing nurses for schools and gained consent from the city's health commissioner and the Board of Education for a 1-month demonstration.

Lina Rogers, a Nurses' Settlement resident, became the first school nurse. She worked with the children in New York City schools and made home visits to instruct parents and follow-up on children excluded or otherwise absent from school. The nurses found that "many children were absent for lack of shoes or clothing, because of malnourishment, or because they were serving their families as babysitters" (Hawkins, Hayes, and Corliss, 1994, p. 417). The school nurse experiment was such a huge success that it became permanent, with twelve more nurses appointed 1 month later. School nursing was soon implemented in Los Angeles, Philadelphia, Baltimore, Boston, Chicago, and San Francisco.

THE PROFESSION COMES OF AGE

Established by the Cleveland Visiting Nurse Association, the publication of the Visiting Nurse Quarterly in 1909 initiated a professional medium of communication for clinical and organizational concerns. In 1911 a joint committee of existing nurse organizations convened, under the leadership of Lillian Wald and Mary Gardner, to standardize nursing services outside the hospital. Recommending formation of a new organization to address public health nursing concerns, 800 agencies involved in community health nursing activities were invited to send delegates to an organizational meeting in Chicago in June 1912. After a heated debate on its name and purpose, the delegates established the **National Organization for Public Health Nursing** (NOPHN) and chose Lillian Wald as its first president (Dock, 1922). Unlike other professional nursing organizations, the NOPHN membership included both nurses and their lay supporters. The NOPHN sought "to improve the educational and services standards of the public health nurse, and promote public understanding of and respect for her work" (Rosen, 1958, p. 381). With greater administrative resources than any of the other national nursing organizations existing at that time, the NOPHN was soon a dominant force in public health nursing (Roberts, 1955).

The NOPHN also sought to standardize community and public health nursing education. Visiting nurse agencies found that graduate nurses were unprepared for home visiting. It became apparent that the basic curriculum of many schools of nursing was insufficient. Because diploma schools of nursing emphasized hospital care of patients, community and public health nurses would require additional education to provide services to the sick at home and to design population-focused programs. In 1914 Mary Adelaide Nutting began the first postgraduate nursing course in public health nursing at Teachers College in New York City in affiliation with the Henry Street Settlement (Deloughery, 1977). The American Red Cross provided scholarships for graduates of nursing schools to attend the public health nursing course. Its success encouraged development of other programs, whose curriculum might seem familiar to today's nurses. Public health nursing did not become a required part of most baccalaureate nursing education programs until the 1950s.

Public health nurses were also active in the **American Public Health Association** (APHA), which was established in 1872 to facilitate interdisciplinary efforts and promote the "practical application of public hygiene" (Scutchfield and Keck, 1997, p. 12). The APHA targeted reform efforts toward contemporary public health issues, including sewage and garbage disposal, occupational injuries, and sexually transmitted diseases. In 1923, the Public Health Nursing Section was formed within the APHA to provide an additional national forum for discussion of strategy for public health nurses within the context of the larger public health organization.

WHAT DO YOU THINK? *Lillian Wald demonstrated an exceptional ability to develop approaches and programs to solve the health care and social problems of her times. How would you apply this creativity to today's health care challenges? If Lillian Wald were looking over your shoulder, what would she recommend?*

PUBLIC HEALTH NURSING IN OFFICIAL HEALTH AGENCIES

The focus of government action for public health nursing was at the local level, in cities, towns, and counties. In the late 1800s, local health departments were formed in urban areas to target environmental hazards associated with crowded living conditions and dirty streets and to regulate public baths, slaughterhouses, and pigsties (Pickett and Hanlon, 1990). By 1900, 38 states had established state health departments, following the lead of Massachusetts in 1869, but the impact of these early state boards of health was very limited. Only three states, Massachusetts, Rhode Island, and Florida, annually spent more than 2 cents per capita for public health services (Scutchfield and Keck, 1997). In 1912, the federal government expanded the role of the U.S. Public Health Service, empowering it to "investigate the causes and spread of diseases and the pollution and sanitation of navigable streams and lakes" (Scutchfield and Keck, 1997, p. 15).

During the 1910s, public health organizations began at the rural level to target epidemics. The Rockefeller Sanitary Commission, active in hookworm control in the southeastern United States, concluded that concurrent efforts for all phases of public health were necessary to successfully address any individual public health problem (Pickett and Hanlon, 1990). For example, in 1911, efforts to control typhoid fever in Yakima County, Washington and to improve health status in Guilford County, North Carolina resulted in the establishment of local health units to serve local populations. Public health nurses were the primary staff members of local health departments. These nurses assumed a leadership role on health care issues through collaboration with local residents, nurses, and other health care providers.

The experience of Orange County, California during the 1920s and 1930s demonstrates the concerns of the public health nurse in the local health department. Following the efforts of a private physician, social welfare agencies, and a Red Cross nurse, the county board created the public health nurse's position to begin in 1922. Presented with a shining new Model T car sporting the bright orange seal of the county, the nurse first addressed the serious communicable disease problems of diphtheria and scarlet fever. Typhoid became epidemic when a drainage pipe overflowed into a well, infecting those who drank the water and those who drank raw milk from an infected dairy. Almost 3000 residents were immunized. Weekly baby conferences provided an opportunity for mothers to learn about care of their infants, and the infants were weighed and received immunizations. Children with orthopedic and other disabilities were identified and referred for medical care in Los Angeles. At the end of this successful first year, the Rockefeller Foundation and the California Health Department provided funding for more public health professionals.

WORLD WAR I AND THE IMPORTANCE OF PUBLIC HEALTH NURSING

In 1918 during World War I, the Vassar Camp School for Nurses started as a unique and patriotic aspect of nursing education. The American Red Cross and the Council of National Defense jointly supported this novel program, which proposed that nursing education could be shortened from 3 years to 2 years for college graduates. The Vassar Camp School, modeled after the Plattsburg Military Camp in New York, gave intensive training to college graduates so that they could become army reserve officers and meet urgent wartime needs. A total of 435 graduates of this program represented many colleges across the United States. The program ended when peace was declared (Buhler-Wilkerson, 1989; Kalisch and Kalisch, 1995; Wilner, Walkey, and O'Neill, 1978).

The personnel needs of World War I in Europe depleted the ranks of public health nurses, yet the NOPHN identified a need for second and third lines of defense at home. Jane Delano of the Red Cross, who was sending 100 nurses a day to the war, agreed that despite the sacrifice, the greatest patriotic duty of public health nurses was to stay at home. Soon after, a world-wide influenza epidemic swept from the Atlantic to the Pacific coast within 3 weeks and was met by a coalition of the NOPHN and the Red Cross. Houses, churches, and halls were turned into hospitals, with loss of life also among nurse volunteers. The NOPHN also loaned a nurse to the U.S. Public Health Service to establish a public health nursing program for military outposts, which led to the first federal government sponsorship (Shyrock, 1959; Wilner, Walkey, and O'Neill, 1978).

PAYING THE BILL FOR COMMUNITY AND PUBLIC HEALTH NURSES

The major obstacle to extending nursing services in the community was limitations on adequate funding. Most early visiting nurse associations sought charitable contributions from wealthy and middle-class supporters. Even poor families were encouraged to pay a small fee for nursing services, reflecting social welfare concerns against promoting economic dependency by providing charity. In 1909, as a result of advocacy by Lillian Wald, the **Metropolitan Life Insurance Company** began a cooperative program with visiting nurse organizations to provide care for sick policyholders. By 1912, 589 Metropolitan Life nursing centers provided care through existing agencies or through visiting nurses hired directly by Metropolitan Life. In 1918, Metropolitan Life calculated an average decline of 7% in the mortality rate of policyholders and almost a 20% decline in the mortality rate of children under age 3. The insurance company attributed this improvement and the reduced costs for the insurance company to the work of visiting nurses (see Research Brief).

RESEARCH *Brief*

The relationship between the nursing profession and Metropolitan Life Insurance Company is both interesting and reflective of a range of historical events in nursing. Metropolitan Life led the insurance industry in the provision of nursing care in the home for its policyholders. Lee Frankel, a friend of Lillian Wald, headed the welfare department at Metropolitan Life. She proposed that nurses could assess illness, teach health practices, and effectively collect data from policyholders. On June 9, 1909 the first Henry Street nurse made a home visit to a policyholder. By 1914 Metropolitan Life provided home nursing care to policyholders in 1804 cities. The original idea was for the company to contract for services with existing nursing agencies. However, in 1910 the Metropolitan Visiting Nurse service was established in St. Paul, Minnesota, and these nurses became "Met nurses." They not only provided care to policy-holders that may have lengthened their lives but also collected immense amounts of data that were invaluable to the insurance industry.

The author describes the relationship among the insurance company, nurses, and policyholders in the study of tuberculosis that began in Framingham, Massachusetts in 1916. The article is not about tuberculosis but is about nursing and how since the early 1900s other groups have tried to be in control.

Hamilton D: Research and reform: community nursing and the Framingham tuberculosis project, 1914-1923, *Nurs Res* 41(1):8, 1992.

EFFORTS TO SHAPE PUBLIC POLICY

Community and public health nurses' efforts to influence public policy bridged World War I and included advocacy for the Children's Bureau and the Sheppard-Towner Program. Responding to lengthy advocacy by Lillian Wald and other nurse leaders, the Children's Bureau was established in 1912 to address national problems of maternal and child welfare. Children's Bureau experts conducted extensive scientific research on the effect of income, housing, employment, and other factors on infant and maternal mortality, leading to federal child labor laws and the 1919 White House Conference on Child Health.

Problems of maternal and child morbidity and mortality spurred the Maternity and Infancy Act (often called the **Sheppard-Towner Act**) in 1921, which provided federal matching funds to establish maternal and child health divisions in state health departments. Education during home visits by public health nurses stressed promoting the health of mother and child, as well as seeking prompt medical care during pregnancy. Although credited with saving many lives, the Sheppard-Towner Program ended in 1929 in response to concerns by the American Medical Association and others that the legislation gave too much power to the federal government and too closely resembled socialized medicine (Pickett and Hanlon, 1990).

In contrast to significant changes in public support for community and public health nursing, some innovations were the result of individual commitment and private financial support. In 1925 the **Frontier Nursing Service** (FNS) was established by **Mary Breckinridge** based on systems of care used in the Highlands and islands of Scotland (Box 2-2, Fig. 2-4). Breckinridge introduced the first nurse-midwives into the United States. The unique pioneering spirit of the FNS influenced development of public health programs geared toward improving the health care of the rural and often inaccessible population in the Appalachian sections of southeastern Kentucky (Browne, 1966; Tirpak, 1975) (Fig. 2-5). FNS nurses were trained in nursing, public health, and midwifery, resulting in reduced pregnancy complications for their patients, and one-third fewer stillbirths and infant deaths in an area of 700 square miles (Kalisch and Kalisch, 1995). Today the FNS continues to provide comprehensive health and nursing services to the people of that area and supports the Frontier School of Midwifery and Family Nursing.

BETWEEN THE TWO WORLD WARS: ECONOMIC DEPRESSION AND THE RISE OF HOSPITALS

A continuing challenge to community and public health nursing was the tension between preventive care and care of the sick and the related question of whether nursing interventions should be directed toward groups and communities or toward individuals and their families. Although each nursing agency was unique and services varied from region to region, voluntary visiting nurse as-

BOX 2-2 Mary Breckinridge and the Frontier Nursing Service

Born in 1881 into the fifth generation of a Kentucky family, Mary Breckinridge devoted her life to the establishment of the Frontier Nursing Service (FNS). Learning from her grandmother, who used a large part of her fortune to improve the education of southern children, Breckinridge later used money left to her by her grandmother to start the FNS (Browne, 1966).

Tutored in childhood and later attending private schools, Mary Breckinridge did not consider becoming a nurse until her husband died. In 1907 she began studying nursing at St. Luke's Hospital School of Nursing in New York. She later married for a second time and had two children. Her son died at the age of 4 years, and her daughter died at birth. From the time of her son's death in 1918, she devoted her energy to promoting the health care of disadvantaged women and children (Browne, 1966).

After World War I and work in postwar France, she returned to the United States passionate about helping the neglected children of rural America. To prepare herself for what would become her life's work, she studied for 1 year at Teacher's College, Columbia University to learn more about public health nursing (Browne, 1966).

Early in 1925 she returned to Kentucky. She decided that the mountains of Kentucky were an excellent place to demonstrate the value of community health nursing to remote, disadvantaged families. She thought that if she could establish a nursing center in rural Kentucky, this effort could then be duplicated anywhere. The first health center was established in a five-room cabin in Hyden, Kentucky. Establishing the center took not only nursing skills but also the construction of the center and later the hospital and other buildings; it required extensive knowledge about securing a water supply, disposing of sewage, get-

ting electric power, and securing a mountain area in which landslides occurred (Browne, 1966). Despite many obstacles inherent in building in the mountains, six outpost nursing centers were built between 1927 and 1930. The FNS hospital in Hyden, Kentucky was completed in 1928, and physicians began entering service. Payment of fees ranged from labor and supplies to funds raised through annual family dues, philanthropy, and fund-raising efforts of Mary Breckinridge (Holloway, 1975).

The FNS established medical, surgical, and dental clinics; provided nursing and midwifery services 24 hours a day; and served nearly 10,000 people spread out over 700 square miles. At the suggestion of a supportive physician, baseline data were obtained on infant and maternal mortality rates before beginning services. The reduced mortality rate after the inception of the FNS is especially remarkable considering the environmental conditions in which these rural Kentuckians lived. Many homes had no heat, electricity, or running water. Often physicians were located over 40 miles from their patients (Tirpak, 1975).

During the 1930s, nurses lived and saw patients from one of the six outposts and often had to make their visits on horseback. Like her nurses, Mary Breckinridge traveled many miles through the mountains of Kentucky on her horse, Babette, providing food, supplies, and health care to mountain families (Browne, 1966).

Over the years several hundred nurses have worked for the FNS. Despite the fact that Mary Breckinridge died in 1965, the FNS has continued to grow and provide needed services to people in the mountains of Kentucky. This service continues today as a vital and creative way to deliver community health services to rural families.

sociations tended to emphasize care of the sick, whereas official public health agencies provided more preventive services. Not surprisingly, this splintering of services led to rivalry between "visiting," or community, and "public health" nurses, which further impeded development of comprehensive community nursing services (Roberts and Heinrich, 1985). In addition, it was possible for one household to receive services from several community nurses representing several agencies (e.g., visits for a postpartum woman and new baby, for a child sick with scarlet fever, and for a elderly person sick in bed). Community health nurses saw this as confusing to the families and as a duplication of scarce nursing resources.

One solution was the "combination service," the merger of sick care services and preventive services into one comprehensive agency, which was most often administered by a public agency. However, compared with visiting nurse organizations, community health nurses in official agencies might have less control over the program because physicians and politicians determined services and assignment of personnel. The "ideal program" of the combination agency proved difficult to administer, and many

of the combination services implemented between 1930 and 1965 later retrenched into their former divided structures.

The economic crisis during the Depression of the 1930s deeply influenced nursing. Not only were agencies and communities unprepared to address the increased needs and numbers of the impoverished, but decreased funding for nursing services reduced the number of employed nurses in hospitals and in the community. The Federal Emergency Relief Administration (FERA) supported nurse employment through increased grants-in-aid for state programs of home medical care. FERA often purchased nursing care from existing visiting nurse agencies, thus supporting more nurses and preventing agency closure. Some Depression-era federal programs built new services; public health nursing programs of the Works Progress Administration (WPA) were sometimes later incorporated into state health departments. In West Virginia, the Relief Nursing Service sought to assist unemployed nurses and provide nursing care for families on relief. Fundamental services included "(1) providing bedside care and health supervision for the family in the home; (2) arranging for

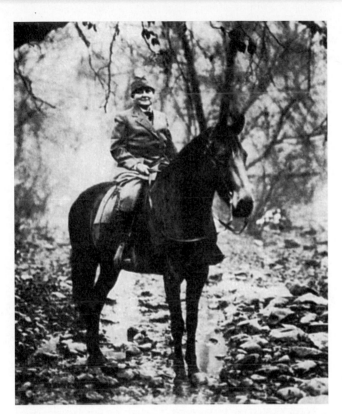

FIG. 2-4 Mary Breckinridge, founder of the Frontier Nursing Service. (Courtesy the Frontier Nursing Service of Wendover, Ky.)

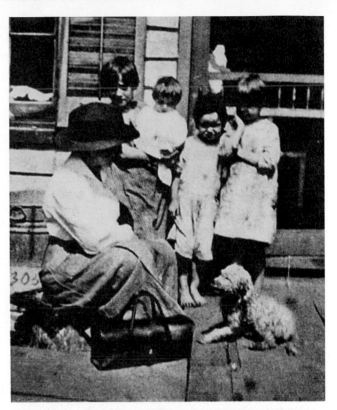

FIG. 2-5 Early public health nurses provided a range of services for families. (Courtesy Instructional Visiting Nurse Association of Richmond, Va.)

medical and hospital care for emergency and obstetric cases; (3) supervising the health of children in emergency relief nursery schools; and (4) caring for patients with tuberculosis" (Kalisch and Kalisch, 1995, p. 306).

Over 10,000 nurses were employed by the Civil Works Administration Programs (CWA) and assigned to official health agencies. "While this facilitated rapid program expansion by recipient agencies and gave the nurses a taste of public health, the nurses' lack of field experience created major problems of training and supervision for the regular staff" (Roberts and Heinrich, 1985, p. 1162). A 1932 survey of public health agencies found that only 7% of nurses employed in public health were adequately prepared (Roberts and Heinrich, 1985). Basic nursing education focused heavily on the care of individuals, and students received limited information on groups and the community as a unit of service. Thus new graduates were inadequately prepared to work in public health and required considerable agency orientation and teaching (National Organization for Public Health Nursing, 1944).

INCREASING FEDERAL ACTION FOR THE PUBLIC'S HEALTH

Changes at the federal level affected the structure of community health resources. Credited as "the beginning of a new era in public nursing" (Roberts and Heinrich, 1985, p. 1162), in 1933 Pearl McIver became the first nurse employed by the U.S. Public Health Service to provide consultation services to state health departments. McIver was convinced that the strengths and ability of each state's director of public health nursing would determine the scope and quality of local health services. Together with Naomi Deutsch, director of nursing for the federal Children's Bureau, and with the support of nursing organizations, McIver and her staff of nurse consultants influenced the direction of public health nursing. Between 1931 and 1938, over 40% of the increase in public health nurse employment was in local health agencies. Even so, over one-third of all counties nationally still lacked local public health nursing services.

The **Social Security Act of 1935** attempted to overcome the national setbacks of the Depression. Title VI of this act provided funding for expanded opportunities for health protection and promotion through education and employment of public health nurses. Over 1000 nurses completed educational programs in public health in 1936. Title VI also provided $8 million to assist states, counties, and medical districts in the establishment and maintenance of adequate health services, as well as $2 million for research and investigation of disease (Buhler-Wilkerson, 1985; Buhler-Wilkerson, 1989; Kalisch and Kalisch, 1995).

A categorical approach to federal funding for public health services reflected the U.S. Congress' preference for funding specific diseases or specific groups. In categorical

A Historical Overview of Community and Public Health Nursing in Canada

Karon Foster, Toronto Public Health and Ryerson Polytechnical University

The history of community and public health nursing in Canada is best described according to the important periods in Canada's history: pre-confederation, post-confederation, and the twentieth century.

PRE-CONFEDERATION

Canada was first settled by the French in 1534 and was called "New France." Life in New France was hard, and the settlers suffered from infectious diseases, malnutrition, inadequate clothing, inadequate shelter, and injuries. Jesuit priests initially provided care to the sick and dying. As more families immigrated, lay women in the community provided care to the sick, midwifery, and bonesetting (setting fractures). One of the first lay healers was Marie Rollet Hébert of Quebec, who cared for the sick in their homes or in her own home. The first nurses in Canada were male attendants stationed at the sick bay in a French garrison in 1629.

Hospitals were not built for another 10 years. The Duchess d'Aiguillon and three nuns from Hospitalières de la Misèricorde de Jèsus are credited with establishing a hospital in Quebec City in 1639. These nuns cared for the sick in the hospital and also went into settlers' homes to provide care. Jeanne Mance and Paul de Chomédy de Sieur Maissoneuve were asked by La Société de Notre Dame de Jésus to build the Hotel Dieu hospital on the Island of Montreal. At Hotel Dieu, care was provided to the sick, and shelter was provided to the poor and to new immigrants.

The first community visiting nurses were the Grey Nuns of Montreal, founded by Marguerite d'Youville in 1738. The focus of their work was to provide direct care and education. The Grey Nuns were also responsible for setting up houses of refuge for the elderly and infirm and for establishing hospitals. In 1844, they established health services in the Red River Settlement (now Manitoba). Health services were also established in Bytown (now Ottawa) in 1845, and in the 1860s they expanded health services to Saskatoon and the Northwest Territories.

In the 1700s, concern for the health of the community was evident by measures to control the spread of infectious diseases. Public health measures such as laws requiring meat inspection, building inspections, and quarantines were initiated. These measures were not always effective, and epidemics of disease continued. In the 1830s, boards of health were established to deal with epidemics. The Public Health Act of 1831 provided legal directives concerning personal and environmental cleanliness, quarantine, and the handling of contaminated objects or bodies.

On July 1, 1867, the provinces of Nova Scotia, New Brunswick, Quebec, and Ontario formed the Dominion of Canada. The British North America Act of 1867 outlined the responsibilities of the federal and provincial governments in relation to health care. The federal government was responsible for maintenance of marine hospitals and quarantines, and the provinces were responsible for the maintenance of hospitals, asylums, and welfare services. This decision explains why health care developed differently in each of the provinces.

POST-CONFEDERATION

During the late 1800s and early 1900s the major threats to health were contagious diseases, maternal deaths, and deaths from childhood diseases. Economic expansion and immigration resulted in more settlers living in urban areas. The cities became overcrowded, and many lived in unsanitary conditions. Public support grew for comprehensive public health programs. In the late 1800s the first permanent boards of health were established in Ontario. Every municipality appointed a board that was responsible for control of communicable diseases and the promotion of health. In 1874, the Mack School was instituted at the General Marine Hospital in St. Catharines as the first training school for nurses in Canada. Other nursing schools were established in the late 1800s in association with the development of hospitals.

In the late 1800s Lady Ishbel, the Countess of Aberdeen and wife of the Governor General, was concerned about the health needs of women and the poor in cities and isolated settlements. She proposed the formation of a group of untrained workers to provide care to these populations, but doctors and nursing groups were opposed to this idea. She revised her plan, and nurses with extra training in midwifery and home visiting were hired. The organization was called the Victorian Order of Nurses (VON). These nurses provided care in the home and were even involved in the Klondike gold rush. The first offices were set up in Halifax, Montreal, Ottawa, and Toronto. Charlotte MacLeod became the Chief Lady Superintendent of the VON and was credited with establishing many branches and training schools during her tenure.

TWENTIETH CENTURY

After World War I, the Canadian Red Cross became instrumental in promoting public health measures and training nurses to work in this area. They developed educational programs about public health, hygiene, and immunization. Programs such as these became the responsibility of the official public health agencies and resulted in the creation of the public health nurse (PHN) position. These nurses became the front-line workers in community health promotion and the maintenance of health. Nursing divisions were developed within public health agencies in the early 1900s in Ontario, Manitoba, Alberta, and British Columbia. The Canadian Red Cross provided grants to six Canadian universities to develop courses in public health. These programs eventually led to the development of baccalaureate programs in nursing.

A Historical Overview of Community and Public Health Nursing in Canada—cont'd

Since the 1950s, the role of the community health nurse (CHN) has continued to evolve. The CHN's role may include direct care to individuals and families. It can also include prevention efforts and promotion of health to individuals, families, groups, or communities. Today community nurses practice in a variety of settings including public health, home care, occupational health, community health centres, and agencies providing health promotion and care to the homeless.

Bibliography

Allemang M: Development of community health nursing in Canada. In Stewart MJ, editor:
Community health nursing: promoting Canadians health, ed 2, Toronto, 1995, WB Saunders.
Baumgart A: Evolution of the Canadian health care system. In Baumgart A, Larsen J, editors:

Canadian nursing faces the future, ed 2, St Louis, 1992, Mosby.
Chalmers K, Kristjanson L: Community health nursing practice. In Baumgart A, Larsen J, editors:
Canadian nursing faces the future, ed 2, St Louis, 1992, Mosby.
Kerr Ross J: The growth of community health nursing in Canada. In Ross J, MacPhail J, editors:
An introduction to issues in community health nursing in Canada, St Louis 1996, Mosby.
Pringle D, Roe D: Voluntary community agencies: VON Canada an example. In Baumgart A, Larsen J, editors: *Canadian nursing faces the future*, ed 2, St Louis, 1992, Mosby.

Canadian spelling is used.

funding, funding is directed toward specific priorities rather than toward a comprehensive community health program. When funding is directed by established national preferences, it becomes more difficult to respond to local and emerging problems. Even so, local health departments shaped their programs according to the pattern of available funds (e.g., maternal and child health services and crippled children [1935], venereal disease control [1938], tuberculosis [1944], mental health [1947], industrial hygiene [1947], and dental health [1947]) (Scutchfield and Keck, 1997). This pattern of funding continues to be an element of the federal approach to health policy.

WORLD WAR II: EXTENSION AND RETRENCHMENT IN COMMUNITY AND PUBLIC HEALTH NURSING

The onset of World War II in 1941 accelerated the need for nurses, both for the war effort and at home. The Nursing Council on National Defense was a coalition of the national nursing organizations that sought to plan and coordinate activities for the war effort. National interests prioritized the health of military personnel and workers in essential industries. Many nurses joined the Army and Navy Nurse Corps. Through the influence and leadership of U.S. Representative Frances Payne Bolton of Ohio, substantial funding was provided by the Bolton Act of 1943 to establish the Cadet Nurses Corps, which increased enrollment in schools of nursing at undergraduate and graduate levels. Under management by the U.S. Public Health Service, the Nursing Council for National Defense received $1 million to expand facilities for nursing education. Training for Nurses for National Defense, the GI Bill, the Nurse Training Act of 1943, and Public Health and Professional Nurse Traineeships provided additional educational funds that expanded both the total number of nurses and the number of nurses with preparation in public health nursing (McNeil, 1967).

The war-related reduction in acute care services as a result of the depletion of nursing and medical personnel from civilian hospitals increased the trend to shift responsibility for patient care to families and others. Non-nursing personnel assumed roles formerly held by registered nurses both at home and in hospitals. "By the end of 1942, over 500,000 women had completed the American Red Cross home nursing course, and nearly 17,000 nurse's aides had been certified" (Roberts and Heinrich, 1985, p. 1165). By the end of 1946, over 215,000 volunteer nurse's aides had received certificates.

In some cases, community health nursing expanded its scope of practice during World War II. For example, community health nurses increased their presence in rural areas, and many official agencies began to provide bedside nursing care (Buhler-Wilkerson, 1985; Kalisch and Kalisch, 1995). The federal Emergency Maternity and Infant Care Act of 1943 (EMIC) provided funding for medical, hospital, and nursing care for wives and babies of servicemen, but only when the services met the tough standards of the U.S. Children's Bureau. In other situations, community health nursing roles were constrained by wartime and postwar nursing shortages. For example, the Visiting Nurse Society of Philadelphia ceased assisting with home births, drastically reduced industrial nursing care, and deferred care for the long-term chronically ill patient.

Reflecting the complex social changes of the war years, local health departments were faced immediately after the war with increased service needs, including sudden increases in client demand for care of emotional problems, accidents, alcoholism, and other responsibilities new to the domain of official health agencies. Changes in medical technology offered new possibilities for screening and treatment of infectious and communicable diseases, such as antibiotics to treat rheumatic fever and venereal diseases and photofluorogram for mass casefinding for pulmonary tuberculosis. Local health departments expanded, both to address underserved areas and to expand types of services, and they often fared better economically than the voluntary agencies.

Job opportunities for public health nurses grew because they constituted a large proportion of the staff in these health departments. Between 1950 and 1955, the proportion of U.S. counties with full-time local health services increased from 56% to 72% (Roberts and Heinrich, 1985). With more than 20,000 nurses employed in health departments, visiting nurse associations, industry, and schools, community and public health nurses continued to be important in translating the advances of science and medicine into saving lives and improving health.

In 1946, representatives of agencies interested in community health met to improve coordination of various types of community nursing and to prevent overlap of services. The resulting guidelines proposed that a population of 50,000 be required to support a public health program and that there should be one nurse for every 2200 people. Community health nursing functions should include health teaching, disease control, and care of the sick. Com-

munities should adopt one of the following organizational patterns (Desirable organization, 1946):

1. Administration of all community health nurse services by the local health department
2. Provision of preventive health care by health departments and provision of home visiting for the sick by a cooperating voluntary agency
3. A combination service jointly administered and financed by official and voluntary agencies with all services provided by one group of nurses

Table 2-2 highlights significant milestones in community and public health nursing from the mid-1800s to the mid-1900s.

THE RISE OF CHRONIC ILLNESSES

Between 1900 and 1955, the national crude mortality rate decreased by 47%. Many more Americans survived childhood and early adulthood to live into the middle and older ages. By mid-century, the leading causes of death were heart disease, cancer, and cerebrovascular disease. Public health

TABLE 2-2 Milestones in History of Community Health and Public Health Nursing: 1866-1945

YEAR	MILESTONE
1866	New York Metropolitan Board of Health established
1872	American Public Health Association established
1873	New York Training School opens at Bellevue Hospital, New York City, as first Nightingale-model nursing school in United States
1877	Women's Board of the New York Mission hires Frances Root to visit the sick poor
1885	Visiting Nurse Association established in Buffalo
1886	Visiting nurse agencies established in Philadelphia and Boston
1893	Lillian Wald and Mary Brewster organized a visiting nursing service for the poor of New York, which later became the famous Henry Street Settlement; Society of Superintendents of Training Schools of Nurses in the United States and Canada was established (in 1912 became known as the National League for Nursing)
1895	Associated Alumnae of Training Schools for Nurses established (in 1911 became the American Nurses Association)
1902	School nursing started in New York (Lina Rogers)
1903	First nurse practice acts
1909	Metropolitan Life Insurance Company provides first insurance reimbursement for nursing care
1910	Public health nursing program instituted at Teachers College, Columbia University, in New York
1912	National Organization for Public Health Nursing formed with Lillian Wald as first president
1914	First undergraduate nursing education course in public offered by Adelaide Nutting at Teacher's College
1918	Vassar Camp School for Nurses organized; U.S. Public Health Service (PHS) establishes division of public health nursing to work in the war effort; worldwide influenza epidemic begins
1919	Textbook, *Public Health Nursing,* written by Mary S. Gardner
1921	Maternity and Infancy Act (Sheppard-Towner Act)
1925	Frontier Nursing Service using nurse-midwives established
1934	Pearl McIver becomes first nurse employed by PHS
1935	Passage of Social Security Act
1941	Beginning of World War II
1943	Passage of Bolton-Bailey Act for nursing education and Cadet Nurse Program established; Division of Nursing begun at PHS; Lucille Petry appointed chief of Cadet Nurse Corps
1944	First basic program in nursing accredited as including sufficient public health content

nurses had contributed to reductions in communicable diseases through immunization campaigns, improved nutrition, and better hygiene and sanitation. Additional factors included improved medications, better housing, and innovative emergency and critical care services. The aged population grew from 4.1% in 1900 to 9.2% of the total in 1950. With increased prevalence of chronic illness, extended life span, and increased duration of life after diagnosis with chronic illness, community and public health nurses faced new challenges related to chronic illness care, long-term illness and disability, and chronic disease prevention.

Studies such as the National Health Survey of 1935-1936 documented the national transition from communicable to chronic disease as the primary cause of significant illness and death. However, public policy and community-oriented nursing services were diverted from addressing the emerging problem, first by the 1930s Depression and then by World War II.

In **official health agencies,** categorical programs focusing on a single chronic disease emphasized narrowly defined services, which might be poorly coordinated with other agency programs. Some visiting nurse associations adopted coordinated home care programs to provide complex, long-term care to the chronically ill, often after long-term hospitalization. These home care programs established a multidisciplinary approach to complex patient care. For example, beginning in 1949, the Visiting Nurse Society of Philadelphia provided care to patients with stroke, arthritis, cancer, and fractures using a wide range of services, including physical and occupational therapy, nutrition consultation, social services, laboratory and x-ray procedures, and transportation services. During the 1950s, often in reaction to family needs and the shortage of nurses, many visiting nurse agencies began experimenting with auxiliary nursing personnel, variously called *housekeepers, homemakers,* or *home health aides.* These innovative programs provided a substantial basis for an approach to sickness care that would be reimbursable by private health insurance and later Medicare and Medicaid.

FAILURE OF FINANCING FOR COMMUNITY-ORIENTED NURSING

Hospitals gradually became the preferred place for illness care and childbirth during the 1930s and 1940s. Improved technology and the concentration of physicians' work in the acute care hospital were influential, but the development of health insurance plans such as Blue Cross provided a way for the middle class to seek care outside the traditional arena of the home. Federal health policy after World War II supported the growth of institutional care in hospitals and nursing homes over community-based alternatives.

Financing for voluntary agencies was greatly reduced in the early 1950s when both the Metropolitan and John Hancock Life Insurance Companies ceased to fund visiting nurse services for the care of their policyholders. The life insurance companies had found nursing services financially beneficial when communicable disease rates were high 30 years before, but reductions in communicable disease rates, improved infant and maternal health, and increased prevalence of chronic illness reduced financing and sponsor interest in home visiting. The American Red Cross also discontinued its programs of direct nursing service by mid-1950. Voluntary nursing agencies developed a variety of initiatives to secure health insurance reimbursement for nursing services. Blue Cross and other hospital insurance programs gradually adopted a formula that traded unused days of hospitalization coverage for postdischarge nursing care at home. The nursing profession also contributed substantially to securing federal medical insurance for the aged, which was implemented as the Medicare program in 1966.

CONSOLIDATION OF NATIONAL NURSING ORGANIZATIONS

Despite the success of the NOPHN, by the late 1940s its membership had declined and financial support was weak. At the same time, the vision of the nursing profession as a whole was to reorganize the national organizations to improve unity, administration, and financial stability. Three existing organizations—the NOPHN, the National League for Nursing Education, and the Association of Collegiate Schools of Nursing—were dissolved in 1952. Their functions were distributed primarily to the new **National League for Nursing,** while the **American Nurses Association,** which merged with the National Association of Colored Graduate Nurses, continued as the second national nursing organization. Despite the optimism of the reorganization and its success in other areas, the subsequent loss of leadership and focus in public health nursing resulted in a weakened specialty.

> **DID YOU KNOW?** *Nurses, including public and community health nurses, interested in the history of nursing can join the American Association for the History of Nursing (AAHN), which holds annual research meetings. Look for the AAHN on the Internet. It can be accessed through the WebLinks of this book's website at www.mosby.com/MERLIN.*

The National League for Nursing enthusiastically adopted the recommendations of Esther Lucile Brown's 1948 study of nursing education, reported as *Nursing for the Future.* Her recommendations to establish basic nursing preparation in colleges and universities was consistent with the NOPHN's goal of including public health nursing concepts in all basic baccalaureate programs. The NOPHN believed that this would remedy the problems of training found in nurses new to community-oriented nursing practice and would thus upgrade the profession. Unfortunately, the implementation of the plan fell short, and training programs in public health nursing concepts for college and university faculty were very brief. The population focus of public health nursing toward the group and larger community was compromised and became less distinct in the hands of educators more familiar with the one-on-one caregiving traditions of clinical, acute care nursing. As a result there became two levels of community-oriented nursing: public health and community health.

NEW FORMS OF PAYMENT FOR COMMUNITY-ORIENTED NURSING

Beginning in earnest in the late 1940s but based on advocacy begun in the late 1910s, policymakers and social welfare representatives sought to establish national health insurance. In 1965, Congress amended the Social Security Act to include health insurance benefits for the elderly (Medicare) and increased care for the poor (Medicaid). Unfortunately, the revised Social Security Act did not include coverage for preventive services, and home health care was compensated for only when ordered by the physician. However, this latter coverage prompted the rapid proliferation of home health care agencies. Many local and state health departments rapidly changed their policies to allow them to provide reimbursable home care. This often resulted in reduced health promotion and disease prevention activities. Between 1960 to 1968, the number of official agencies providing home care services grew from 250 to 1328, and the number of for-profit agencies also mushroomed (Kalisch and Kalisch, 1995).

COMMUNITY ORGANIZATION AND PROFESSIONAL CHANGE

A revolution in health care during the 1960s and 1970s influenced the direction of public health and community-oriented nursing. "The emerging civil rights movement shifted the paradigm from a charitable obligation to a political commitment to achieving equality and compensation for racial injustices of the past" (Scutchfield and Keck, 1997, p. 328). New programs sought to address economic and racial differences in health care services and delivery. Funding was increased for maternal and child health, mental health, mental retardation, and community health training. Beginning in 1964, the Economic Opportunity Act provided funds for neighborhood health centers, Head Start, and other community action programs. Neighborhood health centers increased community access for health care especially for maternal and child care. The work of Nancy Milio in Detroit, Michigan is an example of this commitment to action for the community. Milio built a dynamic decision-making process that included neighborhood residents, politicians, the Visiting Nurse Association and its board, civil rights activists, and church leaders. The Mom and Tots Center emerged as a neighborhood-centered service to provide maternal-child health services and a day care center (Milio, 1971).

New personnel also added to the flexibility of the community-oriented nurse to address the needs of communi-

ties. Beginning in 1965 at the University of Colorado, the nurse practitioner movement opened a new era for nursing's involvement in primary care, which had an impact on the delivery of services in community health clinics. Initially, the nurse practitioner was a public health nurse with additional skills in the diagnosis and treatment of common illnesses. Although some nurse practitioners chose to practice in other clinical areas, those who remained in community health made sustained contributions to providing primary care to people in rural areas, inner cities, and other medically underserved areas (Roberts and Heinrich, 1985). As evidence of the effectiveness of their services grew, nurse practitioners became increasingly accepted as cost-effective providers of a variety of primary care services.

COMMUNITY AND PUBLIC HEALTH NURSING FROM THE 1970S TO THE PRESENT

During the 1970s, nursing was viewed as a powerful force for improving the health care of communities. Nurses made significant contributions to the hospice movement, the development of birthing centers, day care for elderly and disabled persons, drug abuse programs, and rehabilitation services in long-term care. Federal evaluation of the effectiveness of care was emphasized (Roberts and Heinrich, 1985).

During the 1980s, concern grew about the high costs of health care in the United States. Health-promotion and disease-prevention programs received less priority as funding was shifted to meet the escalating costs of acute hospital care, medical procedures, and institutional long-term care. The use of ambulatory services including health maintenance organizations was encouraged, and the use of nurse practitioners was increased. Home health care weathered several threats to adequate reimbursement and, by the end of the decade, began to increase its impact on the care of the sick at home. Individuals and families assumed more responsibility for their own health status because health education, always a part of community health nursing, became increasingly popular. Advocacy groups representing both consumers and professionals urged laws to prohibit unhealthy practices in public such as smoking and driving under the influence of alcohol. As federal and state funds grew scarce, the presence of nurses in official public health agencies diminished. Committed and determined to improve the health care of Americans, nurses continued to press for greater involvement in official and private agencies (Kalisch and Kalisch, 1995; Roberts and Heinrich, 1985).

WHAT DO YOU THINK? *The emphasis of public and community health nursing has been varied and has changed over time. Given this chapter's review of the important issues that nursing can address, what priorities would you set for the work of the contemporary public and community health nurse?*

Establishment of the National Center for Nursing Research (NCNR) in 1985 within the National Institutes of Health in Washington, DC had a major impact on promoting the work of nurses. Through research, nurses document the scope and quality of care provided by examining the outcomes and cost-effectiveness of nursing interventions. With the concerted efforts of many nurses, the NCNR was approved for official institute status within the National Institutes of Health in 1993, becoming the National Institute of Nursing Research (NINR).

By the latter part of the 1980s, public health as a whole had declined significantly in terms of effectiveness in implementing its mission and affecting the health of the public. The seriousness of reduced political support, financing, and impact was vividly described in the landmark report by the Institute of Medicine (IOM), *The Future of Public Health* (1988). The IOM study group found the state of public health in the United States to be in disarray and concluded that, although there was widespread agreement about what the mission of public health should be, there was little consensus on how to translate that mission into action. Not surprisingly, the IOM reported that the mix and level of public health services varied from place to place in the United States (Williams, 1995).

The IOM report emphasized the core functions of public health as assessment, policy development, and assurance (see Chapter 1). Two additional U.S. Public Health Service documents, *Healthy People 2000: National Health Promotion and Disease Prevention Objectives* (1991b) and *Healthy Communities 2000: Model Standards* (1991a), sought to influence goal setting in public health. *Healthy People 2000* proposed a national strategy to improve the health of the public significantly by using strategies to prevent major chronic illness, injuries, and infectious diseases. Specific goals and objectives were established, and time frames for accomplishing them were determined. Strategies recommended in *Healthy People 2000* are summarized in Appendix A.1. Implementation of these strategies has had considerable influence on community-oriented nursing, and many of the objectives and strategies for their accomplishment are described in chapters throughout this text. *Healthy People 2010* will further delineate strategies for public health nurses to use in the care of communities.

The 1990s debate about health care has focused on central issues of cost, quality, and access to direct care services. Despite considerable interest in universal health insurance coverage, neither individuals nor employers are willing to pay for this level of service. The core debate of the economics of health care—who will pay for what—has emphasized reform of medical care rather than comprehensive reform of health care. In 1993, a blue-ribbon group assembled by President Clinton, with First Lady Hillary Rodham Clinton serving as chair, proposed the American Health Security Act. Although this act received insufficient Congressional support, it addressed a wide range of issues and concerns in health care, especially the organization and delivery of medical care with an emphasis on managed care. Consideration

of the act stimulated considerable activity both at the state level and within the private sector to reform health care. However, the aims of public health were never clearly considered in the proposed program, leaving a void in the design of a comprehensive program for health care.

In 1991 the American Nurses Association, the American Association of Colleges of Nursing, the National League for Nursing, and more than 60 other specialty nursing organizations joined to support health care reform. The document resulting from this historic joint effort incorporated the key health care issues of access, quality, and cost, and it set forth a range of efforts designed to build a healthy nation through improved primary care and public health efforts. Professional nursing support for revisions in health care delivery and extension of public health services to prevent illness, promote health, and protect the public continues (Table 2-3).

COMMUNITY AND PUBLIC HEALTH NURSING TODAY

Public health nursing celebrated "A Century of Caring" in 1993 to mark the centennial of the establishment of the Henry Street Settlement. Several organizations and professional groups reflected on the many contributions made by nurses in community health and public health nursing. Two excellent photo essays, *A Century of Caring: A Celebration of Public Health Nursing in the United States, 1883-1993* (U.S. Public Health Service, Division of Nursing, 1993) and *Healing at Home: Visiting Nurse Service of New York, 1893-1993* (Denker, 1994) provide visual evidence of the courage, caring, and commitment of public health nurses over the past 100 years. These volumes trace the specific contributions made by community-oriented nurses, often with minimal support and few resources, who sought to serve people with even overwhelming health problems. Public health nursing, historically and in the present, can be characterized by its reaching out to care for the health of people in need (U.S. Public Health Service, 1993).

DID YOU KNOW? *Many colleges and universities offer courses on the history of nursing, history of medicine, and the history of health care.*

One contemporary leader in public health nursing whose philosophies were influenced by the past was Ruth Freeman (Box 2-3). Today, community and public health nurses look to their history for inspiration, explanation, and prediction. Information and advocacy are used to promote a comprehensive approach to the multiple needs of the diverse populations served. Community-oriented nurses will seek to learn from the past and to avoid known pitfalls as successful strategies to meet the complex needs of today's risk groups are sought. As plans for the future are made, the public health challenges that remain unmet are acknowledged, as is the sustaining vision of what community-oriented nursing can accomplish.

TABLE 2-3 Milestones in History of Community Health and Public Health Nursing: 1946-1995

YEAR	MILESTONE
1946	Nurses classified as professionals by U.S. Civil Service Commission; Hill-Burton Act approved, providing funds for hospital construction in underserved areas and requiring these hospitals to provide care to poor people; passage of National Mental Health Act
1950	25,091 nurses employed in public health
1951	National organizations recommend that college-based nursing education programs include public health content
1952	National Organization for Public Health Nursing merges into the new National League for Nursing; Metropolitan Life Insurance Nursing Program closes
1964	Passage of Economic Opportunity Act; public health nurse defined by the ANA as a graduate of a BSN program; Congress amended Social Security Act to include Medicare and Medicaid
1965	ANA position paper recommended that nursing education take place in institutions of higher learning
1977	Passage of Rural Health Clinic Services Act, which provided indirect reimbursement for nurse practitioners in rural health clinics
1978	Association of Graduate Faculty in Community Health Nursing/Public Health Nursing (later renamed as Association of Community Health Nursing Educators)
1980	Medicaid amendment to the Social Security Act to provide direct reimbursement for nurse practitioners in rural health clinics; both ANA and APHA developed statements on the role and conceptual foundations of community and public health nursing respectively
1983	Beginning of Medicare prospective payments
1985	National Center for Nursing Research established in National Institutes of Health (NIH)
1988	Institute of Medicine publishes *The Future of Public Health*
1990	Association of Community Health Nursing Educators publishes *Essentials of Baccalaureate Nursing Education*
1991	Over 60 nursing organizations joined forces to support health care reform and publish a document entitled *Nursing's Agenda for Health Care Reform*
1993	American Health Security Act of 1993 published as a blueprint for national health care reform; the national effort, however, failed, leaving states and the private sector to design their own programs
1994	NCNR becomes the National Institute for Nursing Research, as part of the National Institutes of Health
1996	Public health nursing section of American Public Health Association, *The Definition and Role of Public Health Nursing* updated
1998	*The Public Health Workforce: An Agenda for the 21st Century* published by the U.S. Public Health Service to look at the current workforce in public, health, educational needs, and use of distance learning strategies to prepare the future public health workers
1999	The Public Health Nursing Quad Council through the American Nurses Association works on a new scope and standards of public health nursing document, which differentiates between community-oriented and community-based nursing practice

BOX 2-3 Ruth Freeman: Public Health Educator, Administrator, Consultant, Author, and Leader of National Health Organizations

Public health nursing by the 1940s had emerged from its pioneer experiences and begun to develop into a professional discipline capable of functioning in an increasing complex health care system. To meet the challenges of providing health services to diverse communities, nursing needed leaders who possessed the necessary intellectual and political capabilities to keep the profession in the forefront of the national public health care movement. Ruth Freeman was one of these leaders.

Born in Methune, Massachusetts on December 5, 1906, Ruth was the oldest of three children in a middle class family. Encouraged by an aunt to become a nurse, Ruth entered the Mount Sinai Hospital in New York City in 1923. As a student, she discovered that nursing was not only about caring for people, but it was also intellectually challenging and offered many professional opportunities. After graduation in 1927, Ruth accepted a staff position at the Henry Street Visiting Nurse Service. This position profoundly influenced her career and view of the power of nursing to help people deal with their illnesses and social problems. Recalling these formative years, Ruth noted that the families taught her an important nursing lesson: "that dying wasn't a calamity, that 'making do' was not demeaning, and helping was not controlling" (Safier, 1977, p. 68). Her Henry Street mentors, including Lillian Wald, reinforced her developing philosophy that the family was the principal decision-maker in their health activities, and that patience and optimism were essential characteristics of an effective nurse (Safier, 1977).

Recognized by faculty in her Columbia University baccalaureate program for her ability to lead, Ruth began her teaching career at the New York University Department of Nursing in 1937. She moved to the University of Minnesota School of Public Health to teach and learn how health care was provided in rural communities. Ruth's insistence that she remain actively engaged in public health work allowed her opportunities to integrate the newly emerging social and biological knowledge into the direct care of clients. Her ability to use this information to alleviate health problems in the community enriched her students' education, and through her many articles and national presentations, she greatly influenced the practice of public health nurses and physicians in the nation.

Ruth's reputation as an innovative thinker and effective administrator led to a position as director of nursing at the American Red Cross and consultant to the National Security Board in Washington, DC (1946 to 1950). This experience solidified her belief in the interdisciplinary nature of community health services and the need for professional nurses to serve as administrators of health agencies and organizations. To ensure her own academic competency, she acquired an MA degree from Columbia University in 1939 and an EdD from New York University in 1951 (Kaufman, 1988).

A new position at the Johns Hopkins University School of Hygiene and Public Health (1950 to 1971) led to Dr. Freeman becoming a professor of public health administration and coordinator of the nursing program. During her tenure at Hopkins, her talents as a teacher, author, consultant, and organizational leader flourished. Author of over 50 publications, several of her books, including *Public Health Nursing Practice, Administration in Public Health Services* (with E.M. Holmes), and *Community Health Practice*, became widely used texts in nursing programs. Her ability to provide insightful leadership led to Dr. Freeman's election and appointment to numerous national posts including president of the National League of Nursing (1955 to 1959), president of the National Health Council (1959 to 1960), and many of the major committees of the American Public Health Association. Dr. Freeman also served as a member of the 1958 White House Conference on Children and Youth and as a consultant to the World Health Organization and the Pan American Health Organization (Bullough, 1988).

The numerous national and international awards bestowed on her acknowledged Ruth Freeman's unique contributions to the professionalization of nursing and the improvement of public health services. These included the prestigious American Nurses Association's Pearl McIver Award, the American Public Health Association's Bronfman Prize, and the Florence Nightingale Medal given by the International Red Cross. She was named, in 1981, an honorary member of the American Academy of Nursing, and in 1984, 2 years after her death, she was awarded American nursing's highest honor, election to the American Nurses Association's Nursing Hall of Fame (Bullough, 1988; Kaufman, 1988; Safier, 1977).

Contributed by Barbara Brodie, PhD, RN, FAAN, Director of the Center for Nursing Historical Inquiry, University of Virginia, Charlottesville.

clinical application

Mary Lipsky has worked for a visiting nurse association in a major urban area for almost 2 years. Her nursing responsibilities include a variety of services, including caring for older and chronically ill clients recently discharged from hospitals, new mothers and babies, mental health clients, and clients with long-term health problems, such as chronic wounds.

When she leaves the field to return to her own home each evening, she finds that she holds her clients in her thoughts. Why is it so difficult for mothers and new babies to qualify for and receive WIC (Women, Infant, Children Nutrition) services? Why must she limit the number of visits and length of service for clients with chronic wounds? Why are there so few services for clients with behavioral health problems? She especially has on her mind the burdens and challenges that families and friends face in caring for the sick at home.

A. Why might it be difficult to solve these problems at the individual level, on a case by case basis?
B. What information would you need to build an understanding of the policy background for each of these various populations?

Answers are in the back of the book.

KEY POINTS

- An historical approach can be used to increase understanding of public and community health nursing in the past, as well as its contemporary dilemmas and future challenges.
- The history of public and community health nursing can be characterized by change in specific focus of the specialty but continuity in approach and style of the practice.
- Public and community health nursing is a product of various social, economic, and political forces; it incorporates public health science in addition to nursing science and practice.
- Federal responsibility for health care was limited until the 1930s when the economic challenges of the Depression permitted re-examination of local responsibility for care.
- Florence Nightingale designed and implemented the first program of trained nursing, while her contemporary, William Rathbone, founded the first district nursing association in England.
- Urbanization, industrialization, and immigration in the United States increased the need for trained nurses, especially in public and community health nursing.
- Increasing acceptance of public roles for women permitted public and community health nursing employment for nurses, as well as public leadership roles for their wealthy supporters.
- The first trained nurse in the United States, who was salaried as a visiting nurse, was Frances Root, who has hired in 1887 by the Women's Board of the New York City Mission to provide care to sick persons at home.
- The first visiting nurses associations were founded in 1885 and 1886 in Buffalo, Philadelphia, and Boston.
- Lillian Wald established the Henry Street Settlement, which became the Visiting Nurse Service of New York City, in 1893. She played a key role in innovations that shaped public and community health nursing in its first decades, including school nursing, insurance payment for nursing, national organization for public health nurses, and the United States Children's Bureau.
- Founded in 1902 with the vision and support of Lillian Wald, school nursing sought to keep children in school so that they could learn.
- The Metropolitan Life Insurance Company established the first insurance-based program in 1909 to support community health nursing services.
- The National Organization for Public Health Nursing (founded in 1912) provided essential leadership and coordination of diverse public and community health nursing efforts; the organization merged into the National League for Nursing in 1952.
- Official health agencies slowly grew in numbers between 1900 and 1940, accompanied by a steady increase in public health nursing positions.
- The innovative Sheppard-Towner Act of 1921 expanded community health nursing roles for maternal and child health during the 1920s.
- Mary Breckinridge established the Frontier Nursing Service in 1925, which influenced provision of rural health care.
- Tension between the community health nursing roles of caring for the sick and of providing preventive care, and the related tension between intervening for individuals or for groups, has characterized the specialty since at least the 1910s.
- As the Social Security Act attempted to remedy some of the setbacks of the depression, it established a context in which community health nursing services expanded.
- The challenges of World War II sometimes resulted in extension of community health nursing care and sometimes in retrenchment and decreased public health nursing services.
- By mid-twentieth century, the reduced incidence of communicable diseases and the increased prevalence of chronic illness, accompanied by large increases in the population over 65 years of age, led to examination of the goals and organization of community health nursing services.
- Between the 1930s and 1965, organized nursing and community health nursing agencies sought to establish health insurance reimbursement for nursing care at home.
- Implementation of Medicare and Medicaid programs in 1966 established new possibilities for supporting community-based nursing care but encouraged agencies to focus on post-acute care services rather than prevention.
- Efforts to reform health care organization, pushed by increased health care costs during the last 40 years, have focused on reforming acute medical care rather than on designing a comprehensive preventive approach.
- The 1988 Institute of Medicine report documented the reduced political support, financing, and impact that increasingly limited public health services at national, state, and local levels.
- In the late 1990s, federal policy changes dangerously reduced financial support for home health care services, threatening the long-term survival of visiting nurse agencies.
- *Healthy People 2000* and *Healthy People 2010* have brought renewed emphasis on prevention to public and community health nursing.

critical thinking activities

1. Interview nurses at your clinical placement about the changes they have seen during their years in a public or community health nursing practice.
2. Identify the visible record of public and community health nursing agencies in your community. Note the buildings, plaques, display cases, and more that are records of the past provision of nursing care in community settings.
3. Interview older relatives for their memories of public and community health nursing care received by them, their families, and their friends. When they were younger, how was the public health nurse perceived in their community?
4. What element or aspect of the history of public and community health nursing would you like to know more about? At your nursing library, review a period of 10 years of one journal to identify trends in how this element or aspect was addressed.
5. The work and impact of several nursing leaders is reviewed in this chapter. Of these leaders, which one strikes you as most interesting? Why?

Bibliography

Backer BA: Lillian Wald: connecting caring with action, *Nurs Health Care* 14:122, 1993.

Brainard A: *Evolution of public health nursing,* Philadelphia, 1922, Saunders.

Browne H: A tribute to Mary Breckinridge, *Nurs Outlook* 14:54, May 1966.

Buhler-Wilkerson K: Public health nursing: in sickness or in health? *Am J Pub Health* 75:1155, 1985.

Buhler-Wilkerson K: Left carrying the bag: experiments in visiting nursing, 1877-1909, *Nurs Res,* 36:42, 1987.

Buhler-Wilkerson K: *False dawn: the rise and decline of public health nursing, 1900-1930,* New York, 1989, Garland Publishing.

Bullough V, Bullough B: *The emergence of modern nursing,* New York, 1964, MacMillan.

Bullough V, Church OM, Stern A: *American nursing: a biographic dictionary,* New York, 1988, Garland Publishing.

Cohen IB: Florence Nightingale, *Sci Am* 250(3):128, 1984.

Craven, FSL: *A guide to district nursing,* New York, 1984, Garland Publishing (originally published London, 1889, MacMillan and Company).

Deloughery GL: *History and trends of professional nursing,* ed 8, St Louis, 1977, Mosby.

Denker EP, editor: *Healing at home: Visiting Nurse Service of New York, 1893-1993,* New York, 1994, The Carl and Lily Pforzheimer Foundation.

Desirable organization for public health nursing for family service, *Pub Health Nurs* 38:387, 1946.

Dock LL: The history of public health nursing, *Pub Health Nurs* 14:522, 1922.

Dock LL, Stewart IM: *A short history of nursing,* ed 4, New York, 1938, GP Putnam's Sons.

Dolan J: *History of nursing,* ed 14, Philadelphia, 1978, WB Saunders.

Frachel RR: A new profession: the evolution of public health nursing, *Pub Health Nurs* 5(2):86, 1988.

Hawkins JW, Hayes ER, Corliss CP: School nursing in America—1902-1994: a return to public health nursing, *Pub Health Nurs* 11(6):416, 1994.

Holloway JB: Frontier Nursing Service 1925-1975, *J Ky Med Assoc* 13:491, 1975.

Institute of Medicine: *The future of public health,* Washington, DC, 1988, National Academy of Science.

Kalisch PA, Kalisch BJ: *The advance of American nursing,* ed 3, Philadelphia, 1995, J.B. Lippincott.

Kalisch PA, Kalisch BJ: *The advance of American nursing,* ed 2, Boston, 1986, Little, Brown & Company.

Kaufman, M, editor: *Dictionary of American nursing biography,* New York, 1988, Greenwood Press.

McNeil EE: *Transition in public health nursing,* John Sundwall Lecture, University of Michigan, Feb 27, 1967.

Milio N: *9226 Kercheval: the storefront that did not burn,* Ann Arbor, MI, 1971, University of Michigan Press.

National Organization for Public Health Nursing: Approval of Skidmore College of Nursing as preparing students for public health nursing, *Pub Health Nurs* 36:371, 1944.

Nightingale, F: Sick nursing and health nursing. In Billings JS, Hurd HM, editors: *Hospitals, dispensaries, and nursing,* New York, 1984, Garland Publishing (originally published in Baltimore, 1894, Johns Hopkins Press).

Nightingale, F: *Notes on nursing: what it is, and what it is not,* Philadelphia, 1946, Lippincott.

Nutting MA, Dock LL: *A history of nursing,* New York, 1935, G. P. Putnam's Sons.

Palmer IS: *Florence Nightingale and the first organized delivery of nursing services,* Washington, DC, 1983, American Association of Colleges of Nursing.

Pellegrino ED: Medicine, history, and the idea of man, *Ann Am Acad Pol Soc Sci* 346:9, 1963.

Pickett G, Hanlon JJ: *Public health: administration and practice,* St. Louis, 1990, Mosby.

Roberts DE, Heinrich J: Public health nursing comes of age, *Am J Pub Health* 75:1162, 1985.

Roberts M: *American nursing: history and interpretation,* New York, 1955, Macmillan.

Rodabaugh JH, Rodabaugh MJ: *Nursing in Ohio: a history,* Columbus, Ohio, 1951, Ohio State Nurses Association.

Rosen G: *A history of public health,* New York, 1958, MD Publications.

Safier, G: *Contemporary American leaders in nursing: an oral history,* New York, 1977, McGraw-Hill.

Scutchfield FD, Keck CW: *Principles of public health practice,* Albany, NY, 1997, Delmar Publishers.

Shyrock H: *The history of nursing,* Philadelphia, 1959, WB Saunders.

Swinson A: *A history of public health,* Exeter, England, 1965, A Wheaton Co.

Tirpak H: The Frontier Nursing Service—fifty years in the mountains, *Nurs Outlook* 33:308, 1975.

US Public Health Service, Division of Nursing: *A century of caring: a celebration of public health nursing in the United States, 1893-1993,* Washington, DC, 1993, US Government Printing Office.

US Public Health Service: *Healthy communities 2000: model standards,* Washington, DC, 1991a, US Government Printing Office.

US Public Health Service: *Healthy people 2000: national health promotion and disease prevention objectives,* Washington, DC, 1991b, US Government Printing Office.

Waters Y: *Visiting nursing in the United States,* New York, 1909, Charities Publication Committee.

Williams, C.A.: Beyond the Institute of Medicine report: a critical analysis and public health forecast. *Fam Community Health,* 18(1):12, 1995.

Wilner, DM, Walkey RP, O'Neill EJ: *Introduction to public health,* ed 7, New York, 1978, Macmillan.

Zerwekh JV: Public health nursing legacy: historical practical wisdom, *Nurs Health Care* 13:84, 1992.

Public Health and Primary Health Care Systems and Health Care Transformation

SUSAN B. HASSMILLER

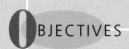 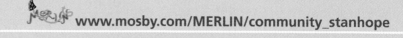

OBJECTIVES

After reading this chapter, the student should be able to do the following:

- Analyze three trends in the United States that are affecting health care.
- Define *public health, primary care, primary health care,* and *community-oriented primary care.*
- Differentiate between primary care and primary health care, including the workforce of each.
- Evaluate the significance of Alma Ata as the basis for primary health care.
- Analyze two of the most common health care systems that manage the personal care of Americans.
- Describe the current public health system in the United States.

- Compare and contrast the responsibilities of the federal, state, and local public health systems.
- Examine community health nursing roles in selected government agencies.
- Analyze the transformation of the U.S. health care system.
- Describe the steps of the community-oriented primary care (COPC) model.
- Compare and contrast COPC with primary care and public health.
- Discuss the importance of community participation in the COPC process or in any system of care.
- Define the nursing role in a COPC system of care.

KEY TERMS

advanced practice nurses
community-based care
community nursing
  centers
community-oriented
  primary care (COPC)
community participation

cost shifting
Declaration of Alma Ata
Health Maintenance
  Organizations (HMOs)
managed care
National Health Service
  Corps

nurse midwifery
physician assistants (PAs)
Preferred Provider
  Organizations (PPOs)
primary care
primary care generalists
primary health care (PHC)

U.S. Department of
  Health and Human
  Services (USDHHS)

See Glossary for definitions

CHAPTER OUTLINE

Current Health Care System in the
  United States
  Cost
  Access
  Quality
Trends Affecting the Health Care
  System
  Demographic Trends
  Social Trends

Economic Trends
  Health Workforce Trends
  Technological Trends
Organization of the Health Care
  System
  Primary Health Care System
  Primary Care System
  Public Health System
  Federal System

State System
  Local System
Transformation of the Health
  Care System
A Comprenhensive Model:
  Integration of Public Health and
  Primary Care
  Community-Oriented Primary
  Care (COPC)

The American health care system has done a remarkable job in many ways in providing health care to the American people, particularly in technology development and skilled provider training. Today's health care facilities would defy the imagination of our predecessors. Although public and private health insurance programs protect most Americans from the financial ravages of illness, the system has some serious liabilities related to cost, access, and quality of health care.

This chapter describes the current primary care and public health systems in the United States and the trends that affect these systems. These systems are compared and contrasted both with one another and with the concept of primary health care. Box 3-1 presents a definition of terms used in this chapter. Current concepts of health care transformation are described as a prelude to a discussion of what an emerging health care system might look like. This chapter describes a reformed health care system as one that weaves primary care and public health into a single integrated system. The role of the nurse is presented in all of the systems, current and future.

CURRENT HEALTH CARE SYSTEM IN THE UNITED STATES

Although the U.S. health care system can take credit for improving the life span of most Americans through advances in medical technology, science, and pharmaceuticals, the system is also plagued with issues related to cost, access, and quality of health care. These issues are at the center of health care debates around the country.

Cost

In 1997, Americans spent $1.092 trillion dollars, nearly 14% of the gross domestic product (GDP) on health care (HFCA, 1998a). This percentage is 40% higher than in Canada, the country that spends the next largest amount. Based on projections, by 2007, health care expenditures will account for nearly 17% of the United States GDP. Projections from the Health Care Financing Administration (HCFA) forecast that health care expenditures will increase by more than 7% annually between 2001 and 2007, and health care expenditures in 2007, $2.133 trillion, will almost double those of 1997. Per capita health care expenditures, expected to increase every year over the next decade, are estimated to be $4093 in 1998 and almost $7100 in 2007 (HCFA, 1998b). The cost-containment efforts that have been instituted since 1983 have attempted to curb the growth of costs, but they have not solved this tremendous problem. See Chapter 5 for details about the economics of health care.

Access

Increasing costs have been accompanied by another significant problem: poor access to health care. According to the Center for Studying Health System Change (1997), nearly one quarter of all Americans report that it has be-

BOX 3-1 Selected Health Care Definitions

Community-Oriented Primary Care (COPC). A community-responsive model of health care delivery that integrates aspects of both primary care and public health. It combines the care of individuals and families in the community with a focus on the community and its subgroups when services are planned, provided, and evaluated (Abramson, 1984).

Disease Prevention. Activities that have as their goal the protection of people from the ill-effects of actual or potential health threats.

Health. A state of complete physical, mental, and social well-being; not merely the absence of disease or infirmity (WHO, 1986a, p. 1).

Health Promotion. Activities that have as their goal the development of human resources and behaviors that maintain or enhance well-being.

Primary Care. Personal health care services that provide for first contact, continuous, comprehensive, and coordinated care. Care is directed primarily at an individual's pathophysiologic process (Starfield, 1992).

Primary Health Care. Essential care made universally accessible to individuals and families within a community through their full participation and provided at a cost that the community and country can afford (WHO, 1978).

Primary Prevention. Actions designed to prevent a disease from occurring; reduces the probability of a specific illness occurring and includes active protection against unnecessary stressors or threats (i.e., health promotion activities).

Public Health. Organized community efforts aimed at the prevention of disease and promotion of health. It links disciplines and rests upon the scientific core of epidemiology (Institute of Medicine, 1988, p. 4).

Secondary Prevention. Early diagnosis and prompt treatment; includes activities such as screening for diseases (e.g., hypertension, breast cancer, blindness, and deafness).

Tertiary Prevention. Treatment, care, and rehabilitation of people to prevent further progression of the disease (Pender, 1996).

come increasingly difficult to receive health care. The American health care system is described as a two-class system: private and public. People with insurance or those who can personally pay for health care are viewed as receiving superior care when compared with people whose only source of care depends upon public funds. This second category includes the working poor who do not qualify for public funds either because they make too much money to qualify or they are illegal immigrants. In 1996, 41.7 million Americans (15.6% of the total population) were uninsured (Haupt and Kane, 1997). The rate of uninsured people is currently rising at the rate of 750,000 people per year and will reach an estimated 44 million people by the year 2002, at which time the average rate of increase will decline partly because of the shifting age structure in the overall population (Institute for the Future, 1997). Young adults 18 to 24 years of age (28.9% of all uninsured) are more likely than other age groups to lack coverage, and the elderly (1.1% of all uninsured) are the least likely to lack coverage (US Census Bureau, 1996a).

Finally, the gradual erosion of public health services has compounded the access problem in the United States. For example, funding to clinics in rural and heavily populated urban areas has been reduced, leading many uninsured people to seek care in the emergency room. To continue to care for the uninsured, hospitals automatically charge more for their services to those who have insurance. This process of making up for lost revenue by charging more to those who are able to pay is called **cost shifting.**

Quality

Quality of care is the third major concern in the United States. Although managed care has succeeded in controlling health care costs, many would say that it has been at the expense of quality. Consumer advocates believe that employers and managed care plans are more concerned with reducing costs than offering needed services (Copeland, 1998). At the other extreme, when care is delivered that is medically unnecessary, the impact on quality of care is as significant as providing insufficient care. Federal and state health insurance plans (e.g., Medicare, Medicaid, and private managed care plans) have incorporated ways to improve the quality of care that they deliver. The best known private group, the National Committee for Quality Assurance (NCQA), has developed a set of standard performance measurements that most managed care organizations are using. The HCFA, home to Medicare and Medicaid, is moving toward similar quality mechanisms for the populations they serve (Wilensky, 1997). The presidentially commissioned committee on consumer health quality recently completed its final report in which it recommended a "Consumer Bill of Rights and Responsibilities." Still to be determined is whether the Bill will be implemented voluntarily or through legislation (Older Americans Report, 1998).

TRENDS AFFECTING THE HEALTH CARE SYSTEM

Because of the national concern for the cost, access, and quality of health care, significant change is expected in the next decade. Several trends, including demography, technology, and economics, will affect how these changes will evolve.

Demographic Trends

The population of the world is growing as a result of fertility and mortality rates. The most explosive growth is occurring in underdeveloped countries accompanied by decreased growth in the United States. Both size and the characteristics of the population contribute to the changing demography.

Size of the population

The Census Bureau reports that the U.S. population increased by 22 million between 1980 and 1990, an increase of 9.8%. This is the second lowest growth spurt in census history (Haupt and Kane, 1997). Immigration, both legal and illegal, also plays a major role in shaping the U.S. population. Nearly 500,000 legal immigrants enter the United States each year (Haupt and Kane, 1997).

The U.S. birth rate has fluctuated greatly in the last 50 years going from the "baby boom" between 1946 and 1964 to the "baby bust" of the 1970s, when the population reached its lowest rate of growth in 1976. It was thought that the rise in birth rates experienced in the late 1970s would level or decline as "baby boom" women passed through childbearing age. However, with women having children at a more advanced aged, birth rates did not begin to decrease until 1991 and then continued to decline throughout the 1990s (National Center for Health Statistics, 1998). It is anticipated that birth rates will continue to decline until 2000 when they are expected to level and remain stable through 2150 (U.S. Census Bureau, 1996b).

Characteristics of the population

The average age in the United States is increasing. Demographers predict a 74% increase in the number of people 50 years of age or older by the year 2020, whereas the number of people under 50 will only grow by only 1% (Exter, 1990). The elderly population will increase slowly during the next 20 years, and then rapidly for the following 20 years. From 2010 to 2030, the number of people 65 years of age and older will increase substantially when the first "baby boomers" turn 65 in 2011. The number of people over 85 years of age is growing so rapidly that by 2050 they will comprise approximately 24% of the elderly population.

The middle-age population will also continue to increase since nearly one-third of Americans were born between 1945 and 1960. The entire "baby boom" generation will be over 35 years of age by the turn of the century.

African-Americans are currently the largest minority group in the United States but will be surpassed by Hispanics by the year 2015 (US Census Bureau, 1996b). Asian-Americans, although the smallest minority group in America, will have the greatest influence. They understand and blend in with the American way of life more quickly than any other minority, are more educated, and make more money per capita than Caucasians or any other minorities (Miller, 1991).

The U.S. household composition is also changing. Families constitute about 71% of all households, down from 81% in 1970 (US Census Bureau, 1996b). Single parents, usually the mother, head 3 out of 10 families. Single-parent families constitute 19% of all Caucasian families, 31% of Hispanic families, and 54% of African-American families (US Census Bureau, 1996b).

In the last decade, mortality rates for both sexes in all age groups have declined (US Census Bureau, 1996b). As a result of medical progress, the leading causes of death have changed from infectious diseases to chronic and degenerative diseases. Substantial gains against infectious diseases have resulted in steady declines of mortality among children. The mortality rates for older Americans have also declined, especially during the 1970s and 1980s. However, people 50 years of age and older have higher rates of chronic illness, and they consume a larger portion of health care services than other age groups.

Social Trends

In addition to the size and changing age distribution of the population, other factors also affect the health care system. Several social trends that influence health care include changing lifestyles, a growing appreciation of the quality of life, changing composition of families and living patterns, rising household incomes, and a revised definition of quality health care.

Historically, U.S. citizens have been driven by the "American dream" that emphasized hard work, getting a good education, and achieving a better life than the previous generation. However, the drive to achieve these goals has diminished, and there have been major shifts in American values and lifestyles. Replacing the work ethic is an increasing emphasis on an improved quality of life and the fulfillment of personal goals (Miller, 1991). This shift in values is reordering the relative importance of economic success.

Americans spend more money on health care, nutrition, and fitness (Miller, 1991), and there is a growing emphasis on the belief that people are responsible for their own health accompanied by an awareness that health is a valuable asset and efforts should be taken to improve it. Currently, it is estimated that 80% to 95% of all health problems are managed at home through self-care measures (Ory and Defriese, 1998). In addition, centers for promoting all aspects of health and self-care are developing in response to this movement.

Economic Trends

About 60 years ago, income was distributed in such a way that a relatively small proportion of households earned high incomes; a somewhat larger proportion of families was in the middle-income range; and the largest proportion of households was at the lower end of the income scale. By the 1970s, household income had risen and income was more evenly distributed, largely as a result of dual-income families. There has always been and continues to be income disparity between Caucasian and minority groups, excluding Asian-Americans (Johnson, 1992; Miller, 1991).

More than 12 million families—about 20% of households—receive only 5% of the total income. In addition, high costs and lower real wages, especially for African-American women, continue to add to the difficulty of rising out of poverty (Johnson, 1992). This means that a sizable proportion of low-income Americans will continue to rely on public support to maintain a minimum standard of living. Chapter 5 provides a detailed discussion of the economics of health care and how financial constraints influence decisions about public health services.

Health Workforce Trends

The emphasis on physician specialization and specialists' tendency to charge more and order more tests than primary care physicians has added to the spiraling health care costs (Greenfield et al, 1992). In the 1990s there was a call for health care cost containment, which demanded a workforce that would help keep costs in line while maintaining quality and increasing accessibility. Efforts by government agencies, such as the Bureau of Health Professions of the U.S. Department of Health and Human Services (USDHHS), and private foundations, such as the Robert Wood Johnson Foundation, provided money for programs to increase the primary care workforce. These strategies included increasing the number of both primary care physicians and advanced practice nurses, such as nurse practitioners and certified nurse midwives. To date there is an adequate number of primary care providers in the United States for all but the most underserved areas, such as the inner cities and very rural areas. Increasing the number of primary care providers and decreasing specialty physician salaries, in addition to the general cost-savings measures instituted by managed care, has helped stabilize escalating health care costs.

Historically, nursing care has been provided in a variety of settings, primarily in the hospital. Currently, 60% of all registered nurses are employed in hospitals (USDHHS, 1996); however, with an emphasis on cost containment and a greater orientation to **community-based care,** hospitals are downsizing their acute care facilities. Although it is estimated that by 2000 about 1.8 million nursing personnel will be needed, it is predicted that many nurses working in acute care will face job loss or job uncertainty. One of the few exceptions will be those nurses working in gerontology.

Increasing minority representation in nursing remains a priority. "Shortages of such individuals adversely affect access, quality of care, and costs" (USDHHS, 1993, p. 15). For example, persons from minority groups, especially where language is a barrier, are more comfortable with and more likely to access care from a provider of their own minority group. Although minorities comprised 27.7% of the U.S. population in 1996, minority nursing school enrollments accounted for only 9.7% (USDHHS, 1996). Nursing will continue to compete with the other health professions to recruit from the same pool of minorities.

Technological Trends

Improved technology is rapidly changing the health care system and is having both positive and negative effects. Technology costs are expected to reach $18 billion dollars in the year 2000 (Copeland, 1998). On the positive side, technological advances promise improved health care services and reduced costs. Reduced costs come from a more efficient means of delivering care as well as replacing people. Contradictory as it may seem, cost is also the most significant negative aspect of advanced health care technology. The more high-tech equipment and computer programs become available, the more they are used. High-technology equipment is expensive, quickly becomes outdated when newer developments occur, and often requires highly trained personnel.

DID YOU KNOW? *The same sensors that are being developed for automobiles, video cameras, and all other electronics will become cheap enough to be used in medical devices for the purpose of remote telemetry. Examples include monitoring vital signs with wireless heart monitors, respiratory meters, blood pressure cuffs, blood glucose monitors, and alerts from pill dispensers that a needed pill has not been taken. Built into the sensors will be the software's capabilities to analyze, report, and react to the presence or absence of abnormal results, which will ensure appropriate follow-up by a nurse (Institute for the Future, 1997).*

Unquestionably, advances in medical technology will continue. However, it is anticipated that the emphasis will shift away from expensive diagnostic and therapeutic technologies. Efforts will focus on devising simpler, cheaper, and more mobile tests and procedures that are less oriented to tertiary care and can be used in nonhospital settings.

ORGANIZATION OF THE HEALTH CARE SYSTEM

An enormous number and range of facilities and providers make up the health care system. These include physicians' and dentists' offices, hospitals, health maintenance organizations (HMOs), nursing homes and other related inpatient facilities, mental health centers, ambulatory care centers, rehabilitation centers, and local, state and federal official and voluntary agencies. In general, however, the American health care system is divided into two somewhat distinct components: a private or personal care component and a public health component, with some overlap, as discussed in the following sections. Although the personal care component is comprised of primary, secondary, and tertiary care, primary health care and primary care will receive the most elaboration in this chapter.

Primary Health Care System

There is considerable controversy over what constitutes primary care and primary health care. Primary health care can be distinguished from primary care in several important ways. **Primary health care (PHC),** generally defined more broadly than primary care, includes a comprehensive range of services including public health, prevention, diagnostic, therapeutic, and rehabilitative services. PHC is essential care made universally accessible to individuals and families in a community. Health care is made available to them

through their full participation and is provided at a cost that the community and country can afford. Full participation means that individuals within the community help in defining health problems and developing approaches to address the problems. The setting for primary health care is within all communities of a country and permeates all aspects of society (World Health Organization, 1978).

PHC encourages self-care and self-management in health and social welfare aspects of daily life. People are educated to use their knowledge, attitudes, and skills in activities that improve health for themselves, their families, and their neighbors. A PHC strategy seeks to ensure individual, family, and community self-reliance and competence.

Primary health care workforce

The primary health care workforce consists of a multidisciplinary team of health care providers. Team members include generalist and public health physicians, nurses, dentists, pharmacists, optometrists, nutritionists, community outreach workers, mental health counselors, and other allied health professionals. Community members are also considered important to the team.

Primary health care movement

The primary health care movement officially began in 1977 when the 30th World Health Organization (WHO) Health Assembly adopted a resolution accepting the goal of attaining a level of health that permitted all citizens of the world to live socially and economically productive lives. At the international conference in 1978 in Alma Ata, USSR, it was determined that this goal was to be met through PHC. This resolution, the **Declaration of Alma Ata,** became known by the slogan "Health for All (HFA) by the Year 2000" and captured the official health target for all of the member nations of the WHO.

In 1981 the WHO established global indicators for monitoring and evaluating the achievement of HFA. In the *World Health Statistics Annual* (1986b), these indicators are grouped into four categories: health policies, social and economic development, provision of health care, and health status. An important part of the global indicators is the emphasis on health as an objective of socioeconomic development (Mahler, 1981). In this context, health improvements are a result of efforts in many areas including agriculture, industry, education, housing, communications, and health care. Because PHC is as much a political statement as a system of care, each UN member country interprets PHC in the context of their own culture, health needs, resources, and system of government.

Although the original definition of PHC has at times been misunderstood, it is important to understand the Alma Ata declaration as the basis for PHC and the global evolvement of this strategy over the past 10 to 15 years. For this reason the complete declaration is presented in Appendix A-4.

Promoting Health/Preventing Disease: Year 2000 Objectives for the Nation

As a WHO member nation, the United States has endorsed primary health care as a strategy for achieving the goal of health for all by the year 2000. However, PHC with its emphasis on broad strategies, **community participation,** self-reliance, and a multidisciplinary health care delivery team is not the primary strategy for improving the health of the American people. The national health plan for the United States focuses more on disease prevention and health promotion in the areas of most concern in the nation.

This focus is exemplified by the health objectives for the nation, *Promoting Health/Preventing Disease: Year 2000 Objectives for the Nation* (USPHS, 1991). These objectives were published by the U.S. Public Health Service of the USDHHS after gathering data from health professionals and organizations throughout the country. The objectives focus on three overarching goals:
- Increase the lifespan of healthy Americans
- Reduce health disparities among Americans and provide all Americans with access to preventive services
- Decrease the race-based disparity in life expectancy.

Specific areas of concern for each of these goals are as follows:
- *Health promotion.* Nutrition; physical activity and fitness; consumption of tobacco, alcohol, and other drugs; family planning; violent and abusive behavior; mental health; and educational and community-based programs
- *Health protection.* Environmental health, occupational safety and health, accidental injuries, food and drug safety, and oral health
- *Preventive services priorities.* Maternal and infant health, immunizations and infectious diseases, HIV infection, sexually transmitted diseases, heart disease and stroke, cancer, diabetes, other chronic disabling conditions; and clinical preventive services for these; also chronic disorders and mental and behavioral disorders
- *System improvement priorities.* Health education and preventive services and surveillance and data systems (USPHS, 1991).

There is considerable overlap between the essential elements of PHC and the areas of concern stated in the Year 2000 objectives. Table 3-1 relates the eight essential elements of PHC to the priority areas as defined by the Public Health Service.

Primary Care System

Primary care, or what some refer to as *primary medical care,* is a personal health care system that provides for first contact, continuous, comprehensive, and coordinated care. It addresses the most common needs of clients within a community by providing preventive, curative, and rehabilitative services to maximize their health and well-being. Although primary care practitioners are encouraged to consider the client's social and environmental attributes in diagnosing, interventions are directed primarily toward an individual's *pathophysiological* process (Starfield, 1992). Table 3-2 presents a comparison of primary health care and primary care.

Primary care is an essential component of an overall primary health care system, so much so that the Institute of Medicine (IOM) has recently focused its attention on a 24-month study to provide guidance for augmenting and improving primary care as an essential component of an effective and efficient health care system. The IOM's *Primary Care: America's Health in a New Era* (1996) report defined primary care and the roles of primary care providers and provided a comprehensive strategic plan of action for increasing the emphasis on primary care in the United States.

Primary care delivery system

Primary care is delivered in a variety of accessible community settings such as physician offices, managed care organizations, community health centers, and **community nursing centers.** With the emphasis on cost containment the health care delivery system is focusing its efforts on **managed care** as an increasingly large segment of the pri-

TABLE 3-1 Year 2000 Objectives and Elements of Primary Health Care (PHC)

Eight Essential Elements of PHC	Year 2000 Objectives
Health education	Physical activity and fitness; tobacco, alcohol, and other drugs; mental health; surveillance and data systems; violence and abusive behavior
Proper nutrition	Nutrition
Maternal and child health care; family planning	Maternal and infant health; family planning
Safe water and basic sanitation	Environmental health
Immunization	Immunization and infectious diseases
Prevention and control of locally endemic diseases	HIV infection; chronic disorders; cancer; heart disease and stroke; sexually transmitted diseases; immunization and infectious diseases; clinical preventive services
Treatment of common diseases and injuries	Unintentional injuries; occupational safety and health
Provision of essential drugs	

TABLE 3-2 How to Differentiate Between Primary Care and Primary Health Care

PRIMARY CARE	PRIMARY HEALTH CARE
Individual-focused	Community-focused
Preventive, rehabilitative, with emphasis on curative	Curative, rehabilitative, with emphasis on preventive
Care provided by generalist physicians, nurse practitioners, nurse midwives, and physician assistants with help of ancillary team members	Care provided by a wide variety of health care team members such as physicians, community health nurses, community outreach workers, nutritionists, sanitation experts
Professional dominance	Self-reliance

mary care system. **Health Maintenance Organizations (HMOs;** also called *Managed Care Organizations*) and **Preferred Provider Organizations (PPOs)** are two of the most common systems that manage the care for a specified population. In 1997 more than 65 million Americans were enrolled in HMO plans and nearly 100 million Americans were enrolled in PPOs (Institute for the Future, 1997; Peterson, 1997).

HMOs in one form or another have existed for over 30 years. Each HMO operates as an organized system of health care that, for a fixed fee, provides primary care services, emergency and preventive treatment, and hospital care to people who have agreed to obtain their medical care from the HMO for a specified period of time. An HMO can be a building in which all health care workers are direct employees, or the organization or plan can consist of a more loosely organized system whereby providers contract with the HMO on a fee-for-service basis. Specialty care is received (and paid for) only upon the recommendation of a primary care provider, sometimes referred to as the *gatekeeper.* Some HMOs, however, are allowing their patients to bypass the primary care provider and receive certain aspects of specialty care as a result of "the hassle factor" of the gatekeeper system and a general consumer demand for specialty services. HMOs keep costs under control by encouraging prevention, keeping referrals to a minimum, and reducing unnecessary hospitalization.

WHAT DO YOU THINK? *A primary care provider in a health maintenance organization should refer patients to specialists only as outlined in the referral guidelines set forth by their employing organization, whether they agree with the guidelines or not.*

A PPO is an organization of providers that contracts on a fee-for-service basis with third-party payers, such as an HMO, to provide comprehensive medical services to subscribers. The agreement between the PPO and the third-party payer allows subscribers to receive medical services at lower-than-usual rates (Roble, Knowlton, and Rosenberg, 1984). Physicians and other primary care providers can be-

long to several preferred provider plans. Other health care delivery organizations include community nursing centers and community health centers.

Efforts are currently underway by the HCFA to apply the same kind of cost-control mechanisms to the Medicare and Medicaid programs that exist for the general population. To make the transition easier for the elderly population, the HCFA has given them a choice of joining HMOs or continuing with their fee-for-service plans. To make it attractive, the HCFA is offering incentives for those choosing to join HMOs, such as reduced prescription copayments. Medicaid recipients are currently being organized into HMOs on a state-by-state basis but generally without the opportunity for choice or incentive programs.

Primary care workforce

Primary care developed in the 1960s as the need to reexamine the role of the general practitioner arose. The Millis Commission (Millis, 1966) expressed concern that a knowledge explosion, development of new technologies, and an increasing number of new specialties were threatening the role of the general practitioner. The specialty of family practice and the arrival of nurse practitioners (NPs) and physician assistants emerged in response to the need to provide primary care.

Currently, primary care providers include generalists who possess skills in health promotion and disease prevention, assessment and evaluation of undiagnosed symptoms and physical signs, management of common acute and chronic medical conditions, and identification and appropriate referral for other needed health care services (USDHHS, 1992). The health care personnel trained as **primary care generalists** include family physicians, general internists, general pediatricians, NPs, physician assistants, and nurse midwives. Some physicians with special training in preventive medicine and public health and obstetrics/gynecology also deliver primary care (USDHHS, 1992).

NPs and certified nurse midwives (CNMs), both considered **advanced practice nurses,** are vital members of the primary care and primary health care team. NPs receive advanced training usually at the masters level, with most taking a certification examination in a specialty

RESEARCH *Brief*

A study of the use of emergency room services of a population of public housing residents determined that a significant number of emergency room visits were for needs that could be more appropriately met in primary care settings. The study found that 68% of the emergency room visits made by this population were between 7:00 AM and 7:00 PM when primary care services were readily available. These daytime emergency room visits tended to be less acute, suggesting that those who used the emergency room as a source of non-urgent care were more likely to do so during the day. The study also found wide variation in the amount of services consumed during an emergency room visit; however, of all visits by this population, 41% consumed no services. In consuming no services, the visit likely consisted of either health assessments, counseling, or patient education, suggesting a need for primary care services to address one's ability to cope with the problems of daily living. Age was a strong predictor of emergency room use, with the very young and very elderly consuming the most services. The author points out that to serve children better, primary care services should focus on prompt treatment of infectious diseases, and to serve the elderly better, primary care should focus on health promotion and chronic disease management.

This study found that a large percentage of emergency room visits among low-income groups were not urgent and required no immediate assistance. Previous studies have revealed that the most significant barrier to seeking primary care services is the lack of an accessible primary care provider. To address this barrier, this study endorses the use of community-based primary care clinics. If primary care clinics are more accessible and available, it can be hypothesized that inappropriate use of the emergency room will decline, which will allow for lower costs and more efficient and effective use of health care resources.

Glick DF, MacDonald Thompson K: Analysis of emergency room use of primary care needs, *Nursing Economics* 15(1):42, 1997.

area, such as pediatrics, adult, gerontology, obstetrics/gynecology, or family. Training emphasizes clinical medical skills (history, physical, and diagnosis) and pharmacology, in addition to the traditional psychosocial- and prevention-focused attributes that are normally ascribed to nursing. Studies have shown that 60% to 80% of primary care, traditionally done by physicians, can be delivered by an NP for less money and with equal or better quality (Office of Technology Assessment, 1986).

Nurse midwifery is defined as "the independent management and care of essentially normal newborns and women antepartally, intrapartally, postpartally, and gynecologically, occurring within a health care system that provides for medical consultation, collaborative management, and referral . . ." (Rooks and Haas, 1986, p. 9). The mother is the primary focus of care for nurse midwives, who spend the majority of their time on prenatal care, labor, delivery, and postpartum care, as well as family planning services. Nurse midwives receive advanced training either at the master's level or by attending a school of nurse midwifery. All CNMs are certified by a national examination.

Physician assistants (PAs) operate under the license of a physician, which is different from NPs and CNMs who operate as independent practitioners. Most PAs receive their training at the baccalaureate level and are able to sit for their certification boards once they have graduated. PAs assist or substitute for physicians in the performance of specific medical tasks. Like NPs, PAs are proficient in history, physicals, and the diagnosing and treating of uncomplicated medical conditions. Both are trained in prescribing a limited numbers of drugs, but the scope of their prescriptive authority depends on the state laws where they live. In the past, CNMs and NPs have received considerable pressure to limit their practice to avoid infringing on what physicians perceive as their role. Many state practice laws have changed, however, with pressure from the federal government, NPs, CNMs, and consumers to practice independently, prescribe, and receive third-party reimbursement.

Public Health System

Although the goal of the public health system is to ensure that the health of the community is protected, promoted, and assured, there is overlap between this system and the personal care system. The overlap comes not only from the personal care system providing health promotion and disease prevention, but also through the public health system providing personal care services for those who cannot afford to receive their care elsewhere. For example, the US-DHHS provides a commissioned corps of uniformed health personnel, the **National Health Service Corps,** to serve residents of medically underserved areas.

The public health system is mandated through laws that are developed at the national, state, or local level. An example of public health laws instituted to protect the health of the community includes mandatory immunizations for all children entering kindergarten and constant monitoring of the local water supply.

Organization of the public health system

The public health system is organized into multilevels composed of the federal, state, and local systems. Although not all local governmental units are involved in health care, most are. For example, school districts are responsible for health education and first aid, with many schools having onsite clinics that are responsible for a comprehensive array of the student's health, including mental health and family planning.

Federal System

U.S. Department of Health and Human Services

The **U.S. Department of Health and Human Services (USDHHS)** is the agency most heavily involved with the health and welfare concerns of U.S. citizens. The organi-

zational chart of the USDHHS (Fig. 3-1) depicts the office of the Secretary, eleven agencies, and a program support center. Although not shown on the organizational chart, David Satcher, M.D. was confirmed in 1998 as the U.S. Surgeon General, a position that has been combined with

U.S. Department of Health and Human Services

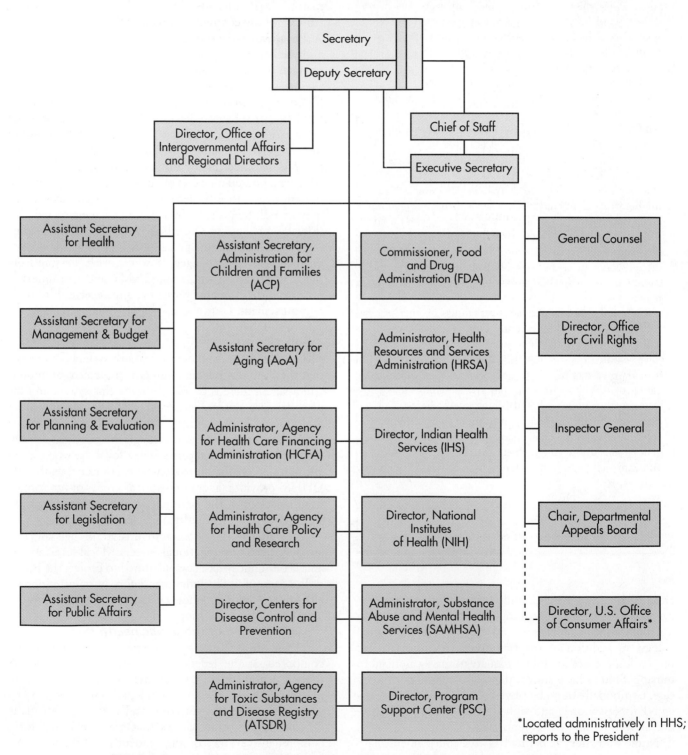

FIG. 3-1 Organization of the U.S. Department of Health and Human Services. (From U.S. Department of Health and Human Services organization chart [www.hhs.gov/about/orgchart. html].)

that of the Assistant Secretary for Health. The USDHHS is charged with regulating health care and overseeing the health status of Americans.

The USDHHS is the largest health program in the world. Its mission is to protect and advance the health of the American people through the following (USPHS, 1994):
- Medical research
- Disease tracking and identification
- Health care to American Indians and Alaskan Natives and medically underserved populations
- Alcohol, drug abuse, and mental health programs
- Identification and correction of health hazards
- Promotion of exercise and healthy habits
- Protection of the nation's food and drug supply
- Medical assistance after disasters

The major components of the USDHHS are shown in Figure 3-1. The USDHHS, directed by the Secretary for Health, is organized into twelve functional units:

1. Administration for Children and Families (ACF)
2. Agency on Aging (AoA)
3. Health Care Financing Administration (HCFA)
4. Agency for Health Care Policy and Research (AHCPR)
5. Centers for Disease Control and Prevention (CDC)
6. Agency for Toxic Substances and Disease Registry (ATSDR)
7. Food and Drug Administration (FDA)
8. Health Resources and Services Administration (HRSA)
9. Indian Health Service (IHS)
10. National Institutes of Health (NIH)
11. Substance Abuse and Mental Health Services Administration (SAMHSA)
12. Program Support Center (PSC)

The PCS supports the Secretary and all of the agencies listed. Ten regional offices are maintained to provide more direct assistance to the states. Their locations are shown in Table 3-3. The HRSA of the USDHHS contains the Bureau of Health Professions, which includes separate divisions for Nursing, Medicine, Dentistry, and Allied Health Professions.

Division of Nursing. The federal government looks to the Division of Nursing to provide the competence and expertise for administering nurse education legislation, interpreting trends and needs of the nursing component of the nation's health care delivery system, and maintaining a liaison with the nursing community and with international, state, regional, and local health interests. As the federal focus for nursing education and practice, the Division identifies current and future nursing issues. The Division works collaboratively with other federal agencies and with national nursing organizations (Division of Nursing, 1993).

National Center for Nursing Research. In late 1985, Congress overrode a presidential veto allowing the creation of the National Center for Nursing Research within the National Institutes of Health. The research and research-related training activities previously supported by the Division of Nursing were transferred to this new center. In 1993 it was renamed the National Institute for Nursing Research. The Institute is the focal point of the nation's nursing research activities. It promotes the growth and quality of research in nursing and patient care, provides important leadership, expands the pool of experienced nurse researchers, and serves as a point of interaction with other bases of health care research.

Agency for Health Care Policy and Research. A significant addition to the USDHHS in 1990 was the creation of the Agency for Health Care Policy and Research (AHCPR). This agency is charged with conducting research on effectiveness of medical services, interventions, and technologies, including research related to nursing interventions and outcomes that contribute to the improved health status of the nation.

Other federal government agencies

The USDHHS has primary responsibility for federal health functions. The cabinet departments of the federal

TABLE 3-3 Regional Offices of the U. S. Department of Health and Human Services

REGION	LOCATION	TERRITORY
1	Boston	Connecticut, Maine, Massachusetts, New Hampshire, Rhode Island, Vermont
2	New York	New Jersey, New York, Puerto Rico, Virgin Islands
3	Philadelphia	Delaware, District of Columbia, Maryland, Pennsylvania, Virginia, West Virginia
4	Atlanta	Alabama, Florida, Georgia, Kentucky, Mississippi, North Carolina, South Carolina, Tennessee
5	Chicago	Illinois, Indiana, Michigan, Minnesota, Ohio, Wisconsin
6	Dallas	Arkansas, Louisiana, New Mexico, Oklahoma, Texas
7	Kansas City	Iowa, Kansas, Missouri, Nebraska
8	Denver	Colorado, Montana, North Dakota, South Dakota, Utah, Wyoming
9	San Francisco	American Samoa, Arizona, California, Guam, Hawaii, Nevada, N. Mariana Islands, Trust Territories
10	Seattle	Alaska, Idaho, Oregon, Washington

government carry out certain functions related to the health of the nation. Those departments include Commerce, Defense, Labor, Agriculture, and Justice.

Department of Commerce. Within the Department of Commerce, the Census Bureau provides health care information. Established in 1902, this bureau conducts a census of the population every 10 years. Also a part of this department is the National Oceanic and Atmospheric Administration, which provides special services in support of controlling urban air quality, a major factor in community health today.

Department of Defense. The Department of Defense delivers health care to members of the military and their dependents. The Assistant Secretary of Defense for Health Affairs administers the Civilian Health and Medical Program of the Uniformed Services (CHAMPUS). The departments within Defense (Army, Navy, Air Force, and Marines) each have a surgeon general. Health services, including community health services for members of the military, are delivered by a health services command in each department. In each command, nurses of high military rank are part of the administration of health services.

Department of Labor. The Department of Labor has two agencies with health functions: the Occupational Safety and Heath Administration (OSHA) and the Mine Safety and Health Administration. Both are charged with writing safety and health standards and ensuring compliance in the workplace. This includes conducting inspections, investigating complaints, and issuing citations if necessary. Each agency coordinates its activities with state departments of labor and health.

Department of Agriculture. The Department of Agriculture is involved in health care primarily through administering the Food and Nutrition Service. Although plant, product, and animal inspection by the Department of Agriculture is also related to health, the Food and Nutrition Service oversees a variety of food assistance activities. This service collaborates with state and local government welfare agencies to provide food stamps to needy persons to increase their food purchasing power. Other programs include school breakfast and lunch programs; the Supplemental Food Program for Women, Infants, and Children (WIC); and grants to states for nutrition education training.

Department of Justice. Health services to federal prisoners are administered within the Department of Justice. The Medical and Services Division of the Bureau of Prisons includes medical, psychiatric, dental, and health support services. It also administers environmental health and safety, farm operations, and food service, along with commissary, laundry, and other personal services for inmates.

State System

Although state health departments vary widely in their roles, they have a substantial role in health care financing (such as Medicaid), providing mental health and professional education, establishing health codes, licensing facil-

ities and personnel, and regulating the insurance industry (Brecher, 1990). State systems also have a substantial role in direct assistance to local health departments, including ongoing assessment of health needs. Box 3-2 provides a list of typical state health department programs.

As in international and federal agencies, nurses serve in many capacities in state health departments such as consultation, direct services, research, teaching, supervision, planning, and evaluation of health programs. Many health departments have a division or department of community health nursing.

Every state has a board of examiners of nurses. The board may be found either in the department of licensing boards of the health department or in an administrative agency of the governor's office. Created by legislation known as a *state nurse practice act*, the examiners' board is made up of nurses and consumers. A few states have other providers or administrators as members. The functions of this board are described in the practice act of each state and generally include licensing and examination of registered nurses and licensed practical nurses; approval of schools of nursing in the state; revocation, suspension, or denial of licenses; and writing of regulations about nursing practice and education.

Local System

The local health department has direct responsibility to the citizens in their community or jurisdiction. Services and programs offered by local health departments vary greatly depending on the state and local health codes that must be followed, the needs of the community, and available funding and other resources. For example, one health department might be more involved with public health education programs and environmental issues, whereas an-

---

BOX 3-2 Typical Programs Found in a State Health Department

Legal services
Service to the chronically ill and aging
Juvenile services
Medical assistance: policy, compliance operations
Mental health and addictions
Mental retardation and developmental disabilities
Environmental programs
Departmental licensing boards
Division of vital records
Media and public relations and educational information
Health services cost review
Case management
Sexually transmitted diseases (screening and treatment)
AIDS services
Referrals to resources
Quality assurance
Health planning and development
Preventive medicine and medical affairs

other health department might emphasize direct client care. Local health departments vary in their level of involvement with sick care or even primary care. A list of health department programs, taken from an urban-suburban county health department in a mid-Atlantic state, is shown in Box 3-3. At the local level, as at the state level, coordination of health efforts between health departments and other county or city departments is essential. For example, local boards of education and departments of social services are an integral part of activities of local governments. More often than at other levels of government, community health nurses at the local level provide direct services. Some community health nurses deliver special or selected services, such as follow-up of contacts in cases of tuberculosis or venereal disease, or providing child immunization clinics. Other community health nurses have a more generalized practice, delivering services to families in certain geographic areas. This method of delivery of nursing services involves broader needs and a wider variety of nursing interventions.

TRANSFORMATION OF THE HEALTH CARE SYSTEM

The rising costs of health care in the United States, uneven access for consumers, and dissatisfaction of both consumers and health care professionals have created an at-

mosphere conducive to rapid change. There are four important competing forces that are helping to shape the health care system: consumers, employers (purchasers), managed care systems including HMOs and hospital systems, and state and federal legislation.

First, consumers want low-cost, high-quality health care without limitations and greater choice in accessing the providers that they want to see. They are becoming more knowledgable about appealing health care decisions that are being made for them and are joining and appealing to consumer groups to help them fight their battles in and outside of the court room. Consumer groups, especially those that are involved with creating managed care "report cards," will continue to play a major role in helping to shape the future health care system.

Second, employers (purchasers of health care), want accessible basic health care plans at reasonable costs. They put continual pressure on HMOs to decrease costs and are always threatening to change plans if their costs are not low enough or their benefits do not fit the needs of their employees. Employers are increasingly expecting their employees to pick up a greater share of this cost and continue to drop health care coverage for family members.

WHAT DO YOU THINK? *Mandating small business owners to purchase health insurance for their employees (employer mandates) is a reasonable way to help ensure that the health needs of this nation, especially the working poor, will be taken care of.*

Managed care plans and other major health care systems continue to strive for a balance between consumer and purchaser demands, while always keeping a close eye on their own bottom line expenditures. To maintain profitability while providing quality care, HMOs and other health care systems have had to down-size and create alliances, mergers, and other joint ventures.

Finally, legislation, especially concerning access and quality issues continues to be debated and enacted, thus creating yet another force helping to shape a health care system based on incremental changes. Legislators are pressured by a variety of groups, which include the following:

1. Constituents who seek changes because of an unsatisfactory experience with a health care system or provider
2. Consumer groups representing the uninsured
3. Employers who continually fight against mandated coverage for their employees
4. The managed care industry that is trying to remain profitable in the face of rising costs

Other examples of a health care system in transformation include the following:

• Regionalization of managed health care in both the private and public (Medicare and Medicaid) sectors based on a competitive pre-paid capitated system. Local initiatives will continue to be needed to address the

BOX 3-3 Examples of Programs Provided by Local Health Departments

Addiction and alcoholism clinics
Adult health
Birth and death records
Child daycare and development
Child health clinics
Crippled children's services
Dental health clinic
Environmental health
Epidemiology and disease control
Family planning
Geriatric evaluation
Health education
Home health agency
Hospital discharge planning
Hypertension clinics
Immunization clinics
Information services
Maternal health
Medical social work
Mental health
Mental retardation and developmental disabilities
Nursing
Nursing home licensure
Nutrition
Occupational therapy
School health
Speech and audiology

needs of their homeless, underserved, and uninsured populations.

- Enormous growth in the home health care industry, with a 60% increase in spending between 1993 and 1994 alone. Increased fraud within the last couple of years may cause Medicare to cut back on payments and cause the industry to slow or even decrease.
- Consumers of health care will continue to feel empowered to make changes in the health care system. This will lead to healthier people in healthier communities. Consumers of health care will also become more informed and involved in their own health care.
- Advances in diagnostic and surgical technology may lead to higher survival rates and less time spent in sick care. This will be counterbalanced by the fact that Americans still make health behavior choices such as smoking, not exercising, and excessive eating that keep them from living a long and healthful existence. In addition, leading-edge technology and surgical procedures will still only benefit those who will be able to afford them.
- Experimentation in health personnel staffing will increase in an attempt to save costs and find new opportunities to substitute technology for human labor.
- Continuing shortage of primary care providers in underserved areas such as rural and inner-city will exist.
- Efforts by health care personnel to bring back the "caring" side of health care as a revolt against the stringent cost-cutting efforts instituted by managed care in the 1990s will be seen.
- Increasing emphasis will be placed on population-based health care, not only as a cost-savings mechanism, but also to promote disease prevention and to meet the health care needs of many people at one time.
- Emphasis will be placed on delivering care leading to the best possible outcomes. This so-called "evidence-based care" is done in an effort to ensure quality.
- Information systems, including the electronic medical record, will save time and effort and will help ensure the delivery of appropriate care. Innovations in the field of information technology are also creating much debate and forthcoming legislation regarding "right to privacy."
- Major shifts of nurses from the acute care setting to the community will continue. Continuing education needs will expand to help nurses learn to transfer skills.

> **DID YOU KNOW?** *The Balanced Budget Act of 1997 provided $20 billion for children's health coverage to be distributed to the states and used over a 5-year period. Children to be covered by the State Children's Health Insurance Program (SCHIP) must be under age 19 in families with incomes up to 200% of the federal poverty level, must not be covered by Medicaid, and must not be receiving coverage under a group or individual insurance plan (White House Press Office, 1999).*

A COMPREHENSIVE MODEL: INTEGRATION OF PUBLIC HEALTH AND PRIMARY CARE

What is needed to improve health care?

1. Delivery systems, as they strive to deliver the most cost-effective care possible, must also find ways to improve access and quality in the communities they serve, especially to the underserved.
2. Students must be prepared to work together with other health professionals to understand the needs of the community and how to promote prevention.
3. Documents such as *Healthy People 2000* and the WHO's *Health For All by the Year 2000* call for increased attention to population-based preventive activities as a means of increasing the health status of Americans.
4. The systems must also become integrated in order to control the cost of personal health care (Lee, 1994).
5. Health professions education should become more responsive to preparing students to better understand the needs of the community and prevention-oriented care (O'Neil, 1993). One model for integrating the public health and primary care systems is called *community-oriented primary care.*

Community-Oriented Primary Care

Community-oriented primary care (COPC), a community-responsive model of health care delivery, integrates aspects of both primary care and public health. It combines the care of individuals and families in the community with a focus on the community and its subgroups when services are planned, provided, and evaluated (Abramson, 1984). This model contends that allocating more resources into community care will ultimately save money, increase access, and create better health outcomes in personal care (Hattis, 1993). As former USDHHS Assistant Secretary for Health, Philip Lee, M.D. has emphasized, "When the public health system is not maintained and falls into disrepair, the health of the community suffers and, inevitably, the health risks, volume of care, and cost of care to the individual increases as well" (Ketter, 1994, p. 17).

Wright (1993), in speaking of health care transformation and the evolving competitive marketplace, states that COPC is the most effective model for emphasizing prevention, using a planning process that targets resources to high-priority needs, and for empowering communities to encourage individual responsibility. Wright (1993) describes the tools required to use the COPC model as follows:

1. A community-based primary care practice
2. An identifiable population or community for which the practice assumes responsibility for effecting change in health status
3. A planning, monitoring, and evaluation process for identifying and resolving health problems.

Although COPC systems in the United States may attempt to invite and maintain community participation,

The Canadian Health Care System and Primary Health Care

Lianne Jeffs, Registered Nurses Association of Ontario and University of Toronto

In Canada, although wide variations exist by geographic (e.g., underserved and rural areas), ethnic (e.g., native Indians), and socioeconomic (e.g., low-income families) variables, the overall health of Canadians is rising. Canada has a lower infant mortality rate of 6 per 1000 as compared with the United States, which has 8 infant deaths per 1000 live births. Canadians also live longer than Americans do. From 1990 to 1995 the gap in life expectancy between Canadians and Americans increased from 2 to 2.8 years for men and from 1.6 to 1.9 years for women (Anderson, 1997).

HEALTH CARE REFORM

Over the last 2 decades fundamental changes have occurred and continue to occur in the Canadian health care system that are rooted in a shift from treating disease to improving health care and a desire for effectiveness and efficiency in the health care system. This has resulted in decentralisation and regionalisation of health care services; a move from acute, institutional care to community-based care; and an increased emphasis on primary health care. Health care reform has occurred in response to a variety of trends including increased health care costs, advances in technology, an aging population, increased chronic illness, increased acuity of clients, continuing costs of cardiovascular diseases and cancer, re-emergence of communicable diseases, and environmental health problems (Stewart, 1995). Another major trend is increased consumer involvement. Canadians want a wellness-oriented health care system with a health promotion/disease prevention focus that is evidence-based.

Other trends in health care reform include a reduction in transfer payments to provinces, delisting of health care services, and user fees. Diminished power and downloading of responsibilities of community health care, including public health services, from federal to provincial to local and regional authorities have occurred without sufficient funding, staffing, and authority to perform the job. From 1985 to 1992, there was only a 2.7 increase in community health nursing positions, which is a relatively small percentage of human resources growth compared with the magnitude of the shift from hospital to community health care services (Rodger and Gallagher, 1996). Moreover, health care needs in both the hospital and community sectors are growing in Canada when investment in these services is decreasing. This coupled with the increased rate of poverty, unemployment, and cuts in government spending threatens not only the social safety net and health care system, but also the overall health status of Canadians (Canadian Public Health Association, 1996).

PRIMARY HEALTH CARE

For over a decade, health professionals, health planners, and decision makers in Canada have emphasised the need for comprehensive and accessible primary health care as outlined by the Alma Ata Declaration (see Appendix A-4). The primary health care system has multidisciplinary teams made up of a variety of health professionals including physicians, nurse practitioners, registered nurses, social workers, dieticians, physiotherapists, dentists, and health promoters who practise in a variety of settings such as public health units, community health centres, and health service organisations. These agencies provide an integrated and coordinated approach to meeting the complex health needs of the individuals and families within the community to which they provide services. Another component of primary health care is public health services, and programs such as the Healthy Cities Project, Best Start, and Better Beginnings reflect the underlying principles of primary health care. Similar to the United States, the struggle to clearly differentiate between primary care and primary health care and operationalization of primary health care principles into the health care system continues in Canadian health care reform.

PUBLIC HEALTH SERVICES

Underlying public health practice in Canada is the legislative mandate designed to protect the public interest relative to communicable diseases and environmental risks. Public health services in Canada are administered primarily through government departments such as departments of health, Ministries of Health and Social Services, and/or departments of public health. Variation of structures occurs across the provincial and territorial jurisdictions as well as in municipal/regional agencies including health units and autonomous agencies. These agencies are responsible for providing basic public health services of communicable disease control, regulation and enforcement of environmental standards, and health promotion and illness and injury prevention programs.

ROLE OF THE REGISTERED NURSE IN THE PRIMARY HEALTH CARE SYSTEM

Registered nurses are key to the provision of comprehensive and effective primary health care services. The value of the registered nurse as a high-quality, cost-effective provider in the primary health care system is well documented. There are many roles for the registered nurse in the primary health care system, depending on educational preparation and experience, including public health nurse, community health nurse, health promotion nurse, primary health care nurse practitioner (legislated in Ontario only), and nursing administrator. Within each of these roles the

Continued

The Canadian Health Care System and Primary Health Care—cont'd

registered nurse can function as an educator, consultant, community developer, facilitator, leader, enabler, advocate, communicator, coordinator, collaborator, researcher, social marketer, and policy formulator.

For the health status of Canadians to improve, there needs to be a strong commitment to the principles of comprehensive and accessible primary health care. This commitment will strengthen the contribution of the multidisciplinary primary health care team, including the registered nurse, in the provision of care to individuals, families, and communities, which will ultimately lead to the overall effectiveness of the Canadian health care system.

Bibliography
Anderson GF: In search of value: an international comparison of cost, access, and outcomes, *Health Affairs* 16(6):163, 1997.
Braunstein J, Young HJ, Beanlands HJ: Administration in public health nursing. In Stewart MJ, editor: *Community nursing: promoting Canadians' health*, Toronto, 1995, WB Saunders Canada.
Canadian Public Health Association: *Action statement for health promotion in Canada*. Ottawa, 1996, the Association.
Cradduck GR: Primary health care practice. In Stewart MJ, editor: *Community nursing: promoting Canadians' health*, Toronto, 1995, WB Saunders Canada.
Registered Nurses Association of Ontario: *RN effectiveness project: clinical, financial, and systems outcomes*, Toronto, 1998, the Association.
Rodger GL, Gallagher SM: The move toward primary health care in community nursing: In Stewart MJ, editor: *Community nursing: promoting Canadians' health*, Toronto, 1995, WB Saunders Canada.
Stewart MJ, editor: *Community nursing: promoting Canadians' health*, Toronto, 1995, WB Saunders Canada.

Canadian spelling is used.

this aspect of the plan cannot be overemphasized. The COPC process of inviting participation by members of the community, although effective, differs from what has generally been called the "community-based" health care approach, which is a process that has been initiated by members of the community themselves. The most effective and most sustainable individual and system changes come when there has been active participation by the people who live in the community regardless of who begins the process. This is an important element in primary health care as well.

The W.K. Kellogg Foundation (1993), a foundation that financially supports efforts to improve the health of communities, states that a community-based practice must involve community members by allowing them to set their own priorities and solutions. Kellogg has found that when the right tools, such as power, information, and financial support, are shared with community members, they become more actively involved in the process. Building a consensus among the many diverse community leaders who have a vested interest in the process will help ensure a more accurate and comprehensive representation of the community's health needs as well as a wider array of solutions to these needs. In this context, it must be remembered that health care cannot be separated from the broader scope of community development, such as housing and economic development. Consider the example of a young mother who has been scolded by a health professional for presenting her child with several infected insect bites without ever addressing the issue of the unavailability of window screens in the family's apartment.

The strategies for using COPC are similar to the nursing process, using the community as the client. The steps of COPC are as follows:
1. Define and characterize the community. Use personal knowledge (including observations) of the community with data obtained from community leaders. Data should include morbidity and mortality rates, existing health care services and accessibility, transportation services, cultural diversity, environmental issues, and more.
2. Identify a list of community health problems and needs, and from that list formulate a community diagnosis. The process of formulating a diagnosis should develop as a consensus from key members of the delivery team and community leaders who truly represent the diverse needs and resources of the community.
3. Assist community leaders in the development of interventions corresponding to the community diagnosis. This includes personal care services as well as health promotion and disease prevention activities. Encourage interdisciplinary teamwork to gain maximum benefits from human resources. Maintain community input to determine feasibility and resources.
4. Coordinate and manage services. Work in partnership with social service agencies, health professionals, and community leaders to provide comprehensive care, and encourage networking.
5. Evaluate the interventions with the input of community leaders. The system should allow for continuous feedback to allow for intermittent modification and redirection of resources.

Role of the nurse in COPC

Since nurses move in and are trusted in the community like few other professionals, they are ideally suited to practice using a COPC model. They can be found in schools, homes, churches, and on street corners developing relationships, collecting data, assessing needs, and providing care. In addition, with the knowledge that nurses have regarding community resources, they make excellent case managers (Bower, 1992).

> **NURSING TIP**
>
> *Many nurses in the United States are practicing illness-oriented care as a result of public need and the revenue attached to these services (Miller et al, 1993). Salmon (1993) states this is a case of mistaken identity because this role has diverted public health nurses away from their central roles in assessment; surveillance; policy and health promotion; and disease and injury prevention activities.*

Although they will continue to be used for some hands-on services, a generalist, prevention-oriented, public health background will allow the public and community health nurse to bridge the gap between personal care and the health of the community.

 clinical application

During a well-child clinic visit, Jenna Wells, RN, met Sandra Farr and her 24-month-old daughter, Jessica. The Farrs had recently moved to the community. Mrs. Farr stated that she knew that Jessica needed the last in a series of immunizations, and because they did not have health insurance, she brought her daughter to the public health clinic. Upon initial assessment, Mrs. Farr told the nurse that her husband would soon be employed, but the family would not have any health care coverage for the next 30 days. The Farrs also need to decide which health care package they want. Mr. Farr's company offers a preferred provider option (PPO), a health maintenance organization (HMO), and a community nursing clinic plan to all employees. Neither Mr. or Mrs. Farr have ever used an HMO or a community nursing clinic, and they are not sure what services are provided.

Mrs. Farr asks Nurse Wells what she should do. Nurse Wells should do which of the following?

A. Encourage Mrs. Farr to choose the HMO because it will pay more attention to the family's preventive needs, *and* direct Mrs. Farr to other sources of health care should the family need to see a provider while they are uninsured.

B. Encourage Mrs. Farr to choose the PPO because it will have a greater number of qualified providers to choose from, *and* direct Mrs. Farr to other sources of health care should the family need to see a provider while they are uninsured.

C. Encourage Mrs. Farr to choose the local community nursing center because it is staffed with nurse practitioners who are well qualified to provide comprehensive health care with an emphasis on health education, *and* direct Mrs. Farr to other sources of health care should the family need to see a provider while they are uninsured.

D. Explain the differences between a PPO, HMO, and community nursing clinic, and encourage Mrs. Farr to discuss the options with her husband, *and* direct Mrs. Farr to other sources of health care should the family need to see a provider while they are uninsured.

Answers are in the back of the book.

KEY POINTS

- Health care in the United States is comprised of a personal care system and a public health system, with overlap between the two systems.
- Primary care is a personal health care system that provides for first contact, continuous, comprehensive, and coordinated care.
- Primary health care is essential care made universally accessible to individuals and families in a community. Health care is made available to them through their full participation and is provided at a cost that the community and country can afford.
- Primary care is part of primary health care.
- Although primary care practitioners are encouraged to consider the client's biopsychosocial needs, interventions are directed primarily at the pathophysiologic process.
- *Public health* refers to organized community efforts designed to prevent disease and promote health.
- Several important trends affecting the health care system are demographic, social, economic, political, and technological trends.
- There are approximately 42 million uninsured people in the United States and many more who simply lack access to adequate health care.
- Many federal agencies are involved in government health care functions. The agency most directly involved with the health and welfare of Americans is the U.S. Department of Health and Human Services (USDHHS).
- Most state and local jurisdictions have government activities that affect the health care field.
- Health care reform measures seek to make changes in the cost, quality, and access of the present system.
- Because of the current emphasis on community-based care, it is predicted that many nurses who are now working in acute care will continue to face job loss and uncertainty.
- With an increasing emphasis on cost containment, the health care delivery system is focusing its efforts on developing managed care systems.
- Community-oriented primary care (COPC) is a model that emphasizes important aspects of both primary care and public health, and therefore is more consistent with the principles of primary health care.
- Strategies for using COPC can be likened to the nursing process, using the community as the client.

- The most sustainable individual and system changes come when there has been active participation from the people who live in the community.
- Building a consensus among the many diverse community leaders will help ensure a more accurate and comprehensive representation of the community's health needs as well as the solutions to address the needs.
- Nurses are more than able to fill the gap between personal care and public health since they have skills in assessment, health promotion, and disease and injury prevention; knowledge of community resources; and ability to develop relationships with community members and leaders.

critical thinking activities

1. Compare the local and state services where you live with those that have been presented in this chapter.
2. Debate the following: The major problem with the health care system is (choose one of the following topics):
   a. Escalating costs (including those from increased technology)
   b. Fragmentation
   c. Access to care
   d. Quality of care
3. Interview a nurse practitioner and a physician assistant to determine any philosophical differences in their scope of practice.
4. If you were asked to plan a disease prevention program in your community, what would you do? Describe the plan you would implement.
5. If there is an HMO in your community, interview three providers and three consumers to determine what each sees as the advantages and disadvantages of this type of care delivery system.
6. Visit your local health department and determine how its services fit into a primary care, public health, or COPC model of care.
7. Determine whether any agency in your community is using the principles of COPC to deliver health care. Identify which principles they are using and those they could be using.
8. Describe three factors that might discourage the COPC approach to care in your community or in the United States.

Bibliography

Abramson, JH: Application of epidemiology in community oriented primary care, *Public Health Rep* 99(5):437, 1984.

Altman SH: *What can we learn from other countries about the mix and interrelationships of primary care and specialty care on access, quality, and cost?* Paper presented at the National Primary Care Conference, March, 1992, Washington D.C.

Bennefield RL: Health insurance coverage: 1996. In *Current population reports of the Census Bureau,* Washington, DC, 1997, U.S. Department of Commerce, Economics and Statistics Administration.

Bower KA: *Case management by nurses.* Kansas City, MO, 1992, American Nurses Publishing.

Brecher C: The government's role in health care. In Kooner AR, editor: *Health care delivery in the United States,* New York, 1990, Springer.

Center for Studying Health Systems Change: *Data bulletin from the Community Tracking Study,* Washington, DC, 1997, Author.

Copeland C: Issues of quality and consumer rights in the health care market, *Employee Benefit Research Institute Issue Brief,* April, 1998 p. 196.

Curley T, Orloff TM, Tymann B: *Health professions education linkages: community-based primary care training,* Washington, DC, 1994, National Governor's Association.

Division of Nursing: *Information booklet on the Division of Nursing,* Rockville, Md, 1993, USDHHS

Exter T: Demographic forecast, *American Demographics* 12(2):55, 1990.

Glick DF, MacDonald Thompson K: Analysis of emergency room use of primary care needs, *Nursing Economics* 15(1):42, 1997.

Greenfield S, Nelson EC, Zubkoff M et al: Variations in resource utilization among medical specialties and systems of care: results from the medical outcomes study. *JAMA* 267(12):1624, 1992.

Hattis PA: Retooling for community benefit, *Health Progress* 74(7):38, 1993

Haupt A, Kane TT: *The Population Reference Bureau's population handbook,* ed 4, Washington, DC, 1997, Population Reference Bureau.

Health Care Financing Administration: *Table 1: national health expenditures aggregate and per capita amounts, percent distribution, and average annual percent growth, by source of funds: selected calendar years 1960-97,* November, 13 1998, www.hcfa.gov/stats/NHE-Proj/tables/t01.htm

Health Care Financing Administration: *Table 1: national health expenditure amounts, percent distribution, and average annual percent growth, by source of funds: selected calendar years 1970-2007,* November 6, 1998, www.hcfa.gov/stats/NHE-Proj/tables/t01.htm

Institute for the Future: *Piecing together the puzzle: the future of health and health care in America,* December, 1997, a commissioned report to the Robert Wood Johnson Foundation.

Institute of Medicine: *Primary care: America's health in a new era,* Washington, DC, 1996, National Academy Press.

Institute of Medicine: *The future of public health,* Washington, DC, 1988, National Academy Press.

Johnson T: *Changing demographics in minority populations of the United States in caring for the emerging majority: creating a new diversity in nurse leadership.* Washington, DC, 1992, U.S. Department of Health and Human Services.

Ketter J: Is there a cure for our ailing public health system? *American Nurse* June, 17, 1994.

Lee P: Shattuck lecture. Delivered at the annual meeting of the Massachusetts Medical Society, 1994. Unpublished white paper.

Mahler H: The meaning of "Health for all for the year 2000" *World Health Forum* 2(1):5, 1981.

Miller CA et al: Longitudinal observations on a selected group of local health departments: a preliminary report, *J Public Health Policy* Spring, 34, 1993.

Miller E: *Future vision,* Naperville, Illinois, 1991, Sourcebooks Trade.

Millis JS: *The graduate education of physicians: report of the citizens commission on graduate medical education,* Chicago, 1966, American Medical Association.

National Center for Health Statistics: *Monthly Vital Statistics Report,* 46(11):5, 1998.

Office of Technology Assessment (OTA): *Nurse practitioners, physicians' assistants, and certified nurse-midwives: a policy analysis* (Health Technology Case Study No. 37), Washington, DC, 1986, U.S. Government Printing Office.

Older Americans Report: *Commission on Healthcare wraps up: doesn't endorse bill of rights,* Silver Spring, Md, 1998, Business Publications.

O'Neil EH: *Health professions education for the future: schools in service to the nation,* San Francisco, 1993, Pew Health Professions Commission.

Ory MG, DeFriese GH: *Self care in later life: research, program and policy perspectives,* New York, 1998, Springer Publishing Co.

Pender NJ: *Health promotion in nursing practice,* ed 3, Norwalk, Conn, 1996, Appleton & Lange.

Peterson MA: Health care into the next century, *J Health Polit Policy Law* 22(2):291, 1997.

Rooks J, Haas JE, editors: *Nurse midwifery in America: a report of the American College of Nurse Midwives Foundation,* Washington, DC, 1986, American College of Nurse Midwives Foundation.

Salmon ME: Public health nursing: the opportunity of a century. *Am J Public Health* 83(12):1674, 1993.

Shalala DE: Health care reform isn't dead. *The Washington Post* A23, October 10, 1994.

Starfield B: *Primary care: concept, evaluation and policy,* New York, 1992, Oxford University Press.

Trafford A, Rich S: Health care reform in congress? *The Washington Post* 12, September 20, 1994.

U.S. Census Bureau: *Household and family characteristics: March 1995,* P20-488, Washington, DC, 1996a, Author.

U.S. Census Bureau: *Population projections of the United States by age, sex, race and Hispanic origin (1995-2050),* Washington, DC, 1996b, Author.

U.S. Department of Health and Human Services: *Health personnel in the United States: eighth report to Congress 1991* [DHHS Pub. No. HRS-P-OD-92-1], Washington, DC, 1992, U.S. Government Printing Office.

U.S. Department of Health and Human Services: *An agenda for health professions reform,* Rockville, Md, 1993, Health Resources and Services Administration.

U.S. Department of Health and Human Services: *The registered nurse population,* Rockville, Md, 1996, Health Resources and Services Administration.

U.S. Public Health Service: *Healthy people 2000: national health program and disease prevention.* Washington, DC, 1991, U.S. Government Printing Office.

U.S. Public Health Service: *Keeping America healthy* [Brochure], Washington, DC:, 1994, U.S. Government Printing Office.

White House Press Office: *White House fact sheet on CHIP programs,* April 20, 1999.

Wilensky GR: Promoting quality: a public policy view, *Health Affairs* 16:77, 1997

WK Kellogg Foundation: *Lessons learned in community-based health programming,* Battle Creek, Mich, 1993, the Foundation.

World Health Organization: *Primary health care,* Geneva, 1978, WHO.

World Health Organization: *Basic documents,* ed 36, Geneva, 1986a, WHO.

World Health Organization: *World health statistics annual,* Geneva, 1986b, WHO.

Wright RA: Community-oriented primary care: the cornerstone of health care reform, *JAMA* 269(19):2544, 1993.

CHAPTER 4

Perspectives on International Health Care

KATHLEEN HUTTLINGER

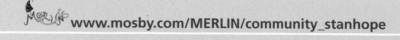
OBJECTIVES

After reading this chapter, the student should be able to do the following:

- Identify the major aims and goals for world health that were presented at the International Conference on Primary Health Care at Alma Ata.
- Analyze the role of public and community health nursing in international health care.

- Evaluate the relationship between economic development and the status of health in developed and lesser developed countries.
- Describe at least five organizations that are involved in international health.
- Discuss some of the major international health concerns in developed and lesser developed countries.

KEY TERMS

developed country
disability-adjusted life
  years (DALYs)
global burden of disease
  (GBD)
governmental
  organizations
health commodification

Health for All by the Year
  2000 (HFA2000)
intergovernmental
  organizations
lesser developed country
Pan American Health
  Organization (PAHO)
philanthropic
  organizations

primary health care
private and commercial
  organizations
private voluntary
  organizations
professional and technical
  organizations
religious organizations
secular organizations

United Nations Children's
  Fund (UNICEF)
World Bank
World Health
  Organization (WHO)

See Glossary for definitions

CHAPTER OUTLINE

Overview of International Health
International Health and the Role
  of Primary Health Care
Major International Health
  Organizations
    Private Voluntary
    Philanthropic
    Professional and Technical

Private and Commercial
Governmental
Intergovernmental
International Health and
  Economic Development
Health Care Systems
    United Kingdom
    Canada

Sweden
China
Major World Health Problems
  and the Burden of Disease
    Communicable Diseases
    Maternal and Women's Health
    Diarrheal Disease
    Nutrition and World Health

This chapter describes some of the major public health problems of the world and the role of nurses in international public settings. In particular, it discusses the role of primary health care in international health and presents examples of different health systems. Also discussed are ways that nurses are involved in world health. Finally, it explains the relationship of economic development to health care throughout the world.

OVERVIEW OF INTERNATIONAL HEALTH

In 1977, attendees at the annual meeting of the World Health Assembly maintained that a major social goal for all of its member agencies should be "the attainment by all citizens of the world by the year 2000 a level of health that will permit them to lead a socially and economically productive life" (World Health Organization, 1986a, p. 65). The goal of **Health for All by the Year 2000 (HFA2000)** has been promoted by numerous health-related conferences held around the world. It was also reinforced at the International Conference on Primary Health Care that was held in Alma Ata, Kazakhstan in 1978 in what was then Soviet Central Asia. The conference was sponsored by the World Health Organization (WHO) and the United Nations Children's Fund (UNICEF). The participants in this conference, who represented 143 countries and 67 organizations, adopted a resolution that proclaimed that the major key to attaining HFA2000 was the worldwide implementation of primary health care (Basch, 1990; Lucas, 1998).

Since the conference at Alma Ata and as the twenty-first century begins, interest in world health and how best to attain it has grown. People around the world want to know and understand the issues and concerns that affect health on a global basis. This is important since many countries have not yet experienced the technological growth in their health care systems that has been realized by more developmentally advanced countries such as the United States, Canada, and several countries in Western Europe. Many terms are used to describe nations that have achieved a high level of industrial and technological advancement (along with a stable market economy) and those that have not. For the purposes of this chapter, the term **developed country** refers to those countries with a stable economy and a wide range of industrial and technological development. Examples of such countries are the United States, Canada, Japan, the United Kingdom, Sweden, France, and Australia. A country that is not yet stable with respect to its economy and technological development is referred to as a **lesser developed country.** Examples of countries considered lesser developed are Bangladesh, Zaire, Haiti, Guatemala, countries in sub-Sahara Africa, and the island nation of Indonesia. Both developed and lesser developed countries are found in all parts of the world and in all geographic and climatic zones (Evlo and Carrin, 1992).

Health problems exist throughout the world, but lesser developed countries are often faced with health care problems such as *leishmaniasis, schistosomiasis, pediculosis, typhus, yellow fever,* and *malaria.* Ongoing health problems in need of control in lesser developed countries include measles, mumps, rubella, and polio, whereas the current health concerns of the more developed countries reflect ongoing struggles with hepatitis, the appearance of new viral strains like the *hantavirus,* and larger social yet health-related issues such as violence and substance abuse (Crompton & Savioli, 1993). For example, in 1995 war broke out in the lesser developed East African country of Rwanda. In less than 3 months, an estimated 500,000 to 1 million people died, and hundreds of thousands fled to the neighboring countries of Zaire, Uganda, Tanzania, and Burundi. These fleeing people, many of whom were women and children, became the victims of rape and other violent acts in addition to the relocation problems of lack of housing, food, and sanitation and communicable disease (Porta, 1996).

With the inception of HFA2000, countries realized that they needed to improve their economic development and therefore began to request monetary assistance and technological expertise from wealthier and more developed countries (Collado, 1992; Lucas, 1998; World Bank, 1992, 1993). According to the WHO, HFA is a strategic process that can lead to progressive improvement in the health of people and is not a single, finite goal (WHO, 1998). It is a call for social justice and solidarity. As economic agreements between countries remove financial and political barriers, growth and development are stimulated. Simultaneously, global health problems that once seemed distant are brought closer to people all over the world, political and economic barriers between countries fall, and the movement of population groups increases, as does the risk of exposure to numerous kinds of diseases and health risks (Basch, 1990; Howson, Fineberg, and Bloom, 1998). For example, in 1997 a deadly bird flu epidemic in Hong Kong had potential worldwide involvement (Hong Kong Chicken Ban, 1998).

Not only do world travelers serve as hosts to various types of disease agents, but travelers may expose themselves to diseases and environmental health hazards that are unknown or rare in their home country (Fig. 4-1). Two examples of diseases from recent years that were once fairly isolated and rare but are now wide-spread throughout the world are acquired immunodeficiency syndrome (AIDS) and drug-resistant forms of tuberculosis (TB) (Howson, Fineberg, and Bloom, 1998).

Despite efforts by individual governments and international health organizations to improve the general economy and welfare for all countries of the world, many health problems continue to exist, especially among the poor. In many countries, there is a lack of political commitment to health care, a lack of recognition of basic human rights issues, a failure to achieve equity in access to primary health care, inappropriate use of and allocation of resources for high-cost technology, and persistently low status of women (WHO, 1998) (Fig. 4-2). Currently, the lesser developed countries experience high infant and child mortality rates, with diarrheal and respiratory diseases as major contributory factors (Lucas, 1998; WHO, 1998; World Bank, 1993). Other major worldwide health problems include nutritional deficiencies among all age groups, women's health and fertility problems, sexually transmitted diseases (STDs) and illnesses related to the human immunodeficiency virus (HIV), malaria, TB, drug-resistant diseases, occupational and environmental health hazards, and abuses of tobacco, alcohol, and drugs.

In 1995, because of these continuing problems, the World Health Assembly requested that the director-general of the WHO take all of the necessary steps and actions to renew the policy of HFA. The WHO was challenged to develop a new and holistic health policy that would be based on the concepts of equity and solidarity with an emphasis on the individual's, family's and community's responsibility for health. HFA2000 was a priority at the WHO's executive board meeting in January, 1998 and was an open discussion at the general assembly in May, 1998. Strategies for achieving this goal included building on past accomplishments and the identification of global priorities and targets for the first 20 years of the twenty-first century (WHO, 1998).

HOW TO *Stay Current About World Health*

One of the ways that you can stay current with the world's health problems and advances is by reading your daily newspaper and those that cover international news. Examples of newspapers that cover international health are the Wall Street Journal, USA Today, and the New York Times.

Being informed about world health is important, especially for nurses. Many of the world's health problems directly affect the health of individuals who live in America. For example, the 103rd U.S. Congress passed the North American Free Trade Agreement (NAFTA), which has opened the trade borders between the United States, Canada, and Mexico. An opening of the borders in 1994 allowed an increased movement of products and people (Fig. 4-3). Along the United States/Mexico border, an influx of undocumented immigrants in recent years has raised concerns for the health of people who live along the border. Many immigrants have settled on unincorporated land, known as *colonias*, outside of the major metropolitan areas in California, Arizona, New Mexico, and Texas. For the most part, the colonias have no developed roads, transportation, water, and electrical services. The result has been an increase in numerous disease conditions associated with poverty, poor sanitation, and overcrowded conditions including amebiasis, respiratory and other diar-

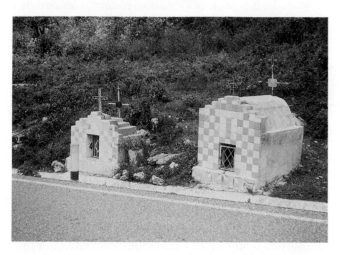

FIG. 4-1 A driver in rural Colombia may be confronted with many road hazards as noted by these roadside shrines. (Courtesy K. Huttlinger.)

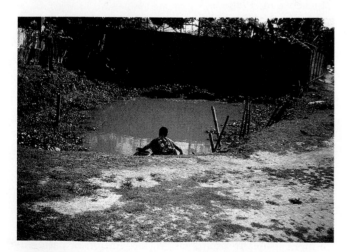

FIG. 4-2 Water holes like this in rural Oman are used for drinking, bathing, and feeding livestock. (Courtesy K. Huttlinger and L. Krefting.)

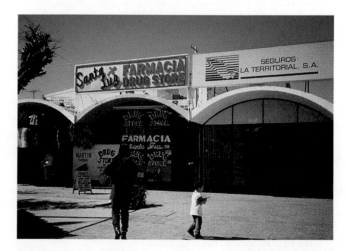

FIG. 4-3 The NAFTA encouraged trade between Mexico, Canada, and the United States. A local farmacia in Nogales, Mexico supplies Americans with lower-cost prescription medicines. (Courtesy K. Huttlinger.)

rheal diseases, and environmental health hazards (Cech and Essman, 1992; Hernandez-Pena et al, 1993).

On a more positive note, the NAFTA has stimulated interest in the government of Mexico to strive for modernization of their medical system in order to respond to the demands of a more global competition. It is anticipated that the implementation of the NAFTA will provide for a more effective enforcement of environmental and health regulations in Mexico as a result of a more rigorous surveillance under conditions of the NAFTA (Ortega-Cesena, Espinosa-Torres, and Lopez-Carillo, 1994). At this time, there is no information that indicates the success or failure of the surveillance system. On the other hand, the Mexican National Academy of Medicine has been active in making recommendations to the government to anticipate the beneficial interactions that can occur between Mexico, Canada, and the United States as part of this trade agreement (Gomez-Dantes, Frenk, and Cruz, 1997).

Nurses play an active role in the international border areas where political and economic boundaries mesh. For example, areas along the U.S.-Mexico border are remote, and health care can be scarce. Nurses supported by private foundations and by local and state public health departments often provide the only health care service in these areas. As such, they contribute to the provision of reliable health care to people in these areas and have served as valuable resources for identifying potential health risks.

INTERNATIONAL HEALTH AND THE ROLE OF PRIMARY HEALTH CARE

The role of **primary health care** in international health is associated with the worldwide conference that was held at Alma Alta and that proclaimed HFA2000 (WHO/ UNICEF, 1978; WHO, 1998). The conference participants proposed that the delivery of primary health care should be made available to people throughout the world and that this care needs to be based on current technology and acceptable practice methods. They also proposed that community members need to be involved in all aspects of the planning and implementation of health services (see Appendix A.4).

Recognizing that there would be differences among countries with respect to the implementation of primary health care because of local customs and environments, it was anticipated that several major components should be included in each plan for health services (WHO/ UNICEF, 1978):

1. An organized approach to health education that involves professional health care providers and trained community representatives
2. Aggressive attention to environmental sanitation, especially food and water sources
3. Involvement and training of community and village health workers in all plans and intervention programs
4. Development of maternal and child health programs that include immunization and family planning

5. Initiation of preventive programs that are specifically aimed at local endemic problems such as malaria and schistosomiasis in tropical regions
6. Accessibility and affordability of services for the treatment of common diseases and injuries
7. Availability of chemotherapeutic agents for the treatment of acute, chronic, and communicable diseases
8. Development of nutrition programs
9. Promotion and acceptance of traditional medicine

The aim of participants of the Alma Ata conference was to emphasize universal access and participation and to encourage a reallocation of resources, if needed, to reduce the inequality of health care that existed among the nations of the world. They encouraged community participation in all aspects of health care planning and implementation and the delivery of health care that was "scientifically sound, technically effective, socially relevant and acceptable" (WHO/ UNICEF, 1978, p. 2). These aims continue to be reinforced and remain an integral part of the goals of the WHO to include essential health care that is accessible to all people of the world at a cost that the community and country can afford (WHO, 1998).

An example of a country that has made a particular effort to implement primary health care services is Mexico. Mexico has initiated a module program that is administered through the Ministry of Health and is characterized by village-based health posts. Each of the health posts is operated by a community volunteer and a health committee. The volunteer and committee are supervised by a nurse who operates from a regional health center. It is believed that this module system can address community needs and will ultimately lead to better use of services and resources.

DID YOU KNOW? *In 1997, UNICEF issued a report that summarized national achievements in child health, nutrition, education, water, sanitation, and progress for women: 44 countries have legislated against domestic violence, 17 have made marital rape a criminal offense, 27 have passed sexual harassment laws, and 12 now have laws against female genital mutilation.*

Nurses can and do play important roles in the primary health care team throughout the world. In particular, nurses with community and public health experience can provide much needed knowledge and skill in those countries where nursing is not an organized profession and give guidance not only to the nurses, but also the auxiliary personnel who are part of the primary health care team. In many settings throughout the world, nurses provide direct client care and facilitate the educational and health promotional needs of the community. Unfortunately, in the lesser developed countries, the role of the nurse is poorly defined if at all (Fig. 4-4), and care is often dependent upon and directed by physicians (Waller and Cammuso,

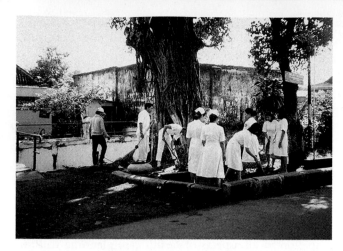

FIG. 4-4 When not providing direct client care, nurses in Indonesia must help keep the hospital grounds clean. (Courtesy K. Huttlinger.)

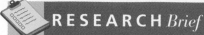

RESEARCH *Brief*

This study describes a survey that was conducted in Uganda to identify what senior nursing personnel perceived their jobs to entail and to determine if their educational preparation helped them in their roles. The researchers also wanted to find out what would strengthen the nursing curricula to better prepare nurses who work in the community health districts. The researchers found out that most of the nurses surveyed were in supervisory and management roles in the community and that these individuals stressed the need for more management skills to be taught as part of their basic nursing education. Interestingly, none of the nurse who were surveyed perceived themselves as leaders, and most displayed an inability to prioritize tasks in the work setting.

Ziegler PB, Anyango H, Ziegler HD: The need for leadership and management training for community nurses: results of a Ugandan district health nurse survey, *J Community Health Nurs* 14(2):119, 1997.

1997). In contrast, in the more developed countries, nursing is often seen as one of the strongest advocates of the principles of primary health care through its social commitment to equality of health care and support of the concepts that are contained in the Alma Ata declaration (Andrews and Gottschalk, 1996).

MAJOR INTERNATIONAL HEALTH ORGANIZATIONS

The number of international health organizations continues to grow and reflects an increasing interest in the world's health. Basch (1990) classifies the organizations that participate and contribute to the world's health as private voluntary, philanthropic, professional and technical, commercial, governmental, and intergovernmental.

Private Voluntary

Private voluntary organizations include both religious and secular groups. **Religious organizations** consist of several denominations and religious interests and support many different kinds of health care programs, including the sponsorship of hospitals in rural and urban areas, refugee centers, orphanages, and leprosy treatment centers. For example, the Maryknoll Missionaries are sponsored by the Roman Catholic Church and carry out health service projects around the world. The many Protestant and Evangelical groups function both as separate entities and as part of the Church World Service, which works jointly with **secular organizations** to improve efforts with health care, community development, and other needed projects. Other private and voluntary groups that assist with the worldwide health effort include CARE, Oxfam, and Third World First. Many of these organizations receive funding from more developed countries including the United States, the United Kingdom, Sweden, Canada, and countries in Western Europe.

Philanthropic

Philanthropic organizations are those that receive funding from private endowment funds. Some of the more active philanthropic organizations that are involved in health care throughout the world include the W.K. Kellogg Foundation, the Milbank Memorial Fund, the Pathfinder Fund, the Hewlett Foundation, the Ford Foundation, the Rockefeller Foundation, and the Carnegie Foundation. The purpose and programmatic goals of each organization differ widely with respect to funding, and purposes often change as governing boards change. Some of the worldwide health care activities that have been sponsored throughout past years include projects in public and preventive health; vital statistics; medical, nursing, and dental education; family planning programs; economic planning and development; and the formation of laboratories to investigate communicable diseases.

Professional and Technical

One of the most famous of the **professional and technical organizations** is the Institut Pasteur, which has been in existence since the 1880s. In particular, its laboratories have facilitated the development of sera and vaccines for countries in need, have disseminated current health information, and have trained and provided fellowships for medical training and study in France.

Private and Commercial

Private and commercial organizations such as Nestle and the Johnson & Johnson Company provide financial and technical backing for investment, employment, and access to market economies and to health care. Several of these organizations have come under sharp criticism because of their promotion of infant formulas, pharmaceuticals, and medical supplies to lesser developed countries. For example, **health commodification** refers to the buying and selling of health and health care products such as pharmaceuticals in all areas of the world. In recent years, the health commodification of pharmaceuticals in Southern India has been criticized for not considering the cultural and social structure of the country and thus interfering with a longstanding traditional medical system. In Southern India, good health and prosperity are related to certain social parameters bestowed to families and communities as a result of their conformity to the sociomoral order that was set down by their ancestors, gods, and patron spirits (Nichter, 1989). The taking of pharmaceutical agents thus disrupts the social and cultural order of things that have been addressed by more traditional practices. Similar controversies in other countries have involved infant formulas and oral rehydration therapies (ORTs).

Governmental

Various **governmental organizations** throughout the world enter into bilateral arrangements with other countries. Most of these arrangements are made between a lesser developed country and one that is more economically advanced. Some of the countries that have provided assistance include the United States, Canada, the United Kingdom, Japan, Sweden, and Germany. Incentives for engaging in formal arrangements may include economic enhancements for the benefit of both countries, national defense of one or both countries, or to enhance and protect the private investments that are carried out by individuals in both nations. Countries with advanced medical systems and technology may enter into a collaborative effort with a lesser developed country to conduct medical research. For example, the Japanese government currently has an active collaborative arrangement with Indonesia to study ways to control the spread of yellow fever and malaria.

Intergovernmental

Four of the best-known **intergovernmental organizations** are the World Bank, the World Health Organization (WHO), the United Nations Childrens Fund (UNICEF), and the Pan American Health Organization (PAHO). These organizations collaborate with a number of governments, private foundations, and other health care efforts on an ongoing basis.

World Bank

The major aim of the **World Bank** is to facilitate significant interventions to improve the health status of individuals living in areas that lack economic development. For example, it supports projects that enable communities to obtain safe and usable water and affordable housing, develop effective sanitation systems, and assist with numerous health care interventions such as family planning. It also provides financial assistance for people seeking careers as health providers. In addition, the World Bank has been involved in projects that deal with the development of economic growth and the improvement of internal infrastructures such as communication systems, roads, and electricity.

The World Bank has collaborated with the WHO from time to time, such as with the recent efforts to control the tropical disease onchocerciasis in West Africa. The World Bank will also lend money to governments and private foundations to develop specific projects to advance the health status of their people.

World Health Organization

The First International Sanitary Conference of the mid 1880s that directed efforts at worldwide control of cholera was a precursor to the **World Health Organization (WHO)** (Basch, 1990). Continued efforts by this and other worldwide agencies resulted in the formation of the WHO in 1946 as an outgrowth of the League of Nations and the charter of the United Nations (UN). The UN charter provided for the formation of a special health agency to address the wide scope and nature of the world's health problems. The WHO headquarters are in Geneva, with six regional headquarters in Copenhagen, Alexandria, Brazzaville, New Delhi, Manila, and Washington, D.C. It is headed by a director general and five assistant generals.

The scope of the WHO is extremely broad and consists of more than 25 major functions with over 100 subfunctions. More than 1000 ongoing health-related projects are occurring at any one time. Some of these projects may be operated and funded by the WHO itself or in collaboration with other governments and health care agencies. However, most of the projects are associated with technical services or services to governments. Requests for assistance are made directly to the WHO by a country for an individual project or as part of a larger collaborative endeavor that involves many regions. Examples of collaborative efforts include comparative family planning programs, applied research on communicable disease and immunization, or the project that investigates the role of midwifery in maternal and child health. However, many of the programs sponsored by the WHO involve individual countries, with emphasis placed on training of medical personnel, development of health services, primary health care, and specific disease control programs.

United Nations Childrens Fund

The **United Nations Childrens Fund (UNICEF)** was formed shortly after World War II to assist children in the war-ravaged countries of Europe. After the war, it became apparent that children throughout the world needed assistance. With financial assistance from the UN General Assembly, programs were developed to control yaws, leprosy, and TB. Other efforts have since been aimed at the provision of safe drinking water, education, and maternal and child health. UNICEF has worked closely with the WHO over the past years as an advocate for women's and children's health.

Pan American Health Organization

Founded in 1902, the **Pan American Health Organization (PAHO)** is one of the oldest continuously functioning international health organizations. This organization focuses its efforts on working to improve health and living standards of the countries of the Americas. It functions to distribute epidemiological information, to provide technical assistance with a wide range of health and environmental issues, to support fellowships, and to promote research and professional education. It serves as the specialized organization for health of the Inter-American System and also as the Regional Office for the Americas of the WHO. Further, it is recognized as part of the United Nations system.

Focusing primarily on reaching people through their communities, the PAHO works with a variety of governmental and non-governmental entities to focus on the priority health issues of the peoples of the Americas. Primary concerns of the PAHO are the fight against the spread of AIDS and improving the health of the most vulnerable groups in this part of the world: mothers and children, workers, the poor, the elderly, and refugees and displaced persons. The PAHO seeks collaboration not only within countries, but also among countries as they work together toward common goals in health.

INTERNATIONAL HEALTH AND ECONOMIC DEVELOPMENT

The health of the world's people is related to economic, industrial, and technological development. Even though several studies of lesser developed countries have indicated that the general demand for health care is related to health production technology, little evidence shows how and under what circumstances this technology affects the use of health care services (Wouters, 1992). Access to services and the removal of financial barriers alone do not account for use of health services. In fact, the introduction of health care technology from more developed countries to lesser developed countries has led to less-than-satisfactory results. For example, during the 1980s in an Eastern Mediterranean country, two-thirds of the high-output x-ray machines were not in use because of a lack of qualified and trained individuals to carry out routine maintenance and repairs (Perry and Marx, 1992). In another example, a hospital in a Latin American country was given a high-technology neonatal intensive care unit by a wealthier and more technologically advanced country. However, 70% of the infants died after discharge because there were no follow-up nutritional and prevention services. Many of the infants experienced malnutrition and complications from dehydration on return to their home communities. More successful programs might have been developed for Eastern Mediterreanean areas, and Latin America focused on general public health and less complex kinds of health care technology (Perry and Marx, 1992). Quite simply the most basic needs were not met nor was recognition given to what resources and services the country could sustain.

Given these two examples, the improvement in the overall health status of a population contributes to the economic growth of a country in several ways (World Bank, 1993; World Bank, 1998a; van der Gaag and Barham, 1998):

- A reduction in production loss that is caused by workers who are absent from work because of illness
- An increase in the use of natural resources that may be inaccessible because of the presence of disease entities
- An increase in the number of children who can attend school and eventually participate in their country's economic growth
- The addition of monetary resources to the economic development of a country that has been otherwise spent on treating disease and illness

However, adequate health care coverage for individuals who reside in lesser developed countries is often lacking because their governments often reallocate financial resources from internal health needs and education and invest it instead in the country's market economy or to develop technology. Many countries also divert resources to develop the underlying infrastructure that they believe is needed for technological and industrial improvement. Unfortunately, when governments experience an economic crisis, household expenditures are affected adversely. Most often, the provision of health services in lesser developed countries depends on the importation of drugs, vaccines, and other health care products (World Bank, 1998a; van de Gaag and Barham, 1998). This provision depends on a network of foreign exchange that is influenced by economic and political factors. Often, lesser developed countries have a difficult time maintaining a balance of payments, which leads to severe shortages of foreign exchange and subsequent reduction in the ability to import goods (Evlo and Carrin, 1992).

Because the economics of international development are complex, it is often difficult to convince governments to direct their resources away from perceived needs such as military and technology and instead place the resources in health and educational programs. Ideally, the role of the more developed countries is to assist lesser developed countries in identifying internal needs and to support cost-efficiency measures and share their technology and industrial expertise (Wouters, 1992).

It is important that nurses who work in international communities not only acknowledge the importance of technology and development but also recognize the political and economic implications. Provision of health services alone will not ease a country's health care plight (Fig. 4-5).

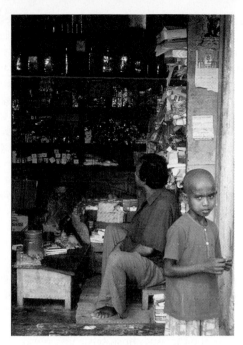

FIG. 4-5 A local pharmacy in rural Bangladesh. (Courtesy K. Huttlinger and L. Krefting.)

NURSING TIP

When carrying out a health assessment interview, always ask if the client has recently traveled out of the United States. Sometimes people bring back diseases that are hard to diagnose.

HEALTH CARE SYSTEMS

The countries of the world present many different kinds of health care systems. However, most health care systems consist of several fundamental elements (Basch, 1990):

- Usership (who can use the system)
- Benefits, or what kind of coverage a citizen might expect
- Providers who deliver health care
- Facilities, or where the provision of health care takes place
- Power, or who controls access and usability of the system

The role of nursing in each of these countries is as diverse as the kind of health care system in which nurses are a part. To help illustrate these concepts, a brief description of several select health systems is provided.

United Kingdom

The United Kingdom has a health system that is owned and operated by the government, and services are available to all of its citizens without cost or for a small fee. Administration of the services is conducted through a system of health authorities. Each health authority plans and pro-

vides services for 250,000 to 1 million people. The services offered by each health authority are comprehensive in that health care is available to all who want it and covers all aspects of general medicine, disability and rehabilitation, and surgery. Although physicians are the primary providers in this system, nurses and allied health professionals are also recognized and used. Services are made available through hospitals, private physicians and allied health professional clinics, health outreach programs such as hospice, boroughs, and environmental health services. Physicians are paid by the number of clients that they serve and not by individual visits. The system is financed by the government through individual and corporate taxation. Although the British system has come under criticism in past years, individual citizens maintain a high level of support for government funding and control of their health services.

One of the hallmarks of the system is a demonstrated reduction in infant mortality. This rate improved from 14.3 deaths per 1000 births in 1975 to 8.8 in 1988. Overall life expectancy in Great Britain also improved during the same period (National League for Nursing, 1992).

Canada

The Canadian health care system is based on a national health insurance program that is operated by each provincial government. One notable feature of this system is that specialists are concentrated in centers, whereas primary care providers are evenly distributed throughout the Canadian provinces. Physicians are the primary providers, although nurses do play an active role in all aspects of health care delivery, including community and public health. Hospitals and other health care agencies have an annual budget that is set by the provincial government. Financing for the system is derived from provincial and federal governments, which receive monies through personal income taxes. Benefits are broad and cover every aspect of health care but limit certain kinds of elective surgeries as well as dental and eye care. As in Great Britain, infant mortality rates have decreased during the past 10 years, and overall life expectancy has increased.

Canada has had an organized system for health care for many years. The original plan for prepaid health care began during World War I when rural municipalities in Saskatchewan employed contract physicians to care for residents. The revenue to hire these general practice physicians came from local property taxes and "premiums" charged to non-property owners (Taylor, 1980, p. 184). The success of this early work in Saskatchewan supported the passage in 1947 of legislation to establish the first compulsory hospital insurance plan in North America by the cooperative Commonwealth Federation Party (Kerr and MacPhail, 1996). Several significant milestones in the development of a Canadian health plan included the following:

- **1949** *National Health Grants Act.* Funded hospital construction much like the Hill-Burton Act in the United States.

- **1957** *Hospital Insurance and Diagnostic Services Act.* Prepaid universal coverage for all residents including both inpatient and outpatient care; this was on a 50-50 cost sharing basis between the province and federal funds.
- **1966** *Medical Care Insurance Act.* Expanded prepaid hospital coverage to include medical care; this also began in Saskatchewan.
- **1977** *Fiscal Arrangements and Established Programs Financing Act.* Replaced the increasingly expensive 50-50 cost sharing with block grants; the federal contribution was reduced to 25%; physicians became dissatisfied with their levels of reimbursement and began using copayments and extra billing.
- **1984** *Canada Health Act.* Disallowed extra billing and copayment fees and added a clause for federal reimbursement for "health practitioners," which opened the door for nurse practitioners to provide primary care.

Five basic principles of health care form the basis for the Canadian national health insurance system. These principles are similar to those proposed in the unsuccessful health reform plan in the 1990s in the United States:
- *Universality.* Coverage to the entire population.
- *Comprehensiveness.* Coverage for all medically necessary services.
- *Accessibility.* Because of the relatively sparsely populated, rural areas across Canada, providing accessibility has been a challenge. As in the United States, physicians prefer to work and live in urban, not rural, areas.
- *Portability.* Coverage for residents who require health services soon after they move to a different province or during a visit outside their home province.
- *Public administration.* Nonprofit administration of services by an organization fiscally responsible to the provincial government.

As can be seen from what is reimbursed, this system supports hospital and physician dominance. Health care services are provided through the private sector on a fee-for-service basis, and the vast majority of hospitals are owned and operated by nonprofit groups including municipalities, voluntary agencies, and religious groups. Although these institutions employ some physicians, most of the medical staff is composed of private physicians who are granted admittance privileges by each of the facilities (Sokolovsky, 1993). Hospitals and other health care agencies have an annual budget that is set by the provincial government. Financing for the system is derived from provincial and federal governments, which receive monies through personal income taxes. The federal government does provide block grants to help defray the cost. Most of the provinces have instituted some kind of expenditure target or limit to control the amount spent on physician services (Sokolovsky, 1993). Home and community care were not initially eligible for federal reimbursement. Like health care in the United States, in Canada there is a maldistribution of physicians, and nurses are underused. Nursing education entered the university after World War II, and Canada currently has excellent baccalaureate, masters, and doctoral programs in nursing.

As their health care system continues to be examined, it is likely that nurses in Canada can carve out a greater role in a more cost-effective system. This will be especially true if the goal of HFA2000 is achieved. For the last decade, Canadian provinces have examined the way they can incorporate principles of primary health care (PHC). There are unlimited opportunities for nurses to play key roles in a community-based primary health care system. Such a system is consistent with what nurses learn in baccalaureate education in both Canada and the United States.

Sweden

Health care in Sweden is made available to all its citizens. The system is based on a national health service that is operated almost completely by the Swedish government. County councils hire physicians to operate the health systems on a local basis, with hospitals being run by either local or area agencies and with budgets determined by the area's medical needs. The role of nurses in the health care delivery system is not as pronounced as in the United States, Canada, or Great Britain, but there are indications that nurses are gaining in their professional role and autonomy. The financial basis for the Swedish health care delivery system is derived from a proportional wage tax of 13.5%, with 35% of the total costs generated by federal revenues. The remaining 4% is obtained through direct patient fees (National League for Nursing, 1992). The services that are provided for in this system are comprehensive and range from all hospital expenses to preventive services, physician services, prescription drugs, dental and eye care, and psychiatric care. During the past 10 years, infant mortality has decreased and life expectancy has increased.

China

Great advances in public and community health have been the hallmark of the People's Republic of China since it was founded in 1949 (CIA, 1992). Examples of public health advances that were made in China include controlling contagious diseases such as cholera, typhoid, and scarlet fever and the reduction of infant mortality (Wei, 1992). These accomplishments in public health were credited to the political system that was and is largely socialistic and featured a health care system that is described in socialistic terms as collective. The Chinese collective system emphasized the common good for all people, not individuals or the needs of special groups. This system was financed through cooperative insurance plans. The collective health care system was owned and controlled by the state and was characterized by the use of barefoot doctors who were medical practitioners trained at the community level and who could provide a minimal level of health care throughout the country. Barefoot doctors combined Western medicine with traditional techniques such as acupuncture and herbal remedies. An emphasis was placed on improving the quality of water supplies and on disease prevention and massive public health campaigns against sanitation problems like flies, mosquitos, and the snails that spread schistosomiasis.

The current Chinese government has made health care a priority and has set goals to provide medical care to all of its citizens. Today, health care in China is managed by the Ministry of Public Health, which sets national health policy. Local and provincial governments implement directives from the Ministry. As of 1992 (CIA, 1992), the Ministry supervised approximately 207,000 medical organizations including public health, 620,000 hospitals, and 3600 epidemic-prevention stations throughout China. The Ministry is also actively involved in medical and nursing education and sets standards for the curricula in schools and for placing graduates (CIA, 1992; World Bank, 1998b). During the 1970s, a series of economic reforms and changes took place that have resulted in the privatization of some of the medical care. This is a dramatic change away from the previous socialistic system. China continues to strive toward a system that improves health services while keeping rising costs under control. This is occurring at a time when the entire social services system is undergoing remarkable change. The model that China is using currently for medical care combines private medical accounts and pooled resources with a large burden of cost being placed on employers (World Bank, 1998b).

MAJOR WORLD HEALTH PROBLEMS AND THE BURDEN OF DISEASE

As described previously, present indicators of world health demonstrate that critical health care needs still exist throughout the world despite earnest attempts to attain good health. As world economies lagged during the late 1970s, 1980s, and into the 1990s, the amount of debt that was incurred by lesser developed countries increased, and the money that was once used for health care was used to pay off the debt. Therefore even though attempts have been made by lesser developed countries to address their health care needs, major health problems still exist. Communicable diseases that are often preventable are still common throughout the world but are more common in lesser developed countries. In addition, both developed and lesser developed countries have to find ways to cope with the aging of their populations, which presents governments with the burden of providing care for people who become ill with more expensive noncommunicable and chronic forms of diseases and disabilities. Illnesses such as AIDS have emerged to raise new issues and concerns throughout the world, whereas some longstanding diseases such as TB and malaria still

persist and add to a growing burden of overextended health care delivery systems.

Mortality statistics do not adequately describe the outlook of health in the world. The WHO and the World Bank (1993, 1998a) have developed an indicator called the **global burden of disease (GBD).** The GBD combines losses from premature death and losses of healthy life that result from disability. *Premature death* is defined as the difference between the actual age at death and life expectancy at that age in a low-mortality population. People who have debilitating injuries or diseases must be cared for in some way, most often by family members, and thus no longer can contribute to the family's or community's economic growth (World Bank, 1993, 1998a). The GBD represents units of **disability-adjusted life years (DALYs)** (World Bank, 1993, 1998a). In 1990, for example, 1.36 billion DALYs were lost worldwide, which equates to 42 million deaths of newborn children or of 80 million deaths of people who reach age 50. Approximately 12.4 million children under age 5 died during the same year in developing countries, which represents a tremendous loss of future human potential. If these children could face the same risks as those in countries with developed market economies, the deaths would decrease by 90% to 1.1 million. This example serves to demonstrate the importance of having accessible and affordable health prevention programs for children around the world (World Bank, 1993, 1998c). Overall, premature deaths throughout the world during the 1990s accounted for 66% of all DALYs lost, with debilitating injuries and diseases accounting for 34%.

Comparably, in the lesser developed countries, 67% of all DALY loss during the 1990s was attributed to premature death. In contrast, the more developed countries reported only 55% from this same cause. Communicable diseases still account for the greatest proportion of calculated DALYs worldwide for both males and females, followed by noncommunicable diseases and injuries. Research studies have indicated that infections and parasitic diseases remain a threat to the health of many population groups. Results from these studies demonstrate continuing need for intervention with infectious and other kinds of communicable diseases. Conditions that contribute to one quarter of the GBD throughout the world include diarrheal disease, respiratory infections, worm infestations, malaria, and childhood diseases such as measles. In 1992, sub-Sahara Africa demonstrated a GBD of 43% DALYs lost, largely because of preventable diseases among children. Other countries with comparable DALYs are India (28%) and the Middle Eastern crescent (29%). In adults, STDs and TB combine to account for 70% of the world's GBD (World Bank, 1993, 1998a).

Determining the total amount of loss even using the GBD is difficult because many consequences of disease and injury are hard to measure. For example, measuring the social and cultural impact of the disfigurements that result from accidents or debilitating diseases such as leprosy and river blindness is difficult. Likewise, it is problematic to measure social conditions such as familial and marital dysfunction, war, and familial violence.

As described previously, communicable diseases still contribute substantially to the world's disease burden. The following sections describe those selected communicable diseases that still present problems worldwide: TB, AIDS, and malaria. Other health problems discussed include maternal and women's health, diarrheal disease in children, and nutrition.

Communicable Diseases

One example of the long-term benefits of immunizing children against communicable disease is the successful campaign against smallpox that was carried out during the 1960s and 1970s by the WHO. Smallpox has been virtually eliminated throughout the world, with only occasional and incidental reportings. The systematic and planned smallpox program formed the basis for a series of worldwide efforts that are now being implemented to control and eradicate other infectious and communicable diseases. In 1974 the WHO formed the Expanded Programme on Immunization, which sought to reduce morbidity and mortality from diphtheria, pertussis, tetanus, TB, measles, and poliomyelitis throughout the world (Schild and Assad, 1983; WHO, 1986b). The major aim of immunization is to induce an immunity to a disease without experiencing the actual disease (Thanassi, 1998).

Tuberculosis

It is estimated that 80 million new cases of TB will occur worldwide during the late 1990s and into the early years of 2000. Of these 80 million cases, 4 million will be associated with HIV (Lienhardt and Rodrigues, 1997). Predictions also indicate that 30 million people will die of TB during the same period (Dolin, Raviglione, and Kochi, 1994). At present, TB represents the largest cause of death from a single infectious agent and strikes nearly 3 million people each year. This particular statistic represents 25% of premature adult deaths in lesser developed countries that might have been prevented (WHO, 1992a). The growth of the world's population, including an increase in the number of aged individuals and the adverse effects of HIV, contributes to the large projected estimations of TB (Dolin, Raviglione, and Kochi, 1994).

A third of the world's population, or 1.7 billion people, harbor the TB pathogen *Mycobacterium tuberculosis*. Clinical manifestations of the disease include pulmonary TB, which is the most widespread form; TB meningitis, which is a leading cause of childhood mortality; and TB of a variety of other organs. The WHO (1992a) reported that of the 8 million new cases reported in 1992, 3.6 million were of the pulmonary TB form, and these numbers have remained constant during the late 1990s (Lienhart and

Rodrigues, 1997; World Bank, 1998a). Even though the disease affects all age groups, the heaviest toll is among young adults.

The presence of disease-causing bacilli in sputum examination is not evident in all forms of pulmonary TB. About half the cases are detectable by sputum smear examination, and these are of the infectious pulmonary type. Chemotherapy undoubtedly reduces the number of individuals who die from TB. However, many lesser developed countries do not have organized treatment and prevention programs and therefore lose more people each year to TB than either malaria or measles (Lienhardt and Rodrigues, 1997; WHO, 1992a).

Although TB is known worldwide, the greatest number of cases are seen in sub-Sahara Africa, where the incidence is 260 cases per 100,000 people. This area is followed by the dense population centers in Southeast Asia and Western Pacific regions, with reportable cases of TB accounting for 60% of the new cases each year worldwide. As might be expected, the largest declining rates for TB are seen in the highly industrialized countries of the world. Worldwide, approximately 2.53 million deaths were attributable to TB in 1990, which exceeds the number of deaths that resulted from measles and malaria. The case fatality ratio for untreated TB is greater than 50%. Of these deaths, 1.1 million occurred in Southeast Asia and 0.6 million in the Western Pacific. Also in 1990, 116,000 TB deaths could be attributed to HIV infection, with most of these deaths occurring in sub-Sahara Africa (Dolin, Raviglione, and Kochi, 1994). Additional estimates have indicated that one-quarter of adult deaths that could be avoided in lesser developed countries are caused by TB. This equates to a tremendous loss of social and economic potential for these countries.

Two factors are a threat to TB control and eradication. The first is the appearance of the HIV virus, which is one of the highest risk factors associated with latent TB. HIV-associated TB infections most often progress to an active disease. Information currently available suggests that 5% to 10% of individuals infected with HIV and *M. tuberculosis* will develop TB each year. This can be compared with 2% of people infected with *M. tuberculosis* but not HIV who will develop TB (Dolin, Raviglione, and Kochi, 1994; Lienhardt and Rodrigues, 1997). The appearance of HIV has added to the difficulty of treatment programs in both developed and lesser developed countries. For example, in Africa, almost half of those individuals who are HIV seropositive are also infected with TB, and it is estimated that nearly 5% to 8% of these individuals will develop the clinical manifestations of TB. More importantly, HIV-positive individuals with infectious TB increase the possibility of transmission of TB to their families and to the community, thus increasing the prevalence of this condition (Murray, 1997).

The second factor that poses a threat to the control and eradication of TB is the growing resistance of TB bacillus to isoniazid and rifampin, the two drugs that are currently used to treat TB. Resistance to these drugs is already evident around the world, including the Mexico/Texas border communities (Quiroga, 1995). The WHO and other organizations maintain that a high priority needs to be given to TB control and eradication programs around the world. They advocate a short-term chemotherapy of smear-positive patients as being one of the most cost-effective health interventions available.

Bacille Calmette-Guérin (BCG) consists of a series of vaccines that induce active immunity. These are used to prevent TB and have been available since the 1920s. Although the effectiveness of BCG is still questionable, research studies have demonstrated that it is effective in preventing the more lethal forms of TB, including meningitis and miliary disease in children (WHO, 1992a). These same studies have demonstrated that more than 80% of the infants in lesser developed countries have been vaccinated, with lesser coverage in sub-Sahara Africa. However, more studies are needed worldwide to determine the effect that BCG can have on the more infectious types of TB. Present indications are that BCG does not reduce the transmission of infectious types of TB.

The standard chemotherapeutic treatments used in many countries for TB are isoniazid, thioacetazone, and streptomycin and are effective at reducing sputum-positive cases to noninfectious. The drug and the combinations that are used vary from country to country. To be effective, however, treatment must be carried out on a consistent basis. Many lesser developed countries have difficulty getting patients to comply with any treatment regimen, and many of the TB intervention programs in these countries have been unable to carry out curative programs following standard treatment regimens (Pio et al, 1997; WHO 1992a). In 1990, the WHO Global Tuberculosis Program (GTB) promoted the revision of national tuberculosis programs to focus on short-course (SCC), directly observed treatment (DOTS). The introduction of DOTS programs has been successful in several lesser developed countries, including Malawi, Mozambique, Nicaragua, and Tanzania, producing a cure rate of approximately 80%. The SCC program involves aggressive administration of chemotherapeutic drugs combined with short-term hospitalization. Short-term chemotherapy uses a combination of drugs over 6 to 8 months and costs about $50 to $80 (United States) per patient. The long-term program involves two to three drugs taken over 12 to 18 months for a cost of $10 to $15 (United States) per patient. However, only 30% of patients complete the 12- to 16-month program, whereas more than 60% complete the SCC program. The key to the program lies in a well-managed system with regular supply of antituberculosis drugs to the treatment centers, follow-up care, and rigorous reporting and analysis of patient information (WHO, 1992a). Despite these efforts, little progress and international support have been given to place TB control programs as a number-one priority worldwide.

Acquired Immunodeficiency Syndrome

As is discussed in Chapter 39, acquired immunodeficiency syndrome (AIDS) has rapidly become a major cause of morbidity and mortality throughout the world (Heyward and Curran, 1988; Kalibala and Anderson, 1993). Once infected, the HIV remains with individuals for the remainder of their lives. The virus may produce no symptoms for years, but risk increases with the threat of a breakdown of the immune system and the subsequent infections that may occur. Worldwide prevention programs are important because failing to control this virulent disease will result in damaging and costly consequences for all countries in the future.

In 1987, 100 countries reported the existence of HIV, which causes AIDS, with estimates of 5 to 10 million people who had already contracted the disease (Basch, 1990). Current estimates of the spread of AIDS indicate that more than 150 million people presently carry the virus throughout the world, and of these, 590,000 include children (Carrington, 1994; HIV, 1998). It is estimated that by the year 2000, AIDS will contribute to 3.3% of the global burden of disease and that 1.8 million people will die of AIDS each year (World Bank, 1993). This is particularly significant because recent reports indicate that infection rates for AIDS double rapidly in lesser developed countries. The threat of AIDS doubling or tripling these projections by the year 2000 is realistic and frightening. In fact, a new strain of HIV uncovered recently in West Africa is alarming health officials because it is so different from other known strains and is easily escaping detection by standard blood screening methods (New strain of HIV found in West Africa considered very rare, 1998).

In lesser developed countries, AIDS is associated with poverty. Approximately 80% of the individuals currently infected with HIV live in lesser developed countries. For example, countries in sub-Sahara Africa lie in one of the areas of the world that is most affected by AIDS, and reports indicate that more than 8 million adults exhibit signs of infection. Based on population totals, this amounts to 1 in every 40 adults infected with HIV, with certain urban areas accounting for infection rates as high as 1 in every 3 adults. Unfortunately, this statistic is also evidenced by increases in childhood mortality when decreases were previously noted. UNICEF issued a report in 1990 that predicted that up to 5.5 million children would be orphaned during the 1990s in East and Central Africa as a result of parents with AIDS dying and leaving a child behind (Kalibala and Anderson, 1993).

Present efforts to control the spread of AIDS are directed toward prevention. AIDS spreads rapidly in the absence of prevention, particularly among high-risk or core groups such as prostitutes (both male and female) and intravenous (IV) drug users. From these core groups, AIDS spreads in a slow but accelerated manner to the rest of the general population. An increasing concern is the number of HIV-positive children emerging worldwide (Foster, 1998; Gibbons, 1997). Therefore prevention and intervention programs that target core population groups are essential because their effectiveness diminishes as the infection moves out of high-risk and high-transmission core groups (World Bank, 1993).

The consequences of AIDS in terms of cost to the individual, family, community, and country are tremendous. AIDS affects adults in their most productive years. Since many AIDS victims are heads of households or major economic household contributors, a negative economic effect is experienced by families, communities, and countries. Those countries with the highest HIV infection and AIDS disease rates have discovered that their health systems quickly become overburdened. AIDS patients, with their related infection, tax even the most economically sound health care systems, let alone those striving to stay economically stable. If the spread of AIDS is left unchecked, many countries will experience an accelerated demand for health services that will infringe on the health care of non-infected HIV patients.

The WHO has established a program with collaborative governments that is directed at education at the individual and community levels, providing for safe blood transfusions and injections and care for those who have the disease (Basch, 1990). It is clear that many gaps are present in the understanding of AIDS and the HIV infectious process. Priorities to investigate more efficient and effective means by which to control the spread of HIV are being developed throughout the world, but much more needs to be done. Nurses can assist in this global effort by conducting research and intervention studies that address many of the identified problem areas involving AIDS, particularly at the individual, family, and aggregate levels. Nurses are in key positions to develop intervention programs with target core populations, including young adults and women, and to participate in playing an active role in meeting this worldwide challenge.

Malaria

Malaria continues to be one of the most prevalent communicable diseases in the world. Ninety countries and areas are considered malaria ridden (Thanassi, 1998; WHO, 1994). Countries where the disease is most endemic are those that lie in the tropical areas of Asia, Africa, and Latin America. It is estimated that 300 to 500 million people develop clinical cases of malaria each year, with more than 90% of these occurring in equatorial Africa (WHO, 1994). This current situation exists despite worldwide efforts to eradicate and control the spread of malaria over the past 50 years.

There are two primary modes of malarial control—vector reduction and chemotherapy (Basch, 1990). The methods of vector control vary widely, from the larvae-eating fish tilapia to the use of insecticidal sprays and oils.

Needless to say, the latter poses a potential threat to the environment, where other potential hazards such as lumbering and mining already threaten the delicate ecosystem of the tropical areas involved. Countries that do not have strict environmental laws continue to use DDT sprays to control mosquito populations despite the advent of DDT-resistant mosquitoes. The non-DDT insecticide sprays, such as malathion, generally cost more and present an extra financial cost to lesser developed countries. Other methods for control and eradication that are being considered by malaria-ridden countries are environmental management, reduction and control of the source, and elimination of the adult mosquito.

Chemotherapeutic agents can be used for both protection and treatment of the disease. Drugs for treatment and prophylaxis are expensive and often cause side effects. However, current evidence suggests that the *Plasmodium sporozoites* are becoming resistant to both treatment and preventive chemotherapeutic agents. Efforts are presently underway to develop an antimalarial vaccine, but so far the results have been unsuccessful. Individuals who live or travel to Anopheles-infected areas are urged to protect themselves with mosquito netting, clothing that protects vulnerable parts of the body, and repellents for both their bodies and their clothes.

Maternal and Women's Health

The WHO and UNICEF have begun a global initiative to reform the health care received by women and children in developing countries (Heiby, 1998). However, studies on women's health indicate that most deaths to women around the world are related to pregnancy and childbirth. Most these deaths occur in lesser developed countries (AbouZahr and Royston, 1992; Heiby, 1998; Tomlinson, 1996). Throughout the world, women between 15 and 44 years of age account for approximately one-third of the world's disease burden and one-fifth of the burden for women 45 to 59 years of age. This burden comprises diseases and conditions that are either exclusive or predominantly found among women, including maternal mortality and morbidity, cervical cancer, anemia, STDs, osteoarthritis, and breast cancer (World Bank, 1993). Although most of these conditions can be dealt with by cost-effective prevention and screening programs, many lesser developed countries have ignored women's health issues other than those directly related to pregnancy and childbirth. Emphasis for health programs appears to be directed to those that favor male children and adult males over adult females (Ganatra and Hirve, 1994).

Furthermore, lesser developed countries presently account for 87% of the world's births. However, statistics from many lesser developed countries indicate that prenatal services and safe birthing services are unavailable, inaccessible, and unaffordable to women throughout the world, with the continent of Africa exhibiting the highest maternal mortality rates (Anderson, 1996). An African woman's risk of dying from pregnancy-related causes is 1 in 20 (AbouZahr and Royston, 1992; Andrews, 1996). Africa is followed by the countries of Bangladesh, Pakistan, and India. These three countries account for nearly half of the world's maternal deaths but only 29% of the world's births. In fact, these three countries have more maternal deaths each week than Europe has in a single year (Basch, 1990). Still, an accurate reporting of maternal deaths is difficult to obtain because many of the women who die live in remote areas of the world, they are poor, and their deaths are considered by many to be unimportant (Kestler, 1993).

The primary causes of maternal mortality, particularly in lesser developed countries, are varied. Most of the causes that are directly related to maternal mortality include hemorrhage, infection, convulsions, and coma caused by eclampsia and obstructed labor, and infections from unsanitary conditions and nonsterile and poorly performed abortions. Risk factors for maternal mortality include poor nutritional status, disease conditions, high parity, and age below 20 and above 35 years.

To date, little attention has been paid to the problem of maternal mortality, even though the reported statistics are high throughout the world. There has been, however, a movement to address the issue by the WHO and by the UN Fund for Population Activities (UNFPA). These two organizations have called for government initiatives and actions to address direct obstetric deaths as well as those that arise from indirect causes. The WHO and UNFPA have argued that their initiatives and their call for action for programs addressing maternal health are associated with the health of infants and children.

In support of the recommendations of the WHO and UNFPA, the World Health Assembly's Technical Discussions on Women, Health, and Development in 1992 presented several suggestions to the WHO, including the following (WHO, 1992b):

- Assisting governments to initiate legislation that addresses women's health problems
- Supporting research that addresses socioeconomic implications of diseases in women
- Developing proactive strategies to intervene and reduce health problems among women

Even so, safe motherhood initiatives undoubtedly are drastically needed throughout the world. These initiatives need to include accessible family planning services, access of prenatal and postnatal health care services, ensuring access to safe abortion, and improving the nutritional status of all women.

WHAT DO YOU THINK? *By law and custom, women in Uganda are not allowed to own property and have virtually no means by which to earn an income on their own.*

Diarrheal Disease

Diarrhea is one of the leading causes of illness and death in children under 5 years of age throughout the world and is most prominent in the lesser developed countries despite recent initiatives by the WHO to correct this problem (Heiby, 1998). For example, Guerrant (1986, 1992) indicates that diarrheal disease accounted for more than half of all the causes of death among children in Brazil. The prevalence of diarrheal disease was so pervasive in 1978 that the World Health Assembly established a global program to reduce mortality and morbidity in infants and young children who suffered from all forms of the disease. This program continues today (Lucas, 1998).

Diarrhea is a symptom of a variety of different illnesses, and the definitions and perceptions of it vary greatly from country to country. For example, in Bangladesh, diarrhea is defined as more than two watery or loose stools in 24 hours, whereas Indonesians define it as four loose stools in 24 hours (Basch, 1990). Definitions are complicated by the observable presence of blood, mucus, or parasites. The age of the individual who is experiencing the diarrhea also complicates definitions.

Causes of diarrhea are just as varied and diverse as its definitions and perceptions. Some of the causes include (1) viruses such as the rotavirus and Norwalk-like agents; (2) bacteria, including *Campylobacter jejuni, Clostridium difficile, Escherichia coli, Salmonella,* and *Shigella;* (3) environmental toxins; (4) parasites such as *Giardia lamblia* and *Cryptosporidium;* and (5) worms. Nutritional deficiencies can also cause diarrhea and are most often secondary to infectious agents. Of these, the rotavirus has emerged as a major world concern, hospitalizing 55,000 American children and killing 1 million children in the world each year (Diarrhea vaccine OK'd, 1998).

Dehydration is an immediate result of diarrhea and leads to a loss of fluid and electrolytes. The loss of up to 10% of the body's electrolytes can lead to shock, acidosis, stupor, and failure of the body's major organs (e.g., kidney, heart). Persistent diarrhea often leads to loss of body protein and increased susceptibility to infection. Prevention and control of diarrheal disease, especially in infants and children, should therefore be a major aim of countries around the world. In addition, many countries have developed diarrhea control programs that improve childhood nutrition. These programs focus on the promotion of breast-feeding, weaning practices, promotion of oral rehydration therapy (ORT), and supplementary feeding programs (Briscoe, 1984). However, all these programs must be considered in conjunction with improving the social and economic conditions that contribute to safe environmental, sanitary, and general living conditions of populations around the world (Basch, 1990).

Nutrition and World Health

Good nutrition is an essential part of good health. Poor nutrition by itself or that associated with infectious disease accounts for a large portion of the world's disease burden (World Bank, 1993). Those environmental and economic conditions that are related to poverty contribute to under-consumption of nutrients, especially those nutrients that are needed for protein building, such as iodine, vitamin A, and iron. Worldwide, women and children suffer dispro-portionately from nutrition deficits, especially of the mi-cronutrients just mentioned (Caballero and Rubinstein, 1997; Humphrey, West, and Sommer, 1992).

One of the effects of poor nutrition is stunting, or low height and weight for a given age. Stunting is most fre-quently the result of eating foods that do not provide enough energy and those foods that do not contain enough protein (World Bank, 1993). Since protein foods are usually more expensive than nonprotein food sources, many households cut back or unconsciously eliminate protein-rich foods to save money. Several countries where populations are most affected by stunting are India (65%), Asia (50%, not including India and China), China (40%), and sub-Sahara Africa (40%) (World Bank, 1993).

: WHAT DO YOU THINK? *Nutritional support through continued breast feeding and improved weaning prac-tices using high-density, easily digestible, local foods is especially important during and after episodes of diarrhea.*

Iron deficiencies are also common in lesser developed countries and severely affect women and children. A defi-ciency of iron in the diet reduces physical productivity and affects the capacity of children to learn in school. Iron deficiency in the diet also affects a person's appetite, caus-ing many individuals, especially children, to experience a lessened desire to eat, which in turn affects overall food in-take and growth over a prolonged time.

Women are most susceptible to iron deficiency as a re-sult of menstruation and child bearing. Women who expe-rience iron deficiency can develop a severe shortage of iron in their blood that results in anemia. Anemia in-creases a woman's risk of hemorrhage during childbirth. A World Bank report (1993) indicates that 88% of all preg-nant women in India are anemic, compared with 60% of the pregnant women in other parts of Asia. This statistic is compared with the developed, market economy countries, where only 15% of the population of pregnant women ex-perience iron-deficiency anemia (Caballero and Rubin-stein, 1997).

Other common dietary deficiencies observed through-out the world include iodine, vitamin A, and calcium de-ficiencies. The total impact of malnutrition and dietary de-ficiencies cannot be underestimated. Any malnourished condition among a population can increase susceptibility to illness. For example, the principal causes of death among malnourished persons are measles, diarrheal and respiratory disease, TB, pertussis, and malaria. The loss of

life from these diseases can be measured as 231 DALYs worldwide, with one-fourth of the 231 being directly at-tributable to malnourishment and dietary deficiencies.

Worldwide initiatives that have been directed at over-coming nutritional deficits have included the following (World Bank, 1993):
• Control of infectious diseases
• Nutritional education
• Control of intestinal parasites
• Micronutrient fortification of food
• Food supplementation
• Food price subsidies

In addition to contributions by individual governments, the organizations that have been most active in assisting with these initiatives have included the International Red Cross, the WHO, and many international religious and private foundations.

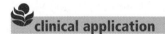

clinical application

The role of nurses in international health varies dramati-cally from country to country, as does the role of profes-sional nursing. It is not surprising to learn that nursing plays a more active role in health care delivery in the more technologically advanced countries such as the United States, Canada, Australia, New Zealand, the United King-dom, and other countries in Western Europe. The more developed countries have a defined role for nurses, whereas the role is less defined, if at all, in lesser devel-oped countries

During the last decade, developing countries have im-plemented primary health care programs directed at pre-vention and management of important public health prob-lems. With the increasing migration between and within countries because of war and famine, a greater need for nursing's expertise in alleviating suffering of refugees and displaced persons has emerged. Starvation, disease, death, war and migration underscore the need for support from wealthier nations of the world.

More than 30 million refugees and internally displaced persons in developing countries are currently dependent on international relief assistance for their survival. Mortal-ity rates in these populations during the acute phase of dis-placement have been up to 60 times the expected rates. Displaced populations in Ethiopia and Southern Sudan have suffered the highest mortality rates. In Afghanistan infectious diseases accounted for one half of all admissions to the hospital—mostly malaria and typhoid fever. The greatest mortality rate has been in children 1 to 14 years old. The major causes of death have been measles, diar-rheal diseases, acute respiratory infections, and malaria.

Nurses from abroad are often used to combat the major mortality in refugee camps—malnutrition, measles, diar-rhea, pneumonia, and malaria. Nurses are following the principles of primary health care and are promoting adequate food, safe drinking water, shelter, environmental sanitation, and immunizations. These life-saving practices have been implemented in the following countries: Thailand (Myanmar refugees), Rwanda, Zaire, Angola, Afghanistan, the Sudan, and the former Yugoslavia.

You are sent to a country ravaged by war in which many people are refugees. You are asked to work side-by-side with other nurses, both foreign and native to the country.

A. What would you do first to develop this group of nurses into a functioning team?
B. Which health and environmental problems would you attempt to handle early in your work?
C. Identify second-stage interventions and prevention once the initial crisis stage is relieved.

Answers are in the back of the book.

KEY POINTS

- Health for all the world's people is a collective goal of its nations and is promoted by the major world health organizations.
- As the political and economic barriers between countries fall, the movement of people back and forth across international boundaries increases. This movement increases the spread of various disease entities throughout the world.
- Nurses can and do play an active role in the identification of potential health risks at U.S. borders, with immigrant populations throughout the nation, and as participants in international health care delivery.
- Primary health care is one of the major keys in the provision of universal access of health care for the world's populations.
- The major organizations that are involved in world health include (1) private voluntary, (2) philanthropic, (3) professional and technical, (4) private and commercial, (5) governmental, and (6) intergovernmental.
- The health status of a country is related to its economic and technical growth. More technologically and economically advanced countries are referred to as *developed*, whereas those that are striving for greater economic and technological growth are termed *lesser developed*. Many lesser developed countries often divert financial resources from health and education to other internal needs such as defense or economic development that are not aimed at the poor.
- The global burden of disease (GBD) is a way to describe the world's health. The GBD combines losses from premature death and losses that result from disability. The GBD represents units of disability-adjusted life years (DALYs).
- Critical world health problems still exist and include communicable diseases such as tuberculosis, measles, mumps, rubella, and polio; maternal and child health; diarrheal diseases; nutritional deficits; malaria; and AIDS.

critical thinking activities

1. In your class, divide into small groups and discuss how you might find out if there are immigrant communities in your area. You might want to contact your local health department, area social workers, or community social organizations and churches.
   a. Discuss how you might gain access to one of these immigrant groups. Once gaining access, how would you go about determining what specific kinds of services they may need? What are their beliefs about health and health care? What customs regarding health were followed in their country of origin? How does the American health care system differ from the health care system in their country?
   b. As a nurse, what kinds of interventions might you consider implementing with these immigrant populations? What special skills or knowledge might you need to provide care to these populations?
2. Write to one of the major international health organizations and obtain their mission and goal statements. What kinds of health-related activities do they focus on? Does the organization that you identified have a specific role defined for nurses? How can a nurse who is interested become involved in their program and activities.
3. Pick a country or area of the world outside of the United States that interests you. Go to the library and obtain information about the following:
   a. Status of health care in that country
   b. Major health concerns
   c. GBD (global burden of disease)
   d. Whether this country is developed or lesser developed
   e. Which, if any, international health care organizations are involved with the delivery of health care in that country
4. Determine the role of primary health care in developed and lesser developed countries. Describe the role of community and public health nursing in primary health care in both types of countries.
5. Choose one or more of the following countries, and find out from your local or state health department the health risks that are involved in visiting that country: Indonesia, Zaire, Paraguay, Bangladesh, Kuwait, Kenya, Mexico, China, and Haiti.

Bibliography

AbouZahr C, Royston E: Excessive hazards of pregnancy and childbirth in the Third World, *World Health Forum* 13:343, 1992.

Anderson CM: Women for women's health: Uganda, *Nursing Outlook* 44:141, 1996.

Andrews CM, Gottschalk J: An international community-based nurse education program, *J Community Health Nurs* 13(1):59, 1996.

Basch PF: *Textbook of international health*, New York, 1990, Oxford University Press.

Briscoe J: Water supply and health in developing countries, *Am J Public Health* 74:1009, 1984.

Bibliography—cont'd

Caballero B, Rubinstein S: Environmental factors affecting nutritional status in urban areas of developing countries, *Arch Latinoam Nutr* 47(2 Suppl 1):3, 1997.

Carrington T: AIDS pulls together the young and old in Ugandan villages, *Wall Street Journal,* Dec 29, 1994.

Cech I, Essman A: Water sanitation practices on the Texas-Mexico border: implications for physicians on both sides, *South Med J* 85(11):1053, 1992.

Central Intelligence Agency (CIA): *China: evolution of its ministries and commissions, 1949-1992,* Washington, DC, 1992, CIA.

Collado C: Primary health care: a continuing challenge, *Nurs Health Care* 13(8):408, 1992.

Crompton D, Savioli L: Intestinal parasitic infections and urbanization, *Bull World Health Organ* 71(1):1, 1993.

Diarrhea vaccine OK'd, *San Francisco Chronicle.* Sept 1,1998.

Dolin P, Raviglione M, Kochi A: Global tuberculosis incidence and mortality during 1990-2000, *Bull World Health Organ* 72(2):213, 1994.

Evlo K, Carrin G: Finance for health care: part of a broad canvas, *World Health Forum* 13:165, 1992.

Foster G: Today's children: challenges to child health promotion in countries with severe AIDS epidemics, *J Assoc Nurses AIDS Care* 10(Suppl 1):S17, 1998.

Ganatra B, Hirve S: Male bias in health care utilization for under-fives in a rural community in western India, *Bull World Health Organ* 72(1):101, 1994.

Gibbons M: Global issues in HIV/AIDS in children, *J Assoc Nurses AIDS Care* 8(3):69, 1997.

Gomez-Dantes O, Frenk J, Cruz C: Commence in health services in North America within the context of the North American Free Trade Agreement, *Rev Panam Salud Publica* 1(6): 460, 1997.

Guerrant R: Unresolved problems and future considerations in diarrheal research, *Pediatr Infect Dis J* 5:S155, 1986.

Guerrant R et al: Diarrhea as a cause an effect of malnutrition: diarrhea prevents catch-up growth and malnutrition increases diarrhea frequency and duration, *Am J Trop Med Hyg* 47(1):28, 1992.

Heiby JR: Quality improvement and the integrated management of childhood illness: lessons from developed countries, *Qual Improv* 24(5):264, 1998.

Hernandez-Pena P et al: The free trade agreement and environmental health in Mexico, *Salud Publica Mex* 35(2):119, 1993.

Heyward W, Curran J: The epidemiology of AIDS in the U.S., *Sci Am October* 72, 1988. HIV: 590,000 children newly infected worldwide in 1997, *Dtsch Med Wochenschr* 123(1-2):A12, 1998.

Hong Kong chicken ban, *West Contra Costa Times,* Feb 8, 1998.

Howson CP, Fineberg HV, Bloom BR: The pursuit of global health: the relevance of engagement for developed countries, *Lancet* 351(9102):586, 1998.

Humphrey J, West K, Sommer A: Vitamin A deficiency and attributable mortality among under-5-year-olds, *Bull World Health Organ* 70(2):225, 1992.

Kalibala S, Anderson S: AIDS in Africa: a family disease, *World Health* 6:8, 1993.

Kerr JR, MacPhail J: *An introduction to issues in community health nursing in Canada,* St Louis, 1996, Mosby.

Kestler E: Wanted: better care for pregnant women, *World Health Forum* 14:356, 1993.

Lienhardt C, Rodrigues LC: Estimation of the impact of the human immunodeficiency virus infection on tuberculosis: tuberculosis risks re-visited? *Int J Tuberc Lung Dis* 1(5):196, 1997.

Lucas A: WHO at country level, *Lancet* 351(9104):743, 1998.

Murray JF: Tuberculosis and HIV infection: global perspectives, *Respirology* 2(3):209, 1997.

National League for Nursing: Comparison of national health care systems, *Nurs Health Care* 13(4):202, 1992.

New strain of HIV found in West Africa considered very rare, *Washington Post,* September 1, 1998.

Nichter M: Pharmaceuticals, health commodification, and social relations: ramifications for primary health care. In Nichter M, editor: *Anthropology and international health,* Boston, 1989, Kluwer Academic Publishers.

Ortega-Cesena J, Espinosa-Torres F, Lopez-Carillo L: Health risk control for organophosphate pesticides in Mexico: challenges under the Free Trade Treaty, *Salud Publica Mex* 36(6):624, 1994.

Perry S, Marx ES: What technologies for health care in developing countries? *World Health Forum* 13:356, 1992.

Pio C et al: National tuberculosis programme review: experience over the period 1990-1995, *Bull World Health Organ* 75(6):569, 1997.

Porta C: Rwanda's two wars, *Reflections* 22(4):20, 1996.

Quiroga M: Personal communication, director of nursing, El Paso City/County Health Department, 1995.

Schild GC, Assad F: Vaccines: the way ahead, *World Health Forum* 4:353,1983.

Sokolovsky J: *CRS report for Congress: Education and Public Welfare Division,* Washington, DC, 1993, Library of Congress.

Taylor, MG: The Canadian health insurance program. In Meilicke CA, Storch JL, editors: *Perspectives on Canadian health and social services policy: history and emerging trends.* Ann Arbor, Mich, 1980, Health Administration Press.

Thanassi WT: Immunizations for international travelers, *West J Med* 168(3):197, 1998.

Tomlinson AJ: Maternal health in developing countries, *Lancet* 347(9003):769, 1996.

van der Gaag J, Barham T: Health and health expenditures in adjusting and nonadjusting countries, *Soc Sci Med* 46(8):995, 1998.

Waller AJ, Cammuso BJ: Health care in the new Russia: a Western perspective, *Nurs Forum* 32(3):27, 1997.

Wei H: Child development in China, *Beijing Review* 35(32):24, 1992.

World Bank: *World development report 1992: development and the environment,* New York, 1992, Oxford University Press.

World Bank: *World development report 1993: investing in health,* New York, 1993, Oxford University Press.

World Bank: *World development indicators 1998,* New York, 1998a, Oxford University Press.

World Bank: *China 2020,* New York, 1998b, Oxford University Press.

World Bank: *Annual review of development effectiveness,* New York, 1998c, Oxford University Press.

World Health Organization/United Nations Children's Fund: *Primary health care,* Geneva, 1978, WHO/UNICEF.

World Health Organization: *Twelve yardsticks for health,* New York, 1986a, WHO.

World Health Organization: *WHO-CDD: research on vaccine development* [WHO Document CDD/IMV/86.1], Geneva, 1986b, WHO.

World Health Organization: Tuberculosis control and research strategies for the

1990s: memorandum from a WHO meeting, *Bull World Health Organ* 70(1):17, 1992a.

World Health Organization: Women, health and development, *Int Nurs Rev* 40(1):29, 1992b.

World Health Organization: World malaria situation in 1991, *World Health Bull* 72:160, 1994.

World Health Organization: *Health for all: origins and mandate, special publication: the World Health Report: life in the 21st century— vision for all,* Geneva, Switzerland, 1998, WHO.

Wouters AV: Health care utilization in developing countries: role of the technology environment in "deriving" the demand for health care, *Bull World Health Organ* 70(3):381, 1992.

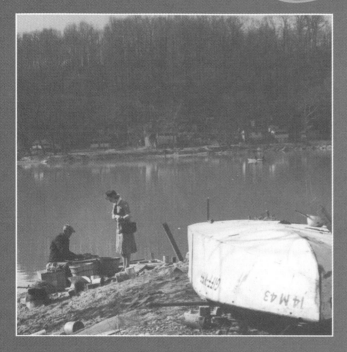

PART Two

Influences on Health Care Delivery and Community-Oriented Nursing

In recent years the U.S. health care system has been criticized for its rapidly rising health care costs, inconsistency in the level and quality of services provided from one area of the country to another, and a general inconsistency in accessibility of health services. With 43.4 million Americans uninsured and 12% of the remaining population underinsured, it has been recognized that equal access to health care services is not a right, as most Americans think it should be. The inconsistency in health care is more significant when cost is considered. Specifically, health care costs in the United States increased from $24 million in 1960 to over $1 trillion in 1996.

These factors have led to major health care reform debates at the national and state levels. The health care delivery system has moved into a managed care system that seeks to control costs. As a result of the debates, legal, economic, ethical, social, cultural, political, and health-policy issues have become extremely important. Now more than ever in the history of community and public health nursing, nurses must understand how these issues affect their practice and the outcomes of care.

In health care reform, public health is redefining its role in improving the nation's health. Nurses, as the largest public health provider workforce, must be a force in redefining the renewed public health system. Understanding the issues that affect decisions about health care priorities is imperative. Knowledge is power.

The chapters in Part Two provide the community and public health nurse with an understanding of the economic, ethical, cultural, environmental, and policy issues that affect nursing in general and community and public health nursing specifically.

Concern currently exists that the environment's effects on health and social conditions are causing an increase in the rate of infectious diseases. Community and public health nurses must be concerned with prevention, control, case-finding, reporting, and maintenance strategies as they relate to both communicable and infectious disease processes and to environment-related problems. Technological advances increasingly influence the environment and make it a potential threat to many aspects of health maintenance. Nurses must help others recognize how their actions as individuals, as well as in a composite group (aggregate) or community, are destroying vital parts of the environment.

Economics of Health Care Delivery

CHERYL BLAND JONES & KAREN MACDONALD THOMPSON

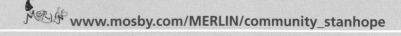

OBJECTIVES

After reading this chapter, the student should be able to do the following:

- Relate economics to nursing and health care.
- Describe the economic theories of microeconomics and macroeconomics.
- Trace the evolution of health care service delivery.
- Identify major factors influencing national health care spending.
- Analyze the role of government and other third-party payers in health care financing.

- Identify mechanisms for financing health care services delivery.
- Discuss the implications of health care rationing from an economic perspective.
- Analyze the relationship between poverty and health care financing.
- Evaluate primary prevention relative to health economics.

KEY TERMS

benefit-cost analysis (BCA)
budget constraint
business cycles
capitation
consumer price index
cost-effectiveness analysis (CEA)
demand
diagnosis related groups (DRGs)

economic growth
economics
effectiveness
efficiency
fee-for-service
gross domestic product (GDP)
gross national product (GNP)
health economics

human capital
inflation
macroeconomic theory
managed care
managed competition
Medicaid
Medicare
microeconomic theory
opportunity costs

prospective reimbursement
retrospective reimbursement
supply
third-party payment
utility
willingness to pay

*See **Glossary** for definitions*

CHAPTER OUTLINE

The views expressed in this chapter are those of the authors and do not necessarily reflect those of the Agency for Health Care Policy and Research.

The authors acknowledge the important foundational work for this chapter developed by Dr. Marcia Stanhope in previous editions of this book.

The historical evolution of the nation's health care delivery system has given way to a health care market that is constrained and polarized. Although the U.S. health care system once supported and encouraged much expansion, unlimited spending, and a booming job market, the system at the turn of the century is very different. Today's health care system is constantly changing, increasingly competitive, limited in resource availability, and restricting in resource use, service availability, and access to technological advances. Furthermore, the current system encourages providers to deliver care outside of traditional setting and disciplinary boundaries. The changing nature of health care has subsequently polarized various groups that come into contact with the system—clinicians, administrators, providers, payers, consumers, and policy makers—in reaction to and in anticipation of further system problems.

McCloskey (1995) notes that the health care system repeats that focus on either cost or quality. Looking back over time, these cycles are apparent. For example, during the 1960s when Medicare and Medicaid were implemented, the social and health care emphasis was on providing quality health care for the elderly and poor; during the late 1980s and early 1990s the focus was on containing the increasing costs of health care. In between these periods, the system has cycled, to varying degrees, between cost and quality.

With the emphasis in health care over time shifting between cost and quality, nurses are challenged to implement changes in practice and participate in research and policy activities designed to provide the best return on investment of health care dollars (i.e., to design models of care, at a reasonable price, that improve the quality of care delivered). These activities require a basic understanding of economics and the health care system and awareness of the effects of nursing practice on the delivery of cost-effective care (Pew Health Professions Commission, 1993).

Economics is the area of social science concerned with the allocation of scarce resources and provides the means to evaluate the attainment of society's wants and needs in relation to resource constraints (Cleland, 1990). Subsequently, **health economics** is concerned with the allocation of scarce resources within the health care sector and focuses on resource allocation issues related to producing and distributing health care. Economic evaluations in health care often create policy challenges. The provision of health care to society requires the allocating of public resources to produce needed services. The allocating of public money is a sensitive issue and often meets resistance from individuals and groups within society, given that allocating money to health goods limits the amount of money available for other public needs, such as education, transportation, recreation, and defense.

This chapter provides an overview of important economic issues in health care. These issues are particularly relevant to community and public health nurses whether they work with individuals and families or communities and programs: these nurses are intricately involved in problem solving and decision making through their roles as designers, planners, coordinators, and evaluators of quality, cost-effective health care programs for society.

ECONOMIC THEORIES

Two branches of economics are relevant to understanding and making application within health care: microeconomics and macroeconomics. **Microeconomic theory** deals with the behaviors of individuals and organizations and the effect of those behaviors on prices, costs, and the allocating and distributing of resources. Within economics, behaviors are based on 1) individual or organizational choices and the level of satisfaction from consuming a particular good (product) or service, or **utility,** and 2) the amount of money available to an individual or organization to spend on a particular good or service, or **budget constraint.** Microeconomics applied to health care examines the behaviors of individuals and organizations that result from trade-offs in utility and budget constraints.

Two basic principles of microeconomic theory are **supply** and **demand,** both of which are affected by price. A simple illustration of the relationship between supply and demand is provided in Figure 5-1. The upward-sloping supply curve represents the seller's side of the market, and the downward-sloping demand curve reflects the buyer's desire for a given product. As shown here, suppliers are willing to offer increasing amounts of a good or service in the market for an increasing price (Folland, Goodman, and Stano, 1993). The demand curve represents the amount of a good or service the consumer is willing to purchase at a certain price. This curve illustrates that when lesser quantities of a good or service are available in the marketplace, the price tends to be higher than when larger quantities are available. The point on the curve where the supply and demand curves cross is the equilibrium, or the point where producer and consumer desires meet. Supply and demand curves can shift up or down as a result of competition for a good or service, an increase in the costs of materials used to make a product, technological advances, a change in consumer preferences, or other concerns (Folland, Goodman, and Stano, 1993).

This oversimplified process is, in reality, quite complex. For example, when there are lesser quantities of a specific good available in the market, yet consumers want to purchase more of the good, the quantity of the good that they desire often is not readily available. Producers of the good or service need time to make and offer the amount of the item demanded. Consequently, the price of the good or service typically is high to offset the costs of producing the increased quantity and quickly getting a product to market. As more of the good or service is offered in the marketplace, consumers respond, the demand for the item falls, the supply increases, and the price goes down. A good example of this process is the supply, demand, and

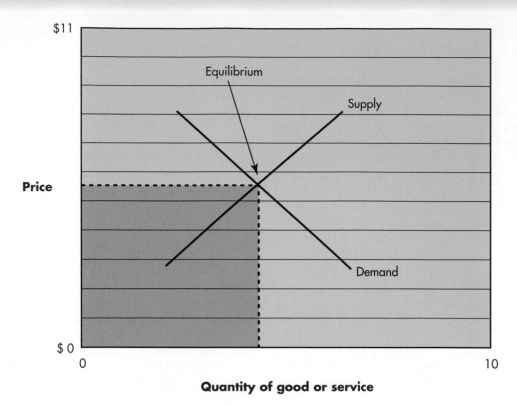

FIG. 5-1 Supply and demand curves.

price of microcomputers over the past 10 years. As more microcomputers and producers of microcomputers have entered the market, the supply of microcomputers has increased and the price of microcomputers has declined.

The willingness of consumers to pay for a product or service also influences supply and demand. The amount of money the individual person or organization is willing to pay, to a degree, reflects consumer choice and decision making. Specifically, **willingness to pay** for a good or service reflects the consumer's choice to make a "trade-off," or to purchase a particular good or service, and not other things (Folland, Goodman, and Stano, 1993). Thus willingness to pay reflects individual desires, choices, and the level of satisfaction (i.e., utility) that is expected for a good or service. Willingness to pay for a good or service can be determined directly through surveys or indirectly by examining purchasing behaviors (Gold et al, 1996).

Other decisions that affect supply and demand are based on the concept of **human capital.** Human capital is a way of measuring the value society places on the worth of individuals. Human capital values health in terms of the productive value of people in the economy (Gold et al, 1996). The value is quantified and expressed in dollar amounts, and it constitutes a real limit on how much money either people or society will pay for health care. This method of decision making usually focuses on possible losses of people that result from not investing in a health program or service, such as to death or poor health.

Consumer choice and decision making also reflect the **opportunity costs** associated with purchasing a good or service, where opportunity costs reflect the dollar value of other goods and services not purchased (Folland, Goodman, and Stano, 1993). For example, when a community health clinic invests money in renovating and equipping a new examination room to expand the clinic's ability to care for more clients, the investment reflects an administrative decision about willingness to spend the clinic's money. The clinic administration's willingness to invest in expanding suggests that the expense is worth the cost (i.e., the opportunity costs, or money spent on expanding that could have been spent in other ways, are expected to be less than the potential gains). Ultimately, this decision reflects the philosophy and values held by the clinic's administration, strategic plan, and organizational goals.

Two other terms are relevant to a discussion of microeconomics: efficiency and effectiveness. **Efficiency** refers to producing maximum output, such as a good or service, using a given set of resources or inputs, such as labor, time, and available money (Folland, Goodman, and Stano, 1993). Efficiency suggests that resources or inputs are combined and used in such a way that there is no better way to produce the service or output and that no additional improvements can be made. The word *efficiency* often emphasizes time, or speed in performing tasks, and the minimizing of any waste or unused input during production. Although these notions are true, efficiency depends

BOX 5-1 Efficiency versus Effectiveness

To illustrate the differences between efficiency and effectiveness, consider the case of a nurse who is designing a community outreach program to educate high-risk, first-time mothers about the importance of childhood immunization. The most efficient method to disseminate the information to a large number of mothers might be to have the child health team from the public health department hold an evening educational session at the health department open to the public. However, if the goals of the program are to change behaviors—increase community mothers' knowledge and awareness of infectious diseases, reduce the incidence of preventable infections in the community, and decrease the number of hospital admissions—the most effective means of offering the program might be to link public health nurses with new mothers for one-on-one, in-home counseling, demonstration, and follow-up.

BOX 5-2 Contribution of Health Care to the Economy

When the media refers to "the economy," the phrase typically is used as a macroeconomic term to describe the wealth and financial performance of the nation in aggregate. Health care contributes to the economy through goods and services produced and employment opportunities.

upon not simply tasks but rather the processes of producing a good or service and whether all possible improvements have been made.

Effectiveness, on the other hand, refers to the extent to which a health care service meets some established, pre-set goal or objective. In short, effectiveness means how well a program or service achieves what the developers intended. For example, the effectiveness of a medication is related to how well that medication treats the clinical problem for which it is intended. Box 5-1 discusses the differences between efficiency and effectiveness.

Macroeconomic theory focuses on the "big picture" (i.e., behaviors such as growth, expansion, and/or decline of an aggregate). The level of interest in microeconomics is the individual or organization, whereas the level of interest in macroeconomics is the total, or aggregate, of all individuals and organizations. The aggregate typically reported is a country or nation and includes factors such as levels of income, employment, general price levels, and rate of economic growth. This aggregate approach reflects, for example, the contribution of all organizations and groups within health care, or all industry within the United States, including health care, on the nation's economic outlook.

Health care macroeconomic issues are concerned with issues such as the influences of health care costs, quality, access, and policies on the overall U.S. economy. Aggregate and industry factors are examined in considering health care financing, national health insurance, rationing, and managed care and in comparing the U.S. health care system with that of other countries (Cleland, 1990). Box 5-2 provides a brief overview of the economy and the contribution of health care.

The primary focus of macroeconomics is business cycles and economic growth (Boyes, 1992). **Business cycles**

are natural, recurring expansions and contractions within business. These cycles can be brought about by a number of influences, such as political changes (a new president is elected), policy changes (a new legislation is implemented), knowledge and technological advances (a new medication to treat depression is placed on the market), or simply the belief by a recognized business leader that the cycle is shifting, or should shift, in another direction (a noted Harvard economist predicts that the United States is entering a recession). These fluctuations can have an effect on the lives of individuals and operations of organizations (Boyes, 1992).

Economic growth reflects an increase in the output of a nation, as opposed to a decline in output (Boyes, 1992). Two common measures of economic growth are **gross national product (GNP)** and **gross domestic product (GDP)**. GNP is the total market value of all goods and services produced in an economy during a period of time (e.g., quarterly or annually) (Boyes, 1992). GDP is the total market value of the output of labor and property located in the United States (USDHHS, 1998). GDP reflects only national output, whereas GNP reflects national output *plus* income earned by U.S. businesses or citizens (Boyes, 1992). This discussion focuses on GDP because U.S. health care spending reports are based on GDP.

DID YOU KNOW? *The use of GNP versus GDP depends on whether labor and property used to produce a good or service are located in the United States. If labor and property are located in the United States, then output will be counted in the GDP; if labor and property are located outside of the United States, then output is not included in GDP.*

Nurses face microeconomic and macroeconomic issues everyday. For example, they are influenced by microeconomics when referring clients for available services, informing clients and others of the cost of services, assessing community need for a particular service, evaluating client access to services, and determining health provider and agency response to client needs. Nurses who work with aggregates of individuals and communities are faced with macroeconomic issues such as health policies that make the development of new programs possible; local, state, and federal budgets that support certain programs; and the total effect that services will have on improving the health of the community. In short, an economic perspective enhances nurses' ability to understand and argue a position for meeting society's needs.

Is Health Care Resistant to Principles of Economics?

It is often argued that unique aspects of the health care sector make the application of economic theories impossible or inappropriate. These arguments, often made by passionate health care professionals include the following (Folland, Goodard, and Stano, 1993):

- The health care consumer is "captive" because the health care market is not competitive; there is not enough information in health care such that consumers cannot adequately make decisions.
- The financing of health care in the United States does not allow consumers to make trade-offs in costs and quality of care.
- The political nature of health care decision making makes the industry subject to the influence of special interest groups.
- Uncertainty in health care services cannot be explained in economic evaluations.
- Illness and vulnerability are too sensitive to do economic analyses.

The counter to these arguments is that the unique qualities of health care are not that unique from other markets and that these unique qualities of health care actually make economic principles relevant. Furthermore, many individuals wrongly misinterpret economics as only focusing on costs without fully appreciating that economics emphasizes the contrast of cost *and* quality and the identification of "best" solutions to improve social welfare.

During the late 1980s and early 1990s, the health care industry became increasingly competitive, imposed cost constraints, and a slow-down in health care spending occurred. Unfortunately, many of the changes in health care adopted during that time were implemented while only partially applying economic theory and emphasizing costs. Economics shows that in a truly competitive market, producers of services compete for customers on the basis of product price and quality; only more recently have quality issues been seriously discussed in health care.

Economic Analytical Tools

Two techniques are commonly used in economic analyses to examine costs and aid in resource decision making: benefit-cost analysis and cost-effectiveness analysis. These tools are particularly useful to nurses as they conduct community needs analyses and develop, propose, implement, and evaluate programs to meet identified community health needs. In both cases, costs of a program or intervention are weighed against expected outcomes.

Benefit-cost analysis (BCA) (or cost-benefit analysis, CBA) is a method of comparing the monetary gains and expenses associated with a health care program or service, including start-up and maintenance costs (Gold et al, 1996). This technique provides a way to estimate overall program and social benefits, the net of costs. Dollar benefits and other costs typically are determined for health care programs by identifying direct income and outlays expected and by determining willingness to pay for services plus human capital costs (Gold et al, 1996). The dollar figures for benefits and costs are then "discounted" to reflect the time value of money.

DID YOU KNOW? *The value of money varies over time, such that $1 today is worth more than $1 tomorrow as a result of inflation, interest rates, etc.*

A positive net benefit indicates that the program is worthwhile. Benefit-cost estimates should be made for all alternative programs (including the standard mode of delivering care), and the program with the greatest net social benefit is the program of choice. The Research Brief illustrates how BCA can be used in health care.

BCA requires that all costs and benefits are known and can be quantified in dollars; herein lies the major problem with its use. Although it is fairly easy to estimate the direct dollar costs of a health care program, it is often very difficult to quantify the non-dollar benefits and indirect costs. For example, benefits or gains could come in the form of increased financial income and expenses, which are fairly easy to measure. More difficult to measure are benefits such as improved community welfare attributable to a particular program and costs that would result without a particular program, such as the value of potential lives lost because of lack of access to health care services. Furthermore, because estimates of expected benefits and costs that would be averted or lost through, for example, a community AIDS prevention program depend on data available and assumptions made, the results from the BCA may be challenged by others who question data sources and/or hold different assumptions.

Cost-effectiveness analysis (CEA) compares the costs of alternative programs or interventions relative to objectives. In this case, no attempt is made to quantify the dollar benefits of programs or interventions or to compare non-dollar benefits with costs. In fact, CEA assumes that outcomes cannot be quantified in dollars. Instead, costs are compared with some other measure of intervention or program objective. An objective commonly used in health care CEAs is improvement in *quality adjusted life years* (QALYs) for those who would be affected by the program. QALYs are the sum of years of life multiplied by the quality of life in each of those years. The QALY assigns a weight ranging between zero (death) and one (perfect health) to reflect quality of life during a given period (Gold et al, 1996). The value of a year in less than perfect health

RESEARCH *Brief*

AN EXAMPLE OF A BENEFIT-COST ANALYSIS

Mauskopf, Bradley, and French (1991) performed a BCA of a proposed OSHA hepatitis B vaccine program for health care workers exposed to the hepatitis B virus 12 or more times per year. The cost of vaccinating the 5.3 million high-risk workers is estimated at $60.4 million dollars. The value of avoided medical treatment, lost productivity, and prophylaxis associated with the estimated 5000 to 6500 cases of acute and chronic hepatitis B prevented per year is listed below. The program was estimated to provide a net benefit of $48.6 to $84.6 million. A second analysis estimated the value of avoided pain and suffering at a net benefit of $518.6 to $716.6 million.

Vaccination of High Risk Workers	Program Cost (million $)	Benefits (million $)	Net Benefit (Benefit-Cost)
Benefits include avoided medical treatment, lost productivity, and prophylaxis after exposure	>−60.4	+109 to 145	+ 48.6 to 84.6
Benefits include avoided medical treatment, lost productivity, prophylaxis after exposure, and pain and suffering	−60.4	+575 to 773	+518.6 to 716.6

Additionally, it was estimated that, since the dollar value of avoiding one case of hepatitis B is approximately $117,000, an expanded program to include low-risk workers (at a cost of $17.95 per worker) would only have to avoid one or more cases per year per 6517 low-risk workers to be cost-effective ($117,000/$17.95).

Hocking (1992) questioned the model under which Mauskopf, Bradley, and French (1991) conducted their BCA, noting that if an industry model were used, costs and benefits to the employer would have to be estimated. This would include the value to the employer from reduction in absenteeism in addition to avoided medical costs.

Mauskopf JA, Bradley CJ, French MT: Benefit-cost analysis of hepatitis B programs for occupationally exposed workers, *J Occup Med* 33(6):691, 1991.

---

is assigned a value between 0 and 1 (Haddix et al, 1996). In this case, the costs of program or intervention alternatives are compared with real or anticipated improvements in clients' QALYs. Box 5-3 highlights the steps involved in conducting a CEA.

CEA is not without problems, however. Like BCA, the results of a CEA can be challenged because of data problems and assumptions made in conducting analyses. Furthermore, depending on program or intervention goals, the most effective means of providing a service may not necessarily be the least costly, particularly over the short-run. This notion is particularly true in public health, when the cost effectiveness of a preventive service may not be known for some time in the future and/or if service effectiveness is difficult or impossible to measure. For example, the total cost savings of a community AIDS prevention program might be difficult to project 20 years into the future. There is also concern about comparing cost alternatives to QALYs because of the subjectivity associated with determining the value of quality of life and equating that value to health.

HEALTH SYSTEM EVOLUTION: THE CONTEXT OF CARE DELIVERY

From the 1800s through the late 1900s, the U.S. health care delivery system experienced four developmental stages with differing emphasis on health care economics. A

BOX 5-3 Steps in Cost Effectiveness Analysis (CEA)

1. Establishment of program or service goals and objectives before implementation
2. Consideration of all possible alternatives to achieve the goal or objectives
3. Analysis of costs for each alternative, discounted over the lifetime of the project to account for the time value of money
4. Ranking of alternatives from least to most costly
5. Selection of the least costly alternative, relative to established goals or objectives

developmental framework for health services is useful to describe the evolution of the organization of health care delivery and to provide the context for a discussion of health economics. Figure 5-2 illustrates the four basic components included in the framework for health services delivery: *service needs and intensity, facilities, technology,* and *labor.* Intensity is the use of technologies, supplies, and health care services by or for the client. Intensity includes and is a partial measure of the use of technologies (Banta, 1995a). *Medical technology* refers to "the set of techniques, drugs, equipment, and procedures used by health care professionals in delivering medical care to individuals and the system within which such care is delivered" (Banta, 1995a).

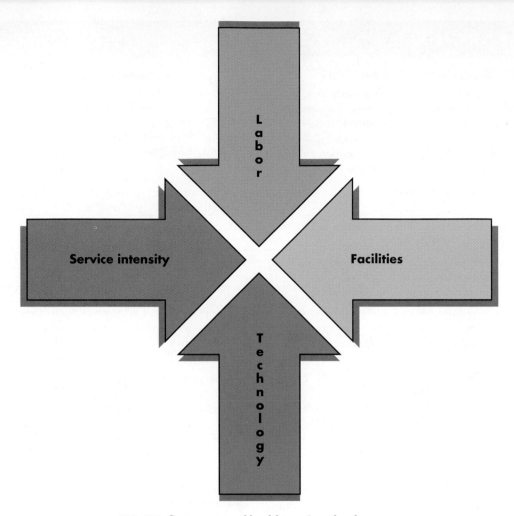

FIG. 5-2 Components of health services development.

Developmentally, the health services delivery framework acknowledges that the four framework components have changed over time, reflecting macrolevel, or societal, changes in morbidity and mortality rates, national health policy, and economics. Developmental aspects of the framework are captured in four time periods, or stages, as shown in Figure 5-3. Each element of the framework is used to show changes within stages to illustrate the growth and development of the U.S. health care system.

The *first developmental stage* (1800 to 1900) was characterized by epidemics of infectious diseases, such as cholera, typhoid, smallpox, influenza, malaria, and yellow fever. Health concerns at the time also related to social and public health, including contamination of food and water supplies, inadequate sewage disposal, and poor housing conditions (Banta, 1995b; Pickett and Hanlon, 1990). Most health care was provided in the home by family and friends. Hospitals were few in number and characterized by overcrowding, disease, and unsanitary conditions. Sick persons who were cared for in hospitals often died from poor hospital conditions, and most people avoided being cared for in a hospital unless there was no alternative. In

this first developmental phase, health care was paid for by individuals who could afford health care, through bartering with physicians, or through charitable contributions from individuals and organizations.

Technology to aid in disease control was very basic and practical but in keeping with knowledge development of the time. The physician's "black bag" contained the few medicines and tools available for treatment. While the types of health care providers and numbers of practitioners influence the economics of health care, the labor force was composed mostly of physicians and nurses who attained their skills through apprenticeships, or on-the-job training. Nurses in the United States were predominantly female, and education was linked to religious orders, with expectations of service, dedication, and charity (Kovner, 1995). The focus of nursing was primarily to support physicians and assist clients with activities of daily living.

The *second developmental stage* (1900 to1945) of U.S. health care delivery focused on the control of acute infectious diseases. Environmental conditions influencing health began to improve, with major advances in water purification, sanitary sewage disposal, milk and water quality, and

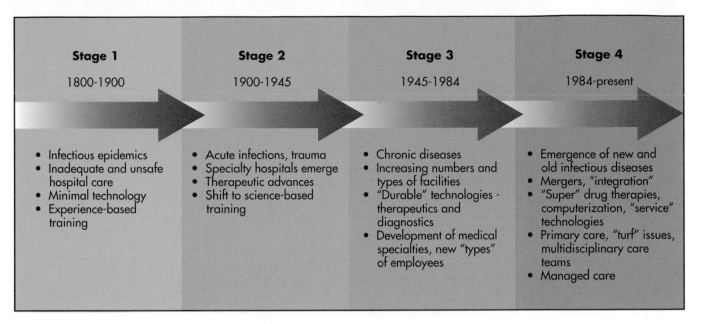

Stage 1	**Stage 2**	**Stage 3**	**Stage 4**
1800-1900	1900-1945	1945-1984	1984-present
• Infectious epidemics • Inadequate and unsafe hospital care • Minimal technology • Experience-based training	• Acute infections, trauma • Specialty hospitals emerge • Therapeutic advances • Shift to science-based training	• Chronic diseases • Increasing numbers and types of facilities • "Durable" technologies - therapeutics and diagnostics • Development of medical specialties, new "types" of employees	• Emergence of new and old infectious diseases • Mergers, "integration" • "Super" drug therapies, computerization, "service" technologies • Primary care, "turf" issues, multidisciplinary care teams • Managed care

FIG. 5-3 Developmental framework for health services delivery: service needs and intensity, facilities, technology, and labor.

urban housing quality. The health problems of the era changed from mass epidemics to individual acute infections or traumatic episodes (Pickett and Hanlon, 1990).

Hospitals and health departments experienced rapid growth during the late 1800s and early 1900s as technological advances in society were made (Kovner, 1995). In addition to private and charitable financing of health care, city, county, and state governments were beginning to contribute to health care by providing services for poor persons, state mental institutions, and other specialized hospitals, such as tuberculosis hospitals. Public health departments were emphasizing case finding and quarantine. While health care was paid for primarily through individuals, the Social Security Act of 1935 signified the federal government's increasing interest in addressing social welfare problems.

Clinical medicine entered its "golden age" during this period. Major technological advances in surgery and childbirth and the identification of disease processes such as the cause of pernicious anemia enhanced the ability to diagnose and treat diseases. The discovery and development of pharmacologic advances, such as insulin in 1922 for control of diabetes, sulfa drugs in 1932 for treatment of infectious diseases, and antibiotics such as penicillin in the 1940s, eradicated certain infectious diseases, increased treatment options, and decreased morbidity and mortality rates (Rice, 1994).

Technological and knowledge advances shifted physician education away from apprenticeships to scientifically based college education, which occurred after the publication of the Flexner Report in 1910. Nurses were trained primarily in hospital schools of nursing, with an emphasis on following and executing physicians' orders. Nurses in training were unmarried and under the age of 30 and provided the bulk of care in hospitals (Kovner, 1995). Public health nurses who tracked infectious diseases and implemented quarantine procedures worked more collegially with physicians (Kovner, 1995). This period saw the emergence of university-based nursing programs established to accommodate the expanding practice base of nursing. Client education was assumed as a nursing function early in the development of the health care delivery system. There were roughly 40 types of other health care providers before 1940, such as pharmacists.

The *third developmental stage* (1945 to 1984) included a shift away from acute infectious health problems of previous stages toward chronic health problems such as heart disease, cancer, and stroke, resulting from increasing affluence and lifestyle changes in the United States. To meet society's needs, the number and types of facilities expanded to include, for example, hospital clinics and long-term care facilities. The Joint Commission on Accreditation of Hospitals, established in 1951 and later renamed the Joint Commission on Accreditation of Health Care Organizations, focused on the safety and protection of the public and the delivery of quality care (Weitzman, 1990).

Changes in the overall health of American society also shifted the focus of technology, research, and development. Major technological advances included the development of chemotherapeutic agents; immunizations; anesthesia; electrolyte and cardiopulmonary physiology; expansion of diagnostic laboratories and complex equipment such as the computerized tomography (CT) scanner; organ and tissue transplants; radiation therapy; laser surgery; and specialty units for critical care, coronary care, and intensive care. The first "test tube baby" was born via in vitro fertilization, and other fertility advances soon emerged.

Health care providers constituted more than 5% of the total U.S. workforce during this period. The three largest health care employers were hospitals, convalescent institutions, and physicians' offices. Between 1970 and 1984 alone, the number of persons employed in the health care industry grew by 90%. The number of personnel employed in the community also increased. The expansion of care delivery into other sites, such as community-based clinics, increased not only the number but also the types of health care employees. For example, physician assistants were trained under the supervision of physicians and employed to assist physicians in delivering routine medical care.

Technological advances brought about increased specialialty training for physicians and nurses, and care was organized around these specialties. The repeating shortage of nurses throughout the century was being acknowledged as themes of nursing shortages in the 1970s and early 1980s emerged. Nursing education expanded from hospital-based diploma and university-based baccalaureate training to include associate degree preparation at the entry level. As the closure of nursing diploma schools began in the early-to-mid 1980s, the number of baccalaureate and associate degree programs began to increase. Graduate nursing education expanded to include nurse practitioner (NP) and clinical nurse specialty (CNS) training to meet increasing societal demands, specialization, and technological advances. The first doctoral programs in nursing were instituted to build the scientific base for nursing, and to increase the number of nursing faculty members.

The role of the commercial health insurance industry increased, and a strong link between employment and the provision of health care benefits emerged. Furthermore, the federal government's role expanded through landmark policy making that would affect health care delivery well into the twenty-first century. Specifically, the passage of Titles XVIII and XIX of the Social Security Act in 1965 created the Medicare and Medicaid programs, respectively. The health care system appeared to have unlimited resources for growth and expansion.

The *fourth developmental stage* (1984 to present) is a period of limited resources, with emphasis on cost containment, restricted growth in the health care industry, and reorganization of care delivery. Escalating health care costs and limited public and private resources have taken priority in policy discussions, with increasing interest in the financing of health care. For example, amendments were made to the Social Security Act in 1983 creating diagnostic-related groups and a prospective system of paying for health care provided to Medicare recipients. The 1997 Balanced Budget Act legislated additional federal mandates for Medicare and Medicaid. Private-sector employer concerns about the rising costs of health care for employees and fear of profit losses spurred a major

change in the delivery and financing of health care known as *managed care*.

Subsequently, this period included drastic change in the settings and organization of health care delivery. Transformation in health care organizations became commonplace, and buzz words of the period were *reorganization, reengineering, restructuring,* and *downsizing.* Organizational mergers occurred at an accelerated rate in an effort to consolidate care, find economies of scale in the management of care, and coordinate care across the continuum (i.e., from "cradle to grave"). Merger discussions focused on horizontal integration, which indicated the union of similar agencies (e.g., acute care hospital mergers) and vertical integration, or a merger between different types of organizations (e.g., an acute care hospital, a long-term care facility, and a home health facility).

These pressures brought about hospital closings and a shifting of care once delivered exclusively in hospitals to other settings, such as ambulatory and community-based clinics and specialty diagnostic centers that offer technologies like magnetic resonance imaging (MRI) and sonography. Rehabilitative, restorative, and palliative care once delivered in the traditional hospitals was shifted to other settings, such as sub-acute care hospitals, specialty rehabilitation hospitals, long-term care, and even to individual homes. Although the basis of care delivery was no longer the traditional acute care hospital, the nature of the care delivered in hospitals changed remarkably, as evidenced by the following:

- Patients admitted to hospitals were more acutely ill.
- Length of stay for patients admitted to hospitals declined.
- Care delivery became more intense as a result of both of the above.

Technological advances, such as the widespread use of computers and the Internet, have enabled society to become increasingly sophisticated about health. The public's increasing knowledge about health care and awareness of health care advances have influenced their demand for health care, such as diagnostic and therapeutic services for treatment. Furthermore, pharmaceutical companies and other technological suppliers actively market their products through television, printed advertisements, the Internet, and other sources so that clients rapidly become aware of the availability of new technologies.

Health professionals are dependent upon technology to care for clients. Distance as a barrier to the diagnosis and treatment of disease has been overcome through the use of telehealth. Health care professionals, along with payers, have become the principal purchasing agents of technology for the client. They, in essence, often make decisions about when and if a certain technology will be used in a given situation. Nurses have become dependent upon technologies to monitor client progress, make decisions about client care, and deliver care in new and innovative ways.

Health professionals of this stage were forced to consider alternative models of care delivery that run counter to traditional approaches. The consideration of these alternatives was prompted by economic and policy pressures to correct for the excesses of the health care system created during the previous developmental periods. The shift away from traditional hospital-based care to the community and the need to consider new models of care brought about an increased emphasis on primary care, the development of care delivery teams, and collaboration in practice and education. The substituting of one type of health personnel for another was occurring to control care delivery costs at two major levels: the substitution of NPs for primary care providers and the substitution of unlicensed personnel for staff nurses in hospitals and long-term care facilities. This substitution fueled discipline debates and territorial, or "turf," battles.

The increase in specialization of health professionals has led to changes in certification, qualifications, education, and standards of care in health professions. These factors, in turn, contributed to the increased number and kinds of providers to meet the demands of the health care system. Between 1990 and 1996 alone, health service employment increased by 19%, more than twice the increase of the total U.S. workforce, despite an intense focus on cost containment and threats of workforce shifts and downsizing (USDHHS, 1998). Moreover, the number of types of health care personnel has risen to more than 200. In 1996, approximately 45% of all health employees worked in hospitals (down from 50% in 1990), 16% were employed in nursing homes, and 13% were employed in physicians' offices. The Bureau of Labor Statistics (BLS) predicts that two sectors of health care employment will be among the top ten industries with fast employment growth between 1996 and 2006: the health services sector in general is ranked second (behind computer and data processing services) with a projected job growth of 68%, and offices of health practitioners are ranked ninth, with a projected growth of 47% (Bureau of Labor Statistics, 1998). Box 5-4 presents the numbers of certain active health care professionals in 1995.

BOX 5-4 Number of Health Care Professionals in the United States

In 1995, the numbers of active health professionals included the following:
- 672,859 physicians
- 28,900 optometrists
- 182,300 pharmacists
- 10,300 podiatrists
- 2,115,800 registered nurses

From USDHHS: *Health: United States, 1998*, DHHS Pub No (PHS) 98-1232, Washington, DC, 1998, U.S. Government Printing Office.

The registered nurse labor market is the largest sector of health care professionals, representing 2.6 million practicing registered nurses (Moses, 1997). Of those practicing nurses, approximately 13% were employed in community and public health. The nursing profession is identified as one of five occupations projected to have the largest number of new jobs going into the twenty-first century, with above average anticipated earnings (Bureau of Labor Statistics, 1998). The loss of nursing jobs from hospital downsizing was reported in the early 1990s, and nursing positions were threatened by new models of care delivery that used unlicensed personnel. However, this fear was short-lived, and by the late 1990s, concerns of another nursing shortage were reported in the popular press in spite of the fact that the supply of nurses was at an all-time high (Aiken, Sochalski, and Anderson, 1996). An increasing number of advanced practice nurses capatalized on expanding employment opportunities of the mid-to-late 1990s, such as primary care providers and care managers. The continuing shift in emphasis on preventive health care and health promotion is clearly in line with community and public health nursing and an increasing role for nursing within community settings and care delivery programs such as managed care.

Finally, during this period the United States experienced an increase in the number and types of communicable, infectious, and environmental illnesses. Infant mortality is at a record low in the United States, and life expectancy is at a record high. Chronic illnesses resulting from environmental and lifestyle influences are increasing. With the resurgence of communicable and infectious diseases, such as tuberculosis, acquired immunodeficiency syndrome (AIDS), and new strains of streptococcus, major challenges in health care delivery are anticipated in the twenty-first century. These realities of the current health care delivery system likely will spill over into the next millennium, and the health care industry will face many new and recurring themes during future developmental phases.

TRENDS IN HEALTH CARE SPENDING

Much has been written in the popular and scientific literature about the costs of U.S. health care and how society makes decisions about allocating available and scarce resources. Given that economics in general and health care economics in particular are concerned with resource allocation and decision making, any discussion of the economics of health care must consider past and current health care spending. The trends documented here reflect past public and private decisions about health care and health care delivery. Past spending reflects past decision making; likewise, past decisions reflect the values and beliefs held by society and policy makers that undergird policy making at any given point in time.

Figure 5-4 shows U.S. health care expenditures between 1960 and 1996. Spending for health care increased from approximately $24 million in 1960 to over $1 trillion in

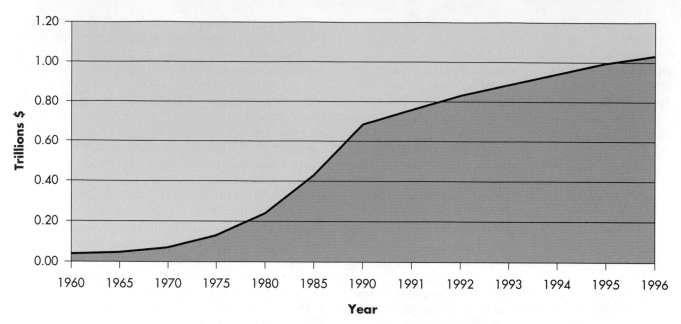

FIG. 5-4 National health expenditures for selected years from 1960 to1996. (Data from Levit KR et al: National health expenditures, 1996, *Health Care Fin Rev* 19[1]:161, 1997; USDHHS: *Health: United States, 1998,* DHHS Pub No [PHS] 98-1232, Washington, DC, 1998, U.S. Government Printing Office.)

1996, the first time in U.S. history that health care spending extended above this point (Levit et al, 1997). These numbers reflect per-person spending amounts of $124 in 1960 and $3759 in 1996 (Levit et al, 1997), an increase of over 3000%. Interestingly, the general U.S. population during this same period increased by approximately 48% (USDHHS, 1998).

Figure 5-5 provides a breakdown of the distribution in health care expenses for 1996 (USDHHS, 1998). The largest proportions of health care expenses were for hospital care and physician services, 34% and 19%, respectively. Although percentages for both of these categories have fluctuated over time, it is interesting to note that the percentages of both of these categories are now close to the 1960 percentages of 34.5% and 19.7%, respectively (USDHHS,1998). Only a small fraction of health care dollars was spent on home health, public health, and research and construction, each receiving roughly 3% of total health care funds in 1996. For historical reference, these categories were funded accordingly at 0.2%, 1.4%, and 6.3% in 1960 (USDHHS, 1998), suggesting that home health and public health have increased slightly in societal value while research has declined.

The GDP is useful in determining the contribution of the health care sector relative to all other sectors of production in the United States. Figure 5-6 illustrates the proportion of GDP attributable to health care between 1960 and 1996 (USDHHS, 1998). Health care spending represented approximately 14% of the GDP between 1993 and 1996, or almost $14 of every $100 spent in the United

States went to pay for health care services (Levit et al, 1997).

Increases in health care expenditures—in total and as percentage of GDP—slowed between 1993 and 1996, the first time in 37 years that health care spending remained relatively stable for 3 consecutive years (Levit et al, 1997). This period of relative stability within the health care sector likely can be attributed to the prospective payment system, the focus on managed care, reorganization and reengineering efforts, and the general focus on cost containment as described previously.

The basic indicator of inflation typically found in discussions of health care spending is the **consumer price index** (CPI). The CPI measures inflation by comparing prices overall and for categories of consumed goods and services purchased by urban wage earners and their families over a certain time period (e.g., quarterly or yearly). The index is standardized to prices in a typical, or base, year, and changes over time are related to the base year as a point of reference. Although the base year chosen is arbitrary, the index is useful to examine trends in price changes over time. The medical care component of the CPI compares selected prices of hospital, medical, dental, and pharmaceutical products and services and documents price changes for these services (USDHHS, 1998).

Figure 5-7 shows changes in the CPI between 1960 and 1996. Inflation began to decline in 1985, and with this overall decline in prices came the lowest annual increase in health care prices since 1960. By 1993 health care costs were twice the overall inflation rate of the United States (USDHHS, 1993). In 1996, the medical care component

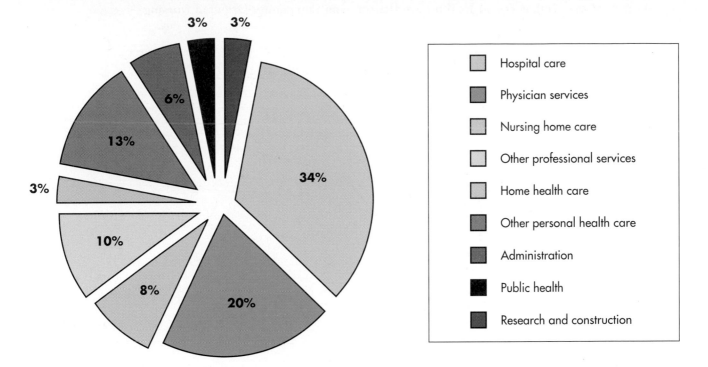

■	Hospital care
■	Physician services
■	Nursing home care
■	Other professional services
■	Home health care
■	Other personal health care
■	Administration
■	Public health
■	Research and construction

Notes: 1) Percentages have been rounded upward to add to 100. 2) "Other professional services" includes dental and other non-physician health care services. 3) "Other personal services" includes drugs and other non-durable health care goods, vision products and other durable health care goods, and any other personal health care.

FIG. 5-5 Distribution of U.S. health care expenditures, 1996. (Data from Levit KR et al: National health expenditures, 1996, *Health Care Fin Rev* 19[1]:161, 1997; USDHHS: *Health: United States, 1998,* DHHS Pub No [PHS] 98-1232, Washington, DC, 1998, U.S. Government Printing Office.)

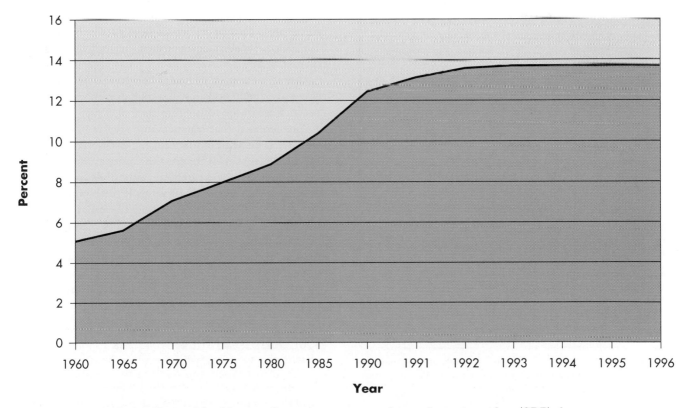

FIG. 5-6 National health expenditures as percentage of gross domestic product (GDP), for selected years from 1960-1996. (Data from Levit KR et al: National health expenditures, 1996, *Health Care Fin Rev* 19[1]:161, 1997; USDHHS: *Health: United States, 1998,* DHHS Pub No [PHS] 98-1232, Washington, DC, 1998, U.S. Government Printing Office.)

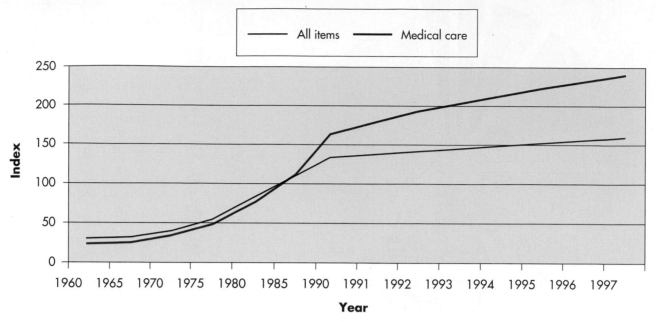

All items ——— Medical care

* Data are shown in 5 year intervals between 1960 and 1990; annual data are reported for 1990 through 1997

FIG. 5-7 Consumer price index for selected years from 1970-1996. (Data from USDHHS: *Health: United States, 1998,* DHHS Pub No [PHS] 98-1232, Washington, DC, 1998, U.S. Government Printing Office.)

BOX 5-5 Predicted Changes in Health Care Spending

Researchers predict that between 1996 and 2007, health care spending will change in the following ways:
- Hospital spending growth will be less than aggregate spending.
- Spending for physician services will be substantial, increasing from 2.9% in 1996 to an estimated 7.3% by the year 2000.
- Spending on pharmaceuticals is expected to accelerate through 1998 and sustain an annual growth rate below 6% during the period.
- Spending for nursing home care will initially accelerate, then decelerate to an average of 5.1% during the period.
- Home health care spending will be greater than aggregate spending growth.
- Annual spending for specialist such as podiatrists, optometrists, and chiropractors will increase from 6.8% in 1996 to 8.3% by 2001.
- The overall costs of health care benefits will increase faster than the growth in total compensation, suggesting that the numbers of uninsured will grow as individual employees increasingly become more responsible for benefit payments.

Based on data from Smith et al: The Health Expenditures Projection Team: the next ten years of health spending: what does the future hold? *Health Affairs* 17(5):128, 1998.

of the CPI was 3.5% compared with 2.9% spending in the United States overall. Personal health care expenses increased only 4.4%, a decline in the CPI (Levit et al, 1997). Hospitals and physicians are the two major recipients of health care dollars, receiving approximatelly 40% and 22% of personal health expenditures, respectively, in 1996 (Levit et al, 1997).

Although the costs of health care have decelerated in recent years, predictions suggest that health care spending may increase in the future (Smith et al, 1998). The basis of this prediction is that possible cost savings from managed care have been achieved or in some cases exceeded. Smith and colleagues suggest that health care spending may reach $2.1 trillion by the year 2007, almost doubling current spending within less than 10 years. If these projections are true, health care will represent approximately 17% of GDP. Future health care spending increases also can be partially attributed to public concern for quality health care and input into decision making and demand for correction by public policy makers. See Box 5-5 for a more in-depth overview of predicted changes in health care spending

WHAT DO YOU THINK? *Projections indicate that health care spending will increase, perhaps even double, in less than 10 years and that health care will represent approximately 17% of GDP. If this happens, what impact will this increase have on the U.S. society and economy? Is spending 17% of GDP on health care a concern? Provide rationale for your position.*

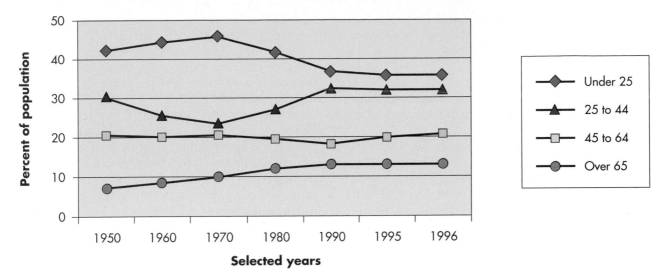

FIG. 5-8 U.S. population by age group for selected years from 1950-1996. (Data from USD-HHS: *Health: United States, 1998*, DHHS Pub No [PHS] 98-1232, Washington, DC, 1998, U.S. Government Printing Office.)

Factors Influencing Health Care Costs

Health economists, providers, payers, and politicians have explored various explanations for the rapid rate of increase in health expenses relative to population growth. The explanation that individuals, over time, have consumed more health care is not sufficient. A more plausible possibility is that the health care consumed by individuals became more expensive for a combination of complex reasons. The following factors frequently are attributed to total and per capita health care spending increases over the past 40 years (Levit et al, 1997): inflation, changes in population demography, and technology and intensity of services. An in-depth discussion of each factor is presented here.

Price inflation

Price **inflation** in health care has been a recurring concern since the 1950s, especially since there is the pervasive belief, usually backed up by documented proof, that increasing amounts and proportions of public resources have been allocated to health care rather than to other societal investments. Inflation occurs when there is a sustained upward trend in the prices of goods and services (Boyes, 1992). General inflation in the U.S. economy affects the prices of all goods and services in the United States, including health care. However, there is a certain amount and/or proportion of inflation that is specific to the health care industry.

Changes in demographics

Another factor often associated with rising health care costs is the change in demographics. The changing demographics, in turn, impact the ways in which health care resources are allocated and technologies are developed. The first notable demographic change is that the U.S. population, in general, has increased in size. This means that, across all age groups and segments of society, the sheer number of people requiring health services has increased.

Second, while all age groups are increasing in number, an important demographic shift is the aging of the society. In 1996, approximately 13% of the U.S. population was over the age of 65; the same age group comprised approximately 9% of the total U.S. population in 1960 (USDHHS, 1998). By the year 2030, the over-65 age group will comprise roughly 20% of the U.S. population (HCFA, 1998). The proportion of the population in the 25- to 44-year-old age group increased from 26% in 1960 to 32% in 1996, and the proportion of the population in the 45- to 64-year-old age group remained relatively stable at 20%. Interestingly, the proportion of the population under the age of 25 has steadily declined from a high of 46% in 1970 to 35% 1996 (USDHHS, 1998). This shift in the age of the population, shown in Figure 5-8, places increasing pressure on society to allocate and spend more money on age-related health issues, including long-term care, research, and prevention and treatment of chronic diseases.

This trend will continue and become more profound as the baby boom generation ages. The *baby boom generation* refers to individuals born between 1946 and 1964. The first of the baby boomers have turned 50 years old. This well-educated generation is more oriented to preventive health care and is just beginning to move into the time of life when long-term care will be needed. Just as this group increased the need for pediatric health care in the 1950s, they now will increase the need for long-term care for chronic conditions (Pew Health Professions Commission, 1993). The financing of long-term care is a growing issue as the aging of the baby boomers nears. In 1996 the cost of 1 year in a nursing home averaged over $37,500

(USDHHS, 1998). To receive Medicaid long-term care benefits, elderly persons must "spend down" their life savings, including selling their homes, to poverty levels. The decreasing size of the younger and college-aged population, usually the healthiest group requiring less health care service, will mean fewer persons to contribute toward paying for the cost of elder care (Pew Health Professions Commission, 1993).

Other demographic factors potentially will add to increasing health care costs. There has been an increase in racial diversity within the United States. Table 5-1 documents this trend of increasing diversity in the population: the proportion of Caucasians has decreased, and the proportion of all other racial groups has increased. Recent reports suggest that the ethnic mix in the United States will continue to shift as, for example, the proportion of Hispanics surpasses the proportion of African-Americans in the year 2010 (U.S. Census Bureau, 1996). Given that racial diversity varies by state and geographic region, the emphasis and relative importance of these issues also varies across the United States. For example, in 1994 California voters passed the controversial Proposition 187, an initiative that restricts the use of public-supported services by illegal immigrants.

Increased racial diversity presents certain health care challenges. Individuals of other nationalities often immigrate to the United States to escape social hardships within their country of origin, many of which, such as poor sanitation and over-crowding, are known detriments to health. Thus some in these groups have entered the United States in poor health, lived in poverty and under poor circumstances after arriving, and have not had access to needed health care services. Beyond those just entering the United States, there are U.S.-born individuals of all racial and ethnic groups who live in poverty, receive little or no educa-

tion, have a low-paying or no job, are homeless, and/or lack access to needed health care services.

When these demographic issues coexist, many health care problems often exist. As a result, individuals across all racial groups will continue to need services to meet even the most basic of health care necessities. Providing access to such services adds to the overall health care costs (Pew Health Professions Commission, 1993) and creates an important, yet fundamental, question for the society: How can and should the United States allocate its money to get the best return on investment? There are complexities and strong opposing viewpoints that surround this question, making it historically difficult for the nation to take a definitive stand on this sensitive issue.

Technology and intensity

The introduction of new technologies enhances the delivery of care, but it also has the potential to increase the costs of care. As new and more complex technology is introduced into the system, the cost is typically high. However, clients often demand access to the technology, and providers want to use the technology. In an effort to keep health care costs down, however, payers have attempted to restrict use and availability of certain technologies. For example, the drug Viagra, developed for the treatment of impotence by Pfizer Pharmaceuticals, is an example of a controversial technological advancement that, upon immediate availability to the public, was in high demand and prescribed by providers, yet restricted in use by payers.

The adoption of new technologies demands investment in personnel, equipment, and facilities. Furthermore, new technology adds to administrative costs, especially if the federal government provides financial coverage for the service or is involved in regulation of the technology. Table 5-2 outlines federal regulations that have, over time, contributed to the use of technology.

TABLE 5-1 U.S. Population (in thousands) by Ethnicity (%)

Year	All Persons	Caucasian	African-American	American Indian or Alaska Native	Asian Pacific Islander	Hispanic White	Non-Hispanic
1950	150,697	134,945 (90%)	15,045 (10%)	—	—	—	—
1960	179,323	158,832 (89%)	18,872 (11%)	—	—	—	—
1970	203,212	177,749 (87%)	22,580 (11%)	—	—	—	—
1980	226,546	194,712 (86%)	26,683 (12%)	1,420 (0.6%)	3,729 (2%)	14,609 (6%)	180,907 (80%)
1990	248,710	208,704 (84%)	30,483 (12%)	2,065 (0.8%)	7,457 (3%)	22,354 (9%)	188,300 (76%)
1995	262,755	218,086 (83%)	33,141 (13%)	2,242 (0.9%)	9,286 (4%)	26,994 (10%)	193,523 (74%)
1995	265,284	219,748 (83%)	33,503 (13%)	2,288 (0.9%)	9,743 (4%)	28,269 (11%)	193,978 (73%)

Adapted from USDHHS: *Health: United States, 1998*, DHHS Pub No (PHS) 98-1232, Washington, DC, 1998, U.S. Government Printing Office.

A health care problem that has contributed to the overall cost of health care through medical care, research, development of new technologies, and cash assistance to clients is AIDS. AIDS is a problem that has affected a large number of people requiring a wide array of services (intensity), expensive treatments (technologies), and care. Expenditures by the federal government alone for AIDS increased from approximately $6 million in 1982 to approximately $8.5 billion in 1997 (USDHHS, 1994, 1998). Expenditures for AIDS have also exacerbated already existing concerns about health care financing and the amount of money that has been spent on research, development, and treatment.

Chernew and colleagues (1998) identify technology as the "predominant factor" behind health care cost increases. Interestingly, they note that managed care plans, while restricting use of certain technologies, have failed to contain the health care cost increases.

Figure 5-9 summarizes the influence of demographic changes, service intensity and technology, and inflation on health care costs (USDHHS, 1998). In the early 1980s, the influence of economy-wide inflation reached its peak, although the influence of this factor has increased in recent years. Medical inflation, in contrast, remained below 20% throughout the period. The influence of intensity vacillated during the period, although its influence was at an all-time low in 1995 and 1996. Population influences, which reached a low-point around 1980, increased in 1995 and 1996 to near 1960 levels. These factors will undoubtedly change in the future as political, social, economic, and health care forces evolve.

FINANCING OF HEALTH CARE

Health care financing has evolved during the twentieth century from a system supported primarily by consumers to a system financed by third-party payers, publicly by state and federal governments, and privately through insurers and managed care. Figure 5-10 shows changes in the percentages of financing by source. From 1950 to 1990, out-of-pocket spending decreased, philanthropic payments increased slightly, and third-party public and private insurance payments increased dramatically. Combined state and federal government contributions are currently higher than those of private payers. In 1996, public contributions equaled about 46% of health care payments, private health insurance contributed approximately 32%, and other private sources contributed approximately 4%; consumers paid approximately 19% of health care payments with out-of-pocket money.

Public Support

The federal government became involved in health care financing for population groups early in U.S. history. In 1798 the federal government created the Marine Hospital Service to provide medical service for sick and disabled

TABLE 5-2 Examples of Federal Regulatory Mechanisms Contributing to Technology Costs and Control

YEAR	FEDERAL REGULATION
1906	Prescription drug regulation passes (Food, Drug, and Cosmetic Act [now FDA])
1938	Manufacturers are required to prove drug safety (Food, Drug, and Cosmetic Act)
1952	Hill-Burton Act provides construction monies for new hospitals
1965	Amendments made to Social Security Act providing Medicare and Medicaid to support health care services provided to certain groups
1972	Social Security Act amendments: 1) extend coverage for end-stage renal disease to provide payment for use of treatment technologies; and 2) provide for professional standards review organizations to review appropriateness of hospital care for Medicare/Medicaid recipients
1974	Health Planning and Resources Development Act introduces certificate-of-need to limit major health care expansion at local and state levels
1976	Medical devices amendments regulate safety and effectiveness of medical equipment, such as pacemakers
1978	Medicare End-Stage Renal Disease Amendment provides home dialysis and kidney transplantation; Health Services Research, Health Statistics, and Health Care Technology Act establishes national council on health care technology to develop standards for use
1982	Tax Equity and Fiscal Responsibilities Act establishes prospective payment system for hospitalized Medicare patients by DRG category
1989	Omnibus Reconciliation Act created: 1) physician resource-based fee schedule to be implemented by 1992, with emphasis on high-tech specialities of surgery; and 2) the Agency for Health Care Policy and Research to perform research on effectiveness of medical services, interventions, and technologies, including nursing
1996	Health Insurance Portability and Accountability Act enacted to protect health insurance coverage for laid-off or displaced workers
1998	Third-party reimbursement for Medicare Part B services under Public Law 105-33 for NPs and CNS

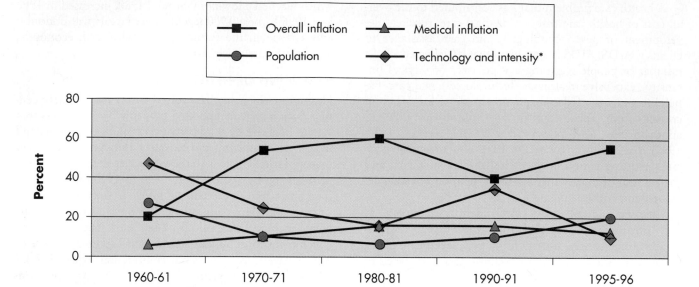

* Residual of growth that cannot be attributed to price increases or population growth; represents changes in use or kinds of services and supplies

FIG. 5-9 Factors affecting growth of health care expenditures. (Data from USDHHS: *Health: United States, 1998,* DHHS Pub No [PHS] 98-1232, Washington, DC, 1998, U.S. Government Printing Office.)

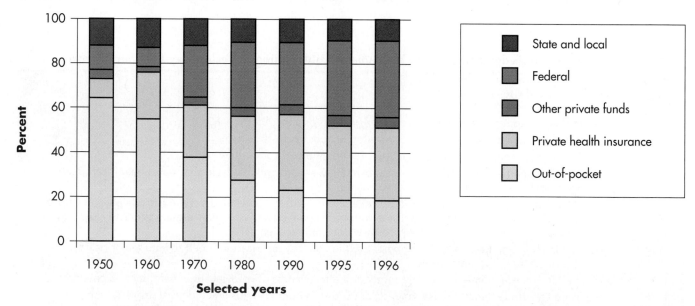

FIG. 5-10 Personal health care expenditures by source of funds. (Data from USDHHS: *Health: United States, 1998,* DHHS Pub No [PHS] 98-1232, Washington, DC, 1998, U.S. Government Printing Office.)

sailors and to protect the nation's borders against the importing of disease through seaports. The Marine Hospital Service is considered the first national health insurance plan in the United States. The original plan cost each sailor 20 cents per month in a payroll deduction for illness care.

The National Health Board was established in 1879. The board was later renamed the United States Public Health Service (PHS). Within the PHS, the federal government developed a public health liaison with state and local health departments for the purpose of controlling communicable diseases and improving sanitation. Additional health pro-

TABLE 5-3 Comparison of Medicare and Medicaid Programs

FEATURE	MEDICARE	MEDICAID
Obtain information	Local Social Security Administration office	State welfare office
Recipients	People who are 65 years old, are disabled, or have permanent kidney failure	Certain low-income and needy people, including children; the aged, blind, and/or disabled; and those eligible to receive federally assisted income
Type of program	Insurance	Insurance
Government affiliation	Federal	Joint federal/state partnership
Availability	All states	All states
Financing of hospital insurance	Medicare Trust Fund, mandatory payroll deductions (1.45% employed persons; 2.9% self-employed); recipient deductibles; trust fund interest	Federal and state governments
Financing of medical insurance	Recipient premium payments ($43.80 per month in 1998); general revenue of the U.S. Treasury	Federal and state governments
Types of coverage	Inpatient and outpatient hospital services, skilled nursing facilities, home health services, hospice care, physician services, medical and health services equipment and supplies	Inpatient and outpatient hospital services; prenatal care; vaccines for children; physician, dental, NP, and nurse midwifery services; skilled nursing facility services for persons 21 years of age or older; family services; rural health clinic services; diagnosis; and treatment of children under 21 years of age

grams were also developed to meet obligations to federal beneficiaries, including American Indians (Indian Health Service), the armed forces (Department of Defense), and veterans of wars (Veterans Administration).

Today, the U.S. government is involved in health care research, training, financing, and delivery and provides funding for the following:

- Research on health care issues with broad national interest (e.g., AIDS research)
- Delivering care to special groups (e.g., mothers, infants, and the aged)
- Special problems or programs (e.g., food and drug safety through the U.S. Food and Drug Administration [FDA] requirements and food inspection)
- International health through its affiliation with the World Health Organization (WHO)
- Training health professionals, such as nurses and physicians

Medicare and Medicaid, two federal programs administered by the Health Care Financing Administration (HCFA), account for the majority of public health care spending. The HCFA is the federal regulatory agency within the USDHHS that is responsible for overseeing and monitoring Medicare and Medicaid spending. This agency routinely collects and reports actual health care use and spending and projects future spending trends.

Table 5-3 provides an overview and comparison of these programs. Through these programs, the federal gov-

ernment purchases health care services for population groups provided through independent health care systems, such as managed care organizations, private physicians, and hospitals.

Medicare

The **Medicare** program, established in Title XVIII of the Social Security Act of 1965, provides hospital insurance and medical insurance to elderly persons, permanently and totally disabled persons, and people with end-stage renal disease. Currently 38.1 million people are enrolled in Medicare, or more than 10% of the total U.S. population (USDHHS, 1998).

The hospital insurance package, Part A, is available to all elderly individuals who have paid Social Security taxes. Estimates indicate that 98% of the elderly population are covered by Part A, which provides payment for hospital services, home health services, and extended care facilities. Part A requires a deductible from recipients of $764 for the first 60 days of services and a coinsurance payment of $191 for 61 to 90 days of service based on a rate equal to a 1-day stay in the hospital. That deductible has increased over the years as daily hospital costs have increased (HCFA, May 1999).

The medical insurance package, Part B, is available to all eligible people who wish to pay a monthly premium for the coverage. Approximately 96% of the elderly population is covered. The premium cost was $43.80 per month in 1998 (HCFA, May 1999). Part B provides coverage for services other than hospitalization, such as physician care, outpatient hospital care, outpatient physical therapy, home health care not covered by Part A, laboratory services, ambulance transportation, prostheses, equipment, and some supplies. After a deductible, up to 80% of reasonable charges are paid for these services. Part B resembles the major medical insurance coverage of private insurance carriers.

Figure 5-11 shows total expenses of the Medicare program from 1967 to 1996. Since the passage of the Medicare amendments to the Social Security Act in 1965, the cost of Medicare has increased dramatically. Hospital care continues to be the major factor contributing to Medicare costs; however, with shorter hospital stays, home health and nursing home costs have increased dramatically.

As a result of increasing costs, Congress passed a law in 1983 that radically changed Medicare's method of payment for hospital services. The Social Security amendments of 1983 (PL98-21) mandated an end to cost-plus reimbursement by Medicare and instituted a 3-year transition to a prospective payment system (PPS) for inpatient hospital services. The purpose of the new hospital payment scheme was to shift the financial incentives away from the provision of more care, the use of more technology, and the use of more hospital care. Reimbursement is based on a fixed price per case for clients in 468 **diagnosis related groups (DRGs).** The objective of this system was to reduce hospital costs while maintaining quality health care and access. Although this type of reimbursement originally was mandated for hospitals only, prospective payment for other health care services has been instituted. The Balanced Budget Act (BBA) of 1997 determined that pay-

ments to Medicare skilled nursing facilities (SNFs) would be made based on the PPS, effective July 1, 1998. The PPS payment rates cover SNF services, including routine, ancillary, and capital-related costs 1998 (HCFA, 1998). Payments to physicians, home health, and ambulatory care continues to be considered, with suggestions to reduce the coverage and have the client pay a portion of the cost of, for example, home health care.

Elderly persons spend approximately $54 billion per year, or 20% of their income, on health care, and 66% of Medicare fee-for-service beneficiaries purchase private supplemental health insurance premiums (HCFA, 1998). This is due to limits in coverage, including certain preventive care, payment of Medicare premiums, the need to have additional insurance for coverage gaps, and the limited number of physicians and agencies who accept Medicare and Medicaid payment. Aged persons then are left to cover the difference between Medicare services and additional costs.

Medicaid

The **Medicaid** program, Title XIX of the Social Security Act of 1965, provides financial assistance to states and counties to pay for medical services for the aged poor, the blind, the disabled, and families with dependent children. The Medicaid program is jointly sponsored and financed with matching funds from the federal and state governments. Currently, 36 million people are enrolled in Medicaid (USDHHS, 1998). Medicaid expenditures from 1972 to 1996 are shown in Figure 5-12.

Full payment for five types of service was provided at the inception of Medicaid (USDHHS, 1993, 1998):

1. Inpatient and outpatient hospital care

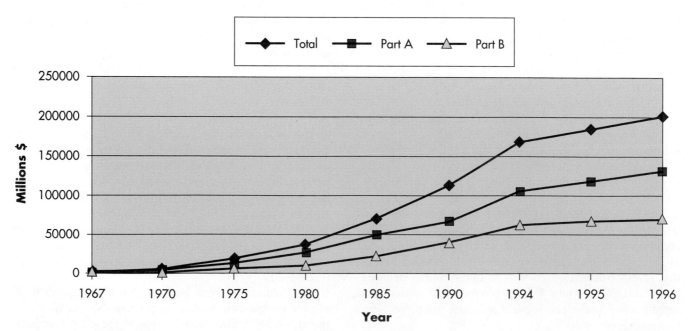

FIG. 5-11 Medicare expenditures for selected years from 1967-1996. (Data from USDHHS: *Health: United States, 1998,* DHHS Pub No [PHS] 98-1232, Washington, DC, 1998, U.S. Government Printing Office.)

2. Laboratory and radiology services
3. Physician services
4. Skilled nursing care at home or in a nursing home for people over 21 years of age
5. Early periodic screening and childhood development (EPSDT) services for those under 21 years of age

The 1972 Social Security amendments added family planning to the list of full-pay services. Prescriptions, dental services, eyeglasses, intermediate care facilities, and coverage for the medically indigent are allowable program options. By law, the medically indigent are required to pay a monthly premium.

Any state participating in the Medicaid program is required to provide the six basic services to participants who are below state poverty income levels. The optional programs are provided at the discretion of each state. In 1989, changes in Medicaid required states to provide care for children under 6 years of age and to pregnant women under 133% of the poverty level. For example, if the poverty level were $12,000, a pregnant woman could have a household income as high as $16,000 and still be eligible to receive care under Medicaid. These changes also provided for pediatric and family NP reimbursement. In the 1990s, states were allowed to petition the federal government for a waiver. If the waiver was approved, the states could use their Medicaid monies for programs other than the six basic services. The first waiver to be approved was given to Oregon for their health care reform plan. Other states have received waivers to develop Medicaid managed care programs for special populations.

The major expense categories for the Medicaid program historically have been skilled and intermediate nursing home care and inpatient hospital care. When combined, today these two categories account for 49% of all costs to the program (USDHHS, 1998). Because of increasing emphasis on preventive care and community-based care, home health and other care, such as EPSDT, family planning, and clinics, are increasing in cost.

Public health

Most public government agencies operate on an annual budget and plan for costs by estimating salaries, expenses, and costs of services for a year. Public health agencies, such as health departments and WIC programs, receive primary funding from tax revenues, with additional money for select goods and services through private third-party payers. Selected public health programs receive reimbursement for services as follows: through grants given by the federal government to states for prenatal and child health; through Medicare and Medicaid for home health, nursing homes, WIC programs, and EPSDT; and through collection of fees on a sliding scale for select client services, such as immunizations.

In 1996, only 3.4% of all health care-related federal funds were expended for federal health programs, such as WIC, versus 97% for other types of health and illness care. In addition to this 3.4% allotment, public health funds also come through states and territorial health agencies. State and local governments contributed 11.1% to public and general assistance, maternal-child health, public health activities, and other related services in 1965; in 1996, the pro-

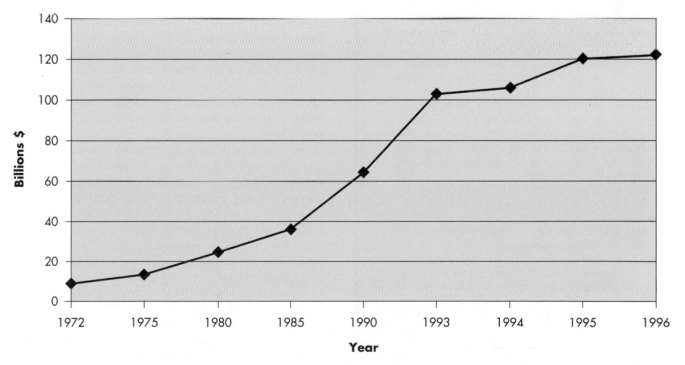

FIG. 5-12 Medicaid expenditures for selected years from 1972-1996. (Data from USDHHS: *Health: United States, 1998,* DHHS Pub No [PHS] 98-1232, Washington, DC, 1998, U.S. Government Printing Office.)

portion contributed to health care through state and local governments had declined to 5.7%. While this proportion fluctuated during the period, the average state and local contribution ranged between 6% and 7% (USDHHS, 1998).

Other public support

The U.S. government also contributes funds to health care through the military medical care system, the Civilian Health and Medical Program of the Uniformed Services (CHAMPUS), the Veteran's Administration (VA), and the Indian Health Service (IHS) (Box 5-6). These programs are very important in providing needed health care services for certain populations, yet combined, these programs represented only approximately 13% of public health care spending in 1996, less than spending for either Medicare or Medicaid alone (Levit et al, 1997).

Private Support

There are several private health care payer sources: insurance, employers, managed care, and individuals. Although insurance and consumers have been prominent health care payment sources for some time, the role of employers and managed care has become increasingly prominent and powerful during the last two decades of the twentieth century.

Insurance

Insurance for health care was first offered by the private sector in 1847 by a commercial insurance company. The purpose of the insurance was to provide security and in-demnity for health care services to individuals. The idea behind insurance was that it provided security, guaranteeing (within certain limits) monies to pay for health care services to defray potential financial losses from unexpected illness or injury related to accidents, catastrophic communicable diseases, such as smallpox and scarlet fever, and recurring (but unexpected) chronic illnesses.

A comprehensive study in the 1920s by the Committee on the Costs of Medical Care showed that a small portion of the population was paying most of the costs of medical care for the majority of the people. The Depression of the 1930s, rising medical costs, and the need to spread financial risk across communities spurred the development of the **third-party payment** system.

The system began as a major industry in the 1930s with the Blue Cross system, which initially provided prepayment for hospital care. It was modeled on the Baylor University prepayment plan established in 1929 to provide teachers with hospital coverage. In 1939 Blue Shield created plans to provide physician payment. The Blue Cross plans began as tax-free, nonprofit organizations established under special enabling legislation in various states.

In the 1940s and 1950s hospital and medical-surgical coverage increased substantially. Employee group coverage appeared, and profit-making commercial insurance underwriters began offering health insurance packages with competitive premiums. The commercial insurance companies could offer lower premium rates because of the methods used to set rates. Insurance and premium setting, in general, are based on the notion of risk pooling (i.e., insurance companies were willing to risk the unlikely occurrence that all or even a large portion of individuals covered under a plan would need payment for health services at any given time) (Folland, Goodman, and Stano, 1993). Blue Cross used a community rate, establishing a similar premium rate for all subscribers regardless of illness possibilities. In contrast, the commercial companies used an experience rate in which the premium was based on an estimate of the illness risk or the number of claims to be made by the subscriber.

Premium competition, the offering of health insurance as a fringe benefit, and the use of health insurance as a negotiable collective bargaining item led to an increase in covered benefits, payment of higher portions of medical care expenses, and increased employer-paid premiums. In turn, these factors pushed up premium costs and health care costs and enabled insurance plans to financially cover high-risk segments of the population, such as aged, poor, or disabled persons.

The needs of high-risk populations led to the passage of Medicare and Medicaid legislation. These and other national health programs targeted health care coverage for specific population groups. These programs, with related federal regulations, and insurance company reimbursement methods contributed to increased costs. Because these programs directed additional money into the health

---

BOX 5-6 Other Public Health Care Programs

- *Military Medical Care System.* Provides health care coverage to military personnel and their dependents at no direct cost to the recipient. The system is composed of hospitals and clinics, typically located at military bases.
- *Civilian Health and Medical Program of the Uniformed Services (CHAMPUS).* Provides coverage for military families and dependents to obtain private sector care if service is unavailable in the military system. The program is provided, financed, and supervised by the military system.
- *Veterans Administration (VA).* Health care system provided as a benefit for retired, disabled, and other specified categories of military service veterans. The system is composed of 172 hospitals and more than 200 outpatient departments.
- *Indian Health Service (IHS).* An agency within the Public Health Service that provides direct care to improve the health status of native Americans living on reservations. This agency operates approximately 50 hospitals and 340 clinics to serve over 1 million Native Americans.

Adapted from USDHHS: *Health: United States, 1998,* DHHS Pub No (PHS) 98-1232, Washington, DC, 1998, U.S. Government Printing Office.

care system to subsidize care, there were financial incentives to encourage the use of services by providers (i.e., the more services ordered, the more money received); the use of services by clients (i.e., the more available the payment for services that might otherwise have gone unused, the more services requested); and more access to a wide variety of new technologies, support for research and development, and increased intensity of services provided. However, because many people do not have access to insurance (i.e., coverage through a private or public source), there is growing concern about the number of uninsured individuals in the United States.

The Congressional Budget Office projects that private insurance premiums will on average increase about 5.1% per year between 1996 and 2007 (Congressional Budget Office, 1999). However, a greater increase in premiums may occur in the future as a result of pressure from employers, consumers, and policy makers. Driving forces behind this pressure are quality of care and clients' rights and the concern that these areas are being compromised in the current climate of managed care. Furthermore, the initial cost savings from managed care may have been realized, and costs will have to be increased to simply maintain coverage, not to mention engaging in activities to increase availability of current or new services and technologies.

Employers

Since the beginning of Blue Cross and Blue Shield, health insurance became tied to employment and the business sector. This tie was strengthened during World War II to compensate, attract, and retain employees (Folland, Goodman, and Stano, 1993). Since that time, employers have become increasingly prominent in determining health insurance benefits.

Receiving health insurance through an employer is unlike the way an individual gets other types of insurance (Folland, Goodman, and Stano, 1993). For example, automobile insurance is a product that individuals purchase out of pocket and choose a plan by making comparisons among insurers, specific plans offered and levels of coverage, premiums required, and individual needs. The link between health insurance and employers causes difficulties, for example, when one loses a job, changes jobs, or is between jobs.

In 1995, private businesses paid for 62.4% of health care expenditures, compared with approximately 79% in 1965. Of this 62.4%, 26% was paid through employer contribution to private health insurance premiums, up from approximately 16% in 1965 (USDHHS, 1998). This substantial contribution to health care by the private business sector gives the purchaser considerable health care buying power and gives the private business sector clout in the policy-making arena.

Although employers originally offered health benefits to attract and retain employees, there is an important explanation for providing health benefits by employers: the U.S. tax system provides incentives to employees and employers for providing health benefits to employees. Specifically, individuals are not taxed on health benefits received, and employees are effectively better off because "after-tax" wages that would otherwise pay for health benefits are not used (Folland, Goodman, and Stano, 1993). Any additional insurance that individuals choose to purchase, above and beyond that which the employer provides, usually comes out of "pre-tax" dollars, such that employees taxable wages are reduced. Employers, on the other hand, can deduct employee health insurance premiums as a cost of doing business, which reduces taxable income. The net effect is that both employees and employers, to a certain degree, are better off if the employer purchases health insurance, as long as the costs of providing benefits does not become too costly for the employers, outweighing the tax benefits of doing so.

Employers, in essence, add another "layer" to the health care payment scheme: individuals gain access to insurance to pay for health care services through their employers; employers make decisions about the level of care and plan of coverage that will be offered to employees; insurers make decisions about services that will be covered through various plan options offered to employers; and providers deliver care to individuals within these parameters. One can argue that with the addition of each "layer" comes added costs and less choice by the client.

Employers have incentives to keep costs down. Additional costs of doing business decrease profits, decrease their ability to make investments, and decrease pay-outs to stock-holders. In an effort to bypass the costs added by insurers, some employers have found it less costly to "self-insure," an arrangement whereby an employer contracts directly with providers to provide health care services to employees rather than going through health insurance companies to purchase employee insurance. Some large businesses directly employ onsite providers for care delivery or offer onsite wellness programs. These programs within the private sector offer opportunities for nurses to provide wellness programs, provide health assessments, and screen and monitor employees and their families. This move to self-insure has resulted in savings to companies and has reduced overall sick care costs (Knickman and Thorpe, 1999).

These and other efforts by employers have strengthened their health care buying power. In fact, employers' quest to keep health care costs and employee benefit costs down brought about the increase in managed care in the United States.

Managed care

Managed care is a philosophy of health care that integrates the financing, delivery, and use of care. This philosophy often gets misinterpreted as a source of financing exclusively because the managed care movement has overemphasized costs and underemphasized quality, and subsequently, reports in the popular press have focused on resultant denials of care to individuals, clients' dissatisfaction with care, and a general lack of trust in the system of care. Negative press has also focused on the costs of providing administrative support to oversee managed care plans, providers, and others involved in the delivery of managed care.

Managed care offers a set of services to purchasers, such as employers or Medicare, for a set fee. This fee, in turn, is used to pay providers through predetermined arrangements for services delivered to covered individuals (USDHHS, 1998). The concept of managed care is based on the notion that the use of costly care could be reduced through consumer education on illness prevention and health maintenance. Therefore managed care is also based on the underlying values of disease prevention, health promotion, wellness, and consumer education, all of which are important principals that often get overlooked.

Types of arrangements commonly used in managed care are health maintenance organizations (HMOs) and preferred provider organizations (PPOs). Box 5-7 provides an overview of HMOs and PPOs. Although HMOs and PPOs seem like relatively new entrants in health care and

> ### BOX 5-7 Types of Managed Care
>
> 1. *Health Maintenance Organization* (HMO) is a provider arrangement whereby comprehensive care is provided to plan members for a fixed, "per member per month" fee. Common features include the following:
>   a. Capitation
>   b. Use of designated providers
>   c. Point-of-service care, or receiving care from non-designated plan providers
>   d. One of the following models:
>   1) *Staff model,* whereby physicians are HMO employees
>   2) *Group model,* whereby a physician group practice contracts with the HMO to provide care
>   3) *Individual practice association* (IPA), whereby the HMO contracts with physicians in solo, small group practices, or physician networks to provide care
>   4) *Mixed model,* whereby the HMO uses a combination group/IPA arrangement.
> 2. A *Preferred Provider Organization* (PPO) is a provider arrangement whereby predetermined rates are established for services to be delivered to members. Common features include the following:
>   a. Hospital and physician providers
>   b. Discounted rate setting
>   c. Financial incentives to encourage plan members to select PPO providers
>   d. Expedited claims payment to providers

From Folland S, Goodman AC, Stano M: *The economics of health and health care,* New York, 1993, Macmillan Publishing Co; USDHHS: *Health: United States, 1998,* DHHS Pub No (PHS) 98-1232, Washington, DC, 1998, U.S. Government Printing Office.

to many recipients of care, HMOs have actually been around since the 1940s. The Health Maintenance Organization Act was enacted in 1972, and since that time, the number of individuals receiving care through HMOs and other types of managed care organizations has increased considerably: between 1976 and 1997, the number of individuals enrolled in an HMO increased from 6 million to almost 67 million, while the percentage of the population enrolled in an HMO increased from approximately 3% to 25% (USDHHS, 1998).

Managed care involves the use of utilization review, or processes to determine the necessity of care and the appropriate use of resources to deliver care. The process of utilization review often includes the use of second opinions to ensure that care is necessary, preauthorization of selected hospital admissions, and concurrent review of care (Thorpe, 1995).

Managed care is based, in part, on the principals of managed competition. Managed competition was introduced in health care in the late 1980s and early 1990s as a means of addressing the increasing costs of health care and to introduce quality into the forefront of discussions. **Managed competition** simply means that individuals make decisions, or trade-offs, about the quality or type of care they wish to receive based on 1) knowledge and information about health care problems, care, and providers; and 2) the costs of care (Enthoven, 1993).

Several basic issues, however, prevent the full implementation of managed competition in health care:
1. "Information assymetry" exists in health care, whereby consumers do not have full knowledge of a health problem or health care delivery options, nor do they always want that knowledge. While access to the Internet and the increase in health care news in the media have increased awareness of certain health care problems, all information is not currently available or accessible by many individuals.
2. The costs of care are not openly shared. Providers are hesitant to give out cost information, and consumers do not know if the price is consistent with the level or quality of care received.
3. Information on outcomes and quality of care delivered by providers and health plans is not readily available, and even when related information is available, it is often overlooked in decision making. For example, a recent survey report of the Commonwealth Fund finds that information is not frequently used by employers to make decisions about selection of managed care plans: accreditation data is required by only 9% of employers, and quality of care data is used by only 6% of employers (Commonwealth Fund, 1998). Furthermore, only 1% of surveyed employers pass information on health plan quality to their employees.
4. Financial incentives for employees, employers, providers, and payers foster market resistance to

change in the delivery and financing of health care. For example, labor unions want health benefits to remain a part of employment compensation, and employers have tax incentives to continue providing health benefits.

5. Adequate and sufficient data upon which to base health care decisions are not available.

Although managed care has been credited with some success in decreasing costs by reductions in hospital use, lengths of hospital stays, and shifting the providing of care outside of the hospital setting (Knickman and Thorpe, 1999), the full impact of managed care cannot be determined because of "bad data" (O'Connor, 1998). These "bad data" primarily consist of financial claims data. Attempts to collect practice, provider, and outcomes data have been made, yet it is often impossible to link administrative, financial, practice, provider, and client outcomes databases. Data inadequacies are partially due to the fact that implementing an information system is expensive in terms of the initial purchase of hardware, software, and training; the ongoing commitment of system maintenance and upgrade; and human resources needed to collect, enter, analyze, and interpret data. An even bigger potential expense is taking action to remedy problems uncovered by these data systems and determining accountability and responsibility for taking such action.

DID YOU KNOW? *A major obstacle in the implementation of managed care or managed competition relates to issues of knowledge development, technology, and information systems. Knowledge and technology have developed rapidly in health care, and information systems play an increasingly important role in decision making. Howeverm currently, the full integration of knowledge, technology, and information systems in health care is costly and slow. Data about cost and quality in health care typically are not collected by health care organizations, data that are collected is not useful, reports are not provided to purchasers, and information is not available for purchasers or consumers to make decisions and trade-offs about costs and quality of care. In fact, O'Connor (1998) notes that health care is experiencing a case of "bad data," whereby the wrong data, such as claims data, are being used to make decisions. Subsequently, any cost savings that have been realized by managed care cannot be linked to managed care. Existing health information systems do not meet organizational, consumer, and payer needs for information on outcomes of care; are difficult to maintain and upgrade; and are often outdated when they become available.*

In short, health care is a complex market and not one whereby information about health care, health problems, and the costs of care are openly exchanged. Nonetheless, managed care represents a step toward managed competition without fully embracing and realizing all aspects of managed competition.

Individuals

Before 1930 and the beginning of Blue Cross, the client, or consumer of health care, had more control and influence over health care costs because nearly all health care costs were paid using out-of-pocket money. In this scenario, consumers had to make decisions about how they would spend their money, making certain "trade-offs", for example, about the type and price of health care they were willing to buy. Furthermore, entering the system was restricted in large part to those who could afford to pay for care or to those few who could find care financed through charitable and philanthropic organizations. However, with the beginning of the U.S. health care third-party payer system and up until the late 1980s, health care was for the most part a seller's market. Control over the services offered and price was held by the provider, who decided the type and level of care or service that would be offered.

In the purest sense, "consumer" implies that money is exchanged for goods and services purchased and used. Under the third-party system, however, this meaning becomes blurred because the one making purchasing and payment decisions for health care services is typically not the person receiving care. Specifically, the third party makes decisions about the level and type of care that will be purchased for recipients and determines how payment will be made, and the recipient has a limited influence on how services will be reimbursed. However, the consumer does affect the provider and payment through political channels.

In 1996, individuals paid out-of-pocket for approximately 17% of total health expenditures, including approximately 15% of physician services and 3% of hospital care (Levit et al, 1997). However, these figures do not reflect the amount of money the consumer pays in taxes to finance government-supported programs such as Medicare and Medicaid, insurance premiums coming out of paid wages that decrease the size of paychecks, or the direct insurance premiums paid for supplemental insurance to plug the gaps in the primary health insurance policy and Medicare (USDHHS, 1993, 1998).

The average monthly cost for private health insurance increased by approximately 64% between 1988 and 1993 for single coverage and by 79% for family coverage (Levit et al, 1997). This increase brought the average range of employees' contributions to health insurance premiums between $39 to $49 per month for individual coverage and $151 to $190 per month for family coverage (USDHHS, 1998). Levit, Lazenby, and Braden (1998) note that these premiums reflected a shift of the health care cost burden from employers to employees, with the percentage of employer contributions to health care declining. The decrease in employer contribution to health insurance premiums parallels the move away from traditional insurance plans by small and large employers to managed care plans.

The shift in responsibility for health insurance premiums is not necessarily bad. In theory, this shift should mean that control over health care decision making, such as the price a consumer is willing to pay for a particular type of health care service and quality, rests with the person buying and receiving health care. Furthermore, if employers no longer include health care benefits as a part of total employee salary and benefits, wages should increase sufficiently to cover the costs that employers have generally contributed. Whether these expectations occur remains to be seen. Shifting responsibility for health insurance premiums and the changing demographics of the workforce in general are bringing about a decline in employee enrollments in health insurance plans (i.e., employees are choosing to use their resources in other ways and are willing to assume the risks of having an illness for which they may have to pay) (Ginsberg, Gabel, and Hunt, 1998).

Given that access to health insurance is tied to employment, there was growing concern in the late 1980s and early 1990s about employment layoffs and downsizing occurring in private business. Those who lost their jobs lost their ability to pay for health insurance and to qualify to purchase insurance privately. The Health Insurance Portability and Accountability Act of 1996 (HIPAA) was enacted to protect health insurance coverage for workers and families after a job change or loss (HCFA, Feb 1999). Although increasing the number of people who have access to health insurance and health care, there are claims that individual premiums are high, that insurance companies have lost their ability to pool risks, and that the HIPAA is just one more federal control mechanism (Nichols and Blumberg, 1998).

Another insurance reform discussion at the political level concerns medical savings accounts (MSAs). MSAs are touted as a way of turning health care decision-making control over to individuals receiving care. MSAs are tax-exempt accounts available to individuals who work for small companies, established usually through a bank or insurance company, that enable individuals to save money for future medical needs and expenses (IRS, 1998). Money contributed to an MSA comes out of "pre-tax" dollars and employer contributions, so initial set-aside money does not come out of taxable income. Furthermore, interest earned in MSAs are tax-free, and any unused money in an MSA can be held in the account from year to year until the money is used. MSAs, in theory, would allow individuals to make cost/quality "trade-offs" but would mean that individuals become knowledgeable about health care, become involved in health care decision making, and take responsibility for the decisions made. Providers, in turn, must be willing to provide and disclose information to individuals and relinquish control of health care decision making. The HIPAA and MSAs are examples of current health insurance reform efforts, and these efforts will likely remain in the forefront of political discussions for some time to come.

WHAT DO YOU THINK? *Americans report concern about the U.S. health care system, particularly managed care reform, yet they are generally satisfied with the care they receive personally (HMO reform, 1998). What are possible explanations for this conflicting information?*

Health Care Financing and the Costs of Health Care

Third-party pay reimbursement is often blamed for rising health care costs. Historically, third-party payers provided better coverage for more expensive hospital services than for ambulatory care, home health care, or nursing home care. This practice encouraged provider and consumer use of more costly hospital care because the client's bill was paid by the insurer. Given a choice between hospital and home care, hospital care typically was chosen. Furthermore, simply having payment coverage for services encouraged consumers to demand services. In turn, provider incentives to use less-costly services were lacking because government or private insurers paid most hospital and physician bills. Third-party reimbursement for surgery, diagnostic procedures, and other technological interventions also encouraged the use of these services, regardless of their necessity.

The financing of health care in the United States is complex. Through the mid-1980s, consumer demands placed pressures on the private business sector to increase and strengthen health benefits offered and on policy makers to expand government programs for the aged and poor. However, the late 1980s and 1990s brought about a different turn of events. The public and private sectors became very focused on the increasing costs of health care and containing those costs. This period was a time of employee downsizing and organizational restructuring in the private business sector, which meant that businesses had a greater effect on health benefits offered. Through their political clout, employers influenced public policy making. The results have been multidimensional: cut backs in employee health insurance benefits offered through employers; increasing employee responsibility for health insurance premiums; streamlining of the Medicare and Medicaid programs; more emphasis on home and community care; and a dramatic shift to managed care. Collectively, changes of the 1980s and 1990s have brought about changes in how payments are made to health care providers.

HEALTH CARE PAYMENT SYSTEMS

Several methods have been used by public and private sources to pay health care providers for health care services. These include retrospective and prospective reimbursement for paying health care organizations and fee-for-service and capitation for paying health care practitioners (Knickman and Thorpe, 1999).

Paying Health Care Organizations

Retrospective reimbursement is the traditional reimbursement method whereby fees for the delivery of health care services in an organization are set after services are delivered (Knickman and Thorpe, 1999). In this scenario, reimbursement is based on either organizational costs or charges. The *cost method* reimburses organizations based on the cost per unit of service (e.g., home health visit, patient day) for treatment and care. Costs include all or a percentage of added, allowable costs. Allowable costs are negotiated between the payer and provider and include items such as depreciation of building, equipment, and administrative costs (e.g., administrative salaries, utilities, and office supplies) (Knickman and Thorpe, 1999). For example, the unit of service in home health is the visit, and the agreed-on price is a set amount of money that the home health agency will be paid for a home visit in the region of the United States in which the home care agency is located.

The *charge method* reimburses organizations based on the price set by the organization for delivering a service (Knickman and Thorpe, 1999). In this case, the organization determines a charge for providing a particular service, provides the service to a client, and submits a bill to the payer, and the payer in turn provides payment for the bill. With this method the charge may be greater than the actual cost to the agency to deliver the service. When the charge method is used, the client often has to pay the difference between what the third party pays and what the agency has charged. Often the third party will only pay the cost of the service rather than what the agency charges.

Prospective reimbursement is a more recent method of paying an organization whereby the third-party payer establishes the amount of money that will be paid for the delivery of a particular service before offering the services to the client (Knickman and Thorpe, 1999). Since the establishment of prospective payment in Medicare in 1983, private insurance has followed suit by requiring preapprovals before clients can receive certain services, such as hospital admission or mammograms more than once per year (Knickman and Thorpe, 1999). Under this payment scheme, the third-party payer reimburses an organization based on what the payer predicts costs to deliver a particular service will be; these predictions vary by case mix and/or client diagnoses and geographic location.

Prospective payment was aimed at controlling government health care costs for Medicare recipients. Amendments to the Social Security Act created the prospective system of paying for hospital care received by Medicare recipients within certain diagnosis groups, known as diagnosis related groups (DRGs) (Knickman and Thorpe, 1999). Similarly, ambulatory care services received by Medicare recipients are classified into Ambulatory Payment Classes (APCs), which reflect the type of ambulatory clinical services received and resources required (HCFA, March

1999). Prospective payment to skilled nursing facilities is also adjusted for case mix and geographic variations (HCFA, April 1999).

Positive and negative incentives are built into these reimbursement schemes. The retrospective method of payment encourages organizations to inflate their prices in one area to offset agency losses in another. Furthermore, this system gives little incentive to providers to keep service costs low. In fact, prices under retrospective reimbursement often exceed the actual costs of delivering a service to include an additional amount to cover losses in other areas. These losses can result from providing service to nonpaying clients or from providing care to clients covered under plans that do not cover the total costs of delivering a service (Knickman and Thorpe, 1999). The major disadvantage of this system is that little regard is given to the costs involved. This practice of charging a payer at a higher rate to cover losses in the provision of care is referred to as *cost-shifting*.

Prospective cost reimbursement encourages agencies to stay within budget limits and adds an incentive for providing less service to contain or reduce costs. This method clearly provides financial incentives to agencies that keep costs and risks low. If an organization provides care to a particular patient or group of patients by keeping the costs of delivering the service lower than the amount of reimbursement, the provider keeps the difference; however, if the provider's costs exceed the reimbursement, the provider must assume the risk and pay the difference. The major disadvantage of this method is that organizations tend to overemphasize cost containment and risk compromising quality of care.

A growth in contracting for health care services, designed to create incentives for providers to compete on price, has occurred as managed care has increased in health care markets. For example, contracting, or competitive bidding, has been used in states to provide Medicaid services to eligible recipients. Hospitals and other health care providers who do not have a contract with the state to provide services are not eligible to receive Medicaid payments for client care. Managed care organizations also use this approach to negotiate with health care organizations, such as hospitals, for coverage of services to be provided to covered enrollees, often called *covered lives*.

Paying Health Care Practitioners

The traditional method of paying health care practitioners is known as **fee-for-service** (Knickman and Thorpe, 1999) and is analogous to the retrospective method described above. The practitioner determines the costs of providing a service, delivers the service to a client, and submits a bill for services delivered to a third-party payer, and the payer pays the bill. This method is based on usual, customary, and reasonable (UCR) charges for specific services in a given geographic region, determined by periodic re-

Economic Delivery of Health Care in Canada

Lianne Jeffs, Registered Nurses Association of Ontario and University of Toronto

HEALTH EXPENDITURES AND HEALTH STATUS

Health expenditures continue to rise in Canada, which ranks second among Organisation for Economic Cooperation and Development (OECD) countries in total health care spending, with 7.4% of its Gross Domestic Product (GDP) spent on health care (OECD, 1995). Health expenditures expressed as a percentage of GDP are a measurement of the proportion of a country's wealth that is devoted to the health of its population. Despite its high ranking, Canada's level of public health expenditure is similar to several European countries. In addition to direct public expenditures on health, public spending on income security, education, and labour market programs are also influential on the health status of a nation's population. The level of public spending on income security programs, provision of social welfare, public pensions, and unemployment benefits in Canada total 11.9% of the GDP, which is below the average of other OECD countries (OECD, 1994a, 1994c). The state of health of Canadians is among the best in the world, with long life-expectancy rates (77.63 years) and a low infant mortality rate of 0.67 per 100 births (OECD, 1994b).

In the late 1960s and early 1970s, concern that health care expenditures were increasing above inflation was the driving force behind several national reports (e.g., Commission of Inquiry on Health and Social Development, 1972; Hastings, 1973; Lalonde, 1975). These reports emphasised the need for greater efficiency and provision of less-expensive health care services. Currently, Canada's national health care system is based on two statutes: the Canada Health and Social Transfer (CHST) and the Canadian Health Act (CHA). The CHST is the vehicle through which funds are transferred from the federal government to provinces in support of hospital and medical insurance programs defined by the CHA. The CHA outlines the cost-sharing agreement between the federal and provincial governments. Following is a list of the major federal financial initiatives related to the Canadian health care system. At first glance, the CHA appears to take a broad definition of health; however, it is restricted to care provided in hospitals and by physicians. Public health is not formerly a part of the CHA, which places community health-promotion and disease-prevention programs and public health services at risk.

FINANCING OF THE CANADIAN HEALTH CARE SYSTEM

Financing of health care in Canada shifted from the private to the public sector in 1957. For over 40 years, mainly taxes and premiums collected by federal and provincial governments have financed the publicly funded health care system. The shortage of resources in the health care system and pressures of globalisation and trade liberalisation have opened the door to private initiatives, which threatens the viability of a publicly funded health care system. Financing of the Canadian health care system has both public and private sources. The methods of funding in the public sector are the result of a redistribution of public funds to institutions. Public sources include consolidated revenue funds, earmarked taxes, intergovernmental transfers, employer-based taxes, and volunteer and federal expenditures. Private sources include private insurance, point-of-service charges, philanthropic donations, lotteries, and premiums.

In Canada, governments have five main methods of payment to finance activities of their institutions: payment by global budget, per capita payment, payment by episode of care, fee-for-service payment, and per diem payment. Funding is distributed from the provincial governments' central health budget directly to individual and institutional providers within the municipalities or regions in a single-payer funding mechanism. Community health centres (CHCs), health service organizations (HSOs), and Community Care Access Centres (CCACs) receive global funding from the provincial government, and the funds are allocated for salaries, services, and operating costs according to the needs of the community they serve. With the recent downloading of public health services to the municipalities in the provinces, public health units will be receiving the majority or entire funding from regional sources.

FEDERAL, PROVINCIAL, AND MUNICIPAL ROLES IN THE ECONOMIC DELIVERY OF HEALTH CARE

Because health care is under provincial jurisdiction, the federal government has no direct power or influence on ensuring that provincial insurance plans cover health care services of other health care providers and outside hospitals and in the community and public health sectors. This has become a problem because technological advances have allowed for more care to be provided in the community and in home settings delivered mainly by registered nurses and other nonphysician providers. Some of the provinces have made attempts to shift institution-based services to community-based services; however, resources have not always followed. With the current funding arrangements, it is difficult to shift funds from one organisation to another. At the provincial level, health insurance acts and other legislation define what each health plan will pay for and under what conditions. Several provinces have extended their funding umbrella to provide for a fairly inclusive and comprehensive public health and health promoting system; however, coverage varies among provinces and territories. The recent change in legislation that has shifted public health services to the municipalities has ma-

Economic Delivery of Health Care in Canada–cont'd

jor implications for the funding of public health programs and services. Of particular importance are those programs with a health promotion and illness- and injury-prevention focus because municipalities that are faced with competing needs may opt to eliminate these services to provide other public health services such as garbage removal and sewage.

FEDERAL FINANCIAL INITIATIVES RELATED TO THE CANADIAN HEALTH CARE SYSTEM

1948 Grants for hospital construction and some general services

1953 Child and Maternal Health Care Act (social needs grants fixed amounts per unit of activity; payment was contingent on provincial reporting to the federal government)

1958 Hospital Insurance and Diagnostic Services Act (funding based on 25% of national per capita costs in the specific province × the provincial population; specified expenditures, no ceiling, and no conditions on provincial financing arrangements)

1968 Medical Care Act (Medicare) (funding based on 50% of national per capita cost × provincial population; provinces had to comply with four conditions: universality, comprehensiveness, public administration, and portability)

1976 Ceilings places on growth of Medicare grant (ceiling limit = population growth + 13% in 1976 and 10.5% in 1977)

1977 Established Programs Financing Act (equal per capita payment, block funding)

1984 Canada Health Act (provinces receive full federal payments if they comply with the principles of the CHA: portability, public administration, accessibility, universality, and comprehensiveness).

1996 Canada Health and Social Transfer (amalgamated EPF and Canada Assistance Plan into one cash transfer, fixed cash transfer for 1996 to 97 and 1997 to 98)

Bibliography

Deber R et al: The public private mix in health care. In *Striking a balance, volume 4: health care systems in Canada and elsewhere*, Quebec, 1998, Minister of Public Works and Government Services.

Maslove AM: National goals and the federal role in health care. In *Striking a balance, volume 4: health care systems in Canada and elsewhere*, Quebec, 1998, Minister of Public Works and Government Services.

Organization for Economic Cooperation and Development: *Employment outlook*, Paris, 1994a, OECD.

Organization for Economic Cooperation and Development: *Health data*, Paris, 1994b, OECD.

Organization for Economic Cooperation and Development: *New directions in social policy*, Paris, 1994c, OECD.

Organization for Economic Cooperation and Development: *Income distribution in OECD countries*, Paris, 1995, OECD.

Scott G: International comparison of the hospital sector. In *Striking a balance, volume 4: health care systems in Canada and elsewhere*, Quebec, 1998, Minister of Public Works and Government Services.

Canadian spelling is used.

gional evaluations of physician charges across specialties (Knickman and Thorpe, 1999). Historically, Medicare, Medicaid, and private insurance companies have used this method of reimbursing physicians.

A major effort to regulate and control the costs of physician fees was introduced in 1990 in the Omnibus Reconciliation Act. After a study by the Physician Payment Review Commission established by Congress, the resource-based relative value scale (RBRVS) was established. The RBRVS method reimburses physicians for specific services provided and the amount of resources required to deliver the service (Knickman and Thorpe, 1999). Resources are defined broadly and include not only the costs of providing the service, but also the training that is required to provide a particular service and the time required to perform certain procedures, including client diagnosis and treatment. The RBRVS method of reimbursement, adopted by Medicare in 1991, acknowledges the breadth and depth of knowledge required by primary care physicians in the community to provide services aimed at prevention, health promotion, teaching, and counseling.

Capitation is similar to prospective reimbursement for health care organizations. Specifically, third-party payers determine the amount that practitioners will be paid for a unit of care, such as a client visit, before the delivery of the service, thereby placing a limit on the amount of reimbursement received per patient (Knickman and Thorpe, 1999). In contrast to a fee-for-service arrangement, where the practitioner determines services that will be provided to clients and the charges for those services, practitioners being paid through capitation mechanisms are given the rate they will be paid for a client's care, regardless of specific services provided. Therefore, for example, physicians and other practitioners are aware, in advance, of the payment they will receive to perform a routine, uncomplicated physical examination or a more complex, detailed physical examination, diagnosis, and treatment (Knickman and Thorpe, 1999).

In capitated arrangements, physicians and other practitioners are paid a set amount to provide care to a given client or group of clients for a set period of time and amount of money. This arrangement, typically used by managed care organizations, is one whereby the practitioner contracts with the managed care organization to provide health care services to plan members for a predetermined and negotiated fee. The agreed-upon fee is negotiated between the practitioner and the managed care organization before the delivery of services and is set at a discounted rate, and the practitioner and managed care organization come to a legal agreement, or contract, for the delivery and payment of services. The managed care organization pays the predetermined fee to the practitioner, often before the delivery of services, to provide care to plan members for a set period of time (Knickman and Thorpe, 1999).

Practitioner reimbursement methods also have built-in incentives that affect service use and access. Fee-for-service arrangements place control over the number and kinds of services provided for a client in the hands of practitioners. Furthermore, the use of UCR charges encourages practitioners to charge maximum fees to the UCR charge schedule within a specific geographic area. Practitioners reimbursed through capitation have incentives to focus on efficiency, and in an effort to maximize reimbursement, to provide services to an increasing number of clients. The consumer, in turn, often is left responsible for any practitioner fees over the amount reimbursable through third-party coverage.

Reimbursement for nursing services

Historically, practitioners eligible to receive reimbursement for health care services included physicians only. However, nurses who function in certain capacities, such as NPs, clinical specialists, and midwives, also provide primary care to clients and receive reimbursement for their services. However, being recognized as primary care providers and eligible to receive reimbursement has not been an easy achievement.

Hospital nursing care costs traditionally have been included as part of the overall patient room charge and reimbursed as such. Other agencies, such as home health care agencies, include nursing care costs with administrative costs, supplies, and equipment costs. Nursing organizations, such as the American Nurses Association, have long advocated that nursing care should become a separate budget item in all organizations so that cost studies can show the efficiency and effectiveness of the nursing profession. Major efforts have been directed toward costing out nursing services and identifying the contributions of nursing to the system (Grimaldi et al, 1982; McKibbin et al, 1985; Melby, 1998; Stanhope, 1990; Thompson, 1984).

Spurred by efforts to control the costs of medical care, effective January 1, 1998, NPs and CNSs were granted third-party reimbursement for Medicare Part B services only under Public Law 105-33 (ANA, 1999b). This new law sets reimbursement for NPs and CNSs at 85% of physician rates for the same service, an extension of previous legislation that allowed the same reimbursement rate to NPs and CNSs practicing in rural areas.

NURSING TIP

The Rural Health Clinic Services Act of 1977 provided indirect reimbursement for NPs in rural health clinics, with payment going to clinics for nurses' salaries. The 1980 and 1989 Medicaid amendments to the Social Security Act provided direct reimbursement for nurse midwives, pediatric NPs, and family NPs. The 1989 amendments allow these nurses to provide services without physician supervision. In the 1990 Omnibus Budget Reconciliation Act, Medicare amendments included a provision for direct reimbursement of NPs and CNSs working in collaboration with a physician for services provided in rural areas. Direct reimbursement is also available to these nurses.

Enactment of this law was brought about by years of work in this area, including research documenting NP and CNS contributions to health care delivery and client outcomes and active lobbying efforts by professional nursing organizations. For example, landmark studies released by the Center for National Health Care Technology that provided support for the cost-effectiveness of NPs as primary care providers (Congress of the United States, Office of Technology Assessment, 1986; Leroy and Solkowitz, 1981). In recent years, other studies have provided further support for the cost-effectiveness of NPs and the cost-benefit ratio, efficiency, efficacy, and effectiveness of nursing services (Brown and Grimes, 1995; Burgel, 1993; Safriet, 1992).

Additionally, data about the cost-benefit ratio, efficiency, and effectiveness of nursing care in general has been made (Congress of the United States, Office of Technology Assessment, 1990; Stanhope, 1990).

Today, nurse-managed clinics provide health care services to individuals in the United States who might not otherwise have access to health care, such as the elderly, homeless, and school children. All of these events have moved the discipline toward more autonomous nursing practice and are serving as an impetus for evaluating and documenting nurses' contributions to health care delivery.

OTHER FACTORS AFFECTING RESOURCE ALLOCATION IN HEALTH CARE

The allocation of health care is affected largely by the way in which health care is financed in the United States. Third-party coverage, whether public or private, greatly affects distribution of health care. In addition to insurance status, socioeconomic status affects health care consumption through the ability to either purchase insurance or purchase services directly out-of-pocket. There are also other barriers to access to care. The effects of these factors and those of health care rationing on the allocation of health care are discussed.

The Uninsured

In 1996, 68% of the total U.S. population had private health insurance. An additional 15% received insurance through public programs, and 17%, or 37 million, were uninsured. In 1999 the number of uninsured has increased to 43.7 million. Of those under 65 years of age (nearly all of the elderly are covered through Medicare), 69% are covered through private insurance, 12% are covered by public insurance, and 19% are uninsured (Agency for Health Care Policy and Research, 1998). The typical uninsured person is a member of the workforce or their dependent. Uninsured workers, numbering 22 million individuals, or 17% of the workforce, are likely to be in low-paying jobs, part-time or temporary jobs, or jobs at small businesses (Kaiser Commission on Medicaid and the Uninsured, 1998). These uninsured workers cannot afford to purchase health insurance, and/or their employers may not offer health insurance as a benefit. Others who are typically uninsured are young adults, especially males, minorities, persons under 65 years of age in good or fair health, and the poor or near poor. These individuals may be unable to afford insurance, lack access to job-based coverage, or because of their age and/or good health status, may not perceive the need for insurance. Because of the eligibility requirements for Medicaid, the near-poor are actually more likely to be uninsured (27%) than the poor (23%).

The Poor

"Health disparities between poor people and those with higher incomes are almost universal for all dimensions of health" (USDHHS, 1991, p. 29). In fact, socioeconomic status (SES) is inversely related to mortality and morbidity for almost every disease. Poor Americans with an income below $10,000 a year have a mortality rate nearly three times that of Americans with incomes of $30,000 or more even after accounting for age, gender, race, education, and risky health behaviors (smoking, drinking, overeating, and lack of exercise) (Lantz et.al, 1998). Historically, the link between poor health and SES resulted from poor housing, malnutrition, inadequate sanitation, and hazardous occupations. Today, explanations for this phenomenon include the cumulative effects of a constellation of characteristics that explain the concept of "poverty." These characteristics include low educational levels, unemployment or low occupational status ("blue collar" or unskilled laborer), and low wages.

Access to Care

Medicaid is intended to improve access to health care for the poor. Although Medicaid recipients have improved access (approximately twofold) when compared with the uninsured, Medicaid recipients are only about half as likely to obtain needed health services (medical/surgical care, dental care, prescription drugs, and eyeglasses) as the privately insured (Berk and Schur, 1998). Specifically, "the poorest Americans have Medicaid insurance, yet they also have the worst health" (Income and health, 1998).

Insurance coverage is often used as a ticket to access to health care (i.e., insurance coverage gives one opportunity to get health services). In reality, access to care extends beyond insurance coverage. The poor and near poor are more likely to lack a usual source of care, more likely to postpone needed medical care, less likely to use preventive services, and consequently, more likely to be hospitalized for avoidable conditions than those who are not poor (USDHHS, 1998).

The primary reasons for delay, difficulty, and/or failure to access care include inability to afford health care (59.9%) and insurance-related reasons (19.5%), including insurer not approving, covering, or paying for care; having preexisting conditions; and doctors' refusing to accept the insurance plan. Other barriers include lack of transportation, physical barriers, communication problems, child care needs, lack of time or information, or refusal of services by providers (Weinick, Zuvekas, and Drilea, 1997). Additionally, lack of after-hours care, long office waits, and long travel distance are cited as access barriers (Forrest and Starfield, 1998). Community characteristics also contribute to individuals' ability to access care. For example, the prevalence of managed care and the number of safety net providers, as well as the wealth and size of the community, affect accessibility (Cunningham and Kemper, 1998).

Because reimbursement for services provided to Medicaid recipients is low, physicians are discouraged from providing services to this population. Thus people on Medicaid frequently have no primary care provider and often rely on the emergency department for primary care services (McNamara, Witte, and Koning, 1993; Nadel, 1993). Although physicians can respond to monetary incentives in client selection, emergency depatments are required by law to evaluate every client regardless of ability to pay. Emergency department copayments are modest and are frequently waived if the client is unable to pay (Kellerman, 1994). Thus low out-of-pocket client costs provide incentives for Medicaid clients and the uninsured to use emergency depatments for primary care services (Gill, 1994). Consequently, the uninsured and people on Medicaid and Medicare use disproportionately more emergency depatment services than those who have private third-party coverage (Nadel, 1993). Additionally, members of racial and ethnic minority groups and those of low SES are often dependent upon emergency depatments as a regular source of care. Such inappropriate use of services is inefficient and costly.

Health Care Rationing

Escalating health care spending has spurred renewed interest in health care rationing. As health care costs continue to grow, the opportunity costs of health care, or money available to spend on other needs, increases. With unsuccessful attempts at cost containment and cost reduction, new plans are being considered to control the use of services and technologies.

Rationing is not new to health care. For decades the uninsured and those who do not qualify for federal programs have been denied care or have been eligible only for limited services. The absence of universal health care and federal program eligibility criteria are other examples of health care rationing.

By 1990, Oregon had passed the Basic Health Services Act to ensure basic health care to all state citizens. This plan, recognized as a model health plan, used a priority ranking system of health services according to their effectiveness and benefit. High-cost technologies that produced only marginal benefit were not provided under the plan (Dougherty, 1991).

The key point in the Oregon plan is that a minimum set of covered services was established. Through limiting coverage to basic services, cost increase is managed. Opponents to this system argue that specialty services not covered by the plan can only be consumed by those residents who can purchase those services out-of-pocket either directly or through supplemental insurance. Efforts have been made (in Oregon and elsewhere) to expand coverage to include additional services; however, critics against state and federal mandates to expand insurance coverage for more services (such as chiropractors and podiatrists) argue that expansion of coverage beyond basic services increases costs (American HealthLine, 1998). As a result, individuals and employers refuse to pay for insurance coverage, and the number of uninsured rises.

Since demands for health care are insatiable while resources are limited, decisions regarding distribution of care must be made. Although there is still social support for national universal coverage for basic services, no agreement in terms of implementing such a plan has emerged. As a result, decisions regarding resource allocation are predominately based on how the care of individuals is financed.

Rand Corporation studies have shown that clients and providers will make choices based on who pays. The ability and willingness of individuals to pay through a fee-for-service system, or any cost sharing such as an insurance deductibles, decrease contact with the health care system (client self-rationing). "Free care" results in quicker decisions by clients to seek health care. Conversely, when the client is paying, quicker decisions are made by the provider to offer more complex care. Such provider practices are often affected, however, in a managed care system with set capitation payments. Insurers also determine allocation of care through preexisting condition clauses and through selective coverage of individuals and services. The ability of an individual to receive a certain medical technology, such as laser angioplasty, may depend upon the health plan in which they are enrolled since health insurance plans vary dramatically in their coverage of new technologies (Steiner et al, 1997). Additionally, insurance companies may either deny coverage or increase premiums based on lifestyle risks such as lack of seat belt use, drinking, and smoking habits.

Rationing health care in any form implies reduced access to care and potential decreases in acceptability and quality of services offered. Managed care offers the possibilities of more appropriate allocation of health care and better organized care to meet basic health care needs of the total population. A shift in the general approach to health care in the United States from a reactionary, acute-care orientation toward a proactive, primary prevention orientation is necessary to achieve not only a more cost-effective but also a more equitable health care system.

PRIMARY PREVENTION

While improving access to care is and has been a focus of health care reform and a worthy goal to accomplish, the benefits of reducing access to care differences will only affect health outcomes to the extent that health care services affect health outcomes. As noted by Pincus and colleagues (1998), access to medical services is critical to outcomes of acute processes but seems limited in its capacity to affect outcomes of outpatient care. To support the argument that access to care and consumption of health care plays only a small role in affecting health status, Pincus and colleagues (1998) note that in the United Kingdom, where there is universal access through the National Health Service, health differences by SES widened between 1970 and 1980.

Society's investment in the health care system has been based on the premise that more health services equal better health. There are, however, other non–health care factors that affect health. There are four major factors that affect health levels: personal behavior/lifestyle, environmental factors (including physical, social, and economic environments), human biology, and the health care system. Of these four major factors, medical services are said to have the least effect on health. Attempts to quantify the effect of these four factors on health reveals that behavior and lifestyle have the greatest effect on health, followed by environment and biology accounting for 70% of all illnesses (USDHHS, 1991). Despite the significant role of behavior and environment on health, estimates indicate that 97% of health care dollars is spent on secondary and tertiary care. Such a reactionary, secondary-care system results in high cost, high technology, and disease-specific care and is consistent with the U.S. system's historical emphasis on "sickness care." A more proactive investment in disease prevention and health promotion targeted at improving health behaviors, lifestyle, and the environment has the potential to improve health status, thereby improving quality of life while reducing health care costs. The USDHHS has argued that a higher value should be placed on primary prevention. The goal of this approach is to preserve and maximize human capital through providing health promotion and social practices that result in less disease. An emphasis on primary prevention may reduce dollars spent and increase quality of life.

The reality is that health care resources are limited, and this has resulted in health care rationing. The return on investment in primary prevention through gains in human capital has, unfortunately, not been acknowledged. Consequently, significant investments in primary prevention and public health care have not been made. Reasons given for lack of emphasis on prevention in clinical practice and lack of financial investment in prevention include the following (Young, Griffith, and Kamerow, 1994):
• Provider uncertainty concerning which clients should receive services and at what interval
• Lack of education about preventive services
• Negative attitudes about the importance of preventive care
• Lack of time for delivery of preventive services
• Delayed or absent feedback regarding success of preventive measures
• Lack of reimbursement for these services
• Lack of organization to deliver preventive services
Additionally, C. Everett Koop (Fries et al, 1998), former U.S. Surgeon General, notes that greed in the health care industry is a significant factor in the lack of investment in primary prevention.

A focus on prevention could mean a reduction in the need for and use of medical, dental, hospital, and health provider services. Under fee-for-service payment, this would mean that the health care system, the largest employer in the United States, would be reduced in size and would become less profitable. However, with the increasing costs of health care, consumer demand, and changes in financing mechanisms, there is a new trend toward financing more preventive care services. Today, the third-party payers are beginning to cover preventive services, recognizing that the growth of the health care system can no longer be supported. Under capitated health plans, health care providers stand to make money by keeping clients healthy and reducing health care use. Only through aligning client interests with financial interests of the health care industry will primary prevention and public health be raised to the status and priority of acute care and chronic care.

Although critical in building the argument for making the investment, quantifying the cost-effectiveness of prevention is challenging, imprecise, and filled with criticisms. Often, indirect evidence must be used to demonstrate effectiveness of an intervention. Also, it is often necessary to demonstrate potential effects through estimating attributable risk (the amount of disease or injury that could be eliminated if the risk for that disease or injury were avoided) and prevented fraction (the amount of a health problem that has actually been avoided by a prevention strategy). Other factors also must be considered, such as variations in compliance, use, and efficacy (Haddix et al, 1996). The time lag between intervention, improvements in health status, and effects on overall health and

costs of care also runs counter to the American quick-fix, immediate-gratification culture (Fries et al, 1998).

Despite difficulties, methods for determining prevention effectiveness are becoming standardized and used more widely, such as cost-effectiveness and benefit-cost analysis. Regardless of the method, prevention effectiveness analyses are outcome oriented. This area of research seeks to link interventions with health outcomes and economic outcomes and reveal the trade-offs between the two.

Theoretical support for increasing national investment in primary prevention is sound and long-standing. Since the public health movement of the mid nineteenth century, public health officials, epidemiologists, and public health nurses have been working to advance the agenda of primary prevention to the forefront of the health care industry. Today, these efforts continue across a number of disciplines and in both the public and private sectors, as shown in Box 5-8.

ECONOMICS AND THE FUTURE OF COMMUNITY AND PUBLIC HEALTH NURSING PRACTICE

The failure of sweeping health care reform during the 1990s opened the door to the market-driven growth of managed care. The American Nurses Association notes that managed care offers the potential of bringing improvements in the health care delivery system, such as eliminating waste and redundancy, a greater focus on health promotion and disease prevention, more attention to chronic illness, and a focus on accountability of providers, practitioners, and payers. This potential has gone unrealized. An overt emphasis on profit-making, "bottom-line" approaches that often appear to come at the expense of quality and access has highlighted managed care as it exists today (ANA, 1999a).

Accounts of mistreatments in health care frequently are reported in the press. In response, numerous bills were introduced at the state and federal levels in 1996 and 1997 to regulate managed care and/or consumer protection. Notable enactments include the Patient Protection Act (Box 5-9) and the HIPAA. The President's Advisory Commission on Consumer Protection and Quality in the Health Care Industry in1998 also developed a Consumer Bill of Rights and Responsibilities, and current congressional efforts are underway to protect the public against unsafe service delivery practices and to ensure quality.

The balance of interest within society and health care will continue to shift toward a focus on quality in the remainder of the twentieth century. Health care system concerns of the twenty-first century are expected to focus on examining the quality of health care relative to the costs of care delivered (i.e., the value derived from various care delivery models and providers and organizing and prioritizing available health care resources). These changes will result from continued efforts of both the public and private sectors to reform the U.S. health care system. The current era of health care delivery will be noted as a time of vast changes in all sectors of health care delivery.

BOX 5-8 How to Promote the Health and Well-Being of the American People

PEW CHARITABLE TRUSTS

Pew's Health and Human Services program's (*Public Voices, Public Choices*) foci:
- Public health
- Bioethics
- Health care delivery systems
- Welfare reform
  Pew Health Professions Commission
- Access to care for all
- Cost-effective use of resources
- Market efficiency coupled with public compassion
- Orientation to health rather than medical care
- Participation by the public, both individually and collectively
- Evidence-based decision making

FEDERAL RECOMMENDATIONS

Public Health Service: *Healthy People* (US Department of Health, Education, and Welfare, 1979)
- Elimination of cigarette smoking
- Reduction of alcohol use
- Moderate dietary changes to reduce intake of excess calories, fat, salt, and sugar
- Moderate exercise
- Periodic screening for major causes of morbidity and mortality, such as cancer
- Adherence to speed laws and use of seat belts

Public Health Service: *Healthy People 2000* (USDHHS, 1991)
- Health promotion
- Family planning
- Mental health
- Health protection

NURSING'S AGENDA FOR HEALTH CARE REFORM*
- Restructured health care system emphasizing access, primary care, and community care
- Use of cost-effective providers
- Personal health and self-care
- A standard package of essential health care services for all citizens, phased in
- Planned health care services representing national demographics
- Steps to reduce health care costs based on managed care
- Case management
- Long-term care
- Insurance reforms
- No payment at point of care
- Establishing a public or private review to monitor the system

*American Nurses Association. *Nursing's agenda for health care reform.* Washington, DC, 1991, American Nurses Publishing.

BOX 5-9 Elements of the Patient Protection Act

Guaranteeing a Patient Right-to-Know will allow free and open communications between patients and doctors in order to make fully-informed decisions about the best course of treatment. This is commonly referred to as lifting "gag rules" placed on medical providers.

Ensuring Access to Emergency Care by Applying Prudent Layperson Standards will guarantee that patients will be treated in emergency departments when they need care most by prohibiting health plans from arbitrarily refusing to pay for covered emergency benefits.

Providing Direct Access for OB/GYNs will allow women the opportunity to bypass the insurance company's gatekeeper and go directly to their provider.

Disclosing Plan Information will make it easier for patients to learn what their health plan covers specifically, including benefits, doctors, and facilities. It also enables patients to better compare coverage information between health plans.

Expediting Internal Review will hold insurance companies accountable by giving patients access to immediate decisions from doctors about what is covered for emergency, urgent, and routine services without preventing legal options already provided under current law.

Providing Independent Medical Expertise in External Appeals will guarantee unprecedented patient protection by requiring that an independent doctor decides if a requested service is medically necessary, if originally turned down by internal review.

Creating Association Health Plans will provide avenues so small businesses can pool together for their employees to enjoy the kinds of coverage afforded in big businesses.

Guaranteeing Patient Choice of Doctors will allow new avenues to health care coverage where quality and choice are unavailable by requiring health plans to offer point-of-service options.

Improving Medical Savings Accounts will make it easier for patients to increase access to health care services and have greater control over their health care dollars.

Creating HealthMarts will increase consumer choice by serving as a cooperative group marketplace where working families may choose from a menu of benefit options.

Creating Community Health Organizations will promote expansion of health coverage to all patients within their communities.

Reforming Health Care Lawsuits will hold down costs by ensuring that doctors are free to practice medicine responsibly without the fear of unnecessary litigation, excessive legal damages, or greedy trial lawyers.

Safeguarding Medical Record Confidentiality will protect personal and sensitive health care data from abuse.

From HR 4250 Patient Protection Act of 1998, 105th US Congress, July 16, 1998.

Nurses must plan for future changes in health care financing by becoming aware of the costs of nursing services, identifying aspects of care where cost savings can be safely achieved, and developing knowledge on how community nursing practice affects and is affected by the principles of economics. In this century, nursing must continue to focus on improving the overall health of the nation, defining its contribution to the health of the nation, deriving the value of nursing care, and ensuring its economic viability within the health care marketplace. Nurses must effect health care system change by providing leadership in developing new models of care delivery that provide effective, high-quality care and assuming a greater role in evaluating client care and nurse performance. It is through their leadership that nurses will contribute to improved decision making about the allocation of scarce health care resources.

clinical application

Connie, a community health nursing student, has identified a case load of five families in a home health nursing program offered by the local public health department. She is interested in assessing the costs of care to her clients and to the agency. Connie approaches the public health nurse administrator and asks the following questions:

A. How is the agency reimbursed for home health visits?
B. How is the payment for the visit determined?
C. Are nursing care costs known?
D. Are visits rationed to clients?

Answers are in the back of the book.

KEY POINTS

- From 1800 to the 1980s the U.S. health care delivery system experienced three developmental stages, with different emphasis on health care economics. Since 1985, the health care delivery system has entered a fourth developmental stage.
- Four basic components provide the framework for the development of health care services delivery: service needs and intensity, facilities, technology, and labor (workforce).
- Three major factors have been associated with the growth of the health care delivery system: price inflation, changes in population demographics, and technology and service intensity.
- Health care financing has evolved through the twentieth century from a system financed primarily by the consumer to a system financed primarily by third-party payers.
- To solve the problems of rising health care costs, a number of plans for future payments of health care are being considered; all include some form of rationing.
- Excessive and inefficient use of goods and services in health care delivery has been viewed as the major cause of rising health care costs.
- The concept of human capital has evolved in economics as a way to measure the value society places on the worth of an individual.

- The goal of health economics is maximum benefits from services of health providers, leading to health and wellness of the population.
- Economics is concerned with use of resources, including money, to fulfill society's unlimited wants.
- Health economics is concerned with the problems of producing services and programs and distributing them to clients.
- The goal of public health is providing the most good for the most people.
- Nurses need to understand basic economic principles to avoid contributing to rising health care costs.
- The GNP reflects the market value of goods and services produced by the United States.
- The GDP reflects the market value of the output of labor and property located in the United States.
- Microeconomic theory shows how supply and demand can be used in health care.
- Macroeconomic theory helps one to look at national and community issues that affect health care.
- Social, economic, and communicable disease epidemics mark the problems of the twenty-first century.
- Medicare and Medicaid are two government-funded programs that help meet the needs of high-risk populations in the United States.
- Health care reform focused primarily on health insurance reform will change the way health care is delivered and financed in the twenty-first century.
- 68% of the U.S. population has health insurance. The remaining uninsured represents millions of people, mostly the working poor, elderly persons, and children.
- Poverty has a detrimental effect on health.
- Health care rationing has always been a part of the U.S. health care system.
- Nurses are cost-effective providers and must be an integral part of managed care.
- *Healthy People 2000* is a document that has established U.S. health objectives.
- Human life is valued in health economics, like money. An emphasis on changing lifestyles and preventive care will reduce the unnecessary years of life lost to early and preventable death.

critical thinking activities

1. Define the following terms in your own words: economics, health economics, gross national product, gross domestic product, consumer price index, and human capital.
2. Compare the advantages and disadvantages of applying economics to public health care issues.
3. Compare and contrast efficiency and effectiveness, with reference to community health.
4. Apply the concepts of supply and demand to an example from community health.
5. Review Chapter 6. Debate in the class the ethical implications of the goal of rationing. Focus your debate on the implications for nursing practice.
6. Invite a public health nurse administrator to meet with your class or clinical conference group. Ask how inflation, changes in population, and technology have changed the public health care delivery system and nursing practice.

Bibliography

Agency for Health Care Policy and Research: *Medical Expenditure Panel Survey highlights: health insurance coverage in America 1996* (AHCPR Pub. No. 98-0031), Rockville, Md, 1998, AHCPR.

Aiken LH, Sochalski J, Anderson GF: Downsizing the hospital nursing workforce, *Health Affairs* 15(4):88, 1996.

American Nurses Association: *Managed care legislation–1997,* May 1999a (www.nursingworld.org/gova/hod97/mgdcare.htm)

American Nurses Association: *Medicare reimbursement for NPs and CNSs, May 1999b* (www.nursingworld.org/gova/medreimb.htm)

American Nurses Association. *Nursing's agenda for health care reform.* Washington, DC, 1991, American Nurses Publishing.

Banta HD: Technology assessment in health care. In Kovner A, editor: *Health care delivery in the United States,* New York, 1995a, Springer.

Banta HD: What is health care? In Kovner A, editor: *Health care delivery in the United States,* New York, 1995b, Springer.

Berk ML, Schur CL: Access to care: how much difference does Medicaid make? *Health Affairs* 17(3):169, 1998.

Boyes WJ: *Macroeconomics intermediate theory and policy,* ed 3, Cincinnati, Ohio, 1992, South-Western Publishing.

Brown SA, Grimes DE: *Nurse pracitioners and certified nurse-midwives: a meta-analysis of studies on nurses in primary care roles,* Washington, DC, 1995, American Nurses Publishing.

Bureau of Labor Statistics, US Department of Labor: *Occupational outlook handbook, 1998-99 Edition,* Washington, DC, 1998, Superintendent of Documents, U.S. Government Printing Office (Bulletin 2500).

Burgel BJ: *Innovation at the worksite: delivery of nurse-managed primary health care services.* Washington, DC, 1993, American Nurses Publishing.

Chernew ME et al: Managed care, medical technology, and health care cost growth: a review of the evidence, *Medical Care Research & Review* 55(3):259, 1998.

Cleland V: *The economics of nursing,* Norwalk, Conn, 1990, Appleton & Lange. Commonwealth Fund: *When employees choose health plans: do NCQA accreditation and HEDS data count? Sept 1998, Media Center news release* (www.cmwf.org/media/releases/gabel293-0915.asp)

Congress of the United States, Office of Technology Assessment: *Health Care in rural America,* Washington, DC, 1990, US Government Printing Office.

Congress of the United States, Office of Technology Assessment: *Nurse practitioners, physician assistants, and certified nurse midwives: quality, access, cost and payment issues,* Health Program, 1986 (unpublished report).

Congressional Budget Office: *Major contributors to the revenue and spending projections: the economic and budget outlook, fiscal years 1998-2007, January 1999* (www.cbo.gov/showdoc.ctm?index=2&sequence=14&from=S)

Cunningham PJ, Kemper P: Ability to obtain medical care for the uninsured: how much does it vary across communities? *JAMA* 280(10):921, 1998.

Dougherty CJ: Setting health care priorities: Oregon's next step, *Hastings Center Report* 21(3):1, 1991.

Enthoven AC: The history and principles of managed competition, *Health Affairs* 12(Suppl):24, 1993.

Folland S, Goodman AC, Stano M: *The economics of health and health care,* New York, 1993, Macmillan.

Forrest CB, Starfield B: Entry into primary care and continuity: the effects of access, *American Journal of Public Health* 88(9):1330, 1998.

Fries JF et al: Beyond health promotion: reducing need and demand for medical care, *Health Affairs* 17(2):70, 1998.

Gill JM: Nonurgent use of the emergency department: appropriate or not? *Annals of Emergency Medicine* 24(5):953, 1994.

Ginsberg PB, Gabel JR, Hunt KA: Tracking small-firm coverage, 1989-1996, *Health Affairs* 17(1):167, 1998.

Gold MR et al: *Cost-effectiveness in health and medicine,* New York, 1996, Oxford University Press.

Grimaldi P et al: RIMs and the cost of nursing care, *Nurs Management* 13, 1982.

Haddix AC et al: *Prevention effectiveness: a guide to decision analysis and economic evaluation,* New York, 1996, Oxford University Press.

Health Care Financing Administration: *1998 Medicare chartbook: a profile of Medicare* (www.hcfa.gov/pubforms/chartbk.htm).

Health Care Financing Administration: *Case mix prospective payment for SNF's Balanced Budget Act of 1997, June 24, 1998* (www.hcfa.gov/medicare/overview.html)

Health Care Financing Administration: *HIPAA: the Health Insurance Portability and Accountability Act of 1996, Feb 22, 1999* (www.hcfa.gov/HIPAA/HIPAAHm.htm)

Health Care Financing Administration: *Hospital outpatient prospective payment system, March 11, 1999* (www.hcfa.gov/medicare/hopsmain.htm)

Health Care Financing Administration: *Medicare: a brief summary, May 1999* (www.hcfa.gov/medicare.ormedmed.htm#E13E1)

Health Care Financing Administration: *SNF prospective payment system,* April 8, 1999 (www.hcfa.gov/medicare/snfpps.htm)

Health insurance coverage: national consensus needed, *American HealthLine,* Oct 1, 1998.

HMO reform: still high on voters' list of concerns, *American HealthLine,* Sept 17, 1998.

Income and health: poor are left behind in health gains, *American HealthLine,* July 30, 1998.

Internal Revenue Service: *Understanding MSAs,* Nov 19, 1998 (www.irs.gov/forms_pubs/pubs/p96901.htm)

Kaiser Commission on Medicaid and the Uninsured: *Uninsured facts: the uninsured and their access to health care,* Washington, DC, 1998, the Commission.

Kellerman AL: Nonurgent emergency department visits: meeting an unmet need, *Journal of the American Medical Association* 271(24):1953, 1994.

Knickman J, Thorpe K: Financing for health care. In Kovner A, editor: *Health care delivery in the United States,* New York, 1999, Springer.

Kovner C: The health care workforce in the United States. In Kovner A, editor: *Health care delivery in the United States,* New York, 1999, Springer.

Lantz PM et al: Socioeconomic factors, health behaviors, and mortality: results from a nationally representative prospective study of US adults, *JAMA* 279(21):1745, 1998.

Leroy L, Solkowitz S: *The implications of cost-effectiveness analysis of medical technology,* US Congress, Office of Technology Assessment, Case Study no. 16, Washington, DC, 1981, US Government Printing Office.

Levit KR et al: National health expenditures, 1996, *Health Care Fin Rev* 19(1):161, 1997.

Levit KR, Lazenby HC, Braden BR: National health spending trends in 1996, *Health Affairs* 17(1):35, 1998.

Mauskopf JA, Bradley CJ, French MT: Benefit-cost analysis of hepatitis B programs for occupationally exposed workers, *J Occup Med* 33(6):691, 1991.

McCloskey J: Breaking the cycle. *J Prof Nurs* 11(2):67, 1995.

McKibbin R et al: *DRGs and nursing care,* HCFA grant No 15-C-98421/7-02, Kansas City, Mo, 1985, Center for Research, American Nurses Association.

McNamara P, Witte R, Koning A: Patchwork access: primary care in EDs on the rise, *Hospitals* 67(10):44, 1993.

Melby C: Physician and nurse reimbursement. *Online Journal of Issues in Nursing* (www.nursingworld.org/ojin/tpc6/tpc6_3.htm), June 10, 1998.

Moses EG: *The registered nurse population, findings from the national sample survey of registered nurses, March 1996,* Washington, 1997, Division of Nursing, Bureau of Health Professionals, Health Resources and Services Administration, PHS, USDHHS.

Nadel MV: *Emergency departments: unevenly affected by growth and change in patient use* (GAO/HRD-93-4), Washington, DC, 1993, U.S. General Accounting Office, Human Resources Division.

National Center for Health Statistics: *Healthy People 2000 review, 1997,* Hyattsville, Md, 1997, Public Health Service (PHS) 98-1256.

Nichols LM, Blumberg LJ: A different kind of 'new federalism'? the Health Insurance Portability and Accountability Act of 1996, *Health Affairs* 17(3):25, 1998.

O'Connor K: A disaster on the health care horizon. *Washington CEO* 9(4):12, 1998.

Pew Health Professions Commission: *Contemporary issues in health professions, education and workforce reform,* San Francisco, 1993, UCSF Center for the Health Professions.

Pickett G, Hanlon J: *Public health administration and practice,* St Louis, 1990, Mosby.

Pincus T et al: Social conditions and self-management are more powerful determinants of health than access to care. *Annals of Internal Medicine* 129:406, 1998.

Rice D: The health status and national health priorities. In Lee P, Estes C, editors: *The nation's health,* ed 4, Boston, 1994, Jones & Bartlett.

Safriet BJ: Health care dollars and regulatory sense: the role of advanced practice nursing, *Yale J Regulation* 9(2):417, 1992.

Smith S et al: The Health Expenditures Projection Team: the next ten years of health spending: what does the future hold? *Health Affairs* 17(5):128, 1998.

Stanhope, M. *An innovative approach to nursing care of the homeless/very poor,* Washington, DC, 1990, TSNI.

Steiner CA et al: Technology coverage decisions by health care plans and considerations by medical directors, *Medical Care* 35(5): 472, 1997.

Thompson J: The measurement of nursing intensity. In USDHHS: *Health Care Financing Review: 1984 annual supplement,* Baltimore, 1984, Health Care Financing Administration.

Thorpe K: Health care cost containment. In Kovner A, editor: *Health care delivery in the United States,* New York, 1995, Springer.

US Census Bureau: *Resident population of the United States: middle series projections 2006-2010 by sex, race, and Hispanic origin with median age, March 1996* (www.census.gov/population/projections/nation/nsrh/nprh0610.txt)

USDHHS: *Health: United States, 1993,* DHHS Pub No (PHS) 94-1232, Washington, DC, 1994, U.S. Government Printing Office.

USDHHS: *Health: United States, 1998,* DHHS Pub No (PHS) 98-1232, Washington, DC, 1998, U.S. Government Printing Office.

USDHHS: *Healthy People 2000: national health promotion and disease prevention objectives,* Washington, DC, 1991, USDHHS, Public Health Service.

US Department of Health, Education, and Welfare: *Healthy People: the Surgeon General's report on health promotion and disease prevention,* DHEW Pub No (PHS) 79-55071, Washington, DC, 1979, USDHEW.

Weinick RM, Zuvekas SH, Drilea SK: *Access to health care: sources and barriers, 1996,* Rockville, MD, 1997, Agency for Health Care Policy and Research. MEPS Research Findings No. 3. AHCPR Pub. No. 98-0001.

Weitzman BC: The quality of care: assessment and assurance. In Kovner A, editor: *Health care delivery in the United States,* New York, 1990, Springer.

Young S, Griffith H, Kamerow D: *Put prevention into practice: a program for community health centers, 1994* (www.hhs.gov/cgibin/waisgate?WAISdocID=870041254+1+0+0&WAISaction=retrieve).

Ethics in Commmunity-Oriented Nursing Practice

SARA T. FRY

OBJECTIVES

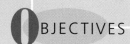 www.mosby.com/MERLIN/community_stanhope

After reading this chapter, the student should be able to do the following:

- Describe professional responsibilities in community health care.
- Identify the relationship of ethical rules, principles, and theories in community oriented nursing decisions.

- Discuss the application of ethical principles, including their potential conflicts.
- Apply the concept of accountability.
- Discuss clients' rights in today's health care system.
- Develop a nursing care plan that takes into account principles of ethics.

KEY TERMS

accountability	Code for Nurses	informed consent	right to health care
advance directive	codes of ethics	justice	rule of utility
advocacy	coercive health measures	maximin theory	rules
autonomy	confidentiality	Patient's Bill of Rights	theories
beneficence	egalitarian theory	principles	utilitarian theory
caring	entitlement theory	public health ethic	veracity
clients' rights	ethical decision making	right to health	*See Glossary for definitions*

CHAPTER OUTLINE

Community and public health nurses experience many ethical conflicts in today's health care delivery system. The nursing profession has traditionally upheld the rights and needs of the individual client. Today, however, this focus is difficult to maintain when nurses have the additional goal of improving the health of populations at risk. The traditional focus is also difficult to maintain when nursing resources are influenced by legislation and funding for specific population groups. One result of this latter difficulty is that other populations identified as being at risk are not adequately served by community-oriented nursing efforts because of the lack of funds. Nurses who experience this conflict between the individualistic focus of the professional ethic and the aggregate focus of public health recognize the dilemma of professional nursing in community health settings.

The purpose of this chapter is to analyze traditional ethics of professional nursing and apply these principles to the practice of community-oriented nursing. Since the client is the focus of all nursing actions, clients' rights are discussed first.

Not all nursing actions are simply related to clients' rights. General ethical principles, moral rules, and the various theories of social justice also influence health care delivery and nursing services. These principles, their definitions, and applications in community-oriented nursing are presented, and their priority in nursing is discussed. *Accountability*—being answerable to someone for what has been done in the nursing role—is a strong value in nursing, directing the nurse to practice professional skills and expertise in a certain way. Thus the development of methods to measure accountability is also a high priority in nursing. It is a priority because nursing must not only demonstrate the cost effectiveness of its services in promoting health and preventing illness, but it also must show how it meets normal requirements for professional practice. If nursing can demonstrate its ability to increase the community's health while meeting requirements for accountability to clients, great gains will be made in the name of community-oriented nursing services.

ETHICAL DECISION MAKING

Ethical decision making in the clinical area involves many variables. It can be enhanced by an orderly process that considers ethical principles, client values, and professional obligations. The need for this orderly process is demonstrated by the increasing use of ethical decision-making frameworks in nursing practice (Thompson and Thompson, 1985). Although such frameworks should not be used as foolproof formulas for ethical decision making, they help individual nurses explore moral issues and relevant values to arrive at specific decisions (Fry, 1989, 1994a).

Jameton's Method for Resolving Nursing Ethics Problems is a representative framework that can be used in community-oriented nursing practice (1984). His framework involves six steps and is summarized in the How To box that follows. The use of ethical decision-making frameworks can assist the community-oriented nurse in situations laden with conflicting values. They are not used to "solve" the moral conflict, but they do provide an orderly means for considering the issues involved.

:HOW TO *Make an Ethical Decision*

1. Identify the problem. *The nurse should clarify what is at issue: values, conflicts, and matters of conscience.*
2. Gather additional information. *The nurse should decide who the main decision maker is and what the clients or their surrogate decision makers want.*
3. Identify all the options open to the decision maker. *All possible courses of action and their outcomes should be considered. The likelihood of whether future decisions might have to be made should also be evaluated.*
4. Think the situation through. *Consider the basic values and the professional obligations involved. Explore the ethical principles and relevant rules.*
5. Make the decision. *The decision maker should choose the course of action that reflects his or her best judgment.*
6. Act and assess the decision and its outcomes. *The nurse should compare the actual outcomes of the situation with the projected outcomes. Can the process of decision making be improved for further situations having similar characteristics? Can this decision be generalized to other client care situations?*

Modified from Jameton A: *Nursing practice: the ethical issues,* Englewood Cliffs, NJ, 1984, Prentice-Hall.

There are a number of typical case situations found in the community and throughout this chapter. Jameton's Method for Resolving Nursing Ethics Problems should be used to analyze the issues and clarify the decision-making process. These questions will help in applying the moral concepts and ethical principles in this chapter to the nurse-client relationship. The cases are placed throughout the chapter to assist the reader to better understand the content of the chapter.

:HOW TO *Manage an Ethical Conflict*

Discuss the client care situation with the following:
• *Another nurse*
• *Nursing leadership*
• *A representative from the Ethics Committee*
• *The client or the client's family*
• *The client's physician*
• *A religious counselor*

CLIENTS' RIGHTS AND PROFESSIONAL RESPONSIBILITIES IN COMMUNITY HEALTH CARE
Clients' Rights

A right to health and a right to health care are often considered extensions of basic human rights. However, the recognition of other **clients' rights,** such as rights to informed consent, to refusal of treatment, or to privacy, have apparently been aided by consumer groups and health care providers such as the American Hospital Association (AHA) (Annas, 1996).

DID YOU KNOW? *One of the earliest recognitions of a right to health was made by the National Convention of the French Revolution in 1793. The leaders of the revolution declared that there should be only one patient to a bed in hospitals and that hospital beds should be placed at least 3 feet apart.*

Right to health

A **right to health** has been historically recognized as one of the basic human rights. When introducing the Public Health Act of 1875 to the British Parliament, Prime Minister Disraeli noted that "the health of the people is really the foundation upon which all their happiness and all their powers of state depend" (Brockington, 1956, p. 47). In modern times, the right to health has been considered comparable to the rights of life and liberty. The right to health obligates "the State to prevent individuals from depriving each other of their health" (Szasz, 1976, p. 478).

In the United States, early nineteenth-century public health measures, such as sanitation and water supply regulations to control the spread of disease, demonstrate early protective laws concerning human health and hygiene. However, most of these measures protected a negative right to health: the right to not have one's health endangered by the actions of others.

Positive obligations to provide services may seemingly "flow from negative rights" (Beauchamp and Faden, 1979, p. 124): The negative right to be free to enjoy good health may lead to the positive right to obtain certain services or have community health safeguards. For example, the negative right not to have one's health endangered by others led to public health measures concerning sewage disposal, water supplies, and the regulation of prostitution (Brockington, 1956). This negative right has even led to regulations concerning housing and measures protecting children's health. More recently, it has encouraged some health advocates to propose broad, federally supported programs and services to protect citizens against preventable diseases and disability (in particular, alcoholism and smoking-related illness) caused, in part, by social conditions (Beauchamp, 1985).

Thus, *advocacy,* in the guise of protecting a negative right to health, has helped open the door to consideration of the right to health as a positive right. It has been aided by documents such as the *Universal Declaration of Human Rights of the United Nations Assembly.* This document acknowledges the right of all persons to a standard of living adequate to provide for health and well-being and the right "to food, clothing, housing, and medical care" (UNESCO, 1949). This document suggests that persons have not only a strong negative right to health but also a strong positive right to health care. It suggests that persons are entitled to certain services, programs, and goods to maintain or achieve health as a basic human right.

Right to health care

Even though one may think that the "right to health" means "right to health care" (Daniels, 1979), the two terms explain different kinds of rights. The right to health is a negative right to a natural human good, which can be of various degrees. It is a right not to have one's health interfered with by others. However, the **right to health care** is a positive right to goods and services to maintain and improve whatever state of health exists. It is a rights claim against the state or its agencies to provide specific health care services. For example, immunization programs, kidney dialysis services, home health services for Medicare and Medicaid recipients, and federally funded prenatal and family planning services all recognize the positive right to specific health care services.

The distinction between the two terms is often blurred for two reasons. First, the World Health Organization (WHO) defines *health* as "a state of complete physical, mental, and social well-being and not merely the absence of disease or infirmity" (WHO, 1958, p. 459). The emphasis on complete physical, mental, and social well-being in this definition suggests that one is unhealthy without complete well-being. However, persons experience varying degrees of health but are not necessarily "unhealthy." Services must be provided to bring about physical, mental, and social well-being for one to possess complete health. Thus in recognizing a right to health, the right to health care services to achieve *complete* health must also be recognized.

This is obviously a mistake. The WHO definition of health should merely be considered an ideal state of health, one that very few persons actually possess or maintain over a long time. As a definition of an ideal state of health, it has no bearing on the provision of health care services as a right of all persons and should not be construed as a situation that must, in fact, exist.

A second reason why the distinction between the terms *right to health* and *right to health care* has become blurred stems from the recent advances of modern medicine and the willingness of government to support medical treatment for specific disorders such as renal disease (P.L. 92-603, 1972) and some genetic disorders (P.L. 92-278, 1976). This tendency has created an increase of expectations in terms of services to achieve optimal health. It seems as if government, in recognizing a right of citizens to be as healthy as possible, must necessarily recognize a right of citizens to have those services to achieve optimal health. Therefore by supporting treatment of some diseases and genetic disorders, government has created the idea that the right to health means a right to good health, a state that can only be achieved through the providing of specific health care services.

NURSING TIP

When protecting the rights of clients to receive high-quality health care (such as when requesting authorization from the health care insurer for more nursing care visits to a client), clarify the nurse's ethical responsibilities to the client using good communication and negotiation skills.

Yet this idea is clearly wrong. In an analysis of Szasz's position (1976), Bell points out that "the right to health does not include a right to health care because it does not include a right to good health (only a right to good health if I already have it)" (Bell, 1979, p. 162). Recognizing the right to health does not mean simply that the state is obligated to initiate health services to maintain health or improve it. Although there may be other reasons why the differences between the right to health and the right to health care are not clear, these two reasons are certainly important.

DID YOU KNOW? *In 1972 the AHA issued its study entitled the Patient's Bill of Rights. Soon, health care facilities began to use this document for health care providers to communicate rights to their clients. The bill affirmed the basic human rights of all clients who seek health care services (AHA, 1973). It included the rights to (1) receive considerate and respectful care, (2) obtain complete medical information, (3) receive information necessary for giving informed consent, (4) refuse treatment, (5) request services, (6) refuse participation in research projects, (7) expect reasonable continuity of care, (8) be informed of institutional regulations, (9) have privacy, (10) have personal information and medical records treated confidentially, (11) be provided with information on other institutions and individuals related to care and treatment, and (12) examine and obtain explanations of financial charges.*

Other rights

The rights to health and health care are not the only basic human rights of clients recognized by the health care delivery system. The basic human right of all clients to refuse treatment was formally legislated by the Omnibus Budget Reconciliation Act (OBRA) of 1990. The Patient Self-Determination Act (PSDA) became effective December 1, 1991. This act requires all health care institutions receiving Medicare or Medicaid funds to inform clients that they have the right to refuse medical and surgical care. Clients also have the right to initiate a written **advance directive,** a written or oral statement by which competent

persons make known treatment preferences and/or designate a surrogate decision maker if they should become unable to make medical decisions on their own behalf.

Home health care agencies and managed care organizations are required to make this information available in writing when the client comes under an agency's care. Box 6-1 lists the specific requirements of the PSDA.

Societal Obligations

The issue of client rights is a problem in health care delivery because society does not make clear its obligations to citizens regarding health. As a result, health care providers fail to recognize and protect clients' basic rights. To correct this problem, health professionals need to consider what society's obligations are to citizens regarding health and what kind of responsibilities health care providers have in response to client rights?

Discrepancies in availability of health services according to income or place of residence were reported by the President's Commission for the Study of Ethical Problems in Medicine and Biomedical and Behavioral Research in a lengthy document entitled *Securing Access to Health Care* (President's Commission, 1983). The commission reached several conclusions concerning current patterns of access to health care and made significant recommendations for changes.

The cornerstone of these conclusions is that "society has an ethical obligation to ensure equal access to health care for all" (President's Commission, 1983, p. 4). Commission members noted that this obligation "rests on the special importance of health care and is derived from its role in relieving suffering, preventing premature death, [and] restoring functioning" (p. 29). Considering these obligations, the commission recommended that costs for

BOX 6-1 Requirements of the Patient Self-Determination Act (PSDA)

- Provide written information to adult clients about their rights to make medical decisions, including the right to accept or refuse treatment and the right to formulate advance directives.
- Document in each client's record whether the client has previously executed an advance directive.
- Implement written policies regarding the various types of advance directives.
- Ensure compliance with state laws regarding medical treatment decisions and advance directives.
- Refrain from discriminating against individuals regarding their treatment decision specified in an advance directive.
- Provide education for staff and the community on issues and the law concerning advance directives.

From Omnibus Budget Reconciliation Act of 1990, sections 4206 and 4751, PL 101-508, Nov 5, 1990.

health care for those unable to pay ought to be spread equally at the national level and that costs should not be "allowed to fall more heavily on the shoulders of residents at different locations" (p. 30). The commission further recommended that the federal government assume ultimate responsibility for ensuring that equal access to health care for all is achieved "through a combination of public and private sector arrangements" (p. 29). These conclusions and recommendations are summarized in Box 6-2.

CASE 1   What Are Society's Obligations to the Client?

Mr. H is a 48-year-old man referred to the visiting nurse association for evaluation and treatment of stasis ulcers on his legs and for maintenance of a weight-reduction program for both Mr. H and his wife. Mr. H is 6 feet tall and weighs more than 380 pounds. Mr. And Mrs. H have a 27-year-old mentally retarded son.

When she visited the home, Karla Lowe, the visiting nurse, found large, oozing, sticky areas of raw tissue on Mr. H's legs. Ms. Lowe cleaned and dressed the ulcers and continued visiting them every other day for the next 3 months. As the ulcers began to heal, Ms. Lowe attempted to engage them in discussion about nutrition and hygiene and to encourage them to start a weight-reduction program. Mr. and Mrs. H were not interested and chose not to participate in any type of weight-reduction program.

BOX 6-2   Ethical Framework of the President's Commission

The Commission concluded the following:
- Society has an ethical obligation to ensure equitable access to health care for all.
- The societal obligation is balanced by individual obligations.
- Equitable access to health care requires that all citizens be able to secure an adequate level of care without excessive burdens.
- When equity occurs through the operation of private forces, there is no need for government involvement, but the ultimate responsibility for ensuring that society's obligation is met, through a combination of public- and private-sector arrangements, rests with the federal government.
- The cost of achieving equitable access to health care should be shared fairly.
- Efforts to contain rising health care costs are important but should not focus on limiting the attainment of equitable access for the least-served portion of the public.

From President's Commission for the Study of Ethical Problems in Medicine and Biomedical and Behavioral Research: *Securing access to health care, vol 1: report on the ethical implications of differences in the availability in health services,* Washington, DC, 1983, US Government Printing Office.

Several months went by, and Mr. H's ulcers stopped healing. When they began to deteriorate, he was hospitalized. Within a few weeks, they had healed enough that he could return home. Ms. Lowe visited his home to change dressings as before, but despite her efforts the ulcers deteriorated once again. It was too soon for him to return to the local hospital under his Social Security Supplemental Income benefits, so it was arranged to have him admitted to the state hospital. Two days later he signed himself out of this hospital. "It was too far away, and I didn't know anybody. Besides, they were too rough on me," he stated.

Angered by Mr. H's decision, his physician refused to continue treating him, and Ms. Lowe was left without any current physician orders. This meant that she could no longer give Mr. H physical care or receive reimbursement for her visits. Mr. H's unwillingness to cooperate in the development of "healthy behaviors" made him ineligible for the agency's health maintenance program. When Ms. Lowe explained the situation to her client, Mr. H said that Mrs. H could wash his legs and apply the medicine that Ms. Lowe had been applying. Besides, he did not think that his physicians had really helped him, and he had no intention of ever going to one again. He would miss Ms. Lowe's visits but thought he would manage. Ms. Lowe left a number to call if they ran into any unforeseen problems.

Nearly a year passed. One summer day Mrs. H called Ms. Lowe. She said that Mr. H was "awful sick" and had been in bed for nearly a month. The Visiting Nurse Association (VNA) policy allowed a one-time evaluation visit, so Ms. Lowe visited the home. She found Mr. H's legs alive with the larvae of the summer flies attracted to the steamy bedroom. She urged Mr. H to seek hospitalization. He would not be turned away, even if he no longer had a physician. Mr. H agreed, an ambulance was called, and Mr. H was transported to the local hospital. Because of the condition of his legs, a bilateral leg amputation was performed.

When news of Mr. H's general condition got out (he had created quite a sensation in the emergency department of the local hospital), the people of the small town were aghast. How could a man be allowed to rot away? Where were all the services? Who was responsible? The mayor appointed a special task force to investigate the matter. Months (and endless newspaper columns) later "no fault" was found, and it was announced that the town's health services "had sufficient mechanisms to prevent such a thing from ever happening again." Mr. H recovered, obtained prostheses, and moved to another state where he had family to help him.

Yet Ms. Lowe was not satisfied. Did the system fail clients such as Mr. H? Did clients have an obligation to accept the services offered to them and the recommendations of health workers who took care of them? If they refused to follow recommendations, did it mean that health care services should be totally withdrawn? Could the amputations have been prevented if Ms. Lowe had at least continued her visits and prevented the extreme condition of Mr. H's legs before his last hospitalization?

Discussion Questions

1. What are society's health care obligations to Mr. H?
2. What are the VNA's obligations to Mr. H according to the Patient Self-Determination Act?
3. Can the conclusions in the report of the President's Commission, *Securing Access to Health Care* (1983), help Ms. Lowe?
4. Is it reasonable for clients such as Mr. H to refuse treatments in advance by executing a written advance directive? Why or why not?

Professional Responsibilities

In response to clients' rights, health care professionals have particular duties or responsibilities, as illustrated in Figure 6-1. Some of these duties are supported by professional codes of ethics and correlate with the client's basic liberty rights.

Code duties

Professional **codes of ethics** are statements encompassing rules that apply to persons in professional roles. Two questions generally arise concerning the importance of these codes in health care delivery (Beauchamp and Walters, 1994):

1. What is their relation to universal moral principles?
2. What is their relation to legal requirements for professional practice?

In answering the first question, consider the rules contained in professional codes of ethics for nurses to be specific applications of more universal moral principles. Some professional codes of ethics are merely statements about professional etiquette or conduct between profes-

sional groups and have no relation to external principles. This is not the case in nursing. The professional code of ethics for nurses prescribes moral behavior and actions based on moral principles (Fry, 1994b). Thus the professional nurse has a moral obligation to follow the rules in a code of ethics such as the *Code for Nurses with Interpretive Statements* of the American Nurses Association (ANA, 1985).*

CASE 2 | **The Visiting Nurse and the Obstinate Client: Are Professional Responsibilities Ever Limited?**

Mr. Jeff Williams, team leader in Home Health Care Services at the county health department, was preparing to visit Mr. Chisholm, a 59-year-old client recently diagnosed as having emphysema. Well known to the health department, Mr. Chisholm was unemployed because of a farming accident several years earlier. Hypertensive and overweight, he was also a heavy long-term cigarette smoker despite his decreased lung function. Mr. Williams visited Mr. Chisholm to find out why the client had missed his latest chest clinic appointment. He also wanted to find out if the client was continuing his medications as ordered.

As Mr. Williams parked his car in front of his client's house, he could see Mr. Chisholm sitting on the front porch smoking a cigarette. A flash of anger made him wonder why he continued trying to teach Mr. Chisholm reasons for not smoking and why he took the time from his busy home care schedule to follow up on Mr. Chisholm's missed clinical appointments. This client certainly did not seem to care enough about his own health to give up smoking.

During the home visit, Mr. Williams determined that Mr. Chisholm had discontinued the use of his prophylactic antibiotic and was not taking his expectorant and bronchodilator medication on a regular basis. Mr. Chisholm's blood pressure was 210/114 mm Hg, and he coughed almost continuously. Although he listened politely to Mr. Williams's concerns about his respiratory function and the continued use of his medications, Mr. Chisholm simply made no effort to take responsibility for his health care. Even so, another clinic appointment was made, and Mr. Williams encouraged the client to attend.

As he drove to his next home visit, Mr. Williams wondered to what extent he was obligated as a nurse to spend time on clients who took no personal responsibility for their health. He also wondered if there was a limit to the amount of nursing care a noncooperative client could expect from a community health service.

Discussion Questions

1. What are Mr. Williams's professional responsibilities for Mr. Chisholm's rights to health care?

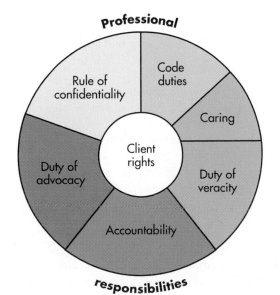

FIG. 6-1 Client rights and professional responsibilities.

---

*Hereafter referred to as *Code for Nurses.*

2. Is there a limit to the amount of care nurses should be expected to give to clients?

3. What authority defines the moral requirements and moral limits of nursing care to clients?

Modified from Veatch RM, Fry ST: *Case studies in nursing ethics*, Philadelphia, 1987, JB Lippincott.

In answering the second question, some of the rules in the **Code for Nurses** have legal ties to licensure requirements concerning professional acts. For example, the rules of respecting client confidentiality and accountability are mentioned in the *Code for Nurses* as both morally obligatory and legally required.

Codes of ethics also prescribe duties that are required of the professional in response to clients' rights (Fry, 1994b). The duties of veracity and advocacy are specifically mentioned in the *Code for Nurses* as correlating with clients' rights.

Veracity

Truthfulness has long been regarded as fundamental to the existence of trust among human beings. **Veracity** is a duty to tell the truth and not lie or deceive others. In health care relationships, several arguments are usually given in support of veracity (Beauchamp and Childress, 1994).

One argument claims that veracity is part of the respect that is owed other persons. Persons are respected because they are self-determining, or autonomous, individuals with all the rights and privileges of autonomous persons. These include the right to be told the truth and not be lied to or deceived. Because one respects persons and their autonomy, nurses have a duty of veracity. An example is being truthful to clients regarding the nature of the care they are receiving.

CASE 3 **When the Family Asks the Nurse Not to Tell the Truth**

Ralph Bradley, a recently widowed man in his mid-60s, was discharged from the hospital after exploratory surgery that disclosed colon cancer with metastasis to the lymph nodes. His physician referred him to a home health agency for nursing care follow-up. In reading the referral, the nurse learned that Mr. Bradley had been living with a married daughter and her family since his wife's death. An unmarried daughter apparently lived nearby, visiting him regularly and helping with his daily care. The referral did not explain what, if anything, the client had been told by his physician concerning his condition.

During the first home visit, it became apparent that Mr. Bradley did not know that the tumor removed from his body had been diagnosed as cancerous or that it had metastasized to the lymph nodes. He did not realize the seriousness of his condition, but he did express concern about his health. He complained of vague pain in the abdomen, asked for information about the results of the tests performed before

discharge from the hospital, and wanted to know how soon he would be able to return to his work as a cabinetmaker. When the nurse avoided a direct answer to these questions, Mr. Bradley asked directly, "Is everything all right?" The married daughter, who was present when her father was asking these questions, assured him that everything was all right and that he would soon be up and around.

Walking the nurse to her car when the visit was over, the married daughter confided that it was the family's wish that their father not be told how serious his condition was. She said that her mother's recent death had been very difficult for him to accept. They did not want him to be further burdened with the knowledge of his condition. The nurse listened, acknowledging the difficulties posed by the wife's recent death and the father's serious condition. She told the daughter, however, that it would be very difficult, if not impossible, for anyone from her agency to continue to provide nursing care to Mr. Bradley without his knowledge of his condition.

When she returned to her office, the nurse discussed Mr. Bradley's situation with her supervisor. The nurse did not want to continue visiting the client knowing he was being deceived by the physician and family. The supervisor suggested that she consult with the attending physician as soon as possible and explain that Mr. Bradley was asking questions about his condition. Luckily, the nurse was able to reach the physician before it was time to make the next home visit. She asked the physician what the client had been told about his condition. The physician said that at the family's request, Mr. Bradley had not been told that he had cancer. He said he agreed with the family that Mr. Bradley could probably not withstand the anxiety of knowing he had a terminal illness so soon after his wife's death. The physician also expressed concern about Mr. Bradley's daughters who, as he put it, "need a little time to accept the mother's death, as well as accept the impending death of the old man." The physician said that he would consider any act of disclosure on the nurse's part at this time to be inappropriate to her role as a visiting nurse and inconsistent with the well-being of the client and his family.

Discussion Questions

1. What is the professional duty of veracity?

2. What reasons might the nurse give for telling Mr. Bradley the truth?

3. What reasons might the nurse give for not telling Mr. Bradley the truth?

4. How does not telling the truth constrain nursing care in the community?

Modified from Veatch RM, Fry ST: *Case studies in nursing ethics*, Philadelphia, 1987, JB Lippincott.

A second argument claims that the duty of veracity is derived from, or is a way of expressing, the duty of keeping promises (Ross, 1930). Communicating with the client creates an implicit contract to tell the truth and not lie or deceive. The contract between client and nurse creates the expectation that nurses will, in interacting with the client, speak truthfully.

A third argument claims that relationships of trust are necessary for cooperation between clients and health care professionals. After all, not to tell the truth or to deceive clients will, in the long run, undermine relationships and cause undesirable consequences for future relationships with clients. Thus the nurse has a responsibility to maintain truthful relationships with clients to protect and strengthen other health care relationships in general.

However, nurses often have difficulty heeding or observing a duty of veracity. The truth is sometimes withheld or filtered because a nurse may think certain information will cause a client anxiety. Nurses also withhold information because they think that clients, particularly if very sick or dying, do not really want to know the truth about their conditions. However, this belief is not substantiated by surveys of sick and dying clients.

Regardless of the reasons for not telling the truth to clients or withholding information, it is clear that health professionals have a duty of veracity. As the *Code for Nurses** notes, "Clients have the moral right ... to be given accurate information, and all the information necessary for making informed judgments" (ANA, 1985, p. 2). In fact, the duty not to lie or deceive is a stronger moral duty than the duty to disclose information.[†] The duty of veracity correlates with the client's right to know and includes a strong moral obligation not to lie or deceive.

Confidentiality

In general social interaction, certain information is regarded as confidential. Regarding information as confidential enables control of the disclosure of personal information and limits the access of others to sensitive information (Fry, 1994a).

In community health care relationships, **confidentiality** of information is maintained for several reasons. If health care professionals did not follow a rule of confidentiality, clients might not seek help when they needed it. They would not reveal necessary information that would facilitate treatment. For example, family-planning clients might not reveal information about their reproductive history that would encourage appropriate and safe nursing care and follow-up treatment. Maintaining confidentiality helps protect the nurse-client relationships.

Another reason for maintaining confidentiality is that privacy is recognized as a basic human right. Because persons are self-determining moral agents, they have a right to determine how personal information, especially health information, is communicated. As the *Code for Nurses* points out, "The nurse safeguards the client's right to privacy by judiciously protecting information of a confidential nature" (ANA, 1985, p. 4). Because of respect for persons, nurses respect clients' rights to privacy by maintaining the moral rule of confidentiality.

In health care relationships, however, the duty to observe the rule of confidentiality is not always absolute. It is merely a *prima facie* duty (i.e., it may be overridden when in conflict with other duties that are morally stronger). The duty to observe confidentiality may be overridden for several reasons:

1. *When in conflict with other duties toward the client.* For example, the duty to preserve life may outweigh the duty to respect confidential information concerning self-destructive wishes of the client.
2. *When in conflict with duties toward identified others.* For example, if a mental health client tells the nurse of intent to harm or kill another member of the community, the nurse's duty to protect others by warning the intended victim will override the duty of confidentiality. This action may even be required by law (Tarasoff, 1976).
3. *When in conflict with duties toward unidentified others or the rights and interests of society in general.* For example, the law requires communicable diseases such as tuberculosis or venereal disease to be reported regardless of the confidential nature of that information. Another example includes health records used for epidemiological research without the client's knowledge. Of course, stringent constraints are placed on the use of this information by epidemiologists in health research (Gordis and Gold, 1980; Kelsey, 1981). In general, however, the duty to increase or protect the health of the community through research outweighs the duty to respect the confidentiality of health records.

CASE 4   The Nurse Who Could Not Protect the Client's Right to Confidentiality

Jane Sanborn was the occupational health nurse in a federal health agency. Among her responsibilities was the completion of the health status section of a form that included both personal and health history for periodic health examinations of the facility's employees. The physician completed the medical portion of the health report, recorded a decision about the employee's fitness for work, and returned the report to Ms. Sanborn, who maintained a confidential file for employees' health reports and records. Employees were asked to sign a statement on the health report that information in the report relating to employee fitness for the job could be shared with the employer as necessary.

One day Ms. Sanborn received a memo directing her to send a copy of an employee's health report to Washington,

---

*Quotations from *Code for Nurses* reprinted with permission of the ANA.

[†]The duty to disclose information evolves from special relationships between agents. In such relationships, one agent can claim a right to information that the other agent would not be obligated to provide to a stranger. The duty not to lie, however, does not depend on special relationships. Lying threatens any relationship because lying is telling something false to deceive a person.

D.C. for filing in a centralized data bank. Ms. Sanborn questioned the request and asked for an explanation of the purpose of the centralized file. No explanation was provided, and the original request was repeated. Ms. Sanborn responded that she would send the health record as soon as she obtained the consent of the employee. The employee's original consent was to share information only with his immediate employer. Before she could contact the employee, however, Ms. Sanborn was again asked to send the health record immediately; additional consent from the employee was not required. When she discussed the matter with the physician and the administrator of the health facility, Ms. Sanborn was told that she should comply with the request because it was the accepted practice to send any requested employee health records to the centralized file without obtaining consent from employees. Under pressure from both the physician and the administrator, she sent the health record to the centralized data bank.

Discussion Questions

1. Why did Jane Sanborn break confidentiality in this situation?

2. Is there a morally justifiable reason to override the employee's right to confidentiality in this case situation?

3. Why is the rule of confidentiality important in community health nursing?

Modified from Veatch RM, Fry ST: *Case studies in nursing ethics*, Philadelphia, 1987, JB Lippincott.

Advocacy

The nursing profession recognizes a strong duty of **advocacy** where the care or safety of clients is concerned. As the *Code for Nurses* states, ". . . the nurse must be alert to and take appropriate action regarding any instances of incompetent, unethical, or illegal practice by any member of the health care team or the health care system, or any action on the part of others that places the rights or best interests of the client in jeopardy" (ANA, 1985, p. 6). In the role of advocate, the nurse speaks for or in support of the best interests of the individual client or vulnerable client populations.

The role of advocate can be difficult for the nurse.

1. Clients should always determine what is in their best interests. Doing what the nurse thinks is in the best interests of clients can lead to paternalism when the wishes of clients are never ascertained.

2. The duty of advocacy extends to populations at risk, which may bring the public health nurse into conflict with health policy or established professional practices within a community or institution. Nurse advocates who have experienced this kind of conflict have sometimes found their jobs and other professional relationships in jeopardy. Positions of advocacy can be difficult to maintain when they conflict with accepted professional practices.

3. Does the duty of advocacy require nurses to put their own job, health, or professional standing at risk on behalf of advocacy for the client? According to Beauchamp and Childress (1994), this is not a moral requirement of the principle of beneficence. The nurse must fulfill the primary commitment to client care and safety by protecting the client from harm. The implicit contract of the nurse-client relationship does, in general, require positive acts of benefiting from care rendered. However, strictly speaking, this contract does not extend to the role of advocate. Thus the community health nurse is only required, in the role of advocate, to protect, speak for, and support the interests of the client not to be harmed by providing health care services.

⋮ CASE 5   The Nurse Epidemiologist and Newborn Morbidity Statistics

Sharon Smith was the public health nurse responsible for interpreting mortality and morbidity statistics for her county public health department. Based on a preliminary listing of figures, she initiated a comparative study of newborn morbidity from the death certificates of infants delivered at five county hospitals. The study revealed that one hospital had a high rate of newborn deaths. On closer observation, the nurse found that the interns and residents of this hospital were using a particular kind of instrument-assisted delivery. When she presented her findings to the county health officer, he shelved the report. She persisted and eventually went public with her findings. Despite eventual investigation into the matter and a change of the procedures at the hospital in question, Ms. Smith was labeled "a traitor" by officials at her health department, and she lost the support of nurse colleagues employed by the county public health agency. After several months of this treatment, she resigned her position.

Discussion Questions

1. What does the duty of advocacy mean in this case situation?

2. What is the appropriate action for the nurse in protecting the health, welfare, and safety of the client?

3. Does the duty of advocacy override personal concerns of the nurse? Why or why not?

Modified from Veatch RM, Fry ST: *Case studies in nursing ethics*, Philadelphia, 1987, JB Lippincott.

Caring

The value of **caring** is widely recognized as important to the nurse-client relationship (Fry, 1994a). Caring behavior is expected of the nurse and is generally considered fundamental to the nursing role. Leininger (1984), for example, argued that caring has a direct relationship on human health. Her research demonstrates that all cultures and communities practice caring behaviors that reduce intercultural stresses and conflicts and protect human survival.

Recent feminist interpretations of human caring relate it to ethical behaviors and choices. Noddings (1984) states that ". . . to care may mean to be charged with the protection, welfare, or maintenance of something or someone" (p. 9). Nurse caring is specifically directed toward the protection of the health and welfare of clients in the community. When caring is valued as important to the nursing role, it indicates a commitment toward the protection of human dignity and the preservation of human health.

Pellegrino (1985) also characterized caring as a moral obligation or duty among health professionals. He believed that one is obligated to promote the good of another with whom a special relationship exists. Since nurses have special relationships with their clients, they are called upon and expected to provide caring behaviors to those who have health needs. Caring is a form of involvement with others that is directly related to concern about how other individuals experience their world (Benner and Wrubel, 1989). Caring is therefore always practiced within some context, and its significance is interpreted in terms of the special duties or obligations between individuals within that context (Fry, 1994a).

CASE 6 The Client Who Did Not Want to Be Clean

Marion Downs, a community health nurse, must decide whether to refer her client, 72-year-old Sadie Jenkins, to the community court fiduciary for consideration of conservatorship and guardianship. Miss Jenkins has no living relatives and lives alone in a one-room apartment furnished with a bed, refrigerator, table, chair, lamp, and small sink. Since she does not have a stove, two meals per day are supplied by her landlord. With the support of her Social Security check and food stamps, she has adequate money for her needs and has lived for more than 10 years in these arrangements. She is also in good physical health.

Marion has made four home visits to Miss Jenkins to check her vital signs and medication routine after recent treatment in the Health Center's Hypertension Clinic. Although Miss Jenkins has made excellent progress and no longer requires visits from the community health nurse, her landlord, the other residents of her small apartment building, and her immediate neighbors are urging the nurse to "do something" about Miss Jenkins. Admittedly, Miss Jenkins's apartment has a strong odor from the long-term accumulation of dust, dirt, and mold. There are visible cockroaches in the apartment, and an unemptied bedpan is often sitting next to Miss Jenkins's bed (it is "too much trouble," Miss Jenkins stated, to walk to the hall bathroom shared by Miss Jenkins and two other tenants). Marion has noticed that Miss Jenkins has worn the same soiled clothes every time she has been to her apartment. It is also obvious that Miss Jenkins has not bathed for a long time, her hair is unwashed, and she apparently does not clean her nails and dentures. In addition, her toenails are so long that they

have perforated the canvas of her tennis shoes, apparently the only shoes that she likes to wear.

However, Miss Jenkins is comfortable with her lifestyle and does not want to change her living arrangements. Although Marion has offered to contact agencies to help Miss Jenkins, homemaker service, counseling, and senior citizens, Miss Jenkins says that she is comfortable and does not want or need help from anyone.

Discussion Questions

1. Should Marion use her role of community health nurse to create an arrangement by which Miss Jenkins would lose the right to control her person, her financial resources, and her environment?
2. Can an individual in the community be forced to be clean and to live in a clean environment?
3. How far should a nurse go in providing "good" for a client, and who determines what is "good"?

Modified from Veatch RM, Fry ST: *Case studies in nursing ethics,* Philadelphia, 1987, JB Lippincott.

Accountability

Nursing has long recognized the need for moral accountability in responding to basic human rights in practice. In the *Code for Nurses,* accountability is defined as "being answerable to someone for something one has done" (ANA, 1985, p. 8). **Accountability** includes providing an explanation to oneself, the client, the employing agency, and the nursing profession for what one has done in the role of nurse. It is an obligation that has both moral and legal components and implies a contractual agreement between two parties. When a nurse enters into a contractual agreement to perform a service for a client, the nurse will be held answerable for performing this service according to agreed-upon terms, within an established time period, and with stipulated use of resources and performance standards. The nurse as contractor is responsible for the quality of the services rendered and is accountable to the individual client, the health service agency, the nursing profession, and even his or her own conscience for what has been done (Fry, 1994a).

The moral obligation of accountability corresponds to the client's right to an accepted level of competent nursing care and the right to self-determination in health care. As a moral obligation, accountability directs the professional to act in a particular way according to moral norms (Fry, 1994a).

In nursing, and especially in community-oriented nursing, accountability appears to be what defines the kinds of relationships among client, nurse, other professionals, and the public at large that form the moral foundations of the professional ethic (Fry, 1994a). Furthermore, since accountability correlates to clients' rights to competent levels of nursing care, it is responsive to the human traditions that can be found in nursing's history. Accountability enables the nurse to achieve the protection of the client's human dignity and right to self-determination in health matters.

CASE 7 When Aging Parents Can No Longer Live Independently

Joyce Fisher, a home health agency nurse, has just received a telephone call from the daughter of a client, 82-year-old Mr. Sims, whom she had visited some months before. The daughter was very distraught, telling Joyce that her father had fallen at home but refused to be seen by a physician. Ms. Sims's mother had called her at her place of business and pleaded with her to come to the home and stay with them. The daughter was exasperated by the frequency of these types of phone calls from her parents in recent weeks and was appealing to Joyce for help in making some long-term decisions for the care and safety of her parents.

Joyce clearly remembers the conversations that she had with Mr. and Mrs. Sims and their daughter several months ago after Mr. Sim's last hospitalization. Mr. and Mrs. Sims live alone in a small home and are frequently visited by the daughter, who buys their groceries and takes them to their various health appointments. Mr. Sims has always been the decision maker of the family but allows this amount of assistance from the daughter "for Mama's sake." Another daughter lives in a nearby city but has chronic health problems that prohibit her active involvement in the affairs of her parents. A son lives on the west coast and travels constantly in his line of business. He supports his parents by sending money for their expenses to his sister (Mr. Sims has refused direct financial aid from any of the children). All three children are concerned about the future welfare of their parents but have been unsuccessful in persuading them to change their mode of living.

The present problem exists because Mr. and Mrs. Sims are losing their ability to live independently and make their own decisions. Mr. Sims's unexplained falls are also increasing, a continued source of worry for Mrs. Sims and a genuine concern for their daughter. They all look toward Joyce Fisher as the person who can help them make and support a decision that will preserve some autonomy for the aging parents and respect their choices and lifestyle. However, Joyce doubts that what is best for all concerned can avoid infringing on the choices and self-respect of the parents.

Discussion Questions

1. What is the role of the home health nurse in assisting individuals to reach a decision with which they can live?
2. What does it mean to respect Mr. and Mrs. Sims as autonomous individuals?
3. Do clients really have the right to refuse services or treatment from the community health nurse? Does such refusal limit future treatment? Why or why not?
4. Is there any happy medium for aging parents when they can no longer live independently?

Modified from Veatch RM, Fry ST: Case studies in nursing ethics, Philadelphia, 1987, JB Lippincott.

ETHICAL PRINCIPLES IN COMMUNITY HEALTH
Relationship of Ethical Rules, Principles, and Theories

In making moral decisions, various rules, principles, or theories apply (Fig. 6-2). **Rules** state that certain actions should (or should not) be performed because they are right (or wrong). An example would be that "Nurses ought to always tell the truth to clients." **Principles** are more abstract than rules and serve as the foundation of rules. For example, the ethical principle of autonomy is the foundation for such rules as "Always support the right to informed consent," "Tell the truth," and "Protect the privacy of the client." Likewise, the principle of justice serves as the foundation of rules such as "Treat equals equally" and "Divide your time on the basis of needs." **Theories,** however, are collections of principles and rules. They provide theoretical foundations for deciding what to do when principles or rules conflict. Examples of a few major theories are *utilitarianism, deontology,* and *natural law.*

Within theories, the various moral rules and principles are arranged according to their importance or ability to be justified. For example, in utilitarianism the principle of beneficence often carries more weight than the ethical principles of autonomy or justice. However, ethical principles are not absolute. Each ethical principle is always morally significant but may not always prevail when in conflict with other principles. Ethical theories simply suggest which ethical principles will more likely prevail when moral decisions have to be made.

But what makes some judgments moral and others nonmoral? Moral judgments are evaluations of what is good or bad, right or wrong, and have certain characteristics that separate them from nonmoral evaluations such as personal preferences, beliefs, or matters of taste. The difference between the evaluations lies in the reasons for or the characteristics of the judgments themselves (Frankena, 1973). Moral judgments are generally made concerning human actions, institutions, or character traits.

Nurses frequently make moral judgments. When the nurse decides to arrange a home visiting schedule on the basis of need or seriousness of illness, a moral judgment is made. When the nurse decides to refer a client to a physician for further evaluation based on the expressed wishes of the client and his or her condition, a moral judgment is made. When in response to a request for an abortion a nurse decides, regardless of personal beliefs, to inform the client of all the options available, a moral judgment is made. When a nurse, resisting pressure from other individuals, decides not to participate in political activities

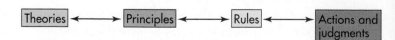

FIG. 6-2 The relationship of ethical theories, principles, and rules.

that might lessen health care coverage for vulnerable populations, a moral judgment is made.

Principle of Beneficence

Definition

The principle of **beneficence** is that "we ought to do good and prevent or avoid doing harm" (Frankena, 1973, p. 45). Beneficence is a duty to help others gain what is of benefit to them but does not carry the obligation to risk one's own welfare or interests in helping others. Some theorists maintain that beneficence does not morally require the nurse to always benefit others even when one can do so. Rather, nurses are only morally required to prevent harm, which may be true in general social interactions among persons. However, the implicit contract underlying the nature of the nurse-client relationship seems to indicate that positive benefiting or acts of beneficence should take place.

The need for health care forms the basis of the relationship between nurse and client and imposes a moral duty on the nurse to benefit the client through nursing actions. However, there may be limits on the amount of beneficial nursing care a client should expect. Certainly nurses should not be expected to provide nursing care to individual clients or client populations if they are putting themselves at risk. Care also should not be expected if clients' needs infringe either upon nurses' personal lives or upon their responsibilities to other clients or their own families. Although the duty to prevent harm to clients is a stringent one, the claim to positive benefiting is limited.

Application in community-oriented health care

In nursing, the principle of beneficence can be applied in (1) balancing harms and benefits to client populations and (2) the use of cost-benefit analyses in decisions affecting client populations.

Balancing harms and benefits. Service that brings about the greatest balance of good over evil, or benefit over harm, is in accordance with a **rule of utility.** This rule is derived from the principle of beneficence and includes a moral duty to weigh and balance benefits against harms to increase benefits and reduce the occurrence of harms (Beauchamp and Childress, 1994).

In public health a rule of utility may be the basis for deciding whether to fund certain health programs more than others, conduct screening programs for communicable diseases, or conduct research projects in which individual rights to privacy may be concerned. In each example, the decision is made by balancing the possible harms and benefits of several alternative courses of action. The nurse should accurately assess the known benefits and harms to clients from the point of view of nursing care and should present them with other relevant facts that might enter into the decision-making process.

Cost-benefit analysis. Cost-benefit analysis is a specific application of the principle of beneficence. It measures the harms and benefits of various health programs while figuring the costs of potential trade-offs in certain courses of actions. Examples of factors taken into consideration include lives saved, costs averted, taxes saved, and illness prevented. All of these are eventually converted into one common unit, usually money, to measure the benefits and costs of alternative approaches to a problem or to decide how to distribute health program funds (see Chapter 21).

Problems and conflicts

Decision making in community settings on the basis of a principle of beneficence and of weighing harms and benefits raises moral questions concerning (1) paternalism in health care decisions and (2) the extent of the rule of utility in decision making.

Paternalism. Paternalism is a liberty-limiting principle that is frequently invoked to override people's actions or expressed wishes for their own good or best interests. Parents may override a child's desire to play with the interesting knobs on a stove because they do not want the child to get burned. Nurses may override clients' expressed wishes "not to hear any bad news" by telling them the results of laboratory testing so that their health status can be treated and improved. Nurses do this because they feel it is in clients' best interests to know the status of their health.

It is morally justified to restrict a person's liberty when not doing so could cause possibly life-threatening physical harm. However, it is more difficult to justify paternalistic actions for perceived psychological harms. For example, it might seem morally justified to override a teenager's desire to participate in a research project that may have a potential health risk. However, it is not morally justifiable to withhold information of a defective fetus from a woman who is 6 months pregnant because it might cause her psychological harm and grief during the remaining months of pregnancy.

It is also difficult to justify paternalistic actions for benefiting the person whose liberty is restricted. For example, it is difficult to morally justify forcibly giving medication to a mental health client who has refused chemotherapy simply because the medication will benefit him by reducing paranoia or irrational fears. However, health care practitioners often carry out paternalistic actions. Are there some acts of paternalism that are morally justified, and if so, what are the criteria for justified paternalism in health care decisions?

Since paternalism always violates the moral principle of autonomy and the moral rule to treat persons as self-determining moral agents, justified paternalism is a very limited area. According to Gert, Culver, and Clouser (1997), paternalism is justified only if (1) the evils that would be prevented are much greater than the evils, if any, that would be caused by the violation of the moral rule and (2) if one would be willing to universally allow the violation of the moral rule in these same circumstances and be able to publicly advocate this kind of violation. Thus justified paternalism seems to be limited to those acts that prevent persons from committing some grave bodily harm to themselves, such as self-mutilating or self-destructing behaviors, and acts committed out of ignorance, such as unknowingly ingesting harmful substances. Beyond these and similar acts, it is difficult to justify paternalism.

Extent of the rule of utility. Attempting to bring about the greatest possible balance of benefit over harm may lead to two problems. The first is the potential overriding of individual liberties and values for the common good. For example, in calculating the benefits of a health policy in terms of tax savings and other economic benefits, the health needs of individual citizens may be overlooked or simply not deemed as important. Human needs and wants that cannot be easily or accurately converted into money units may simply be left out in deciding on the greatest amount of overall benefit. In the final analysis, cost-benefit strategies may not truly represent the value choices of individuals. Thus policy decisions based on the rule of utility as expressed in cost-benefit analysis may be inaccurate and irrelevant to the health needs of individuals.

A second problem arises when the rule of utility is applied in health policy decisions having long-term effects. For example, it is often unclear how short-term harms and benefits should be weighed against long-term consequences in cost-benefit analysis. If the benefits and harms to individual health or economic savings in the future are judged more important than present savings or health conditions, individual and collective interests in health may be sacrificed for future benefits.

Principle of Autonomy

Definition

Autonomy refers to freedom of action that an individual chooses. Persons who are autonomous are capable of choosing and acting on plans they themselves have selected. To respect persons as autonomous individuals is to acknowledge their personal rights to make choices and act accordingly (Fry, 1994a). They are respected as self-determining moral agents or persons. Thus when nurses respect persons as moral agents, they are acting in accordance with the requirements of the moral principle of autonomy.

Application in community-oriented health care

The principle of autonomy is applied in (1) respect for persons; (2) protection of privacy; (3) provision of informed consent; (4) freedom of choice, including treatment refusal; and (5) protection of diminished autonomy.

> **DID YOU KNOW?** *Some ethical conflicts experienced by nurses have been the same over time. For example, in an early research study about nurses' ethical conflicts conducted by Vaughan in 1935, 2265 moral problems, 67 problems of etiquette, and 110 questions about ethical behavior were found in the diaries of 95 nurses working in various localities in the United States. This was an average of 23.4 moral problems experienced by*

each nurse over a period of 3 months. The most frequently mentioned problem was cooperation—between nurses and physicians, among nurses in general, with and among supervisors, between nurses and clients' relatives, in giving medications and treatments, and in maintaining asepsis. In a 1994 study of ethical conflicts experienced by 462 practicing nurses in the state of Maryland, Fry and Damrosch (1994b) found that 40% of the nurse participants had direct involvement with ethical issues either 1 to 4 times weekly or daily to almost daily. One of the most frequent experienced ethical issues was conflict in the nurse-physician relationship.

Respect for persons. Clients are respected because they are persons and have the right to determine their own plan of life. Community health nurses acknowledge respect by seriously considering the opinions and choices of clients and not obstructing their actions unless they are harmful to themselves or others. Denying clients freedom to act on their own judgments or withholding information necessary to make judgments demonstrates a lack of respect for clients.

Elderly clients provide an example. Community health nurses often find it easier and quicker to communicate with family members than with the clients themselves. They may simply tell the client what treatment has to be performed, not giving them choices or even involving them in deciding on the treatment plan. Age, however, does not render a client less worthy of respect (Fig. 6-3). Elderly persons have the right to determine their life and health plans insofar as they have the capacity to do so. To deny them the opportunity to choose according to their capacities demonstrates a lack of respect for persons and is an infringement on the principle of autonomy.

Protection of privacy. Community health nursing care involves close observation of clients, physical touching, and access to personal health and economic information about clients and their families. All of these aspects of nursing care may invade the privacy of clients or threaten their right to control personal information.

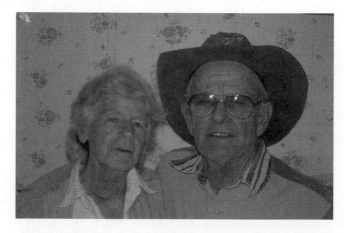

FIG. 6-3 Age does not render clients less worthy of respect.

Since the relationship between nurse and client is built on trust, the nurse has a responsibility to protect the privacy of clients and their families insofar as their health is concerned. Personal information gathered in the home assessment of clients must be recorded in a manner that acknowledges respect for clients' privacy and is communicated only to those directly concerned with client care.

When personal economic information must be shared with third parties for payment of nursing care, clients have the right to authorize or withhold disclosure of information. Even though the information may be essential for continuity of nursing care services, the client retains control of all information.

When clients' records are examined for quality assurance purposes, or when notes about home or clinic visits are included in research studies, the protection of privacy may be a genuine problem. Using health records in determining funding levels for community-oriented nursing services does not justify using nurse-generated information about the client without the client's knowledge and permission. Health record information can only be used for quality assurance purposes or research studies. This information can be shared with others only under clearly defined policies and written guidelines protecting client privacy. Community-oriented nursing services are also responsible for making sure that policies and guidelines appropriately protect client privacy. These services must ensure that clients are informed of this protection *before* their personal information is released to any source. Only then can an agency meet the requirements of the ethical principle of autonomy.

Provision of informed consent. The principle of autonomy requires that clients be given "the opportunity to choose what shall or shall not happen to them" (National Commission, 1978, p. 10). Clients are provided this opportunity when adequate disclosure standards for **informed consent** are included in the contract for nursing services. Three elements are essential for adequate informed consent:

- *Information.* The nurse must disclose information about treatment procedures, their purposes, any discomforts and anticipated benefits, alternative procedures for therapy, and options for questioning procedures or ending the contract at any time. Clients should also be adequately informed about how confidentiality of their health records will be maintained.
- *Comprehension.* The manner and context in which information is conveyed to clients is also important for informed consent requirements. Clients must be allowed time to consider information provided by the nurse and time to ask questions. If the client is unable to comprehend because of a language barrier, the nurse must provide an interpreter. The client must be competent to understand and make decisions rationally. Competent clients can understand a treatment procedure or proposed care plan, weigh its discomforts and

benefits, and then make decisions about undertaking the procedure or plan.
- *Voluntariness.* Any contract or agreement with the client constitutes valid consent only if it is given voluntarily and is free of coercion or undue influences. Voluntariness includes the freedom to choose one's own health goals without the controlling influence of another person or certain conditions, such as debilitating disease, psychiatric disorders, and drug addictions (Beauchamp and Childress, 1994). Again, the principle of autonomy is the main ethical principle guiding this provision.

These three elements—information, comprehension, and voluntariness—constitute informed consent in nursing practice. Informed consent is not valid without all elements, and no contract between client and nurse is ethically acceptable without valid informed consent.

Individual freedom of choice. Respecting the client's right to self-determination includes respecting a decision to refuse treatment. Factors the nurse must weigh include the client's personal freedom, the potential harm to the client or other citizens, the cost of treatment refusal, and the values of society. As long as a client is judged competent to make this kind of decision, however, it is difficult to infringe on autonomy by not allowing treatment refusal. The right of the client to refuse treatment and the right to initiate written advance directives are protected by the Patient Self-Determination Act (1990).

In nursing, respect for the client's or guardian's right to refuse treatment may hinge on the nurse's judgment of the client's decision-making ability. The physical competency of the elderly or severely ill client, the psychological competency of former clients with mental illness, and the maturity or legal competency of minors may, in part, rely on the assessment of client abilities by the community health nurse. In some situations the nurse may need to assess whether an advance directive is an accurate statement of what the client wants, whether a client has fully taken into account the consequences of a treatment decision before completing an advance directive, and whether a surrogate decision maker is inappropriately making decisions for a client with intact decision-making capacity (Mezey et al, 1994).

In situations of questionable competency, decisions have generally been made opting for the preservation of life (Beauchamp and Childress, 1994). In situations in which competency to make decisions has been established, other factors such as obligations to others (e.g., dependent children) may determine whether autonomy of choice will be respected. No hard-and-fast rule on treatment refusal can be made. However, nurses should recognize that respect for persons may involve allowing clients and their legal guardians to make decisions concerning their lives and health that may be very difficult for the nurses to accept.

Protection of diminished autonomy. The principle of autonomy is generally applied only to persons capable of autonomous choice. Factors such as immaturity or physical or psychological incapacities may diminish one's autonomy. In such cases, it is sometimes considered justifiable to interfere with the actions of these individuals to protect them from harmful results of their choices and actions. This interference, however, requires appeals to other principles, such as beneficence (see Research Brief).

The nurse may have difficulty recognizing when diminished capacities render clients incapable of self-determination. The capacity for self-determination is relative to maturity, chronological age, the presence or absence of illness, mental disability, or social factors. However, respect for the principle of autonomy requires that practitioners recognize when persons lack the capacity to act autonomously and therefore are entitled to protection in health care delivery (Fig. 6-4).

Problems and conflicts

Respecting the ethical principle of autonomy can be difficult in nursing practice. Those areas creating the most conflict for nurses include (1) carrying out **coercive health measures** and (2) invasions of privacy for health reasons.

Coercive health measures. Clients consulting a community agency may have a communicable disease that not only is harmful to themselves if untreated but also may affect the health of family members, neighbors, or coworkers. The client may not want to receive treatment and may even refuse to take medications or attend follow-up care recommended for the illness. For example, many areas of the United States still require clients diagnosed with active tuberculosis to be confined until their disease is no longer considered active or communicable to others. Clients have no choice in the matter. They must be admitted and must take treatment, regardless of their own wishes, choices, or life plans.

The public health nurse may be the one to enforce these regulations or be the agent to override a client's expressed wishes in this matter. Thus nurses may find themselves forced to choose between individual rights to self-determination in health matters and the protection of the community's health.

Invasions of privacy. In protecting the health of vulnerable populations, the public health nurse may infringe on rights to privacy by actively gathering private information. For example, a sharp rise in the incidence of venereal disease among a high-school population may require interviewing teenagers diagnosed with the disease and accurately following up with all named contacts. This action may lead to invasions of individual privacy through discussion of sexual habits and preferences and potential disclosures to adults, including parents.

RESEARCH *Brief*

In a descriptive study of 332 certified nephrology nurses (CNNs) practicing in dialysis settings in four eastern states and the District of Columbia, the researchers found that the most common practice context for ethical conflicts involved decisions about discontinuation or initiation of dialysis (69%). Study participants described dialysis being initiated on patients with terminal cancer or multisystem organ failure or who were comatose with no chance of survival. Some patients were dialyzed to the moment of death. The CNNs saw dialysis as prolonging painful deaths with additional painful and invasive procedures for patients. Other ethical conflicts involved competent patients who requested discontinuation of dialysis but who were dialyzed at the family's request, providing dialysis to chronically noncompliant patients, providing dialysis to HIV-positive patients with dementia who were abusive to nursing staff and other patients, and practicing under unsafe working conditions.

More than half of the conflicts described were experienced as moral dilemmas (two or more ethical principles apply but support mutually inconsistent courses of action) and a significant number (34%) were experienced as moral distress (knowing the right thing to do but not being able to do so because of various constraints or lack of decision-making authority). About 44% of the ethical conflicts were not resolved, and 18% of the conflicts were only resolved by the patient's death. CNNs who had ethics education in their basic preparation for nursing were more likely to experience ethical conflict as a moral dilemma, whereas those without ethics education were more likely to experience conflict as more distress.

This study is the first known systematic description of ethical conflicts experienced by CNNs practicing in dialysis settings. The conflicts reported may indicate that there are significant issues in patient care regarding patients' decisions to discontinue dialysis and the dialysis of terminally ill patients.

Redman BK, Hill MN, Fry ST: Ethical conflicts reported by certified nephrology nurses (CNNs) practicing in dialysis settings, *ANNA J* 24(1):23, 1997.

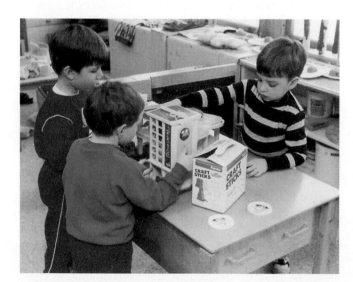

FIG. 6-4 Children have diminished autonomy and are entitled to protection in health care delivery. (From Wong: *Nursing care of infants and children,* ed 6, St Louis, 1999, Mosby.)

All of these actions infringe on self-determining behavior but are considered justifiable because of potential harm to others. Nonetheless, it is the nurse's responsibility to inform those whose privacy is invaded that information will be recorded and communicated in a way that does not infringe on their future privacy.

Privacy may also be invaded by the assessment and recording of personal client information. For example, the community health nurse may record information about the social habits and lifestyles of pregnant women. Subsequently, that information may be used in research studies correlating neonatal mortality and morbidity with social habits during pregnancy. This type of personal information is often freely communicated because of the trust relationship between nurse and client. It may also be recorded in the client's record without full understanding of the potential impact of this information if, in fact, a child is born with anomalies related to social habits or lifestyles during pregnancy. The presence of this information in prenatal records means that it might eventually be shared with other health professionals and members of the client's family, constituting further invasion of the client's right to privacy of personal information.

These invasions of privacy may be justified because they prevent harm to innocent third parties. However, communicating this information while remaining sensitive to the client's right to privacy may create conflicts of interest for the nurse.

Requests for euthanasia or assistance to commit suicide. Clients frequently ask nurses for information about euthanasia and/or assistance in bringing about their own deaths. Such a request may create conflict for a nurse, especially when the nurse feels that the client has a right to decide when and how he or she dies or the nurse does not think that the client's quality of life is very good. Nurses must remember that euthanasia (i.e., any action that intentionally brings about the client's death for reasons of mercy) and professionally assisted suicide (i.e., providing assistance to a client in ending his or her own life) are very controversial acts for the nurse. The ANA *Code for Nurses* states that it is unethical and illegal to participate in acts of euthanasia. It is also considered unethical for a nurse to assist a client to end his or her life (although some states have enacted legislation permitting clients, under certain circumstances, to legally make such requests from health professionals).

WHAT DO YOU THINK? *In public opinion surveys about professional aid in dying, 50% to 75% of adults favor allowing health care professionals to euthanize or to assist the suicide of those who are terminally ill. Nurses, however, are ethically and legally prohibited from assisting the suicide of anyone and participating in acts of euthanasia. What should the nurse do when a terminally ill and suffering client asks the nurse to help him die?*

Little is known about the practices of nurses regarding euthanasia or clients' requests for assistance to end their own lives. In one recent study (Matzo and Emanual, 1997) of oncology nurses, it was found that 71% of the nurses had been asked by clients to provide euthanasia or assistance in commiting suicide, but only 1% of the nurses actually provided assistance in suicide while 4.5% participated in an act of euthanasia (i.e., injecting a drug to intentionally end a client's life). Further study is needed to learn how nurses respond to clients' requests for euthanasia or assistance in bringing about their own deaths or how such requests create ethical conflict in nursing practice.

Principle of Justice

Definition

The formal principle of **justice** holds that equals should be treated equally and that those who are unequal should be treated differently according to their differences (Beauchamp and Childress, 1994). In consideration of a community's health, material principles of justice are considered (i.e., need, merit, contributions to society) to determine which social burdens and benefits, including health goods, should be distributed among all individuals in the community.

Application in community-oriented health care

Different theories of justice may be considered in deciding how to distribute health care resources. These theories include the entitlement theory, utilitarian theory, maximin theory, and egalitarian theory. Each theory has its advantages and disadvantages in distributing health goods in the community.

Entitlement theory. The **entitlement theory** claims that everyone is entitled to whatever they get in the natural lottery at birth. The theory assigns no responsibility to government or its agencies to improve the lot of those less fortunate than others. If people are healthy and rich and have been able to acquire possessions by purchase, gift, or legitimate exchange, they are entitled to what they have. They may also increase their possessions in any way possible, as long as they do not cheat others (Nozick, 1974). It is unfortunate that some people are mentally or physically disabled, but others have no obligation to give money to those with disabilities to make their lives more comfortable. Aiding the unfortunate is simply an act of charity of community members.

In this theory, inequalities between individuals in health, position, and wealth are tolerated. Only aggression or harm against others and the unjust acquisition of goods are prohibited. Thus the actual distribution of goods seems more in line with a principle of autonomy or right to liberty than a principle of justice (Veatch, 1981).

Utilitarian theory. The **utilitarian theory** of justice holds that the best way to distribute resources among citizens is to decide how spending or using resources will achieve the greatest good and serve the largest number of people (Mill, 1957). In times of limited resources, when all that is needed or wanted cannot be provided in the community, this method of distribution is appealing. Although it does tend to overlook the needs and wants of individuals, it manages to maximize net benefits over costs and serves the greatest number of people.

In this theory the needs and wants of some individuals will not be satisfied, and they may actually be harmed in the process. This is unfortunate. However, by distributing limited resources so that "the greatest good for the greatest number" is achieved, government and its agencies would fulfill their obligations to citizens. It is easy to see that the principle of beneficence dominates other considerations in utilitarianism. Justice is served by benefiting the greatest number at the least cost.

Maximin theory. The **maximin* theory** of justice first identifies the least advantaged members of the community and decides how they might be benefited rather than deciding on greatest net aggregate benefit. It then permits free exercise of liberty by all citizens. At the same time, it allows social and economic inequalities to evolve so that these inequalities benefit the least advantaged or least well-off members of society (Rawls, 1971). Many kinds of inequalities in health, health care resources, and possession of economic benefits will be tolerated and considered as long as the position of the least advantaged is improved or benefited. For example, health professionals can charge high fees or receive substantial salaries as long as they also serve the interests of disadvantaged persons. In a similar manner, costly health care resources such as kidney dialysis, magnetic resonance imaging (MRI) scans, and artificial hearts can be developed and purchased by those who can afford them, as long as the lot of the least advantaged persons is also improved in the process.

Obviously, distributing health goods according to this theory will create problems in times of limited resources. Providing benefit first to the least advantaged persons is a constraint on the expansion of health care resources and technological advancement. Thus it is possible that technological advancement and the development of more sophisticated health care goods cannot be made widely available to the public in times of limited economic resources. The result is that interests and needs in matters of health may not be satisfied within this system of justice.

Egalitarian theory. The **egalitarian theory** of justice holds that justice requires the "equality of net welfare for individuals" (Veatch, 1981, p. 265). In this theory the distribution of goods in the community takes the needs of all citizens into account equally. Thus everyone would have a claim to an equal amount of all goods and resources, including health care.

Clearly, this is a goal that cannot be achieved. It would be virtually impossible for any system of justice to guarantee equality of goods and resources for everyone, let alone

equal health care. At least with respect to health care, the egalitarian theory must be amended. Instead of health care being a good that everyone should have in equal amounts, basic health care should be viewed as a good to which all should have equal access. Everyone should have equal access to those basic health goods and resources to improve their health according to need (Veatch, 1981).

This system respects the autonomy of individuals to seek the health services they need or want and gives equal consideration to the positive benefiting of individuals in improved health. Most important, it is just because it follows the dictates of a principle of justice while, at the same time, not limiting the liberty of anyone in terms of basic health needs. It treats equals equally and unequals unequally and provides a just manner for the distribution of health resources in the community.

Problems and conflicts

The application of a principle of justice creates conflicts in two areas. First, it generates considerable challenges about establishing priorities for the distribution of basic goods and health services in the community. Second, it creates conflicts in determining which population or individuals should obtain available health goods and nursing services.

Distributing basic goods and services. In deciding how to distribute basic health care assets or resources within a community, there are several decisions to be made:

1. *How should priorities be set?* Should the protection and promotion of health be the main consideration, or should a major portion of resources be set aside for other social goods, such as housing or education? If community leaders agree that everyone has a right to equal access to basic health care according to need and that this right must be satisfied for justice to be served, then enough community assets and financial resources will be allotted to meet the requirements of this basic right (Milio, 1975).

2. *What are the most effective and efficient methods of meeting this basic right while preventing catastrophic events that need immediate and more concentrated attention?* Such events may lead to death or disability. Should the emphasis be placed on direct health care services (e.g., clinics, programs) to care for illness, or should indirect services (e.g., health education, transportation services) to prevent illness or promote health receive equal emphasis?

3. *What is the appropriate relationship between rescue services and preventive services?* Is it more effective to concentrate on kidney dialysis and terminal cancer services, or should concentrated effort and economic resources be devoted to prevention of disease and disability through, for example, hypertension and diabetes screening?

4. *Should certain diseases or categories of illness receive more emphasis than others?* For example, should the preven-

---

*Maximin is an abbreviation for "maximizing the minimum position in society."

tion and treatment of coronary heart disease take precedence over the prevention and treatment of venereal disease? Decisions in this area may result in allocating money and services to certain socioeconomic or racial groups. Such delicate decisions will require careful consideration to avoid conflicts of interest.

5. *In establishing certain priorities, will these priorities compromise important values or principles?* For example, preventive strategies aimed at discouraging alcohol use or smoking may involve emphasis on behavioral change or the altering of lifestyles. The nurse might question whether these preventive strategies would have a substantial impact on the autonomy of community members, particularly regarding their choice to engage in behaviors that are health risks.

Clearly, acting on certain priorities may create conflicts of interest among health care providers, with subsequent influence on the actual delivery of needed nursing care. These conflicts of interest continue into the next area of decision making.

> **‖ NURSING TIP**
>
> *Clearly articulate value conflicts in describing an ethical conflict in client care. Once the value conflicts are stated clearly, it is easier to resolve ethical conflict.*

Distributing nursing resources. Once the priorities for health are designated, nurses needs to decide how to deliver health care equally according to client needs. There are several strategies that can be implemented:

1. *Focus services on those who have the most reasonable chance of benefitting from services.* Examples are children and childbearing families. This is a utilitarian approach to distributing services aimed at providing the greatest overall benefit. It is questionable whether this strategy meets the moral requirements of a principle of justice, which holds that everyone has a claim of equal access to basic health care services according to need. Certainly a strategy that focuses on one age group in the community will overlook many individual needs and cannot be considered just.

2. *Provide basic services in all categories in limited amounts, and accommodate requests for nursing care services on a first-come, first-served basis.* This approach may certainly cost more in terms of services provided. It may even overlap with similar services provided in the community through health maintenance organizations (HMOs) or group practices of private family physicians. It does meet the basic requirement of providing the opportunity for everyone to have equal access to services, even though they may have to wait a long time to be served. However, it may not be the most efficient means of disbursing nursing resources according to the needs of clients.

3. *Focus nursing services on those who are most able to pay for services.* This approach is all too frequently used in today's health care delivery system. This approach has been fostered by legislation and funding by government and its agencies. Unfortunately, this approach may have limited relevance to the needs of a particular community. For example, focusing the majority of nursing resources on a home health care program because of Medicare reimbursements would be unjust to other community health needs if the community had only a small elderly population.

4. *Categorize those in the community according to health needs, and decide who should receive first priority.* Those who cannot survive without nursing resources (those receiving kidney dialysis or respiratory therapy at home) have first priority. Those who can be assisted to prevent long-term disability (e.g., populations at high risk, preeclamptic clients, children with minor cardiac anomalies) would come next. Last priority would be given to those who do not have an acute disabling illness or are not at risk of long-term disability (e.g., school-age children, the elderly, or some persons with chronic diseases). Other groups who may be given a high priority include those whose health needs can be easily met and who can benefit the health of others (e.g., women with uncomplicated pregnancy, mothers with children under 2 years of age). This approach has a decidedly utilitarian twist, and it limits the access of some groups to nursing services according to their priority (Fig. 6-5). Although it distributes nursing resources according to who can benefit the most, some clients (e.g., dying cancer clients) would have no access to the system at all. This can hardly be considered just if the principle of justice is adopted (rather than a utilitarian principle of beneficence) as the guiding principle for distributing health goods.

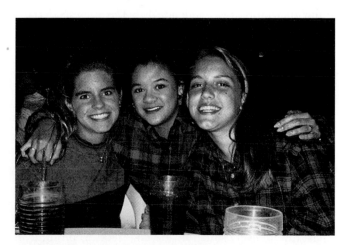

FIG. 6-5 Teenage populations have a low priority in the allocation of health and nursing services. (From Wong: *Nursing care of infants and children*, ed 6, St Louis, 1999, Mosby.)

As can be demonstrated by all of these various approaches to distributing nursing care resources, the moral requirements of justice create numerous conflicts of interest for health practitioners when they face specific choices.

APPLICATION OF ETHICS TO COMMUNITY-ORIENTED NURSING PRACTICE
Priority of Ethical Principles

In community-oriented nursing, ethical principles direct and guide nursing actions with individuals and aggregate groups. The professional ethic in most nursing actions places a greater emphasis on the observance of the principles of autonomy and beneficence than on the principle of justice. For example, in the *Code for Nurses*, respect for the principle of autonomy is emphasized by such statements as "the nurse provides services with respect for human dignity and the uniqueness of the client," that "clients have the moral right to determine what will be done with their own person," and that "the nurse's respect for the worth and dignity of the individual human being applies irrespective of the nature of the health problem" (ANA, 1985, pp. 2, 3). All of these statements indicate a high respect for client autonomy or claim that the nurse has a strong, primary duty to respect the client's right to self-determination.

The ethical principle of beneficence is given slightly less emphasis in the *Code for Nurses*. For example, the code claims that "the nurse's primary commitment is to the health, welfare, and safety of the client"; that "the nurse safeguards the client's right to privacy by judiciously protecting information of a confidential nature"; and that "nurses are responsible for advising clients against the use of products that endanger the client's safety and welfare... The nurse may use knowledge of specific services or products in advising an individual client, since this may contribute to the client's health and well-being" (ANA, 1985, pp. 4, 6, 15). Acts of beneficence may even include overriding the autonomy of individuals in the interests of other clients. The *Code for Nurses* justifies this action whenever "the nurse recognizes those situations in which individual rights to autonomy in health care may temporarily be overridden to preserve the life of the human community" (ANA, 1985, pp. 2, 3).

However, the principle of justice is not strongly emphasized in the professional code of ethics. The *Code for Nurses* notes in passing that nursing practice is not influenced by age, sex, race, color, personality, or other personal attributes or individual differences in customs, beliefs, or attitudes. The code states that "nursing care is delivered without prejudicial behavior"; that "the nurse adheres to the principle of nondiscriminatory, nonprejudicial care in every situation and endeavors to promote its acceptance by others"; and that "the setting shall not determine the nurse's readiness to respect clients and to ren-

der or obtain needed services" (ANA, 1985, pp. 3, 4). Clearly, these statements related to the moral requirements of the principle of justice are not as strong as those related to the moral requirements of the principles of autonomy and beneficence.

In the community, nursing actions are guided not only by the professional ethic and its priority of ethical principles, but also by the **public health ethic,** which has a different priority of principles. This ethic is strongly modeled on the priority of the principle of beneficence and follows the rule of utility in disease detection and prevention and in health maintenance. Following a rule of utility in matters of health might influence the practice of community-oriented nursing. For example, it might encourage the nurse to identify the needs of aggregates in order to provide population groups with net benefit over possible health harms (Fry, 1994). This emphasis on the moral requirements of the principle of beneficence does not easily align with the highly individualistic approach of the *Code for Nurses*, with its emphasis on respect for client autonomy.

Accountability in Community-Oriented Nursing

Moral accountability in nursing practice means that nurses are answerable for how they promote, protect, and meet the health needs of clients while respecting individual rights to self-determination in health care. In community-oriented nursing, where the greater emphasis is on aggregates rather than individual clients, moral accountability means being answerable for how the health of aggregate groups has been promoted, protected, and met (Fig. 6-6).

The moral requirements of the principles of autonomy and justice are still important in community-oriented nursing, but they are less important than the requirements of the principle of beneficence. In community-oriented nursing, the emphasis of the professional ethic is slanted toward benefit to aggregates, which implies following a rule of utility in planning, implementing, and evaluating population-focused nursing services.

WHAT DO YOU THINK? *Meeting accountability requirements in community and public health nursing will be different than meeting accountability requirements in other spheres of nursing practice. For example, the professional ethic clearly indicates that all nurses are morally accountable for how they respect the client's right to self-determination and provide health services with respect for "the uniqueness of the client." However, in community and public health, nurses are also morally accountable for how they provide health services to maximize total net health in population groups. Rather than being primarily accountable for how the moral requirements of the principle of autonomy are met in individual client care, the public health nurse is accountable for maximizing the total net health benefits of the community.*

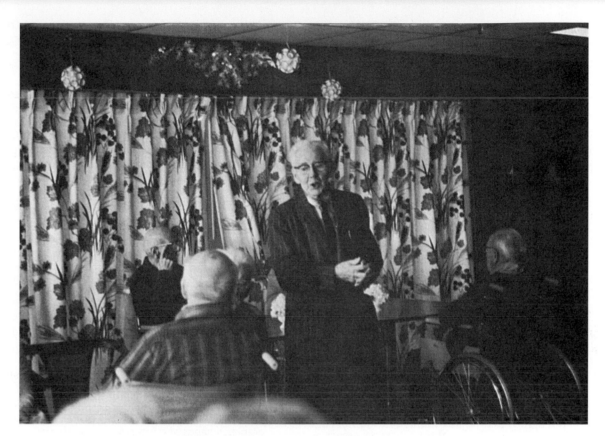

FIG. 6-6 Community health nurses are accountable for the health of aggregate groups, such as elderly clients in a nursing home.

Future Directions in Community-Oriented Nursing

The emphasis on the moral requirements of a principle of beneficence in community-oriented nursing has two implications. Since community-oriented nursing derives its theoretical direction from both public health services and professional nursing theories for the purpose of improving the health of the entire community, it is important that the planning, implementation, and evaluation of nursing services in the community be clearly differentiated from the provision of nursing services in other spheres of health care delivery. Community-oriented nursing is a synthesis of the sciences of both public health and nursing. However, there must be a clear understanding of how the ethical components of professional practice, including the observance of clients' rights and professional responsibilities, are considered in the provision of nursing services. Clarity and agreement on the priority of ethical principles in community-oriented nursing are also necessary. Improving the health of the entire community by identifying aggregates and directing resources to them indicates an orientation toward meeting health needs according to the rule of utility. Is the ethical prin-

ciple of beneficence the principle that should primarily guide community-oriented nursing practice? The moral underpinnings of community-oriented nursing clearly need to be given careful consideration in any statement defining the role of the discipline.

The second implication concerns the evaluation of accountability. Certainly nursing has been affected by changes in both the health care delivery system and nursing practice in recent years. Accountability requirements have likewise been affected by changes in public and professional expectations and the scope of nursing practice. For example, the expanded role of the nurse has increased the legal accountability of the nurse practitioner, who is certified to function as an independent caregiver. Thus there is a current and future need for periodic assessment of the moral and legal requirements of accountability in all nursing services.

One must also determine how accountability will be measured in community-oriented nursing and how existing programs and services will be evaluated to determine the effectiveness of various nursing services in meeting accountability requirements. This task has yet to be accomplished by today's community-oriented nursing leaders.

clinical application

Sharon Lloyd, employed by a private, for-profit home care agency, has been authorized to make three home visits to Mrs. Callahan, recently discharged from the hospital after surgery for excision of a nonmalignant abdominal mass. Mrs. Callahan needed wound care and instruction in how to provide her own wound care. Mrs. Callahan was very obese and had difficulty seeing the abdominal incision to provide wound care and also too weak to be responsible for her care. Sharon instructed her husband, who seemed willing to help, in providing the wound care. However, he disliked looking at the wound and did not follow through with Sharon's instructions. Although she spent considerable time instructing Mr. Callahan in how to care for his wife, he forgot what should be done each time Sharon asked him to show her how he would clean the wound and reapply a dressing.

Sharon judged that more home visits were needed to prevent infection in the wound and to help Mrs. Callahan assume her own care. Sharon then called the case manager at the Callahan's HMO and requested three more home visits. The case manager would not authorize the visits claiming that Mr. Callahan was willing to do the care for his wife. Sharon agreed that he was willing but was not capable of doing so. Her clinical judgement was that more time was needed to prevent harm from occuring to Mrs. Callahan. Again, the case manager refused to authorize more nursing care visits to the client. What should Sharon do?

A. What options does Sharon have to obtain authorization for more home visits to Mrs. Callahan?
B. Should Sharon say she has done what she could, the Callahan's will have to cope the best they can, and go onto her next client? Why or why not?
C. How can home care nurses advocate for quality of client care in a managed care environment?

Answers are in the back of the book.

KEY POINTS

- Because clients have rights, health care professionals have responsibilities to tell the truth, respect confidentiality, function as client advocates, and accept accountability for providing proper health care.
- The development of methods to measure accountability is a high priority in nursing.
- A right to health has been historically recognized as a basic human right.
- The negative right to be free to enjoy good health may lead to the positive right to obtain certain services or community health safeguards.
- "Right to health" and "right to health care" are different kinds of rights and should be kept separate.

- Health care providers do not often communicate rights to their clients. However, the Patient's Bill of Rights has been criticized for several reasons.
- Clients have the right to accept or refuse treatment and the right to formulate advance directives.
- According to a recent presidential commission, "society has an ethical obligation to ensure equitable access to health care for all."
- The professional code of ethics for nurses prescribes moral behavior and actions based on moral principles.
- The need for moral accountability within nursing practice has been recognized since Florence Nightingale began her nurse training program.
- The ethical principles operable in community-oriented nursing are beneficence, autonomy, and justice.
- The four major theories of justice used to decide the allocation of health care resources are the entitlement theory, the utilitarian theory, the maximin theory, and the egalitarian theory. The moral requirements of justice create numerous conflicts of interest for health practitioners when specific choices must be made.
- The professional ethic generally places a greater emphasis on observance of the principles of autonomy and beneficence than on the principle of justice in most nursing actions.
- In community-oriented nursing, moral accountability means being answerable for how the health of aggregate groups has been promoted, protected, and met.
- Clients' rights to equal access to health care and the aggregate's needs and interests in health matters will often compete for the attention and services of the nurse.

critical thinking activities

1. Hold a conference among two or three nursing students and two or three practicing community and public health nurses. Discuss how these nurses assume responsibility and accountability for individual nursing judgments and actions in their areas of practice. Be sure to distinguish moral accountability from legal accountability.
2. Suggest three ways by which nursing might extend the scope of accountability for nurses in delivering nursing care services to aggregate groups in the community.
3. Select an aggregate group at risk in your community. Formulate a plan of nursing care delivery in response to a health care need using a specific theory of distributive justice.
4. Determine how client's rights to privacy are respected and protected in a community health care agency. To what extent do nurses contribute to the protection of client privacy? Are client records used in research studies? If so, how is personal information about the client protected? Suggest two methods by which client privacy could be more adequately protected. What would be the relative costs and benefits of your proposed methods?
5. Discuss the role of nurses in discussing and implementing advance directives in community health settings.

Bibliography

American Hospital Association: Statement on a patient's bill of rights, *Hospitals* 47:41, 1973.

American Nurses' Association: *Code for nurses with interpretive statements,* Kansas City, Mo, 1985, the Association.

Annas GJ: Patients' rights movement. In Reich WT, editor: *Encyclopedia of bioethics,* ed 2, New York, 1996, Simon & Schuster.

Beauchamp DE: Public health and individual liberty, *Ann Rev Public Health* 1:121, 1980.

Beauchamp DE: Community: the neglected tradition of public health, *Hastings Center Rep* 15:28, 1985.

Beauchamp TL, Childress JF: *Principles of biomedical ethics,* ed 4, New York, 1994, Oxford Press.

Beauchamp TL, Faden RR: The right to health and the right to health care, *J Med Philos* 4:118, 1979.

Beauchamp TL, Walters L: Rights and responsibilities. In Beauchamp TL, Walters L, editors: *Contemporary issues in bioethics,* ed 4, Belmont, Calif, 1994, Wadsworth.

Bell NK: The scarcity of medical resources: are there rights to health care? *J Med Philos* 4:158, 1979.

Benner P, Wrubel J: *The primacy of caring: stress and coping in health and illness,* Menlo Park, Calif, 1989, Addison-Wesley.

Brockington C: *A short history of public health,* London, 1956, Churchill.

Daniels N: Rights to health care and distributive justice: programmatic worries, *J Med Philos* 4:174, 1979.

Feinberg J: *Social philosophy,* Englewood Cliffs, NJ, 1973, Prentice-Hall.

Frankena WK: *Ethics,* Englewood Cliffs, NJ, 1973, Prentice-Hall.

Fry ST: Rationing health care: the ethics of cost containment, *Nurs Econ* 1:165, 1983.

Fry ST: Ethical decision making. Part I. Selecting a framework, *Nurs Outlook* 37:248, 1989.

Fry ST: *Ethics in nursing practice: a guide to ethical decision making,* Geneva, 1994a, International Council of Nurses.

Fry, ST, Damrosch, S: Ethics and human rights issues in nursing practice: a survey of Maryland nurses, *Maryland Nurse* 13(7):11, 1994b.

Gert B, Culver CM, Clouser KD: *Bioethics: a return to fundamentals,* New York, 1997, Oxford University Press.

Gordis L, Gold E: Privacy, confidentiality, and the use of medical records in research, *Science* 207:153, 1980.

Jameton A: *Nursing practice: the ethical issues,* Englewood Cliffs, NJ, 1984, Prentice-Hall.

Kant I: *Groundwork of the metaphysic of mortals,* New York, 1964, Harper & Row. (Translated by Paton HJ; originally published in 1785.)

Kelsey JL: Privacy and confidentiality in epidemiological research involving patients, *IRB* 3:1, 1981.

Leininger MM: *Care: the essence of nursing and health,* Detroit, 1984, Wayne State University Press.

Matzo ML, Emanual EJ: Oncology nurses practices of assisted suicide and patient requested euthanasia. *Oncol Nur Forum* 24(10):1725, 1997.

Mezey M et al: The Patient Self-Determination Act: sources of concern for nurses, *Nurs Outlook* 42:30, 1994.

Milio N: *The care of health in communities: access for outcasts,* New York, 1975, Macmillan.

Mill JS: *Utilitarianism,* New York, 1957, Bobbs-Merrill. (Edited by Priest, O; originally published in 1863).

National Commission for the Protection of Human Subjects of Biomedical and Behavioral Research: *The Belmont report: ethical principles and guidelines for the protection of human subjects of research,* DHEW Pub No (OS) 78-0012, Washington, DC, 1978.

Noddings N: *Caring: a feminine approach to ethics and moral education,* Berkeley, 1984, University of California Press.

Nozick R: *Anarchy, state, and utopia,* New York, 1974, Basic Books.

Omnibus Budget Reconciliation Act of 1990, sections 4206 and 4751, PL 101-508, Nov 5, 1990.

Pellegrino E: The caring ethic: the relation of physician to patient. In Bishop AH, Scudder JR, editors: *Caring, curing, coping: nurse, physician, patient relationships,* Birmingham, Ala, 1985, University of Alabama Press.

President's Commission for the Study of Ethical Problems in Medicine and Biomedical and Behavioral Research: *Securing access to health care, vol 1: report on the ethical implications of differences in the availability in health services,* Washington, DC, 1983, US Government Printing Office.

Public Law 92-603, Social Security amendments of 1972, 92nd Congress, Oct 30, 1972.

Public Law 92-278, The national sickle cell anemia, Cooley's anemia, Tay-Sachs and Genetic Disease Act, Title IV, 90 stat, Section 410, 1976.

Rawls J: *A theory of justice,* Cambridge, Mass, 1971, Harvard University Press.

Rosen G: *Preventive medicine in the United States: 1900-1975,* New York, 1975, Science History Publishers.

Ross WD: *The right and the good,* Oxford, 1930, Oxford University Press.

Szasz T: The right to health. In Gorovitz S et al, editors: *Moral problems in medicine,* Englewood Cliffs, NJ, 1976, Prentice-Hall.

Tarasoff v. Regents of The University of California, 131 Cal Rptr 14, 551P2d 334, 1976.

Thompson JB, Thompson HO: *Bioethical decision making for nurses,* Norwalk, Conn, 1985, Appleton-Century-Crofts.

UNESCO: *Human rights, a symposium,* New York, 1949, Allan Wingate.

Vaughan, RH: *The actual incidence of moral problems in nursing: a preliminary study in empirical ethics* (Thesis), Washington, D.C., 1935, Catholic University of America.

Veatch RM: *A theory of medical ethics,* New York, 1981, Basic Books.

Veatch RM, Fry ST: *Case studies in nursing ethics,* Sudbury, Mass, 1995, Jones & Bartlett.

World Health Organization: *The first ten years of the World Health Organization,* New York, 1958, WHO.

Cultural Diversity and Community-Oriented Nursing Practice

CYNTHIA E. DEGAZON

OBJECTIVES

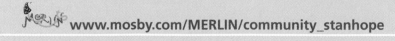

www.mosby.com/MERLIN/community_stanhope

After reading this chapter, the student should be able to do the following:

- Analyze the effect of culture on nursing practice.
- Describe major barriers to developing cultural competence.
- Compare and contrast the effects of cultural organizational factors on health and illness among culturally diverse groups in a community.
- Examine issues related to minority access and use of cultural health practices.
- Conduct a cultural assessment of a person from a cultural group other than one's own.
- Evaluate culturally competent nursing interventions to help clients promote health and prevent disease.
- Analyze the role of the nurse as an advocate for culturally competent nursing care.

KEY TERMS

cultural accommodation
cultural awareness
cultural blindness
cultural competence
cultural conflict
cultural encounter

cultural imposition
cultural knowledge
cultural preservation
cultural relativism
cultural repatterning
cultural skill

culture
culture brokering
culture shock
ethnicity
ethnocentrism
prejudice

race
racism
stereotyping

See Glossary for definitions

CHAPTER OUTLINE

Caring for culturally diverse groups has been a focus of nursing from its beginning. As early as 1893, public health nursing was started by nurses in New York City who provided home care to immigrants, particularly recent arrivals (Denker, 1994). These nurses were not from the same cultural background as the immigrants and had to deal with the cultural differences between themselves and the persons in their care.

The United States has always been a multicultural society. Recent changes in immigration laws have increased migration and the volume of cultural groups entering the United States (Battle, 1998). The 1965 amendment of the Immigration and Nationality Act changed the quota system that discriminated against individuals from Southern and Eastern Europe, and the Refugee Act of 1980 provided opportunities to immigrate for those who needed to escape political persecution (e.g., Cubans, Vietnamese, Laotians, Cambodians, and Russian Jews). Table 7-1 summarizes the immigration patterns of these groups over the past 30 years. More recently, the 1986 Immigration Reform Control Act permitted illegal immigrants already living in the United States an opportunity to apply for legal status if they met certain requirements (Louden, 1996).

If the current immigration trend continues, the United States will consist of a greater variety of cultural groups. About 51.1% of the total population, or more than 135 million people, will be of a culture other than Caucasian and comprise the nation's majority (USDOC, 1997). About 25% of them will speak languages other than English at home.

There is great diversity among the cultural groups in values and beliefs. In turn, their beliefs of health and illness also differ. Therefore the workplace offers enormous challenges for nurses who want to understand beliefs of health and illness of clients as they provide interventions that promote and maintain wellness.

In many instances, especially in home care, nurses must assist ill persons from various cultures over a period of weeks or months to adjust to changes in health status, adapt individual and family behaviors to improve health status, and overall, to develop health promoting patterns. It is essential for nurses to know the pathophysiology of the illness and the cultural views that have an effect on the illness. However, an obstacle to helping clients promote and maintain their wellness is an insufficient number of nurses who understand the experiences and needs of diverse cultural groups (Bernal, 1993).

The purpose of this chapter is to explore cultural competence among community oriented nurses. A nurse who cares for clients (individuals, families, and communities) who are culturally different from himself or herself will be able to apply strategies that are beneficial, appropriate, and useful to the client. In this chapter, emphasis is on four cultural groups: African-Americans, Asian-Americans, Hispanic-Americans, and Native Americans. These groups have been consistently identified in the literature as having more economic difficulties, poorer health, and less-accessible health care than other groups (Giger and Davidhizar, 1999; Spector, 1996).

DID YOU KNOW? *As human beings, we have more similarities than differences with one another.*

CULTURE, RACE, AND ETHNICITY

The concepts of culture, race, and ethnicity play a strong role in understanding human behavior. In everyday living, these three concepts are often used incorrectly. Nurses are expected to understand the meaning of each when providing culturally relevant health care to clients of diverse cultures.

Culture

Culture is a learned set of ideals, values, and assumptions about life that are widely shared among a group of people (Leininger, 1995). It is a dynamic process that develops over time and changes with difficulty. In response to the needs of its members and their environment, culture provides guidance to help them solve life's problems.

Individuals learn about their culture during the process of language learning and being socialized, usually as children (Battle, 1998). Parents and family, the most important sources for the transfer of traditions, teach both explicit and implicit behaviors of the culture. The explicit behaviors, such as language, interpersonal distance, and kissing in public, can be observed and allow the individual to identify the self with other persons of the culture. This way people share traditions, customs, and lifestyles with others. The implicit behaviors are less visible and include the way individuals perceive health and illness, body language, difference in language expressions, and the use of titles. These behaviors are subtle and may be difficult for persons to articulate and explain, yet they are very much a part of the culture. For example, deferring to the elderly, standing when they enter the room, or offering them a seat in which to sit suggests a cultural value related to the elderly. Another example of an implicit aspect of culture is the use of language to communicate. For example, in one culture a sign might read "No smoking is permitted." In another culture the sign might read "Thank you for not smoking." The former statement represents a culture that values directness, whereas the latter values indirectness.

Each culture has an organizational structure that distinguishes it from another and provides the structure for what members of the cultural group determine as appropriate or inappropriate behavior. Such organizational elements include child-rearing practices, religious practices, family structure and values, and attitudes (Locke and Hardaway, 1992). In the case of language, there are idiomatic expressions unique to each language (Phillips, Luna de Hernandez, and Torres de Ardon, 1994). The organizational elements of various cultures have been described by Andrews

TABLE 7-1 Immigrants by Country of Birth: 1981 to 1995 (in thousands; for fiscal years ending in year shown)

CONTINENT/COUNTRY	1981-1990	1991-1993	1994	1995
All countries	7338.1	3705.4	804.4	720.5
Europe[1]	705.6	438.9	160.9	128.2
France	23.1	8.6	2.7	2.5
Germany	70.1	23.7	7.0	6.2
Greece	29.1	5.8	1.4	1.3
Ireland	32.8	30.6	17.3	5.3
Italy	32.9	7.7	2.3	2.2
Poland	97.4	72.5	28.0	13.8
Portugal	40.0	9.4	2.2	2.6
Romania	38.9	20.2	3.4	4.9
Soviet Union, former[2]	84.0	159.2	63.4	54.5
Armenia	NA	NA	4.0	2.0
Azerbaijan	NA	NA	3.8	1.9
Belarus	NA	NA	5.4	3.8
Moldova	NA	NA	2.3	1.9
Russia	NA	NA	15.2	14.6
Ukraine	NA	NA	21.0	17.4
Uzbekistan	NA	NA	3.4	3.6
United Kingdom	142.1	52.7	16.3	12.4
Yugoslavia	19.2	8.1	3.4	8.3
Asia[1]	2817.4	1073.5	292.6	267.9
Afghanistan	26.6	8.5	2.3	1.4
Bangladesh	15.2	17.7	3.4	6.1
Cambodia	116.6	7.5	1.4	1.5
China	388.8[3]	137.5	54.0	35.5
Hong Kong	63.0	30.0	7.7	7.2
India	261.9	121.9	34.9	34.7
Iran	154.8	47.6	11.4	9.2
Iraq	19.6	9.7	6.0	5.6
Israel	36.3	13.8	3.4	2.5
Japan	43.2	23.0	6.1	4.8
Jordan	32.6	13.0	4.0	3.6
Korea	338.8	63.9	16.0	16.0
Laos	145.6	25.9	5.1	3.9
Lebanon	41.6	17.3	4.3	3.9
Pakistan	61.3	39.5	8.7	9.8
Philippines	495.3	188.1	53.5	51.0
Syria	20.6	8.7	2.4	2.4
Taiwan	(3)	43.9	10.0	9.4
Thailand	64.4	21.1	5.5	5.1
Turkey	20.9	7.2	1.8	2.9
Vietnam	401.4	192.7	41.3	41.8
North America[1]	3125.0	1896.4	272.2	231.5
Canada	119.2	45.9	16.1	12.9
Mexico	1653.3	1286.5	111.4	89.9

NA, Not available.   *Continued*

[1]Includes countries not shown separately.

[2]Includes other republics and unknown republics not shown separately.

[3]Data for Taiwan included with China.

[4]Includes Australia, New Zealand, and unknown countries.

Data from US Census Bureau: *Statistical abstract of the United States: 1997,* ed 117, Washington, DC, 1997, Author.

TABLE 7-1 Immigrants by Country of Birth: 1981 to 1995 (in thousands; for fiscal years ending in year shown)—cont'd

CONTINENT/COUNTRY	1981-1990	1991-1993	1994	1995
Caribbean[1]	892.7	337.0	104.8	96.8
Cuba	159.2	35.8	14.7	17.9
Dominican Republic	251.8	128.8	51.2	38.5
Haiti	140.2	68.6	13.3	14.0
Jamaica	213.8	60.0	14.3	16.4
Trinidad and Tobago	39.5	22.0	6.3	5.4
Central America[1]	458.7	226.8	39.9	31.8
El Salvador	214.6	100.4	17.6	11.7
Guatemala	87.9	47.9	7.4	6.2
Honduras	49.5	25.3	5.3	5.5
Nicaragua	44.1	33.9	5.3	4.4
Panama	29.0	9.7	2.4	2.2
South America[1]	455.9	189.2	47.4	45.7
Argentina	25.7	10.6	2.3	1.8
Brazil	23.7	17.5	4.5	4.6
Chile	23.4	6.6	1.6	1.5
Colombia	124.4	45.7	10.8	10.8
Ecuador	56.0	24.6	5.9	6.4
Guyana	95.4	29.1	7.7	7.4
Peru	64.4	36.6	9.2	8.1
Venezuela	17.9	7.7	2.4	2.6
Africa[1]	192.3	91.0	26.7	42.5
Egypt	31.4	12.7	3.4	5.6
Ethiopia	27.2	15.0	3.9	7.0
Nigeria	35.3	16.9	4.0	6.8
South Africa	15.7	6.6	2.1	2.6
Other countries[4]	41.9	16.4	4.6	4.7

and Boyle (1998), Giger and Davidhizar (1999), Leininger (1995), and Spector (1996). It is important that nurses know these organizational elements to provide appropriate care to persons of diverse cultures. This does not mean, however, that one should overlook or fail to incorporate the individuality of any person within any culture when developing a plan of care. Just as all cultures are not alike, all individuals within a culture are not alike. Each individual should be viewed as a unique human being with differences that are respected. Box 7-1 summarizes factors that may contribute to individual differences within cultures.

Race

Race is primarily a social classification that relies on physical markers such as skin color to identify group membership (Bhopal and Donaldson, 1998). Individuals may be of the same race but differ in culture. For example African-Americans are usually born in Africa, the Caribbean, or North America. Although they are a heterogeneous group, they are often viewed as culturally and racially homogeneous. A frequent consequence of this is that the many

cultural differences of these individuals from different countries are overlooked because of their similar racial characteristics (Snowden and Holschuh, 1992). This often blurs understanding of this culturally diverse group.

Another factor highlighting race's diminishing importance in comparison to ethnic identity is the interracial family. Physical changes in biracial and multiracial generations lead to changes in physical appearances of individuals and make race less important in ethnic identity.

Ethnicity

Ethnicity is the shared feeling of peoplehood among a group of individuals (Gordon, 1964). Ethnicity reflects cultural membership and is based on individuals sharing similar cultural patterns (such as values, beliefs, customs, behaviors, and traditions) that over time create a common history that is exceedingly resistant to change. Ethnicity represents the identifying characteristics of culture, such as race, religion, or national origin. It is influenced by education, income level, location, and association with ethnic groups other than one's own. Therefore there is a recipro-

BOX 7-1 Factors Influencing Individual Differences Within Cultural Groups

Age
Religion
Dialect and language spoken
Gender identity roles
Socioeconomic background
Geographic location in the country of origin
Geographic location in the current country
History of the subcultural group with which clients identify in their current country of residence
History of the subcultural group with which clients identify in their country of origin
Amount of interaction time among older and younger generations
The degree of assimilation in the current country of residence
Immigration status*
Conditions under which migration occurred*

Except where noted with an asterisk (*), from Orque M: Orque's ethnic/cultural system: a framework for ethnic nursing care. In Orque MS, Bloch B, Monrroy LSA, editors: *Ethnic nursing care: a multicultural approach*, St Louis, 1983, Mosby.

cal relationship between the individual and society. Members of an ethnic group give up aspects of their identity and society when they adopt characteristics of the group's identity. However, when there is a strong ethnic identity, the group maintains the values, beliefs, behaviors, practices, and ways of thinking.

CULTURAL COMPETENCE

Many people are taught by and have knowledge of a dominant culture (Brislin, 1993). As long as the person is operating within that culture, response occurs without thinking to a variety of situations and does not require examination of the cultural content of the behavior in order to make a response. However, in today's climate of multiculturism, nurses are caring for a greater number of culturally diverse clients than ever before. The nurse must understand cultural competence to provide nursing care that meets the needs of these persons.

Cultural competence is a set of knowledge-based and interpersonal skills that nurses use to effectively care for the client (individual, family, and community) (Campinha-Bacote, Yahle, and Langenkamp, 1996; Frei et al, 1994). Cultural competence reflects a higher level of knowledge than cultural sensitivity, which was once thought to be all that was needed for nurses to effectively care for their clients.

Culturally competent nursing care is guided by four principles (AAN Expert Panel, 1992):
1. Care is designed for the specific client.
2. Care is based on the uniqueness of the person's culture and includes cultural norms and values.

3. Care includes self-empowerment strategies to facilitate client decision making in health behavior.
4. Care is provided with sensitivity based on the cultural uniqueness of clients.

Nurses must be culturally competent for the following reasons:
1. *The nurse's culture often differs from that of the client.* Nurses come from a variety of cultural backgrounds and have their own cultural traditions. Each nurse has a unique set of cultural experiences that gives meaning and understanding to his or her behavior. Since the nursing profession is a subsystem of the U.S. health care system, many nurses also bring biomedical beliefs and values to the practice environment that may differ from client's beliefs and values. With such differences of beliefs and values, when the client and the nurse interact they may have a different understanding as to the meaning of the problem and different expectations about what to do to promote and protect health. In these circumstances, cultural competence helps nurses engage strategies that respect client's values and expectations without diminishing the nurses' own values and expectations.
2. *Care that is not culturally competent may further increase the cost of health care and decrease opportunities for positive client outcomes.* In the current health care climate of economic constraints, the health care industry is very focused on cost effectiveness. Cost effectiveness means that there is a balance between cost and quality (Irvine, Sidani, and Hall, 1998). Quality of care means that positive health outcomes are achieved. Care that is not focused on the clients' values and ideas is likely to increase cost and diminish quality. For example, when clients are using both folk medicine and traditional medicine and nurses fail to assess and use this information in teaching, the clients may not get the full benefits of the treatment protocol. This suggests that positive outcomes, which are indicators of quality, may not be met. When quality is compromised, additional resources may be needed to achieve the health care outcomes. Increased use of resources means that cost is increased.
3. *Specific objectives for persons of different cultures need to be met as outlined in Healthy People 2010.* Achievement of *Healthy People 2010* objectives requires that clients' lifestyle and personal choices be considered. For example, the American health care system views excessive drinking as a sign of disease. In 1994, 28.0 per 100,000 Native Americans died of alcohol-related motor vehicle accidents, a rate that is four times higher than the general population (USDHHS, 1998). The national goal is to reduce these deaths by 46% by the year 2010. However, many Native Americans view the use of alcohol consumption as an acceptable way to participate in family celebrations and tribal ceremonies (Orlandi, 1992). Refusal to drink with family may be

TABLE 7-2 Selected Risk Reduction 2010 Objectives for Target Groups

OBJECTIVES	1995 BASELINE
1. Increase years of healthy life to at least 66 years	63.9
Target group: African-American	56.0
2. Reduce homicides to less than 7.2 per 100,000 people	9.2 (age adjusted)
Target group: African-American male 15 to 34 years of age	114.6
3. Decrease coronary heart disease deaths to no more than 51 per 100,000	108.0
Target group: African-American	147.0
4. Decrease hepatitis B rates to 0 per 100,000 in persons less than 25 years of age (except perinatal infections)	
Target group: Asian/Pacific Islander	29.4
5. Reduce to 13% the proportion of adults (18 and older) who use tobacco products	24.7
Target group: Native American	36.2

From US Department of Health and Human Services, Office of Public Health and Science: *Healthy people 2010 objectives: draft for public comment*, Washington, 1998, US Government Printing Office.

TABLE 7-3 The Cultural Competence Framework: Stages of Competence Development

	CULTURALLY INCOMPETENT	CULTURALLY SENSITIVE	CULTURALLY COMPETENT
Cognitive dimension	Oblivious	Aware	Knowledgeable
Affective dimension	Apathetic	Sympathetic	Committed to change
Skills dimension	Unskilled	Lacking some skills	Highly skilled
Overall effect	Destructive	Neutral	Constructive

From Orlandi MA: Defining cultural competence: an organizing framework. In Orlandi MA, editor: *Cultural competence for evaluators*, Washington, DC, 1992, USDHHS.

viewed as a sign of rejection. In Western culture alcoholism is viewed as a mental illness. In the Native American culture, it may be viewed as a disharmony between the individuals and their spirit world and treated through traditional medicine. West (1993, p. 234) asserts that "if the government sends Indians to a health clinic where personnel do not understand the holistic health practices of Indians and where young white people serve as caregivers and authority figures, failure is likely to result." To have successful outcomes, nurses who develop population-based programs to reduce alcohol-related deaths must respect the cultural uniqueness of Native Americans. Table 7-2 gives examples of health promotion objectives for selected minority groups who are at risk.

Developing Cultural Competence

Developing cultural competence is an ongoing life process. It is challenging and at times painful as the nurse struggles to break with the old and adopt new ways of thinking and performing (Frei et al, 1994). Nurses develop cultural competence in different ways, but development occurs mainly through experiences with clients of other cultures and through the nurses' awareness of these experiences. Since there are varying degrees of cultural competence, not all nurses may reach the same level of development.

As summarized in Table 7-3, Orlandi (1992) suggests a three-stage process for developing cultural competence: culturally incompetent, culturally sensitive, and culturally competent. Each stage is based on four dimensions that include an overall effect of cognitive (thinking), affective (feeling), and psychomotor (doing) skills on nursing care. *Stop now and describe your cultural competence with persons of a culture different from your own by staging each of these four dimensions.*

Campinha-Bacote, Yahle, and Langenkamp (1996) offer a model to explain the development of cultural competence. The components of the model are as follows:

- Cultural awareness
- Cultural knowledge
- Cultural skill
- Cultural encounter

Cultural awareness

Cultural awareness is an appreciation of and sensitivity to the client's values, beliefs, practices, lifestyles, and problem-solving strategies (Campinha-Bacote, Yahle, and

Langenkamp, 1996). To be aware suggests that nurses are receptive to learning about the cultural dimensions of the client. Cultural awareness includes an examination of the nurse's personal values and biases (Misener et al, 1997). Nurses who are culturally aware understand the basis for their own behavior and how it helps or hinders the delivery of competent care to persons from cultures other than their own (AAN Expert Panel, 1992). Culturally aware nurses recognize that health is expressed differently across cultures and that culturally competent care can be delivered in a variety of modes consistent with the client's health values. For example, at a community outreach program, the nurse was teaching a racially mixed group the screening protocol for breast and cervical cancer detection. An African-American woman in the group refused to give the return demonstration for breast self-examination. When encouraged to do so, she said "my breasts are much larger than those on the model. Besides, the models are not like me. They were all white." After hearing the client's comments, the nurse realized that she had made no reference in her talk to the influence of culture or race on screening for breast and cervical cancer.

The nurse talked with the client, asked for her recommendations, and encouraged her to return the demonstration. The nurse coached the client through the self-examination process while pointing out that regardless of breast size, shape, and color, the technique is the same for feeling the tissue and squeezing the nipple to make certain that there is no discharge. Because this nurse was culturally aware, she did not become angry with herself or with the client and she did not impose her own values on the client. Rather, she encouraged the client to talk about her culture so that she could learn the appropriate intervention strategies to help the client meet her cultural needs. In contrast, if the nurse was not culturally aware, she may have misunderstood the client's concerns and acted in a defensive manner. Such an interaction, most likely, would have ended in a confrontation that would not have been helpful to the client or the nurse. Box 7-2 identifies a number of questions on which nurses may focus as they try to know their own culture and the implications of their own cultural values.

Cultural knowledge

Cultural knowledge is another component that is essential to caring for a multicultural society. Cultural knowledge provides nurses with organizational elements of cultures and current information on what is necessary to provide effective nursing care. Emphasis is on learning about the clients' worldview from an emic (native) perspective. Knowledge of the client's culture decreases misinterpretations by the nurse and supports the client's cooperation with the health care regimen (Leininger, 1995). Leininger (1995) points out that nurses who lack cultural knowledge may develop feelings of inadequacy and helplessness because they are often unable to effectively help

their clients. In a study involving 150 community health nurses, Bernal and Froman (1987) found that the nurses indicated they did not feel confident in caring for African-Americans, Puerto Ricans, and Southeast Asians. Nurses with more education were not more culturally competent than those with less education. Similarly, Eliason (1998) reported in a study that there is a significant positive relationship between students' comfort level and the amount of experience they have had in caring for culturally diverse clients. This supports the need for nurses' education to include exposure to a variety of cultures. When knowledge of the client's culture is missing or inadequate, it can also lead to negative situations such as lack of cooperation of clients with the health care regimen and inadequate use of health services (Leininger, 1995). It is unrealistic to expect that nurses will have knowledge of all cultures. Instead they should be aware of and know how to obtain the knowledge of cultural influences that affect groups with whom they interact.

Cultural skill

The third component in developing cultural competence is **cultural skill.** Cultural skill reflects the effective integration of cultural awareness and cultural knowledge to meet clients' needs. When interacting, culturally skillful nurses use appropriate touch during conversation, modify the physical distance between self and others, and use

---

BOX 7-2 Early Cultural Awareness

- Think about the first time you had contact with someone you realized was culturally different from you.
- Briefly describe the situation/event.
  How old were you?
  What were your feelings?
  What were your thoughts?
- What did your parents and other significant adults say about those who were culturally different from your family?
  What adjectives were used?
  What attitudes were conveyed?
- As you got older, what messages did you get about minority groups from the larger community or culture?
- As an adult, how do others in the community talk about culturally different people?
  What adjectives were used?
  What attitudes were conveyed?
  How does this reinforce or contradict your earlier experience?
- What parts of this cultural baggage make it difficult to work with clients from different cultural groups?
- What parts of this cultural baggage facilitate your work with clients?

From Randall-David E: *Culturally competent HIV counseling and education,* McLean, VA, 1994, The Maternal and Child Health Clearinghouse.

strategies to avoid cultural misunderstandings while meeting mutually agreed-upon goals.

Cultural encounter

A **cultural encounter** is the final step in becoming culturally competent. In this step, nurses integrate at all levels of care the importance of culture as they make changes to meet the culturally unique needs of the client. Cultural encounters involve all interactions, not only those that are health related (Jezewski, 1993). The most important encounters are those where nurses learn directly from clients about their life experiences and the significance of these experiences for health (Leininger, 1995).

DID YOU KNOW? *Nurses can assist clients to develop cultural encounters with clients of other cultures who are recovering from similar illnesses. In these educational groups, clients learn from each other survival strategies and ways of integrating themselves back into families, community, and workplace.*

In some communities, nurses may have few opportunities to develop cultural competence by working directly with persons of other cultures. When nurses come into contact with persons who are culturally different from themselves, they should adapt general cultural concepts to the situation until they are able to learn directly from the clients about their culture (Fig. 7-1). Developing cultural competence also comes from reading about, taking courses

on, and discussing within multicultural settings on different cultures. Nurses should be aware that having cultural competence is not the same as being a cultural expert on a group that is different from their own. A successful encounter may be judged based on four aspects (Brislin, 1993):

1. Nurses should feel successful with established relationships with the client.
2. Clients feel that the interactions were warm, cordial, respectful, and cooperative.
3. The tasks are done efficiently.
4. Nurse and client experience little or no stress.

Dimensions of Cultural Competence

Nurses integrate their professional knowledge with the client's knowledge and practices to negotiate and promote culturally relevant care for a specific client. Leininger (1995) suggests three modes of actions, based on negotiation between the client and nurse, that guide the nurse to deliver culturally competent care: cultural preservation, cultural accommodation, and cultural repatterning. When these decisions and actions are used with cultural brokering, the nurse is able to fulfill the various roles vital to providing holistic care for culturally diverse clients.

Cultural preservation

The goal of **cultural preservation** is to support the use by clients of those aspects of the client's culture that promote healthy behaviors. For example, Ms. Lin, a 73-year-old Chinese woman, is discharged to home care after

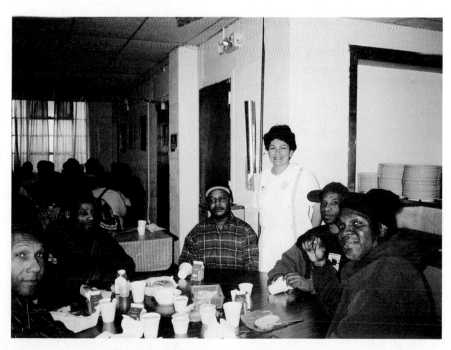

FIG. 7-1 An Hispanic nursing student interacting with African-American men at a nutritional center. To interact in a culturally competent manner, the student needs to have an awareness of and knowledge about the differences between her culture and the men's culture and the skill to portray this in her behavior toward them.

surgery for cancer of the large intestine. The nurse found her at home alone with her 76-year-old husband. After the physical assessment, the nurse discussed making a referral for Ms. Lin to have a home health aide to assist her with physical care and light housekeeping chores. The family was gracious but seemed hesitant to accept the referral. The nurse knew that the Chinese value the extended family network and family decision making. She asked the couple if they would like to discuss the situation with their daughters. Both the client and her husband seemed pleased with the idea, and the nurse promised to get back to them the next day. When the nurse returned for her visit, one of Ms. Lin's daughters was present and told the nurse that the family could manage without additional help. The three daughters had made a schedule to take turns in caring for their parents. The nurse demonstrated acceptance and support for the family's decision and told them that if they decide at a later time to have the home health aide, they should call the agency. She then gave them the telephone number and scheduled the next follow-up visit with them.

Cultural accommodation

Cultural accommodation means that the nurse negotiates with clients to include aspects of their folk practices with the traditional health care system to implement essential treatment plans. The emphasis should be to make sure that the practice is not harmful, is safe, and has health benefits for the client. For example, Ms. Etienne is a 36-year-old Haitian woman who is pregnant and diagnosed with hypertension. For each of her last three visits at the neighborhood health clinic, the client was hypertensive. When questioned, Ms. Etienne confided in the nurse that she was drinking special teas that were prescribed by her voodoo priest to support her having a "strong baby." The nurse asked for the names of the herbs that she was using. The nurse than scheduled a conference with the pharmacist to discuss the specific ingredients in the herbs and ways that they might help the client to meet her cultural needs. The nurse found out that one of the herbs led to the client's high blood pressure and negotiated with the client not to take the specific tea.

Cultural repatterning

Cultural repatterning means that the nurse works with clients to make changes in health practices when these behaviors are harmful or decrease the clients' well being. For example, a culturally competent nurse knows of the high incidence of obesity among Mexican-American women 20 years of age and over (USDHHS, 1998). While respecting the client's tradition, the nurse must teach the client about weight loss and about ways of including cultural foods that would support a healthier lifestyle (see Research Brief).

Culture brokering

Culture brokering is another action used by culturally competent nurses to make certain that clients receive culturally appropriate care (Jezewski, 1993). **Culture brokering** is advocating, mediating, negotiating, and intervening between the health care culture and the client's culture on be-

half of clients. Culturally competent nurses are in a position to understand both cultures and may use knowledge to resolve or lessen problems that may have resulted from individuals in either culture not understanding the other person's values. To illustrate, migrant workers tend to have high occupational mobility; many are poor and may have limited formal education. They may only seek health care when they are ill and cannot work. Whenever nurses interact with them, they should use every opportunity to teach them about prevention and health maintenance, environmental sanitation, and nutrition because it may be the only opportunity that the nurse will ever have to treat a particular migrant worker. Nurses should also advocate for the rights of the migrant worker to receive quality health care. For example, the nurse may contact the Migrant Health Services for follow-up or referral care for the migrant worker.

INHIBITORS TO DEVELOPING CULTURAL COMPETENCE

When nurses fail to provide culturally competent nursing care, it may be because they have had minimal opportunity for learning about transcultural nursing, their supervi-

RESEARCH *Brief*

A study was conducted in South Carolina to determine differences in functional status, health status, and use of community services between elderly African-Americans and Caucasians diagnosed with diabetes. Data were collected over an 8-year period from the agency records for a four-county non-retirement and non-resort region. Results showed that there were no significant differences between the groups in functional status or health status. However, the elderly Caucasian had significantly more difficulty in specific activities of daily living, such as house cleaning, food preparation, and transportation. Although both groups underused the community services, the use of services was significantly lower for the African-Americans elders. Community services included case management, outreach, congregate meals, home-delivered meals, commodity distribution, recreation, and transportation.

Underuse of community services is a significant finding, particularly as it relates to the elderly who live alone. The elderly who do not use community services are likely to be at an increased risk for developing diabetic complications, a poorer quality of life, and as a consequence, increased mortality. The findings suggest that nurses should explore reasons for the failure to use and develop interventions that would increase use of services, especially to vulnerable groups such as elderly African-Americans with diabetes.

Witucki J, Wallace DC: Differences in functional status, health status, and community-based service use between Black and White diabetic elder, *J Cult Divers* 6(3), 94, 1998.

sors are pressuring them to increase productivity by increasing their case loads, or they are pressured by colleagues who are not knowledgeable about cultural concepts and are offended when others use the concepts. Any of these factors may result in nurse behaviors such as stereotyping, prejudice and racism, ethnocentrism, cultural imposition, cultural conflict, and cultural shock.

Stereotyping

Stereotyping is the basis for ascribing certain beliefs and behaviors about a group to an individual without giving adequate attention to individual differences (Brislin, 1993). Stereotyping blocks the willingness of a person to be open and to learn about specific individuals or groups. When information is not immediately available, nurses frequently generalize about a group's behavioral pattern as a guide until they have had time to observe and assess the client's behavior. This is a problem. With added data, nurses may not be willing to include new and specific data about the client. New information may be distorted to fit with preconceived ideas. The generalizing that was a beginning point for understanding the individual becomes a final point where the individual is stereotyped based on the group's behavior (Galanti, 1997).

Stereotypes can be positive, but they are often negative. For example, Asians are positively stereotyped as the "model" minority group, so there is the expectation that they will always behave in ways that reinforce the stereotypical notion. Other groups are stereotyped as "industrious and hard working." Nurses use negative stereotypes when they label a Native American who complains of abdominal pain as an alcoholic because they know that there is a high incidence of alcoholism in the group. Similarly, nurses may label a young African-American woman who is complaining of abdominal pain as having a sexually transmitted disease because women in this group may be believed to be sexually permissive. When clients perceive that they are being stereotyped, they may respond with anger and hostility. This in turn perpetuates the stereotype and creates barriers for some members of this group to seeking health care. Nurses should always avoid using stereotypes, and to minimize their use they should become more aware of their biases about other groups and recognize the effect of socialization on individual differences.

Prejudice and Racism

Prejudice is the emotional manifestation of deeply held beliefs (stereotypes) about other groups (Brislin, 1993). It usually refers to negative feelings conjured up as a result of prejudging, limited knowledge about, or limited contact with the individual. Those who are prejudiced deny individuals, based on race, skin color, ethnicity, or social standing, the opportunity to benefit fully from society's offerings of education, good jobs, and community activities.

Racism is a form of prejudice and refers to the belief that persons who are born into a particular group are inferior, for example, in intelligence, morals, beauty, and self-worth (Brislin, 1993). The Tuskegee Syphilis Study is a well-known example of racism directed at a specific racial group (Gamble, 1997). This study was conducted by the Public Health Service to observe the effects of syphilis on African-American men over a period of 40 years. African-American men with syphilis were recruited for the study but were not told that they had syphilis. These men were told that they were being treated for "bad blood." However, the treatment for syphilis was being withheld. As a result, hundreds of men lost their lives because of the effects of syphilis. The consequence of such racism has contributed to the belief among some African-Americans that research might be designed to harm them and that all care might be a part of a research study, especially government programs, designed to harm.

WHAT DO YOU THINK? *A 90-year-old South American woman refuses to have her nursing care provided by an African-American nurse. Should the community agency assign a nurse from another racial group to care for the client or should the client be transferred to another community health agency?*

Prejudice and racism can be understood using a two-dimensional matrix: overt versus covert and intentional versus unintentional. Locke and Hardaway (1992) depict four types of prejudice/racism that result from this matrix: overt intentional, covert intentional, overt unintentional, and covert unintentional. Since nurses are members of society, they too can exhibit prejudice and racism. *Overt intentional* prejudice/racism means that the behavior is both apparent and purposeful. The nurse is aware of personal biases and beliefs and integrates them into a plan of action to negatively manage client problems. With *overt unintentional*, the behavior is apparent but not purposeful and no harm is intended. *Covert intentional* means that the behavior is subtle and purposeful and the person tries to avoid being viewed as prejudicial or racist. *Covert unintentional* means that the behavior is neither apparent or purposeful. The person is unaware of the behavior. Regardless of the type of prejudice or racism, the behavior is harmful to the client. Nurses may also be the recipient of prejudicial or racist acts. Nurses do not have to endure such behavior and should avoid internalizing the behavior, set limits with clients, and share the behavior with other colleagues (Miles, 1997). An example of each type of prejudice/racism is presented in Box 7-3.

Ethnocentrism

Ethnocentrism, or cultural prejudice, is the belief that one's own group determines the standards for behavior by which all other groups are to be judged. Ethnocentric nurses are unfamiliar and uncomfortable with that which is different from their culture. They devalue experiences of others and judge them to be inferior, and they treat those who are different from themselves with suspicion or hostility (Andrews and Boyle, 1998). This behavior is in con-

---

BOX 7-3 Types of Prejudice/Racial Behaviors

OVERT INTENTIONAL PREJUDICE/RACISM

Two homeless women, one African-American and the other Irish, are clients at the neighborhood health care center. Both women are having financial difficulty. The African-American client's husband was laid off 4 years ago after his company merged with another company. The Irish client is undergoing radiation treatment for metastatic cancer and has lost her job as a result of her prolonged illness. Both women are without health insurance. The nurse referred the Irish client to social services but did not refer the African-American woman. The nurse believed that minority clients have direct experience with some local and national government programs. Therefore this client knows about available resources and can negotiate the social system for herself and family. By contrast, the nurse believed that the Irish woman had a catastrophic illness, she had no prior experience negotiating government programs, and the nurse needs to advocate for her. The nurse, not knowing the health-seeking behaviors of either client, stereotyped both women and intentionally played out her stereotypes about the two racial groups.

OVERT UNINTENTIONAL PREJUDICE/RACISM

The nurse was assigned to make an initial visit to two clients recently discharged from the hospital with a diagnosis of hypertension. The nurse performed physical assessments on both clients. She developed an extensive culturally relevant teaching plan with the Filipino client that included information on sodium restriction and the effect on kidney functioning, ways to integrate cultural foods into the diet, and support in lifestyle changes. With the Puerto Rican client, the nurse performed a routine physical assessment and did not discuss the client's culturally special dietary requirements. The nurse believed that the Puerto Rican client was not capable of understanding such complex information and was going to continue to seek help from her cuarandera (a folk practitioner) to manage

the hypertension. At the end of his visit, the nurse says to this client, "Take care of yourself. See you next time." In this situation, the nurse did not realize that he had stereotyped the client and that his actions were hurtful. He believed that he was providing quality care based on the client's needs.

COVERT INTENTIONAL PREJUDICE/RACISM

A Native American nurse works in a home health agency within a diverse community and is very concerned about her client care assignment. She has observed that her clients are always among the poorest and live in the most unsafe areas of the community. Her nonminority colleagues are not assigned to those sections of the community. In a recent staff meeting she raised the concerns with her supervisors. On hearing her observations, the nursing supervisors looked at her in a skeptical manner and asked what she was talking about. This is covert racism because the nursing supervisors were aware of the informal policy that they assign minority nurses to clients in a particular area of the community. They had discussed the practice among themselves but would never admit to it. The supervisors felt that the best way for minority clients to be the recipients of culturally competent care was to assign a minority nurse to care for them.

COVERT UNINTENTIONAL PREJUDICE/RACISM

A middle-class family has a physically and mentally challenged child. The parents' insurance refuses to pay for the child's medical care. The nurse, who has been working for the agency for many years, is aware but failed to tell the parents that the baby can qualify for Medicaid through the handicapped insurance program, even though both parents work and their income is above the Medicaid guidelines limit. This nurse demonstrated prejudice against the mentally ill child.

---

trast to **cultural blindness,** in which the tendency is to ignore all differences between cultures and to act as though the differences do not exist.

Cultural Imposition

The belief in one's own superiority, or ethnocentrism, may lead to **cultural imposition.** Cultural imposition is the process of imposing one's values on others. Nurses impose their values on clients when they forcefully promote Western medical traditions while ignoring the clients' value of non-Western treatments such as acupuncture, herbal therapy, or spiritualistic rituals. A goal for nurses is to develop an approach of **cultural relativism,** where they recognize that clients have different approaches to health care and each approach should be judged on the client's beliefs.

Cultural Conflict

Cultural conflict is a perceived threat that may arise from a misunderstanding of expectations between clients and

nurses when either group is not aware of cultural differences (Andrews and Boyle, 1998). Although cultural conflicts are unavoidable, the goal for nurses should be to manage conflicts so that they do not affect the delivery of culturally competent nursing care (Brislin, 1993).

Culture Shock

Culture shock is the feeling of helplessness, discomfort, and disorientation experienced by an individual attempting to understand or effectively adapt to a different cultural group because of differences in practice, values, and beliefs.

Nurses may experience culture shock when they interact with a client whose culture is different from their own. It may be a normal reaction to beliefs and practices of clients' cultures that are not allowed or disapproved of in the nurse's own culture (Andrews and Boyle, 1998). Culture shock is brought on by anxiety that results from losing familiar signs and symbols of social interaction. As nurses change their practice environments and leave the safety of the hospital for community settings, they may experience heightened discomfort and feelings of powerlessness as they confront differences between themselves and clients. This is especially true when the nurse has little knowledge or exposure to the culture from which the client comes. Being aware of the clients' own cultural beliefs and having knowledge of other cultures may help nurses to be less judgmental and more accepting of cultural differences.

CULTURAL NURSING ASSESSMENT

A cultural nursing assessment is "a systematic identification of the culture care beliefs, meanings, symbols, and practices of individuals or groups within a holistic perspective including the worldview, life experiences, environmental context, ethnohistory, and social structure factors" (Leininger, 1995, p. 118). Nurses use a component of data collection to help them identify and understand clients' beliefs about health and illness. By adopting a relativistic approach, nurses avoid judging or evaluating the client's beliefs and values in terms of their own culture.

A nonjudgmental approach toward the client's culture is helped through such skills as listening, explaining, acknowledging, recommending, and negotiating (Berlin and Fowkes, 1982). It is vital that nurses listen to clients' perceptions of their problems and, in turn, that nurses explain to clients their own perceptions of problems discussed. Nurses and clients should acknowledge and discuss similarities and differences between the two perceptions to develop suggestions for management of problems. Nurses also negotiate with clients on nursing care actions to meet clients' needs.

A variety of tools is available to assist nurses in conducting cultural assessments (Andrews and Boyle, 1998; Leininger, 1995; Ludwig-Beymer et al, 1998; Tripp-Reimer, Brink, and Saunders, 1997). The focus of such tools varies, and selection is determined by the dimensions of culture to be assessed.

During initial contacts with clients, nurses should perform a cultural assessment that may be brief or the beginning of an indepth assessment (Tripp-Reimer, Brink, and Saunders, 1997). In a brief cultural assessment, nurses ask clients about their ethnic background, religious preference, family patterns, food patterns, and health practices. Such basic data helps nurses understand the client from the client's point of view and recognize the uniqueness of the client, thus avoiding stereotyping. Data from a brief assessment help determine the need for an in-depth cultural assessment.

An in-depth cultural assessment should be conducted over a period of time and should not be restricted to the first encounter with the client. This gives both clients and nurses time to get to know each other and, especially for clients, to see nurses in helping relationships. Tripp-Reimer, Brink, and Saunders (1997) suggest that an indepth cultural assessment should be conducted in two phases: a data collection phase and an organization phase.

The *data collection phase* consists of three stages.
1. The nurse collects self-identifying data similar to those collected in the brief assessment.
2. The nurse raises a variety of questions that seek information on clients' perception of what brings them to the health care system, the illness, and treatments expected.
3. After the nursing diagnosis is made, the nurse identifies cultural factors that may influence the effectiveness of nursing care actions.

In the *organization phase*, data are routinely examined, and areas of difference between the client's cultural needs and the goals of Western medicine are identified. Nurses may use Leininger's (1995) three actions (discussed previously in this chapter) to guide them in selecting and discussing culturally appropriate interventions with clients.

Members of minority groups may distrust and fear the Western medical health care system of which nurses are a part. Persons from these cultures may initially have difficulty discussing their beliefs, values, and practices with nurses. This is especially so when they do not know how nurses will receive the information.

The key to a successful cultural assessment lies in nurses being aware of their own culture. Randall David (1989) developed a variety of principles that may be helpful as nurses conduct cultural assessments. Nurses should do the following:
1. Always be aware of the environment. They should look around and listen to what is being said and understand nonverbal communications before taking action.
2. Know about community social organizations such as schools, churches, hospitals, tribal councils, restaurants, taverns, and bars.
3. Know the specific areas that they want to focus on before they begin the cultural assessment.
4. Select a strategy to help them gather cultural data. Strategies may include in-depth interviews, informal conversations, observations of everyday activities or specific events of the client, survey research, and a case method approach to study certain aspects of a client.
5. Identify a confidante who will help "bridge the gap" between cultures.
6. Know the appropriate questions to ask without offending the client.
7. Interview other nurses or health care professionals who have worked with the specific client to get their input.
8. Talk with formal and informal community leaders to gain a comprehensive understanding about significant aspects of community life.
9. Be aware that all information has both subjective and objective aspects, and verify and cross check the information that is collected before acting on it.
10. Avoid pitfalls in making premature generalizations.
11. Be sincere, open, and honest with themselves and the clients.

HOW TO *Select and Use an Interpreter* _____

1. When feasible, select an interpreter who has knowledge of health-related terminology.
2. Use family members with caution because it may be inappropriate to discuss intimate health matters in the presence of certain family members (Tripp-Reimer and Afifi, 1989).
3. The gender of the interpreter may be of concern, particularly when asking questions about sexuality or child birth (Brown, 1990). In some cultures women may prefer a female interpreter and men may prefer a male.
4. The age of the interpreter may also be of concern. For example, older clients may want a more mature interpreter. Children tend to have limited language skills, and when used as interpreters, they may have difficulty interpreting the information.
5. Differences in socioeconomic status, religious affiliation, and educational level between the client and the interpreter may lead to problems in translation of information.
6. Identify the client's birth origin and language or dialect spoken before selecting the interpreter. For example, Chinese clients speak different dialects depending on the region in which they were born.
7. Avoid using an interpreter from the same community as the client to avoid a breach of confidentiality.
8. Avoid using professional jargon, colloquialisms, abstractions, idiomatic expressions, slang, similes, and metaphors (Randall-David, 1989). Speak slowly and use words that are common in the client's culture.
9. Clarify roles with the interpreter.
10. Introduce the interpreter to the client, and explain to the client what the interpreter will be doing
11. Review the situation and information to be translated before and at the end of each health care encounter (Hatton, 1992).
12. Observe the client for non-verbal messages, such as facial expressions, gestures, and other forms of body language (Giger and Davidhizar, 1999). If the client's responses do not fit with the question, the nurse should check to be sure that the interpreter understands the question.
13. Increase accuracy in transmission of information by asking the interpreter to translate the client's own words, and ask the client to repeat the information that was communicated.
14. At the end of the interview, review the material with the client to ensure that nothing has been missed or misunderstood.

Using an Interpreter

Communication with the client or family is required for a cultural assessment. When nurses do not speak or understand the client's language, they should make every effort to obtain assistance from an interpreter. Hatton's (1992) research findings suggest that nurses should be aware of the powerful role that interpreters play in determining information shared between clients and nurses. Interpreters may emphasize their personal preferences by influencing both nurses' and clients' decisions to select and participate in treatment modalities. Nurses may minimize this by learning basic words and sentences of the most commonly spoken languages in the community. Strategies that nurses may use to select and effectively use an interpreter are listed in the How To box.

DID YOU KNOW? *Health care agencies have a responsibility to effectively communicate with their clients. When an interpreter is not available to translate, the client may view this behavior as unacceptable and bring legal action against the agency.*

VARIATIONS AMONG CULTURAL GROUPS

Although all cultures are not the same, all cultures have the same basic organizational factors (Giger and Davidhizar, 1999). These factors should be explored in a cultural assessment because of their potential for differences among groups. They are communication, space, social organization, time, environment control, and biological variations. Some of these differences among cultural groups are presented in Table 7-4.

Communication

Understanding variations in patterns of verbal and nonverbal communication is the basis for achieving therapeutic goals. Variations among cultures are reflected in verbal styles, such as pronunciation, word meaning, voice quality, and humor, and in nonverbal styles, such as eye contact, gestures, touch, interjection during conversation, body posture, facial expression, and silence. For example, when gathering data from an Hispanic woman, the nurse should be aware that the style may be low-keyed and she may avoid eye contact and be hesitant to respond to questions. This behavior should not be interpreted as lack of interest or inability to relate to others (Randall-David, 1989). An example of this occurred when a nurse gave instructions to Asian clients on taking antituberculin drugs. The clients smilingly responded with "yes, yes." The nurse interpreted this response to mean that the clients understood the instructions and that they were accepting of the treatment protocol. One week later, when the clients returned for a follow-up visit, the nurse discovered that the medications had not been taken. The nurse knew that acceptance by and avoidance of confrontation or disagreement with those in authority are important behaviors in the Asian culture;

TABLE 7-4 Variations Among Selected Cultural Groups

	AFRICAN-AMERICANS	ASIANS	HISPANICS	NATIVE AMERICANS
Verbal communication	Asking personal questions of someone that you have met for the first time is seen as improper and intrusive	High level of respect for others, especially those in positions of authority	Expression of negative feelings is considered impolite	Speaks in a low tone of voice and expects the listener to be attentive
Non-verbal communication	Direct eye contact in conversation is often considered rude	Direct eye contact among superiors may be considered disrespectful	Avoidance of eye contact is usually a sign of attentiveness and respect	Direct eye contact is often considered disrespectful
Touch	Touching one's hair by another is often considered offensive	It is not customary to shake hands with persons of the opposite sex	Touching is often observed between two persons in conversation	A light touch of the person's hand instead of a firm handshake is often used when greeting a person
Family organization	Usually have close extended family networks; women play key roles in health care decisions	Usually have close extended family ties; emphasis may be on family needs rather than individual needs	Usually have close extended family ties; all members of the family may be involved in health care decisions	Usually have close extended family; emphasis tends to be on family rather than on individual needs
Time	Often present oriented	Often present oriented	Often present oriented	Often past oriented
Perception	Harmony of mind, health, body, and spirit with nature	When there is a balance between the "yin" and "yang" energy forces	Balance and harmony among mind, body, spirit, and nature	Harmony of mind, body, spirit, and emotions with nature
Alternative healers	"Granny," "root doctor," voodoo priest, spiritualist	Acupuncturist, acupressurist, herbalist	Curandero, espiritualista, yerbero	Medicine man, shaman
Self-care practices	Poultices, herbs, oils, roots	Hot and cold foods, herbs, teas, soups, cupping, burning, rubbing, pinching	Hot and cold foods, herbs	Herbs, corn meal, medicine bundle
Biological variations	Sickle cell anemia, mongolian spots, keloid formation, inverted "T" waves, lactose intolerance, skin color	Thalassemia, drug interactions, mongolian spots, lactose intolerance, skin color	Mongolian spots, lactose intolerance, skin color	Cleft uvula, lactose intolerance, skin color

interventions were adjusted accordingly. The nurse repeated the medication instructions and gave the clients an opportunity to raise questions and concerns and to repeat the instructions that were given. The nurse also discussed the cultural meaning and treatment of tuberculosis.

NURSING TIP

Respect all information that a client shares with you even though the information may be in conflict with your own value system.

Space

Personal space is the area that persons need between themselves and others to feel comfortable. When this space is violated, the client may experience discomfort. Findings from early research indicate that European-American nurses have specific spatial preferences related to an intimate zone (personal distance, social distance, and public distance) that may be observed when they care for clients.

Other cultural groups also have spatial preferences. To illustrate, Hispanics tend to be comfortable with less space because they like to touch persons with whom they are speaking. Filipinos may view touching strangers as inappropriate; therefore nurses may stand farther away from Filipinos than from Hispanics. Nurses should take cues from clients to place themselves in the appropriate spacial zone and avoid misinterpretation of clients' behavior as they handle their spatial needs. On the other hand, clients who are comfortable with closer distances may experience discomfort when nurses stand farther away and interpret the behavior as rejecting.

Social Organization

Social organization, especially that of the family, also is defined differently across cultural groups. In African-American culture, for example, family may include individuals who are unrelated or remotely related. Members of families depend on the extended family and kinship networks for emotional and financial support in times of crises. Mothers and grandmothers play important roles in African-American culture and may need to be included in health care decisions and socioeconomic groups. The significance of family also varies across cultures. This is particularly so in Hispanic and Asian cultures. Members of these groups tend to believe that the needs of the family come before those of the individual. In the Native American family, members honor and respect their elders and look to them for leadership, believing that wisdom comes with increasing age (West, 1993). When working with clients from these cultures, nurses should be aware that it may be futile to exclude family involvement in decision making. At the same time, nurses should advocate for the individual, so that when families make decisions, the individual's needs are also being considered.

Time Perception

The perception of time also differs across cultures. Cultures are considered either future oriented, present oriented, or past oriented. The American middle-class culture tends to be future oriented, and individuals are willing to delay immediate gratification until future goals are accomplished. Clients valuing longevity may moderate their dietary intake and engage in exercise activities to minimize future health risks. In contrast, African-American and Hispanic families may place greater value on quality of life and view present time as being more important than future time. The future is unknown, but the present is known. When nurses discuss health promotion and disease prevention strategies with persons from a present orientation, they should focus on the immediate benefits these clients would gain rather than emphasize future outcomes. That is not to say that clients cannot or would not learn about preventing future problems, but the nurse needs to connect her teaching to the "here and now."

In cultures that focus on a past orientation (e.g., the Vietnamese culture), individuals may focus on wishes and memories of their ancestors and look to them to provide direction for current situations (Giger and Davidhizar, 1999). In a past-oriented culture, time is viewed as being more flexible than in a present-oriented culture. It has less of a fixed point, and individuals are not offended by being late or early for appointments. Nurses socialized in the Western culture may view time as money and equate punctuality with goodness and being responsible. Working with clients who have a different time perception than the nurse can be problematic. Nurses should clarify the clients' perception to avoid misunderstanding. It is not feasible to expect that clients will change their behavior and adopt the nurse's schedule. Nurses should explain the importance of keeping appointments from the Western perspective. For example, the nurse can communicate a willingness to be flexible in scheduling appointments and explain to the client that the time will be set aside specifically for that client. Along with culture, socioeconomic status and religion may influence perception of time.

Environmental Control

Environmental control refers to the relationships between humans and nature. Cultural groups might perceive humans as having mastery over nature, being dominated by nature, or having a harmonious relationship with nature.

Individuals who perceive mastery over nature believe that they can overcome the natural forces of nature. Such individuals would expect a cure for cancer through the use of medications, antibiotics, surgical interventions, radiation, and chemotherapy. They are willing to do whatever it takes to achieve health.

In contrast, those who view nature as dominant (e.g., African-Americans and Hispanics) believe that they have little or no control over what happens to them. They may not adhere to a cancer treatment protocol because of the belief that nothing will change the outcome because it is their destiny. These individuals are less likely than those of other world views to engage in illness prevention activities.

Persons who view a human harmony with nature (e.g., Asians and Native Americans) may perceive that illness is disharmony with other forces and that medicine is only able to relieve the symptoms rather than cure the disease. They would look to find the treatment for the malignancy from the mind, body, and spirit connection where healing comes from within. These groups are likely to look to naturalistic solutions, such as herbs, acupuncture, and hot and cold treatments, to resolve or cure a cancerous condition (Fig. 7-2).

DID YOU KNOW? *Some clients may view their illness as punishment for misdeeds and may have difficulty accepting care from nurses who do not share their belief.*

Biological Variations

Biological variations distinguish one racial group from another. They occur in areas of growth and development, skin color, enzymatic differences, and susceptibility to disease (Andrews and Boyle, 1998; Giger and Davidhizar, 1999). For example, Western-born neonates are slightly heavier at birth than those born in non-Western cultures. Another variation is mongolian spots that are present on the skin of African-American, Asian, Hispanic, and Native American babies. These are bluish discolorations that may be mistaken for bruises.

Other common and obvious variations include eye shape, hair texture, adipose tissue deposits, shape of ear lobes, thickness of lips, and body configuration. Variations

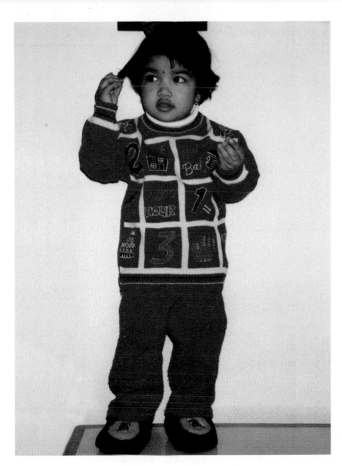

FIG. 7-2 A child from Nepal living in the United States. The child has a black dot on her forehead to protect her from the "evil eye."

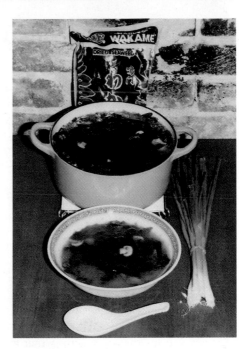

FIG. 7-3 Mi-Yuk Kook (seaweed soup) is a Korean dish eaten by postpartum women to stop bleeding and to clean up body fluids. It is also eaten every birthday.

in growth and development may be influenced by environmental conditions such as nutrition, climate, and disease. Research findings suggest that Asian men have a greater sensitivity than Caucasian Europeans to codeine and experience significantly weaker effects from the drug (Wu, 1997). These men are missing an enzyme called CYP2D6, which allows the body to metabolize codeine into morphine, which is responsible for the pain relief provided by codeine. When an individual is missing the enzyme, no amount of codeine will lessen the pain and other pain reducing medicines should be explored. A more common enzyme deficiency is glucose-6-phosphate dehydrogenase (G-6-PD), which is responsible for lactose intolerance in many ethnic groups (Giger and Davidhizar, 1999).

EFFECTS OF CULTURE ON NUTRITION

Nutritional practices are an integral part of the assessment process for all families, especially since they play a prominent role in health problems of some groups (Greenberg et al, 1998). Efforts to understand dietary patterns of clients should go beyond relying on membership in a defined group. Knowing clients' nutrition practices makes it possible to develop treatment regimens that would not conflict

BOX 7-4 Assessment of Dietary Practices and Food Consumption Patterns

- What is the social significance of food in the family?
- What foods are most frequently bought for family consumption? Who makes the decision to buy the food?
- What foods, if any, are taboo or prohibited for the family?
- Does religion play a significant role in food selection?
- Who prepares the food? How is it prepared?
- How much food is eaten. When is it eaten and with whom?
- Where does the client live and what types of restaurants does he or she frequent?
- Has the family adopted foods of other cultural groups?
- What are the family's favorite recipes?

with their cultural food practices (Fig. 7-3). Box 7-4 identifies several questions that nurses should ask when conducting a nutritional assessment.

In mutual goal setting with the client and nutritionist to change harmful dietary practices, the nurse might need to consult culturally oriented magazines. A number of popular magazines, such as *Essence, Ebony,* and *Latina,* have created new dishes from old family recipes using healthier ingredients. These dishes are very tasty and resemble old traditions, yet they are not as harmful.

TABLE 7-5 Selected Food Preferences and Associated Risk Factors Among Selected Cultural Groups

CULTURAL GROUP	FOOD PREFERENCES	NUTRITIONAL EXCESS	RISK FACTORS
African-Americans	Fried foods, greens, bread, lard, pork, rice, foods with high sodium and starch content	Cholesterol, fat, sodium, carbohydrates, calories	Coronary heart disease, obesity
Asians	Soy sauce, rice, pickled dishes, raw fish, tea, balance between yin (cold) and yang (hot) concepts	Cholesterol, fat, sodium, carbohydrates, calories ulcers	Coronary heart disease, liver disease, cancer of the stomach,
Hispanics	Fried foods, beans and rice, chili, carbonated beverages, high fat and sodium foods	Cholesterol, fat, sodium, carbohydrates, calories	Coronary heart disease, obesity
Native Americans	Blue corn meal, fruits, game and fish	Carbohydrates, calories	Diabetes, malnutrition, tuberculosis, infant and maternal mortality

Data from Andrews MM, Boyle JS: *Transcultural concepts in nursing care*, ed 3, Philadelphia, 1998, J.B. Lippincott; Giger JN, Davidhizar R: *Transcultural nursing: assessment and intervention*, ed 3, St Louis, 1999, Mosby.

Table 7-5 lists various dietary practices that are prevalent among some cultural groups in American society. Many of these practices may have their origin in religious as well as cultural traditions. Religion may become a barrier by causing additional tensions in the nurse-client relationship as nurses negotiate with clients to meet their health needs.

SOCIOECONOMIC FACTORS AND CULTURE

Socioeconomic factors contribute greatly to understanding perceptions of health and illness among minority groups. These groups may not have similar opportunities for education, occupation, income earning, and property ownership as the dominant group. According to the U.S. Census Bureau (USDOC, 1997), there are more Caucasian families than minorities below the poverty level. However, the concentration of minority families is greater. For example, Caucasian families represent 8.5% of those in poverty, whereas African-Americans represent 26.4% and Hispanics represent 27.0%. Consequently, minority families are disproportionately represented on the lower tiers on the socioeconomic ladder. Poor economic achievement is also a common characteristic found among populations at risk, such as those in poverty, the homeless, migrant workers, and refugees.

Socioeconomic status is a critical factor in determining access to health care and the development of some chronic health problems (Kington and Smith, 1997). Nurses should be able to distinguish between culture and socioeconomic class issues and not misinterpret behavior as having a cultural origin, when in fact it should be attributed to socioeconomic class. Data suggest that when nurses and clients come from the same social class, it is likely that they operate from the same health belief model, and consequently there is less opportunity for misinterpretation and communication problems.

There is also danger in believing that certain cultural behaviors, such as folk practices, are restricted to lower socioeconomic classes. Roberson (1987) found that health professionals, such as nurses and physicians, also used folk systems in conjunction with the biomedical system to promote their health and prevent disease. Therefore nurses must conduct a cultural assessment for all individuals when they first come in contact with them. Nurses should have guidance in integrating cultural concepts with other aspects of client care to meet their clients' total health care needs.

clinical application

Mr Nguyen, a 64 year old from rural Vietnam, entered the United States with his family 3 years ago through the displaced persons program. Mr. Nguyen was a farmer in his homeland, and since his arrival he has been unable to obtain a stable job that allows him to adequately care for his family. His financial resources are limited and he has no insurance. He speaks enough English to interact directly with people outside his family and community. His oldest daughter, Shu Ping, is enrolled in a 2-year program to become a registered nurse.

The Nguyen family attends the neighborhood church where there are other Vietnamese families. Mr. Nguyen has also been attending the clinic at the hospital but refuses to discuss with his family, even with Shu Ping, the reason for these visits. Shu Ping became increasingly concerned as she observed her father having insomnia, retarded motor activity, an inability to concentrate, and weight loss. However, Mr. Nguyen denied that he was not well. Shu Ping decided to discuss her concerns with a nurse, with whom she had developed an attachment, at the church. She invited the nurse to her home for lunch on a Saturday so the nurse could meet her father and validate her impressions.

After several visits with the family, the nurse was able to establish a close enough relationship with Mr. Nguyen so that she could engage him in a discussion of his health. Because of her extensive work with other Vietnamese immigrants, the nurse was familiar with themes of loss and decided to focus her conversation with Mr Nguyen on his adjustment to the new community living, gains and losses as a result of immigration, and coping strategies. After several discussions with Mr. Nguyen, he confided in the nurse that he feared that he was dying because he had been diagnosed with cancer of the small intestine. He further revealed that he did not share the diagnosis with the family as he did not want them to know of his "bad news." Mr. Nguyen had refused treatment because he knew that people never got better after they had cancer; they always died.

Which of the following actions best characterizes the nurse's willingness to provide culturally competent care to Mr. Nguyen and his family?

A. Discuss with the client his understanding of his diagnosis.
B. Discuss with the client the prognosis for a person diagnosed with cancer of the small intestine in Vietnam.
C. Discuss with the client the prognosis for a person diagnosed with cancer of the small intestine in the United States.
D. Discuss the medical treatment and surgical intervention for cancer of the small intestine.

Answer is in the back of the book.

KEY POINTS

- The United States is an increasingly diverse population, and it is key that nurses, particularly community-oriented nurses, learn about the culture of the individuals for whom they give care.
- Culture is a learned set of behaviors that are widely shared among a group of people that helps guide individuals in problem solving and decision making.
- Nurses should include the clients' cultural beliefs and practices to improve the clients' health status and reduce health care costs.
- Culturally competent nursing care is designed for a specific client, reflects the individual's needs and experiences, and is provided with sensitivity.
- *Culturally competent* means that the nurse is culturally aware, culturally knowledgeable, and able to use cultural skills with culturally diverse clients.
- There are four modes of action that nurses may use to negotiate with clients and promote culturally compe-

tent care: cultural preservation, cultural accommodation, cultural repatterning, and culture brokering.
- Barriers to providing culturally competent care are stereotyping, prejudice and racism, ethnocentrism, cultural imposition, cultural conflict, and culture shock.
- Nurses should complete a cultural assessment on every client with whom they interact. They use cultural assessments to help them understand clients' perspectives of health and illness and to guide them in discussing culturally appropriate interventions with the client. The needs of clients are based on age, education, religion, and socioeconomic status.
- When nurses do not speak or understand the client's language, they should make every effort to obtain assistance from an interpreter. In selecting an interpreter, nurses should consider the clients' cultural needs and respect their right to privacy.
- Dietary practices are an integral part of the assessment data. Efforts to understand dietary practices should go beyond relying on membership in a defined group and include nutritional practices and religious requirements.
- Members of minority groups are greatly represented on the lower tier of the socioeconomic ladder. Poor economic achievement is also a common characteristic among populations at risk, such as those in poverty, the homeless, migrant workers, and refugees. Nurses should be able to distinguish between culture and socioeconomic class issues and not interpret behavior as having a cultural origin when in fact it is attributed to socioeconomic class.

critical thinking activities

1. Describe what it has felt like to be put in an inferior position or have disparaging remarks made about you. How could you use this experience to become more culturally competent?
2. Identify some positive and negative stereotypes that are used to describe groups in your community. What are the implications of these stereotypes in health teaching and for these groups?
3. How has socialization to your community influenced your selection of friends and colleagues.
4. Interview an older person. What folk practices does he or she use to promote health and prevent disease? How could you use these practices to assist him or her in health promotion and disease prevention?
5. Identify major values of the dominant American group. How do these values differ from the values of other minority cultural groups? What is the significance of these differences for nurses?.
6. What strategies would you use when caring for clients who do not speak your language and for whom no translator is readily available?

Bibliography

AAN Expert Panel on Culturally Competent Health Care: Culturally competent health care, *Nurs Outlook* 40:277, 1992.

Andrews MM, Boyle JS: *Transcultural concepts in nursing care*, ed 3, Philadelphia, 1998, J.B. Lippincott.

Battle DE: *Community disorders in multicultural populations*, ed 2, Boston, 1998, Butterworth-Heinemann

Berlin E, Fowkes W: A teaching framework for cross-cultural health care, *West J Med* 139:934, 1982.

Bernal H: A model for delivering culture-relevant care in the community, *Public Health Nurs* 10(4):228, 1993.

Bernal H, Froman R: The confidence of community health nurses in caring for ethnically diverse populations, *Image* 19:201, 1987.

Continued

Bibliography—cont'd

Bhopal R, Donaldson L: White, European, Western, Caucasian, or what? inappropriate labeling in research on race, ethnicity, and health, *Am J Public Health* 88(9):1303, 1998.

Brink PJ: Value orientations as an assessment tool in cultural diversity, *Nurs Res* 33:198, 1984.

Brislin R: *Understanding culture's influence on behavior,* Fort Worth, Texas, 1993, Harcourt Brace.

Brookins GK: Culture, ethnicity, and bicultural competence: implications for children with chronic disease and disability, *Pediatrics* 92:1056, 1993.

Brown BJ: A world view of nursing practice. In Chaska NL, editor: *The nursing profession,* St Louis, 1990, Mosby.

Bucher L, Klemn P, Adepoju J: Fostering cultural competence: a multicultural care plan, *J Nurs Educ* 36(7):334, 1996.

Campinha-Bacote J, Yahle T, Langenkamp M: The challenge of cultural diversity for nurse educators, *J Contin Educ Nurs* 27:59, 1996.

Caudle P: Providing culturally sensitive health care to Hispanic clients, *Nurse Pract* 18(12):40, 1993.

Chachkes E, Christ G: Cross cultural issues in patient education, *Patient Educ Couns* 27:13, 1996.

Clinton JF: Cultural diversity and health care in America: knowledge fundamental to cultural competence in baccalaureate nursing students, *J Cult Divers* 3(1):4, 1996.

Degazon CE: Coping, diabetes and the older African American, *Nurs Outlook* 43:254, 1996.

Denker EP, editor: *Healing at home: visiting Nurse Service of New York, 1893-1993,* Dalton, Mass, 1994, Studley Press.

Donley R: The alternative health revolution, *Nurs Econ* 16(6):298, 1998.

Eliason MJ: Ethics and transcultural nursing care. In Spradley BW, Allender JA, editors: Readings in community health, ed 5, Philadelphia, 1997, J.B. Lippincott.

Eliason J: Correlates of prejudice in nursing students, *J Nurs Educ* 37(1):27, 1998.

Fielo S, Degazon CE: When cultures collide: decision making in a multicultural environment, *N&HC Perspectives on Community* 18:238, 1997.

Frei F et al: *Work design for the competent organization,* Westport, Conn, 1994, Quorum Books.

Galanti GA: *Caring for patients from different cultures,* ed 2, Philadelphia, 1997, University of Pennsylvania Press.

Gamble VN: Under the shadow of Tuskegee: African Americans and health care, *Am J Public Health* 87:1773, 1997.

Giger JN, Davidhizar R: *Transcultural nursing: assessment and intervention,* ed 3, St Louis, 1999, Mosby.

Giger JN, Davidhizar R, Cherry B: Biological variations in the Black patient, *Imprint* 32(2):95, 1991.

Gordon MM: *Assimilation in American life,* New York, 1964, Oxford University Press.

Greenberg MR et al: Region of birth and Black diets: the Harlem household survey, *Am J Public Health* 88:1199, 1998.

Hatton DC: Information transmission in bilingual, bicultural contexts, *J Community Health Nurs* 9(1):53, 1992.

Irvine D, Sidani S, Hall LM :Finding value in nursing care: a framework for quality improvement and cultural evalutation, *Nurs Econ* 16(3):110, 1998.

Jezewski MA: Culture brokering as a model for advocacy, *Nurs Health Care* 14(2):78, 1993.

Kington RS, Smith JP: Socioeconomic status and racial ethnic differences in functional status associated with chronic diseases, *Am J Public Health* 8(5):805, 1997.

Leininger MM: *Transcultural nursing: concepts, theories, research, and practices,* New York, 1995, McGraw Hill.

Lester N: Cultural competence: a nursing dialogue, *Am J Nurs* 98(8):26, 1998.

Lester N: Cultural competence: a nursing dialogue 2, *Am J Nurs* 98(9):36, 1998.

Lipson JG, Dibble SL, Minarik PA, editors: *Culture and nursing care: a pocket guide,* San Francisco, 1996, UCSF Nursing Press.

Locke DC, Hardaway YV: Moral perspectives in interracial settings. In Cochrane D, Manley-Casimir M, editors: *Moral education: practical approaches,* New York, 1992, Praeger.

Louden D: Our diverse population: the emerging reality, *NLN Research and Policy PRISM,* 1996.

Ludwig,-Beymer P et al: Community assessment in a suburban Hispanic community: a description of method, *J Transcultural Nurs* 8(10):19, 1998.

Maclachlan M: *Culture and health,* New York, 1997, John Wiley & Son.

Miles A, Awong L: When the patient is a racist, *Am J Nurs* 97(8):72, 1997.

Misener TR et al: Sexual orientation: a cultural diversity issue for nursing, *Nurs Outlook* 45:178, 1997.

Narayan MC, Rea H: The South Asian client, *Home Healthcare Nurse* 15(7):461, 1997.

Orlandi MA, editor: *Cultural competence for evaluators,* Washington, DC, 1992, USDHHS.

Orque M: Orque's ethnic/cultural system: a framework for ethnic nursing care. In Orque MS, Bloch B, Monrroy LSA, editors: *Ethnic nursing care: a multi-cultural approach,* St Louis, 1983, Mosby.

Phillips LA, Luna de Hernandez I, Torres de Ardon E: Focus on psychometrics: strategies for achieving cultural equivalence, *Res Nurs Health* 17:149, 1994.

Randall-David E: *Strategies for working with culturally diverse communities and clients,* Bethesda, Md, 1989, Association for the Care of Children's Health.

Roberson MHB: Folk health beliefs of health professionals, *West J Nurs Res* 9:257, 1987.

Smith LS: Concept analysis: cultural competence, *J Cult Divers* 5(1):4, 1998.

Snowden LR, Holschuh J: Ethnic differences in emergency psychiatric care and hospitalization is a program for the severely mentally ill, *Community Ment Health* J 28:281, 1992.

Spector RE: *Cultural diversity in health and illness,* ed 4, Norwalk, 1996, Appleton & Lange.

Talabere L: Meeting the challenge of culture care in nursing: diversity, sensitivity, competence and congruence, *J Cult Divers* 3(2):53, 1996.

Talbot L, Curtis L: The challenges of assessing skin indicators in people of color, *Home Healthcare Nurse* 14(3):167, 1996.

Tripp-Reimer T, Afifi LA: Cross-cultural perspectives on patient teaching, *Nurs Clin North Am* 24(3):613, 1989

Tripp-Reimer T, Brink PJ, Saunders JM: Cultural assessment: content and process. In Spradley BW, Allender JA, editors: Readings in community health, ed 5, Philadelphia, 1997, J.B. Lippincott.

U.S. Department of Commerce: *Statistical abstract of the United States,* ed 117, Washington, DC, 1997, US Government Printing Office.

US Department of Health and Human Services, Office of Public Health and Science: *Healthy people 2010 objectives: draft for public comment,* Washington, 1998, US Government Printing Office.

West EA: The cultural bridge model, *Nurs Outlook* 41:229, 1993.

Witucki J, Wallace DC: Differences in functional status, health staus, and community-based service use between Black and White diabetic elders, *J Cult Divers* 5(3):94, 1988.

Wu C: Drug sensitivity varies with ethnicity, *Science News* 152:165, 1997.

CHAPTER 8

Environmental Health

ANN H. CARY & LILLIAN H. MOOD

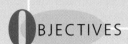BJECTIVES ——————— 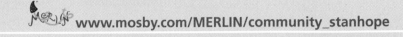 www.mosby.com/MERLIN/community_stanhope

After reading this chapter, the student should be able to do the following:

- Explain the relationship between the environment and human health and disease.
- Apply the nursing process to the practice of environmental health.

- Describe legislative and regulatory policies that have influenced the impact of the environment on health and disease patterns in communities.
- Explain and compare the roles and skills for nurses practicing in the field of environmental health as well as those practicing in many other fields.
- Incorporate environmental principles in practice.

KEY TERMS

bioaccumulation
biodegradation
compliance
dermal absorption
dilution
dose
enforcement

environmental media
estuaries
incineration
ingestion
inhalation
landfilling
land use planning

leachate
non-point sources (NPSs)
outrage factors
permitting
plume
receptor population
remediation

risk assessment
risk communication
route of exposure
source of harm
waste minimization
water discharge
See Glossary for definitions

CHAPTER OUTLINE

The authors acknowledge the contributions of Max Lum, Beth Hibbs, Lynelle Phillips, and Diane Narkunas to this chapter in the previous edition of this text.

Why should a textbook for nurses have a chapter on environmental health? It would not be too dramatic to say that the reason is because lives depend on it. From the smallest one-cell organisms in the food chain to the global issues of warming, ozone depletion, the loss of living species, and deforestation, the environment affects and alters lives.

HUMAN DEPENDENCE ON THE ENVIRONMENT

The science of public health has long recognized environment as a primary determinant of health (Pope, Snyder, and Mood, 1995). Dependence of the human species can be seen through the lens of each of the environmental media: air, water, soil, and food.

Life is dependent upon the purity of air. The pollutant load carried in the air affects its breathable quality and life and health. Life is dependent upon the oxygen exchange with green leafy trees and on the temperature of the air. Scientists know that even a 1° change in the average temperature on the planet makes a difference in the melting of glaciers, water temperatures, sea levels, and plant life. The recent experience with El Niño, the weather phenomenon created by the warming of the Pacific waters, made evident the planet-wide effect of changes in temperatures of water and air.

There is lack of consensus in the scientific community on global warming, but in the book *Earth in the Balance,* then Senator, now Vice President, Al Gore could have been writing for nurses when he said, "Global warming is the fever that accompanies a victim's desperate effort to fight off an invading virus whose waste products have begun to contaminate the metabolic processes of the host" (Gore, 1993, p 216).

Water is necessary for all life forms. Human bodies are made up of 75% water. Only 2.5% of the water on this planet is freshwater, not salt water. Much of the freshwater is in the ice of the polar icecaps; groundwater makes up most of what remains, leaving only 0.01% in lakes, creeks, streams, rivers, and rainfalls (Gore, 1993). Life is dependent upon freshwater resources and water's drinkable quality to survive.

Water is necessary for the production of food and is also necessary for life. Rudy Mancke, a noted naturalist, notes that humans are not a chlorophyll-producing lifeform but consumers on this planet (Mancke, 1998). The quality of the soil in which plants grow is essential to the safety of the food chain. The quality of the soil is affected by its water supply and by the potential for deposition of contaminants from the air. Soil that is free from harmful contaminants and pathogens is basic to life and health.

Human actions affect basic ecological shifts. One example is the destruction of forests, which disrupts the basic oxygen exchange and the stability of soil and pollutes water bodies with sediment. Human actions contribute to environmental impacts or insults. Industry discharges into the air impact its quality, as do individually controlled dis-

charges, such as automobile exhaust, which is the largest contributor to ground-level ozone pollution (SCDHEC, 1998), which can negatively affect the human respiratory system.

Discharges into water bodies from industries and from wastewater treatment systems contribute to destruction of water quality. Water quality is also affected by **non-point sources (NPSs)** of pollution, such as stormwater run-off from paved roads and parking lots, erosion from clear-cut tracts of land for timbering and mining, run-off from chemicals added to soils as fertilizers and pesticides (whether as large-scale farming operations or from individual lawns and gardens). Animal waste from wildlife or confined animal operations for food production (swine and poultry) can get into nearby water bodies and result in coliform contamination and nutrient overload. The result can be illness from ingestion of contaminated water and the creation of conditions amenable to toxic algae growth, such as *Pfiesteria piscicida* (SC Task Group on Toxic Algae, 1998).

The chain of potential damage continues in the additives to farm produce and to animal diets, such as antibiotics, which become secondary additives to humans who consume the end products. Food preparation, washing, cooking temperatures, and time have an effect that has been all too evident in foodborne outbreaks and public health scares related to alar in apples and salmonella and *Eschericha coli* 057 in chicken, eggs, and hamburger (APHA, 1995). The preparation link in the chain is important whether it takes place in home kitchens, in public eating places, or in the handling of food and milk in canning, freezing, and packaging for consumption.

> ▌**DID YOU KNOW?** *The number of waterborne outbreaks from infectious agents and chemical poisoning increased in the 1990s.*

The bottom line is that life depends on the environment, and what humans do collectively affects that vital resource for present and future generations. A central concept in Native American cultures is that humans are stewards, not proprietors, of the environment. Native Americans make the "Rule of Seven" central to all environmental decisions: What will be the effect on the seventh generation? This long view is essential to environmental health.

HEALTHY PEOPLE 2000 OBJECTIVES AND ENVIRONMENTAL HEALTH

Environmental health is one of the 22 priority areas of the *Healthy People 2000* objectives. The federal government has long recognized the relationship between the importance of environmental risks and the underlying factors contributing to diseases. Therefore 17 environmental health objectives are found in this report (Box 8-1). As of the mid-1990s, three of the objectives were progressing in the cor-

BOX 8-1 Targets of Environmental Health Improvements in *Healthy People 2000*

Asthma hospitalizations

Prevalence of serious mental retardation

Waterborne diseases

Blood lead levels exceeding 15 and 25 µg/dl

Counties not exceeding standards for air pollution

Radon testing

Toxic agent releases

Solid waste production and disposal

Safe drinking water

Impaired surface waters: rivers, lakes, estuaries

Home testing for lead-based paint

Construction standards to minimize radon levels

State disclosure laws for radon levels and lead-based paint

Health risks from hazardous waste sites

Household hazardous waste collection

State laws and funds to track sentinel environmental diseases

Children's exposure to tobacco smoke at home

rect direction: 1) more people with clean air in their communities, 2) more people with radon-tested houses, 3) and elimination of the incidence of children with blood lead levels of 25 µg/dl (USDHHS, 1995).

DID YOU KNOW? *Factors contributing to the reduction of lead levels in the United States include reduced lead in gasoline, a reduction in the number of manufactured foods and drink cans and household plumbing components containing lead solder, lead screening laws, and lead paint abatement programs in communities.*

PROTECTING THE ENVIRONMENT

The evolution of formal government structures for environmental protection began in most places with sanitarians or civil engineers, usually addressing safe management of wastewater. The additions of other disciplines of expertise (e.g., hydrogeologists, chemists, biologists, climatologists) to the environmental health team enhanced the ability to make progress. Nurses and other disciplines with medical and community expertise, bring an essential additional dimension to the interdisciplinary work of environmental health. There is some variation among states in the organization and approach to environmental protection, but the common essential strategies of prevention, control, environmental standards, and monitoring are found in every state.

Prevention

As in every public health intervention, prevention is a basic value. Preventing problems is less costly whether the cost is measured in resources consumed or human effects. Education is a primary preventive strategy. State and local environmental protection agencies are involved in educating individuals, groups, and communities about environmental concepts and ways to prevent environmental problems.

Examples of education interventions are numerous. Environmental staff meet with and speak to individuals, neighborhood and civic organizations, and schools. Educational materials are developed and distributed on a wide range of topics and tailored to the needs of various segments of the population. In some states (e.g., South Carolina) curricula for teaching environmental protection have been developed with classroom teachers from the kindergarten level through high school, and training in its use is provided to school districts.

Camps that offer hands-on experience and learning about the environment are offered by partnerships between government and voluntary environmental organizations. Recognition and incentive programs target school groups that develop and implement environmental protection projects. Community coalitions are enlisted as partners in environmental monitoring (e.g., Riverwatch, Waterwatch) and in preventing environmental contamination from NPSs.

Waste minimization efforts range from encouraging the use of less material in packaging and use of non-disposable items like diapers and napkins to the composting of organic matter. Many initiatives to reduce the production of wastes that require disposal target the general population, but some states also have organized units to assist industry, in a nonregulatory capacity, to identify ways to reduce wastes of their operations. In South Carolina a waste minimization unit of the Department of Health and Environmental Control is staffed with retired industrial and environmental engineers who respond to industry requests for in-depth analysis of their operations and recommend changes to reduce waste. Industries participate because they recognize that less waste means more efficient operations and less cost for waste disposal, both of which are good for their bottom line.

One industry's waste can frequently become someone else's raw material, with economic benefits to both. An example is cement industry boilers that are fueled with soil contaminated by leaking underground gasoline tanks. The post-burning decontaminated soil is then used as raw material in making cement. This innovative solution has been prohibited by the Environmental Protection Agency (EPA), refusing to allow the burning of contaminated soils for fuel in cement kilns. In the past, excessive secretiveness and confidentiality of business information has blocked communication about the use of this concept. Industry partners can be linked by health and environmental professionals with the knowledge of potential mutual benefits.

Land use planning is another effective prevention strategy. Authority for planning and zoning of land use is usually given to local (city and county) governments. Conscientious and thoughtful attention to divisions between industrial and residential areas; preservation of green space with parks, greenways, and land trusts; and limits on types of industries recruited and welcomed can result in more livable and sustainable communities. Good planning can also expand the opportunity for co-location of industries that can partner in the exchange of waste and raw materials.

Federal and state initiatives can support local planning processes. For example, federal legislation encourages redevelopment of existing industrial and contaminated sites rather than using pristine green areas for industrial development (SCDHEC, 1998). State initiatives, like Maryland's "Smart Growth," promote planning through incentives to reduce urban sprawl (Glendening, 1998). Both state and federal support for mass transit systems can prevent pollution from a proliferation of automobiles with harmful emissions.

WHAT DO YOU THINK? *Waste materials from outside the United States should be accepted into the landfills in the United States as one method of increasing revenue sources for state budgets.*

Control

Potentially harmful pollution that cannot be prevented must be controlled. The first step in the process of controlling pollution is **permitting.** Industries and businesses whose processes will result in releases (discharges, emissions) that have the potential for harm are required to obtain environmental permits to construct and operate. A range of permits may be required (e.g., stormwater control, construction, operating for air and wastewater discharges, and waste management). It is in the permitting process that maximum opportunities to incorporate some of the previously mentioned prevention strategies can be exercised. For example, waste minimization can be included as a permit condition, with the agreement of the industry, even if it is not required by law or regulation. Once a condition exists in the permit, it has the force of law.

The permitting process includes submission of an application, which includes a required range of details on the proposed operation. Plans are studied, engineering processes are modeled and validated, and other technical requirements are reviewed by appropriate regulatory experts. There is usually some form of public participation required or included voluntarily. The public involvement can include public notice, public comment, and public meetings and hearings initiated by the regulatory agency. Public involvement can also take the form of voluntary agreements and dispute resolution between the industry and the community, which may or may not involve a government entity. Limits on what an industry or business can release or emit lawfully are based on environmental standards.

Environmental Standards

The primary goal of environmental standards is the protection of human health. Other factors, such as cost and feasibility, enter into the final decisions on acceptable standards. Examining the potential sources for environmental standards highlights the dilemma of ensuring human safety and protection. It is obvious that standards protective of human health cannot be developed through broad population experiments, using standard scientific methods, with one segment of the population exposed to various doses and another matched community used as controls. Thus the options for setting standards that are protective of human health and safety are several, albeit all imperfect. These options are more limited than is the case with drug studies. Environmental standard setting must use wide-scale epidemiology, which is expensive and frequently impractical. The first method for arriving at environmental standards is using laboratory animal experiments. This option has the advantage of a relatively short time line, which is also one of the drawbacks. In laboratory experiments, small animals are exposed to large doses of chemicals over a short time period and results are observed and measured. The outcomes must then be extrapolated to large animals (humans), exposed to small doses over an extended period of time.

A second option is using data from worker studies. Again, extrapolation is required, from data on relatively healthy adults who work with chemicals at close range in enclosed environments for a limited time during a day, to a population, varying in age and health status, living 24 hours a day at some distance in an open environment subject to variables in weather.

The third method for developing environmental standards is to learn from the progressive effects on persons exposed through unintended releases and disasters. Examples would be tracking the health effects of persons exposed to radionuclides from the World War II bombing of Hiroshima and the more recent nuclear accident at Chernobyl in the former Soviet Union. In large-scale events such as these, where populations cannot be relocated, health professionals study effects of exposure while trying to mitigate effects through diet (e.g., limiting intake of milk from exposed cows or eating plants with high uptake of contaminants).

The uncertainty in conclusions from any of these methods requires that a significant safety factor be built into the standard, usually of several degrees of magnitude beyond the safe level indicated by the data. For example, if the data indicates a safe level of exposure to be 10 parts per billion (ppb), the standard may be set at 1 ppb. Environmental standards may be expressed as a permitted level of emissions, a maximum contaminant level (MCL) allowed, an action level for environmental clean-up, or a risk-based calculation (Table 8-1).

A standard is often reflective of a level of pollution that will limit the number of excess deaths at a given level of

TABLE 8-1 Examples of Environmental Standards

EXPRESSION OF STANDARD	EXAMPLE
Maximum contaminant level (MCL)	Total trihalomethanes allowed as a by-product of chlorination of drinking water = 1 mg/L
Permitted emission	20% opacity in air emissions
Action level	Lead level for environmental clean-up of soil in residential areas = 400 ppm (parts per million)
Risk-based calculation	1,1,2,2-Tetrachloroethane = 110 μg/liter for a cancer risk of 10^{-5}, or 1 in 100,000 wastewater discharges into streams

exposure over a specified period of time. For example, the MCL for a contaminant in drinking water may be the level of exposure that would produce one excess (over the expected rate) cancer death if a person drank one liter of the water a day for 70 years. Cancer deaths have been the most frequently used outcome measure in environmental standards, but the risk calculations are now expanding to include birth defects, reproductive disorders, immune function disorders, and morbidity (kidney, liver, respiratory, neurotoxic) (Pope, Snyder, and Mood, 1995) (Tables 8-2 and 8-3). There is no place where the need for research is more evident as an undergirding tool for determinants of health (see the Canadian model in Figure 8-2 later in this chapter) than in setting environmental standards. The costs for meaningful studies are very high.

Monitoring

Once environmental standards are set, both as a basis for permitting and in individual facility permits, the next step in control is monitoring. Any monitoring process must use methods approved by the EPA or scientific consensus. Monitoring procedures must follow accepted protocols (e.g., maintaining a documented chain of custody of samples of soil to ensure accuracy and protection from post-sampling contamination at the laboratory).

Environmental monitoring takes two main forms. One is actual inspections of permitted facilities to observe first-hand whether the plans submitted in the permit application are being implemented as approved. In addition to unannounced inspections, continuous monitoring of data and operating procedures required in permits are studied for any variations from what is allowed. Finally, periodic measures of the facility outputs in air and water emissions are calculated or measured directly to ensure compliance with laws and regulations. An alternative or adjunct monitoring method is self-reported data from the regulated agency. Factors must be considered in deciding how much of the monitoring requirement can be met through self-reporting, such as costs, reliability, public trust, and acceptance.

Beyond the monitoring of individual permitted facilities, official regulatory agencies design sampling net-

TABLE 8-2 Percentage of Cancer Deaths Attributable to Different Factors

FACTOR	RANGE OF BEST ESTIMATES	BEST ESTIMATES (%)
LIFESTYLE		
Tobacco	25-40	30
Diet	10-70	35
Infection	1	10
Reproduction and sexual behavior	1-13	7
Alcohol	2-4	3
TOTAL	39-100	85
SOCIETAL		
Occupation	2-8	4
Industrial products	<1-2	<1
Food additives	2	<1
Medicines and medicinal procedures	0.5-3	1
TOTAL	4-15	6
ENVIRONMENTAL		
Pollution	<1-5	2
Geophysical factors	2-4	3
Cumulative attributable risks	3-9	5
TOTAL	46-100	96

Based on data from Doll R, Peto R: Causes of cancer: quantitative estimate of avoidable risks of cancer in the United States today, *J Nat Cancer Inst* 66:1191, 1981.

works for measuring the quality of water and air throughout the geographic area for which they have responsibility. Routine samples are taken at designated monitoring sites and analyzed for criteria pollutants measured nationwide (Box 8-2) and for pollutants resulting from activity specific to the area (e.g., types of local industrial operations) (Box 8-3).

Compliance and enforcement are the next building blocks in controlling environmental damage. **Compliance**

TABLE 8-3 Environmental Agents Implicated in Adverse Reproductive Outcomes

EXPOSURE	KNOWN/SUSPECTED EFFECT
Anesthetic compounds	Infertility, spontaneous abortion, fetal malformations, low birth weight
Antineoplastics	Infertility, spontaneous abortion
Dibromochloropropane	Sperm abnormalities, infertility
Ionizing radiation	Infertility, microcephaly, chromosomal abnormalities, childhood malignancies
Lead	Infertility, spontaneous abortion, developmental disabilities
Manganese	Infertility
Organic mercury	Developmental disabilities, neurologic abnormalities
Organic solvents	Congenital malformations, childhood malignancies
PCBs, PBBs	Fetal mortality, low birth weight, congenital abnormalities, developmental disabilities

From Aldrich T, Griffith J: *Environmental epidemiology and risk assessment*, New York, 1993, Van Nostrand Reinhold.

BOX 8-2 Criteria Air Pollutants (National Ambient Air Quality Standards)

Ozone (ground level)
Sulfur dioxide
Nitrogen dioxide
Particulate matter
Carbon monoxide
Lead

BOX 8-3 Routine Water Analysis (Private Well)

BACTERIOLOGICAL

Total coliform
Fecal coliform
Chlorine residual

CHEMICAL

Lead
Hardness
Nitrates
Chloride
Alkalinity
Iron
pH
Copper
Calcium
Manganese
Magnesium
Zinc

refers to the processes for ensuring that permitting requirements are met. When permit or other legally defined violations are found, the first effort is to get quick, voluntary compliance from the violator. Incentives in the form of reducing or eliminating fines and penalties may be ne-

gotiated in return for rapid and effective action to correct the problem. Formal **enforcement** actions are taken when voluntary compliance is not achieved. The range of enforcement tools that may be employed include fines or penalties, suspended specific operations, or closure of the facility. If the violation is deemed to be willful and with full knowledge that it was unlawful, criminal law may provide for incarceration of the owners/operators in addition to the other consequences.

Enforcement processes may also include provision for public involvement, although this is less common. The public often does not feel included at the level they desire in enforcement or permitting procedures. Rationale for excluding the public can range from a goal of early correction of the problem to a concern that time required for public comment/forums or industry guarding of information for fear of private party lawsuits will delay a solution. Another view, however, is that public involvement is essential to ensure aggressive enforcement.

Clean-up or **remediation** of environmental damage is the final control step. The authority to direct and ensure adequate restoration of environmental quality may be done directly by state or federal government agencies, depending on authority or jurisdiction in law or regulations, or contracted out to private companies, with official oversight. For example, a contaminated site may meet the requirements for the federal "Superfund" National Priority List (Comprehensive Environmental Response Compensation and Liability Act [CERCLA]). In this case the EPA would assume the lead responsibility for clean-up. In contrast, a site where an operating-regulated facility is the violator may be cleaned up with the state taking the lead, either through authority under state law or delegated program responsibility from the EPA.

Public information and involvement processes, such as citizen advisory panels or community forums, are integral to remediation, where implications for future land use and remedies acceptable to the affected community are part of the decision process.

CITIZEN ROLES

Where do nurses enter this picture? It is best to begin with the basic roles of nurses as informed citizens and the personal actions each takes to protect and conserve water and trees, to reduce waste, to recycle, and to prevent and clean up litter in the environment.

In the citizen role, nurses are respected and trusted messengers. There are several examples where community groups depend on nurses for accurate information and as spokespersons on environmental issues. Surveys have shown that nurses and doctors are considered by the public to be the most reliable sources of environmental health information (USC, 1990). In the personal experience of the author, a citizen group led by a nurse was organized to protect the quality of the air. This group not only had an effect on a local industry but also was instrumental in the passage of a state air toxics law. In another community a nurse organizer and spokesperson influenced a county council land use decision that prevented the location of an asphalt plant in the neighborhood.

Nurses can take another step as citizens by using skills as citizen-advocates in communities to affect public policy, laws, and regulations that protect a life-supporting environment. As informed citizens, nurses can foster community action to address environmental threats and thus threats to health.

NURSING'S ENVIRONMENTAL HERITAGE

Within the profession, there is widespread recognition that nurses, like physicians, are taught very little about the environment and environmental threats to health. This recognition and the concern it generates led to two separate studies by the Institute of Medicine (IOM) in the National Academy of Science. The IOM conducted a study of environmental medicine (Warren, 1988) and a study of nursing, which produced the report *Nursing, Health, and Environment* (Pope, Snyder, and Mood, 1995).

> **NURSING TIP**
>
> *"Freedom from illness or injury is related to lack of exposure to toxic agents and other environmental conditions that are potentially detrimental to human health"* *(Pope, Snyder, and Mood, 1995, p. 3).*

The IOM nursing study recognized early that the environment, as a determinant of health, is deeply rooted in nursing's heritage. Pictures of and quotes from Florence Nightingale are used throughout the report, not only because she is a recognized symbol of nursing (i.e., the lady with the lamp), but also because of the central focus of environment in her practice.

> **NURSING TIP**
>
> *"In watching diseases, both in private homes and in public hospitals, the thing which strikes the experienced observer most forcibly is this, that the symptoms or the sufferings generally considered to be inevitable and incident to the disease are very often not symptoms of the disease at all, but of something quite different—of the want of fresh air, or of light, or of warmth, or of quiet, or of cleanliness, or of punctuality and care in the administration of diet, of each or of all of these. . ."* *(Nightingale, 1859, p. 8).*

Florence Nightingale is well known for her work in Crimea and is called by some "the mother of biostatistics" for her skilled use of data, both her own observations and the aggregate compilation of information, to compel action on conditions affecting health. Lillian Wald, who coined the name "public health nurses," spent her life improving the environment of the Henry Street neighborhood and working her broad network of influential contacts to make changes in the physical environment and social conditions that had direct health impacts.

A twentieth-century nurse leader, Virginia Henderson offered a definition of nursing that many nurses were taught in their first "fundamentals" course. That definition provided a broad and reliable direction for practice that fostered prevention and building on strengths toward self-sufficiency, two key elements in environmental health.

> **NURSING TIP**
>
> *"The unique function of the nurse is to assist the individual, sick or well, in the performance of those activities contributing to health or its recovery (or to a peaceful death) that the client would perform unaided if he/she had the necessary strength, will, or knowledge. It is likewise the function of nurses to help people gain independence as rapidly as possible"* *(Henderson, 1966, p. 15).*

DETERMINANTS OF HEALTH

"The mission of public health is fulfilling society's interest in ensuring conditions in which people can be healthy" (Yordy and Remington, 1988, p. 7). As discussed in Chapter 5, there are four major health determinants. In this chapter two are discussed—genetics and environment. These two factors together make clear the enormous impact of surroundings on well being. The interaction between these two major determinants is the focus of some of the most cutting-edge research in cancer and in links between deviant and aggressive behavior, learning difficulties, and toxic burden (EPA, 1996).

The model of the public health/epidemiology triangle of agent, host, and environment forms the basis for com-

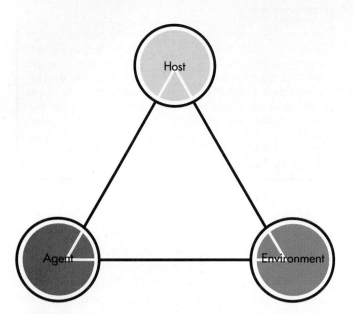

FIG. 8-1 The epidemiologic triangle. For a disease process to occur, there must be a unique combination of events (i.e., a harmful agent that comes into contact with a susceptible host in the proper environment). The occurrence of a disease can be blocked by intersecting the triangle at any of its three sides. A disease or outcome is never caused by one event but rather a chain of events that form a web (epidemiologic web), which because of its complexity, can never be fully understood. (From Cassens BJ: *Preventive medicine and public health,* New York, 1992, ed. 2, John Wiley & Sons.)

municable disease prevention and control (Fig. 8-1). The history of public health has many examples of gains in population health achieved through modifying environments with sanitary practices, such as protecting drinking water from contamination from human wastes, pasteurization of milk, and refrigeration of food (Pickett and Hanlon, 1990).

Canada further explained the determinants of health in a document prepared in 1994 for the Ministers of Health (Federal, Provincial, and Territorial Advisory Committee, 1994). Their expanded list includes physical environments and points out the necessary tools of research, information, and public policy for population health (Fig. 8-2).

All of these perspectives from the past and present are reminders of the richness and necessity of the interdisciplinary nature of public health practice if a broad definition of health is the goal. In order to have a healthy population, there must exist a healthy planet.

ENVIRONMENTAL HEALTH COMPETENCIES FOR NURSES

If the evidence convinces nurses that they belong in the picture of environmental health, what do nurses need to know to be effective partners in the enterprise? The 1995 IOM study *Nursing, Health, and Environment* (Pope, Snyder, and Mood, 1995) identifies four general environmental health competencies for nurses, which are presented in Box 8-4 and detailed in the following sections.

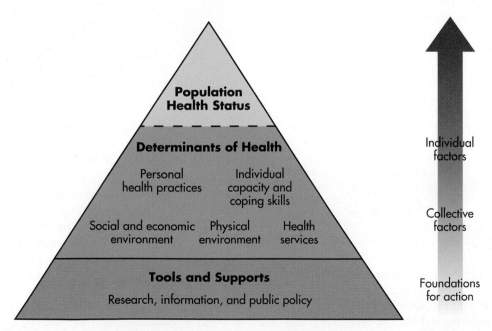

FIG. 8-2 Canadian model of determinants of health. (From Federal, Provincial, and Territorial Advisory Committee on Population Health: *Strategies for population health: investing in the health of Canadians,* Ottawa, Ontario, 1994, Health Canada.

Environmental Health In Canada

Catherine Clarke, Toronto Public Health

FEDERAL RESPONSIBILITIES

The two government agencies responsible for environmental health matters at the federal level are Environment Canada and Health Canada. Environment Canada is concerned with protecting and conserving the natural environment and promoting sustainable development. Health Canada provides national leadership in the development of health policy and the enforcement of health regulations. Both departments are involved in research into health and environmental issues and the preparation and dissemination of technical and public education materials related to human health and the environment.

PROVINCIAL AGENCIES

At the provincial level, Ministries of the Environment are responsible for establishing, monitoring, and enforcing requirements to protect the quality of the natural environment and encourage the efficient use and conservation of resources. Ministries of Health administer provincial health care systems that include community and public health as well as health promotion and disease prevention programs and services. They provide authority to local and regional boards of health and establish guidelines for the provision of programs and services that protect and promote health, including environmental health. Ministries of Labour set standards regarding environmental exposure levels in the workplace. All ministries administer relevant legislation, maintain databases, and publish technical and public education materials related to their areas of responsibility.

LOCAL/REGIONAL BOARDS OF HEALTH

These agencies are responsible for enforcing local by-laws, conducting complaint investigations and risk assessments, and inspecting premises to ensure compliance with pertinent legislation. Staff are often 'first responders' to community concerns, and liaise with, or refer to, provincial ministries responsible for monitoring and enforcement when appropriate. Their emphasis is on the provision of primary prevention strategies. The degree to which local and regional boards of health provide secondary prevention strategies, including screening and monitoring programs, varies considerably across regions and provinces.

CANADIAN RESOURCES

There are Canadian equivalents to each of the categories listed in Box 8-5 of this chapter. The following is a list of some specific sources of Canadian environmental health information:

Federal

Health Canada—Environmental Health Program
Health Canada—Great Lakes Health Effects Program
Health Canada—Laboratory Centre for Disease Control
Environment Canada
Canadian Mortgage and Housing Association

Provincial

Ministries of Health, Environment, Labour
Provincial public health associations

Local/Regional

Boards of health
Poison control centres

Nongovernmental

Canadian Institute for Environmental Law and Policy
Canadian Environmental Law Association
Canadian Institute for Child Health
Canadian Association of Physicians for the Environment
Canadian Public Health Association
Pollution Probe
Learning Disabilities Association of Canada

Bibliography
Sutcliffe PA, Deber RB, Pasut G: Public health in Canada: a comparative study of six provinces, *Can J Public Health* 87(4):246, 1997.

Canadian spelling is used.

Basic Knowledge

No single chapter in a book can provide all the environmental science needed for competent nursing practice. The science base is too expansive and is constantly undergoing change. Interdisciplinary practice makes it unnecessary for the nurse to be an in-depth expert in environmental science. It is essential to have a basic understanding of four particular principles and how they are manifested in environmental threats to health and environmental protection and to have a working knowledge of how to access more detailed information as the situation demands.

Environmental principle 1: Everything is connected to everything else

This principle was introduced in elementary school science, in which students are taught about the water cycle of evaporation and condensation. Further evidence of the truth of this principle can be found in the effects of burn-

BOX 8-4 General Environmental Health Competencies for Nurses

BASIC KNOWLEDGE AND CONCEPTS

All nurses should understand the scientific principles and underpinnings of the relationship between individuals or populations and the environment (including the work environment). This understanding includes the basic mechanism and pathways of exposure to environmental health hazards, basic prevention and control strategies, the interdisciplinary nature of effective interventions, and the role of research.

ASSESSMENT AND REFERRAL

All nurses should be able to successfully complete an environmental health history, recognize potential environmental hazards and sentinel illnesses, and make appropriate referrals for conditions with probably environmental causes. An essential component is the ability to access and provide information to clients and communities and to locate referral sources.

ADVOCACY, ETHICS, AND RISK COMMUNICATION

All nurses should be able to demonstrate knowledge of the role of advocacy (case and class), ethics, and risk communication in client care and community intervention with respect to the potential adverse effects of the environment on health.

LEGISLATION AND REGULATION

All nurses should understand the policy framework and major pieces of legislation and regulations related to environmental health

From Pope AM, Snyder MA, Mood LH, editors: *Nursing, health, and environment*, Washington, DC, 1995, Institute of Medicine, National Academy Press.

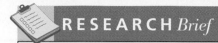

RESEARCH *Brief*

This is a case study of childhood lead exposure in a family living at the poverty level. It is known that child lead exposure is endemic among those living in poverty and substandard housing. Children and families living along the U.S.-Mexico border experience multiple exposures to environmental hazards, especially lead. The impact of lead exposure on fetuses, infants, and children is dramatically compounded by poor nutrition, extreme poverty, inadequate access to health care, hazardous occupational exposures of other family members, social isolation, language and legal barriers, high-risk home environments, lead-laden herbal home remedies, and medicinal and cultural practices.

In this case of Hispanic children and their families, the authors found evidence to support exposure to lead for many of the reasons listed above as well as likely exposure pathways, such as inhaling and ingesting lead-laden dust from auto repair, wire recycling, and paint chips. This research supports the role that public health nurses can play in doing routine assessments of populations known to be at risk and providing community health services to reduce the long-term effects of lead exposure.

Amaya MA et al: Childhood lead poisoning on the US-Mexico border: a case study in environmental health nursing lead poisoning, *Public Health Nurs* 14(6):353, 1997.

ing fossil fuel and domestic and hospital wastes that can result in air transport of mercury. The mercury is deposited on the surface of bodies of water, often in quantities that are not detectable or barely detectable. The chemistry of the water can change the chemical form of the mercury from organic to methyl. Plants growing in the sediment of the river or lake bottoms take up the methyl mercury, fish eat the plants, and larger fish eat the smaller fish. Unlike humans, fish reatain the mercury. **Bioaccumulation** is magnified through the food chain, resulting in harmful concentrations of mercury in some fish species that are consumed by humans. Mercury intake by humans can be devastating to the formation and development of the central nervous systems (CNS) of fetuses, infants, and children and can cause CNS symptoms and problems in adults if eaten frequently and in large enough quantities (ATSDR, 1989).

Warnings of the consequences of this unbroken chain of connections are found in fish consumption advisories in more than 40 states (SCDHEC, 1998). Communicating this complex message and the need for advice over time is a challenge in itself.

Another familiar example of the consequences of the connectedness of our environment is that of lead in paint, banned in 1978 but still present in older homes in poor neighborhoods and in restored homes in more affluent communities. More than 80% of U.S. homes built before 1978—some 64 million—contain lead paint (EPA, 1996). The lead-containing paint chips are scraped, become airborne in breathing space for a brief time, and then end up in nearby soil. Children play in the soil where their hand-to-mouth activity results in exposure to lead that has developmental and behavioral effects, both known and being discovered through research (ATSDR, 1990) (see the Research Brief about lead poisoning).

Lead poisoning is a top environmental health hazard in young children, affecting as many as 1.7 million children 5 years of age and under (EPA, 1996). The remedies for lead contamination have a required chain of their own: education for prevention, screening (both the victim and the source), mitigation or treatment (in the individual and the environment), and authority for regulatory and remedial action in public policy. The principle of connectedness is the essence of tracking exposures and risks.

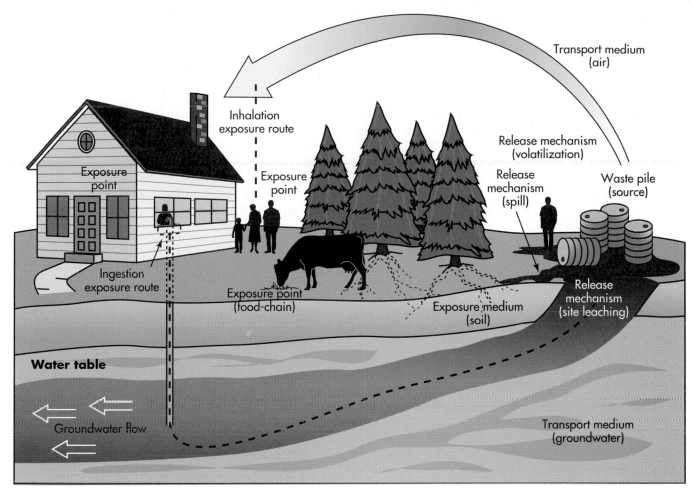

FIG. 8-3 Exposure pathways. (From Agency for Toxic Substances and Disease Registry, 1992.)

For persons to be harmed by something in the environment, several factors must be in place and connected (Fig 8-3):

- A **source of harm** must exist, which has chemical and/or physical properties that make it persistent and/or transportable (volatile, water-soluble) in the environment.
- An **environmental media** is necessary for transport—air, water (surface and/or groundwater), or soil.
- A **receptor population** must be within the exposure pathway for harm to human health. Potential population exposures are important if the contaminant is persistent and land/property use changes over time.
- A **route of exposure** is an essential element. Humans can only be exposed to environmental contaminants through three routes: inhalation, ingestion, and dermal absorption. **Inhalation** requires the contaminant to be within the breathing space. **Ingestion** may occur through drinking contaminated water or milk. Contaminants may also be ingested by eating plants that have taken up the contaminant, eating animals that have eaten contaminated plants or smaller animals (as in the earlier mercury example), or putting contaminated soil

into the mouth (illustrated in the lead example). **Dermal absorption** requires direct contact with a contaminant that can be absorbed through the skin.

- The final ingredient for exposure is **dose.** This element is familiar to nurses. There must be an adequate amount of the chemical to result in human harm. Almost any chemical can be harmful in large enough doses. Nurses practice the dosing principle by giving careful instructions to clients regarding prescribed medications. The converse is also true; very small amounts of even the most toxic materials can do no or immeasurably small harm.

A citizen calls the local health department to report that his drinking water, from a private well, "smells like gasoline." A water sample is collected, and analysis reveals the presence of petroleum products. A nearby rural store and service station has removed its old underground gasoline storage tanks and replaced them, as required by law. Contaminated soil from the old leaking tank has been removed, and a well to monitor groundwater contamination is scheduled for installation. Sandy soil has allowed more rapid movement of the contamination through the groundwater, and the **plume** has reached the neighbor's drinking-water well in levels that exceed the drinking-water standard. Possible responses to the problem are short-term alternate drinking water (bottled), long-term extension of water lines from a nearby municipality, monitoring and clean-up of the contaminated groundwater (including testing other wells), testing children for lead poisoning, and informing the community of the risks and remedies.

The necessity for every element of an exposure pathway to be present in sufficient quantity for harm is a powerful illustration of the principle of connectedness. A quote attributed to Chief Seattle, a nineteenth-century Native American, summarizes the first environmental principle eloquently: "Whatever befalls the earth befalls the sons of the earth. Man did not weave the web of life; he is merely a strand in it. Whatever he does to the web, he does to himself." The second principle is related to the first.

Environmental principle 2: Everything has to go somewhere

Again this principle can be traced to science taught in elementary education: matter cannot be created or destroyed. Once waste products are generated, they must be disposed of in one of three ways. **Incineration** can change the chemical composition through heat, but the products of burning—ash, air emissions—must be controlled and disposed of in one of the other options. A second option is **water discharge.** To interrupt the exposure pathway, the products to be disposed of in water must be treated to ensure that the dosage in the water is not great enough to cause harm or to alter the waste product to a less toxic

form. The third option is burial in the soil, or **landfilling.** Again, the chemical properties must be considered and protections put in place, such as liners and **leachate** pumps and monitors, to avoid migration of harmful dosages into groundwater or air.

Each of these options intends to either 1) provide an opportunity to alter the waste product to a less toxic form through chemical intervention, or **biodegradation,** or 2) store the product in a bio-unavailable form or place. Since either of the options for disposal can be a problem, the option of prevention becomes more appealing (e.g., changing a process from an oil base to a water base, and eliminating oil-containing waste products). Waste minimization can be seen as secondary prevention: reduce, reuse, and recycle. The range of choices involved in producing, packaging, and purchasing products indicates that citizens and industries can make powerful differences in the environmental problem of waste disposal. Just keep in mind that everything has to go somewhere and that it will be connected to humans in some way.

The principles of connectedness and matter occupying space are magnified in importance when the issues of population growth and density are considered, as shown in Figure 8-4. One surprising conclusion may be that family planning could be an important nursing intervention in environmental health. Family planning helps to control the population growth and therefore affects the environmental consequences. One additional point of emphasis is that human effects are intensified in the most sensitive,

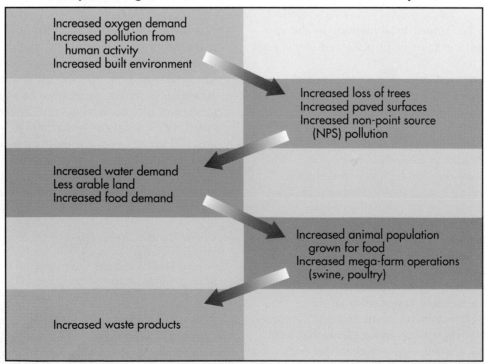

Population growth

Increased oxygen demand
Increased pollution from
    human activity
Increased built environment

Increased water demand
Less arable land
Increased food demand

Increased waste products

Environmental consequences

Increased loss of trees
Increased paved surfaces
Increased non-point source
    (NPS) pollution

Increased animal population
    grown for food
Increased mega-farm operations
    (swine, poultry)

FIG. 8-4 Connectedness of population growth and environmental consequences.

vulnerable environments, such as **estuaries,** the nurseries for much of sea and coastal plant and animal life.

Some of the most valued food sources are also the most sensitive to pollution. Shellfish are very efficient filters of contaminants in the water in which they live. For example, oysters filter and retain almost all contaminants from the water in which they grow. It is impossible to rid them of contaminants after harvesting. The only protection for human consumption is to grow oysters in environments free from harmful contamination. This is why shellfish beds are closed to harvesting after significant rainfall—to protect comsumers from the NPS pollution caused by the run-off of rainfall from surrounding land into surface water. Safe seafood depends on clean water. This example leads to the third principle.

Environmental principle 3: The solution to pollution is dilution

Reflecting on the element of dosage in human exposure reveals the truth in this principle. The use of this principle can be seen in historic environmental and sanitation measures. Garbage was moved from streets to the nearest body of water. Early industries went from dumping wastes outside their buildings to piping them to the nearest stream or river. Human wastes followed the same paths and pipelines. The problem with this principle was that it was tied to a world view that saw the environment as an unlimited resource, a limitless repository for whatever was useless. The **dilution** capacity of large rivers and certainly the ocean seemed boundless. The belief in the capacity of air to dilute resulted in such "solutions" as taller smoke stacks to release pollutants higher into the atmosphere. The reality, more evident every day, is that this planet and its capacity to assimilate byproducts of human civilization is far from limitless. It is, in fact, fragile and delicately balanced, and the knowledge and practice about how to live peacefully within that balance without doing harm is far from adequate. The fourth principle reflects this insight.

Environmental principle 4: Today's solution may be tomorrow's problem

As in almost every aspect of life, environmental scientists and regulators are dealing with incomplete information and insufficient science. The relatively brief history of organized environmental protection is filled with examples. Garbage that went from the streets into unlined landfills is now a source of groundwater contamination. Gasoline tanks that were buried underground to avoid an ugly landscape were found to leak over time. New solutions of lined landfills and double-walled storage tanks, with sensors for leaks and monitoring wells, have emerged, as has the increasing work of cleaning up the earlier "mistakes."

It needs to be emphasized that what can now be called mistakes were not necessarily the result of malicious carelessness or insensitivity. There were simply public policy decisions based on the best information available at the time. The "best information" is often likely to be incomplete and imperfect. That is why research, highlighted in

the Canadian model of determinants of health (see Fig. 8-2), continues to be such an essential tool. Science-based decisions remain a public policy goal. An encouraging trend in industry's new product development is engineering analysis of the full life-cycle of the product, from raw material to waste disposal. Up-front consideration of the costs and effects throughout the cycle can lead to choices that prevent future problems.

One of the greatest challenges and a major source of concern in today's environmental picture are solutions themselves. The growing number and complexity of chemicals that are part of everyday life exemplify this. Citizens have enthusiastically embraced "better living through chemistry" with more than 65,000 new chemical compounds introduced into the environment between 1950 and 1984 (Pope, Snyder, and Mood, 1995), and an estimated 1000 or more have been added each year since. The uses range from industrial to household to medical, and there is no doubt that chemicals have been a part of the solution to numerous problems.

The problem with the enormous growth in chemical production is that the effects of new chemicals on the environment are unknown. A relatively small proportion of the chemicals in use have been well-researched and have defined health effects (Pope, Snyder, and Mood, 1995). Even those with substantial data supporting individual effects have unknown effects when questions of cumulative and synergistic effects of exposures to small quantities of a wide array of substances over time need to be answered. Neighborhoods that are in close proximity to industrial parks express concern that, even when only allowable levels of each chemical are released at each regulated facility, no one is able to say what the negative effects of exposure to the combination of small amounts of chemicals may be over time.

The prospect of grasping and recalling all that is known about chemicals and incorporating that knowledge into practice is staggering. Fortunately, chemicals group themselves into "families" so that it is possible to understand the actions and risks associated with those groupings. Examples are metals and metallic compounds (arsenic, cadmium, chromium, lead, mercury); hydrocarbons (benzene, toluene, ketones, formaldehyde, trichloroethylene); irritant gases (ammonia, hydrochloric acid, sulfur dioxide, chlorine); chemical asphyxiants (carbon monoxide, hydrogen sulfide, cyanides); and pesticides (organophosphates, carbamates, chlorinated hydrocarbons, bipyridyls).

With the ever-changing landscape of chemicals to consider, this is a time when technology is part of the solution. The National Library of Medicine (NLM) databases are now accessible on the Internet and are increasingly user friendly. The NLM website provides choices of the medical databases (PubMed, GratefulMed) previously only accessible through professional Medline searches. The databases can be searched for possible environmental linkages to illnesses using illness and symptom search terms. The most recent public access point to the NLM toxicology databases is a website on the Internet. Using chemical name search terms and health effects display options, one can both understand and rule out some potential environmental threats to health. (The NLM website can be accessed through the Weblinks component of this textbook's website at www.mosby.com/MERLIN.)

Other databases are available through the EPA and the Centers for Disease Control and Prevention (CDC) websites. The EPA is developing geo-mapped displays of regulated facilities, and the CDC makes local health statistics accessible through the Internet.

One challenge growing from increased public access through the Internet is the demand for interpretation from health professionals by citizens. Nurses may find themselves fielding questions on cause and effect linkages where citizens have found co-existing factors, such as an industry with regulated air emissions in a neighborhood experiencing several cases of breast cancer. Such requests for interpretation of data will highlight the need for nurses to be well grounded in principles of epidemiology and risk communication.

Assessment and Referral

The second general environmental health competency cited in the IOM study is assessment and referral. Both of these activities are familiar components of nursing practice, but their scope and implementation have specific meaning in environmental health.

Assessment activities of nurses can range from individual health assessments to being a full participant in community assessment or a partner in a specific environmental site assessment. The skills and tools may range from developing and using computer-assisted geographic information systems (GIS) to small area analysis or individual exposure history. This section focuses on assessing environmental factors for potential and actual effects on an individual's health and incorporating these factors into all health histories and physical examinations.

There are numerous forms and formats for taking environmental exposure histories. One form is shown in Appendix J.7. The key questions in any assessment should cover past conditions in work, home, and community environments (Pope, Snyder, and Mood, 1995):

1. What are your longest held jobs, current and past?
2. Have you been exposed to any radiation or chemical liquids, dusts, mists, or fumes?
3. Is there any relationship between current symptoms and activities at work or at home?

Referral resources may vary in communities. One starting point may be the environmental epidemiology or toxicology unit of the state health department or environmental agency. Another local or state resource may be environmental medicine experts in medical schools. The Association of Occupational and Environmental Clinics is a network of specialty clinics, housed in medical schools and available for consultation or assessment of individual

---

 BOX 8-5 Information and Guidance Sources for Referrals

FEDERAL AGENCIES

Agency for Toxic Substances and Disease Registry (ATSDR)
Centers for Disease Control and Prevention (CDC)
Consumer Product Safety Commission
Environmental Protection Agency (EPA)
   Office of Children's Environmental Health
Food and Drug Administration (FDA)
National Institute for Occupational Safety and Health
National Institute of Environmental Health Sciences
National Institutes of Health (NIH)
   National Cancer Institute
   National Institute of Nursing Research
Occupational Safety and Health Administration (OSHA)

STATE AGENCIES

State Health Departments
State Environmental Protection Agencies

ASSOCIATIONS AND ORGANIZATIONS

National Environmental Education and Training Foundation, Inc.
Association of Occupational and Environmental Clinics
Society for Occupational and Environmental Health (SOEH)
American Association of Poison Control Centers
Pesticide Education Center
Teratogen Exposure Registry and Surveillance
American Cancer Society
American Lung Association
American College of Occupational and Environmental Medicine

---

cases and for provision of educational programs for health professionals.

Local resources include local health and environmental protection agencies; poison control centers; agricultural extension offices (pesticides); and occupational and environmental departments in schools of medicine, nursing, and public health. Some local and state agencies have developed topical directories to assist in accessing the appropriate staff for specific questions. Many of the resources have websites that allow ready access through the Internet and can be located by using any of the popular search methods. Box 8-5 lists many general referral sources. Table 8-4 lists several major toxic agents and symptoms that may be associated with past exposure to them. Further investigation is needed to determine the exact connection between exposure and manifestation.

Advocacy, Ethics, and Risk Communication
Advocacy

In environmental health, nurses are called on to expand their traditional advocacy of individual clients to speaking and acting on behalf of groups and communities concerning their environment.

TABLE 8-4 Toxic Agents and Symptoms that May be Associated with Past Exposure to Them

AGENT	PRIMARY MANIFESTATIONS
Arsenic	Peripheral neuropathy, sensory-motor; nausea and vomiting, diarrhea, constipation; dermatitis, finger and toenail striations, skin cancer; nasal septum perforation; lung cancer
Lead	Anemia; nephropathy; abdominal pain ("colic"); palsy ("wrist drop"); encephalopathy, behavioral abnormalities; spontaneous abortions
Mercury (organic)	Dermatitis; sensorimotor changes, visual field constriction, tremor
Benzene	Acute CNS depression; leukemia, aplastic anemia; dermatitis
Formaldehyde	Irritant and contact dermatitis; eye irritation; respiratory tract irritation, asthma
Trichloro-ethylene (TCE)	Acute CNS depression; peripheral and cranial neuropathy; irritation; dermatitis; arrhythmias
Ozone	Delayed pulmonary edema (generally 6 to 8 hours after exposure)

Adapted from Pope AM, Snyder MA, Mood LH, editors: *Nursing, health, and environment*, Washington, DC, 1995, Institute of Medicine, National Academy Press.

Carolyn Needleman, a social worker and member of the IOM study committee on environment, writes of advocacy at the policy level. She quotes Jack Rothman, who wrote in the 1960s of policy advocacy as "community organization practice," and she describes three types (Pope, Snyder, and Mood, 1995, p. 256):

1. Needleman defines *locality development* as mobilizing resources and energizing interested people around a common concern, where a high degree of consensus already exists, and gives the example of a nurse working with a rural community to monitor the quality of well water. She describes interactions as "warm and process-oriented," the effort as "inclusive and cooperative," and conflicts settled through empathy and compromise. Skills she cites as important are organizing, program development, communications and public speaking, coalition building, and mediation.

2. *Social planning* also occurs within a climate of consensus on the problem. The effort is often highly technical and interdisciplinary in nature, such as a program to address radon exposure in a neighborhood. Interaction is more task oriented and impersonal. Conflicts are usually resolved on the basis of expert opinion. Skills given as important to this type of advocacy are scientific expertise, program planning, and evaluation research.

3. *Social action* takes place in situations with strong disagreement, serious interest conflicts, and large power imbalances among factions with a stake in the issue. The issue of environmental justice, where communities of minority populations and low-income communities see themselves as bearing a disproportionate burden of pollution, is a prime example in environmental health. The nurse advocate may be working from the community group base to organize, articulate the concerns, document evidence of harm, persuade public decision makers, or enlist legal and media assistance to achieve a remedy defined by the community.

The nurse advocate may also work from an agency base to get visibility for community concerns, provide or arrange forums where the community can have its voice heard, provide information on technical matters as well as on the decision process, and speak on behalf of the community in policy discussions when community members may not be present. Whatever the base of action, the community interests involve civil rights and social justice, and their effort is passionate and often emotional. Needed skills common to working from a community or agency base are communication, group facilitation, mediation, and conflict resolution.

One of the real challenges for nurse advocates in social action is to move the interaction from an adversarial relationship to a collaborative effort. Skills in finding common ground are necessary to create and maintain communication, to keep people together, and to find workable solutions in the midst of areas of disagreement. Chapter 19 offers a model of collaborative actions.

Public participation or citizen involvement in regulatory decisions that affect them is often a requirement of environmental law and regulation. Affected communities and the public in general can be eloquent and passionate advocates for the protection of their health, their homes, and their neighborhoods. They may see threats to their safety and quality of life in proposed new or expanded industry and many times do not see equivalent benefits, much less benefits that outweigh the risks. They may be openly vocal about their distrust of the government charged with protecting them. The reality may be that the benefits and costs of the proposed project or facility are different for each group.

Because forums for public participation are historically adversarial and conflict-laden and can become verbally abusive, regulatory agencies have sometimes looked for ways to avoid or minimize the opportunities to hear directly from the public. The nurse can be a welcomed partner in facilitating the public input process, which may be the activity and interaction that is most uncomfortable for environmental scientists. The public generally has known and had experience with nurses as empathetic listeners and professionals with the community's interests at heart. Having a nurse as a facilitator of the dialogue allows people to relax a little, knowing they will be heard. Increased civility and respectful attention can lead to better outcomes in public dialogue.

The skillful nurse advocate and facilitator can be instrumental in shifting the organizational culture of regulatory agencies and regulated industries to view public participation as valued rather than required, where new and useful information leads to better decisions. A shift can occur in seeing public input processes as saving time rather than taking time when lengthy adversarial legal appeal processes are prevented. The most positive outcome may be opening the communication between the community and the industry as neighbors, all interested in the well-being of their surroundings.

Ethics

A grounding in ethics is essential for nurses making their own choices, in describing issues and options within groups, and in advocating for ethical choices. When the sticking points are around competing "goods" such as jobs versus environmental protection, or production versus conservation, the skillful nurse can change the discussion from "either/or" to "both" by opening new possibilities for both ethical and mutually satisfactory outcomes. Ethical issues likely to arise in environmental health decisions are as follows:

- Who has access to information and when?
- How complete and accurate is the available information?
- Who is included in decision making and when?
- What and whose values and priorities are given weight in decisions?
- How are short- and long-term consequences considered?

Risk communication

Risk communication is both an area of practice and a skill that is a composite of two separate words: "risk" and "communication." *Risk* is a familiar term in nursing practice. It is recognized in counseling regarding risks of pregnancy, communicable disease (especially sexually transmitted disease), unintentional injury, and personal choices (such as smoking, alcohol consumption, and diet). Risk assessment in environmental health has focused on characterizing the hazard (the "source"), its physical and chemical properties, its toxicity, and the presence of or potential for the other elements in the exposure pathways—mode of transmission, route of exposure, receptor population, and dose. Risk has traditionally been formulated as *magnitude*

(the size, severity, extent of area, or population affected) multiplied by the *probability* (how likely exposure or damage is to occur (Sandman, Chess, and Hane, 1991) (Box 8-6). For example, an environmental risk assessment of a contaminated site would involve a calculation of the dose that might be received through all routes of exposure, the toxicity of the chemical, the size and vulnerability (age, health) of the population potentially exposed (resident, future resident, transient), and the likelihood of exposure.

Sandman, Chess, and Hane (1991) noted, in their experience, that the reaction to things that scare people and the things that kill people are often not related to the actual hazard. They have gone further to probe what is behind those differences and identified a list of 20 **outrage factors** to explain people's responses to risk (Table 8-5). They maintain that the outrage is just as predictable and open to intervention as the science of addressing the hazard.

"Communication" of risk involves understanding the outrage factors relevant to the risk being addressed so they can be incorporated in the message—the information—to either reduce unnecessary fear or create action to ensure safety or prevent harm. An example of raising outrage to produce action can be seen in the shift from emphasis on smokers (voluntary) to victims of passive smoking (involuntary) to stimulate public policy that limits or bans smoking in public places. When the emphasis on risk went from a voluntary choice of smokers to an involuntary exposure of nonsmokers, the outrage level of the nonsmoking public became high enough to result in legislation guaranteeing smoke-free public spaces (e.g., public buildings, airplanes, and restaurants) (see the Research Brief about smoking).

Conversely, outrage diminishes when people get information on the situation from a trusted source, and doctors and nurses are often cited in surveys as trusted sources of information on environmental risks (USC, 1990). The public trust is a compelling incentive to match professional knowledge and skills to a community's expectations. The outrage factor can also be a driving force in

---

BOX 8-6 Definitions of Risk

RISK = MAGNITUDE X PROBABILITY

There is a growing body of literature from practitioners and researchers who have studied the human reaction to risk, real and perceived. Sandman, Chess, and Hane (1991) have written and spoken extensively on the factors related to risk that produce public "outrage." They propose a different formula for risk:

RISK = HAZARD + OUTRAGE

Addressing only the hazard is doing only half of the necessary work; addressing the response (outrage) is equally important.

From Sandman PM, Chess C, Hane BJ: *Improving dialogue with communities,* New Brunswick, NJ, 1991, Rutgers University.

building credibility and trustworthiness in every person whose work involves interacting with the public.

Risk communication includes all the principles of good communication in general. It is a combination of the following:

- *The right information.* Accurate, relevant, in a language that audiences can understand. The hazard assessment (toxicity, dosage, volatility, and solubility—all components of the formal environmental risk assessment described previously) is essential information for shaping the message.
- *To the right people.* Those affected and those who are worried but may not be affected. Information on the community is essential: the geographic boundaries, who lives there (demographics), how they get information (flyers or newspapers, radio, television, word of mouth), where they get together (school, church, community center), and who within the community can help plan the communication.
- *At the right time.* For timely action or to allay fear.

Five themes recur in interactions with the public as presented in the How To feature on p. 174.

These are good quality indicators in risk communication and a means of becoming a trustworthy source of information in the public's eyes. These actions can be controlled, and they always make a difference. Consider the situation that occurred in a neighborhood of apartment residents with a stream nearby where children played. During a routine sample testing of the stream water, a local environmental staff discovered a chemical known to be used by a neighboring industry. The industry was notified and immediately began a search for the source. A sign was posted that warned persons to avoid contact with the stream—"No swimming or wading." The apartment management was contacted, and a meeting with residents was arranged.

The early meeting meant that a lot of information was not yet known—how the chemical got into the stream, how much had been released or spilled, and how long it would take to restore the stream to a safe level. However, the rapid response, the obvious concern of the industry, the availability of a qualified toxicologist skilled in public interactions, and the rationale for early contact ("We thought it would be irresponsible not to alert you early, to protect your children's safety, even though we do not have full information on the problem to give to you.") resulted in a reassured rather than an outraged community. Plans were made for what would be done, and arrangements

TABLE 8-5 Outrage Factors: Characteristics of Risk that Contribute to the Public's Feeling of Outrage

Safer = Less Outrage	Less Safe = More Outrage
12 PRINCIPAL OUTRAGE COMPONENTS	
Voluntary	Involuntary (coerced)
Natural	Industrial (artificial)
Familiar	Exotic
Not memorable	Memorable
Not dreaded	Dreaded
Chronic	Catastrophic
Knowable (detectable)	Unknowable (Undetectable)
Individually controlled	Controlled by others
Fair	Unfair
Morally irrelevant	Morally relevant
Trustworthy sources	Untrustworthy sources
Responsive process	Unresponsive process
8 SECONDARY OUTRAGE COMPONENTS	
Affects average populations	Affects vulnerable populations
Immediate effects	Delayed effects
No risk to future generations	Substantial risk to future generations
Victims statistical	Victims identifiable
Preventable	Not preventable (only reducible)
Substantial benefits	Few benefits (foolish risk)
Little media attention	Substantial media attention
Little opportunity for collective action	Much opportunity for collective action

RESEARCH *Brief*

The purpose of this study was to look at differences in environmental tobacco smoke exposure between smokers and nonsmokers. The study method used a diary of 1 full day's activities. The presence of smoke in their environment was reported on in this way by 1579 Californians. Active smoke and passive smoke from tobacco are chemically similar.

This study concluded that clients who smoke incur greater exposure to the harmful effects of smoking since they report up to four times more passive smoke exposure than nonsmokers. Smokers tend to associate with other smokers and/or spend more exposure time in the company of others who smoke. Therefore they are exposed to the chemical effects of their own active smoking as well as the passive smoking of others. There smokers have two risk factors from the ill effects of tobacco: 1) the number of tobacco products they actively use and 2) the passive smoke inhalation from other smokers.

A suggestion may be that the workplace construct separately ventilated smoking lounges to meet the needs of the smoking workforce and to protect the health of nonsmoking workers

Robinson JP, Switzer P, Ott W: Daily exposure to environmental tobacco smoke: smokers vs nonsmokers in California, *AJPH* 86(9):1303, 1996.

HOW TO *Interact with the Public to Get Action*

1. *Listen. Really listen; do not just wait your turn to speak.*
2. *Take the public seriously. Even when the hazard is minimal. Their concern is real and deserves a serious response.*
3. *Treat the public with respect. Even, perhaps especially, when outrage is high. Underlying the loud voices and the anger will almost always be feelings of fear and powerlessness. Do not give away your power as a knowledgeable, caring, and responsible professional by reacting to anger or blaming with anger or defensiveness.*
4. *Given the public "straight" information. What is known, when it was known, what is not known, and what is being done to learn more. Always provide information in a language that is understandable.*
5. *Do what you say you will do. From returning phone calls to taking major action steps.*

From Mood LH: Environmental health policy: environmental justice. In Mason, Leavitt, editors: *Policy and politics in nursing and health care*, ed 3, Philadelphia, 1998, WB Saunders.

were made for updating the residents as new information became available. The citizens left the meeting knowing that their government was acting quickly in their best interests and that their industry neighbors were taking their responsibility for correcting the problem seriously. Using the language of the risk formula, the outrage was addressed before the hazard itself could be resolved.

WHAT DO YOU THINK? *Access to information on the existence of toxic substances leaching into the water table of a community should be withheld from the public until the government completes negotiations with the party responsible for the toxic substance.*

Legislation and Regulation

The fourth general competency in environmental health practice is familiarity with the laws and regulations that form the policy framework for environmental health. Some environmental laws, primarily related to sanitary practices, have been a part of public health for a long time. The EPA was not established until 1970, and the major federal environmental laws, such as the Clean Air Act and the Safe Drinking Water Act, the "Superfund" legislation (providing funding for environmental clean-up of the most seriously contaminated sites where no responsible party can be held accountable), and their amendments, have all followed during the mid-1970s without a real effect until the 1980s (EPA, 1993) (Box 8-7).

Sources of laws and ordinances bring variety to regulation among states and local areas. State laws supplement federal laws in addressing water quality, air quality, and waste management and may impose more stringent requirements than federal statutes, with some exceptions, but may

BOX 8-7 Major Federal Environmental Laws

Clean Air Act (CAA)
Clean Water Act (CWA)
Safe Drinking Water Act (SDWA)
Comprehensive Environmental Response, Compensation, and Liability Act (CERCLA)
Resource Conservation and Recovery Act (RCRA)
Federal Insecticide, Fungicide, and Rodenticide Act (FIFRA)
Toxic Substances Control Act (TSCA)
Marine Protection, Research, and Sanctuaries Act (MPRSA)
Uranium Mill Tailings Radiation Control Act (UMTRCA)
Pollution Prevention Act (PPA)

not be more lenient. Local ordinances can impose additional requirements to protect communities from environmental hazards of pollution and growth. Some state statutes require that local requirements be met before consideration of permit applications. For example, a state law may specify that no environmental permit application will be considered that is inconsistent with local zoning ordinances.

Environmental laws are primarily written separately for each media (air, water, and soil) and have been enacted and amended at different times. The patchwork result means that there may be inconsistencies among laws and regulations, particularly in public participation requirements, and there may be gaps where no specific law or rule exists. A working knowledge of environmental laws and regulations is essential if the nurse is to provide or facilitate access to accurate information for communities, guide communities through public participation and decision-making processes, inform communities of their rights, and recognize policy gaps for attention and advocacy.

ROLES FOR NURSES IN ENVIRONMENTAL HEALTH

Nurses can be involved in a number of roles in environmental health, in full-time work, as an adjunct to existing roles, and as informed citizens:

- *Community involvement/public participation.* Organizing, facilitating, and moderating. Making public notices effective, public forums accessible and welcoming of input, information exchange understandable, and problem solving acceptable to culturally diverse communities are valuable assets a nurse contributes. Skills in community organizing and mobilizing can be essential to a community having a meaningful voice in decisions that affect them.
- *Individual and population* **risk assessment.** Using nursing assessment skills to detect potential and real exposure pathways and outcomes for clients cared for in the acute, chronic, and healthy communities of practice.

- *Risk communication.* Interpreting, applying principles to practice. Nurses may serve as skilled risk communicators within agencies, working for industries, or working as independent practitioners. Amendments to the Clean Air Act require major industrial sources of air emissions to have risk management plans and to inform their neighbors of specifics of the risks and plans (Clean Air Act, 1996).

HOW TO *Apply the Nursing Process to Environmental Health*

If you suspect that a client's health problem is being influenced by environmental factors, follow the nursing process and note the environmental aspects of the problem in every step of the process:

1. *Assessment. Include inventories and history questions that have environmental items as a part of the general assessment.*
2. *Diagnosis. Relate the disease and the environmental factors in the diagnosis.*
3. *Goal setting. Include outcome measures that mitigate and eliminate the environmental factors.*
4. *Planning. Look at community policy and laws as methods to facilitate the care needs for the client; include environmental health personnel in planning.*
5. *Intervention. Coordinate medical, nursing, and public health actions to meet the client's needs*
6. *Evaluation. Examine criteria that include the immediate and long-term responses of the client as well as the recidivism of the problem for the client*

- *Epidemiologic investigations.* Nurses need to have the skills to respond in scientifically sound and humanly sensitive ways to community concerns about cancer, birth defects, and stillbirths that citizens fear may have environmental causes.
- *Policy development.* Proposing, informing, and monitoring action from agencies, communities, and organization perspectives.
- *Teaching others.* The public, other nurses, and other disciplines. Teaching may be done in informal sessions, in structured learning experiences in agencies, and in formal academic settings. There are a number of existing skills that nurses bring to the work of environmental health:
  - Listening (nursing is one of the few professions systematically taught how to listen)
  - Group facilitation
  - Knowledge of human response to illness and health
  - Advocacy
  - Epidemiology
  - Systems theory (how community and institutional systems work)
  - Building constructive working relationships
  - Using the nursing process to address concerns

Some skills need to be enhanced and expanded, such as advocacy, group facilitation, working across systems, and leadership. Models of leadership that are collaborative and non-hierarchical fit best into the community focus of environmental health.

Nurses already skilled in public health practice will find the interdisciplinary work of environmental health familiar and supportive. The partners will expand from doctors, social workers, health educators, and epidemiologists to include chemists, hydrogeologists, biologists, climatologists, and other scientists and engineers. The skills in valuing and building teamwork and synergy among a variety of experts are essential to effective work on environmental issues. Other content may require new knowledge and skills (e.g., environmental science and risk communication).

The assimilation of the concepts of environmental health into a nurse's daily practice gives new life to traditional public health values of prevention, building community, and social justice. There is great congruence with many personal, religious, and spiritual values of stewardship of creation, preserving the gifts of nature, and decision making that provides for quality of life for present and future generations. It is a context for practice where nurses are welcomed and valued for their contribution.

clinical application

At the county health department, a 3-year-old boy named Billy presents with gastric upset and behavior changes. These symptoms have persisted for several weeks. Billy's parents report that they have been renovating their home to remove lead paint. They had been discouraged from routinely testing their child because their insurance does not cover testing and they could not find information on where to have the test done. Their concern has heightened with the persistent symptoms in their child.

You test Billy's blood-lead level and find 45 ug/dl. You research lead poisoning and discover that children are at great risk because of their inclination to absorb lead into their central nervous systems. You also find that chronic lead poisoning may have long-term effects, such as developmental delays and impaired learning ability. You refer Billy to his primary care physician. On further investigation, you find that Billy's home was built before 1950 and is still under renovation. The sanitarian tests the interior paint and finds a high lead content. Ample amounts of sawdust from sanding are noted in various rooms of the home. You determine that a completed exposure pathway exists.

A. What would you include in an assessment of this situation?
B. What prevention strategies would you use to resolve this issue?
  - At the individual level?
  - At the population level?

Answers are in the back of the book.

KEY POINTS

- Nurses have responsibilities to be informed consumers and to be advocates for citizens in their community regarding environmental health issues.
- Models describing the determinants of health acknowledge the role of the environment in health and disease.
- Proving a connection allows for the identification of risk and exposure in environmental health.
- Correlates of harm include source, environmental media, a receptor population, route of exposure, and dose.
- Incineration, discharge, and landfills allow waste products to be altered to a less toxic or bio-unavailable form.
- For many substances there is a lack of scientific evidence of the health effects of new and existing chemical compounds.
- Prevention activities include education, waste minimizing, and land use planning.
- Control activities include environmental permitting, environmental standards, monitoring, compliance and enforcement, and clean up and remediation.
- Every nursing assessment should include questions and observations concerning intended and unintended environmental exposures.
- Environmental databases facilitate the easy and immediate access to environmental data useful in assessment, diagnosis, intervention, and evaluation.
- Both case and class advocacy are important skills for nurses in environmental health practice.
- Risk communication is an important skill and must acknowledge the outrage factor experienced by communities with environmental hazards.

- Federal, state, and local laws and regulations exist to protect the health of citizens from environmental hazards.
- Environmental health practice engages multiple disciplines, and nurses are important members of the environmental health team.
- Environmental health practice includes principles of health promotion, disease prevention, and health protection.
- *Healthy People 2000* and *Healthy People 2010* objectives both address targets for the reduction of risk factors and diseases related to environmental causes.

critical thinking activities

1. Explain why the source of drinking water is important to investigate in the assessment of an unusually high number of cancer cases in a community; in increased lead levels in children from a certain school; and in an outbreak of a gastrointestinal epidemic in an agricultural community.
2. Discuss the differences and similarities between the Canadian Model and the Epidemiological Triangle in explaining the determinants of health.
3. Discover if your jurisdiction has a law or regulation for the disclosure of radon levels for personal property as part of the act of sale for real estate. If your community does not, investigate with the government officials of the community the reasons for the lack of disclosure requirement.

Bibliography

Agency for Toxic Substances and Disease Registry (ATSDR): *Lead toxicological profile,* Atlanta, Ga, 1990, USDHHS, PHS.

Agency for Toxic Substances and Disease Registry (ATSDR): *Mercury toxicological profile,* Atlanta, Ga, 1989, USDHHS, PHS.

Aldrich T, Griffith J: *Environmental epidemiology and risk assessment,* New York, 1993, Van Nostrand Reinhold.

Amaya MA et al: Childhood lead poisoning on the US-Mexico border: a case study in environmental health nursing lead poisoning, *Public Health Nurs* 14(6):353, 1997.

American Public Health Association: *Control of communicable diseases manual,* ed 16, Washington, DC, 1995, the Association.

Clean Air Act, Risk Management Programs, Section 112(r)(7), Federal Register, Part III EPA, 40 CFR, Part 68, June 20, 1996.

Comprehensive Environmental Response Compensation and Liability Act (CERCLA), 42 U.S.C. 9601 (Federal Code of Law), December 11, 1980.

Environmental Protection Agency: *Access EPA,* EPA Publication 220-B-93-008, Washington, DC, 1993, EPA.

Environmental Protection Agency: *Environmental health threats to children,* Washington, DC, 1996, EPA.

Federal, Provincial, and Territorial Advisory Committee on Population Health for Canadian Ministers of Health: *Strategies for population health,* Halifax, Nova Scotia, 1994, the Committee.

Glendening PN: *Smart growth and neighborhood conservation,* Annapolis, Md, 1998, Maryland Office of Planning (www.op.state.md.us/smart growth).

Gore A: *Earth in the balance,* New York, 1993, Penguin Books.

Henderson V: *The nature of nursing,* New York, 1966, McMillan .

Mancke R: Nature walk lecture, Congaree Swamp National Monument, SC, April, 1998.

Mood LH: Environmental health policy: environmental justice. In Mason DJ, Leavitt JK, editors: *Policy and politics in nursing and health care,* ed 3, Philadelphia, 1998, WB Saunders.

Nightingale F: *Notes on nursing: What it is and what it is not,* London, 1859, Harrison.

Pickett GE, Hanlon JJ: *Public health administration and practice,* St Louis, 1990, Mosby.

Pope AM, Snyder MA, Mood LH, editors: *Nursing, health and environment,* Washington, DC, 1995, Institute of Medicine, National Academy Press .

Robinson JP, Switzer P, Ott W: Daily exposure to environmental tobacco smoke: smokers vs nonsmokers in California, *AJPH* 86(9):1303, 1996.

Sandman PM, Chess C, Hane BJ: *Improving dialogue with communities,* New Brunswick, NJ, 1991, Rutgers University.

South Carolina Department of Health and Environmental Control: *Quality of the environment in South Carolina,* Columbia, SC, 1998, SCDHEC.

South Carolina Task Group on Toxic Algae: State task group studies *P. fiesteria,* 1(1), 1998.

University of Southern California College of Business Administration, Division of Research: *USC Report on the Survey on Environmental Issues,* Columbia, SC, 1990, USC.

USDHHS: *Healthy People 2000: midcourse review and revisions,* Washington, DC, 1995, USDHHS, Public Health Service.

Warren JV, Goldstein BD: *Role of the primary care physician in occupational and environmental medicine,* Washington, DC, 1988, Institute of Medicine, National Academy Press.

Yordy KD, Remington RD: *The future of public health,* Washington, DC, 1988, Institute of Medicine, National Academy Press.

Policy, Politics, and the Law

JOYCE BONICK

www.mosby.com/MERLIN/community_stanhope

OBJECTIVES

After reading this chapter, the student should be able to do the following:

- Describe the trends and roles of several levels of government.
- Identify the impact of changing governmental roles and structures on health care.
- Describe the major governmental functions in health care.

- Discuss nursing roles in selected governmental agencies.
- Shape health policy by participating in the regulation-making process and the political arena.
- Describe selected laws that affect nursing practice, both generally and in special areas of practice.
- Conduct a brief exercise in legal research as one means of staying informed about current law.

KEY TERMS

block grant	legislative process	politics	*Scorpio*
Code of Regulations	*Lexis*	precedent	sovereign immunity
constitutional law	National Institute for	private sector	U.S. Department of
Division of Nursing	Nursing Research	professional negligence	Health and Human
Federal Register	nurse practice acts	Public Health Service	Services (USDHHS)
government	Occupational Safety and	(PHS)	World Health
health policy	Health Administration	public sector	Organization (WHO)
judicial and common law	(OSHA)	regulations	
law	police power	respondeat superior	
legislation	policy	scope of practice	*See Glossary for definitions*

CHAPTER OUTLINE

The author acknowledges the contribution of Cynthia Northrop and Marcia Stanhope to the content of this chapter.

Nurses are affected significantly by the political system and the government of the United States, state and local governments, and other institutions responsible for implementing health policy. This chapter provides descriptions of the institutions, including the organization and primary functions of governments, governmental regulation, and the influence of politics on nursing practice. This chapter concludes with an overview of laws affecting community and public health nursing practice.

DEFINITIONS

To understand the relationship between health policy, politics, and laws, one must first understand the definitions of the terms. **Policy** is a settled course of action to be followed by a government or institution to obtain a desired end. **Health policy** is a set course of action to obtain a desired health outcome, either for an individual, family, group, community, or society. Policies are made not only by governments but also by such institutions as a health department or other health care agency, a family, or a professional organization.

Politics plays a role in the development of such policies. Politics is found in families, professional and employing agencies, and governments. **Politics** is the art of influencing others to accept a specific course of action. Therefore political activities are used to arrive at a course of action (the policy). **Law** is a system of privileges and processes by which people solve problems based on a set of established rules; it is intended to minimize the use of force. Laws govern the relationships of individuals and organizations to other individuals and to government. Through political action a policy becomes a law. After a law is established, regulations further define the course of action (policy) to be taken by organizations or individuals in reaching an outcome. **Government** is the ultimate authority in society and is designated to enforce the policy whether it is related to health, education, economics, social welfare, or any other society issue. The following discussion explains the role of government in health policy.

GOVERNMENTAL ROLE IN HEALTH CARE

In the United States, the federal and most state governments are composed of three branches: the executive branch is composed of the President (or governor), cabinet, and regulatory units, such as the U.S. Department of Health and Human Services (USDHHS); the legislative branch is made up of two houses of Congress: the Senate and the House of Representatives; and the judicial branch is composed of the Supreme Court. Each of these branches plays a significant role in development and implementation of health policy. The executive branch administers and regulates policy. For example, the Division of Nursing of the USDHHS writes criteria to fund nursing education. The legislative branch passes laws that become policy (e.g., the Medicare amendments of the 1966 Social

Security Act). The judicial branch interprets laws and the meaning of policy, as in its interpretation of states' rights to grant abortions.

WHAT DO YOU THINK? *Government has too much influence on the way health care services are delivered and on who receives care.*

One of the first constitutional challenges to congressional legislation in the area of health and welfare came in 1937, when Congress established unemployment compensation and old-age benefits. Although Congress had created other health programs, its legal basis for doing so had never been challenged before. The Supreme Court interpreted the meaning of the Constitution and decided that such federal government action was within congressional powers to promote the general welfare. Most legal bases for congressional action in health care are found in Article I, Section 8 of the U.S. Constitution, including the following:

1. Provide for the general welfare.
2. Regulate commerce among the states.
3. Raise funds to support the military.
4. Provide spending power.

These statements have been interpreted by the Court to include a wide variety of federal powers and activities.

State power concerning health care is mostly **police power.** This means that states may act to protect the health, safety, and welfare of their citizens. Such police power must be used fairly, and the state must show that it has a compelling interest in taking actions, especially actions that might infringe on individual rights. Examples of a state using its police powers include requiring immunization of children before school admission and requiring casefinding, reporting, follow-up care, and treatment of tuberculosis. These activities protect the health, safety, and welfare of state citizens.

Trends and Shifts in Governmental Roles

Governmental involvement in health care at both the state and federal levels began gradually. Many historical events correspond closely with the role that has developed. Wars, economic instability, depressions, different viewpoints, and political parties all have shaped the governmental role. Before the 1930s the only major governmental action relating to health was the creation in 1798 of the Public Health Service (PHS). In 1930 federal laws were passed to promote the public health of merchant seamen and Native Americans. The Social Security Act of 1935 was a substantial piece of legislation. It has grown to include not only the aged and unemployed but also survivors' insurance for widows and children, child welfare, health department grants, maternal and child health projects, Medicare, and Medicaid. In 1934 Senator Wagner of New York initiated the first national health insurance bill. In 1946 Congress enacted a mental health bill and the Hospital Survey and

Construction Act and created the National Institutes of Health (NIH) in 1948. These legislative acts created entities that became part of the executive branch, now within the USDHHS. The USDHHS, a regulatory agency known until 1980 as the Department of Health, Education, and Welfare (DHEW), was not created until 1953.

In a democracy the role of government in the area of health care depends on the beliefs of its citizens. Strong beliefs of self-determination and self-sufficiency mixed with beliefs about social responsibilities are hallmarks of a multiple approach to solving society's problems. Political party platforms demonstrate how different beliefs yield different approaches to problems. A good example of this was the debate in the 1990s between the Democratic and Republican parties over health care reform. The Democratic platform called for a health care system that was universally accessible and affordable. The Republican platform supported continuing the current system and reducing government's role in health care delivery through cuts in Medicare and Medicaid benefits. However, in an effort to begin health care reform, both parties passed the Health Portability and Accountability Act. This act became law in 1997 and is designed to ensure that workers will have health insurance coverage when they change or lose employment, even if they have preexisting medical conditions.

Nurses are becoming more aware of the influence of political parties on health care delivery. In 1991 the American Nurses Association, the National League for Nursing, the American Association of Colleges of Nursing, and more than 60 nursing specialty organizations published nursing's agenda for health care reform. This "white paper" was the profession's response to the political party's attempts to reform health care, indicating the direction in which organized nursing wanted to see the new policy develop.

Before the current response to reform, a major effort of the Reagan administration was to shift federal government activities to the states. In addition, passage in 1985 of the Gramm-Rudman Act, which was designed to decrease the federal budget deficit, not only promoted the continued shift of federal programs to states but also resulted in significant cutbacks in health and social programs. This effort continued in 1995 as the Republican-controlled Congress wanted to cut maternal and child health programs and school lunch programs at the federal level. They wanted to give a sum of money to the states in the form of block grants to continue the programs in the states. The public was rightfully concerned about this approach because the states would not have to spend the money on the school lunch program, for example, but could choose to spend the money instead on other programs that may not be as beneficial to children in poverty.

This discussion has focused primarily on trends and shifts within and among different levels of government. An additional aspect of government responsibilities is the relationship between government and individuals. Freedom of individuals must be balanced with government powers. Citizens express their views on the amount of governmental interference that will be tolerated. For example, the issue of sex education in public schools shows at least two viewpoints on the government-individual relationship:

- Ever since the legislative branch of government established a system of education, some citizens believe that education should include content on sex.
- Some citizens believe that sex education belongs in the family and should not be interfered with by public schools, which are governmentally established.

RESEARCH *Brief*

The purpose of this study was to determine whether there has been a shift in popular attitudes toward federal policies that corresponds with an increasing political interest in health care reform. Survey data collected between 1975 and 1989 were used to answer the following questions:

1. Who supports and who opposes an active federal role in health care reform?
2. How do those who support such policies differ from those who oppose them?
3. How do patterns of public support for health care compare with patterns of support for social policy?
4. How are these differences changing over time?

This study concluded that there is a higher level of popular support for government action in health care and it is distributed among population groups differently than for other federal policies.

Support for federal health policy has grown over time. The gaps in support between rich and poor, educated and uneducated, old and young are reduced for health policy. Characteristics that make a difference in how one responds to federal policies are age, gender, race, education, marital status, income level, employment status, and rural vs. urban residence. Gaps in support for antipoverty programs and general domestic policies still exist.

There is some evidence that growing support for health policy may be a result of the political ideology of the Reagan and Bush administrations. Support for such policy does not translate into a willingness to pay for new health programs.

Nurses can use this study to form strategies for promoting health care reform. Nurses will want to show others (clients, communities, legislators) how health care reform is an investment in society by improving the health of the nation, that health care reform promotes equal opportunity for all citizens to have health care, and that supporting investments in health care for all will eventually reduce the cost of health care for every citizen.

Schlesinger M, Lee TK: Is health care different? popular support of federal health and social policies, *J Health Polit Policy Law* 18(3 part 2):551, 1993.

These are only two of the views expressed in the literature. There are strong feelings about this issue, and the example shows how opinions about government versus individual responsibilities can be divided.

Governmental Health Care Functions

Federal, state, and local governments all carry out four general categories of health care functions: direct services, financing, information, and policy setting.

Direct services

Federal, state, and local governments provide direct health services to certain individuals and groups. For example, the federal government provides health care to Native Americans, members and dependents of the military, veterans, and federal prisoners. State and local governments employ nurses to deliver services to individuals and families, usually based on financial need. State and local governments also may provide direct, specific services to all individuals, such as hypertension or tuberculosis screening, immunizations for children, and primary care for inmates in local jails or state prisons.

Financing

Governments pay for some health care services, training of personnel, and research. Financial support in these areas has significantly affected consumers and health care providers. State and federal governments finance the direct care of clients through the Medicare, Medicaid, and Social Security programs. Many nurses have been educated with government funds; schools of nursing have been built and equipped through federal capitation funds. Governments also have financially supported other health care providers. Monies in the form of grants have been given by governments for specific research and demonstration projects. One of the best-known centers of medical research is the federally funded NIH. In 1993 the National Institute of Nursing Research was established by Congress to promote nursing research. This provides a substantial sum of money to the discipline of nursing for the purpose of defining the knowledge base of nursing.

Information

All branches and levels of government have collected, analyzed, and made available data about health care and health status in the United States. An example is the annual report, *Health: United States,* compiled by the USDHHS (1999). Collection of vital statistics, including mortality and morbidity data, gathering of census data, and sponsoring of health care status surveys are all government activities. Table 9-1 lists examples of available international and federal government data sources on the health status of the total U.S. population. These sources are available in the government documents sections of most large libraries. This information is especially important because it can

---

TABLE 9-1 International and National Sources of Data on the Health Status of the U.S. Population

ORGANIZATION	DATA SOURCE
INTERNATIONAL	
United Nations	Demographic Yearbook
World Health Organization	World Health Statistics Annual
FEDERAL	
Public Health Service	National Vital Statistics System
	National Survey of Family Growth
	National Health Interview Survey
	National Health Examination Survey
	National Health and Nutrition Examination Survey
	National Master Facility Inventory
	National Hospital Discharge Survey
	National Nursing Home Survey
	National Ambulatory Medical Care Survey
	National Morbidity Reporting System
	U.S. Immunization Survey
	Surveys of Mental Health Facilities
	Estimates of National Health Expenditures
	AIDS Surveillance
	Abortion Surveillance
	Nurse Supply Estimates
Department of Commerce	U.S. Census of Population
	Current Population Survey
	Population Estimates and Projections
Department of Labor	Consumer Price Index
	Employment and Earnings

help nurses understand the major health problems in the United States and those in their own state.

Policy setting

Policy setting relates to all government functions. Decisions about health care are made by governments at all levels and within all branches. Governments often show preference between groups when giving financial support. Such decisions affect the health care resources of each group and show the influence of government policy setting. Health policy decisions, or courses of action, usually have broad implications for financial growth, resource use, and development in the health care field. Examples of policy setting include the passage of amendments to the Social Security Act that established Medicare and the Professional Standards Review Organization (PSRO) in 1972 to monitor the quality of care given to hospitalized Medicare clients. The law that has had the most significant impact on the development of public health policy, public health nursing, and social welfare policy in the United States is the Sheppard-Towner Act of 1921.

In 1912 the Child Health Bureau was established as part of the U.S. PHS. In 1917 the Bureau published a report, *Public Protection of Maternity and Infancy,* to highlight findings of studies on infant and maternal mortality and consequently on the plight of women and children in the United States. In 1918 the first congresswoman, Jeanette Rankin, introduced a bill that later became the Sheppard-Towner Act. This act made nurses available to provide health services for women and children, offered well-child and child-development services, provided adequate hospital services and facilities for women and children, and provided grants-in-aid for the establishment of maternal and child welfare programs.

The Sheppard-Towner Act helped establish precedent and set patterns for the growth of modern-day public health policy. It established the federal government's involvement in health care and the system for federal matching grants-in-aid awarded to states. The Act set the role of the federal government in creating standards to be followed by states in conducting *categorical programs* such as today's Women, Infants, and Children program (WIC) and Early Periodic Screening and Developmental Testing program (EPSDT). Also established was the position of the consumer in influencing, formulating, and conducting public policy; the government's role in research; a system for collecting national health statistics; and the integrating of health and social services (Pickett and Hanlon, 1990). This policy established the importance of prenatal care, anticipatory guidance, client education, and nurse-client conferences, all of which are viewed today as essential nursing responsibilities.

Healthy People—an example of current national health policy

In 1979, the Surgeon General issued a report that began a 20-year focus on promoting health and preventing disease for all Americans. The report, entitled *Healthy People,* used morbidity rates to track the health of individuals through the five major life cycles of infancy, childhood, adolescence, adulthood, and older age.

In 1989, *Healthy People 2000* became a national effort of representatives from government agencies, academia, and health organizations. Their goal was to present a strategy for improving the health of the American people. Their objectives are being used by public health organizations to assess current health trends, health programs, and disease prevention programs.

Throughout the 1990s, all states used *Healthy People 2000* objectives to identify emerging public health issues. The success of the program on a national level was accomplished through state and local efforts. Surveys early in the 1990s from public health departments indicated that 8% of the national objectives had been met and progress on an additional 40% of the objectives was noted. In the mid-course review published in 1995, it is noted that 50% of the objectives are making significant progress toward being met.

Using the progress made in the past decade, the committee for *Healthy People 2010* proposed two goals:
- To increase years of healthy life
- To eliminate health disparities among different populations

They hope to reach these goals by such measures as promoting healthy behaviors, increasing access to quality health care, and strengthening community prevention. *Healthy People 2010* will be presented to the World Health Organization (WHO) as one model for WHO's "Health for All" program. Community health programs will continue to be influenced by *Healthy People* policies as they identify health care needs and standards necessary to meet them within states and local areas. Box 9-1 presents one example of the integration of *Healthy People 2000* objectives into the proposed framework of *Healthy People 2010.*

ORGANIZATION OF GOVERNMENT AGENCIES

Nurses are actively involved with many levels of international and national government. This section discusses international organizations and roles of nurses in different national government agencies.

International Organizations

In June, 1945 many national governments joined together to create the United Nations (UN). Aims and goals described in its charter include several dealing with human rights, world peace, security, and promotion of economic and social advancement of all people. The UN is headquartered in New York City and is made up of six principal subgroups. Several other subgroups and many specialized agencies and autonomous organizations are also within the system. One of the special autonomous organizations is the **World Health Organization (WHO).**

Established in 1946, the WHO relates to the UN through the Economic and Social Council to attain its

BOX 9-1 Health Status Model: An Integration of *Healthy People 2000* Objectives into *Healthy People 2010* Categories

INCREASE YEARS OF HEALTHY LIFE
Lung cancer deaths (16.2)*
Breast cancer deaths (16.3)
Cardiovascular disease deaths (15.1)

PROMOTE HEALTHY BEHAVIORS
Overweight (7.3)
AIDS incidence (18.1)
Syphilis incidence (19.3)
Teen pregnancies (5.1)
Cigarette smoking prevalence (3.4)
Alcohol and drug misuse (4.4, 4.8)

PROTECT HEALTH
Motor vehicle crash deaths (9.3)
Work-related injury deaths (10.1)
Air quality exposure (11.5)

ASSURE ACCESS TO QUALITY HEALTH CARE
Infant mortality (14.1)
Measles incidence (20.1)
Tuberculosis incidence (20.4)
Low birth weight prevalence (14.5)
First trimester prenatal care (14.11)
Pneumonia/flu immunization (20.11)
Cervical cancer screening (16.12)
Mammography screening (16.11)
Hypertension (15.4)
Hypercholesterolemia (15.6)
Suicides (6.1)
Depression (6.15)

STRENGTHEN COMMUNITY PREVENTION
Homicides (7.1)
Childhood poverty (8.3)

*Parentheses indicate related *Healthy People 2000* objective number.
Note: The category names reflect *Healthy People 2010* goals, and the health-related issues are objectives of *Healthy People 2000*.
From USDHHS: *Leading indicators for Healthy People 2010*, Washington, DC, 1998, USDHHS.

goal of the highest possible level of health for all citizens throughout the world. Headquartered in Geneva, Switzerland, the WHO is composed of three main branches: the World Health Assembly, the Executive Board, and the Secretariat (Fig. 9-1). The organization has six regional offices. The office for the Americas is located in Washington, DC and is known as the Pan American Health Organization (PAHO).

The World Health Assembly meets annually and is the policy-making body of the WHO. The WHO provides worldwide services to promote health, cooperates with member countries in promoting their health efforts, and coordinates biomedical research. Its services, which benefit all countries, include a day-to-day information service on the occurrence of internationally important diseases; publication of the international list of causes of disease, injury, and death; monitoring of adverse reactions to drugs; and establishment of world standards for antibiotics and vaccines. Assistance available to individual countries includes support for national programs to fight disease, train workers, and strengthen health services. An example of biomedical research collaboration is a special program to study six widespread tropical diseases: malaria, leprosy, "snail fever," filariasis, leishmaniasis, and "sleeping sickness."

The number of nursing roles in international health is increasing. Besides offering direct health services, nurses serve as consultants, educators, and program planners and evaluators. They focus their work on a variety of public health concepts, including environment, sanitation, communicable disease, wellness, and primary care. At least two of the contributors to this text have been WHO consultants, Dr. Beverly Flynn and Dr. Carolyn Williams.

In 1978 the International Conference on Primary Health Care sponsored by the WHO and held in Alma Ata, USSR, declared that the world community's goal should be the attainment of a level of health by the year 2000 that would permit all people to live socially and economically productive lives (WHO, 1978). The conference resolved that primary health care was the key to attaining this goal (see Appendix A-4). At about the same time, the WHO Expert Committee on Community Health Nursing convened and outlined the broad role of community health nurses in primary health care. The WHO is encouraging strengthened regulation of nursing education and practice related to primary health care, and it is in support of nurses in their efforts to become forces in attaining the goal of "health for all" (WHO, 1986). This is an example of an international organization and policy that is certain to affect the future of nursing education and community-oriented nursing practice.

Federal Agencies

Many federal agencies are involved in governmental health care functions. Legislation passed by Congress may be delegated to any regulatory agency within the executive branch for implementation, surveillance, regulation, and enforcement. Congress decides which agency will monitor specific laws. For example, most health care legislation is delegated to the USDHHS; however, legislation concerning the environment or occupational health would probably be monitored by the Environmental Protection Agency (EPA) or the Labor Department. Examples of those departments most involved with health care are included in the following discussion.

U.S. Department of Health and Human Services

The **U.S. Department of Health and Human Services (USDHHS)** is the agency most heavily involved with the health and welfare concerns of U.S. citizens. It touches

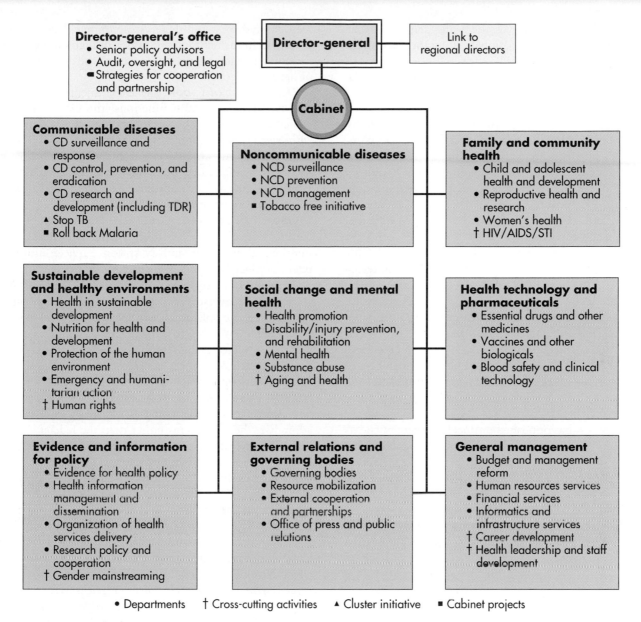

FIG. 9-1 Structure of the World Health Organization. (Used with permission of the Office of Publication, Geneva, 1999, WHO.)

more lives than any other federal agency. As mentioned previously, the organizational chart of the USDHHS (see Figure 3-1 on page 50) depicts the office of the Secretary and four principal operating components: the Social Security Administration, the Health Care Financing Administration, the Administration for Children and Families, and the PHS. The PHS is charged with regulating health care and overseeing the health status of Americans.

Public Health Service

The **Public Health Service (PHS)** has been a long-standing, significant contributor to the improved health status of Americans. The Health Resources and Services Administration (HRSA) of the PHS contains the Bureau of Health Professions (BHPr), which includes a Division of Nursing, as well as Divisions of Medicine, Dentistry, and Allied Health Professions.

The **Division of Nursing** has these specific goals (USDHHS, HRSA, BHPr, Division of Nursing, 1995):
- Enhancing nursing's contribution to primary health care and public health.
- Developing and promoting innovative practice models for improved and expanded nursing services.
- Enhancing racial and ethnic diversity and cultural competency in the nursing workforce.
- Promoting improved and expanded linkages between education and practice.
- Improving and expanding nursing services to high-risk and underserved populations.
- Enhancing nursing's contributions to achieving the *Healthy People 2000* objectives and health care reform.
- Capacity building for meeting the nursing service needs of the nation.

In late 1985 Congress overrode a presidential veto, allowing the creation of the National Center for Nursing Research within the NIH. In 1993 the Center became one of the National Institutes of Health and was renamed the **National Institute of Nursing Research.**

The research and research-related training activities previously supported by the Division of Nursing were transferred to this new Institute. The National Institute of Nursing Research is the focal point of the nation's nursing research activities. It promotes the growth and quality of research in nursing and client care, provides important leadership, expands the pool of experienced nurse researchers, and serves as a point of interaction with other bases of health care research.

A significant addition to the PHS in 1990 was the creation of the Agency for Health Care Policy and Research (AHCPR). This agency is charged with conducting research on effectiveness of medical services, interventions, and technologies, including research related to nursing interventions and outcomes that contribute to the improved health status of the nation. The AHCPR conducted focus groups to look at research showing positive outcomes of care for specific client problems (e.g., incontinence, pain management) that showed nursing's influence in positive outcomes for clients.

The AHCPR has published protocols for care of clients with a variety of health problems. These protocols will become the future standards of health care delivery. In addition, the AHCPR has a project called "Put Prevention Into Practice" to promote the use of standardized protocols for primary care delivery for clients across the age span (see Appendix A-2). These protocols can be used by nurses in planning disease prevention and health promotion activities for their clients.

Other federal government agencies

The USDHHS has primary responsibility for federal health functions. Several other cabinet departments of the federal government carry out certain other health-related functions. These departments include Commerce, Defense, Labor, Agriculture, and Justice.

Department of Commerce. Within the Department of Commerce (DOC) is the Census Bureau, which carries out an information function in health care. Established in 1902, the Bureau conducts a census of the population every 10 years. Also a part of the DOC is the National Oceanic and Atmospheric Administration, which provides special services in support of controlling urban air quality, a major factor in community health today.

Department of Defense. The Department of Defense delivers health care to members of the military and their dependents. The Assistant Secretary of Defense for Health Affairs administers the Civilian Health and Medical Program of the Uniformed Services (CHAMPUS). Each department within Defense (Army, Navy, Air Force, and Marines) has a Surgeon General. Health services, including community health services for members of the military, are delivered by a health services command in each department. In each command, nurses of high military rank, including brigadier general, are part of the administration of health services.

Department of Labor. The Department of Labor has two agencies with health functions: the OSHA and the Mine Safety and Health Administration. Both are charged with writing safety and health standards and ensuring compliance in the workplace. This includes conducting inspections, investigating complaints, and issuing citations if necessary. Each agency coordinates its activities with state departments of labor and health.

Department of Agriculture. The Department of Agriculture is involved in health care primarily through administering the Food and Nutrition Service. Although plant, product, and animal inspection by the Department of Agriculture is also related to health, the Food and Nutrition Service oversees a variety of food assistance activities. This service collaborates with state and local government welfare agencies to provide food stamps to needy persons to increase their food purchasing power. Other programs include school breakfast and lunch programs, WIC, and grants to states for nutrition education and training. These programs are examples of some that could be negatively affected if Congress decides that states will administer these programs rather than the federal government. Monies are given to the states as block grants. A **block grant** is a sum of money given to a state or local government whereby the federal government offers a general purpose for the use of the money but allows the state or local area to spend the money without meeting specific conditions. A general purpose might be nutrition. The state could then determine where the nutrition money would go. It may not go to the programs just mentioned, which have been successful.

Department of Justice. Health services to federal prisoners are administered within the Department of Justice. The Medical and Services Division of the Bureau of Prisons includes medical, psychiatric, dental, and health support services. It also administers environmental health and safety, farm operations, and food service, along with commissary, laundry, and other personal services for inmates.

State and Local Government Departments

Most state and local (county and city) areas perform governmental activities that affect the health care field. At the state level, three executive branch departments are described: health, education, and corrections. The organization of a local health department is outlined, and community health roles are discussed.

Selected health departments

In most state health departments, nurses serve in capacities similar to those in international and federal agencies: consultation, direct services, research, teaching, supervision, planning, and evaluation of health programs. Most health departments have a division or department of

Policy, Politics, and the Law in Canada

Lianne Jeffs, Registered Nurses Association of Ontario and University of Toronto

POLICY AND POLITICAL ACTION

To continue to have an influential role in the health care system, nurses will need to have a more global view of health care, an understanding of political processes, and an understanding of the issues impacting the health of Canadians. Public policy in Canada is largely influenced by the prevailing dominant ideologies and societal values. Current ideologies include cost effectiveness and efficiency, individual freedom, regional and geographic sensitivity, national identity and unity, and equality. Public policy is commonly defined as what governments choose to do or not to do, since both decisions and indecision represent policy action. Policymaking is a process by which choices are made to allocate limited resources and is usually in the form of policy committees. These committees include representation from various levels of elected or appointed government official and bureaucrats, representatives of organised societal groups, and influential individuals.

CANADIAN POLITICAL SYSTEM

Canada is a confederation of 10 provinces and 2 territories that was established by the British North America (BNA) Act of 1867. This organisational structure divided power between the federal and provincial governments. The Canadian government is grounded in British parliamentary roots. The power resides in the sovereign of their representative (governor general at the federal level and lieutenant governor at the provincial/territorial level). The Canadian democratic electoral system is based on single member constituencies in which the candidate with the most votes wins the electoral district. The leader of the party with the most votes becomes the prime minister (federal) or the premier (provincial/territorial). The prime minister selects an executive council, known as the *cabinet*, from the elected legislature, and each cabinet member is assigned a portfolio (department or ministry) of government.

LEGISLATIVE PROCESS IN CANADA

The legislative process in Canada starts with a bill—a proposal to create a new law or change an existing one. Most bills considered by Parliament are public bills. There are two types of public bills: 1) government public bills introduced and sponsored by a minister and 2) a bill sponsored by a private member. A bill can be introduced in the House of Commons (C-bills) or the Senate (S-bills). Most public bills start in the House of Commons. A bill can be passed, amended, delayed, or defeated. Once both houses have approved a bill, it is presented for royal assent and becomes law. The passing of a bill goes through several stages before becoming law. This process is detailed below. Nurses have experience influencing federal legislation, as evidenced by strong lobbying efforts led by the Canadian Nurses Association, which resulted in an amendment to the Canada Health Act of 1984 that enabled provincial health plans to fund services of nurses and other health professionals on a direct reimbursement basis.

REGULATION OF NURSING PRACTICE IN CANADA

Registered nurses practice within an ethical and standards-of-practice framework. The nursing profession is regulated at the provincial level. Each province and territory has passed statutes and regulations with respect to the governance of nursing, authority to establish educational requirements, prerequisites for entry to the practice of nursing, fees, complaints, and disciplinary procedures. A fairly uniform system exists in most jurisdictions of Canada. Ontario, however, has both the Regulated Health Professions Act of 1991, which is responsible for the overall supervision of health professions, and the Nursing Act of 1991 to influence nursing practice in the province. The provincial and territorial regulatory body exists with the primary focus of protecting the welfare of the public relative to the nursing profession. All nursing regulatory bodies in Canada require applicants for membership to have graduated from an approved school of nursing and have passed the requisite nursing registration examination before they are admitted as members of the association.

IMPLICATIONS FOR COMMUNITY AND PUBLIC HEALTH NURSING PRACTICE

The community health nurse should have an understanding of the standards of practice that their respective provincial regulatory body requires and of the federal, provincial, and municipal legislation that directly impacts their practice. The practice of public health is based on provincial public health acts. Other legislation includes mental health acts, communicable disease legislation, nursing acts, health unit acts, hospital acts, medical professional acts, and occupational health and safety acts. Community health nurses should also be aware of general legal principles including consent to treatment, negligence, confidentiality, documentation of client care, criminal law, and family and child violence. Registered nurses who are employed by an official governmental health unit work with medical officers of health and public health inspectors to carry out the legislation and regulations by providing health services to community residents.

HOW A BILL GETS PASSED IN THE CANADIAN GOVERNMENT

1. First reading in either House of Commons or Senate
2. Second reading (debate and vote on principle of the bill)
3. Parliamentary committee hearings and clause-by-clause examination

continued

Policy, Politics, and the Law in Canada—cont'd

4. Report to the House of Commons or Senate
5. Report stage debate; vote on amendments from committee
6. Third reading (bill is debated for a final time and voted on)
7. Introduction of the bill into other House of Parliament (repetition of process)
8. Royal assent (the bill becomes law)

Bibliography

Canadian Nurses Association: *Canadian Nurses Association's getting started: a political action guide for Canada's registered nurses.* Ottawa, 1997, the Association.

Keating M, Smith O: *Ethical and legal issues in Canadian nursing*, Toronto, 1995, WB Saunders Canada.
Larson J, Baumgart AJ: Overview: shaping of public policy. In Baumgart AJ, Larsen J, editors: *Canadian nursing faces the future*, ed. 2, St Louis, 1992, Mosby.
Miller C: Legal issues. In Stewart M et al.: *Community health nursing in Canada*, Toronto, 1985, Gage.

Canadian spelling is used.

BOX 9-2 Selected Programs Within a Typical State Health Department

Legal services
Services to the chronically ill and aging
Juvenile services
Medical assistance: policy, compliance, operations
Mental health and addictions
Mental retardation and developmental disabilities
Environmental programs
Departmental licensing boards
Division of vital records
Health services cost review
Health planning and development
Preventive medicine and medical affairs

---

public health nursing. Box 9-2 lists typical programs in a state health department.

Every state has a board of examiners of nurses. The board may be found either in the department of licensing boards of the health department or in an administrative agency of the governor's office. Created by legislation known as a *state nurse practice act,* the examiner's board is made up of nurses and consumers. A few states have other providers or administrators as members. The functions of this board are described in the practice act of each state and generally include licensing and examination of registered nurses and licensed practical nurses; approval of schools of nursing in the state; revocating, suspending, or denying of licenses; and writing of regulations about nursing practice and education. **Nurse practice acts** will be discussed later in a section on the scope of nursing practice.

State education departments

Some state departments of education coordinate health curricula and services provided within local school systems. Other state legislatures mandate that services be coordinated solely within the health department or jointly

between the health and education departments. Often liaison groups or councils are formed to facilitate joint coordination. These councils develop policy and guidelines for school health services and health education. Nurses often represent health and education departments at these councils and help shape health policy. Nurses also serve in departments of education in capacities similar to those in health departments.

State departments of corrections

Nurses work in state departments of corrections as planners and coordinators and sometimes as supervisors of health and nursing services for inmates in state prisons. Nurses in such state positions also may coordinate the health service efforts of local jails. Local jails may hire nurses directly or use the services of nurses in local health departments.

Local health departments

Depending on funding and other resources, programs offered by local health departments vary greatly. A fairly comprehensive list of such programs, taken from an urban-suburban county health department in a mid-Atlantic state, is shown in Box 9-3. At the local level, as at the state level, coordinating health efforts between health departments and other county or city departments is essential. For example, local boards of education and departments of social services are an integral part of activities of local governments. More often than at other levels of government, nurses at the local level provide direct services. Some nurses deliver special or selected services, such as follow-up of contacts in cases of tuberculosis or venereal disease or providing child immunization clinics. Other nurses have a more generalized practice, delivering services to families in certain geographic areas.

Social Welfare Programs

In addition to health programs, federal, state, and local governments also provide social welfare programs. Generally these programs provide money to the poor, elderly, disabled, and unemployed.

BOX 9-3 **Examples of Programs Provided by Local Health Departments**

Addiction and alcoholism clinics
Adult health
Birth and death records
Child day care and development
Child health clinics
Crippled children's services
Dental health clinic
Environmental health
Epidemiology and disease control
Family planning
Geriatric evaluation
Health education
Home health agency
Hospital discharge planning
Hypertension clinics
Immunization clinics
Information services
Maternal health
Medical social work
Mental health
Mental retardation and developmental disabilities
Nursing
Nursing home licensure
Nutrition division
Occupational therapy
Physical therapy
School health
Speech and audiology
Vision and hearing screening

The federal Social Security Act established a number of programs, including the social insurance programs, Social Security, unemployment insurance, and welfare. The Social Security Administration, which is within the USDHHS, administers the following programs:

- Old Age Survivors and Disability Insurance (OASDI)
- Aid to Families with Dependent Children (AFDC)
- Supplemental Security Income (SSI)

OASDI provides monthly benefits to retired and disabled workers, their spouses and children, and survivors of insured workers. AFDC, which is a federal and state program, helps needy families with children. AFDC subsidizes children deprived of the financial support of one of their parents as a result of death, disability, absence from the home, or in some states, unemployment. SSI is a federal program for the aged, blind, and disabled that may be supplemented by state support. The funds for these programs are provided by contributions from employees, employers, and self-employed individuals. These contributions are pooled into a special trust fund that is paid upon a worker's retirement, death, or disability as partial replacement of the earnings the family has lost.

In 1965, amendments to the Social Security Act created Medicare and Medicaid. These programs are administered by the HCFA within the USDHHS; in the case of Medicaid the administration is done in conjunction with state governments (see Chapter 5 for additional discussion of Medicare and Medicaid programs).

In addition, there are human development services coordinated by the Division of Administration for Children and Families within USDHHS. Programs are focused on the aging, children, youth and families, Native Americans, and the developmentally disabled. For example, the Older Americans Act is designed to promote the welfare and needs of older people. Through this act the federal government promotes the development of state-administered community-oriented systems of comprehensive social services for the elderly. Social programs focused on children and families include programs on adoption opportunities, Head Start services, runaway-youth facilities, child-abuse prevention and treatment, juvenile justice, and delinquency prevention. Other programs promote the social and economic development of Native Americans.

The Administration for Developmental Disabilities assists states in increasing the provision of quality services to persons with developmental disabilities. Grants are administered that support projects aimed at removing physical, mental, social, and environmental barriers for these disabled individuals. Social welfare policies and programs affect nursing practice. Community resources that improve the quality of life for specific populations help nurses assist clients in attaining optimal health.

Impact of Governmental Health Functions and Structures on Nursing

The variety and range of functions of government agencies has had a major impact on the practice of nursing. Funding in particular has shaped roles and tasks of community-oriented nurses. The designation of money for specific needs has led to special, more narrowly focused nursing roles. For example, funds assigned to communicable disease programs or family planning usually will not support home care services. Therefore nurses develop specialty roles related to these funded programs (e.g., immunization nurses, family planning nurses).

Training grants from the USDHHS Division of Nursing for nurse practitioners (NPs) in primary care have provided incentives to individual nurses to attend programs and develop new nursing roles within the health care system. School, adult, and pediatric NPs emerged primarily because of the funding provided by government agencies.

Other health policy information, funding, and direct services functions of government have influenced nursing. Legislatures have identified special needs and programs to meet the needs of special populations, such as migrant workers, pregnant women, homeless persons, or at-risk children. Often nurses are called upon to implement these programs. Vital statistics and other epidemiological data collected by government agencies have influenced the location, workforce, planning, and evaluation of nursing services.

According to the evolving policies of the federal government administrations of the 1980s, federal money given to the states was in the form of block grants. The block grant had a great impact on community-oriented nursing. Having less money in special programs resulted in a shift of nursing roles toward more general practice. Whether community health nursing should be a specialty or a general practice is an age-old debate. The purpose of mentioning the debate here is to show how government funding has shaped the functions of community health nurses within all levels of government. When governments give money to special programs, community health nursing roles become specialized and take care of the needs of certain clients only, such as the immunization of children. When governments give money to states to spend as they wish, community health nursing roles become generalized, and the nurse takes care of all client needs (e.g., pregnant mothers, sick children, and homeless men's health assessment are all provided in one clinic).

THE NURSE'S ROLE IN THE POLITICAL PROCESS

The number and types of laws influencing health care are increasing. Because of this, involvement in the political process at all possible points is important to nursing.

> **NURSING TIP**
>
> The nurse's basic understanding of the political process should include knowing who the lawmakers are, how bills become laws, the regulation-writing process, and methods of influencing the process and shaping health policy. With this knowledge nurses can shape nursing practice. See Figure 9-2 on how a bill becomes a law.

The federal and state legislatures are composed of two houses: an assembly, or house, and a senate. Representatives and senators are elected by the people within geographic jurisdictions. Each state has two federal senators and one or more representatives, depending on the state's population. Each state has its own rules for deciding on the number of senators and representatives within the state for the state legislature.

Although Congress meets throughout the year, state legislatures have sessions of varying lengths. Each legislature has its own leadership, usually dominated by either the Democratic or Republican party. Roles include the presiding officer, party floor leaders, and committee chairpersons.

An important part of this **legislative process** is the work of the staffs of the legislatures. These individuals do the legwork, research, paperwork, and other activities that move policy ideas into bills and then into law. In addition to the individual legislators' staffs, committee staffs are also important. Both of these can provide valuable information for citizens and their legislators. Nurses often serve as staff to legislators or are constituents (citizens) of a legislator and will want to give to or get information from that legislator about health policy. The legislative process begins with ideas that are developed into bills. After a bill is drafted, it is introduced to the legislature, given a number, read, and assigned to a committee. Hearings, testimony, lobbying, education, research, and informal discussion follow. If the bill is passed from the committee, the entire house hears the bill, amends it as necessary, and votes on it. A majority vote moves the bill to the other house, where it is read, amended, and voted on. Nurses can be involved in this process at any point. Many professional nursing associations have professional lobbyists, legislative committees, and political action committees (PACs) to shape health policy.

Common methods of lobbying include face-to-face encounters, personal letters, mailgrams, telegrams, telephone calls, testimony, petitions, reports, position papers, fact sheets, letters to the editor, news releases, speeches, coalition-building, demonstrations, and law suits. Depending on the issue, each of these can be equally effective. Tips on communication are provided in the How To boxes. Tips on writing to and visiting legislators and general tips on political action are presented in Boxes 9-4, 9-5, and 9-6.

> **HOW TO**   *Build a Professional Image*
>
> *What images do you have of yourself: strong, assertive, confident, competent, powerful? To be politically influential requires being an effective image shaper. What images do you convey in the workplace, the community, the government, and professional organizations? The following checklist will help you identify some of your messages.*
>
> - *In your daily encounters with clients and their families, do your verbal and nonverbal behaviors convey your professional pride and confidence?*
> - *Do you carry business cards to facilitate contacts with persons you meet?*
> - *Do you share your expertise through the local and national media?*
> - *Do you thoroughly document your nursing care?*
> - *Do you spend time every day teaching and listening to the concerns of your clients and their families?*
> - *At staff meetings, do you set the tone for serious collaboration by asking questions and giving your opinions?*
> - *Do you regularly communicate your ideas, concerns, and suggestions to your supervisors, public officials, and organizational leaders?*
> - *Do you vote in every national and local election?*
> - *What does your body language communicate?*
> - *Do you call or write to supervisors, community people, public officials, and organizational leaders to thank them when they have helped you with a problem or issue?*
> - *Does your attire communicate that you are a serious, businesslike professional?*
>
> From Mason DJ, Talbott SW, Keavitt JK: *Policy and politics for nurses: action and change in the workplace, government, organizations, and community,* ed 2, Philadelphia, 1993, WB Saunders.

The Federal Level

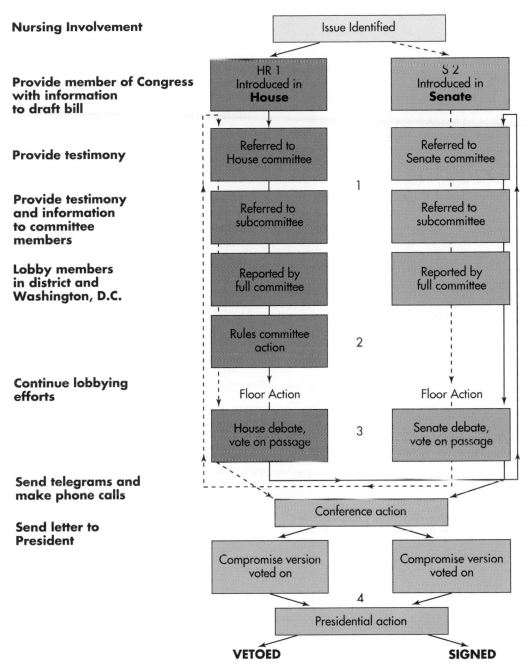

Nursing Involvement

Provide member of Congress with information to draft bill

Provide testimony

Provide testimony and information to committee members

Lobby members in district and Washington, D.C.

Continue lobbying efforts

Send telegrams and make phone calls

Send letter to President

Issue Identified

HR 1 Introduced in **House**

S 2 Introduced in **Senate**

Referred to House committee

Referred to Senate committee

Referred to subcommittee

Referred to subcommittee

Reported by full committee

Reported by full committee

Rules committee action

Floor Action

Floor Action

House debate, vote on passage

Senate debate, vote on passage

Conference action

Compromise version voted on

Compromise version voted on

Presidential action

VETOED   **SIGNED**

1 A bill goes to full committee first, then to special subcommittees for hearings, debate, revisions, and approval. The same process occurs when it goes to full committee. It either dies in committee or proceeds to the next step.

2 Only the House has a Rules Committee to set the "rule" for floor action and conditions for debate and amendments. In the Senate, the leadership schedules action.

3 The bill is debated, amended, and passed or defeated. If passed, it goes to the other chamber and follows the same path. If each chamber passes a similar bill, both versions go to conference.

4 The President may sign the bill into law, allow it to become law without his signature, or veto it and return it to Congress. To override the veto, both houses must approve the bill by a 2/3 majority vote.

FIG. 9-2 How a bill becomes a law. (From Mason DJ, Talbott SW, Keavitt JK: *Policy and politics for nurses: action and change in the workplace, government, organizations, and community,* ed 2, Philadelphia, 1993, WB Saunders.)

HOW TO *Refine Your Communication Skills*

Since communication is a key aspect of political activity and policy development, it is imperative to possess finely honed skills:

- *Get assistance in developing your writing and speaking; they are indispensable in sending messages that will be taken seriously.*
- *Attend continuing education sessions on public speaking, writing, and media training.*
- *Volunteer to speak at programs in your workplace, at nursing association meetings, and in the community.*
- *Testify at public hearings.*
- *Write short articles in your areas of expertise for your local newspapers and workplace newsletters.*
- *Team up with colleagues when you visit legislators, write an article, testify, or speak on a radio show or at a workshop. You will learn from the shared experience and bolster each other's confidence.*
- *Learn invaluable influence skills through committee work and involvement in nursing organizations, work-related committees, political action committees, multidisciplinary and consumer groups, and political clubs.*
- *Vote and get others to vote.*

From Mason DJ, Talbott SW, Keavitt JK: *Policy and politics for nurses: action and change in the workplace, government, organizations, and community*, ed 2, Philadelphia, 1993, WB Saunders.

Behind the scenes of this process lies the political party activity in which nurses should be involved. A wide variety of activities are available, including voting, participating in the party organization, registering voters, getting out the vote, fundraising, building networks or communication links, and participating in political action committees.

The passage of the National Health Research Extension Act of 1985 is one example of how nurses can use their influence. This act included the establishment of the National Center for Nursing Research. The Center began as the idea of a small group of nurses who worked to gain the support of colleagues and major national nursing organizations. Individual nurses provided testimony to Congress on the importance of nursing research. Some visited their congressional representatives to lobby for the bill. Many wrote letters and provided position papers and fact sheets to help legislators understand the need for the Center. Although the process took several years, the idea became a reality. Both the nursing profession and the client will benefit from the research and the knowledge base developed through the Center, now one of the National Institutes of Health.

More recently, the American Nurses Association, through its national organization and state nursing associations, was a strong lobbyist for the Patient Safety Act of 1997. This law requires health care facilities to make pub-

---

BOX 9-4 Tips for Writing to Legislators

1. Use your own stationery, not hospital or agency stationery. A letter is better than a postcard or telegram. Use your own words; form letters are not as effective as original ones.
2. Identify your subject clearly. State the name (and bill number if possible) of the legislation you are writing about.
3. Be brief, giving the reasons that you are for or against the legislation.
4. Explain how the issue would affect you, the nursing profession, clients, and/or your community.
5. Know what committees your legislators serve on and indicate in the letter if the bill will be brought before any of those committees. Know the current status of the bill (where it is in the legislative process).
6. Sign your name with "R.N." after it. Be sure your correct address is on the letter and the envelope. (Envelopes sometimes get thrown away before the letter is answered.)
7. Be courteous. A rude letter neither makes friends nor influences the legislator. Be sure to express your appreciation for work well done, a good speech, a favorable vote, or fine leadership in committee or on the floor.
8. Timing is important. Try to write your positions on a bill while it is in committee. Your legislators will usu-

ally be more responsive to your appeal at that time rather than later, when the bill has already been dealt with by a committee.
9. Limit your letter to one issue.
10. Keep a copy of all correspondence for your files. Send a copy of your letter and any response from the legislator to the government relations' staff at your professional nursing organization.
11. Address written correspondence as follows (the same general format applies to state and local officials):

U.S. Senator	U.S. Representative
Honorable Jane Doe	Honorable Jane Doe
United States Senate	House of Representatives
Washington, DC 20510	Washington, DC 20515
Dear Senator Doe:	Dear Representative Doe:

12. Mailgrams, which take 2 days, and telegrams, which are faster, can be ordered through Western Union's toll-free number: 1-800-325-6000.
13. You may be able to send a facsimile transmission (fax) to your legislator if you both have the necessary technology. This technique offers speed and conveys a sense of urgency. If you choose this method, follow up by sending the original letter through the mail.

From Mason DJ, Talbott SW, Keavitt JK: *Policy and politics for nurses: action and change in the workplace, government, organizations, and community*, ed 2, Philadelphia, 1993, WB Saunders.

BOX 9-5 Tips for Visiting Legislators

1. Call ahead to make an appointment to meet with the legislator. If the legislator is unavailable, ask to meet with the staff person who handles health issues.
2. Prepare. Know the background of the legislator and the history of the bill or issue you are discussing. Contact the government relations staff at your professional nursing organization to let them know about the visit. They may be able to provide important information about the issue, the political climate, your legislator's previous record on this issue, and the overall lobbying strategy on this issue.
3. At the beginning of the visit, introduce yourself and state what you want to discuss. Specify the issues and bills.
4. Ask the legislator what his or her position is on the issue or bill.
5. Many legislators and staff may not be familiar with nursing practice or legislative concerns. Be prepared to discuss them in basic terms. If possible, be prepared with facts about nursing practice in your state or district.
6. Ask if he or she has heard from others who support this issue or bill. Ask what the supporters are saying.
7. Ask if he or she has heard from opponents. Ask who the opponents are and what their arguments are.
8. Offer to provide additional information if you do not have data at hand, but do not make promises you cannot keep. It is better to admit that you do not know than to promise and not deliver or to convey erroneous information.
9. Follow up with a thank-you note, and share your reflections on the visit.
10. Keep a written record of your visit. Notify government relations staff of your professional nursing organization so that they can follow up with the legislator.
11. Spend more time with your legislators even if their position is not in agreement with yours. You might lessen the intensity of their positions and maintain contact for subsequent issues.
12. Invite legislators to meet you and your colleagues at your worksite to help expand their understanding of nursing and health care issues.

From Mason DJ, Talbott SW, Keavitt JK: *Policy and politics for nurses: action and change in the workplace, government, organizations, and community*, ed 2, Philadelphia, 1993, WB Saunders.

BOX 9-6 Tips for Action

- Get to know your legislators and the chair of your state board of nursing. Make sure you meet the governor and know the governor's chief executive aide.
- Apply the problem-solving and negotiation skills you have developed in nursing to the process of making and implementing laws. They are the same skills you use to convince a diabetic client to let you help him or her develop a care plan.
- Cultivate relationships with people who make the rules or pass the laws.
- Run for office.
- Develop a bipartisan nurse advisory council to assist your local legislator. (One state organized a statewide advisory group for a U.S. Senator. This group previewed U.S. health legislation for the Senator, and several nurses testified before the U.S. Senate Appropriations Subcommittee on Health and Human Services.)
- Spend an hour or two a week to upgrade your knowledge of political developments, health policy initiatives, legislators, and state government executives.

From Mason DJ, Talbott SW, Keavitt JK: *Policy and politics for nurses: action and change in the workplace, government, organizations, and community*, ed 2, Philadelphia, 1993, WB Saunders.

RESEARCH *Brief*

The purpose of this observational research study was to do a case analysis to look at the policies and the potential implications for seven states who, by 1995, had made legislative changes to reform their health care systems: Florida, Hawaii, Massachusetts, Minnesota, Oregon, Vermont, and Washington. Common problems across states were identified, as were common factors that helped states survive. Three major factors appeared to lead to success in reforming health policy:

1. Taking advantage of a window of opportunity (i.e., people must be ready for change)
2. A need for policy entrepreneurship (i.e., an individual citizen, nurse, or legislature must be willing to emerge as a leader in the legislative process and must have a passion for change, understanding of the issue, having a positive, objective outlook, and be willing to take a risk)
3. Involvement of key persons and groups affected by the change

Nurses can use these three factors in promoting legislation, regulatory change, or in introducing new public health policy.

Paul-Shaheen P: The states and health care reform: the road traveled and lessons learned from seven that took the lead, *J Health Polit Policy Law* 23(2), 1998.

lic some information on nurse staff levels, staff mix, and outcomes, and requires the USDHHS to review and approve all health care acquisitions and mergers. All of these requirements are to determine any long-term effect on the health and safety of clients, communities, and staff. On a more local level, in 47 states the passage of prescriptive authority for advanced practice nurses was achieved by individual nurses, state nurses associations, and various specialty groups lobbying state legislators (Pearson, 1999).

PRIVATE SECTOR INFLUENCE ON REGULATION AND HEALTH POLICY

In each level of government the executive branch can, and in most cases must, prepare regulations. These regulations are detailed, and they establish, fix, and control standards and criteria for carrying out certain laws. Figure 9-3 shows the steps in the typical regulation-writing process.

When the legislature passes a law and delegates its administration to an agency, it gives that agency the power to make regulations. Because regulations flow from legislation, they have the force of law.

The **private sector,** which includes everyone that is not part of the government or **public sector,** can influence and shape legislation through many means. Through the same means, the private sector also influences the writing of regulations. This part of the chapter describes the process of regulation writing and ways to influence it. Nursing students and clinicians are members of the private sector and are influenced by regulations that affect nursing practice.

Process of Regulation

After a law is passed, the appropriate executive department begins the process of regulation by studying the topic or issue. Advisory groups or special task forces, including nondepartmental members, are sometimes formed to provide the content of the regulations. As the work of the groups or individual department members progresses, initial drafts of the proposed regulations are written. Nurses, including students, can influence these regulations by writing letters to the regulatory agency in charge or by speaking at public hearings.

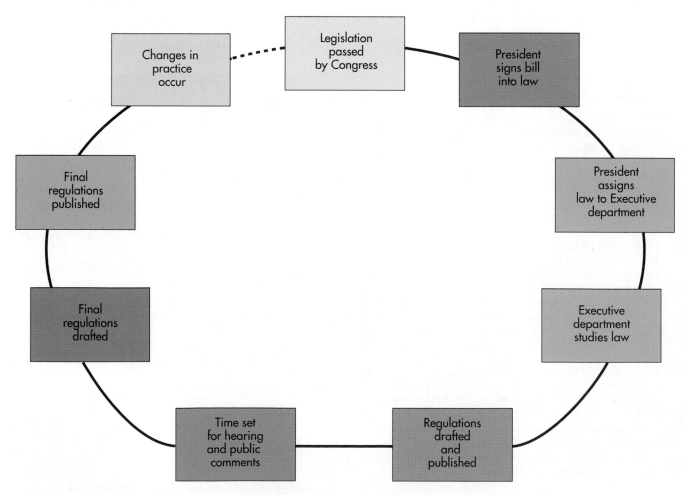

FIG. 9-3 The regulation writing process.

After rewriting, the proposed regulations are put into final draft form and printed in the legally required publication, which at the federal level is the *Federal Register.* Similar registers exist in most states where regulations from state departments, including state health departments, are published. The publication of proposed regulations includes notice about a time period within which public comment will be accepted. Public comment is usually in written form. The notice also may give a date, time, and place for a hearing that is open to the public. Anyone may attend; if one wishes to speak at the hearing, published rules for that procedure must be followed. This usually involves notifying the agency of an intent to speak and limiting the length of testimony as specified by the agency.

Revisions made to the proposed regulations are based on public comment and public hearing. Depending on the amount and content of the public reaction, final regulations are prepared or more study of the area and issues is conducted. Final published regulations carry the force of law. The date when regulations become effective also is published. It is at this point that practice is changed to conform to the new regulations. Close monitoring by and participation of the private sector in regulation writing can begin as soon as a law is passed and delegated to an executive branch agency. Government manuals, updated at least yearly, list names and phone numbers of individuals within the executive branch. Early contact and expression of interest in how a particular law gets administered may result in membership on a task force or advisory board. The membership of such groups is public information, and these members can be contacted to determine their thoughts on the direction that the regulations will take.

Regular surveillance of the *Federal Register* or state registers is essential. Once proposed resolutions are published, members of the private sector may influence regulations by attending the hearings, providing comments, testifying, and engaging in lobbying aimed at individuals involved in the writing. Concrete, written suggestions for revision submitted to these individuals are usually persuasive. A good example of how nurses can influence regulations occurred in one state in 1997 when the Cabinet for Health Services wrote regulations to charge a 2% tax on nurses' and other health providers' salaries to recover the cost of the Medicaid program. Nurses filled the 200-seat auditorium at the state capitol and provided testimony, wrote letters of protest, and contacted key officials personally. They were able to show that they were being double-taxed on their salaries by the state and being penalized for providing care to underserved populations.

Final regulations, published in a *Code of Regulations* (both federal and state), usually lead to changes in practice. Regulations need to be made available to all individuals whose practice is affected. This dissemination can be helped by private sector involvement. Regulations need to be included in manuals of policies and procedures of the agencies affected by them. For example, Medicare regulations setting standards for nursing homes and home health are incorporated into these agencies' manuals.

LAWS AFFECTING COMMUNITY-ORIENTED NURSING PRACTICE

Community-oriented nursing combines nursing practice and public health practice. The community-oriented nurse is subject to the laws relating to nursing practice and public health practice. This section discusses the various types of laws, how they affect nurses, and the legal resources available.

Types of Laws

Several definitions of *law* are available. However, many of these tend to describe what law is not rather than what it is. Definitions of *law* include the following:
- A rule established by authority, society, or custom
- The body of rules governing the affairs of people within a community or among states; social order; the common law
- A set of rules or customs governing a discrete field or activity (e.g., criminal law, contract law)
- The system of courts, judicial process, and legal officers, or lawyers, giving effect to the laws of a society

These definitions reflect the close relationship of law to community and to society's customs and beliefs. Since community-oriented nursing reflects society's beliefs and customs, law has had a major impact on this practice. Although community-oriented nursing practice emerged from individual voluntary activities, society soon recognized the need for it. Through legal mandates, positions and functions for nurses in community settings were created. These functions in many instances carry with them the "force of law." For example, if the nurse discovers a person with smallpox, the law directs the nurse and others legally designated in the community to take specific action. This is just one example of how the law has shaped nursing practice.

WHAT DO YOU THINK? *As a former Speaker of the House of Representatives noted, "all politics is local." Therefore should nurses focus their political activities only in the local community?*

There are three types of law in the United States: constitutional law, legislation and regulation, and judicial and common law.

Constitutional law
Constitutional law emerges from federal and state constitutions. From this type of law nurses can get answers to

questions in selected practice situations. For example, on what basis can the state require quarantine or isolation of individuals with tuberculosis? The answer to this question can be found in constitutional law. The U.S. Constitution specifies explicit and limited functions of the federal government. All other powers and functions are left to the individual states. The major power of the states relating to nursing practice is the right to intervene in a reasonable manner to protect the health, safety, and welfare of the citizenry. As described previously in this chapter, the state's "police power" is not without limitation. First, it must be a "reasonable" exercise of power. Second, if the power interferes or infringes on individual rights, the state must demonstrate that there is a "compelling state interest" in exercising its power. Therefore isolating an individual or separating one from a community because he or she has a communicable disease has been deemed an appropriate exercise of state powers. The state can isolate an individual even though it infringes on individual rights (freedom, autonomy) under the following conditions:

1. The isolation is done in a reasonable manner.
2. There is a compelling state interest in the prevention of an epidemic.
3. The isolation is necessary to protect the health, safety, and welfare of individuals in the community or the public as a whole.

WHAT DO YOU THINK? *The community's rights are more important than the individual's rights when there is a threat to the health of the public.*

The legal and medical communities and AIDS activists reject the social quarantine of individuals with AIDS. This is an example of how individual freedom and autonomy of the individual come before "compelling state interest."

Legislation and regulation

Legislation is the type of law that comes from the legislative branches of federal, state, or local government. Much legislation has an effect on nursing. **Regulations** are very specific statements of law that relate to individual pieces of legislation. For example, state legislators have enacted laws (statutes) establishing boards of nursing and defining terms such as *licensed registered nurse* and *nursing practice*. The boards of nursing, through regulation, enforce the statutory law by writing rules on how to become a licensed registered nurse and such practice issues as delegation and continuing education requirements. Nurses often are employed by the executive branch through the state or local health department. Therefore nursing interventions are often directed at implementing legislation and regulations.

Nurses employed in other community settings, those with no governmental responsibilities or legal mandates, are nevertheless often subject to legislation and regulations. For example, nurses employed by private agencies who are giving home health care must deliver care according to federal Medicare legislation and regulations or state Medicaid legislation and regulations for the agency to be reimbursed for those services. Private and public health care services rendered by nurses are subject to many government regulations.

Judicial and common law

Judicial and common law is the last group of laws having an impact on nursing. Judicial law is based on court or jury decisions. The opinions of the courts are judicial opinions and are referred to as *case law.* The court uses other types of laws to make its decisions, including previous court decisions or cases. **Precedent** is one principle of common law. Judges are bound by previous decisions unless they are convinced that the "old law" is no longer relevant or valid. This process is called *distinguishing* and usually involves a demonstration of how the currently disputed situation differs from the previously decided situation. Other principles of common law are part of a court's rationale and the basis of making a decision. Such principles include justice, fairness, respect for individuals, autonomy, and self-determination. These play an important role in decisions made by courts (see Chapter 6).

General Community-Oriented Nursing Practice and the Law

Despite the broad nature and varied roles of nursing practice, two legal aspects apply to most practice situations. The first aspect is professional negligence, or malpractice; the second is the scope of practice defined by custom and state practice acts.

Professional negligence

Professional negligence, or malpractice, is defined as an act or failure to act on behalf of a client that leads to injury of that client. To prove that a nurse was negligent, the client must prove all of the following:

1. The nurse owed a duty to the client or was responsible for the client's care.
2. The duty to act as a reasonable, prudent nurse or as another nurse would act under the circumstances was breached or not fulfilled.
3. The failure to be reasonable under the circumstances led to the alleged injuries.
4. The injuries provided the basis for a monetary claim through the legal system.

Reported cases involving negligence and community-oriented nurses are almost nonexistent. As one example, a case involving an occupational health nurse is discussed. Although occurring some years ago, this example clearly represents the four criteria that must be present to prove negligence. Since nurses still use standing orders, a similar problem could happen to a nurse today.

DID YOU KNOW? *In the eyes of the law, the "prudent nurse" used as an example, or standard, to judge the competency of a nurse's practice can be practicing anywhere in the United States and not just in the community in which you work.*

The California case of Cooper versus Motor Bearing Co., 288P 2d 581, involved an occupational health nurse who negligently implemented standing orders on an injury involving a puncture wound. The nurse, by her own testimony, did not examine or probe the wound, nor did she refer the worker to a physician; she simply swabbed and bandaged it. Only after 10 months, in which time there were many documented visits to the dispensary and complaints by the worker that the wound was not healing, did the nurse refer him to the company doctor. On referral, basal cell carcinoma was found and surgery followed.

The fact that the nurse was employed by the industry to render first aid established the first element of negligence: a duty was owed to the worker. The nurse acknowledged that it was her duty to refer any unfamiliar or questionable condition or injury to the doctor for diagnosis. The standard of good nursing care in the community was to examine the wound for the presence of foreign bodies. The nurse knew that the normal healing time was 1 to 2 weeks. If a wound persisted and did not heal, proper nursing care would indicate referral to a physician. Testimony was given that the practice of an occupational health nurse in this particular type of industry is to probe wounds for foreign bodies. According to the nurse's education and experience, she should have been aware of the possibility of foreign objects being present in such a wound.

In this case the nurse's failure to detect the foreign body was the proximate cause of the basal cell carcinoma. The pain, suffering, lost time and wages, and bodily disfigurement were all injuries that could be calculated and totaled as a monetary amount. The nurse and the company were found negligent by the California Court.

An integral part of negligence suits is the question of who should be sued. Obviously, those who made the mistakes should be sued, but part of the consideration has to do with who can best pay for the injuries. When a nurse is employed and functioning within the scope of that job, the employer is responsible for the nurse's negligent actions. This is referred to as the doctrine of **respondeat superior.** By directing a nurse to carry out a particular function, the employer becomes responsible for negligence, along with the individual nurse. The scope of employment is usually more inclusive than a job description but does not include criminal activities. Because employers are usually better able to pay for the injuries suffered, they are sued more often than the nurses themselves.

Nurses employed by government agencies need to ascertain whether that agency has **sovereign immunity.** Under this doctrine the agency may be exempt from suit for particular kinds of actions, such as negligence. However, sovereign immunity will not protect nurses who are acting under the auspices of the government when the negligence occurs. Public health nurses may have personal immunity for particular practice areas, such as giving immunizations. In some states the legislature has granted personal immunity to nurses employed by public agencies to cover all aspects of their practice.

Nursing students need to be aware that they are governed by the same laws and rules governing the professional nurse. Students are expected to meet the same standard of care of any licensed nurse practicing under the same or similar circumstances. Lower standards of care by students are not acceptable. Students are expected to be able to perform all tasks and make clinical decisions based on the knowledge they have gained or been offered, according to their progress in their educational programs. If a faculty member gives a student an assignment based on the student's progress in the program, the faculty member is not considered liable for the student's actions.

Scope of practice

The issue of **scope of practice** involves differentiating among the practices of physicians, nurses, and other health care providers. Scope of practice is assessed by 1) examining the usual and customary practice of a profession and 2) taking into account how legislation defines the practice of a particular profession in a jurisdiction. The issue is especially important to community-oriented nurses who have traditionally practiced with much autonomy.

The usual and customary practice of nursing can be determined through a variety of sources, including the following:

1. Content of nursing educational programs, general and special
2. Experience of other practicing nurses (peers)
3. Activities and statements, including standards, of nursing professional organizations
4. Policies and procedures of agencies employing nurses
5. Needs and interests of the community
6. Literature, including books, texts, and journals

All of these sources can describe and help determine the scope of the usual practice of a nurse. Every nurse should know and follow closely the proposed changes in practice acts in nursing, medicine, pharmacy, and other related professions. These pieces of state legislation define the scope of practice for professionals in these areas. The nurse should always examine all definitions related to nursing practice. For example, a review of the Pharmacy Act will let the nurse know whether to question the right to dispense medications in a family planning clinic in a local health department. Defining *scope* forces one to clarify both independent and dependent nursing functions. The failure to know one's limitations could lead, for example, to charges of practicing as a pharmacist without a license, with fines and possible suspension or revocation of license. Just as practice acts vary, so do the issues of scope of practice. It is best to refer directly to practice acts for a particular state code.

Because of the variety of legal aspects, the following section deals with areas of practice having special focuses.

Special Community-Oriented Nursing Practice and the Law

Legal aspects of community-oriented nursing vary depending on the setting where care is delivered, the clinical specialty, and the functional role. Four special areas of practice and their respective legal aspects are discussed to illustrate how the law affects specific practice areas: school and family health, occupational health, home care and hospice services, and correctional health. Examples of legislation and judicial opinions affecting nurses within these selected areas are included.

School and family health

School and family health nursing may be delivered by nurses employed by health departments or boards of education. School health legislation establishes a minimum of services that must be provided to children in public and private schools. For example, most states require that children be immunized against certain communicable diseases before entering school. Children must have had a physical examination by that time, and most states require at least one physical at a later time in their schooling. Legislation also specifies when and what type of health screening will be conducted in schools (e.g., vision and hearing testing).

Legislation treating child abuse and neglect makes a large impact on nursing practice within schools and families. Most states require nurses to notify police or a social service agency of any situation in which they suspect a child is being abused or neglected. This is one instance in which society permits a professional to breach confidentiality to protect someone who may be in a helpless and vulnerable position. There is civil immunity for such reports, and the nurse may be called as a witness in any court hearing. The majority of legal cases involving community-oriented nurses concern child abuse.

Other examples of federal legislation affecting nursing practice with regard to schools and families are Head Start, early diagnostic screening programs, nutritional programs, services for the handicapped, and special education. Most of this legislation, although written by the U.S. Congress, requires cooperative federal and state funding, planning, and implementation. Each nurse working within a service based on legislation should be oriented to the legislation. It is advisable that the legislation and its regulations be included in the nursing agency's manual of policies and procedures so that the nurse may refer to it.

Occupational health

Occupational health is another special area of practice that is affected greatly by state and federal laws. The **Occupational Safety and Health Administration (OSHA)** imposes many requirements on industries. These requirements shape the functions of nurses and the types of services given to workers. The OSHA also establishes a reporting system for workers exposed to toxic agents in the workplace. A record-keeping system required by the OSHA greatly affects health records in the workplace. Each state has an agency similar to the OSHA that also monitors and inspects industries, as well as the health services rendered to them by nurses. Most states have a "worker's right to know" law requiring employers to provide employees with information concerning the nature of toxic substances they may encounter in the workplace during their employment. In addition, all states have workers' compensation statutes that provide a legal opportunity for claims of workers injured on the job. Access to records, confidentiality, and the use of standing orders are legal issues of great significance to nurses employed in industries.

Home care and hospice

Home care and hospice services rendered by nurses are affected greatly by state laws that require licensing and certification. Compliance with these laws is directly linked to the method of payment for the services. For example, a service must be licensed and certified to obtain payment for services through Medicare. Federal regulations implementing Medicare have an effect on much of nursing practice, including how nurses record details of their visits.

Many states have passed laws requiring nurses to report elder abuse to the proper authorities. Legislation affecting home care and hospice services has related to such issues as the right to death with dignity, rights of residents of long-term facilities and home-health clients, definitions of death, and the use of living wills, specifically advance directives that now must be given to and signed by all clients of nurses. The legal and ethical dimensions of nursing practice are particularly important in this area of practice. Individual rights, such as the right to refuse treatment, and nursing responsibilities, such as the legal duty to render reasonable and prudent care, may often be in conflict in delivering home and hospice services. Much case discussion, sometimes including outside consultation, is required when rights and responsibilities are in conflict and a decision must be made to resolve that conflict.

Correctional health

Nursing practice in correctional health systems is controlled by federal and state laws and regulations and by recent Supreme Court decisions. The laws and decisions relate to the type and amount of services that must be provided for incarcerated individuals. For example, physical examinations are required of all prisoners after they are sentenced. Regulations specify basic levels of care that must be provided for prisoners, and care during illness is particularly addressed. Court decisions requiring adequate health services are based on constitutional law. If minimum services are not provided, it is a violation of a prisoner's right to freedom from cruel and unusual punishment. Such decisions provide a framework that strongly influences the setting of nursing priorities. For example, providing sick calls would take priority over nutritional classes.

Each of the preceding areas of special community-oriented nursing practice is shaped significantly by legislation and judicial opinion. Those nurses responsible for setting and implementing program priorities need to identify and monitor laws related to each special area of practice.

> **DID YOU KNOW?** *Persons with communicable diseases such as tuberculosis may be confined to a prison hospital if they are considered a threat to their community by failing to follow their treatment regimen.*

Legal Resources

In addition to seeking legal counsel, nurses can actively remain current with respect to nursing-related laws and regulations. There are many resources in public libraries and law libraries, including the following:

- State bar association publications
- State code
- State annotated code
- Indexes to codes
- Supplements to codes and indexes
- *Federal Register* and state registers
- *Code of Regulations* (federal and state)
- Administrative agency rules and decisions
- Case law
- Opinions of attorney generals
- Legal dictionaries
- Legislative histories
- Legal periodicals

To use these legal resources, begin by reviewing the topical index to each source. As the headings are reviewed, several can be identified and related to the content areas of practice (such as immunizations or family planning) and the types of clients (e.g., minors, adolescents, and children) served by the nurse. Computer search tools are often available. One legal computerized search tool is called *Lexis.* The Library of Congress has a service called *Scorpio.* Both services will search not only books and journals but also recent case laws, bills, amendments, and legislation. One of the best ways to stay informed is to read the area newspaper.

🌱 clinical application

Larry was in his final rotation in the Bachelor of Science in Nursing program at State University. He was anxious to complete his community health nursing course because upon graduation he would begin a position as a staff nurse specializing in school health at the local health department. His wife was expecting their first child, and she had been receiving prenatal care at the health department.

Larry was aware that a few years ago the federal government had, by law, provided block grants to states for primary care, maternal child health programs, and other health care needs of states. He had read the *Federal Register* and knew that the regulations for these grants had been written through USDHHS departments. He was aware that these regulations did not require states to fund specific programs.

Larry read in the local paper that the health department was closing its prenatal clinic at the end of the month. When this state had received its block grant, they decided to spend its money for programs other than prenatal care. Larry found that a 3-year study in his own state showed improved pregnancy outcomes as a result of prenatal care. The results were further improved when the care was delivered by community health nurses.

Larry was concerned that, as a student, he would have little influence. However, he decided to call his classmates together to plan a course of action.

What would such an action plan include?

Answer is found in the back of the book.

🔑 **KEY POINTS**

- Many historical events have been significant in developing the role of government in health care.
- The legal basis for most congressional action in health care can be found in Article I, Section 8 of the U.S. Constitution.
- The four major health care functions of the federal government are direct service, financing, information, and policy setting.
- The goal of the World Health Organization is the attainment by all people of the highest possible level of health.
- Many federal agencies are involved in government health care functions. The agency most directly involved with the health and welfare of Americans is the U.S. Department of Health and Human Services (USDHHS).
- Most state and local jurisdictions have government activities that affect the health care field.
- The variety and range of functions of government agencies have had a major impact on nursing. Funding in particular has shaped the role and tasks of nurses.
- The private sector can influence legislation in many ways, especially through influencing the process of writing regulations. Nurses are a part of the private sector.
- The number and types of laws influencing health care are increasing. Because of this, involvement in the political process is important to nurses.
- Professional negligence and the scope of practice are two legal aspects particularly relevant to nursing practice.
- Nurses must consider the legal implications of their own practice in each clinical encounter.
- The federal and most state governments are composed of three branches: the executive, the legislative, and the judicial.
- Each branch of government plays a significant role in health policy.
- The U.S. Public Health Service was created in 1798.
- The first national health insurance bill was introduced in Congress in 1934.
- The political party platforms are good sources of information to find out how a government will respond to a health policy issue.

continued

KEY POINTS—cont'd

- *Health: United States* is an important source of data about the nation's health care problems.
- In 1912 the Child Health Bureau was established.
- In 1921 the Sheppard-Towner Act was passed and had an important influence over child health programs and community health nursing practice.
- The Division of Nursing, the National Institute of Nursing Research, and the Agency for Health Care Policy and Research are governmental entities important to nursing.
- Nurses through state and local health departments function as consultants, direct care providers, researchers, teachers, supervisors, and program managers.
- The state governments are responsible for regulating nursing practice within the state.
- Federal and state social welfare programs have been developed to provide monetary benefits to the poor, elderly, disabled, and unemployed.
- Social welfare programs affect nursing practice. These programs improve the quality of life for special populations, thus making the nurse's job easier in assisting the client with health needs.
- The nurse's scope of practice is defined by legislation and by standards of practice within a specialty.

critical thinking activities

1. Conduct an interview with the local health officer. Ask for information from a 10-year period. See if you can see trends in population size and needs and corresponding roles and activities of government that were implemented to meet these changes.
2. Examine a current health department budget and compare it with a budget from previous years. Has there been any impact on health care because of changes in government spending?
3. Select a community or public health nursing role you would like to examine more closely. Interview a person in that role, asking questions about job function, organizational structure, agency goals, salary, mobility within the agency, and potential contributions of this role to the health of the community.
4. Locate your state register or other documents, such as newspapers, that publish proposed regulations. Select one set of proposed regulations and critique them. Submit your opinion in writing as public comment, or attend the hearing and testify on the regulations. Be sure to submit something in writing. Evaluate your participation by stating what you learned and whether the proposed regulations were changed in your favor.
5. Find and review your state nurse practice act and define your scope of practice.
6. Contact your local public health agency to discuss the state's official powers in regulating epidemics, such as the recent AIDS outbreak. Explore the state's right to protect the health, safety, and welfare of the citizens. Ask about the conflict between the state's rights and individual rights and how such issues are resolved. Ask about the standards of care that apply to this issue and how it is decided which services offered to clients should be mandatory and which should be voluntary. Explore how the role of public health differs in these epidemics compared with the past epidemics of smallpox and tuberculosis.

Bibliography

American Nurses Association: *Code for nurses,* Kansas City, Mo, 1995, the Association.

American Nurses Association: *Nursing's social policy statement,* ed 2, 1995, the Association.

American Public Health Association: *The definition and role of public health nursing,* Washington, DC, 1996, the Association.

Aroskar M: Legal and ethical issues: politics and ethics in nursing—implications for education, *J Prof Nurs* 10(3):129, 1994.

Bacon D, Davidson R, Keller M: *The encyclopedia of the United States Congress,* New York, 1995, Simon & Schuster.

Chapman E: Putting the case for the nurse: handling and avoiding clinical negligence claims, *J Prof Nurs* 9(7):443, 1994.

Davis A: *Ethical dilemmas and nursing practice,* ed 4, New York, 1997, Appleton & Lange.

Division of Nursing, Bureau of Health Professionals, Health Services and Resources Administration, Public Health Service: *The division of nursing,* Hyattsville, Md, 1993, the Division.

Eskreis T: Seven common legal pitfalls in nursing, *Am J Nurs* 98(4):34, 1998.

Gittler J, Bayer R: Public health policy and TB, *J Health Polit Policy Law* 9(1):149, 1994.

Gittler J, Boubjer R: The importance of public health for the 21st century, *J Health Polit Policy Law* 19(1):155, 1994.

Grad F: *The public health law manual,* ed 2, Washington, DC, 1990, APHA.

Green J: The $147,000 misunderstanding: repercussions of overestimating the costs of AIDS, *J Health Polit Policy Law* 19(1):69, 1994.

Guido GW: *Legal issues in nursing,* ed 2, Stamford, Conn, 1997, Appleton & Lange.

Hudson-Rodd N: Public health: people participating in the creation of healthy places, *Public Health Nurs* 11(2):119, 1994.

Jacobs LR: Health reform impasse: the politics of American ambivalence toward government, *J Health Polit Policy Law* 18(3 part 2):629, 1993.

Mason DJ, Talbott SW, Leavitt JK: *Policy and politics for nurses: action and change in the workplace, government, organizations, and community,* ed 2, Philadelphia, 1998, WB Saunders.

Pearson L: Annual update of how each state stands on legislative issues affecting advanced nursing practice, *Nurse Pract* 24(1), 1999.

Pickett G, Hanlon J: *Public health administration and practice,* St Louis, 1990, Mosby.

Sharpe N: All politics is local and other rules, *Nurs Manage* 25(3):22, 1994.

Sullivan G: Home care: more autonomy, more legal risks, *RN* 57(5):1, 1994.

Thomas PA: Teaching students to become active in public policy, *Public Health Nurs* 11(2):75, 1994.

United Nations: *Basic facts about the UN,* New York, 1990, UN.

United States Congressional Budget Office: *Analysis of Clinton health care reform plan,* Washington DC, 1994, Bureau of National Affairs.

U.S. Department of Health and Human Services, HRSA, BHPr, Division of Nursing: Washington, DC, 1995, USDHHS.

U.S. Department of Health and Human Services: *Health: United States,* 1998, DHHS Pub No (PHS) 99-123(2), Hyattsville, Md, 1999, USDHHS.

U.S. Department of Health and Human Services: *Healthy People 2000 Review 1997,* DHHS Pub No (PHS) 98-1256, Hyattsville, Md, 1994, USDHHS.

U.S. Department of Health and Human Services: *Leading indicators for Healthy People 2010,* Washington, DC, 1998, USDHHS.

World Health Organization, United Nations Children's Fund: *Primary health care: a joint report,* Geneva, 1978, WHO.

World Health Organization: Primary health care needs: conclusion and recommendations of a WHO study group, *Int Nurs Rev* 34(2):52, 1987.

World Health Organization: *The work of WHO, 1988-1990: biennial report of the Director-general,* Geneva, 1990, WHO.

World Health Organization: *Technical report series,* 738, Geneva, 1986, WHO.

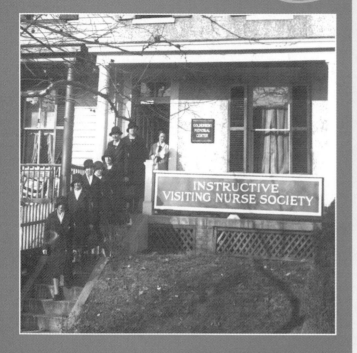

PART Three

Conceptual Frameworks Applied to Community-Oriented Nursing Practice

In 1988 the National Center for Nursing Research (NCNR) was established under the National Institutes of Health to facilitate nursing research. In 1993 the U.S. Congress expanded the scope and functions of the NCNR and made it one of the National Institutes of Health and renamed it the National Institute of Nursing Research (NINR). The NINR is crucial to the profession's movement to build a stronger base for practice. Although no conceptual or theoretical model will meet the needs of all community or public health nurses, several nursing and public health models serve as frameworks for organizing educational programs and for making practice decisions.

In 1988 the Institute of Medicine report on the Future of Public Health identified the three primary or core functions of public health: 1) assessment through data collection and sharing of information; 2) policy development for family, community, and state level health policies; and 3) ensurance of the availability of necessary health services for clients. In 1993 the Public Health Nursing Directors of Washington State developed a model showing how public health/community health nurses perform the three core functions with all clients: individuals, families, and communities.

The scientific base provided by public health as a specialty remains the foundation for community-oriented nursing. In Part Three, five chapters provide information about how to use conceptual models, epidemiology, research, and principles of education to organize community-oriented practice to meet the core functions of public health. Each chapter provides both theory and practical application of the specific topic to the clinical area. This section provides readers with tools that can be used to influence public health and community health nursing practice.

It has been estimated that the effect of the medical care system on usual indices for measuring health is about 10%. The remaining 90% is determined by factors over which health care providers have little or no direct control, such as lifestyle and social and physical environmental conditions. This text focuses on the processes and practices for promoting health, principally by the nurse, who is considered to be an ideal person to demonstrate and teach others how to promote health. To be effective, health promotion requires that people cease focusing on how to "fix" themselves and others only when they detect physical and emotional disequilibriums and that they instead assume personal responsibility for health promotion. Such a change in emphasis requires that health care providers incorporate health promotion techniques into their practice.

Organizing Frameworks Applied to Community Health Nursing

LOIS W. LOWRY & KAREN S. MARTIN

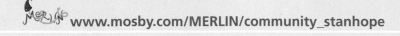 www.mosby.com/MERLIN/community_stanhope

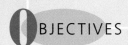BJECTIVES

After reading this chapter, the student should be able to do the following:

- Define the terms *theory, model, concept,* and *conceptual model.*
- Differentiate between conceptual model and theory.
- Identify at least three uses of conceptual models in nursing.
- Differentiate between the ANA and the APHA models of community health nursing.

- Describe key components of the Neuman Systems Model and the Omaha Classification System.
- Apply the Neuman Systems Model to community and public health practice.
- Apply the Omaha System to community and public health practice.
- Describe how the Neuman Systems Model and Omaha Systems complement each other

KEY TERMS

assurance activities	flexible line of defense	nursing diagnosis	Omaha System Problem
boundary	general systems theory	nursing intervention	Rating Scale for
client problem	hypotheses	nursing practice	Outcomes
concepts	information management	nursing process	Omaha System
conceptual model	intervention	Omaha System	openness
documentation	lines of resistance	Intervention Scheme	organization
entropy	model	Omaha System Problem	theory
environment	negentropy	Classification Scheme	wholeness
evaluation	Neuman Systems Model		
feedback	normal line of defense		*See Glossary for definitions*

CHAPTER OUTLINE

The authors of this chapter acknowledge the contributions of Jeanette Lancaster.

Community and public health nursing blends nursing and public health theory into a population-focused practice to promote and preserve the health of communities. Community and public health nursing practice focuses on the care of individuals, families and groups within the context of promoting and preserving the health of the community as a whole.

This chapter provides an overview of concepts, models, and theories that are important for community and public health nursing practice. First, theory and theory development are discussed, followed by a description of the competencies and essential functions of community and public health nursing. Next, two models for organizing data and guiding community and public health nursing practice are presented in detail: the Neuman Systems Model and the Omaha Classification System. Over the last decade, these two models have demonstrated usefulness for nurses. This in no way implies that these are the only two models that effectively guide community and public health nursing practice; however, there are data to show that these models are frequently used with positive outcomes. Also, both models are used to guide curriculum design for courses in community and public health nursing and are guides for nursing practice in service agencies.

DEFINING CONCEPTS, MODELS, AND THEORIES

A **theory** is a construct that accounts for or organizes phenomena. A nursing theory explains or describes a specific phenomenon of nursing (Barnum, 1994). A theory focuses on one or more concrete, specific concepts and statements that link the concepts. Theory provides a starting point to collect facts in a systematic way so that phenomena can be described, explained, or predicted (Fawcett, 1997). Theories vary in scope from grand theories that are very broad to mid-range and can be tested through research.

Models are ways of viewing real phenomena. Models can be physical, symbolic, or mental. A physical model is a specific, observable replica of the real structure. For example, when a new health department building is about to be constructed, the architect may assemble a small replica that is simply a scaled version of the proposed new structure. Symbolic models have a higher level of abstraction than do physical models. For example, signs have symbolic meanings to those who read them. A "No smoking" sign signifies that the readers should refrain from certain actions. Mental models have an even greater level of abstractness than do both physical and symbolic models since they convey a mental image, not a real picture. For example, the term *nursing* has different meanings to each person. Nursing is considered an abstract concept that is included in conceptual models.

A **conceptual model** is a set of images and thought patterns that are conveyed by language. Conceptual models in nursing provide a distinctive frame of reference for the discipline based on four central concepts: person, environment, health, and nursing. These **concepts** are agreed upon as the metaparadigm of nursing; the most abstract component of the structural hierarchy of contemporary nursing knowledge (Fawcett, 1993). A metaparadigm consists of highly abstract concepts that identify the phenomena of interest to the discipline.

Most disciplines have one metaparadigm and multiple conceptual models (Fawcett, 1997). Each conceptual model provides a unique view of the metaparadigm concepts formulated from the values, experiences, philosophy, and worldview of the author of the model. Conceptual models with the greatest usefulness in community health nursing view people as being in continuous interaction with a dynamic environment. The environment may affect the health of persons or be affected by actions of persons. Environment provides the context within which community and public health nursing is practiced. The focus of care is the aggregate. The goal of care is the promotion of health and prevention of illness.

Although the terms *model* and *theory* are often used interchangeably, they differ in several ways. One main difference is in the level of abstraction. A conceptual model is a highly abstract system of global concepts and propositional statements. In contrast, a mid-range theory focuses on one or more concrete, specific concepts and statements. A second difference involves the ability to test the model or theory. A conceptual model cannot be tested directly because the concepts are not operationally defined and the relationships are not observable. On the other hand, a mid-range theory is clearly stated and operationally defined, and **hypotheses** are formulated so they can be tested through research. Conceptual models constitute a key stage in theory development by providing focus, identifying relevant concepts, and ruling out unrelated variables. Table 10-1 defines several key terms useful in understanding the language of theory.

USING CONCEPTUAL MODELS

Conceptual models that are most useful to community and public health nursing portray people as being in continuous interaction with the environment. The environment is dynamic and can be either positive or negative. The unique feature of community and public health nursing is the emphasis on assisting individuals, families, groups, and communities to maintain their highest possible level of health. To accomplish this, the community is viewed from a holistic perspective as a motivator or disrupter of health. The nursing goal is to assess, plan, implement, and evaluate ways to make the community a healthier place to live.

To some extent, everyone has developed a conceptual model because all people have assumptions and beliefs about how the world operates. Everyone has a unique set of concepts guiding how ideas and information are categorized, how situations are viewed, and how responses are selected. A person's conceptual model influences behavior either consciously or subconsciously. In particular, a model

TABLE 10-1 Key Terms to Understanding The Language of Theory

TERM	DEFINITION
Conceptual model	A set of concepts that provides a frame of reference for members of a discipline to guide their thinking, observations, and interpretations; propositions of a conceptual model are abstract and general.
Concepts	The building blocks of theory; they describe mental images of phenomena and can be concrete (chair) or abstract (fear).
Constructs	Concepts that describe phenomena that are not directly observable, such as society, intelligence, and age.
Propositions	Statements that describe the relationship between concepts (e.g., "Persons and their environment are in constant interaction").
Theory	A set of interrelated constructs (concepts), definitions, and propositions that present a systematic view of phenomena by specifying relationships among variables, with the purpose of explaining and predicting phenomena.

Based on data from Kerlinger F: *Foundations of behavioral research*, ed 4, New York, 1986, Holt, Rinehart & Winston.

directs one's worldview. The *worldview* refers to philosophical assumptions about the nature of interactions between a person and the environment. That is, a person's conceptual model determines what is considered relevant, what is eliminated, which concepts or constructs are identified, and how they are defined. For example, Neuman's worldview claims that environment is a source of stressors that can have positive and negative effects on the health of persons (Neuman, 1995). On the other hand, Rogers' (1980) worldview of person and environment regards them as irreducible wholes, changing continuously, mutually, creatively, and inseparably. Each model states unique assumptions about the worldview that it represents.

In addition to reflecting diverse worldviews, conceptual models of nursing can be classified according to their origins, such as human development, needs, interaction, or systems theory (Marriner-Tomey, 1998; Meleis, 1991). Most nursing models fall within these classifications because each suggests a way to interpret and link the four metaparadigm concepts of the discipline of nursing—person, environment, health, and nursing—according to a specific school of thought. That is, all models identify *person* as an integrated biopsychosocial being but may use different definitions. For instance, *person* may be defined as an adaptive system (Roy and Andrews, 1991), an energy field (Rogers, 1980), or a behavioral system (Johnson, 1990). *Environment* is often identified as all internal and external influences that surround persons. *Health* may be presented as a continuum from illness to wellness or a value or a dichotomy of stability versus instability. The concept of *nursing* is also defined, and nursing actions are described to represent a specific viewpoint of the model (Fawcett, 1995). A nursing model sometimes reflects more than one viewpoint; it is then classified within the most dominant category.

Many nurses use one particular nursing model to guide practice; others merge more than one model into a unique guide for their practice. Most often nurses select nursing models that are supported by theories borrowed from other disciplines, such as psychology, sociology, and the biological sciences. Nurse educators use conceptual models to guide curriculum development and research studies. Later in this chapter, examples of the Neuman Systems Model are given as a guide for an undergraduate nursing course and nursing practice.

In nursing, specific theories are used to describe, explain, and predict client manifestations of actual or potential health problems (Fawcett, 1995). A model, like a blueprint for building a house, describes the structure of how parts are related, whereas a theory moves beyond description to explain relationships among the parts and to predict outcomes. By using models in practice, nurses can identify problems from which hypotheses can be generated. These hypotheses can then be tested in practice and education to validate or refute the theory from which they are derived.

Scope and Standards of Public Health Nursing

A revised definition of *public health nursing* has been set forth by the leaders of the Quad Council of Public Health Nursing Organizations, which is made up of the American Nurses Association, Council of Community, Primary, and Long Term Care; the American Public Health Association, Section of Public Health Nursing; the Association of Community Health Nursing Educators; and the Association of State and Territorial Directors of Nursing. They define *public health nursing* as population-focused, community-oriented nursing practice. The goal of public health nursing in this definition is the prevention of disease and disability. Practice includes assessment, policy development, and assurance activities of nurses working in partnerships with nations, states, communities, organizations, groups, and individuals. Appendix E.1 provides a list of the Standards of Practice and the Standards of Professional Performance.

DID YOU KNOW? *Public health nurses provide a critical linkage between epidemiological data and clinical understanding of health and illness.*

The focus of public health nursing is on the prevention of illness and the promotion and maintenance of health. The major goal of the public health nurse, as pointed out in Chapter 1, is the preservation and improvement of the community's health. This overall objective is accomplished in two ways: direct primary care and population-focused practice.

Direct primary care

Direct primary care focuses on individuals, families, and groups within a designated community. Community health nurses work directly with clients to promote optimal health and, where health has been disrupted, to assist in restoration and stabilization of chronic conditions. The pattern of practice takes place through clinics, home health care, and group work with clients having common health needs. Practice is collaborative with other members of the health care team, is holistic in orientation, and emphasizes the evaluation of nursing care to individuals, families, and the community. Specific ways in which community health nurses provide direct primary health care include the following:

- Immunizing children and conducting well-child clinics
- Providing nursing care to clients with diseases such as tuberculosis, acquired immunodeficiency syndrome (AIDS), and sexually transmitted diseases
- Conducting primary care clinics in locations such as migrant camps, school-based clinics, work sites, shelters, and correctional facilities

Population-focused practice

The goal of population-focused practice is to enable communities to be healthy. Goal achievement requires a collaborative, interdisciplinary process of assessment, policy development, and assurance activities. An example of community assessment is evaluation of the potential health risk factors and disease indicators in a community. For example, the problem of improper waste disposal or stagnant water near a residential area would be considered a community and public health nursing problem in terms of how this environmental condition influences the morbidity and mortality of the residents. Nurses would engage in policy development to establish partnerships with other agencies to reduce the identified problem of environmental pollution (i.e., improper waste disposal or the presence of stagnant water). The nurse would advocate for the health needs of the residents and serve as a catalyst to effect change in the community.

Assurance activities refer to monitoring access to health services, determining the effectiveness of the services provided in relation to the needs of the people, and working to improve the quality of the health services continually. Population-focused practice, as opposed to direct primary care, focuses on the community as a client, and the goal is to assist communities to identify health needs, establish priorities, plan and implement actions, and identify and intervene in factors affecting the health of the community as a whole. This mode emphasizes the ongoing interaction between people and their environment in which each is affected by the other.

WHAT DO YOU THINK? *Responsibility and accountability for the provision of basic health services to the entire population must include public and private providers.*

American Public Health Association Definition of Public Health Nursing

The Public Health Nursing section of the American Public Health Association (APHA) has defined *public health nursing* as follows (APHA, 1996, p. 4): "Public health nursing is the practice of promoting and protecting the health of populations using knowledge from nursing, and social and public health sciences." Specific examples of public health nurse activities include the following:

- Participation in interdisciplinary programs that monitor, anticipate, and respond to public health problems
- Evaluation of health trends and risk factors of population groups to determine priorities for interventions
- Policy development to reduce health problems
- Assessment and evaluation of health care services
- Provision of health education, care management, and primary care to individuals and families who are members of vulnerable populations and high-risk groups

Public health nursing is a population-focused practice, and the goal is to promote healthy communities. This is the central feature that differentiates public health nursing from all other specialty areas. Promotion of population-focused practice requires a collaborative, interdisciplinary process of assessment, policy development, and assurance activities to promote healthy outcomes in a community (APHA, 1996, p. 4).

Historically, both the ANA and the APHA definitions have emphasized the blending of nursing and public health knowledge as a foundation for determining the scope of practice. They have both acknowledged that public and community health nursing efforts are directed toward all people, whether they are cared for as individuals, as part of a family, in a community, or as a community at large. Each definition emphasized a multidisciplinary role for the successful implementation of public health practice and focused on the increasing priority of health promotion. The APHA definition emphasizes primary care more than the ANA definition has done, and it emphasizes the need to determine those groups within a community that are at greatest risk for health disruption so that nursing interventions can target them to prevent the onset of disease.

Systems Models in Community and Public Health Nursing

As mentioned previously, a variety of conceptual models can be used to guide nursing actions. However, community and public health nursing as defined by both the ANA and the APHA can be logically understood from a systems perspective. Systems theory can be used to describe and explain the behaviors of individuals, groups, and communities. It emphasizes how each isolated part affects the whole and how the whole affects each part. Conceptual models based on systems theory, known as *systems models,* are especially useful in community and public health nursing. Communities, made up of multiple subsystems and groups that interface and influence each other, can be analyzed, interpreted, and understood from a systems theory perspective.

Systems models focus on organization, interaction, interdependency, and integration of parts and subparts. Systems models are based on **general systems theory** as described by von Bertalanffy (1952, p. 11), who wrote that "every organism represents a system, by which term we mean a complex of elements in mutual interaction." Concepts frequently discussed in relation to general systems theory are wholeness, organization, openness, boundary, entropy, negentropy, and equifinality. **Wholeness** refers to that condition in which a collection of parts responds as an integrated single part. The arrangement of the elements and their relationship to each other represent their **organization.**

The **openness** of a system refers to the extent to which it exchanges energy with the environment. An open system is affected by the environment (receives input) and in turn affects the environment by its output. In an open system, a continuous give-and-take relationship occurs with the environment. In contrast, in a closed system, no energy is exchanged and no interaction occurs with the environment. All living systems are open; the use of the term *closed system* actually indicates a relative expression, since at present it is impossible to demonstrate a totally closed system.

Boundary refers to a line or border that defines what elements constitute the system. In biological terms the cell membrane is a boundary encompassing the contents of a cell. In social systems the boundary is more like an imaginary line that groups certain individuals together. Thus a boundary can be physical or may be designated by roles and expectations. Simply stated, a boundary is similar to a fence around the system. Another way to view boundary is to consider it as a filter that permits the exchange of elements, information, or energy between the system and its environment. The more porous the filter, the greater the degree of interaction that is possible between the system and its environment.

Each system requires a specific form of energy to continue functioning. Entropy is a concept based on the second law of thermodynamics, which states that elements in a closed environment will proceed toward greater randomness or less order. **Entropy** is also described as disordered energy, or energy that is bound and cannot be converted to work. **Negentropy** is the energy that is "free," can be used for work, and tends toward order. Because living systems are open systems, they make use of negentropy rather than entropy. In systems theory, equifinality means that the end state of the open system is independent of the beginning state. For example, an infant born before 40 weeks' gestation may take longer to achieve developmental milestones, but eventually the child will grow into an adult.

All systems function through four processes: input, output, throughput, and feedback. **Feedback** is the process whereby the output of the system is redirected as input to the same system. The body, as a physiological system, uses feedback to regulate temperature, heart rate, and respiration. Feedback serves to regulate the system so that it remains stable.

Communities can be understood from a systems perspective in the following way. According to systems theory, the *community* is an open system that exchanges materials such as energy, goods and services, values, and ideals with the environment inside and outside the community. The community as a system has boundaries, the most obvious being geographic lines such as mountains or rivers. The imaginary boundary is one that encompasses all the subsystems in the community and identifies what is inside and outside the subsystem. Entropy can describe landfill garbage dumps, which disintegrate and the results of which may not be converted to something useful. Negentropy can describe the resources, health, wealth, and altruistic values of the people. These are sources of energy that promote well-being in the community. Equifinality indicates the community's attempt to attain or maintain balance and beauty. For example, after a storm or other natural disaster that may destroy part of the community, the members will mobilize to restore stability. Communication is the means within the community that helps subsystems relate to each other and to the entire community to keep functions in tact.

The community is a social system made up of interrelated and interdependent subsystems. The subsystems are economics, education, religion, health care, politics, welfare, law enforcement, energy, and recreation. When any one of the subsystems is affected, it affects the community as a whole. One subsystem that immediately affects the whole community is the economic system. If a major employer in the community lays off workers, the entire community, including its economic, social, educational, and health care institutions, are affected.

Systems thinking, popularized in the 1960s, remains relevant in today's world. Several nurse theorists, including Johnson (1990), King (1981), Roy and Andrews (1991), Neuman (1995), Rogers (1980), and Orem (1991), developed conceptual models of nursing based on systems theory. Table 10-2 summarizes the definitions of *person*

TABLE 10-2 Definitions of *Person, Environment, Health,* and *Nursing*

Person (Client)	Environment	Health	Nursing Goals
An adaptive can be a person or group system (Roy and Andrews, 1991, p. 28).	"The world around and within persons that is the source of stimuli: focal, contextual, residual, or groups" (Roy and Andrews, 1991, p. 39).	"A reflection of adaptation with a goal of becoming integrated whole"(Roy and Andrews, 1991, p. 20).	"Promotion of adaptation in each of four modes, thus contributing to health, quality of life, and death with dignity" (Roy and Andrews, 1991, p. 20).
"Unitary man—a four-dimensional, negentropic energy field identified by pattern and organization and manifesting characteristics and behaviors that are different from those of the parts and which cannot be predicted from knowledge of the parts" (Rogers, 1980, p. 332).	A four-dimensional, negentropic energy field identified by pattern and organization and encompassing all that is outside any given human field (Rogers, 1980, p. 332).	Health not specifically defined; however, disease and pathology are value terms (Rogers, 1980, p. 336) and since values change, phenomena perceived as disease (e.g., hyperactivity) may change over time and not be perceived as disease.	Goal of nursing is that individuals achieve their maximum health potential through maintenance and promotion of health, prevention of disease, nursing diagnosis, intervention, and rehabilitation (Rogers, 1970, p. 86).
Behavioral system (Johnson, 1990, p. 24).	Malfunctions in behavioral systems are frequently caused by sudden internal or external environmental change (Johnson, 1990, p. 26; refers to human interaction with environment).	It seems reasonable to assume that health would be considered behavior that is patterned, orderly, purposeful, predictable, and functionally efficient and effective (Johnson, 1990, p. 25).	Goal of nursing is to preserve the organization and integration of behavioral system balance and dynamic stability at the highest possible level for the individual" (Johnson, 1990, p. 29).
"A provider of self-care or one providing care to another" (Orem, 1991, p. 117).	Although not explicitly defined, speaks to the role of the nurse in providing a developmental environment that promotes personal growth (Orem, 1991, p. 14).	"The state of wholeness and integrity of developed human structures and of bodily and mental functioning" (Orem, 1991, p. 179).	"Deliberate helping service to bring about humanely desirable conditions in persons and their environments" (Orem, 1991, p. 187).
"An wholistic being composed of the interrelationship of the five variables (physiologic, psychologic, sociocultural, developmental, and spiritual) that are always present" (Neuman, 1995).	"All internal and external forces that could affect life and development" (Neuman, 1995, p. 12); "consists of the internal and external forces surrounding man at any point in time. Created environment represents an open system exchanging energy with both the internal and external environments" (Neuman, 1995, p. 31).	"Health or wellness is the condition in which all parts and subparts (variables) are in harmony with the whole of man." Disharmony "reduces the wellness state" (Neuman, 1995, p. 32). Health is equated with system stability. The wellness-illness continuum implies energy flow is continuous between client system and environment (Neuman, 1995).	"Nursing can use this model to assist individuals, families, and groups to attain, retain, and maintain a maximum of total wellness by three modes of prevention as intervention" (Neuman, 1995, p. 33).
"A social, sentient, rational, reacting, perceiving, controlling, purposeful, action-oriented, and time-oriented being (King, 1981, p. 143).	Writes about environment, but does not define it; "the internal environment of human beings transforms energy to enable them to adjust to continuous external environmental changes . . ." (King, 1981, p. 5).	"Dynamic life experiences of a human being, which implies continuous adjustment to stressors in the internal and external environment through optimum use of one's resources to achieve maximum potential for daily living" (King, 1981, p. 5).	"Nursing is perceiving, thinking, relating, judging, and acting vis-a-vis the behavior of individuals who come to a nursing situation" (King, 1981, p. 2). "Nursing is a process of human interactions between nurse and client whereby each perceives the other and the situation; and through communication, they set goals, explore means, and agree on means to achieve goals."

(client), *environment, health,* and *nursing* according to these theorists. Although all these models are applicable to community and public health nursing, the Neuman Systems Model is a particularly good fit and is discussed in detail in the next section.

NEUMAN SYSTEMS MODEL

Betty Neuman developed the Health Care Systems Model as an organizing framework for graduate students to facilitate their understanding of client needs within a holistic viewpoint (Neuman and Young, 1972). Neuman defines, describes, and links together the four concepts of nursing's metaparadigm (person, environment, health, nursing) within the model from worldviews of reciprocal interaction (Fawcett, 1995). Neuman uses the systems approach to provide organization while maintaining the potential to accommodate change in the system. Neuman believes that as nursing becomes more complex and comprehensive, a broad, flexible, expansive structure is required. Systems thinking enables nurses to focus on clients, themselves, and their surrounding environment in an interactive, creative way. The system provides an organizational structure that maintains relative stability during the process of change (Neuman, 1995).

The **Neuman Systems Model** depicts an open system in which persons and their environments are in dynamic interaction (Neuman, 1995). The client system is composed of five interacting variables: physiological, psychological, sociocultural, developmental, and spiritual. These variables have a basic core structure unique to the individual but with a range of responses common to all human beings. Client systems may be individuals, families, groups, or communities.

The model, as seen in Figure 10-1, shows the client system as concentric rings surrounding the basic core. The outer ring is a broken circle indicating an open system that exchanges energy with the environment. This ring, called the **flexible line of defense,** protects the system in a dynamic way, expanding when more protection is provided and contracting when less protection is available. The second ring, the **normal line of defense,** represents the usual wellness level of the client system. This line of defense is the result of previous system behavior and defines the stability and integrity of the system. As with the flexible line of defense, the normal line of defense is dynamic and may expand or contract when under the influence of stressors in order to maintain system stability. A series of inner circles between the normal line of defense and the basic core, known as **lines of resistance,** contain factors that support the defense lines and protect the basic structure. The lines of resistance are activated when stressors invade the system to assist the system in reconstituting. If lines of resistance are ineffective in their efforts, system energy is depleted and death of the system may occur (Neuman, 1995).

In the model, **environment** is defined as all internal and external influences surrounding and affecting the client system. The client may influence or be influenced by environmental forces, either positively or negatively, at any given point in time. The processes of input, output, and feedback between the client and environment are circular and reciprocal. Stressors occurring within and outside the client system can create instability. Thus the lines of resistance and defense are activated to defend the system in the presence of stressors. When system stability is attained, maintained, or retained, the result is a healthy system. Figure 10-1 shows stressors invading the lines of defense and classifies stressors as intrapersonal, interpersonal, or extrapersonal factors.

Optimal system stability is the best possible health state at any given time when all system variables are in balance within the client system. Variance from wellness occurs when the system gets out of balance (Neuman, 1995). For example, client system energy levels are affected by actual or potential stressors that can increase energy with positive stress (eustress) or decrease energy with distress or negative stress. High-level wellness is evidenced by abundant energy within a client system. When more energy is generated than used, the client system moves toward negentropy; conversely, when more energy is required than generated, movement is toward entropy or illness.

The major goal of nursing in the Neuman Systems Model is to keep the client system stable through accurate assessment of actual and potential stressors, followed by implementation of appropriate interventions. Three intervention modalities are suggested: 1) primary prevention strategies are implemented to strengthen the lines of defense by reducing risk factors and preventing stress, 2) secondary prevention begins after the occurrence of symptoms to strengthen the lines of resistance by establishing relevant goals and interventions to reduce the reaction, and 3) tertiary prevention can be initiated at any point after treatment when some degree of system stability has occurred. Reconstitution at this point depends on the successful mobilization of client resources to prevent further stressor reaction or regression (Neuman, 1995). Figure 10-1 depicts the three intervention strategies targeted toward the client system.

The three prevention-as-intervention modalities can be used separately or simultaneously to direct nursing actions. Within the systems perspective, all modalities lead back toward primary prevention in a circular fashion. Health promotion, therefore, becomes a specific goal for nursing action in the Neuman model. For example, before or after stressor invasion, intervention goals include education and mobilization of support resources to bolster lines of defense, reduce the effect of a stressor, and increase client resistance. Health promotion efforts support secondary and tertiary goals to promote optimal wellness.

Health promotion within the Neuman Systems Model makes the model useful in meeting the objectives of *Healthy People 2000* (USDHHS, 1992). Specifically, *Healthy People 2000* not only provides objectives to reduce the

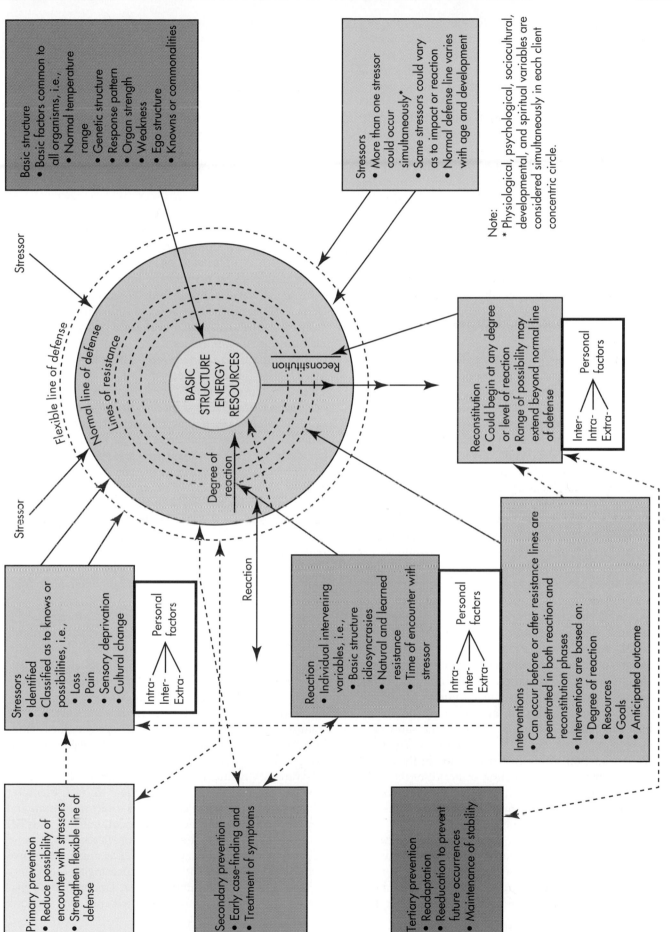

FIG. 10-1 The Neuman Systems Model. (Copyright 1970, Betty Neuman.)

prevalence of risks to health but also emphasizes the prevention of suffering and disease within a cost effective framework. Neuman's model with guidelines for primary, secondary, and tertiary interventions presents a theoretical framework for the implementation of the national goals.

Furthermore, the Neuman Systems Model has been adopted by nurses in 14 countries to guide curriculum development and nursing practice with individuals, families, and communities. Recently, several community nursing centers have adopted the model as their framework. The familiar vocabulary of the model, its systems perspective, and the integration of multiple psychosocial theories that support the model's propositions increase the usefulness of this model. The comprehensive nature of the model encourages other health care disciplines, such as physical therapy, social work, and public health, to use it. Indeed, the Neuman Systems Model facilitates a multidisciplinary approach to providing quality care at an efficient cost.

Application of the Neuman Systems Model to Communities

As mentioned previously, the Neuman Systems Model is used frequently and successfully by nurses in the United States, Canada, and some European countries. In some cases, the nurses consider clients or families within the community as the focus of care. Clients may be in their homes, at community clinics, or at other sites.

In other instances, the community itself is the client. As described in Chapter 15, the community is considered the client only when the focus of care is an aggregate population in the community. Interventions would result in healthful change that benefits the entire community.

Community-as-client goals often emphasize health promotion and health maintenance. When the community is the focus of service, the nurse and community must form a partnership to achieve mutual goals. In community partnerships the members and professionals who have vested interests in the success of the effort actively participate in collaborative decision making (Goeppinger and Shuster, 1992). Assessment, diagnoses, planning, intervention, and evaluation focus on the entire community or aggregates within it. (For more information on community as client, refer to Chapter 15.) In the Neuman Systems Model, the community is seen as a system of interfacing subsystems. Optimal functioning within and between the subsystems results in optimal functioning of the whole system. Conversely, dysfunction within or between any of the subsystems can compromise the function or health of the entire system. Stressors that affect any subsystem and create instability for the community must be assessed so that appropriate interventions can be designed to reduce these stressors and promote health. This process is interactive and collaborative between the nurses and the community.

Three types of prevention as intervention can be used. Primary prevention is appropriate to identify community risk factors and to plan mutually for health education programs with the community leaders. Health promotion and disease prevention are foci within primary prevention. Secondary prevention interventions begin when one or more normal defenses of the community have been invaded, resulting in the development of specific health problems. At this point, nurses assist the community in identifying the stressors and begin treatment to correct the problem as well as initiate interventions to strengthen the lines of resistance to prevent further dysfunction within the community system. For example a flu epidemic would require implementation of secondary intervention strategies.

Tertiary prevention, the third intervention strategy, is most appropriate within a community that has become chronically dysfunctional over time. For example, a major disaster such as a hurricane or flood (external stressor) can create multiple health problems for the community and leave it severely compromised. A community that is isolated from other areas so that sufficient food is not available to be transported is vulnerable to disease and malnutrition. Communities losing a major source of employment (e.g., coal mining, steel manufacturing) or having a high incidence of heart disease are other examples. Over time, chronic health problems develop because of these stressors and lead to poor nutrition, postponement of medical care, and depression, and ultimately a chronically ill community results. The nurse, partnering with the community, assists in readaptation and reeducation to prevent further instability within the community. The nurse also initiates primary intervention strategies to reduce the possibility of further encounters with stressors and to strengthen community lines of defense. All three types of interventions may be initiated one at a time or concurrently after the stressors have been identified and the degree of reaction has been assessed. The community and health care professionals set goals and determine resources to meet the goals.

As seen in Figure 10-1, the core or basic structure of the community as client represents the energy, resources, and basic factors common to the infrastructure of the community. These can be classified as physiological, psychosocial, sociocultural, developmental, and spiritual variables (Neuman, 1995). Table 10-3 provides a definition and example of each variable; for instance, physiological community variables are the structure (e.g., geographic boundaries, rural or urban) and functions (e.g., local government, police and fire protection) of the community. Each of the five variables is interdependent with the other variables; flexible boundaries exist between them. In fact, examples of some factors could be categorized under more than one variable, such as health beliefs (sociocultural and spiritual) or aging (developmental and physiological). The purpose of categorizing in this way is to provide a comprehensive framework for assessment, thus eliminating the possibility of overlooking any community area. Understanding that the variables are interactive and interdependent supports

TABLE 10-3 Definitions and Examples of Community Variables

VARIABLE	DEFINITION	EXAMPLES
Physiological	Structures and functions of community	• Urban, rural, suburban • Geographic boundaries/location • Water, sewage systems • Safety systems (police, fire) • Government • Transportation system
Psychological	Cognitive and affective characteristics	• Happy/depressed town • Intelligence level • Isolation vs. sensory overload
Sociocultural	Social, economic, demographic, political, recreational, and health characteristics and communication patterns among subsets	• Communication patterns • Liberal vs. conservative • Poor/middle class/affluent • Race, ethnicity • Type of industry • Day care for elderly/children • Ambulance service • Clinics/hospitals
Spiritual	Moral, religious, and value systems of community	• Churches • Health beliefs • Burial and birth practices • Adult bookstores
Developmental	History, stage, and evolution of subsystems and aggregates in community	• National registry of homes • Aging/adolescent populations • Deteriorating/emerging city

the idea of a community gestalt (wholeness) as the Neuman Systems Model proposes.

As with people, however, communities do not function optimally all the time. Stressors, either positive or negative, affect one or more parts of the community, thus affecting the whole. As systems theory indicates, a change in one subsystem or part will affect the entire system. Stressors can be defined as intracommunity (originating from within one or more subsystems or the whole), intercommunity (originating from adjacent areas), or extracommunity (imposed from structures outside the community). For example, a hazardous waste dump adjacent to an elementary school would be an intracommunity stressor, whereas racial tension between in-town residents and out-of-town residents would be an intercommunity stressor. Examples of extracommunity stressors could be new industries encroaching on farm lands surrounding the community, an interstate highway system planned through town, or decreased federal funding for community health services. Table 10-4 provides further examples of stressors within each variable of community as client.

Nurses create partnerships between subgroups within the community resources and intracommunity and extracommunity resources to help the community maintain health. Communication is the medium by which information is exchanged and plans are formulated to raise health standards. Sometimes the nurse must motivate the community to change and must provide the leadership for implementing change. The nurse begins the change process by becoming familiar with the basic structure of the community and developing a database of community variables. Assessment of the infrastructures that protect the community is paramount. For example, police and fire protection, health and illness services, and the penal system represent the lines of resistance within the community established to protect, stabilize, and maintain a steady state for the community. These are depicted as broken lines in concentric circles surrounding the core in the Neuman Systems Model (see Fig. 10-1).

Neuman's normal line of defense represents the usual range of responses developed over time that mark the unique aspects of any community. These could include the type of politics and government structure, ways of doing business to maintain a stable economy, and communication lines within and among groups and organizations. The normal line of defense could also be viewed as the usual coping behaviors the community uses to maintain balance. The normal line of defense is protected by the flexible line of defense, which acts as a buffer zone so that the normal state of community wellness is maintained. If the community is stable, the flexible line of defense can expand to provide more services for citizens, greater economic opportunities for industry, or more recreational parks within the community. On the other

TABLE 10-4 Stressors Affecting Community-as-Client Variables

PHYSICAL	PSYCHOLOGICAL	SOCIOCULTURAL	DEVELOPMENTAL	SPIRITUAL
INTRACOMMUNITY				
Increased infant mortality rate Hazardous waste dump Water supply contaminated	Insufficient health education about AIDS Increased divorce rate Potential for decreased emotional health in public housing areas	Homes crowded in downtown Park land bought by developer Decreased family income	High teen pregnancy rate Potential need for more child care centers Deteriorating inner city community	Many religious sects Health beliefs influenced by folk wisdom
INTERCOMMUNITY				
Poor roads connecting town or regional medical center Distribution of Physicians uneven	Anger between political parties Potential for isolation of elderly rural persons Inadequate communication system between rural and urban areas	Racial tension between migrants and townspeople	Historical significance of town Young vs. old Communities	Diverse value system between rural and urban sectors
EXTRACOMMUNITY				
Interstate highway system planned through town Nuclear power plant site outside town Flu epidemic Decreased state funding for services	Belief system of national political party in opposition to community's beliefs Fear of environmental contamination	Failure of industry that employs people Potential for unemployment related to industrial plant closing Influx of ethnic groups	New industry encroaching on farm land Potential for increase in young families to support new industry Potential growth in schools	New morality in opposition to community values Community selected as headquarters site for national denomination

hand, if the community experiences a minor emergency, such as a fire or disease outbreak, the flexible line of defense contracts to protect the community. The lines of resistance then mobilize to protect the infrastructure of the community.

Using the Neuman Systems Model perspective as just described, the nurse can develop a mental image of the community as client that includes variables that represent its structure and the lines of defense. A database can be established at this point that includes all the important aspects of the community. Each identified community subsystem is subsumed under one of the five variables.

The next step is to identify community stressors that affect each subsystem and to assess the degree of community or aggregate reaction to the stressors. Appropriate interventions are then targeted. For example, primary prevention might include giving immunizations, supporting positive coping strategies of a group of AIDS clients, and providing health education seminars. Secondary interventions will include early case finding followed by appropriate referrals and counseling about high-risk behaviors. Implementing treatment for an epidemic outbreak are also

secondary interventions. Assisting the community to readapt after a major epidemic or period of debilitation would constitute tertiary intervention. Common to all three models of intervention are client advocacy, coordination of health resources, and provision of information to maintain or regain system stability.

Use of the Neuman Systems Model for Community Outcomes

An example of the use of the Neuman Systems Model in community health nursing education and practice follows. Nursing faculty at Lander University in Greenwood, South Carolina have used the model as the conceptual basis for the curriculum since 1985. One project (called *TEAM MED*) provides learning opportunities in a "real world" clinical laboratory that is shared by faculty members and students who work collaboratively under the guidance of an occupational health nurse to promote health for employees of the South Carolina Department of Transportation (SCDOT). TEAM MED provides a program of health promotion, early detection, and disease prevention for SCDOT employees and is a collaborative effort between the SCDOT and universities throughout the state.* Lander University assumes responsibility for the employees (about 425) in seven counties in upstate South Carolina (Freese, Natvig, and Douglas, 1997).

The TEAM MED project, based on the Neuman Systems Model, is used in several courses in the nursing curriculum. For example, in the Wellness Nursing course, students learn primary prevention as intervention by providing flu shot clinics for SCDOT employees. Likewise in the Public Health Nursing course, students learn how to assess a community as client by working with SCDOT employees as an aggregate client. Students of the Nursing Research course learn how to develop research proposals that are based on problems identified from TEAM MED and framed within the Neuman Systems Model. Senior and registered nurse students coordinate TEAM MED assessments and follow-up for junior students working with the project in the Leadership and Management course.

Individual client in community

Through their learning activities with TEAM MED, students learn how to apply the Neuman Systems Model at both individual and community-as-client levels. At the individual level, the client is the employee of the SCDOT. The normal line of defense is the state of health of the employee that evolved over time. Students collect data on the employee's normal line of defense by assessing wellness factors in the areas of general health status, exercise habits and preferences, eating habits, alcohol and drug patterns, stress and coping, safety habits, and health maintenance habits (such as dental care).

Follow-up health care for individual employees emphasizes health promotion through primary and secondary prevention; however, services are offered at all three levels of Neuman's typology. Primary prevention as intervention includes a comprehensive risk assessment for each employee-client, with individual counseling based on his or her results. Secondary prevention as intervention includes treating symptoms (such as elevated cholesterol) appropriately and referring medical problems that require physician attention. Tertiary prevention as intervention is involved for the occasional employee who has required major medical intervention (such as coronary bypass surgery) followed by rehabilitation. Students assist with planning and implementing rehabilitation programs.

Aggregate client in community

Students also learn how to view SCDOT employees as an aggregate client, defined by the policies and employment expectations that they share as employees of the SCDOT. Based on the work of Beddome (1989, p. 569), when the Neuman Systems Model is applied to an aggregate community client, the intrasystem is the group of people who share one or more characteristics. For the TEAM MED project, the intrasystem includes an "immediate caregiving system." For TEAM MED, the intersystem includes the SCDOT occupational health nurse working in a community-university partnership with nursing faculty and students. The aggregate extrasystem includes eight interdependent subsystems: communication, transportation, health and safety, economies, education, law and politics, sociocultural, religion, and recreation (Anderson, McFarlane, and Helton, 1986). Interaction among these subsystems can affect the health of the aggregate community either positively or negatively. TEAM MED focuses on assessing and strengthening the health and safety subsystem, such as providing education on seat belt usage and safe lifting techniques.

The community client's normal line of defense is the system's state of health developed over time. For SCDOT employees as an aggregate client, data from assessment of each employee's wellness factors are compiled into an aggregate form. Then each county is analyzed and wellness factors are listed by county. These reports are used to implement projects to improve employee health and safety.

The community client's flexible line of defense is composed of programs and activities that protect the client's normal state of wellness by serving as a buffer system. The TEAM MED program is one component of the flexible line of defense for the aggregate community of SCDOT employees. Prevention-as-intervention strategies described previously (such as health assessment, teaching, and medical referrals) serve to promote client system stability as an occupational workforce.

This example illustrates a seamless process of education and practice. Students educated from a model perspective are prepared to practice in a community that is also familiar with the model's worldview. Thus the ultimate goal, positive health outcomes, can be achieved.

OMAHA SYSTEM

Nurses and administrators in community settings face urgent practice, documentation, and information management challenges (Martin and Scheet, 1992a; Westra, Martin, and Swan, 1996). The scope of community and public health nursing practice has always been complex, diverse, and independent. However, because of the magnitude and speed of current health care system changes, nurses and administrators have critical needs in three areas:

1. Timely, valid, and reliable data that describe clients' demographic characteristics, severity and acuity of their illnesses, type and location of services, and reimbursement issues
2. Timely, valid, and reliable data that quantify the clients receiving care, the services they receive, and the costs and outcomes of that care

---

* The information collected in this publication was accomplished through the efforts of TEAM MED, a collaborative program that provides a wellness program the South Carolina Department of Transportation personnel with participation from Clemson University Joseph F. Sullivan Center, School of Nursing and the Department of Public Health; University of South Carolina, College of Nursing; University of South Carolina–Spartanburg, School of Nursing; University of South Carolina–Aiken, School of Nursing.

3. Verbal and written methods for collaboration among nurses and between nurses and other professionals

According to Clark and Lang (1992, p. 27), "If we cannot name it, we cannot control it, finance it, teach it, research it or put it into public policy." Counting data must be added to naming data in Lang's statement to address urgent practice, documentation, and data management challenges.

The ANA established a Steering Committee on Data Bases in 1991 to explore interrelated concerns involving changing nursing practice, standardized nursing language, and automation. Since then, the ANA committee decided to 1) recognize five diverse classification systems that met their research, practice, and information system criteria; 2) publicize the systems and the related issues in a monograph; and 3) collaborate with the National Library of Medicine to include the systems in the Metathesaurus, a database that is available internationally (Johnson and Maas, 1999; Zielstorff et al, 1993). The five systems are the North American Nursing Diagnosis Association (NANDA), the Omaha System, the Iowa Nursing Interventions Classification, the Iowa Nursing Outcomes Classification, and the Home Health Care Classification. The NANDA consists of nursing diagnoses that have been used most frequently in acute care settings (Carroll-Johnson and Parquette, 1994). The Omaha System includes nursing diagnoses, interventions, and an outcome rating scale; it is used most frequently in community settings (Martin and Scheet, 1992a, 1992b). Because the Iowa Nursing Interventions Classification and the Iowa Nursing Outcomes Classification were designed for use with the NANDA, they are also used in many acute care settings (Johnson and Maas, 1999; McCloskey and Bulechek, 1996). The Home Health Care Classification focuses on interventions generated by home health care agencies and includes some of the NANDA nursing diagnoses (Saba et al, 1991). Table 10-5 compares the five systems. The Omaha System's Problem Classification Scheme, Intervention Scheme, and Problem Rating Scale for Outcomes are described in detail later in this section.

Definitions

Although the following concepts have been defined in various ways, their similarities involving evolution and interchangeable use are emphasized in this chapter. The concepts are nursing diagnosis and client problem; nursing intervention, action, and activity; and evaluation and outcome measurement. All concepts can be applied to different situations and populations. The concepts can be incorporated into community health programs as well as acute and long-term care programs. The concepts can apply to the client as a single individual, family, group, or community.

Nursing diagnosis is a clinical judgment about individual, family, or community responses to actual and potential health problems and life processes. It provides the basis for selection of nursing interventions to achieve outcomes for which the nurse is accountable (Carroll-Johnson, 1990).

Client problem is a matter of difficulty or concern that historically, presently, or potentially adversely affects any aspect of the client's well-being; accurate problem identification enables the professional to focus interventions (Martin and Scheet, 1992a).

Intervention describes activity that follows a thought process or written exercise, usually referred to as *planning*. It is an action or activity implemented to address a specific

TABLE 10-5 Comparison of Classification Systems

SYSTEMS AND ORIGINS	TAXONOMIC STRUCTURE AND ORGANIZATION	SETTINGS WHERE ESPECIALLY APPLICABLE
North American Nursing Diagnosis Association (NANDA) (early 1970s)	Nursing diagnoses with nine human response patterns	Hospitals, ambulatory care, nursing homes
Iowa Nursing Interventions Classification (mid-1980s)	Nursing interventions with six domains	Hospitals, ambulatory care, nursing homes
Iowa Nursing Outcomes Classification (early 1990s)	Nursing outcomes with specific indicators and measurement scales	Hospitals, ambulatory care, nursing homes
Home Health Care Classification (1987)	Some NANDA nursing diagnoses; nursing interventions with four categories	Home care
Omaha System (early 1970s)	Nursing diagnoses/client problems with four domains; interventions with four categories; rating scale with three concepts and Likert-type scale	Community, including home care, public health, schools, nursing centers, emerging health delivery settings

client problem and to improve, maintain, or restore health or prevent illness (Martin and Scheet, 1992a).

A **nursing intervention** is any treatment based upon clinical judgment and knowledge that a nurse performs to enhance client outcomes. These treatments include direct and indirect care and nurse- and/or physician-initiated and other provider initiated treatments (McCloskey and Bulechek, 1996).

Evaluation is a process designed to determine a value or amount or to compare accomplishments with some standards. Donabedian's (1966) structure, process, and outcome framework is considered classic and has provided nurses with an evaluation model. Evaluation based on client outcomes assumes that changes in client health status and behavior result from or are consequences of care. Evaluation has been defined as measurement of client progress by comparing client knowledge, behavior, and status ratings at admission, regular intervals, and dismissal (Martin and Scheet, 1992a).

Concepts of the Nursing Process

Nursing diagnosis is an essential component of the **nursing process.** Nursing diagnosis follows the data collection or assessment phase. The identification of accurate nursing diagnoses or client problems is critical to the success of nursing care. Plans and interventions, the next phases of the nursing process, reflect the art and science of nursing. Interventions should be based on research evidence. The nurse's skill in selecting and implementing optimal interventions is crucial to achieving the best possible outcomes. The final phase of the nursing process, evaluation, often receives little attention from clinicians or administrators in the practice setting. Without examining the results of care during and at the end of nursing service, accurate conclusions about the efficiency and effectiveness of care are not possible. Fortunately, heightened interest in evaluation and measurement of client outcomes is occurring because of new accreditation and federal regulations, legislation, escalating health care costs, and increasingly vocal consumers.

It is important for the nurse to recognize that the nursing process exists within a larger perspective. In addition to nursing, other disciplines that require logical, scientific thinking and systematic nomenclature also employ a problem-solving approach. The problem-solving process includes generalized information gathering, problem identification, and analysis, as well as decision making based on fact, intuition, and experiences. Physicians employ a medical diagnostic process that is similar to the nursing process and the problem-solving approach. Table 10-6 illustrates the relationship of the nursing process to the medical diagnostic and problem-solving processes.

Description of the Omaha System and Its Application to Practice

The staff and administrators of the Visiting Nurse Association (VNA) of Omaha, Nebraska began addressing **nursing practice, documentation,** and **information management** concerns as early as 1970. They began to convert their narrative method of documentation to a problem-oriented approach. At that time, no systematic nomenclature or classification of client problems existed that could be used with a problem-oriented record system. This realization provided the impetus for initiating research at the VNA of Omaha.

With the assistance of community health nursing educators, the VNA of Omaha staff conducted three research projects between 1975 and 1986 that were funded by contracts with the U.S. Department of Health and Human Services (USDHHS) Division of Nursing. The results of these projects were the Problem Classification Scheme, the Intervention Scheme, and the Problem Rating Scale for Outcomes (Martin and Scheet, 1992a, 1992b). A fourth research project was funded by a 1989-1993 grant from the National Institute of Nursing Research, National Institutes of Health. That research was designed to examine reliability, validity, and usability of the Omaha System among diverse test agencies (Martin, Leak, and Aden, 1992; Martin and Norris, 1996, in press; Martin, Scheet, and Stegman, 1993). A summary of the purpose, methods, sample size, and test sites of the article by Martin and colleagues is included in the Research Brief.

Concepts included in the nursing process and clinical judgment provide the theoretical framework for the **Omaha System.** As depicted in Figure 10-2, when the three Omaha System schemes are considered collectively, they are equivalent to the nursing process. The client as an individual, family, or community appears at the center of the model, a location that illustrates the numerous ways

---

TABLE 10-6 Relationship of Nursing Process to Problem-Solving and Medical Diagnostic Processes

NURSING PROCESS	PROBLEM-SOLVING PROCESS	MEDICAL DIAGNOSTIC PROCESS
Data collection	Information gathering	History and physical examination
Nursing diagnosis	Problem	Diagnosis
Plan	Plan	Plan
Intervention	Action	Treatment
Evaluation	Evaluation	Evaluation

RESEARCH *Brief*

A study between 1989 and 1993 was designed to provide descriptive data about the characteristics of home health clients, the services that nurses provide to those clients, and the outcomes of those services. Few similar studies have been conducted. The study examined 2403 home health clients served by four agencies in Nebraska, New Jersey, and Wisconsin. Demographic, health history, and clinical data were analyzed. The Omaha System was used as the model for describing and measuring data specific to clients' health-related problems, nursing interventions, and outcomes of care. Results of the study included the following: 1) the median age of the clients was 68.6 years; 2) nurses conducted 70% of all home visits, identified 9107 client problems, and provided more than 96,000 interventions; and 3) clients' knowledge, behavior, and status improved on problem-specific outcome subscales. These data depict important characteristics of home health clients in a large national sample and suggest that community health services do make a difference. Findings also support the usefulness of the Omaha System in describing and quantifying nursing practice in community settings.

Martin KS, Scheet NJ, Stegman MR. Home health clients: characteristics, outcomes of care, and nursing interventions, *Am J Public Health* 83(12):1730, 1993.

the Omaha System can be used and the essential partnership between the client and the clinician.

Staff from the VNA and seven test agencies located in Iowa, Delaware, Texas, Indiana, New Jersey, Wisconsin, and Nebraska participated in the research projects to develop and refine the three interrelated components of the Omaha System. An inductive approach was used throughout the research projects. Empirical data gathered by practicing community health nurses provided the basis for development and refinement. Approximately 600 nurses were directly involved in gathering data and evaluating the system.

The Omaha System is the only system developed by and for practicing community health nurses. Nurses who practice in diverse community settings need comprehensive tools to manage client data. Nurses, however, are not the only members of community-oriented health care delivery teams. The goals of the Omaha System research were 1) to develop a structured and comprehensive system that could be both understood and used by members of various disciplines and 2) to foster collaborative practice. Therefore the Omaha System was designed to guide practice decisions, sort and document pertinent client data uniformly, and provide a framework for an agency-wide, multidisciplinary clinical data management information system capable of meeting the needs of clinicians, supervisors, and administrators (Martin and Martin, 1997). Marek's research (1996) is an example of projects conducted by faculty and practitioners to extend the initial Omaha Systems research (see the Research Brief).

FIG. 10-2 Conceptualization of the family nursing process. (Modified from Martin KS, Scheet NJ: *The Omaha System: applications for community health nursing,* Philadelphia, 1992, W.B. Saunders.)

RESEARCH *Brief*

This study was designed to identify, from routinely collected health care record data, characteristics that describe home clients' health needs and to explain variation in home health care use. Retrospective data were obtained from 317 home health care client records from one home health care agency. Outcome variables of care included number of visits and hours of care. Predictor variables included nursing diagnoses, medical diagnoses, and client demographic variables. Nursing diagnoses were classified using the Omaha System. Nursing diagnoses explained a significant amount of variance over and above the demographic and medical diagnosis variables in both the number of nursing visits and hours of nursing care. The results of this study suggest that data related to nursing diagnoses are a valuable source of information when examining home health care nursing resource use.

Marek KD: Nursing diagnosis and home care nursing utilization, *Public Health Nurs* 13(3):195, 1996

When Omaha System surveys were conducted nationally, approximately 250 sites indicated that they used the system. The number of employees using the Omaha System ranged from 1 to 600 persons in a site (Martin and Scheet, 1992a). Users included nurses and members of many disciplines: home care and public health agencies, nursing centers, clinics, schools, ambulatory care centers, correctional facilities, and nursing education programs. Another first occurred in 1997 when the faculty of a major college of nursing implemented a revised curriculum based on the Omaha System (Merrill et al, 1998). Since the Omaha System books were released in 1992, the number of users has dramatically increased, but no systematic survey has been conducted to count them.

Problem Classification Scheme

The **Omaha System Problem Classification Scheme** is a client-focused taxonomy of nursing diagnoses comprised of simple and concrete terms. The language of the scheme is organized at four discrete levels of abstraction, a characteristic that increases its power. The vocabulary of each of the four levels is consistent and parallel. Because the scheme is not intended to be exhaustive, terms that are consistent with the scheme's classification rules can be added where the place-holder term "Other" appears. The levels of the scheme are 1) domains, 2) problems, 3) modifiers, and 4) signs and symptoms. The content and relationship of the domain and problem levels are depicted in Box 10-1 and are further illustrated by the case example in the Clinical Application at the end of this chapter.

The four domains define the scope of practice. These domains are 1) environmental, 2) psychosocial, 3) physiological, and 4) health-related behaviors. Understanding the meaning of and relationship among the domains is a prerequisite to implementing the scheme accurately.

The 40 client problems are the second level of the Problem Classification Scheme (excluding "Other"; see Box 10-2). These client problems or nursing diagnoses are the most critical portion of the scheme. Problems identified by the nurse are always documented in the client record.

Two sets of modifiers represent the third level of the scheme and are used in conjunction with each client problem. Modifiers selected by the nurse are 1) family or individual and 2) actual, potential, or health promotion. Using two modifiers with a problem enhances application across the health-illness continuum and adds an important degree of specificity and precision. Some nurses have expanded the "individual" and "family" modifiers to include groups and communities.

The fourth level of the Problem Classification Scheme involves a cluster of signs and symptoms specific to each problem. Clues and cues are produced as the nurse gathers, sorts, and prioritizes data. These suggest signs and

---

BOX 10-1 Domains and Problems of the Omaha System Problem Classification Scheme

I. Environmental Domain
   01. Income
   02. Sanitation
   03. Residence
   04. Neighborhood/workplace safety
   05. Other
II. Psychosocial Domain
   06. Communication with community resources
   07. Social contact
   08. Role change
   09. Interpersonal relationship
   10. Spirituality
   11. Grief
   12. Emotional stability
   13. Human sexuality
   14. Caretaking/parenting
   15. Neglected child/adult
   16. Abused child/adult
   17. Growth and development
   18. Other
III. Physiological Domain
   19. Hearing
   20. Vision
   21. Speech and language

22. Dentition
23. Cognition
24. Pain
25. Consciousness
26. Integument
27. Neuromusculoskeletal function
28. Respiration
29. Circulation
30. Digestion-hydration
31. Bowel function
32. Genitourinary function
33. Antepartum/postpartum
34. Other
IV. Health-Related Behaviors Domain
   35. Nutrition
   36. Sleep and rest patterns
   37. Physical activity
   38. Personal hygiene
   39. Substance use
   40. Family planning
   41. Health care supervision
   42. Prescribed medication regimen
   43. Technical procedure
   44. Other

BOX 10-2 Categories of the Omaha System Intervention Scheme

I. HEALTH TEACHING, GUIDANCE, AND COUNSELING

Health teaching, guidance, and counseling are nursing activities that include giving information, anticipating client problems, encouraging client action and responsibility for self-care and coping, and assisting with decision making and problem solving. The overlapping concepts occur on a continuum with the variation due to the client's self-direction capabilities.

II. TREATMENTS AND PROCEDURES

Treatments and procedures are technical nursing activities directed toward preventing signs and symptoms, identifying risk factors and early signs and symptoms, and decreasing or alleviating signs and symptoms.

III. CASE MANAGEMENT

Case management includes nursing activities of coordination, advocacy, and referral. These activities involve facilitating service delivery on behalf of the client, communicating with health and human service providers, promoting assertive client communication, and guiding the client toward use of appropriate community resources.

IV. SURVEILLANCE

Surveillance includes nursing activities of detection, measurement, critical analysis, and monitoring to indicate client status in relation to a given condition or phenomenon.

symptoms that, in turn, suggest the presence of actual client problems.

Intervention Scheme

The **Omaha System Intervention Scheme** is a systematic arrangement of nursing actions or activities designed to help nurses and other health care professionals document both plans and interventions. The scheme is intended for use with nursing diagnoses. Using the same taxonomic principles as described for the Problem Classification Scheme, the language is organized into three levels of abstraction or specificity: 1) categories, 2) targets, and 3) client-specific information. The content and relationship of the category and target levels are depicted in Box 10-2 and are further illustrated with the case example in the Clinical Application.

The four intervention categories represent the essence of community health practice. When viewed collectively, the categories describe the clinician's primary functions in relation to importance and time. The categories are 1) health teaching, counseling, and guidance, 2) treatments and procedures, 3) case management, and 4) surveillance.

The second level of the Intervention Scheme is an alphabetical listing of 62 targets (excluding "Other"; Box

10-3). *Targets* are the objects of nursing interventions. The targets are used to delineate a problem-specific intervention category by offering a more specific level of detail.

The third level of the Intervention Scheme is designed for client-specific information. Pertinent, concise words or short phrases are documented by clinicians as they develop plans or document care provided to a specific client. Although not part of the research projects, the VNA of Omaha Staff organized their suggestion into care planning guides specific to each of the 40 problems of the Problem Classification Scheme (Martin and Scheet, 1992b). Box 10-4 gives examples of problems and the signs and symptoms that help to identify the problem.

Problem Rating Scale for Outcomes

The **Omaha System Problem Rating Scale for Outcomes** is a five-point Likert-type scale that offers a systematic, recurring way of measuring client progress throughout the time of service. It was designed for use with any client problem in the Problem Classification Scheme. In addition, the scale provides both a guide for practice and a method of documentation. When establishing the initial ratings for client problems, the nurse creates an independent data baseline, capturing the condition and circumstances of the client at a specific point in time. This admission baseline is used to compare client's ratings at later intervals and at dismissal. The content and relationship of the concepts and numerical ratings are depicted in Table 10-7 and further illustrated by the case example in the Clinical Application.

The Problem Rating Scale for Outcomes comprises three summated or Likert-type ordinal scales, for knowledge, behavior, and status. *Knowledge* involves what a client knows and understands about a specific health-related problem. *Behavior* involves the client's practices, performances, and skills. *Status* involves what a client is and how the client's conditions or circumstances improve, remain stable, or deteriorate. Although the three concepts are interrelated, they represent three distinct dimensions of client outcomes. The three dimensions of the scale are equal in importance, although they may not be equally important when used with a specific client.

The ratings have characteristics of ordinal scales: 1) mutually exclusive classes or categories, 2) each continuum collectively exhaustive, and 3) categories that fit into a specific order or sequence. Each scale has a continuum of five categories or degrees for response; very positive and negative categories are located at the ends of each continuum.

COMPLEMENTARITY OF THE NEUMAN SYSTEMS MODEL AND THE OMAHA SYSTEM

Neuman and Martin foresee possibilities for nurses to use the Neuman Systems Model and Omaha System together to describe, implement, measure, and evaluate their practice. The Neuman Systems Model effectively provides the "wide umbrella" or theoretical, general framework, whereas the more specific codes of the Omaha System offer a

BOX 10-3 Second Level of the Omaha System Intervention Scheme: Targets

01. Anatomy/physiology
02. Behavior modification
03. Bladder care
04. Bonding
05. Bowel care
06. Bronchial hygiene
07. Cardiac care
08. Caretaking/parenting skills
09. Cast care
10. Communication
11. Coping skills
12. Day care/respite
13. Discipline
14. Dressing change/wound care
15. Durable medical equipment
16. Education
17. Employment
18. Environment
19. Exercises
20. Family planning
21. Feeding procedures
22. Finances
23. Food
24. Gait training
25. Growth/development
26. Homemaking
27. Housing
28. Interaction
29. Lab findings
30. Legal system
31. Medical/dental care
32. Medication action/side effects

33. Medication administration
34. Medication set-up
35. Mobility/transfers
36. Nursing care, supplementary
37. Nutrition
38. Nutritionist
39. Ostomy care
40. Other community resources
41. Personal care
42. Positioning
43. Rehabilitation
44. Relaxation/breathing techniques
45. Rest/sleep
46. Safety
47. Screening
48. Sickness/injury care
49. Signs/symptoms—mental/emotional
50. Signs/symptoms—physical
51. Skin care
52. Social work/counseling
53. Specimen collection
54. Spiritual care
55. Stimulation/nurturance
56. Stress management
57. Substance use
58. Supplies
59. Support group
60. Support system
61. Transportation
62. Wellness
63. Other

BOX 10-4 Examples of Problems, Modifiers, and Signs/Symptoms from the Omaha System Problem Classification Scheme

01. Income
    Health promotion
    Potential deficit
    Deficit
    01. Low/no income
    02. Uninsured medical expenses
    03. Inadequate money management
    04. Able to buy only necessities
    05. Difficulty buying necessities
    06. Other
33. Antepartum/postpartum
    Health promotion
    Potential impairment
    Impairment
    01. Difficulty coping with pregnancy/body changes
    02. Inappropriate exercise/rest/diet/behaviors
    03. Discomfort
    04. Complications
    05. Fears delivery procedure
    06. Difficulty breast-feeding
    07. Other
08. Role change
    Health promotion
    Potential impairment
    Impairment

01. Involuntary reversal of traditional male/female roles
02. Involuntary reversal of dependent/independent roles
03. Assumes new role
04. Loses previous role
05. Other
35. Nutrition
    Health promotion
    Potential impairment
    Impairment
    01. Weighs 10% more than average
    02. Weighs 10% less than average
    03. Lacks established standards for daily caloric/fluid intake
    04. Exceeds established standards for daily caloric/fluid intake
    05. Unbalanced diet
    06. Improper feeding schedule for age
    07. Nonadherence to prescribed diet
    08. Unexplained/progressive weight loss
    09. Hypoglycemia
    10. Hyperglycemia
    11. Other

TABLE 10-7 The Omaha System Problem Rating Scale for Outcomes

CONCEPT	1	2	3	4	5
KNOWLEDGE The ability of the client to remember and interpret information	No knowledge	Minimal knowledge	Basic knowledge	Adequate knowledge	Superior knowledge
BEHAVIOR The observable responses, actions, or activities of the client fitting the occasion or purpose	Not appropriate	Rarely appropriate	Inconsistently appropriate	Usually appropriate	Consistently appropriate
STATUS The condition of the client in relation to objective and subjective defining characteristics	Extreme signs/symptoms	Severe signs/symptoms	Moderate signs/symptoms	Minimal signs/symptoms	No signs/symptoms

method of describing the detailed level of problem identification, intervention, and outcome measurement. Used together, the two systems give the practitioner an organizing theoretical framework and a set of tools that facilitate evidence-based quality care.

Both systems are firmly grounded in a systems approach and the nursing process, which require critical thinking, correct identification of the client's perceptions, and negotiation between providers and clients. Both systems can be used to promote wellness and interdisciplinary collaboration.

In recognizing that the two systems are complementary, the authors' intent is to maintain the integrity of each system when using them in concert. Several people who have identified the compatibility and complementary features of the two systems are proceeding with pilot projects in academic and service settings to test their use together (Martin and Neuman, personal communication, 1998).

Application of the Two Systems

The following example illustrates how the Neuman Systems Model and the Omaha System Intervention Scheme were used together in planning and documenting care for senior citizens at a Community Nursing Center (CNC) in southeastern Pennsylvania. Diana Newman, associate professor at Neumann College and Coordinator of the CNC, developed a data collection instrument that organizes data according to the variables of the Neuman Systems Model and the categories of the Omaha System Intervention Scheme. The model provides the comprehensive framework that is theory based and wellness focused, whereas the Omaha System intervention scheme organizes the nursing actions according to the primary functions of clinicians. In other words, the Neuman Systems Model is the structure at an abstract level that includes all the client variables for which data is needed, and the Intervention Scheme provides both categories from which the nurse selects specific strategies for care and a problem rating scale to track client progress.

Community sites

The data collection instrument, which is a work in progress (Newman, 1998), is used by nurse clinicians and students at two CNC sites. The sites provide health promotion activities for underserved senior citizens from an apartment complex and a senior center. Usually senior clients come voluntarily to the center; however, home visits are offered to those with mobility problems and often referrals are made from local hospitals and community home care agencies. The CNC's goals are to provide community-oriented, integrated, cost effective, safe, and accessible health care. First, unmet needs of seniors are identified, then activities are provided to meet the needs. Further, data are collected for planning purposes. This CNC is a result of collaborative efforts between two nursing schools and a citizens' advisory committee and is funded by a local philanthropic organization.

Instrument description

The data collection instrument was developed to reflect the goals of the CNC to provide health promotion and preventive services to clients. Client care episodes, responses to preventive services, and the costs of these services are recorded on the instrument. The client data is

TABLE 10-8 Data Collection Instrument Sample Items

VARIABLE	DIMENSION	QUESTIONS

Physiological	Elimination	How often do you have a bowel movement?
		  a. Every day ___
		  b. More than once per day ___
		  c. Every third day ___
		  d. Less than once every third day ___

	Neurological/
	  musculoskeletal
		Perform an assessment of the client's deep tendon reflexes:
		  a. Biceps ___
		  b. Triceps ___
		  c. Knee ___
		Key: 4+ = Brisk
		      3+ = More brisk than normal
		      2+ = Normal
		      1+ = Diminished
		       0 = No response

Developmental	Housing	Please check the type of housing client lives in.
		Please add further information in the comments section.
		1. Client lives in:
		  a. An apartment ___
		  b. Own home ___
		  c. Lives with his or her family (please describe) ___
		  d. Other (please describe) ___
		2. How many rooms does the client have? ___
		3. Please check yes or no to the following statements:
		                             YES NO
		  a. Heat and ventilation are present ___ ___
		  b. Safety hazards are present ___ ___
		  c. Insect infestation is present ___ ___
		  d. Housing is clean ___ ___
		  e. Housing is well lit ___ ___
		  f. Elevator is present ___ ___
		  g. Walk up
		4. Comments:

Psychological		1. What is the client's mood? 2. Ask the client to describe his or her family structure. 3. Draw a genogram to document the family structure.
Sociocultural	Education	What is the client's level of education (please circle): 0 1 2 3 4 5 6 7 8 9 10 11 12 13 14 15 16 17 18 19 20 Grade School High School College Grad School

	Financial security	What is the client's source of financial security? (Check all that apply)
		  a. Employment ___
		  b. Retirement income ___
		  c. Public income ___
		  d. Savings ___
		  e. Family ___
		  f. Other ___

Spiritual	Religion	What is the client's religion?
		  a. Jewish ___
		  b. Protestant ___
		  c. Roman Catholic ___
		  d. Other ___

	Spiritual beliefs, support, and access	1. What are the spiritual beliefs of the client? 2. What spiritual support is available to the client? 3. How does the client access spiritual support?

BOX 10-5 Primary, Secondary, and Tertiary Preventions Within the Omaha Scheme

PRIMARY PREVENTIONS

1. Health teaching, guidance and counseling:
   a. Information given ___
   b. Anticipatory guidance ___
   c. Encouraging self-care and coping ___
   d. Assistance with decision making and problem solving ___

Specific Action Taken:

Client Response:

PRIMARY AND SECONDARY PREVENTIONS

2. Treatments and procedures:
   a. Prevention of signs and symptoms ___
   b. Identifying risk factors ___
   c. Decreasing and alleviating signs and symptoms __

Specific Action Taken:

Client Response:

PRIMARY AND TERTIARY PREVENTIONS

3. Case management:
   a. Coordination, advocacy, and referral ___

   b. Facilitate service delivery on behalf of the client by:
      1) Communicating with health and human service providers ___
      2) Promoting assertive client communication ___
      3) Guiding the client toward the use of appropriate community resources___

Specific Action Taken:

Client Response:

4. Surveillance: Please check which action(s) were taken to indicate client status in relation to a given condition or phenomenon.
   a. Detection ___
   b. Measurement ___
   c. Critical analysis ___
   d. Monitoring ___

Specific Action Taken:

Client Response:

---

used to plan individual and aggregate health promotion activities. Also, the instrument provides statistical data to help managers make informed decisions about programs and to expedite the agency billing process.

The data collection instrument is divided into 11 sections with a total of 331 items. Each section includes specific questions based on the Neuman variables and client stressors, strengths, and perceptions. Nursing diagnoses and goals lead to the interventions selected from the Omaha Scheme. A brief outline of the instrument follows:

- Background data (20 items): Demographics, sources of health care
- Health history (24 items): Diseases, surgeries, immunizations, and health behavior screening
- Variables:
  - Physiological (200 items): Divided into 11 subsections based on physiological functions
  - Developmental (33 items): Activities of daily living, functional status, safety, risk factors, housing
  - Psychological (9 items): Mood, support systems, life transitions
  - Sociocultural (6 items): Race, ethnicity, education, occupation, financial level
  - Spiritual (4 items): Religion, beliefs
- Summary: Client stressors, strengths, and perceptions
- Nursing diagnoses
- Nursing goals

- Intervention scheme
  - Health teaching (6 items)
  - Treatments and procedures (5 items)
  - Case management (7 items)
  - Surveillance (6 items).
- Follow-up visits and signatures.

Specific questions to elicit information about client health status and functional ability are shown in Table 10-8. The sample questions illustrate how the data collection instrument is organized according to Neuman variables and the subsets of information under each variable. Box 10-5 illustrates how the intervention scheme is used. Appropriate interventions are classified according to the Omaha categories and also listed as primary, secondary, or tertiary interventions. Both the Omaha categories and Neuman interventions direct nursing actions.

The process

A request for client medical information is sent out to the client's primary care provider after the client is enrolled in the CNC. This form includes authorization by the client to obtain information such as medical diagnoses, medications, diet, and activity from the primary care provider, who in turn signs and returns the form to the CNC. Client data are collected over several visits until the data collection instrument is complete. Nursing interventions are classified using the Interventions Scheme (Martin, Sheet, and Stegman, 1993) and then placed in the

TABLE 10-9 Section of Bear Family Case Using the Omaha System

DOMAIN	CLIENT DATA	PROBLEMS AND SIGN/SYMPTOMS	RATINGS*	INTERVENTIONS
Health-related behaviors	5'6", AP 170 lb, gained 30 lb Diet: high Na and canned foods. Referred to low- Na diet as punishment	35. Nutrition 01. Weighs 10% more than average 04. Exceeds established standards for daily caloric/ fluid intake 05. Unbalanced diet 07. Nonadherence to prescribed diet	K=3 B=2 S=2	I 23 III 37

*K, Knowledge; B, Behavior; S, Status. See also Table 10-7 and Boxes 10-2 to 10-5 for Omaha System.

appropriate intervention—primary, secondary, or tertiary—of the Neuman Systems Model (Neuman, 1995). The Neuman preventions are subsumed within the health teaching, guidance, and counseling section of the Omaha Intervention Scheme. The Omaha system is useful for coding primary, secondary, and tertiary preventions within the current Physician Terminology Codes (Krischner, et al, 1997) and the International Classification of Disease (Baierschmidt et al, 1996). All data are recorded in a format that is compatible with statistical computer programs such as SPSS+.

This data collection instrument demonstrates the complementary nature of the Neuman Systems Model and the Omaha Intervention Scheme. The systems approach of the Neuman Model provides the theoretical framework, whereas the Omaha Scheme provides the specific classifications for coding reportable data. Used the two systems together illustrates the components of the structural hierarchy of nursing knowledge (i.e., a conceptual-theoretical-empirical framework that is useful for practice and research). The conceptual model concepts supported by theoretical knowledge and real world indicators (Omaha System) provide the comprehensive structure that drives the nursing process, which leads to quality care and cost-effective outcomes.

clinical application

Julie Bear is a composite of many clients served by the staff of the Polk County Health Department, Balsam Lake, Wisconsin. Julie came to the County WIC Clinic for food and resource information. She was a 15-year-old Native American who lived with her family, had no source of personal income, and did not know how to obtain tribal health services. Julie was 5 months pregnant and a primipara. She had no visible edema but had proteinuria. Her blood pressure was 140/92 mm Hg. She weighed 170 pounds and had gained 30 pounds since becoming pregnant. Julie had just seen a family practice physician who diagnosed ne-

phrotic syndrome and prescribed a low-sodium, high-protein diet. Based on her diagnosis, prenatal questionnaire scores, and financial status, she qualified for WIC and the agency's public health nursing program for case management and home visits.

When the nurse, Lucy Benson, made an admission visit, she observed and heard extensive data. Based on the data, Lucy identified five problems in the Bear family, including nutrition as an problem specific to Julie.

Which approach would be most appropriate for Lucy to use as she gathered and documented pertinent nutritional data for Julie?

A. Identify Julie's eating patterns in relation to standardized assessment materials that are designed for all pregnant women and are based on the six groups of the food guide pyramid.
B. Base Julie's nutritional assessment on Lucy's own balanced diet and experience with her own problem-free pregnancy last year.
C. Use no guidelines for completing the nutritional assessment, but record all data that Julie volunteers.
D. Use the Omaha System as a tool to explore Julie's current and prepregnancy weight, eating patterns, and attitudes about food while being sensitive to her heritage, cultural values, and economic resources, as shown in Table 10-9 below.

Answer is in the back of the book.

K EY POINTS

- Models can be physical, symbolic, or mental ways of viewing real phenomena.
- Conceptual models guide members of a discipline in their thinking, observing, and interpreting.
- Community and public health nursing is population focused, and the goal is to improve the health of the community.
- Community and public health nursing practice is interdisciplinary and includes assessment, policy development, and a wide range of actions designed to promote healthy outcomes in a community.

continued

KEY POINTS—cont'd

- Systems models have particular usefulness for guiding education, practice, and research in community and public health nursing.
- The Neuman Systems Model can be effectively used to guide community and public health nursing education and practice.
- The Neuman Systems Model depicts an open system where people are in dynamic interaction with the environment in regard to physiological, psychological, sociocultural, developmental, and spiritual variables.
- The Neuman Systems Model includes primary, secondary, and tertiary intervention modalities, which make it especially useful in community health.
- The Omaha System was developed and refined through a process of research. Reliability and validity were established for the entire system.
- The Omaha System is unique in that it is the only complete system of nursing language developed inductively by and for practicing community health nurses.
- The Omaha System was designed to follow taxonomic principles. The system consists of a Problem Classification Scheme, Intervention Scheme, and Problem Rating Scale for Outcomes.
- The system includes language and codes for nursing diagnoses, nursing interventions, and client outcomes.
- The Omaha System offers benefits in three principal areas: practice, documentation, and data management. These areas are of concern to community health educators and students as well as community health clinicians and administrators.

- The Neuman Systems Model and Omaha System are complementary systems that can be used in concert while retaining the integrity of each.

critical thinking activities

1. Identify several concepts in nursing that you think are related and that guide actions. Using the concepts, try to construct a conceptual framework for your practice.
2. Debate one of these issues:
   a. Conceptual models should (should not) guide nursing practice
   b. Conceptual models help (hinder) community health nursing practice.
3. Choose a clinical experience where you have visited a family in their home, or create a fictitious family. Analyze their situation, including your nursing care plan, using the Neuman Systems Model.
4. Accompany an experienced home health, public health, or school health nurse on a home, clinic, or school visit. Observe and discuss if that nurse uses a nursing diagnosis, intervention, or outcome measurement system or framework.
5. Work with a partner or in a small group. Select a community client whom you have visited or think of a fictitious client. List typical referral and first-visit data. Independently apply the three parts of the Omaha System to the client data. Compare each portion of your selections with your partner or group members. Discuss.
6. Use the Neuman Systems Model and Omaha Intervention Scheme to prepare a data collection form.

Bibliography

American Nurses Association: *A conceptual model of community health nursing practice,* Kansas City, Mo, 1980, The Association.

American Nurses Association: *Scope and standards of public health nursing practice,* Washington, DC, 1999, the Association.

American Nurses Association: *Standards of community health nursing practice,* Kansas City, Mo, 1986, The Association.

American Public Health Association: *The definition and role of public health nursing: a statement of the public health nursing section the delivery of health care,* Washington, DC, 1996, The Association.

Anderson E, McFarlane J, Helton A: Community-as-client: a model for practice, *Nurs Outlook* 34(5):220, 1986.

Association of Community Health Nursing Educators: *Essentials of baccalaureate nursing education for entry level practice in community health nursing,* Louisville, Ky, 1990, the Association.

Baierschmidt C et al, editors: *International classification of diseases,* ed 5, Salt Lake City, 1996, Medicode.

Barnum BJS: *Nursing theory: analysis, application, evaluation,* ed 3, Philadelphia, 1994, JB Lippincott.

Beddome G: Application of the Neuman Systems Model to the assessment of community-as-client. In Neuman B, editor: *The Neuman Systems Model: application to nursing education and practice,* ed 2, East Norwalk, Conn, 1989, Appleton & Lange.

Carroll-Johnson RM: Reflections on the 9th biennial conference, *Nurs Diagnosis* 1(1):49, 1990.

Carroll-Johnson RM, Parquette M, editors: *Classification of nursing diagnoses: proceedings of the tenth conference,* Philadelphia, 1994, JB Lippincott.

Clark J, Lang N: An international classification for nursing practice, *Int Nurs Rev* 39(4):109, 1992.

Donabedian A: Evaluating the quality of medical care, *Milbank Memorial Fund Q* 44(2):166, 1966.

Fawcett J: *Analysis and evaluation of conceptual models of nursing,* ed 3, Philadelphia, 1995, Davis.

Fawcett J: *Analysis and evaluation of nursing theories,* Philadelphia, 1993, Davis.

Fawcett J: The structural hierarchy of nursing knowledge: components and their definitions. In King IM, Fawcett J, editors: *The language of theory and metatheory,* Indianapolis, Ind, 1997, Center Nursing Press.

Freese BT, Natvig D, Douglas M: *TEAM MED,* 1997 (unpublished manuscript).

Goeppinger J, Shuster GF: Community as client: using the nursing process to promote health. In Stanhope M, Lancaster J, editors: *Community health nursing,* ed 3, St Louis, 1992, Mosby.

Johnson DE: The behavioral system model for nursing. In Parker ME, editor: *Nursing theories in practice,* New York, 1990, National League for Nursing.

Johnson M, Maas M: Nursing-sensitive patient outcomes: development and importance for use in assessing health care effectiveness. In Cohen E, DeBack V, editors: *The outcomes mandate: case management in health care today.* St. Louis, 1999, Mosby.

Kerlinger FN: *Foundations of behavioral research,* ed 3, New York, 1986, Holt, Rinehart, & Winston.

King I: *A theory for nursing: systems, concepts, process,* New York, 1981, Wiley.

Krischner CG et al, editors: *Physicians current procedural terminology,* ed 4, Chicago, 1997, American Medical Association.

Marek KD: Nursing diagnosis and home care nursing utilization, *Public Health Nurs* 13(3):195, 1996.

Marriner-Tomey A, Alligood MR, editors: *Nursing theorists and their work,* ed 4, St Louis, 1998, Mosby.

Martin KS, Norris J. Psychometric analysis of the problem rating scale for outcomes, *Outcomes Manag Nurs Pract* 3(1)20, 1999.

Martin KS, Martin DL: How can the quality of nursing practice be measured? In McCloskey JC, Grace HK, editors: *Current issues in nursing,* ed 5, St Louis, 1997, Mosby.

Martin KS, Leak GK, Aden CA: The Omaha System: a research-based model for decision making, *J Nurs Adm* 22(11):47, 1992.

Martin KS, Norris J: The Omaha System: a model for describing practice, *Holist Nurs Pract* 11(1):75, 1996.

Martin KS, Scheet NJ, Stegman MR: Home health clients: characteristics, outcomes of care, and nursing interventions, *Am J Public Health* 83(12):1730, 1993.

Martin KS, Scheet NJ: *The Omaha System: applications for community health nursing,* Philadelphia, 1992a, WB Saunders.

Martin KS, Scheet NJ: *The Omaha System: a pocket guide for community health nursing,* Philadelphia, 1992b, WB Saunders.

McCloskey JC, Bulechek GM, editors: *Nursing interventions classification,* ed 2, St Louis, 1996, Mosby.

Meleis AI: *Theoretical nursing,* ed 2, Philadelphia, 1991, JB Lippincott.

Merrill AS et al: Curriculum restructuring usually the practice-based Omaha system, *Nurse Educ* 23(3):41, 1998

Neuman B: *The Neuman Systems Model: application to nursing education and practice,* ed 3, Norwalk, Conn, 1995, Appleton & Lange.

Neuman B, Young RJ: A model for teaching total person approach to patient problems, *Nurs Res* 21:264, 1972.

Newman D: *Development of an instrument based on the Neuman Systems Model and Omaha System,* 1998 (unpublished manuscript).

Orem D: *Nursing: concepts of practice,* ed 4, St Louis, 1991, Mosby.

Rogers ME: *An introduction to the theoretical basis of nursing,* Philadelphia, 1970, Davis.

Rogers ME: Nursing: a science of unitary man. In Riehl JP, Roy CS, editors: *Conceptual models for nursing practice,* New York, 1980, Appleton-Century-Crofts.

Roy C, Andrews HA: *The Roy Adaptation model,* Norwalk, Conn, 1991, Appleton-Lange.

Saba VK et al: A nursing intervention taxonomy for home health care, *Nurs Health Care* 12(6):296, 1991.

US Department of Health and Human Services: *Healthy People 2000: national health promotion and disease prevention objectives,* Washington, DC, 1992, USDHHS, Public Health Service.

von Bertalanffy L: *Problems of life: an evaluation of modern biological and scientific thought,* New York, 1952, Harper.

Westra BL, Martin KS, Swan AR: Recognizing the needs for standardized documentation and classifying patient needs, *Home Health Care Management and Practice* 8(5):24, 1996.

Zielstorff RD et al: *Next-generation nursing information systems,* Washington, DC, 1993, American Nurses Association/National League for Nursing.

CHAPTER 11

Epidemiologic Applications

ROBERT E. MCKEOWN & SALLY P. WEINRICH

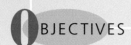 BJECTIVES

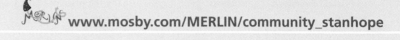 www.mosby.com/MERLIN/community_stanhope

After reading this chapter, the student should be able to do the following:

- Define *epidemiology* and describe its essential elements and approach.
- Describe the history of epidemiology and how its scope and methods have evolved.
- Discuss the elements and interactions of the epidemiologic triangle.
- Explain the relationship of the natural history of disease to the various levels of prevention and to the design and implementation of community interventions.

- Interpret basic epidemiologic measures of morbidity and mortality.
- Discuss descriptive epidemiologic parameters of person, place, and time.
- Describe the features of common epidemiologic study designs.
- Describe essential characteristics and methods of evaluating a screening program.
- Explain the most common sources of bias in epidemiologic studies.
- Evaluate epidemiologic research and apply findings to community-oriented nursing practice.

KEY TERMS

agent	descriptive epidemiology	incidence rate	risk
analytic epidemiology	determinants	levels of prevention	screening
attack rate	distribution	natural history of disease	secular trends
bias	ecologic fallacy	negative predictive value	sensitivity
case-control study	ecologic study	point epidemic	specificity
causality	environment	positive predictive value	surveillance
cohort study	epidemic	prevalence rate	validity
confounding	epidemiology	rates	web of causality
cross-sectional study	host	reliability	*See Glossary for definitions*

CHAPTER OUTLINE

The authors acknowledge the contributions of Carol Garrison to this chapter in the previous edition of this text.

What and who is an epidemiologist? The editors of the *American Journal of Public Health* raised that question in 1942 (Editorial, 1942) and elicited a wide range of responses from readers. More recent articles and editorials continue to address the nature, scope, and direction of epidemiology (Koopman, 1996; Pearce, 1996; Susser and Susser, 1996a, 1996b; Winkelstein, 1996). Even now the question may not be settled, yet since 1942, epidemiology has made major contributions to 1) understanding the factors that contribute to health and disease, 2) the development of health promotion and disease prevention measures, 3) the detection and characterization of emerging infectious agents, 4) the evaluation of health services and policies, and 5) the practice of community and public nursing.

DEFINITION AND DESCRIPTION

Epidemiology has been defined as "The study of the *distribution* and *determinants* of health-related states or events in specified populations, and the application of this study to control of health problems" (Last, 1995, p. 55). As the scope of epidemiology has broadened in the twentieth century, the definition has changed. The term originally referred to epidemics that were primarily infectious in origin. However, now it includes chronic diseases, such as cancer and cardiovascular disease, and more recently, mental health and other health-related events, such as accidents, injuries and violence, occupational and environmental exposures and their effects, and positive health states. In addition, epidemiologic methods now are used to study health-related behaviors, such as diet and physical activity (Brownson, Remington, and Davis, 1998), and they are used in health services research (Brownson and Petitti, 1998) and to investigate such things as the association between poverty and poor living conditions with increased risk of infection, chronic diseases, and violence (NCHS, 1998). Epidemiologic methods are used extensively to determine to what extent the goals of *Healthy People 2000* (USDHHS, 1991), the United States' health objectives, have been accomplished and to monitor progress toward the *Healthy People 2010* objectives.

Epidemiology investigates the **distribution** or patterns of health events in populations and the determinants that influence those patterns. Epidemiologists characterize health outcomes in terms of what, who, where, when, and why: What is the disease? Who is affected? Where are they? When do events occur? This focus of epidemiology is called **descriptive epidemiology,** which seeks to describe a disease entity according to person, place, and time. The **determinants** of health events are those factors, exposures, characteristics, behaviors, and contexts that determine (or influence) the patterns: How does it occur? Why are some affected more than others? Determinants may be individual, relational or social, communal, or environmental. This focus on investigation of causes and associations is called **analytic epidemiology,** which is directed toward understanding the etiology (or origins and causal factors) of the disease. The results of these investigations are used to guide or evaluate policies and programs that improve the health of the community.

The first step in the epidemiologic process is to define a health outcome (the case definition, usually cases of disease, but also of injuries, accidents, or even wellness). Epidemiology has played important roles in the refinement of the case definition for AIDS and in the development of precise diagnostic criteria for psychiatric disorders. Epidemiologic methods are then used to quantify the frequency of occurrence and characterize both the case group and the population from which they come (i.e., describing the distribution, or the who, where, and when) and to search for factors that explain the pattern or risk of occurrence (i.e., determinants, or why and how). These are the two foci of description and analysis described previously that constitute two major categories of epidemiology.

The World Health Organization (WHO) defines health as "a state of complete well-being, physical, social, and mental, and not merely the absence of disease or infirmity" (IOM, 1988, p. 39). The Institute of Medicine's (IOM) 1988 study *The Future of Public Health* defined the mission of public health as "the fulfillment of society's interest in assuring conditions in which people can be healthy" and noted "the substance of public health [is]: organized community efforts aimed at the prevention of disease and promotion of health" (IOM, 1988, p. 40). This definition implies establishment of public policies and programs and the delivery of specific services to individuals, but it also suggests that the policies, programs, and services go beyond a narrow biomedical model of health. Public health activity is channeled in three directions: community prevention (proactive), disease control (reactive), and personal and community health (proactive and reactive) services. The IOM report notes that epidemiology is the core science of public health, which is described as a constellation of disciplines with a common mission: optimal health for the whole community. Nursing's definition of health as "the diagnosis and treatment of human responses to actual or potential health problems" coincides well with epidemiologic principles (ANA, 1995, p. 6). This holistic approach for understanding health is particularly appropriate for community and public health nursing professionals. The concept of health employed clearly influences nursing practice (see Chapter 14).

The IOM report cautions, however, that this broad understanding of health and the role of public health professionals and agencies forces "practitioners to make difficult choices about where to focus their energies and raises the possibility that public health could be so broadly defined so as to lose distinctive meaning" (IOM, 1988, p. 40). Nurses are especially well suited to address this concern because of their holistic view of health and broad, interdisciplinary approach to intervention. For that reason, the insight and training of nurses are critical to collaboration among health professionals, including epidemiologists, in order to ensure conditions to support health.

Epidemiology builds on and draws from other disciplines and methods, including clinical medicine and laboratory sciences, social sciences, quantitative methods (especially biostatistics), and public health policy and goals, among others. Epidemiology differs from clinical medicine, which focuses on the diagnosis and treatment of disease in *individuals*. The focus of epidemiology is the study of *populations* in order to understand the determinants of health and disease in communities and to investigate and evaluate interventions to prevent disease and maintain health. Effective community and public health nursing bridges these disciplines in its focus on individual clients and services provided for them as well as on the broader context in which they live and the complex interplay of social and environmental factors that affect their well-being. This task involves using epidemiologic methods and findings in community health programs and preventive measures.

HISTORY

Some writers cite Hippocrates in the fourth century BC as an ancient precursor of epidemiology (Timmreck, 1994; Winkelstein and French, 1972). He maintained that to understand health and disease in a community one should look to geographic and climatic factors, the seasons of the year, the food and water consumed, and the habits and behaviors of the people. His approach anticipates in a general way the major categories of descriptive epidemiology: namely the distribution of health states by personal characteristics, place, and time. However, modern epidemiology only emerged within the last two centuries and developed as a discipline with a distinctive identity and method in the twentieth century (Susser, 1985).

Notable events in the history of epidemiology are listed in Table 11-1. This section highlights a few major developments. In the nineteenth century, germ theory developed with the isolation of organisms, including a number of infectious agents, induction of disease in susceptible hosts, and development of the idea of specificity in the relation of organism and outcome. These successes led to increased emphasis on the role of the agent in the genesis of disease. There is a parallel today in the emphasis on molecular studies in epidemiology. Pasteur also recognized the role of personal characteristics, such as immunity and host resistance, in explaining differential susceptibility to disease (Susser, 1973; Vandenbroucke, 1990). Furthermore, the accomplishments of the sanitary movement in reducing disease contributed to the acceptance of germ theory while emphasizing the importance of environmental influences for disease rates and variability by person, place, and time (IOM, 1988).

Two refinements in research methods in the eighteenth and nineteenth centuries were critical for the formation of epidemiologic methods: 1) use of a comparison group and 2) the development of quantitative techniques (numeric measurements or counts). One of the most famous studies using a comparison group is the pivotal mid-nineteenth century investigation of cholera by John Snow, who some call the "father of epidemiology" (Lilienfeld and Stolley, 1994; Susser, 1973; Timmreck, 1994). By mapping cases of cholera that clustered around a single public water pump in one outbreak, Snow demonstrated a connection between water supply and cholera. He later observed that cholera rates were higher among households supplied by water companies whose water intakes were downstream from the city than among households whose water came from further upstream, where it was subject to less contamination. Because in some areas households in close proximity to each other had different sources of water, differences observed in rates of cholera could not be attributed to location or economic status. Snow showed that households receiving water from the Lambeth Company, whose intake had been moved away from sewage contamination, had rates of cholera substantially lower than those supplied by Southwark and Vauxhall, a company whose intake was still in a contaminated section of the river (Table 11-2). Snow realized that his investigation was an example of what is called a "natural experiment," which added credibility to his argument that foul water was the vehicle for transmission of the agent that caused cholera.

Another of what Lilienfeld called the "threads of epidemiology" (Lilienfeld and Lilienfeld, 1980) is found in the increased emphasis on a quantitative approach. One prominent example of the use of quantitative methods to study large public health problems was Edwin Chadwick's 1842 *Report on the Sanitary Conditions of the Laboring Population of Great Britain,* in which mortality (vital statistics) and morbidity data demonstrated the association between mortality rate and environmental conditions: poor sanitation, overcrowding, and contaminated water (Chadwick, 1842). Chadwick recognized that the mortality rate was an indicator of a larger morbidity rate (i.e., the number who die from a disease is but "an indication of the much greater number" who suffer from the disease but survive) (Lilienfeld, 1984). Even today, research indicates that income distribution is an important factor in variation of mortality rates (Lynch et al, 1998).

In the twentieth century, development and application of epidemiologic methods were stimulated by changes in society brought on by such factors as the Great Depression, World War II, a rising standard of living for many but horrible poverty for others, improved nutrition, new vaccines, better sanitation, the advent of antibiotics and chemotherapies, and declines in infant and child mortality and birth rates. The result of these changes was increased longevity and a shift in the age distribution of the population, which meant an increase in age-related diseases: coronary heart disease (CHD), stroke, cancer, and senile dementia (Susser, 1985). Figure 11-1 shows the 10 leading causes of death in the United States in 1900 and in 1997 with the percentage of all deaths attributed to each.

TABLE 11-1 Significant Milestones in the History of Epidemiology

YEAR	RESPONSIBLE PERSON/ ORGANIZATION	SIGNIFICANT EVENT
1662	John Graunt	Used Bills of Mortality (forerunner of modern vital records) to study patterns of death in various populations in England. Published early form of life table analysis.
1747	James Lind	Studied scurvy using observation and comparison of response to various dietary treatments (early precursor of clinical trial).
1760	Daniel Bernoulli	Used life table technique to demonstrate that smallpox innoculation conferred life-long immunity.
1775	Percival Pott	First "cancer epidemiologist." Noted that a high proportion of patients presenting with cancer of the scrotum were chimney sweeps. Inferred that exposure to soot was the cause. (Lack of a comparison group would reduce validity of inference by today's standards.)
1798	Edward Jenner	Demonstrated effectiveness of smallpox vaccination.
1798	Marine Hospital Service	Forerunner of U.S. Public Health Service (1912)
1836	Pierre Charles- Alexandre Louis	Comparative observational studies to demonstrate ineffectiveness of bloodletting. Emphasized the importance of statistical methods ("la méthode numerique"). Influenced many of the pioneers in epidemiology in England and the United States.
1836		Establishment of Registrar-General's Office in England as registry for births, deaths, and marriages.
1840s	William Farr	Developed forerunner of modern vital records system in Registrar-General's Office. Study of mortality in Liverpool led to significant public health reform. Pioneered mortality surveillance and anticipated many of the basic concepts in epidemiology. His data provided much of the basis for Snow's work on cholera
1850		Founding of London Epidemiological Society. Known for influential reports on smallpox vaccination and studies of cholera.
1850	Lemuel Shattuck	Reported on sanitation and public health in Massachusetts
1850s	John Snow	Epidemiologic research on transmission of cholera. Used mapping and natural experiment, comparing rates in groups exposed to different water supplies.
1870-1880s	Robert Koch	Discovered causal agents for anthrax, tuberculosis, and cholera; development of causal criteria.
1887	Joseph Kinyuon	Founded "Laboratory of Hygiene," forerunner of the National Institute of Health (1930).
1921	Wade Hampton Frost	Founded first U.S. academic program in epidemiology at Johns Hopkins University.
1942		Office of Malarial Control in War Areas established; became Communicable Disease Center (CDC) in 1946; then Centers for Disease Control (1973); now Centers for Disease Control and Prevention.
1948		Framingham cohort study of cardiovascular disease begins.
1950s	A. Bradford Hill and Richard Doll	Pioneering studies on smoking and lung cancer.

From IOM: *The future of public health*, Washington, DC, 1988, National Academy Press; Lilienfeld DE, Stolley PD: *Foundations of epidemiology*, ed 3, New York, 1994, Oxford University Press; USDHHS: *Public health service fact sheet*, Washington, DC, 1984, USDHHS, Public Health Service; Susser M: Epidemiology in the United States after World War II: the evolution of technique, *Epidemiol Rev* 7:147, 1985; Timmreck TC: *An introduction to epidemiology*, Boston, 1994, Jones & Bartlett.

TABLE 11-2 Household Cholera Death Rates by Source of Water Supply in John Snow's 1853 Investigation

COMPANY	NUMBER OF HOUSES	DEATHS FROM CHOLERA	DEATHS PER 10,000 HOUSEHOLDS
Southwark and Vauxhall	40,046	1263	315
Lambeth	26,107	98	37
Rest of London	256,423	1422	59

From Snow J: On the mode of communication of cholera. In *Snow on cholera*, New York, 1855, The Commonwealth Fund.

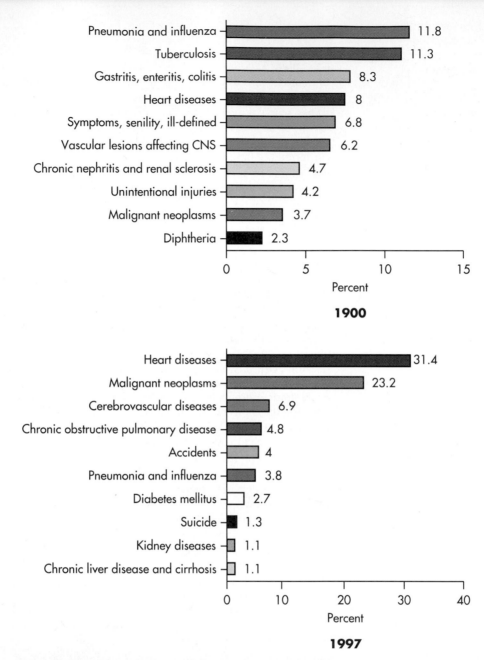

FIG. 11-1 Ten leading causes of death as a percentage of all deaths, United States, 1900 and 1997. (Data from Brownson et al: *Chronic disease epidemiology and control*, Washington, DC, 1993, American Public Health Association; Ventura SJ et al: Births and deaths: preliminary data for 1997, *National Vital Statistics Reports* 47(4):1998.)

There was an associated shift from looking for single agents, such as the infectious agent that causes cholera, to seeking multifactorial etiology (i.e., many factors or combinations of factors contributing to disease, such as the complex of factors that cause cardiovascular disease). The possibility that behavioral and environmental causes existed for many conditions formerly thought to be degenerative diseases of aging raised the possibility of prevention or delay of onset (Susser, 1985). In addition, the development of genetic and molecular techniques (such as genetic

markers for increased risk of breast cancer and sophisticated tests for antibodies to infectious agents or for other biologic markers of exposures to environmental toxins, such as lead or pesticides) have markedly increased the epidemiologist's ability to classify persons in terms of exposures or inherent susceptibility to disease. These two expansions of epidemiologic investigation—upward toward consideration of broader environmental contexts and community level factors (termed *eco-epidemiology* by some; Susser and Susser, 1996a, 1996b) and downward to the

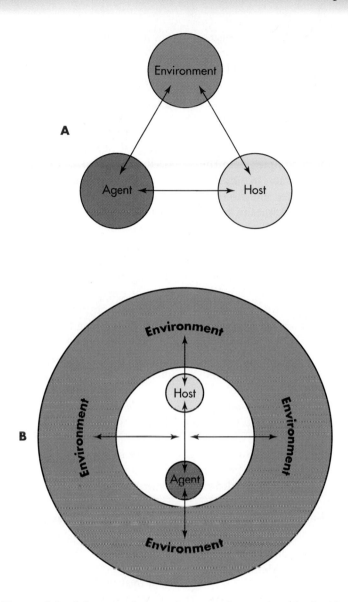

FIG. 11-2 Two models of the agent-host-environment interaction (the "epidemiologic triangle").

molecular and genetic levels—have prompted some to call for a renewed look at both epidemiologic theory (Krieger, 1994; Krieger and Zierler, 1995) and methods incorporating multilevel analysis (Diez-Roux, 1998) in epidemiologic investigations. These developments are of particular interest to nurses who are in contact with people in their living and work environments and understand the role of those environments (even beyond chemical or biologic exposures) to their well-being. Further, nurses in the community are able to assess a broad range of health outcomes as well as factors that contribute to wellness and illness.

In recent years, new infectious diseases, such as Lyme disease, Legionnaire's disease, and HIV/AIDS, and new forms of old diseases, such as resistant strains of tuberculosis (TB), have emphasized the importance of infectious disease epidemiology. As noted previously, epidemiologic

methods also have been applied to a broader spectrum of health-related outcomes, including accidents, injuries and violence, occupational and environmental exposures, psychiatric and sociologic phenomena, health-related behaviors, and health services research. This demonstrates again the collaborative and multidisciplinary nature of epidemiologic investigations (Susser, 1985).

BASIC CONCEPTS IN EPIDEMIOLOGY
Epidemiologic Triangle: Agent, Host, and Environment

Epidemiologists understand that disease results from complex relations among causal agents, susceptible persons, and environmental factors. These three elements—**agent, host,** and **environment**—are called the *epidemiologic triangle* (Fig. 11-2, *A*). Changes in one of the elements of the triangle can influence the occurrence of disease by increasing or decreasing a person's risk for disease. Risk is understood as the probability that an individual will become ill (Last, 1995). As Figure 11-2, *B* suggests, both agent and host, as well as their interaction, are influenced by the environmental context in which they exist while they may influence the environment itself. Some examples of these three components are listed in Box 11-1.

Causal relationships are often more complex than the epidemiologic triangle conveys. It is common to speak of a **web of causality,** recognizing the complex interrelationships of numerous factors interacting, sometimes in subtle ways, to increase (or decrease) risk of disease. Furthermore, associations are sometimes mutual with lines of causality going in both directions.

A common example of complex factors in a causal web is depicted for cardiovascular disease in Figure 11-3. Fortunately, effective interventions to disrupt causal pathways and prevent disease are often possible without a complete understanding of all causal elements in their interrelations. Some authors use the term *black box epidemiology* to refer to research of associations without understanding how factors and outcomes are related (Susser, 1996a, 1996b). Recently some researchers have advocated a new paradigm that goes beyond the two-dimensional causal web to consider multiple levels of factors that affect health and disease (Diez-Roux, 1998; Krieger, 1994). This approach expands epidemiologic studies both upward to broader contexts (such as neighborhood characteristics) and downward to the genetic and molecular level. This multilevel analytic approach should provide insight into the myster-

ies inside the "black box" even if public health practitioners continue to apply successful interventions in the absence of clear understanding of underlying processes and relationships. The determination of what is successful will often also rely on epidemiologic studies.

Stages of Health and Intervention

The goal of epidemiology is to understand causal factors well enough to devise interventions to prevent adverse events before they start (prevent initiation of the disease process or prevent injury). Public health professionals speak of three levels of prevention tied to specific stages in the **natural history of disease.** The natural history of disease is the course of the disease process from onset to resolution (Last, 1995). Table 11-3 illustrates the relationship among the stages of disease and **levels of prevention.** Nurses can play a leading role in understanding and implementing primary and secondary preventive measures and in supplying tertiary prevention services.

Primary prevention

Primary prevention involves interventions that promote health and prevent disease processes from developing. These activities are aimed at individuals who are susceptible to disease but have no discernible pathology (prepathogenesis). Diet and exercise are examples of primary prevention for cardiovascular disease. Nurses are key players in primary prevention programs, such as immunizations, provision of and training in the use of barrier contraceptives, and health education in areas such as diet and physical activity and parenting.

Secondary prevention

Secondary prevention aims to detect disease in the early stages (early pathogenesis) before clinical signs and symptoms manifest in order to intervene with early diagnosis and treatment. The goal is to reverse or reduce the severity of the disease or provide a cure. Early stages of cardiovascular disease may be detected by treadmill stress tests or screening for hypertension. Screening programs, such as blood pressure checks or Pap smears to detect cervical dysplasia, are often used to detect early disease in symptom-free persons. Family counseling might be viewed as another form of secondary prevention, designed to intervene before problems become serious. Because of the important role that nurses play in secondary prevention, a more detailed discussion of screening programs is presented later in the chapter.

Tertiary prevention

Tertiary prevention is directed toward persons with clinically apparent disease. The aim is to ameliorate the course of disease, reduce disability, or rehabilitate. Persons with diagnosed heart disease may undergo coronary artery bypass surgery or enter cardiac rehabilitation programs. Other examples include treatment of clients with TB, the use of physical therapy to prevent contractures in clients with stroke or head or spinal cord injuries, or rehabilitation of an injured worker to return to work. Rehabilitative

---

BOX 11-1 Examples of Agent, Host, and Environmental Factors in the Epidemiologic Triangle

AGENT
Infectious agents (bacteria, viruses, fungi, parasites)
Chemical agents (heavy metals, toxic chemicals, pesticides)
Physical agents (radiation, heat, cold, machinery)

HOST
Genetic susceptibility
Immutable characteristics (age and gender)
Acquired characteristics (immunologic status)
Lifestyle factors (diet and exercise)

ENVIRONMENT
Climate (temperature, rainfall)
Plant and animal life (agents or reservoirs or habitats for agents)
Human population distribution (crowding, social support)
Socioeconomic factors (education, resources, access to care)
Working conditions (levels of stress, noise, satisfaction)

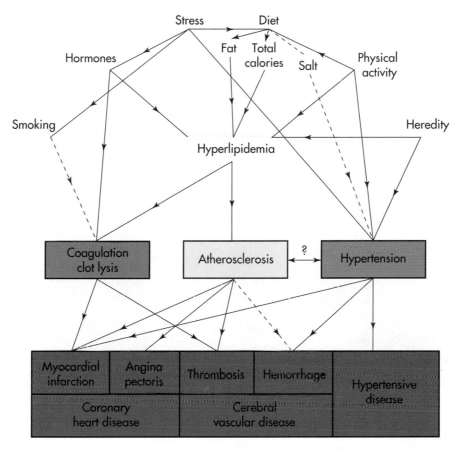

FIG. 11-3 An example of a web of causality for cardiovascular disease. (From Stallones RA: *Cerebrovascular disease epidemiology: a workshop,* Public Health Monograph No 76, Pub No 1441, Washington, DC, 1966, US Public Health Service.)

TABLE 11-3 Relationship of the Stages of Disease to Levels of Prevention

STAGE OF DISEASE PROCESS			
Pre-pathogenesis ↓ Susceptibility	Pathogenesis ↓ Preclinical	↓ Clinical	Resolution ↓ Death, disability, recovery
LEVEL OF PREVENTION			
Primary prevention	Secondary prevention		Tertiary prevention
EXAMPLES OF INTERVENTION RELATED TO CARDIOVASCULAR DISEASE			
Diet and exercise	Blood pressure and cholesterol screening, treadmill stress test		Cardiac rehabilitation, medication, surgery
OTHER EXAMPLES OF INTERVENTIONS			
Immunization, water treatment	Pap smear, screening for HIV		Physical therapy, surgery, medical treatment

job training with counseling for juvenile offenders is another form of tertiary prevention. Nurses often play a critical role in monitoring compliance and in providing services that contribute to recovery or enhanced quality of life for persons affected by disease or injury.

Primary, secondary, and tertiary prevention have been the standard classification of preventive measures in public health. More recently there has been a reformulation that reflects the target population for preventive interventions (Fig 11-4). The IOM publication on pre-

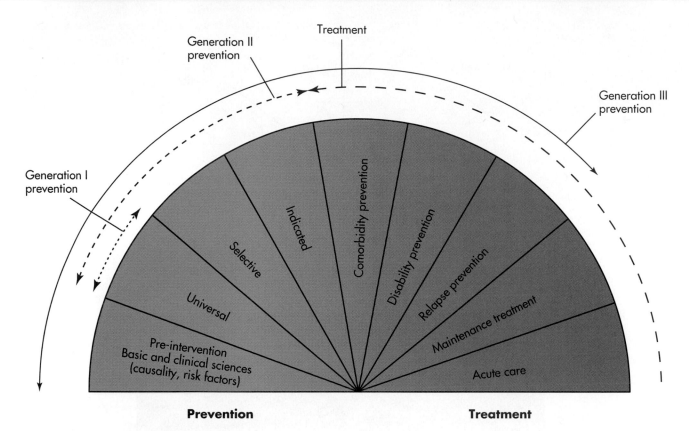

FIG. 11-4 Health intervention spectrum. (From National Institute of Mental Health: *Priorities for prevention research at NIMH: a report by the National Advisory Health Council Workgroup on Mental Disorders Prevention Research,* Pub No. 98-4321, Washington, DC, 1998, NIH.)

vention research in mental disorders (Mrazek and Haggerty, 1994) classifies intervention as *universal* when it is directed to the general population and provides general benefit with little risk at low cost; *selective* when it is directed toward persons or groups who are at increased risk for developing a problem, with risk and harms justified on the basis of the potential reduction in adverse outcomes; and *indicated* when more costly and higher-risk interventions target high-risk persons who already evidence a problem. This report reserves the term *prevention* only for those interventions that occur before onset of disorder. Treatment interventions involve two components: *case identification* and *standard treatment for known disorders.* Finally, the components of maintenance in continuing disorder are *compliance with long-term treatment* and *provision of after-care services, including rehabilitation.* Clearly these categories can be applied to other health outcomes. For example, nurses are often involved in various preventive interventions directed toward reducing the incidence of TB. They also participate in programs for identification of cases and initiation of standard therapy. Given the emergence of new drug-resistant strains of TB, nurses design and implement programs to increase long-term compliance and provide after-care for identified clients.

BASIC METHODS IN EPIDEMIOLOGY
Sources of Data

One of the first issues to address in any epidemiologic study is how the data will be obtained (Kelsey et al, 1996). There are three major categories of data sources commonly used in epidemiologic investigations:

1. Routinely collected data, such as census data, vital records (birth and death certificates), and surveillance data (systematic collection of data concerning disease occurrence) as carried out by the Centers for Disease Control and Prevention (CDC)
2. Data collected for other purposes but useful for epidemiologic research, such as medical, health department, and insurance records
3. Original data collected for specific epidemiologic studies

Routinely collected data
The United States census is conducted every 10 years and provides population data, including demographic distribution (age, race, sex), geographic distribution, and additional information about economic status, housing, and education. These data provide denominators for various rates.

Vital records are the primary source of birth and mortality statistics. Although registration of births and deaths is mandated in most countries, providing one of the most complete sources of health-related data, the quality of specific information varies. For example, on birth certificates, sex and date of birth are fairly reliable, whereas gestational age, level of prenatal care, or smoking habits of the mother during pregnancy are less reliable. On death certificates, the quality of the cause of death information varies over time and from place to place, depending on diagnostic capabilities and custom. Vital records are readily available in most areas; they are inexpensive, convenient, and allow study of long-term trends. Mortality data, however, are only informative for fatal diseases.

Data collected for other purposes

Hospital, physician, health department, and insurance records provide information on morbidity, as do **surveillance** systems, such as cancer registries and health department reporting systems, which solicit reports of all cases of a particular disease within a geographic region. Other information, such as occupational exposures, may be available from employer records.

Epidemiologic data

The National Center for Health Statistics sponsors periodic health surveys and examinations in carefully drawn samples of the U.S. population. These surveys provide information on the health status and behaviors of the population. For many studies, however, the only means of obtaining the needed information is to collect the required data in a study specifically designed to investigate a particular question. The design of such studies is discussed in the next section.

Measures of Morbidity and Mortality Rates

Rates in epidemiology

Epidemiologic studies usually rely on **rates,** a measure of the frequency of a health event in a defined population during a specified period of time (Last, 1995). Epidemiology focuses on the distribution of health events. Because people differ in their probability or risk of disease, the primary concern is how they differ. Mapping cases of a disease in an area, as John Snow mapped cases of cholera in one area of London and as many epidemiologists now map various health-related events, can be instructive, especially if other factors, such as industrial development, show similar patterns. However, mapping cases is limited in what it can reveal. A higher number of cases may simply be the result of a larger population with more people who are potential cases. Any description of disease patterns should take into account the size of the population at risk for the disease (i.e., look not only at the numerator, the number of cases, but also at the denominator, the number of people in the population at risk). For example, 50 cases of influenza might be viewed as a serious epidemic in a population of 250 but would indicate a rather low rate in a population of 250,000. Using rates instead of simple counts of cases takes the size of the population at risk into account.

An **epidemic** occurs when the rate of disease, injury, or other condition is clearly in excess of the usual (endemic) level of that condition. There is no specific threshold of incidence that indicates an epidemic exists. Because smallpox has been eradicated, any occurrence of smallpox might be considered an epidemic by this definition. In contrast, given the high rates of ischemic heart disease in the United States, an increase of many cases would be needed before an epidemic was noted, although some might argue that the very high rates that exist compared with earlier periods already indicate an epidemic.

Risk

Risk refers to the probability that an event will occur within a specified time period, and a population at risk is the population of persons for whom there is some finite probability (even if small) of that event. For example, although the risk of breast cancer in men is small, a few men do develop breast cancer and therefore could be considered part of the population at risk. There are some outcomes for which certain people would never be at risk (e.g., men cannot be at risk of ovarian cancer, nor can women be at risk of testicular cancer). A high-risk population, on the other hand, would include those persons who, because of exposure, lifestyle, family history, or other factors, are at greater risk for disease than the population at large. For example, as far as is known, all persons are susceptible to HIV infection. Therefore everyone is in the population at risk for HIV and AIDS. Persons who have multiple sexual partners without adequate protection or who use IV drugs are in the high-risk population for HIV infection.

> **WHAT DO YOU THINK?** *Genetic testing is becoming more common, but most tests for disease indicate only susceptibility to disease, not certainty. Similarly, screening tests are never perfect, so there is always some probability of misclassifying a person. How should these difficult concepts of probability and uncertainty be presented to clients when interpreting test results?*

Mortality rates

There are a number of mortality rates with which the student should be familiar (Table 11-4). Note that many commonly used mortality rates are not true rates but proportions (Gordis, 1996). Although measures of mortality reflect serious health problems and changing patterns of disease, they are limited in their usefulness. They are only informative for fatal diseases and do not provide direct information about either the level of existing disease in the population or the risk of getting any particular disease. Furthermore, it is not uncommon for a person who has one disease (e.g., prostate cancer) to die from a different cause (e.g., stroke).

Because the population changes during the course of a year, it is useful to take an estimate of the population at midyear as the denominator for annual rates. The *crude annual mortality rate* is an estimate of the risk of death for a person in a given population for that year. These rates are multiplied by a scaling factor, usually 100,000, to avoid small fractions. The result is then expressed as the number

TABLE 11-4 Common Mortality Rates

RATE/RATIO	RATE PROPORTION/EQUATION
Crude mortality rate	Usually an annual rate that represents the proportion of a population who die from any cause during the period. **Example:** In 1991 there were 2,169,518 deaths in a total population of 252,177,000.
Age-specific rate	$\dfrac{\text{Number of deaths among persons of given age group}}{\text{Midyear population of that age group}}$ **Example:** 1991 age-specific rate for 15 to 24 year olds: $\dfrac{36,452}{36,399,000} = 100.1$ deaths per 100,000 15 to 24 year olds
Cause-specific rate	$\dfrac{\text{Number of deaths from a specific cause}}{\text{Midyear population}}$ **Example:** 1991 cause-specific rate for HIV: $\dfrac{29,555 \text{ HIV deaths}}{252,177,000} = 11.7$ per 100,000
Case-fatality rate	$\dfrac{\text{Number of deaths from a specific disease in a given period}}{\text{Number of persons diagnosed with that disease}}$ **Example:** If 87 of every 100 persons diagnosed with lung cancer dies within 5 years, the 5-year case fatality rate is 87%. The 5-year survival rate is 13%.
Proportionate mortality ratio	$\dfrac{\text{Number of deaths from a specific disease}}{\text{Total number of deaths in the same period}}$ **Example:** In 1991 there were 720,862 deaths from diseases of the heart out of 2,169,518 deaths from all causes. $\dfrac{720,862}{2,169,518} = 0.332$, or 33.2%, of all deaths were due to heart disease
Infant mortality rate	$\dfrac{\text{Number of infant deaths under 1 year of age in a year}}{\text{Number of live births in the same year}}$ **Example:** In 1991 there were 36,766 deaths under 1 year of age and 4,110,907 live births: $\dfrac{36,776}{4,110,907} = 0.0089$, or 8.9 deaths per 1000 live births
Neonatal mortality rate	$\dfrac{\text{Number of infant deaths under 28 days of age in a year}}{\text{Number of live births in the same year}}$ **Example:** In 1991 there were 22,978 neonatal deaths and 4,110,907 live births: $\dfrac{22,978}{4,110.907} = 5.59$ per 1000
Postneonatal mortality rate	$\dfrac{\text{Number of infant deaths from 28 days to 1 year in a year}}{\text{Number of live births in the same year}}$ **Example:** In 1991 there were 13,788 postneonatal deaths and 4,110,907 live births: $\dfrac{13,788}{4,110,907} = 3.35$ per 1000

From National Center for Health Statistics (NCHS): *Health, United States, 1998*, Hyattsville, Md, 1998, Public Health Service.

of deaths per 100,000 persons. Although a crude mortality rate is calculated easily and represents the actual death rate for the total population, it has certain limitations. It does not reveal specific causes of death, which change in relative importance over time. Also, it is affected by the age distribution of the population because older people are at much greater risk of death than younger people.

Mortality rates also are calculated for specific groups (e.g., age-, sex-, or race-specific rates). In these instances, the number of deaths occurring in the specified group is divided by the population at risk, now restricted to the number of persons in that group. This rate may be interpreted as the risk of death for persons in the specified group during the period of observation.

The *cause-specific mortality rate* is an estimate of the risk of death from some specific disease in a population. It is the number of deaths from a specific cause divided by the total population at risk, usually multiplied by 100,000. Two related measures should be distinguished from the cause-specific mortality rate. The *case fatality rate* (CFR) is the proportion of persons diagnosed with a particular disorder (i.e., cases) who die within a specified period of time. The CFR may be interpreted as an estimate of the risk of death within that period for a person newly diagnosed with the disease (e.g., the proportion of persons with breast cancer who die within 5 years). Since the CFR is the proportion of diagnosed persons who die within the period, 1 minus the CFR yields the survival rate. For example, if the 5-year CFR for lung cancer is 86%, then the 5-year survival rate is only 14% (Brownson et al, 1998). Persons diagnosed with a particular disease often want to know the probability of surviving. These rates provide that information.

The second measure to be distinguished from the cause-specific mortality rate is the *proportionate mortality ratio* (PMR), the proportion of all deaths that are due to a specific cause. The denominator is not the population at risk of death but the total number of deaths in the population; therefore, the PMR is not a rate, nor does it estimate the risk of death. The magnitude of the PMR is a function of both the number of deaths from the cause of interest and the number of deaths from other causes. If deaths from certain causes decline over time, deaths from other causes that remain fairly constant may have increasing PMRs. For example, motor vehicle accidents accounted for 5.2 deaths per 100,000 persons 5 to 14 years of age in the United States in 1996. This was 24% of all deaths in this age group (the PMR). By comparison, motor vehicle accidents caused 23.0 deaths per 100,000 persons 65 years of age and older in 1996, which was less than 0.5% of all deaths in the older age group (Peters et al, 1998). This demonstrates that, although the *risk* of death from a motor vehicle accident was over four times as great in the older group (based on the rates), such accidents accounted for a far greater proportion of all deaths in the younger group (based on the PMR). The reason has to do with the much greater risk of death from other causes in the older group.

Health professionals also are interested in measures of infant mortality which are used around the world as an indicator of overall health and availability of health care services. The most common measure, the *infant mortality rate,* is the number of deaths to infants in the first year of life divided by the total number of live births. Because the risk of death declines rather dramatically during the first year of life, *neonatal* and *postneonatal mortality rates* are also of interest.

Rate adjustment

Although rates are of central importance in epidemiologic studies, rates can be misleading when compared across different populations. For example, the risk of death increases rather dramatically after 40 years of age, so a higher crude death rate is expected in a population of older people compared with a population of younger people (Gordis, 1996). Comparing the overall mortality rate in an area with a large elderly population to the rate in a younger population would be misleading. Methods that adjust for differences in populations can be used to compare death rates. Age adjustment is based on the assumption that a population's overall mortality rate is a function of the age distribution of the population and the age-specific mortality rates.

Age adjustment can be performed by direct or indirect methods. Both methods require a "standard population," which can be an external population, such as the U.S. population for a given year; a combined population of the groups under study; or some other standard chosen for relevance or convenience.

A *direct* adjusted rate applies the age-specific death rates from the study population to the age distribution of the standard population. The result is the (hypothetical) death rate of the study population if it had the same age distribution as the standard population.

The *indirect* method, as the name suggests, is more complicated. The age-specific death rates of the standard population applied to the study population's age distribution produce an index rate that is used with the crude rates of both the study and standard populations to produce the final indirect adjusted rate, which is also hypothetical. The indirect method may be required when the age-specific death rates for the study population are unknown or unstable (i.e., based on relatively small numbers).

Often, instead of an indirect adjusted rate, a standardized mortality ratio (or SMR) is calculated. This is the number of observed deaths in the study population divided by the expected number of deaths, based on the age-specific rates in the standard population and the age distribution of the study population (Gordis, 1996).

Although this discussion has focused on age-adjustment, the process can be used to adjust for any factor that might vary from one population to another. For example, to compare infant mortality rates across populations with differing birth-weight distributions, these methods may be used to produce birth-weight-adjusted infant mortality rates. Note that all adjusted rates are fictitious rates. They may resemble crude rates if the distribution of the study sample is similar to the distribution of the standard population. The magnitude of adjusted rates is dependent on the standard population used. The choice of a different standard would produce a different adjusted rate.

Measures of morbidity

Prevalence rate. Epidemiologists and other health professionals are interested in measures of morbidity, especially prevalence and incidence rates, which provide information concerning the levels of disease in a population, the rate of disease development, and the risk of disease. The **prevalence rate** is a measure of existing disease in a population at a particular time (i.e., the number of existing cases divided by the current population). One also can calculate the prevalence of a specific risk factor or exposure. For example, a health department and community hospital might jointly institute an intensive, broad-based screening program in an area characterized by over-crowded housing, limited access to services, and under-use of preventive health practices. Their program includes physical examinations; tuberculin skin tests followed up by chest x-ray examinations where indicated; cardiovascular, glaucoma, and diabetes screening; and mammography for women and prostate screening for men over 45 years of age. Of the 8000 women screened, 35 had previously been diagnosed with breast cancer, and 20 who had no history of breast cancer were later found to have cancer of the breast. The prevalence of breast cancer in this population of women would be as follows:

$$\frac{55}{8000} = 0.006875, \text{ or } 687.5 \text{ per } 100,000$$

A prevalence rate is not an estimate of the risk of *developing* disease because it is a function of both the rate at which new cases of the disease develop and how long those cases remain in the population. In this example, the prevalence of breast cancer in this population of women is a function of how many new cases develop and how long women live with the cancer. The duration of a disease is affected by case fatality and cure. (For simplicity, in this example, women with a history of the disease are counted in the prevalence rate even though they may have been cured.) A disease with a short duration (e.g., an intestinal virus) may not have a high prevalence rate even if the rate of new cases is high, because cases do not accumulate (see Point Epidemic section in this chapter.) A disease with a long course will have a higher prevalence rate than a rapidly fatal disease that has the same rate of new cases.

Incidence rate. The **incidence rate** reflects the number of *new* cases developing in a population at risk during a specified time. A cumulative incidence rate estimates the risk of developing the disease in that population during that time. The population at risk is considered to be persons without the disease but who are at risk of acquiring it. Note that existing (or prevalent) cases are excluded from the population at risk for this calculation, since they al-

ready have the condition and are no longer at risk of developing it. Incidence counts new cases in a disease-free group (or cohort) of persons who are followed for some period. The risk of disease is a function of both the rate of new disease development and the length of time the population is at risk. To continue with the example given previously, one could follow the 7945 women in whom no breast cancer was detected and note the number of new cases of breast cancer detected over the following 5 years. Assuming no losses to follow-up, if 44 women were diagnosed over the 5-year period, then the 5-year cumulative incidence of breast cancer in this population would be as follows:

$$\frac{44}{7945} = 0.005538, \text{ or } 553.8 \text{ per } 100,000$$

Incidence and prevalence compared. Because the prevalence rate measures existing cases of disease and is roughly proportional to the incidence multiplied by the duration of disease, it is affected by factors that influence risk and by factors that influence survival or recovery. In mathematical notation,

$$P \approx I \times D$$

where P = prevalence, I = incidence, and D = duration

HOW TO *Quantify a Health Problem in the Community*

Planning for resources and personnel often requires quantifying the level of a problem in a community. For example, to know how different districts compare in the rates of very-low-birth-weight infants, one would calculate the prevalence of very-low-birth-weight births in each district:

1. *Determine the number of live births in each district from birth certificate data obtained from the vital records division of the health department.*
2. *Use the birth weight information from the birth certificate data to determine the number of infants born weighing less than 1500 grams in each district.*
3. *Calculate the prevalence of very-low-birth-weight births by district as the number of infants under 1500 grams at birth divided by the total number of live births.*
4. *If the number of very-low-birth-weight births in each district is small, use several recent years of data to obtain a more stable estimate.*

For that reason, prevalence measures are less useful when looking for factors related to disease etiology. Because prevalence rates reflect duration in addition to the risk of getting the disease, it is difficult to sort out what factors are related to risk and these risk factors may be masked by differences in survival or cure. For example, the 5-year survival rate for breast cancer is about 85%, but the 5-year survival rate for lung cancer in women is only about 15%. Even if the incidence rates of breast and lung cancer were the same in women (and they are not), the prevalence rates would differ because, on average, women live longer with breast cancer (i.e., it has a longer duration). Incidence rates, on the other hand, are the measure of choice to study etiology because incidence is affected only by factors related to the risk of developing disease and not to survival or cure. Prevalence is useful in planning health care services because it is an indication of the level of disease existing in the population and therefore of the size of the population in need of services. In the previous example of screening, the health department would want to know both the existing level of TB in the area (the prevalence) in order to plan services and direct prevention and control measures and the rate at which new cases are developing (the incidence) in order to study risk factors and evaluate the effectiveness of prevention and control programs.

Attack rate. One final measure of morbidity, often used in infectious disease investigations, is the **attack rate,** a form of incidence rate defined as the proportion of persons who are exposed to an agent and develop the disease. Attack rates are often specific to an exposure; food-specific attack rates, for example, are the proportion of persons becoming ill after eating a specific food item.

Comparison Groups

The use of comparison groups is at the heart of the epidemiologic approach. Incidence or prevalence rates in groups that differ in some important characteristic must be compared to gain clues about which factors influence the distribution of disease (disease determinants or risk factors). Observing the rate of disease only among persons exposed to a suspected risk factor will not show clearly that the exposure is associated with increased risk until the rate observed in the exposed group is compared with the rate in a group of comparable unexposed persons. To illustrate, one might investigate the effect of smoking during pregnancy on the rate of low birth weight by calculating the rate of low-birth-weight infants born to women who smoked during their pregnancy. However, the hypothesis that smoking during pregnancy is a risk factor for low birth weight is supported only when the low-birth-weight rate among smoking women is compared with the (lower) rate of low-birth-weight infants born to nonsmoking women.

⋮ HOW TO's *of Community and Public Health Nursing*

Epidemiologic concepts are used in an ongoing assessment of both community and individual health problems. The assessment of health problems in a community needs to start with the community's incidence, morbidity, and mortality rates for specific diseases. Major causes of hospitalization and emergency department visits need to be included. Additional areas for community assessment are outlined in the next section. Similarly, individual health problems need to incorporate evaluations of health risk based on lifestyle patterns along with the standard history and clinical examinations.

⋮ HOW TO *Assess Health Problems in a Community*

1. *Identify major causes of disease through incidence, morbidity, and mortality rates.*
2. *Evaluate major causes of hospitalizations and emergency department visits.*
3. *Ask key community leaders to discuss critical community health problems.*
4. *Hold focus groups with community groups involved in health.*
5. *Analyze community environmental health hazards and pollutants (e.g., water, sewage).*
6. *Examine community knowledge and practice of preventive health (e.g., use of infant car seats, safe playgrounds, lighted streets for safety).*
7. *Identify cultural priorities and beliefs about health.*
8. *Assess community's interpretation of and degree of trust in federal, state, and local assistance programs.*
9. *Conduct community surveys to assess specific problems.*

⋮ HOW TO *Assess Health Problems in an Individual*

1. *Obtain history of physical and mental health problems.*
2. *Ask individual to identify major health problems. Always start interventions with what individual views as important.*
3. *Obtain family history of diseases. Identify possible genetic link based on early age of disease and/or multiple family members with disease.*
4. *Perform clinical examination, including laboratory work.*
5. *Evaluate health risk based on lifestyle. Include smoking status, dietary patterns of fiber and fat, exercise patterns, stress factors, and risk-taking behaviors.*
6. *Identify immediate and long-range safety concerns.*
7. *Assess individual's cultural beliefs about health.*
8. *Assess social support.*
9. *Examine knowledge and practice of preventive health care.*
10. *Provide appropriate age-based screening (e.g., cancer screening, hypertension screening).*

DESCRIPTIVE EPIDEMIOLOGY

Descriptive epidemiology describes the distribution of disease, death, and other health outcomes in the population according to person, place, and time, providing a picture of how things are or have been—the who, where, and when of disease patterns. Analytic epidemiology, on the other hand, searches for the determinants of the patterns observed—the how and why. That is, epidemiologic concepts and methods are used to identify what factors, characteristics, exposures, or behaviors might account for differences in the observed patterns of disease occurrence. Descriptive and analytic studies are observational, meaning the investigator observes events as they are or have been and does not intervene to change anything or to introduce a new factor. Experimental or intervention studies, on the other hand, include interventions to test preventive or treatment measures, techniques, materials, policies, or drugs.

Person

Personal characteristics of interest in epidemiology include race, sex, age, education, occupation, income (and related socioeconomic status), and marital status. As noted previously, the most important predictor of overall mortality is age. The mortality curve by age drops sharply during and after the first year of life to a low point in childhood, then begins to increase through adolescence and young adulthood (Gordis, 1996).

There are also substantial differences in mortality and morbidity rates by sex. Female infants have a lower mortality rate than comparable male infants, and the survival advantage continues throughout life. (NCHS, 1998; Peters et al, 1998). However, patterns for specific diseases vary. For example, women have lower rates of CHD until menopause, after which the gap narrows. For rheumatoid arthritis, the prevalence among women is greater than among men (Brownson et al, 1998).

Although the concept of race as a variable for public health research has come under scrutiny (CDC, 1993; Fullilove, 1998), there are clear differences in morbidity and mortality rates by race in the United States (Peters et al, 1998; NCHS, 1998). The 1996 U.S. age-adjusted death rate for African-Americans was 1.6 times higher than for Caucasian Americans. Death rates were also higher among African-Americans for 12 of the 15 leading causes of death in 1996 (Peters et al, 1998). The infant mortality rate for African-American infants, though declining, is still more than twice as high as the rate among Caucasian. The NCHS report *Health, United States, 1998* provides further insight into health disparities across socioeconomic levels.

Place

When considering the distribution of a disease, geographic patterns come to mind: Does the rate of disease differ from place to place (e.g., with local environment)? If there were no effects of geography on disease occurrence, random geographic patterns might be seen, but that is often not the case. For example, at high altitudes there is lower oxygen tension, which might result in smaller babies. Other diseases reflect distinctive patterns by place. For example, Lyme disease is more likely to be found in areas where there are reservoirs of the disease, a large tick population is the vector for transmission to humans, and contact between the human population and the tick vectors (Benenson, 1995).

In general, one expects variations by geographic location (place) to be due to differences in the chemical, physical, or biologic environment. However, variations by place also may result from differences in population densities or customary patterns of behavior and lifestyle or other personal characteristics. For example, one might find variations by place because of high concentrations of a re-

ligious, cultural, or ethnic group who practice certain health-related behaviors. The high rates of stroke found in the southeastern United States are likely a result of a number of social and personal factors that may have little to do with geographic features per se. Recent research has also focused on neighborhood level variables, such as unemployment and crimes rates, social cohesion, and access to important services (O'Campo et al, 1995; Sampson, Raudenbush, and Earls, 1997). These are factors that may be of particular interest to nurses, who are in a unique position to assess their effect on the health of communities.

Time

Secular changes

The third component of descriptive epidemiology is time: Is there an increase or decrease in the frequency of the disease over time or are other temporal patterns evident? Long-term patterns of morbidity or mortality rates (i.e., over years or decades) are called **secular trends.** Secular trends may reflect changes in social behavior or practices. For example, the increase in lung cancer mortality rate that has been observed in recent years is a delayed effect of increases in smoking in prior years, and the decline in cervical cancer deaths is primarily due to widespread screening using a Pap test (Brownson et al, 1998).

DID YOU KNOW? *Lung cancer has now surpassed breast cancer as the leading cause of cancer mortality among women. The rapidly increasing rate of lung cancer deaths in women mirrors the patterns of increased rates of smoking among women and increased cigarette advertising directed toward women.*

Some apparent secular trends may be the result of increased diagnostic capability or changes in survival (or case fatality) rather than in incidence. For example, case fatality from breast cancer has decreased in recent years while the incidence of breast cancer has increased. Some, though not all, of the increased incidence is due to improved diagnostic capability. These two trends result in a breast cancer mortality curve that is flatter than the incidence curve (Brownson et al, 1998; Holleb, Fink, and Murphy, 1991). Relying on the mortality data alone does not accurately depict the true situation. Changes in case definition or revisions in the coding of a disease according to the International Classification of Diseases (ICD) also affects secular trends. Such changes can produce an artificial change in the rate (Peters et al, 1998).

Point epidemic

One temporal and spatial pattern of disease distribution is the **point epidemic.** This time-and-space-related pattern is particularly important in infectious disease investigations, but it is also recognized as a significant indicator for toxic exposures in environmental epidemiology. A point epidemic is most clearly seen when the frequency of cases is graphed against time. The sharp peak characteristic of such graphs indicates a concentration of cases about some short interval of time. The peak often indicates the response of the population to a common source of infection or contamination to which they were all simultaneously exposed. Knowledge of the incubation or latency period (the time between exposure and development of signs and symptoms) for the specific disease entity can help to determine the probable time of exposure. A common example of a point epidemic is an outbreak of gastrointestinal illness from a food-borne pathogen. Nurses alert to a sudden increase in the number of cases of a disease can chart the outbreak, determine the probable time of exposure, and by careful investigation, isolate the probable source of the agent.

Cyclical patterns

In addition to secular trends and point epidemics, there are also cyclical time patterns of disease. One common type of cyclical variation is seasonal fluctuation in a number of infectious illnesses. Seasonal changes may be influenced by changes in the agent itself, changes in population densities or behaviors of animal reservoirs or vectors, or changes in human behaviors resulting in changing exposures (being outdoors in warmer weather and indoors in colder months). There also may be artificial seasons created by calendar events, such as holidays and tax-filing deadlines, which may be associated with patterns of stress-related illness. Patterns of accidents and injuries also may be seasonal, reflecting differing employment and recreational patterns. Some disease cycles, such as influenza, have patterns of smaller epidemics every few years, depending on strain, with major pandemics occurring at longer intervals (Benenson, 1995). Workers in community health can prepare to meet increased demands on resources by careful attention to these cyclical patterns.

Event-related clusters

A third type of temporal pattern is nonsimultaneous, event-related clusters. These are patterns in which time is not measured from fixed dates on the calendar but from the point of some exposure, event, or experience presumably held in common by affected persons, though not occurring at the same time. An example of this pattern would be vaccine reactions in an ongoing immunization program. Clearly, if vaccinations are being given on a regular basis, one might see nonspecific symptoms, such as fever, headaches, or rashes, fairly consistently over time, making identification of a cluster related to the vaccinations difficult. If, however, the occurrence of symptoms is plotted against the time since the vaccination, vaccine reactions are likely to show up as a peak in the number of cases at some period after the immunization.

ANALYTIC EPIDEMIOLOGY

Descriptive epidemiology deals with the *distribution* of health outcomes, whereas *analytic* epidemiology seeks to discover the *determinants* of outcomes, the how and the why (i.e., the factors that influence observed patterns of health and disease and increase or decrease the risk of adverse outcomes). This section deals with analytic study designs and the related measures of association derived from them. Table 11-5 summarizes the advantages and disadvantages of each design.

DID YOU KNOW? *Epidemiologic studies conducted by nurse researchers have direct application to all areas of nursing?*

Ecologic Studies

An epidemiologic study that is a bridge between descriptive epidemiology and analytic epidemiology is the **ecologic study.** The descriptive component involves examining variations in disease rates by person, place, or time. The analytic component lies in the effort to determine if there is a relationship of disease rates to variations in rates for possible risk (or protective) factors or characteristics. The identifying characteristic of ecologic studies is that only aggregate data, such as population rates, are used rather than data on individuals' exposures, characteristics, and outcomes. For example, information on per capita cigarette consumption might be examined in relation to lung cancer mortality rates in several countries, in several groups of people, or in the same population at different times. Other examples include comparisons of rates of breast feeding and of breast cancer, average dietary fat content and rates of CHD, or unemployment rates and level of psychiatric disorder.

Ecologic studies are attractive because they often make use of existing, readily available rates and are therefore quick and inexpensive to conduct. They are subject, however, to **ecologic fallacy** (i.e., associations observed at the group level may not hold true for the individuals that comprise the groups, or associations that actually exist may be masked in the grouped data). This may be the result of other factors operating in these populations for which the ecologic correlations do not account. For that reason, ecologic studies may be suggestive but require confirmation in studies using individual data (Gordis, 1996; Lilienfeld and Stolley, 1994). However, recent studies have shown that ecologic data can add important information to analyses even when individual level data are available (Lynch et al, 1998; O'Campo et al, 1995)

Uncertainty concerning the temporal sequence of events is a disadvantage of ecologic studies shared with cross-sectional study designs (discussed in the next section). For example, in the study of unemployment rates and psychiatric disorder, it is unclear whether unemployed persons are at higher risk for psychiatric problems or persons with existing psychiatric problems are more likely to be unemployed. Although determining whether one event precedes or succeeds another may seem at first to be a simple matter, in practice it may be difficult to confirm.

TABLE 11-5 Comparison of Major Epidemiologic Study Designs

STUDY DESIGN	ADVANTAGES	DISADVANTAGES
Ecologic	1. Quick, easy, and inexpensive first study 2. Uses readily available existing data 3. May prompt further investigation; suggest other/new hypotheses 4. May provide information about contextual factors not accounted for by individual characteristics	1. Ecologic fallacy: the associations observed may not hold true for individuals 2. Problems in interpreting temporal sequence (cause and effect) 3. More difficult to control for confounding, and "mixed" models (ecologic and individual data) more complex statistically
Cross-sectional (correlational)	1. Gives general description of scope of problem; provides prevalence estimates 2. Often based on population (or community) sample, not just those who sought care 3. Useful in health service evaluation and planning 4. Data obtained at once; less expense and quicker than cohort because no follow-up 5. Baseline for prospective study or identify cases and controls for case-control study	1. No calculation of risk; prevalence, not incidence 2. Temporal sequence unclear 3. Not good for rare disease or rare exposure unless large sample size or stratified sampling 4. Selective survival can be major source of selection bias; surviving subjects may differ from those who are not included (death, institutionalization, etc.) 5. Selective recall or lack of past exposure information can create bias
Case-control (retrospective, case comparison)	1. Less expensive than cohort; smaller sample required 2. Quicker than cohort; no follow-up 3. Can investigate more than one exposure 4. Best design for rare diseases 5. If well designed, can be important tool for etiologic investigation 6. Best suited to diseases with relatively clear onset (timing of onset can be established so that incident cases can be included)	1. Greater susceptibility than cohort studies to various types of bias (selective survival, recall bias, selection bias in choice of both cases and controls) 2. Information on other risk factors may not be available, resulting in confounding 3. Antecedent-consequence (temporal sequence) not as certain as in cohort 4. Not well suited to rare exposures 5. Gives only an indirect estimate of risk 6. Limited to a single outcome because of sampling on disease status
Prospective cohort (concurrent cohort, longitudinal, follow-up)	1. Best estimate of disease incidence 2. Best estimate of risk 3. Fewer problems with selective survival and selective recall 4. Temporal sequence more clearly established 5. Broader range of options for exposure assessment	1. Expensive in time and money 2. More difficult organizationally 3. Not good for rare diseases 4. Attrition of participants can bias estimate 5. Latency period may be very long; may miss cases 6. May be difficult to examine several exposures
Retrospective cohort (nonconcurrent cohort)	1. Combines advantages of both prospective cohort and case-control 2. Shorter time (even if follow-up into future) than prospective cohort 3. Less expensive than prospective cohort because relies on existing data 4. Temporal sequence may be clearer than case-control	1. Shares some disadvantages with both prospective cohort and case-control 2. Subject to attrition (loss to follow-up) 3. Relies on existing records that may result in misclassification of both exposure and outcome 4. May have to rely on surrogate measures of exposure (such as job title) and vital records information on cause of death

Cross-Sectional Studies

The **cross-sectional study** provides a snap shot, or cross section, of a population or group (Gordis, 1996; Lilienfeld and Stolley, 1994). Information is collected on current health status, personal characteristics, and potential risk factors or exposures all at once. The cross-sectional study is characterized by the simultaneous collection of information necessary for the classification of exposure and outcome status, although there may be historical information collected (e.g., on past diet or history of radiation exposure).

Cross-sectional studies are sometimes called *prevalence studies* because they provide the frequency of existing cases of a disease in a population (Kelsey et al, 1996). One way

RESEARCH *Brief*

This correlational survey research described an educational program on prostate cancer and free prostate cancer screening that was given to 179 men at work sites. There were significant increases in prostate cancer screening after the educational program. Only 16% of the African-American men had obtained a digital rectal examination in the last 12 months; 44% of the men participated in the free screening, an almost fourfold increase. Similarly, only 6% of the African-American men had received a PSA screen in the last 12 months, yet 42% obtained PSA screening after the educational program, a sevenfold increase.

The role of nurses includes identifying at-risk individuals and advocating screening and preventive health practices. Occupational health nurses could use the model of empowerment through education at work sites. Most professional health organizations (e.g., American Cancer Society, American Heart Association) have audiovisual and written materials that nurses could use at no cost. Work sites could be targeted based on the health prevention practice being taught. For example, work sites associated with occupational exposure to prostate cancer, such as sites that use or manufacture cadmium, batteries, and pesticides, could be targeted. In addition to practicing preventive health on the individual level, nurses need to advocate at the community level for policies and reimbursement that support at-risk populations.

Weinrich S et al: Work sites: effective sites for recruitment of African American men into prostate cancer screening. *J Community Health Nurs* 15(2):113, 1998.

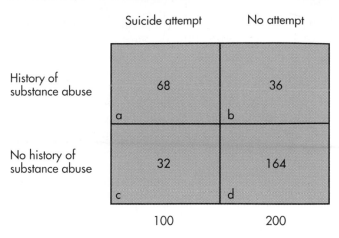

FIG. 11-5 Case-control study.

for inclusion). Suppose that physical activity not only reduced the risk of CHD but also markedly improved survival among those with CHD. Sedentary persons with CHD would then have higher fatality rates than physically active persons who did develop CHD. One might observe higher rates of physical activity in a group of persons surviving with CHD than in a general population without CHD, both because of the survival advantage and participation of survivors in cardiac rehabilitation programs. It could erroneously appear that physical activity was a risk factor for CHD. A cross-sectional study is discussed in the Research Brief.

Case-Control Studies

In the **case-control study,** design subjects are enrolled because they *are* known to have the outcome of interest (cases) or they are known *not* to have the outcome of interest (controls). Case-control status is verified using a clear case definition and some previously determined method or protocol (e.g., by an examination, laboratory test, or medical chart review). Information is then collected on the exposures or characteristics of interest, frequently from existing sources, subject interview, or questionnaire (Armenian, 1994; Kelsey et al, 1996; Schlesselman, 1982). The question in a case-control study is, "Do persons with the outcome of interest (cases) have the exposure characteristic (or a history of the exposure) more frequently than those without the outcome (controls)?"

Given the way subjects are selected for a case-control study, neither incidence nor prevalence can be calculated directly. In a case-control study, an odds ratio tells how much more or less likely the exposure is to be found among cases than among controls. The odds of exposure among cases (a to c in Fig. 11-5) are compared with the odds of exposure among controls (b to d in Fig. 11-5). The ratio of these two odds provides an estimate of the relative risk.

Suppose a research group wanted to study risk factors for suicide attempts among adolescents. They were able to

cross-sectional studies evaluate the association of a factor with a health problem is to compare the prevalence of the disease in those with the factor (or exposure) with the prevalence in the unexposed. The ratio of the two prevalence rates indicates an association between the factor and the outcome. If the prevalence of CHD in smokers were twice as high as the prevalence among nonsmokers, the prevalence ratio would be 2. If a factor is unrelated to the prevalence of a disease, the prevalence ratio will be close to 1. A value less than 1 may suggest a protective association. For example, the prevalence of CHD is lower among those who are physically active than among sedentary persons, so the prevalence ratio for the association between physical activity and CHD should be less than 1. Prevalence ratios require caution in interpretation because the prevalence measure is affected by cure, survival, and migration and does not estimate the risk of *getting* the disease.

Cross-sectional studies are subject to bias resulting from selective survival (i.e., existing cases who have survived to be in the study may be different from cases diagnosed about the same time who have died and are not available enroll 100 adolescents who had attempted suicide and selected 200 adolescents from the same community with no history of suicide attempt. One of the factors they want to investigate is a history of substance abuse (SA). Through a questionnaire and other medical records, they were able to determine that 68 of the 100 adolescents who had attempted suicide had a history of substance abuse, while 36 of the 200 adolescents with no suicide attempt had such a history. The information could be presented as shown in Figure 11-5.

The odds of a history of substance abuse among suicide attempters is a/c, or 68/32, whereas the odds of substance abuse among controls is b/d, or 36/164. The odds ratio (equivalent to ad/bc) is as follows:

$$\frac{68 \times 164}{36 \times 32} = 9.68$$

This would be interpreted to mean that adolescents who attempted suicide are almost 10 times more likely to have a history of substance abuse than adolescents who have not attempted suicide. Note that, as with the prevalence ratio, an odds ratio of 1 is indicative of no association (i.e., the odds of exposure are similar for cases and controls). An odds ratio less than 1 suggests a protective association (cases are less likely to have been exposed than controls).

Because the number of cases is known or actively sought out, case-control studies do not demand large samples or the long follow-up time that is often required for prospective cohort studies. That is why many of the influential cancer studies have been of the case-control design.

Case-control studies are, however, prone to a number of biases. (See further discussion in Bias section of this chapter.) Because these studies begin with existing cases, differential survival can produce biased results. The use of recently diagnosed, or "incident," cases may reduce this bias. Because exposure information is obtained from subject recall or past records, there may be errors in exposure assessment or misclassification. As a result of the sampling on disease status, case-control studies are limited to a single outcome, although they may investigate a number of potential risk factors.

Cohort Studies

In epidemiology, the term *cohort* is used to describe a group of persons who are born at about the same time, or in analytic studies, a group of persons, generally sharing some characteristic of interest, who are enrolled in a study and followed over a period of time to observe some health outcome. Because of this ability to observe the development of new cases of disease, **cohort study** designs allow for calculation of incidence rates and therefore estimates of risk of disease. Cohort studies may be prospective or retrospective (Kelsey et al, 1996; Rothman and Greenland, 1998).

Prospective cohort studies

In a prospective cohort study (also called a *longitudinal* or *follow-up study*), subjects determined to be free of the

outcome under investigation are classified on the basis of the exposure of interest at the beginning of the follow-up period. The subjects are then followed for some period of time to ascertain the occurrence of disease in each group. The question is, "Do persons with the factor (or exposure) of interest develop (or avoid) the outcome more frequently than those without the factor (or exposure)?"

For example, one might recruit a cohort of subjects classified as physically active ("exposed") or sedentary ("not exposed"). One might further quantify the amount of the "exposure" if there is sufficient information. These subjects would then be followed over time to determine the development of CHD. This study design avoids the problem of selective survival seen in the earlier example of a cross-sectional study of physical activity and CHD. The cohort study also has the ability to estimate the risk of acquiring disease for those who are exposed compared with those who are unexposed (or less exposed). This ratio of cumulative incidence rates is called the *relative risk*.

For example, suppose 1000 physically active and 1000 sedentary middle-aged men and women were enrolled in a prospective cohort study. All were free of CHD at enrollment. Over a 5-year follow-up period, regular examinations detect CHD in 120 of the sedentary men and women and in 48 of the active men and women. Assuming no other deaths or losses to follow-up, the data could be presented as shown in Figure 11-6.

The incidence of CHD in the active group is a/(a+b), or 48/1000, and the incidence of CHD in the sedentary group is c/(c+d), or 120/1000. The relative risk is as follows:

$$\frac{48/1000}{120/1000} = 0.4$$

As in the example of prevalence ratio, because physical activity is protective for CHD, the relative risk is less than 1. The interpretation for this hypothetical example is that, over a 5-year period, the risk of CHD in persons who are physically active is about 0.4. If the risk were greater for those exposed, the relative risk would be greater than 1. For example, if the relative risk of CHD for smokers compared

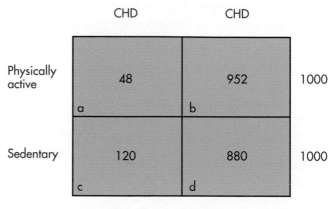

FIG. 11-6 Cohort study.

with nonsmokers is 3.5, it would be interpreted to mean that the risk of CHD among smokers is 3.5 times the risk of nonsmokers. The null value indicating no association is 1, since the incidence rates and thus the risk would be equal in the two groups if there were no association.

Because subjects are enrolled before onset of disease, the cohort design can study more than one outcome, calculate incidence rates and estimate risk, establish the temporal sequence of exposure and outcome with greater clarity and certainty, and may avoid many of the problems of the earlier study designs with selective survival or exposure misclassification. On the other hand, large samples are often necessary to ensure that enough cases are observed to provide statistical power to detect meaningful differences between groups. This is complicated by the long period required for some diseases to develop (the latency period). Also, the number of subjects required to observe sufficient cases makes longitudinal studies unsuitable for very rare diseases unless they are part of a larger study of a number of outcomes.

Retrospective cohort studies

Retrospective cohort studies combine some of the advantages and disadvantages of case-control studies and prospective cohort studies. One relies on existing records, such as employment, insurance, or hospital records, to define a cohort who is classified as having been exposed or unexposed at some time in the past. The cohort is followed over time using the records to determine if the outcome occurred. Retrospective cohort studies (also called *historical cohort*) may be conducted entirely using past records or may include current assessment or additional follow-up time after study initiation. The obvious advantage of this approach is the time savings because one does not have to wait for new cases of disease to develop. The disadvantages are largely related to the reliance on existing historical records. Retrospective cohort studies frequently are used in occupational epidemiology where industrial records are available to investigate work-related exposures and health outcomes.

EXPERIMENTAL STUDIES

The study designs discussed so far are called *observational studies* because the investigator observes the association between exposures and outcomes as they exist but does not intervene to alter the presence or level of any exposure or behavior. Studies in which the investigator initiates some treatment or intervention that may influence the risk or course of disease are called *intervention,* or *experimental,* studies. Such studies test whether interventions are effective in preventing disease or improving health. Like observational studies, experimental studies generally use comparison (or control) groups, but unlike observational studies there is the possibility of randomly allocating persons to a particular intervention group and determining the type or level of the "exposure" (the treatment or intervention). Intervention studies are of two general types:

clinical trials and community trials (Lilienfeld and Stolley, 1994; Meinert, 1986).

WHAT DO YOU THINK? *Epidemiologic studies are often inconclusive concerning causal associations. The same may be true for epidemiologically based evaluations of prevention programs. Should there be a difference in how we interpret results for purposes of designing future research as opposed to recommending guidelines? Should there be a difference in interpretation and application of epidemiologic results for individuals and for community or public policy?*

Clinical Trials

In clinical trials, the research issue is generally the efficacy of a medical treatment for disease, such as a new drug or existing drug used in a new or different way, surgical technique, or other treatment. The preferred method of subject allocation in clinical trials is randomization (i.e., assigning treatments to clients so that all possible treatment assignments have a predetermined probability but neither subject nor investigator determines the actual assignment of any participant). Randomization avoids the bias that may result if subjects self-select into one group or the other or if the investigator or clinician chooses subjects for each group.

A second aspect of treatment allocation is the use of masking, or "blinding," treatment assignments. The optimal design for most situations is the double-blind study in which neither the subject nor the investigator knows who is receiving which treatment. The aim of blinding is to reduce the bias from overestimating therapeutic benefit for the experimental treatment when it is known who is receiving it.

Clinical trials generally are thought to provide the best evidence of causality because of the assignment of treatment and the greater control over other factors that could influence outcome. Like cohort studies, clinical trials are prospective in direction and provide the clearest evidence of temporal sequence.

However, clinical trials are generally conducted in a contrived situation, under controlled conditions, and with select client populations. That means that treatment may be less effective when applied under more realistic clinical or community conditions in a more diverse client population. There are also ethical considerations in experimental studies that go beyond those that apply to observational studies. Also, clinical trials tend to be costly in time, personnel, facilities, and other factors.

Community Trials

Community trials are similar to clinical trials in that an investigator determines the exposure or intervention, but in this case the issue is often health promotion and disease prevention rather than treatment of existing disease. The intervention is usually undertaken on a large scale, with the unit of treatment allocation being a community, region, or group rather than individuals. Although a pharmaceutical product may be involved in a community trial, such as fluoridation of water or mass immunizations, community trials often involve educational, programmatic, or policy interventions. Studying the effect on diabetes rates of providing exercise programs and facilities and increasing availability of healthy, fresh foods are examples of community interventions.

Although community trials provide the best means of testing whether changes in knowledge or behavior, policy, programs, or other mass interventions are effective, they are not without problems. For many interventions, it may take years for the effectiveness of the intervention to be evident. In the meantime, other factors also may influence the outcome either positively (making the intervention look more effective than it really is) or negatively (making the intervention look less effective than it really is). Comparable community populations without similar interventions for comparative analysis are often difficult to determine. Even when comparable comparison communities are available, especially when the intervention is improved knowledge or changed behavior, it is difficult and unethical to prevent the control communities from making use of generally available information, effectively making them less different from the intervention communities. Also, because community trials are often undertaken on a large scale and over long periods of time, they can be expensive, requiring large staff, complicated logistics, and extensive communication resources.

SCREENING

Screening is the application of a test to people who are as yet asymptomatic for the purpose of classifying them with respect to their likelihood of having a particular disease. Screening may be a component of secondary prevention efforts. From a clinical perspective, the aim of screening is early detection and treatment when there is a more favorable prognosis. From a public health perspective, the objective is to sort out efficiently and effectively those who probably have the disease from those who probably do not, again to detect early cases for treatment or begin public health prevention and control programs. A screening test is not a diagnostic test. Screening programs require referral and diagnostic evaluation for those who screen positive to determine if they actually have the disease and need treatment.

Successful screening programs have several characteristics that depend on both the tests and population screened (Box 11-2). Among the desirable traits are the availability of reliable and valid screening tests (Gordis, 1996).

Reliability and Validity
Reliability

All measurements need to be concerned about the precision or **reliability** of the measure (its consistency or repeatability) and the accuracy of the measure (Is it really measuring what we think it is and how closely?). Suppose you want to do a blood pressure screening in a community. You will take blood pressures on a large number of people, perhaps following up with repeated measures for individuals with higher pressures.

If the sphygmomanometer used for the screening varies in its readings so that one does not get the same reading twice in a row, then it lacks precision. The instrument would be unreliable even if the overall mean of repeated measurements were close to the true overall mean for the persons measured. The problem would be that the readings would not be reliable for any individual, which is what a screening program requires.

On the other hand, suppose the readings are reproducible, but unknown to you, tend to be about 10 mm Hg too high. This instrument is producing precise and reliable readings. However, the uncorrected (or uncalibrated) instrument lacks accuracy (does not give a valid reading). In short, a measure can be consistent without producing valid results.

There are three major sources of error affecting the reliability of tests:
- Variation inherent in the trait itself (e.g., blood pressure that changes with time of day, activity, level of stress, and other factors)
- Observer variation, which can be divided into intraobserver reliability (consistency by the same observer) and interobserver reliability (consistency from one observer to another)
- Inconsistency in the instrument, which includes the internal consistency of the instrument (e.g., do all items in a questionnaire measure the same thing) and the stability (or test-retest reliability) of the instrument over time

Validity: sensitivity and specificity

Validity in a screening test is measured by sensitivity and specificity. **Sensitivity** quantifies how accurately the test identifies those *with* the condition or trait. In other

---

BOX 11-2 Characteristics of a Successful Screening Program

1. *Valid (accurate).* There is a high probability of correct classification of persons tested.
2. *Reliable (precise).* Gives consistent results from time to time, place to place, and person to person.
3. *Capable of large group administration.*
   a. Fast in both the administration of the test and obtaining of the results.
   b. Inexpensive in both personnel required and in the materials and procedures used.
4. *Innocuous.* There are few if any side effects, and the test is minimally invasive.
5. *High yield.* The test is able to detect enough new cases to warrant the effort and expense. *Yield* is defined as the amount of previously unrecognized disease that is diagnosed and treated as a result of screening.

words, sensitivity represents the proportion of persons with the disease whom the test correctly identifies as positive (true positives). High sensitivity is needed when early treatment is important and when identification of every case is important.

Specificity indicates how accurately the test identifies those *without* the condition or trait (i.e., the proportion of persons without the disease whom the test correctly identifies as negative [true negatives]). High specificity is needed when rescreening is impractical and when reducing false positives is important (see the Research Brief).

The sensitivity and specificity of a test are determined by comparing the results from the test with results from a definitive diagnostic procedure (sometimes called the *gold standard*). For example, the Pap smear is a common screening procedure for detection of cervical dysplasia and carcinoma. The definitive diagnosis of cervical cancer requires a biopsy with histologic confirmation of malignant cells. The ideal for a screening test is 100% sensitivity and 100% specificity, meaning that 100% of those who actually have the disease are positive on the test and the test is negative

for all those who do not have the disease. In practice, sensitivity and specificity are often inversely related. That is, if the test results are such that one can choose some point beyond which a person is considered positive (a "cutpoint"), as in a blood pressure reading to screen for hypertension or a serum glucose reading to screen for diabetes, then moving that critical point to improve the sensitivity of the test will result in a decrease in specificity or an improvement in specificity can be made only at the expense of sensitivity.

Table 11-6 shows a typical table for classification and calculation of sensitivity and specificity. Some writers refer to a false-positive rate, which is 1 minus the specificity, and a false-negative rate, or 1 minus the sensitivity. These "rates" are simply the proportions incorrectly classified among nondiseased and diseased subjects, respectively.

A third measure associated with sensitivity and specificity is the predictive value of the test. The **positive predictive value** is the proportion of persons with a positive test who actually have the disease, interpreted as the probability that an individual with a positive test has the disease. The **negative predictive value** is the proportion of persons with a negative test who are actually disease-free. Although sensitivity and specificity are relatively independent of the prevalence of disease, predictive values are affected by the level of disease in the screened population and by the sensitivity and specificity of the test. When the prevalence is very low, the positive predictive value will be low, even with tests that are sensitive and specific. Additionally, lower specificity produces lower positive predictive values because of the increase in the proportion of false-positive results.

Consideration of the human and economic costs of missing true cases by lowering the sensitivity versus the cost of falsely classifying noncases by lowering the specificity is necessary in setting cutpoints. Factors to be considered in-

RESEARCH *Brief*

Race- and age-specific values for prostate specific antigen (PSA) have been advocated. The race- and age-specific distribution of serum PSA in South Carolina was compared with distributions obtained in data from the Olmsted County study and from the Walter Reed Army Medical Center/ Center for Prostate Disease Research study. The sample was 1127 healthy African-American and Caucasian males from 40 to 69 years of age from a cross-section of the general population in 11 counties of central South Carolina. The subjects, who participated in a prostate cancer educational program, subsequently obtained a physical examination including PSA determination.

Higher PSA levels were found in older men and among African-American subjects. Within each of the three studies, there were substantial race- and age-related differences in serum PSA levels, and for that reason, each lends credence to the use of race- and age-normed reference ranges for normal PSA that are specific to the population from which the norms are derived.

Nurses need to be aware that reference ranges for normal serum PSA levels may vary from setting to setting. Men with questionable PSAs need to be referred, especially if they have the increased risk factors for prostate cancer of African-American race and/or family history of prostate cancer. Nurses need to advocate for screening and prevention programs targeted to the at-risk populations.

Weinrich M. et al: General population reference ranges for serum prostate specific antigen in Black and White men without cancer. *Urology* 12(6), 1998.

TABLE 11-6 Classification of Subjects According to True Disease State and Screening Test Results for Calculation of Indices of Validityable to Different Factors

RESULT OF SCREENING TEST	DISEASE STATE	
	DISEASE	NO DISEASE
Positive	True positive (TP)	False positive (FP)
Negative	False negative (FN)	True negative (TN)

Sensitivity = TP / (TP + FN)
Specificity = TN / (TN + FP)
False negative "rate" = 1 − Se = FN / (FN + TP)
False positive "rate" = 1 − Sp = FP / (TN + FP)
Positive predictive value = TP / (TP + FP)
Often multiplied by 100 and expressed as a percentage.

clude the importance of capturing all cases, the likelihood that the population will be rescreened, the interval between screenings relative to the rate of disease development, and the prevalence of the disease. A low prevalence typically requires a test with high specificity, otherwise the screening will produce too many false positives in the large nondiseased population. On the other hand, a disease with a high prevalence usually requires high sensitivity, otherwise too many of the real cases will be missed by the screening (false negatives).

Two or more tests can be combined to enhance sensitivity or specificity. They may be combined in series or in parallel.

In *series* testing one is considered positive only if positive on *all* tests in the series, and one is considered negative if negative on *any* test. For example, if a blood sample were screened for HIV, a positive ELISA test might be followed up with a Western blot, and the sample would be considered positive only if *both* tests were positive. Series testing enhances specificity, producing fewer false positives, but sensitivity may be low. In series testing, sequence is important; one often uses a very sensitive test first to pick up all cases plus false positives, then a second test that is very specific to eliminate false positives.

In *parallel* testing one is considered positive if positive on *any* test and is considered negative only if negative on *all* tests. To return to the example of a blood sample being tested for HIV, a blood bank might consider a sample positive if it were positive on *either* the ELISA *or* the Western blot. Parallel testing enhances sensitivity, leaving fewer false negatives, but specificity may be low.

CAUSALITY

Statistical Associations

One of the first steps in assessing the relationship of some factor with a health outcome is determining whether a statistical association exists. If the probability of disease seems unaffected by the presence or level of the factor, no association is apparent. If, on the other hand, the probability of disease does vary according to whether the factor is present, then there is a statistical association. The earlier discussion of null values is pertinent at this point. When an observed measure of association (such as a relative risk) does not differ from the null value, it may not be assumed that there is an association between the factor and outcome under investigation.

To say that a result is statistically significant means that the observed result is unlikely to be due to chance. Note that statistical significance is also determined by sample size. In other words, the difference between 34.3% and 35.9% in a study group of 1000 is not statistically significant at the 0.05 level of significance. However, in a much larger sample, a difference of this amount would be significant.

Bias

One also may observe a statistically significant result because of **bias,** a systematic error resulting from the study design, execution, or confounding. For example, if there were a gum ball machine with colors randomly mixed and three red ones in a row came out, that would be due to chance. If, however, the person loading the gum ball machine had poured in a bag of red ones first, then green ones, then yellow, it would not be surprising to get three red ones in a row because of the way the machine was loaded. In epidemiologic studies, results are sometimes seen because of the way the study was "loaded" (i.e., the way the study was designed or subjects were selected or information collected and subjects classified). Although the types of bias are numerous, there are three general categories of bias.

Bias attributable to the way subjects enter a study is called *selection bias*. It has to do with selection procedures and the population from which subjects are drawn. It may involve self-selection factors as well. For example, are teenagers who agree to complete a questionnaire on alcohol, tobacco, and other drug use representative of the total teenage population?

Bias attributable to misclassification of subjects once they are in the study is *information*, or *classification* (or misclassification), *bias*. It is related to how information is collected, including the information that subjects supply or how subjects are classified.

Bias resulting from the relationship of the outcome and study factor with some third factor not accounted for is called **confounding.** For example, there is a well-known association between maternal smoking during pregnancy and low-birth-weight babies. There is also an association between alcohol consumption and smoking that is not due to chance nor is it causal (i.e., drinking alcohol does not cause a person to smoke, nor does smoking cause a person to drink alcohol). If one were to investigate the association of alcohol consumption and low birth weight, smoking would be a confounder because it is related to both alcohol consumption and low birth weight. Failure to account for smoking in the analysis would bias the observed association between alcohol use and low birth weight. In practice one can often identify potentially confounding variables in order to adjust for them in analysis.

Criteria for Causality

The existence of a statistical association does not necessarily mean that there is a causal relationship. As the previous sections have shown, the observed association may be a random event (due to chance) or may be due to bias from confounding or in the study design or execution. Statistical associations, although necessary to an argument for **causality,** are not sufficient proof. The criteria for causality, originally established to evaluate the link between an infectious agent and a disease, have been revised and elaborated to apply also to other outcomes. Although various lists of criteria have been proposed, there is fairly general agreement on the seven criteria that are listed in Box 11-3 (Gordis, 1996; Lilienfeld and Stolley, 1994). Some have questioned the use of lists of criteria as misleading, espe-

BOX 11-3 Criteria for Causality

1. *Strength of association.* A strong association between a potential risk factor and an outcome supports a causal hypothesis (i.e., a relative risk of 7 provides stronger evidence of a causal association than a relative risk of 1.5).
2. *Consistency of findings.* Repeated findings of an association with different study designs and in different populations strengthen causal inference.
3. *Biologic plausibility.* Demonstration of a physiologic mechanism by which the risk factor acts to cause disease enhances the causal hypothesis. Conversely, an association that does not initially seem biologically defensible may later be discovered to be so.
4. *Demonstration of correct temporal sequence.* For a risk factor to cause an outcome, it must precede the onset of the outcome. (See the discussion of this issue in the section on study designs.)
5. *Dose-response relationship.* The risk of developing an outcome should increase with increasing exposure (either in duration or quantity) to the risk factor of interest. For example, studies have shown that the greater the amount a woman smokes during pregnancy, the greater the risk of delivering a low-birth weight infant.
6. *Specificity of the association.* The presence of a one-to-one relationship between an agent and a disease (i.e., the idea that a disease is caused by only one agent and that agent results in only one disease lends support to a causal hypothesis, but its absence does not rule out causality). This criterion grows out of the infectious disease model, where it is more often, though not always, satisfied and is less applicable in chronic diseases.
7. *Experimental evidence.* Experimental designs provide the strongest epidemiologic evidence for causal associations, but they are not feasible or ethical to conduct for many risk factor-disease associations.

cially because only temporal sequence is necessary (Rothman and Greenland, 1998). Although no single epidemiologic study can satisfy all criteria, epidemiology relies on the accumulation of evidence and the strength of individual studies to provide a basis for effective public health interventions and policies.

APPLICATIONS OF EPIDEMIOLOGY IN COMMUNITY AND PUBLIC HEALTH NURSING*

Nurses work in a range of settings and agencies providing direct services and interaction with individual clients and their families, as well as leadership in community-level organizations including visiting nurse associations, community maternity and child health or mental health centers,

*This section is an adaptation of the application section, The Epidemiological Model Applied in Community Health Nursing, by Linda Shortridge and Barbara Valauiso, found in the third edition of this book.

alcohol and drug intervention programs, health maintenance organizations, and nursing centers. Nursing in occupational health settings must consider family resources and needs in planning care even when contact is limited to the individual worker. Nurses employed in administrative positions, such as the director of a visiting nurse association or the nursing administrators in a health department, may be involved in planning and evaluating services of the agency or in coordinating the services of a variety of community agencies. Similarly, nurses serving on community boards will need to be concerned with coordination of existing services and planning to meet currently unmet needs. Regardless of the agency or the nurses' position, epidemiologic methods provide essential resources for planning, conduct, and evaluation of their work.

Care of clients and families is based on the following steps of the nursing process: 1) assessment, 2) planning, 3) implementation, and 4) evaluation. The same process is used in providing care for communities. In both instances, epidemiology furnishes the baseline information for assessing needs, identifying problems, formulating appropriate strategies for study of the problems, setting priorities in development of a plan of care, and evaluating the effectiveness of care.

NURSING TIP

Epidemiology uses a process similar to the nursing process.

Agencies that provide care to communities relate to agencies whose primary purpose is the provision of direct services to clients through referrals, required reporting, and feedback mechanisms. If such information is available at all levels with a common basis of understanding and interpretation, then the referral and reporting system within a community will be facilitated and the system should respond effectively to a need. To assess needs, the nurse providing direct care requires data on the presence or absence of risk characteristics, including family composition and relationships, socioeconomic and cultural factors, environmental factors, and medical and health history. The nurse involved in planning services for the community requires parallel data, including the presence and distribution of risk characteristics; population composition by age, race, and socioeconomic and cultural factors; environmental factors; and medical and health histories.

Assessment of health needs based on sound quantitative and qualitative measurement (descriptive epidemiology), understanding factors that influence health and disease (analytic epidemiology), and evaluation of treatment interventions and program and policy implementation (analytic and experimental epidemiology and health services research) (Brownson and Petitti, 1998; Gordis, 1996) are essential for nurses at all levels to plan and provide appropriate care. Epidemiologic concepts, such as the web of causality; the natural history of disease; and primary, secondary, and tertiary prevention, provide a unifying approach for studying and understanding disease processes and interventions. Measures of morbidity and mortality rates provide a standard means of quantifying both the extent of health problems and the risk of specific outcomes. Study design methods provide the tools for extending an understanding of factors that place persons at increased risk or, conversely, provide protection from adverse outcomes. These examples represent some of the ways the practice of community and public health nursing is enhanced by the understanding and application of epidemiologic concepts and methods.

clinical application

You are a nurse at a local health department where Sam, a 46-year-old African-American male, comes for a routine blood pressure check. He mentions that his father recently died from prostate cancer and that he is worried about himself. Further assessment reveals that his father was diagnosed with prostate cancer when he was 52, and Tom's uncle, who is 56 years old, was recently diagnosed with prostate cancer. You know from Tom's health history that Tom smokes 1 pack of cigarettes a day and eats fried food frequently.

Which action would be your best choice?

A. Give Tom a digital rectal examination (DRE) and prostate specific antigen (PSA) immediately to screen for prostate cancer.

B. Do not discuss or provide prostate cancer screening with Tom since he is under 50 years old.

C. Advise Tom to be tested immediately for the prostate cancer gene because of his family history.

D. Inform Tom of the risks and benefits of prostate cancer testing as well as his increased personal risk of prostate cancer because of his family history, smoking, and dietary habits. Involve Tom in the decision-making process about prostate cancer screening.

Answer is in the back of the book.

KEY POINTS

- Epidemiology is the study of the distribution and determinants of health-related events in human populations and the application of this knowledge to improving the health of communities.
- Epidemiology is a multidisciplinary enterprise that recognizes the complex interrelationships of factors that influence disease and health at both the individual and community levels and provide basic tools for the study of health and disease in communities.
- Epidemiologic methods are used to describe health and disease phenomena and to investigate the factors that promote health or influence the risk or distribution of disease. This knowledge can be useful in planning and evaluating programs, policies, and services and in clinical decision making.

- Basic concepts important to epidemiology are the interrelations of agent, host, and environment (the "epidemiologic triangle"); interactions of factors, exposures, and characteristics in a causal web affecting risk of disease; and levels of prevention corresponding to stages in the natural history of disease.
- Primary prevention involves interventions to reduce the incidence of disease by promoting health and preventing disease processes from developing.
- Secondary prevention includes programs (such as screening) designed to detect disease in the early stages before signs and symptoms are clinically evident in order to intervene with early diagnosis and treatment.
- Tertiary prevention provides treatments and other interventions directed toward persons with clinically apparent disease with the aim of lessening the course of disease, reducing disability, or rehabilitating.
- Basic epidemiologic methods include the use of existing data sources to study health outcomes and related factors and the use of comparison groups to assess the association of exposures or characteristics to health outcomes.
- Epidemiologists rely on rates to quantify levels of morbidity and mortality. Prevalence rates give a picture of the level of existing cases in a population at a given time. Incidence rates measure the rate of new case development in a population and provide an estimate of the risk of disease.
- Descriptive epidemiologic studies provide information on the distribution of disease and health states according to personal characteristics, geographic region, and time. This knowledge enables practitioners to target programs and allocate resources more effectively and provides a basis for further study.
- Analytic epidemiologic studies investigate associations between exposures or characteristics and health or disease outcomes, with a goal of understanding the etiology of disease. Analytic studies provide the foundation for understanding disease causality and for developing effective intervention strategies aimed at primary, secondary, and tertiary prevention.
- Epidemiologic methods also are used in the planning and design of screening (secondary prevention) and community health intervention (primary prevention) strategies and in the evaluation of their effectiveness.

critical thinking activities

1. Look at a recent issue of the *Final Mortality Statistics* from the National Center for Health Statistics or the most recent issue of *Health: United States*. Examine the trends in cause-specific mortality and choose one or two of the leading causes of death.
   a. On the basis of current epidemiologic evidence, what factors have contributed to the observed trend in mortality rates for this disease? Changes in survival? Changes in incidence?
   b. Are the changes due to better (or worse) primary, secondary, or tertiary prevention? Are there modifiable factors, such as health behaviors, that lend themselves to better prevention efforts? What would they be?

2. Examine the leading causes of infant death in the United States.
   a. What differences in intervention approaches are suggested by the various causes of death?
   b. How would you design an epidemiologic study to examine risk factors for specific causes of neonatal and postneonatal death? What types of epidemiologic measures would be useful? What study design(s) would be appropriate?
   c. How would you use the information from your study to develop an intervention program and to define the target population for your intervention?
3. Find a report of an epidemiologic study in one of the major public health, nursing, or epidemiology journals. How do the findings of this study, if valid, affect your nursing practice? How do you incorporate the results of epidemiologic research into your nursing practice?

Bibliography

American Cancer Society: *Cancer facts and figures–1998*, Atlanta, 1998, the Society.

American Nurses Association: *Nursing's social policy statement*, Washington, DC, 1995, American Nurses Publishing.

American Nurses Association: *Standards of community health nursing practice*, Washington, DC, 1986, the Association.

Armenian HK, editor: Applications of the case-control method, *Epidemiol Rev* 16(1):1, 1994.

Benenson AS: *Control of communicable diseases in man*, ed 16, Washington, DC, 1995, American Public Health Association.

Brownson RC, Petitti DB, editors: *Applied epidemiology: theory to practice*, New York, 1998, Oxford University Press.

Brownson RC, Remington PL, Davis JR: *Chronic disease epidemiology and control*, ed 2, Washington, DC, 1998, APHA.

Centers for Disease Control and Prevention (CDC): Use of race and ethnicity in public health surveillance: summary of the CDC/ATSDR workshop, *MMWR Morb Moral Wkly Rep* 42(No RR-10), 1993.

Centers for Disease Control and Prevention (CDC): Addressing emerging infectious disease threats: a prevention strategy for the United States (Executive Summary), *MMWR Morb Moral Wkly Rep* 43(No RR-5):1, 1994.

Chadwick E: *Report on the sanitary conditions of the laboring population of Great Britain*, Edinburgh, 1842, University Press.

Diez-Roux AV: Bringing context back into epidemiology: variables and fallacies in multilevel analysis, *Am J Public Health* 88(2):216, 1998.

Editorial. *Am J Public Health* 32:414, 1942.

Fox SH, Koepsell TD, Daling JR: Birth weight and smoking during pregnancy-effect modification by maternal age, *Am J Epidemiol* 139:1008, 1994.

Fullilove MT: Comment: abandoning "race" as a variable in public health research: an idea whose time has come, *Am J Public Health* 88(9):1297, 1998.

Gordis L: *Epidemiology*, Philadelphia, 1996, WB Saunders.

Holleb AI, Fink DJ, Murphy GP: *American Cancer Society textbook of clinical oncology*, Atlanta, 1991, American Cancer Society.

Institute of Medicine (IOM): *The future of public health*, Washington, DC, 1988, National Academy Press.

Kelsey JL et al: *Methods in observational epidemiology*, ed 2, New York, 1996, Oxford University Press.

Koopman JS: Comment: emerging objectives and methods in epidemiology, *Am J Public Health* 86(5):630, 1996.

Krieger N: Epidemiology and the web of causation: has anyone seen the spider? *Soc Sci Med* 39(7):887, 1994.

Krieger N, Zierler S: What explains the public's health? a call for epidemiologic theory, *Epidemiology* 7(1):107, 1995.

Last JM: *A dictionary of epidemiology*, ed 3, New York, 1995, Oxford University Press.

Lederberg J et al, editors: *Emerging infections: microbial threats to health in the United States*, Washington, DC, 1992, National Academy Press.

Lieberman E et al: Low birthweight at term and the timing of fetal exposure to maternal smoking, *Am J Public Health* 84(7):1127, 1994.

Lilienfeld AM: Epidemiology and health policy: some historical highlights, *Public Health Reports* 99(3):237, 1984.

Lilienfeld AM, Lilienfeld DE: The 1979 Heath Clark lectures: the epidemiologic fabric–weaving the threads, *Int J Epidemiol* 9(3):199, 1980.

Lilienfeld DE, Stolley PD: *Foundations of epidemiology*, ed 3, New York, 1994, Oxford University Press.

Lynch JW et al: Income inequality and mortality in metropolitan areas of the United States, *Am J Public Health* 88(7):1074, 1998.

Mrazek PJ, Haggerty RJ, editors: *Reducing risks for mental disorders: frontiers for preventive intervention research*, Committee on Prevention of Mental Disorders, Washington, DC, 1994, Institute of Medicine, National Academy Press.

Meinert CL: *Clinical trials: design, conduct and analysis*, New York, 1986, Oxford University Press.

National Center for Health Statistics (NCHS): *Health, United States, 1998*, Hyattsville, Md, 1998, Public Health Service.

O'Campo P et al: Violence by male partners against women during the childbearing year: a contextual analysis, *Am J Public Health* 85(8):1092, 1995.

Pearce N: Traditional epidemiology, modern epidemiology, and public health, *Am J Public Health* 86(5):678, 1996.

Peters KD, Kochanek KD, Murphy SL: *Deaths: final data for 1996: national vital statistics reports*, Hyattsville, Md, 1998, National Center for Health Statistics.

Rothman KJ, Greenland S: *Modern epidemiology*, ed 2, Philadelphia, 1998, Lippincott-Raven.

Sampson RJ, Raudenbush SW, Earls F: Neighborhoods and violent crime: a multilevel study of collective efficacy, *Science* 277(15):918, 1997.

Schlesselman JJ: *Case-control studies: design, conduct, analysis*, New York, 1982, Oxford University Press.

Snow J: On the mode of communication of cholera. In *Snow on cholera*, New York, 1855, The Commonwealth Fund.

Stallones RA: *Cerebrovascular disease epidemiology: a workshop*, Public Health Monograph No 76, Pub No 1441, Washington, DC, 1966, US Public Health Service.

Susser M: *Causal thinking in the health sciences*, New York, 1973, Oxford University Press.

Susser M: Epidemiology in the United States after World War II: the evolution of technique, *Epidemiol Rev* 7:147, 1985.

Susser M, Susser E: Choosing a future for epidemiology: I. eras and paradigms, *Am J Public Health* 86(5):668, 1996a.

Susser M, Susser E: Choosing a future for epidemiology: II. from black box to Chinese boxes and eco-epidemiology, *Am J Public Health* 86(5):674, 1996b.

Timmreck TC: *An introduction to epidemiology*, Boston, 1994, Jones & Bartlett.

U.S. Department of Health and Human Services: *Healthy People 2000: national health promotion and disease prevention objectives*, Washington, DC, 1991, USDHHS, Public Health Service.

U.S. Department of Health and Human Services: *Public health service fact sheet*, Washington, DC, 1984, USDHHS, Public Health Service.

continued

Bibliography—cont'd

Vandenbroucke JP: Epidemiology in transition: a historical hypothesis, *Epidemiology* 1(2):164, 1990.

Ventura SJ et al: Births and deaths: preliminary data for 1997, *National Vital Statistics Reports* 47(4):1998.

von Eschenbach AC et al. American Cancer Society guideline for the early detection of prostate cancer: update 1997, *CA Cancer J Clin* 47:261, 1997.

Weinrich S et al: Social support and psychological correlates of high school students who use illicit drugs in response to stress, *J Wellness Perspective* 13:17, 1997.

Weinrich S et al: Work sites: effective sites for recruitment of African American men into prostate cancer screening. *J Community Health Nurs* 15(2):113, 1998.

Weinrich M et al: General population reference ranges for serum prostate specific antigen in Black and White men without cancer, *Urology* 12(6), 1998.

Winkelstein W, French FE, editors: *Basic readings in epidemiology,* ed 3, New York, 1972, MSS Educational Publishing.

Winkelstein W: Editorial: eras, paradigms, and the future of epidemiology, *Am J Public Health* 86(5):621, 1996.

Xu J et al: Evidence for a prostate cancer susceptibility locus on the X chromosome. *Nat Genet* 20:175, 1998.

Research Applications

BEVERLY C. FLYNN & JOYCE S. KROTHE

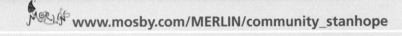 www.mosby.com/MERLIN/community_stanhope

OBJECTIVES

After reading this chapter, the student should be able to do the following:

- Discuss priority areas for research in community and public health nursing with particular attention to primary health care and health promotion.
- Describe the stages of the research process, including methodologic considerations.
- Describe the role of the CHN and others and issues in research.

- Evaluate several community and public health nursing research studies employing both quantitative and qualitative methods.
- Explain ways in which the practicing community and public health nurse can participate in the research process.

KEY TERMS

assumptions
health promotion

human subjects review
  committees
limitations

national health objectives
practice-based research
primary health care

qualitative methods
quantitative methods
research process
See Glossary for definitions

CHAPTER OUTLINE

Research for community and public health nursing has increased over the years. However, nurses must continue to expand the scientific knowledge base unique to their practice to provide high-quality services and creative, scientifically oriented solutions to today's health problems. This is especially important in an environment in which community-oriented practice is increasing.

What is the best way to structure such research? Primary health care, as defined by the World Health Organization (WHO, UNICEF, 1978), is an appropriate framework to guide research and to develop concepts in community and public health nursing. **Practice-based research** questions and the key concepts of primary health care and health promotion, as defined by the World Health Organization (Ottawa Charter, 1986; WHO, UNICEF, 1978), also form an appropriate research framework. This chapter focuses on selected research issues, the roles and functions of the researcher and collaborators, and examples of research from community and public health nursing practice.

RELATIONSHIP OF COMMUNITY AND PUBLIC HEALTH NURSING TO PRIMARY HEALTH CARE

All countries that sent representatives to a world conference in Alma Ata, Russia endorsed primary health care as the best approach for reaching the goal of "health for all by the year 2000" (WHO, UNICEF, 1978). **Primary health care** is essential health care based on practical, scientifically sound, and socially acceptable methods and technology made universally accessible to individuals and families in the community through their full participation and at a cost that the community and country can afford to maintain at every stage of their development in the spirit of self-reliance and self-determination.

Health promotion further supports primary health care. **Health promotion** is "the process of enabling people to increase control over, and to improve, their health" (Ottawa Charter, 1986, p. 1). Five major aspects of health promotion, in order of priority, are 1) building health-promoting public policy, 2) creating supportive environments, 3) strengthening community action, 4) developing personal skills, and 5) reorienting health services.

Community and public health nursing, primary health care, and health promotion are linked to one another. Each incorporates community-oriented practice, involvement of the community in health care decisions and goal setting, a focus on disease prevention and health promotion, and use of an interdisciplinary and multisectoral approach in planning and implementing appropriate solutions to health problems. Because community and public health nursing, primary health care, and health promotion are complementary, research conducted by community and public health nurses can make a significant contribution to primary health care practice.

In response to the complex issues in health care reform, Buhler-Wilkerson (1993) suggests that nurses revisit Lillian Wald's vision of the role of community-oriented nursing.

Community-oriented nursing provides care responsive to clients' needs while "encouraging public responsibility, and providing a unifying structure for the delivery of comprehensive, equally available health care" (Buhler-Wilkerson, 1993, p. 1785). Focusing on individual needs within a social and economic context—a multisectoral approach—is consistent with the philosophy of primary health care and serves as a conceptual framework for research.

Although the past decade has witnessed a renewed emphasis on research-based nursing practice, the roots of nursing research can be traced to Florence Nightingale. Her early emphasis was on careful observation of clients and adaptation of nursing care based on systematic observation rather than trial and error. Nightingale's methodology provided the foundation for the evolution of nursing science and a unique body of research-based nursing knowledge (Brockopp and Hastings-Tolsma, 1994).

THE RESEARCH PROCESS

The nursing process, epidemiologic process, and research process are all problem-solving methods of scientific inquiry. Each involves assessment, planning, implementation, evaluation, and action. The action phase leads to ongoing reassessment, followed by additional planning and implementation. The epidemiologic and research processes develop knowledge. The nursing process uses knowledge in providing health and health-related services to individual clients, families, groups, and communities. The nursing process and the epidemiologic processes as applied to community and public health nursing are discussed elsewhere in this text. The stages of the **research process** are summarized in Box 12-1.

Although the listing is sequential, the researcher actually works back and forth among the various stages of the research process. Decisions made in any one stage must be consistent with decisions made in other stages. All stages are viewed as part of the total study and are arrived at logically and systematically. The following nursing practice examples clarify each stage of the research process.

Assessment/Conceptual Stage

The assessment/conceptual stage involves translating a hunch or curiosity about a clinical problem into a research question. For example, a nurse may wonder why some elderly people in the community can live independently while others enter a nursing home. The nurse reviews related research literature to gain an overview of the situation and the current stage of research in this area. This initial literature review helps the nurse select a purpose and scope for the study. In the example given, the nurse would decide that the purpose of the study is to determine how community and public health nursing services assist elderly persons to live in the community. Next, characteristics of the study population are clearly defined. For example, the study population may include elderly people within a specific age range and who live within a specified

BOX 12-1 Stages of the Research Process

ASSESSMENT/CONCEPTUAL STAGE

Identify a problem for study
Review related literature
Identify the purpose of the research
Choose the population to be studied

PLANNING/DESIGN STAGE

State the research problem
Continue review of related literature
Select a conceptual framework
Select a research design and appropriate methodology
Design the data collection plan
Finalize and review the research plan
Implement human subjects approval process
Implement pilot studies and revisions in design

IMPLEMENTATION/EMPIRICAL STAGE

Invite community members to participate
Implement data collection plan
Prepare data for analysis

EVALUATION/ANALYTICAL STAGE

Analyze the data
Interpret the results
Draw conclusions

ACTION/DISSEMINATION STAGE

Communicate the research findings
Use the findings in practice
Inform health policy makers
Take action for social change
Plan additional research

Selected stages of the research process are modified from Polit DF, Hungler BP: *Essentials of nursing research: methods, appraisal, and utilization*, Philadelphia, 1993, JB Lippincott.

geographic area served by a particular community or public health nursing agency.

Planning/Design Stage

Once a relevant purpose, scope, and study population are selected, the researcher begins the planning/design stage. This is a logical, organized process that proceeds consistently step by step. Planning involves critical thinking and communicating ideas in a clear and logical way, consistent with the format required by potential funding sources.

Designing a research project is a problem-solving process. After identifying a problem for study and formulating a question about the problem, the researcher continues to review related literature, decide on a methodology consistent with the research question, and write a clear proposal. Tornquist and Funk (1990) provide a helpful resource for writing a research proposal. Brink and Wood (1994) point out that not all questions can or need to be answered by research. They define a researchable question

as "an explicit query about a problem or issue that can be challenged, examined, and analyzed and that will yield useful new information" (p. 2). Potential topics for research stem from the thoughts, observations, and practice experiences of the nurse and can be investigated using quantitative or qualitative methods.

In the planning stage, the specific research focus is stated. In the previous example, the nurse decides that the problem to be investigated is a lack of information about the relationship between community and public health nursing services and the ability of elderly people to live independently in the community.

Next, key terms are defined. In the example, the nurse decides that for the purpose of the study, elderly people will be defined as persons 75 years of age or older who live in the geographic area served by a specific community or public health nursing agency. Literature review can be used to define terms and assist in further developing a scientific body of knowledge for nursing practice. In addition, through an extensive literature review, the nurse identifies conceptual frameworks and analyzes how research and data analysis were carried out in previous research studies. Of particular concern is what has been applied in practice based on findings of previous research studies.

The nurse also must select a conceptual framework that is appropriate for the problem to be investigated. In the example, the nurse selects an ecological conceptual framework that can be adapted from the health services research field. This framework incorporates environmental concerns, health services, and client characteristics that are congruent with the basic premise of primary health care.

Next, the nurse outlines specific research questions or hypotheses for the research. These statements include the key variables of the study. The **national health objectives** may be helpful in specifying and defining key variables (USDHHS, 1997). The national health objectives indicate major health concerns for different age groups and provide specific standards that researchers can use to evaluate program progress.

In this example, the nurse questions whether the range of community and public health nursing services for elderly people will enable them to live independently in the community. The national health objectives specify that independence is preserved when there are no more than 90 per 1000 people 65 years of age or older who have difficulty performing two or more personal care activities (USDHHS, 1997). It is hypothesized that the greater the range of community and public health nursing services available, the more elderly people are able to live independently in the community. The key variables are the range of community and public health nursing services and elderly people's performance of personal care activities.

The nurse next selects a research approach appropriate to the phenomenon being investigated; it may be historical, survey, or experimental. Each approach creates different requirements for a research design. Considerations include whether the data will be collected at one point in time or longitudinally and whether the data will be collected from a single group or across various groups in the population. In the example, the nurse decides that a historical approach, or a review of past information, will not adequately address the problem. An experimental approach is not feasible because the study cannot be conducted under controlled conditions. Instead, the nurse decides that a survey is the most appropriate approach for comparing elderly people living independently in the community with use of community and public health nursing services. This approach permits a research design for collecting data during one time period.

Planning also should include consideration of methodologies appropriate to the research question. **Quantitative methods** have been the dominant methodology in nursing research. However, there is a growing acceptance of nursing science as a composite of different perspectives and varied research methodologies. Although recognition of **qualitative methods** as a tool of science is rather recent in the nursing literature, its tradition in the United States began during the late 1800s. "At that time, qualitative strategies were used to disclose the rapidly developing social problems in cities pursuant to industrialization, urbanization, and mass immigration. Qualitative descriptions encouraged social change by making urban problems visible to the public" (Munhall and Boyd, 1993, p. 72).

Traditional scientific inquiry is usually referred to as *quantitative research.* This method advocates objectively gathering data that can be verified by another researcher and generalized to other populations. These methods are characterized by deductive reasoning, objectivity, quasi-experiments, statistical techniques, and control.

Although many nursing research questions are amenable to traditional methodologies, others require a different approach. Qualitative methods may be more compatible with a particular phenomenon being studied. This method is characterized by inductive reasoning, subjectivity, discovery, description, and the meaning of an experience to an individual or group (Brockopp and Hastings-Tolsma, 1994).

"One of the most obvious differences between qualitative and quantitative studies is the apparent absence of standardized procedures to follow when using particular qualitative methods. The hallmark of good qualitative methodology is its variability, rather than its standardization." (Popay, Rogers, and Williams, 1998, p. 346). This statement does not preclude the fact that there are explicit methods to draw upon when conducting a qualitative study.

DID YOU KNOW? *Although the dominant methodology used in nursing research has been quantitative, there is a growing acceptance of nursing science as a composite of different perspectives and thereby of quantitative and qualitative research methodologies (Munhall and Boyd, 1993)*

Munhall and Boyd (1993) suggest that nurse researchers will find a congruence between nursing's philosophical embrace of humanism and holism and qualitative methodologies. At the same time, "not every research interest can be accommodated by the qualitative perspective, nor should nursing . . . adopt a single method for developing knowledge about . . . the multi-dimensional world of nursing" (Munhall and Boyd, 1993, p. 74).

Sarter (1988) noted that during the 1980s the paths to nursing knowledge were broadened to include qualitative methods. This broadening affords nurse scholars access to human experience. Many nurse theorists think it is important to understand the clients' perspective in order to provide appropriate nursing care.

Once the researcher has considered methodologic options, the next stage involves selecting a data-gathering method, such as observing, measuring, or interviewing. The researcher identifies specific techniques or instruments that are consistent with the research design. For example, if a questionnaire is considered for data collection, a specific instrument can be selected, such as picture questionnaires instead of print for subjects who cannot read.

Since decisions need to be made about a data-gathering method for each of the major variables in the research study, the researcher may decide to use more than one instrument. In the example described previously, the nurse may decide to use both observing and interviewing methods. The nurse researcher will observe community and public health nurses who provide services to elderly people to determine the scope and range of services provided. To avoid making nurses and clients feel uncomfortable about being observed, the nurse researcher can use qualitative methodology and participant observation in working with the nurses. Thus the nurse researcher will participate in a natural situation for data collection. In addition to observation, a quantitative method, such as an interview questionnaire, may be used to determine the level of physical functioning of elderly people.

The research questions and methodologies chosen guide the plan for data analysis. It is useful to identify the computer software available to assist with data analysis and also to decide how findings will be presented. For example, the researcher may want to design sample tables for the data once they are collected. These tables will help ensure that all the data necessary to answer the research questions have been collected.

The research questions and plan for data analysis guide sample selection. The research method to be used directs the sample size. There are many methods of sample selection, but two will be considered here: random and deliberate sampling. Random sampling means that every case or participant has an equal opportunity to be included in the study. Deliberate sampling means that specific persons are invited to participate in the study. Choice of research methodologies will determine the characteristics of the sample population.

In this example the nurse decides to study elderly persons within the geographic boundaries served by a nursing agency. After consultation with a statistician, the nurse decides that the sample should consist of 100 persons over 75 years of age living in the community. This figure is based on an estimated sample size required for the statistics selected. The researcher may use power analysis software that can help determine sample size. Of course, it is impossible to know the exact number of elderly people living in the community, so the nurse estimates the total elderly population based on census data. A deliberate sample of persons 75 years of age and older is selected until 100 are included in the sample.

Important in the design phase is research approval by the institutional **human subjects review committees.** These are groups of representatives of various related disciplines or departments brought together to review research proposals. Their major concerns are protecting human research participants from physical or mental harm, as well as protecting the researcher from undue complaints. This process also satisfies a number of funding agencies and federal, state, and institutional regulations.

In the example, the local health department has a committee that reviews research proposals involving health department services. The nurse researcher must obtain approval from the committee before the research begins. The first step is to communicate clearly in writing to the review committee what is planned, how participants will be involved in the research, and whether their participation will put them at risk for physical or mental harm. The researcher is ethically responsible for carrying out these plans as directed or approved by the committee. Changes that occur in the plans need to be reported to the committee for further sanctioning.

Pilot studies can be used to test data-gathering methods and to apply the data analysis plan. A pilot study is especially important when the data-gathering technique is unfamiliar to the researcher: the instrument may be new, it may not have been used with the population under study, or the study may be conducted in an unfamiliar environment. The nurse researcher in the example decides to pilot test the study with five elderly clients from a neighboring county after obtaining permission from both the nurse and the clients.

Next, the assumptions and limitations of research need to be identified. **Assumptions** are characteristics of the research situation that are not explored, usually because they have been well demonstrated in previous research. An assumption of the fictitious study is that some community services enable elderly people to live independently in the community.

Limitations are uncontrollable elements of the research. They limit the certainty of the findings or their applicability to the population in general. In this study, a limitation is that deliberate sampling does not ensure that all elderly people are equally represented. As a result, the study findings may not be applicable beyond the study sample.

Implementation/Empirical Stage

The implementation/empirical stage of the research plan refers to the carrying out of the research procedures. This stage includes inviting the sample group members to participate, obtaining their informed consent, collecting and verifying the data, and analyzing the data. The nurse researcher may send a letter to potential participants inviting them to participate. After a follow-up phone call, an appointment is arranged with the client and the nurse. At this meeting the participants, both the client and the nurse, are asked to give their signed informed consent to participate in the study.

The nurse researcher then collects data through observation and interviews. Information collected in qualitative studies is validated with the participants. Depending on methodologic choices, data analysis occurs concomitantly with data collection (qualitative methodology) or at the conclusion of the data collection phase (quantitative methodology).

Regardless of methodologic considerations, data collection and analysis follow specified guidelines. "Like empirical method, each qualitative approach requires certain steps, in a certain order, according to certain rules, and is thus subject to certain measures of the value of research findings. Merely interviewing people does not place a study in the qualitative paradigm" (Munhall and Boyd, 1993 p. 90). Qualitative research is characterized by prolonged contact with the phenomenon being studied, thus capturing the insider's or emic construction. It is holistic and contextual, meaning that a particular phenomenon is not isolated for study but examined in the natural setting. The researcher must be aware of the guidelines of all methodologies used.

Evaluation/Analytical Stage

The evaluation/analytical stage includes analyzing the findings and comparing them with previous research results. Conclusions are then drawn, building on a body of previous knowledge. Research reports should provide clear documentation of what was done and when. The results of the research for the specific problem, research questions, or hypotheses under study are presented. If the research design is quantitative, hypotheses that were not supported also need to be reported. Recommendations for future research should be clear and consistent with the study results. The need for replication studies should be specified. Replication studies with other populations are useful because recommendations for practice should be based on more than one set of study results. The research findings are presented to professional colleagues; to persons in decision-making positions, such as administrators, policy makers, and legislators; and to the general public, which might be affected by any decisions made.

In the hypothetical research example, the study findings indicated that the greater the range of community or public health nursing services, the greater the ability of elderly people to live independently. Future research should include information regarding severity of health problems. The nurse researcher presented the findings to the administrators and staff at the local health department, to the county-wide senior citizen organization, to professional colleagues at their annual meeting, to a reporter for an article in a local paper, and to the state legislative committee responsible for formulating policy for community care.

Action/Dissemination Stage

The results of nursing research should be used in practice. Nurses must make specific recommendations based on research findings to improve the health of the community. By applying research results in practice, nurses can institute social change. Policy makers, other professionals, and the community learn that the research findings are relevant and applicable to practice. For example, based on findings of a research study of the needs of elderly people, policy implications for community long-term care are suggested (Krothe, 1997).

The results of such a study could support the expansion of community or public health nursing services. The economic difference between maintaining elderly clients in their homes and placing them in an institution could be a compelling argument in support of expanded home health care services. Research documenting the cost effectiveness of nursing care is vitally needed. Such effectiveness is measured in many ways beyond cost, including quality of care, client satisfaction, and the ability to maintain independence.

Research results can help agencies develop research programs within their organizations. The results should be presented to clinical audiences. Research experiences can mobilize staff nurses to build a program of research around common clinical problems. Reporting the results of research outcomes in professional journals and at professional meetings also facilitates the growth and use of nursing knowledge (Brockopp and Hastings-Tolsma, 1994). Consistent with primary health care and health promotion approaches, relevant research findings must also be reported to community groups. This information can become part of the community's educational experience and help the community make appropriate decisions based on local needs.

HOW TO *Apply Research Findings in Practice*

One way to provide quality community and public health nursing services is to apply research findings in practice. Some ways to do this are as follows:

1. *Read journals that report research relevant to practice, for example* Public Health Nursing, Nursing Research, *the* American Journal of Public Health, *or* Family and Community Health.
2. *Begin a research discussion group with colleagues, and identify who is responsible for reviewing research in these journals.*
3. *Form a journal club.*
4. *Discuss the quality of research studies.*
5. *Obtain research assistance, such as with statistical analysis and research methods, if needed.*
6. *Identify research findings that can be applied to practice.*
7. *Discuss clinical practice situations in which the findings can be applied.*
8. *Apply the findings and evaluate results.*
9. *Discuss what has been found.*
10. *Describe the research findings and the application to practice to nursing administrators and policy makers.*
11. *Post brief summaries of research findings in prominent locations in the work place.*
12. *Distribute research findings that have application to practice to colleagues via electronic mail.*

Data-based information from nursing research should be communicated to policy makers at the local, state, and national levels. Research findings thus inform health policy makers and create responsive policy formulation (Flynn, Rider, and Ray, 1991).

PRACTICE-GENERATED QUESTIONS FOR RESEARCH

Significant questions for research can be generated from community and public health nursing practice in response to everyday observations in the field. Brink and Wood (1994) identify the point at which observation ceases to be an everyday occurrence and becomes genuine research: "It stops being a normal part of everyday life and becomes research if it is systematically planned and recorded. This makes the difference between simply observing the world around you and collecting research data through observation" (p. 147).

Practicing nurses often have difficulty identifying potential questions for research that arise from their practice. They may not consider research as part of their practice.

NURSING TIP

Research is problem solving with empirical evidence. You can identify researchable problems by asking yourself what scientific or theoretical basis you have for how you are doing things.

The following discussion focuses on examples of questions for research that are generated in practice. These questions are grouped by the concepts of primary health care: accessibility, community involvement, disease prevention and health promotion, appropriate technology, and multisectoral approach.

Accessible Health Care

Accessibility of health services refers to the extent to which community and public health nursing services reach people who need them the most and how equitably these services are distributed throughout the population. A question for research related to this concept is whether nursing services are accessible to those in greatest need (see Research Brief about the epidemiologic survey done in Ontario):

- Are the services available to groups of people most in need of them in terms of time, location, and personnel?
- Are these services available in both urban and rural areas?
- Who uses and who does not use the nursing services?
- What are the health care needs of the people who use the service compared with those who do not?
- What are the barriers to the use of services?
- Are the costs too high?
- Are the services relevant to consumers' perceived needs?
- Are nurses sensitive to the concerns of consumers?
- Do consumers have transportation to reach the services?
- Are services offered at times when those most in need of them are able to access them?

RESEARCH *Brief*

This study explores the mental and physical health status and use of services among the informal caregivers of the chronically ill, elderly, disabled, and mentally ill in Ontario, Canada. Research participants were identified by stratification and multistage probability sampling of respondents in the Ontario Health Survey, a community-oriented epidemiologic survey. The main objectives of the study were to compare characteristics of caregivers with noncaregivers in the community and determine whether being a caregiver is associated with various physical or mental health problems and use of services. The following statistical tests were used: chi-square statistic; t tests; and proportions (95% confidence intervals around the proportions). The results of the study indicated that caregivers had higher rates of mental health disorders than noncaregivers and used mental health services at twice the rate of noncaregivers. It provided important information about potential unmet needs of caregivers, as well as implications for nursing practice and policy considerations for governments that increasingly advocate community care.

Cochrane JJ, Goering PN, Rogers JM: The mental health of informal caregivers in Ontario: an epidemiological survey, *American Journal of Public Health* 87(12):2002, 1997.

HOW TO *Identify Researchable Problems*

Community and public health nursing practice presents daily problems and successes. The following are questions that can help identify researchable problems:

1. *What examples from your clinical practice seem to lead to successful outcomes?*
2. *Are there examples from your clinical practice that continue to cause problems?*
3. *What differences are there in access to health services or health status in the population you are serving? Why do these differences exist?*
4. *What can be done to address these discrepancies?*
5. *What Healthy People national health objectives standards pertain to populations you work with?*
6. *What does the research literature say about identifying problems for research? What has worked or not worked in practice?*
7. *What questions for research come to mind? How would you compare two or more different approaches for dealing with the same problem. How would you design a study with a control group.*
8. *What are the ethics of such a comparison? Can you offer different services to different populations without jeopardizing the quality of care?*

Community Involvement

Community involvement is concerned with the level of participation of community residents in health care decision making. To promote community development and self-reliance, residents need to participate in decisions about the community's health. Residents and health providers need to work together to identify problems and seek solutions.

Questions for research generated from practice relate to the level and mechanism of community involvement in health decision making. For example, to what extent is the community involved in the various stages of assessing health care needs, planning, management, and monitoring nursing services? What mechanisms and processes can people use to be actively involved and to take joint responsibility, along with nurses, for decisions? In particular, what decisions involving the community have been implemented and evaluated? Is use of nursing services improved as a result?

Disease Prevention and Health Promotion

Community and public health focuses on health promotion and prevention of disease rather than on curative services. Examples are activities that include physical exercise, seat belt use, smoking cessation, and other healthful lifestyle changes (see Research Brief about health promotion for immigrant women).

Priority questions for research include the following: What are the major preventable health problems in the community? For example, are there high rates of automobile accidents or heart disease in a particular community? Are problems being addressed by preventive and health-

RESEARCH *Brief*

The author examines the health promotion beliefs and practices of immigrant women and how their cultural values influence their health promotion behaviors. The methodology for the research study was a descriptive ethnographic study, permitting an emic view yielding data within a cultural context that could not be gained from a standardized survey instrument. Health promotion activities were found to be closely tied to activities of daily living and contextually related to the health and well-being of the entire family, rather than for individual well-being per se. The effects of migration were found to interfere with women's ability to continue some health promoting behaviors; for example, climatic changes between India and Canada significantly decreased walking activities. Nurses should be aware of the effects of migration and culture on health behaviors and integrate these into health promotion activities.

Choudhry UK: Health promotion among immigrant women from India living in Canada, *Image J Nurs Sch* 30(3):269, 1998

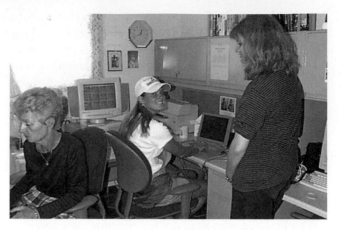

FIG. 12-1 Computerized nursing record systems are an example of technological changes that affect nursing practice and research.

by their users, and are in harmony with the environment" (p. 1).

The overriding questions include the following:
- Do the services use the simplest and least costly technology available?
- Are the services acceptable to the community?
- Are they affordable initially and over time?
- What is the cost effectiveness of alternative approaches or strategies for nursing services?
- Are family home visits as effective as working with families in groups?
- Are nonprofessionals, such as home health aides and community health workers, effective in providing some aspects of nursing services?
- What are the most effective management and supervisory techniques for nonprofessionals and professionals within a nursing agency?

There are technology changes that affect nursing practice and research. For example, more people have access to computers. Nurses may have computerized record systems that offer new opportunities for data collection and analysis (Fig. 12-1).

promoting measures? What measures are being taken to reduce or control these problems? Are they culturally relevant? Do the nursing services include recommendations for infant car seat use, programs to reduce alcohol intake among drivers, smoking cessation programs, and programs that promote health in schools?

DID YOU KNOW? *Nurses conduct research that addresses significant issues in the broader environment. The Institute of Medicine's study of Nursing Health and the Environment (Pope, Snyder, and Mood, 1995) reported that nursing research focused on populations at risk for health problems, including agricultural workers, industrial workers, health service providers, pregnant women, new mothers, and disabled people. Health hazards studied by nurses included pesticides, accidents, lead exposure, and natural disasters.*

Appropriate Technology

Appropriate technology refers to health care that is both relevant and acceptable to people's health needs and concerns. It includes issues of cost and affordability of services within the context of existing resources, such as the number and type of health professionals and other providers, equipment, and supplies and their pattern of distribution throughout the community. The National Science Foundation's definition (1979) of *appropriate technology* summarizes these considerations: "Appropriate technologies are defined as those which are decentralized, require low capital investment, conserve natural resources, are managed

Multisectoral Approach

The health of a community cannot be improved by intervention only within the health sector. Other sectors are equally important in promoting the community's health and self-reliance. For example, education, business, environment, the faith community, industry, housing, and nutrition are interrelated with health. Therefore these sectors need to work together to coordinate their goals, plans, and activities to ensure that they contribute to the health of the community and to avoid conflicting or duplicating efforts (see Research Brief about health care delivery in faith communities).

Relevant questions for research include the following:
- What mechanisms exist that promote or hinder multisectoral collaboration?

RESEARCH *Brief*

The authors trace commonalities in philosophies of the nursing profession and faith communities through history to empower people and enhance their self-care capacity to the present day model of parish nursing. They note an absence in the literature of evidence-based research on parish nursing and outcome-based practice. The purpose of this exploratory study was to document implementation by parish nurses of the *Healthy People 2000* objectives to build partnerships to enhance the health of the community. The method used was a descriptive retrospective study using monthly parish nurse reports and interviews with parish nurses. Implementation of *Healthy People 2000* objectives were identified across the life span from retrospective review of reports and validation during interviews. Community partnerships developed, for example, when parish nurses addressed the *Healthy People 2000* objectives 9.6 and 9.17 related to home and fire safety and formed a partnership with firefighters to secure smoke detectors for individuals who needed them. Results of this study support parish nursing as a model to address challenges set forth in *Healthy People 2000* for effective delivery of health services in the community and building community coalitions to address health needs.

Weis D, Matheus R, Schank MJ: Health care delivery in faith communities: the parish nurse model, *Public Health Nursing* 14(6):368, 1997.

- Do the committees or task forces that address community-wide concerns represent various fields, such as education, industry, housing, transportation, and health?
- What are examples of multisectoral efforts in seeking solutions to community problems?
- How were successful solutions derived in the past?
- What factors contributed to their success?
- What conflicts exist across sectors?
- How are conflicting activities across the various sectors resolved?
- What are the gaps in efforts across the various sectors in solving community health problems?

ROLES AND ISSUES IN RESEARCH

Although some of the roles of the nurse researcher and the issues related to research are presented in other sections of this chapter, additional aspects are worthy of consideration.

Relationships

The practicing nurse may conduct research or work with a researcher within an organization to carry out a study. The practicing nurse, the administrator of nursing services, and the researcher can also be partners in a joint endeavor.

Partners each have their own areas of expertise, but they benefit from the expertise of the others. The nurse, as an expert in practice, can identify problems that must be researched and the feasibility of various research designs. The administrator can help identify policy issues related to the research and can provide organizational and financial support. The researcher can help develop practice problems into researchable questions, suggest appropriate research methods, and collect and analyze data.

The nurse may also work with the community group concerned with the research problem. Citizens, professionals, and other persons interested in community health may identify a priority problem for research. In this case, persons in the group have expertise about the community, and the researcher and the nurse work as resources to the group in conducting the research.

Involving others in the research process is not without problems. Perhaps the most difficult aspect for researchers is sharing activities that usually fall under their domain, such as involving others in identifying the important questions to be researched. Because nursing research often takes place in a dynamic setting in which the chief responsibility is health care (e.g., a neighborhood clinic), priority may be given to clinical commitments rather than to research. For example, access to records and files may be controlled by others, and client information may be withheld by the agency. As a result, the research itself may become part of the politics of the situation. Researchers need to be aware of these dynamics and use their expertise to ensure that the research is conducted with proper attention to sound principles. Skills in communication and collaboration are essential to the process.

Communication

Communication with participants, co-researchers, nursing practitioners, administrators, community residents, and policy makers is important throughout the research process. Communication can take many forms. The researcher needs to consider the appropriateness of verbal, written, and visual aids in clarifying information being presented. Often the researcher has an academic background and appointment and has been socialized differently from practitioners and community citizens. Because researchers in nursing are often practitioners first, this gap may be closed. Even so, the researcher must carefully consider how the information is presented, including the level of understanding of the reader or listener, and be attentive to issues of concern to the audience being addressed. The format of presentation will vary depending on whether the audience is a group of academic researchers, practicing nurses, policy makers, or community citizens.

Information must be disseminated about the research early in the study and throughout the project. Negative findings, such as the discovery that nursing intervention did not reduce costs, must be presented along with positive results. A focus on concepts rather than on the specific program being studied may facilitate the acceptance of negative findings.

Ethics and the Researcher Role

Ethical issues need careful attention when research of any type is conducted. Ethical issues arise out of conflicting social pressures between the profession and society. For example, should one publish the results of research when the findings reflect negatively on a particular group? This information may be taken out of context and used to limit government funding of services to a particular group. In addition it may promote victim blaming.

WHAT DO YOU THINK? *The nurse researcher has an ethical responsibility to report both positive and negative results of research regardless of the consequences to nursing programs being studied.*

Ethical issues also must be considered in designing a study. For example, nurses may wish to evaluate the effectiveness of a home health agency's policies for the care of clients with acquired immunodeficiency syndrome (AIDS). It would be unethical to assign a group of clients with AIDS as a control group if that meant withholding information about the diagnosis from the nurses providing nursing services to these clients.

Dilemmas may arise over ensuring the confidentiality of responses, disclosing the actual purpose of the research to the respondents, or even disseminating results of the research to the respondents. As noted previously, research plans are under close scrutiny by human subjects review committees in institutions today. The researcher is ethically responsible for carrying out these plans as directed or approved by the committee. Changes that occur in research plans must be reported to the committee for further sanctioning.

There are also ethical considerations in data reporting. This issue is important in nursing research because few replication studies exist. Fraudulent research data and results of health-related research have been published. The effects of this can be widespread, affecting not only the profession but also, more importantly, persons in the community and policy formulation.

Position of Researcher in Employment Setting

Those who employ the researcher and potential uncertainties about the authority structure are often major sources of concern for the nurse researcher. In an academic setting the researcher may be a faculty member who also has responsibilities for classroom teaching, clinical supervision of students, academic advising, and committee work. To be involved in a major research effort, the faculty member typically will need to be relieved of some of these responsibilities. Consideration can be given to a semester of full-time research, a reduction in teaching responsibilities and committee work, or some combination of these for the du-

ration of the project. Support of release time is often facilitated when researchers obtain external funding for a portion of their salary.

It may be possible to establish more innovative employment opportunities in research: status as a visiting scholar or visiting researcher within a community organization or university, shared positions between universities and other organizations, or the promotion of sabbatical leave opportunities between service and academic institutions. When researchers are hired by community organizations, they should clarify their research role. Questions should include the following:

- What are the other expectations for this position (e.g., service, administration, or other research)?
- How will the results be disseminated if they reflect negative features of a service program or a professional group?
- If the organization chooses not to disseminate a research report, what happens to the researcher's work?
- Does the researcher have continued access to the data?
- Can the researcher prepare papers for presentation at professional meetings and in the professional literature?

Researchers need to establish a clear understanding with their employers and administrators about the organization of and expectations for their work, as well as the organization's authority in relation to publication and the researcher's access to data for professional purposes.

Another aspect that needs to be reemphasized relates to the action phase of the research process. For example, after completing an investigation, the results are found to be significant for nursing practice. The researcher must use the results in practice. He or she also must see that the findings are clearly understood by relevant others, such as administrators, nurses, legislators, or citizens in the community. The nurse researcher may need to communicate research findings to legislators so that appropriate policies and legislation are enacted. At this point, the link between research and practice can become reality.

Funding of Research

A final issue is obtaining funds for research. Some federal funding is available for nursing research through agencies such as the National Institute of Nursing Research and the Agency for Health Care Policy and Research. However, obtaining money for research, especially federal funding, is increasingly competitive. For this reason, the pursuit of funding from voluntary foundations and organizations should not be overlooked. Private foundations, such as the Robert Wood Johnson Foundation or the W.K. Kellogg Foundation, offer program funding that can include evaluation research.

State and local funding sources include community foundations, local chapters of Sigma Theta Tau, regional nursing research societies, the March of Dimes, the American Heart Association, the American Cancer Society, hospitals, and corporations. Universities may offer small grants for faculty members to initiate research. Local and state health departments offer program grants through maternal child health or various preventive block grants that have evaluation research components. Employers can sometimes grant release time from work so that educators, administrators, consultants, and practitioners can conduct research.

Table 12-1 provides a summary of selected examples of funding sources. Researchers need to explore alternative funding sources, be aware of new funding initiatives, and design creative financing options.

Mechanisms for collaborative research also need to be established and funded. Research institutes and centers with connections between community groups, health care organizations, industries, and universities can facilitate research in community and public health nursing. Such institutes can promote interdisciplinary collaboration to study community health problems and practice issues. The institutes also provide a unique environment for the de-

lineation and articulation of the various research roles. The institutes afford collaborative opportunities for community residents, students, educators, and service personnel to seek solutions to community health problems. Joint financing could be arranged between a community group, a service agency, and a university for research.

SUGGESTIONS FOR PARTICIPATION IN RESEARCH

Practicing nurses can participate in each stage of the research process. They are in key positions to identify clinical problems to be researched. Nurses can take anecdotal notes about clinical situations that will help in identifying key variables for study. They also can read research on the topic of concern and discuss observations with other nursing colleagues, including researchers. Frequently, nurse researchers work in universities and are more than willing to collaborate in joint research efforts. Practicing nurses can assist researchers in securing institutional approval to conduct research and in facilitating access to research participants. They also may be involved in data collection, whether for pilot studies, replication studies, or original research. The nurse may be a participant in research by answering questionnaires and participating in interviews or by being observed in practice.

> **WHAT DO YOU THINK?** *Baccalaureate nursing students can participate in the research process. They can be involved in planning and implementing research studies with faculty guidance and mentoring.*

Nurses can provide valuable insights into study findings, often explaining relationships, or a lack thereof, to researchers. They can apply relevant research findings in practice. They also can explain or report on research findings to community members, administrators, policy makers, and others, thus initiating action for social change.

Nurses work with community members in improving their health. They can help seek and identify scientifically oriented solutions to health and nursing problems; thus they are in a key position to develop knowledge that can be used in practice and that has implications for health policy.

clinical application

Laura and Jennifer, two senior baccalaureate nursing students in the community health nursing course, had their clinical experience at an outreach site of a rural nurse managed clinic. They were involved with the owner of a local sock factory in planning for disease prevention and health promotion activities for the employees. After consulting with the faculty members responsible for the course and the nurse managed clinic, they designed a survey to distribute to employees to assess their needs for health education programming. The students submitted the survey

continued

TABLE 12-1 Examples of Funding Sources for Research

Level of Funding	Funding Source
NATIONAL	
Federal	National Institutes of Health
	National Institute for Nursing Research
	National Cancer Institute
	Agency for Health Care Policy and Research
Private/voluntary	W.K. Kellogg Foundation
	Robert Wood Johnson Foundation
	Pew Charitable Trusts
	Rockefeller Foundation
	American Cancer Society
	American Heart Association
	American Diabetes Foundation
STATE	
Public	State department of health
	Department of family and social services
	State universities
Private/voluntary	March of Dimes
	State hospital association
	State cancer society
	State heart association
	State nurses association
	Corporations
LOCAL	
Public	Health department
Private/voluntary	Sigma Theta Tau chapters
	Regional nursing research societies
	March of Dimes
	Business and industry

clinical application—cont'd

to the university's institutional review board for approval before distributing it to the employees.

One of the employee priorities identified from the survey data was to establish a smoking cessation program for factory employees. The students met with the factory owner, the faculty members, and a representative of the local chapter of the American Lung Association to plan for implementation of this initiative. A time line was established to notify employees of an opportunity to participate in the smoking cessation program. This included notices distributed in employee paychecks and signs posted in prominent locations throughout the factory.

The students discussed plans for conducting a research study related to implementation and evaluation of the smoking cessation program with the faculty members. Which action would be a logical first step in planning for the research study?

A. Distribute written materials to all employees summarizing the harmful health effects of smoking.

B. Design a data-collection plan to gather a smoking history from participants before they enroll in the program.

C. Discuss with the factory owner incentives for employees who complete the program.

D. Implement a phase-in plan for a smoke free work environment, including a smoke-free lounge.

Answer is found in the back of the book.

KEY POINTS

- Although research for community and public health nursing practice has developed over the years, community and public health nurses need to increase their scientific research base.
- Community and public health nursing, primary health care, and health promotion are complementary. Research conducted by community and public health nurses can make a significant contribution to nursing practice and also to primary health care.
- The research process is a problem-solving process. It involves assessment, planning, implementation, evaluation, and action.

- Significant questions for research can be generated from community and public health nursing practice and linked with the key concepts of primary health care.
- Community participation is a key concept of primary health care and is concerned with the level of citizen involvement in health decision making.
- Potential questions to be answered by research address the basic concepts of primary health care and health promotion.
- The ethical issues in research need thoughtful attention by the nurse researcher.
- The issue of who employs the researcher and potential uncertainties about the authority structure are often major sources of concern for the nurse researcher.
- Federal money for research is competitive. Researchers and others need to locate alternative funding sources and use creative financing options.
- Clinical applications of selected community and public health nursing studies are suggested to improve services and promote policy change.

critical thinking activities

1. Identify one priority problem that has relevance to community and public health nursing practice that could be researched in the community.
2. From your community and public health nursing experiences, specify a research question that you can relate to one of the concepts of primary health care.
3. Identify a research study in the literature relevant to community and public health nursing, and identify the strengths and limitations of the research.
4. Talk with a community member, a community or public health nurse, a researcher, and an administrator who have been involved in research. Ask them about their roles and functions in research. What were the sources of role strain?
5. Identify three funding sources for research in community and public health nursing.
6. From the literature, identify research findings, one in a research study that uses quantitative methods and one that uses qualitative methods, that can be applied in community and public health nursing practice.
7. Identify a researchable topic based on your community and public health nursing practice that has implications for health care reform.
8. Communicate the findings of a nursing research study that support community care to a policy maker at the local, state, or national level.

Bibliography

Ahljevych K, Bernhard L: Health-promoting behaviors of African American women, *Nurs Res* 43(2):86, 1994.

Black ME et al: The impact of a public health nurse intervention on influenza vaccine acceptance, *Am J Public Health* 83(12):1751, 1993.

Brink PJ, Wood MJ: *Basic steps in planning nursing research: from question to proposal*, Boston, 1994, Jones & Bartlett.

Brockopp DY, Hastings-Tolsma MT: *Fundamentals of nursing research*, Boston, 1994, Jones & Bartlett.

Buhler-Wilkerson K: Bringing care to the people: Lillian Wald's legacy to public health nursing, *Am J Public Health* 83(12):1778, 1993.

Choudhry UK: Health promotion among immigrant women from India living in Canada, *Image J Nurs Sch* 30(3):269, 1998.

Cochrane JJ, Goering PN, Rogers, JM: The mental health of informal caregivers in Ontario: an epidemiological survey, *Am J Public Health* 87(12):2002, 1997.

Flynn BC, Rider M, Ray DW: Healthy cities: the Indiana model of community development in public health, *Health Educ Q* 18(3):331, 1991.

Hansell MJ: Sociodemographic factors and the quality of prenatal care, *Am J Public Health* 81(8):1023, 1991.

Jemmott LS, Jemmott JB: Increasing condom-use intentions among sexually active black adolescent women, *Nurs Res* 41(5):273, 1992.

Krothe JS: Giving voice to elderly people: community-based long-term care, *Public Health Nursing* 14(4):217, 1997.

Long KA, Boik RJ: Predicting alcohol use in rural children: a longitudinal study, *Nurs Res* 42(2):79, 1993.

Munhall PL, Boyd CO: *Nursing research: a qualitative perspective,* New York, 1993, National League for Nursing.

National Science Foundation: *NSF announcements for December, NSF bulletin,* Washington, DC, 1979, the Foundation.

Polit DF, Hungler BP: *Essentials of nursing research: methods, appraisal, and utilization,* Philadelphia, 1993, JB Lippincott.

Popay J, Rogers A, Williams G: Rational and standards for the systematic review of qualitative literature in health services research, *Qualitative Health Research* 8(3), 341, 1998.

Pope AM, Snyder MA, Mood L, editors: *Nursing health and environment: strengthening the relationship to improve the public's health,* Washington, DC, 1995, National Academy Press.

Rickelman BL, Gallman L, Parra H: Attachment and quality of life in older, community-residing men, *Nurs Res* 43(2);68, 1994.

Sarter B, editor: *Paths to knowledge: innovative research methods for nursing,* New York, 1988, National League for Nursing.

Tornquist EM, Funk SG: How to write a research grant proposal, *Image J Nurs Scholarship* 22:44, 1990.

US Department of Health and Human Services: *Developing objectives for Healthy People 2010,* Washington, DC, 1997, USDHHS, Office of Disease Prevention and Health Promotion.

Weis D, Matheus R, Schank MJ: Health care delivery in faith communities: the parish nurse model, *Public Health Nursing* 14(6):368, 1997

World Health Organization: *Ottawa Charter for health promotion,* Copenhagen, 1986, WHO.

World Health Organization, UNICEF: *Primary health care: a joint report,* Geneva, 1978, WHO.

Educational Theories, Models, and Principles Applied to Community and Public Health Nursing

LISA L. ONEGA

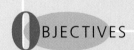 **O**BJECTIVES

www.mosby.com/MERLIN/community_stanhope

After reading this chapter, the student should be able to do the following:

- Evaluate six educational theories as they relate to community and public health nurse educators.
- Analyze three models for effective health education.
- Discuss three categories of educational principles.

- Explain the five steps of the educational process.
- Describe the importance of evaluating the educational product.
- Design an educational plan for an identified high-risk community group.

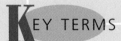 **K**EY TERMS

affective domain	critical theory	humanist theory	short-term evaluation
behavioral theory	developmental theory	long-term evaluation	social learning theory
cognitive domain	health belief model	PRECEDE-PROCEED model	
cognitive theory	health promotion model	psychomotor domain	*See Glossary for definitions*

CHAPTER OUTLINE

General Educational Theories
  Behavioral Theory
  Social Learning Theory
  Cognitive Theory
  Humanist Theory
  Developmental Theory
  Critical Theory
Health Education Models
  PRECEDE-PROCEED Model
  Health Belief Model
  Health Promotion Model

Nurses' Application of Health
  Education Models
Educational Principles
  Nature of Learning
  Events of Instruction
  Effective Educator
Educational Process
  Identify Educational Needs
  Establish Educational Goals
   and Objectives

Select Appropriate Educational
  Methods
Implement the Educational
  Plan
Evaluate the Educational
  Process
Educational Product
  Evaluation of Health and
   Behavioral Changes
  Short-Term Evaluation
  Long-Term Evaluation

The author wishes to thank Douglas C. Forness for his assistance with designing and developing the boxes, figure, and tables for this chapter.

ealth education is a vital part of community and public health nursing. The promotion, maintenance, and restoration of health requires that community and public health clients receive a practical understanding of health-related information. Community and public health clients include individuals, families, and communities. An individual is any person regardless of age, gender, or other characteristic. Families are a group of individuals linked by ancestry, marriage, or household and may consist of nuclear, extended, biological, adoptive, or another alternative makeup. A community may be a small group, support system, club, church, school, neighborhood, or loosely tied and widely scattered group with a common interest or cause.

Because nurses see clients with varying needs and abilities in a variety of settings, they are in key positions to deliver health education. The information that nurses provide enables clients to make knowledgeable decisions, cope more effectively with alterations in their health and lifestyles, and assume greater personal responsibility for their health (Graham, 1992).

In a time of growing health care costs and increasing collaboration between health service providers and consumers, clients are increasingly sharing responsibility for their own health maintenance. Nurses educate consumers about ways to manage their own health processes more effectively (Clarke, Beddome, and Whyte, 1993). As people live longer, they often experience the chronic illnesses related to aging that require complex changes in diet, exercise, lifestyle, and medical treatments. Health education becomes crucial to health care because of such social changes (Annand, 1993). Also, attainment and maintenance of the objectives of *Healthy People 2000* depend heavily on community-oriented programs to promote healthy habits and lifestyles (USDHHS, 1991).

Healthy People 2000 sets forth a strategy for improving national health by describing objectives that, if attained and maintained, are designed to prevent major chronic illness, injuries, and infectious diseases. Education, a primary strategy in assisting people to change their habits, is provided in a wide variety of community health settings including schools, homes, the workplace, and ambulatory and inpatient health care facilities (USDHHS, 1991).

While the accomplishment and maintenance of a number of the objectives of *Healthy People 2000* relies on educational strategies, several objectives specifically address health education (USDHHS, 1991). These are listed in Box 13-1. Currently, *Healthy People 2010* is being developed to establish national health objectives for the next decade. Two overarching goals of *Healthy People 2010* are 1) to increase quality of years and healthy life and 2) to eliminate health disparities. Objectives are organized into four categories with each requiring health education:
1. Promote healthy behaviors
2. Promote healthy and safe communities

BOX 13-1 *Healthy People 2000* Educational Objectives

- Increase to at least 75% the proportion of people 10 years of age or older who have discussed issues related to nutrition, physical activity, sexual behavior, tobacco, alcohol, other drugs, or safety with family members on at least one occasion during the preceding month.
- Increase to at least 50% the proportion of counties that have established culturally and linguistically appropriate community health promotion programs for racial and ethnic minority populations.
- Increase to at least 90% the proportion of hospitals, health maintenance organizations, and large group practices that provide client education programs and to at least 90% the proportion of community hospitals that offer community health promotion programs addressing the priority health needs of their communities.
- Increase to at least 75% the proportion of local television affiliates in the top 20 television markets that have become partners with one or more community organizations around one of the health problems addressed by the *Healthy People 2000* objectives.

From USDHHS: *Healthy people 2000: national health promotion and disease prevention objectives*, Washington, DC, 1991, USDHHS, Public Health Service.

---

3. Improve systems for personal and public health
4. Prevent and reduce diseases and disorders

The ability to apply learning theories in a variety of educational settings is essential to guide the thinking, decision making, and practice of nurses. To promote the health of clients, it is necessary to teach health concepts and self-care skills in understandable ways.

Learning is defined in a variety of ways. Most definitions of the learning process include a measurable change in behavior that persists over time. Newly learned knowledge and behaviors are practiced and thus are repeatedly reinforced (Padilla and Bulcavage, 1991). Although many theories and principles related to learning are applicable to community and public health nursing, only samples of the most useful and readily adaptable ones are included here. A solid theoretical foundation of health education enables the nurse to educate clients successfully. Figure 13-1 presents the sequence of actions that a nurse follows when developing an educational program.

GENERAL EDUCATIONAL THEORIES

Educational theories help nurses understand how people learn and how to design and implement client education. Table 13-1 provides an overview of six major educational theories useful in community and public health nursing. It is important to understand each of these educational theories and to be able to choose and then apply the most appropriate theory to a wide variety of health education sit-

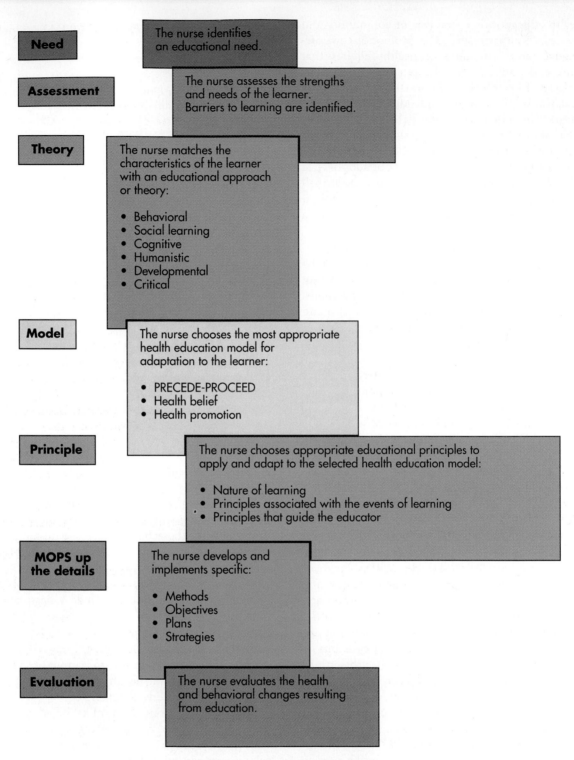

FIG. 13-1 The sequence of actions that a nurse follows when developing an educational program.

uations. Often it is necessary to combine a number of these perspectives in the education process.

Behavioral Theory

Behavioral theory approaches the study of learning by concentrating on behaviors that can be observed and mea-sured. The goal of behavioral approaches to learning is be-havioral change. A *target behavior*, which the educator seeks to either increase or decrease, is identified. To increase a behavior, one identifies and consistently uses a *reinforcer* to modify the target behavior. To decrease a behavior, one identifies and consistently uses *withdrawal of a reinforcer*

TABLE 13-1 Overview of Six General Educational Theories

THEORY	FOCUS	METHOD
Behavioral	Change behavior	Reinforcement or punishment
Social learning	Change expectations and beliefs	Link information, beliefs, and values
Cognitive	Change thought patterns	Variety of sensory input and repetition
Humanist	Use feelings and relationships	Learners will do what is best for themselves (self-determination)
Developmental	Consider human developmental stage	Educational opportunities match readiness to learn
Critical	Increase depth of knowledge	Ongoing dialogue and open inquiry

Data from Driscoll MP: *Psychology of learning for instruction*, Boston, 1994, Allyn & Bacon; Edwards L: Health education. In Edelman CL, Mandle CL, editors: *Health promotion throughout the lifespan*, ed 5, St Louis, 1998, Mosby.

(punishment) to modify the target behavior (Dembo, 1994; Dignam, 1992; Driscoll, 1994).

The behavioral approach is useful when the educator has full control over the reward/consequences environment (i.e., the feedback system). This approach is also useful when the learner has cognitive limitations because the behavioral approach requires only the most rudimentary use of cognition.

For example, a nurse working in a school system might want to decrease the number of adolescent deaths associated with alcohol use. The nurse identifies the target behavior as use of a designated driver. He or she works to increase the use of designated drivers for transporting students from school-related functions. Therefore after every school-related sporting or social event, four trained adults sit at the exit doors, evaluate the sobriety of designated drivers, and assign designated drivers to cars. Designated drivers each receive $10 for gasoline from raised funds, have their names printed in the weekly school newspaper, and become eligible for a weekly prize drawing of $20.

Social Learning Theory

Social learning theory builds on the principles of behavioral theory and contends that behavior is a function of an individual's expectations about the value of an outcome (Do I want the outcome?) or self-efficacy (Can I achieve the outcome?). If clients believe that an outcome is desired and attainable, they are more likely to change their behavior to achieve that goal. Thus educators may use this theory to change behaviors by enabling clients to either change their expectations about the value of a certain outcome, their ability to achieve the desired outcome, or both (Blair, 1993; Dembo, 1994; Padilla and Bulcavage, 1991).

For example, if a nurse wants to help a group of obese women lose weight, the nurse instructs the women to eat less, select healthful foods, and exercise more. By providing scientific data describing balanced eating and the positive effects of exercise, the nurse helps the women believe that decreased food intake and increased exercise will result in weight loss. Thus through case study presentations

and before-and-after photos, the nurse helps the women change their expectations about their power to achieve the goal of weight loss. Without belief in their ability to change, the women may be unable to remain motivated to change their target behaviors.

Cognitive Theory

Cognitive theory maintains that by changing thought patterns and providing information, learners' behavior will change. This theory claims that people's thought patterns undergo constant change as they interact with their environment. Thus the educator seeks to provide information in a variety of ways that will change clients' thought patterns and ultimately will be followed by changes in behavior (Dembo, 1994; Dignam, 1992; Driscoll, 1994).

For example, if a woman does not perform a monthly breast self-examination (BSE), the nurse instructs the client to begin doing so. The nurse tries to change the woman's thought patterns by providing information about BSE in a variety of ways. The nurse verbally teaches the client about the procedure and explains the reasons for doing BSE. The nurse next shows the woman a video about BSE. The nurse then observes as the client practices BSE on a breast model. The nurse then gives the woman a handout with the procedure written and depicted on it. The nurse instructs the client to hang the handout next to the bathroom mirror to remind her to do monthly BSEs. Thus by using a variety of environmental cues and sensory input, the client's thought patterns can be changed, thereby influencing her behavior related to BSE.

Humanist Theory

Humanist theory describes the influence that feelings, emotions, and personal relationships have on behavior. Humanistic theorists believe that learners should be encouraged to examine their feelings and engage in various forms of self-expression. In addition, humanists think that people need to be aware of and able to clarify their values. If people are given free choice, they will do what is best for themselves. Humanists encourage health educators not to be overly controlling and restrictive with learners, but rather to help them grow and develop according to their natural inclinations (Dembo, 1994; Dignam, 1992).

For example, if members of a retirement community want to develop a health promotion program, they may invite a nurse to schedule meetings to assist them in furthering this goal. At the meetings, the nurse facilitates group discussion about the goals and strategies of the program and provides a variety of handouts related to health promotion. The nurse also answers questions and offers encouragement to group members as they develop their own health promotion program.

Developmental Theory

Developmental theory maintains that learning occurs in concert with developmental stages. Each stage is a major transformation from the previous stage; therefore learning occurs differently in each developmental period. Readiness to learn depends on the individual's developmental stage (Hancock and Mandle, 1998).

For example, to help a family with a toddler prevent accidents in the home, the nurse educates the parents about safety practices. The nurse also teaches the parents how to educate the toddler simply and clearly about safety according to the toddler's developmental stage and readiness to understand concepts and behavioral patterns. The nurse recognizes that the parents' and the toddler's levels of readiness to learn are different. Since the toddler cannot reach the stovetop, teaching about the dangers of a hot stove at this stage of physical development is unnecessary. However, the toddler is at risk for accidental poisoning. Although the parents may teach the toddler not to open bottles and jars without their help, all poisons must be removed from the toddler's reach as a necessary precaution. The risk of poison ingestion is incomprehensible to the toddler because of the stage of both language and cognitive development.

Critical Theory

Critical theory approaches learning as an ongoing dialogue. An individual holds a belief about a health matter. The educator attempts to change this belief by questioning the learner. As the learner answers the questions, the learner's beliefs begin to change, new questions arise, and the learner then asks the educator questions. The educator responds to these questions. This process of discourse ultimately changes thinking and behavior (Dignam, 1992; Welton, 1993).

For example, the nurse would like a newly diagnosed group of diabetic clients to assume responsibility for the management of their diabetes. The nurse asks the clients what they know about diabetes. The clients demonstrate that they can check their own blood sugar levels and prepare their own insulin injections. However, on further questioning, it is discovered that the clients are not familiar with the long-term complications of diabetes. The nurse then educates them about these complications. As a

---

BOX 13-2 PRECEDE and PROCEED Acronyms

PRECEDE IS AN ACRONYM FOR:
Predisposing,
Reinforcing, and
Enabling
Causes in
Educational
Diagnosis and
Evaluation

PROCEED IS AN ACRONYM FOR:
Policy,
Regulatory, and
Organizational
Constructs in
Educational and
Environmental
Development

Based on data from Green LW, Kreuter MW: CDC's planned approach to community health as an application of PRECEDE and an inspiration for PROCEED, *J Health Educ* 23(3):140, 1992.

---

result, the clients begin to go to an ophthalmologist every year and check their feet daily for changes in skin color or integrity.

HEALTH EDUCATION MODELS

Conceptual models organize global ideas and simplify complete systems of thought into succinct formats. Thus conceptual models provide meaningful descriptions to guide the thinking, observations, and practice of educators (Driscoll, 1994; Edwards, 1998). Three health education models are described in this section:
- PRECEDE-PROCEED
- Health belief
- Health promotion

These three models are directly applicable to the nurse's educational role and provide a practical way of viewing the process of health education.

PRECEDE-PROCEED Model

The *PRECEDE-PROCEED model* focuses primarily on planning and evaluating community health education programs. The PRECEDE-PROCEED acronym is explained in Box 13-2. Additionally, the nine phases of the model are outlined in Table 13-2.

One strength of the PRECEDE-PROCEED model is that it consistently involves the client in a problem-solving approach to provide health education for an identified area of need. The PRECEDE-PROCEED model focuses on helping communities change their behaviors. It begins by assessing the environment in which the group lives and considering the social factors that influence health behaviors. Next, the model examines both the internal and environmental factors of the group that predispose it to certain behaviors or health problems (PRECEDE). The model then

TABLE 13-2 The Nine Phases of the PRECEDE-PROCEED Model

PHASE	TITLE	DESCRIPTION
1	Social diagnosis	The social concerns of the community are identified.
2	Epidemiological diagnosis	Epidemiological data are used to suggest health problems.
3	Behavioral and environmental diagnosis	Behavioral and environmental risk factors that seem to affect health are identified.
4	Educational and organizational diagnosis	Predisposing, reinforcing, and enabling factors are identified.
5	Administrative and policy diagnosis	Planning related to health education and policy regulations occurs.
6	Implementation	The health education program is implemented.
7	Process evaluation	The education process is evaluated in an ongoing fashion.
8	Impact evaluation	The immediate effects or objectives of the educational program are evaluated.
9	Outcome evaluation	The short-term and long-term effects of the educational program are evaluated.

Data from Green LW, Kreuter MW: CDC's planned approach to community health as an application of PRECEDE and an inspiration for PROCEED, *J Health Educ* 23(3):140, 1992; Green LW, Ottoson JM: *Community health*, ed 7, St Louis, 1994, Mosby; Hawe P, Degeling D, Hall J: *Evaluating health promotion: a health worker's guide*, Philadelphia, 1990, MacLennan & Petty.

calls for the identification of factors that will help the group to adopt healthy actions. Priorities are set. The program is developed, implemented, and evaluated (PROCEED). The PRECEDE-PROCEED model is easy to use; its steps serve as a checklist for ensuring that all stages of the problem-solving process are followed (Edwards, 1998; Green and Kreuter, 1992; Padilla and Bulcavage, 1991).

Health Belief Model

The **health belief model** was developed to provide a framework for understanding why some people take specific actions to avoid illness, whereas others fail to protect themselves. When the model was developed, both public and private health sectors were concerned that people were reluctant to be screened for tuberculosis, to have Pap smears to detect cervical cancer, to be immunized, or to take other preventive measures that were either free or available at a nominal cost. The model was designed to predict which people would use preventive measures and to suggest interventions that might reduce client reluctance to access health care (Padilla and Bulcavage, 1991; Salazar, 1991). Box 13-3 outlines the three major components of the health belief model: individual perceptions, modifying factors, and variables affecting the likelihood of action. In addition, cues to action such as mass media campaigns, advice from others, reminder postcards from health care providers, illnesses of family members or friends, and newspaper or magazine articles may help motivate clients to take action (Salazar, 1991).

The health belief model is beneficial in assessing health protection or disease prevention behaviors. It is also useful in organizing information about clients' views of their state of health and what factors may influence them to change their behavior. The health belief model, when used appropriately, provides organized assessment data about

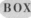 **BOX 13-3 The Three Major Components of the Health Belief Model**

INDIVIDUAL PERCEPTIONS

Person's *beliefs* about his or her own *susceptibility* to disease
PLUS
The *seriousness* with which he/she views the disease
EQUALS
The *perceived threat* of an illness for each person

MODIFYING FACTORS
Demographic Variables

Age
Gender
Race
Ethnicity

Sociopsychological Variables

Personality
Social class
Peer pressure

Structural Variables

Knowledge about the disease
Prior contact with the disease

VARIABLES AFFECTING THE LIKELIHOOD OF INITIATING ACTION

Person's *perceived benefits* of action
MINUS
His or her *perceived barriers* to accomplishing action
EQUALS
The *likelihood* that a person will take action to change his or her behaviors

Based on data from Salazar MK: Comparison of four behavioral theories, *AAOHN J* 39(3):128, 1991.

BOX 13-4 Three Categories of Determinants of Health Promoting Behavior

COGNITIVE-PERCEPTUAL FACTORS

Definition of health
Importance of health
Perceived health *status*
Perceived *control* of health
Perceived *self-efficacy*
Perceived *benefits* of health-promoting behavior
Perceived *barriers* to health-promoting behavior

MODIFYING FACTORS

Demographic Factors

Age
Gender
Race
Ethnicity
Education
Income

Biological Characteristics

Body weight
Body fat
Height

Interpersonal Influences

Expectations of significant others
Family patterns of health care
Interactions with health professionals

Situational (Environmental) Factors

Access to care

Behavioral Factors

Cognitive and psychomotor skills necessary to carry out healthy behaviors

VARIABLES AFFECTING THE LIKELIHOOD OF INITIATING ACTION

Variables affecting the likelihood of action depend on internal and external cues:
• The desire to feel well
• Individualized health teaching
• Mass media health promotion campaigns

Data from Palank CL: Determinants of health-promotive behavior: a review of current research, *Nurs Clin North Am* 26(4):815, 1991; Simmons SJ: The Health-Promoting Self-Care System Model: directions for nursing research and practice, *J Adv Nurs* 15(10):1162, 1990.

---

clients' abilities and motivation to change their health status. Health education programs can then be developed to better fit the needs of clients (Salazar, 1991).

Health Promotion Model

The **health promotion model** was developed as a complement to other health-protecting models such as the health belief model. The health promotion model explains the likelihood that healthy lifestyle patterns or health-promoting behaviors will occur (Palank, 1991; Simmons, 1990). Box 13-4 outlines the three major categories of determinants of health-promoting behavior: cognitive-perceptual factors, modifying factors, and variables affecting the likelihood of action. Although these three categories are similar to the three factors of the health belief model, the health promotion model expands and modifies them.

This model, as with the health belief model, is useful to the nurse as a framework for client assessment. However, the health promotion model expands the principles of the health belief model and states that individuals are likely to change their behavior to feel better physically, psychologically, socially, and spiritually.

Nurses' Application of Health Education Models

It is up to the nurse to select the most appropriate model for educational programs. For example, when providing educational programs to communities, the nurse may use the PRECEDE-PROCEED model to organize the teaching program. However, when delivering education to individuals or families, the nurse may use the health belief model or the health promotion model to identify the specific beliefs, behaviors, or cultural factors that must be modified to change behavior.

The health belief model is particularly useful in assessing the likelihood that clients will change their health behaviors and in developing concrete plans aimed at changing health beliefs. The health promotion model borrows concepts from general education theories and other health education models. It provides a broad base for assessing health perceptions and attempting to help clients modify their health behaviors by changing their perceptions of the factors affecting health. Many other health education models may also be used by the nurse to plan educational interventions.

DID YOU KNOW? *One in four adolescents in the United States suffers as a result of pregnancy, drug use, dropping out of school, depression, suicidal thoughts, or violence. Statistics show that of all U.S. high school students, 54% have had sexual intercourse, 72% do not always wear seat belts, 51% are not enrolled in physical education, 42% were in a physical fight during the last year, 31% had five or more alcoholic drinks on one occasion in the past month, and 28% smoked cigarettes in the past month. These statistics indicate that community health education reform is needed to improve the health of the nation's teens. Comprehensive health education programs need to begin in the early school years (Andrews, 1994).*

TABLE 13-3 Steps in the Cognitive Domain as Compared with the Affective Domain

STEP	COGNITIVE DOMAIN	AFFECTIVE DOMAIN
Knowledge	Requires *recall* of information	Learner *receives* the information
Comprehension	*Combines* recall with understanding	Learner *responds* to what is being taught
Application	Takes new information and *uses it in a different way*	Learner values the information
Analysis	Breaks down communication into constituent parts in order to understand the parts and their *relationships*	Learner *makes sense* of the information
Synthesis	Builds on the previous four levels by putting the parts back together into a *unified whole*	*Learner* organizes the information
Evaluation	*Judges the value* of what has been learned	Learner *adopts behaviors* consistent with the new value system

Data from Dembo MH: *Applying educational psychology*, ed 5, New York, 1994, Longman.

EDUCATIONAL PRINCIPLES

A variety of educational principles can be used to guide the selection of health information for individuals, families, and communities. Three of the most useful categories of educational principles include those associated with the nature of learning, the events of instruction, and guidelines for the effective educator.

Nature of Learning

One way to think about the nature of learning is to examine the cognitive, affective, and psychomotor domains of learning (Dembo, 1994; Rankin and Stallings, 1996). Each domain has specific behavioral components that form a hierarchy of steps or levels, and each level builds on the previous one. Understanding these three learning domains is crucial in providing effective health education.

Cognitive domain

The **cognitive domain** includes memory, recognition, understanding, and application and is divided into a hierarchical classification of behaviors. Learners master each level of cognition in order of difficulty (Dembo, 1994). For health education to be effective, the instructor must first assess the cognitive abilities of the learner so that the instructor's expectations and plans are directed toward the correct level. Teaching above or below the client's level of understanding may lead to frustration and discouragement.

Affective domain

The **affective domain** includes changes in attitudes and the development of values. In affective learning, nurses consider and attempt to influence what individuals, families, and communities think, value, and feel. Since the values and attitudes of nurses may differ from those of their clients, it is important to listen carefully to detect clues to feelings that may influence learning. As with cognitive learning, affective learning consists of a series of steps (Dembo, 1994). Steps in the affective domain as compared with the cognitive domain are listed in Table 13-3. It is dif-

BOX 13-5 Levels of Psychomotor Learning

Reflex movements. Occur in response to a stimulus without conscious awareness
Basic movements. Develop from a combination of reflex movements
Perceptual abilities. Transfer visual stimuli into appropriate movements
Physical abilities. Combine basic body movements by incorporating endurance, strength, flexibility, and agility
Skilled movements. Indicative of a degree of proficiency
Nondiscursive communication. Complex movements are used to communicate feelings, needs, or interests to others

Adapted from Dembo MH: *Applying educational psychology*, ed 5, New York, 1994, Longman.

ficult to change deep-seated characteristics such as values, attitudes, beliefs, and interests. To make such changes, people need support and encouragement from those around them to reinforce new behaviors.

Psychomotor domain

The **psychomotor domain** includes the performance of skills that require some degree of neuromuscular coordination. Clients are taught a variety of psychomotor skills including giving injections, taking blood pressure, measuring blood sugar levels, bathing infants, changing dressings, and walking with crutches. The levels of psychomotor learning from the simplest to the most complex level of observable movements are outlined in Box 13-5.

Three conditions must be met before psychomotor learning occurs (Dembo, 1994):

1. The learner must have the *necessary ability*. For example, the nurse may find that a client with Alzheimer's disease may only be capable of following instructions

of one or two steps. Therefore the nurse must adapt the education plan to fit the client's abilities.

2. The learner must have a *sensory image* of how to carry out the skill. For instance, when educating a group of pregnant women about techniques to manage labor, the nurse asks the clients to visualize themselves in calm control of their delivery.

3. The learner must have *opportunities to practice* the new skills being learned. Practice sessions should be provided during the program because many clients will not have the facilities, motivation, or time to practice what they have learned at home.

To facilitate skill learning, the educator should show the learner the skill either in person, on a video, or with pictures. Then the educator should allow the learner to practice and immediately correct any errors in performing the skill.

In assessing a client's ability to learn a skill, the educator should evaluate physical, intellectual, and emotional ability. For example, a tremulous person with poor eyesight may be incapable of learning insulin self-injection. Similarly, some clients do not have the intellectual ability to learn the steps that make up a complex procedure. The nurse should teach at the level of the learner's ability.

Events of Instruction

To educate others effectively, the nurse needs to understand the basic sequence of instruction. When nurses consider the following nine steps of instructing others, they can systematically plan health education so that learners gain as much as possible from the instruction (Driscoll, 1994).

1. *Gaining attention.* Before learning can take place, the educator must gain the learner's attention. One way to do this is by convincing the learner that the information about to be presented is important and beneficial to the learner.

2. *Informing the learner of the objectives of instruction.* Before teaching begins, the major goals and objectives of instruction should be outlined so that learners develop expectations about what they are supposed to learn.

3. *Stimulating recall of prior learning.* The educator should have learners recall previous knowledge related to the topic of interest. This helps learners link new knowledge with prior knowledge.

4. *Presenting the stimulus.* The essential elements of a topic should be presented in a clear, organized, and simple manner and in a way that is congruent with the learner's strengths, needs, and limitations.

5. *Providing learning guidance.* For long-lasting behavioral changes to occur, learners must store information in long-term memory. With guidance from the educator, a learner can transform general information that has been presented into meaningful information that the learner can recall.

6. *Eliciting performance.* Learners should be encouraged to demonstrate what they have learned, and by doing so, learners can correct errors and improve skills.

7. *Providing feedback.* Educators should provide feedback to learners to help them improve their knowledge and skills. Learners can then modify their thinking and behaviors based on this feedback.

8. *Assessing performance.* Learning should be evaluated. Knowledge and skills should be formally assessed with the expectation that new information has been understood.

9. *Enhancing retention and transfer of knowledge.* Once a baseline level of knowledge and skills has been attained, educators should help learners apply this information to new situations.

By using these instructional principles, nurses can help clients maximize learning experiences. If steps of this process are omitted, superficial and fragmented learning may not occur.

Effective Educator

Nurse educators must be effective teachers. Six basic principles that guide the effective educator are listed in Box 13-6 and are discussed in this section.

Sending a clear message

Regardless of the importance of the content or the interest level of the learner, if the material is not presented in a clear and organized manner, the learner will not receive or retain an optimum level of information. At various stages in the educational process, the educator must reassess learner readiness and be aware of possible barriers to effective communication (Hamachek, 1995). Emotional stress and physical illness are only two factors that may limit the amount of information a learner can absorb. The nurse educator must be aware of various factors affecting the learner and recognize that the needs and barriers influencing the learner's receptivity may vary from session to session. Educational strategies and activities can be developed and adjusted to fit the dynamic needs of the learner.

The educator is responsible for providing information that is understandable. Medical jargon and technical terms

---

BOX 13-6 Six Principles that Guide the Educator

Message. Send a clear message to the learner.
Format. Select the most appropriate learning format.
Environment. Create the best possible learning environment.
Experience. Organize positive and meaningful learning experiences.
Participation. Engage the learner in participatory learning.
Evaluation. Evaluate and give objective feedback to the learner.

Adapted from Knowles M: *The adult learner: a neglected species*, ed 5, Houston, 1998, Gulf.

may interfere with the clarity of the intended message (Damrosch, 1991). For example, in helping clients understand diet control for hypertension, the nurse might use the phrase "high blood pressure" rather than the term "hypertension" to tailor the message to the learner's ability to understand. Box 13-7 presents communication guidelines in educational interactions.

Selecting the learning format

The educator must decide how to teach. The educator selects an appropriate learning format, or strategy, for implementing the learning program. A format should be chosen that matches the goals and objectives of the program and should be adapted to meet the learning needs of the client. In addition, teaching tools such as printed materials or audio-visual aids that will enhance learning should be selected (MacDonald, 1999). Three examples of learning formats are outlined in Box 13-8.

Creating the best learning environment

Educational programs quickly lose their effectiveness if the environment is not conducive to learning. The nurse can begin to establish an appropriate learning climate for an educational event when announcements of the program are made. The tone and appearance of letters, flyers, and media messages announcing the program draw a mental picture for participants of what the activity will be like. By carefully considering program objectives and information about the culture, beliefs, and educational level of learners, the nurse can develop preparatory materials that appeal to the target population (Knowles, 1998). During the program, it is important to create a positive, supportive, and pleasant atmosphere for the client so that learning can be maximized. Three environmental realms that should be considered are described in Box 13-9.

WHAT DO YOU THINK? *The nurse educator needs to consider the setting in which community education will take place. Currently, school, work, and health care settings are common sites of health education. The educational setting has an impact on the teaching plan; cost-effectiveness; individual, family, and community behavioral changes; participation; and health care education policies (Mullen et al, 1995).*

Organizing learning experiences

Regardless of the educator's level of knowledge or the quality of the interpersonal relationship that the educator has developed with the learner, sound organization of the

---

BOX 13-7 Communication Guidelines for Educational Interactions

Begin strongly. People remember the first point.

Use a clear, direct, and succinct style. This helps the learner to remain focused.

Use the active voice. For example, the educator may say, "We will discuss relaxation techniques" instead of "Relaxation techniques will be discussed."

Accentuate the positive. For example, the educator may say, "The majority of individuals are able to lose weight with a well-balanced diet and exercise" instead of "A few people have not been able to lose weight with a well balanced diet and exercise."

Use vivid communication, not statistics or jargon. Specific case histories are often more meaningful than general, nonspecific terms or dry statistics.

Refer to trustworthy sources. For example, "the surgeon general" is a more credible source than "some people."

Base strategies on a knowledge of the audience. Be aware of the perceptions and perspectives of the audience.

Make points explicitly. Be direct and give clear instructions.

End strongly. The last point made is likely to be remembered.

Adapted from Damrosch S: General strategies for motivating people to change their behavior, *Nurs Clin North Am* 26(4): 833, 1991.

BOX 13-8 Examples of Learning Formats

1. The client is a large class of university students studying communicable diseases. The selected format is a lecture to be followed by a question and answer period.
2. The client is a group from a shelter for victims of domestic violence. The chosen format is an informal, small-group, open discussion after a short poster presentation.
3. The client is a family with a newly diagnosed insulin-dependent diabetic 6-year-old child. The objectives are different for each family member. Therefore the format must be adapted to each member as well. The child requires materials appropriate to his or her developmental stage. The objectives for the child are to overcome fear of injections and to begin to deal with possible lifestyle changes. The material will be presented in the form of a picture book and storytelling that provides a realistic yet nonthreatening look at both the illness and the treatment. The objectives for the parents are to understand both the short- and long-term ramifications of their child's disease and to learn the specific skills needed to manage the illness at home.
   a. Informational handouts will be gathered, and several medical journal articles will be copied and given to the parents to read.
   b. Insulin injection demonstrations and practice sessions will be provided.
   c. The nurse will provide the phone number to the clinic for follow-up questions as well as phone numbers for several diabetes associations.
   d. The family will be introduced to a local chapter of a support group appropriate to their specific needs. This will help them process their fears and concerns.

material is essential for learning to occur. Materials should be presented in a logical and integrated manner, from simple foundational concepts to more complex ideas. These should represent building blocks in a well-designed structure with a clear and unambiguous blueprint. The educator should reduce difficult or confusing concepts to their component parts and show the learner how to reassemble them one at a time. The pace of the presentation should match the ability of the learner and leave adequate pause for the learner to absorb the material.

The principles of continuity, sequence, and integration are important for the organization of educational programs. A lack of *continuity* causes a break in the flow of logical thought and may confuse the learner. Repeated emphasis of essential points helps the learner maintain continuity.

In *sequencing,* each learning experience builds on the previous one and requires a higher level of functioning. Learning activities should be sequenced so that participants start with simple, easy-to-master exercises or materials and progress to more complex ones requiring greater skill, coordination, or understanding.

BOX 13-9   Environmental Realms

PHYSICAL REALM

This realm includes setting up the program and positioning the presenter and the clients in a physical relationship to one another. It also includes lighting and temperature of the room, volume of amplification equipment, furniture, and bathroom facilities. The more subtle effects of environment are those that create a stimulating setting, allow for few external distractions, and assist the learner in concentration and attention.

INTERPERSONAL REALM

This realm consists of human relationships and should be therapeutic, supportive, and conducive to producing quality educational interactions. The interpersonal dynamic should be one in which learners experience a clear sense that the educator cares about their progress and needs. Learners also can contribute to the interpersonal environment by showing interest in the subject and remaining responsive to both peer and group interactions.

ORGANIZATIONAL REALM

This realm entails the administrative aspects of the educational program. Beginning with scheduling, announcements, and other preparations, this is the realm that makes the components of the program merge into an effective learning session. Arrangements for parking, delivery of audio-visual materials, ensuring readability of printed or projected materials, and responsiveness to ongoing learner needs and requests are a few examples of organizational aspects of environment.

Adapted from Knowles M: *The adult learner: a neglected species,* ed 5, Houston, 1998, Gulf.

Integration of various aspects of the material demonstrates how each component fits into the whole. Without integration, the learner is left with a puzzle of disjointed facts or concepts that is difficult to assimilate in a productive way (Knowles, 1998).

Encouraging participatory learning

People learn better when they are actively involved in the learning process. Participation increases motivation, flexibility, and learning rate. Participatory learning is not limited to the psychomotor domain. The cognitive and affective domains also call for a teaching strategy in which the instructor enlists the active involvement of the learner. Verbal response or feedback, as long as it engages the learner, is participatory. Merely sitting and listening is not as effective as discussion, even when the presentation is stimulating, interesting, and dynamic. Role play, acting out an experience, storytelling, "hands-on" training, and similar activities are good examples of participatory learning. Immediate feedback, an important advantage of participatory learning, ensures that errors are corrected before problematic habits or misconceptions develop. Computer-assisted learning provides immediate feedback to learners (Knowles, 1998).

The educator can structure learning activities and the environment to facilitate participatory learning. Using proper teaching materials, learners can be provided with adequate prompting and modeling to ensure their ability to practice and to demonstrate mastery of the material. By using the principle of participatory learning, the material becomes more accessible and meaningful to learners and is more likely to be retained and used in the future (Knowles, 1988) (see Research Brief about learner readiness).

Providing evaluation and feedback

It is essential to evaluate learning and provide constructive and helpful feedback to the learner throughout the educational process to avoid discouraging or offending the learner. Through clear and behaviorally focused feedback, clients can monitor their progress, level of knowledge, and

---

RESEARCH *Brief*

Most psychiatric nurses know that learner readiness is an important part of client education; however, many psychiatric clients deny their illness, refuse treatment, are unable to concentrate, or may appear disinterested. Freed used a phenomenologic method to evaluate the stories that 12 psychiatric nurses told about educating psychiatric clients who did not exhibit typical signs of learner readiness. She identified that the major pattern that emerged from these psychiatric nurses' stories was perseverance. She determined that perseverance is composed of elements of trust, patience, acceptance, caring, and hope.

Freed PE: Perseverance: the meaning of patient education in psychiatric nursing, *Arch Psychiatr Nurs* 2:107, 1998.

learning needs. The educator may use tools such as quizzes, tests, completed study sheets, observation of skills, small-group tasks, and competency rating scales to evaluate learning outcomes. Not only should learners receive feedback, but the educator should also elicit feedback from learners throughout the educational process. Based on the feedback that the educator receives from learners, modifications in the implementation and presentation of the educational program can be made (Knowles, 1998).

EDUCATIONAL PROCESS

In addition to understanding the nature of learning, the events of instruction, and strategies for effective education, knowledge of the educational process is essential for the nurse. Interestingly, the educational and nursing processes are similar, and both are used at the individual, family, and community levels (Bigbee and Jansa, 1991). A comparison of the two processes is outlined in Table 13-4. Additionally, each step of the educational process is discussed in this section.

Identify Educational Needs

Nurses learn about the health education needs of their clients by performing a systematic and thorough client needs assessment. The steps of a needs assessment are listed in Box 13-10. Once needs have been identified, they are prioritized so that the most critical educational needs are met first (Strodtman, 1984).

> **┇ NURSING TIP**
>
> *Client-centered education is a term used to define education based on what individuals, families, or communities identify that they need to learn. Traditionally, health care professionals have designed educational programs based on their agenda, not on that of their clients.*

TABLE 13-4 A Comparison of the Nursing and Educational Processesable to Different Factors

NURSING PROCESS	EDUCATIONAL PROCESS
Assessment	Identify educational needs.
Diagnosis	Establish educational goals and objectives.
Planning	Select appropriate educational methods.
Implementation	Implement the educational plan.
Evaluation	Evaluate the educational process and product.

Data from Edwards L: Health education. In Edelman CL, Mandle CL, editors: *Health promotion throughout the lifespan*, ed 5, St Louis, 1998, Mosby; Hawe P, Degeling D, Hall J: *Evaluating health promotion: a health worker's guide*, Philadelphia, 1990, MacLennan & Petty; Strodtman LK: A decision-making process for planning patient education, *Patient Educ Counseling* 5(4): 189, 1984.

A variety of factors influence clients' learning needs and their ability to learn. Demographic, physical, geographic, economic, psychological, social, and spiritual characteristics of learners should be considered when identifying learning needs.

> **┇ WHAT DO YOU THINK?** *Nurse educators need to establish health education agendas for various special populations including children, adolescents, elders, women, men, and underserved groups (McLeroy KR et al, 1996).*

Educators need to understand how the learner's existing knowledge, skills, and motivation influence learning. Resources for and barriers to learning should be identified. Resources include printed materials, equipment, agencies, and other individuals. Barriers include lack of time, money, space, energy, confidence, and organizational support (Edwards, 1998; Rankin and Stallings, 1996). Communication barriers may result from cultural and language differences between the nurse and the client or from printed materials that are inappropriate to the client's reading level. Such adverse influences on the learning process can be minimized with a vigilant awareness of both initial and newly developing barriers during the educational process (Volker, 1991).

Establish Educational Goals and Objectives

Once learner needs are determined, goals and objectives to guide the educational program can be identified. Goals are broad, long-term expected outcomes such as, "Mr. Williams will become independently able to take care of his ostomy bag within 3 months." Goals of the program should directly address the client's overall learning needs (Rankin and Stallings, 1996).

Objectives are specific, short-term criteria that need to be met as steps toward achieving the long-term goal such as, "Mr. Williams will properly reattach his own ostomy bag, after the nurse has cleaned the site five consecutive times within 2 weeks." Objectives are written statements of

> **BOX 13-10 Steps of a Needs Assessment**
>
> 1. Identify what the client wants to know.
> 2. Determine how the client wants to learn.
> 3. Identify what will enhance the client's ability and motivation to learn.
> 4. Collect data systematically from the individual, family, community, and other sources to assess learning needs, readiness to learn, and situational and psychosocial factors influencing learning.
> 5. Analyze assessment data to identify cognitive, affective, and psychomotor learning needs.
> 6. Encourage client participation in the process.
> 7. Assist the client in prioritizing learning needs.

Based on data from Volker DL: Patient education: needs assessment and resource identification, *Oncol Nurs Forum* 18(1):119, 1991.

TABLE 13-5 Four Parts of an Objective

Question	Example • String all "A" phrases together as one sentence for one example. • String all "B" and "C" phrases together in like manner.
Who is to exhibit the behavior?	a. Each member of the Jones family b. Ms. Smith c. Eighty percent of the target population
What behavior is expected?	a. will give an insulin injection to Billy b. will perform a blood sugar test on herself c. will take their children to receive immunizations
Conditions and qualifiers of behavior	a. with accuracy regarding dosage b. with accuracy regarding the blood sugar reading c. within 1 month of the immunization due date
Standards of behavior or performance	a. 100% of the time for ten consecutive trials. b. within 10 points of the educator's reading for ten consecutive trials.

Data from Green LW, Ottoson JM: *Community health*, ed 7, St Louis, 1994, Mosby; Hawe P, Degeling D, and Hall J: *Evaluating health promotion: a health worker's guide*, Philadelphia, 1990, MacLennan & Petty.

BOX 13-11 Strategies to Enhance Learning

Printed materials
Audio-visual materials
Computer-assisted learning
Demonstrations
Guest speakers
Role play
Field trips
Peer presentations
Peer counseling and tutoring

Adapted from Knowles M: *The adult learner: a neglected species*, ed 5, Houston, 1998, Gulf.

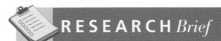

RESEARCH *Brief*

Printed educational materials are among the most convenient and economical methods of health education. Estey, Musseau, and Keehn evaluated reading materials developed at both the fifth- and the ninth-grade levels with general medical and surgical clients. They used the Wide Range Achievement Test-Revised (WRAT-R) to assess the reading levels of clients and the Cloze test to determine the reader's level of comprehension. They found that more subjects were able to understand the materials written at the fifth-grade reading level than those written at the ninth-grade level.

Estey A, Musseau AI, Keehn L: Comprehension levels of patients reading health information, *Patient Educ Counseling* 18:165, 1991.

an intended outcome or expected change in behavior and should define the minimum degree of knowledge or ability needed by a client (Green and Ottoson, 1994; Hawe, Degeling, and Hall, 1990; Rankin and Stallings, 1996; Strodtman, 1984). Objectives must be stated clearly. Expected outcomes must be defined in measurable terms. The four parts of an objective are outlined in Table 13-5.

Select Appropriate Educational Methods

Educational methods should be chosen to facilitate the efficient and successful accomplishment of program goals and objectives. The methods should also be appropriately matched to the client's strengths and needs. Caution should be used to avoid complex methodologic designs. The educator should choose the simplest, clearest, and most succinct manner of presentation. The educator should be able to use a broad array of tools designed to convey information (Knowles, 1988). A few examples of strategies that may be used to enhance learning are listed in Box 13-11.

When nurses select educational methods, they should consider developmental disabilities, age, educational level,

knowledge of the subject, and size of the group. Matching media and other tools to the needs of the learner is an important skill for educators to develop. (see Research Brief about research comprehension levels).

For example, clients with a visual impairment may need more verbal description. Clients with hearing impairments may need increased visual material. Speakers who can use sign language may be necessary. Also, limitations in attention and concentration require creative methods and tools for keeping the learner focused. Such methods and tools include frequent breaks; austere, nondistractive surroundings; small-group interactions that keep the learner involved and interested; and the use of "hands-on" equipment such as mannequins, models, and other materials that the learner can physically manipulate. Comprehension and retention are related to the depth or intensity of the learner's involvement. The educator tries to involve the learner appropriately and creatively in a variety of ways and as actively as possible.

> **NURSING TIP**
>
> *A resource manual or directory that organizes information on community education programs and materials enables nurses to access educational information quickly and efficiently.*

Implement the Educational Plan

Once educational methods have been selected, they should be implemented through management of the educational process. Implementation entails the following:

1. Control over starting, sustaining, and stopping each method and strategy in the most effective and appropriate time and manner
2. Coordination and control of environmental factors, the flow of the presentation, and other contributory facets of the program
3. Keeping the materials logically related to the core theme and overall program goals

The educator must be flexible. He or she must modify educational methods and strategies to meet unexpected challenges that may confront both the educator and the learner. External influences such as time limitations, expense, administrative and political factors, and learner needs require an ongoing evaluation of their effect on the educational program (Knowles, 1998; Strodtman, 1984). Thus implementation is a dynamic element in the educational process.

> **HOW TO** *Effectively TEACH Clients*
>
> *T*une in. *Listen before you start teaching. Client's needs should direct the content.*
> *E*dit information. *Teach necessary information first. Be specific.*
> *A*ct on each teaching moment. *Teach whenever possible. Develop a good relationship.*
> *C*larify often. *Make sure your assumptions are correct. Seek feedback.*
> *H*onor the client as a partner. *Build on the client's experience. Share responsibility with the client.*
>
> Adapted from Hansen M, Fisher J: Patient-centered teaching from theory to practice, *Am J Nurs* 98(1):56, 1998.

Evaluate the Educational Process

Evaluation is as important in the educational process as it is in the nursing process. Evaluation provides a systematic and logical method for making decisions to improve the educational program. Educational evaluation involves three areas (Hawe, Degeling, and Hall, 1990):

- Educator evaluation
- Process evaluation
- Product evaluation

Both educator and process evaluation are described in this section. Product evaluation is described in the next section.

Educator evaluation

Feedback to the educator allows for modifications in the teaching process and enables the nurse to better meet the learner's needs. The learner's evaluation of the educator occurs continuously throughout the educational program. The educator may receive feedback from the learner in written form, such as an evaluation sheet. The educator may also receive feedback verbally or nonverbally, as in return demonstrations and by facial expressions (Knowles, 1998).

The educator should assume that inadequate learner responses reflect an inadequate program, not an inadequate learner. If evaluation reveals that the learning objectives are not being met, the nurse must determine why the instruction is not effective. It is then the educator's responsibility to present the material creatively and meaningfully in new ways that will increase learner retention and the learner's ability to apply the new knowledge (Hawe, Degeling, and Hall, 1990; Knowles, 1998). Ultimately, the educator must assume responsibility for the success or failure of the educational process and the development of learner knowledge, skills, and abilities.

Process evaluation

Process evaluation examines the dynamic components of the educational program. It follows and assesses the movements and management of information transfer and attempts to keep the objectives on track. Process evaluation is necessary throughout the educational program to determine whether goals and objectives are being met and the time required for their accomplishment. Ongoing evaluation also allows the teacher to correct misinformation, misinterpretation, or confusion.

Goals and objectives also should be periodically reconsidered. The nurse must ask if the desired health behavior change is really necessary. Such a question inevitably leads back to the original learning objectives and encourages the nurse to rethink the practicality and merit of each of the objectives. Factors that influence learner readiness and motivation should be reassessed if teaching seems to be ineffective. Process evaluation uses information gathered from the educator as well as from learner evaluations and assesses the dynamics of their interactions (Hawe, Degeling, and Hall, 1990; Knowes, 1990).

> **DID YOU KNOW?** *When evaluating teaching and program effectiveness, keep in mind the concept of the curve of normal distribution. In any group of learners, about 2% will be extremely negative and 2% will be extremely positive when they evaluate the program. Another 14% will be fairly negative, and 14% will be quite enthusiastic. The majority of participants (68%) will be somewhat neutral in their responses. Therefore even though the nurse should consider the extremely negative responses, avoid alarm or discouragement until the proportion of extremely negative responses exceeds 16% (Knowles, 1988).*

EDUCATIONAL PRODUCT

The educational product is the outcome of the educational process. The product is measured both qualitatively and quantitatively. For instance, a qualitative assessment should answer the question, "How well does the learner appear to understand the content?" A quantitative assessment should answer the question, "How much of the content does the learner retain?" Thus the quality of the product is measured by improvement and increase, or the lack thereof, in the learner's knowledge, skills, and abilities related to the content of the educational program.

In nursing, the educational product is assessed as a measurable change in the health or behavior of the client. Evaluation of the educational product can be divided into three components:
1. Evaluation of health and behavioral changes
2. Short-term evaluation
3. Long-term evaluation

Evaluation of Health and Behavioral Changes

A variety of approaches, methods, and tools can be used to evaluate health and behavioral changes. These include questionnaires, surveys, skills demonstrations, testing, subjective client feedback, and direct observation of improvements in client mastery of materials. Qualitative or quantitative strategies may be used, depending on the nature of the expected educational outcome. Evaluation of outcomes measured includes changes in knowledge, skills, abilities, attitudes, behavior, health status, and quality of life (Hawe, Degeling, and Hall, 1990).

Approaches to evaluating health education effects will vary, depending on the situation. For example, when considering a client's ability to perform a psychomotor skill, such as changing a dressing, viewing the actual performance of the skill is the most appropriate means of evaluation. Another more complex example is the nurse's completion of the implementation phase of a family education program. The nurse might use a specific tool, such as the Family Assessment Device, a self-report instrument designed specifically to evaluate the effects of clinical interventions for families, to measure learning. The family functioning components that the Family Assessment Device measures are problem solving, communication, roles, affective responsiveness, affective involvement, behavior control, and general functioning (Reeber, 1992). This type of evaluation tool is necessary to measure a wide array of variables; when working with families, educational outcomes may sometimes be manifested in unexpected ways.

If evaluation of the educational product shows positive changes in health status and health-related behaviors, the educator can expect good results in similar health educational programs. If evaluation of the educational product shows that either no changes or negative changes in health status and health-related behaviors resulted, then various components of the educational process can be examined and modified to produce better results in the future (Redman, 1993).

Short-Term Evaluation

It is important to evaluate short-term health and behavioral effects of health education programs and to determine if they are really caused by the educational program. Short-term objectives are often easy to evaluate (Edwards, 1998; Green and Ottoson, 1994; Hawe, Degeling, and Hall, 1990). For example, a **short-term evaluation** of whether a client can perform a return demonstration of breast self-examination requires minimal energy, expense, or time; skill mastery can be determined within a matter of minutes. If the short-term objective is not met, the nurse determines why and identifies possible solutions so that successful learning can occur. If the short-term objective is met, the nurse can then focus on long-term evaluation designed to assess the lasting effects of the education program, in this case, that of ongoing monthly breast self-examinations performed by the learner independently at home.

Long-Term Evaluation

The ultimate goal of health education is to help clients make lasting behavioral changes that will improve their overall health status. Long-term follow-up with clients is a challenging task. Even though clients make positive behavioral changes and their health status improves, they often no longer use the health care services of the nurse (Redman, 1993). Some of the other reasons long-term evaluation can be challenging are listed in Box 13-12.

Long-term evaluation is geared toward following and assessing the status of an individual, family, or community over time. The tools of evaluation are designed to assess whether specific goals and objectives were met. Also, the extent and direction of changes in health status and health behaviors that the client has experienced are monitored (Redman, 1993).

For nurse educators, the goal of long-term evaluation is to analyze the effectiveness of the education program, not the specific health status of the individual client. Nurses track the client's (who may be an entire community) performance of objectives over time. They do not track individual community members themselves. Thus in a changing population, long-term evaluation of the results of an education program is still possible. The percentage of objectives and goals met by sampling the target population gives valid statistics for program assessment, even though the individual population may have experienced a complete turnover.

For example, a nurse notes that according to annual health department data, 60% of all pregnant women in the nurse's catchment area received some prenatal care. Wanting to increase this percentage to 100%, the nurse tries an educational intervention in which radio and television stations make public service announcements about the importance and availability of prenatal services.

BOX 13-12 Why Long-Term Evaluation Is Challenging

COOPERATION

Clients may not adhere with return appointments or calls.

Clients may show a lack of interest in their own health care.

Clients may think it is too time-consuming or expensive to follow up.

TIME

Follow-up requires making phone calls, evaluating clients, and reviewing and analyzing the results of the evaluation.

ENERGY

Follow-up requires the educator to keep track of clients and to relocate those who have moved.

The nurse must obtain the cooperation of clients.

The nurse must balance long-term evaluation responsibilities with other demands.

EXPENSE

Travel, phone calls, mail, and staff time are all expenses related to long-term evaluation.

Based on data from Redman BK: Patient education at 25 years; where we have been and where we are going, *J Adv Nurs* 18(5):725, 1993.

After 1 year, the nurse discovers that 80% of all pregnant women now receive prenatal care. The nurse continues to use public service announcements the following year because good results are evident. However, the long-term goal of the education program to influence the behavior of 100% of the pregnant women in the community has not yet been met. Therefore the nurse also enlists volunteers to put informational posters in shopping malls, grocery stores, public transportation stops, laundries, and on public transportation vehicles. The second year after implementing the revised educational program, again using the statistics from the health department, the nurse finds that 95% of all pregnant women in the target area now receive prenatal care. The nurse can thus evaluate and modify a community educational program over time to increase the rate, range, and consistency of progress made toward meeting the long-term goals of the project.

clinical application

During an initial survey of a community, the nurse finds in local school records that an unusually large percentage of elementary school children are not receiving standard immunizations for communicable childhood diseases. The nurse identifies education about immunizations as a need in the community.

The nurse then performs an assessment, which shows that the majority of the parents are of a certain ethnic group, are single, work full time, and are of a lower socioeconomic status. The nurse designs a simple verbal questionnaire that includes questions about attitudes and beliefs related to immunizations and assigns several pollsters to speak with a sampling of the parents. The following barriers to learning are identified:

• Lack of awareness about the need for and the benefits of immunization
• Belief that immunizations can be harmful to children
• Belief that immunizations are expensive
• Inability to get time off from work to have children immunized

The nurse next develops a strengths-and-needs list from the information gathered in the survey. Strengths that the nurse finds in the community members are their desire to be good parents and their involvement in the parent/teacher organization. The survey also demonstrates that the average education of the parents is at a tenth-grade level. The nurse identifies the following as client needs:

• Knowledge about the existence and benefits of immunization
• Valid information about the risks of immunization
• Knowledge that immunizations are free
• Information about the availability and accessibility of immunizations through the school system

Using a town meeting format, the nurse explains that the community has a mobile immunization unit that operates in the evenings for families with infants and preschoolers and for families who do not have transportation available to them.

The nurse next matches the characteristics of the learner to an educational theory. In this case, the nurse educator chooses to combine and apply three theories to the educational situation. *Social learning theory* is chosen because of the desire to influence the parents' beliefs and expectations. *Cognitive theory* is chosen because the nurse believes that the parents will respond to a variety of information. *Humanistic theory* is selected because the client is a close-knit, supportive community and is strongly devoted to its children.

The nurse educator selects a health education model for adaptation to the learner. The health belief model is chosen because of the need to change many of the parents' beliefs about immunizations. Based on the principles of this model, the nurse expects that the behaviors of the parents will change once their beliefs change.

The nurse considers educational principles and determines that the educational format should be that of a "town meeting." The most convenient environment conducive to the concentration and comfort of the group is the local high-school theater. To complete the design of the format, the nurse plans an informal lecture about immunizations. A local family physician who grew up in the neighborhood and has family still living in the community

continued

clinical application—cont'd

will give the lecture. After the talk, parents will be invited to ask questions and discuss issues. The program will conclude by asking parents to enjoy snacks and socialize with each other. Small discussion groups will be encouraged to develop into community action groups of those who think that Immunizations are important.

The nurse also organizes other educational methods, objectives, plans, and strategies (MOPS). For example, the nurse may ask interested parents to volunteer in the arrangement of further meetings. Once the previously listed plans and strategies have been developed, the nurse then implements them. First, the nurse arranges a meeting with as many of the target group as possible through the local parent/teacher organization. The meeting is widely advertised through direct mailing to the target group and through notices that the children take home with their report cards. Public service announcements on the local television news and radio broadcasts are made. Carpools and shuttle vans are arranged for those who call for assistance with transportation. The date and time of the program are made as convenient as possible.

Soon after the strategies for these objectives have been implemented, the nurse educator develops an evaluation program for 3 months, 6 months, 9 months, and 1 year after the initiation of the educational program to evaluate the success of the program. The central criterion for the determination of success is the number of children receiving immunizations. Thus even as the specific individuals change over time, the program evaluation process can be applied far into the future without the need for fundamental revision.

A. What aspect(s) of this clinical application indicate that the nurse educator needs to have a solid foundation in community and public health nursing?
B. How would the program have differed if the nurse had used behavioral theory to understand how individuals learn instead of social learning theory, cognitive theory, and humanistic theory?
C. What strategy might the nurse use to determine whether the program attendees enjoyed and benefited from the program?
D. Would the evaluation process be adequate if long-term evaluation were omitted?

Answers are in the back of the book.

KEY POINTS

- Health education is a vital component of community and public health nursing because the promotion, maintenance, and restoration of health rely on clients' understanding of health care requirements.

- Six important general educational theories used to guide the practice of the nurse educator are behavioral, social learning, cognitive, humanist, developmental, and critical theories.
- Three current and useful models for organizing health education are the PRECEDE-PROCEED, health belief, and health promotion models.
- Three domains of learning are cognitive, affective, and psychomotor. Depending on the needs of the learner, one or more of these domains may be important for the nurse educator to consider as learning programs are developed.
- Nine principles associated with instruction are gaining attention, informing the learner of the objectives of instruction, stimulating recall of prior learning, presenting the stimulus, providing learning guidance, eliciting performance, providing feedback, assessing performance, and enhancing retention and transfer of knowledge.
- Principles that guide the effective educator include message, format, environment, experience, participation, and evaluation.
- The five phases of the educational process are identifying educational needs, establishing educational goals and objectives, selecting appropriate educational methods, implementing the educational plan, and evaluating the educational process and product.
- Evaluation of the product includes the measurement of short-term and long-term goals and objectives related to improving health and promoting behavioral changes.

critical thinking activities

1. Review the general theories of learning summarized in the chapter. Decide which one would most effectively fit the learning needs of an individual who has been recently diagnosed with lung cancer, a family caring for an individual with Alzheimer's disease, and a community in which adolescent cigarette smoking is on the rise.
2. Recall an educational interaction with a client that did not seem to go well. Identify what might have been the problem based on educational principles. Develop a plan for ways in which the interaction could have been improved, again based on educational principles.
3. Recall a learning experience in which either the message, format, environment, experience, participation, or evaluation were problematic. Then develop a plan for how the problem could have been overcome and turned from a negative or neutral learning situation into a positive one.
4. Review the phases of the educational process. Apply this process to an individual with hypertension, a family with a child who has attention deficit disorder, and a community in which tuberculosis is on the rise.

Bibliography

Andrews DJ: Comprehensive health education: primary prevention's best hope, *J Med Assoc Ga* 83:397, 1994.

Annand F: A challenge for the 1990s: patient education, *Today's OR Nurse* 15(1):31, 1993.

Bigbee JL, Jansa N: Strategies for promoting health protection, *Nurs Clin North Am* 26(4):895, 1991.

Blair JE: Social learning theory: strategies for health promotion, *AAOHN J* 41(5):245, 1993.

Clarke HF, Beddome G, Whyte NB: Public health nurses' vision of their future reflects changing paradigms, *Image J Nurs Scholarship* 25(4):305, 1993.

Damrosch S: General strategies for motivating people to change their behavior, *Nurs Clin North Am* 26(4):833, 1991.

Dembo MH: *Applying educational psychology,* ed 5, New York, 1994, Longman.

Dignam D: Cinderella and the four learning theories, *Nurs Prax N Z* 7(3):17, 1992.

Driscoll MP: *Psychology of learning for instruction,* Boston, 1994, Allyn & Bacon.

Dunbar CN: Developing a teaching program, *Am J Nurs* 98(8):16B, 1998.

Edwards L: Health education. In Edelman CL, Mandle CL, editors: *Health promotion throughout the lifespan,* ed 5, St Louis, 1998, Mosby.

Estey A, Musseau A, Keehn L: Comprehension levels of patients reading health information, *Patient Educ Counseling* 18:165, 1991.

Freed PE: Perseverance: the meaning of patient education in psychiatric nursing, *Arch Psychiatr Nurs* 2:107, 1998.

Gallagher S, Zeind SM: Bridging patient education and care, *Am J Nurs* 98(8):16AAA, 1998.

Graham KY: Health care reform and public health nursing, *Public Health Nurs* 9(2):73, 1992.

Green LW, Kreuter MW: CDC's planned approach to community health as an application of PRECEDE and an inspiration for PROCEED, *J Health Educ* 23(3):140, 1992.

Green LW, Ottoson JM: *Community health,* ed 7, St Louis, 1994, Mosby.

Hamachek D: *Psychology in teaching, learning, and growth,* ed 5, Boston, 1995, Allyn & Bacon.

Hancock LA, Mandle CL: Overview of growth and developmental framework. In Edelman CL, Mandle CL, editors: *Health promotion throughout the lifespan,* ed 5, St Louis, 1998, Mosby.

Hansen M, Fisher J: Patient-centered teaching from theory to practice, *Am J Nurs* 98(1):56, 1998.

Hawe P, Degeling D, Hall J: *Evaluating health promotion: a health worker's guide,* Philadelphia, 1990, MacLennan & Petty.

Jasovsky DA, Webb EM: Where are your patient education resources? *Am J Nurs* 98(4):16AAA, 1998.

Knowles M: *The adult learner: a neglected species,* ed 5, Houston, 1998, Gulf.

Knowles MS: *The modern practice of adult education: from pedagogy to andragogy,* ed 5, Chicago, 1988, Follett.

MacDonald RE: *A handbook of basic skills and strategies for beginner teachers: facing the challenge in today's schools,* Reading, Mass, 1999, Addison Wesley Longman.

McLeroy KR et al: Creating capacity: establishing a health education research agenda for special populations, *Health Educ Q* 22(3):390, 1995.

Mullen PD et al: Settings as an important dimension in health education/promotion policy, programs, and research, *Health Educ Q* 22(3):329, 1995.

Padilla GV, Bulcavage LM: Theories used in patient/health education, *Semin Oncol Nurs* 7(2):87, 1991.

Palank CL: Determinants of health-promotive behavior: a review of current research, *Nurs Clin North Am* 26(4):815, 1991.

Rankin SH, Stallings KD: *Patient education: issues, principles, practices,* ed 3, New York, 1996, J.B. Lippincott.

Redman BK: Patient education at 25 years: where we have been and where we are going, *J Adv Nurs* 18(5):725, 1993.

Reeber BJ: Evaluating the effects of a family education intervention, *Rehabil Nurs* 17(6):332, 1992.

Salazar MK: Comparison of four behavioral theories, *AAOHN J* 39(3):128, 1991.

Simmons SJ: The Health-Promoting Self-Care System Model: directions for nursing research and practice, *J Adv Nurs* 15(10):1162, 1990.

Strodtman LK: A decision-making process for planning patient education, *Patient Educ Counseling* 5(4):189, 1984.

USDHHS: *Healthy people 2000: national health promotion and disease prevention objectives,* Washington, DC, 1991, USDHHS, Public Health Service.

Volker DL: Patient education: needs assessment and resource identification, *Oncol Nurs Forum* 18(1):119, 1991.

Welton MR: The contribution of critical theory to our understanding of adult learning. In Merriam SB, editor: *An update on adult learning theory,* San Francisco, 1993, Jossey-Bass.

Community Health Promotion: An Integrative Model for Practice

PAMELA A. KULBOK, SHIRLEY C. LAFFREY, & JEAN GOEPPINGER

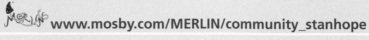 www.mosby.com/MERLIN/community_stanhope

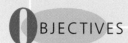
OBJECTIVES

After reading this chapter, the student should be able to do the following:

- Compare and contrast definitions of health.
- Evaluate how one's definition of health influences nursing practice.
- Contrast the health paradigm and the pathogenic paradigm as the basis for health promotion and illness prevention interventions.
- Analyze the interrelationship of individual, family, aggregate, and community as the target of health promotion strategies.

- Evaluate the methods used to assess the health risks of individuals, families, aggregates, and community groups.
- Explain multilevel approaches to promote health; prevent illness and reduce risk; and treat illness in individuals, families, aggregates, and community groups.
- Analyze why community and public health nursing roles are essential to health promotion and illness prevention.

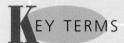
KEY TERMS

client system	disease self-management	health maintenance	multilevel intervention
community	focuses of care	health promotion	risk appraisal
community health	health	illness prevention	self-care
disease management	health behavior	lifestyle	*See Glossary for definitions*

CHAPTER OUTLINE

Lifestyle is a critical factor influencing the health of Americans. Interest in healthy lifestyles is reflected in the growing body of scientific evidence linking lifestyle, health, and the public's recent emphasis on self-care, as well as the continued emphasis on public health programming for vulnerable populations. People in many countries recognize the need to exercise regularly, maintain their weight at recommended levels, and manage stress in their lives. Increasingly, people are driving more slowly, drinking and smoking less, and paying more attention to their lifestyles. Others jog or walk, participate in structured physical fitness programs, and engage in a variety of relaxation techniques at home and at work. Despite this increased interest in health, nurses, other health professionals, and the public increasingly recognize that initiating and maintaining a healthy lifestyle is difficult and requires different kinds of activities directed toward individuals, families, and the environments in which they live.

This chapter describes an integrative model for community and public health nursing practice (Laffrey and Kulbok, 1998). This integrative model can help nurses plan care for clients in the community and for the whole community. The model synthesizes knowledge from public health, nursing, and the social sciences. This chapter also defines some of the basic concepts with which community and public health nurses are concerned and describes the historical roots of these concepts including how health and health promotion are defined for individuals, families, groups or aggregates, and communities. The concepts of community, illness care, illness prevention, risk reduction, self-care, and disease management are also discussed. These concepts and their linkages determine the direction and methods for community and public health nursing practice. The chapter describes studies that illustrate multilevel care. The application of the integrative model of community and public health nursing shows that the way the concepts are viewed is important in the nurse's approach to practice.

SHIFTING EMPHASIS FROM ILLNESS AND DISEASE MANAGEMENT TO WELLNESS

Nurses clearly recognize the need to shift the emphasis of health care from illness to wellness. In community and public health nursing practice, it is abundantly clear that although illness and disease affect the health of individuals, families, groups, and communities, so do many other factors. The biomedical model of health, defined as absence of disease, cannot explain why some individuals exposed to illness-producing stressors remain healthy, while others, who appear to be in health-enhancing situations, become ill. Nurses assist clients in identifying their health potential and in taking measures that enhance their health.

Health is more than the absence of disease or illness. However, viewing clients from the perspective of the biomedical model alone makes it difficult to identify health potential beyond the absence of disease. For example,

most people over 65 years of age have at least one diagnosed chronic disease. Limiting the definition of health potential to the absence of disease or illness would result in these persons never being healthy. This is a pessimistic definition; nursing actions can help elderly and chronically ill persons become healthier if a broader definition of health is used.

Studies show that there is no better way to promote healthy aging and improve the quality of life of older persons than through basic health habits such as exercise, balanced nutrition, a positive outlook, and not smoking (Rosenberg, 1994). The goal of health care must be directed toward helping older clients identify their health potential and providing nursing care that helps them move toward their health potential.

Laffrey, Loveland-Cherry, and Winkler (1986) describe two paradigms from which the key concepts of nursing science (e.g., persons, health, environment) and nursing could be viewed.

1. *Pathogenic, or disease, paradigm.* Health is defined as the absence of disease. The pathogenic paradigm assumes that human beings are composed of organ systems and cells and that health care focuses on identifying what is not working properly with a given system and repairing it. Within this paradigm, health behavior is based on how the client complies with the recommendation of the health professional.

2. *Health paradigm.* Health is more subjectively defined and is a "fluid, flexible process" (Laffrey, Loveland-Cherry, and Winkler, 1986, p. 97). Human beings are defined as complex and interconnected with the environment and are different from and greater than the sum of their parts. Health behavior within the health paradigm involves the human being's total lifestyle and interaction with the environment and is therefore not judged simply by compliance with a prescribed regimen. The health paradigm is based on a holistic view of human beings and is consistent with high-level wellness as defined by Dunn (1973).

Both paradigms support the specific aims and processes of community and public health nursing (Laffrey, Loveland-Cherry, and Winkler, 1986). The pathogenic approach directs nursing toward disease prevention, risk reduction, prompt treatment, and disease management, whereas the health approach directs community and public health nursing practice toward promotion of greater levels of positive health. If health is defined broadly as the life process, taking into account the mutual and simultaneous interaction of humans and their environment, then disease and illness can be seen as potential manifestations of that interaction. Therefore the health paradigm does not exclude any part of the life process and, as such, includes disease prevention and disease treatment.

The recent growth of managed health care has encouraged an integrated focus on health promotion, disease prevention, and illness care. This integration is generally intended when the term *disease management* is used. **Disease management** is a clinical care process for individuals with chronic conditions, which crosses the continuum from primary prevention to long-term health maintenance (Johnson, 1996, p. 54); it "pushes" managed care from treatment to prevention. Disease management is no longer specific to the disease being managed; rather, it is viewed as a process that has "brought the consumer into health management and squeezed the dollars out of high-cost conditions" (Johnson, 1996, p. 53).

The first generation of managed care produced case management programs to manage high-cost, high-volume catastrophic diseases. The second generation expanded the focus of programs to include comprehensive analysis of resources and alternative settings for treatment for a broader range of chronic diseases. The third generation of managed care has been described as "proactive health management or preventive care—trying to keep people healthy" (Johnson, 1996, p. 54), which some see as stages of maturity (Johnson, 1996). Others acknowledge that the roots of case management are in public health and district (Issel, 1997; Utz and Kulbok, 1998). Whether the label is health management or disease management, the characteristics of community and public health nursing practice include the meaning of health and the actions taken by nurses and clients to optimize health potential.

Confusion will continue to exist, despite the fact that a broader idea of health is becoming generally accepted, if indicators of health promotion continue to be concerned only with disease and illness. Downie, Tannahill, and Tannahill (1996) argue against medicalizing health promotion because this leads to a "new generation of experts dominating the media with the high-pressure selling of positive health" (p. 196). Tillich (1961) argues that health care workers imply that ordinary people are not able to manage their own health but that expert professionals can do so with medical technology and pills. Therefore to simply incorporate health promotion into existing models of health care might violate the premises on which community and public health nursing is based.

Shifting Emphasis from Individual to Multilevel Interventions

Because the individual ultimately makes decisions to engage in healthy or risky behaviors, lifestyle improvement efforts typically focus on the individual as the target of care (Jeffrey, 1989; Von Korff et al, 1992). However, Jeffrey (1989) pointed out that there are different perspectives associated with risky behaviors. When individuals make decisions about their behaviors, they generally focus on immediate personal rewards or threats. However, from a public health perspective, even though the individual might believe that the risk from a behavior such as smoking is low, the estimated deaths attributable to smoking in the United States are substantial (e.g., 400,000 in 1990 [McGinnis and Foege, 1993]) and the cost to society is

great. Moreover, from the public health perspective, it is clear that health behaviors have multilevel determinants both internal and external to the individual. Tobacco use by a child is associated with personal attributes of the child (e.g., self-esteem), family characteristics (e.g., parental attitudes toward smoking), aggregate characteristics (e.g., peer pressure to smoke), community factors (e.g., availability of cigarettes), and other social factors (e.g., taxation of cigarettes) (Von Korff et al, 1992). Therefore interventions to initiate or maintain health behavior must be systematically directed toward the multiple targets of the individual, family, group or aggregate, community, and society.

Downie, Tannahill, and Tannahill (1996) and Lowenberg (1996) argued that it is not realistic to emphasize individual responsibility for health behavior while excluding community. They cautioned against the danger of "victim blaming" by placing the responsibility for health behavior on the individual. Likewise, expecting the community to be solely responsible for people's health behaviors is a patronizing, "top-down" attitude that leads people to feel as if they have no power or control. Thus making either the individual or the community solely responsible for health results in people feeling victimized. Downie, Tannahill, and Tannahill propose a "new sense of community responsibility" (1996, p.199). "Community responsibility empowers individuals to be knowledgeable . . . about their own health, and at the same time, empowers the community to provide needed leadership and professional assistance for community development—to work with and through the community to promote health. Health and well-being are, in the end, a set of relationships among citizens" (p. 170). The World Health Organization (WHO, 1984) also support this approach, which considers both the individuals within the community and the community itself in its emphasis on full (public) participation in health-promoting activities as described in Chapter 17.

An Integrative Model for Community Health Promotion

Laffrey and Kulbok (1998) developed a model for community health promotion to guide community and public health nursing. This model, shown in Figure 14-1, is based on two complementary paradigms for nursing: the health paradigm and the pathogenic (disease) paradigm as described previously (Laffrey, Loveland-Cherry CJ, and Winkler, 1986). The health paradigm focuses on promoting health as a dynamic, creative, and positive quality of life and includes the promotion of physical, mental, emotional, functional, spiritual, and social well-being. The pathogenic paradigm includes both the care and prevention of illness, disease, and disability and focuses on reducing known risks and threats to health and preventing disease. Although clinical strategies may be similar within the two paradigms, the ultimate goal of each is fundamentally different. This difference can be seen in the specific purpose of the nursing care and whether it is aimed

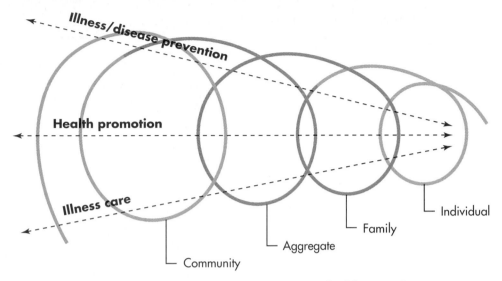

FIG. 14-1 An integrative model for community health promotion.

at resolving a disease or illness or promoting greater health.

The integrative model includes two major dimensions: client system and focus of care. The **client system** is multidimensional and includes various levels of clients toward which community and public health nursing care is targeted. The client system becomes more complex, beginning at its most delimited target, the individual. When the individual is the client, the environment includes the family, population group, and the community of which the individual is a part. The nurse is concerned with how these environments affect the individual.

The level of client can also be the family, aggregate, or community. As the nurse focuses on the family, the aggregate and community are the environment for the family. When the client is the aggregate, the community is the environment. Different kinds of assessments and nursing interventions appropriate at each level of client within the system are discussed later in this chapter. It is important to note that nursing is holistic in nature and addresses multiple levels of client within the total system.

The **focuses of care** in the model include *health promotion, illness (disease or disability) prevention,* and *illness care.* Each focus is appropriate for some aspects of nursing. Even more important is the awareness that the goal of all care is a healthier community, and this is achieved through health promotion interventions. No matter where community and public health nursing care begins, it leads to health promotion of the community. This does not mean that one nurse provides all levels of care, but it does underscore the need for nurses to have a good understanding of care requirements at all of the client levels. The individual, family, aggregate, and community each has characteristics, strengths, and health needs that are unique and that differ from the other levels.

The integrative community health promotion model reflects the basic beliefs and values of community and public health nursing. The model depicts continuity and expansiveness of the client systems and focuses of care. The central axis, or core, of the model is health promotion. At its narrowest focus, illness care is provided to individuals. At the model's broadest level of care, the nurse works with community leaders and lay people to plan programs to promote optimal health of its citizens. The goals of nursing actions in the integrative model, at any client level from the individual to the community, are to achieve the maximal health potential through an active partnership between the nurse and the client system. When nurses facilitate an active partnership with the client system, whether the focus of care is health promotion, illness prevention, or illness care, they involve clients in every step of the process of managing health care from the assessment of health needs to implementation and evaluation of outcomes.

NURSING TIP

Nurses facilitate an active partnership with clients by involving them in every step of the process of managing health care from the assessment of their health needs to planning, implementing, and evaluating health outcomes.

DEFINITIONS, HISTORICAL PERSPECTIVES, AND METHODS
Health and Health Promotion
Historical perspectives

Health is the pivotal term in a model for community and public health nursing practice. Beginning with Nightingale's efforts to discover and use the laws of nature to enhance humanity, nursing has always taken an active role in promoting the health of populations and the total community. How one defines health shapes the entire process of nursing, including making the decision of what is to be assessed and with what level of client and the decision of how to evaluate the outcomes of care. When health is defined as alleviating illness symptoms, the assessment consists of the duration, intensity, and frequency of the specific symptoms. Intervention is aimed at symptom relief and perhaps treatment of the cause of the symptoms. Evaluation consists of a determination of whether the symptoms are alleviated. On the other hand, if health is defined as maximizing a community's physical recreation opportunities, the assessment then focuses on existing recreation facilities, accessibility to the population, and beliefs and knowledge related to recreation and land use in the community.

Descriptions of the nature of health have puzzled human beings from the earliest times. The ancient Greeks viewed health as the influence of environmental forces such as living habits; climate; and quality of air, water, and food on human well-being. This holistic view of health is not new. For instance, in Greek literature the goddess Hygeia represented the belief that humans could remain healthy if they lived rationally. Certain activities of daily living, such as exercise, were considered essential to the maintenance of health. Similarly in Judeo-Christian times, food laws were instituted that promoted health. Box 14-1 lists health perspectives over time.

Scientific medicine emerged slowly from the sixteenth to the nineteenth centuries. Resistance to scientific discoveries, such as the germ theory of disease and the principle of antisepsis, hindered the application of new medical science to medical practice. However, in the twentieth century, medical science grew in power, and the rate of scientific progress was described as a revolution (Somers and Somers, 1961). With the development of the scientific approach toward disease, self-care was ignored in favor of professional care.

The South African philosopher Jan Christian Smuts introduced the holistic view of health in 1926. Holism was a way to understand whole organisms and systems as being greater than and different from the sum of their parts (Smuts, 1926). The holistic perspective of health was overshadowed by the scientific view of disease as being a deviation from the biochemical norm. A focus on treatment and cure, with its dependence on health professionals, continued to overshadow self-care, health promotion, and illness prevention. Despite a growing emphasis on self-care, the biomedical emphasis continues to this day.

During the last four decades, the idea of self-care as derived from a positive idea of health has reemerged and may compete with professional care. Some proponents of self-care emphasize lay diagnosis and self-treatment, as opposed to professional diagnosis and collaborative management. Other versions of self-care focus on teaching people

---

BOX 14-1 Health Perspectives Over Time

ANCIENT GREEK VIEW
- Health was the totality of environmental forces influencing human well-being.
- Ways of living were essential to maintain health.

1700S TO 1800S
- Opposition to scientific discoveries existed (e.g., germ theory of disease and principle of antisepsis).
- Translation of new medical science into medical practice impeded emphasis on self-care.

EARLY TO MID-1900S
- Holistic view of health was reintroduced as an antidote to the medical science model.
- Scientific and biologic view of disease dominated.
- Self-care was deemphasized.

LATE 1900S
- Reemergence of the ideal of self-care was accelerated by the climate of political activism.
- An increased recognition that people produce health by what they do and do not do for themselves emerged.
- Collaboration existed between consumers and providers, and renegotiation of professional roles in health care emerged.
- New models of chronic disease self-management under managed care were developed.

---

how to work with their health care providers. In both cases, the health care system is changing; roles are being renegotiated emphasizing collaboration between consumers and providers.

The self-care movement was accelerated by the political climate of the 1960s and 1970s. Racial minorities began to demand their rights in the 1960s, and women and the elderly began to make their demands public in the 1970s. A challenge to professional health care, which many believe exemplifies elite rather than democratic control, is illustrated clearly in the ideology of self-care. Illich wrote, "The medical establishment has become a major threat to health. The disabling impact of professional control over medicine has reached the proportions of an epidemic" (1976, p. 3). He warned that politicians and legislators might promote self-care because of their interest in cost containment rather than a genuine belief in individuals' abilities to preserve health. More than 20 years later the same warning can be made about the cost-driven managed care movement.

Many health professionals contend that the individual is in a position to produce health. Fuchs (1974) suggests that the "greatest potential for improving health lies in what we do and don't do for and to ourselves" (p. 55). Other self-care advocates believe that modern medicine has been given too much credit for improvements in

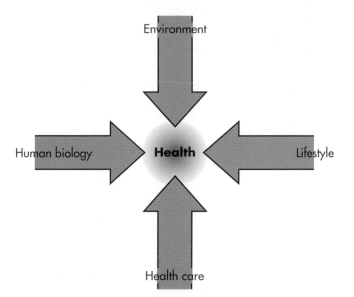

FIG. 14-2 Determinants of health. (Adapted from LaLonde M: *A new perspective on the health of Canadians,* Ottawa, 1974, Government of Canada.)

BOX 14-2 **Landmark Health Promotion/Disease Prevention Initiatives**

- *1974* LaLonde's *New Perspectives on the Health of Canadians*
- *1976* Forward Plan for Health, FY 1978-82
- 1979 The Surgeon General's Report *Healthy People*
- 1989 *Guide to Clinical Preventive Services*
- 1990 *Healthy People 2000*
- *1991* Nursing's Agenda for Health Care Reform
- 1994 *Put Prevention into Practice* (PPIP)
- 1995 *Guide to Clinical Preventive Services,* edition 2
- 1997 *Healthy People 2010* framework opened for public comment.

health. Wildavsky (1977) asserts that the medical system affects only 10% of the variability in health indicators such as infant mortality, disability days, and adult mortality. He attributes the remaining 90% to factors over which physicians lack control, "from individual lifestyle (smoking, exercise, worry), to social conditions (income, eating habits, physiological inheritance), to the physical environment (air and water quality)" (p. 105).

In the political arena, these conclusions were introduced by LaLonde in *A New Perspective on the Health of Canadians* (1974). As the Canadian Minister of National Health and Welfare, LaLonde urged a more comprehensive approach to health care. He identified four major determinants of health: human biology, environment, lifestyle, and health care (Fig. 14-2). In 1976 policy makers in the United States echoed LaLonde's ideas. Efforts to improve health habits and the environment were viewed as the best hope of achieving any significant extension of life expectancy (USDHEW, 1976, p. 69). Box 14-2 lists some landmark initiatives in health promotion and disease prevention.

The U.S. Public Health Service first established national objectives involving disease prevention, health protection, and health promotion strategies in the Surgeon General's report *Healthy People* (USDHEW, 1979). Disease prevention strategies focused on services such as family planning and immunizations delivered in clinical settings. Health protection strategies were directed to environmental measures to ". . . significantly improve health and the quality of life for this and future generations of Americans . . ." (p. 101), including occupational health and accidental injury control. Health promotion strategies were designed to achieve well-being through community and individual lifestyle

change measures. Health promotion was described as beginning with basically healthy people who are seeking to improve their lifestyles. The Surgeon General's report (USDHEW, 1979) also described inherited biological factors, the environment, and behavioral factors as the three categories of risks to health, which are identical to LaLonde's first three major determinants of health.

Although a national initiative for health promotion was gaining momentum, disease prevention continued to be the main focus for intervention. However, interesting shifts were evident: 1) emphasis was placed on health promotion and education of at-risk groups and the general population, and 2) prevention of complications of hypertension was emphasized through adherence to medical treatment (Marston-Scott, 1988). The USDHHS report in 1991 on national health objectives, *Healthy People 2000,* emphasized health promotion first, then health protection, and finally preventive services (Kulbok and Baldwin, 1992). The objectives listed in *Healthy People 2000* also addressed the determinants of health as originally described by LaLonde.

The politics of the existing illness care system poses a major difficulty for promoting holistic health. Health care is big business and often prefers to keep the biomedical model in place. *Nursing's Agenda for Health Care Reform* (ANA, 1991) challenges the utility of the medical care system. More than 60 nursing and allied health care organizations, representing 1 million nurses, health professionals, and consumers, endorsed a landmark reform agenda for a true "health" care system (Reifsnider, 1992). Historically, nurses have been leaders in providing primary health care (Stanhope, 1995). As the twentieth century draws to a close, health professionals have once again been called upon to provide expertise for *Healthy People 2010.* Many nursing organizations, including the Association of Community Health Nursing Educators (ACHNE) and the Public Health Nursing (PHN) Section of the American Public Health Association, participated in the initial process of development of new priorities and health directions. These nursing organizations will help shape the health promotion and disease prevention objectives for the year 2010.

Definitions of health

The WHO (1958), in its classic definition of health as a state of complete physical, mental, and social well-being and not merely the absence of disease and infirmity, reflected a holistic perspective. This definition was considered both visionary and idealistic. However, the WHO perspective had definition and measurement problems (Kulbok, 1983). In 1975 Terris noted that epidemiologists considered the WHO definition to be "vague and imprecise with a Utopian aura" (p. 1037). He expanded the definition: "Health is a state of physical, mental and social well-being and the ability to function and not merely the absence of illness and infirmity" (p. 1038). In adding "ability to function" and deleting the word "complete" from the WHO definition, the WHO definition was placed in a more realistic context, providing an important and useful framework for health promotion.

Smith (1981) suggests that the idea of health directs the nature of nursing practice, education, and research. She clarifies the idea of health by observing that, in the literature, health was described as a comparative concept, allowing for "more" or "less" health, or degrees of health, along a health-illness continuum. Smith proposed four models of health, ordered from narrow and concrete to broad and abstract. These models were clinical health, or the absence of disease; role performance health, or the ability to perform one's social roles satisfactorily; adaptive health, or flexible adaptation to the environment; and eudaemonistic health, or self-actualization and the attainment of one's greatest human potential.

It is important for nurses to examine their personal definition of health and recognize how the nursing care they provide is directed by their health definition. A nurse who defines health as the absence of disease is likely to focus primarily on physical and biological signs and symptoms of disease with minimal attention to the quality of social roles and evidence of subjective well-being. A nurse who broadly defines health as self-actualization is more likely to consider indicators of physical health, social health, and the potential for maximum well-being when planning nursing care. Nurses have contributed to the ongoing discussion of the nature of health in individuals and communities by emphasizing positive health and health promotion, while acknowledging the importance of illness and disease.

Definitions of health promotion

Health promotion is an accepted aim of nursing practice, although it is rarely defined and is not often differentiated from disease prevention or health maintenance (Brubaker, 1983). Leavell and Clark (1965) strongly influenced the evolution of health promotion and disease prevention strategies through their classic definitions of primary, secondary, and tertiary levels of prevention that were rooted in the biomedical model of health and epidemiology. The application of preventive measures, according to Leavell and Clark, corresponds to the natural history of disease. Primary preventive measures are directed toward "well" individuals in the prepathogenesis period to promote their health and to provide specific protection from disease. Secondary preventive measures are applied to diagnose or to treat individuals in the period of disease pathogenesis. Tertiary prevention addresses rehabilitation and the return of people with chronic illness to a maximal ability to function (Table 14-1).

Even though primary, secondary, and tertiary levels of prevention had their origins in the medical model, Leavell and Clark moved beyond the medical model. They conceptualized primary prevention as two distinct components: health promotion and specific protection. Health promotion focuses on positive measures such as education for healthy living and promotion of favorable environmental conditions as well as periodic selective examinations such as well child developmental assessment and health education. The other aspect of primary prevention, specific protection, includes measures to reduce the threat of specific diseases such as hygiene and the elimination of workplace hazards (Kulbok and Baldwin, 1992).

When health promotion and specific protection are used as subconcepts of primary prevention, they appear to stem from a definition of health as the absence of disease. However, differences in health promotion and specific protection strategies suggest that they are not the same. Some terms used to describe health promotion are linked to a positive view of health (e.g., health habits), whereas other terms are linked to the negative view of the absence of disease (e.g., disease prevention). The confusion in terminology is increased when actions to promote health, protect health, and prevent disease are used interchangeably as indicators of preventive behavior (Kulbok and Baldwin, 1992).

Kasl and Cobb (1966) presented classic definitions to distinguish health behavior from illness and sick role behavior. **Health behavior** is any action to prevent or detect disease in the asymptomatic stage undertaken by people who consider themselves to be healthy. This definition was a beginning focus on prevention, but because it was restricted to actions to prevent or detect disease, it did not include health promotion or wellness. Illness behavior is any action undertaken by a person to eliminate a symptom of illness. Sick role behavior is any activity undertaken to facilitate recovery from illness (Kasl and Cobb, 1966).

An equally important definition (Harris and Guten, 1979) described self-reported behaviors used by adults to protect their health. Health protective behavior (HPB) is behavior that individuals perform to protect their health,

TABLE 14-1 Levels of Application of Preventive Measures in the Natural History of Disease

THE NATURAL HISTROY OF ANY DISEASE OF MAN				
PREPATHOGENESIS PERIOD		PERIOD OF PATHOGENESIS		
HEALTH PROMOTION	SPECIFIC PROTECTION	EARLY DIAGNOSIS AND PROMPT TREATMENT	DISABILITY LIMITATION	REHABILITATION
Health education Good standard of nutrition adjusted to developmental phases of life Attention to personality development Provision of adequate housing, recreation, and agreeable working conditions Marriage counseling and sex education Genetics Periodic selective examinations	Use of specific immunizations Attention to personal hygiene Use of environmental sanitation Protection against occupational hazards Protection from accidents Use of specific nutrients Protection from carcinogens Avoidance of all allergens	Case-finding measures, individual and mass Screening surveys Selective examinations *Objectives:* To cure and prevent disease processes To prevent the spread of communicable diseases To prevent complications and sequelae To shorten period of disability	Adequate treatment to arrest the disease process and to prevent further complications and sequelae Provision of facilities to limit disability and to prevent death	Provision of hospital and community facilities for retraining and education for maximum use of remaining capacities Education of the public and industry to utilize the rehabilitated As full employment as possible Selective placement Work therapy in hospitals Use of sheltered colony
PRIMARY PREVENTION		SECONDARY PREVENTION		TERTIARY PREVENTION
LEVELS OF APPLICATION OF PREVENTATIVE MEASURES				

From Leavell HF, Clark EG: *Preventive medicine for the doctor in his community: an epidemiologic approach*, New York, 1965, McGraw-Hill.

regardless of their actual or perceived health status and whether the behavior is proved effective. Thus HPB moved beyond the realm of medically prescribed behaviors (i.e., behaviors that the medical community accepts as effective). Kulbok (1985) built on Harris and Guten's (1979) definitions and presented the term *preventive health behavior* to describe behaviors that promote health and prevent disease. Later, Kulbok et al (1997) studied a group of five national health promotion experts and found differences between the terms health promotion and health promotion behavior. The group defined health promotion as activities undertaken by health professionals to promote health in their clients and includes health education and counseling. Health promotion behavior, on the other hand, was defined as behavior that an individual performs to promote his or her health and well-being.

Kulbok (1985) proposed a Resource Model of Health Behavior, in which social and health resources were viewed as correlates of health behaviors. Two major findings were reported in studies to test this model (Kulbok, 1985; Kulbok et al, 1998; Kulbok, Kirkwood, and Hulton, 1997). First, health behavior is multidimensional, and there are several categories of health behavior including positive behaviors (e.g., diet, exercise) and avoidance behaviors (e.g., substance use). Second, different health and social resources are asso-

ciated with different health behaviors. Strategies to promote well-being often focus on helping clients practice new, healthy behaviors or to change unhealthy behaviors. Successful intervention is more likely when nurses understand how social and health resources are related to health behaviors of individuals and how personal and community resources may affect behavior choices.

Laffrey (1990) differentiated among health promotion, illness prevention, and health maintenance. Health promotion is behavior directed toward achieving a greater level of health. **Illness prevention** is behavior directed toward reducing the threat of illness or disease, and **health maintenance** is directed toward keeping a current state of health. This definition of health maintenance is similar to tertiary prevention (Leavell and Clark, 1965). Applying these definitions requires that one assess not only the behavior but also the basis on which one makes a choice to perform a given behavior. In a study of community-residing men and women with and without chronic diseases, Laffrey (1990) asked subjects to identify their five most important health behaviors. For each behavior reported, subjects were asked the major reason they usually performed that behavior. Responses indicated that behaviors were performed for each of the three reasons. For example, one individual reported that he exercises because he has several risk factors for coronary artery disease. Exercise, for him, is an illness-preventing behavior. Another person reported that he exercises because regular, vigorous exercise makes him feel more energetic and he functions at a higher level than he did when he was sedentary. For this individual, exercise is a health promotion behavior. A third individual who reported exercising regularly to maintain her weight used exercise as a health maintenance behavior.

Pender (1996) also differentiated between health-protecting and health-promoting behaviors. Health protection refers to behaviors that decrease one's probability of becoming ill, whereas health promotion refers to behaviors that increase well-being of either an individual or a group. Although health protection and health promotion are complementary, health promotion is a broader concept that encompasses both individuals and groups.

The WHO described health promotion as "the process of enabling people to increase control over, and improve their health" (1984, p. 3). According to the Ottawa Charter, health promotion combines both individual and community level strategies including "building healthful public, creating supportive environments, strengthening community action, developing personal skills, and reorienting health services" (Bracht, 1990, p.38). Health is a resource for daily living. For individuals or communities to realize physical, mental, and social well-being, they must become aware of and learn to use the social and personal resources available within their environment. Kulbok's (1985) model of health resources, Laffrey's (1990) health behavior choices, and Pender's (1996) definition of health promotion are congruent with the WHO process of health promotion. Health promotion and self-care are consistent with the goals of community and public health nursing.

Definitions of self-care and disease self-management

The term **self-care** has influenced how nurses approach health promotion. Orem (1995) has developed a nursing model in which self-care describes activities that individuals initiate and perform on their own behalf to maintain life, health, and well-being. According to Orem, individuals are not always able to be completely self-sufficient in their self-care. Consequently, although self-care is a lay responsibility, professional care may be required to enhance an individual's capability for self-care. Within this model, nursing care depends on the capability of individuals and can range from total care to partial care to education and support of individuals to assist them increase their self-care capability. Orem's self-care focus is on the individual. Her idea of self-care includes a full range of activities that individuals can do for themselves in a variety of health and illness matters.

Goeppinger (1982) notes that self-care activities may be carried out by the individual, the community, or the society and are based on scientific, religious, philosophical, and cultural influences. The care provided by nurses and other primary care workers may be directed toward the individual by changing health beliefs and behaviors. From a public health and political perspective, it is important that self-care also emphasize community responsibility and social change. For example, the WHO definition of health promotion noted earlier included one's use of personal and social resources within the environment to promote health and well-being. An important precursor to the use of resources by the population is to develop adequate resources within the environment to enhance the health of the population.

There is no question that self-care practices promote healthy lifestyles and prevent the onset of disease. However, it is also clear that individuals with chronic conditions can influence their comfort, ability to function, and other illness outcomes through self-care practices (Marston-Scott, 1988). The term **disease self-management** evolved in part from an expanded definition of self-care, which includes persons with chronic conditions. For example, under managed care, new buzzwords—chronic disease self-management (Lorig, 1996)—and disease management (Johnson, 1996)—are viewed as more than just a trend. The most expansive definition of disease management includes partnerships between the managed care organization, the client, and the provider. Disease management focuses on assisting the client to self-manage the disease process by learning about the disease and various treatment options and outcomes (Johnson, 1996). This approach is reinforced by the current changes in reimbursement policies that emphasize disease treatment and prevention (i.e., disease "self-management").

Lorig (1996) argues, as chronic disease increases, a self-management model where professionals and clients are partners in care, learning to manage day-to-day living is essential. An effective self-management model is directed toward the subjective consequences of illness, focuses on client-centered decision-making, and creates partnerships between clients and providers (Lorig, 1996). Education to enhance a client's capacity for self-care practices and self-management of chronic conditions is an intervention that is consistent with the integrative model for community health promotion. Interventions are directed toward multiple client levels, supporting the individual's capacity for adopting self-care practices (e.g., knowledge and skills related to diabetes self-management) and maximizing environmental resources needed to sustain them (e.g., family support for dietary changes and affordable prescriptions, blood glucose testing equipment).

Methods for disease prevention and risk reduction

Health providers use the disease prevention strategy of risk appraisal and risk reduction to help individuals and groups maximize their self-care activities. It compares information supplied by individuals about their health-related practices, health habits, demographic characteristics, and personal and family medical history with data from epidemiological studies and vital statistics. It uses these comparisons to predict individuals' risks of morbidity and mortality and to suggest areas in which disease risks may be reduced. The goal of **risk appraisal** and reduction is to prevent disease or detect disease in its earliest stages. The knowledge base for risk appraisal and reduction is the scientific evidence, which relates risk factors and disease and the effectiveness of interventions in reducing both mortality and risks of mortality.

Since the early 1970s, risk appraisal and reduction gained popularity among health professionals. This trend was influenced by the emphasis on health promotion and disease prevention, epidemiological studies that provided an empirical database for making predictions from risk appraisal methods, and a proliferation of risk appraisal tools for use in clinical practice. The health insurance industry recognized the potential of risk reduction for cost containment and promoted the approach in occupational and health care settings.

In health risk appraisal (HRA), data about health risks experienced by an individual or group are collected and analyzed, and a health risk profile is generated. Health risk appraisal may be done at both individual and community levels. A clinical approach is used to identify risks in individuals, and an epidemiological approach is frequently used to identify risks at the population level. Both of these approaches are important to nurses. In this section, the methods of individual and community health risk appraisal are discussed. Later in the chapter, some influential community and epidemiological studies are reviewed.

Box 14-3 lists the three most common types of health risk appraisal approaches used to assess individuals. Each type of risk appraisal is complex, and only the basic concepts and selected procedures are described in this chapter. More complete explanations are found in the references cited at the end of the chapter. An example of a risk appraisal tool and clinical guidelines are shown in Appendixes A-2 and G.

Health risk appraisal. Robbins and Hall (1970) approached an individual's health from the perspective of what was likely to occur rather than what had already occurred. They recognized that most chronic diseases have a predictable sequence and that the characteristic precursors of many diseases can be monitored and controlled. Robbins and Hall put the concept of prospective medicine into practice by developing a method to profile risk called the *health hazard appraisal.*

BOX 14-3 Health-Risk Appraisal Approaches

- The health-hazard appraisal and its many versions
- Clinical guidelines and recommendations for preventive services
- Wellness appraisals or inventories

HOW TO *Profile Client Risk*

1. Assess the total risks to a client's health based on knowledge of the client
2. Assess the natural history of certain diseases and the major causes of mortality for aggregates of the client's age, sex, race, and family history
3. Assist the health provider in the initiation of lifestyle changes in the client to avoid health threats or to prevent complications
4. Institute treatment or lifestyle changes early in the course of disease
5. To accomplish these objectives, data are collected with a self-administered questionnaire, basic laboratory tests, and clinical examination.
6. The questionnaire asks information about personal characteristics and behaviors known to predict disease.
7. These data are compared with data compiled from the 10 major causes of death of an aggregate of the same age, sex, and race as the client.
8. Based on the comparison, the client's appraisal age and achievable age are calculated.
9. The appraisal age is the health age of the average person in the client's age, sex, and race aggregate with a similar risk profile. For example, a 20-year-old Caucasian woman might have an appraisal age of 15 years if she has good health habits and no family history of chronic disease. Another 20-year-old Caucasian woman might have an appraisal age of 26 years if she smokes, fails to wear a seat belt while driving, does not perform regular breast self-examinations, and has a family history of hypertension. The second woman's achievable age could be lowered considerably if she were to modify her behavior.
10. Achievable age refers to the health age the client could achieve by modifying health hazards.

Risk appraisal instruments are convenient tools that determine individual health risks. One of the most comprehensive HRAs is the Healthier People Questionnaire (HPQ) developed by the Carter Center at Emory University and the Centers for Disease Control and Prevention (CDC). The CDC, along with a network of state health departments and universities, based the HPQ on a decade of development work and on the Risk Factor Update Project (Breslow et al, 1985). The HPQ is computer scored and is available to the public. In 1991 the Healthier People Network (HPN) took responsibility for the ongoing scientific integrity of the health risk appraisal instrument. A newly released Version 6 (now called the HPN Health Risk Appraisal) was updated using 1990 mortality and census data. In addition, a new risk appraisal for older adults (55 to 90 years of age) addresses issues of functional status and morbidity. Current program information is available from the HPN. See this book's website for information about how to contact the HPN.

The Lifestyle Assessment Questionnaire (LAQ) from the National Wellness Institute (NWI, 1989) includes the

HPQ, a wellness inventory, and a personal growth section. Users are provided with a Personal Wellness Report, which summarizes their LAQ results and provides them with a sample action plan for increasing wellness behaviors. Also, the NWI offers age-specific risk appraisals and wellness inventories. See this book's website for information about how to contact the NWI.

Clinical preventive services guidelines. Gradual acceptance of scientific evidence of the benefits associated with key preventive measures led to the development of clinical practice guidelines in the late 1970s. For example, Breslow and Somers (1977) proposed the lifetime health-monitoring program, which also uses clinical practice guidelines and epidemiological data to identify specific needs for health care. They provided a list of recommendations for preventive measures appropriate for each of 10 age groups.

In 1989 the U.S. Preventive Services Task Force published the first *Guide to Clinical Preventive Services* based on review of the scientific evidence on 169 clinical preventive services for 60 target conditions. The Guide included information about the appropriate content of periodic health examinations (Griffith and Diguiseppi, 1994). Clinical preventive services refer to disease prevention and health promotion services delivered to individuals in health care settings, including immunizations (e.g., influenza, pneumococcus, and childhood vaccines), screening (e.g., blood pressure measurement, Papanicolaou smear, mammogram), counseling (e.g., smoking cessation, diet, and exercise guidance), and chemoprophylactic regimens (e.g., hormone replacement and aspirin). Many of these preventive measures are routine nursing interventions. The second edition of the *Guide* was published in 1996.

To ensure implementation of the Clinical Preventive Services Guidelines, the Public Health Service of the U.S. Department of Health and Human Services (USDHHS), provider organizations, and major health-related groups collaborated to develop a program entitled "Put Prevention into Practice" (PPIP). The PPIP program is designed to influence the health promotion and disease prevention practices of health care professionals and the public. The PPIP program uses materials designed to improve delivery of preventive services including the *Child Health Guide* and the *Adult Personal Health Guide,* which are passport-size, consumer-held minirecords (Griffith and Diguiseppi, 1994). The PPIP program is designed to influence the health promotion and disease prevention practices of health care professionals and consumers. PPIP materials are available in English and Spanish from the U.S. Government Printing Office.

Wellness inventories. Wellness inventories differ from health risk appraisal instruments and guidelines for preventive services by defining health risks more broadly and leading to health enhancement or promotion as well as prevention and risk reduction. Typical wellness instruments include questions related to self-responsibility, nutrition awareness, physical fitness, stress management, and environmental sensitivity (Ardell, 1977). Travis' Wellness Self-Evaluation (1977) includes a Life Change Index, Eating Habits Survey, Wellness Inventory Symptom Checklist, Medical History, Purpose in Life Test, Stress Assessments, and Creativity Index. The Wellness Inventory of the LAQ (NWI, 1989) described previously covers six dimensions: physical, social, emotional, intellectual, occupational, and spiritual.

Advantages and disadvantages. There are certain advantages and disadvantages to using health risk appraisals. They support individuals' self-care behaviors and provide direction for nurses to counsel and educate clients about healthy behaviors. Individuals become more aware of their health risks (Avis, Smith, and McKinlay, 1989; Shultz, 1984), more willing to discuss their health behaviors (Skinner et al, 1985), and more likely to initiate recommended changes (Shultz, 1984). Another advantage of HRAs is that they are used to measure the outcomes of risk reduction interventions. By completing HRAs, individuals and groups receive immediate feedback about how their behavioral changes influence their health risks and life expectancy.

Despite these advantages, it is important to know the limitations of risk appraisal tools. Some of these limitations are inherent in the tools themselves, whereas others relate more to problems in usage (Kirscht, 1989). Actual tool limitations are questionable validity and reliability of the instruments. Also, there may be an overemphasis on lifestyle factors and lack of attention to other important risks, such as environmental hazards and inadequate health care (Meeker, 1988; Smith, McKinlay, and McKinlay, 1989; Smith, McKinlay, Thorington, 1987). When selecting an HRA tool, it is important to assess strengths and limitations of the tool overall and for specific populations.

The best results are obtained by using health risk appraisals in conjunction with clinical observation and assessment. Although an educational message may have a great impact on some individuals, others may deny the message or avoid its implications (Becker and Janz, 1987). Even when individuals are motivated by health appraisal feedback, they may not have the behavioral skills necessary to initiate and sustain changes in lifestyle. This is especially true regarding those behaviors that are difficult to change, such as smoking habits.

Another limitation of health risk appraisals is that they are probably more suitable for use with middle-age people than for those younger than 35 or older than 65 years of age (Doerr and Hutchins, 1981). Health risk appraisals provide little incentive to the very young to change poor health habits because the effects of lifestyle on illness are usually not detected until middle to late adulthood. In addition, because they were developed and tested with Caucasian, middle-class populations, existing appraisals are probably less useful with blue-collar workers (Shy et al,

1985). Their use with minorities is compromised by the inadequacy of epidemiological data on risk factors, such as the lack of available and accessible health services for the poor. An individual's ability to change lifestyle is limited by living in a system that may restrict participation in decision making and economic and educational opportunities or by living in an environment where external threats to health, such as violence, are common (Rowley, 1985).

Community

Historical perspectives

After health and health promotion, the third major concept in an integrated model for nursing is **community.** The emphasis on community as the focus of practice has been gaining attention since the mid-1970s. McKinlay and McKinlay (1977) attributed declining mortality and morbidity rates to better standards of living, such as sanitation, clean air and water, and availability of healthy foods. The Institute of Medicine's (IOMs) report on *The Future of Public Health* also emphasized community by stating that the "mission of public health is to assure conditions in which people can be healthy by generating organized community effort to . . . prevent disease and promote health (IOM, 1988, p. 7).

As discussed previously, the national health goals in *Healthy People* (USDHEW, 1979) and *Healthy People 2000* (USDHHS, 1991) emphasized the environment and the community as central to achieving health. In 1991 the American Public Health Association (APHA) published *Healthy Communities 2000: Model Standards for Community Attainment of the Year 2000 National Health Objectives.* The objectives in *Healthy People 2000* are included in these model standards, and a practical outline is provided for each objective. Communities can tailor the outlines to their own local needs, and health department managers work with these model standards to develop programs that fit the needs and resources of their own communities. Nurses participate in this process through community assessments, community development activities, and identification of key persons in the community with whom to build partnerships for health programs. Model standards provide a link between the national health objectives in *Healthy People 2000* and community-wide program planning.

The model standards provide an opportunity for nurses to participate in community-wide health care. Edwards and Dees (1990) argued that the contribution of community and public health nursing to problems of the environment lies in the ability to integrate concepts of health and disease, individual and aggregate, public health and nursing, and health promotion and disease prevention. This integration means that nurses must consider the complex relationship between the personal and environmental forces that affect health. About 20 years ago, Milio (1976) offered a set of propositions for improving health behavior by considering personal choices in the context of available societal resources. These propositions (Box 14-4) con-

stitute a fitting model for health promotion that addresses both personal and societal resources as nursing moves into the new millenium.

For nurses, therefore, it is important to realize that individuals make choices about various health practices. The degree of freedom in the personal choices of individuals is affected greatly by others in the family and peer group, options available within the immediate environment, and the norms and values within the community. Behavior change is based on interventions targeted to the person within the environment but must also include interventions targeted to the immediate and surrounding environment.

Community models and frameworks

The theoretical frameworks developed within nursing primarily are oriented to individuals. There is an assumption in the nursing profession that simply changing the word "man" or "human being" to "aggregate" or "community" is sufficient (Hanchett, 1988). Moe (1977) defined community as people and the relationships that emerge among them, developing and using common institutions and physical environment. Nurses become aware that the community is more than the sum of the individuals, families, and aggregates within it and that interaction among the individuals, families, aggregates, and organizations must be considered for any real change to occur.

Despite a community-oriented ideal, the concept of the community as client is not easily integrated into practice. Consequently, nursing practice directed to the community has been neglected in favor of providing care to ill and disadvantaged individuals in the community. Chopoorian (1986) argues that a lack of consciousness of community may "contribute to the peripheral role of nurses in the larger arena of social, economic, and political affairs" (p. 42). Nurses strengthen their position with the community

---

BOX 14-4 Milio's Propositions for Improving Health Behavior

- Health status of populations is a function of the lack or excess of health-sustaining resources.
- Behavior patterns of populations are related to habits of choice from actual or perceived limited resources and related attitudes.
- Organizational decisions determine the range of personal resources available.
- Individual health-related decisions are influenced by efforts to maximize valued resources in both the personal and societal domains.
- Social change is reflective of a change in population behavior patterns.
- Health education will impact behavior patterns minimally without new health-promoting options for investing personal resources.

Adapted from Milio N: A framework for prevention: changing health-damaging to health generating life patterns, *Am J Public Health* 66(5):435, 1976.

by looking not at the profession or to individual clients as objects of reform, but rather at the environment, which can be re-conceptualized as social, economic, and political structures; as human social relations; and as everyday life (Chopoorian, 1986). This dynamic perspective leads to interventions targeted to public health policy.

Several authors described community from a systems perspective (Anderson and McFarlane, 1995; Blum, 1981; Hanchett, 1979, 1988; Salmon-White, 1982) by viewing human beings within a hierarchy of natural systems and health as a function of harmonious interrelationships among various levels of the hierarchy. Movement in one level of the hierarchy has a corresponding movement in all levels. If individual, family, aggregate, community, and society are different levels of the system's hierarchy, then any change in one level has a corresponding change in all other levels.

Hanchett (1979, 1988) notes that people in relation to one another, to their geographic location, and to available services and resources are the elements of the community system with which the nurse must be concerned. Hanchett states the importance of considering the whole community as more than and different from the sum of its people and their interrelations. She moves beyond definitions of a community as structure or process to one that incorporates a wholeness of energy. Hanchett notes that "**community health** is a function of the energy, the individuality, and the relationships of the community as a whole, and of the individuals and groups within the community" (p. 34).

Anderson and McFarlane (1995) and Salmon-White (1982) developed models based on the assumption that assessing the various components of the system facilitates a healthy community. The community-as-partner model includes eight major community subsystems (Anderson and McFarlane, 1995). The basic core of the community, according to these authors, is its people, their values, beliefs, culture, religion, laws, and mores. Within a community system, the people interact with the other subsystems. A community health assessment must obtain information about the subsystems and the pattern of interactions among the subsystems and of the total community with the systems external to it.

The model created by Salmon-White (1982) is based on the public health mission of organized efforts to protect, promote, and restore health. It proposes that community and public health nursing includes prevention, protection, and promotion strategies. The model embraces multiple health determinants and is consistent with the Canadian Framework for Health (LaLonde, 1974).

In these two models, interventions are planned at the system level by participating with relevant subsystems. Although these models provide guidance for assessing community and aggregate systems, they cannot easily be used to direct interventions. Furthermore, these models focus on stability and equilibrium by protecting the community from specific disease risks; less attention is directed toward factors that promote an optimally healthy community. Nevertheless, several major community-wide studies have drawn on concepts such as those presented in these models. These community and epidemiological studies are described next.

Multilevel community studies

Two influential community studies of health risks, morbidity, and mortality are the Framingham Heart Study, initiated in 1949, and the Human Population Laboratory's longitudinal survey in Alameda County, California, initiated in the early 1970s. In the Framingham Heart Study, 5209 adults in a small town in Massachusetts agreed to be followed over their lifespans to identify factors contributing to coronary heart disease and high blood pressure. Periodic health assessments were done, and morbidity and mortality data were collected. Heart disease was found to be more prevalent among smokers and those with elevated blood pressure, cholesterol levels, or low levels of exercise. Obesity contributed to high blood pressure and elevated cholesterol levels and thus to heart disease (Haynes, Feinlieb, and Kannel, 1980).

The Alameda County Study was designed to follow a sample of 6928 individuals over a 4-year period (Breslow, 1972). Social and behavioral factors were studied in relation to mortality. The health behaviors studied included eating three meals daily, eating breakfast, sleeping 7 to 8 hours a night, using alcohol moderately, exercising regularly, not smoking, and maintaining a desirable height-to-weight ratio (Belloc, 1973). Smoking, alcohol use, physical exercise, hours of sleep, and weight in relation to height were found to be related to mortality (Berkman and Breslow, 1983). Social networks (Renne, 1974) (e.g., contact with friends and relatives, church and group membership) was inversely related to mortality. These findings led to the inclusion of social and environmental variables, as well as personal behaviors, in health risk appraisals. Later studies verified the early findings (Kotler and Wingard, 1989).

Findings from these early large-scale surveys prompted a number of public health multilevel programs. Examples of community-oriented risk-reduction interventions were the Stanford Heart Disease Prevention Program (Farquhar et al, 1990), the North Karelia Study (Puska et al, 1983), the Pawtucket Study (Lasater et al, 1984), and the Minnesota Heart Health Program (Luepker et al, 1994; Perry et al, 1992).

The findings of the Stanford Three-City Program were encouraging (Maccoby et al, 1977). A media campaign was provided alone in one community and in conjunction with face-to-face instruction in two other communities. Reductions in cigarette smoking, blood pressure, and serum cholesterol levels were greater in the two communities that received the combined program than in the community that received only the mass media campaign.

The Stanford Five-City Project began in 1979 with a 6-year community health education program aimed at reducing cardiovascular (CV) risk factors. The program was delivered through multiple channels (Winkleby et al, 1996). Two treatment cities received a low-cost, comprehensive program based on social learning theory (Perry, Baranowski, and Parcel, 1990), communication theory, behavior change theory, community organization, and social marketing. Once again, improvements in serum cholesterol levels, blood pressure, smoking rate, and resting pulse were observed in these cities after the program (Farquhar et al, 1990; Winkleby, 1994; Winkleby, Flora, and Kraemer, 1994; Winkleby et al, 1996). A survey to evaluate the long-term effects of the intervention indicated that the changes after the intervention were sustained in the treatment cities. CV and all-cause mortality rates were maintained or improved in the treatment cities, whereas they leveled out or worsened in the comparison cities (Winkleby et al, 1996).

Positive changes were also found in the North Karelia Study (Puska et al, 1983). Citizens of North Karelia, a rural area in Finland, were selected for this program because they had a high mortality rate from CV disease in the early 1970s. More than half of the North Karelia men smoked, consumed large amounts of animal fats, and had elevated serum cholesterol levels. In addition, many had untreated hypertension. The government directed the program at an individual and community level to help the citizens modify their high-risk behaviors. The North Karelia Project involved retraining of health professionals, reorganization of public health services, production of low-fat and low-salt dairy products and meat, and community health education. Follow-up studies demonstrated that the three major risk factors for CV disease decreased much more in North Karelia than in a comparison county (Puska et al, 1983).

The Pawtucket Study is an ongoing project in a Rhode Island community that traditionally has had high rates of CV disease. The interventions are directed toward both individuals and the community to help individuals adopt new behaviors and to create a supportive environment (Carlton et al, 1995, p. 777). Churches, social groups, the business community, and volunteers provided the education intervention. The food industry offered "Heart Healthy" food items and menus, and media campaigns informed citizens about their cholesterol levels and other CV risk factors (Carlton et al, 1995). A follow-up survey $8\frac{1}{2}$ years after the beginning of the program indicated no differences between Pawtucket and the comparison city in blood pressure, cholesterol levels, or smoking prevalence. Obesity levels were lower for the Pawtucket residents. The authors concluded that possible national media exposure, high levels of unemployment, and stress during the time of the study might have contributed to the lack of difference between the two cities. During the peak time of the intervention, a significant increase was seen in the Pawtucket population in heart healthy behaviors, suggesting that community interventions can reach a large number of people.

The Minnesota Heart Health Program (Luepker et al, 1994) was initiated in 1980 with 400,000 persons in six Midwest communities. Three communities received the program, and three served as controls. Risk factor improvements were seen in all six communities, and only modest differences were found between the treatment and control cities (Luepker et al, 1994). Favorable health risk changes were found across age and education groups and gender. Winkleby (1994) notes that these findings reflect the contemporary health promotion movement. Future programs must combine public policy initiatives and community-wide health education strategies with interventions directed to specific high-risk populations (Luepker et al, 1994).

WHAT DO YOU THINK? *There are some community-wide health promotion studies, such as the federally funded heart disease prevention trials, that show only modest differences between the intervention and comparison communities. Researchers suggest that this may be due to the contemporary health promotion movement and national media attention to healthy lifestyles.*

These programs and others provide beginning scientific knowledge for the implementation of risk appraisal and reduction programs. However, the relative effectiveness of specific interventions in reducing risk is unclear (Frank et al, 1993; Luepker et al, 1994). The program descriptions make it clear that multiple levels of intervention (**multilevel intervention**) are needed to reach the community in a meaningful way. Nurses have a close relationship with individuals, families, high-risk groups, and organizations such as schools and workplaces. They are positioned to contribute to risk reduction, disease and illness prevention, and health promotion by participating in community projects such as the ones described here. It is important that nurses develop health programs and document improved outcomes for high-risk groups with whom they interact.

NURSING TIP

Although an important starting point may be the care of the failure-to-thrive child, the nurse recognizes that solving the immediate problem is not sufficient. The care of one child needs to be used to identify the magnitude of the problem to develop programs to improve outcomes at this special population level.

APPLICATION TO COMMUNITY AND PUBLIC HEALTH NURSING
Multilevel Community Projects

The aim of community and public health nursing is to create partnerships with individuals, families, groups, and communities to promote their health. Chapter 15 describes types of partnership. In a passive partnership, nurses develop and direct interventions for the benefit of individuals or communities. As the partnership becomes more active, community members become more involved in assessing, planning, implementing, and evaluating change. In an active partnership, both professionals and community residents determine health needs. As residents increase their awareness, they are better able to determine what they want for themselves, their families, and their community and more likely to direct program development using the health professionals as consultants. Some examples from community studies, which address multiple levels of clients and focuses of care, are described in this section. These projects show expanded opportunities for assessment, planning, intervention, and evaluation.

Stoner, Magilvy and Schultz (1992) demonstrated active partnership in their assessment of several communities in Colorado. In response to an invitation from each community, the authors and their students collected existing data, interviewed key informants about their perceptions of the community's health needs, and presented their findings in town meetings. The population was thus able to give feedback on which to base health goals for the community.

Flick and colleagues (1994) and Van Hook (1997) describe other community partnerships. In the first, a partnership was developed by nurses with an urban neighborhood in St. Louis, Missouri to enhance its capacity to improve its own health (Flick et al, 1994). This project, conducted over 7 years, was based on a community-organizing model; mobilization occurred through community participation and control, with health professionals serving as a resource to the community. The second partnership included East Tennessee State University and two counties in Tennessee (Van Hook, 1997). It was designed to meet the service needs of underserved rural citizens and provide educational experience for health professional students. Faculty members, students, and community leaders served on advisory boards. Based on a community assessment, the School of Nursing opened a rural health clinic and provided a range of health services.

At the aggregate level of client system, a smoking reduction program in San Francisco targeted Vietnamese men (Jenkins et al. 1997). A media campaign included articles in Vietnamese newspapers and magazines, television coverage, bumper stickers, posters, brochures, and anti-tobacco billboards and anti-tobacco presentations. Materials were distributed to Vietnamese physicians to give to clients, and anti-tobacco activities were developed in language schools. Smoking control ordinances and no-smoking signs were also provided to Vietnamese restaurants. Two years later, smoking rates were significantly lower, especially for young men and students, as compared with Vietnamese men in a comparison city.

Another program by Perry and colleagues (1998) was directed to a healthy aggregate. This program was designed to increase fruit and vegetable consumption among fifth graders in 20 elementary schools in St. Paul, Minnesota. The program consisted of a school curriculum, parental education, school food services changes, education of food services staff, and involvement of the food industry in supplying nutritious foods. Eating habits were measured through dietary recalls, observation of eating patterns during school lunch, and telephone surveys to the parents. After the intervention, fruit consumption and combined fruit and vegetable consumption increased for all of the children at lunch; vegetable consumption was increased only for girls. Total 24-hour recall indicated an increase in daily fruit and a decrease in fat consumption by both the girls and boys.

Amaya and colleagues (1997) reported a project targeted to the individual and family levels of the client system. In this family living on the U.S.-Mexico border, two children were found to have elevated blood lead levels. The assessment of the family indicated that the exposure was probably related to the home and occupational environment. Risk factors included living near a waste dump, no sewage system or running water, peeling lead-based paint on the window sills, and auto parts and oil spills in the yard. In addition, the adults were employed in auto repair and recycling, and the family lacked access to health care and was socially isolated. The intervention included screening and education of individuals about hand-washing and family education regarding risk factors on the property and in the home. The authors recommended that a screening program be developed for the population living on the border and that programs be tailored to their needs.

The projects described in the previous paragraph show the importance of multiple approaches to reaching the population. Cassano and Frongillo (1997) argue that a multilevel approach to community-oriented programs requires that one attend to all client levels. For example, in nutritional programs, it is important to address the individual, household, grocery store accessibility and environment, the community, and the food environment. No one individual can address all of these levels, but there is increasing emphasis on working in teams and partnerships consisting of health providers and residents. Nurses have an opportunity to work with and to lead these multidisciplinary teams to conduct assessments, develop strategies with the community and its populations, and facilitate the empowerment of community residents. As the twenty-first century draws near, it is increasingly important that nurses incorporate these strategies into their practice (see Research Brief).

Application of the Integrative Model for Community Health Promotion

One example of community and public health nursing care that reflects the four client systems and multiple focuses of care is shown in Table 14-2. The health problem

RESEARCH *Brief*

Community development theory was used to assess the need for a nurse-managed clinic. Citizen participation was paramount in identifying the health needs of residents of public housing. Faculty members at the University of Virginia School of Nursing provided clinical experiences for undergraduates at public housing for the elderly and disabled for 10 years. Faculty members' concerns about the need for consistent services to high-risk residents and a request by the local housing authority to expand services to a second site (where 98% were female and 55% were children) provided the impetus for seeking grant funding for a community nursing center.

A comprehensive community health needs assessment was done by faculty members and students using existing epidemiological and census data, neighborhood windshield surveys, face-to-face interviews about the health and social problems of residents, and focus groups with residents and community leaders. The survey instrument was adapted from Neuber's Community Oriented Needs Assessment Model. The findings indicated that health problems of indigent residents far exceeded those of the state (e.g., in 1989 the infant mortality rate of minorities in Charlottesville, Virginia was 24.3 per 1000, compared with rate of 10 per 1000 in Virginia as a whole). Residents identified individual problems such as hypertension and obesity, neighborhood problems related to drug and alcohol use, problem behavior among children, and barriers to health care (e.g., transportation, cost). Community leaders were concerned about teen pregnancy, drug abuse, and poverty. When these leaders were asked what services were most needed from a nursing clinic, they listed well-child screening, parenting education, and medication management. Faculty members and students will continue to collaborate and partner with community members in all project phases from assessment to intervention and outcome evaluation.

Glick DF et al: Community development theory: planning a community nursing center, *JONA* 26(7/8):1, 1996.

that comes to the nurse's attention in this example is a young child with a diagnosis of failure to thrive.

Illness care

The nurse initiates care at the individual level with a goal of resolving the failure to thrive. The child's health is assessed and monitored, and the mother is taught principles of nutrition, feeding, and care of the ill child. At the family level, the nurse assesses the presence of malnutrition within the family and refers other family members for care as needed. Also, the family is referred for counseling to relieve the stress related to the child's illness. At the aggregate level, the nurse assesses the community for the prevalence of failure-to-thrive children or teaches classes to raise awareness in the community about this condition and to educate groups about referral and emergency food sources. At the community level, the nurse works with key leaders and citizens to assess the prevalence of nutrition-related illnesses in the community.

Illness/disease prevention

At the individual level, well-balanced nutrition and childcare is taught to mothers to prevent recurrence of malnutrition in the child. A health risk appraisal and recommendations from the *Guide to Clinical Preventive Services* provide direction for age-specific periodic health examination, assessment, and counseling interventions. In addition, the nurse selects an appropriate health risk appraisal tool for use with clinical observation and assessment. The high-risk family is taught nutrition principles and assisted to incorporate healthy food into their diets to prevent nutrition-related problems. Using an aggregate approach, the nurse assesses the community for aggregates at risk for malnutrition (e.g., schoolchildren, poor persons, the elderly, and the homeless), analyzes health-risk data, and works with others to institute programs to reduce their risk, thereby preventing malnutrition. Community multimedia education for malnutrition risk reduction and lobbying for legislation to promote resources for adequate nutrition within the community are examples of a community approach.

Health promotion

At the individual level, the nurse helps the individual adopt a healthy lifestyle as appropriate to his or her age, culture, and resources. For the young child, this includes educating and supporting the parent to provide health-enhancing care. Within a family client perspective, the approach includes the entire family and planning with the family on how to adopt healthy lifestyle activities. These activities range from balanced nutrition to planning for relaxation activities for the family. A wellness inventory helps the nurse design an intervention targeted to the family's awareness of personal self-care. At the aggregate level, the nurse educates school personnel regarding healthy lunches for the aggregate of students or teachers. Regardless of the level of health need or client system at which care begins, the ultimate goal of the nurse is health promotion of the total community and its constituents. Participating with community leaders and citizens to establish nutrition education or exercise classes is an example of a community level approach.

Although an important starting point is the care of the failure-to-thrive child, the nurse recognizes that solving the immediate problem is not sufficient. The child's health problem is viewed within a broader context of an optimally healthy child, family, aggregate of children, and community. This approach necessitates that the nursing intervention not be limited to solving the immediate problem of weight gain, but rather that care be oriented toward interventions that promote optimal health for the child,

TABLE 14-2 Community Health Levels of Care: Malnutrition/Failure to Thrive

| FOCUS OF CARE | CLIENT SYSTEM | | | |
	INDIVIDUAL	FAMILY	AGGREGATE	COMMUNITY
Illness care	Weigh and measure the child Monitor the child's symptoms Teach mother basic nutrition and child care for failure-to-thrive child	Teach signs and symptoms of malnutrition to high-risk family members Refer family for care for nutrition-related problems	Assess prevalence of failure to thrive children in the community Teach classes about emergency food sources and referral sources for aggregate of failure to thrive children	Assess community for accessibility and adequacy of care providers to treat malnutrition and failure to thrive in the community
Illness/disease prevention	Teach mother well-balanced nutrition and child care to prevent recurrence of malnutrition and failure to thrive	Teach nutrition to high-risk family members to prevent nutrition-related problems	Assess community for prevalence of children at risk of malnutrition Develop classes about reducing risks of malnutrition in aggregate of high-risk children	Participate in providing community-wide multimedia education for reduction of malnutrition Lobby for legislation to promote resources to ensure adequate nutrition to the community
Health promotion	Support individual efforts to adopt health promotion lifestyle, including healthy nutrition	Plan with family to adopt a healthy lifestyle and incorporate healthy foods into daily eating patterns	Educate school personnel regarding healthy school lunches for aggregate of school children	Work with community leaders and citizens to establish nutrition education programs in the community

family, aggregate of high-risk children, and the total community.

In summary, the concepts of *health, health promotion,* and *community* are inextricably linked. As described throughout this chapter, it is difficult to talk of one without including the others. It is also important that nurses examine their definitions and beliefs about each concept as the basis for their practice. The essence of the community and public health nursing perspective is the ability to see the totality of community while addressing its component parts and, at the same time, to see the total needs for health promotion, health protection, illness and disease prevention, and illness care and management. It is the integrative relationship among all these levels that distinguishes community and public health nursing from nursing in more circumscribed settings, such as hospitals and clinics.

clinical application

A rural health outreach program serves indigent and other vulnerable populations. The program's goals include increased knowledge about risk factors, services, and self-care; improved community health; increased access and affordability of individual and community health promotion services; and reduced barriers to health services. The program offers health promotion and disease prevention educational materials and classes throughout the region in churches, schools, community centers, and fire departments. In addition, clinics have been established in eight local sites across the county. Clinic services include health risk appraisal, disease screening, immunizations, health education, counseling, and referral. Funding from a variety of public and private sources supports the program. It is essential that the program show effective outcomes if it is to sustain its funding.

Mary Ann is a BSN-prepared nurse working for the outreach program. She is a member of a group tasked to evaluate whether the outreach program (including the eight clinics) is effective in meeting the stated objectives.

A. Using the integrative model for community health promotion as a guide, how might you organize a comprehensive approach to assessment and data collection?
B. What are sources of baseline data including individual, aggregate, and community health indicators?
C. What is the value of interviewing clinic participants about their perception of health and the value of health services?
D. Who else can you interview to elicit important information about the usefulness of the outreach program?

E. What strategies can be employed to promote citizen participation and partnership among concerned health professionals and community residents and to ultimately sustain the program?

Be creative and comprehensive in your approach, and consider cultural factors associated with rural populations in the United States. Today, with continued spending limits placed on federal and state programs for health promotion and disease prevention, many nurses are confronted with issues of outreach and sustainability of important health programs. Future success of community health promotion programs is based on demonstrating outcomes.

Answers are in the back of the book.

KEY POINTS

- Community and public health nursing is concerned with promoting the health of populations and of the total community. The concept of health shapes the process of nursing practice from assessment of health-related needs of individuals, families, aggregates, and communities to evaluation of behavioral outcomes.
- The greatest benefits in public health are likely to accrue from efforts to improve individual lifestyle, social conditions, and the physical environment. Long-term benefits may very well result from the findings of genetic research.
- Nurses have a history of commitment to primary health care and to enhancing levels of wellness in populations. Rich opportunities to guide health care reform endeavors await nurses, especially future community and public health nursing leaders.
- It is important for nurses to examine their own personal definition of health and to recognize how nursing care is directed by this health definition. A nurse who defines health broadly as self-actualization is more likely to consider multiple indicators of physical health, social health, the ability to adapt to the changing environment, and potential for maximum well-being when planning nursing care.
- The goal of risk appraisal and reduction is the prevention or early detection of disease. The knowledge base for this approach is the scientific evidence regarding the relationship between risk factors and mortality and the effectiveness of planned interventions in reducing both risks and mortality.
- Health risk appraisal is used to assess the total risks to an individual's health. Knowledge of the risks may be used to initiate disease-preventing lifestyle changes and to institute treatment and lifestyle changes as early in the course of disease as possible.
- Clinical preventive guidelines use clinical and epidemiological data to identify specific individual health risks, and they provide a detailed list of recommendations for preventive measures appropriate to different age groups.
- Wellness inventories define health risks broadly and emphasize empowerment of individuals to achieve health.
- Clinical observation, assessment, and nursing interventions used in conjunction with health-risk appraisals are essential to obtain the best results. Although educational messages have an impact on some individuals, others may not respond. Even when individuals are motivated by health-appraisal feedback, they may not have the behavioral skills necessary to initiate and sustain changes in lifestyle.
- The Stanford Heart Disease Prevention Program, the North Karelia Study, the Pawtucket Study, and the Minnesota Heart Health Program provided a beginning scientific knowledge base for the design and implementation of risk-appraisal and risk-reduction programs.
- Community and public health nursing care must extend beyond resolving a specific illness to preventing the illness and promoting optimal health for the individual, the family, the aggregate, and the total community. All of these levels are important to the health of the community and its populations.

critical thinking activities

1. State your personal definition of health, and interview a nurse, client, and physician about their definitions of health. Discuss the range of definitions using Smith's four models of health as a frame of reference.
2. Compare and contrast definitions of *health promotion, disease prevention,* and *health maintenance.* Discuss whether the same strategies (e.g., a physical fitness or stress management program) can be defined as health promoting, disease preventing, or health maintaining?
3. Define community health promotion, and provide examples of health promotion indicators for a specified community.
4. Develop a nursing care plan for adolescent substance abuse using Milio's (1976) propositions as a frame of reference.
5. Use the integrative model for community health promotion to develop a community-wide plan for adolescent substance abuse.
6. Analyze the role of partnership with the community in various practice settings such as school health, public health, and home health.
7. Describe community health levels of care including the client system and the focus of care:
   a. For teenage pregnancy, beginning with health promotion at the individual level
   b. For breast cancer, starting from the level of community illness/disease prevention

Bibliography

Amaya MA et al: Childhood lead poisoning on the US-Mexico border: a case study in environmental health nursing lead poisoning, *Public Health Nursing* 14(6):353, 1997.

American Nurses Association: *Nursing's agenda for health care reform,* Washington, DC, 1991, the Association.

American Public Health Association: *Healthy Communities 2000: model standards for community attainment of the year 2000 national* health objectives, ed 3, Washington, DC, 1991, the Association.

Anderson E, McFarlane J: *Community-as-partner: theory and practice in nursing,* Philadelphia, 1995, Lippincott.

continued

Bibliography—cont'd

Ardell DB: *High level wellness: an alternative to doctors, drugs, and disease,* Emmaus, Pa, 1977, Rodale.

Avis NE, Smith KW, McKinlay JB: Accuracy of perceptions of heart attack risk: what influences perceptions and can they be changed? *Am J Public Health* 79(12):1608, 1989.

Becker MH, Janz NK: Behavioral science perspectives on health hazard/health risk appraisal, *Health Services Res* 22(4):537, 1987.

Belloc NB: Relationship of health practices and mortality, *Prev Med* 2(1):67, 1973.

Berkman LF, Breslow L: *Health and ways of living, the Alameda County Study,* New York, 1983, Oxford University Press.

Blum HL: *Planning for health,* ed 2, New York, 1981, Human Sciences.

Bracht N, editor: *Health promotion at the community level,* Newbury Park CA, 1990, Sage.

Breslow L: A quantitative approach to the World Health Organization's definition of health: physical, mental, and social well-being, *Int J Epidemiol* 1(4):347, 1972.

Breslow L, Somers AR: The lifetime health-monitoring program: a practical approach to preventive medicine, *N Engl J Med* 296(11):601, 1977.

Breslow L et al: *Risk Factor Update Project: final report,* Atlanta, 1985, USDHHS.

Brubaker BH: Health promotion: a linguistic analysis, *Adv Nurs Sci* 5(3):1, 1983.

Carlton RA et al: The Pawtucket heart health progarm; community changes in cardiovascular risk factors and projected disease risk, *Am J Public Health* 85(6):777, 1995.

Cassano PA, Frongillo EA: Annotation: developing and validating new methods for assessing community interventions, *Am J Public Health* 87(2):157, 1997.

Chopoorian TL: Reconceptualizing the environment. In Moccia P, editor: *New approaches to theory development,* Pub No 15-1992, New York, 1986, National League for Nursing.

Doerr BT, Hutchins EB: Health risk appraisal: process, problems, and prospects for nursing practice and research, *Nurs Res* 30(5):299, 1981.

Downie RS, Tannahill C, Tannahill A: *Health promotion models and values,* ed 2, New York, 1996, Oxford University Press.

Downie RS, Fyfe C, Tannahill A: *Health promotion models and values,* New York, 1990, Oxford University Press.

Dunn HL: *High-level wellness,* Arlington, Va, 1973, Beatty.

Edwards LH, Dees RL: Environmental health: the effects of life-style on the world around us. In Wold SJ, editor: *Community health nursing: issues and topics,* East Norwalk, Conn, 1990, Appleton & Lange.

Farquhar JW et al: Effects of community-wide education on cardiovascular disease risk factors: the Stanford five-city project, *JAMA* 264:359, 1990.

Flick LH et al: Building community for health: lessons from a seven-year-old neighborhood/university partnership, *Health Educ Q* 21(3):369, 1994.

Frank E et al: Cardiovascular disease risk factors: improvements in knowledge and behavior in the 1980s, *Am J Public Health* 83(4):590, 1993.

Fuchs V: *Who shall live,* New York, 1974, Basic Books.

Glick DF et al: Community development theory: planning a community nursing center, *JONA* 26(7/8):1, 1996.

Goeppinger J: Changing health behaviors and outcomes through self-care. In Lancaster J, Lancaster W, editors: *Concepts for advanced nursing practice: the nurse as a change agent,* St Louis, 1982, Mosby.

Griffith HM, Diguiseppi C: Guidelines for clinical preventive services: essential for nurse practitioners in practice, education, and research, *Nurse Pract* 19(9):25, 1994.

Hanchett ES: *Community health assessment: a conceptual tool kit,* New York, 1979, Wiley.

Hanchett ES: *Nursing frameworks and community as client: bridging the gap,* East Norwalk, Conn, 1988, Appleton & Lange.

Harris DM, Guten S: Health protective behavior: an exploratory study, *J Health Soc Behav* 20:17, 1979.

Haynes SG, Feinleib M, Kannel WB: The relationship of psycho-social factors to coronary heart disease in the Framingham Study III: eight year incidence of coronary heart disease, *Am J Epidemiol* 111(1):37, 1980.

Illich I: *Medical nemesis: the expropriation of health,* New York, 1976, Random House.

Institute of Medicine: *The future of public health,* Washington, DC, 1988, National Academy Press.

Issel LM: Measuring comprehensive case management interventions: development of a tool, *Nurs Case Manag* 2(4):132, 1997.

Jeffery RW: Risk behaviors and health: contrasting individual and population perspectives, *Am Psychol* 44(9):1194, 1989.

Jenkins CNH et al: The effectiveness of a media-led intervention to reduce smoking among Vietnamese-American men, *Am J Public Health* 87(6):1031, 1997.

Johnson SK: The state of disease management, *Case Review* 2(4):53, 1996.

Kasl SV, Cobb S: Health behavior, illness behavior and sick-role behavior [review], *Arch Environ Health* 12(4):531, 1966.

Killeen ML: What is the health risk appraisal telling us? *West J Nurs Res* 11(5):614, 1989.

Kirscht JP: Process and measurement issues in health risk appraisal, *Am J Public Health* 79(12):1598, 1989.

Kotler P, Wingard DL: The effect of occupational, marital and parental roles on mortality: the Alameda County Study, *Am J Public Health* 79(5):607, 1989.

Kulbok PA: A concept analysis of preventive health behavior. In Chinn PL, editor: *Advances in nursing theory development,* Rockville, Md, 1983, Aspen.

Kulbok PA: Social resources, health resources, and preventive health behavior: patterns and predictors, *Public Health Nurs* 2(2):67, 1985.

Kulbok PA, Baldwin JH: From preventive health behavior to health promotion: advancing a positive construct of health, *Adv Nurs Sci* 14(4):50, 1992.

Kulbok PA, Kirkwood B, Hulton L: *Predictors of health behavior in young adults.* Paper presented at the American Public Health Association Annual Meeting, Indianapolis, Ind, November 1997.

Kulbok PA et al: Advancing discourse on health promotion: beyond mainstream thinking, *Adv Nurs Sci* 20(1):12, 1997.

Kulbok PA et al: *The inventory of multidimensional behavior for health promotion* (under review).

Laffrey SC: An exploration of adult health behaviors, *West J Nurs Res* 12(4):434, 1990.

Laffrey SC, Dickinson D: *How community health nurses view their roles* (submitted for publication).

Laffrey SC, Kulbok PA: *An integrative model for community nursing* (under review).

Laffrey SC, Loveland-Cherry CJ, Winkler SJ: Health behavior: evolution of two paradigms, *Public Health Nurs* 3(2):92, 1986.

Laffrey SC et al: Assessing Arab-American health care needs, *Soc Sci Med* 29(7):877, 1989.

LaLonde M: *A new perspective on the health of Canadians,* Ottawa, 1974, Government of Canada.

Lasater T et al: Lay volunteer delivery of a community-based cardiovascular risk factor change program: the Pawtucket Experiment. In Matarazzo JD et al, editors: *Behavioral health: a handbook of health enhancement and disease prevention,* Silver Spring, Md, 1984, Wiley.

Leavell HR, Clark EG: *Preventive medicine for the doctor in his community: an epidemiological approach,* ed 3, New York, 1965, McGraw-Hill.

Lorig K: Chronic disease self-management: a model for tertiary prevention, *Am Behav Scientist* 39(6):676, 1996.

Lowenberg JS: Health promotion and the "ideology of choice," *Public Health Nurs* 12(5):319, 1996.

Luepker RV et al: Community education for cardiovascular disease prevention: risk factor changes in the Minnesota Heart Health Program, *Am J Public Health* 84(9):1383, 1994.

Maccoby N et al: Reducing the risk of cardiovascular disease: effects of a community-based campaign on knowledge and behavior, *J Community Health* 3(2):100, 1977.

Marston-Scott M-V: The use of knowledge. In Hardy ME, Conway ME, editors: *Role theory: perspectives for health professionals,* ed 2, Norwalk, Conn, 1988, Appleton-Century-Crofts.

McGinnis JM, Forge WH: Actual causes of death in the United States, *JAMA* 270(18):2207, 1993.

McKinlay JB, McKinlay SM: The questionable contribution of medical measures to the decline of mortality in the United States in the twentieth century, *Milbank Q* 55(3):405, 1977.

Meeker WC: A review of the validity and efficacy of the health risk appraisal instrument, *J Manipulative Physiol Ther* 11(2):108, 1988.

Milio N: A framework for prevention: changing health-damaging to health-generating life patterns, *Am J Public Health* 66(5):435, 1976.

Minkler M: Improving health through community organization. In Glanz K, Lewis FM, Rimer BK, editors: *Health behavior and health education: theory, research, and practice,* San Francisco, 1990, Jossey-Bass.

Moe EV: Nature of today's community. In Reinhardt AM, Quinn MD, editors: *Current practice in community health nursing,* St Louis, 1977, Mosby.

National Wellness Institute: *Lifestyle Assessment Questionnaire,* Stevens Point, Wis, 1989, The Institute.

Orem D: *Nursing: concepts of practice,* ed 5, St Louis, 1995, Mosby.

Pender N: *Health promotion in nursing practice,* ed 3, East Norwalk, Conn, 1996, Appleton & Lange.

Perry CL, Baranowski T, Parcel GS: How individuals, environments, and health behavior interact: social learning theory. In Glanz K, Lewis FM, Rimer BK, editors: *Health behavior and health education: theory, research, and practice,* San Francisco, 1990, Jossey-Bass.

Perry CL et al: Changing fruit and vegetable consumption among children: the 5-a-Day Power Plus program in St. Paul, Minnesota, *Am J Public Health* 88(4):603, 1998.

Perry CL et al: Community-wide smoking prevention: long-term outcomes of the Minnesota Heart Health Program and the Class of 1989 Study, *Am J Public Health* 82(9):1210, 1992.

Puska P et al: Change in risk factors for coronary heart disease during 10 years of a community intervention programme (North Karelia Project), *Br Med J* 287(6408):1840, 1983.

Reifsnider E: Restructuring the American health care system: an analysis of nursing's agenda for health care reform, *Nurse Pract* 17(5):65, 1992.

Renne KS: Measurement of social health in a general population survey, *Soc Sci Res* 3(1):25, 1974.

Robbins LC, Hall JN: *How to practice prospective medicine,* Indianapolis, 1970, Methodist Hospital of Indiana.

Rosenberg IH: Keys to a longer, healthier, more vital life, *Nutr Rev* 52(8 Pt 2):S50, 1994.

Rowley DL: Are current health risk appraisals suitable for black women? In Society of Prospective Medicine: *Proceedings of the 21st Annual Meeting of the Society of Prospective Medicine,* Bethesda, Md, 1985, the Society.

Salmon-White M: Construct for public health nursing, *Nurs Outlook* 30(9):527, 1982.

Shultz CM: Lifestyle assessment: a tool for practice, *Nurs Clin North Am* 19(2):271, 1984.

Shy CM et al: Project to modify the CDC Health Risk Appraisal for blue collar workers. In Society of Prospective Medicine: *Proceedings of the 21st Annual Meeting of the Society of Prospective Medicine,* Bethesda, Md, 1985, the Society.

Skinner HA et al: Lifestyle assessment: just asking makes a difference, *Br Med J* 290(6463):214, 1985.

Smith JA: The idea of health: a philosophical inquiry, *Adv Nurs Sci* 3(3):43, 1981.

Smith KW, McKinlay SM, McKinlay JB: The reliability of health risk appraisals: a field trial of four instruments, *Am J Public Health* 79(12):1603, 1989.

Smith KW, McKinlay SM, Thorington BD: The validity of health risk appraisal instruments for assessing coronary heart disease risk, *Am J Public Health* 77(4):419, 1987.

Smuts JC: *Holism and evolution,* New York, 1926, Macmillan.

Somers HM, Somers AR: *Doctors, patients and health insurance: the organization and financing of medical care,* Washington, DC, 1961, The Brookings Institute.

Stanhope MK: Primary health care practice: is nursing part of the solution or the problem? *Fam Community Health* 18(1):49, 1995.

Stoner MH, Magilvy JK, Schultz PR: Community analysis in community health nursing practice: the GENESIS model, *Pub Health Nurs* 9(4):223, 1992.

Terris M: Approaches to an epidemiology of health, *Am J Public Health* 65(10):1037, 1975.

Tillich P: The meaning of health, *Perspect Biol Med* 5(Autumn):92, 1961.

Travis JW: *Wellness workbook for health professionals,* Mill Valley, Calif, 1977, Wellness Resource Center.

US Department of Health, Education, and Welfare: *Forward plan for health, FY 1978-82,* DHEW PHS Pub No (OS) 76-50046, Washington, DC, 1976, US Government Printing Office.

US Department of Health, Education, and Welfare: *Healthy People: the surgeons general's report on health promotion and disease prevention,* DHEW Pub No 79-55071, Washington, DC, 1979, US Government Printing Office.

US Department of Health and Human Services: *Healthy People 2000: national health promotion and disease prevention objectives,* DHHS Pub No 91-50212, Washington, DC, 1991, US Government Printing Office.

US Preventive Services Task Force: *A guide to clinical preventive services: an assessment of the effectiveness of 169 interventions,* Baltimore, Md, 1989, Williams & Wilkins.

Utz S, Kulbok PA: Managing care through advanced nursing practice. In Lancaster JL, Lancaster W, editors: *Nursing issues in leading and managing change,* St Louis, 1998, Mosby.

Van Hook RY: East Tennessee State University: preparing health professionals for practice in Appalachia. In USDHHS (HRSA): *The third national primary care conference: community-based academic partnerships, case studies,* Washington, DC, 1997, USDHHS.

Von Korff M et al: Multi-level analysis in epidemiologic research on health behavior and outcomes, *Am J Epidemiol* 135(10):1077, 1992.

Wildavsky A: Doing better and feeling worse: the political pathology of health policy, *Daedalus* 106:105, 1977.

Winkleby MA: The future of community-based cardiovascular disease intervention studies, *Am J Public Health* 84(5):1369, 1994.

Winkleby MA, Flora JA, Kraemer HC: A community-based heart disease intervention: predictors of change, *Am J Public Health* 84(5):767, 1994.

Winkleby MA et al: The long-term effects of a cardiovascular disease prevention trial: the Stanford five-city project, *Am J Public Health* 86(12):1773, 1996.

World Health Organization: *The first ten years of the World Health Organization,* New York, 1958, WHO.

World Health Organization: *Health promotion: a discussion document on the concept and principles,* Copenhagen, 1984, WHO Regional Office for Europe.

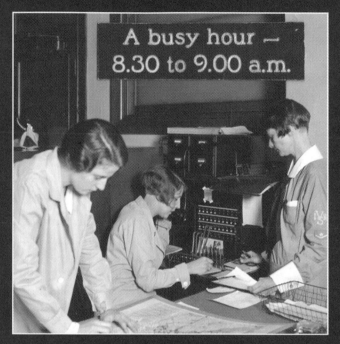

A busy hour —
8.30 to 9.00 a.m.

Four

Issues and
Approaches in
Community-
Oriented Health
Care

The primary orientation of health care delivery has been toward care and cure of the individual. There is increasing evidence that lifestyle and personal health habits influence the health of individuals, families, groups, and communities.

Although it is necessary to identify health-risk factors among individuals and groups in the community, it is of paramount importance that community and public health nurses learn to identify and work with health problems of the total community. This may be referred to as an aggregate approach or a population focused approach to health care delivery. Healthy communities provide greater resources for growth and nurturing of individuals and families than do their unhealthy counterparts.

Certainly, community-oriented nurses use a public health approach to work with individuals and familes in promoting health, intervening in disease onset or progression, and assisting with rehabilitation. Likewise, nurses often find that strategies used to introduce health behaviors directed at illness prevention and lifestyle changes are applicable to groups in the community and the community at large. Group concepts promoting health behaviors through groups, identifying community groups and their contributions to community life, and helping groups work toward community health goals are essential to community-oriented nursing practices.

Healthy communities/healthy cities is an organized approach to helping communities organize and move to provide environments for healthful living for their populations. In this approach, health is described as encompassing the physical and mental health of individuals and families plus the social, political, economic, educational, cultural, and environmental settings of the total community.

The nurse will be able to help communities attain their health goals by understanding the organization of communities, the effects of rural versus urban settings on health issues, how and why programs are managed, and how to evaluate programs for quality and effectiveness. A community assessment provides the basis for helping communities establish their goals. The use of a nurse-managed clinic is one approach community-oriented nurses have found to be successful in meeting the needs of aggregates, or vulnerable at-risk populations, whose needs must be considered when trying to improve the health of a community. Case management is an approach that has been used by community and public health nurses since its inception to match the most appropriate services and health care delivery interventions to population needs.

Although all communities strive to protect their populations and provide a safe living environment, natural and person-made disasters may occur; community and public health nurses can play a significant role in helping a community through such a crisis. The chapters in this section of the text help the nurse learn how to work with aggregates and to develop healthy communities.

Community as Client: Using the Nursing Process to Promote Health

GEORGE F. SHUSTER & JEAN GOEPPINGER

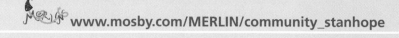

www.mosby.com/MERLIN/community_stanhope

OBJECTIVES

After reading this chapter, the student should be able to do the following:

- Decide whether nursing practice is community oriented.
- Illustrate selected concepts basic to community-oriented nursing practice—community, community client, community health, and partnership for health.
- Understand the relevance of the nursing process to community-oriented nursing practice.
- Decide which methods of assessment, intervention, and evaluation are most appropriate in selected situations.
- Develop a community-oriented nursing care plan.

KEY TERMS

aggregate
APEXPH
change agent
change partner
community
community assessment
Community-as-Partner
  Model
community competence
community health
community health
  problem
community health
  strength

community-oriented
  practice
community partnership
confidentiality
database
data collection
data gathering
data generation
early adopters
evaluation
goals
implementation
informant interviews
interacting groups

interdependent
intervention activities
late adopters
lay advisors
mass media
mediating structures
nominal groups
objectives
participant observation
partnership
PATCH
probability
problem analysis
problem correlates

problem prioritization
Program Planning Model
role negotiation
secondary analysis
surveys
target of practice
typologies
value
windshield surveys

See Glossary for definitions

CHAPTER OUTLINE

Although in the past nurses have viewed the community as a client, many public and community health nurses consider the community their most important client and, more recently, their partner (Anderson and McFarlane, 1995). This chapter clarifies community concepts and provides a guideline for nursing practice with the community client, emphasizing the use of the nursing process from assessment through evaluation to promote community health. This process begins with community assessment, which involves getting to know the community. It is a logical, systematic approach to identifying community needs, clarifying problems, and identifying community strengths and resources.

COMMUNITY DEFINED

The concept of *community* varies widely. The Expert Committee Report on community health nursing of the World Health Organization (WHO, 1974, p. 7) includes this definition: "A community is a social group determined by geographic boundaries and/or common values and interests. Its members know and interact with one another. It functions within a particular social structure and exhibits and creates norms, values and social institutions."

Other theorists and writers present **typologies,** which involve classification of communities by category rather than single definitions. One such typology of community was described by Blum in the 1974 edition of his classic text, *Planning for Health.* The categories, or types of communities, include communities defined by geopolitical boundaries, their interactions (such as between schools, social services, and governmental agencies), and their ability to solve problems. Some types of communities are listed in Box 15-1.

Blum's work (1974) shows the complexity of modern society. Nurses working in communities quickly learn that society consists of many different kinds of communities. Some of the communities listed in Box 15-1 are communities of place because interactions occur within a specific geographic area. Neighborhood and face-to-face communities are two examples of this type of community. Other

BOX 15-1 Types of Communities

Face-to-face community
Neighborhood community
Community of identifiable need
Community of problem ecology
Community of concern
Community of special interest
Community of viability
Community of action capability
Community of political jurisdiction
Resource community
Community of solution

From Blum HL: *Planning for health,* New York, 1974, Human Sciences Press.

communities, such as communities of special interest or resource communities, are spread out across widely scattered geographic areas. They are brought together by common concerns and interests that can be long term or short term in nature. An example of another type of community is a community of problem ecology, which is created when environmental problems like water pollution affect a widespread area. For instance, a problem such as water pollution can bring people together from areas that would not normally share a common interest. Nurses also may work in partnership with political communities, such as school districts, townships, or counties. Because the nature of each type of community varies, nurses planning interventions with communities must take into account the characteristics of that specific community. Each community is unique, and its defining characteristics will affect the nature of the partnership.

In most definitions, the concept of *community* includes three dimensions: people, place, and function. The *people* are the community residents. *Place* refers both to geographic and time dimensions, and *function* refers to the aims and activities of the community. Community-oriented nurses regularly need to examine how the personal, geographic, and functional dimensions of community shape their nursing practice. They can use both a conceptual definition and a set of indicators for the concept of *community* in their practice.

In this chapter, the following conceptual definition is used: **Community** is a locality-based entity, composed of systems of formal organizations reflecting society's institutions, informal groups, and aggregates. As defined in Chapter 1, an **aggregate** is a collection of individuals who have in common one or more personal or environmental characteristics. The components of community are **interdependent,** and their function is to meet a wide variety of collective needs. This definition of community includes personal, geographic, and functional dimensions and recognize interaction among the systems within a community. Indicators of the dimensions of this definition are listed in Table 15-1.

If the community is where community-oriented nurses practice the nursing process, and the community is the client of that practice, then nurses will want to analyze and synthesize information about the boundaries, components, and dynamic processes of the client community. The next section describes the community as client: it is both the setting for practice and the target of practice for the public and community health nurse.

COMMUNITY AS CLIENT

Community and public health nursing has often been considered unique because of its **target of practice.** The idea of health-related care being provided within the community is not new. At the turn of the century most persons stayed at home during illnesses. As a result, the practice environment for all nurses was the home rather than the hospital.

TABLE 15-1 The Concept of Community Specified

DIMENSIONS	INDICATORS
Space and time	Geopolitical boundaries Local or folk name for area Size in square miles, acres, blocks, or census tracts Transportation avenues such as rivers, highways, railroads, and sidewalks History Physical environment such as land use patterns and condition of housing
People or person	Number and density of population Demographic structure of population such as age, sex, socioeconomic, and racial distributions; rural and urban character, and dependency ratio Informal groups such as block clubs, service clubs, and friendship networks Formal groups such as schools, churches, businesses, industries, government bodies, unions, and health and welfare agencies Linking structures (intercommunity and intracommunity contacts among organizations)
Function	Production, distribution, and consumption of goods and services Socialization of new members Maintenance of social control Adapting to ongoing and expected change Provision of mutual aid

As the range of community nursing services expanded, many different kinds of agencies were started, and their services often overlapped. For instance, both privately established voluntary agencies and official local health agencies worked to control tuberculosis. The nurses employed by these agencies were called *community health nurses, public health nurses,* or *visiting nurses.* Nurses practiced in clients' homes and not in the hospital. Early public health nursing textbooks included lengthy descriptions of the home environment and tools for assessing the extent to which that environment promoted the health of family members. Health education about the domestic environment was often a major part of home nursing care.

By the 1950s, schools, prisons, industries, neighborhood health centers, as well as homes, had all become areas of practice for community nurses. Many of the new community nurses did not consider the environments in which they practiced. Although their practices took place within the community, they focused on the individual client or family seeking care. The care provided was not community oriented; rather, it was oriented toward the individual or family who lived in the community, or what is now called *community-based nursing practice.* This commitment to direct "hands-on" clinical nursing care delivered to individuals or families in community settings has been and remains a more popular concept of community nursing practice than the idea of the whole community as the target of nursing practice. This remains true despite the American Public Health Association, Public Health Nursing Section definition of public health nursing as "the practice of promoting and protecting the health of populations using knowledge from nursing, social, and public health sciences" (APHA, PHN Section, 1996, p. 1). When the location of the practice is the community and the focus of the practice is the individual or family, then the client remains the individual or family, not the whole community.

Therefore the community is considered the client only when the nursing focus is on the collective or common good instead of individual health. Community-oriented practice seeks healthful change for the whole community's benefit (Shiell and Hawe, 1996). Although the units of service may be individuals, families or other interacting groups, aggregates, institutions, and communities, the resulting changes are intended to affect the whole community. For example, an occupational health nurse's target might be preventing illness and injury and maintaining or promoting the health of an entire company workforce. Because of this focus, the nurse not only would help the individual disabled worker seeking service become independent in activities of daily living but also would become involved with promoting vocational rehabilitation and seeking reasonable employment policies for all disabled workers.

WHAT DO YOU THINK? *Many nurses believe that home health nursing is focused on the individual and it therefore should not be considered a part of community health nursing. Other nurses argue that home health nursing focuses on the family, takes place in the community, and should be considered a part of community health nursing.*

Community Client and Nursing Practice

Population-focused care is experiencing a rebirth, and the community as client is relevant to nursing practice for several reasons. The concept of community as client makes direct clinical care an aspect of population-focused community health practice (Abraham and Fallon, 1997). For instance, sometimes direct nursing care is provided to individuals and family members because their health needs represent common community-related problems rather than problems that are unique to their situations. Changes in their health will affect the health of their communities (Courtney et al, 1996). In such cases, decisions are made at the individual level because the individual's health is related to the health of the population as a whole and because the individual has an effect on community health. Improved health of the community remains the overall goal of nursing intervention. Interventions to stop spouse and elder abuse are two examples of nursing interventions done primarily because of the effects of abuse upon society and therefore upon the population as a whole.

The concept of community as client also highlights the complexity of the change process. Change for the benefit of the community client often must occur at several levels, ranging from the individual to society as a whole. In his classic work, Ryan (1976) points out that the "victim" cannot always be blamed and expected to correct the problem without changes also being made at the same time in the helping professions and public policy. For instance, lifestyle-induced health problems, such as smoking, overeating, and speeding, cannot be solved simply by asking individuals to choose health-promoting habits. Society also must provide healthy choices. Most individuals cannot change their habits alone; they require the support of family members, friends, community health care systems, and relevant social policies.

A commitment to the health of the community client requires a process of change at each of these levels. Both collaborative practice models involving the community and nurses in joint decision making and specific nursing roles are required for each of the units of service (Courtney et al, 1996). One nursing role emphasizes individual and direct personal care skills. Another nursing role focuses on the family as the unit of service. A third focuses on the community as a unit of service, especially constituent community groups (Russell, 1992).

Viewing the community as client and thus as the target of service means embracing two key concepts: community health and partnership for community health. Together these form not only the goal but also the means of community-oriented practice.

GOALS AND MEANS OF COMMUNITY-ORIENTED PRACTICE

In **community-oriented practice** the nurse and community seek healthful change together (Shiell and Hawe, 1996). Their common goal of community health involves an ongoing series of health-promoting changes rather than a fixed state. The most effective means of completing healthy changes in the community is through this same partnership. Specific examples of partnership between the nurse and the community (Jefferson County) are provided throughout this chapter.

Community Health

Like the concept of community, community health has three common characteristics, or dimensions: status, structure, and process. Each dimension has a unique effect on a community's health as the goal of community-oriented practice.

Status

Community health in terms of status or outcome is the most well-known and accepted approach; it involves biological, emotional, and social components. The *physical component* of community health often is measured by traditional morbidity and mortality rates, life expectancy indices, and risk factor profiles. The question of exactly which risk factors are most important has been a matter of ongoing controversy. In an effort to help resolve this question, *Morbidity and Mortality Weekly Report* published the work of a consensus committee involving representatives from a number of community-health-related organizations. This committee identified by consensus 18 community health status indicators (Box 15-2).

The *emotional component* of health status can be measured by consumer satisfaction and mental health indices. Crime rates and functional levels reflect the *social component* of community health. Other status measures, such as worker absenteeism and infant mortality rates, reflect the effects of all three components.

Structure

Community health, when viewed from the structure of the community, is usually defined in terms of *services* and *resources*. A structural perspective also defines the characteristics of the community structure itself. Indicators used to measure community health services and resources include service use patterns, treatment data from various health agencies, and provider/client ratios. These data provide information, such as the number of available hospital beds or the number of emergency room visits to a particular hospital. The problems with using these measures are serious. For instance, problems with access to care and quality of care are well known through stories reported in local newspapers. Less well known, but of equal concern, is the false belief that providing health care improves health. Such problems require cautious use of health services and resources as measures of community health.

Attributes of the community structure are commonly identified as social indicators, or correlates, of health. Measures of community structure include demographic characteristics, such as socioeconomic and racial distributions, and educational levels. Their relationships to health status have been thoroughly documented. For instance, studies have repeatedly shown that health status decreases with age and improves with higher socioeconomic levels.

BOX 15-2 Consensus Set of Indicators* for Assessing Community Health Status

INDICATORS OF HEALTH STATUS OUTCOME

1. Race/ethnicity-specific infant mortality, as measured by the rate (per 1000 live births) of deaths among infants less than 1 year of age

Death rates (per 100,000 population)† for:

2. Motor vehicle crashes
3. Work-related injury
4. Suicide
5. Lung cancer
6. Breast cancer
7. Cardiovascular disease
8. Homicide
9. All causes

Reported incidence (per 100,000 population) of:

10. Acquired immunodeficiency syndrome
11. Measles
12. Tuberculosis
13. Primary and secondary syphilis

INDICATORS OF RISK FACTORS

14. Incidence of low birth weight, as measured by percentage of total number of live-born infants weighing less than 2500 g at birth
15. Births to adolescents (females 10 to 17 years of age) as a percentage of total live births
16. Prenatal care, as measured by percentage of mothers delivering live infants who did not receive prenatal care during first trimester
17. Childhood poverty, as measured by the proportion of children less than 15 years of age living in families at or below the poverty level
18. Proportion of persons living in counties exceeding U.S. Environmental Protection Agency standards for air quality during previous year

*Position or number of the indicator does not imply priority.

†Age-adjusted to the 1940 standard population.

From Consensus set of health status indicators for the general assessment of community health status—United States, *MMWR Morb Mortal Wkly Rep* 40(27):449, 1991.

Process

The view of community health as the *process* of effective community functioning or problem solving is well established. However, it is especially appropriate to community-oriented nursing because it directs the study of community health to promote effective community action for health promotion, which is an important aim of community-oriented nurses. Kristjanson and Chalmers (1990) have presented a model of community level practice that reflects the process dimension. They call it the *Health Promotion Model* and describe it as "a mediating, enabling, and advocacy strategy that aims to develop community systems and make health a politically accountable issue."

The concept of community competence, defined originally in a classic work by Cottrell (1976), provides a basic understanding of the process dimension of community health. **Community competence** is a process whereby the components of a community—organizations, groups, and aggregates—"are able to collaborate effectively in identifying the problems and needs of the community; can achieve a working consensus on goals and priorities; can agree on ways and means to implement the agreed-on goals; and can collaborate effectively in the required actions" (Cottrell, 1976, p. 197). Cottrell (1976) also proposes eight essential conditions of competence. The conditions are listed and defined in Table 15-2.

The term **community health** as used in this chapter is the meeting of collective needs by identifying problems and managing interactions within the community itself and between the community and the larger society (Hemstrom, 1995). This definition emphasizes the process

dimension but also includes the dimensions of status and structure. Indicators for all three dimensions are listed in Table 15-3.

The use of status, structure, and process dimensions to define community health, as illustrated in Table 15-3, is an effort to develop a broad definition of community health, involving indicators that are often not included when discussions focus only on risk factors as the basis for community health. Nevertheless, epidemiological data related to health risks of aggregates and communities, commonly expressed as rates and confidence intervals, are vital indicators of health status (Dever, 1997). Data about the structure of the community and its processes provide different information that is complementary to the health risk data and therefore necessary for the development of a clear understanding of the community (Shiell and Hawe, 1996).

Healthy People 2000

One important guideline that is available for nurses working to improve the health of the community is *Healthy People 2000*, a publication from the U.S. Department of Health and Human Services (USDHHS, 1991) that offers a vision of the future for public health and specific objectives to help attain that vision. The *Healthy People 2000* vision recognizes the need to work collectively, in community partnerships, to bring about the changes that will be necessary to fulfill this vision. "The final message of this report is one of shared responsibility among the many partners in prevention. It is what we do collectively and personally that will move us as individuals and as a Nation towards a healthier future" (USDHHS, 1991, p.88).

TABLE 15-2 The Eight Essential Conditions of Community Competence

CONDITION	DEFINITION
Commitment	The affective and cognitive attachment to a community "that is worthy of substantial effort to sustain and enhance" (Cottrell, 1976, p. 198)
Awareness of self and others and clarity of situational definitions	The lucid and realistic perception of one's own and other persons' community components, identities, and positions on issues
Articulateness	The technical aspects of formulating and stating one's views in relation to other persons' views
Effective communication	The accurate transmission of information based on the development of common meaning among the communicators
Conflict containment and accommodation	The inventive and effective assimilation and management of true or realistically perceived differences
Participation	Active, community-oriented involvement
Management of relations with larger society	Adeptness at recognizing, obtaining, and using external resources and supports and, when necessary, stimulating the creation and use of alternative or supplementary resources
Machinery for facilitating participant interaction and decision making	Flexible and responsible procedures (formal and informal), facilities interaction, and decision making

From Goeppinger J, Lassiter PG, Wilcox B: Community health is community competence, *Nurs Outlook* 30(8):464, 1982.

TABLE 15-3 Concept of Community Health Specified

DIMENSION	INDICATORS
Status	Vital statistics (live births, neonatal deaths, infant deaths, maternal deaths) Incidence and prevalence of leading causes of mortality and morbidity Health risk profiles of selected aggregates Functional ability levels
Structure	Health facilities such as hospitals, nursing homes, industrial and school health services, health departments, voluntary health associations, categorical grant programs, and prepaid health plans Health-related planning groups Health manpower, such as physicians, dentists, nurses, environmental sanitarians, social workers, and others Health resource use patterns, such as bed occupancy days and client/provider visits
Process	Commitment Awareness of self and others and clarity of situational definitions Articulateness Effective communication Conflict containment and accommodation Participation Management of relationships with society Machinery for facilitating participant interaction and decision-making

Healthy People 2000 provides the foundation for a national illness-prevention strategy built on three main goals: "increasing the span of healthy life for Americans, reducing health disparities among Americans, and achieving access to preventive services for all Americans" (National Center for Health Statistics, 1996, p.1). Because *Healthy People 2000* is a dynamic rather than static, the Public Health Service (PHS) continues to review progress. In 1995 the PHS published a midcourse review of the objectives with changes that included 19 new objectives, revisions of language in existing objectives for clarity, and new special population targets, which focus on groups with the highest risk of premature death, disease, or disability (National Center for Health Statistics, 1996, p.1).

DID YOU KNOW? *There is a valuable* Healthy People 2000 *website that can be accessed on the Internet through the WebLinks of this book's website (www. mosby.com/MERLIN). From the* Healthy People 2000 *site, information can be obtained about priority areas, lead agencies, fact sheet, midcourse review, progress review, publications list, midcourse review, and* Healthy People 2010.

Strategies to Improve Community Health

Healthy People 2000 has stimulated a number of joint efforts to develop strategies for achieving its goals. These efforts have involved such organizations as the Centers for Disease Control and Prevention (CDC), the American Public Health Association (APHA), the Association of State and Territorial Health Officials (ASTHO), and the National Association of County Health Officials (NACHO). The results of these efforts are a number of publications and guidelines that provide detailed strategies for achieving the objectives in *Healthy People 2000.* These publications include *Healthy Communities 2000: Model Standards, Assessment Protocol for Excellence in Public Health (APEXPH),* and *Planned Approach To Community Health (PATCH).* Each of these three approaches offers step-by-step guidelines for community interventions. *Healthy Communities 2000: Model Standards,* for example, is a guidebook using an 11-step process written to help plan community public health services. It emphasizes health outcomes, a community focus, and a government presence at the local level that is often in the form of a local public health agency.

APEXPH and *PATCH* are two planning tools that can be used to help implement the *Healthy Communities 2000: Model Standards.* **APEXPH** is a process emphasizing local level activity and focuses on improving the public health of communities by increasing the capacity of the local health care agencies to provide core functions, such as assessment and policy development. **PATCH** materials focus more on the prevention of identified chronic disease and health promotion programs and their planning and implementation processes (APHA, 1994; APHA Model Standards, 1993). Readers interested in contacting these organizations can refer to Box 15-3.

The World Health Organization's (WHO) Healthy Cities initiative offers yet another approach to community-oriented health promotion. First initiated in Europe during the middle 1980s, Healthy Cities has become a movement on a global scale with hundreds of Healthy Cities initiatives. Healthy Cities initiatives are based on the belief that the health of the community is affected by political, economic, environmental, and social factors. The Healthy Cities approach emphasizes community development through broad-based local citizen involvement to address local problems (Flynn, 1997). Healthy Cities efforts focus on social change, including developing supportive environments; developing personal skills; and re-

BOX 15-3 Information You Can Use

MODEL STANDARDS

American Public Health Association
1015 15th Street, NW
Washington, DC 20005
(202) 789-5618

APEXPH

National Association of County Health Officials
1100 17th Street, NW
2nd Floor
Washington, DC 20036
(202) 783-5550

PATCH

National Center for Chronic Disease Prevention and Health Promotion
Centers for Chronic Disease Control and Prevention
4770 Buford Hwy NE, Mailstop K-46
Atlanta, GA 30341-3717
(404) 488-5426

See also WebLinks on this book's website at www.mosby.com/MERLIN.

orienting health care services, health policy, and community action (Flynn,1997).

Several different community-oriented health promotion approaches have been noted here, but regardless of what approach is taken, specific strategies to improve community health often depend on whether the status, structure, or process dimension of community health is being emphasized (Courtney et al, 1996; Freudenberg et al, 1995). If the emphasis is on the status dimension, the best strategy is usually at the levels of primary or secondary prevention because the objective is either to prevent a disease or treat it in its early stages. Immunization programs are an example of a nursing intervention at the primary prevention level.

Nursing intervention strategies focused on the structural dimension are directed to either health services or demographic characteristics. Intervention aimed at altering health services might include program planning. Interventions aimed at affecting demographic characteristics might include community development.

When the emphasis is on the process dimension, the best strategy is usually health promotion, also a primary prevention strategy. For example, if family-life education is lacking in a community because of ineffective communication among families, children, school board members, religious leaders, and health professionals, then the most effective strategy may be to open discussion among these groups and help community members develop education programs.

Community Partnerships

Community partnership is crucial because community members and professionals who are active participants in a collaborative decision-making process have a vested interest in the success of efforts to improve the health of their community (Courtney et al, 1996). Consequently, successful strategies for improving community health must include community partnership as the basic means, or key, for improvement (McClowry et al, 1996). Community partnership is a basic focus of such community-oriented approaches as Healthy Cities.

Most changes must aim at improving community health through active partnerships between community residents and health workers from a variety of disciplines. Unfortunately, community residents often are viewed only as data sources and receivers of intervention. This form of partnership is called *passive participation*. In contrast is the lay-professional partnership. This approach specifically emphasizes *active participation*. Power is shared among lay and professional persons throughout the assessment, planning, implementation, and evaluation processes.

In the past, nurses have not been influential in initiating community changes, although they generally have been actively involved in the implementation phase. Intervention by the nurse for the community's benefit, or passive participation, has been a common practice mode (Hatziandreau et al, 1995). Passive participation contrasts with the partnership approach in which all involved are assessing, planning, and implementing needed community changes (Baker et al, 1997).

Partnership means the active participation and involvement of the community or its representatives in healthful change (Eng, Parker, and Harlan, 1997). Partnership is defined here as the informed, flexible, and negotiated distribution (and redistribution) of power among all participants in the processes of change for improved community health. The three main characteristics of partnership are captured by the following adjectives:

1. *Informed.* Lay and professional partners must be aware of their own and other's perceptions, rights, and responsibilities (Jackson and Parks, 1997).
2. *Flexible.* Lay and professional partners must recognize the unique and similar contributions that each can make to a given situation. For example, professionals often contribute important knowledge and skills that laypersons lack. On the other hand, laypersons' definitions of community health problems are often more accurate than those of professionals.
3. *Negotiated.* Because contributions vary and each situation is different, the distribution of power must be negotiated at every stage of the change process.

Partnership, as defined here, is a concept that is as essential for nurses to know and use as are the concepts of community, community as client, and community health. Experienced nurses know that partnership is important because health is not always a reality, but rather it is generated through new and increasingly effective means of lay-professional collaboration. For example, safety is an issue for many urban neighborhoods. Active effects by neighborhood residents can make neighborhoods cleaner and safer places to live (Hemstrom, 1995). However, such changes also require active professional service providers, such as school teachers, public safety officers, and horticulturists. Partnership in identifying problems and setting goals is especially important because it brings commitment from all persons involved, which is essential to successful change.

The significance and effectiveness of partnership in improving community health is supported by a growing body of literature. Studies document the use of partnership models involving urban areas (Parker et al, 1998) and lay advisors (Baker et al, 1997; Schultz et al, 1997). The roles of these partners-in-health have included listening sympathetically, offering advice, making referrals, and starting programs (Aguirre-Molina and Parra, 1995; Bechtel, Garrett, and Grover, 1995; Courtney et al, 1996, Goeppinger et al, 1995). Recent work by Hildebrandt (1996) and Kroeger and colleagues (1997) shows the continuing use of partnership models for improving health in other countries. In international health, partnership models generally are viewed as empowering people, through their lay leaders, to control their own health destinies and lives. In the United States, partnership models have often involved churches and informal community leaders.

Professional health workers often have challenged the notion of partnership, despite data supporting its effectiveness. Unfortunately, passive compliance is more frequently sought than the true collaboration inherent in a partnership. Also, questions often are raised about the ability of health care consumers to determine health needs accurately and to evaluate professional practice (Howell et al, 1998).

COMMUNITY-FOCUSED NURSING PROCESS: AN OVERVIEW OF THE PROCESS FROM ASSESSMENT TO EVALUATION

Most nurses are familiar with the nursing process as it applies to individually focused nursing care. Using it to promote community health makes this same nursing process community focused (Flick, Reese, and Harris, 1996). The phases of the nursing process that directly involve the community as client begin at the start of the contract or partnership and include assessment, diagnosis, planning, implementation, and evaluation. Figure 15-1 provides an overview of the nursing process with the community as client.

The use of the nursing process with the community as client is presented in the following sections with a real case study taken from the practice of a nurse. For clarity, infant malnutrition is the only community health problem used to illustrate application of the nursing process. In reality, several different community health problems were identified by the partnership. Their relative importance was examined, and infant malnutrition was picked as the most important problem from among all of the identified problems before continuing with intervention.

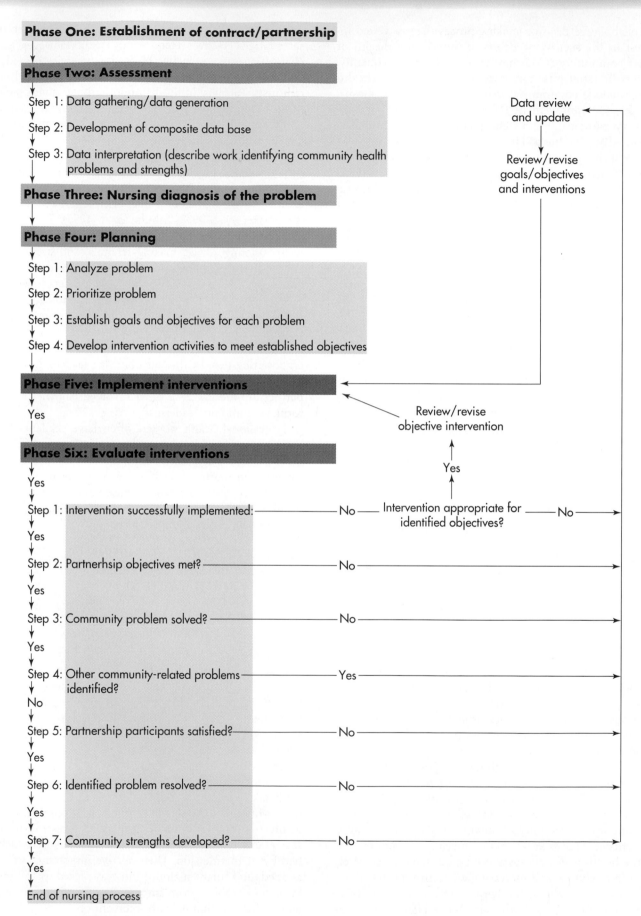

FIG. 15-1 Flow chart illustrating the nursing process with the community as client.

Assessing Community Health

Community assessment is the process of critically thinking about the community and involves getting to know and understand the community as client. The community assessment phase involves a logical, systematic approach to the initial phase of the nursing process. Community assessment helps identify community needs, clarify problems, and identify strengths and resources. There are different types of community assessment. Community assessments can be short and simple or long and complex. One example of a short and simple community assessment is the windshield survey, which is discussed later in this section. In contrast, this section describes the longer and more complex process of a comprehensive community assessment. Comprehensive community assessment is the necessary initial phase of the community nursing process with the community as client.

Assessing community health requires three steps:

- *Step 1.* Gathering relevant existing data and generating missing data
- *Step 2.* Developing a composite database
- *Step 3.* Interpreting the composite database to identify community problems and strengths

Gathering the data and its initial interpretation are the first steps in the assessment phase of the nursing process (see Fig. 15-1).

Data collection and interpretation

The primary goal of **data collection** is to get usable information about the community and its health. The systematic collection of data about community health requires gathering or compiling existing data and generating missing data. These data are then interpreted, and community health problems and community abilities are identified.

Data gathering. Data gathering is the process of obtaining existing, readily available data. These data usually describe the demography of a community: age, sex, socioeconomic, and racial distributions; vital statistics, including selected mortality and morbidity data; community institutions, including health care organizations and the services they provide; and health personnel characteristics. Often these data have been collected by others via structured interviews, questionnaires, or surveys and are available in published reports.

Data generation. Data generation is the process of developing data that do not already exist through interaction with community members or groups. This type of information is harder to get and is generally not statistical in nature. Data that often must be generated include information about a community's knowledge and beliefs, values and sentiments, goals and perceived needs, norms, problem-solving processes, power, leadership, and influence structures. These data are more likely to be collected by interviews and observation (Ludwig-Beymer et al, 1996).

Composite database. Combining the gathered and generated data creates a composite **database.** Data analysis seeks to make sense of the data. First, data are analyzed and synthesized and themes are noted. **Community health problems,** or needs for action, and **community health strengths,** or abilities, are determined. Next, the resources available to meet the needs are identified. Problems are indicated by differences between the nurse's and community's goals for community health and the themes or findings from the data analysis. Strengths, on the other hand, are suggested by similarities between the nurse's and community's concepts of community health and available data. The nurse and community, working in a partnership, identify problems. Next, the resources available to meet the needs are identified. Active community participation is critical for the data interpretation process, particularly in identifying problems.

The **Program Planning Model,** first proposed by Delbecq and Van de Ven (1971), continues to be widely used to encourage lay people to participate in defining problems. The model shows how to use active community participation in problem definition and program planning. It makes the most of the contributions by various groups with diverse interests, skills, and knowledge. This model depends heavily on **nominal groups,** "groups in which individuals work in the presence of one another but do not interact" (Delbecq and Van de Ven, 1971, p. 467); the separation of the individual from collective (or group) problems; and a round-robin process for listing problems without evaluating or elaborating on them at the same time. This model is popularly known as the *nominal group process.*

Other consensus methods, such as the Delphi technique, also are used to define the extent of agreement among content experts, policy makers, and community members about the presence and importance of certain health problems. Experience shows that consensus methods will produce useful results if the following conditions are met (MacLachlan, 1996; Redman et al, 1997):

1. Problems are carefully selected.
2. Participants in the process are deliberately selected and closely monitored.
3. Justified and reasonable levels of consensus are expected.
4. Findings are used as guides to decisions.

Data collection methods

Several methods to collect data are needed. Methods that encourage the nurse to consider the community's perception of its health problems and abilities are as important as those methods structured to identify knowledge that the nurse considers essential.

Five useful methods of collecting data are informant interviews, participant observation, windshield surveys, secondary analysis of existing data, and surveys. These methods can be grouped into two distinct but complementary categories: 1) methods that rely on what is directly observed by the data collector and 2) methods that rely on what is reported to the data collector.

Collection of direct data. Informant interviews, participant observation, and windshield surveys are three methods of directly collecting data. All three methods require sensitivity, openness, curiosity, and the ability to listen, taste, touch, smell, and see life as it is lived in a community. **Informant interviews,** which consist of directed talks with selected members of a community about community members or groups and events, are basic to effective data collection. Also basic is **participant observation,** the deliberate sharing, if conditions permit, in the life of a community. Informant interviews and participant observation are good ways to generate information about community beliefs, norms, values, power and influence structures, and problem-solving processes. Such data can seldom be reported in numbers, so often they are not collected. Even worse, conclusions that are based on intuition and unchecked are sometimes used to replace this type of data. Conclusions from direct data collection methods should be confirmed by those people providing information.

:HOW TO *Identify a Key Informant*

- *Talking to key informants is a critical part of the community assessment.*
- *Key informants are not always people who have a formal title or position.*
- *Key informants often have an informal role within the community.*
- *County health department nurses and church leaders are often key informants.*
- *They also know many community members and can identify other key informants.*

In the example of the community with the infant malnutrition problem, informant interviewing with social workers and religious leaders provided data indicating a community with well-defined clusters of persons with low incomes, concerns about adolescent pregnancy, and worries about the health of its babies. This data, which reflects the concerns and worries of the Jefferson County community, would have been difficult to acquire without personal interviews.

Windshield surveys are the motorized equivalent of simple observation. They involve the collection of data "which will help define the community, the trends, stability, and changes that will affect the health of the community" (Stanhope and Knollmueller, 2000).

: NURSING TIP

If you do a windshield survey as part of your community assessment, go two times: once during the day when people are at work and children are at school, and a second time in the evening after work is done and school is out.

The nurse, driving a car or riding public transportation, can observe many dimensions of a community's life and environment through the windshield. Common characteristics of people on the street, neighborhood-gathering places, the rhythm of community life, housing quality, and geographic boundaries can be observed readily. Again,

using the infant malnutrition example, the windshield survey suggested that the community had a large unemployed population because adults were observed "hanging out" at country crossroads during the day.

Windshield surveys can be used by themselves for short and simple assessments. However, it is used here as one part of the longer, more complex comprehensive community assessment. An example of a windshield survey can be found in Appendix C.2.

:HOW TO *Obtain a Quick Assessment of a Community*

- *One way of getting a quick, initial sense of the community is to do a windshield assessment using a format like the one provided as an example Appendix C.2.*
- *Nurses interested in doing a windshield assessment need to either take public transportation, have someone else drive while they take notes, or plan to frequently stop and write down what they see.*
- *The windshield survey example provided in Appendix C.2 is organized into 15 elements with specific questions to answer that are related to each element.*
- *Nurses who use this approach will have an initial descriptive assessment of community when they are done.*
- *If interventions are planned, the more thorough and more comprehensive process described in this chapter will be necessary.*

Collection of reported data. Secondary analysis and surveys are two methods of collecting reported data. In **secondary analysis,** the nurse uses previously gathered data, such as minutes from community meetings. This type of analysis is extremely valuable because it saves time and effort. Many sources of data are readily available and useful for secondary analysis including public documents, health surveys, minutes from meetings, statistical data, and health records. In the Jefferson County infant malnutrition example, birth records noting low birth weights and health department clinic records of low-weight-for-height children provided information that showed a higher-than-average rate of infant malnutrition.

Surveys report data from a sample of persons. They are equally useful, but they take more time and effort than observational methods and secondary analyses because they require time-consuming and costly data collection. Thus the survey method is not often used by the nurse. However, surveys are necessary for identifying certain community problems (Dever, 1997). For example, a lack of accessible personal health services cannot be documented readily and reliably in any other way.

Assessment guides

Nursing assessment of community health—data collection and interpretation—must be focused. Focus, or perspective, can be provided by detailed assessment guides, which are built on a conceptual framework of definitions of community and community health.

Concepts that can be measured in behavioral or observable terms can serve as assessment guides. The concepts of community and community health have already been defined in such terms. The concept of community has been specified (see Table 15-1). The definition previously given includes three dimensions: people or person, place and time, and function. Several indicators specify each of these dimensions. For example, indicators such as size in square miles and political boundaries represent the geographic dimension.

A detailed description of community health—its status, structure, and process dimensions—is presented in Table 15-3. In the infant malnutrition example, status dimension data were gathered from morbidity and mortality data; structural dimension data were gathered from vital statistics and from informant interviews with social workers; and process dimension data were gathered from informant interviews with community religious leaders. In this way the concepts of community and community health provide the framework for the Assessment Guide in Appendix C.1. Together, the concepts and Assessment Guide constitute the Community Health Assessment Model, the basis of the Community-Oriented Health Record (COHR) (see Appendix C.1). Data, problems, and abilities are all organized by using the Community Health Assessment Model.

The **Community-as-Partner Model** is another example of an assessment guide developed to show that nurses can work with communities as partners (Anderson and McFarlane, 1996). This model illustrates how communities change and grow best by full involvement and self-empowerment. The heart of this model is an assessment wheel that illustrates that the people actually are the community. Surrounding the people, and integral to the community, are eight identified subsystems: housing, education, fire and safety, politics and government, health, communication, economics, and recreation. These subsystems both affect and are affected by the people who make up the community. This model and additional information to understand it can be found in Appendix H.1.

‼ WHAT DO YOU THINK? *In 1998 Howell and colleagues studied the Healthy Start initiative to reduce infant mortality rates and said that there can be problems when communities use a community empowerment model. Community involvement may interfere with the effectiveness of program operations, create goals that differ from the program's original goals, and slow the development of the program down. Should Healthy Start sites use a different approach? Why or why not?*

Assessment issues

Gaining entry or acceptance into the community is perhaps the biggest challenge in assessment. The nurse is usually an outsider and often represents an established health care system that is neither known nor trusted by community members who may therefore react with indifference or even active hostility to the nurse. In addition, nurses may feel insecure about their skills as a community worker, and the community may refuse to acknowledge its need for those skills. Because the nurse's success largely depends on the way he or she is viewed, entry into the community is critical. Often the nurse can gain entry by taking part in community events, looking and listening with interest, visiting people in formal leadership positions, employing an assessment guide, and using a peer group for support.

Once the nurse gains entry at an initial level, **role negotiation** often becomes an issue. The concept of role involves the values, behaviors, or goals that govern an individual's interactions with others. The nurse must decide how long to separate the roles of data collector and intervenor. Effective implementation of the nursing process requires initial collection of an adequate database. The danger of premature response to health needs and social injustice is great. Nurses can assist in role negotiation by a thoughtful and consistent presentation of the reasons for their presence in the community and by sincere demonstrations of their commitment to the community. Keeping appointments, clarifying community members' perceptions of health needs, and respecting an individual's right to choose whether he or she will work with the nurse are often useful techniques.

Maintaining **confidentiality** is also important. Nurses must be very careful to protect the identity of community members who provide sensitive or controversial data. In some cases the nurse may consider withholding data; in other situations the nurse may be legally required to disclose data. For example, nurses are required by law to report child abuse.

Of a less personal nature is the issue of small-area analysis (Dever, 1997). There are potential problems of small-area analysis, although the issue raised here concerns how mistakes can be made when conclusions are based on data gathered from small areas. For example, calculation of mortality rates in a rural county when the denominator is as small as 5000 may be skewed. This issue often raises questions about the validity of many identified health problems. It also reinforces the usefulness of looking at the same problem using several methods, because if similar health problems are identified using several assessment methods, the nurse can be more confident of their validity.

Remember, a community assessment will identify multiple community health problems. Each of these problems must be analyzed and given a priority score to determine which are the most serious problems. In the next sections, the infant malnutrition example is used to illustrate how an identified problem generates a community-focused nursing diagnosis, which is analyzed and assigned a priority score.

Community-Oriented Nursing Diagnosis

The assessment activities and the creation of a composite database will result in a list of community health problems.

Each problem needs to be identified clearly and stated as a community health diagnosis. The statement of the problem in a community health diagnosis format is the third phase of the community-as-client process. The development of the community health diagnosis in this phase of the process helps clarify the problem and is an important first step to planning. In the planning phase, where each diagnosis is analyzed, priorities are established and community-focused interventions are identified. Community diagnoses clarify who gets the care (the community as opposed to an individual), provide a statement identifying problems faced by who is getting the care, and identify factors contributing to the problem.

Although the North American Nursing Diagnosis Association (NANDA) is a familiar nursing diagnosis taxonomy for most students, NANDA's focus has been at the individual rather than the community level of diagnosis. NANDA is not the only accepted system of nursing diagnosis; for example, home health nurses are familiar with the OMAHA system of nursing diagnosis. In this chapter a version of a three-part nursing diagnosis format proposed by Muecke (1984) is used:

1. Risk of _____
2. Among _____
3. Related to _____

"Risk of" identifies a specific problem or health risk faced by the community. "Among" identifies the specific community client with whom the nurse will be working in relation to the identified problem or risk (see Box 15-1). "Related to" describes characteristics of the community and its environment that were identified in the composite database of the assessment phase. Each community has its own unique characteristics. Some of these characteristics are strengths that the nurse can build upon, but other characteristics contribute to the problem identified in the community health diagnosis. The characteristics, or factors, related to the identified problem are listed after the "related to" statement as the third part of the community health diagnosis.

The example being used for illustration in this chapter is infant malnutrition. Based on assessment data the community diagnosis for infant malnutrition using this format would be the following:

1. Risk of infant malnutrition
2. Among families in Jefferson County
3. Related to lack of regular developmental screening; no outreach program to identify at-risk infants; families' lack of knowledge about WIC; confusion among community families about WIC program enrollment criteria; community families' lack of infant-related nutritional knowledge

Frequently, a number of community health diagnoses will be made based on the different problems identified during the assessment data. In the next phase, "Planning for Community Health," weights and priorities are established among the problems identified in the assessment phase, and the problems have now been stated in a community-focused nursing diagnosis format.

Planning for Community Health

The planning phase includes analyzing the community health problems identified in the community nursing diagnoses and establishing priorities among them, establishing goals and objectives, and identifying intervention activities that will accomplish the objectives.

Problem analysis

Problem analysis seeks to clarify the nature of the problem. The nurse identifies the origins and effects of the problem, the points at which intervention might be undertaken, and the parties that have an interest in the problem and its solution. Analysis often requires the development of a problem matrix, in which the direct and indirect factors that contribute to the problem and outcomes of the problem are identified; relationships among the problem are noted; and factors that contribute to the problem and outcomes of the problem are mapped. The matrix is important because the nurse can anticipate that several of the same factors that contribute to a problem and affect the outcomes of a problem also underlie many of the problems. The problem of highest priority may be among the common factors that contribute to the problem and affect the outcomes of the problem.

Problem analysis should be undertaken for each identified problem. It often requires organizing a special group composed of the nurse, persons whose areas of expertise relate to the problem, persons whose organizations are capable of intervening, and representatives of the community experiencing the problem. Both content and process specialists must participate. Together they can identify the **problem correlates,** defined as contributing factors to the problem, and explain the relationships between each correlate and the problem.

This process is seen in Table 15-4 as an example of problem analysis. Problem correlates (factors that contribute to the problem and outcomes of the problem) for infant malnutrition are listed in the first column. Correlates are from all areas of community life. Social or environmental correlates are as appropriate as those oriented to the individual. For example, teenage pregnancy is a social correlate of infant malnutrition, and high unemployment is an environmental correlate. In the second column the relationships between each correlate and the problem are noted. The third column contains data from the community and the literature that support the relationship, using the suspected infant malnutrition example and a few of its correlates.

Infant malnutrition is thought to be correlated with inadequate diet, community norms, poverty, disturbed mother-child relationships, and teenage pregnancy.

Problem priorities

Infant malnutrition represents only one of several community health problems identified by the community as-

TABLE 15-4 Problem Analysis: Infant Malnutrition

NAME OF COMMUNITY: JEFFERSON COUNTY
PROBLEM STATEMENT: INFANT MALNUTRITION IN JEFFERSON COUNTY

PROBLEM CORRELATES (FACTORS CONTRIBUTING TO THE PROBLEM AND OUTCOMES OF THE PROBLEM)	RELATIONSHIP OF CORRELATES TO PROBLEM	DATA SUPPORTIVE TO RELATIONSHIPS (REFER TO APPROPRIATE SECTIONS OF DATABASE AND RELEVANT RESEARCH FINDINGS IN CURRENT LITERATURE)
1. Inadequate diet	Diets lacking in required nutrients contribute to malnutrition.	All county infants and their mothers seen by PHNs in 1997 referred to nutritionist because of poor diets.
2. Community norms	Bottle-fed babies less apt to receive adequate amounts of safe milk containing necessary nutrients.	Area general practitioners and nurses agree that 90% of mothers in county bottle feed.
3. Poverty	Infant formulas are expensive.	60% of new mothers in county are receiving welfare.
4. Disturbed mother-child relationship	Poor mother-child relationship may result in infant's failure to thrive.	Data from nursing charts of 43 mothers with infants diagnosed as "failure to thrive."
5. Teenage pregnancy	Teenage mothers most apt to have inadequate diets prenatally, to bottle feed, to be poor, and to lack parenting skills.	90% of births in 1998 were to women 19 years of age or younger.

sessment. In reality, several community health problems besides infant malnutrition were identified. They included a mortality rate from cardiovascular disease that was higher than the national norm and, as expressed by many residents, a desire to quit smoking.

Each problem identified as part of the assessment process must be put through a ranking process to determine its importance. This ranking process, in which problems are evaluated and priorities established according to predetermined criteria, is termed **problem prioritization.** It takes into account what can be provided by community members, content experts, administrators, and others who can provide resources.

Problem priority criteria. Criteria that have been helpful in ranking identified problems include the following:
1. Community awareness of the problem
2. Community motivation to resolve or better manage the problem
3. Nurse's ability to influence problem solution
4. Availability of expertise to solve the problem
5. Severity of the outcomes if the problem is unresolved
6. Speed with which the problem can be solved
Using the example of infant malnutrition again, these six criteria are listed in the first column of Table 15-5.

Given an acceptable and comprehensive set of criteria and a list of community health problems, the process of assigning priorities is rather simple. Each problem is considered independently, and an overall priority score is calculated. This calculation involves two separate but related weighted factors: the first factor involves criteria related to

the identified problem itself, and the second factor involves the same criteria but is weighted based on the partnership's ability to make a change in each of the criteria in factor one.

Each of the six criteria listed in Table 15-5 is considered separately and independently and then assigned a weight. The criteria are weighted on a scale ranging from a low score of 1 to a high score of 10. Listed in the second column of Table 15-5, these criteria are weighted jointly by the members of the partnership based on the perceived importance of each criterion to the identified community health problem. For instance, when members of the partnership assigned a weight to the first criterion listed in Table 15-5, they had to ask each other, "How important is community awareness of infant malnutrition in Jefferson County for problem resolution?"

The second factor, the importance of each criterion relative to the problem, also must be considered and rated relative to the partnership's ability to resolve the problem. In deciding the rating to be given, the members of the partnership answer questions related to their ability to influence and/or change the situation relative to the criterion. In the infant malnutrition example, they asked each other to identify the extent of the community's awareness of the problem. After members have talked about the criterion's importance and have agreed on its rating, the score is recorded. To understand the difference between the ideas of criteria weight and problem rating, it may be helpful to remember that a criterion could be extremely important in considering priorities, but that criterion might rate low for a particular problem because the mem-

TABLE 15-5 Problem Prioritization: Infant Malnutrition

Criteria	Criteria Weights (1-10)	Problem	Rating (1-10)	Rationale for Rating	Problem Ranking (weight × rate)
1. Community awareness of the problem	5	Infant malnutrition in Jefferson County	10	Health service providers, teachers, and a variety of parents have mentioned problem.	50
2. Community motivation to resolve the problem	10		3	Most believe that this problem is not solvable because most of those affected are indigent.	30
3. Nurse's ability to influence problem resolution	5		8	Nurse are skilled at consciousness raising and mobilizing support.	40
4. Ready availability of expertise relevant to problem resolution	7		10	WIC program and nutritionists are available. A county extension agent is interested.	70
5. Severity of outcomes if problem is left unresolved	8		5	Effects of marginal malnutrition are not well documented.	40
6. Quickness with which problem resolution can be achieved	3		3	Time to mobilize rural community with no history of social action is lengthy.	9
					Total: 239*

*Maximum possible score = 600.

bers of the community partnership believe that it would be difficult to influence or change things relative to that particular criterion. One example of the difference between the perceptions of the nurse and community members is smoking in public buildings; the community nurse might identify smoking as a public health problem, but community members might view smoking as an issue of individual choice and personal freedom.

This process is repeated separately for each identified problem, and a ranking score is determined; then the ranking scores for all of the problems are compared. Priorities among the identified problems are established. The problems with the highest priority scores are the ones selected as the focus for intervention. Arriving at a priority score for each identified problem can appear complicated; however, it helps to recall that the criteria were set up and weighted by the people taking part in the community partnership before prioritizing began. Also, the reasons for rating and each rating score are decided and set up based on active input by all members in the community partnership. Although the number scores are subjective, the active involvement of the nurse and various community representatives helps to ensure that the data used to establish the rationale are real and accurate. Community participation also helps to ensure that the significance of the score for each problem reflects its importance relative to other community health problems.

The process of establishing a total ranking score for the problem of suspected infant malnutrition is called *problem prioritization* and is depicted in Table 15-5 where criterion two, community motivation to resolve the problem, is used as an example. Community motivation to resolve the problem was the criterion weighted as most important to problem resolution as indicated by the criterion weight of 10. However, most community residents believed that the problem could not be solved because of the poverty of those affected and because partnership members did not believe they could actually have an impact on poverty, so they rated their ability to intervene low as indicated by the rating of 3. As a result the relative ranking of this criterion, when applied to the problem of infant malnutrition, was low in comparison with the other criteria. The score of 30 indicates this.

A similar process with the remaining five criteria listed in Table 15-5 yielded a total ranking score of 239 for the suspected infant malnutrition problem. The only ranking shown is for one community problem, which received a ranking of less than 50% of the total score possible. Such a ranking would need to be compared with the ranking of other problems to see the partner's commitment to solving the problem. Assuming that 239 is the highest-ranking score among the several identified community health problems, infant malnutrition is the logical priority problem for intervention.

TABLE 15-6 Goals and Objectives: Infant Malnutrition

NAME OF COMMUNITY: JEFFERSON COUNTY
PROBLEM/CONCERN: INFANT MALNUTRITION
GOAL STATEMENT: TO REDUCE THE INCIDENCE AND PREVALENCE OF INFANT MALNUTRITION

PRESENT DATE	OBJECTIVES (NUMBER AND STATEMENT)	COMPLETION DATE
1-98	1. 80% of infants seen by health department, neighborhood health center, and private physicians will have their developmental levels assessed.	8-98
1-98	2. WIC program eligibility will be determined for 80% of infants seen by health department, neighborhood health center, and private physicians.	5-98
1-98	3. An outreach program will be implemented to identify at-risk infants not now known to health care providers.	8-98
1-98	4. WIC program eligibility will be determined for 25% of at-risk infants.	1-99
1-98	5. 75% of all infants eligible for WIC food supplements will be enrolled in the program.	12-98
1-98	6. 50% of the mothers of infants enrolled in WIC will demonstrate three ways of incorporating WIC supplements into their infants' diets.	5-98

Establishing goals and objectives

Once high-priority problems are identified, relevant goals and objectives are developed. **Goals** are generally broad statements of desired outcomes. **Objectives** are the precise statements of the desired outcomes.

An example of one of the goals and the specific objectives associated with it for the infant malnutrition problem is depicted in Table 15-6. The goal is to reduce the incidence and prevalence of infant malnutrition. *The objectives must be precise, behaviorally stated, incremental, and measurable.* In this example the specific objectives pertain to assessing infant developmental levels, determining Women, Infants, and Children (WIC) Program eligibility, implementing an outreach program, enrolling infants in the WIC program, and providing supplemental foods in existing diets.

As noted previously, establishing these goals and objectives involves collaboration between the nurse and representatives of the community groups affected by both the problem and the proposed intervention. This often requires a great deal of negotiation among everyone taking part in the planning process. One important advantage offered by the continuous active involvement of people affected by the outcomes is that they have a vested interest in those outcomes and therefore are supportive of and committed to the success of the intervention. Once goals and objectives are chosen, intervention activities to accomplish the objectives can be identified.

Identifying intervention activities

Intervention activities, the means by which objectives are met, are the strategies used to meet the objectives, the ways change will be effected, and the ways the problem cycle will be broken. Because alternative intervention activities do exist, they must be identified and evaluated. Sketching out possible interventions and selecting the best set of activities to achieve the goal of documenting and

reducing infant malnutrition are depicted in Tables 15-7 and 15-8.

To achieve the objective related to assessment of infant developmental levels (see Table 15-6, objective 1), five intervention activities are listed in the second column of Table 15-7. Each is relevant to the first objective: 80% of infants seen by the health department, neighborhood health center, and private physicians will have their developmental levels assessed. The first two activities involve WIC program personnel as the principal change agents. The last three involve the nurse, WIC program personnel, and the staff of the health department, neighborhood health center, and private physicians' offices as the change partners.

The expected effect of each of the activities is considered in the third and fifth columns of Table 15-7. The **value,** or the likelihood that the activity will help meet the objective and finally resolve the problem, is noted in the third column. Clearly it is more valuable in the long term to educate others in how to assess infant development (activity 4) than to do it for them (activity 1). It is also valuable to analyze the change process necessary to complete the objective (activity 5). As a result, activities 4 and 5 have higher value scores than activity 1, in which the professional staff alone carries out the intervention.

On the other hand, the **probability,** or the likelihood that the means can be implemented, is highest when only the nurse is involved, because the nurse has more control over self-behavior than over the behavior of others. Therefore activities 1 and 3 have higher probabilities than activities 2, 4, and 5, as recorded in the fifth column. Conditions explaining the numerical scores are noted briefly in the fourth column. A total score is computed by multiplying the value of the activity by the probability. These scores are listed in the last column. The activities with the

TABLE 15-7 Plan: Intervention Activities to Assess Infants' Developmental Levels

NAME OF COMMUNITY: JEFFERSON COUNTY

OBJECTIVE NUMBER 1 AND STATEMENT: 80% OF INFANTS SEEN BY HEALTH DEPARTMENT, NEIGHBORHOOD HEALTH CENTER, AND PRIVATE PHYSICIANS WILL HAVE THEIR DEVELOPMENT LEVELS ASSESSED.

DATE	INTERVENOR ACTIVITIES/ MEANS	VALUE TO ACHIEVING OBJECTIVE (1-10)	ACTIVITY/MEANS SELECTED FOR IMPLEMENTATION	PROBABILITY OF IMPLEMENTING ACTIVITY (1-10)	ACTIVITY RANKING (VALUE × PROBABILITY)
1-98	1. WIC program supplies personnel to assess infant developmental levels.	1	Insufficient personnel and time; existing community resources (potential) are ignored.	10	10
1-98	2. WIC program provides in-service education to staff on assessment of infant development.	5	Antipathy between WIC personnel and other health workers is high. The need for education must be assessed first, and enthusiasm for objectives must be created.	5	25
1-98	3. CN provides in-service education to staff in assessment of infant development.	3	The CN cannot do it alone.	10	30
1-98	4. CN helps WIC personnel identify in-service educational needs of area health care providers about assessment of infant development.	8	Most likely to build on existing community strengths; CN skilled in needs assessment and interpersonal techniques are needed to decrease. antipathy	8	64
1-98	5. CN helps WIC personnel identify driving and restraining forces relative to implementation of objective.	10	Without this, change effort is likely to fail.	8	80

highest total scores become the priority intervention activities because it is important to be able to both affect the objective (value) and carry out the means (probability). In this case, activities 4 and 5, with total scores of 64 and 80 respectively, would be selected.

Although the numbers assigned by the nurse to both value and probability are based on subjective judgment, their products are quite useful. When the scores in the two columns are multiplied, the resulting totals give you a basis for judging which of the potential intervention activities will be most effective in meeting the objectives.

A second example of plan development is shown in Table 15-8. The activities relate to objective 3 of the goals and objectives (see Table 15-6) that involve starting up and carrying out an outreach program. These activities involve using lay advisors, hospital nurses, community and public health nurses, and WIC program personnel. Activity 1 with a total score of 40 and activity 2 with a total score of 48 were selected. Activity 1 builds on existing informal com-

munity leaders, and activity 2 addresses needed changes in the formal health care delivery system.

Implementation for Community Health

Implementation, the fourth phase of the nursing process, involves the work and activities aimed at achieving the goals and objectives. Implementation efforts may be made by the person or group who established the goals and objectives, or they may be shared with or even delegated to others. The issue of having a central authority to oversee the efforts to start up and carry out the plan is important, and the nurse's position on this issue can be affected by a variety of factors.

Factors influencing implementation

Implementation is shaped by the nurse's chosen roles, the type of health problem selected as the focus for intervention, the community's readiness to take part in problem solving, and characteristics of the social change process. The nurse taking part in community-oriented intervention

TABLE 15-8 Plan: Intervention Activities to Implement an Outreach Program

NAME OF COMMUNITY: JEFFERSON COUNTY

OBJECTIVE NUMBER 3 AND STATEMENT: AN OUTREACH PROGRAM IS IMPLEMENTED TO IDENTIFY AT-RISK INFANTS NOT NOW KNOWN TO HEALTH CARE PROVIDERS.

DATE	INTERVENOR ACTIVITIES/ MEANS	VALUE TO ACHIEVING OBJECTIVE (1-10)	ACTIVITY/MEANS SELECTED FOR IMPLEMENTATION	PROBABILITY OF IMPLEMENTING ACTIVITY (1-10)	ACTIVITY RANKING (VALUE × PROBABILITY)
1-98	*1. CN identifies and trains lay advisors in community as case finders.	8	Lay leaders already known, proven to be effective change agents; cannot, however, be paid.	6	48
1-98	*2. Local hospital administrators alter job descriptions of nurses in maternity and pediatrics to include case finding and referral.	8	All babies in Jefferson County born in hospital since 1994. Administrator interested in community. Administration powerful and can alter nurses' job descriptions.	5	40
1-98	3. CN encourages public health nurses to do better job of case finding.	8	Public health nurses have historic role in case finding. CN not well known by PHNs. PHNs reported to be overworked.	2	16
1-98	4. WIC personnel devote one evening per week to case finding.	1	One nurse (nonresident) eager to do this. Does not develop existing community resources.	10	10

has knowledge and skills that the other intervenors do not have; the question is how the nurse uses the position, knowledge, and skills.

Nurse's role. Nurses can act as content experts, helping communities select and attain task-related goals. In the example of infant malnutrition, the nurse used epidemiological skills to determine the incidence and prevalence of malnutrition. The nurse also served as a process expert by increasing the community's ability to document the problem rather than by only providing help as an expert in the area.

Content-focused roles often are considered **change agent** roles, whereas process roles are called **change partner** roles. Change agent roles stress gathering and analyzing facts and implementing programs, whereas change partner roles include those of enabler-catalyst, teacher of problem-solving skills, and activist advocate.

The problem and the nurse's role. The role the nurse chooses depends on the nature of the health, the community's decision-making ability, and on professional and personal choices. Some health problems clearly require certain intervention roles. If a community lacks democratic problem-solving abilities, the nurse may select teacher, facilitator, and advocate roles. Problem solving skills must be explained and modeled. A problem with determining the status of community health, on the other hand, usually requires fact-gatherer and analyst roles. Some prob-

lems, such as the example of infant malnutrition, require multiple roles. In that case, managing conflict among the involved health care providers demanded process skills. Collecting and interpreting the data necessary to document the problem required both interpersonal and analytical skills.

The community's history of taking part in decision making is a critical factor. In a community skilled in identifying and successfully managing its problems, the nurse may best serve as technical expert or advisor. Different roles may be required if the community lacks problem-solving skills or has a history of unsuccessful change efforts. The nurse may have to focus on developing problem-solving capabilities or on making one successful change so that the community becomes empowered to take on the job of promoting change on its own behalf.

Social change process and the nurse's role. The nurse's role also depends on the social change process. Not all communities are open to innovation. Ability to change is often related to the extent to which a community adheres to traditional norms. The more traditional the community, the less likely it is to change. Innovation is often directly related to high socioeconomic status; a perceived need for change; the presence of liberal, scientific, and democratic values; and a high level of social participation by community residents (Rogers 1995). Innovations with the highest adoption rates are seen as better than the other available choices. They also fit with existing values, can be started as a limited trial, and are easily explained or demonstrated. They are also simple and convenient (Rogers 1995). For example, people living in a community might go to an immunization clinic rather than a private physician if the clinic is nearby and less expensive and if the physician is not always available when needed.

Innovations also are easier to accept when the innovation is shared in ways that fit in with the community's norms, values, and customs and when information is spread by the best communication mode (mass media for early adopters and face-to-face for late adopters). Other factors that positively influence acceptance include the support of other communities for the change efforts, identification and use of opinion leaders, and clear, straightforward communication about the innovation (Rogers, 1995).

Many complex factors combine to shape how the change process is started and maintained. Therefore the nurse must be adaptable. The roles required to begin change may differ from those used to maintain or stabilize it. Also, the roles required to initiate, maintain, and stabilize change may vary from community to community and from one intervention to another within the same community. Thus the nurse must be skilled in a variety of implementation mechanisms.

Implementation mechanisms

Implementation mechanisms are the vehicles, or modes, by which innovations are transferred from the planners to the community. The nurse alone is never considered an implementation mechanism. Change on behalf of the community client requires multiple implementation mechanisms. The nurse must identify and appropriately use all of them. Some important implementation mechanisms, or aids, include small interacting groups, lay advisors, the mass media, and health policies.

Small interacting groups. Small **interacting groups,** formal and informal, are essential implementation mechanisms. Many of the formal groups in the community are families, legislative bodies, health-care recipients, and service providers. Some of the informal groups are neighborhoods and social action groups. The common tie among these diverse groups is their location between the community and individuals. Because of their intermediate position, they can and do act both to support and to constrain change efforts at the community and individual levels. They are potentially powerful precisely because they are **mediating structures.**

As a result, the nurse needs to identify which groups view the proposed change as beneficial and which do not. New small groups may need to be formed to encourage the change. Changes may be necessary in the innovation or in how the innovation is spread throughout the community to increase acceptance. At first the innovation may have to be directed to groups with a majority of **early adopters** (those with broad perspectives and abilities to adopt new ideas from mass media information sources)

and to groups whose goals are the same as those of the intervention plan (Eng, Parker, and Harlan, 1997). Using a small group to initiate community-oriented change is illustrated in the Progress Notes in Table 15-9.

Lay advisors. **Lay advisors** are people who are influential in approving or vetoing new ideas and from whom others seek advice and information about new ideas (Eng, Parker, and Harlan, 1997; Eng and Smith, 1995). They often perform a similar function to that of early adopters. Lay advisors, or opinion leaders, can be identified by their agreement with community norms, heavy involvement in formal social groups, specific areas of skill and knowledge, and a slightly higher social status than their followers (Rogers, 1995).

Mass media. Both small interacting groups and lay advisors are particularly useful in instituting change among **late adopters,** those who are last to embrace change. However, groups dominated by early adopters and lay advisors can be reached through the mass media. **Mass media,** like newspapers, television, and radio, represent an impersonal and formal type of communication and are useful in providing information quickly to a large number of people. Using the mass media is efficient because the proportion of resources spent to population covered is low and populations can be targeted. For example, information about teenage pregnancy can be efficiently provided through rock music stations.

In addition to being efficient, the mass media are effective aids in intervention. The Stanford Five-City-Project used mass media as a major portion of the project's education intervention, and recent risk-factor scores for cardiovascular disease have improved as a result (Winkleby, Flora, and Kraemer, 1994).

Health policy. Health policy also can play a critical part in the adoption of healthful community-oriented change (Dever, 1997). The major intent of public policy in the health field is to address collective human needs, and it often serves to limit individual choice for the public good. For instance, drivers have been urged for several years to wear automobile seat belts. However, the incidence of automobile fatalities was not reduced until drivers were required to observe lowered speed limits and, in some states, to wear seat belts and use special restraining seats for children. Obviously health policy can help encourage interventions that promote community health.

If public policy that will encourage or even simply allow health-generating choices is to become law, the nurse must actively lobby for it. See Chapter 9 for a more indepth discussion.

The nurse also must use small groups, lay advisors, and the mass media as aids to getting started. Working with naturally occurring small groups like the family and with lay advisors is familiar to most community-oriented nurses. Working with legislators and the mass media is less familiar, yet all resources must be used to achieve healthful change in the community client.

TABLE 15-9 Progress Notes: Infant Malnutrition

NAME OF COMMUNITY: JEFFERSON COUNTY
GOAL: TO REDUCE THE INCIDENCE AND PREVALENCE OF INFANT MALNUTRITION

DATE	NARRATIVE, ASSESSMENT, PLAN (NAP)*	BUDGET, TIME
2-14-98	**Objective 1, Means 4** *Narrative:* Meeting to develop needs assessment was attended by CN, two WIC personnel, and physicians from health department, neighborhood health center, and local medical society. Consensus rapidly achieved among 5 of 6 participants that goal, objectives, and means (especially Objective 1, Means 4) were appropriate. Physician representing medical society consistently objected, stating vehemently that private sector had long provided adequate medical care for area youngsters. Physician would not recommend that medical society support the effort. CN afraid that this would jeopardize entire effort. Eventually, however, physician left and plans were made to develop and conduct needs assessment and to continue seeking medical society's help. *Agenda:* CN to develop needs assessment tool with WIC personnel and health systems agency planner. Physicians to develop list of providers to be contacted. Neighborhood health center physician to get a place on medical society agenda and attempt to clarify plans. WIC personnel to contact nonphysician health workers to introduce plan and develop provider list. *Assessment:* Plans made to proceed with needs assessment and partner support essential to accomplishment of objective. Group process problematic, and CN ineffective because of discomfort with conflict between physician and WIC staff member. *Plans:* Meeting scheduled for 2-28-98 to deal with agreed-on agenda. Before 2-28 meeting, CN will discuss ways to better handle conflict with consultation group, collaborate in drafting needs assessment, and telephone others to determine their progress. <div align="right">J. Goeppinger, RN, CN</div>	$200, 2 hours meeting and 2 hours of preparation time

*Record both objective and subjective data. Interpret these data in terms of whether the objectives were achieved and whether the intervenor activities used were effective. The plan is dependent on the assessment and may include both new or revised objectives and activities.

No matter what means are used, all efforts to start and maintain changes must be documented. Evaluation, the sixth phase of this process, is also important to determine and improve the ability of community-oriented nursing practice to produce the desired results. Evaluation also increases the knowledge base and improves the rate of success in competing for funds for needed programs to solve community problems.

Evaluating the Intervention for Community Health

Simply defined, **evaluation** is the appraisal of the effects of some organized activity or program. An example of evaluation research is provided in the Research Brief. Evaluation may involve the design and conduct of evaluation research, in which social science research methods are used to determine program effectiveness, efficiency, adequacy, appropriateness, and unintended consequences (Dever, 1997). Evaluation also may involve the more elementary process of assessing progress by contrasting the objectives and the results. This section deals with the basic approach of contrasting objectives and results.

Evaluation begins in the planning phase, when goals and measurable objectives are established and goal-attaining activities are identified. After implementing the intervention, only the accomplishment of objectives and the effects of intervention activities have to be assessed. The progress notes direct the nurse to perform such appraisals concurrently with implementation. In assessing the data recorded there, the nurse is requested to evaluate whether the objectives were met and whether the intervention activities used were effective.

The nurse also must decide whether the costs in money and time were worth the resulting benefits. This process is depicted in the progress notes. In Table 15-9 the nurse has noted progress toward the needs assessed and difficulties encountered in handling conflict among the group members.

Such an evaluation process is oriented to community health because the intervention goals and objectives come from the nurse's and the community's ideas about health. Simple as it appears, it is not without problems. The lack of a comparison community or even adequate baseline information casts doubts about the success or failure of the intervention. Nursing interventions also may have such widespread and therefore weak effects that often the crude statistical measures do not detect them. Models for the practitioner to use in determining cost-benefit and cost-effectiveness figures are complicated and therefore not commonplace. Finally, the lay role in evaluation has never been fully accepted. Professionals have adopted partnership in assessment and implementation more readily than in evaluation. The issue of who has the power to define, judge, and institute change in professional activities is by no means resolved. With evaluation the entire process is open to renegotiation to achieve community health (Fig. 15-2).

Role of outcomes in the evaluation phase

Students using the community-as-client process presented in this chapter must recognize that in a political climate where health resources are limited, the measurement of outcomes is a particularly important part of the evaluation process. This is one reason for placing emphasis on measurable objectives. The Pew Health Professions Commission (1995) reports the need for improving the health of the entire population and the need to focus on outcomes and evidence-based measures. Outcomes measures answer questions about results of the intervention. Dever (1997) emphasizes outcomes questions about appropriate and effective interventions such as: Was the appropriate intervention done ineffectively or effectively? Was an inappropriate intervention done ineffectively or effectively? To answer these and other outcomes questions, Dever emphasizes epidemiology and the correct use of rates and numbers as one means of evaluating intervention outcomes among defined communities. Often data collected over time can also pro-

RESEARCH *Brief*

The elderly are often seen as one group, but in reality, researchers divide them into three groups: the young old (65 to 74), middle old (75 to 84), and old old (85 and older). The purpose of this study was to look at the use of community-focused services among these three groups. Existing data from a regional Area Agency on Aging were used for data analysis. Chi-square statistics and regression analyses were conducted to examine the effects of demographic, socioeconomic, and health status variables on the usage of community-based services.

Overall, case management, congregate meals, home-delivered meals, recreation, and outreach were the most frequently used services. Service usage varied among groups. Differences existed among the young old, middle old, and old old in both the types and the number of services that were used. Study results support planning efforts to tailor community-focused services to specific elderly cohorts rather than treating the young old, middle old, and old old as a homogenous group requiring the same type and mix of services.

Wallace DC, Hirst PK: Community-based service use among the young, middle, and old old. *Public Health Nurs* 13(4):286, 1996.

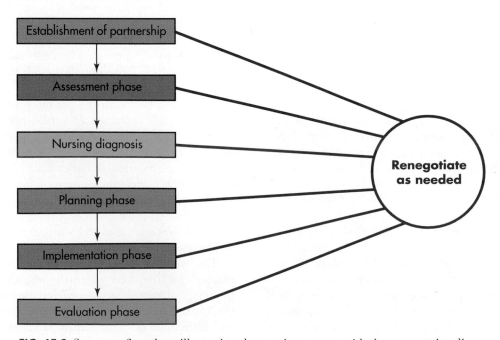

FIG. 15-2 Summary flow sheet illustrating the nursing process with the community client.

vide important outcomes information about health trends within the community. As indicated previously, epidemiological data and trends do not provide the only measure of success, but they do provide important information about the intervention. Nurses need to consider the collection of this type of outcome data for use as part of the evaluation phase.

PERSONAL SAFETY IN COMMUNITY PRACTICE

Personal safety is a prerequisite for effective community-oriented nursing practice, and it should be a consideration throughout the process. An awareness of the community and common sense are the two best guidelines for judgment. For example, common sense suggests not leaving anything valuable on a car seat or leaving your car unlocked. Similar guidelines apply to the use of public transportation. Calling ahead to schedule meetings will help prevent delays or confusion, and it gives the nurse an opportunity to lay the groundwork for the meeting. If there is no telephone or no access to a neighbor's telephone, plan to establish a time for any future meetings during the initial visit. Regardless of whether there has been telephone contact, there are rare situations when a meeting may be postponed because the nurse arrives at a location where people are unexpectedly hanging out by the entrance and the nurse has concerns about personal safety.

For nurses who are either just beginning their careers in community health or who are just starting a new position, there are three clear sources of information that will help answer any questions about personal safety:

1. *Other nurses, social workers, or health care providers who are familiar with the dynamics of a given community.* They can provide valuable insights into when to visit, how to get there, and what to expect because they function in the community themselves.
2. *Community members.* The best sources of information about the community are the community members themselves, and one benefit of developing an active partnership with community members is their willingness to share their insight about day to day community life.
3. *The nurse's own observations.* Knowledge gained during the data collection phase of the process should provide a solid basis for an awareness of day-to-day community activity. Nurses with experience practicing in the community generally agree that if they feel uncomfortable in a situation, they should trust their feelings and leave.

clinical application

Lily, a nurse in a small city, became aware of the increased incidence of respiratory diseases through contact with families in the community and the local chapter of the American Lung Association. During family visits, Lily noticed that many of the parents were smokers. Because most of the families Lily visited had small children, she became concerned about the effects of secondhand smoke on the health of the infants and children among her family caseload.

Further assessment of this community indicated that the community recognized several problems, including school safety and the risk of water pollution, in addition to the smoking problem that Lily had identified during her family visits. Talks with different community members revealed that they wanted each of these identified problems "fixed," although these same community members also remained uncertain of how to start. In deciding which of the three identified problems to address first, which criterion would be most important for Lily to consider:

A. The amount of money available
B. The level of community motivation to "fix" one of the three identified problems
C. The number of people in the community who expressed a concern about one of the three identified problems
D. How much control she would have in the process

Answer is found in the back of the book.

KEY POINTS

- Most definitions of community include three dimensions: (1) networks of interpersonal relationships that provide friendship and support to members; (2) residence in a common locality; and (3) "solidarity, sentiments, and activities."
- A community is defined as a locality-based entity, composed of systems of formal organizations reflecting societal institutions, informal groups, and aggregates that are interdependent and whose function or expressed intent is to meet a wide variety of collective needs.
- A community practice setting is insufficient reason for saying that practice is oriented toward the community client. When the location of the practice is in the community but the focus of the practice is the individual or family, then the nursing client remains the individual or family, not the whole community.
- Community-oriented practice is targeted to the community, the population group in which healthful change is sought.
- Community health as used in this chapter is defined as the meeting of collective needs through identifying problems and managing interactions within the community itself and between the community and the larger society.
- Most changes aimed at improving community health involve, of necessity, partnerships among community residents and health workers from a variety of disciplines.
- Assessing community health requires gathering existing data, generating missing data, and interpreting the database.
- Five methods of collecting data useful to the nurse are informant interviews, participant observation, secondary analysis of existing data, surveys, and windshield surveys.
- Gaining entry or acceptance into the community is perhaps the biggest challenge in assessment.

Continued

KEY POINTS—cont'd

- The nurse is usually an outsider and often represents an established health care system that is neither known nor trusted by community members, who may react with indifference or even active hostility.
- The planning phase includes analyzing and establishing priorities among community health problems already identified, establishing goals and objectives, and identifying intervention activities that will accomplish the objectives.
- Once high-priority problems are identified, broad relevant goals and objectives are developed.
- The goal, generally a broad statement of desired outcome, and objectives, the precise statements of the desired outcome, are carefully selected.
- Intervention activities, the means by which objectives are met, are the strategies that clarify what must be done to achieve the objectives, the ways change will be affected, and the way the problem will be interpreted.
- Implementation, the third phase of the nursing process, is transforming a plan for improved community health into achievement of goals and objectives.
- Simply defined, evaluation is the appraisal of the effects of some organized activity or program.

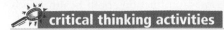

critical thinking activities

1. Observe an occupational health nurse, community or public health nurse, school nurse, family nurse practitioner, or emergency department nurse for several hours. Determine which of the nurse's activities are community oriented, and state the reasons for your judgement.
2. Using your own community as a frame of reference, develop examples illustrating the concepts of *community, community client, community health,* and *partnership for health.*
3. Read your local newspaper and identify articles illustrating the concepts of *community, community client, community health,* and *partnership for health.*
4. Using any two of the conditions of community competence given in the chapter, analyze your own community briefly. Give examples of each condition.

Bibliography

Abraham T, Fallon PJ: Caring for the community: development of the advanced practice nurse role, *Clinical Nurse Specialist* 11(5):224, 1997.

Aguirre-Molina M, Parra PA: Latino youth and families as active participants in planning change: a community-university partnership. In Zambrana RE, editor: *Understanding Latino families: scholarship, policy, and practice,* Thousand Oaks, Calif, 1995, Sage.

Anderson ET, McFarlane J: *Community-as-partner: theory and practice in nursing,* Philadelphia, 1995, J.B. Lippincott.

American Public Health Association, Public Health Nursing Section: *The definition and role of public health nursing,* Washington, DC, 1996, APHA.

American Public Health Association: *Community strategies for health: fitting in the pieces,* Washington, DC, 1994, the Association.

American Public Health Association Model Standards: *The guide to implementing model standards: eleven steps toward a healthy community,* Washington, DC, 1993, the Association.

Baker EA et al: The Latino Health Advocacy Program: a collaborative lay health advisor approach, *Health Educ Behav* 24(4):495, 1997.

Bechtel GA, Garrett C, Grover S: Developing a collaborative community partnership program in medical asepsis with tattoo studios, *Public Health Nurs,* 12(5):348, 1995.

Blum HL: *Planning for health,* New York, 1974, Human Sciences Press.

Bolton LB, Georges CA: National Black Nurses Association community collaboration model, *J Natl Black Nurses Assoc* 8(2):48, 1996.

Coakes SJ, Kelly GJ: Community competence and empowerment: strategies for rural change in women's health service planning and delivery, *Aust J Rural Health* 5(1):26, 1997.

Consensus set of health status indicators for the general assessment of community health status—United States, *MMWR Morb Mortal Wkly Rep* 40(27):449, 1991.

Cottrell LS: The competent community. In Kaplan BH, Wilson RN, Leighton AH, editors: *Further explorations in social psychiatry,* New York, 1976, Basic Books.

Courtney R: Community partnership primary care: a new paradigm for primary care, *Public Health Nurs,* 12(6):366, 1995.

Courtney R et al: The partnership model: working with individuals, families, and communities toward a new vision of health, *Public Health Nurs* 13(3):177, 1996.

Delbecq AL, Van de Ven AH: A group process model for problem identification and program planning, *J Appl Behav Sci* 62:467, 1971.

Dever GEA: *Community health analysis,* ed 2, Gaithersburg, Md, 1991, Aspen.

Dever GEA: *Improving outcomes in public health practice,* Gaithersburg, Md, 1997, Aspen.

Eng E, Parker E: Measuring community competence in the Mississippi Delta: the interface between program evaluation and empowerment: special issue: community empowerment, participatory education, and health: I, *Health Educ Q* 21(2):199, 1994.

Eng E, Parker EA, Harlan C: Lay health advisors: a critical link to community capacity building, *Health Educ Behav* 24(4):413, 1997.

Eng E, Salmon ME, Mullan F: Community empowerment: the critical base for primary health care, *Fam Community Health* 15(1):1, 1992.

Eng E, Smith J: Natural helping functions of lay health advisors in breast cancer education, *Breast Cancer Res Treat* 35(1):23, 1995.

Feuerstein MT: Participatory evaluation: an appropriate technology for community health programmes, *Contact* 55:1, 1980.

Flick LH, Reese C, Harris A: Aggregate/community-centered undergraduate community health nursing clinical experience, *Public Health Nurs* 13(1):36, 1996.

Flynn BC: Partnerships in healthy cities and communities: a social commitment for advanced practice nurses, *Adv Pract Nurs Q* 2(4):1, 1997.

Freudenberg N et al: Strengthening individual and community capacity to prevent disease and promote health: in search of relevant theories and principles, *Health Educ Q* 22(3):290, 1995

Fuchs JA: Planning for community health promotion: a rural example, *Health Values* 12(6):3, 1988.

Gillis AJ: Allocation of healthcare resources: the case for health promotion, *Nurs Forum* 27(4):21, 1992.

Goeppinger J et al: An examination of the effective self-care education for persons with arthritis, *Arthritis Rheum* 32:464, 1989.

Goeppinger J, Lassiter PG, Wilcox B: Community health is community competence, *Nurs Outlook* 30(8):464, 1982

Goeppinger J et al: From research to practice: the effects of the jointly sponsored dissemination of an arthritis self-care nursing intervention, *Appl Nurs Res* 8(3):106, 1995.

Hatziandreu EJ et al: The cost effectiveness of three programs to increase use of bicycle helmets among children, *Public Health Reports* 110(3):251, 1995.

Hemstrom MM: Application as scholarship: a community client experience, *Public Health Nurs* 12(5):279, 1995.

Hettinger BJ, Brazile RP: A database design for community health data, *Comput Nurs* 10(3):109, 1992.

Hildebrandt E: Building community participation in health care: a model and example from South Africa, *Image J Nurs Sch* 28(2):155, 1996.

Howell EM et al: Back to the future: community involvement in the Healthy Start Program, *J Health Polit Policy Law* 23(2):291, 1998.

Hutsell CA et al: Creating an effective infrastructure within a state health department for community health promotion: the Indiana PATCH experience, *J Health Educ* 23(3):164, 1992.

Jackson EJ, Parks CP: Recruitment and training issues from selected lay health advisor programs among African Americans: a 20-year perspective, *Health Educ Behav* 24(4):418, 1997.

Jones ME, Clark DW: Nurse practitioners develop leadership in community problem-solving, *J Am Acad Nurs Pract* 2(4):160, 1990.

Kreuter MW: PATCH: its origin, basic concepts, and links to contemporary public health policy, *J Health Educ* 23(3):135, 1992.

Kristjanson L, Chalmers K: Nurse-client interactions in community-based practice: creating common ground, *Public Health Nurs* 7(4):215, 1990.

Kroeger A et al: Operational aspects of bed-net impregnation for community-based malaria control in Nicaragua, Ecuador, Peru, and Columbia, *Trop Med Int Health* 2(6):589, 1997.

Kyba F, Hathaway W, Okimi P: Health promotion in a museum: a collaborative community partnership, *Nurse Educator* 22(4):32, 1997.

Ludwig-Beymer P et al: Community assessment in a suburban Hispanic community: a description of method, *J Transcult Nurs* 8(1):19, 1996.

MacLachlan M: Identifying problems in community health promotion: an illustration of the Nominal Group Technique in AIDS education, *J R Soc Health* 116(3):143, 1996.

McClowry SG et al: A comprehensive school-based clinic: university and community partnership, *J Soc Pediatr Nurses* 1(1):19, 1996.

McDonald A, Chavasse J: Community care: community participation within an Irish Health Board area, *Br J Nurs* 6(6):341, 1997.

Millar AB, Grucnewald PJ: Use of spatial models for community program evaluation of changes in alcohol outlet distribution, *Addiction* 92, Suppl-83, 1997.

Muecke MA: Community health diagnosis in nursing, *Public Health Nurs* 1(1):23, 1984.

National Center for Health Statistics: *Healthy People 2000 review, 1995-96,* Hyattsville, Md, 1996, Public Health Service.

Parker EA et al: Detroit's East Side Village Health Worker Partnership: community-based lay health advisor intervention in an urban area, *Health Educ Behav* 25(1):24, 1998.

Pew Health Professions Commission: *Critical challenges: revitalizing the health professions for the twenty-first century,* San Francisco, 1995, University of California: San Francisco Center for the Health Professions

Redman S et al: Consulting about priorities for the NHMRC National Breast Cancer Centre: how good is the nomial group technique, *Aust N Z J Public Health* 21(3):250, 1997.

Rivera SJ, Palmer-Willis H: County nursing service assessment tool: an overview, *Public Health Nurs* 8(4):264, 1991.

Rogers E: *Diffusion of innovations,* ed 4, New York, 1995, Free Press.

Russell K: Strengthening Black and minority community coalitions for health policy action, *J Natl Black Nurs Assoc* 6(1):42, 1992.

Ryan W: *Blaming the victim,* New York, 1976, Vintage Books.

Schulz AJ et al: "It's a 24-hour thing . . . a living-for-each-other concept": identity, networks, and community in an urban village health worker project, *Health Educ Behav* 24(4):465, 1997.

Shiell A, Hawe P: Health promotion community development and the tyranny of individualism, *Health Econ* 5(3):241, 1996.

Stanhope M, Knollmueller R: *Handbook of community-based and home health nursing practice,* ed 3, St. Louis, 2000, Mosby.

Urrutia-Rojas X, Aday LA: A framework for community assessment: designing and conducting a survey in a Hispanic immigrant and refugee community, *Public Health Nurs* 8(1):20, 1991.

US Department of Health and Human Services: *Healthy People 2000: national health promotion and disease preventive objectives,* Washington, DC, 1991, USDHHS, Public Health Service.

Wickizer TM et al: Activating communities for health promotion: a process evaluation method, *Am J Public Health* 83(4):561, 1983.

Williams C: Community-oriented population-focused practice: the foundation of specialization in public health nursing. In Stanhope M, Lancaster J, editors: *Community health nursing,* ed 5, St Louis, 2000, Mosby.

Winkleby MA, Flora JA, Kraemer HC: A community-based heart disease intervention: predictors of change, *Am J Public Health* 84(5):767, 1994.

World Health Organization: Community health nursing: report of a WHO expert committee, *Tech Rep Series* No 558, Geneva, 1974, WHO.

Community and Public Health Nursing in Rural Environments

ANGELINE BUSHY

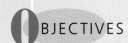

www.mosby.com/MERLIN/community_stanhope

OBJECTIVES

After reading this chapter, the student should be able to do the following:

- Compare and contrast definitions of *rural* as opposed to *urban.*
- Describe residency as a continuum, ranging from farm residency to core inner city.
- Compare and contrast the health status of rural and urban populations on select health measures.
- Analyze barriers to care in health professional shortage areas and for underserved populations.

- Evaluate issues related to delivery of services for rural underserved populations.
- Describe characteristics of rural and small-town residency.
- Examine the role and scope of community and public health nursing practice in rural and underserved areas.
- Evaluate two professional-client-community partnership models that can effectively provide a continuum of care to residents living in an environment with sparse resources.

KEY TERMS

core metropolitan
farm residency
frontier

health professional shortage area (HPSA)
medically underserved

nonfarm residency
rural
rural-urban continuum

suburbs
urban
See Glossary for definitions

CHAPTER OUTLINE

ccess to health care is a national priority, especially in regions with an insufficient number of health care providers. Recruiting and retaining qualified health professionals in underserved communities, particularly the inner city and rural areas of the United States, is difficult. Until recently, however, limited research has been undertaken on the special challenges, problems, and opportunities of nursing practice, especially nursing in rural settings. This chapter presents major issues surrounding health care delivery in rural environments that sometimes differs from that in urban or more populated settings. Common definitions are discussed for the term 'rural', its associated lifestyle, the health status of rural populations, barriers to obtaining a continuum of health care services, and nursing practice issues. Strategies are discussed to help nurses deliver more effective community-oriented services to clients who live in isolated environments with sparse resources. This chapter describes rural nursing practice and can be used by students, nurses who practice in rural health departments, and those who work in agencies located in urban areas that offer outreach services to rural populations in their catchment area.

HISTORICAL OVERVIEW

Formal rural nursing originated with the Red Cross Rural Nursing Service, which was organized in November, 1912. The Committee on Rural Nursing was under the direction of Mabel Boardman (chair), Jane Delano (vice chair), and Annie Goodrich along with other Red Cross leaders and philanthropists (Bigbee and Crowder, 1985). Before, care of the sick in a small community was provided by informal social support systems. When self-care and family care were not effective in bringing about healing, this task was assigned to healing women who lived in the community. Historically, the health needs of rural Americans have been numerous, and although not necessarily unique, they are different from those of urban populations. Consistent problems of maldistribution of health professionals, poverty, limited access to services, ignorance, and social neglect have plagued many rural communities for generations. Over the years, the history of the Red Cross Rural Nursing Services shows a consistent movement away from its initial rural focus, as demonstrated by its frequent name changes. Unfortunately, as with the Rural Red Cross Service, concern for rural health is often temporary and replaced by other areas of greater need (Bigbee and Crowder, 1985). Hopefully health care reform initiatives will soon focus on assuring access to care for rural and urban residents.

DEFINITION OF TERMS
Rurality: A Subjective Concept

Everyone has an idea as to what constitutes rural as opposed to urban residence. However, the two cannot be viewed as two opposing entities. Moreover, with the increased degree of urban influence on rural communities

the differences no longer are as distinct as they may have been even a decade ago (Baer, Johnson, and Gessler, 1997; U.S. Census Bureau, 1998; Cromartie and Swanson, 1995; Gahr, 1993; Gesler, 1997; Gesler and Ricketts, 1992; Hewitt, 1992; Weinert and Boik, 1994). In general, **rural** is defined in terms of the geographic location and population density, or it may be described in terms of the distance from (e.g., 20 miles) or the time (e.g. , 30 minutes) needed to commute to an urban center. Other definitions equate rural with **farm residency** and **urban** with **non-farm residency**. Some consider "rural" to be a state of mind. For the more affluent, rural may bring to mind a recreational, retirement, or resort community located in the mountains or in lake country where one can relax and participate in outdoor activities, such as skiing, fishing, hiking, or hunting. For the less affluent, the term can impose grim scenes. For example, some people may think of an impoverished Indian reservation that is comparable with an underdeveloped country, or it may bring to mind images of a migrant labor camp with several families living in a one-room shanty with no access to safe drinking water or adequate sanitation.

Just as each city has its own unique features, it is also difficult to describe a "typical rural town" because of the wide population and geographic diversity. For example, rural towns in Florida, Oregon, Alaska, Hawaii, and Idaho are different from one another, and quite different from those in Vermont, Texas, Tennessee, Alabama, or California. Furthermore, there can be vast differences among rural areas within one state. Still, descriptions and definitions for rural tend to be more subjective and relative in nature than for urban.

For instance, "small" communities with populations of more than 20,000 have some features that one may expect to find in a city. Then again, residents who live in a community with a population of less than 2000 may consider a community with a population of 5000 to 10,000 to be a city. Although some communities may seem geographically remote on a map, the residents who live there may not feel isolated. Those residents believe they are within easy reach of services through telecommunication and dependable transportation, although extensive shopping facilities may be 50 to 100 miles from the family home, obstetric care may be 150 miles away or nursing services in the district health department in an adjacent county may be 75 or more miles away.

Rural-Urban Continuum

Frequently used definitions to describe and differentiate rural from urban are provided by several federal agencies (Box 16-1) (Braden and Beauregard, 1994; U.S. Census Bureau, 1998; USDC, 1996; USDA, 1995; 1997; USOTA, 1992). These definitions, which in many cases are dichotomous in nature, fail to take into account the relative nature of ruralness. Rural versus urban residency is not an opposing lifestyle. Rather, rural-urban residency must be seen as a

rural-urban continuum ranging from living on a remote farm, to a village or small town, to a larger town or city, to a large metropolitan area with a "core inner city" (Fig. 16-1).

Furthermore, since 1991 there has been a significant population shift in the United States. The fastest growing rural counties are located in rural regions of the nation and along the far edges of larger metropolitan counties. Demographers metaphorically refer to this demographic phenomenon as the "doughnut effect." That is to say, people are moving away from highly populated areas to far-flung **suburbs** of urban centers. Most of the population growth has been in counties with a booming economy, room to grow, and in western and southern states. Since 1990, the U.S. population has increased 0.9% overall. Despite glimmers of an urban renaissance, suburbs that are closer to the metroplitan area grew 1.2% compared with outer and more rural suburbs with a 2.6% increase in population. More specifically, from 1996 to 1997, of the fastest growing counties with 10,000 persons or more, four were located in western states, five in southern states, and one in a midwestern state (Bowers and Cook, 1997; Johnson, 1996; Johnson-Webb, Baer, and Gesler, 1997; Lee, 1991; Nasser, 1998a, 1998b; Woodyard, 1997).

Obviously, population shifts of this nature and size also affect the health status and lifestyle preferences of these communities. As beliefs and values change over time, urban-rural differences narrow in some aspects and enlarge in others. Depending on the definition that is used, the actual rural population might vary slightly. Generally, about 25% of all U.S. residents live in rural settings. For this chapter, rural refers to areas having fewer than 99 persons per square mile and communities having 20,000 or fewer inhabitants.

CURRENT PERSPECTIVES
Population Characteristics

Adding to the confusion about what constitutes rural versus urban residency are the special needs of the numerous underrepresented groups (minorities, subgroups) who reside in the United States. In general, there is a higher proportion of Caucasians in rural areas (about 82%) than in **core metropolitan** areas (about 62%). There are, however, regional variations, and some rural counties have a significant number of minorities. Of the total rural population, nearly 4 million are African-American, almost 2 million are Native American, 34 million are Asian-Pacific Islanders, and 75 million are of other races (U.S. Census Bureau,

---

BOX 16-1 Terms and Definitions

Core Metropolitan: Densely populated counties with more than 1 million inhabitants.

Frontier: Regions having fewer than six persons per square mile.

Farm Residency: Residency outside area zoned as "city limits"; usually infers involvement in agriculture.

Nonfarm Residency: Residence within area zoned as "city limits."

Nonmetropolitan Statistical Area (non-SMSA): Counties that do not meet SMSA criteria.

Other Metropolitan: Fringe counties of core metropolitan; all other metropolitan.

Rural Areas: Communities having less than 20,000 residents or fewer than 99 persons per square mile.

Standard Metropolitan Statistical Area (SMSA): Region with a central city of at least 50,000 residents.

Suburban: Area adjacent to a highly populated city.

Urban Areas: Geographic areas described as nonrural and having a higher population density; more than 99 persons per square mile; cities with a population of at least 20,000 but less than 50,000.

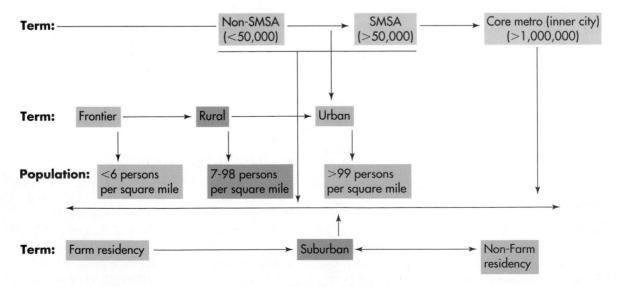

FIG. 16-1 The continuum of rural-urban residency.

1998; NRHA, 1994a; 1994b; 1997a; 1997b). Little is documented on the needs and health status of special rural populations. Anthropologists are quick to report that, within a group, there often exists a wide range of lifestyles. Consequently, even in the smallest or most remote town or village, a subgroup may behave differently and have different values regarding health, illness, and patterns of accessing health care. Their lifestyle too may be associated with health problems that are different from the predominant cultural group within a given community. Background information on those particular populations can be found in other chapters of this text. Table 16-1 presents demographic data comparing rural and urban population.

Demographically, rural communities are described as "bipolar" in age distribution because they have a higher-than-average number of younger and older residents. In other words, one finds a higher proportion of persons between 6 and 17 years of age and over 65 years of age living in rural compared with urban areas. Persons 18 years of age and over living in rural areas are more likely to be, or to have been, married than adults in the three urban categories. As a group, rural people also are more likely to be widowed. As for level of education, adults in rural areas have fewer years of formal schooling than do urban adults.

Rural families tend to be poorer than their urban counterparts. Comparing annual incomes with the standardized index established by the U.S. Census Bureau, more than one-fourth of rural Americans live in or near poverty and nearly 40% of all rural children are impoverished (The 1998 HHS Poverty Guidelines, 1998; Packard Foundation, 1997a, 1997b). Compared with those in metropolitan settings, a substantially smaller percentage of families living in rural and nonmetropolitan areas are at the high end of the income scale. Accompanying the recent population shifts from urban to formerly rural areas, average income level may also be changing; however, no data are available at this time. Regardless, level of income is a critical factor in whether a family has health insurance or qualifies for public insurance. Hence rural families are less likely to have private insurance and more likely to have public insurance or to be uninsured.

The working poor, of which there are many in rural areas, are particularly at risk for being underinsured or uninsured (HRSA, 1997; Mueller et al, 1995; Mueller, Patil, and Boilesen, 1995; NRHA, 1997a, 1998a). In working poor families, one or more of the adults is employed but still cannot afford private health insurance. Furthermore,

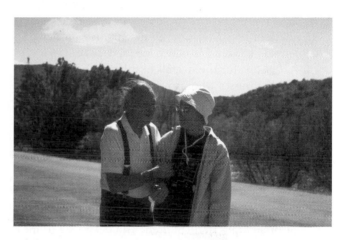

A higher proportion of elderly people live in rural areas compared with urban areas.

TABLE 16-1 Selected Population Characteristics by Place of Residence

	CORE METRO (%)	OTHER METRO (%)	URBAN NONMETRO (%)	RURAL (%)
AGE (YR)				
6-17	15.2	17.3	—	20
25-54	43.3	42.0	40.8	38.3
65	12.0	—	10.0	17.3
MARITAL STATUS (OVER 17 YEARS OF AGE)				
Never married	26.5	21.0	19.3	16.5
Were married	52.7	60.5	61.0	64.6
EDUCATION (YR)				
<12	25.0	25.0	40.0	36.0
>12	40.0	40.0	30.0	24.0
POVERTY RATE				
Below indices	19.0	15.0	22.0	26.0

Data from US Department of Commerce: *Statistical abstract of the United States*, Washington, DC, 1996, U.S. Census Bureau; US Department of Agriculture: *Agriculture fact book*, Washington, DC, 1997, USDA Office of Communications; The 1998 HHS Poverty Guidelines, *Federal Register* 63(36):9235, February 24, 1998.

their annual income is such that it disqualifies the family from obtaining public insurance. A number of reasons are cited to explain why this phenomenon occurs more often in rural settings. For instance, several individuals are self-employed in a family business, such as ranching or farming, or they work in small enterprises, such as a service station, restaurant, or grocery store. Also, an individual may be employed in part-time or seasonal occupations, such as farm laborer and construction in which health insurance often is not an employee benefit. In other situations, a family member may have a preexisting health condition that makes the cost of insurance prohibitive, if it is even available to them.

A few rural families "fall through the cracks" and are unable to access any type of public assistance because of other deterrents. For example, language barriers, being physically compromised, the geographic location of an agency, lack of transportation, or having the status of "undocumented" worker. Insurance, or the lack of it, has serious implications for the overall health status of rural residents and the nurses who provide services to them.

Health Status of Rural Residents

Even though rural communities constitute about one-fourth of the total population, the health problems or the health behaviors of those residents are not fully understood. Even less is known about former urban residents who recently relocated to rural regions. This section, however, summarizes what is known about the overall health status of rural adults and children. The health status measures that are addressed in this section are perceived health status, diagnosed chronic conditions, physical limitations, frequency of seeking medical treatment, usual source of care, maternal-infant health, children's health, mental health, minorities' health, and environmental and occupational health risks (Braden and Beauregard, 1994; Gesler and Ricketts, 1992).

: DID YOU KNOW? *Compared with urban Americans, rural residents have the following:*
- *Higher infant and maternal morbidity rates*
- *Higher rates of chronic illness, including hypertension, cardiovascular disease, cancer, and diabetes*
- *Unique health risks associated with occupations and the environment, such as machinery accidents, skin cancer from sun exposure, and respiratory problems associated with exposure to chemicals and pesticides*
- *Stress-related health problems and mental illness, but the incidence of those conditions is not known*

Perceived health status

In general, rural populations have a poorer perception of their overall health and functional status than their urban counterparts. Specifically, rural residents over 18 years of age assess their health status less favorably than do urban residents. Studies show that rural adults are less likely

to engage in preventive behavior, which increases their exposure to risk. Specifically they are less likely to wear seat belts, have regular blood pressure checks, have Pap smears, and complete self-breast examinations. Ultimately, failure to participate in these lifestyle behaviors affects overall health status of rural residents, their level of function, physical limitations, degree of mobility, and level of self-care activities (Lee, 1998; Long and Weinert, 1989, 1992; Sternbert, 1997; Weinert and Long, 1991, 1993).

Chronic illness

Compared with their urban counterparts, rural adults are more likely to have one or more of the following chronic conditions: hypertension, arthritis/rheumatism, diabetes, cardiovascular disease, or cancer. Nearly half of all rural adults have been diagnosed with at least one of these chronic conditions compared with about a quarter of nonrural adults. More specifically, the prevalence rate of diagnosed diabetes in rural adults is about 7 out of 100 as opposed to 5 out of 100 in nonrural environments. More rural adults have cancer (almost 7%) compared with urban adults (about 5%). Although most AIDS cases still are found in urban areas, the rate is increasing in rural areas (NRHA, 1998b).

: DID YOU KNOW?
- *The AIDS rates are increasing more quickly in rural areas (30%) than in metropolitan areas (25.8%). Rural populations (fewer than 50,000) have the highest rates of increase in AIDS cases, representing 6.7% of all cases in the United States, with heterosexual contact accounting for most cases in many areas (NRHA, 1998a, 1998b)*
- *In rural areas, gay men often are not openly gay and tend to engage in unprotected sex with strangers.*
- *Homophobia, racism, sexism, and AIDS stigma make HIV prevention efforts nearly impossible in some rural areas.*
- *Migration of people from urban to rural areas is cited as one possible contributor to the increased rates in rural areas. Among HIV-infected persons, more interstate than intrastate migration takes place from time of diagnosis until death.*

A higher percentage of rural adults receive medical treatment for both life-threatening illness and degenerative or chronic conditions than do urban adults. Life-threatening conditions include malignant neoplasms, heart disease, cardiovascular problems, and liver disorders. Degenerative or chronic diseases include diabetes, kidney disease, arthritis and rheumatism, and chronic diseases of the circulatory, nervous, respiratory, and digestive systems. In essence, chronic health conditions, coupled with their poor health status, limit the physical activities of a larger proportion of rural residents compared with their urban counterparts (ANA, 1996; Brooks, 1998; Bushy, 1998b; Edelman and Menz, 1996; USDHHS, 1994b; USOTA, 1992; Yawn, 1994).

Physical limitations

Limitations in mobility and self-care are strong indicators of an individual's overall health status. Specifically assessed measures on a national health survey included walking one block, walking uphill or climbing stairs, bending, lifting, stooping, feeding, dressing, bathing, or toileting. More rural adults (9%) experience at least three of these limitations compared with metropolitan adults (6%). The increased prevalence of poor health status and impaired function is not necessarily due to the increased number of older adults found in rural areas. Similar patterns are evident in adults 18 to 64 years of age. Rural adults under 65 years of age are more likely than urban adults to assess their health status as fair to poor, and a greater percentage have been diagnosed with a chronic health condition.

Based on data from national health surveys, the overall health status of rural adults leaves much to be desired. This is attributed to a number of factors, including impaired access to health care providers and services coupled with other rural factors. Hence nurses in rural practice settings play an important role in providing a continuum of care to clients living in these underserved areas. Specifically, nurses can help clients have healthier lives by teaching them how to prevent accidents, engage in more healthful lifestyle behaviors, and reduce the risk of chronic health problems. Once diagnosed with a long-term problem, nurses can help clients in rural environments manage chronic conditions to achieve better health outcomes and functioning.

Patterns of health service use

In measuring the use of health care services, more than three-fourths of adults in rural areas received medical care on at least one occasion during a year. Table 16-2 summarizes the frequency of visits to ambulatory care settings by rural and metropolitan residents (Braden and Beauregard, 1994). Despite their overall poorer health status and higher incidence of chronic health conditions, rural adults seek medical care less often than urban adults. In part this discrepancy can be attributed to scarce resources and lack of providers in rural areas. Other reasons for this phenomenon are discussed in a subsequent part of this chapter focusing on barriers to accessing health care.

> **NURSING TIP**
>
> Nurses must be especially thorough in their health assessment of rural clients who may not receive regular care for chronic health conditions

Availability and access of health care

The ability of a person to identify a usual source of care is considered a favorable indicator of access to health care and a person's overall health status. In essence, a person who has a usual source of care is more likely to seek care when ill and is more compliant with prescribed regimens. Having the same provider of care can enhance continuity of care, as well as a client's perceived perception of the

TABLE 16-2 Annual Number of Visits Per Person to an Ambulatory Care Setting by Place of Residence

PLACE OF RESIDENCE	NUMBER OF VISITS
UNINSURED/PUBLIC COVERAGE	
Rural/nonmetropolitan	7.5 visits
All metropolitan	7.5 visits
PRIVATE INSURANCE	
Rural/nonmetropolitan	6.3 visits
All metropolitan	7.4 visits
NUMBER OF VISITS BY PLACE OF RESIDENCE	
Rural	9.5 visits
Urban nonmetropolitan	10.4 visits
Core metropolitan	12.1 visits
Other metropolitan	10.9 visits

From Braden J, Beauregard K: *National medical expenditure survey-health status and access to care of rural and urban populations,* Research Findings 18, Rockville, Md, 1994, Agency for Health Care Policy and Research, Public Health Service (Pub No 94-0031).

quality of that care. Rural adults (85%) are more likely than urban adults (78%) to identify a particular medical provider as their usual source of care. As for the type of provider who delivers the care, general practitioners and advanced practice registered nurses (APRNs) usually are seen by rural adults, whereas urban adults are more likely to seek care from a medical specialist. However, this trend may be changing as managed care expands. Managed care advocates primary care providers serving as gate keepers and limits consumers' access to specialists (Aitkin, VanArsdale, and Barry, 1990; Christianson and Moscovice, 1993; Conway-Welch, 1991; Minnesota Center for Rural Health, 1996; RICHS, 1994; Schoenman, 1998).

Another measure of access to care is traveling time and/or distance to ambulatory care services. Rural persons who seek ambulatory care are more likely to travel more than 30 minutes to reach their usual source of care. Extended commuting time also may be a factor for residents in highly populated urban areas and those who must rely on public transportation. Upon arriving at the clinic or doctor's office, however, no differences have been found in the waiting time to see the provider between rural and urban residents.

Measure of usual place and usual provider suggests that rural residents are at least as well off as urban residents in regard to access to care. However, caution must be used when making this generalization because 1 out of 17 rural counties is reported to have no physician. Among rural respondents on national surveys the ability to identify a usual site of care or a particular provider often stems from a community or county having only one, perhaps two, health care providers. The limited number of health care facilities is reinforced by the finding that nearly all rural residents (95%) who seek health care use ambulatory services that are provided in a doctor's office as opposed to a clinic, community health center, hospital outpatient department, or emergency department (BPHC, 1997; NRHA, 1998a; ORHP, 1994; Pearson, 1997; RWJF, 1997; USDHHS, 1994a, 1994b).

It is not unusual for rural professionals to live and practice in a particular community for decades. Moreover, in a **Health Professional Shortage Area (HPSA),** a doctor, a nurse practitioner, or a nurse often provides services to residents who live in several counties. In the case of community and public health nursing, one or two nurses in a county health department usually offer a full range of services for all residents in a catchment area, which may span more than 100 miles from one end of a county to the other. Consequently, rural physicians and nurses frequently report, "I provide care to individuals and families with all kinds of conditions, in all stages of life, and across several generations." In turn, it should not come as a surprise that rural respondents who participate in national surveys are able to identify a usual source and usual provider of health care.

Maternal-infant health

There are conflicting reports in the literature regarding pregnancy outcomes in rural areas. Overall, rural populations have higher infant and maternal morbidity rates, especially counties designated as HPSAs, which often have a high proportion of racial minorities (Table 16-3). Here one also finds fewer specialists, such as pediatricians, obstetricians, and gynecologists, to provide care to at-risk populations.

There are extreme variations in pregnancy outcomes from one part of the country to another, even within states. For instance, in several counties located in the north central and intermountain states, the pregnancy outcome is among the finest in the United States. However, in several other counties within those same states, the pregnancy outcome is among the worst. Particularly at risk are women who live on or near Indian reservations, women who are migrant workers, and women who are of African-American descent and live in rural counties of states located in the deep south (Bushy, 1998a; Clark et al, 1995; NRHA, 1994a, 1994b, 1997a, 1998).

Most nurses understand the effects of socioeconomic factors on pregnancy outcomes, such as income level (poverty), education level, age, employment/unemployment patterns, and use of prenatal services. There are other less well-known determinants, such as environmental hazards, occupational risks, and the cultural meaning placed on childbearing and child rearing practices by a community. The effects of these multifaceted factors vary.

Health of children

Reports on the health status of rural children show regional variations and conflicting data. Comparing rural with urban children under 6 years of age on the measures of access to providers and use of services reveals the following (Packard Foundation, 1997a, 1997b):

- Urban children are less likely to have a usual provider but are more likely to see a pediatrician when they are ill.
- Similar to rural adults, rural children also are more likely to have care from a general practitioner who is identified as their usual care giver.

School nurses are an important factor in the overall health status of children in the United States. The availability of school nurses in rural communities also varies from region to region. More specifically, in **frontier** and rural areas of the United States, school nurses usually are scarce. In part, this deficit can be attributed to limited resources associated with low tax revenues and shortages of health personnel in those counties. In other words, there are fewer tax payers living in those large geographic areas. Some frontier areas have fewer than four persons per square mile and a few have less than two persons per square mile.

TABLE 16-3 Residency and Rate of Infant Mortality and Low Birth Weight (per 1000 population)			
	NATIONAL AVERAGE	NON-HPSA	HPSA
Infant mortality rate	10.4	9.1	12.6
Low birth weight	6.8	5.8	8.3

From Braden J, Beauregard K. *National medical expenditure survey-health status and access to care of rural and urban populations,* Research Findings 18, Rockville, Md, 1994, Agency for Health Care Policy and Research, Public Health Service (Pub No 94-0031).

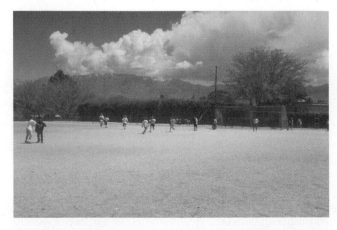

Schools in rural areas do not always have a full-time school nurse. Children living in rural areas do not usually have as much access to health care providers as children living in urban areas.

Consequently, rural county commissioners, like their urban counterparts, are forced to prioritize the allocation of scarce resources among such services as maintaining public utilities, roads, bridges, and schools; supporting a financially suffering county hospital; hiring a county health nurse; and offering school health services. In rural communities there are fewer resources overall, and certain public services must be provided to local residents.

Obviously, creativity is required by both community residents and local health care providers to resolve health care and school nursing needs. Partnership arrangements, for example, have been negotiated by two or more counties that agree to share the cost of a "district" health nurse. Other county commissioners have forged partnerships with an agency in an urban setting and contracted for specific health care services. In both of these situations, it is not unusual for the nurse to provide services to all children attending schools in the participating counties. In some frontier states, schools may be situated more than 100 miles apart and as many miles or more from the district health office. Because of the number of schools and distances between them, the county nurse may only be able to visit each school once, maybe twice, in a school term. Usually the nurse's visit is to update preschool immunizations and perhaps to teach maturation classes to students in the upper grades.

The health status of rural women, infants, and children is less than optimal. In part this can be attributed to inadequate preventive, primary, and emergency services to meet their particular health care needs. On one hand, scarce resources can pose a challenge to a nurse who provides care to rural residents, especially those in underserved areas. On the other hand, resource deficits encourage creativity, innovation, and an espoused characteristic of community and public health nursing in general and of rural nurses in particular.

Mental health

As with other dimensions of the health of rural populations, the facts about their mental health status also are ambiguous and conflicting. Stress, stress-related conditions, and mental illness are prevalent among populations when severe economic difficulties persist. The depressed agriculture, lumber, and mining industries during the 1980s resulted in numerous job losses in rural communities, hence the term *farm stress*. Economic recession also is a contributing factor to a family not having insurance or being underinsured. Interestingly, even if mental health services are available and accessible, rural residents delay seeking care when they have an emotional problem until there is an emergency or a crisis. This phenomenon is reflected in the lower number of annual visits for mental health services and chronic health problems by rural residents.

Mental health professionals who serve rural populations report a persistent, endemic level of depression among residents. They speculate that this condition is associated with the high rate of poverty, geographic isola-

tion, and an insufficient number of mental health services. Depression also may contribute to the escalating incidence of accidents and suicides, especially among rural male adolescents and young men. The incidents have increased dramatically over the last decade and continue to rise in this group, to the point of being epidemic in some small communities (Abraham et al, 1994; AP, 1998a; Human and Wasem, 1991; SAMHSA, 1997; USGAO, 1993). Hopefully the growing national economy of the last 2 or 3 years also is favorably affecting the health status of rural residents. The short- and long-term outcomes, however, remain to be seen.

Reports on the incidence in rural populations of domestic violence and alcohol and chemical substance use and abuse also are conflicting. These behaviors are less likely to be reported in areas where residents are related or personally acquainted. After a period of time, in small, tight-knit communities destructive coping behaviors often come to be accepted as "business as usual for this family." Family problems also may be ignored if formal social services and public health services are sparse or nonexistent and if the community does not trust the professionals who provide services within a local agency. In underserved rural areas there are gaps in the continuum of mental health services, which, ideally, should include preventive education, anticipatory guidance, early intervention programs, crisis and acute care services, and follow-up care. As with other aspects of health care, nurses in rural areas play an important role in community education, case finding, advocacy, and case management of client systems experiencing emotional problems and chronic mental health problems.

Health of Minorities

As mentioned previously, there is a significant number of at risk minority groups in rural America who have some rather unique concerns (in particular, children, the elderly, American Indians, Native Alaskans, Native Hawaiians, migrant workers, African-Americans, and the homeless) (AP, 1998a, 1998b; APHA, 1991, 1996; Brooks, 1998; Mueller et al, 1995; Mueller, Patil, and Boilesen, 1995; NRHA, 1997a; Strickland and Strickland, 1996) (Table 16-4). The rural homeless, for instance, may be seasonal farm workers or families from within a community who had their farm foreclosed. Sometimes the family may be allowed by law to continue living in the house on the farm that once was theirs. The family no longer has a means of livelihood and often remains hidden in the community with insufficient income to purchase food or other necessary services. The particular health problems of these at-risk groups are discussed in other chapters of this text. Nurses should be aware, however, that at-risk and underrepresented groups may experience some unique concerns related to the rural lifestyle, isolation, and sparse resources.

Environmental and occupational health risks

A community's primary industry is an influencing factor in the local lifestyle, the health status of its residents, and the number and types of health care services it may

TABLE 16-4 Health Care Needs and Required Nursing Skills of Special Rural Populations

POPULATION/COMMUNITY	NEEDS/SKILLS
Farmers/ranchers	Advanced life support for cardiac emergencies
	Emergency care for accident/trauma victims
	Environmental hazards
	Perinatal health care
	Farmer's lung
	Dermatitis
	Farm stress/depression
Native Americans	Diabetes
	Alcohol /substance abuse
	Cirrhosis of the liver
	Vehicular accidents
	Hypothermic injuries
	Trauma-related injuries
	Tuberculosis
	Sudden infant death syndrome (SIDS)
	Perinatal health care
African-Americans	Hypertension
	Cardiovascular disease
	Sickle cell anemia
	Perinatal health care
Migrant farm workers	Field sanitation
	Safe drinking water
	Exposure to pesticides, herbicides
	Infectious diseases (e.g., hepatitis, typhoid)
Native Alaskans	Exposure to petroleum by-products
	Toxic residue-contaminated seafood
	Diabetes
	Alcohol/substance abuse
	Cirrhosis of the liver
	Vehicular accidents
	Hypothermic injuries
	Trauma-related injuries
	Tuberculosis
	Sudden infant death syndrome (SIDS)
	Perinatal health care
Coal miners	OSHA standards
	Respiratory diseases (black lung, chronic obstructive pulmonary disease)
	Air/water quality standards
	Substance abuse
	Depression
	Trauma care

need. For instance, four high-risk industries identified by OSHA that are found in predominantly rural environments are forestry, mining, fishing, and agriculture. Associated health risks of these industries are machinery and vehicular accidents, trauma, selected types of cancer, and respiratory disease stemming from repeated exposure to toxins, pesticides, and herbicides (Brasher, 1998; USDA, 1995, 1997).

More specifically, agriculture-type businesses, such as farming and ranching, often are owned and operated by a family. Small enterprises do not fall under OSHA guidelines; therefore safety standards are not enforceable on most farms and ranches. Moreover, small businesses, such as farms, are not covered under workman's compensation insurance. Additional concerns arise because family members participate in the farm or ranch work. This means that some adults and children may operate dangerous farm machinery with minimal operating instructions on the hazards and safety precautions. Consequently, agriculture-related accidents result in a significant number of deaths and long-term injuries, particularly among children and women. The morbidity and mortality rates associated with agriculture vary from state to state. The rising incidence of these injuries and deaths, however, has become a national concern

BOX 16-2 Characteristics of Rural Life

More space; greater distances between residents/ services
Cyclic/seasonal work and leisure activities
Informal social/professional interactions
Access to extended kinship systems
Residents who are related or acquainted
Lack of anonymity
Challenges in maintaining confidentiality stemming from familiarity among residents
Small enterprises (family); fewer large industries
Economic orientation to land and nature (e.g., agriculture, mining, lumbering, fishing)
More prevalent high-risk occupations
Town as center of trade
Churches and schools as socialization centers
Preference for interacting with locals (insiders)
Mistrust of newcomers to the community (outsiders)

BOX 16-3 Barriers to Health Care in Rural Areas

Great distances to obtain services
Lack of personal transportation
Unavailable public transportation
Lack of telephone services
Unavailable outreach services
Inequitable reimbursement policies for providers
Unpredictable weather and/or travel conditions
Inability to pay for care
Lack of "know how" to procure entitlements and/or services
Providers' attitudes and knowledge levels about rural populations
Language barriers; care givers are not linguistically competent
Care and services are not culturally appropriate

(NRHA, 1997b; USOTA, 1992). Nurses in rural settings can help address this problem by including farm safety content in school and community education programs.

In summary, it is risky to generalize about the health status of rural Americans because of their diversity coupled with conflicting definitions as to what differentiates rural from urban residences. There are many vulnerable individuals and families living in rural communities across the United States, but little is known about many of them. This void is a potential research area for nurses who practice in rural environments.

RURAL HEALTH CARE DELIVERY ISSUES AND BARRIERS TO CARE

Although each rural community is unique, the experience of living in a rural area has several common characteristics (AP, 1998c; Ramsbottom-Lucier et al, 1996; Sternbert, 1997) (Box 16-2). Concomitantly, barriers to health care may be associated with these characteristics (i.e., whether services and professionals are available, affordable, accessible, or acceptable to rural consumers).

Availability implies the existence of health services as well as the necessary personnel to provide essential services. Sparseness of population limits the number and array of health care services in a given geographic region. Therefore the cost of providing special services to a few people often is prohibitive, particularly in frontier states where there is an insufficient number of physicians, nurses, and other types of health care providers. Consequently, where services and personnel are scarce, they must be allocated wisely. Accessibility implies that a person has logistical access to, as well as the ability to purchase, needed services. Affordability is associated with both availability and accessibility of care. It infers that services are of reasonable cost and that a family has sufficient resources to purchase them when they are needed. Ac-

ceptability of care means that a particular service is appropriate and offered in a manner that is congruent with the values of a target population. This can be hampered by both the client's cultural preference and the urban orientation of health professions (Conway-Welch, 1991; Gesler and Ricketts, 1992) (Box 16-3).

Providers' attitudes, insights, and knowledge about rural populations are also important. A demeaning attitude, lack of accurate knowledge about rural populations, or insensitivity about the rural lifestyle on the part of a nurse can perpetuate difficulties in relating to those clients. Moreover, insensitivity perpetuates mistrust, resulting in rural clients perceiving professionals as "outsiders to our community." Conversely, some professionals in rural practice express feelings of "professional isolation and community nonacceptance." To resolve these conflicting views, nursing faculty members should expose students to the rural environment. Clinical experiences should include opportunities to provide care to clients in their natural setting (e.g., rural) to gain accurate insight about that particular community.

To design community-oriented programs that are available, accessible, affordable, and appropriate, nurses must design strategies and implement interventions that mesh with a client's belief system (Fuller, 1998; Penney, Gibbons, and Bushy, 1996; Pickard, 1996; Whitener, 1996). This implies that a family and a community are actively involved in planning and delivering care for a member who needs it. Nurses must have an accurate perspective of rural clients. Although the importance of forming partnerships and ensuring mutual exchange seems obvious, to date most of the research about rural communities has been for policy or reimbursement purposes. There are minimal empirical data about rural family systems in terms of their health beliefs, values, perceptions of illness, health care seeking behaviors, and what constitutes appropriate care. Therefore nurses

Rural Community Health Nursing in Canada: Nursing in Canada's Northern Remote Areas

Karon Foster, Toronto Public Health and Ryerson Polytechnical University

CANADA'S FAR NORTH

One of the unique rural areas in Canada is the Far North. The Far North in Canada covers 1.3 million square miles and stretches from the Yukon in the west to Nunavut (Canada's newest territory) in the east and north to the Arctic Circle. The population of 55,000 is distributed among reserves, settlements, villages, towns, and the city of Yellowknife. The population is made up of native groups such as the Metis, the Dene, the Inuit, and non-native residents. Many languages are spoken in this area, some of which are English, French, Inuktitut, Slavey, Dogrib, Chipewyan, Cree, and Gwich'in.

Nurses have traditionally delivered health care in this remote area. The Grey Nuns were the first to provide care, in Fort Providence in 1867. Since 1945 the federal government has been responsible for health care of the natives and inhabitants of the Far North. In 1988 this responsibility was transferred to the territorial governments. Health care is provided in 450 health care facilities, which include hospitals, health centers, and health stations. Health centers include a treatment area, a few inpatient beds, a teaching area, and basic laboratory and x-ray equipment. Nursing stations are located in small communities of 150 to 1500 people and may be staffed with 1 to 5 nurses. Often these health stations are only accessible to larger centers by air.

DIVERSE NURSING ROLES

Like nurses working in other rural areas, nurses in the remote areas of Canada have diverse responsibilities and roles. They provide direct patient care that includes emergency care, monitoring of chronic health problems, prenatal and childcare clinics, and developing and implementing illness prevention and health promotion programs. Non-nursing roles include pharmacist, environmental health officer, clerk, infection control officer, social worker, and x-ray technician. To function effectively in this setting, nurses require many skills. A broad knowledge base is important because they must function as both a generalist and a specialist in acute care and community health. Advanced assessment and diagnostic and prescribing skills are needed to treat acute, chronic, and emergency health problems. Advanced clinical skills such as suturing, application of casts, midwifery, and intravenous therapy are required.

CHALLENGES TO WORKING IN REMOTE AREAS

Nurses face many challenges when they work in these remote areas such as isolation, a scarcity of resources, and a lack of anonymity. Nurses in the health stations face professional isolation because they may be the only health care professional for the community. Communities may not have other health care resources such as Meals on Wheels or public health programs. Support and consultation with other health care workers in larger centers is by phone. Nurses live in the community or the nursing station, so separation of their professional and personal lives is difficult. Even when they are not on duty, they may be stopped and asked for professional advice.

Nurses also face barriers such as culture, language, and a very different living environment. Language barriers can contribute to the social isolation; nurses may only develop relationships with other non-natives in the community. Forming social relationships with non-natives can alienate the community that they serve. New nurses may be overwhelmed by the difference in culture and the harsh environment.

Stress and burnout have been identified as problems for these nurses and may result in a high turnover of staff. Heavy workloads, understaffing, fatigue, culture shock, the challenges of weather, and lack of resources contribute to the high turnover of staff. The community may be left without a nurse, or a pool of relief nurses maybe used until the position is filled. It takes time for members of a community to trust the nurse, and high turnover rates can hamper the development of these relationships.

Ethical, moral, and legal issues can arise. Nurses may have to perform medical procedures for which they have not been adequately trained. They may also have to deliver nursing care to family and friends because they are the only health care provider in the community. As yet, standards that outline the expectations for nurses in expanded roles have not been clearly developed for all areas of Canada.

Bibliography

Brumwell A, Janes C: Primary health care in Rae-Edzo, *Canadian Nurse* 90(3):38, 1994.

Graham R: Inservice education for northern nurses, *Canadian Nurse* 90(3):33, 1994

Gregory D: Nursing practice in native communities. In Baumgart A, Larsen J: *Canadian nursing faces the future*, ed 2, St Louis, 1992, Mosby.

Morewood-Northrop M: Nursing in the northwest territories, *Canadian Nurse* 90(3):26, 1994.

Roberts J: Outpost nurse responds to March column, *Canadian Nurse* 94(6):8, 1998.

Ross D: Nursing up north, *Canadian Nurse* 85(1):22, 1989.

Scott K: Northern nurses burnout, *Canadian Nurse* 87(10):18, 1991.

Canadian spelling is used

BOX 16-4 Characteristics of Nursing Practice in Rural Environments

Variety/diversity in clinical experiences
Broader/expanding scope of practice
Generalist skills
Flexibility/creativity in delivering care
Sparse resources (materials, professionals, equipment, fiscal)
Professional/personal isolation
Greater independence
More autonomy
Role overlap with other disciplines
Slower pace
Lack of anonymity
Increased opportunity for informal interactions with clients/coworkers
Opportunity for client follow-up upon discharge in informal community settings
Discharge planning allowing for integration of formal and informal resources
Care for clients across the life span
Exposed to clients with a full range of conditions/diagnoses
Status in the community; viewed as an occupation of prestige
Viewed as a professional role model
Opportunity for community involvement and informal health education

RESEARCH *Brief*

Nurse researchers at Montana State University proposed the following theoretical concepts and dimensions of rural nursing:

Health. Defined by rural residents as the ability to work. Work and health beliefs are closely related for rural Montana sample.

Environment. Distance and isolation are particularly important for rural dwellers. Those who live long distances neither perceive themselves as isolated nor perceive health care services as inaccessible.

Nursing. Lack of anonymity, outsider/insider, old-timer/newcomer. Lack of anonymity is a common theme among rural nurses who report knowing most people for whom they care, not only in the nurse-client relationship but also in a variety of social roles, such as family member, friend, or neighbor. Acceptance as a health care provider in the community is closely linked to the outsider/insider and newcomer/oldtimer phenomena. Gaining trust and acceptance of local people is identified as a unique challenge that must be successfully negotiated by nurses before they can begin to function as effective health care providers.

Person. Self-reliance and independence in relation to health care are strong characteristics of rural individuals. They prefer to have people they know care for them (informal services) as opposed to an outsider in a formal agency.

Lee H, editor: *Conceptual basis for rural nursing*, New York, 1998, Springer

Long K, Weinert C: Rural nursing: developing a theory base, *Sch Inq Nurs Pract* 3:113, 1989

Long K, Weinert C: Rural nursing: developing the theory base, In Winstead-Fry P, Tiffany J, Shippee-Rice R, editors: *Rural health nursing*, New York, 1992, National League for Nursing.

Weinert C, Long K: Rural families and health care: refining the knowledge base, *J Marriage Fam Rev* 15(1, 2):57, 1990.

must assume a more active role in implementing research on the community nursing needs of rural populations to expand the profession's theoretical base and subsequently implement empirically based clinical interventions.

NURSING CARE IN RURAL ENVIRONMENTS
Theory, Research, and Practice

There is a growing body of literature on nursing practice in small towns and rural environments, and several themes have emerged from it (Box 16-4). Each of these dimensions can be viewed as an opportunity or a challenge by a nurse who practices in this setting.

Researchers from the University of Montana contend that existing theories do not fully explain rural nursing practice (Long and Weinert, 1989, 1992; Weinert and Boik, 1994; Weinert and Long, 1991, 1993). They examined the four concepts pertinent to a nursing theory (health, person, environment, and nursing/caring) and described relational statements that are relevant to clients and nurses in rural environments (see the Research Brief). Since the focus of their research was Anglo-Americans living in the Rocky Mountain area, care must be taken about generalizing those findings to other geographic regions and minorities. They propose that rural residents often judge their health by their ability to work. They consider themselves healthy, even though they may suffer from several chronic

illnesses, as long as they are able to continue working. For them, being healthy is the ability to be productive. Chronically ill people emphasize emotional and spiritual well-being rather than physical wellness.

Distance, isolation, and sparse resources characterize rural life and are seen in residents' independent and innovative coping strategies. Self-reliance and independence are demonstrated through their self-care practices and preference for family and community support. Community networks provide support but still allow for each person's and family's independence. Ruralites prefer and usually seek help through their informal networks, such as neighbors, extended family, church, and civic clubs, rather than seeking a professional's care in the formal system of health care, including services such as those provided by a mental health clinic, social service agency, or health department.

Although nursing is generally similar across settings and populations, there are some unique features associated with practice in a geographically remote area or in small towns where most people are familiar with one another. The subsequent paragraphs highlight a few of the variations that nurses in rural practice report (Aitken, VanArsdale, and Barry, 1990; ANA, 1996; Barger, 1996; Dunkin et al, 1994; Hanson, 1997).

The work and home roles for professional nursing practice in rural areas may not be distinct. In many instances a nurse may have more than one work role in the community, such as a nurse who is also a Sears catalog store owner or a nurse who works at the local hospital or doctor's office and also is actively involved in the management of a family farm. For nurses, this means that many, if not all, clients are personally known as neighbors, friends of an immediate family member, or perhaps part of one's extended family. Associated with the social informality is a corresponding lack of anonymity in a small town. Some rural nurses say, "I never really feel like I am off duty because everybody in the county knows me through my work." In part this can be attributed to nurses being highly regarded by the community and viewed by local people as experts on health and illness. It is not unusual for residents to informally ask a nurse's advice before seeing a doctor for a health problem. Moreover, health-related questions are asked by residents when they see the nurse (who may be a neighbor, friend, or relative) in a grocery store, at a service station, during a basketball game, or at church functions.

Nurses in rural practice must make decisions about individuals of all ages with a variety of health conditions. They assume many roles because of the range of services that must be provided in a rural health care facility. A nurse may assume several roles because of the scarcity of nursing and other health professionals. Stemming from rural residents' expectations of the health care delivery system, the skills needed by nurses in rural practice include technical and clinical competency, adaptability, flexibility, strong assessment skills, organizational abilities, independence, interest in continuing education, sound decision-making skills, leadership ability, self-confidence, skills in handling emergencies, teaching, and public relations. The nurse administrator is also expected to be a "jack-of-all-trades" (generalist) and to demonstrate competence in several clinical specialties in addition to managing and organizing staff within the facility for which he or she is responsible (Bosch and Bushy, 1997b; DeLao, 1992).

There are challenges, opportunities, and rewards in rural community and public health nursing practice. The manner in which each factor is perceived depends on individual preferences and the situation in a given community. Challenges of rural practice include limited educational opportunities, professional isolation, lack of other kinds of health personnel/professionals with whom one can interact, heavy work loads, the ability to function well in several clinical areas, lack of anonymity, and for some, a restricted social life (Stratton, Dunkin, and Juhl, 1995; Stratton et al, 1995).

There are also many opportunities and rewards in rural nursing practice. Those most commonly cited include close relationships with clients and coworkers, diverse clinical experiences that evolve from caring for clients of all ages who have a variety of health problems, caring for clients for long periods of time (in some cases, across several generations), opportunities for professional development, and greater autonomy. Many nurses value the solitude and quality of life found in a rural community personally and for their own family. Others thrive on the outdoor recreational activities. Still others thoroughly enjoy the informal, face-to-face interactions coupled with the public recognition and status associated with living and working as a nurse in a small community.

Community and Public Health Nursing

Although most of the publications about rural health care and nursing focus on hospital practice, much of that information is applicable to community-oriented agencies and community and public health nursing as well (Davis and Droes, 1993; Hamel-Bissel, 1992; Washington State Nursing Network, 1992). The work-related stressors of community and public health nursing have received some attention in the literature. Case (1991) focused on stressful experiences of nurses working in rural Oklahoma health departments (Box 16-5). Similar stressors are cited by nurses who work in urban agencies. However, the rural informants gave anecdotal reports describing the stressors associated with geographic distance, isolation, sparse resources, and other environmental factors that characterize rurality.

BOX 16-5 Work Stressors of Nurses in Rural Practice

Political/bureaucratic problems
Understaffing; overworked
Intraprofessional/interpersonal conflicts
Difficult/unpleasant nurse-client encounters
Unsatisfactory work environment
Relatives who refuse to deliver needed care to client
Clients who are hostile, apathetic, dependent, of low intelligence
Inadequate communication
Fear for personal safety
Difficulty locating clients for care and/or follow-up
"Falling through the cracks"

From Case T: Work stresses of community health nurses in Oklahoma. In Bushy A, editor: *Rural nursing*, vol 2, Newbury Park, Calif, 1991, Sage Publications.

Nursing in rural practice settings is characterized by physical isolation that may lend itself to any one of the following: professional isolation; scarce financial, human, and health care resources; and a broad scope of practice. Because of personal familiarity with local residents, nurses often possess in-depth knowledge about clients and their families. Along with the acknowledged benefits, informal (face-to-face) interactions can significantly reduce a nurse's anonymity in the community and at times be a barrier to completing an objective assessment on a client. Like urban practice, rural community nursing takes place in a variety of locations, including homes, clinics, schools, occupational settings, correctional facilities, and at community events, such as county fairs, rodeos, civic and church-sponsored functions, and school athletic events (Fig 16-2).

Research Needs

There are few empirical studies on rural nursing practice. Much of what exists consists of anecdotal reports by nurses. Several specific areas for research are of particular importance to nursing practice in rural environments.

1. Most nurses indicate that they enjoy practicing in rural areas and are proud of what they do. They believe, however, that their work deserves more recognition by professional nursing organizations. Furthermore, the retention rate of nurses in some practice settings is poor. The perspective of nurses who are dissatisfied with rural nursing is necessary to give a more complete picture of the rural experience. This information can be useful to a variety of people: other nurses who are considering rural practice; nurse managers in need of better screening tools to assess fit of nurse-person-environment when interviewing applicants; planners of continuing nursing education programs; and faculty members who teach community and public health to undergraduate and graduate students.

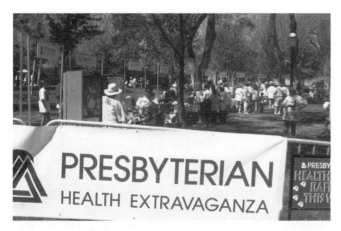

FIG. 16-2 A hospital-sponsored health fair is one example of a community event to provide health services to individuals in a rural area.

2. More information is needed about the stressors and rewards of rural practice. These data could be used to develop stress management techniques by nurses and their supervisors to retain nurses and to improve the quality of their workplace environment.
3. With the increasing number of rural residents in all regions of the United States, empirical data are needed on the particular community nursing needs of rural-client systems, especially under represented groups, minorities, and other at-risk populations that vary by region and state.
4. Since most of the reported research studies on rural nursing have been undertaken with Anglo-Americans living in the intermountain and midwest regions, data is needed from residents in other areas, especially the states east of the Mississippi River.

Preparing Nurses for Rural Practice Settings

Nurses in rural practice must have broad knowledge about nursing theory. Health promotion, primary prevention, rehabilitation, obstetrics, medical-surgical, pediatrics, competency in planning and implementing community assessments, and an awareness and understanding of the particular health concerns in a specific state are important in this practice environment. A community's demographic profile and its principal industry can present a snapshot of some of its social, political, and health risks. From this kind of information, a nurse can anticipate the particular skills that will be needed to care for clients in a catchment area (ANA, 1996; Pan and Straub, 1997; Pearson, 1997).

Stemming from their knowledge of resources and their ability to coordinate formal and informal services, nurses have played and will continue to play an important role in offering a continuum of services for rural clients in spite of sparse resources and fragmentation in the health care delivery system. Preparing nurses to practice in rural environments demands creative and innovative nursing educational opportunities. Collaboration and partnerships must be established between educators, rural nurses, and administrators of health care facilities in rural settings. To meet the demands and expectations of practice in that setting, nursing faculty members must expose students to the rural environment, facilitate the development of generalist skills, and enhance their ability to function in several roles.

WHAT DO YOU THINK? *Within the nursing profession, there is disagreement as to whether rural nursing is a specialty practice.*

FUTURE PERSPECTIVES

Those concerned with rural health, including residents of rural communities, their elected representatives, and the administrators of public and private health care agencies, should be aware of the problems inherent in providing a continuum of care to underserved populations. Typically, media accounts focus exclusively on rural hospitals and the lack of primary care providers. Those reports generally neglect the public health perspective when discussing the continuum of health care in rural environments. Case management and community-oriented primary health care (COPHC), however, have proven to be effective models in helping to address some of those deficits.

Scarce Resources and a Comprehensive Health Care Continuum

The current health care system is fragmented, thereby creating even greater difficulty in providing a comprehensive continuum of care to populations living in areas having scarce resources, such as money, personnel, equipment, and ancillary services. In rural communities, the most critically needed services usually are preventive services, such as health screening clinics, nutrition counseling, and wellness education.

Community and public health nursing needs vary by community. However, there is a prevailing need in most rural areas, especially for the following:

- Shortage areas
- School nurses
- Family planning services
- Prenatal care
- Care for individuals with AIDS and their families
- Emergency care services
- Children with special needs, including those who are physically and mentally challenged
- Mental health services
- Services for the elderly, especially the frail elderly and those with Alzheimer's disease, such as adult day care, hospice, respite care, homemaker services, and meal deliveries to elderly who remain at home

Providing a continuum of care has been hindered by the closure of many small hospitals since 1980. Of those that remain, many report financial problems that could lead to closure (RWJF, 1997; Schoenman, 1998). A shortage or the absence of even one provider, most often a physician or nurse, could mean that a small hospital must close its doors. This phenomenon has a ripple effect on the health of local residents, other health care services, and the economic development efforts in many small communities.

The short supply and increasing demand for primary care providers in general, and nurses in particular, will continue for some time. To help solve this problem, elected officials and policy developers need nurses, especially those in advanced practice roles, to provide vital services in underserved areas. To respond to this opportunity, nurses need to be creative to ensure delivery of appropriate and acceptable services to at-risk and vulnerable populations who live in rural and underserved regions. Nurses must be sensitive to the health beliefs of clients, then plan and provide nursing interventions that mesh with communities' cultural values and preferences.

Healthy People 2000 and *Healthy People 2010* National Health Objectives Related to Rural Health

Since the demographic profile varies from community to community, each state has variations in the health status of its population. *Healthy People 2000* has important implications for nurses in that a significant number of at-risk populations cited in that policy-guiding document live in rural areas across the United States (USDHHS, 1991, 1996). Consequently, priority objectives vary, depending on population mix, health risks, and health status of residents in the state. It is expected that *Healthy People 2010* will emphasize even more the promotion of safe and healthy communities.

At the local level, communities have used *Healthy People 2000* as a guide for action and to identify objectives and establish meaningful goals. *Healthy Communities 2000: Model Standards* (APHA, 1991; APHA, 1996) was designed to help local officials tailor the objectives to their community's needs. This document encourages the establishment of professional-community partnerships. Translating national objectives into achievable community health targets requires integration of the following components to ensure that services will be acceptable and appropriate for rural clients:

- Health statistics must be meaningful, understandable, and include appropriate process objectives that can be measured readily.
- Strategies must be designed that involve the public, private, and voluntary sectors of the community to achieve agreed-upon local objectives.
- Coordinated efforts are needed to ensure that the community works together to achieve the goals.

Consider, for example, these components in developing a health plan for a rural county having a large population of young people. *Healthy People 2000* objectives for the county should target women of childbearing age, children, and adolescents. Priority objectives should include offering accessible prenatal care programs, improving immunization levels, providing preventive dental care instructions, implementing vehicular accident prevention and firearm safety programs, and educating teachers and health professionals for early identification of cases of domestic violence. On the other hand, consider a rural county that has a higher number of individuals over 65 years of age than the national average. Priority objectives in the health plan should target the health risks and problems of the elderly in that community. Specific objectives might include development of health promoting programs to prevent chronic health problems and establishing community programs to meet the needs of those having chronic illness, specifically cardiovascular disease, diabetes, hypertension, and accident-related disabilities.

When implementing community-focused health plans that flow from *Healthy Communities 2000*, consideration always must be given to rural factors, such as sparse population, geographic remoteness, scarce resources, personnel shortages, and physical, emotional, and social isolation. In addition to being actively involved in empowering the community and planning and delivering care, nurses play an important role in representing their community's perspective to local, state, regional, and national health planners and to their elected officials.

BUILDING PROFESSIONAL-COMMUNITY-CLIENT PARTNERSHIPS IN RURAL SETTINGS

Health care reform initiatives are focusing on cutting costs while improving access to care for all citizens, especially vulnerable and underserved populations. The federal Office of Rural Health Policy (1994) emphasizes that community-oriented programming, which actively involves the state and local element, is an essential element for any kind of reform to be successful, especially in rural areas. In other words, professional-client-community partnerships are critical elements for reform to be meaningful at the local level. Two models have been found to be particularly useful in rural environments: case management and COPHC.

Case Management

Case management is a client-professional partnership that can be used to arrange a continuum of care for rural clients, with the case manager tailoring and blending formal and informal resources. Collaborative efforts between a client and case manager allow clients to participate in their plan of care in an acceptable and appropriate way, especially when local resources are few and far between (Bosch and Bushy, 1997a; Bushy, 1997; Goeppinger, 1993). The clinical application at the end of this chapter demonstrates how nursing case management can allow an elderly, rural resident to stay at home if adequate supports can be provided. Outcomes are often remarkably different when case management is used. Additional information on case management is found in Chapter 19.

Community-Oriented Primary Health Care

COPHC is an effective model for delivering available, accessible, and acceptable services to vulnerable populations living in **medically underserved** areas. This model emphasizes flexibility, grass-roots involvement, and professional-community partnerships. It blends primary care, public health, and prevention services, which are offered in a familiar and accessible setting. The COPHC model is interdisciplinary, uses a problem-oriented approach, and mandates community involvement in all phases of the process (Box 16-6).

Building professional-community partnerships is an ongoing process. At various times, nurses, other health professionals, and community leaders must assume the role of advocate, change agent, educator, expert, and/or group facilitator to gain both active and passive support from the

---

BOX 16-6 Community-Oriented Primary Health Care: A Partnership Process

Define and characterize the community.
Identify the community's health problems.
Develop or modify health care services in response to the community's identified needs.
Monitor and evaluate program process and client outcomes.

---

community. Partnerships involve "give and take" by all participants in the negotiations to reach consensus. Essentially, the process begins with professionals gaining entrance into a community, establishing rapport and trust with locals, then working together to empower the community to resolve mutually defined problems and goals. As mentioned previously, *Healthy Communities 2000* is an excellent guide for developing and defining those goals. Stemming from churches' and schools' central importance in a rural community, leaders from those institutions can be key players in building provider-community partnerships. The organizational phase should precede all others. Those efforts lay the foundation for all other activities related to planning, implementing, and evaluating community services.

As with case management for a client, professional-community partnerships allow for more effective identification of existing informal social support systems that are accepted by rural residents. The goal is to integrate community preferences with new or existing formal services. Public input should be encouraged early in the planning process and must continue throughout the process to allow the community to feel that it has "ownership in the project" as opposed to residents viewing it as "an outsider bringing another bureaucratic program into town." Strategies that nurses can use to enhance the building of partnerships in rural environments are listed in the How To box.

Partnership models, such as case management and COPHC, have proven to be highly effective in areas with scarce resources and an insufficient number of health care providers. Individuals and communities who are informed, active participants in planning their health care are more likely to develop consensus about the most appropriate solution for local problems. Subsequently, they are more likely to use and support that system after it is implemented. Partnership models enhance the ability of rural communities to do what they historically have done well (i.e., assume responsibility for the services and institutions that serve its residents). Knowledge about partnership models and the skills to effectively implement them is useful for nurses who coordinate services that are accessible, available, and acceptable for rural populations in their catchment area.

▌HOW TO   *Build Professional-Community-Client Partnerships*

1. *Gain the local perspective.*
2. *Assess the degree of public awareness and support for the cause.*
3. *Identify special interest groups.*
4. *List existing services to avoid duplication of programs.*
5. *Note real and potential barriers to existing resources and services.*
6. *Generate a list of potential community volunteers and professionals who are willing to assist with the project.*
7. *Create awareness among target groups of a particular program (e.g., individuals, families, senior centers, church and recreation groups, health care professionals, law enforcement personnel, and other religious, service, and civic clubs).*
8. *Identify potential funding sources to implement the program.*
9. *Establish the community's health care priority list, and involve large numbers of community members in considering and selecting their health care options.*
10. *Incorporate business principles in marketing the program.*
11. *Measure the health system's local economic impact.*
12. *Educate residents about the important role the local health care system plays in the economic infrastructure of the community and the consequences of a system failure.*
13. *Develop local leadership and support for the community's health system through training and providing experience in decision making.*

clinical application

Ethyl, a 73-year-old widow, was diagnosed more than 10 years ago with progressive Parkinson's disease. Her husband of more than 40 years suddenly died 3 years ago after a serious stroke. Her two married daughters live in California and Illinois. Her small midwestern town has 1000 residents, and the nearest health care is 100 miles away. Her 75-year-old widowed sister, Suzanna, also lives in town. Their brother, Bill (age 71), has recently entered the county nursing home located in a town 20 miles away. Despite her physical rigidity and ataxia, Ethyl manages to live alone in her two-bedroom home with her dog and cat. Ethyl insists that she will not relinquish her private, independent lifestyle as her brother Bill has. Yet, within this past year she has been hospitalized three times for a bad chest cold, for a bladder infection, and after a neighbor found her lying unconscious in the garden. Her doctor says that this last episode was related to "a heart problem."

After discharge, a home health nurse, Liz, was assigned as her case manager. Liz's office is based at the County Senior Center near the nursing home where Bill is a resident. Bill is also one of the clients whom Liz checks on weekly. Liz provides outreach services to all the residents in the county who are referred by a large home health agency in the city. As a case manager, she works closely with the hospital's discharge planners to arrange a continuum of care for clients in the two-county area. Her activities include coordinating formal and informal services for clients, including nutrition, hydration, pharmacologic care, personal care, homemaker services, and routine activities, such as writing checks, home maintenance, and emergency back-up services.

A. Describe the nursing roles that Liz assumes in coordinating a continuum of care for Ethyl in terms of nutrition, transportation, and health care.
B. Identify formal health care and support resources that can be accessed for Ethyl.
C. Identify informal support resources that can be used to ensure that Ethyl is safe.

D. Identify three outcomes that have been achieved by using nursing care management.
E. Select a rural community in your geographic area. Create hypothetical situations, or select real clients with real health problems (e.g., an elderly person with Alzheimer's disease, a middle-age person with cancer requiring end-of life care, a child who is technology-dependent as a result of a farm accident). Prepare a list of services and referral agencies in that community that could be used to develop a continuum of care for each of these cases. How are these the same, or different, from the case described in this chapter?

Answers are found in the back of the book.

▌EY POINTS

- There is great diversity in rural environments across the United States.
- There are variations in the health status of rural populations, depending on genetic, social, environmental, economic, and political factors.
- There is a higher incidence of working poor in rural America than in more populated areas.
- Rural adults 18 years of age and over are in poorer health than their urban counterparts; nearly 50% have been diagnosed with at least one major chronic condition. However, they average one less physician visit each year than healthier urban counterparts.
- About 26% of rural families are below the poverty level; more than 40% of all rural children under 18 years of age live in poverty.
- General practitioners are the usual providers of care for rural adults and children.
- Rural residents often must travel for more than 30 minutes to access a health care provider.
- Nurses must take into consideration the belief systems and lifestyles of a rural population when planning, implementing, and evaluating community services.

- Barriers to rural health care include the availability, affordability, accessibility, and acceptability of services.
- Partnership models, in particular case management and community-oriented primary health care (COPHC) are effective models to provide a comprehensive continuum of care in environments with scarce resources.

3. Discuss economic, social, and cultural factors that affect rural lifestyle and the health care seeking behaviors of residents who live there.
4. Identify barriers that affect accessibility, affordability, availability, and acceptability of services in the health care delivery system.
5. Summarize key nursing concepts as they fit with practice in rural environments.
6. Examine the characteristics of rural community nursing practice and how this differs from practice in more populated settings.
7. Identify challenges, opportunities, and benefits of living and practicing as a nurse in the rural environment.
8. Debate case management and community-oriented primary care as partnership models that can help nurses enhance the continuum of care for clients living in an environment with sparse resources.

critical thinking activities

1. Compare and contrast the terms *urban, suburban, rural, frontier, farm, nonfarm residency, metropolitan,* and *nonmetropolitan.*
2. Describe residency as a continuum, ranging from farm residency to core metropolitan residency.

Bibliography

Abraham I et al: Mental health of rural elderly, *Issues Ment Health Nurs* 15(3):203, 1994.

Aitken T, VanArsdale S, Barry L: Strategies for practice as a clinical nurse specialist in a small setting, *Clin Nurse Spec* 4(1):28, 1990.

American Nurses Association: *Rural/frontier health care task force: rural/frontier nursing: the challenge to grow,* Washington, DC, 1996, the Association.

American Public Health Association: *Healthy communities 2000: model standards,* Washington, DC, 1991, APHA.

American Public Health Association: *Healthy communities 2000: mid-course review,* Washington, DC, 1996, APHA.

Associated Press (AP): Farmworkers' town: hunger striking vegetable pickers seek pay raise, *The Daytona Beach News Journal,* p 2-A, Jan 18, 1998a.

Associated Press (AP): Indian reservation tackles epidemic of teen suicide. *The Daytona Beach News Journal,* p 5-A, Feb 6, 1998b.

Associated Press (AP): 40 below keeps the riff-raff out, *The Daytona Beach News Journal,* p 8-A, Mar 6, 1998c.

Baer K, Johnson M, Gesler W: What is rural: a focus on urban influence codes, *J Rural Health* 13(4):329, 1997.

Barger S: Rural nurses: here today and gone tomorrow, *NRHA Rural Clin Q* 6(3):3, 1996.

Bigbee J, Crowder E: The Red Cross Rural Nursing Service: an innovation of public health nursing delivery, *Public Health Nurs* 2(2):109, 1985.

Bosch D, Bushy A. Case management: implementing homecare in rural areas, *Home Healthcare Consultant* 4(7):19, 1997a.

Bosch D, Bushy A: The 5 As of home care in rural environments, *Caring* 16(1):20, 1997b.

Bowers D, Cook P: Population: nonmetro population rebound continues: socioeconomic conditions issue, *Rural Conditions and Trends* 7(3):6, 1997.

Braden J, Beauregard K. *National medical expenditure survey-health status and access to care* of rural and urban populations, Research Findings 18, Rockville, Md, 1994, Agency for Health Care Policy and Research, Public Health Service (Pub No 94-0031).

Brasher P: Round bales dangerous if not properly handled, *The Bismarck Tribune,* p 10-A, Feb 22, 1998.

Brooks J: Increasing AIDS rates in rural America deserve more attention, *NRHA Rural Clin Q* 8(1):1, 1998.

Bureau of Primary Health Care: *Selected statistics of health professional shortage areas as of September 1996,* Washington, DC, 1997, Division of Shortage Designation, HRSA, USDHHS.

Bushy A. Case management: considerations for coordinating quality services in rural communities, *J Nurs Care Qual* 12(1):26, 1997.

Bushy A: Health issues of women in rural environments: an overview, *J Am Med Womens Assoc* 53(2):53, 1998a.

Bushy A: Rural nursing in the U.S.: where do we stand as we enter the new millennium, *Aust J Rural Health* 6(2):65, 1998b.

Case T: Work stresses of community health nurses in Oklahoma. In Bushy A, editor: *Rural nursing,* vol 2, Newbury Park, Calif, 1991, Sage Publications.

Christianson J, Moscovice I: *Health care reform in rural areas,* Minneapolis, Minn, 1993, University of Minnesota, Rural Health Research Center.

Clark L et al: Prenatal care in non metropolitan and metropolitan America: racial and ethnic differences, *J Health Care Poor Underserved* 6(4):410, 1995.

Conway-Welch C: Issues surrounding the distribution and utilization of nurse nonphysician providers in rural America, *J Rural Health* 7(suppl):388, 1991.

Cromartie J, Swanson L: *Defining metropolitan areas and the rural-urban continuum: a comparison of statical areas based on county and subcounty geography,* Washington, DC, 1995, U.S. Department of Agriculture, Economic Research Division, Rural Economy Division. Staff paper No. AGES-9603.

Davis D, Droes N: Community health nursing in rural and frontier counties, *Nurs Clin North Am* 28(1):159, 1993.

DeLao R: A day in the life of a rural community health nurse: tales from the trenches, *Caring* 11(2):10, 1992.

Dunkin J et al: Characteristics of metropolitan and non metropolitan community health nurses, *Texas J Rural Health* 7(1):18, 1994.

Edelman M, Menz B: Selected comparisons and implications of a national rural and urban survey on health care access, demographics and policy issues, *J Rural Health* 11(3):197, 1996.

Fuller K: The Telecommunication Act and Universal Service, *Rural Heath Education Newsletter,* Kalamazoo, Mich, January 1998, Western Michigan University.

Gahr W: *Rural America: blueprint for tomorrow,* Newbury Park, Calif, 1993, Sage Publications.

Gesler W, Ricketts T: *Health in rural North America: the geography of health care services and delivery,* New Brunswick, NJ, 1992, Rutgers University Press.

Goeppinger J: Health promotion for rural populations: partnership interventions, *Fam Community Health* 16(1):1, 1993.

Hamel-Bissel B: On fear and courage: a first encounter with AIDS in rural Vermont. In Instead-Fry P, editor: *Rural health nursing: stories of creativity, commitment and connectedness,* New York, 1992, NLN Publications.

Hanson M: Rural nurses scarce, *The Bismarck Tribune,* pp 1, 12A, Sept 24, 1997.

Health Resources Services Administration: *Exploratory evaluation of rural applications of telemedicine,* Rockville, Md, 1997, HRSA.

Hewitt M: Defining rural areas. In Gesler W, Ricketts T, editors: *Health in rural North America,* New Brunswick, NJ, 1992, Rutgers University.

Human J, Wasem K: Rural mental health in America, *Am Psychol* 46(3):232, 1991.

Continued

Bibliography—cont'd

Johnson D: Newcomers in porch swings show rural life's on upturn, *New York Times*, p. A1, B6, Sept 6, 1996.

Johnson-Webb K, Baer I, Gesler W: What is rural: issues and considerations, *J Rural Health* 45(2):171, 1997.

Lee H: Definitions of rural: a review of the literature. In Bushy A, editor: *Rural nursing*, vol. I, Thousand Oaks, Calif, 1991, Sage Publications.

Lee H, editor: *Conceptual basis for rural nursing*, New York, 1998, Springer.

Long K, Weinert C: Rural nursing: developing a theory base, Sch Inq Nurs Pract 3:113, 1989.

Long K, Weinert C: Rural nursing: developing the theory base. In Winstead-Fry P, Tiffany J, Shippee-Rice R, editors: *Rural health nursing*, New York, 1992, National League for Nursing.

Minnesota Center for Rural Health: *Getting on the right road to rural health care: a community health development guide*, Duluth, Minn, 1996, Author.

Mueller KJ et al: *Health status and access to care among rural minorities*, Omaha, Neb, 1995, University of Nebraska-Center for Rural Health Research.

Mueller KJ, Patil K, Boilesen E: *The role of uninsurance and race in health care utilization by rural minorities*, Omaha, Neb, 1995, University of Nebraska-Center for Rural Health Research.

Nasser H: Area women flock to doctor in Montana: the only provider for miles around, *USA Today*, p. 7-A, Jan 19, 1998a.

Nasser H: Population moves deeper into suburbs, *USA Today*, p. 3-A, March 18, 1998b.

National Rural Health Association: *A shared vision: building bridges for rural health access*, Conference Proceedings of National Rural Minorities, Kansas City, Mo, 1994a, NHRA.

National Rural Health Association: *Health care in frontier America*, Kansas City, Mo, 1994b, NHRA.

National Rural Health Association: *A national agenda for rural minority health: a strategic planning document*, Kansas City, Mo, 1997a, NHRA.

National Rural Health Association: Fatal rural crashes are focus of new safety plan, *The Nation's Health* (11):9, 1997b.

National Rural Health Associations: *Bringing resources to bear on the changing health care system @ Birmingham, Alabama*, conference proceedings, Kansas City, Mo, 1998a, NRHA.

National Rural Health Association: *Southeastern Conference on Rural HIV/AIDS: issues in prevention and treatment: conference report in rural America @ Atlanta, Georgia*, Kansas City, Mo, 1998b, NRHA.

Newbold KB: Problems in search of solutions: health and Canadian aboriginals, *J Community Health* 23(1):59, 1998.

Office of Rural Health Policy: *Seventh annual report on rural health: recommendations to the Secretary of Health and Human Services*, Washington, DC, 1994, ORHP.

Packard Foundation: *The future of children: welfare to work* 7(1), 1997a.

Packard Foundation: *The future of children: children and poverty* 7(2), 1997b.

Pan S, Straub L: Education for rural health professionals, *J Rural Health* 3(1):78, 1997.

Penney N, Gibbons B, Bushy A: Partners in distance learning: project outreach, *J Nurs Admin* 26(7):27, 1996.

Pickard M: Rural nursing: a decade in review, *NRHA Rural Clin Q* 6(3):1, 1996.

Pearson L: Annual update of how each state stands on legislative issues affecting advanced nursing practice, *Nurse Pract* 22(1):18, 1997.

Ramsbottom-Lucier M et al: Hills, ridges, mountains and roads: geographical factors and access to care in a rural state, *J Rural Health* 12(5):386, 1996.

Robert Wood Johnson Foundation: *State health care reform: looking back toward the future*, Princeton, NJ, 1997, RWJF.

Rural Information Center Health Services (RICHS): *Rural health in brief: nurse practitioners, physician assistants, and certified nurse-midwives: primary care providers in rural areas*, Washington, DC, 1994, US Department of Agriculture Library.

Schoenman J: *Impact of the Balanced Budget Act of 1997 on Medicare risk plan payment rates for rural areas*, Washington DC, 1998, Project Hope-Walsh Center for Rural Health Analysis.

Sternbert S: Study shows yawning gaps in U.S. health care: longevity affected by environment, *USA Today*, p 11-A, Dec 4, 1997.

Stratton T, Dunkin J, Juhl N: Redefining the nursing shortage: a rural perspective, *Nurs Outlook* 43(2):71, 1995.

Stratton T et al: Retainment incentives in three rural practice settings: influence on the job satisfaction of registered nurses, *Applied Nurs Res*, 8(2):73, 1995.

Strickland J, Strickland D: Barriers to preventive health services for minority households in the south, *J Rural Health* 12(3):206, 1996.

Substance Abuse and Mental Health Services Administration, Center for Substance Abuse Treatment: *Bringing excellence to substance abuse services in rural America: 1996 award for excellence papers*, Rockville, Md, 1997, US Government Printing Office, USDHHS Pub. No. (SMA) 97-3134.

The 1998 HHS Poverty Guidelines, *Federal Register* 63(36):9235, February 24, 1998.

U.S. Census Bureau: *Statistical abstract of the United States of 1990: national general population characteristics*, Hyattsville, Md, 1998, Author.

US Department of Agriculture: *Understanding rural America*, Bulletin # 710, Washington DC, 1995, USDA.

US Department of Agriculture: *Agriculture fact book*, Washington, DC, 1997, USDA Office of Communications.

US Department of Commerce: *Statistical abstract of the United States*, Washington, DC, 1996, U.S. Census Bureau.

US Department of Health and Human Services: *Selected statistics on health professional shortage areas as of September 30, 1997*, Washington DC, 1998, USDHHS, HRSA.

US Department of Health and Human Services: *7th Annual report on rural health: recommendations to the Secretary of Health and Human Services by the national advisory committee on rural health*, Hyattsville, Md, 1994a, USDHHS.

US Department of Health and Human Services: *National medical expenditure survey: health status and access to care of rural and urban populations*, Washington, DC, 1994b, USDHHS-AHCPR.

US Department of Health and Human Services: *Healthy people 2000: mid-course review*, Hyattsville, Md, 1996, USDHHS.

US Department of Health and Human Services: *Healthy people 2000: national health promotion and disease prevention objectives*, Washington, DC, 1991, USDHHS, Public Health Service.

US General Accounting Office: *Rural development: profile of rural areas*. Fact Sheet for Congress, Washington, DC, 1993, USGAO.

US Office of Technology Assessment: *Rural health care: defining "rural" areas: impact on health care and policy research*, Washington, DC, 1992, US Government Printing Office.

Washington State Nursing Network: *Celebration of Public Health Nurse Committee: opening doors: stories of public health nursing*, Olympia, Wash, 1992, Washington State Department of Health.

Weinert C, Boik R: MSU Rurality Index: development and evaluation, *Res Nurs Health* 18:453, 1995.

Weinert C, Long K: The theory and research base for rural nursing practice. In Bushy A, editor: *Rural nursing*, vol. I, Newbury Park, Calif, 1991, Sage Publications.

Weinert C, Long K: Support systems for the spouses of chronically ill persons in rural areas, *J Fam Community Health* 16(1):46, 1993.

Whitener L: Telecommunications and rural health care, *J Rural Health* 12(1):67, 1996.

Woodyard C: Rural gold rush: big chains sweep into small towns, *USA Today*, p. 1B, Feb 3, 1997.

Yawn B: Rural medicine practice: present and future. In Yawn B, Bushy A, Yawn R, editors: *Exploring rural medicine*, Thousand Oaks, Calif, 1994, Sage Publications.

Health Promotion Through Healthy Cities

BEVERLY C. FLYNN & L. LOUISE IVANOV

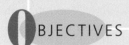

OBJECTIVES

MERLIN www.mosby.com/MERLIN/community_stanhope

After reading this chapter, the student should be able to do the following:

- Trace the Healthy Cities movement.
- Examine the relationship between primary health care, health promotion, and the Healthy Cities movement.
- Describe the steps in the CITYNET-Healthy Cities process.

- Apply the CITYNET-Healthy Cities process to the concepts of health promotion.
- Analyze the role for nursing in a Healthy City.
- Analyze the impact of the CITYNET-Healthy Cities process in health promotion at the community level.

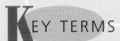

KEY TERMS

appropriate technology
CITYNET process
community participation

equity
health promotion
Healthy Cities

healthy public policy
international cooperation
multisectoral cooperation

primary health care
Healthy People 2010
  objectives
See *Glossary* for definitions

CHAPTER OUTLINE

History of the Healthy Cities
  Movement
Definition of Terms
Models of Community Practice
Healthy Cities Today
  Europe

United States
Canada
Latin America
Future of the Healthy Cities
  Movement
  Facilitators

Barriers
  Healthy Public Policy
Implications for Nursing
Healthy People 2010

The Healthy Cities movement mobilizes local governments, professionals, citizens, and private and voluntary organizations to put health promotion on the political agenda of cities. This is accomplished through application of the World Health Organization's goal of health for all by the year 2000 (WHO and UNICEF, 1978), the strategy of primary care, and the principles of health promotion outlined in the Ottawa Charter for Health Promotion (WHO, 1986). Cities are challenged to do the following (Goldstein and Kickbush, 1996; Tsouros, 1990; Tsouros, 1995):

1. Develop projects that reduce inequalities in health status and access to services
2. Develop healthy public policies at the local level
3. Create physical and social environments that support health, strengthen community action for health, and help people develop new skills for health
4. Reorient health services consistent with the strategy of primary health care and the principles of health promotion

HISTORY OF THE HEALTHY CITIES MOVEMENT

Although the Healthy Cities movement has been labeled "the new public health" (Ashton and Seymour, 1988), others would say that the concept of a healthy city is not new (Hancock, 1993). It is based on the belief that the health of the community is largely influenced by the environment in which people live and that health problems have multiple causes—social, economic, political, environmental, and behavioral. Healthy Cities is consistent with the definition of health promotion that promotes change in the broader environment to support health (WHO, 1986). **Healthy Cities** is based on the recognition that about half of the world's population lives in urban areas, where the human and health-related problems are complex and coupled with increasingly fragmented policy and scarce resources. A key strategy of Healthy Cities is to mobilize the community by developing public, private, and not-for-profit partnerships to address the complex health and environmental problems in the city. The Healthy Cities process involves the following specific steps to conduct community assessments (Tsouros, 1990):

1. Establish priorities, goals, and city-wide action plans
2. Secure resources
3. Establish steering groups to carry out the action
4. Monitor and evaluate progress
5. Review and adjust policies

The Healthy Cities process has been applied to rural and metropolitan areas (Flynn, 1992). Healthy Cities engages local residents for action in health and is based on the premise that when people have the opportunity to work out their own locally defined health problems, they will find sustainable solutions to those problems (Flynn, 1994; Chamberlin, 1996).

The Healthy Cities movement began in the mid-1980s in Toronto, Canada. In 1986 the WHO Regional Office for Europe initiated the WHO Healthy Cities Project. It now has become an international movement involving about 1000 cities. Although 11 cities were selected to participate in the WHO Healthy Cities project in the early years, the current phase includes 35 participating cities. Some of these cities include Camden, England; Horsens, Denmark; Rennes, France; Peco, Hungary; Turku, Finland; and Athens, Greece. In addition, there are 23 national networks and over 650 participating cities and towns throughout Europe. National networks also have developed in Canada, the United States, Australia, Iran, and Egypt. Regional networks are developing in Quebec, Canada; Francophone, Africa; Southeast Asia, and the Western Pacific.

DEFINITION OF TERMS

Healthy Cities is an international movement of cities focused on mobilizing local resources and political, professional, and community members to improve the health of the community. A healthy city is one whose priority is to improve its environment and expand its resources so that community members can support each other in achieving their highest potential.

Guiding the Healthy Cities movement are the principles of health for all (WHO and UNICEF, 1978) and the Ottawa Charter for Health Promotion (WHO, 1986). The principles of health for all include equity, health promotion, community participation, multisectoral cooperation, appropriate technology, primary health care, and international cooperation.

Equity implies providing accessible services to promote the health of populations most at risk for health problems (e.g., the poor, youth, elderly, minorities, homeless, and refugees). Health promotion and disease prevention are focused on providing community members with a positive sense of health that strengthens physical, mental, and emotional capacities. To achieve health for all, individuals within communities must become involved in health promotion. The key to obtaining health for all is through **community participation,** whereby well-informed and motivated community members participate in planning, implementing, and evaluating health programs. In addition, achieving health for all requires **multisectoral cooperation.** This refers to coordinated action by all parts of a community, from local government officials to grass-roots community members. **Appropriate technology** refers to affordable social, biomedical, and health services that are relevant and acceptable to individuals' health, needs, and concerns.

Primary health care, the focus of health care system reform, refers to meeting the basic health needs of a community by providing readily accessible health services. Since health problems transcend international borders, **international cooperation** is needed to ensure that the goal of health for all by the year 2000 is reached.

Health promotion had become a key strategy for the goal of health for all by the time the Ottawa Charter for

Health Promotion was adopted in 1986. This charter provided a clear definition of health promotion and the framework for the Healthy Cities movement (Ashton, 1992; WHO, 1992). *Health promotion* was officially defined as the "process of enabling people to take control over and to improve their health" (WHO, 1986, p. 1). This is accomplished through enabling community members to increase control over and assume more responsibility for health; mediating among public, private, voluntary, and community sectors; and advocating on behalf of people who are powerless to make the necessary changes to promote health.

Five elements make up the strategic framework provided by the Ottawa Charter and are listed in order of priority for health promotion action. These elements are as follows:

1. *Healthy public policy.* Public policy for health that is based on an ecological perspective and multisectoral and participatory strategies (Pederson et al, 1988). Healthy public policy is future oriented and deals with both local health problems and global health issues. In contrast, medical policy is concerned mainly with the existing medical care system and use of technology and biomedical science to treat disease.
2. *Creating supportive environments.* Physical, political, economic, and social systems that support the community's health
3. *Strengthening community action.* Promoting the community's capacity, ability, and opportunity to take appropriate action to protect and improve the health of the community
4. *Developing personal skills.* Helping people develop the lifestyle skills they need to be healthy
5. *Reorienting health services.* Changing the focus of health services toward primary health care, health promotion, disease prevention, and community-oriented care

The CITYNET-Healthy Cities process is an adaptation of the European and Canadian models of Healthy Cities in the United States. The nine-step **CITYNET process** includes the following (Rider et al, 1993):

1. Building the partnership for health
2. Obtaining community commitment
3. Developing the Healthy City Committee
4. Developing leadership in Healthy Cities
5. Assessing the community
6. Community-wide planning for health
7. Community action for health
8. Providing data-based information to policy makers
9. Monitoring and evaluating Healthy City initiatives

DID YOU KNOW? *Implementing the steps of the CITYNET-Healthy Cities process will enable nurses to gain an understanding of the linkages between health, community, and the policy process. Benefits to the community include increased access to services and improved health status, thus promoting equity in health.*

MODELS OF COMMUNITY PRACTICE

The assumptions that professionals have about communities shape the implementation of the Healthy Cities process. Rothman and Tropman (1987) propose three distinct models of community practice:

1. *Locality development* is a process-oriented model that emphasizes consensus, cooperation, and building group identity and a sense of community.
2. *Social planning* stresses rational-empirical problem solving, usually by outside professional experts. The authors note that social planning does not focus on building community capacity or fostering fundamental social change.
3. *Social action,* on the other hand, aims to increase the problem-solving ability of the community along with concrete actions to correct the imbalance of power and privilege of an oppressed or disadvantaged group in the community (Minkler, 1990).

Although it is argued that these models of community practice are not mutually exclusive, efforts generally can be categorized within one model.

Arnstein (1969) depicts a ladder of citizen participation with the lower levels of participation as manipulation, therapy, and informing. The higher levels of participation include partnership, delegated power, and citizen control.

These models of community practice can be summarized as top-down and bottom-up approaches. In a top-down approach, experts and health professionals take the lead in identifying community health problems and implementing programs with little input from the individuals for whom these programs are being planned. A bottom-up approach uses broad-based community problem solving that includes health professionals, local officials, service providers, and other community members, including those at risk for health problems.

DID YOU KNOW? *Community participation can begin at town meetings, city council meetings, crime watch, and other settings where community members, who are people from different walks of life, including health professionals, identify the strengths and health needs of their community and plan appropriate action to address their needs. This is an example of social action, or a "bottom-up" approach to community practice.*

Rothman and Tropman's (1987) locality development and social action are examples of a bottom-up approach in which community participation is evident in all stages of community health planning and practice. Social planning portrays a top-down approach where rational and empirical problem solving usually is conducted by outside experts.

Arnstein's (1969) lower levels of the ladder—manipulation, therapy, and informing—can be equated with a top-down approach in which community practice and action are planned by professionals and experts. The higher levels of the ladder—partnership, delegated power, and citizen control—represent a bottom-up approach, reflecting a multisectoral approach with community participation.

WHAT DO YOU THINK? *Community participation in health decisions is more effective in promoting healthy public policy than decision making by outside professional experts.*

Healthy Cities emphasizes a bottom-up approach with multisectoral planning and action for health. The CITYNET-Healthy Cities process aims at partnerships within the community and focuses on community leadership development for health that is consistent with Rothman and Tropman's (1987) locality development model.

HEALTHY CITIES TODAY

Because cities in Europe and Canada have the longest history in the Healthy Cities movement, examples of Healthy Cities' initiatives from these regions of the world are highlighted first in this section. These examples suggest that different models of community practice are being implemented in the Healthy Cities movement. The locality development and social planning models are used most frequently (Flynn, 1996).

Europe

The largest city in the European Healthy Cities project is St. Petersburg, Russia. In 1992, government officials, health professionals, and consultants from the WHO European Region Healthy Cities Project met to identify the major health problems in St. Petersburg. They decided to begin their health initiative by focusing on programs to decrease the city's high maternal and infant mortality rates. Four projects were developed: a Family Planning Center, a Teen Center, a Maternity Home with rooming in and breast feeding (Baby Friendly Campaign), and a Rehabilitation Center for socially disadvantaged pregnant women (Flynn and Dennis, 1993). A Consensus Conference was held late in 1992 with international consultants to address how to improve the four projects. The local individuals who attended the conference were primarily health professionals, including physicians, nurses, and midwives. This was the first time many of these professionals met together in an interdisciplinary approach to address health problems. The Research Brief details a study of prenatal services done in St. Petersburg.

Horsens Healthy City (Denmark) identified six steps necessary to transform a health promotion idea into action (Bragh-Matzon, 1992). These six steps are as follows:
1. Political commitment and legitimacy
2. Building a small catalyst unit to secure the transformation process
3. Building an infrastructure to secure involvement and legitimization from essential powers in city life

RESEARCH *Brief*

The St. Petersburg, Russia Healthy City Project began its health initiative by focusing on health care services for women primarily because of a high maternal mortality rate and low attendance at prenatal care clinics. This study sought to explain and predict use and satisfaction with prenatal care services in St. Petersburg. A convenience sample of 397 women with uncomplicated pregnancies and normal deliveries was drawn representing an 86% response rate. Survey data were collected retrospectively after women delivered their infants but before they were discharged from the hospital to answer the following questions:

1. Are there characteristics of pregnant women that predict use of prenatal care services and satisfaction with the services?
2. To what extent do predisposing, enabling, and need characteristics contribute to explaining use of prenatal care services and satisfaction with the services?
3. Is there a relationship between use of prenatal care services and satisfaction with the services that explains the start of prenatal care?

Predictors of services use were attitude toward prenatal care, depression, marital status, and employment status. Russian women identified convenience of prenatal care clinics and doctors' behavior as measures of the quality of prenatal care received. Predictors of satisfaction were a regular source of care and negative experiences with health care providers. The findings provide viable alternatives to improve the delivery of prenatal care services in St. Petersburg through a collaborative and multisectoral effort on the part of health policy makers, health care professionals, and educators to encourage early start of prenatal care and provide quality prenatal services.

Ivanov L, Flynn B: Predictors of utilization and satisfaction with prenatal care services in St. Petersburg, Russia, *West J Nurs Res* 21(1):372, 1999.

4. Information, communication, visibility, and public debates on health issues
5. Combining short-term action and long-term planning
6. Promoting and securing the process over time.

The first step involved obtaining a commitment from the city council to support the health-for-all strategy through the Healthy City model. In the second step, the catalyst unit was a small team that bridged the existing government and health structures with the multiple powers and resources within the city. The team included highly experienced professional community members from different disciplines. Nonprofessional community members, or "grassroots" people, were not directly involved in this team. However, their input was sought by professional team members. It was not until the third step that direct community participation occurred. Ordinary citizens were included on a steering committee that became the Health Committee for the city. The function of the Health Committee was to oversee projects and communicate with appropriate individuals and agencies in the city, thereby creating more effective links among politicians, health professionals, and citizens.

Horsens' first health initiative involved conducting a health survey to obtain a health profile for the city. This resulted in the Torsted West Project. The goal of this project was to plan a new residential area along ecological principles. This was accomplished through the six steps mentioned previously. Consultants from other Healthy Cities provided expertise to the project (Draper et al, 1992).

Munich Healthy City in Germany initiated a hospital nutrition project. Input from consultants was sought once the problem was identified by concerned community members (Draper et al, 1992). A concerned group of parents initiated the project. The Parents' Board for Chronically Ill Children was developed. They wrote a proposal on the food needs of hospitalized children to increase community awareness of this problem. They noticed that only medical aspects of diets (e.g., diabetic diets) were being considered during children's hospitalizations rather than providing overall healthy nutrition. The Parents' Board initiated networking with appropriate professionals within the hospital to consider the importance of healthy and child-focused menus. The outcome of collaboration with nurses, doctors, hospital cooks, dietitians, hospital administrators, the city health department, and young clients and their families was improved meals for hospitalized children. This initiative also led to the inclusion of healthy food in nurseries and schools.

Multi-City Action Plans—linking of cities

Multi-City Action Plans (MCAPs) provide platforms for international cooperation in health planning and sharing of professional experts. Groups of Healthy Cities in Europe work together to address common health concerns. This enables smaller cities and those new in the Healthy Cities movement to work together on common health problems, thereby expanding the number of partners and resources available to deal with problems. The goal of the MCAP is to jointly develop, implement, and disseminate innovative models of health promotion. To achieve this goal, a partnership is developed between cities involved in the European Healthy Cities movement. These cities are committed to working together on one common health problem for at least 2 years. The result is open market events that provide forums to present models of successful health promotion projects, exchange information, and monitor progress (Tsouros, 1990).

Examples of health concerns that MCAPs address include AIDS, alcohol, environment and health, diabetes, disability, health-promoting hospitals, nutrition, sports, tobacco-free cities, unemployment, and women's health (World Health Organization, 1994). Specific MCAPs on AIDS activities include surveying user views on existing services and opinions on needed services; encouraging participation of gay or lesbian and other community-based organizations in the HIV/AIDS work and policy development; exchanging educational material and expertise on prevention methods; and developing a guide on services available to travelers with HIV/AIDS. In addition, an MCAP on AIDS newsletter is published and distributed to member cities as a method of communicating and networking.

United States

Healthy Cities in the United States has the longest history in Indiana and California. Healthy Cities Indiana began as a pilot program in 1988 with a grant from the W. K. Kellogg Foundation as a collaborative effort among Indiana University School of Nursing, Indiana Public Health Association, and six Indiana cities. Based on the success of this project, the W.K. Kellogg Foundation funded the dissemination phase called CITYNET-Healthy Cities, in cooperation with the National League of Cities through their network of 19,000 local officials (Flynn, Rider, and Ray, 1991).

The CITYNET process begins with building a partnership and establishing city leaders' commitment to the Healthy City process. Once the commitment is obtained, a Healthy City Committee is established that includes multisectoral representation of the community and citizen participation. Broad multisectoral involvement and citizen participation occur in all the remaining stages of the CITYNET process (leadership development, community assessment, community-wide planning for health, community action, providing data-based information to policy makers, and monitoring and evaluation). CITYNET-Healthy Cities aims at partnerships within the community that require health professionals to recognize that because of the city's complex nature, community problems cannot be medicalized. "Professionalizing" community problems is working at the lowest level of participation—that of providing therapy or treatment rather than community partnership (Arnstein, 1969).

Six cities were initially involved in Healthy Cities Indiana (Gary, Fort Wayne, New Castle, Indianapolis, Seymour, and Jeffersonville). Actions of these cities focused on problems of diverse populations. For example, actions have been directed to local priorities that include problems of children, teen parents, the homeless, access to health care, crime and violence, and the elderly. Action also has been taken on the broader environmental policy issues, including management of solid waste and promotion of air quality. For each of these projects, the CITYNET-Healthy Cities process was followed, thereby providing a broad base of community participation at all stages of community planning (see Research Brief).

During the assessment of their community, the New Castle Healthy City (Indiana) Committee questioned their community's high death rates caused by cancer, chronic

RESEARCH *Brief*

The Healthy Cities process uses action research to empower communities to take action for health. Five concepts that link community empowerment and action research are focus on community, citizen participation, information and problem solving, sharing of power, and quality of life. Two case studies from Healthy Cities Indiana (a pilot program of CITYNET-Healthy Cities) illustrate these concepts. The dynamics of community participation in action research and the successes and barriers to community participation are presented. Outcomes found to empower the community are the extent to which Healthy City projects are initiated, their progress is monitored, continued action in health is supported, resources are obtained, and policies are promoted that contribute to equity in health.

Flynn B, Ray D, Rider M: Empowering communities: action research through healthy cities, *Health Educ Q* 21(3):394, 1994.

obstructive pulmonary disease, and heart disease. The committee asked the following questions: Why were these rates higher than the state and nation? What were the lifestyle choices of community people? What in the environment supported or inhibited healthy choices? They decided to work with CITYNET staff and constructed a survey to obtain baseline data on health behaviors in the community. CITYNET staff trained local volunteers in survey data collection. One thousand surveys were distributed door-to-door using a system to ensure appropriate geographic coverage in the community. They obtained a 50% response rate that demonstrated the community's interest in health concerns. The committee used the national health objectives to compare their findings (USDHHS, 1991). They found high levels of unhealthy behaviors, such as higher cigarette smoking behavior and inadequate exercise than suggested in the national objectives.

The committee then used the survey results to target their Healthy Cities initiatives. The data were used to testify before the County Commissioners on the need for health education and to support the employment of a health educator in the local health department. The cigarette smoking results were used by the committee to testify before the city council in support of an ordinance banning smoking in city buildings. During the last several years, the committee also sponsored community health awareness programs. The 1994 program included a family fitness walk, safety checks of bicycles, and presentations on healthy food preparation emphasizing reduced fat and salt in meals. The committee obtained broad community support and cooperation not only in defining their local problems but also in setting priorities and implementing their initiatives. Their interventions integrated individual lifestyle change and policy change aimed at promoting

supportive environments for health. Plans are underway to repeat the survey to evaluate progress of their Healthy Cities initiatives in reaching the year 2000 health objectives.

The California Healthy Cities project has grown from a few initial cities to the California Network of Healthy Cities funded in part by the State Department of Health Service. It is built on the premise of shared responsibility among community members, local officials, and the private sector. Community participation is the cornerstone of the projects, and the mission is to reduce inequities in health status that exist among diverse populations in cities. The California Endowment to the Center for Civic Partnerships provided funding in 1998 to six communities (Baldwin Park, Berkeley, Montclair, Tulare, Victor Valley, and West Sacramento). Each community received technical assistance, consultation, and funding to achieve their goals. For example, under this program, Berkeley is addressing its high per-capita rate of pedestrian and bicycle injuries and fatalities, and West Sacramento is addressing its high crime rate.

An example of one of the first California Healthy Cities is the Bell Healthy City project. Bell's residents are largely ethnic minorities with an average income of $10,000 per year (Hafey, Twiss, and Folkers, 1992). The City Council voiced concern over the plight of the city and launched a series of Town Hall meetings to learn how to improve the city's quality of life. Community participation was encouraged. A number of goals were set to improve the quality of life in Bell, including developing recreational activities for all age groups; educating the community about graffiti, drug abuse, and vandalism; and providing the community with activities that foster a sense of community pride. Many of these goals currently are being implemented.

Since these initial Healthy Cities efforts in the United States, there are hundreds of Healthy Cities and Communities across the country that are seeking local solutions to complex problems. There are other statewide initiatives of Healthy Communities in states such as Maine, Massachusetts, Colorado, New Mexico, and South Carolina. There is also a national Coalition for Healthier Cities and Communities in which The Hospital Research and Education Trust in Chicago serves as the Coalition Secretariat. Other organizations that support networking among Healthy Cities and Communities include The Healthcare Forum, Healthy Cities and Communities, the Centers for Disease Control and Prevention, and the National Civic League.

Canada

Toronto, Ontario was one of the first cities to become involved in the Healthy Cities movement in North America. The movement began with a strategic planning committee to develop an overall strategy (Hancock, 1992). The committee conducted vision workshops in the community and a comprehensive environmental scan to help identify health needs in Toronto. The outcome was a final report outlining major issues with a strategic mission, priorities, and recommendations for action.

The Toronto Healthy City is involved in a number of projects. One of them is called *Healthiest Babies Possible.* This is an intensive antenatal education and nutritional supplement program for pregnant women who are identified by health and social agencies as high risk. The program includes intensive contact and follow-up of women along with food supplements. It has been successful in decreasing the incidence of low-birth-weight infants.

Another project known as *Parents Helping Parents* identifies children at high risk for neglect or abuse. Parents of these children are linked with specially trained health workers from similar sociocultural backgrounds to help them cope with problems of parenting and learn new and more effective parenting skills. Community participation is especially evident in this program in which community members, frequently from disadvantaged communities, are trained as health workers. The health workers are provided with new skills, a useful role in their communities, and a sense of self-esteem.

The Halton, Ontario Healthy City Project focuses on healthy eating. Through cooperation of community volunteers, community groups, the District Health Council, and the Halton Regional Health Department, Community Kitchens were established (Healthy Lifestyles Take Hold in Halton, 1994). Through pooling of resources (recipes, knowledge, and time), each member of the Community Kitchen is able to take home a variety of prepared meals, thereby reducing food costs. Classes on nutrition, food preparation, and shopping skills are offered to all participants. The spirit of this project spread to the local Salvation Army where ready-to-serve meals for the homeless are made available. In addition, the Girl Scouts Association became involved in Community Kitchens, resulting in a Brownie nutrition badge for girls working at the Kitchens.

Latin America

The Pan American Health Organization is promoting Healthy Municipalities in Central and South America with currently over 1000 Healthy Municipalities reported. Examples of Healthy Municipalities in Latin America are Cienfuegos, Cuba; Mexico City, Mexico; Manizales, Colombia; San Carlos, Costa Rica; and Valdivia, Chile.

FUTURE OF THE HEALTHY CITIES MOVEMENT
Facilitators

The continuance of the Healthy Cities movement is contingent upon several factors that can facilitate the process. The facilitators of the Healthy Cities movement have been identified as follows (Flynn, Rider, and Ray, 1991):

1. Overt and covert political support of the official power structure
2. Participation by smaller cities

3. Broad-based representation on Healthy City committees
4. Committee action that includes affirming values and envisioning common goals, resolving conflict, implementing projects, developing long-term plans that build healthy public policy, and building support for long-term actions
5. Technical support
6. Positive media response

Official political support is important for facilitating the Healthy City committee. Also, the level of political commitment can determine action taken by the committee. The size of the city affects the pace at which a Healthy City project is developed and implemented, with smaller cities typically moving faster. Healthy City committees that obtain broad-based representation are better able to identify community problems, develop and implement appropriate solutions to the problems, and build consensus in the community for support of the solutions. Successful Healthy City committee action enables the committee to continue health promotion action. Technical assistance to research problems and solutions, as well as to evaluate existing programs, facilitates the process. Local media support provides a positive image of the work conducted by the Healthy City committee (Flynn, Rider, and Ray, 1991).

Barriers

Three major barriers are noteworthy:

1. *Lack of political support.* Without support of local political officials, good ideas for health promotion action may not be realized, thereby limiting new health-related policies.
2. *Lack of broad-based representation on the Healthy City committee.* This may lead to action that reflects the needs of a select group within the community rather than comprehensive community health action. Lack of broad-based representation frequently leads to a "top-down" approach in which programs are planned by a few people with little community participation. The outcome of this approach is not likely to change the community's health.
3. *Size of the city.* Larger cities are more complex, making communication across various sectors of the city more difficult and time consuming (Table 17-1).

WHAT DO YOU THINK? *The support of local political officials in planning and implementing health and health-related programs in communities is critical to the development of the Healthy Cities program as well as that of healthy public policies.*

Healthy Public Policy

Healthy public policy is defined as health policies developed through a multisectoral and collaborative process with participation from those community members most

TABLE 17-1 Facilitators and Barriers of the Healthy Cities Movement

FACILITATORS	BARRIERS
Overt and covert political support	Lack of support by local officials
Smaller cities	Larger cities
Broad-based representation on Healthy City Committee	Lack of broad-based representation on Healthy City Committee
Committee action	
Technical support	
Positive media response	

Adapted from Flynn BC, Rider MS, Ray DW: Healthy Cities: the Indiana model of community development in public health, *Health Educ Q* 18(3):331, 1991.

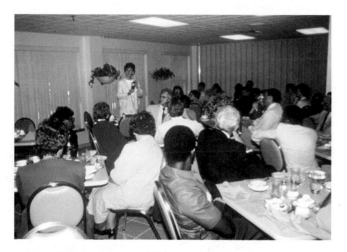

FIG. 17-1 A local-level Healthy Cities network meeting.

affected by the policy (Pederson et al, 1988). Healthy public policy supports health in a broad ecological sense that includes environmental, physical, social, and mental well-being. It transcends traditional departmental and governmental boundaries to include dialogue between policy makers and the public. The health effects of all public decisions are considered. In this sense, healthy public policy proposes a new way of thinking about health and government policy and links policymakers, professionals, and common citizens through a concern for health. Examples of healthy public policies are seat belt legislation, no-smoking policies in public buildings, motorcycle helmet laws, and immunization policies for school-age children. Healthy public policies create supportive environments for health by "making the healthy choices the easy choices" for people to make (Ashton, 1987).

The Healthy Cities movement supports the promotion of healthy public policy at the local level through multisectoral action and community participation (Fig. 17-1). As the Healthy Cities movement spreads worldwide, healthy public policies may become the norm for providing healthier environments in which to live.

IMPLICATIONS FOR NURSING

Nurses can use The CITYNET Manual developed by CITYNET-Healthy Cities staff to guide the community's work in Healthy Cities (Rider et al, 1993). The manual incorporates the nine steps of the CITYNET Healthy Cities process, which, in turn, offer examples of implications for nursing:

- *Step 1: Building the partnership for Healthy Cities.* Nurses can orient community leaders to the Healthy Cities process. Identify key city leaders, politicians, and health providers and talk to them about the health benefits of becoming a Healthy City.

NURSING TIP

Since nurses naturally work with community people from different walks of life and are respected health professionals in the community, they are well suited to promote Healthy Cities. Look for opportunities within existing community partnerships that you work with that are also interested in promoting the community's health. Plan how to introduce them to the Healthy Cities process, and work together to establish ideas about ways to initiate the Healthy Cities process with your combined network of contacts.

- *Step 2: Community commitment.* Nurses can answer policy makers' questions about what political commitment means to the community's health. They also can meet with heads of community agencies to solicit their commitment to the Healthy Cities process.
- *Step 3: Development of the Healthy City committee.* Based on the nurse's knowledge of key community people and populations at risk for problems, nurses can contact community leaders and other citizens to serve on the committee. Nurses can ensure that the committee represents the various sectors of the community. They may serve as a member of the committee, representing the public health sector.
- *Step 4: Leadership development in Healthy Cities.* Nurses recognize that although leaders exist in every community, they may not understand their potential in pro-

moting health. Nurses can recommend relevant consultants, speakers, conferences, workshops, and network sessions that are related to local concerns.

- *Step 5: Community assessment.* Nurses can conduct community assessments, such as windshield surveys and needs assessments. They can be a resource to the committee or work as a member of a team that conducts the community assessment.
- *Step 6: Community-wide planning for health.* Nurses can use group dynamics skills to help the Healthy City Committee identify their priorities and strategically plan for local health action.
- *Step 7: Community action for health.* Nurses can redirect community health services toward local priorities and plans. For example, nurses can facilitate by expanding a community health service, such as an exercise program for the elderly (Fig 17-2).
- *Step 8: Providing data-based information to policy makers.* Nurses may be asked to testify or assist others in preparing testimony that will be given to the city council or county commissioners about issues identified by the Healthy City Committee.
- *Step 9: Monitoring and evaluating progress.* Nurses may be asked by the Healthy City Committee to provide the data relevant to community health services and to assist them in recommending policy changes. Nurses also may coordinate or be part of a research team conducting program evaluation research.

DID YOU KNOW? *Nurses can help community leaders apply the CITYNET Healthy Cities process in their communities. They should begin where the community is, no matter what step of the CITYNET process the community begins with. Many communities begin with Step 5, Community assessment. Nurses often provide information that is used in a community assessment. They can use this as an opportunity to guide community leaders to report their findings back to the broader community. Communities may use the community assessment to not only identify needs and strengths in the community but also to obtain community commitment for participation in the overall Healthy Cities process. Community leaders need to understand that all steps are necessary to sustain Healthy Cities as an ongoing process in their community.*

Although these are examples of the practice of nursing in Healthy Cities, the nurse must recognize that the goal is to promote the community's leadership for health. In other words, he or she must not do for the community what it can do for itself. The role of the nurse and of other health professionals in Healthy Cities is to work in partnership with community leaders (Flynn, 1997). John Ashton (1989), one of the founders of the European Healthy Cities project, summarizes the role of health professionals in Healthy Cities as being "on tap, not on top."

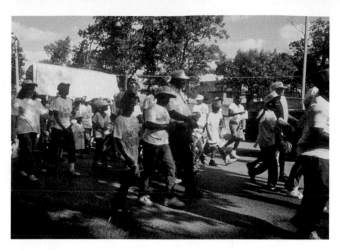

FIG. 17-2 A Healthy Cities-sponsored "Walk Against Drugs."

HOW TO *Organize a Community Meeting about Healthy Cities*

1. Identify who should be included in the community meeting. It is critical that all sectors and population groups in the community be involved.
2. How will they be invited to the meeting? Who will invite them? Allow at least 2 weeks so people can arrange their schedule.
3. Who will convene the meeting?
4. Set the date and time for the meeting and arrange for a neutral meeting place
5. Plan the meeting agenda.
   a. Introduction of participants
   b. Introduction to Healthy Cities
   c. Identification of community people who should be there—Who did we miss?
   d. Questions and discussion about Healthy Cities or community issues that are important
   e. Commitment to the Healthy Cities process
   f. Formation of the Healthy City Committee—obtaining names and addresses of those interested
   g. Other suggestions

HEALTHY PEOPLE 2010

The *Healthy People 2010* **objectives** are health objectives set through collaboration among government, voluntary, and professional organizations, businesses, and individuals as the means of providing access to health for all and improving health outcomes for the nation. The 2010 objectives will focus more on prevention, surveillance and data systems, quality health care, changes in demographics that include an older and more culturally diverse population, and diseases new to the twenty-first century. In addition, there will be greater focus on implementation of community participation and intersectoral collaboration to reflect the Health for All strategy set by the World Health Organization (WHO). The proposed framework for the objectives is titled *Healthy People in Healthy Communities*. This framework incorporates the WHO strategies for Health for All that acknowledges mental, physical, and social well-being as dependent upon health improvements at the individual, family, and community level. Within this framework, the overarching goals for the nation are as follows:

1. Increase years of healthy life plus quality of life
2. Eliminate health disparities

The overarching goals are accompanied by enabling goals that provide guidance to achieving the goals:

1. Promote healthy behaviors
2. Protect health
3. Ensure access to quality health care
4. Strengthen community prevention

The framework is further divided into 22 focus areas that are comparable with those used in the *Healthy People 2000* priority areas. Evaluating progress toward the objectives can be accomplished by measuring health outcomes and behavioral, health service, and community interventions that have been implemented (Poland, 1996). The nurse who understands the Healthy Cities model of health promotion and can implement the steps of the CITYNET-Healthy Cities process will be prepared to use the *Healthy People in Healthy Communities 2010* objectives to improve the health of individuals, families, and communities through community participation and multisectoral cooperation.

clinical application

Since the nurse works in partnership with the community in Healthy Cities, the examples of outcomes of Healthy Cities initiatives reflect that partnership rather than a specific nursing intervention. The principles of health promotion provide a framework for relating examples of outcomes in several Indiana cities that have used the CITYNET-Healthy Cities process.

An example of an outcome related to the first principle, promoting healthy public policy, is found in the New Castle, Indiana Healthy City. Healthy City Committee members provided testimony to the city council and drafted and supported an ordinance that was passed banning cigarette smoking in city buildings. An outcome related to the second principle, creating supportive environments, is found in the Fort Wayne, Indiana Healthy City. Healthy City Committee members collaborated in a community-wide program to address the fact that only 65% of Fort Wayne preschool children were immunized. Access to immunization services was expanded to five sites throughout the city at three different times in a program called "Super Shot Saturday." An example of an outcome related to strengthening community action is the strategy to collect information about health concerns from community residents at local health fairs. Several Healthy Cities committees used this strategy to encourage community participation in es-

tablishing priorities for action. An example of an outcome related to improving personal skills is the Seymour Healthy City's family fitness walk. An example of reorienting health services is the Clark County Community Health Clinic's expansion of services to the uninsured at one urban and two rural sites using nurse practitioners. These services are focused on disease prevention and health promotion of clients with selected chronic illnesses.

Which of the following concepts of primary health care and health promotion do these examples suggest?

A. Equity
B. Community Participation
C. Multisectoral Cooperation
D. Appropriate Technology
E. International Cooperation

Answer is in the back of the book.

KEY POINTS

- Although Healthy Cities began in the mid-1980s in Canada and Europe, it is now an international movement of cities focused on mobilizing local resources and political, professional, and community members to improve the health of the community.
- The principles of primary health care and health promotion guide the Healthy Cities movements.
- The models of community practice most frequently found in the Healthy Cities movement are locality development and social planning and an emphasis on partnerships with the community.
- Examples of Healthy Cities initiatives indicate that a broad range of health problems and issues are being addressed at the local level.
- The continuance of Healthy Cities is contingent upon several facilitators and barriers to the movement.
- As the Healthy Cities movement spreads worldwide, healthy public policies may become the norm for providing healthy environments in which to live.
- Implications of Healthy Cities for nursing can be organized by the steps of the CITYNET-Healthy Cities process.
- Outcomes of Healthy Cities suggest the successes of multisectoral community partnerships formed.
- The *Healthy People 2010* objectives incorporate community participation and intersectoral cooperation in their strategy for improving the health of individuals, families, and communities.

critical thinking activities

1. Evaluate the effectiveness of a current approach to a health problem in your community (e.g., teen pregnancy). Describe how the approach would change with implementation of the CITYNET-Healthy Cities process. Compare and contrast the two approaches in addressing this problem.
2. Discuss the role of the nurse in health promotion.
3. Identify city council members, the president of the Chamber of Commerce, the director of Family Services, the mayor, a religious leader, and other community

leaders who are the "movers and shakers" in getting things done. Generate a list of questions that will help these leaders describe the major strengths and problems of the community. Interview several local leaders and summarize their responses.

4. You are asked by the health commissioner to organize a community coalition for orientation to the Healthy Cities process. Outline the Healthy Cities process.

5. Describe your philosophy of community leadership development for health promotion.

6. Debate the model that is most effective in health promotion: social planning, community development, or social action.

7. Discuss ways in which proposed *Healthy People 2010* objectives can incorporate community participation and intersectoral cooperation. Examples of objectives are as follows:

a. Reduce to no more than 20% the proportion of children 6 years of age and younger who are regularly exposed to tobacco smoke at home. (Baseline: More than 39% in 1986, because 39% of households with one or more children 6 years of age or younger had a cigarette smoker in the household).

b. Increase to 95% the proportion of all females 15 to 44 years of age who use contraception at risk for unintended pregnancy.

Bibliography

Arnstein S: A ladder of citizen participation, *J Am Institute Planners* 35:216, 1969.

Ashton J: Making the healthy choices the easy choices, *Nutrition and Food Science,* Jul/Aug:2, 1987.

Ashton J: *Creating healthy cities.* Paper presented at Healthy Cities Indiana Network Session, Seymour, Indiana, May, 1989.

Ashton J: *Healthy cities,* Milton Keynes, UK, 1992, Open University Press.

Ashton J, Seymour H: *The new public health,* Philadelphia, 1988, Open University Press.

Biagh-Matzon K: Horsens. In Ashton J, editor: *Healthy cities,* Milton Keynes, UK, 1992, Open University Press.

Chamberlin RW: World Health Organization healthy cities and the US family support movements: a marriage made in heaven or estranged bed fellows? *Health Promotion International* 11(2):137, 1996.

Draper R et al: *WHO Healthy Cities project: review of the first five years (1987-1992),* Copenhagen, Denmark, 1993, WHO Regional Office for Europe.

Flynn BC: Healthy cities: a model of community change, *Family and Community Health* 15(1):13, 1992.

Flynn BC: Healthy cities: toward worldwide health promotion. *Annu Rev Public Health* 17:299, 1996.

Flynn BC: Partnerships is healthy cities and communities: a social commitment for advanced practice nurses, *Advanced Pract Nurs Q* 2(4):1, 1997.

Flynn BC: Partners for healthy cities, *Health Forum J* 37(3):55, 1994.

Flynn BC, Dennis LI: Healthy families. In Altergott K, editor: *One world many families,* Minneapolis, 1993, National Council on Family Relations.

Flynn BC, Ray D, Rider M: Empowering communities: action research through healthy cities, *Health Educ Q* 21(3):395, 1994.

Flynn BC, Rider MS, Ray DW: Healthy Cities: the Indiana model of community development in public health, *Health Educ Q* 18(3):331, 1991.

Goldstein G, Kickbush I: A healthy city is a better city, *World Health* 49(1):4, 1996.

Hafey JM, Twiss JM, Folkers LF: California. In Ashton J, editor: *Healthy cities,* Milton Keynes, UK, 1992, Open University Press.

Hancock T: The healthy city: utopias and realities. In Ashton J, editor: *Healthy cities,* Milton Keynes, UK, 1992, Open University Press.

Hancock T: The evolution, impact, and significance of the healthy cities/healthy communities movement, *J Public Health Policy* 14(1):5, 1993.

Healthy lifestyles take hold in Halton, *The Ontario Prevention Clearinghouse Newsletter* 4(3):4, 1994.

Ivanov LL, Flynn BC. Predictors of utilization and satisfaction with prenatal care services in St. Petersburg, Russia, *West J Nurs Res,* in press.

Minkler M: Improving health through community organization. In Glanz K, Lewis FM, Rimer BK, editors: *Health behavior and health education,* San Francisco, 1990, Jossey-Bass.

Pederson AP et al: *Coordinating healthy public policy: an analytic literature review and bibliography,* Canada, 1988, Ministry of National Health and Welfare.

Poland BD: Knowledge development and evaluation in, of, and for healthy community initiatives, Part II: Potential content foci, *Health Promotion International* 11(4):341, 1996.

Rider MS et al: *The CITYNET manual: how communities can (and do!) create healthy cities,* Indianapolis, 1993, Indiana University/Institute of Action Research for Community Health.

Rothman J, Tropman JE: Models of community organization and macro practice: their mixing and phasing. In Cox FM et al, editors: Strategies of community organization, ed 4, Itasca, Ill, 1987, Peacock.

Tsouros AD: *World Health Organization Healthy Cities Project: a project becomes a movement,* Copenhagen, Denmark, 1990, FADL Publishers.

Tsouros AD: World Health Organization Healthy Cities Project: state of the art and future plans, *Health Promotion International* 10(2):133, 1996.

USDHHS: *Developing objectives for Healthy People 2010,* Washington, DC, 1997, USDHHS, Office of Disease Prevention and Health Promotion.

USDHHS: *Healthy People 2000: national health promotion and disease prevention objectives,* Washington, DC, 1991, USDHHS, Public Health Service.

World Health Organization: *Book of abstracts: International Healthy Cities Conference,* Copenhagen, Denmark,1998, World Health Organization Regional Office for Europe.

World Health Organization: *Briefings on multi-city action plans: WHO Healthy Cities Project Phase II 1993-1997,* Copenhagen, Denmark, 1994, WHO Regional Office for Europe.

World Health Organization: *Ottawa charter for health promotion,* Copenhagen, Denmark, 1986, WHO Regional Office for Europe.

World Health Organization: *Twenty steps for developing a healthy cities project,* Copenhagen, Denmark, 1992, WHO Regional Office for Europe.

World Health Organization, United Nations Children's Fund: *Primary health care,* Geneva, Switzerland, 1978, WHO, UNICEF.

The Nursing Center: A Model of Community Health Nursing Practice

KATHERINE K. KINSEY & MARJORIE BUCHANAN

 www.mosby.com/MERLIN/community_stanhope

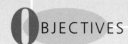BJECTIVES

After reading this chapter, the student should be able to do the following:

- Describe key characteristics of the nursing center model.
- Identify multilevel interventions for health.
- Identify three or more roles for advanced practice nurses in nursing centers.

- List three or more population groups who could be served by a nursing center.
- Discuss the value of community collaboration.
- Evaluate the feasibility of starting a nursing center.
- Analyze the nursing center model for nursing practice and research.

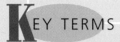EY TERMS

advanced practice nurses
community collaboration
community health
 workers

comprehensive primary
 health care centers
contracts
grants
multilevel interventions

nursing centers
parent organization
special care nursing
 centers
stakeholder

sustainability
wellness centers

See Glossary for definitions

CHAPTER OUTLINE

The authors acknowledge Sara Barger's prior work related to this chapter.

Nursing centers provide new opportunities to improve the health status of communities through direct access to nurses and nursing models of care. Working in partnership with the community, advanced practice nurses and other health professionals reach out to residents and provide comprehensive primary care services, public health programs, and targeted interventions for special needs populations.

In contrast to the prevailing illness-oriented and institution-based care with continuing inadequate health outcomes, nursing centers promoting the well-being of populations are located in accessible and familiar settings for community residents. Nursing centers provide direct access to health-oriented care (Buchanan, 1997). Nurses believe that there is growing evidence that this approach will improve health outcomes over time and contribute to reducing overall costs of care.

However, nursing centers are relatively new in today's health care delivery system. To secure their future, centers must confront and change traditional views held by policymakers, payers, managed care organizations, health systems, and other providers about nurses who provide and manage health care in noninstitutional settings (Lancaster, 1999). Thus advocating for changes in practice regulations, insurance, and payment for care overseen and delivered by nurses, as well as including health promotion and disease prevention in routine health care, are essential. With public and professional support, nursing centers will survive and thrive in the changing health care landscape.

Nursing centers and other community-oriented health services challenge nurses to expand their knowledge and skills. Responsible professionals must direct and manage health care services and possess superb clinical knowledge, skills, political abilities, and a business orientation. Nurses who possess these skills ensure the viability of nursing centers and the future of preventive care in an emerging and ever-changing health care system (Kinsey, 1999).

This chapter provides an overview of nursing centers, their origins, and their evolution to the present. Roles and responsibilities for nurses in delivering services, managing center operations, and providing educational opportunities are discussed. Recommendations for program evaluation and clinical research are presented. Strategies are presented to recognize opportunities that secure the future of nursing centers in the mainstream health care system.

OVERVIEW OF NURSING CENTERS

Over the past 25 years, a range of definitions has described nurse-managed community nursing practices. These descriptions have focused primarily on 1) ensuring direct access to nurses by those in the general public who do not require institutional points of entry, and 2) maintaining control over nursing practice by assuming responsibility and accountability for the following:
• Clinical and community health care in the center

• Multidisciplinary and interorganizational collaboration where appropriate
• High standards of care and monitoring of quality and outcomes
• Center operations, including management of staff, information systems, fundraising, and other fiscal affairs

In recent years, nursing centers have broadened these definitions to emphasize a health-orientation, connections to the communities, local factors that influence everyday life, and personal relationships with those they serve. In 1995, the American Nurses Association (ANA) issued a position paper on health promotion and disease prevention that supports the goals and objectives of individual nursing centers. The paper recognized health promotion strategies as the pivotal points of any health care system designed to control costs and reduce human suffering. The statement acknowledges that nursing's scope of practice includes prevention and that nursing's efforts should focus on health promotion and disease prevention interventions (ANA, 1995).

Nursing centers are strategically positioned to improve the health and well-being of vulnerable populations. They build on the core values and beliefs of the nursing discipline. Trust, health, caring, personal respect, equity and social justice serve as the foundation of a center, from which health is viewed as a resource for everyday life (Buchanan, 1997). Efforts focus on enhancing people's capacity to meet their personal, family, and community responsibilities and interests. As described in Box 18-1, a nursing center's mission, vision, purpose, and goals for services and programs are designed to address the interests and needs of particular populations. Examples of specific nursing center approaches and models are presented in Box 18-2 and Figure 18-1.

BOX 18-1 Elements Included in Nursing Centers

• *Multi-sector community partnerships* in establishing and supporting the center's health efforts
• *Holistic approach* to care based upon complex and interrelated biopsychosocial factors
• *Relationship-based practice* with individuals, families, and communities that fosters understanding of the environment, personal interests, and needs for health care
• *Community-oriented culturally competent care* that is accessible, acceptable, and responsive to the populations being served
• *Multi-level interventions* that acknowledge organizational, environmental, and health and social policy contributions to health, health problems, and issues of access to care
• *Interorganizational and interdisciplinary collaboration* that cross health and human service systems and increase opportunities for comprehensive and seamless services among care providers, agencies, and payers.

BOX 18-2 Overview of the La Salle Neighborhood Nursing Center in Philadelphia, Pennsylvania

MISSION

Through the development and implementation of exemplary health care and educational programs, the La Salle Neighborhood Nursing Center supports and enhances the teaching, learning, and service mission of the School of Nursing and the University.

VISION

The School of Nursing and its Neighborhood Nursing Center will be positioned as a nationally recognized provider of quality health care services in urban settings.

PURPOSE

The organization's general purpose is to provide access to public health nursing, counseling, and primary care services to underserved, urban residents in a multiculturally diverse community. Emphasis is placed on health promotion, disease and injury prevention, screening, detection, early intervention, and rehabilitation.

GOALS

• To improve the health of individuals, families, and their communities
• To provide direct access to primary health care services to underserved individuals, families, and groups
• To emphasize disease prevention and health promotion as well as national health objectives established by *Healthy People 2000* and *Healthy People 2010*
• To involve those who are at highest risk and least likely to be served by existing health care services through outreach and casefinding
• To evaluate program services and population-focused outcomes
• To promote organizational, environmental, and public policy change
• To provide community consultation
• To provide optimal community-based educational experiences for students and clients

From Kinsey K: *La Salle neighborhood nursing center annual report*, Philadelphia, Penn, 1999, La Salle University School of Nursing.

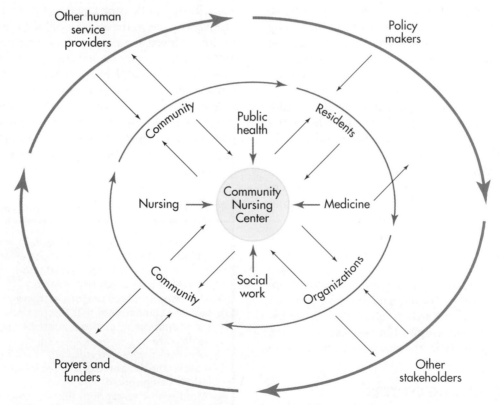

FIG. 18-1 The Lundeen community nursing center model. (From Sally Peck Lundeen, 1997)

HISTORICAL PERSPECTIVE: LOOKING BACK TO LOOK FORWARD

Present day nursing centers emerged from academic nursing programs in the 1970s. At that time, opportunities did not exist within the traditional health care system for faculty members or their new nurse practitioner students to apply their knowledge and skills within a nursing framework of care. Bold initiatives in schools of nursing at the University of Wisconsin–Milwaukee, Arizona State University, and other institutions led to the establishment of practice settings in partnership with nearby communities. These practices simultaneously provided health care to the community and learning experiences for nursing students. The success of these early efforts has generated academic nursing centers in colleges and universities across the country. Interest in this model is growing rapidly among community service organizations, schools, churches, public housing facilities, and many other organizations. Although there is no accurate record of how many nursing centers have been developed and where they are located, it appears that there are centers in nearly every state, and in urban, suburban, and rural communities alike. Most centers are viewed as "safety net providers" and provide care for vulnerable populations who face significant barriers to accessible and affordable health care (National Health Policy Forum, 1998). Many centers are expanding and providing services in multiple satellite sites, or "outposts."

Nursing centers can trace their origins to the beginning of public health nursing in the past century. Poor living conditions and evident health needs of poor and immigrant families provided the driving force for the establishment of the Henry Street Settlement in New York City by Lillian Wald in 1893. Her vision of nursing practice included health teaching and disease prevention for those who were well, care for the sick and infirm, and advocacy for health reforms that included education, industrial safety, housing, and recreation. The Henry Street model engaged the community in both health and social services (Reverby, 1993). Notable outcomes of this model were professional obstetrical care becoming more acceptable, stabilization of family life, and housing improvements. In addition, the comprehensive approach contributed to the decline of infectious diseases and school absenteeism (Buhler Wilkerson, 1993).

DID YOU KNOW? *Nursing centers can trace their origins back to Lillian Wald's public health nursing work and the establishment of the Henry Street Settlement in New York City in 1893.*

In 1916, Margaret Sanger challenged tradition and started the first birth control clinic. She provided women with much needed information about family planning and contraceptive methods with a goal of improving the health of women and their families through health education. In 1925, Mary Breckenridge developed a decentralized model of care in rural Kentucky and opened the first of six sites comprising the Frontier Nursing Services. Bedside nursing, midwifery, infant and preschooler health programs, immunizations, and school health services for isolated rural families were then provided on horseback and today in all terrain vehicles (Glass, 1989). See Chapter 2 for more details about the history of nursing programs and services.

In 1948, the World Health Organization (WHO) provided its first formal definition of health. In 1978, that definition was updated to describe health as a person's state of physical, mental, and social well-being that is adequate to allow the person to live a productive life in the community. Emphasis was placed on the importance of full and organized community participation and ultimate self-reliance, with individuals, families, and communities assuming more responsibility for their own health (WHO, 1978). Commitments were made by nations to strive for primary health care for all by the year 2000.

However, medical care developments during World War II led to postwar creation of institutional facilities and a biomedical infrastructure that began to dominate the health care landscape. As institutional care rose, care in the community diminished until both social and economic concerns began to rise. Limited health care access by the poor and elderly as well as racial differences in health status led to new public policy developments such as Medicare and Medicaid in the 1960s and 1970s. Rising costs of care led to managed care efforts in the 1980s, such as diagnosis-related groups (DRGs) and health maintenance organizations (HMOs). Furthermore, the aging of the population and rising rates of preventable chronic and communicable diseases and other conditions indicated a need to redirect health care priorities, policies, and financing mechanisms away from costly illness-oriented care toward a health-oriented model of care (WHO, 1999) (Fig. 18-2).

The nurse practitioner role was established in 1965. This role enabled nurses to provide primary health care to clients and heralded the beginning of today's nursing centers. Many university-based or academic nursing centers began in the 1970s to provide services, student learning experiences, and sites for faculty practice and research (Murphy, 1995). In the 1970s, nurses were challenged to develop new means for providing nursing care and delivering nursing services by establishing nursing centers in institutional, community, and primary care settings.

M. Lucille Kinlein in 1971 established the first independent nurse practice. She stated, "I became convinced that the only way to identify precisely and meet satisfactorily the nursing needs of people was to change the setting in which I came into contact with persons in need of nursing care" (Kinlein, 1972, p.23).

The first national nursing centers' conference was held in 1982 to share experiences and ideas, followed by a second conference in 1984. A definition of *nursing centers* was agreed upon that encompassed the provision of holistic, client-centered health services using a nursing model. Participants in the third conference in 1986 determined that affiliation with a national nursing organization would further their efforts to promote nursing centers, which led to the group's 1988 integration with the National League for Nursing (NLN). A special practice council within the NLN was formed and named the Council for Nursing Centers, which serves as a communication hub for many centers across the country (Murphy, 1995).

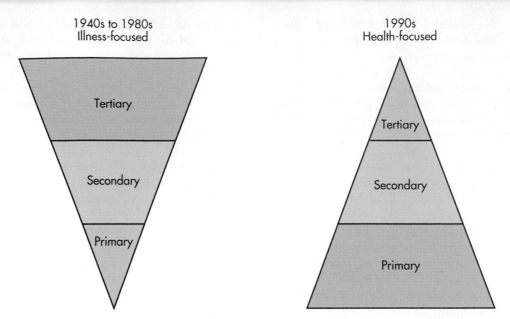

FIG. 18-2 The paradigm shift from illness-focused care in the 1940s through 1980 to health-focused care in the 1990s.

By the mid 1980s, the ANA Nursing Centers Task Force developed the most frequently cited and still current nursing center definition.

Nursing Centers—sometimes referred to as community nursing organizations, nurse managed centers, nursing clinics, and community nursing centers—are organizations that give the client direct access to professional nursing services. Using nursing models of care professional nurses in these centers diagnose and treat human responses to actual and potential health problems, and promote health and optimal functioning among target populations and communities. The services provided in these centers are holistic, client-centered, and reimbursed at a reasonable fee level. Nurses maintain accountability and responsibility for client care and professional practice. Overall accountability and responsibility remain with the nurse executive. Nursing centers are not limited to any particular organizational configuration. They can be freestanding businesses or affiliated with universities or other service institutions like home health agencies and hospitals. The primary characteristic of the organization is responsiveness to the health needs of the population. (Aydelotte et al, 1987, p. 1).

Other elements of nursing center models include health promotion, disease prevention, and multidisciplinary collaboration. Many centers also include student learning, faculty practice, and research.

During the past 2 decades, financial support for nursing centers has come from both the public and private sectors. The Division of Nursing in the U.S. Department of Health and Human Services (USDHHS) has made special project grants to nursing centers since the mid-1970s to improve public access to nurses in noninstitutional community settings. This funding has launched many of the most promising nursing center models. Currently funding 33 centers in various locales across the country, the Division of Nursing

continues to explore challenging nursing center issues and prioritize these issues for funding (Clear, Starbecker, and Kelly, 1998).

Also during the past 2 decades, the W.W. Kellogg and Robert Wood Johnson Foundations have made start-up grants and special project grants to nursing centers. Private foundation support is particularly important for centers that are not academically based and thus ineligible for Division of Nursing funds. Regardless of the type of funding sources available to a nursing center, all require fiscal support for start-up operations as well as the on-going provision of services that are not typically reimbursed with existing health care dollars.

DID YOU KNOW? *Nursing centers can be found in every region of the United States.*

Nursing centers have proliferated throughout the 1990s. In addition to academic-based centers, there is an increasing number of centers established by community organizations, schools, senior centers, churches, and housing and assisted living facilities to serve vulnerable populations. Interest in nursing centers is growing in populations who recognize their need for ready access to care. As the health care system moves toward community health-oriented services, clients' needs and interests in nursing centers will dictate that centers become preferred models for care as the nation moves into the next century. The newest challenge to this model of care will be the conflict between the business side of nursing centers (Kinsey, 1999) in a managed care environment and the commitment to use the *Healthy People 2010* framework in nursing center practice, which is discussed in the next section.

BOX 18-3 *Healthy People 2010* Aims and Focus Areas

The aims of *Health People 2010* are as follows:
- Promote healthy behaviors
- Promote healthy and safe communities
- Improve systems for personal and public health
- Prevent disease and disorders
  Healthy People 2010 focus areas are as follows:
- Physical activity and fitness
- Nutrition
- Tobacco use
- Educational and community-based programs
- Environmental health
- Food safety
- Injury and violence prevention
- Occupational safety and health
- Oral health
- Access to quality health services
- Family planning
- Maternal, infant, and child health
- Medical product safety
- Public health infrastructure
- Health communication
- Arthritis, osteoporosis, and chronic back conditions
- Cancer
- Diabetes
- Disability and secondary conditions
- Heart disease and stroke
- Human immunodeficiency virus
- Immunizations and infectious diseases
- Mental health and mental disorders
- Respiratory disease
- Sexually transmitted diseases
- Substance abuse

From Office of Disease Prevention and Health Promotion: *Developing objectives for Healthy People 2000*, Washington, DC, 1997, USDHHS.

Healthy People 2010

The Healthy People initiative has framed the nation's health promotion and disease prevention agenda since 1980. *Healthy People 2010* builds on *Healthy People 2000*, the 1990 goals, and the lessons learned. It also represents a partnership including government, voluntary, and professional organizations, businesses, and individuals. *Healthy People 2010* goals are to eliminate health disparities and to increase years of quality and healthy life with greater emphasis on healthy communities (USDHHS, 1997).

The context in which *Healthy People 2010* aims and objectives have been developed differs from prior decades (Box 18-3). It accounts for demographic changes in the nation, with its more racially and culturally diverse and older populations, technological advances, worldwide communication systems, and preventive therapies (vaccines and pharmaceuticals). These changes and other worldwide events will continue to alter public health perspectives and professional practices and roles (Shoultz and Amundson, 1998).

TYPES OF NURSING CENTERS AND MULTILEVEL INTERVENTIONS

Each nursing center has a "personality" of its own. Its mission, values, goals, and purpose as well as the commitment to community well-being contribute to any nursing center's profile (Henderson, McManus, and Morris, 1996). Many nursing centers reflect the history and growth of the lead organization, be it academic, freestanding non-profit, visiting nurse, home health, or a proprietary agency. Occasionally, the structure of a nursing center bridges several organizational entities to accommodate the needs of an institution or community (Harris, 1999).

Types of Centers

In many communities, nursing center services are actually **comprehensive primary health care centers.** Services include community outreach; physical and mental/behavioral health; linkages to specialized health care and social support; public health programs that include health education, screening, immunizations, and home visiting; enabling services such as translation, child care; advocacy; and policy development; and program evaluation (IOM, 1998).

Other nursing centers have a particular focus. These centers are viewed by the community as **special care nursing centers** for unique populations or wellness centers. The services of a special care/special population nursing center are carefully designed to respond to the expressed needs of individuals and families. These models are limited in number and are viewed as an adjunct to comprehensive primary health care models (Henderson, McManus, and Morris, 1996). Special care nursing centers include continence programs for women, midwifery services for adolescent mothers, and senior health centers.

On the other hand, **wellness centers** complement the existing primary care services in the community. These centers focus on health promotion and disease prevention and serve as linking agents to community resources. They offer social support and enabling services and ensure that families access and use health care services appropriately.

Regardless of the nursing center service model, the populations involved are diverse and typically have interrelated individual health, social, and community needs. The types of populations served can range from middle-class insured adults and their families to families with no health care coverage. The age grouping of clients can be the focus of the nursing center model (a special population center could serve solely pediatric HIV/AIDS or geriatric clients), or the age of clients can represent a community profile with ages ranging from the very young to the very old. Many nursing centers provide comprehensive services to vulnerable at-risk population groups. Box 18-4 presents some population groups that could benefit from nursing center services in local areas.

These unique populations have varied needs. Personal resources, family supports, and community programs may be lacking. Nurses working in a nursing center environment must be skilled in applying **multilevel interventions** at the individual/family, community, and system levels to make positive change happen for clients and others.

Multilevel Interventions

Nursing center staff may focus their efforts on system issues, community capacity, or building family and individual health care access, or the staff may concentrate program efforts solely at the individual or family level and later address system and community issues (Table 18-1). There is no one approach. Figure 18-3 suggests that this approach should incorporate the "big picture" and that the majority of interventions will take place in community (out of hospital) settings.

Imagine a web of neighborhood-based centers with the following characteristics:
• People can be understood within the context of everyday life.
• Community residents can be encouraged and educated about healthy lifestyles and health care practices through public health education programs.
• Common barriers to care, such as transportation, child care, language, and cultural differences, can be overcome with an array of enabling and supportive services.

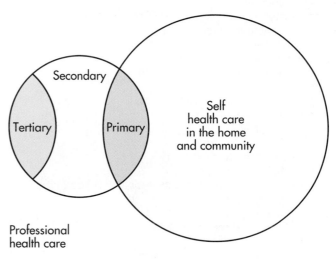

FIG. 18-3 Primary health care model. (Adapted from Goeppinger J: Primary health care: an answer to the dilemmas of community nursing, *Nurs Outlook* 1(3):129, 1984)

BOX 18-4 Populations Served by Nursing Centers

Elderly persons and their families
Culturally and linguistically diverse groups (e.g., Russians, Albanians, Mexicans, Koreans)
Homeless persons
Migrant workers
Children and youth in public and independent schools
Underimmunized children and adults
HIV-positive individuals
Incarcerated persons
Childbearing adolescent and adult women
Minority males with history of hypertension

TABLE 18-1 Focus of Health Efforts at Different Intervention Levels

MULTI-LEVEL INTERVENTION	FOCUS OF EFFORTS FOR HEALTH
Individual and family	Primary care service that is accessible, acceptable, and affordable for people across the age continuum
	Care management within the context of families' everyday lives and with their full participation
	Access to specialty care and treatment programs through institutional and other community providers
	Family centered rather than public health promotion and disease prevention programs and services
	Enabling and supportive services appropriate for each family in overcoming barriers to health and health care
Community	Increased community capacity for health through public awareness and education
	Increased understanding about and strategic interventions regarding environmental factors causing or contributing to health problems
	Linked community and institutional health care resources
	Partnerships with housing, law, education, environmental, and other sectors for improved health and human service delivery
System	Health insurance for all that includes both health and illness care
	Policies and funding that support healthy communities across sectors, such as housing, legal aid, education, child care, and others
	Regulatory and payer recognition of nonphysician providers

- People can enter earlier, with greater ease and confidence, and continue in care long enough to realize positive outcomes.

The implementation of multilevel interventions requires that nursing center staff have the advanced skills and the commitment to work with diverse groups. In addition, the staff must have the administrative support and staff expertise to make constructive contributions to community well-being happen. If applied appropriately, the multilevel intervention approach can help people enter the health care system earlier, with greater ease and confidence, and to continue in care long enough to realize positive outcomes (Fig. 18-4).

WHAT DO YOU THINK? *Is it possible to apply multilevel interventions with one or more clients in any clinical setting?*

ESSENTIAL NURSING CENTER ROLES AND EVOLVING RESPONSIBILITIES

Nursing center models support the development of advanced practice nurses and allied health professionals in the fields of primary care, public health, and specialty care. The nursing center type, or "personality," and its related services determine nursing roles and responsibilities as well as staffing patterns. In addition, funding sources dictate staffing assignments. Furthermore, local community input and resources shape the nursing center services and staff roles. The center's organizational framework evolves from the parent organization's structure (university, health department) as well as the dynamics of programs and staff roles. The framework shows the roles and responsibilities of one or many involved in this model of care.

An essential role shared by every nursing center is that of nurse executive or director. Other positions may include advanced practice nurses such as public health nurses, nurse practitioners, nurse midwives, and community health clinical nurse specialists, as well as onsite ambulatory care staff, students, community health workers, support staff, and other providers and community members.

Director

The director, or nurse executive, is an individual committed to the nursing center model. The director is knowledgeable about the target community and the community receiving service; has the ability and willingness to work with many community organizations and groups; and has a background in organizational planning, administration, and fiscal management. The roles and responsibilities of the nurse executive are dynamic and diverse. The nurse executive is responsible for grantsmanship, oversight of contracts and grants, annual reports, and development of an advisory board or board of directors. If the nurse executive is a faculty member, another role is that of faculty liaison with other university and school faculty members. Frequently this nurse is viewed by community members as the spokesperson on their behalf with other health, social, and educational organizations. In these instances, the director must possess superb communication skills and an established background in policy and program development (Brown, 1997).

Successful nursing centers are directed and managed by nurses who understand the bottom line. These directors dedicate time to the planning processes and develop strategies to keep nursing centers in the business of direct nursing care to community members. The directors use data, collaborative feedback, and existing resources to modify and adjust the overall direction of the nursing center as indicated. Difficult and realistic decisions must be made if funding sources and public policies change and alter the nature of the nursing center's operation (Mackey and McNeil, 1997).

Advanced Practice Nurse

Advanced practice nurses have additional education and training beyond their basic nursing program. This prepares

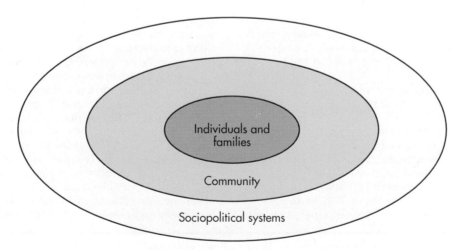

FIG. 18-4 Multilevel intervention.

them to provide an expanded level of health services to individuals and families. Public health nurses, nurse practitioners, mental health specialists, and other clinical nurse specialists such as community health clinical specialists are considered advanced practice nurses. Frequently, advanced practice nurses coordinate one or more service programs. These nurses are responsible for the oversight of other clinical staff as well as planning, coordinating, and evaluating program outcomes. Programs can include pediatric primary care, home visiting for pregnant women, substance abuse counseling for women and their families, and lead poisoning prevention education to caregivers of young children.

Community and Public Health Nurse

Nurses with advanced preparation in community or public health nursing are essential to the advancement of nursing center services. These nurses use nursing and public health principles to promote and sustain the health of populations in neighborhood and community settings. Their work is diverse. It ranges from assessing a population's need and interest in health care to writing a grant for expanding services. These nurses implement group health education classes and screenings and provide case management in community and home settings. Community and public health nurses advocate for changes in community life that will improve the health of residents. Box

18-5 demonstrates the skills of public health nurses to work with community members and a partnering hospital to initiate a nurse-managed center and to engage residents in ongoing primary health care.

Nurse Practitioner

The implementation phase described in Box 18-5 principally uses nurse practitioners for the provision of onsite services. This is the case with some centers. In other centers, nurse practitioners provide both onsite and in-home services (McNeil and Mackey, 1995). Other nursing centers integrate nurse practitioner services with public health services. Because of changes in the Medicare reimbursement regulations, nurse practitioners can now conduct in-home assessments and clinical follow-up of homebound seniors or provide center-based services to people 65 years of age or older in urban and rural settings.

The academic and clinical preparation of the nurse practitioner varies from center to center. A "specialty care" center targeting the frail elderly may only have geriatric nurse practitioners available for services. Comprehensive primary health care centers will have family, adult, and pediatric nurse practitioners available. The staffing pattern for a full complement of nurse practitioners varies depending on client characteristics, patterns of use, community access factors, funding sources, and site environment.

BOX 18-5 "If You Staff It, Residents Will Come to a Nurse Managed Health Center"

One community/home health agency with a 100-year history of providing preventive services and in-home nursing care for individuals of all ages merged its resources with a neighboring hospital. The merging of services evolved into the establishment of a nurse-managed health center in an underserved suburban setting. Public health nurses, employees of the home health agency, and hospital personnel worked with local residents to determine community need and to create plans for the health center. Community members considered the health center to be one aspect of improving their neighborhood through this expansion of their existing community center. Residents had identified three major problems in their neighborhood:
1. Access to services with significant financial and transportation barriers
2. Need for ongoing psychosocial interventions
3. Lack of provider familiarity of the community and home environments

Agency staff, with the assistance of nursing students and faculty members, conducted a door-to-door survey in the two targeted census tracts. Other health problems were identified by the survey, including lack of access to health education and an overuse of hospital emergency departments for episodic care. About 47% of those surveyed reported that they had visited an emergency department between one to seven times within the past 12 months. Based on community interest, documented health needs of the target population, and fiscal commitments by the hospital for site renovation, a nurse-managed center was established at the community center in 1996.

Despite all the work before the center was opened, the collaborative work between the community and the health center staff had just begun. This model was new in this setting; residents were unaccustomed to ongoing care. Trust had to be built. The question initially was "If you build it, will people come?" Two years later, the question has changed to "If you staff it, will people come?" Yes is the resounding answer. Much planning, outreach, and relationship building was required by all parties. Graduate public health and nurse practitioner students and undergraduate nursing students have been involved since the center began. Their contributions have helped the number of clients and use of the primary health care services increase over time. In 2 years, the number of clients and client contacts has exceeded client growth targets per year. Current data document clients' pattern changes in the use of primary health care, the use of emergency departments for episodic care, and community satisfaction with the nursing center in their neighborhood.

Contributed by Marilyn Harris, RN, MSN, Executive Director, Abington Memorial Hospital Home Care, Abington, Pennsylvania.

Nurse Midwife

In primary health care nursing centers, nurse midwives are proven assets. Nurse midwives provide prenatal, childbirth, postpartum and family planning services in the centers or affiliated health care institutions. In addition, they make home visits as needed to adolescent and adult childbearing women. Nurse midwives collaborate with other advanced practice colleagues and together develop initiatives that address the needs of women and their families.

Clinical Nurse Specialist

The roles and responsibilities of a clinical nurse specialist vary with client populations and an individual specialist's educational and practice background. For example, one center may need a clinical nurse specialist for mental health and substance abuse counseling. This specialist may have a master's or doctorate degree in mental health nursing as well as certification as an addictions counselor. Another center may identify a need for a community health ad-

vanced practice nurse with incontinence therapy skills to work with clients and family members concerning incontinence.

Onsite Ambulatory Care Nurse

Nurses with other educational and experiential backgrounds, including baccalaureate preparation, are needed to carry out nursing center core functions. Functions include client assessment and triage, assisting with primary health care services, and initiating onsite educational programs. These programs help clients and their families become more self-reliant. Onsite nurses are often the first contact and link for clients within the nursing center complex. The responsibilities of the ambulatory care nurse are multiple and interrelated. Telephone triage, appointment follow-up, pregnancy testing and counseling, childhood and adult immunizations, linkages with school nurses, data collection, and reports are necessary responsibilities in this practice setting.

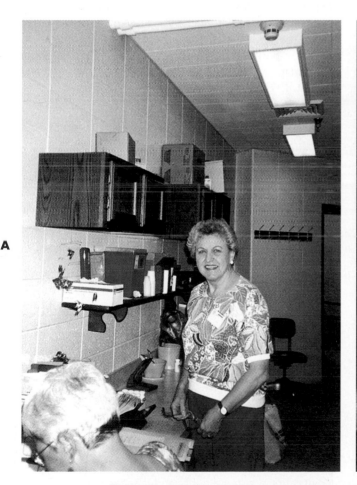
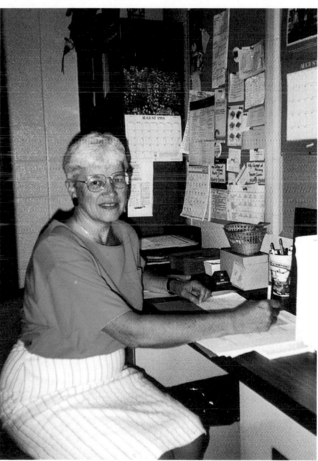

Two staff members at a university nursing center. **A,** Nurse volunteer Agnes Black assists nursing staff in delivery of care at the University of Kentucky College of Nursing's Nurse-Managed Center for the Homeless. **B,** Public Health Clinical Nurse Specialist Ruth Berry serves as nurse director of the University of Kentucky College of Nursing's Nurse-Managed Center for the Homeless.

Community Health Worker

Community health workers are essential staff in many nursing centers in the United States. Community health workers are paraprofessionals who often are neighborhood residents who have completed high school or 2-year associate degree programs. They want to work with others in their community. The workers are trained in community outreach, family case management, or onsite services. The workers are assigned activities that target population groups in specific neighborhoods or core census tracts. For example, a worker could be involved in cancer prevention education with high-risk minority adults in a targeted neighborhood.

Support Staff

The operations of any nursing center require support staff. Typically, the staff includes a business or operations manager and data operations personnel. The **parent organization** may dedicate a portion of staff lines, including human resources and public relations, to assist the director and senior staff. It is ideal if an advanced practice nurse has a business and personnel management background. These are areas that more nurses should be qualified to assume. The operations manager handles the contracts and grant budgets, advertising for staff, personnel hires, and billing. The operations manager often handles personnel management, staffing patterns, site management, and data collection.

Data operations personnel are essential as any nursing center develops. Client- and population-based outcomes are necessary for program evaluation, proposal development, and funding purposes. Documented short- and long-term outcomes are presented to funding agencies, policy makers, community members, and the public.

Other support staff may be involved in public relations and multimedia campaigns to introduce the nursing center model to the general public and to gain support as the center expands. It is important to maintain communication with the local media and to alert the media to new programs. All staff should contribute educational articles to the newspaper for publication.

Other Providers and Community Members

Other providers are engaged in nursing center work as physician collaborators or as administrative and clinical social work and outreach staff of various community organizations. Representation is diverse and variable. Organizations such as local churches, synagogues and mosques, independent and public schools, Head Start programs, day care centers, hospitals, and county health departments have staff that work with nursing center staff, clients, and their extended families.

Students

Students have important roles in these centers. They can work on a particular program or grant-funded project. Nursing students have opportunities to learn about the overall center functions and the interactions of health care economics, service, education, and research (Josten, Aroskar, and Shannon, 1996). Students have varied and challenging work with community members and learn to develop communication strategies that engage community members in determining health practices for themselves and their families (Ryan et al, 1997). Box 18-6 lists roles of students.

COMMUNITY COLLABORATION

Community collaboration influences the development of a nursing center's philosophy, goals, and organizational structure. Successful collaboration relates to the center's capacity to address common purposes with community members. Everyone involved in this process is a critical **stakeholder** interested in community wide benefits and committed to working together. Collaboration includes the staff's ability to share risks, responsibilities, resources, and rewards with others who may be relatively new stakeholders in the collaboration process (William, Greenwald, and Nudelman, 1996). Box 18-7 lists common collaborators. Collaboration enhances the capacity of another person, group, or organization for mutual benefit and achieves a common purpose (Burger et al, 1998). Skills in networking, coordination, and cooperative learning are necessary (Burke, 1997).

BOX 18-6 Student Roles

Advocate
Data collector
Evaluator
Learner
Planner
Collaborator
Educator
Facilitator
Partner
Provider

BOX 18-7 Examples of Community Collaborators

Industries with full- and part-time employees
Small businesses
Local hospitals
Religious organizations
Parish nurses
Home care agencies/visiting nurse associations
Educational systems: public and independent
Recreation centers
Local police district
Juvenile/family court
Senior centers
Public housing for low-income families and seniors

Executive directors, faculty members, staff members, and students need to recognize factors that influence successful collaboration. The factors can also lead to the redesign of a nursing center's organizational framework, mission, and goals. The six factors are environment, membership characteristics, process and structure of the group, communication patterns, purpose of the collaboration, and resources within and outside the group (Mattessich and Monsey, 1992). Table 18-2 provides examples of each factor.

THE BUSINESS OF NURSING CENTERS: GOVERNANCE, START-UP, AND SUSTAINABILITY
Governance

The efforts of community collaboration often influence the governance of nursing centers; therefore the governance structure varies from center to center. It is important to know the governance structure and the persons responsible for decision-making processes on a day-to-day basis as well as overall administrative and fiscal oversight. For example, if the parent organization is a university, its board of trustees is the overall governing body. In this instance, a nursing center will have input by an advisory board or committee. This committee does not have financial responsibilities; the board of trustees does. The advisory committee is responsible for clinical oversight of the programs, professional development, fundraising, and community networking. It is composed of community members, professionals, and representatives of other groups. Members commit to periodic meetings and workgroups

that support the development and growth of the nursing center.

The composition of a board of trustees or an advisory board should reflect the community's demographic profiles. The nomination and selection of members is critical for the future of the nursing center. The members represent diverse work, educational, and professional backgrounds. Quarterly or more frequent meetings are held. Students and staff should have opportunities to attend scheduled meetings and workgroups.

The nursing center development outline displayed in Box 18-8 is a reference for students, faculty members, staff members, and community members. It is one tool to guide the development of a nursing center and is a checklist for established nursing centers.

Start-Up and Sustainability

Several factors must be considered when starting a nursing center (Shaw, Brown, and Bromiley, 1998). Nurses must be willing to seek expert advice and support throughout the exploratory phases. Most importantly, they must understand that this work is a business enterprise in which the art and science of nursing will be practiced. **Sustainability** of a nursing center involves effort and resources needed to deliver health programs and services in an effective, consistent, and reliable manner over time so as to achieve desired outcomes.

Nurses with an understanding of business can use financial advisors as they plan whether to start a nursing center. Final decisions about establishing a nursing center

TABLE 18-2 Factors Influencing the Success of Collaboration

FACTORS RELATED TO:	FACTORS
Environment	History of collaboration or cooperation in the community
	Collaborative group seen as a leader in the community
	Political/social climate favorable
Membership characteristics	Mutual respect, understanding, and trust
	Appropriate cross-section of members
	Members see collaboration as in their self-interest
	Ability to compromise
Process/structure	Members share a stake in both processes and outcome
	Multiple layers of decision making (participative)
	Flexibility
	Development of clear roles and policy guidelines
	Adaptability
Communication	Open and frequent communication
	Established informal and formal communication links
Purpose	Concrete, attainable goals and objectives
	Shared vision
	Unique purpose
Resources	Sufficient funds
	Skilled convener

From Mattessich P, Monsey B: *Collaboration: what makes it work*, St Paul, Minn, 1992, Amherst H. Wilder Foundation.

BOX 18-8 Outline of Essential Elements in the Development of a Nursing Center

I. Organizational development
   A. Governance structure and process guidelines
      1. Governance structure and process (board member composition, roles and responsibilities, subgroups/committees, leadership positions, decision-making process, voting privileges, linkages to program administration and staff, etc.)
      2. Meeting schedule for all groups, committees, etc.
      3. Mechanisms for communicating information, project progress, meetings, etc.
      4. Mechanisms for follow-up action on governing board decisions/actions
   B. Administrative activities
      1. Role and responsibilities of project directors/project administrators/program manager
      2. Fiscal management system and personnel
      3. Information management system and personnel
      4. Oversight of overall project progress, process, outcomes, cost
      5. Personnel policies/supervision of staff
   C. Advisory Committee(s)
      1. Structure (connections to governing board, project administration, program services)
      2. Membership composition; appointment process, term of membership
      3. Leadership positions and process for elections
      4. Roles and responsibilities
      5. Working groups or committees
      6. Meeting schedule
II. Program development
   A. Needs assessment (project director, collaborating partners, and community)
      1. Overview of city
      2. Target populations for each program
      3. Specific community assessments of target populations
   B. Plan for community collaboration and project governance
      1. Model for multi-sector collaboration (health, education, business, law, community residents, etc.) in project governance
      2. System for community communication about the project (public forums, public information campaigns, etc.)
      3. Structures for community advisement on program services (advisory committees, community workers as staff, etc.)
   C. Program plan (nurse practitioner or clinical nurse specialist)
      1. Program goals for improvements in community health status, client services, nursing education, faculty practice and research, and objectives (stated as measurable outcomes)
      2. Program activities to meet objectives and timeline for implementation
      3. Communication with multidisciplinary professional resources (MD, nutritionist, etc.)
      4. Communication with network of referral agencies
      5. Monitoring and coordination of program service delivery (quality management)
      6. Program staff supervision
   D. Administrative/business plan (nurse administrator/business manager)
      1. Ensuring follow-up action to governing board decisions
      2. Overall project oversight (ensuring adherence to policies and procedures, achievement of goals and objectives, etc.)
      3. Systems oversight (fiscal management, information management, program management, collaboration process management, service contracts/linkages with other systems [education or other])
      4. Personnel management
   E. Information management plan (data systems analyst)
      1. Client care records
      2. Aggregate program records
      3. Fiscal records
      4. Health status indicators/project benchmark data
   F. Evaluation plan (nurse evaluator)
      1. Formative (monitoring collaborative process, progress in meeting project goals and objectives, making midcourse corrections)
      2. Summative (measuring degree to which overall goals and objectives were met, their impact on health status [education, or other elements of project], and analysis of outcomes with regard to balance in quality of care, access to care, and cost of care/project)
   G. Sustainability plan (project directors and collaborating partners)
      1. Maintaining balance among quality of care, access to care, and cost of care
      2. Obtaining reimbursement for services
      3. Developing long-term strategic plan
      4. Identifying sources of other support (federal grants, private foundation grants, volunteer development, miscellaneous fundraising activities)

will be made through in-depth exploration of the following areas:
1. Organizational goals, commitments, and resources
2. Community interests, assets, and needs
3. Feasibility study, internal and external to the parent organization
4. Strategic plan
5. Business plan
6. Information management plan and resources
7. Existing social policy and health care financing
8. Legal and regulatory considerations

Assessment phase

The initial work of assessing the interests, resources, and capacity of an organization to establish a nursing center model is interrelated yet separate. For example, a feasibility study may be undertaken before the development of a business plan, but elements of the feasibility study will be incorporated into the business plan. Similarly, a strategic plan builds on feasibility data as well as economic principles and practices. Other considerations include workforce needs, a personnel management plan, public information and outreach campaigns, community capacity, and the health care environment to support funding (Rhyne et al, 1998).

Feasibility study. A feasibility study reveals the strengths, limitations, and capacity of an organization and the community to support a nursing center. It requires interviews with key individuals, surveys, and data-collection methods that yield essential information. The methods include focus groups and community forums.

Epidemiologic, environmental, and other existing community assessments should be examined and interpreted. The feasibility study includes relevant and current data from local public health agencies. Local government, social service agencies, and tertiary care institutions can provide data that indicate health needs and gaps in care for targeted groups. Examination of legal and regulatory criteria must be undertaken. Each state has regulations regarding advanced practice nurses, particularly nurse practitioners. These regulations must be reviewed and understood.

Planners will participate in all review processes and support community collaboration. The overall process supports the development of business plans and strategic plans.

Business plan. A sound business plan ensures that consideration is given to all aspects of establishing a nursing center. This plan describes the development and direction of the nursing center and how goals will be met.

Strategic plan. The strategic plan complements the business plan as it looks into the future and guides the work of the nursing center. Strategic plans should be developed on a regular timeline and changed as indicated by local events and community input. Strategic planning meetings are periodically scheduled to review and refine the plan. The plan includes goals, objectives, and target timelines for implementation and evaluation of projected and ongoing services. Questions that should be addressed in a strategic plan include the following:
- Where will the center be after start-up?
- Where should the center be in 5, 7, 9 years?
- How can the staff move the center in the appropriate direction?
- What resources will be needed?

Feasibility studies, business plans, and strategic plans lay the foundation for strong nursing centers. The plans are crucial to the day-to-day functioning of a newly opened nursing center and reflect the abilities of the management team to build community coalitions and collaboration (McNeil and Mackey, 1995a). Shared resources and like interests across groups and organizations demonstrate a nursing center's credibility in the community, commitment to use community recommendations, flexibility and creativity in working with particular population groups, and functional linkages with organizations and institutions (Rhyne et al, 1998).

As the plans to establish a nursing center develop, cooperative relationships with the local health care and social service providers are established. The common goals of improving community well-being and sharing resources across systems lay the groundwork for working together.

HOW TO Develop a Business Plan

A business plan consists of the following information:
1. Cover page. *This includes date, name, address, phone number of the person(s) responsible for the nursing center, and any consultants to the business plan.*
2. Executive summary. *This is a 1- or 2-page overview of the center and the plan.*
3. Table of contents.
4. Description of the business plan. *This details what the center is and what services it will provide.*
5. Survey of the industry. *This summarizes the past, present, and future of the local and regional health care market.*
6. Market research and analysis. *This description outlines existing competition and the potential market share and identifies target groups.*
7. Marketing plan. *This details how the center will reach its targeted clients.*
8. Organizational chart *with a description of the management team.*
9. List of supporting professional staff, *such as accountants.*
10. Operations plan. *This describes how and where services will be provided.*
11. Research and development. *This projects program improvement and opportunities for new initiatives.*
12. Overall schedule. *The timeline establishes the start date and development phase of the nursing center.*
13. Critical risks and problems. *This examines the internal and external threats to the center and how these will be addressed.*
14. Financial plan. *The fiscal projections for the first 3 to 5 years are presented. A budget, cash-flow forecast, and break-even point are included.*
15. Proposed funding. *Specific sources are listed that can provide funding.*
16. Legal structure of the center. *This describes the status of the center, such as free-standing, corporation, or part of a larger organization.*
17. Appendices and supporting documents.

From Vogel G, Doleysh N: Entrepreneuring: a nurse's guide to starting a business, ed 2, New York, 1994, National League for Nursing.

Medical providers may be unfamiliar with a nursing center model and will need information about the center and its services. The support of the allied health and medical community advances the nursing center model rapidly in some communities.

> **WHAT DO YOU THINK?** *What might happen if an organization drives the motives to establish a nursing center model?*

Considerable work goes into the processes of community assessment, feasibility, business plans, and organizational networking. At this point the initial work may be considered completed, yet there are recurrent themes and questions that deserve review. Key persons should ask the following questions:

- Why would the organization want to do this?
- What will be the immediate and long-term outcomes for the organization and the community?
- Can the investment (staff, money, time, and space) be made?
- Does the community truly want and need a nursing center model?

The desires of the organization cannot be the motivation for the nursing center. If the establishment of a nursing center is solely done from the organization's point of view, the possibility of long-range sustainability may be jeopardized. The final question above is the most critical one. No assessment, study, or plan can ignore this question. If the answer is not clear, more time must be spent to find out if there is a match in need, interest, and a center's potential capacity.

For example, if the community wants to help young women move from public assistance into jobs and the immediate need is day care, a nursing center that offers linkages with day care providers and onsite physical examinations and childhood immunizations will be an essential community resource. If the nursing center moves ahead with initial plans of offering senior citizen services only, the immediate and expressed community in need has been ignored.

> **NURSING TIP**
>
> *There must be a match between services wanted and needed by the community and what is offered by the center.*

Outcome data

Nursing centers are responsible to the community. Client needs and resources change. Trends in health care services, client responses, and changes in community features must be monitored and reported. Sources of ill health, including noncommunicable conditions, are to be assessed. The influences of social, economic, environmental, behavioral, and infectious diseases are factors that affect health. Also it is necessary to measure client needs and apply various strategies to improve health. The evidence about the center needs to be collected, analyzed, and shared through forums such as professional publications, popular press, conferences, and public meetings.

Nursing center administrators and managers need to pay attention to service costs in relation to outcome data. Client-oriented outcome data must highlight projected and actual cost savings. This is particularly important when prevention strategies have eliminated or reduced the need for expensive, tertiary care.

Nursing center administrators must also measure what their consumers and the public in general wants the health care system to do. Nursing center tools should determine how well the provider or the health care system at large is doing (Lansky, 1998). Surveys indicate that the American public has five health care concerns:

- Access and communication (being treated respectfully; understanding what is being said and having access to services and providers)
- Being healthy (through prevention and education)
- Getting better (returning to normal functioning through early intervention)
- Living with a chronic condition (being as functional and as independent as possible)
- Coping with changes resulting from disability and death (having sources of comfort and support)

Outcome measurements can include client access and use of onsite services, childhood and adult immunization patterns, pregnancy outcomes, emergency department and hospital use, other health indices, client satisfaction, and quality-of-life measures (Eddy, 1998). Measurement instruments require technological support and staff expertise. No nursing center can efficiently function and effectively determine client- and population-based outcomes without these resources. Nursing center planners and administrators must factor the expenses involved in data collection up front in any business plan.

Funding

It is challenging for those involved in the planning process to forecast programs, determine service patterns, integrate outcome measures, and project costs. The planning process can be daunting, and sufficient time needs to be devoted to revenue sources. If matters of money are not thoroughly considered, the center's future will be compromised and may not withstand the stresses of funding changes, political decisions, and policy changes. Consequently, planners must responsibly scrutinize funding needs and sources (Kinsey and Gerrity, 1997). These sources are variable and include private, public, and corporate funding.

The business plan provides information that forecasts the minimum funding necessary to start a nursing center and to project income over 1 to 3 years from its beginning. A break-even analysis is essential. Other needed components include existing local financial resources, such as the health department; anticipated changes in health and social service funding; potential client characteristics; and commercial and public reimbursement for advanced practice nurses, including practitioners and community and public health nurses. Areas that must be examined carefully are the managed care reimbursement criteria in a particular state and the state's reimbursement parameters for advanced practice nurses.

NURSING TIP

Find out what your state's current legislation is regarding advanced practice nurses independent and reimbursable practice.

Sources of start-up funding include personal or borrowed funds; grants and contracts from local, state, or federal agencies or foundations; and private contributions (Dees, 1998). The Public Health Service of the U.S. Department Health and Human Services, Division of Nursing, has been a principal source of start-up funding for nursing centers operated by schools of nursing. The U.S. Bureau of Primary Care has been a source of funding for nursing centers located in public housing complexes. Other centers have obtained funding from private philanthropic foundations such as the Robert Wood Johnson Foundation and the W.K. Kellogg Foundation.

Grants are a source of initial and ongoing funding. The funding organization generally releases guidelines as to what the organization will fund. The guidelines are frequently released as a request for proposals (RFP). A proposal developed in response to the RFP specifies how the nursing center would meet the goals of the granting organization in a given timeline. The description of services and client outcomes must be presented to the RFP guidelines.

Contracts are another source of funding. Contracts are drawn up for a particular service with projected outcomes and a given timeline. Contracts represent opportunities for nursing centers to advance service, practice, and education. Identification of sources of contracts is the responsibility of the executive director and senior staff. Contracts can be with the local government, state agencies, or private organizations. For example, the local Head Start organization may ask for nursing center services for admission screening to Head Start. The contract would be for nurse practitioners, ancillary staff, and resources to screen preschool children for Head Start admissions.

Other sources of potential income to the nursing center include fee-for-service, commercial reimbursement, self-pay, and fundraising. Depending on the nursing center model developed and anticipated clients, fee-for-service may be the best economic strategy. Commercial reimbursement includes Medicare and commercial health care insurers with established fee schedules; self-pay may include a sliding fee schedule. Self-pay refers to the client's responsibility to pay for service delivered. Managed care contracts are other sources of income (Berry and Nelson, 1998).

Foundations, charitable contributions, and private pledges may offset the expenses relating to services provided to clients without health insurance or with limited insurance coverage. Fundraising by the center and its parent organization may also support the expenses dedicated to provide health services to those unable to pay. Fundraising can take the form of direct mailings, pledges, and events that raise money.

The establishment of a nursing center is warranted if there are documented reasons for using the model with the target population or in a geographic area, the economic feasibility, the long-term commitment of the planners, and if necessary, the parent organization. Careful planning builds the foundation that supports research and program evaluation and promotes opportunities to secure the nursing center's future.

RESEARCH IN NURSING CENTERS

Research in nursing centers provides the opportunity to answer questions and share the findings with colleagues and the public. The critical questions are about individual and population health status, client outcomes over time, roles and capacities to address health promotion with the existing health system, and the value and affordability of care (Berry and Nelson, 1998). In addition, many nursing centers serve as clinical laboratories for nursing and other health professional students. Centers offer many opportunities for educational research.

Each center needs a research agenda. The WHO's priorities for a common nursing research agenda displayed in Box 18-9 offers a framework. The research focus must include identifying and clarifying client needs, particularly those not engaged in an existing health system; description of nursing interventions and linkage with consumer needs and resources; demonstration of effective interventions that produce appropriate outcomes; and cost analysis and documented cost-effectiveness of services (Hirschfeld, 1998).

Over the past 2 decades, nursing center research has principally focused on the development and characteristics of nursing centers. Descriptive data have been collected about clients, types of services, financial supports, and community relationships. More than descriptive clinical studies are needed now. Efforts are underway to capture and name the unique features of nursing models of care and link them with health outcomes. For example, the significance of psychosocial interventions of nursing practice is being examined, such as listening to, support of, and interpretation of information. Client satisfaction studies document the perceived value by those who use nursing centers. Factors associated with access to services are being examined. These include availability, timeliness, acceptability, and affordability of services. Environmental condi-

BOX 18-9 WHO Priorities for a Common Nursing Research Agenda

- Evaluation of the effects of health care reform on equity, sustainability, and quality care, as well as on the workforce, particularly nursing personnel
- Comparative analysis of supply and demand of the health workforce
- Evaluation of health care organization, work conditions, technology, and supervision on the motivation and productivity of nursing personnel
- Analyses of the feasibility, effectiveness, and quality of education and practice where:
  - nurses have the responsibility for the entire range of care in a given community— promotive, preventive, curative, rehabilitative, long-term, and palliative care (including mental health/illness)
  - the focus of care is on individual versus community/public health versus environment
- Under which conditions are there feasible options, providing sound models of quality service delivery?
- Comparative analysis of the effectiveness of education and quality of services provided by nurses versus the effectiveness of education and quality of services based on different options of skill mix (within nursing and with other professions)
- Action research on delivery modes and necessary context for quality nursing care to vulnerable populations (e.g., homeless, chronically mentally ill, urban slum dwellers)
- Quality of care at different levels of the health care system and to different population groups (e.g., what are the educational and legal requirements for appropriate care to women, minorities, etc.)
- Ethics research related to different population groups and ethical considerations in research
- Culturally appropriate models of care and culturally appropriate human resource recruitment, retention, and deployment strategies
- Specific focus on home care, occupational health, and infection control in light of emerging trends

From Hirschfeld M: WHO priorities for a common nursing agenda, *Image* 30(2), 1998.

RESEARCH *Brief*

This article examines the concept of population characteristics as an organizational unit of analysis in the context of one primary care nursing center with three sites. The article presents the development of population focused assessment and outcome data and the interaction of predisposing, enabling, and need factors. Data analysis documented that the population group who lived in public housing had a decrease in the number of visits to emergency departments over a 3-year period. Use of population-based research supports the development of program planning activities and staffing patterns as well as determining the appropriateness of group interventions, such as health promotion activities, screenings, and immunizations. The authors identified challenges to using this approach if nursing centers have captured only individual client data or have grouped populations across sites. Faulty inferences can be drawn. It is necessary for nursing center researchers and staff to be aware of the strengths and weaknesses of every level and analysis of client- or population-level outcome. Caution is urged when drawing conclusions about findings and to carefully consider the type of data source.

Glick D, Thompson K, Ridge R. Population-based research: the foundation for development, management, and evaluation of a community nursing center, *Fam Community Health* 21(4):41, 1999.

tions, housing, transportation, criminal activities, and welfare-to-work transitions that influence health care access and use patterns are being examined. The Research Brief details one recent nursing center study.

The costs of care are linked to various outcome measures. The analyses of care costs are crucial to long-term sustainability of nursing centers. The effects of nursing models of care must be considered within society's continuing efforts to contain health care costs while improving health status. More refined studies are needed in this area, including studies across nursing centers to document common client outcomes (Buerhaus, 1998).

The essential players in health care continue to change. The purchasers, providers, clients, and commercial and public health care insurers are assuming new roles. Competition in the health care market is evident. The strains of change and competition stress nursing centers' capacity to conduct research and share data in the appropriate forums. The work must continue to capture essential information, conduct appropriate analyses, and share the findings with all stakeholders (Gaus and Fraser, 1996).

The stronger the research agenda, the greater the capacity to collect and manage data and to the degree that key stakeholders are notified, the greater the potential for nursing centers to survive and thrive in the emerging health care environment.

Thus centers must integrate research efforts into all aspects of their operations, and centers must reach out to similar models, share common goals and data, and commit to working with one another. One example of working together is the Regional Nursing Centers Consortium.

Regional Nursing Centers Consortium

The Regional Nursing Centers Consortium was established in 1996 to meet the needs of centers located in Pennsylvania, New Jersey, and Delaware. Since that time, Consortium outreach has expanded. Nursing centers, community health centers, and ambulatory care centers

BOX 18-10 Regional Nursing Centers Consortium (RNCC): Pennsylvania, New Jersey, and Delaware

MISSION

The mission of the Regional Nursing Centers Consortium is to serve its members by fostering greater recognition, using support of nursing centers, and expanding quality health care to vulnerable populations.

VALUES

- Nursing models of care
- Individual, family, and community health
- Community collaboration
- Multidisciplinary health care alliances

PURPOSES

- Foster understanding and recognition of nursing centers
- Promote the use of nursing centers
- Provide a forum for communication and collaboration
- Offer services that enhance members' management capabilities

- Broker open and honest dialogue about nursing center issues

NURSING CENTER CLASSIFICATIONS

- Comprehensive primary health care
- Health promotion/disease prevention and education
- Specialized health care to targeted populations

DEFINITION

Nursing centers are health centers managed by nurses in partnership with the communities they serve. They provide direct access to nurses and high-quality services, including primary health care, health promotion, education, and disease prevention.

From Regional Nursing Centers Consortium: *Mission, values, purposes, classification, and shared definition*, Philadelphia, 1998, Author.

across the United States have been in contact with the Consortium for consultation and support services.

The consortium offers the support and direction needed to sustain centers and to move the primary health care agenda forward in the region and beyond. The mission, purpose, and statement of values listed in Box 18-10 frame the work of the membership organization. The organization uses a definition that describes common characteristics across its members (Regional Nursing Centers Consortium, 1998).

Nurses and other professionals involved in the Consortium can be change agents. In collaboration with other health care providers, community members, and other organizations, nurses can demonstrate innovative community nursing practice models. These models support high-quality, affordable primary health care programs. The Consortium is just one example of what it and others can do when they work together. The potential for far-reaching change has been created. Time will tell the effectiveness and long-lasting community value of nursing centers.

THE FUTURE OF NURSING CENTERS

Nationally, nursing is strategically placed to make significant contributions to the health of people and achieve the *Healthy People 2010* goals of reducing health disparities and increasing years of productive life. The nursing center model offers unique opportunities to develop preventive services to improve the well-being of individuals, families, and communities. Nurses can continue to build community trust, support, and ability necessary to move the nursing center model into the mainstream of health care in the twenty-first century.

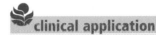

clinical application

The La Salle Neighborhood Nursing Center (LSNNC) has three primary health care sites and a variety of public health and outreach programs available to those who live or work in northwest, north, and northeast Philadelphia neighborhoods (more than 300,000 residents). This is an established center, and programs are based on community needs assessments. More than 300 uninsured children were seen one or more times during the year, and families were uncertain about what resources were available in the community. The local community was and continues to be challenged by the growing number of uninsured. According to the health commissioner, the highest number of uninsured adults, families, and their offspring reside or work in the Philadelphia neighborhoods served by LSNNC. Despite the Pennsylvania Children's Health Insurance Program (CHIP) coverage available to children of low- or modest-income families, LSNNC staff noted an increasing number of children who were uninsured and lacked a primary care "home." The stress on the care providers was evident.

What would be the best strategy to help the community solve the problem?

A. Write a grant and seek funding from a foundation interested in helping children.
B. Establish an advisory group to do a needs assessment to define the problem.
C. Initiate a program targeting the problem.
D. Do a research study to find out why there are so many uninsured children.

Answer is in the back of the book.

KEY POINTS

- Advanced practice nurses engage in a number of roles in nursing centers. These nurses with education beyond the baccalaureate degree are prepared to manage and deliver health care services to individuals, families, groups, communities, and populations. Specific advanced practice nurses include community health clinical nurse specialists, nurse practitioners, public health nurses, nurse midwives, and nurse anesthetists.
- Community collaboration involves the development of a voluntary, strategic alliance of private and nonprofit organizations and groups to enhance one another's capacity to achieve a common purpose by sharing risks, responsibilities, resources, and rewards.
- Comprehensive primary health care services emphasize health promotion and disease prevention, community involvement, multisectoral cooperation, and use of appropriate technology to provide accessible, acceptable, and affordable public and primary care services.
- Multilevel interventions are strategies used for personal, organizational, environmental, and policy development to achieve health goals by addressing the array of causative and contributing factors in health and illness.
- Nursing models of care are health care service delivery models that involve the intersection of persons, environment, health, and nursing and are based on nurses' belief that health is a resource for everyday life.
- Nursing centers are organizations that give the client direct access to professional nursing services. Using nursing models of care, professional nurses diagnose and treat human responses to actual and potential health problems and promote health and optimal functioning among target populations and communities. Their services are holistic, client centered, and reimbursable at a reasonable level.
- Accountability and responsibility for client care and professional practice remain with the professional nurse in a nursing center. Overall accountability and responsibility remain with the nurse executive.
- Nursing centers are not limited to any particular organizational structure. They may be affiliated with universities, community organizations, hospitals, or other service organizations, or they may be free standing.
- The primary characteristic of the organization is responsiveness to the health needs of a population.
- Stakeholders are all of those persons who have an investment or stake in the outcomes of a program and therefore have reasons to be interested in the evaluation of a program.
- Sustainability of a nursing center involves effort and resources needed to deliver health programs and services in an effective, consistent, and reliable manner over time so as to achieve desired outcomes.
- Research is needed to show the effects of nursing centers on client health care outcomes.

critical thinking activities

1. Visit a nursing center in your state or region and determine the model used to organize the center.
2. Review the mission, vision, purpose, goals, organizational structure, advisory committee or board of trustees, composition, and services of one nursing center.
3. Update your knowledge about your state's nurse practice act and advanced practice nurse reimbursement through managed care and public and private service contracts.
4. Identify nursing employment possibilities within the nursing center model.
5. Debate the economic and community sustainability of urban versus rural nursing center models.
6. Identify three or more potential organizations that would be community collaborators with nursing center staff.
7. Describe opportunities for student learning within a nursing center model.

Bibliography

American Nurses Association: *Health promotion and disease prevention: a position statement*, Kansas City, Mo, 1995, ANA.

Anderson E, McFarlane J: *Community as a partner*, Philadelphia, 1996, Lippincott-Raven.

Anderson KH: Establishing and sustaining a family nursing center for families with chronic illness: the Wisconsin experience, *J Fam Nurs* 4(2):127, 1998.

Aydelotte et al: *The nursing center: concept and design*, Kansas City, Mo, 1987, American Nurses Association.

Aydelotte MK, Gregory MS: Nursing practice: innovative models. In National League for Nursing: *Nursing centers: meeting the demand for quality health care*, New York, 1989, NLN.

Beery B, Nelson G: *Evaluating community-based health initiative: dilemmas, puzzles, innovations, and promising directions: making outcomes matter*, Seattle, Wash, 1998, Group Health/Kaiser Permanente Community Foundation.

Brown RE: Leadership to meet the challenges to the public's health, *Am J Public Health* 87(4):554, 1997.

Buchanan M: The new system of care. In National League for Nursing: *Teaching in the community: preparing nurses for the 21st century*, New York, 1997, NLN.

Buerhaus PI: Nursing and cost-effectiveness analysis, *Image* 30(3):202, 1998.

Buhler Wilkerson K: Bring care to the people: Lillian Wald's legacy to public health nursing, *Am J Public Health* 83(12):1778, 1993.

Burger A et al: Notes from the field, *Am J Public Health* 88(5):821, 1998.

Burke JF: Universities should become partners in their communities, *The Philadelphia Inquirer* Sept 15, 1997.

Clear JB, Starbecker M, Kelly DW: Nursing centers and health promotion: a federal vantage point, *Fam Community Health* 21(4):1, 1999.

Dees JR: Enterprising nonprofits, *Harvard Business Review*, pp 55-67, Jan-Feb, 1998.

Eddy DM: Performance measurement: problems and solutions, *Health Affairs* 17(4):7, 1998.

Evans LK et al: *Health care for the 21st century: greater Philadelphia style*. A paper prepared for the Independence Foundation, March 28, 1997.

Gaus CR, Fraser I: Shifting paradigms and the role of research, *Health Affairs* 15(2):235, 1996.

Glass LK: The historical origins of nursing centers. In National League for Nursing: *Nursing centers: meeting the demand for quality health care*, New York, 1989, NLN.

Glick D, Thompson K, Ridge R: Population-based research: the foundation for development, management, and evaluation of a community nursing center, *Fam Community Health* 21(4):41, 1999.

Harris MD: The development of a hospital-sponsored, community-based, nurse-managed health center, *Fam Community Health* 21(4):63, 1999.

Henderson FC, McManus J, Morris A: *The making of a nursing center,* Natchez, Miss, 1996, Natchez Printing.

Hirschfeld MJ: WHO priorities for a common nursing agenda, *Image* 30(2), 1998.

Institute of Medicine. *Defining primary care: an interim report,* Washington, DC, 1998, National Academy Press.

Josten L, Aroskar M, Shannon M: *Educating nurses for public health leadership: project report,* Minneapolis, 1996, University of Minnesota.

Kinlein ML: Independent nurse practitioner, *Nurs Outlook* 21(1):22, 1972.

Kinsey K: *La Salle neighborhood nursing center annual report,* Philadelphia, Penn, 1999, La Salle University School of Nursing.

Kinsey K, Gerrity P: Planning, implementing, and managing a community-based nursing center: current challenges and future opportunities *Handbook of Home Health Care Administration* 77:903, 1997.

Lancaster J: *Nursing issues in leading and managing change,* St Louis, 1999, Mosby.

Lansky D: Measuring what matters to the public, *Health Affairs* 17(4):40, 1998.

Lundeen SP: An alternative paradigm for promoting health in communities: the Lundeen community nursing center model, *Fam Community Health* 21(4):15, 1999.

Mackey TA, McNeil NO: Negotiating private sector partnerships with academic nursing centers, *Nurs Econ* 15(1):Jan-Feb, 1997.

Mattessich P, Monsey B: *Collaboration: what makes it work,* St Paul, Minn, 1992, Amherst H. Wilder Foundation.

McNeil NO, Mackey TA: The consistency of change in the development of nursing faculty practice plans, *J Prof Nurs* 11(4):220, 1995a.

McNeil NO, Mackey TA: *Marketing and teaching strategies for advanced practice nursing: proceedings of the American Association of Colleges of Nursing's Master's Education Conference and Preconference,* San Antonio, Texas, 1995b, University of Texas–Houston Health Science Center.

Murphy B: *Nursing centers: the time is now,* New York, 1995, National League for Nursing Press.

National Health Policy Forum: *Providing community-based primary care: nursing centers, CHCs, and other initiatives: a site visit report,* Washington. DC, 1998, The George Washington University.

Regional Nursing Centers Consortium: *Mission, values, purposes, classification and shared definition,* Philadelphia, 1998, Author.

Reverby S: From Lillian Wald to Hillary Rodman Clinton: what will happen to public health nursing? *Am J Public Health* 83(12):1662, 1993.

Rhyne R et al: *Community-oriented primary care: health care for the 21st century,* Washington, DC, 1998, APHA.

Ryan SA et al: A faculty on the move into the community, *N HC Perspect Community* 18(3):138, 1997.

Shaw G, Brown R, Bromiley P: Strategic stories: how 3M is rewriting business planning, *Harvard Business Review,* p 41, May-June, 1998.

Shoultz J, Amundson MJ: Nurse educators' knowledge of primary health care implications for community-based education, practice, and research, *Nurs Health Care Perspect* 19(3):114, 1998.

US Department of Health and Human Services: *Developing objectives for Healthy People 2010,* Washington, DC, 1997, US Government Printing Office.

Vogel G, Doleysh N: *Entrepreneuring: a nurse's guide to starting a business,* ed 2, New York, 1994, National League for Nursing.

William BL, Greenwald HP, Nudelman PM: Managed care and public health: building a partnership, *Public Health Nurs* 13(5):305, 1996.

World Health Organizatiom: *Health for all policy: origins and renewal,* 1999, WHO (www.who.ch/ppe/policy/origins.htm).

World Health Organization: *Primary health care: report of the International Conference on Primary Health Care, Alma-Ata, USSR 6-12 September,* Geneva, Switzerland, 1978, WHO.

Case Management

ANN H. CARY

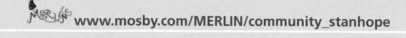

OBJECTIVES

After reading this chapter, the student should be able to do the following:

- Define *continuity of care, care management, case management,* and *advocacy.*
- Describe the scope of practice, roles, and functions of a case manager.

- Compare and contrast the nursing process with processes of case management and advocacy.
- Identify methods to manage conflict and the process of achieving collaboration.
- Define and explain the legal and ethical issues confronting case managers.

www.mosby.com/MERLIN/community_stanhope

KEY TERMS

advocacy	case management	information exchange	outcome criteria
affirming	clarification	process	problem solving
allocation	collaboration	informing	problem-purpose-
amplification	constituency	intermediate criteria	expansion method
assertiveness	coordination	integrative outcomes	promoter
autonomy	cooperation	intercessor	supporting
beneficence	critical paths	justice	timelines
brainstorming	demand management	liability	utilization management
capitation	disease management	life care planning	variance
care management	distributive outcomes	mediator	verification
CareMaps tool		negotiating	*See Glossary for definitions*

CHAPTER OUTLINE

Concepts of Case Management
  Definitions
  Case Management and the
    Nursing Process
  Characteristics and Roles
  Knowledge and Skill
    Requirements

  Tools of Case Managers
Public Health and Community
  Models of Case Management
Advocacy, Conflict Management,
  and Collaboration Skills for Case
  Managers
    Advocacy

Conflict Management
Collaboration
Issues in Case Management
  Legal Issues
  Ethical Issues

The evolving health care systems of today integrate financing, management, and delivery services. To promote population health, the relationship of these three factors is critical. Care may be financed through insurance methods like fee-for-service, **capitation,** or self-pay. Delivery of care may come through a network of providers, such as negotiated contracts with hospitals, physicians and nurse practitioners, pharmacies, ancillary health services, and outpatient centers. Managing the health of populations served by the integrated systems is essential. Population management extends to wellness and health promotion, illness prevention, acute and subacute care, rehabilitation, end-of-life care, and coordinated care. The evaluation of integrated systems shifts the focus of care in important ways (Qudah and Brannon, 1996):

- Emphasis is on population health management across the health care continuum, rather than on episodes of illness for an individual.
- Management shifts from inpatient care as the point of management to primary care providers as points of entry.
- Care management services and programs provide access and accountability for the continuum of health.
- Successful outcomes are measured by the performance of the health care system (rather than limited to individual provider performance) to meet the needs of populations.

The contemporary focus of the integrated health systems defines the nature of the client as a population rather than an individual. In these systems, population management entails: assessing the needs of the population served through health histories, insurance claims, use patterns, and risk factors. Such an assessment creates benefits and network designs to address these needs and to prioritize actions to produce a desired effect on the outcome and the likelihood of success with available resources. Population management also involves selecting and educating the population about programs of wellness, prevention, health promotion, and demand management. It also involves instituting a care management process that coordinates care across the continuum for a population and assigning case managers to clients and primary care physicians. These case managers may work with the hospital-based and specialty case managers, but they maintain accountability across the continuum (Qudah and Brannon, 1996).

Nurse case managers in their practices have as core values 1) increasing the span of healthy life, 2) reducing disparities in health among Americans, and 3) promoting access to care and preventive services, the goals of *Healthy People 2000.* Many of the interventions that nurses use with clients, as well as the design of the health care systems and the number of covered lives in those systems, promote further progress in meeting the *Healthy People 2000* objectives. Case management and care management offer opportunities for nurses to help in meeting the objectives for specific population targets listed in *Healthy People 2000: Midcourse Review* (USDHHS, 1995). Although these objectives are to be met by year 2000, 21% have moved in the wrong direction or have experienced no change. Progress with objectives for special population targets has shown significant problems in achievement of the objectives with 30% of the targets moving in the wrong direction or experiencing no change.

Care management is an enduring process in which a population manager establishes systems and monitors the health status, resources, and outcomes for a targeted segment of the population. The population case manager is the tactical architect for a population's health in the delivery system. The building blocks that are used include risk analysis, data monitoring for health indicators and variances of the population from the norm, epidemiologic investigation of causes of these variances, multidisciplinary development of action plans and programs for the population, and identification of case management triggers or events that promote earlier referrals of high-risk clients when prevention can have dramatic results (Qudah and Brannon, 1996).

Care management strategies were initially developed by health maintenance organizations (HMOs) in the late 1970s to manage the care of different populations while promoting quality of care and ensuring appropriate use and costs. Case management strategies include utilization management, critical paths, disease management, demand management, and case management.

Utilization management attempts to redirect care and monitors the appropriate use of provider care and treatment services for both acute and community/ambulatory services. Providers are offered multiple options for care with differing financial implications.

Critical paths are tools that specify activities that providers use in a timely sequence to achieve desired outcomes for care. The outcomes are measurable and the critical path tools strive to reduce variences in client care. Case management services are used for clients with specific diagnoses who may have high use patterns, are noncompliant, have cost caps, or have a limit on spending ($10,000 or $20,000).

Disease management activities target chronic and costly disease conditions that require long-term care interventions (e.g., diabetes). These strategies address the entire cycle of a disease process typically incorporating primary, secondary, and tertiary care interventions and self-care management activities.

Demand management seeks to control use by providing clients with correct information to empower themselves to make healthy choices, use healthy and health seeking behaviors to improve their health status, and make fewer demands on the health care system (Coleman and Zagor, 1998).

Case management comprises the activities implemented with individual clients in the system. The case manager builds on the basic functions of the traditional role and adapts new competencies for managing transition from one part of the system to another or to home, wellness and prevention, and multidisciplinary teams. Additionally, case managers in care-managed programs are expanding their clinical expertise to embrace the components of disease management, a successful strategy for population outcomes. Specialty case management by masters-prepared clinical nurse specialists is an emerging role in this field.

This chapter guides the reader through the nature and process of case management for individual and family clients. Case management has had a rich tradition in community and public health nursing while assuming more recent prominence in the acute care literature (Cohen and Cesta, 1993). Nursing has maintained the leadership among health care providers in coordinating resources to achieve health care outcomes based on quality, access, and cost. As health care delivery moves to capitation financing with an emphasis on pursuing the most efficient use of services to manage client outcomes, case management emerges as a strong role.

CONCEPTS OF CASE MANAGEMENT
Definitions

Reviewing multiple definitions of case management helps to see how complex the process has become. Weil and Karls (1985) describe case management as a "set of logical steps and a process of interaction within a service network which assures that a client receives needed services in a supportive, effective, efficient and cost-effective manner" (p. 4). Case management is defined by the American Hospital Association (AHA, 1986) as the process of planning, organizing, coordinating, and monitoring services and resources needed by clients while supporting the effective use of health and social services. Bower (1992) describes the continuity, quality, and cost-containing aspects of case management as a health care delivery process whose goals are to provide quality health care, decrease fragmented services, enhance the client's quality of life, and contain costs. Secord (1987) defines case management as a systematic process of assessment, planning, service coordination, referrals, and monitoring that meets the multiple service needs of clients. A focus on collaboration is viewed in the National Case Management Task Force definition: "a collaborative process which assesses, plans, implements, coordinates, monitors and evaluates the options and services to meet an individual's health needs, using communication and available resources to promote quality, cost effective outcomes" (Mullahy, 1998a, p. 9). Case management is defined in the public health nursing literature (Kenyon et al, 1990) as the "ability to establish an appropriate plan of care based on assessment of the client and family and to coordinate the necessary resources and services for the client's benefit" (p. 36). Case management is viewed as only one competency, or skill, that nurses need to provide quality care. Case management is identified as one of the eleven competencies for practice in community health nursing. Knowledge and skills required to achieve

this competency include knowledge of community resources and financing methods, written and oral communication and documentation, negotiation and conflict resolution skills, critical thinking processes to identify and prioritize problems from the provider and client views, and identification of best resources for the desired outcomes.

The complexity of case management practice is further apparent by noting the **coordination** activities of multiple providers, payers, and settings throughout a client's continuum of care. Care provision by many disciplines (the client, family, significant others, and community organizations) must be assessed, planned, implemented, adjusted, and based on mutually agreed-upon goals. Although the nurse may be employed and located in one setting, the nurse will be influencing the selection and monitoring of care provided in other settings by formal and informal care providers. With the use of electronic care delivery through telehealth activities, case management activities are now delivered via telephone, e-mail, fax, and video visits in a clients residence. They may also be delivered to a global network of clients located in different countries.

A particularly challenging problem is the fragmenting of services, which can result in overuse, underuse, gaps in care, and miscommunication. This may ultimately result in costly client outcomes. Parker and colleagues (1992) discuss the unique complexity of case management in rural settings, where fewer organized community-based systems, geographic distance to delivery, population density, finances, pace and lifestyle, values, and social organization differ from more urbanized environments. The complexity is further fueled by chaotic systems, changes in today's health care market in which providers, services, and coverage details are constantly manipulated.

> **DID YOU KNOW?** *Although the activities in case management may differ among providers and clients, the goals are durable in four aspects:*
> - *To promote the quality of the services provided to populations*
> - *To reduce institutional care while maintaining quality processes and satisfactory outcomes*
> - *To manage resource use through protocols, evidence-based decision making, guideline use, and disease-management programs*
> - *To control expenses by managing care processes and outcomes*
>
> Adapted from Flarey DL, Blancett SS, editors: *Handbook of nursing case management: health care delivery in a world of managed care,* Gaithersburg, Md, 1996, Aspen Publishers.

> **WHAT DO YOU THINK?** *When selecting clients to receive telehealth case management services, patient characteristics and individual circumstances must be considered. Identify the sensory and functional indicators of clients that must be assessed and monitored to initiate telehealth case management services appropriately.*

TABLE 19-1 The Nursing Process and Case Management

NURSING PROCESS	CASE MANAGEMENT PROCESS	ACTIVITIES
Assessment	Case finding; identification of incentives for the target population; screening and intake; determination of eligibility; assessment	Develop networks with target population; disseminate written materials; seek referrals; apply screening tools according to program goals and objectives; use written and onsite screens; apply comprehensive assessment methods (physical, social, emotional, cognitive, economic, and self-care capacity); perform interdisciplinary, family, and client conferences
Diagnosis	Identification of the problem	Determine conclusion based on assessment; use interdisciplinary team
Planning/ outcome	Problem prioritizing planning to address care needs	Validate and prioritize problems with all participants; develop activities, timeframes, and options; gain client's consent to implement; have client choose options
Implementation	Advocation of client's interests; arrangement of delivery of service; monitoring of clients during service	Contact providers; negotiate services and price; coordinate service delivery; monitor for changes in client or service status
Evaluation	Reassessment	Examine outcomes against goals; examine needs against service; examine costs; examine satisfaction of client, providers, and case manager

Case Management and the Nursing Process

The community-oriented nurse views the process of case management through the broader health status of the community. Clients and families in service represent the microcosm of health needs within the larger community. Through a nurse's case management activities, general community weaknesses in quality and quantity of health services often are discovered. For example, the management of a severely disabled child by a nurse case manager may uncover the absence of respite services or parenting support and education resources in a community.

NURSING TIP

Use the components of the nursing process when implementing the functions of a case manager with clients.

While managing the disability and injury claims at an industry, the nurse may discover that referrals for home health visits and physical therapy are generally underused by the acute care providers in the community. Through a nurse's case management of brain-injured young adults, the absence of community standards and legislative policy for helmet use by bicyclists and motorcyclists may stimulate the nurse to advocate for a community policy. Case management activities with individual clients and families will reveal the larger picture of health services and health status of the community. Community assessment, policy development, and assurance activities that are the essential core of public health actions are often the next logical steps for a nurse's practice when observed at the individual and family intervention levels through case management. Clearly, the core components of case management and the nursing process are complementary (Table 19-1). Secord's (1987) illustration of case management remains an appropriate picture of the process that nurses use (Fig. 19-1).

Characteristics and Roles

Case management can be labor intensive, time consuming, and costly. Because of the increasing number of clients with complex problems in nurses' caseloads, the intensity and duration of activities required to support the case management function may soon exceed the demands that the direct caregiver can meet. Managers and clinicians in community health are exploring methods to make case management more efficient. In an earlier effort to achieve efficiency, tasks and activities offered to describe the characteristics desired for the effective case manager hold true today (Weil and Karls, 1985):

1. Technical qualifications to understand and evaluate specific diagnoses, generally requiring clinical credentials (and experience) and financial abilities
2. Ability to use language and terminology (able to understand and explain to others in simple terms)
3. Ability to be assertive and diplomatic with people at all levels
4. Ability to assess situations objectively to determine the appropriateness of case management

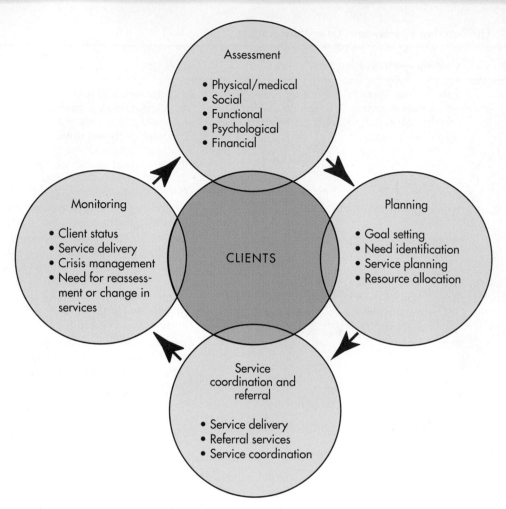

FIG. 19-1 Core components of case management. (From Secord LJ: *Private case management for older persons and their families,* Excelsior, Minn, 1987, Interstudy.)

5. Knowledge of available resources and the strengths and weaknesses of each
6. Ability to act as advocate for the client and third party payer
7. Ability to act as a counselor to clients in providing support, understanding, information, and intervention

Likewise, Coleman and Hagen (1991) and Cary (1998) have described the roles that case managers assume in the practice setting (Box 19-1). The roles demanded of the nurse as case manager are vividly influenced by the forces that support or detract from feasible and creative possible solutions. Figure 19-2 presents factors that demand the attention of both the nurse and the client during the case management process.

Knowledge and Skill Requirements

Adoption of the case management role for a nurse does not happen automatically with position. Knowledge and skills that are developed and refined are essential to successful role implementation. Bower (1992) suggests knowledge domains useful for nurses and systems desiring to im-

plement quality case management roles (Box 19-2). If a nurse seeks a case manager position, some of the skills and knowledge areas will need to be developed through orientation and mentoring experiences.

HOW TO *Learn About Telehealth Interventions for Clients*

1. *Make it a point to learn how telehealth works in your community.*
2. *Consider telehealth as an option when considering available resources.*
3. *Seek continuing education courses that will educate you on the art and science of telehealth application.*
4. *Seek networking opportunities with professional organizations and other case managers about the uses of telehealth.*
5. *Improve your personal interaction skills that will assist in decision making about the use of telehealth services.*

From Wrinn MM: The emerging role of telehealth in health care, *Continuing Care* 17(8):18, 1998a.

BOX 19-1 Case Manager Roles

Facilitator. Supports all parties to work toward mutual goals

Liaison. Provides a formal communication link among all parties concerning the plan of care management

Coordinator. Arranges, regulates, and coordinates needed health care services for clients at all necessary points of services

Broker. Acts as an agent for provider services that are needed by clients to stay within coverage according to budget and cost limits of health care plan

Educator. Educates client, family, and providers about case management process, delivery system, community health resources, and benefit coverage so that informed decisions can be made by all parties

Negotiator. Negotiates the plan of care, services, and payment arrangements with providers; uses effective collaboration and team strategies

Monitor/reporter. Provides information to parties on status of members and situations affecting patient safety, care quality, and patient outcome and on factors that alter costs and liability

Client advocate. Acts as advocate, provides information, and supports benefit changes that assist member, family, primary care provider, and capitated systems

Standardization monitor. Formulates and monitors specific, time-sequenced critical path and CareMap (see text) plans and disease management protocols that guide the type and timing of care to comply with predicted treatment outcomes for specific client and conditions; attempts to reduce variation in resource use; targets deviations from standards so adjustments can occur in a timely manner

Systems allocator. Distributes limited health care resources according to a plan or rationale

From Cary AH: Advocacy or allocation, *Nursing Connection* 11(1):1, 1998.

BOX 19-2 Knowledge Domains for Case Management

- Knowledge of health care financial environment and the financial dimension of client populations that nurses manage
- Clinical knowledge, skill, and maturity to direct quality-induced timing and sequencing of care activities
- Care resources for clients within institutions and communities: facilitating the development of new resources and systems to meet clients' needs
- Transition planning for ideal timing and sequencing of care
- Management skills: communication, delegation, persuasion, use of power, consultation, problem solving, conflict management, confrontation, negotiation, management of change, marketing, group development, accountability, authority, advocacy, ethical decision making, and profit management
- Teaching, counseling, and education skills
- Program evaluation and research
- Performance improvement techniques
- Peer consultation and evaluation
- Requirements of eligibility and benefit parameters by third-party payers
- Legal issues
- Information systems: clinical and management

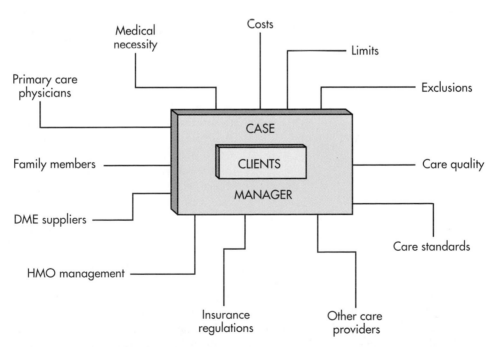

FIG. 19-2 Forces affecting solutions in the case management process. (From Hicks LL, Stallmeyer JM, Coleman JR: *The role of the nurse in managed care*, Washington, DC, 1993, American Nurses Publishing.)

Tools of Case Managers

Case management plans have evolved through a variety of names and methods (e.g., critical paths, critical pathways, CareMaps, multidisciplinary action plans, nursing care plans). Regardless of the term used, standards of client care, standards of nursing practice, and standards of practice for case management serve as a core foundation of case management plans. Likewise, in multidisciplinary action plans, core professional standards of each discipline guide the development of the standards process.

WHAT DO YOU THINK? *The five "rights" of case management are right care, right time, right provider, right setting, and right price. How does the nurse judge the effectiveness of case management?*

As early as 1985 the New England Medical Center in Boston instituted a system of critical path development to guide the case management process in the acute care setting. A critical path is a case management tool composed of abbreviated versions of processes that are specific to each discipline (e.g., nursing midwife); it is used to achieve a measurable outcome for a specific client "case" (Zander, Etheredge, and Bower, 1987). The critical path shows the key "incidents" that must be achieved in a timely manner to produce an appropriate length of stay. In the New England model, key incidents included consults, tests, activities, treatments, medication, diet, discharge planning, and teaching. The paths note the variances produced by clients because all clients may not fit the picture of the ideal progress that a client should follow through the system. However, the critical paths are not revised unless a body of evidence is collected from a number of clients, suggesting that adjustment needs to be made in the expected actions. CareMaps became the second generation of critical paths of care.

As described by Zander (1994), A **CareMaps tool** is a "cause-and-effect grid which identifies expected patient/family and staff behaviors against a time line for a case-type or otherwise defined homogeneous population" (p. 4). The four components of the CareMaps tool are as follows:

1. Index of problems with intermediate and outcome criteria
2. Time line
3. Critical path
4. Variance record

Outcome criteria are the measurable ends to be achieved based on the problems presented by the client's condition of health or illness. **Intermediate criteria** are incremental incidents that serve to monitor progress toward outcomes. **Timelines** are landmarks of an episode of health or illness care from initial encounter to the transfer of accountability to the client or another health care agency. Timelines with standard nursing diagnoses and outcomes (and those of other disciplines) constitute the map. The timeline plan can be in hours, days, weeks, or

months. **Variance** is the difference between what is expected and what is occurring with the client. Cohen and Cesta (1993) describe variances as *operational* (broken equipment, staffing mix, delays, lost documentation), health care *provider* (variance in provider practice, level of expertise/experience), *client* (client refusal, nonavailability, change in status), and *unmet clinical quality indicators*. Variance data are useful in understanding why expected client outcomes and indicators have not been met and allow for early correction of the care process.

The adaptation of the case management care plan is a crucial skill for standardizing the process and outcome of care. It links multiple provider interventions to client responses and offers reasonable predictions for client's progress. Institutions report that sharing of case management plans with clients empowers the client to assume responsibility for monitoring and adhering to the plan of care. Self-responsibility by clients truly links autonomy and self-determination as the core of case management. As a nurse employed to function as a case manager, ample opportunities exists to develop, test, and revise CareMap prototypes for a target population experiencing health deficits.

Disease management is a systematic program of services for all clients with specific conditions such as cancer, depression, asthma or diabetes. For clients with these conditions, disease management programs contain the following (LaPensee, 1997):

- Case management and risk sharing arrangements between payers and providers
- Programs for monitoring the use of prescriptions and treatment interventions to assess outcomes and costs
- Educational initiatives to meet clients' learning needs and providers' knowledge of cost-effective treatments
- Interventions to modify health behaviors and increase compliance with treatment regimens

Chronic disease clients are well-suited to the benefits of a disease management approach to case management because the goals are to interrupt and prevent the continuation of a disease process using secondary and tertiary prevention techniques. Promotion of wellness is paramount to success (McClinton, 1998a). Research has demonstrated that disease management programs promote greater control of signs and symptoms in clients (Solberg et al, 1997). As the science of disease management evolves to predict direct relationships between outcomes and protocols of care, case managers will be able to ensure cost-effective, optimal clinical care across the continuum, a goal of care management for populations. For case managers, disease management strategies, which are part of the care management initiative, shift the client-specific, episodic management functions toward holistic case-management functions that are proactive and population based (Ward and Rieve, 1995; Rieve, 1998).

Life care planning is another tool used in case management that assesses the current and future needs of a client. The life care plan is a customized, medically based document that provides assessment of all present and future needs, services, equipment, supplies, and living arrangements for a client. Life care plans are typically used for clients experiencing catastrophic illness or adverse events as a result of professional malpractice. These plans may be used by plaintiff or defense lawyers to analyze damages, set financial reserves that can be used to pay for care in the future, and create a lifetime-oriented care plan. A systematic process is used, and multiple disciplinary input is required to craft the first phase of the plan, such as thorough assessment of the client, financial/billing agreements, information release signed by a client, and targeted date for the report to be completed. Development of the plan is the second phase. The plan is based on several factors: social situation, leisure activities, educational and employment status, medical history, physical abilities, current status, and assistance required for activities of living. The plan includes projected costs and resources for the frequency and duration of treatments, equipment, supplies, and need for reevaluation. The case manager will obtain multiple price quotes from local and national providers, investigate support services and funding to meet client needs, and use complicated economics projections about future inflation for care as well as present time value of the dollar. Ultimately the life care plan seeks to portray the actual needs of a client that are consistent with the changes in a client's life because of the injury (McKinley and Zasler, 1998).

PUBLIC HEALTH AND COMMUNITY MODELS OF CASE MANAGEMENT

Carondelet St. Mary's, in Tucson, Arizona, has developed a community nursing network (CNN) in which 15,000 enrollees are distributed among 17 community health centers. Professional nurse case managers help older clients attain healthier lifestyles and maintain themselves in the community. Nurses have been successful in delivering services at a cost of less than $5 per month per Medicare enrollee. Through nurse case management services, this nursing health maintenance organization (HMO) has cut the number of inpatient days per 1000 enrollees by one-third at an average cost of $900 per day and a savings of $300,000 for every 1000 enrollees (ANA 1993; ANF, 1993).

Statewide programs in New Jersey use case management methodologies to promote early identification, selection, evaluation, diagnosis, and treatment of children with potentially physically compromised needs. Local case management units provide coordinated and comprehensive care. Collaboration with existing local and regional agencies serving children supports this process. The nurse case manager performs the following services:

1. Provides counseling and education to parents and children on identifying problems and family knowledge level
2. Develops individual plans including multidisciplinary services (education, social, medical development, rehabilitation)

3. Finds appropriate community services
4. Acts as a family resource in crises and when service concerns arise
5. Facilitates communication between child and family
6. Monitors services for outcomes

Interdisciplinary teams include public health nurses and master's-prepared social workers for larger caseloads. A recommended caseload is 300 to 350 children per case manager (Bower, 1992).

The case management program for persons with acquired immunodeficiency syndrome (AIDS) pioneered at San Francisco General Hospital focuses on the support of community-based outpatient services to reduce dependency on unnecessary and more costly services. It follows the public health model of minimizing hospitalizations

RESEARCH *Brief*

An experimental approach to case management was tested to discover the use of child health clinic and immunization services by 98 Medicaid infants from low-income families. The experimental case management condition consisted of a single public health nurse (PHN) providing both case management and preventive child health services. The control condition consisted of multiple nurse providers of child health services to an infant and the segregation of case management delivery from child health services delivery.

Data were collected from health department clinical records to document the PHN interventions, child health clinic visits, immunizations, and demograhics. The health districts' protocols for case management of Medicaid infants and child preventive services were followed for the experimental and control groups. However, the infants in the experimental group received "continuous care" by one PHN, whereas the control-group infants received care from multiple PHN providers, or "fragmented care."

Differences between the preventive services obtained by infants receiving the two approaches were significant, although the study sample immunization rate of 62% is considerably below the national objective of 90% for 2-year-old children by the year 2000 (USDHHS, 1992).

Implications for nursing practice are as follows:

1. Case management delivery by a consistent provider who incorporates case management, delivery of preventive services, and home health visits can result in greater use of age-appropriate services by infants and their families.
2. The use of a consistent (singular) case manager can result in fewer nursing efforts (follow-up contacts) required to achieve adequacy of child preventive services.

Erkel EA et al: Case management and preventive services among infants from low-income families, *Public Health Nurs* 11(5):352, 1994.

and length of stay, using community-based services, and brokering among a strong network of community services: housing, home, hospice delivery, and respite care. The San Francisco Department of Public Health used its positive reputation with the gay community to plan, develop, and evaluate care (Bower, 1992; Foster and Hall, 1986).

Liberty Mutual Insurance Company has used case management principles for more than 30 years in workers' compensation and has expanded services for employees whose conditions were noted as chronic or catastrophic. Box 19-3 lists examples of case-managed conditions. Case managers coordinate all parties and services to reduce excessive expenses caused by lack of coordination, failure to use efficacious alternatives, duplication, and fragmentation (Bower, 1992).

Important guidance in developing a community case management program is found in the United States. Case management is a key component of federally financed and many state-financed delivery systems. The experiences of states over the past 2 decades provides testimony to the importance of case management for populations at risk. For older clients, state-initiated case management provides objective advice and assistance with care needs and provides access to multidisciplinary providers and services. For payers (federal, state, clients), case management serves as a vehicle to ensure that funds are allocated appropriately to those in greatest need.

HOW TO *Ensure High Quality for Clients*

1. *Provide access to easily understood information for each client*
2. *Provide access to appropriate specialists*
3. *Ensure continuity of care for those with chronic and disabling conditions*
4. *Provide access to emergency services when and where needed*
5. *Disclose financial incentives that could influence medical decisions and outcomes*
6. *Prohibit "gag clauses" where providers cannot inform clients of all possible treatment options*
7. *Provide antidiscrimination protections*
8. *Provide internal and external appeals processes to solve grievances of clients*

From McClinton DH: Protecting patients, *Continuing Care* 17(7):6, 1998b.

Case management serves a policy-assurance and accountability function for communities. Within the states, examples of the types of agencies designated to conduct case management are district offices of state government, area agencies on aging, county social services departments, and contractors. States maintain the oversight responsibilities for case management agencies to (1) ensure compliance with program standards, contracts, reporting, and fiscal controls; (2) identify emerging problems and issues to be rectified by additional state policies; and (3) provide

---

BOX 19-3 Examples of Case-Management Conditions

High-risk neonates
Severe head trauma
Spinal cord injury
Ventilator dependency
Coma
Multiple fractures
Acquired immunodeficiency syndrome (AIDS)
Severe burns
Cerebrovascular accident (CVA)
Amputations
Terminal illness
Substance abuse
Transplantation
Chronic diseases and disabilities

---

onsite technical assistance and consultation to improve performance. States' payment methods for case management include daily/monthly rates, hourly/quarterly rates, capped rates for services, and capped aggregate allocation to cover both case management and provider costs (Congressional Research Service, 1993).

These models offer one solution to unnecessary health care expenditures; an estimated one-third of all health care administered in the United States is not needed (Lashley, 1993). Case management offers a method to reduce costs and to use appropriate health care services. Imagine the effect on health status if these saved resources were shifted to primary prevention and health promotion activities.

ADVOCACY, CONFLICT MANAGEMENT, AND COLLABORATION SKILLS FOR CASE MANAGERS

Now that the concept, scope, role, and functions of case management and case managers have been reviewed, three specific skills essential to the role performance of the case manager will be discussed: advocacy, conflict management, and collaboration.

Advocacy

For community-oriented nurses, **advocacy** involves differing activities, ranging from self-reflection to lobbying for health policy. Advocacy is essential for practice with clients and their families, communities, organizations, and colleagues on an interdisciplinary team. The functions of advocacy require scientific knowledge, expert communication, facilitating skills, and problem-solving and affirming techniques. As the Code of Nurses (ANA, 1985) states, "the goal of nursing actions is to support and enhance the client's responsibility and self-determination" (p. I). However, this goal is a contemporary one. As Nelson (1988) indicates, the perspective regarding the advocacy function has shifted through time. The nurse advocate has been described in earlier writings as one who acted on behalf of or interceded for the client. An example of the **intercessor**

RESEARCH *Brief*

The study was designed to measure the effect of coping resources on the amount (hours) of help used by disabled elderly individuals in their homes. These resources enable the disabled elderly to continue living in the community and avoid or postpone nursing home placement. Based on a national sample of 4563 community-dwelling elderly who participated in the 1989 National Long-Term Care survey, the research showed that family help and living arrangements, more than income and public programs, kept elderly, disabled invidiuals in the community. Disabled elderly individuals with a network of family helpers and who lived with a helper received more in-home help than those living alone or without family helpers. The most important coping resources are a combination of family helpers and when helpers reside with the elderly.

Implications for the care manager include the following:

1. The presence of a willing family caregiver provides more hours of care for a disabled elderly client and maintains the client in the community.
2. Even with cash income and third party payments to obtain paid help, these effects are relatively smaller by comparison.
3. With reduced family network availability, more funding for paid help will be necessary to reduce institutionalization.

Boaz RF, Hu J: Determining the amount of help used by disabled elderly persons at home: the role of coping resources, *J Gerontol B Psychol Sci Soc Sci* 52B(6):S317, 1997.

role is the community health nurse who calls for a well-child appointment for a mother visiting the family planning clinic when the mother is capable of making an appointment on her own. The contemporary goal of advocacy would direct the nurse to move clients toward making the call themselves.

The evolution of the advocacy role to that of mediator by the nurse advocate is described as a response to the complex configuration of social change, reimbursers, and providers in the health care system (Winslow, 1984). *Mediation* is an activity in which a third party attempts to provide assistance to those who may be experiencing a conflict in obtaining what they desire. The goal of the nurse advocate as **mediator** is to help parties understand each other on many levels so that agreement on an action is possible. In the instance of a nurse as case manager for an HMO, mediation activities between an elderly client and the payer (HMO) could accomplish the following results: the client may understand the options for community-based skilled nursing care, and the payer may understand the client's desires for a less restrictive environment for

care. Although the case manager as mediator does not decide the plan of action (in contrast to the role of arbitration), he or she facilitates the decision-making processes between the parties so that the desired care can be reimbursed within the range of options available to the client.

In contemporary practice the nurse advocate makes the client's rights the priority. The goal of **promoter** for the client's autonomy and self-determination may result in a high degree of independence in decision making. For example, when a group of young pregnant women is the collective "client," the nurse advocate's role may be to inform the group of the benefits and consequences of breast-feeding their infants. However, if the new mothers decide on formula feeding, the nurse advocate should support the group and continue to provide parenting, infant, and well-child services.

The next proposition shows a different perspective of the nurse advocate as promoter. It holds that the nurse's role as advocate may demand a variety of functions that are influenced by the client's physical, psychologic, social, and environmental abilities. The nurse adapts the advocacy function to the client's dynamic capabilities as the client follows a path to a healthy status. Even clients who desire access to more substantial health promotion activities can benefit from a partnership with the nurse advocate. Examples of advocacy in such cases might include promoting a client group's access to onsite physical fitness programs in the occupational setting or supporting parents' and students' concerns about the high fat content of vending machine cuisine in the school system. With the cost of health care exceeding 1 trillion dollars annually and consumers assuming a larger financial portion of the care they choose, the promoter role of advocacy for those clients capable of autonomy is expected to increase.

> **NURSING TIP**
>
> *For clients who have no health coverage or who do not qualify for other programs, pharmaceutical companies may have a program of free supplies of drugs for these clients. Call a pharmaceutical company for information on eligibility of your client.*

Process of advocacy

The goal of advocacy is to promote self-determination in a **constituency.** The constituency may be a client, family, peer, group, or community. The process of advocacy was defined by Kohnke (1982) to include informing, supporting, and affirming—the third essential part of advocacy. All three activities require self-reflection and skill development by the nurse. It is often easier for the nurse to inform, support, and affirm another person's decision when it matches the nurse's values. However, when clients make decisions within their value systems that are different than the nurse's values, the advocate may feel conflict in contributing to the process of informing, supporting, and affirming those decisions.

Promoting self-determination in others demands a philosophy of free choice once the information necessary for decision making has been discussed.

Informing. Knowledge is essential, but not sufficient, to the outcome of decision making. The interpreting of knowledge is affected by the client's values and the meaning the client assigns to the knowledge. The interpreting of facts is the result of both objective and subjective processing of information. Subjective dimensions greatly influence client decisions.

Informing clients about the nature of their choices, the content of those choices, and the consequences to the client is not a one-way activity. The **information exchange process** is composed of interactions that reflect three subprocesses: amplifying, clarifying, and verifying. **Amplification** occurs between the nurse and client to assess the needs and demands that will eventually affect the client's decision. Information is exchanged from both viewpoints. Although the exchange may be initiated at the objective factual level, it will likely proceed to include the subjective perspectives of both parties.

The information exchanged between the parties is important to consider. Guidelines include the nurse's need to do the following:

1. Assess the client's present understanding of the situation.
2. Provide correct information.
3. Communicate with the client's literacy level in mind, making the information as understandable as possible.
4. Use a variety of media and sources to increase the client's comprehension.
5. Discuss other factors that affect the decision, such as financial, legal, and ethical issues.
6. Discuss the possible consequences of a decision.

The tone of the amplifying process can direct the remainder of the information exchange. It is important to relate with clients in a manner that reflects the advocate's endorsement of their self-determination. Setting aside the time necessary to listen to clients is critical. Clients will sense that they are part of a mutual process if the nurse can engage them during the information exchange with a message that says, "I respect your needs and desires as I share my knowledge with you." Nonverbal behaviors, including using direct eye contact, sitting at the client's level, arriving and leaving at a prescribed time, and using verbal patterns that foster exchange (open-ended statements, questions, probes, reflections of feelings, paraphrasing), convey the active promotion of self-determination.

A client may not desire the exchange of information because of lack of self-esteem, fear of the information, or inability to comprehend the content of the communication. In such a case, the focus is to understand the client's desire for no information and to express to the client the consequences of such inaction. The nurse may invite the client to ask for the information exchange at a later time when the client is ready and can intermittently check with the client whether information exchange and amplification is desired. In these cases the nurse should document the implemented nursing actions to reflect the guidelines just discussed. This can reduce the basis for legal action and misunderstanding by other parties.

Clarification is a process in which the nurse and client strive to understand meanings in a common way. Clarification builds on the breadth and depth of the exchange developed in amplification to determine if the parties understand each other. During this process, misunderstandings and confusions are examined. The goal of clarifying is to avoid confusion between the parties. To foster clarification, nurses can use certain verbal prompts:

- "What do you understand about . . .?"
- "Please tell me more about how you . . ."
- "I don't think I am clear. Let me explain the situation in another way. As an example . . ."
- "What other information would be helpful so that we both understand?"

Verification is the process used by the nurse advocate to establish accuracy and reality in the informing process. If the nurse discovers that a client is misinformed, the nurse may return to the clarification or amplification stage and begin the process again. Verifying produces the chance for the nurse advocate and client to examine "truth" from their perspectives, which may include knowledge, intuition, previous experiences, and anticipated consequences.

In reality, promoting a client's self-determination may take the advocate and client through the information exchange process several times as new dimensions or obstacles to an issue develop. Information exchange is a critical process for advocacy and is applicable to all advocacy clients: individuals, families, groups, and communities.

Supporting. The second major process, **supporting**, involves upholding a client's right to make a choice and to act on the choice. People who become aware of clients' decisions fall into three general groups: supporters, dissenters, and obstructors. Supporters approve and support clients' actions. Dissenters do not approve and do not support clients. Obstructors cause difficulties while clients try to implement their decisions.

Kohnke (1982) and Cary (1998) point to the need for the nurse advocate to implement several actions that fulfill the supporting role. Assuring clients that they have the right and responsibility to make decisions and reassuring them that they do not have to change their decisions because of others' objections are important interventions.

Affirming. The third process in the advocacy role is **affirming**. It is based on an advocate's belief that a client's decision is consistent with the client's values and goals. The advocate validates that the client's behavior is purposeful and consistent with the choice that was made. The advocate expresses a dedication to the client's mission, and a purposeful exchange of new information may occur so the client's choice remains viable. Recognizing that a client's needs may fluctuate with changing resources, the affirming activity must encourage a process of reevaluation and rededication to promote self-determination.

The importance of affirming activities cannot be emphasized strongly enough. Many advocacy activities stop with assuring and reassuring, but affirming is often critical in promoting a client's self-determination. Table 19-2 compares the nursing process with the advocacy process.

The advocate's role in the decision-making process is not to tell the client which option is "correct" or "right." The advocate's role is to provide the opportunity for information exchange, giving clients the tools that can empower them in making the best decision from their perspective. Enabling the client to make an "informed decision" is a powerful tool for building self-confidence. It gives the client the responsibility for selecting the options and experiencing the success and consequences based on current data. Clients are empowered in their decision making when they can recognize events that are beyond their control and can link events that occur by chance with predictable events to make decisions they want.

Nurses can promote client decision making by using the information exchange process, promoting use of the nursing process, including written techniques (contracts, lists), using reflection and prioritizing, and using role playing to "try on" and determine the "fit" of different options and consequences for the client. By engaging clients in the information exchange process and helping them recognize the progression of activities they experience as they build their "informed decision-making base," the nurse advocate is empowering clients with skills that can strengthen their autonomy and confidence in the future.

Advocacy is a process that requires a balance between "doing for" and "promoting autonomy." The process is influenced by the client's physical, emotional, and social abilities. The goal of advocacy is to promote the ultimate degree of self-determination possible for the client given the client's current and potential status; for most clients, this goal can be realized.

When clients are comatose, unborn, or legally incompetent, nurse advocates have unique functions. The advocate's role is usually determined by the legal system; however, in some cases nurses must decide what roles they will play. These are areas requiring intensive self-reflection, research, and collaboration with professionals, family members, and significant others.

Skill development

Skills needed by the nurse advocate are not unique to their profession. Nursing demands technical, relation-building, and problem-solving skills. Advocacy requires applying nursing skills to promote client self-determination. However, several other skills are necessary and well-defined.

Advocates must be open minded and aware of people, society, and social order (Kohnke, 1982). Knowledge of nursing and knowledge from other disciplines is essential for the advocacy role in establishing authority and developing skills. Highly developed communication skills and a strong sense of self-esteem and professional confidence are also needed (Webb, 1987). The capacity for assertiveness for personal rights and the rights of others is essential.

Systematic problem solving

The nursing process—assessment, diagnosis, planning, implementation, and evaluation—constitutes an example of a method of **problem solving** that can be used in the advocacy role. Advocates can be particularly helpful with clients in illuminating values and generating alternatives as described in the following paragraphs.

Illuminating values. People's values affect their behavior, feelings, and goals. In the process of amplifying, clarifying, and validating, the advocate understands a client's values. Through the process of self-revelation, an emerging value (about environment, people, cost, quality) may become more apparent to a client. This can have an impact in two ways. The client may be able to focus on actions consistent with the value, or the value may lend confusion and assist the client in prioritizing action. Values can also change as new or relevant data are processed. The advocate's role is to assist clients in discovering their values, which can be particularly demanding in the information exchange and affirming process.

Generating alternatives. Clients and advocates may feel limited in their options if they generate solutions before completely analyzing the problems, needs, desires, and consequences. Several techniques can be used to generate alternatives, including brainstorming and a technique known as the problem-purpose-expansion method. In **brainstorming,** the nurse, client, professionals, or significant others generate as many alternatives as possible, without critical evaluation. Brainstorming creates a list that can be examined for the critical elements the client seeks to preserve (e.g., environmental preferences, degree of control). The list can be analyzed according to the conse-

TABLE 19-2 Nursing Process and Advocacy Process

NURSING PROCESS	ADVOCACY PROCESS
Assessment/diagnosis	Information exchange Gather data Illuminate values
Planning/outcome	Generate alternatives and consequences Prioritize actions
Implementation	Decision making Support of client Assure Reassure
Evaluation	Affirmation Evaluation Reformulation

Communication that seeks to amplify, clarify, and verify knowledge, beliefs, and behaviors is used throughout both processes.

quences, the probability of chance events occurring, and the effect of the alternatives on self and others.

The **problem-purpose-expansion method** is a way to broaden limited thinking (Volkema, 1983). It involves restating the problem and expanding the problem statement so that different solutions can be generated. For example, if the problem statement is to convince the insurance company to approve a longer hospital stay, the nurse and client have narrowed their options. However, if the problem statement is to make the client's convalescence as optimal and safe as possible, several solutions and options are available, such as the following:

- Obtaining skilled nursing facility placement
- Obtaining home health skilled services
- Arranging physician home visits
- Paying for custodial care
- Paying for private skilled care
- Obtaining informal caregiving

Impact of advocacy

Advocacy empowers clients to participate in problem-solving processes and decisions about health care. Clients try to understand changing opportunities in the health care system for access, use, and continuity of care while nurse advocates promote client control of morale, life satisfaction, self-esteem, and adherence to therapeutic regimens (Kohler, 1988). Clients are part of larger systems: the family, the work environment, and the community. Each system interacts with the client to shape the available options through resources, needs, and desires. Each system also has both confirming and conflicting goals and processes that need to be understood for client self-determination to be successful. For example, the practice of advocacy among minority groups may entail the ability to focus attention on the magnitude of problems caused by diseases affecting minority clients. Whether the client is an individual, family, group, or community, the advocacy function can promote the interest of self-determination that characterizes progressive societies.

Advocacy is not without opposition. Clients and advocates may find barriers to services, vendors, providers, and resources. A community may experience a shortage in nursing home beds, a child care facility may experience staffing shortages, a family may not have the financial resources to keep a child at home, or a client may find that the school system cannot fund a full-time nurse for its clinic. The reality of scarce resources constitutes a difficult barrier for advocates. However, it is often events such as these that stimulate a community's self-determination and innovative actions to correct gaps in service.

Allocation and advocacy: complement or conundrum?

While advocacy holds a traditional role in the nursing profession, **allocation** is a staple of market competition. Nurses perform allocation roles when they triage clients and/or perform the gatekeeping and rationing functions.

The field of medicine has struggled with the allocation debate (Mechanic, 1997). Nurses often reflect that clinical judgments are influenced by their values and ethics and by technology and science (AACN, 1997). When working in organizations, nurses experience allocation demands at the systems level through budgetary decisions and staffing assignments and at the clinical level by establishing and implementing treatment protocols. When nurses act as client advocates by clarifying a client's desires or needs, they may be in conflict with systems procedures for allocating limited resources within these systems. The nurse who has both advocacy and allocation responsibilities in a job position may benefit from a clear understanding of personal and professional values as well as a systematic procedure for mediating conflict between the two competing responsibilities (Cary, 1998).

WHAT DO YOU THINK? *Case management includes the functions of both advocacy and allocation of health care services in the current delivery system. How can these functions pose a professional dilemma for the case manager?*

Conflict Management

Case managers help clients manage conflicting needs and scarce resources. Techniques for managing conflict include the range of active communication skills. These skills are directed toward learning all parties' needs and desires, detecting their areas of agreement and disagreement, determining their abilities to collaborate, and assisting in discovering alternatives and valuable activities for reaching a goal. Mutual benefit with limited loss for everyone is a goal of conflict management.

Conflict and its management vary in intensity and energy in a number of ways. The effort needed to manage a conflict depends on different factors: evidence to support facts and objective and subjective perceptions of the parties involved.

Negotiating is a strategic process used to move conflicting parties toward an outcome. The outcome can vary from one in which one person enlarges their share at another person's expense (**distributive outcomes**) to one in which mutual advantages override individual gains (**integrative outcomes**). Integrative outcomes are usually based on problem-solving and solution-generating techniques (Bisno, 1988).

The process of negotiation can be characterized in three stages: prenegotiation, negotiation, and aftermath. Prenegotiations are activities designed to have parties agree to collaborate. Parties must see the possibility of achieving an agreement and the costs of not achieving an agreement. Preparations must be made as to time, place, and ground rules concerning participants, procedures, and confidentiality.

The negotiation stage consists of phases in which parties must develop trust, credibility, distance from the issue (to limit the feeling of "one best way"), and the ability to retain personal dignity. Bisno (1988) characterizes the phases as the following:

- *Phase 1.* Establishing the issues and agenda. This is accomplished by identifying, clarifying, presenting, and prioritizing the issues.
- *Phase 2.* Advancing demands and uncovering interests. Negotiations center around presenting parties' interests and differentiating among parties' demands and positions.
- *Phase 3.* Bargaining and discovering new options. Debates include gathering facts based on reasoning that will generate understanding and promote relearning. Bargaining reduces differences on issues by giving or removing rewards or desired objects. Creating new solutions or options through brainstorming, reflective thinking, and problem-purpose-expansion techniques is important in achieving options that provide mutual benefits.
- *Phase 4.* Working out an agreement. This may involve settling on some but not all points. Parties can agree to reexamine the issues later, and steps for implementation and follow-up must be clarified.

The aftermath is the period after an agreement in which parties are experiencing the consequences of their decisions. The reality of their decisions may lead to a reevaluation of their values.

Thomas and Kilmann (1974) postulate that in a conflict situation, parties engage in behaviors that reflect the dimensions of assertiveness and cooperation. **Assertiveness** is the ability to present one's own needs. **Cooperation** is the ability to understand and meet the needs of others. Each person uses a predominant orientation and secondary orientation to engage in conflict. Behaviors seen in conflict management are described in Box 19-4. The importance of

---

BOX 19-4 Categories of Behaviors Used in Conflict Management

Competing. An individual pursues personal concerns at another's expense.
Accommodating. An individual neglects personal concerns to satisfy the concerns of another.
Avoiding. An individual pursues neither his or her concerns nor another's concerns.
Collaborating. An individual attempts to work with others toward solutions that satisfy the work of both parties.
Compromising. An individual attempts to find a mutually acceptable solution that partially satisfies both parties.

Modified from Thomas KW, Kilmann RH: *Thomas-Kilmann conflict mode instrument*, New York, 1974, Xicom.

---

the Thomas-Kilmann categories, although written some time ago, is that one can use a variety of orientations and that each orientation can be valuable in a given situation.

Clearly, flexibility in conflict management behavior can encourage an outcome that meets the client's goals. Helping parties navigate the process of reaching a goal requires effective personal relations, knowledge of the situation and alternatives, and a commitment to the process.

WHAT DO YOU THINK? *The health care benefit plan of a client may omit treatments and services that, according to evidence, improve health outcomes. Other complementary health services (e.g., acupuncture) may be omitted from the benefit plan because the evidence to determine health outcomes is not available. What should be the case manager's role with the client, benefit plan administrator, and the provider when services are not eligible to a client from his or her health plan?*

Collaboration

In case management the activities of many disciplines are needed for success. Clients, the family, significant others, payers, and community organizations contribute to achieving the goal. **Collaboration** is achieved through a developmental process. It occurs in a sequence, yet it is reciprocal between those involved (Cary and Androwich, 1989) and can be characterized by seven stages and activities (Fig. 19-3).

The goal of communication in the collaborative development process is to promote amplification, clarification, and verification of all team members' points of view. Although communication is an essential component in collaboration, it is not sufficient to result in or maintain collaboration. Although the collaboration model recognizes the contributions inherent in joint decision making, one member of the team should be accountable to the system, and the client and should be responsible for monitoring the entire process.

Case managers are uniquely positioned to encounter conflict on a daily basis. Competing needs, resources, organizational demands, and professional role boundaries among resources present opportunities and pitfalls for conflict management and collaboration. Box 19-5 lists stages of collaboration.

Teamwork and collaboration clearly demand knowledge and skills about clients, health status, resources, treatments, and community providers. The ability to assess clients' and families' complex needs requires knowledge of intrapersonal, interpersonal, medical, nursing, and social dimensions. The demonstration of team member and leadership skills in facilitating a goal-directed group process is essential. It is unlikely that any single professional has the expertise required in all aspects. It is likely, however, that the synergy produced by all involved can result in successful outcomes.

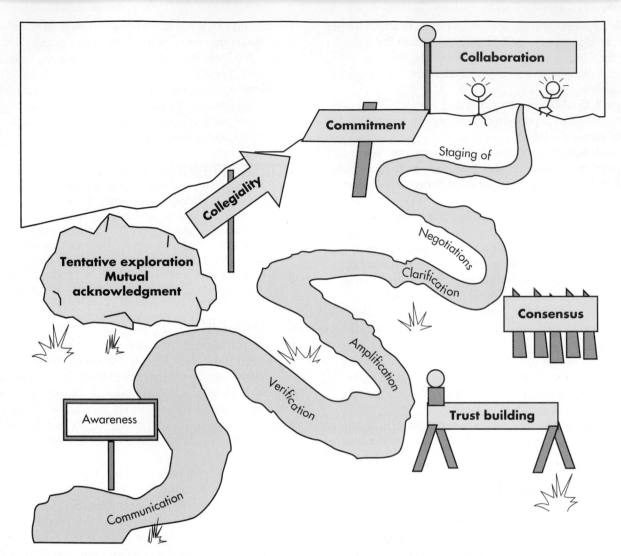

FIG. 19-3 Collaboration is a sequential yet reciprocal process. (From Cary AH, Androwich I: Paper presented at the Association of Community Health Nursing Educators Spring Institute, Seattle, Wash, June, 1989.)

DID YOU KNOW? *Family caregivers may be poorly prepared to assume high-technology care of the client at home. They often receive inadequate information about the client's illness trajectory, likely burdens and benefits of caregiving, economic consequences, and the complex and technical details of a plan of treatment.*

ISSUES IN CASE MANAGEMENT

Legal Issues

Liability concerns of case managers exist when three conditions are met: 1) the provider had a duty to provide reasonable care, 2) a breach occurred through an act or omission to act, and 3) the act or omission caused injury or damage to the client. Case managers must strive to reduce risks, practice wisely within acceptable standards, and limit legal defense costs through professional insurance coverage. Five general areas of risk are reviewed:

1. *Liability for managing care* (Hinden et al, 1994)

a. Inappropriate design or implementation of the case management system
b. Failure to obtain all pertinent records on which case management actions are based
c. Failure to have cases evaluated by appropriately experienced and credentialed clinicians
d. Failure to confer directly with the treating provider at the onset and throughout the client's care
e. Substituting a case manager's clinical judgment for that of the medical provider
f. Requiring the client or his or her provider to accept case management recommendations instead of any other treatment
g. Harassment of clinicians, clients, and family in seeking information and setting unreasonable deadlines for decisions or information
h. Claiming orally or in writing that the case management treatment plan is better than the provider's plan

BOX 19-5 Stages of Collaboration

1. AWARENESS

Make a conscious entry into a group process; focus on goals of convening together; generate definition of collaborative process and what it means to team members.

2. TENTATIVE EXPLORATION AND MUTUAL ACKNOWLEDGMENT

Exploration

Disclose professional skills for the desired process; disclose areas where contributions cannot be made; disclose values reflecting priorities: identify roles and disclose personal values, including time, energy, interest, and resources.

Mutual Acknowledgment

Clarify each member's potential contributions; verify the group's strengths and areas needing consultation; clarify member's work style, organizational supports, and barriers to collaborative efforts.

3. TRUST BUILDING

Determine the degree to which reliance on others can be achieved; examine congruence between words and behaviors; set interdependent goals; develop tolerance for ambiguity.

4. COLLEGIALITY

Define the relationships of members with each other; define the responsibilities and tasks of each; define entrance and exit conditions.

5. CONSENSUS

Determine the issues for which consensus is required; determine the process used for clarifying and decision making to reach consensus; determine the process for reevaluating consensus outcomes.

6. COMMITMENT

Realize the physical, emotional, and material actions directed toward the goal; clarify procedures for reevaluating commitments in light of goal demands and group standards for deviance.

7. COLLABORATION

Initiate a process of joint decision making reflecting the synergy that results from combining knowledge and skills.

Modified from Cary A, Androwich I: *A collaboration model: a synthesis of literature and a research survey.* Paper presented at the Association of Community Health Nursing Educators Spring Institute, Seattle, June 1989; Mueller WJ, Kell B: *Coping with conflict,* Englewood Cliffs, NJ, 1972, Prentice Hall.

    i. Restricting access to otherwise necessary or appropriate care because of cost

    j. Referring clients to treatment furnished by providers that are associated with the case management agency without proper disclosure

    k. Connecting case managers' compensation to reduced use and access

2. *Negligent referrals* (Hyatt, 1994)

    a. Referral to a practitioner known to be incompetent

    b. Substituting inadequate treatment for an adequate but more costly option

    c. Curtailing treatment inappropriately when curtailment caused the injury

    d. Referral to a facility or practitioner inappropriate for the client's needs

3. *Experimental treatment and technology* (Saue, 1994)

    a. Failure to apply the contractual definition of "experimental" treatment found in the client's insurance policy

    b. Failure to review sources of information referenced in the client's insurance policy (e.g., Food and Drug Administration [FDA] determination, published medical literature)

    c. Failure to review the client's complete medical record

    d. Failure to make a timely determination of benefits in light of timeliness of treatment

    e. Failure to communicate how coverage was determined to the insured client or participant

    f. Improper financial considerations determining the coverage

4. *Confidentiality* (Scheutzow, 1994)

    a. Failure to deny access to sensitive information that is awarded special protection by state law

    b. Failure to protect access allowances to computerized medical records

5. *Fraud and abuse* (Sollins, 1994)

    a. Making false statements of claims or causing incorrect claims to be filed

    b. Falsifying the adherence to conditions of participation of Medicare and Medicaid

    c. Submitting claims for excessive, unnecessary, or poor quality services

    d. Engaging in payment, bribes, kickbacks, or rebates in exchange for referral

Legal citings relevant to case management and managed care include negligent referrals, provider liability, payer liability, breach of contract, and bad faith. As in any scope of nursing practice, proactive risk management strategies can lower the provider's exposure to legal liability.

Saue (1994) notes that court cases influence the legal considerations of case managers. When courts find that cost considerations affect medical care decisions, all parties to the decision will be liable for resulting damages. Guidelines to reduce risk exposure include the following:

1. Clear documentation of the extent of participation in decision making and reasons for decisions

2. Records demonstrating accurate and complete information on interactions and outcomes
3. Use of reasonable care in selecting referral sources, which may include verifying of licensure of providers
4. Written agreements when arrangements are made to modify benefits other than those in the contract
5. Good communication with clients
6. Informing clients of their rights of appeal

Ethical Issues

Case managers as nursing professionals are guided in ethical practice by the Code of Ethics for Nursing (ANA, 1985) and the contract expressed in Nursing's Social Policy Statement (ANA, 1995, p. 4):

> Nursing is a caring-based practice in which processes of diagnosis and treatment are applied to the human experiences of health and illness. Nurses are guided by a philosophy of caring and advocacy. Nurses have a high regard for patient self-determination, independence and informed choice in decision making. Recognizing that responses to illness and disability may limit independence and self-determination, nurses focus on the rights of individuals, families and communities to define their own health-related goals and seek out health care that reflects their values.

This contractual philosophy of nursing practice is ideally suited to preserving the principles of autonomy, beneficence, and justice in case management processes. Banja (1994a) describes how case managers may confront dilemmas in each of these areas.

Case management may hamper a client's **autonomy** of individual right to choose a provider if a particular provider is not approved by the case management system. If a new provider must be found who can be approved for coverage, continuity of care may be disrupted. **Beneficence** can be influenced when excessive attention to cost containment supersedes or impairs the nurse's duty to provide measures to improve health or relieve suffering. "If cost containment goals are accomplished by decreasing services, at what point do health providers' behaviors exchange the good of their (clients) for the interests of restraining spending?" (Banja, 1994a, p. 39).

Justice as an ethical principle for case managers considers equal distribution of health care with reasonable quality. Tiers of quality and expertise among provider groups can be created when quality providers refuse to accept reimbursement allowances from the managed system, leaving less-experienced or lower-quality providers as the caregiver of choice for clients being managed.

Standards of practice and care, codes of ethics, licensure laws, and organizational policies and procedures (e.g., ethics committees, risk management units) offer the case manager information and support in managing ethical conflicts and dilemmas in the case management system. Maintaining familiarity with ethical issues published in the case management literature can offer specific assistance for practicing case managers. Boxes 19-6 and 19-7 list credentialing and accreditation options.

BOX 19-6 Credentialing Resources for Case Managers: Individual Certification Options

- National Board for Certification in Continuity of Care: (860) 586-7525—Multidisciplinary, A-CCC (Continuity of Care Certification—Advanced)
- Healthcare Quality Certification Board of the National Association for Healthcare Quality: (818) 286-8074—Multidisciplinary, CPHQ (Certified Professional in Health Care Quality)
- Rehabilitation Nursing Certification Board (800) 229-7530—CRRN (Certified Rehabilitation Registered Nurse)
- National Academy of Certified Case Managers: (800) 962-2260—Multidisciplinary, CMC (Care Manager Certified)
- Commission for Case Manager Certification: (847) 818-0292—Multidisciplinary, CCM (Certified Case Manager)
- Certification of Disability Management Specialists Commission: (847) 394-2106—Multidisciplinary, CDMS (Certified Disability Management Specialist)
- American Nurses Credentialing Center: (800) 284-2378—Nurses, RNCm (Case Management)
- Commission on Disability Examiner Certification (CDEC) —Specialty certification for life care planners.
- Center for Care Management: (508) 651-2600—Case Management Administrators

For further information, see the Weblinks on this book's website at www.mosby.com/MERLIN.

BOX 19-7 Case Management Program Accreditation Options

In January 1998, the American Accreditation Health Care Commission/URAC began developing accreditation standards for case management programs, which typically exist within managed care companies or free-standing companies. The accreditation will establish national standards for the structure and process of case management organizations. See the URAC website (www.urac.org) for contemporary status of accreditation development and implementation.

To access this and other websites, refer to the Weblinks on this book's website at www.mosby.com/MERLIN.

---

clinical application

During her regularly scheduled blood pressure clinic in a local apartment cluster, Mrs. B., a 45-year-old woman, complained of feeling dizzy and forgetful. She could not remember which of her six medications she had taken during the last few days. Her blood pressure readings on reclining, sitting, and standing revealed gross elevation. The nurse and Mrs. B. discussed the danger of her present status and the need to seek medical attention. Mrs. B. called her physician from her apartment and agreed to be transported to the emergency department.

While in the emergency department, Mrs. B. manifested the progressive signs and symptoms of a cerebrovascular accident (CVA, stroke). During hospitalization, she lost her capacity for expressive language and demonstrated hemiparesis and loss of bladder control. Her cognitive function became intermittently confused, and she was slow to recognize her physician and neighbors who came to visit. The utilization review nurse contacted the case manager from the health department to screen and assess for the continuum of care needs as early as possible because she lived alone and family members resided out of town.

It became apparent that family caregiving in the community could only be intermittent because members lived too far away. Mrs. B. had residual functional and cognitive deficits that would demand longer-term care.

As the case manager contracted by the plan, place the following actions in the order of sequence to construct a case management plan:

A. Discuss with the family their schedule of availability to offer care in the clients home.
B. Call the client and introduce yourself as a prelude to working with her.
C. Obtain information on the scope of services covered by the benefit plan for your client.
D. Arrange a skilled nursing facility site visit for the patient and family.

Answer is in the back of the book.

KEY POINTS

- An important role of the community-oriented nurse is that of client advocate.
- The goal of advocacy is to promote the client's self-determination.
- When performing in the advocacy role, conflicts may emerge regarding the full disclosure of information, territoriality, accountability to multiple parties, legal challenges to client's decisions, and competition for scarce resources.
- The functions of advocacy and allocation can pose dilemmas in practice.
- Amplification, clarification, and verification are three communication skills necessary in the advocacy process.
- Additional skills important in fulfilling the role of client advocate include the helping relationship, assertiveness, and problem solving.
- Problem solving is a systematic approach that includes understanding the values of each party and generating alternative solutions.
- Brainstorming and the problem-purpose-expansion method are two techniques to enhance the effectiveness of problem-solving skills.
- During conflict, negotiations can move conflicting parties toward an outcome.
- Prenegotiation, negotiation, and aftermath are three phases of managing a conflict.
- Each individual has a predominant orientation when engaging in conflict: competing, accommodating, avoiding, collaborating, or compromising.

- Collaboration may result by moving through seven stages: awareness, tentative exploration and mutual acknowledgment, trust building, collegiality, consensus, commitment, and collaboration.
- Care management is a strategic program to maintain the health of a population enrolled in a delivery system.
- Continuity of care is a goal of community-oriented nursing practice. It requires making linkages with services to improve the client's health status.
- As the structure of the health care system moves toward delivering more services in the community, the achievement of continuity of care will present a greater challenge.
- Case management is typically an interdisciplinary process in which the client is the focus of the plan.
- Documentation of case management activities and outcomes are essential to community-oriented nursing practice.
- Case management is a systematic process of assessment, planning, service coordination, referral, monitoring, and evaluation that meets the multiple service needs of clients.
- Community-oriented nurses have within their scope of practice advocacy, allocation, and case management functions.
- Nurses functioning as advocates and case managers need to be aware of the ethical and legal issues confronting these components of their practice.
- Standardization of care for predictable outcomes can be achieved through critical paths, disease management protocols, and multidisciplinary action plans.
- Telehealth application provides new alternatives within resource delivery options but must be customized for clients.

critical thinking activities

1. Observe a typical workday of a community health or public health nurse, noting the types of activities that are done in coordination and case management and the amount of time spent in these areas. Interview several staff members to determine whether they perceive that their time spent in case management is changing. To what degree are the staff members involved in care management activities?
2. Initiating, monitoring, and evaluating resources are essential components of community and public health nursing practice. Describe a client situation and the case management process that might occur in the following practices:
   a. School nurse in an elementary school and in a high school
   b. Occupational health nurse in a hospital and in a manufacturing plant
   c. Nurse working in a well-child clinic
   d. Case manager employed by a managed care organization
   e. Care manager employed in a health benefits corporation
3. The values and beliefs held by a community health nurse influence the nurse's ability to be an advocate for clients. Discuss your values and beliefs about rationing health care and how they may effect your ability to be a client advocate.

Continued

critical thinking activities—cont'd

4. Read the following article: Cary A: Advocacy and alloca-tion, *Nursing Connections* 11(1):35, 1988. Discuss your reactions to the following statement: "Allocation always works within the mixed interests of the individual and society" (p.39).

a. What are the mixed values of individuals?
b. What are the mixed values of delivery systems?
c. What are the mixed values of society in the United States? In underdeveloped nations?

Bibliography

Advisory Commission on Consumer Protection and Quality in the Health Care Industry: *Consumer bill of rights and responsibilities—report to the President of the United States,* Washington, DC, 1997, U.S. government Printing Office.

Allen SA: Medicare case management, *Home Health Nurse* 12(3):21, 1994.

American Academy of Nursing: *Managed care and national health care reform: nurses can make it work,* Washington, DC, 1993, American Academy of Nursing.

American Association of Colleges of Nursing: *The essentials of baccalaureate education for professional nursing practice,* Washington, DC, 1997, the Association.

American Hospital Association: *Glossary of terms and phrases for health care coalitions,* Chicago, 1986, AHA Office of Health Coalitions and Private Sector Initiatives.

American Nurses Association: *A statement on the scope of home health nursing practice,* Washington, DC, 1999, American Nurses Publishing.

American Nurses Association: *Code of ethics for nursing,* Washington, DC, 1985, the Association.

American Nurses Association: *Innovation at the worksite,* draft, Washington, DC, 1992b, the Association.

American Nurses Association: *Managed care: cornerstone for health care reform-a fact sheet,* Washington, DC, 1993, the Association.

American Nurses Association: *Nursing's principles for a managed care environment,* Washington, DC, 1998, American Nurses Publishing.

American Nurses Association: *Nursing's social policy statement,* Washington, DC, 1995, the Association.

American Nurses Credentialing Center: *Certification catalogue,* Washington, DC, 1998, American Nurses Publishing.

American Nurses Foundation: *America's nurses: an untapped natural resource,* Washington, DC, 1993, The Foundation.

Arras JD, Dubler NN: Executive summary of project conclusions: the technical tether, an introduction to the ethical and social issues in high-tech home care, *Hastings Center Report,* special supplement, New York, 1994.

Banez-Car M, McCoy N: Training for the transition to case management in home care, *Caring* 13(4):34, 1994.

Banja JD: Ethical challenges of managed care, *Case Manager* 5(3):37, 1994a.

Banja JD: Ethical dimensions of cultural diversity in case management, *Case Manager* 5(4):27, 1994b.

Barkauskas VH: Case management within home care: old ideas and new themes, *Home Health Nurse* 12(1):8, 1994.

Bartling AC: Trends in managed care, *Healthcare Exec* 10(2):6, 1995.

Bisno H: *Managing conflict,* Beverly Hills, Calif, 1988, Sage.

Boaz RF, Hu J: Determining the amount of help used by disabled elderly persons at home: the role of coping resources, *J Gerontol B Psychol Sci Soc Sci* 52B(6):S317, 1997

Bower KA: *Case management by nurses,* Washington, DC, 1992, American Nurses Association.

Cary AH: Advocacy or allocation, *Nursing Connection* 11(1):1, 1998.

Cary AH: Managed care. In Lundy K, James S, Hartman S, editors: *Nursing in the community: continuity of care of individuals, families and populations,* Sudbury, Mass, 1999, Jones and Bartlett.

Cary A, Androwich I: *A collaboration model: a synthesis of literature and a research survey.* Paper presented at the Association of Community Health Nursing Educators Spring Institute, Seattle, June 1989.

Case Management Society of America: *Standards of practice for case management,* Little Rock, Ark, 1995, CMSA

Cohen EL: *Nurse case management in the 21st century,* St Louis, 1996, Mosby.

Cohen EL, Cesta TG: *Nursing case management: from concept to evaluation,* St Louis, 1993, Mosby.

Coleman JR, Hagen E: Collaborative practice: case managers and home care agency nurses, *Case Manager* 2(4):64, 1991.

Coleman JR, Zagor KB: Effective care management, *Continuing Care* 17(7):23, 1998.

Congressional Research Service: *Case management standards in state community-based long-term care programs for older persons with disabilities,* CRS-91-55, Washington, DC, 1993, CRS, Library of Congress.

Deal LW: The effectiveness of community health nursing interventions: a literature review, *Public Health Nurs* 11(5):315, 1994.

Erkel EA et al: Case management and preventive services among infants from low-income families, *Public Health Nurs* 11(5):352, 1994.

Flarey DL, Blancett SS: Case management: delivering care in the age of managed care. In Flarey DL, Blancett SS, editors: *Handbook of nursing case management: health care delivery in a world of managed care,* Gaithersburg, Md, 1996, Aspen Publishers.

Foster J, Hall H: Public health and AIDS, *Caring* 5(6):4, 1986.

Gerson V: Case management accreditation, setting the standard, *Case Manager* 9(5), 1998.

Goodwin DR: Nursing case management activities, *J Nurs Admin* 24(2):29, 1994.

Gustafson DH: The total costs of illness: a metric for health care reform, *Hosp Health Services Admin* 40(1):154, 1995.

Hinden RA et al: Legal hazards on the case management highway, *Case Manager* 5(3):97, 1994.

Hyatt TK: Negligent referral, *Case Manager* 5(3):102, 1994.

James M: At the heart of the disease management revolution, *Case manager* 9(2):47, 1998.

Kenyon V et al: Clinical competencies for community health nursing, *Public Health Nurs* 7(1):33, 1990.

Kohler P: Model of shared control, *J Gerontol Nurs* 14(7):21, 1988.

Kohnke MF: *Advocacy risk and reality,* St Louis, 1982, Mosby.

Lamb GS, Stempel JE: Nurse case management from the client's view: growing as insider-expert, *Nurs Outlook* 42(1):7, 1994.

LaPensee KT: Pricing specialty carve-outs and disease management programs under managed care, *Managed Care Quarterly* 5(2):10, 1997.

Lashley M: The hidden benefits of case management, *Case Manager* 4(3):78, 1993.

Lowery S, editor: Scrambling for CM certification: here's what to know about 6 choices, *Case Management Advisor* 8(1):1, 1997.

May CA, Schraeder C, Britt T: *Managed care and case management: roles for professional nursing,* Washington, DC, 1997, American Nurses Publishing.

McClinton DH: Promoting wellness, *Continuing Care* 17(4):6, 1998a.

McClinton DH: Protecting patients, *Continuing Care* 17(7):6, 1998b.

McKinley LL, Zasler CP: Weaving a plan of care, *Continuing Care* 17(7):19, 1998.

Mechanic D: Muddling through elegantly: finding the proper balance in rationing, *Health Affairs,* 16(5):83, 1997.

Molloy SP: Defining case management, *Home Health Nurse* 12(3):51, 1994.

Mueller WJ, Kell B: *Coping with conflict,* Englewood Cliffs, NJ, 1972, Prentice Hall

Mullahy CM: *The case manager's handbook,* ed 2, Gaithersburg, Md, 1998a, Aspen.

Mullahy CM: *Essential readings in case management,* Gaithersburg, Md, 1998b, Aspen.

Nelson ML: Advocacy in nursing, *Nurs Outlook* 36(3):136, 1988.

Newell M: *Using nursing case management to improve health outcomes,* Gaithersburg, Md, 1996, Aspen.

Parker M et al: Issues in rural case management, *Fam Community Health* 14(4):40, 1992.

Powell SK: *Nursing case management,* Philadelphia, 1996, Lippincott-Raven.

Qudah FJ, Brannon M: Population based case management, *Qual Manag Health Care* 5(1):29, 1996.

Rieve J: Disease management concerns, *Case Manager* 9(2):34, 1998.

Romaine D: Case management challenges, present and future, *Cont Care* 14(1):24, 1995.

Saue JM: Legal issues related to case management. In Fisher K, Weisman E, editors: *Case management: guiding patients through the health care maze,* Chicago, 1994, JCAHO.

Salle SM: Experimental treatment and technology, *Case Manager* 5(3):106, 1994.

Schaffer CL: Case management law, *Contin Care* 13(5):20, 1994.

Scheutzow SO: Confidentiality, *Case Manger* 5(3):108, 1994.

Secord LJ: *Private case management for older persons and their families,* Excelsior, Minn, 1987, Interstudy.

Shwartz M et al: Improving publicly funded substance abuse treatment: the value of case management, *Am J Public Health* 87(10):1659, 1997.

Sollins HI: Fraud and abuse, *Case Manager* 5(3):109, 1994.

Solberg LI et al: Using continuous quality improvement to improve diabetes care in populations: the IDEAL model, *Jt Comm J Qual Improv* 23(11):581, 1997.

Sowell RL, Meadows TM: An integrated care management model: developing standards, evaluation and outcome criteria, *Nurs Admin Q* 18(2):53, 1994.

Thomas KW, Kilmann RH: *Thomas-Kilmann conflict mode instrument,* New York, 1974, Xicom.

Thompson M, Curry MA, Burton D: The effects of nursing case management on the utilization of prenatal care by Mexican-Americans in Rural Oregon, *Public Health Nurs* 15(2):82, 1998.

US Department of Health and Human Services: *Healthy people 2000: midcourse review and 1995 revisions,* Washington, DC, 1995, USDHHS, Public Health Service.

US Department of Health and Human Services: *Healthy people 2000: national health promotion and disease prevention objectives,* Washington, DC, 1992, USDHHS, Public Health Service.

Volkema RJ: *Problem-purpose-expansion: a technique for reformulating problems,* 1983, University of Wisconsin (unpublished manuscript).

Ward MD, Rieve J: Disease management: case management's return to patient-centered care, *J Care Management* 1(4):7, 1995.

Webb C: Professionalism revisited, *Nurs Times* 83(35):39, 1987.

Weil M, Karls JM: Historical origins and recent developments. In Weils M et al, editors: *Case management in human service practice,* San Francisco, 1985, Jossey-Bass.

Winslow GR: From loyalty to advocacy: a new metaphor for nursing, *Hastings Cent Rep* 14:32, 1984.

Wrinn MM: The emerging role of telehealth in health care, *Continuing Care* 17(8):18, 1998a.

Wrinn MM: Stepping up to the plate in 1998, *Continuing Care* 17(1):16, 1998b.

Zander K, editor: *The new definition,* South Natick, Mass, 1994, The Center for Case Management.

Zander K, Etheredge ML, Bower KA: *Nursing case management: blueprints for transformation,* Waban, Mass, 1987, Winslow Printing Systems.

Zander K, McGill R: Critical and anticipated recovery paths: only the beginning, *Nurs Manage* 25(8):34, 1994.

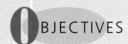

SUSAN B. HASSMILLER

OBJECTIVES

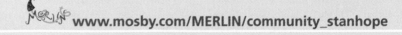
www.mosby.com/MERLIN/community_stanhope

After reading this chapter, the student should be able to do the following:

- Discuss types of disasters, including natural, man-made, and epidemics.
- Evaluate how disasters affect people and their communities.
- Discuss disaster management, including preparedness, response, and recovery.
- Examine the nurse's role in the preparedness, response, and recovery phases of disaster management.

- Describe the priorities in a triage situation.
- Explain the steps for initiating and maintaining a clinic to care for the masses.
- Identify how the community (including voluntary, governmental, and community organizations; business; and labor) works together to prepare for, respond to, and recover from disasters.
- Analyze the role of the American Red Cross in disaster management.

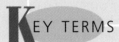

KEY TERMS

delayed stress reaction
disaster
disaster medical
 assistance teams
 (DMATs)

emergency support
 functions (ESFs)
Federal Response Plan
 (FRP)
Level I disaster

Level II disaster
Level III disaster
man-made disasters
mitigation
natural disasters

preparedness
recovery
response
triage
See Glossary for definitions

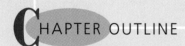

CHAPTER OUTLINE

Disasters
 Defining Disasters
 International Decade for
  Natural Disaster Reduction

Healthy People 2000 and *2010*
 Objectives
 Three Stages of Disaster
  Involvement: Preparedness,
  Response, and Recovery

Preparedness
Response
Recovery

The author wishes to thank the following individuals for their thoughtful review and critique of this chapter: Laurie Willshire, RN, Jane Morgan, RN, and Judy Lee, RN, and all Disaster Services associates who work for the National Headquarters of the American Red Cross. The author also wishes to thank Cyndy Kiely and Brian Castrucci for their thoughtful contributions.

Wherever disaster calls there I shall go. I ask not for whom, but only where I am needed."

From the Creed of the Red Cross Nurse

"We do not expect disasters, but they happen. With living come natural calamities; with industrial and technological advances come accidents; with socioeconomic and political stagnation or change come dissatisfaction, terrorism, and war" (Waeckerle, 1991, p. 820). Although disasters, man-made or natural, are inevitable, there are ways to prevent or manage how people and their communities respond to disasters. This chapter describes management techniques throughout the preparedness, response, and recovery phases of disaster. The nurse's role throughout these phases is highlighted.

WHAT DO YOU THINK? *Much of the destruction caused by natural disasters in the 1990s could have been avoided. In many documented cases, building codes were ignored, warnings were not issued or followed, communities were located in dangerous areas, and plans were forgotten. An "ounce of prevention" or preparedness would have made a real difference (Gerrity and Flynn, 1997).*

DISASTERS

Children often first hear about a natural disaster through the story of Noah and the flood in the Book of Genesis. The fairy tale fashion in which the story is invariably told is inadequate preparation for the destruction and devastation that disasters truly leave behind. Disasters can affect one family at a time, as in a house fire, or they can kill thousands and have economic losses in the millions, as with floods, earthquakes, tornadoes, and hurricanes. Over the last 10 years, major natural disasters have caused a total economic loss of over $400 billion (UNOCHA, 1998b). The loss of life has also been dramatic. Approximately 3 million lives have been lost in the past 20 years as a result of earthquakes, volcanic eruptions, landslides, floods, tropical storms, droughts, and other natural disasters. In addition to the mortality, 1 billion more people have had to cope with the injuries, disease, and homelessness that always follow disasters (UNOCHA, 1998a).

The burden of natural disasters throughout the world fall disproportionately on developing countries. A person living in a developing country is 12 times more likely to perish in a natural disaster than a person living in the United States. This fact is exacerbated by projections suggesting that by 2050, 80% of the world's population will live in developing countries (UNOCHA, 1998a).

The urbanization and overcrowding of cities have increased the danger of natural disasters because communities have been built in areas that are vulnerable to disasters. Increases in population and monetary investment in areas vulnerable to natural disasters have led to the quadrupling of insurance payouts in the United States in every decade.

Projections suggest that by 2050, at least 46% of the world's population will live in areas vulnerable to floods, earthquakes, and severe storms.

Overcrowding and urbanization have also increased man-made disasters. The stress caused by overcrowding has promoted civil unrest and riots. In some parts of the world, modern warfare waged over land rights and space have markedly increased the risk of injury and death from disaster.

The cost of disaster recovery efforts has also risen sharply because of the number of people involved and the amount of technology that must be restored. People in industrialized countries are becoming less self-sufficient because they rely heavily on technology and social and economic systems within their community. People who "live on the brink of disaster" every day, physically, emotionally, and/or economically, are among the first to be affected when calamity strikes.

DID YOU KNOW? *Disasters create the most devastation in developing countries, where the death rate is up to 12 times higher than in developed countries. The poor suffer the most because their houses are less sturdy and they have fewer resources and less means of social security.*

Defining Disasters

A **disaster** is any man-made or natural event that causes destruction and devastation that cannot be alleviated without assistance. The event need not cause injury or death to be considered a disaster. For example, a hurricane may cause millions of dollars in damage without causing a single death or injury. Box 20-1 lists examples of man-made and natural disasters.

Although **natural disasters** will always occur, a lot can be done to prevent further escalation of accidents, death, and destruction after impact. A concise, realistic, and well-rehearsed disaster plan, as well as sustained and open communication among involved organizations and workers, can prevent further damage. Also, many of the **man-made disasters** listed in Box 20-1 can be prevented (e.g., substance abuse that causes major transportation accidents and fires).

International Decade for Natural Disaster Reduction

As the life and economic losses caused by natural disasters increased, the United Nations (UN) declared the 1990s to be the International Decade for National Disaster Reduction (IDNDR). The goal of this UN initiative, located in Geneva as part of the UN Department of Humanitarian Affairs, was to help educate people to reduce their risk of morbidity and mortality caused by natural disasters. To accomplish the program's goals, the IDNDR published a quarterly magazine and regional newsletters and operated

BOX 20-1 Types of Disasters

NATURAL
Hurricanes
Tornadoes
Hailstorms
Cyclones
Blizzards
Drought
Floods
Mudslides
Avalanches
Earthquakes
Volcanic eruptions
Communicable disease epidemics
Lightning-induced forest fires

MAN-MADE
Conventional warfare
Nonconventional warfare (e.g., nuclear, chemical)
Transportation accidents
Structural collapse
Explosions/bombing
Fires
Toxic materials
Pollution
Civil unrest (e.g., riots demonstrations)

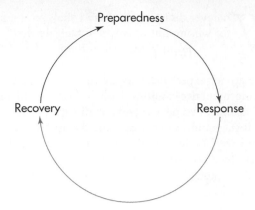

FIG. 20-1 Disaster management cycle (Modified from American Red Cross: *Disasters happen,* Washington, DC, 1993, Author.)

Disasters do play a direct role in the objectives related to unintentional injuries, occupational safety and health, environmental health, and food and drug safety. Professionals, such as those who work at the CDC, study the effects that disasters have on objectives such as the ones listed above and are constantly developing new prevention strategies. Other organizations, such as the American Psychological Association and the American Red Cross, work with communities in the immediate recovery phase of a disaster and sometimes for years thereafter to effect the *Healthy People 2000* objectives related to mental health.

THREE STAGES OF DISASTER INVOLVEMENT: PREPAREDNESS, RESPONSE, AND RECOVERY

Disaster management includes the three stages of a disaster: preparation, response, and recovery. Figure 20-1 depicts the disaster management cycle. A key to disaster **preparedness** is that the plan must be kept realistic yet simple. The reasons for this are that 1) no plan will ever exactly fit the disaster as it occurs, and 2) all plans must be implementable no matter what key members of the disaster team are there at the time (Public health responds to disaster, 1994). The following section elaborates on all three stages, including what the role of the nurse should be.

Preparedness
Personal preparedness

Nurses with client responsibilities can also become disaster victims (Chubon, 1992). Conflict between family- and work-related responsibilities abound. For example, a mother whose child care needs go unmet will not be able to participate fully, if at all, in disaster relief efforts. In addition, the nurse assisting in disaster relief efforts must be as healthy as possible, both physically and mentally. A disaster worker who is not well is of little service to his or her family, clients, and other disaster victims. Personal and family preparation can help ease some of the conflicts that arise and will allow nurses to attend to client needs sooner than one may anticipate.

a public awareness campaign with an annual World Disaster Reduction Day.

From this declaration came a heightened public-private partnering emphasis on **mitigation** (i.e., actions or measures that can either prevent the occurrence of a disaster or reduce the severity of its effects [American Red Cross, 1998a]). Mitigation activities include the following:

1. Awareness and education, such as holding community meetings on disaster preparedness
2. Disaster relief, such as building a retaining wall to divert flood water away from a residence
3. Advocacy, such as supporting actions and efforts for effective building codes and prudent land-use

Dozens of national, state, and local agencies, such as the Institute for Business and Home Safety, American Red Cross, Centers for Disease Control and Prevention (CDC), and local communities of faith, came together during this internationally declared decade for disaster reduction to work proactively to save lives and property.

Healthy People 2000 and *2010* Objectives

Since disasters affect the health of people in many ways, they have an effect on almost every *Healthy People 2000* and *Healthy People 2010* objective. For example, although nutrition and exercise are two important *Healthy People 2000* objectives, they will not take precedence over more pressing needs for people housed in temporary shelter. There are, however, some objectives that are more directly affected.

█HOW TO *Prepare for Safety in a Disaster: Four Steps to Safety* _____

1. Find out what could happen to you
   a. Determine what types of disasters are most likely to happen.
   b. Learn about warning signals in your community.
   c. Ask about postdisaster pet care (shelters usually will not accept pets).
   d. Review the disaster plans at your workplace, school, and other places where your family spends time.
   e. Determine how to help elderly or disabled family members or neighbors.
2. Create a disaster plan
   a. Discuss types of disasters that are most likely to happen and review what to do in each case.
   b. Pick two places to meet, including outside your home and outside your neighborhood.
   c. Choose an out-of-state friend to be your "family contact" to verify location of each family member. After a disaster, it is easier to call long distance than to make local calls.
   d. Review evacuation plans, including care of pets. Identify ahead of time where to go if evacuation is necessary.
3. Complete this checklist
   a. Post emergency phone numbers by telephones.
   b. Teach everyone how and when to call 911.
   c. Determine when and how to turn off water, gas, and electricity at the main switches.
   d. Check adequacy of insurance coverage.
   e. Locate and review use of fire extinguisher.
   f. Install and maintain smoke detectors.
   g. Conduct a home hazard hunt and fix potential hazards.
   h. Stock emergency supplies and assemble a disaster supplies kit.
   i. Acquire first aid and CPR certification.
   j. Locate all escape routes from your home. Find two ways out of each room.
   k. Find the safe spots in your home for each type of disaster.
4. Practice and maintain your plan
   a. Review plan every 6 months.
   b. Conduct fire and emergency evacuation drills.
   c. Replace stored water every 3 months and stored food every 6 months.
   d. Test and recharge fire extinguisher according to manufacturer's instructions.
   e. Test your smoke detectors monthly and change the batteries at least once a year.

█NURSING TIP

Emergency supplies needed in case of disaster:
- A 3-day supply of water (1 gallon per person per day) and food that will not spoil.
- One change of clothing and footwear per person, and one blanket or sleeping bag per person.
- A first-aid kit that includes your family's prescription medications.
- Emergency tools including a battery-powered radio, flashlight, and plenty of extra batteries.
- Candles and matches.
- An extra set of car keys and a credit card, cash, or traveler's checks.
- Sanitation supplies, including toilet paper, soap, feminine hygiene items, and plastic garbage bags.
- Special items for infant, elderly, or disabled family members.
- An extra pair of eye glasses.

The American Red Cross and the Federal Emergency Management Agency (FEMA), two well-known authorities on disaster preparedness, response, and recovery, have devised a personal checklist to help individuals and families prepare for disasters before they strike (FEMA, 1992). The How To box shows an adapted version of the FEMA's recommendations entitled *Four Steps to Safety*. Also, the Nursing Tip lists emergency supplies that should be prepared and stored in a sturdy, easy-to-carry container. Important documents should always be kept in a waterproof container.

Professional preparedness

Professional preparedness requires that nurses become aware of and understand the disaster plans at their workplace and community. Nurses who take disaster preparation seriously will take the time to read and understand workplace and community disaster plans and will participate in disaster drills and community mock disasters. Adequately prepared nurses can function in a leadership capacity and assist others toward a smoother recovery phase. Personal items that are recommended for nurses preparing to help in a disaster include the following (Switzer, 1985):
- Copy of professional license
- Personal equipment, such as a stethoscope
- Flashlight and extra batteries
- Cash
- Warm clothing and a heavy jacket (or weather-appropriate clothing)
- Record-keeping materials
- Pocket-sized reference books

Disaster work is not high tech. Field work, including shelter management, requires that nurses be creative and willing to improvise in delivering care. All workers should be certified in first aid and CPR. In addition, the American Red Cross provides a comprehensive program of disaster training for health professionals to enable them to provide assistance within their own communities and to other stricken communities and countries. The courses teach nurses how to adapt their existing nursing skills to a disaster setting.

Community preparedness

The level of community preparedness for a disaster is only as good as the people and organizations in the community make it. Some communities stay prepared for a possible disaster by having a written disaster plan and by participating in yearly mock disaster drills. Other communities are less vigilant and depend on luck and the fact that they have never been hit before to see them through. Some organizations within the community may be more prepared than others. For example, most health care facilities have written disaster plans and require employees to perform annual mock drills, but many businesses do not have these requirements.

Nurses need to review the disaster history of the community, including how past disasters have affected the health care delivery system and how their particular organization fit into the plan. Understanding these aspects of past disasters influences planning for future disasters. For example, disaster history may reveal that the local disaster services committee has not appropriately used the county's nurses because of a lack of education about their roles. It might be beneficial for this committee to receive an educational program on what nurses do and what role they can play in a disaster. A solid disaster plan requires the talents, coordination, and cooperation of many different people and organizations. Some key community organizations and professionals involved in disaster work include the clergy, morticians, police, fire and rescue personnel, the mayor and other city officials, and the media. Working together cooperatively and with clear role definition before the disaster gives greater ensurance that assistance will be delivered smoothly once a disaster hits.

Finally, the community must have an adequate warning system and a back-up evacuation plan to remove individuals from areas of danger who hesitate to leave their homes. People must be convinced that predisaster warnings are official, serious, and personally relevant before they are motivated to take action. Also, some people mistakenly believe that experience with a particular type of disaster is preparation enough for the next one. Finally, individuals may refuse to leave their homes because they are afraid that their possessions will be lost or destroyed by the disaster and/or from postdisaster looting. It may take a face-to-face encounter with law-enforcement personnel or others in authority to convince individuals to leave their homes and retreat to safer quarters.

Role of the nurse in disaster preparedness

Nurses in disaster preparedness facilitate preparation within the community and place of employment (Fig. 20-2). Within the employing organization the nurse can help initiate or update the disaster plan, provide educational programs and materials regarding disasters specific to the area, and organize disaster drills. The nurse is also in a unique position to provide an updated record of vulnerable populations within the community. For example, when calamity strikes, disaster workers must know what kinds of populations they are attempting to assist. If a tornado strikes a retirement village, the needs will be quite different then if the tornado hits a church with predominantly young families or a center for the physically challenged. In addition to knowing where special populations exist, the nurse should be involved in educating special populations about what impact the disaster might have on them. Individualized strategies should be reviewed, in-

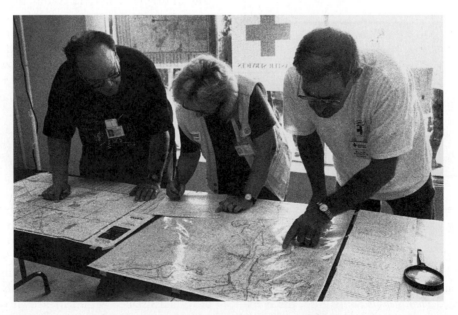

FIG. 20-2 Understanding the community's disaster plan is a key role for nurses who seek greater involvement in disaster management. (Courtesy American Red Cross.)

cluding the availability of specific resources, in the event of an emergency.

The nurse who leads a preparedness effort can help recruit others within the organization who will help if and when a response is required. Although there is no psychological profile of a disaster leader, it is wise to involve persons in this effort who have demonstrated flexibility, decisiveness, stamina, endurance, and emotional stability (Dinerman, 1990). The leader should also possess an intimate knowledge of the institution and familiarity with the individuals who work there. Persons with disaster management training, and especially those who have served during real disasters, also make valuable members of any preparedness team.

Within the community, the nurse may be involved in many roles. As community advocates, nurses help keep a safe environment. Recalling that disasters are not only natural, but man-made as well, the nurse in the community needs to assess for and report environmental health hazards. For example, the nurse should be aware of and report unsafe equipment, faulty structures, and the beginning of disease epidemics such as measles or flu.

The nurse should also understand what the available community resources will be after a disaster strikes, and most important, how the community will work together. A community-wide disaster plan will help the nurse understand what "should" occur before, during, and after the response and his or her role within the plan. The nurse who seeks more involvement or an in-depth understanding of disaster management can become involved in any number of community organizations that are part of the official response team, such as the American Red Cross, Salvation Army, or Emergency Medical System/ Ambulance Corps. The American Red Cross offers classes on disaster health services and disaster mental health services to "help participants identify Disaster Health Services preparedness measures that should take place on the local unit level and to become familiar with Red Cross disaster health services policies, regulations, and procedures that apply on locally administered disaster operations" (American Red Cross, 1989, p. 5). The Red Cross generally requires certification in a disaster health services or a disaster mental health services course before assigning an individual to a disaster site as a Red Cross representative.

For nurses who choose to work with agencies such as the Red Cross, there are many options for involvement. After several hours of disaster training, nurses may wish to take the following steps to get actively involved:
- Join a local disaster action team (DAT).
- Act as a liaison with local hospitals.
- Determine health-related appropriateness for shelter sites; plan with pharmacies, opticians, morticians, and other health personnel to facilitate service for disaster victims.
- Plan for and retain needed supplies.
- Teach disaster nursing in the community.

It is important to keep the nursing and medical protocols and intervention standards, whether they be with the Red Cross or employing institution, up to date and consistent with local public health standards (American Red Cross, 1989). Nurses are needed for national and international disaster assignments as well.

Mass casualty drills or mock disasters

Mass casualty drills or mock disasters are valuable components of any preparedness plan. Whether the drills are carried forth in a desk-top manner or through realistic scenarios, the objectives are as follows (Lehnhof, 1985):
- Promote confidence
- Develop skills
- Coordinate activities
- Coordinate participants

It is critical for those who will be involved in the actual disaster to be involved in the drill (Berglin, 1990). Also, the drill leader needs special skills in disaster management and the ability to coordinate many organizations at one time. Although a successful disaster drill can allow participants to evaluate the rescue plan and make further recommendations, it should not create a misplaced sense of security (Waeckerle, 1991).

Agencies involved in disaster preparedness

Many community agencies contribute to disaster preparedness. Table 20-1 describes the preparedness responsibilities assumed by the American Red Cross, other voluntary organizations, labor business organizations, and local government.

Response

Levels of disaster and agency involvement

There are many small disasters, such as single-family home fires, and even more extensive disasters that do not require the assistance of the FEMA. In this case, the American Red Cross, along with other organizations such as the Salvation Army, works to assist disaster victims. When a presidential declaration has been made, the Red Cross works with the FEMA to assist with recovery efforts. Table 20-2 describes disaster response responsibilities of the American Red Cross, other voluntary organizations, business and labor organizations, and local government.

The response by the FEMA is determined by the level of disaster. Levels are not determined by the number of casualties per se but by the amount of resources needed. According to the FEMA (1998), there are three levels of **response:**
- **Level III disaster.** Considered a minor disaster. The disaster is classified as one that involves a minimal level of damage but could result in a presidential declaration of an emergency or a disaster. A minimal amount of federal involvement may be requested by state and local jurisdictions, in which case the request would be met by existing federal regional resources.
- **Level II disaster.** Considered a moderate disaster, which will likely result in a major presidential disaster

TABLE 20-1 Disaster Preparedness Responsibilities by Agency

AMERICAN RED CROSS	OTHER VOLUNTARY ORGANIZATIONS	BUSINESS AND LABOR ORGANIZATIONS	LOCAL GOVERNMENT
Participates with government in developing and testing community disaster plan. Designates persons to serve as representatives at government emergency operations centers and command posts.	Collaborates in developing and maintaining a local Voluntary Organizations Active in Disaster group to identify roles, resources, and plans for disasters.	Develops disaster plans for business locations and integrates their plans with the community disaster plan.	Coordinates the development of the community plan and conducts evaluation exercises.
Develops and tests local Red Cross disaster plans.	Identifies and trains personnel for disaster response.	Develops procedures to facilitate continuity of operations in times of disaster.	Trains staff to carry out the plan.
Identifies and trains personnel for disaster response.	Identifies community issues and special populations for consideration in disaster preparedness.	Develops plans for assisting business employees after a disaster.	Passes legislation to mitigate the effects of potential disasters.
Collaborates with other voluntary agencies to develop and maintain a local Voluntary Organizations Active in Disaster group to promote cooperation and coordinate resources and people for disaster work.	Makes plans to continue to serve regular clients after a disaster.	Identifies union and business facilities, resources, and people who may be able to support community disaster plans.	Designs measures to warn the population of disaster threats.
Works with business and labor organizations to identify resources and people for disaster work.	Identifies facilities, resources, and people to serve in time of disaster.	Provides volunteers, financial contributions, and in-kind gifts to Red Cross and other voluntary organizations to support disaster preparedness.	Conducts building safety inspections.
Educates the public about hazards and ways to avoid, prepare for, and cope with their effects.	Educates specific client groups on disaster preparedness.	Educates employees and union members about disaster preparedness.	Develops procedures to facilitate continuity of public safety operations in times of disaster.
Acquires material resources needed to ensure effective response.			Identifies public facilities, resources, and public employees for disaster work.
			Educates the public about disaster threats in the community and safety procedures.

From American Red Cross: *Disasters happen* (ARC Pub No 1570), Washington, DC, 1994, ARC.

declaration with moderate federal assistance. Federal regional resources will be fully engaged, and other federal regional offices outside the affected area may be called upon to contribute resources.

- **Level I disaster.** Considered a massive disaster. This disaster involves a massive level of damage, with severe impact or multistate scope. This level of event will result in a presidential disaster declaration, with major federal involvement and full engagement of federal regional and national resources. Hurricane Georges, a catastrophic disaster that devastated parts of the Florida Keys, Mississippi, Louisiana, Alabama, Florida, and several islands in 1998, necessitated a Level I disaster response.

In any large scale or major national disaster, not only do official agencies respond, but many other concerned citizens, including health professionals, come on their own to help as well. At times, so many people come "out

of the woodwork" to help that role conflict, anger, frustration, and helplessness occur. Because of this, it is best that nurses attach themselves to an official agency with assigned disaster management responsibilities (Alson et al, 1993; Switzer, 1985).

The Federal Response Plan

Once a federal emergency has been declared, the **Federal Response Plan (FRP)**, also known as public law 93-288, may take effect depending on the specific needs of the disaster. The FRP is "based on the fundamental assumption that a significant disaster or emergency will overwhelm the capability of State and local governments to carry out the extensive emergency operations necessary to save lives and protect property" (FEMA, 1992, p. 1). Box 20-2 lists the purpose of the FRP.

Within the FRP there are twelve **emergency support functions (ESFs)**, each one headed by a primary agency. Each primary agency is responsible for coordinating efforts

TABLE 20-2 Disaster Response Responsibilities by Agency

AMERICAN RED CROSS	OTHER VOLUNTARY ORGANIZATIONS	BUSINESS AND LABOR ORGANIZATIONS	LOCAL GOVERNMENT
Operates shelters. Provides feeding services. Provides individual and family assistance to meet immediate emergency needs. Services include providing the means to purchase groceries, clothing, and household items. Provides disaster health services, including mental health support. Handles inquiries from concerned family members outside the area. Coordinates relief activities with other agencies, business, labor, and government. Informs the public of services available. Seeks and accepts contributions from those wanting to help.	Provides services that are identified in predisaster planning. Provides regular services to ongoing client groups. Identifies unanticipated needs and provides resources to meet those needs. Acts as advocates for their client groups. Coordinates services with all other groups involved with the disaster response. Seeks and accepts donations from those wanting to help.	Takes action to protect employees and to ensure the safety of the facility. Advises public safety forces of hazardous conditions. Identifies resources such as union halls, generators, and heavy equipment that are available to support the disaster response. Provides volunteers, financial contributions, and gifts of goods and services to the relief effort.	Provides for coordination of the overall relief effort. Advises the public on safety measures such as evacuation. Provides public health services. Provides fire and police protection to the affected area. Inspects facilities for safety and health codes. Provides ongoing social services for the community. Repairs public buildings, sewage and water systems, streets, and highways.

From American Red Cross: *Disasters happen* (ARC Pub No 1570), Washington, DC, 1994, ARC.

in a particular area with all of its designated support agencies. In all, 26 federal agencies and the American Red Cross must respond if called upon. For example, in a presidentially declared disaster, all ongoing health and medical services fall under the auspices of the U.S. Public Health Service. The U.S. Public Health Service divides its responsibilities among its own agencies as needed. The CDC, for instance, may "assist in establishing surveillance systems to monitor the general population and special high-risk population segments; carry out field studies and investigations; monitor injury and disease patterns and injury control measures and precautions" (FEMA, 1992, ESF #8-10). Sheltering, feeding, emergency first aid, providing a disaster welfare information system, and coordinating bulk distribution of emergency relief supplies is the mass care ESF, of which the American Red Cross is the primary agency. It is conceivable that the nurse could be involved with any of the above response efforts within the local community or, with appropriate training, on a national basis.

The National Disaster Medical System (NDMS) is part of the ESF of Health and Medical Services. In a presidentially declared disaster, including overseas war, the U.S. Public Health Service can activate **disaster medical assistance teams (DMATs)** to an area to supplement local and state medical care needs. DMATs can also be activated by the assistant secretary for health upon the request of a state health

BOX 20-2 Purpose of the Federal Response Plan

- Establishes fundamental assumptions and policies
- Establishes a concept of operations that provides an interagency coordination mechanism to facilitate the immediate delivery of federal response assistance
- Incorporates the coordination mechanisms and structures of other appropriate federal plans and responsibilities into the overall response
- Assigns specific functional responsibilities to appropriate federal departments and agencies
- Identifies actions that participating federal departments and agencies will take in the overall federal response in coordination with the affected state

Federal Emergency Management Agency: *The Federal Response Plan (FRP)*, Washington, DC, 1992, FEMA.

officer. Teams of specially trained civilian physicians, nurses and other health care personnel can be sent to a disaster site within hours of activation. DMATs can provide triage and continuing medical care to victims until they can be evacuated to a national network of hospitals prearranged by the NDMS (FEMA, 1992; Waeckerle, 1991).

In reality, because of the nature of this country's disasters since the initiation of DMATs, these teams have been

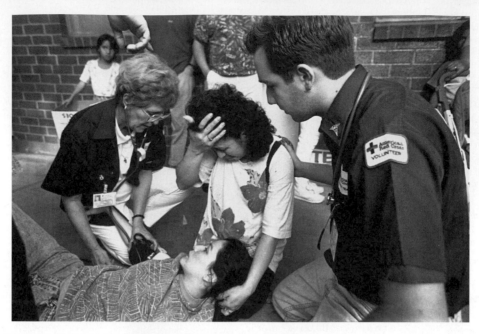

FIG. 20-3 Individuals react to the same disaster in different ways. (Courtesy American Red Cross. All rights reserved in all countries.)

used primarily to staff community health outpatient clinics in the affected areas.

How disasters affect communities

People in a community can be affected physically and emotionally depending on the type, cause, and location of the disaster; its magnitude and extent of damage; its duration; and the amount of warning that was provided. For example, an earthquake may not cause any deaths; however, the structural damage to buildings and the continuous aftershocks that may last for weeks can cause intense psychological stress. In addition, the longer it takes for structural repairs and other clean-up, the longer the psychological effects can last.

The bombing of the Alfred P. Murrah Building in Oklahoma City in 1995 created extreme anger and grief, but this act of terrorism also led many to perform extraordinary acts of compassion (Walsh, 1995). Thousands of people helped, from donating blood and money to rescuing victims from the building to volunteering for the "Compassion Center," a place where family members could go to receive support. One nurse, Rebecca Anderson, paid the ultimate price for her altruism. She was killed by a fall while attempting to rescue survivors inside the gutted building. Although known as the worst man-made disaster in American history, the Oklahoma City bombing will also be remembered as the disaster that brought out the soul and character of the American people.

Individuals react to the same disaster in different ways depending on their age, cultural background, health status, social support structure, and their general adaptability to crisis (Fig. 20-3). Gerrity and Flynn (1997) state that the sequencing of reactions and level of intensity depend to

some extent on the characteristics of the disaster, such as the suddenness of impact, duration of the event, and probability of reoccurence. Box 20-3 describes common adult and child reactions to disasters. The typical first reaction to a disaster is an extreme sense of urgency (Chubon, 1992). Victims become obsessed with personal losses. Other initial reactions include fear, panic, disbelief, reluctance to abandon property, disorientation and numbing, difficulty in making decisions, need for information, seeking help for self and family, and offering help to other disaster victims (American Red Cross, 1991a). Disturbances in bodily functions, such as gastrointestinal upsets, diarrhea, and nausea and vomiting, are also common (Gerrity and Flynn, 1997).

Anger, especially blaming and scapegoating, is common among victims soon after a disaster (Chubon, 1992; Gerrity and Flynn, 1997). Cohen and Ahearn (1980) note that anger and blaming stem from an increasing awareness of what has been lost, physical fatigue, emotional stress, and a continuing change in personal comfort. Victims being interviewed on television after a disaster often say that FEMA or the American Red Cross simply did not do all that was possible. Later responses include difficulty in sleeping, headaches, apathy and depression, moodiness and irritability, anxiety about the future, domestic violence, feelings of being overwhelmed, frustration and feelings of powerlessness over one's own future, and guilt over not being able to prevent the disaster (American Red Cross, 1991a).

An exacerbation of an existing chronic disease is also common. For example, the emotional stress of being a disaster victim may make it difficult for people with diabetes to control their blood sugar levels. Jealousy and resent-

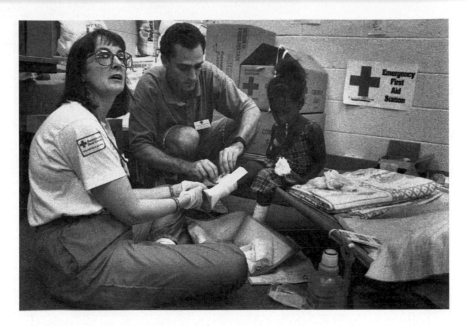

FIG. 20-4 The effects of a disaster on young children can be especially disruptive. (Courtesy American Red Cross. All rights reserved in all countries.)

ment abound, even over fellow victims in the same community. Although poor people are often the most severely affected disaster victims, a group of nurses in South Carolina expressed anger after becoming victims of hurricane Hugo because the poor were receiving added support and attention while they continued to struggle for assistance (Chubon, 1992).

The effects on young children can be especially disruptive (Fig. 20-4). Regressive behaviors such as thumb sucking, bed wetting, crying, and clinging to parents can occur (American Red Cross, 1991b). Fantasies that the disaster never occurred and nightmares are common as well. School-related problems may also occur, including an inability to concentrate and even refusal to go back to school (Gerrity and Flynn, 1997).

WHAT DO YOU THINK? *Is it reasonable for people to drop off chronically ill family members, especially those suffering from Alzheimer's disease, at Red Cross shelters for extended periods of time during the preparedness, response, and recovery phases of disaster?*

An elderly person's reaction to disaster depends a great deal on physical health, strength, mobility, self-sufficiency, and income source and amount (American Red Cross, 1993) (Fig. 20-5). They react more deeply to loss of personal possessions because of the high sentimental value attached to the items and the limited time left to replace them (Gerrity and Flynn, 1997). Anticipatory guidance may help the elderly person who has to move into a nursing home, either temporarily or permanently, or who must adjust to moving in with an adult child. The need for relocation depends on the extent of damage to their home

BOX 20-3 Common Reactions to Disasters by Adults and Children

ADULTS
Extreme sense of urgency
Panic and fear
Disbelief
Disorientation and numbing
Reluctance to abandon property
Difficulty in making decisions
Need to help others
Anger and blaming
Blaming and scapegoating

Delayed Reactions

Insomnia
Headaches
Apathy and depression
Sense of powerlessness
Guilt
Moody and irritable
Jealousy and resentment
Domestic violence

CHILDREN
Regressive behaviors (bed wetting, thumb sucking, crying and clinging to parents)
Fantasies that disaster never occurred
Nightmares
School-related problems, including an inability to concentrate and refusal to go back to school

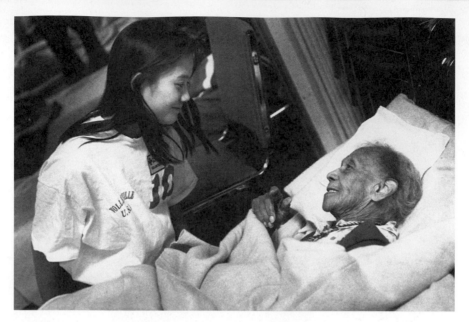

FIG. 20-5 Elderly persons' reactions to a disaster depend greatly on their physical health, strength, mobility, self-sufficiency, and income source and amount. (Courtesy American Red Cross. All rights reserved in all countries.)

BOX 20-4 **Special Population Groups at Greatest Risk for Disruption from a Disaster**

Persons with disabilities
Persons living on a low income, including the homeless
Non-English speaking persons and refugees
Persons living alone
Single-parent families
Persons new to the area
Institutionalized or those with chronic mental illness
Previous disaster victims or victims of traumatic events

---

or their compromised health. An elderly person may hide the seriousness of their losses out of fear of loss of independence (American Red Cross, 1993). Box 20-4 lists other populations at risk for severe disruption from a disaster.

Role of the nurse in disaster response

The role of the nurse during disaster depends a great deal on the nurse's experience, role in institution and community preparedness, specialized training, and special interest. The most important attribute for anyone working in a disaster, however, is that of flexibility (Public health responds to disaster, 1994). If there is one thing certain about disaster, it is that change is a constant (Gaffney, Schodorf, and Jones, 1992).

Although valued for their expertise in community assessment, casefinding and referring, prevention, health education, surveillance, and working with aggregates, there may be times when the nurse is the first to arrive on the scene. In this situation, it is important to remember that all life-threatening problems take precedence. Once rescue

workers begin to arrive at the scene, immediate plans for triage should begin.

Triage is the process of separating casualties and allocating treatment based on the victim's potential for survival. Highest priority is always given to victims who have life-threatening injuries but who have a high probability of survival once stabilized (Dixon, 1986). Second priority is given to victims with injuries with systemic complications that are not yet life threatening but who would be able to wait up to 45 to 60 minutes for treatment. Last priority is given to those victims with local injuries without immediate complications and who can wait several hours for medical attention.

Nurses working as members of an assessment team need to feed back accurate information to relief managers to facilitate rapid rescue and recovery. Often nurses will make home visits to gather needed information. Types of information in initial assessment reports include the following (Lillibridge, Noji, and Frederick, 1993):

- Geographic extent of disaster's impact
- Population at risk or affected
- Presence of continuing hazards
- Injuries and deaths
- Availability of shelter
- Current level of sanitation
- Status of health care infrastructure

These assessments help to match available resources to a population's emergency needs. Lillibridge, Noji, and Frederick (1993) also point out that disaster assessment priorities are related to the type of disaster that has occurred. For example, sudden-impact disasters, such as tornadoes and earthquakes, are more concerned with ongoing hazards, injuries and deaths, shelter requirements, and potable water. Gradual-onset disasters, such as famines, are most concerned with mortality rates, nutritional status, immunization status, and environmental health.

Lack of or inaccurate information regarding the scope of the disaster and its initial effects contributes to the misuse of resources. For example, after hurricane Andrew, a well-meaning general public continued to ship thousands of pounds of clothing to South Florida, well beyond what it could ever hope to use. Much of the clothing eventually had to be burned because there was inadequate onsite personnel to sort and distribute the clothing and the piles eventually became a public health nuisance. Local and regional emergency and public health resources can be readjusted as assessment reports continue to come in. Prioritizing needs that benefit the largest aggregate of imperiled individuals with the most correctable problems is consistent with the most basic tenets of triage (Waeckerle, 1991).

Ongoing assessments or surveillance reports are just as important as initial assessments. Surveillance reports indicate the continuing status of the affected population and the effectiveness of ongoing relief efforts. They continue to inform relief managers of needed resources. Nurses involved in ongoing surveillance can use the methods listed in the How To box to gather information. Surveillance continues into the recovery phase of a disaster.

HOW TO *Gather Disaster Information*

1. Interview
2. Observation
3. Physical examination
4. Health and illness screening
5. Surveys (sample and special health)
6. Records (census, school, vital statistics, and disease reporting)

From Switzer KH: Functioning in a community health setting. In Garcia LM, editor: *Disaster nursing: planning, assessment, and intervention*, Rockville, Md, 1985, Aspen.

Shelter management

Shelters are generally the responsibility of the local Red Cross chapter, although in massive disasters the military may be used to set up "tent cities" for the masses who need temporary shelter. Nurses, because of their comfort with delivering aggregate health promotion, disease prevention, and emotional support, make ideal shelter managers and team members. Although there may be physical health needs to attend to, especially among the elderly and chronically ill, many of the predominant problems in shelters revolve around stress. The shock of the disaster itself, loss of personal possessions, fear of the unknown, living in close proximity to total strangers, and even boredom can cause stress.

Common-sense approaches to working with victims dealing with stress work best. Basic measures that can be taken by the shelter nurse include the following (American Red Cross, 1991a, 1991c):

- Listen to victims tell and retell their feelings related to the disaster and their current situation.
- Encourage victims to share their feelings with one another if it seems appropriate to do so.
- Help victims make decisions.
- Delegate tasks (reading, crafts, and playing games with children) to teenagers and others to help combat boredom.
- Provide the basic necessities (food, clothing, rest).
- Attempt to recover or gain needed items (prescription glasses, medication).
- Provide basic compassion and dignity (privacy when appropriate and if possible).
- Refer to a mental health counselor if the situation warrants.

The American Red Cross provides specialized training in disaster mental health services. Its objective is "assisting the worker or client to understand disaster-related stress and grief reactions, develop adaptive coping and problem-solving skills, and return to a predisaster state of equilibrium or seek recommended further treatment" (American Red Cross, 1991c, p. 5). Highly trained mental health counselors, such as psychologists, psychiatrists, psychiatric social workers, and nurses, are always available in large-scale disasters. They are important members of any disaster team, no matter what the level of disaster, and their services should be used as often as necessary.

Nurses are also involved in the shelter functions of assessment and referral, ensurance of medical needs (prescription glasses, medications), first aid, meal serving, keeping client records, ensuring emergency communications and transportation, and providing a safe environment (American Red Cross, 1988a). The Red Cross provides training for shelter management and expects those trained to follow appropriate protocols.

International relief efforts

Obviously disasters do not occur just in industrialized countries. Other countries, especially those involved with political upheavals, suffer not only from natural disasters but from man-made disasters as well. Civil strife leads to war, famine, and communicable disease outbreaks. Sometimes disaster or relief workers are sent to these international calamities at the request of the affected country's government. At other times workers are not welcomed but instead may go with the support of the UN. When workers are not welcomed, their lives may be in danger, even though they go as peace-keeping agents of the Federation of Red Cross and Red Crescent Societies and the International Committee of Red Cross or as health representatives from the World Health Organization. International disaster or relief workers generally have intense training and preparation before embarking on a mission.

Psychological stress of disaster workers

Psychological stress among victims and workers during disasters is well-documented (Cohen and Ahearn, 1980; Demi and Miles, 1983; Gerrity and Flynn, 1997). The degree of worker stress depends on the nature of the disaster, role in the disaster, individual stamina, and other environmental factors (Richtmeier and Miller, 1985). Environmental factors include noise, inadequate work space, physical danger, and stimulus overload, especially exposure to death and trauma. Other sources of stress may emerge when workers do not think that they are doing enough to help, from the burden of making life and death decisions, and the overall change in living patterns (Errington, 1989; Laube-Morgan, 1992).

When the nurse is from the same community in which disaster has struck, role-conflict from organizational chaos, including the organization being cut off from their usual support systems, also causes stress (Errington, 1989). Nothing has the potential for causing more stress and role-conflict, however, than when the disaster nurse worker is also a victim of the disaster (Laube-Morgan, 1992). Anger and resentment may occur as the job demands time away from one's own calamitous situation. Studies indicate, however, that the nurses' emotional responses do not interfere with their effectiveness in helping others (Chubon, 1992; Laube, 1973).

Symptoms of early stress and burn-out include minor tremors, nausea, loss of concentration, difficulty thinking, and problems with memory (Laube-Morgan, 1992). Suppressing feelings of guilt, powerlessness, anger, and other signs of stress will eventually lead to symptoms such as irritability, fatigue, headaches, and distortions of bodily functions (Errington, 1989). It is normal to experience stress, but it must be dealt with. The worst thing anyone can do is to deny that it exists.

The American Red Cross (1993) recommends the following strategies for dealing with stress while working at the disaster:

- Get enough sleep
- Take time away from the disaster (i.e., breaks)
- Avoid alcohol
- Eat frequently in small amounts
- Use humor to break the tension and provide relief
- Use positive self-talk
- Take time to defuse or debrief
- Stay in touch with people at home
- Keep a journal
- Provide mutual support

Delayed stress reactions, or those that occur once the disaster is over, include exhaustion and an inability to adjust to the slower pace of work or home (American Red Cross, 1991b). Other emotions out of the ordinary may be evident but are normal for someone who has been involved with a disaster. Disappointment may be felt if family members and friends do not seem as interested in what the worker has been through and because the homecoming, in general, does not live up to expectations.

Frustration and conflict may occur as the worker's needs seem totally inconsistent with those of the family and coworker. Frustration and conflict also occur as a result of having left the disaster site, when there remains a real or perceived belief that much more could have been done (Gaffney, Schodorf, and Jones, 1992). Issues or problems that once seemed pressing may now seem trivial. Anger may emerge as others present problems that seem trivial compared with those faced by the victims who were left behind. Disaster workers may fantasize about returning to the disaster site if they think that their actions are appreciated more than at home or the office. Mood swings are common and serve to resolve conflicting feelings. Feelings or actions that persist or that the worker perceives are interfering with daily life should be dealt with by a trained mental health professional (American Red Cross, 1991b). (See the Research Brief.)

Recovery

The stage of disaster known as **recovery** occurs as all involved agencies pull together to restore the economic and civic life of the community (American Red Cross, 1993). For example, the government takes the lead in rebuilding efforts, whereas the business community attempts to provide economic support. Many religious organizations help with rebuilding efforts as well. The Internal Revenue Service educates victims as to how to write off losses and the Housing and Urban Development Department provides grants for temporary housing. The CDC provides continuing surveillance and epidemiological services. Voluntary agencies continue to assess individual and community needs and meet those needs as they are able.

DID YOU KNOW? *The best time to start thinking about the lessons learned from a recent disaster is during the recovery phase of the disaster cycle (Gerrity and Flynn, 1997).*

Role of the nurse in disaster recovery

The role of the nurse in the recovery phase is as varied as in the preparedness and response phases of a disaster. Flexibility remains important for a successful recovery operation. Community clean-up efforts can incur a host of physical and psychological problems. For example, the physical stress of moving heavy objects can cause back injury, severe fatigue, and even death from heart attacks. In addition, the continuing threat of communicable disease will continue as long as the water supply remains threatened and the living conditions are crowded (Gaffney, Schodorf, and Jones, 1992). Nurses must remain vigilant in teaching proper hygiene and making sure immunization records are up to date.

Acute and chronic illnesses can be exacerbated by the prolonged effects of disaster. The psychological stress of clean-up and/or moving can cause feelings of severe hopelessness, depression, and grief (Fig. 20-6). Recovery can be impeded by short-term psychological effects eventually

RESEARCH *Brief*

The aftermath of a natural disaster presents many challenges to health care workers. Most epidemiological investigations after natural disasters have focused on physiological problems and infectious disease outbreak and containment. However, these investigations tend to neglect the long-term effects of natural disasters on effected populations, specifically the long-term mental health effects. Two months after hurricane Andrew struck Dade County, Florida the Centers for Disease Control and Prevention (CDC) and the State of Florida surveyed the affected community to gauge various mental health indicators. As a result of this survey, a community outreach program for mental health and crisis counseling was initiated. The purpose of this study was to assess the effectiveness of this model for delivering mental health referrals to those experiencing long-term mental health effects as a result of a natural disaster.

The study found that certain households were more likely to experience symptoms of mental health distress. These households included those who had incomes less than $20,000, had trouble affording food, failed to see a doctor because of cost, poor health, a job change, job loss, crime or violence in their community after the disaster; and reported that their living situation was worsened by the event. The hypothesis was that the community health outreach program would help families more easily find and access mental health services as compared with those who were not visited by an outreach team.

This study found that community health outreach teams were not an effective method of referring clients to mental health services. Of those contacted by the outreach teams, 70% received referrals or instructions on how to receive the mental health care that they needed. However, those households who were contacted by the team were no more likely than those households not contacted to be referred for help. This suggests that the goal of the community outreach team was not met.

The authors suggest that alternatives to the community outreach team approach should be explored because this is an expensive, labor intensive intervention with limited benefit (e.g., linking victims with familiar neighborhood organizations such as fire departments, schools, and churches). The long-term mental health needs of an affected community should not be neglected. Even though agreement is lacking on the most efficient, cost-effective model for referring people to necessary services, health care providers in postdisaster areas must strive to ensure that all people receive the care they need.

McDonnell SL et al: Long-term effects of hurricane Andrew: revisiting mental health indicators, *Disasters* 19(3):235, 1995.

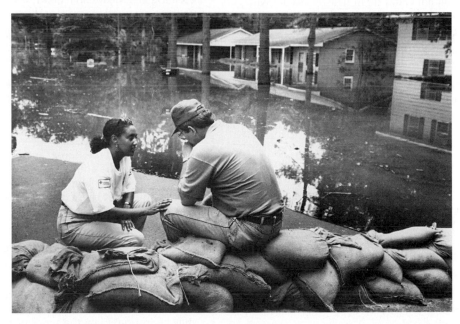

FIG. 20-6 The psychologic stress of cleanup and moving can bring about feelings of severe hopelessness, depression, and grief. (Courtesy American Red Cross. All rights reserved in all countries.)

merging with the long-term results of living in adverse circumstances (Richman, 1993). In some cases, stress can lead to suicide and domestic abuse (Gaffney, Schodorf, and Jones, 1992). Although the majority of people eventually recover from disasters, mental distress may persist in those vulnerable populations who continue to live in chronic adversity (Goenjian, 1993). Referrals to mental health professionals should continue as long as the need exists.

Nurses need to be alert for environmental health hazards during the recovery phase of a disaster. During home visits, nurses may uncover situations such as a faulty housing structure or lack of water or electricity. Objects may have been blown into the yard from a tornado or floated in from a flood that are dangerous and must be removed. Also, the nurse should assess the dangers of live or dead animals and rodents that are harmful to a person's health. An example of this would be finding snakes in and around homes once the waters from a flood start to recede. The role of case finding and referral remains critical during the recovery phase and will continue, in some cases, for a long time. For example, for a full 2 years after the Oklahoma City bombing of the Alfred P. Murrah Federal Building, the American Red Cross supported the Bombing Recovery Project (American Red Cross, 1998b). Follow-up home visits were made for all those in need, although the recovery process for some will last for years. In the end, all of the nurses and organizations in the world can only provide partnerships with the victims of a disaster. Ultimately, it is up to individuals to recover on their own.

clinical application

Paula, a nurse in a medium-sized public health department in Lincoln, Nebraska, was called to serve on her first national disaster assignment. Her disaster skills were tested when a Level I hurricane hit Miami and its surrounding areas. Paula left Lincoln, Nebraska to help manage a shelter in an elementary school cafeteria in nearby Homestead, Florida.

The devastation that Paula saw enroute to the school had a negative effect on her. Paula was assigned to help with client intake. She patiently listened to the disaster victims, referred many of her most distraught clients to the mental health counselor, and prioritized other needs as they arose. For example, she found that many of her clients left their medications behind and needed therapy. Other needs included diapers and formulas for infants, prescription eye glasses, and clothing. By identifying their needs, Paula helped to ensure that the master "need list" was complete.

As the days went on, the stress level in Paula's shelter began to intensify. The crowded living conditions and lack of privacy began to take its toll on the residents. Around the tenth day of Paula's assignment she began to experience pounding headaches and was finding it difficult to concentrate. Paula believed she would be fine, but the mental health counselor told Paula that she was experiencing a stress reaction.

Which action would likely be the most useful for Paula to take:

A. Share her feelings with the onsite mental health counselor on a regular basis.
B. Call home to share her feelings with family members.
C. Meet the needs of her clients to the best of her ability, and accept the fact that stress is a part of the job.

Answer is in the back of the book.

KEY POINTS

- The number of natural disasters has remained constant, but the number of man-made disasters and ensuing deaths continues to rise sharply.
- The cost to recover from a disaster has risen sharply because of the amount of technology that must be restored.
- The Director-General of the World Health Organization made the decade of the 1990s the International Decade for Natural Disaster Reduction based on a worldwide need for disaster education and a curtailment of the fatalistic approach to disasters that so many people take.
- Professional preparedness entails an awareness and understanding of the disaster plan at work and in the community.
- To counteract a historical lack of use or misuse of nurses in disaster planning, response, and recovery, nurses must get involved in their community's planning efforts.
- Disaster health and disaster mental health training from an official agency such as the American Red Cross will help prepare nurses for the many opportunities that await them in disaster preparedness, response, and recovery.
- The response to a disaster is determined by its assigned level. Levels are not determined by the number of casualties per se but by the amount of resources needed.
- Helping clients maintain a safe environment and advocating for environmental safety measures in the community are key roles for the nurse during all phases of disaster management.
- Becoming knowledgeable about available community resources, especially for vulnerable populations, during the preparedness stage of disaster management will ensure smoother response and recovery stages.
- The Federal Response Plan may be activated if a disaster is so significant in its effect that it will overwhelm the capability of state and local governments to carry out the extensive emergency operations needed for community restoration. In all, 26 federal agencies and the Red Cross have specific functions to carry out in such an event.
- People in a community react differently to a disaster depending on the type, cause, and location of the disaster; its magnitude and extent of damage; its duration; and the amount of warning that was provided. Individual variables that cause people to react differently include their age, cultural background, health status, social support structure, and their general adaptability to crisis.
- A great deal of stress is exhibited by nurses who are not only caring for clients but are also disaster victims themselves.
- Disaster shelter nurses are exposed to a variety of physical and emotional complaints, including stress. Stress may be instigated by the shock of the disaster, loss of personal possessions, fear of the unknown, living in close proximity to strangers, and boredom.
- The degree of worker stress during disasters depends on the nature of the disaster, role in the disaster, individual stamina, noise level, adequacy of work space, potential for physical danger, and stimulus overload, especially being exposed to death and trauma.
- Symptoms of worker stress during disasters include minor tremors, nausea, loss of concentration, difficulty think-

ing and remembering, irritability, fatigue, and other somatic disorders.

- A key attribute in aiding disaster victims is flexibility.
- The stage of disaster known as recovery occurs as all involved agencies pull together to restore the economic and civic life of the community.

critical thinking activities

1. Select a vulnerable population within your community and determine what special needs the group would have in time of disaster. What community resources are currently available to help this group?
2. Describe the role of the nurse in the preparedness, response, and recovery stages of disaster.
3. Interview a nurse who has participated in a disaster to determine what role was played and the reaction to that role.
4. Conduct an interview with an official from the fire department, civil defense department, American Red Cross, or other agencies involved with disaster preparation and response to determine what your community's plan is.
5. Discuss the advantages and disadvantages of serving on a disaster, either in your own community or another community. Decide whether you would be a good candidate to serve on a disaster.
6. Contact your local public health department to determine its role in a local disaster, including the role of the nurses that work there.
7. Find out what the disaster plan is for your place of employment.

Bibliography

Alson R et al: Analysis of medical treatment at a field hospital following hurricane Andrew, 1992, *Ann Emerg Med* 22(11):78, 1993.

American Red Cross: *Coping with disaster: emotional health issues for victims* (ARC Pub No 4475), Washington, DC, 1991a, ARC.

American Red Cross: *Coping with disaster: returning home from a disaster assignment* (ARC Pub No 4473), Washington, DC, 1991b, ARC.

American Red Cross: *Disaster health services I: instructor manual* (ARC Pub No 3076-1), Washington, DC, 1989, ARC.

American Red Cross: *Disaster mental health services* (ARC Pub No 3050M), Washington, DC, 1991c, ARC.

American Red Cross: *Disaster mental health services I* (ARC Pub No 3077-1A), Washington, DC, 1993, ARC.

American Red Cross: *Disasters happen* (ARC Pub No 1570), Washington, DC, 1994, ARC.

American Red Cross: The American Red Cross and mitigation, *Disaster Services News Sheet*, Feb 3, 1998a.

American Red Cross: Oklahoma city bombing recovery project: answering the call: Roberta Flynn offers encouragement to victims, *Disaster Services News Sheet*, Feb 27, 1998b,.

Berglin SL: Emergency nurses in community disaster planning, *J Emerg Nurs* 16(4):290, 1990.

Chubon SJ: Home care during the aftermath of hurricane Hugo, *Public Health Nurs* 9(2):97, 1992.

Cohen RE, Ahearn FL: *Handbook for mental health care of disaster victims*, Baltimore, 1980, Johns Hopkins University.

Demi AS, Miles MS: Understanding psychologic reactions to disaster, *J Emerg Nurs* 9:11, 1983.

Dinerman N: Disaster preparedness: observations and perspectives, *J Emerg Nurs* 16(4):252, 1990.

Dixon M: Disaster planning, medical response: organization and preparation, *AAOHN J* 34:580, 1986.

Errington G: Stress among disaster nurses and relief workers, *Int Nurs Rev* 36(3):80, 1989.

Federal Emergency Management Agency: *The Federal Response Plan (FRP)*, Washington, DC, 1992, FEMA.

Federal Emergency Management Agency: *Job aid: disaster levels, classifications and conditions*, Washington, DC, 1998, FEMA.

Federal Emergency Management Agency, American Red Cross: *Your family disaster plan*, Washington, DC, 1992, FEMA, ARC.

Gaffney JK, Schodorf L, Jones G: DMATs respond to Andrew and Iniki, *Journal of Emergency Medical Services*, p. 76, Nov, 1992.

Gerrity ET, Flynn BW: Mental health consequences of disasters. In Noji EK, editor: *The public health consequences of disasters*, New York, 1997, Oxford University Press.

Goenjian A: A mental health relief program in Armenia after the 1988 earthquake, *Br J Psych* 163:230, 1993.

Laube J: Psychological reactions of nurses in disaster, *Nurs Res* 22:343, 1973.

Laube-Morgan J: The professional's psychological response in disaster: implications for practice, *J Psychosoc Nurs* 30(2):17, 1992.

Lehnhof DB: Planning mass casualty drills. In Garcia LM, editor: *Disaster nursing: planning, assessment, and intervention*, Rockville, Md, 1985, Aspen.

Lillibridge SR, Noji EK, Frederick MB: Disaster assessment: the emergency health evaluation of a population affected by a disaster, *Ann Emerg Med* 22(11):72, 1993.

McDonnell S et al: Long-term effects of hurricane Andrew: revisiting mental health indicators, *Disasters* 19(3):235, 1995.

Office of US Foreign Disaster Assistance: *Disaster history:significant data on major disasters worldwide, 1990-present*, Washington, DC, 1990, Author.

Orr SM, Robinson WA: The Hyatt Regency skywalk collapse: an EMS-based disaster response, *Ann Emerg Med* 12:601, 1983.

Pickens S: The decade for natural disaster reduction: the role of health care workers, *Nurs Health Care* (13)4:192, 1992.

Public health responds to disaster: the Los Angeles earthquake, *The Nation's Health*, p. 1, March, 1994.

Richman N: After the flood, *Am J Public Health* 83(11):1522, 1993.

Richtmeier JL, Miller JR: Psychological aspects of disaster situations. In Garcia LM, editor: *Disaster nursing: planning, assessment, and intervention*, Rockville, Md, 1985, Aspen.

Switzer KH: Functioning in a community health setting. In Garcia LM, editor: *Disaster nursing: planning, assessment, and intervention*, Rockville, Md, 1985, Aspen.

United Nations Office for the Coordination of Humanitarian Affairs: *Natural disasters and sustainable development: linkages and policy options*, OCHA-Online, Nov 6, 1998a http://156.106.192.130/dha_ol/programs/idndr/presskit/options.html).

United Nations Office for the Coordination of Humanitarian Affairs: *The role of the insurance industry in disaster reduction*, OCHA-Online, Nov 6, 1998b (http://156.106.192.130/dha_ol/programs/idndr/presskit/role.html).

Waeckerle JF: Disaster planning and response, *N Engl J Med*, 324(12):815, 1991.

Walsh KT: The soul and character of America, *US News and World Report* 118(18):10, 1995.

CHAPTER 21

Program Management

MARCIA STANHOPE

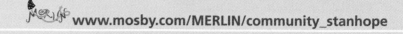
www.mosby.com/MERLIN/community_stanhope

OBJECTIVES

After reading this chapter, the student should be able to do the following:

- Compare the program management process to the nursing process.
- Analyze the program planning process and its application to public and community health nursing.
- Compare and contrast a program planning method to use in community-oriented nursing practice.

- Identify the benefits of program planning.
- Analyze the components of program evaluation and application to nursing practice.
- Identify evaluation methods and techniques.
- Name program evaluation sources.
- Describe types of program evaluation measures.
- Describe types of cost studies applied to program management.

KEY TERMS

assessment of need
case register
cost accounting
cost benefit
cost effectiveness
cost efficiency
cost studies

evaluation
evaluation of program effectiveness
formative evaluation
health index
health planning
health program planning

needs assessment
outcome
planning
process
program
program evaluation
strategic planning

structure
summative evaluation
tracer method

See Glossary for definitions

CHAPTER OUTLINE

Program management consists of assessing, planning, implementing, and evaluating a program. This chapter focuses primarily on planning and evaluation. Although presented in separate discussions, these factors are related and dependent processes that work together to bring about a successful program. This chapter does not deal with implementing programs because most chapters in the text focus on implementation.

The program management process is like the nursing process. One is applied to a program, whereas the other is applied to clients. The process of program management, as with the nursing process, consists of a rational decision-making system designed to help nurses know when to make a decision to develop a program (*problem identification*), where they want to be at the end of the program (*assessment*), how to decide what to do to have a successful program (*planning*), how to develop a plan to go from where they are to where they want to be (implementation), how to know that they are getting there (*formative evaluation*), and what to measure to know that what they are doing is appropriate (*summative evaluation*).

There is more emphasis on accountability for nursing actions and client outcomes today. The introduction of prospective payment systems, health care reform, and managed care has changed the focus of nursing. Planning for nursing services is necessary today if the nurse is to survive in the field of health care delivery.

This chapter examines how nurses can act instead of react by planning programs that can be evaluated for their effectiveness. This discussion focuses on the historical development of health planning and evaluation, a generic program planning and evaluation method, the benefits of planning and evaluation, the elements of planning and evaluation, and how cost studies are applied to program evaluation. Sections of this chapter can be used by undergraduate students whereas other sections are more appropriately used by graduate students.

DEFINITIONS AND GOALS

A **program** is an organized approach to meet the assessed needs of individuals, families, groups, or communities by reducing the effect of or eliminating one or more health problems. Examples of specific programs in public health nursing are home health programs, immunization programs, health-risk screening programs for industrial workers, and family planning programs. These specific programs are usually conducted under the direction of a total program plan of a local health department or a managed care agency. More broadly based group and community programs are the community school health program, the occupational health and safety program, the environmental health program, and community programs directed at specific illnesses through special interest groups (e.g., American Heart Association, American Cancer Society, March of Dimes).

Planning is defined as the selecting and carrying out of a series of actions to achieve stated goals (Kropf, 1995).

The goal of planning is to ensure that health care services are acceptable, equal, efficient, and effective. **Evaluation** is defined as the methods used to determine whether a service is needed and likely to be used, whether it is conducted as planned, and whether the service actually helps people in need (Posavac and Carey, 1997). Evaluation for the purpose of assessing whether objectives are met or planned activities are completed is referred to as **formative evaluation.** This type of evaluation begins with an assessment of the need for a program. Evaluation to assess program outcomes or as a follow-up of the results of the program activities is called **summative evaluation.**

Program evaluation is an ongoing process from the beginning of the planning phase until the program ends. The major goals of program evaluation are to determine the relevance, progress, efficiency, effectiveness, and impact of program activities (Veney and Kaluzny, 1998).

HISTORICAL OVERVIEW OF HEALTH CARE PLANNING AND EVALUATION

As the health care delivery system has grown in the past 70 years, emphasis on **health planning** and evaluation has increased. Factors that have increased interest in planning and evaluation are advances in health care technology and consumer education, increased consumer expectations, third-party payers, budget pressures, increased professional conflicts, focus on preventive care, new focus on health care as a business, unionizing of health care workers, urbanization, increased health risks, personnel shortages, and increased health care costs. In the 1920s to 1940s there were specific actions taken that related to health planning. Table 21-1 outlines the development of health planning.

The post-World War II era after 1944 brought an interest in evaluating program effectiveness. As government and third-party payers began to finance health care services and money became more plentiful, public demand for health services grew. As a result, numbers and kinds of health care agencies increased; laws were passed to increase the scope of and control over health care, and the health care delivery system was beginning to be held accountable for its actions. During this time, legislation was passed to require health care providers and consumers to work together in groups to address issues in health care.

Through the 1970s, laws were passed that changed over time to provide a more comprehensive structure and more power over federal program funds. However, there still existed little authority to carry out some of the more critical tasks of improving the health of clients, increasing accessibility and quality of services, restraining costs, and preventing unnecessary duplication of services. Power over the private health care sector continued to be absent.

As new federalism became the catch phrase of the 1980s and emphasis was placed on cost shifting, reducing costs, and more competition within the health care system, President Ronald Reagan proposed doing away with the federal government's role in health planning. In 1981, with

TABLE 21-1 Historical Development of Health Planning and Evaluation

YEAR	ACTOR	ACTION
1920	Committees on administrative practice and evaluation of American Public Health Association	Called for public health officers to engage in better program planning Reduce haphazard methods used to develop public health programs
1920s	Committee on costs of medical care	Studied social and economic aspects of health services Cited the need for comprehensive health care planning because of rising costs and unequal health care services to target populations
1944	American Hospital Association	Established committee on post-war planning Began region planning for health services nationwide
1946	Federal government, Congress	Passed the Hospital Survey and Construction Act (Hill Burton Act) to legislate health planning, which resulted in growth of number of hospitals
1963	Federal government, Congress	Emphasis on Great Society Programs Community Mental Health Centers Act (P.L. 88-464) was passed to provide mental health programs in the states; defined the role of consumers in making decisions and professionals as advisors in the planning process
1965	Federal government, Congress	Passed Regional Medical Program legislation (P.L. 89-239); upgraded quality of tertiary health care services for the leading causes of death Coined the term "Partnership for Health"
1965	USDHHS	Office of Health Planning opened No direct authority for health planning given
1966	Federal government, Congress	Passed the Comprehensive Health Planning (CHP) and Public Health Services amendments (P.L. 89-749) Developed a national health planning system
1974	Federal government, Congress	Passed National Health Planning and Resources Development Act (P.L. 93-641), which provided specific directions for developing the structure, process, and functions of a national health planning system
1993	President Clinton	Introduced the Health Security Act to provide for health care reform and planning based on population needs
1994-1999	States	Introduced legislation for health care reform based on planning and evaluating state population needs (Kentucky, Hawaii, Minnesota, Oregon, Florida, California, Washington, New York)

cutbacks in federal spending, states began the takeover or dismantling of their own health planning systems. The national health planning system came to a halt. The federal, state, and consumer partnership for health care was nonexistent.

In 1993, with President Clinton's emphasis on health care reform, the decision was made that the government would continue not to be involved in health planning but would use its power to set limits on health insurance costs and limit overall health care spending. In this way it would influence health planning decisions made by the private health care agencies and providers (Kropf, 1995). Although national health care reform did not occur, many states are engaged in reforming their systems.

The process of health planning today is in the control of hospitals, physicians, pharmaceutical companies, equipment companies, insurance companies, and managed care organizations. The outcome of the national and state health care reform effort is often influenced by the political party in power. The nurse must be involved in aspects of health planning for the community in which he or she lives to influence the direction of health care reform.

In addition to health planning in the external environment, internal health care agency planning is necessary to meet the goals and objectives of providing efficient, effective health care services to the client at a reasonable cost. Community health personnel have a responsibility to participate in internal planning and evaluation to solve the problems of a client population. Internal health care agency planning is often affected by the health care planning within the community as well as national health care planning.

BENEFITS OF PROGRAM PLANNING

Systematic planning for meeting client needs benefits clients, nurses, and the employing agencies. Planning focuses attention on what the organization and health provider are attempting to do for clients. Planning assists in identifying the resources and activities that are needed to meet the objectives of client services. Planning reduces role ambiguity (uncertainty) by giving responsibility to specific providers to meet program objectives.

Planning also reduces uncertainty within the program environment and increases the abilities of the provider and the agency to cope with the external environment. Everyone involved with the program can anticipate what will be needed to implement the program, what will occur during implementation, and what the program outcomes will be. Planning helps the provider and the agency anticipate events. Also, planning allows for quality decision making and better control over the actual program results. Today this type of planning is referred to as **strategic planning** and involves the successful matching of client needs with specific provider strengths and competencies and agency resources.

The planning process reflects the desires to implement a reality-based program that can be readily evaluated and can reduce the number of unexpected events from occurring.

PLANNING PROCESS

Health program planning is affected by governmental control over licensure and funding, by society, and by the culture and belief system of the population in which the program must function. Program planning is required by federal, state, and local governments; by philanthropic organizations; and by the employing agency. Planning programs and planning for the evaluation of programs are two very important activities, whether the program being planned is a national health insurance program such as Medicare, a state health care program such as early childhood developmental

TABLE 21-2 Basic Planning Process

BASIC PLANNING	ELEMENTS
1. Formulation	Client identifies problems.
2. Conceptualization	Provider group identifies solutions.
3. Detailing	Client and provider analyze available solutions.
4. Evaluation	Client, providers, and administrators select best plan.
5. Implementation	Best plan is presented to administrators for funding.

screening programs, or a local program such as vision screening for elementary schoolchildren. Regardless of the type of program, the planning process is the same.

Nutt (1984) describes a basic planning process that is reflected in the steps of most planning methods. The process includes five planning stages: formulation, conceptualization, detailing, evaluation, and implementation (Table 21-2).

Basic Program Planning Model
Formulation

The initial and most critical step in planning for a health program is defining the problem and assessing client need. This stage in the planning process can be *preactive*, projecting a future need; *reactive*, defining the problem based on past needs identified by the client or the agency; *inactive*, defining the problem based on the existing health state of the population to be served; or *interactive*, describing the problem using past and present data to project future population needs.

Needs assessment is a key ingredient in the planning process. The target population, or client to be served, by any program must be identified and involved in designing the program development. Program planners must verify that a current health problem exists and is being ignored or being unsuccessfully treated in a client group. Data will provide the rationale to establish a new program or revise existing programs to meet the needs of the client group. The **assessment of need** is defined as a systematic appraisal of type, depth, and scope of problems as perceived by clients, health providers, or both.

The needs assessment process includes six steps (Fig. 21-1). The *client population* may be identified as a community or group, as families, or as individuals. The client population should be defined specifically by its biological and psychosocial characteristics, by geographic location, and by the problems to be addressed. For example, in a community with a large number of preschool children who require immunizations to enter school, the client population may be described as all children between 4 and 6 years of age residing in Central County who have not had up-to-date immunizations.

HOW TO *Develop a Program Plan*

A. Formulate the plan
   1. Assess client need
      a. Who is the client?
      b. What is the need to be met?
      c. How large is the client population to be served?
      d. Where are they located?
      e. Are there other programs addressing the same need? (describe)
      f. Why is the need not being met?
   2. Establish program boundaries
      a. Who will be included in the program?
      b. Who will not be included? Why?
      c. What is the program goal?
   3. Program feasibility
      a. Who agrees that program is needed (administrators, providers, clients, funders)?
      b. Who does not agree?
   4. Resources (general)
      a. What personnel are needed? What personnel are available?
      b. What facilities are needed? What facilities are available?
      c. What equipment is needed? What equipment is available?
      d. Is money needed? Is money available?
      e. Are resources being donated (printing, paper, medical supplies)?
         (1) Type
         (2) Amount
   5. Tools used to assess need
      a. Census data
      b. Key informants
      c. Community forums
      d. Existing program surveys
      e. Surveys of client population
      f. Statistical indicators (e.g., morbidity/mortality data)
B. Conceptualize the problem
   1. List the potential solutions to the problem
   2. What are the risks of each solution?
   3. What are the consequences?
   4. What are the outcomes to be gained from the solutions?
   5. Draw a decision tree to show the problem-solving process used.
C. Detail the plan
   1. What are the objectives for each solution to meet the program goal?
   2. What activities will be done to conduct each of the alternative solutions listed under B1 and based on objectives.
   3. What are the differences in the resources needed for each of the alternative solutions?
   4. Which of the alternative solutions would be chosen if the resources described under A4 were the only resources available?
D. Evaluate the plan
   1. Which of the alternative solutions is most acceptable:
      a. to the clients
      b. to the agency administrator
      c. to you
      d. to the community
   2. Which of the alternative solutions appears to have the most benefits to:
      a. client
      b. agency administrator
      c. you
      d. the community
   3. Based on costs, which alternative solution would be chosen by:
      a. client
      b. agency administrator
      c. you
      d. the community
E. Implement the program plan
   1. Based on data collected, which of the solutions has been chosen?
   2. Why should the agency administrator approve your request? Give rationale
   3. When can the program begin? Give date.

NURSING TIP

The needs to be met for the client population must be identified by both the client and the health provider. If the client population does not recognize the need, the program will usually fail.

A health education program may be necessary to alert the population to the existing need. In the example of the need for immunization of preschool children, public service announcements on television and radio and in newspapers may be used to alert parents to laws requiring immunizations, to the continued existence of communicable diseases, and to communicable diseases, such as smallpox, that have been successfully eradicated by immunization programs. A good example of the use of media is the 1990 outbreak of rubella in Los Angeles. Local and national television was used to bring attention to the problem, to encourage parents to have children immunized, and to encourage other communities to launch campaigns to prevent other outbreaks.

Specifying the size and distribution of a client population for a program involves more than counting the number of persons in the community who may be eligible for the program. More specifically, it involves defining the number of persons with the problem who are unserved by existing programs and the number of eligible persons who have and have not taken advantage of existing services. For

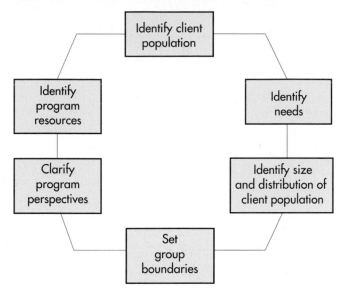

FIG. 21-1 Steps in the needs assessment process.

example, consider again the community need for a preschool immunization program. In planning the program, the estimates of numbers of preschool children in the county may be obtained from census data or birth certificates. The nurse then must determine the number of children unserved and the number of children who have not used services for which they are eligible.

Boundaries for the client population are primarily established by defining the size and distribution of the client population. The boundaries will stipulate who is included and who is excluded in the health program. If the fictional immunization program were designed to serve only preschool children of low-income families, all other preschool children would be excluded.

Perspectives on the program, or what people think about the need for a program, might differ among health providers, agency administrators, policy makers, and potential clients. Collecting data on the opinions and attitudes of all persons directly or indirectly involved with the program's success is necessary to determine the program's feasibility, the need to redefine the problems, or the decision to develop a new program or expand an existing program. For example, policy makers in the 1970s decided that neighborhood health clinics were the answer to providing service for low-income residents. They discovered that their perspectives were not the same as those of most health providers or clients who were not supportive of developing neighborhood clinics. The neighborhood health clinics failed because the clients would not use them. If the policy makers had explored the perspectives of the clients when planning the program, they might have chosen another type of service to offer.

Before implementing a health program, one must also *identify available resources.* Program resources include personnel, facilities, equipment, and financing. The number

and kinds of personnel available to implement a program must be determined. The availability of supplies and up-to-date equipment is as essential a resource for implementing a program as the source and amount of funds. If any one of the four categories of resources is unavailable, the program is likely to be inadequate to meet the needs of the client population.

A number of *needs assessment tools* exist to assist the nurse in the needs assessment process. The major tools used for needs assessment, summarized in Table 21-3, are census data, key informants, community forums, surveys of existing community agencies with similar programs, surveys of residents of the community to be served (client population), and statistical indicators (Rossi and Freeman, 1999).

Conceptualization

The need and demand for a program are determined through the formulation process. The conceptualization stage of planning creates options for solving the problem and considers several solutions. Each option for program solution is examined for its uncertainties (risks) and consequences, leading to a set of outcomes.

When considering alternative solutions to the problem, some will have more risk or uncertainties than others. The nurse must decide between the solution that involves more risk and the solution that is free of risk. A "do nothing" decision is always the decision with the least risk to the provider. When choosing a solution, the nurse looks at whether the desired outcome can be achieved. After careful thought about each possible solution to the problem, the nurse rethinks the solutions. The information collected from census data, key informants, community forums, surveys of existing community agencies, and statistical indicators should be used to develop these alternative solutions.

Decision trees are useful graphic aids that will give a picture of the solutions and the consequences and risks of each solution. Such a picture graph of the process of identifying a solution helps clients and administrators understand why one solution may be chosen over another. Figure 21-2 shows the process of conceptualizing using a decision tree.

In the immunization example, the best consequence would be for families to provide for immunizations. One must consider the value of this action to the parents, the odds that immunizations will be given if a formal clinic is not available, the cost to the parents versus the taxpayer, and the cost to the community. Costs to the community include the possibility of increased incidence of communicable disease or mortality and increased need for more expensive services to treat the diseases if children are not immunized. If the parents provide the immunizations, costs to the taxpayer and to the community are low.

Detailing

In this phase the provider, with client input, considers the possibilities of solving a problem using one of the so-

TABLE 21-3 Summary of Needs Assessment Tools

NAME	DEFINITION	ADVANTAGES	DISADVANTAGES
Community forum	Community, group, organization, open meeting	Low cost Learn perspectives of large number of persons	Limited data Limited expression of views Discourages less powerful Becomes arena to discuss political issues
Key informant	Identify, select, and question knowledgeable leaders	Provides picture of services needed	Bias of leaders Community characteristics may be incorrectly perceived by informants
Indicators approach	Existing data used to determine problem	Excellent data on problems and location of client groups	Data may be obsolete Growth and change in population may make data outdated
Survey of existing agencies	Estimates of client population via services used at similar community agencies	Easy method to estimate size of client group Know extent of services offered in existing programs	Records and data may be unreliable All cases of need may not be reported Exaggeration of services may occur
Surveys/census	Measurement of total or sample client population by interview or questionnaire	Direct and accurate data on client population and their problems	Expensive Technically demanding Need many interviews or observations

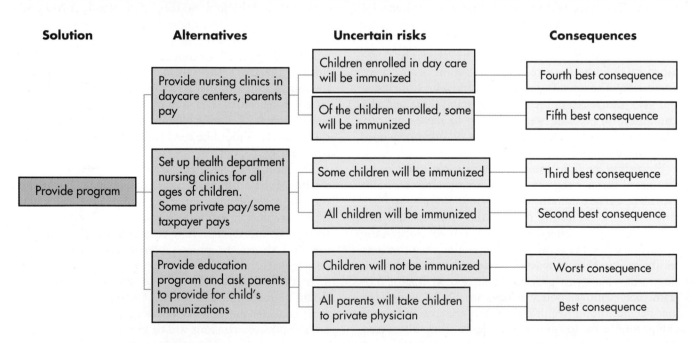

FIG. 21-2 Ranking of solutions to problem: providing a preschool immunization program to low-income children using a decision tree.

lutions identified. The provider details the costs, resources, and program activities needed to choose one of the solutions from the conceptualizing phase. For each of the three proposed alternatives in Figure 21-2, the program planner must list activities that would need to be implemented to use each of the alternatives. To illustrate, con-

sider again the immunization scenario. Using the proposed solution of encouraging the parents to provide the immunizations (the best consequence), examples of activities include developing a script for a health education program and implementing a television program to encourage parents to take children to the physician. If the second, third, or fourth best consequence was chosen, offering a clinic 8 hours per day at the health department and providing a mobile clinic to each daycare center for 4 hours each day to provide the immunizations would be possible activities.

For each alternative the nurse lists the resources needed to implement each activity. The resources to be considered include all costs of personnel, supplies, equipment, facilities, and the potential acceptance by the clients and the administrators of the program. In the example, personnel could include nurses, volunteers, and clerks; supplies might include handouts, Band-Aids, medications, records, and consent forms; equipment might include syringes, needles, stethoscopes, and blood pressure cuffs; and facilities might include a television studio for a media blitz on the education program and a room with examination tables, chairs, and emergency carts. The costs of each solution must be considered by listing the costs of personnel, supplies, equipment, and facilities for each solution. As indicated, clients should review each solution for acceptance.

Evaluation

In the evaluation phase of the plan, each alternative is weighed to judge the costs, benefits, and acceptance of the idea to the client, community, and provider. The information outlined in the detailing phase would be used to rank the solutions for choice by client and provider based on cost, benefit, and acceptance. Consideration must be given to the solution that will provide the desired outcomes. Looking at available information through literature reviews or interviews might suggest whether each of the options had been tried before in another place or by someone else. The results from other sources would be helpful in deciding whether a chosen solution would be useful.

Implementation

In the implementation phase of the planning process, the clients, providers, and administrators select the best plan to solve the original problem. Change theory is useful to help create an environment in which the best solution may be supported. Providing reasons why a particular solution was chosen will help the provider get the approval of administration for the plan. Involving clients and administrators throughout the planning process helps to promote acceptance of the plan. Upon approval the plan is implemented.

PROGRAM EVALUATION
Benefits of Program Evaluation

The major benefit of program evaluation is that it shows whether the program is fulfilling its purpose. It should answer the following questions:

- Are the needs for which the program was designed being met?
- Are the problems it was designed to solve being solved?

This is critical information for funding agencies, top-level decision makers, program accreditation reviews, and the community at large. Evaluation data may be used to justify expanding the program, reducing the program, or even closing it.

Quality assurance programs are prime examples of program evaluation in health care delivery. Evaluation data are used to justify continuing programs in community health. Program evaluation focuses on whether goals were met and the efficiency and effectiveness of program activities. Many methods of program evaluation are described in the literature. The primary method of evaluation used in health care today is Donabedian's Evaluative Framework. The tracer method and case register are other methods applied to program evaluation.

Program records and community indexes serve as the major source of information for program evaluation. Surveys, interviews, observations, and diagnostic tests are ways to assess consumer and client response to health programs. Cost studies help identify program benefits and effectiveness.

As financial resources become scarce, nursing and the health care system must be able to justify their existence, prove that their services are responsive to client needs, and show their professional concern for accountability. Planning and evaluation will assist in meeting these objectives.

Planning for the Evaluation Process

Planning for the evaluation process is an important part of program planning. When the planning process begins, the plan for evaluating the program should be developed. All persons to be involved implementing a program should be a part of the plan for program evaluation. An example of what has been defined as formative evaluation is the assessment of need. The basic questions to be answered, after carefully considering the data collected from census, key informants, community forums, surveys, or health statistics indicators, are as follows:

- Will the objectives and resources of this program meet the identified needs of the client population?
- Is the program relevant?

Once need has been established and the program is designed the nurse must continue plans for program evaluation (see the Research Brief).

As a part of the planning process, Posavac and Carey (1997) describe six steps to use for continuing program evaluation (Fig. 21-3):

1. Identify the relevant people for evaluation. Program personnel, program funders, and the clients of the program should be included in planning for evaluation.
2. Arrange preliminary meetings to discuss the question of how the group wants to evaluate the program and where to start. If the program planners and others agree on an evaluation, the resources needed to do the evaluation must be identified. Evaluation is necessary even though some may not be interested in it. Public health nurses can help others see that without evalua-

RESEARCH *Brief*

The purpose of the project was twofold: 1) to develop a program to prevent diabetes and hypertension among the Chinese population in Chinatown, Hawaii and 2) to develop a relationship with the Chinese Community Association. This article provides evaluation of the program, which was a collaborative effort between the community, the public health nurse, and diabetes nurse educators. The authors used several approaches to developing the program: volunteers helped them access the community, the community association identified participants for the program, and surveys of participants were conducted to determine interest. The authors used techniques of community education and health promotion to implement this self-care management program with 200 Chinese residents of the community. Case studies, laboratory diagnostic tests, blood pressure monitoring, and surveys were used to evaluate the outcomes of the program. The evaluation showed the effectiveness of the education, counseling, support, and outreach approaches used in the program to improve blood glucose and blood pressure levels in the population.

The nurse can use this study to find appropriate ways to work with culturally diverse groups and ways to provide culturally sensitive health care programs.

Wang C, Abbott L: Development of a community based diabetes and hypertension prevention program, *Public Health Nurs* 15(6):406, 1998.

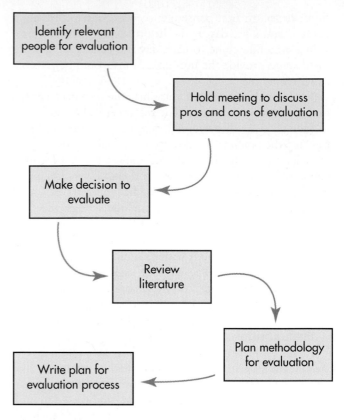

FIG. 21-3 Six steps in planning for program evaluation.

5. Plan the method to be used, including decisions about what items will be measured, how they will be measured, and on what population.
6. Write a plan that outlines the purpose and goals of the overall program, the type of evaluation to be done, the operational measure to be used to evaluate the program goals, the choice of internal or external evaluators, the available resources for conducting the evaluation, and the readiness of the organization, personnel, and clients for program evaluation.

WHAT DO YOU THINK? *Nurses at all levels of education and preparation can participate in program planning and evaluation.*

Evaluation Process

The evaluation process presented by Rossi and Freeman (1999) is explained in this section. It is very similar to the steps in the planning process:

1. *Goal setting.* The value and beliefs of the agency, the providers, and the clients provide the basis for goal setting and should be considered at every step of the evaluation process. In the preschool immunization scenario, the fact that children should not be exposed to early childhood diseases would lead to a program goal to decrease the incidence of early childhood diseases in the county where the program is planned.

tion, money to support programs will not be available or need for a new nurse to help with the work cannot be justified. In health care today there is great emphasis on outcomes of care. The only way to see outcomes is through evaluation.

3. After the relevant people have met and considered the questions in the previous steps, they are ready to begin the evaluation process. Even though evaluation may be desired, the decision to conduct the evaluation may be an administrative one, based on available resources and existing circumstances. For example, if a program evaluation were attempted in a situation in which program personnel wanted it and clients chose to be uncooperative, evaluation efforts would fail.

4. Examine the literature for suggestions about the appropriate methods and techniques for evaluation and their usefulness in program evaluation. If an agency has chosen to use an external evaluator, this person may make suggestions regarding the questions to be answered in the evaluation process. These questions are based on the program goals. If the literature has been reviewed by the public health nurse and others affected by the evaluation, they can determine whether the evaluation suggestions are appropriate for their situation.

2. *Determining goal measurement.* In the case of the previous goal, disease incidence would be an appropriate goal measurement.
3. *Identifying goal-attaining activities,* which includes such activities as media presentations urging parents to have their children immunized.
4. *Making the activities operational,* which involves the actual administration of the immunizations.
5. *Measuring the goal effect,* which consists of reviewing the records and summarizing the incidence of early childhood disease before and after the program.
6. *Evaluation of the program,* which involves determining whether the program goal was achieved. Keep in mind that only one program goal is used in this example. Most programs have multiple goals (Fig. 21-4).

Formulation of Objectives

The most important step in the evaluation process is the writing of program objectives. The objectives set the stage for conducting the program and provide the mechanism for evaluating the activities and the total program. The following discussion helps in the development of clear, concise objectives. Development of program objectives coincides with the initial phases of program planning.

Specification of objectives (goals)

If the objectives are too general, program evaluation becomes impossible. The objectives must be specific and stated so that anyone reading them could conduct the program without further instruction. To be truly effective, objectives must be very specific and should begin with a general program goal and move on to specific objectives that will help meet the program goal.

Useful program objectives include a statement of the specific behaviors, accomplishments, and success criteria, or expected result, for the program. Each program objective requires a *strong, action-oriented verb to specify the behavior, a statement of a single purpose, a statement of a single result, and a time frame for achieving the expected result.* In this continuing example, a program objective that meets these criteria may be to decrease (*action verb*) the incidence of early childhood disease in Center County (*result*) by providing immunization clinics in all schools (*purpose*) between August and December of 2005 (*time frame*).

As objectives are developed, an operational indicator for each objective should be considered so the evaluator knows when and if the objective has been met. For instance, an operational indicator for the previous objective would be a 10% to 25% decrease in the incidence rates of the most frequently occurring childhood vaccine-preventable illnesses in Center County. Such indicators provide a target for persons involved with program implementation. A review of *Healthy People 2000* and *Healthy People 2010* objectives will give the reader examples of objectives that include all the elements listed above.

Levels of program objectives

It is customary for objectives to be stated in levels from general to specific. The first level consists of general and

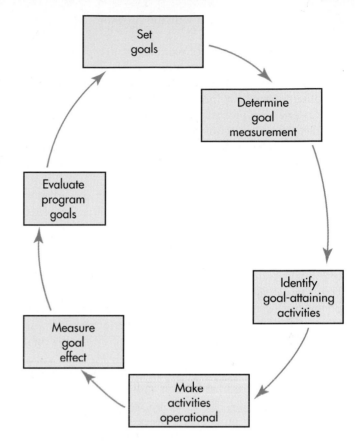

FIG. 21-4 The evaluative process.

broad objectives that are sometimes called *goals.* Their purpose is to focus on the major reason for the program.

A general program objective (*goal*) may be to reduce the incidence of low-birth-weight babies in Center County by 2005 by improving access to prenatal care. The specific objectives, or subgoals, describe a measurable behavior, the circumstances under which the behavior is observed, and the minimal acceptable standard for the performance of the behavior. A specific objective for this program may be to open a prenatal clinic in each health department within the county by January 2000 to serve the population within each census tract of the county.

Specific program activities are then planned to meet each specific objective; resources, such as number of nurses, equipment, supplies, and location, are planned for each of the objectives. It is assumed that as each specific objective is met, the general program objective will also be achieved. Remember that several specific objectives are required to meet a general program objective or goal.

Sources of Program Evaluation

Major sources of information for program evaluation are program participants, program records, and community indices. The program participants, or clients of the service, have a unique and valuable role in program evaluation. Whether the clients, for whom the program was designed, accept the services will determine to a large extent whether the program achieves its purpose. Thus their reactions, feelings, and judgments about the program are very important to the evaluation.

To assess the response of participants in a program, the evaluator may use a written survey in the form of a questionnaire or an attitude scale. Interviews and observations are other ways of obtaining feedback about a program. Attitude scales are probably used most often, and they are usually phrased in terms of whether the program met its objectives. The client satisfaction survey is an example of an attitude scale often used in the health care delivery system to evaluate the program objectives.

The second major source of information for program evaluation is program records, especially clinical records. Clinical records provide the evaluator with information about the care given to the client and the results of that care. To determine whether a program goal has been met, one might summarize the data from a group of records. For example, if one overall goal is to reduce the incidence of low-birth-weight babies through prenatal care, records would be reviewed to obtain the number of mothers who received prenatal care and the number of low-birth-weight babies born to them.

A third major source of evaluation is a community **health index.** Health and illness indicators, such as mortality and morbidity data, are probably cited more frequently than any other single index for program evaluation. Health and illness indicators are useful in evaluating the effects of health care programs on the total community. Incidence and prevalence are also valuable indices used to measure program effectiveness and impact (see Chapter 11 for further discussion of rates and ratios).

An example of a national program based on a needs assessment of the U.S. population is the national health objectives program called *Healthy People 2000* (USDHHS, 1991b). *Healthy People 2000* has three overall goals and 300 specific health status objectives, which include an action verb, a result, a time frame (10 years), and an operational indicator (see Appendix A-1). Each health status objective is accompanied by a risk reduction objective, which further defines the result of the health status objective, and a services objective, which gives the purpose of the objective. Box 21-1 provides an example. *Healthy Communities 2000: Model Standards* (USDHHS, 1991a) suggests activities to evaluate the national health objectives. These activities are listed in Box 21-2.

Aspects of Evaluation

The aspects of program evaluation include the following (Kaluzny and Veney, 1999):
1. *Evaluation of relevance.* Need for the program
2. *Progress.* Tracking of program activities to meet program objectives
3. *Efficiency.* Relationship between program outcomes and the resources spent
4. *Effectiveness.* Ability to meet program objectives and the results of program efforts
5. *Impact.* Long-term changes in the client population

BOX 21-1 *Healthy People 2000:* Example of National Health Objective Combining Health Status, Risk Reduction and Service Goal, and Possible Activities to Meet Objectives

9.1 Reduce (*action verb*) deaths caused by unintentional injuries (*result*) to no more than 29.3 per 100,000 people (*target*) by increasing the use of helmets to at least 80% of motorcyclists and at least 50% of bicyclists (*objective indicator*) by extending to 50 states laws requiring helmet use for all ages (*purpose*) by the year 2000 (*time frame*).

BOX 21-2 *Healthy Communities 2000:* Example of Activities to Evaluate Objective 9.1 to Reduce Deaths Caused by Unintentional Injuries

FOCUS OF OBJECTIVE
Deaths from injuries

OBJECTIVE
Reduce deaths caused by unintentional injuries

EVALUATION INDICATOR
Change in unintentional injury
Number of hospital admissions (increasing or decreasing)
State law changed
Percentage wearing helmets

DID YOU KNOW? Healthy People 2000, *the national program to improve the health of all Americans in 10 years, used key informants, census data, statistical indicators, forums, and surveys of existing programs to establish the goals and objectives of the program.*

Relevance
Evaluation of relevance is an important component of the initial planning phase. As money, providers, facilities, and supplies for delivering health care services are more closely monitored, the needs assessment done by the public health nurse will determine whether the program is needed.

Progress
The monitoring of program activities, such as hours of services, number of providers used, number of referrals made, and amount of money spent to meet program objectives, provides an evaluation of the progress of the program. This type of evaluation is an example of formative evaluation and occurs on an ongoing basis while the program exists. This provides an opportunity to make effective day-to-day management decisions about the operations of the program. Progress evaluation occurs pri-

:::HOW TO *Do a Program Evaluation* _____

A. Program relevance: needs assessment (formative)
   1. Use answers to all questions listed in section A of How To Develop a Program Plan
   2. Based on needs assessment, was program necessary?

B. Program progress (formative)
   1. Monitor activities (circle which this reflects: daily, weekly, monthly, annually)
      a. Name the activities provided.
      b. How many hours of service provided?
      c. How many clients have been served?
      d. How many providers?
      e. What types of clients have been served?
      f. What types of providers were needed?
      g. Where have services been offered (home, clinic, organization)?
      h. How many referrals have been made to community sources?
      i. Which sources have been used to provide support services?
   2. Budget
      a. How much money has been spent to carry out activities?
      b. Will more/less money be needed to conduct activities as outlined?
      c. Will changes need to be made now to objectives and activities to keep the program going?
      d. What changes do you recommend and why?

C. Program efficiency (formative and summative)
   1. Costs
      a. How do the costs of this program compare with those of a similar program to meet the same goal?
      b. Do the activities outlined in B1 compare with the activities in a similar program?
      c. Although this program costs more/less than expected, is it needed? Why?
   2. Productivity (may use national or state averages for comparison)
      a. How many clients does each type of staff see per day (public health nurses, community health nurses, nurse practitioners)?
      b. How does this compare with similar programs?
      c. Although the productivity level of this program is low/high, is the program needed? Why?
   3. Benefits
      a. What are the benefits of the program to the clients served?
      b. What are the benefits to the community?
      c. Are the benefits important enough to continue the program? Why? (Look at cost, productivity, and outcomes of care)

D. Program effectiveness (summative)
   1. Satisfaction
      a. Is the client satisfied with the program as designed?
      b. Are the providers satisfied with the program outcomes?
      c. Is the community satisfied with the program outcomes?
   2. Goals
      a. Did the program meet its stated goal?
      b. Are the client needs being met?
      c. Was the problem solved for which the program was designed?

E. Impact (summative)
   1. Long-term changes in health status (one year or more)
      a. Have there been changes in the communities' health?
      b. What are the changes seen (e.g., morbidity or mortality rates, teen pregnancy rates, pregnancy outcomes)
      c. Have there been changes in individuals' health status?
      d. What are the changes seen?
      e. Has the initial problem been solved or has it returned?
      f. Is new or revised programming needed? Why?
      g. Should the program be discontinued? Why?

marily while implementing the program. The nurse who completes a daily or weekly log of clinical activities (e.g., number of clients seen in clinic or visited at home, number of phone contacts, number of referrals made, number of community health promotion activities) is contributing to progress evaluation of the nursing service.

Efficiency

If the reason for evaluation is to examine the efficiency of a program, it may occur on an ongoing basis as formative evaluation or at the end of the program as a summative evaluation. The evaluator may be able to determine whether the program provides better benefits at a lower cost than a sim-

ilar program or whether the benefits to the clients, or number of clients served, justify the costs of the program.

Effectiveness and impact

An **evaluation of program effectiveness** may help the nurse evaluator determine both client and provider satisfaction with the program activities, as well as whether the program met its stated objectives. However, if evaluation of impact is the goal, long-term effects such as changes in morbidity and mortality must be investigated. Both effectiveness and impact evaluations are usually summative evaluation functions primarily performed as end-of-program activities.

ADVANCED PLANNING METHODS AND EVALUATION MODELS

After the need and the client demand for a program have been determined through the needs assessment process, the next step in the development of the program is to choose a procedural method that will assist the nurse in planning the program to be offered. *The following is offered for students who are more advanced in their career and need to consider several methods of program planning plus more extensive evaluation models for program management.*

Five planning methods are discussed in this section:
1. Planning, Programming, and Budgeting System (PPBS)
2. Program Planning Method (PPM)
3. Program Evaluation Review Technique (PERT)
4. Critical Path Method (CPM)
5. Multi-Attribute Utility Method (MAUT)

PPM and PPBS are more general approaches to program planning, whereas PERT, CPM, and MAUT offer guidelines for identifying and tracking specific program activities essential to program success. All of these approaches establish the basis for program evaluation.

Planning, Programming, and Budgeting System

PPBS is a procedural tool initially developed for use by the Department of Defense and other government agencies. PPBS is an outcome-oriented accounting system, the effect of which is to determine the most efficient method of resource allocation to attain measurable objectives.

PPBS is an economic method of describing a program plan and is compared with the Nutt Model of Program Planning. Steps of PPBS are listed in Box 21-3. In PPBS, planning represents formulation of objectives and conceptualization or identification of alternatives and methods for accomplishing objectives; programming represents detailing of resources (personnel, facilities, equipment, and financing) for each identified alternative; and budgeting represents the assignment of dollar values to resources required for the program implementation or the evaluation of program costs and benefits (Fig. 21-5).

PPBS is widely used for planning broad-scale government programs. It is a system that can also be used to plan programs for an agency or for client groups. For example, PPBS could be used to develop the annual program plan

for the health department or a prenatal program for the local community. A nurse could also use this method to develop a health education program for the school population on sexually transmitted diseases. PPBS's use of objectives that are operationally defined by nursing standards, or performance criteria, is a system that lends itself to effective program evaluation.

Program Planning Method

PPM is a technique employing the nominal group technique of Delbecq and Van de Ven (1971). The nurse can use this method to involve clients more directly in the planning process. PPM is a five-stage process to identify program needs and focuses on three levels of planning groups composed of clients, providers, and administrators. The client or consumer group relays a list of problems to the provider group, who in turn aids the client group in presenting the solution to the problem to the administrative group (Nutt, 1984).

The stages of PPM are compared with Nutt's planning process in Table 21-4. The five stages are as follows:
1. *Problem diagnosis.* Each client in the group works with all other members of the group to develop a written problem list, one problem at a time. After all problems have been shared and recorded, they are dis-

---

BOX 21-3 Steps Involved in PPBS

1. Setting program goals
2. Defining measurable program objectives
3. Identifying and evaluating alternatives to accomplish program objectives
4. Choosing the method for accomplishing the objectives
5. Developing a program budget with justification for minimizing costs while maximizing program benefits

---

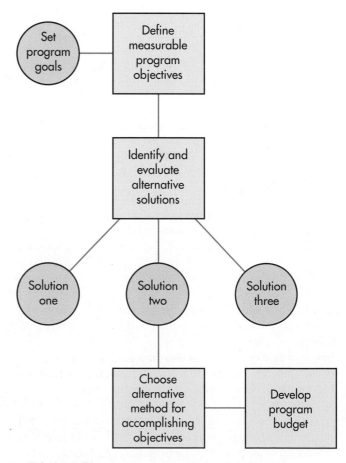

FIG. 21-5 Planning, programming, and budgeting system.

cussed by the total client group. After the discussion, clients select the problems with the highest priority by voting on the ranking of each problem.

2. *Expert provider group identifies solutions for each of the problems identified by the clients.*

3. *Client and provider groups present their problems and suggested solutions* to the administrative group to determine the possibilities of developing a program to resolve one or more of the problems using one or more of the solutions. In this phase, clients and providers are seeking acceptance from the administrators who control the program resources.

4. *Alternative solutions to the problem are identified, and the pros and cons of each are analyzed.*

5. *Client, providers, and administrators select the best plan for program implementation.* In this phase the link between the planned solutions and the problem are evaluated, pointing out strengths and limitations of the proposed program plan.

The nurse may use this technique for developing school health services within the total community or in one school. The nurse working with a senior citizens group may also use this method to identify their priority needs for nursing clinic services at the health department. It is important to note that this method is used to get consensus among all persons involved in the program: clients, providers, and administrators. Consensus is most helpful in having a successful program.

Program Evaluation Review Technique

PERT is a network programming method developed in the 1950s through a joint effort of the United States Navy, Lockheed Aircraft Corporation, and Booz-Allen and Hamilton, Inc. The method was developed for planning and controlling the program activities involved in developing the Polaris missile.

The PERT method is primarily useful for large-scale projects that require planning, scheduling, and controlling a large number of activities. PERT is mentioned here to introduce the reader to the concept of network, or systems, planning. Its objectives are listed in Box 21-4. PERT as a planning method has been used successfully in hospitals to plan for the development of nursing services such as primary care services and for designing projects such as the installation and use of computers for organizing and providing nursing services.

PERT involves the concepts of time and events. The basic tool used in the technique is the network or flow plan, which is a series of circles, ovals, or squares representing the program events, or goals, and their relationships with the activities of the program. The program activities are the time-consuming events of the program and are represented by arrows that connect the program accomplish-

---

BOX 21-4 Major Objectives of PERT

- Focus attention on the key developmental parts of a program
- Identify potential program problems that could interfere with movement toward program goals
- Evaluate program progress toward goal attainment
- Provide a prompt reporting method
- Facilitate decision making

TABLE 21-4 Planning Methods Compared with Basic Planning Process

BASIC PLANNING	PPBS	PPM	PERT/CPM	MAUT
Formulation	Identify the goals and define in measurable terms	Problems identified by client	Identify program activities	Identify target population and program objectives
Conceptualization	Identify alternatives	Provider group identifies solution	Explore time and events required to meet program activities	Identify alternative problem solutions
Detailing	Evaluate alternatives for use of resources	Analyze available solutions	Determine sequencing of events and resources to meet activities	Identify criteria for choice; rank and weight; calculate value
Evaluation	Choose method for accomplishing objectives and develop budget to evaluate costs vs. benefits	Clients, providers, and administrators select best plan	Select appropriate events	Choose best alternatives
Implementation		Best plan presented to administrators for funding		

ments or goals (Fig. 21-6). Note in the flow plan that it may take several activities to attain a program event (goal) and that some events (goals) must be accomplished before other events may be attained. The relationship of several program events (sub-goals) may be essential to attain the ultimate program event (goal).

Another element in PERT is the estimate of the time it will take to implement activities leading to program goals. In PERT, three estimates of activity time are given: the optimistic time it will take to complete activities, given minimal difficulties; the most likely time it will take to complete activities, given experiences with normal development of such activities; and the pessimistic time it will take to complete activities, given maximum difficulties. From the time estimates, a simple formula can be applied to indicate the probability of completing a project in a given time period. The numbers appearing along the arrows in Figure 21-6 are the estimated number of days required for completion of activities leading to a particular event.

Critical Path Method

CPM is a network programming planning method that is described by some authors as a technique in itself and by others as an element of PERT (Rakich, Longest, and Darr,

1992). CPM is a technique that focuses the program planner's attention on the program activities, the sequencing of activities for the best use of time and resources, and the estimated time it will take to complete the project from beginning to end. Using this method the planner can determine the amount of time it will take to accomplish each activity and can identify those activities that may take longer. The planner can then determine the amount of resources needed (personnel, money, facilities, and supplies) to accomplish tasks at given points in time along the program's critical path.

CPM allows for frequent review of progress by program planners. Problems can be identified early in the program implementation, and corrective action can be taken or alternative activities can be substituted for activities that are not meeting program requirements. The amount of time and resources being used during program implementation can be assessed, and time and resources can be increased or decreased as necessary and can be compared with initial estimates of program need.

Hospital nursing services and home health agencies are beginning to use CPM to develop protocols for caring for clients with specific health problems (e.g., breast cancer, hypertension, or total hip replacement). These are called *critical paths,* or *CareMaps.* The CPM protocols identify the estimated number of days the client will be in the hospital and nursing care activities for each day the client is hospitalized, from admission to discharge. The CPM extends to the home, estimating nursing care activities and rehabilitation in the home (see Chapter 19). Nurses must document reasons why activities may not have been accomplished. These notes are used to change nursing care plans and set new goals for clients.

PERT and CPM use the five generic stages of planning described by Nutt. However, these two methods focus on specific activities, times, and events essential to program success. The emphasis in these two models is on detailing and evaluation (see Table 21-4).

The Multi-Attribute Technique

MAUT is a planning method based on decision theory (Edwards, Guttentag, and Snapper, 1975). This method can be adapted for making decisions about the care of a single client or about national health care programs. The purpose of MAUT is to separate all elements of a decision and to evaluate each element separately for its effects on the overall decision considering available options.

If money is no object, then the option with the highest use value is the best decision. However, if this option exceeds the budget, the next highest option may be the alternative to choose. The steps of MAUT (listed in Box 21-5) relate closely to the basic planning process described by Nutt (1984) as shown in Table 21-4.

Steps 1 and 2 of MAUT relate to problem formulation. Step 3 involves conceptualization of the program alternatives, and Steps 4 through 9 focus on detailing and the im-

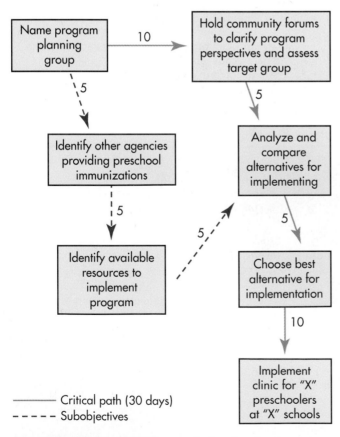

— Critical path (30 days)
----- Subobjectives

FIG. 21-6 Simplified PERT network, for planning a preschool immunization program. Numbers represent days required for completion of activities.

plications of each option. Step 10 involves the evaluation phase of planning or the choice of the best solution as identified in Steps 4 through 9. Placing quantitative values on solutions to meet program needs is most helpful in the implementation phase of planning (e.g., convincing administrators of the need for such a program). However, caution must be taken in using all planning methods since the best solution reflects the bias of the planner.

Evaluation Models and Techniques

Structure-process-outcome evaluation

The method for evaluation of programs by Donabedian (1982) was initially directed primarily toward medical care but is applicable to the broader area of health care. He describes three approaches to assessment of health care: structure, process, and outcome.

Structure refers to settings in which care occurs and includes materials, equipment, qualification of the staff, and organizational structure (Donabedian, 1982). This approach to evaluation is based on the assumption that, given a proper setting with good equipment, good care will follow. However, this assumption is not strongly supported.

Process refers to whether the care that was given was "good" (Donabedian, 1982), competent, or preferred. Use of process in program evaluation may consist of observation of practice but more likely consists of review of records. The review may focus on pathology reports to ascertain whether the number of surgeries was strongly indicated or questionable. The review could focus on whether documentation of preventive teaching was on the clinical record. Audits using specific criteria are examples of the use of process.

Outcome refers to client recovery and restoration of function and survival (Donabedian, 1982), but it is also used in the sense of changes in health status or changes in health-related knowledge, attitude, and behavior. Thus program outcomes may be expressed in terms of mortality, morbidity, and disability for given populations, such as infants, but could be expressed in a broader sense through health promotion behaviors such as weight control, exercise, and abstinence from tobacco and alcohol.

Donabedian's model of evaluating program quality is a popular model and is widely used for evaluation in the health care field. It can be useful in evaluating program effectiveness. The Health Care Financing Administration and other third party payers are currently placing more emphasis on outcome evaluation. It is essential that nurses begin to develop outcome criteria for client interventions.

Tracer method

The board on medicine of the National Academy of Sciences developed a program to evaluate health service delivery called the tracer method (Veney and Kaluzny, 1998). The **tracer method** of evaluation of programs is based on the premise that health status and care can be evaluated by viewing specific health problems called *tracers*. Just as radioactive tracers are used to study the thyroid gland, specific health problems are selected to evaluate the delivery of health and nursing services. Examples of con-

---

BOX 21-5 Ten Basic Steps of the MAUT Method

1. *Identify the person or aggregate for whom a problem is to be solved.* Who is the client for whom the program is being planned?
2. *Identify the issue(s) or decision(s) that are relevant.* This step involves the identification of the program objectives.
3. *Identify the options to be evaluated.* The program planner identifies the available options or action alternatives to accomplish the program goals.
4. *Identify the relevant criteria related to the value of each option.* The program planner places a value on competing options or alternatives or identifies criteria to be considered to make a choice between them.
5. *Rank the criteria in order of importance.* The program planner decides which of the criteria are most important and which are least important for meeting program goals.
6. *Rate criteria in importance.* In this step the program planner assigns an arbitrary rating of 10 to the least important criteria. In considering the next least important criteria, the planner decides how many times more important it is than the least important criteria. If it is considered twice as important, the dimension will be assigned a 20. If it is only considered half as important, it will be assigned a 15. If it is considered

four times as important, it will be assigned a 40. The process is continued until all criteria have been rated.
7. *Add the importance rate, divide each by the sum, and multiply by 100.* This process is called "normalizing" the weights. It is recommended that the number of criteria be kept between 6 and 15. Therefore in this initial process the planner can be concerned with only general criteria for choosing action alternatives.
8. *Measure the location of the option being evaluated by each criteria.* The planner may ask a colleague or expert to estimate on a scale of 0 to 100 the probability that a given option from Step 3 will maximize the value of the criteria from Step 4.
9. *Calculate use of options.* The program planner will obtain the usefulness of each identified action alternative by multiplying the weight for each criterion (Step 7) by the rating of an option for each criterion (Step 8) and adding the products. The sum of the products for each action is termed the "aggregate utility."
10. *Decide on best alternative to meet program objective.* The action alternative with the highest aggregate use is considered the best decision for meeting the program objectives.

ditions selected as tracers are middle ear infection and associated hearing loss, vision disorders, iron deficiency anemia, hypertension, urinary tract infections, and cervical cancer. This approach can be used to compare the following:

- Health status among different population groups
- Health status in relation to social, economic, medical care, nursing care, and behavioral variables
- Various arrangements for health care delivery.

The tracer method is a useful technique for looking at efficiency, effectiveness, and effect of a program.

Case register

Systematic registration of contagious disease has been a practice for many years. Denmark began a national register of tuberculosis in 1921 (Friis, 1999). Its contribution to the reduction in the incidence of contagious diseases has been widely recognized. **Case registers** are also used for acute and chronic disease (e.g., cancer and myocardial infarction).

Registers collect information from defined groups, and the information may be used for evaluating and planning services, preventing disease, providing care, and monitoring changes in patterns and care of diseases. The method is described here because of its use in evaluation of services. The answers to the questions listed in Box 21-6 before and after implementing a program give information about the effects of the program. A tuberculosis register indicates the degree to which infection is being controlled. Cancer registers make state, regional, national, and international comparisons possible, and they provide clues to causes of disease.

BOX 21-6 Examples of Questions Asked About Cases

1. What is the incidence of disease? What differences in incidence are there between one community and another?
2. What percentage of clients recover? What percentage die?
3. Where does death occur?
4. How long do clients wait before contacting a health care provider?
5. How long is it before they see a health care provider?
6. How many cases are associated with other major risk factors?
7. How many cases are associated with environmental factors such as water hardness or air pollution?
8. What happens after clients leave the hospital and when they return to work? Are there rehabilitation programs?
9. How many had been seen by a health care provider shortly before the problem occurred? What prevention measures are taken for persons considered susceptible?

COST STUDIES APPLIED TO PROGRAM MANAGEMENT

Although cost must be considered in planning and evaluating, it is particularly significant in programs involving nursing services. The major types of **cost studies** primarily applied to health care industry are cost accounting, cost benefit, cost efficiency, and cost effectiveness. A discussion of the types of cost studies is presented to give the reader an idea of the kinds of questions that can be answered with such studies. Nurses must be willing to answer these questions to help show the actual costs of nursing programs and the relevance of the programs to the clients they have served.

Cost Accounting

Cost accounting studies are performed to find the actual cost of a program. A question answered by this method could be, "What is the cost of providing a family planning program in Anytown, USA?" To answer the question, the total costs of equipment, facilities (*rental*), personnel (*salaries and benefits*), and supplies used over a period are calculated. The total program costs are divided by the number of clients participating in the program during that time. The total program cost per client is the end product. Thus a cost accounting study can provide data about total program costs and about total cost per client, which makes program management easier. A simple example of cost accounting is what one does each month when balancing a checkbook. One looks at the costs of providing food, shelter, and clothing for a family based on the family income.

Cost Benefit

Cost benefit studies are a way of assessing the desirability of a program by placing a specific dollar amount on all costs and benefits. If benefits outweigh the costs, the program is said to have a net positive impact. The major problem with cost benefit analysis is placing a quantifiable value on all benefits of the program. Can a dollar value be placed on human life, on safety, on the relief of pain and suffering, or on prevention of illness? These are all program benefits. If an attempt is made to perform cost benefit analysis of a hospice program, can a dollar amount be placed on the family and client support and comfort provided or on the relief of pain of the terminally ill client? Can such benefits be weighed against costs to justify continuing the program? Should the program be continued despite costs?

It is recognized that public health programs have net positive impacts because preventing morbidity with illness prevention programs such as hypertension screenings reduces the future cost of chronic long-term illnesses such as cerebrovascular accident (stroke) or cardiovascular disease. To do a cost benefit study for a program, it must be decided which costs and which benefits are to be included, how the costs and benefits are to be valued, and what constraints are to be considered legal, ethical, social, and economic. For example, in a home health care program funded by the state health department to offer care to clients with acquired immunodeficiency syndrome (AIDS), the mortality rate would continue to be high because a cure is not available. Would the program be considered to have a low cost-benefit ratio (*negative impact*) because clients cannot be cured? The program would be considered to have a high cost-benefit ratio (*positive net impact*) if the cost of home health care services was less expensive than providing similar care in the hospital. The benefits of the program would include reducing the costs to the client and reducing the hospital services (Rossi and Freeman, 1999).

In *Healthy People 2000,* information is presented on the costs and benefits of prevention of illness versus an available medical intervention if the illness had been prevented (Table 21-5). The cost per client to use the intervention is considered a negative net impact because the nation has had to spend money on illness that could be prevented and there have been lost work productivity and lost lives (increased mortality rate) as a result of the preventable illness.

Cost Effectiveness

Cost effectiveness analysis, a measure of the quality of a program as it relates to cost, is the most frequently used analysis in nursing. Cost effectiveness is a subset of cost benefit analysis and is designed to provide an estimate of costs to achieve an outcome. A cost effectiveness study can answer several questions: Did the program meet its objectives? Were the clients and nurses satisfied with the effects of the interventions? Are things better as a result of the interventions? (Kaluzny and Veney, 1999). In cost benefit analysis, both costs and outcomes are quantitative, whereas in cost effectiveness analysis the outcomes are qualitative and quantitative. Outcome measures addressed by cost effectiveness might identify the increase in client knowledge after health teaching, change in the client's condition after treatment, difference in graduates of two nursing programs with similar goals, and the ability of two hearing screening programs to detect hearing loss.

A **cost effectiveness** study requires collecting baseline data on clients before the program is implemented and eval-

TABLE 21-5 *Healthy People 2000:* The Economics of Prevention—Costs of Treatment for Selected Preventable Conditions

CONDITION	OVERALL MAGNITUDE	AVOIDABLE INTERVENTION*	COST PER PATIENT†
Heart disease	7 million with coronary artery disease 500,000 deaths/yr 284,000 bypass procedures/yr	Coronary bypass surgery	$30,000
Cancer	1 million new cases/yr 510,000 deaths/yr	Lung cancer treatment Cervical cancer treatment and rehabilitation	$29,000 $28,000
Cerebrovascular accident (stroke)	600,000 strokes/yr 150,000 deaths/yr	Hemiplegia treatment and rehabilitation	$22,000
Injuries	2.3 million hospitalizations/yr 142,500 deaths/yr 177,000 persons with spinal cord injuries in United States	Quadriplegia treatment and rehabilitation Hip fracture treatment and rehabilitation Severe head injury treatment and rehabilitation	$570,000 (lifetime) $40,000 $310,000
Human immunodeficiency (HIV) infection	1-1.5 million infected 118,000 AIDS cases (as of January 1990)	AIDS treatment	$75,000 (lifetime)
Alcoholism	18.5 million abuse alcohol 105,000 alcohol-related deaths/yr	Liver transplant	$250,000
Drug abuse	Regular users 1-3 million, cocaine 900,000, IV drugs 500,000, heroin Drug-exposed babies 375,000	Treatment of cocaine-exposed baby	$66,000 (5 years)
Low-birth-weight baby (LBWB)	260,000 LBWBs born/yr 23,000 deaths/yr	Neonatal intensive care for LBWB	$10,000
Inadequate immunization	Lacking basic immunization series 20%-30%, ages 2 and younger 3%, ages 6 and older	Congenital rubella syndrome treatment	$354,000 (lifetime)

From USDHHS: *Healthy people 2000: national health promotion and disease prevention objectives,* Washington, DC, 1991, USDHHS, Public Health Services.
*Examples (other interventions may apply).
†Representative first-year costs, except as noted. Not indicated are nonmedical costs, such as lost productivity to society.

uation. This occurs after the program is completed. Box 21-7 shows the procedure for completing a cost effectiveness study. There are several potential outcomes of a cost effectiveness study. For example, a nurse is interested in comparing two methods for implementing a program to teach diabetic clients self-care techniques. The nurse chooses self-teaching modules and a group instruction program for comparison. There are several potential outcomes of comparing the two teaching methods. Of the potential outcomes in a cost effectiveness study, the program of choice would be the most effective teaching method for the least cost. However, if the most costly program demonstrates superior outcomes, it may be chosen. If the least costly program is of poor quality, a more costly program would be appropriate.

Cost Efficiency

Cost efficiency analysis is the actual cost of performing a number of program services. To determine cost efficiency of a program, its productivity must be analyzed. Productivity is the relationship between what the nurse does and how much it costs him or her to do it.

To determine the nurse's activities with a group of clients, one is primarily concerned with a nurse's workload, including direct client care and indirect care activities such as charting, phone calls, client care conferences, and travel. The functions are then related to the client load, client need, and the number of nurses available to meet the needs of all clients served by a program.

Figure 21-7 shows an example of the cost efficiency of a home health agency. The graph indicates that as the number of client visits per year increases, the cost per client visit decreases. The graph assumes that the number of nurses from the beginning to the end of the time period is the same, that the nurses' workloads were necessary to provide home health services, that caseloads were assigned based on staff mix and client need, and that the organizational structure helped nurses be highly productive.

All cost studies have three major tasks: financial, research, and statistical. The financial tasks involve identifying total program costs and breaking them down into smaller parts. To identify the costs of a nurse's participation in a teaching program, the costs for facilities, equipment, supplies, and salaries would have to be examined. All costs associated with the program, such as the nurse's time and use of facilities, equipment, and supplies, should be compared with the total program costs. The statistical tasks involve the identification of appropriate quantifiable measures for analyzing data, and the research tasks involve

> **WHAT DO YOU THINK?** *The combination of prenatal care programs delivered by nurses and the Women, Infants, and Children (WIC) supplemental nutritional program produces better pregnancy and postnatal outcomes for mothers and babies than traditional medical care.*

setting up an appropriate study design to answer the questions of benefit, efficiency, or effectiveness.

Nurses with varying educational backgrounds may be involved in cost studies with the assistance of people knowledgeable in research statistics and accounting techniques. Nurses with undergraduate degrees may be involved in the actual implementation of a cost study, whereas nurses with graduate degrees may be involved in planning, designing, implementing, analyzing, and evaluating study results related to program management.

Cost studies are essential to show the worth of nursing in the marketplace of the future, and nurses should be familiar with the results of cost studies so that sound decisions may be made about future program management. Nurses must be ready to identify appropriate program out-

---

BOX 21-7 Steps in Cost Effectiveness Analysis

1. Identify the program goals or client outcome to be achieved.
2. Identify at least two alternative means of achieving the desired outcomes.
3. Collect baseline data on clients.
4. Determine the costs associated with each program activity.
5. Determine the activities each group of clients will receive.
6. Determine the client changes after the activities are completed.
7. Combine the costs (Step 4), the amount of activity (Step 5), and outcome information (Step 6) to express costs relative to outcomes of program goals.
8. Compare cost outcome information for each goal to present cost effectiveness analysis.

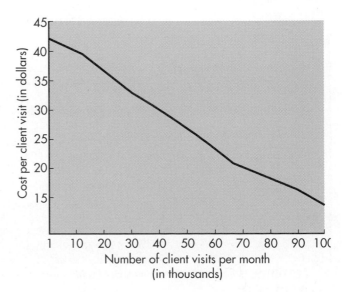

FIG. 21-7 Cost per client visit at a home health agency.

comes, client outcomes, the roles that graduates have in health care delivery, and the requirements to perform nursing procedures so that appropriate decisions about program management will be made based on adequate information.

clinical application

The following is a real-life example of the application of the program management process by an undergraduate community health nursing student. This activity resulted in the development and implementation of a nurse-managed clinic for the homeless. This example shows how students as well as providers can make a difference in health care delivery. It also shows that no mystery surrounds the program management process.

Eva was listening to the radio one Sunday afternoon and heard an announcement about the opening of a soup kitchen within the community for the growing homeless population. She was beginning her community health nursing course and wanted to find a creative clinical experience that would benefit herself as well as others. The announcement gave her an idea. Although it mentioned food, clothing, shelter, and social services, nothing was said about health care.

Eva was interested in finding a way to provide nursing and health care services at the soup kitchen. Which of the following should she do?

A. Talk with key leaders to determine their interest in her idea.
B. Review the literature to find out the magnitude of the problem.
C. Survey the community to find out if others were providing services.
D. Discuss the idea with members of the homeless population.
E. Consider potential solutions to the health care problems.
F. Consider where she would get the resources to open a clinic.
G. Talk with church leaders and community health nursing faculty members to seek acceptance for her idea.

Answer is in the back of the book.

KEY POINTS

- Planning and evaluation are essential elements of program management and vital to the survival of the nursing discipline in health care delivery.
- A program is an organized approach to meet the assessed needs of individuals, families, groups, or communities by reducing or eliminating one or more health problems.
- Planning is defined as selecting and carrying out a series of actions to achieve a stated goal.
- Evaluation is defined as the methods used to determine if a service is needed and will be used, whether a program to meet that need is carried out as planned, and whether the service actually helps the people it intended to help.

- To develop quality programs, planning should include four essential elements: problem diagnosis and assessment of need, identification of problem solutions, analysis and comparison of alternative methods, and selection of the best plan and planning methods.
- The initial and most critical step in planning a health program is assessment of need.
- Some of the major tools used in needs assessment are census data, community forums, surveys of existing community agencies, surveys of community residents, and statistical indicators.
- The major benefit of program evaluation is to determine whether a program is fulfilling its stated goals. Quality assurance programs are prime examples of program evaluation.
- Plans for implementing and evaluating programs should be developed at the same time.
- Program records and community indices serve as major sources of information for program evaluation.
- Planning programs and planning for their evaluation are two of the most important ways in which nurses can ensure successful program implementation.
- Cost studies help identify program benefits, effectiveness, and efficiency.
- The program management process, like the nursing process, is a rational decision-making process.
- The health care delivery system has grown in the past 70 years, making health planning and evaluation very important.
- Comprehensive health planning grew out of a need to control costs.
- Program planning helps nurses and agencies focus attention on services that clients need.
- Planning helps everyone involved understand their role in providing services to clients.
- The assessment of need process provides an evaluation of the relevance that a new service may have to clients.
- A decision tree is a useful tool to choose the best alternative for solving a problem.
- Setting goals and writing objectives to meet the goals are necessary to evaluate program outcomes.
- *Healthy People 2000* is an example of a national program based on needs assessment that has stated goals and objectives on which the program can be evaluated.
- Cost accounting studies are similar to balancing a checkbook and help to determine the actual cost of a program.
- Cost benefit studies are used to assess the desirability of a program by examining costs and benefits, such as the value of human life.
- Cost effectiveness studies measure the quality of a program as it relates to cost.
- Cost efficiency studies examine the actual cost of performing program services and focus on productivity versus cost.
- Program planning models include PPBS, PERT, CPM, and MAUT.
- Program evaluation includes assessing structure, process, and outcomes of care.
- Tracer methods and case registers are two methods of program evaluation.
- The critical path method of evaluating care is a popular model.

critical thinking activities

1. Choose the definitions that best describe your concept of a program, planning, and evaluation.
2. Apply the program planning process to an identified clinical problem for a client group with whom you are working in the community.
   a. Assess the client need.
   b. Choose tools appropriate to the assessment of needs.
   c. Analyze the overall planning process of arriving at decisions about implementing program.
   d. Summarize the benefits for program planning that apply to your situation.
3. Given the situation just described, choose three or four of your classmates to work with on the following projects.

   a. Plan for evaluation of the program in activity 2.
   b. Apply the evaluation process to the situation.
   c. Name the measures you will use to gather data for evaluating your program.
   d. Name the sources you will tap to gain information for program evaluation.
   e. Analyze the benefits of program evaluation that apply to your situation.
   f. Talk with a public or community health nurse or administrator about the application of program planning and evaluation processes at the local agency. Compare their answers to your readings.

Bibliography

Ammerman A, Parks CO: Preparing students for more effective community interventions: assests assessment, *Fam Community Health* 21:1, 1998.

Barclay R: Get the best from your program planners, *Adult Learning* 9(1):12, 1997.

Baron M: Developing an effective community education program through strategic planning, *Community Educ J* 22(2):7, 1995.

Beausejour P: A journey into program management: clinical perspectives, *Leadersh Health Serv* 4(5):36, 1995.

Brown NL et al: A process evaluation of condom availability in the Seattle, Washington public schools, *J Sch Health* 67(8):336, 1997.

Committee on the Costs of Medical Care: *Medical care for the American people,* Chicago, 1932, University of Chicago Press. Reprinted, Washington, DC, 1970, Department of Health, Education, and Welfare.

Davis TM, Allensworth DD: Program management: a necessary component for the comprehensive school health program, *J Sch Health* 64(10):400, 1994.

Dees JP, Garcia MA: Program planning: a total quality approach . . . based on the Plan, Do, Check, Act (PDCA) Cycle developed by Deming (1982), *AAOHN J* 43(5):239, 1995.

Delbecq A, Van de Ven A: A group process model for problem identification and program planning, *J Appl Behav Sci* 7(4):466, 1971.

Donabedian A: *Explorations in quality assessment and monitoring,* vol 2, Ann Arbor, Mich, 1982, Health Administration Press.

Edwards W, Guttentag M, Snapper K: A decision-theoretic approach to evaluation research. In Struening E, Guttentag M, editors: *Handbook of evaluation research,* Beverly Hills, Calif, 1975, Sage.

Feinberg EA et al: Program evaluation and strategic planning in early intervention: general principles and a case example, *Infants Young Child* 8(4):41, 1996.

Foerster S et al: The California Children's 5-a-day-power-play: evaluation of a large scale social marketing initiative, *Fam Community Health* 21(1), 1998.

Fortmann S et al: Effect of community health education on plasma cholesterol levels and diet: the Stanford five-city project, *Am J Epidemiol* 137(10):1039, 1993.

Friis R, Sellers T: *Epidemiology for public health practice,* Gaithersburg, Md, 1999, Aspen.

Garofalo K: Worksite wellness-rewarding healthy behaviors, *AAOHN J* 42(5):236, 1994.

Heinzer M et al: A program evaluation approach to drug administration education, *Nurse Educ* 22(4):25, 1997.

Hickson L et al: Planning a communication education program for older people, *Educational Gerontology* 22(3):257, 1996.

Hostick T et al: Evaluation of stress prevention and management workshops in the community, *J Clin Nurs* 6(2):139, 1997.

Iszler J et al: Formative evaluation for planning a nutrition intervention: results from focus groups, *J Nutr Educ* 27(3):127, 1995.

Kaluzny A, Veney J: Evaluating health care programs and services. In Williams S, Torrens P, editors: *Introduction to health services,* New York, 1999, Wiley.

Kovner A, editor: *Health care delivery in the United States,* New York, 1995, Springer.

Kropf R: Planning for health services. In Kovner A, editor: *Health care delivery in the United States,* New York, 1995, Springer.

Krueger JC: Establishing priorities for evaluation and evaluation research, *Nurs Res* 29:115, 1980.

Kuennen J, Moss V: Community program planning: a clinical outcome, *J Nurs Educ* 34(8):387, 1995.

Lieberman LD: Evaluating the success of substance abuse prevention and treatment programs for pregnant and postpartum women in their infants, *Womens' Health Issues* 8(4):218, 1998.

Meade M: How to plan a project, *Pract Nurse* 12(1):50, 1996.

Moore S: Organizational and managerial supports for service quality in health and human services, *Fam Community Health* 21(2), 1998.

Murray N et al: Development of an intervention map for a parent education intervention to prevent violence among Hispanic middle school students, *J Sch Health* 68(2):46, 1998.

Neild M et al: Evaluation: closing the loop, *Nurs Manage* 29(5):35, 1998.

Norgan GH et al: A program plan addressing carpal tunnel syndrome: the utility of King's goal attainment theory, *AAOHN J* 43(8):407, 1995.

Nutt P: *Planning methods for health and related organizations,* New York, 1984, Wiley.

Pickett G, Hanlon J: *Public health administration and practice,* St Louis, 1990, Mosby.

Posavac EJ, Carey RG: *Program evaluation: methods and case studies,* Englewood Cliffs, NJ, 1997, Prentice Hall.

Price JH et al: Evaluation of a three-year urban elementary school tobacco prevention program, *J Sch Health* 68(1):26, 1998.

Public Law 79-725: *Hospital survey and construction act,* Aug 13, 1946.

Public Law 89-749: *Comprehensive health planning and public services amendments of 1966,* Nov 3, 1966.

Public Law 93-641: *National health planning and resources development act,* Jan 4, 1975.

Rakich J, Longest B, Darr K: *Managing health services organizations,* Baltimore, 1992, Health Professions Press.

Resnicow K, Allensworth D: Conducting a comprehensive school health program . . . school health coordinator, *J Sch Health* 66(2):59, 1996.

Rossi P, Freeman H: *Evaluation: a systematic approach,* Beverly Hills, Calif, 1999, Sage.

Sanson-Fisher R et al: Developing methodologies for evaluating community-wise health promotion, *Health Promot Int* 11(3):227, 1996.

Scheirer MA et al: Measuring the implementation of health promotion programs: the case of the Breast and Cervical Cancer Program in Maryland, *Health Educ Res* 10(1):11, 1995.

Star LM: An effective CPR home learning system: a program evaluation, *AAOHN J* 46(6):289, 1998.

Stein AM: Focus: using structure, process, and outcome for total program evaluation in continuing nursing education, *J Nurs Staff Dev* 11(6):322, 1995.

Suchman EA: *Evaluative research,* New York, 1967, Russell Sage Foundation.

US Department of Health and Human Services: *Healthy communities 2000: model standards,* ed 3, Washington, DC, 1991a, American Public Health Association.

US Department of Health and Human Services: *Healthy people 2000: national health promotion and disease prevention objectives,* Washington, DC, 1991b, USDHHS, Public Health Services.

US Department of Health and Human Services: *Program management: a guide for improving program decisions,* Atlanta, 1989, Centers for Disease Control and Prevention.

Valdiserri R: Applying the criteria for the development of health promotion and education programs to AIDS risk reduction programs for gay men, *J Community Health* 12(4):199, 1987.

Veney J, Kaluzny A: *Evaluation and decision making for health service programs,* Englewood Cliffs, NJ, 1998, Prentice Hall.

Wang C, Abbott L: Development of a community based diabetes and hypertension prevention program, *Public Health Nurs* 15(6):406, 1998.

Quality Management

JUDITH LUPO WOLD

OBJECTIVES

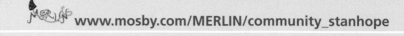

www.mosby.com/MERLIN/community_stanhope

After reading this chapter, the student should be able to do the following:

- Explain total quality management (TQM)/continuous quality improvement (CQI).
- State the goals of TQM/CQI in a health care system.
- Define quality assurance/quality improvement (QA/QI).
- Evaluate the role of QA/QI in continuous quality improvement.
- Analyze the historical development of the quality process in nursing and the changes developing under managed care.
- Evaluate approaches and techniques for implementing continuous quality improvement.
- Examine the ways that managed care is changing the way quality is ensured in health care
- Plan a model QA/QI program.
- Identify the purposes for the types of records kept in community health agencies.
- Evaluate a method for documentation of client care in community and public health nursing.

KEY TERMS

accountability
accreditation
audit process
certification
charter
concurrent audit
credentialing
evaluative studies
licensure

malpractice litigation
managed care
outcome
partnerships
process
Professional Review
  Organization (PRO)

Professional Standards
  Review Organization
  (PSRO)
quality assurance/quality
  improvement (QA/QI)
recognition
records
retrospective audit
risk management

staff review committees
structure
total quality management
  (TQM)/continuous
  quality improvement
  (CQI)
utilization review

See Glossary for definitions

CHAPTER OUTLINE

In a dynamic health care market, the demand for quality seems to be a rallying point for health care consumers. All consumers, including private citizens, insurance companies, and the federal government, are concerned with the highest quality outcomes for the lowest cost (Young, 1998). In addition to the demand for quality and lower cost, the public wants health care delivered with greater accessibility, **accountability,** efficiency, and effectiveness. **Total quality management (TQM)/continuous quality improvement (CQI),** a management style that encompasses quality assurance, or quality control, is one method used to ensure that the client is getting quality care at top value for money spent. Although relatively new in health care, the concept of TQM/CQI has been tried and proven in the industrial sector. The terms *total quality management, continuous quality improvement, total quality,* and *organization-wide quality improvement* often are used synonymously. These terms refer to a management philosophy that focuses on the processes by which work is done with the goal of continuously improving those processes. By obtaining factual information about work processes (e.g., all the steps in certifying a child for the Women, Infants, and Children's [WIC] program), it is possible to discover which steps are unnecessary (i.e., non-value adding) and to eliminate the steps to produce better health outcomes for individuals and communities (Tindall and Stewart, 1993; Verhey, 1996). Box 22-1 presents several abbreviations that are commonly used in health care and quality management.

Both consumers and providers have a vested interest in the quality of the health care system. According to Jonas (1986), the health care provider has three basic reasons to be concerned about health care quality:

1. The principle of nonmalfeasance (above all, do no harm) has been a basic principle of the health care system since the writing of the Hippocratic oath.
2. The principle of beneficence (do good work) is a basic principle of professionalism.
3. The strong social work ethic in our culture places a high value on "doing a good job."

Jonas says that in health care there is a direct link between doing a good job and individual and professional survival. Health care providers pride themselves on individual achievement and responsibility for good client outcomes (Kovner and Jonas, 1998)

The United States is entering a new era of community-oriented, community-controlled delivery of care in which managed care organizations (MCOs) play an integral role (Weiss, 1997). MCOs are entities designed to monitor and deliver health care services within a specific budget (Halverson, Kaluzny, and McLaughlin, 1998). Weiss (1997) states that "in the future, quality will be measured based on the health status of both MCO-enrolled populations and the community or population served as well as individual perceptions of health status" (p 29). As a part of the pursuit of quality health care in communities, health de-

---

BOX 22-1 Commonly Used Abbreviations

AACN	American Association of Colleges of Nursing
ANA	American Nurses Association
ACHNE	Association of Community Health Nursing Educators
APHA	American Public Health Association
CCNE	Commission on Collegiate Nursing Education
CHAP	Community Health Accreditation Program
CQI	Continuous Quality Improvement
JCAHO	Joint Commission on Accreditation of Healthcare Organizations
MCO	Managed Care Organization
NLN	National League for Nursing
PRO	Professional Review Organization
QA	Quality Assurance
QI	Quality Improvement
TQI	Total Quality Improvement
TQM	Total Quality Management

---

partments are examining their place in promoting this quality (Joint Council Committee on Quality in Public Health, 1996). Community and public health nurses are in a perfect position to implement strategies called for in the shift to community-oriented health status improvement. Community assessments, identification of high-risk individuals, targeted interventions, case management, and management of illnesses across the continuum are strategies suggested as part of the focus on improving the health of communities (Weiss, 1997). These strategies have long been used by community and public health nurses.

The growth of the **managed care** industry has changed the face of health care in the United States both in how health care is delivered and how it is received by consumers. Consumers are forming **partnerships** in communities to counter the power of MCOs by holding them accountable for health outcomes in relation to costs. Partnerships are using data-based community assessments to improve health and to ensure that communities receive quality services (Al Assaf, 1998; Bushy, 1997; Lasker, 1997).

Because of managed care and consumer demands for quality nursing, objective and systematic evaluation of nursing care is a priority for the nursing profession. Since nursing is committed to direct accountability, evolving as a scientific discipline, and concerned about how costs of health services limit access, it demands delivery and evaluation of quality service aimed at superior client outcomes (Lindsey, Henly, and Tyree, 1997; Martin, Scheet, and Stegman, 1993; Stevens-Barnum and Kerfoot, 1995).

Records are maintained on all health care system clients to provide complete information about the client and to show the quality of care being given to the client within the system. Records are one necessary part of a CQI process, as are the tools and methods for evaluating quality.

DEFINITIONS AND GOALS

Quality is defined as continuous striving for excellence and a conformance to specifications or guidelines (Davis, 1994). The Institute of Medicine (IOM) defines *quality health care* as "the extent to which health care services . . . have a net benefit. . . That benefit is expected to reflect considerations of client satisfaction and well-being, broad health status and quality of life outcomes, and the processes of client-provider interaction and decision making. The values of both individuals and society are explicitly to be considered. How care is provided should reflect appropriate use of the most current knowledge about scientific, clinical, technical, interpersonal, manual, cognitive, and organizational and management elements of health care" (Lohr, 1990, p. 4).

TQM/CQI, used here synonymously, is a process-driven, customer-oriented management philosophy that includes leadership, teamwork, employee empowerment, individual responsibility, and continuous improvement of system processes to yield improved outcomes (Berwick, 1989). Under TQM/CQI, quality is defined as customer satisfaction. Quality assurance/quality improvement (QA/QI) is the promise or guarantee that certain standards of excellence are being met in the delivery of care (Lalonde, 1988). The quality assurance, or quality control, process does three things (Kinney, Freedman, and Cook, 1994; Maibusch, 1984):

1. Sets standards for care
2. Evaluates care provided based on the standards
3. Takes action to bring about change when care does not meet standards

Quality assurance is concerned with the accountability of the provider and is only one tool in achieving optimum client outcomes (Davis, 1994). Accountability means being responsible for care and answerable to the client (Meisenheimer, 1989). Under QA/QI, quality may have varying definitions.

Quality traditionally has been a prime issue in the delivery of healthcare, and quality assurance programs historically have ensured this accountability. According to Jonas (1995), the goals of quality assurance and improvement are 1) to ensure the delivery of quality client care and 2) to demonstrate the efforts of the health care provider to provide the best possible results. However, standards are a static measurement and do not provide incentive for improvement beyond that standard (Tindall and Stewart, 1993). Under a CQI philosophy, quality assurance and improvement is but one of the many tools used to ensure that the health care agency fulfills what the client thinks are the requirements for the service. Quality assurance focuses on finding what providers have done wrong in the past (e.g., deviations from a standard of care found through a chart audit). CQI focuses on the sources of variation in the ongoing process of health care delivery (i.e., steps in the appointment process) and seeks to improve the process (Tindall and Stewart, 1993).

The process of health care includes two major components: technical interventions (e.g. how well procedures are accomplished, diagnostic accuracy, and treatment effectiveness) and interpersonal relationships between practitioner and client. Both contribute to quality care, and both can be evaluated (Donabedian, 1990). Hart (1993) says that TQM/CQI exists on a continuum with manufacturing and professional services at opposite ends. Although the industrial and health care perspectives on quality are similar, the industrial model does not recognize the intricacies of the practitioner-client relationship. Because of its focus on process as cause of poor outcomes, it downplays both practitioner knowledge and skills and the need for practitioner retraining or censure in case of a standard's violation. Several approaches and techniques are used in quality programs. Approaches are methods used to ensure quality, and techniques are tools for measuring deviations from quality (Kovner and Jonas, 1998).

The term **quality assurance/quality improvement (QA/QI)** is used in place of quality assurance in this chapter to more accurately reflect the current thinking in this field (Schmele, 1993). Traditional approaches to quality focus on assessing or measuring performance, ensuring that performance conforms to standards, and providing remediation if those standards are not met. Such a definition of quality is too narrow in health care systems that try to meet the needs of many clients, both internal and external to the agency (Donabedian, 1990). Many agencies use some of the TQM/CQI concepts, such as client satisfaction questionnaires, but have not adopted the entire management philosophy. However, because QA/QI methods traditionally have been used and are still in use in many agencies, the QA/QI concept will be covered.

HISTORICAL DEVELOPMENT

Improving the quality of care has been a part of nursing since the days of Florence Nightingale. In 1860 Nightingale called for the development of a uniform method to collect and present hospital statistics to improve hospital treatment. Nightingale was a pioneer in setting standards for nursing care. The impetus for establishing nursing schools in the United States came in the late 1800s from a desire to set standards that would upgrade nursing care. In the early 1900s efforts were begun to set similar standards for all nursing schools. From 1912 to 1930 interest in quality nursing education led to the development of nursing organizations involved in accrediting nursing programs. Licensure has been a major issue in nursing since 1892. By 1923 all states had permissive or mandatory laws directing nursing practice.

After World War II, the attention of the emerging nursing profession focused on establishing a scientific method of practice. The nursing process was the chosen method and included evaluation of how nursing activities helped clients (Maibusch, 1984). QA/QI is the evaluative step in the nursing process.

The 1950s brought the development of tools to measure quality assurance. One of the first tools was Phaneuf's nursing audit method (1965), which has been used extensively in community and public health nursing practice.

In 1966 the American Nurses Association (ANA) created the Divisions on Practice. As a result of this, in 1972 the Congress for Nursing Practice was charged with developing standards to institute quality assurance programs. The Standards for Community Health Nursing Practice were distributed to ANA Community Health Nursing Division members in 1973. In 1986 and 1999 the standards were revised.

In 1972 the Joint Commission on Accreditation of Hospitals (JCAH) clearly stated the responsibilities of nursing in its description of standards for nursing services. The JCAH called on the nursing industry to clearly plan, document, and evaluate nursing care provided. In the mid-1980s JCAH became the Joint Commission on Accreditation of Healthcare Organizations (JCAHO) and began developing quality control standards for hospital and home health nursing. JCAHO presently incorporates continuous quality improvement principles in its standards.

Also in 1972, the Social Security Act (Public Law 92-603) was amended to establish the **Professional Standards Review Organization (PSRO)** and to mandate the process review of the delivery of health care to clients of Medicare, Medicaid, and maternal and child health programs. The PSRO program was modified to become the **Professional Review Organization (PRO)** by 1983 Social Security Amendments. The purpose of the PROs is to monitor implementation of the prospective reimbursement system for Medicare clients. Although PSROs were only for physicians, PROs have made quality improvement a primary issue for all health care professionals.

In response to increasing charges of malpractice the government responded with the National Health Quality Improvement Act of 1986. Not funded until 1989, the two major provisions of the act encouraged consumers to become informed about their practitioner's practice record and created a national clearinghouse of information on the malpractice records of providers. The emphasis of this act continued to be on structure rather than process or outcome (NAHQ, 1993).

Efforts to strengthen community health nursing practice include the development of frameworks for nursing practice by both the ANA (1982) and the American Public Health Association (APHA, 1996). Chapter 10 discusses these two models. The quality of nursing education is a major concern of the Association of Community Health Nursing Educators (ACHNE), which was established in 1978. In 1991 and 1993, three reports published by this organization identified the curriculum content required to prepare community nursing students for practice (ACHNE, 1991a, 1991b, 1993). In 1997 the Quad Council (ANA, APHA Public Health Nursing Section, ACHNE, and the Association for State and Territorial Directors of Nursing [ASTDN]) reviewed scopes and standards of population-focused (public health) and community-based nursing practice to guide the profession in obtaining the best health outcomes for the populations they serve. QA/QI programs remain the enforcers of standards of care for many agencies who have not elected to engage in a program of CQI. These activities are called "assurance activities" because they make certain that those policies and procedures are followed so that appropriate quality services are delivered.

WHAT DO YOU THINK? *Critics of professional licensure cite licensing as a "market barrier." Historically licensure has protected the public by ensuring at least a beginning level of proficiency.*

APPROACHES TO QUALITY IMPROVEMENT

Two basic approaches exist in quality improvement: general and specific. The general approach involves a large governing or official body's evaluation of a person's or agency's ability to meet criteria or standards. Specific approaches to quality improvement are methods used to manage a specific health care delivery system in an attempt to deliver care with outcomes that are acceptable to the consumer. QA/QI programs that evaluate provider and client interaction through compliance with standards historically have been used alone to monitor quality care. In a TQM/CQI management approach, QA/QI methods are an integral, but not the only, tool for ensuring quality or customer satisfaction.

General Approaches

General approaches to protect the public by ensuring a level of competency among health care professionals are credentialing, licensure, accreditation, certification, charter, recognition, and academic degrees. Although there has been a long history of public oversight of quality in the United States, this public oversight increasingly involves the private sector. Jost (1995) says that public oversight for quality emerged when the private market failed to focus on health care quality. Some critics cite licensure as a market barrier (Jennison, Young, and Brown, 1993). Diminishing public involvement in quality could leave gaps in external quality assurance mechanisms of the United States (Young, 1998).

Credentialing generally is defined as the formal recognition of a person as a professional with technical competence (Cary, 1989) or of an agency that has met minimum standards of performance. These mechanisms are used to evaluate the agency structure through which care is provided and the outcomes of care given by the provider. Credentialing can be mandatory or voluntary. *Mandatory credentialing* requires statutory laws. State nurse practice acts are examples of mandatory credentialing. *Voluntary credentialing* is performed by an agency or institution. The certification examinations offered by the ANA are examples of voluntary credentialing. Licensing, certification, and accreditation are all examples of credentialing.

Licensure is one of the oldest general quality assurance approaches in the United States and Canada. Individual licensure is a contract between the profession and the state. Under this contract the profession is granted control over entry into and exit from the profession and over quality of professional practice.

The licensing process requires that written regulations define the scope and limits of the professional's practice. Job descriptions based on these regulations set minimum and maximum limits on the functions and responsibilities of the practitioner. Licensure of nurses has been mandated by law since 1903. Today all 50 states have mandatory nurse licensure, which requires all who practice nursing for compensation to be licensed.

Accreditation, a voluntary approach to quality control, is used for institutions. Since 1954 the National League for Nursing (NLN), a voluntary organization, has established standards for inspecting nursing education programs. In 1997 the American Association of Colleges of Nursing (AACN), also a voluntary organization for baccalaureate and higher degree programs, established an affiliate, the Collegiate Commission on Nursing Education (CCNE), to accredit baccalaureate and higher degree nursing programs. In 1966 community health/home health program standards were established by the NLN for the purpose of accrediting these programs through their Community Health Accreditation Program (CHAP). In addition, state boards of nursing accredit basic nursing programs so that their graduates are eligible for the licensing examination.

The accreditation function is quasi-voluntary. Although appearing to be a voluntary participatory program, accreditation often is linked to governmental regulation that encourages programs to participate in the accrediting process. Examples include the federal Medicare regulations restricting payments only to accredited public health and home health care agencies and JCAHO for other health care providers.

Accreditation provides a means for effective peer review and an opportunity for an in-depth review of program strengths and limitations (Cary, 1989). In the past the accreditation process primarily evaluated an agency's physical structure, organizational structure, and personnel qualification. However, beginning in 1990 more emphasis was placed on evaluation of the outcomes of care and on the educational qualifications of the person providing the care.

Certification, another general approach to quality, combines features of licensure and accreditation. Certification usually is a voluntary process within professions. Educational achievements, experience, and performance on an examination determine a person's qualifications for functioning in an identified specialty area. The American Nurses Credentialing Center provides certification in several areas. For example, to become a certified community health nurse, one must have a baccalaureate degree in nursing and 2 years of practice as a community health nurse immediately before application.

Although usually a voluntary process, certification also can be a quasi-voluntary process. For example, to function as a nurse practitioner in some states, one must show proof of educational credentials and take an examination to be "certified" to practice within the boundaries of the state.

Major concerns exist about certification as a quality assurance mechanism. Data are lacking about the clinical competence of the practitioner at the time of certification because clinical competency usually is measured by a written test. There are also insufficient data about the quality of the practitioner's work after the certification process. Except for occupational health nurses and nurse anesthetists, certification has not been recognized by employers as an achievement beyond basic preparation, so financial rewards are few. Although the nursing profession has accepted the certification process as a mechanism for recognizing competence and excellence, certifying bodies must help nurses communicate the significance of certified nurses to the public.

Charter, recognition, and academic degrees are other general approaches to quality assurance. **Charter** is the mechanism by which a state government agency, under state laws, grants corporate status to institutions with or without rights to award degrees (e.g., university-based nursing programs). **Recognition** is defined as a process whereby one agency accepts the credentialing status of and the credentials conferred by another. An example is when state boards of nursing accept nurse practitioner credentials that are awarded by the ANA or by one of the specialty credentialing agencies. *Academic degrees* are titles awarded to individuals recognized by degree-granting institutions as having completed a predetermined plan in a branch of learning. There are four academic degrees awarded in nursing, with some variations at each degree level: Associate of Arts/Science; Bachelor of Science in Nursing; Master of Science in Nursing and Master of Nursing; and Doctor of Philosophy, Doctor of Nursing Science, Doctor of Science in Nursing, and Doctor of Nursing.

Specific Approaches

Historically, quality assurance programs conducted by health care agencies have been a measurement or assessment of the performance of individuals and their conformity to standards set forth by accrediting agencies. TQM/CQI is a management philosophy and method that incorporates many tools, including quality assurance, to maximize customer satisfaction with quality care. Quality care has four components: "professional performance, efficient use of resources, minimal risk to the client of illness or injury associated with care, and patient satisfaction" (Davis, 1994, p. 6). TQM/CQI seeks to eliminate errors in process before negative outcomes can occur rather than waiting until after the fact to correct individual performance. Health care agencies have only recently paid heed to the tenets of TQM/CQI, although Donabedian's early conceptualizations of quality bear a striking resemblance to writings of the industry's TQM leaders. This management philosophy has been incorporated into Japanese industry since the post-World War II era when W. Edwards Deming was invited to Japan to help rebuild its broken economy. In addition to Deming, names associated with the total quality concept are Walter Stewart, who first published in this area, Joseph M. Juran, Armand F. Feigenbaum, Phillip B. Crosby, Genichi Taguchi, and Kaoru Ishikawa. Unlike traditional quality assurance programs, the focus of CQI is the "process" of delivering health care. This process focus avoids assigning personal blame for less than perfect outcomes. Applying TQM in health care allows management to look at the contribution of all systems to outcomes of the organization. Additional distinguishing characteristics of TQM/CQI are the following (McLaughlin and Kaluzny, 1994, p. 4):

1. Empowering clinicians and managers to analyze and improve processes
2. Adopting a norm whereby customer preferences are the primary determinants of quality, and the term *customer* includes both the client and provider in the process
3. Developing a multidisciplinary approach that goes beyond conventional departmental and professional lines
4. Providing the motivation for a rational, data-based, cooperative approach to process analysis and change

Deming's guidelines are summarized by his 14-point program (Deming, 1986, p. 23):

1. "Create and publish to all employees a statement of the aims and purposes of the company or other organization. The management must demonstrate constantly their commitment to this statement.
2. Learn the new philosophy, top management and everybody.
3. Understand the purpose of inspection, for improvement of processes and reduction of cost.
4. End the practice of awarding business on the basis of price tag alone.
5. Improve constantly and forever the system of production and service.
6. Institute training.
7. Teach and institute leadership.
8. Drive out fear. Create trust. Create a climate for innovation.
9. Optimize toward the aims and purposes of the company the efforts of teams, groups, staff areas.
10. Eliminate exhortations for the work force.

11a. Eliminate numerical quotes for production. Instead, learn and institute methods for improvement.
11b. Eliminate management by objective. Instead, learn the capabilities of processes and how to improve them.
12. Remove barriers that rob people of pride of workmanship.
13. Encourage education and self-improvement for everyone.
14. Take action to accomplish the transformation."

Deming's first point emphasizes that an organization must have purpose and values. Health care providers have a clear idea of their values and have been committed to quality in the past as demonstrated by codes of ethics and standards of care. However, successful TQM/CQI processes rely on a cultural change within an organization and the full support of management. With respect to providing quality health care, a paradigm shift from individual provider responsibility to team responsibility must occur (Kaluzny, McLaughlin, and Simpson, 1992). A guiding principle is a customer orientation focused on positive health outcomes and perceived satisfaction. Customer satisfaction surveys must be done for both internal and external users of services.

Personnel policies that are motivating and continuous training/learning opportunities are crucial to any quality improvement program. Deming's eighth point addresses driving out fear. Fear in this context means the fear of being fired for being innovative or taking risks. In the CQI process, individuals are not blamed for failures in the system and therefore are motivated through the group to continually look for problems and improve system performance.

TQM/CQI exists best in a flat organizational structure. This organization operates with a multidisciplinary team approach and a separate but parallel management quality council that monitors strategy and implementation. Teams are empowered to solve problems and locate opportunities for system improvement. Shewhart's circular *Plan/Do/Check/Act* cycle serves as a guideline for the team approach to problem solving. Steps include the following (Deming, 1986, p. 88):

1. "What could be the most important accomplishments of this team? What changes might be desirable? What data are available? Are new observations needed? If yes, plan a change or test. Decide how to use the observations.
2. Carry out the change or test decided upon.
3. Observe the effects of the change.
4. Study the results. What did we learn? What can we predict?
5. Repeat cycle"

A suggested way to start the problem-solving process with a team in Step 1 is "brainstorming" (Al-Assaf, 1993). Brainstorming is getting everyone's input about a possible process situation with no team member criticizing the suggestion. Because TQI organizations are data driven, moving to Step 2 requires that ongoing statistics are collected. Variations from the mean or norm are detected through consistent use of tools, such as the flow chart, the Pareto Chart, cause-and-effect diagrams, checksheets, histograms, control charts, regression, and other statistical analyses (e.g., quality assurance data and techniques, risk management data, risk-adjusted outcome measures, and cost-effectiveness analysis) (McLaughlin and Kaluzny, 1994). Steps 3, 4, and 5 are self-explanatory.

Joseph Juran built on Deming's initial quality work and became a proponent of building quality into all processes. The Juran Trilogy provides an effective comparison of the tasks of quality planning, quality control, and quality improvement. Quality planning involves determining who the clients are, the needs of those clients, the service that fulfills the need, and the process to produce that service. Quality control evaluates the performance of that service, compares it with the service goals, and then makes corrections if necessary. Quality improvement makes sure the infrastructures exist to enable individuals to identify improvement projects. Management of quality improvement establishes project teams and provides those teams with the resources needed to carry out improvement projects (Juran, 1998).

TQM/CQI IN COMMUNITY AND PUBLIC HEALTH SETTINGS

Public health agencies can implement TQM/CQI because of the existing guidelines provided by the 1991 APHA Model Standards. These guidelines "link standards to meeting the health goals for the nation in the year 2000" (Kaluzny, McLaughlin, and Simpson, 1992, p. 258). *Healthy People 2000* and APHA Model Standards (1991) provide not only a prioritized list of health objectives for the nation but also the most current statistics and scientific knowledge about health promotion and disease prevention. These objectives with their stated targets provide measurement tools and reflect intended performance expectations (Durch, Bailey, and Stoto, 1997). *Healthy People 2010*, now being finalized, builds on its predecessor and contains modifications and additional objectives for promoting health and preventing disease. An integral part of the framework of this new document is assuring access to quality health care for all. Additionally, the Assessment Protocol for Excellence in Public Health (APEXPH) (NACHO, 1991) and APEXPH in Practice (NACCHO, 1995) provide a method of assessing community needs and how well departments are operating to meet existing standards. As health care reform evolves, public health facilities face competition in an open market and are moving more rapidly toward corporate forms of management.

A promising outcome of reform is the Community Health Improvement Process (CHIP) described by the Institute of Medicine (Durch, Bailey, and Stoto, 1997) in their report *Improving Health in the Community: A Role for Performance Monitoring*. This report describes how health care and public health can come together in a community-level effort to monitor performance to improve health. Recognizing the multifactorial causes of health problems and the fragmentation that continues to exist in the health care system, this public-private collaborative framework involves many stakeholders, including public health, in monitoring the health of entire communities. *Performance monitoring* is defined as "a continuing community-based process of selecting indicators that can be used to measure the process and outcomes of an intervention strategy for health improvement . . . making the results available to the community as a whole . . . to inform assessments of the effectiveness of an intervention and the contributions of accountable entities" (Durch, Bailey, and Stoto, 1997, p. 418). The performance indicators developed by a CHIP (Fig. 22-1) relate to TQM/CQI. These indicators would measure processes or states that contribute to health and thus the processes are potentially alterable.

Home health care agencies have increasingly adopted quality improvement programs because of the competition that exists. Congruent with the TQM/CQI philosophy, meeting customer expectations is essential for home health care agencies. Davis (1994) presents a quality productivity model for home health care based on Deming's work (Fig. 22-2). Under the first step, labeled *specifier*, Davis specifies that straightforward definitions of requirements and processes are necessary before embarking on a CQI process. This reinforces the need for the continuing learning process called for under Deming's 14 points. The model then proceeds with quality control, quality assurance, and quality continuation processes that should result in quality improvement. Quality control is a proactive process and flows from specifiers being written in measurable terms and taught to all employees. Quality assurance activities are implemented through a proactive quality continuation sequence. Quality assurance retrospectively validates measures of policies, procedures, and standards set forth under quality control. In addition to the quality assurance function, it is important to eliminate errors before they happen. Quality assurance can alert organizations to unwanted trends. The quality continuation sequence is an "alignment of quality policy, procedure, practice, hiring criteria, training, rewards, and recognition" (Davis, 1994, p. 11). Quality improvement results from all preceding activities and is an ongoing process with continuing higher standards for achievement reintroduced into the system.

Other models for QA/QI in home health care have been developed to improve the quality of care in TQM/CQI frameworks emphasizing processes, empowerment and collaboration, consumers, data and measurement, and standards and outcomes (Verhey 1996). One model is a provider partnership that emphasizes processes and systems developed by Care Home Health Services

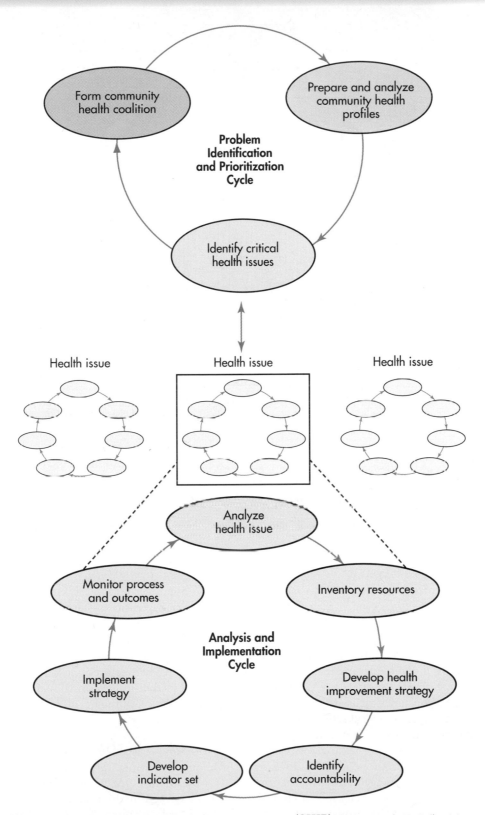

FIG. 22-1 The community health improvement process (CHIP). (From Durch JS, Bailey LA, Stoto M, editors: *Improving health in the community: a role for performance monitoring,* Washington, DC, 1997, National Academy Press.

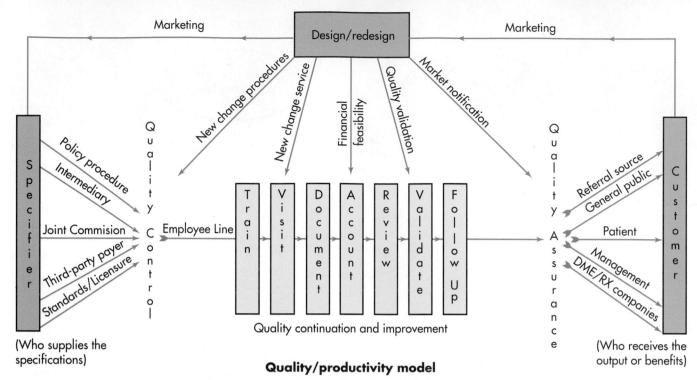

Quality/productivity model

1. Quality control: Measurable process stated in written terms (policy and procedure)
2. Quality assurance: Standard by which the measurable process is validated (audits)
3. Quality continuation: Constant self-measurement by known standards
4. Quality improvement: Culmination of control, assurance, and continuation

DME, Durable medical equipment; Rx, treatment.
NOTE: Model modified from work of W. Edwards Deming—Japan Management, 1950.

FIG. 22-2 Quality productivity model. (From Davis ER: *Total quality management for home care,* Gaithersburg, Md, 1994, Aspen.)

(CHH-Northern California Region). CHH evaluated eight system and process categories, which included condition, availability and courtesy of service, timeliness of response, accuracy of paperwork, promise keeping, cost, and overall satisfaction. Implementation of this model led to increased satisfaction of the provider partners and increased revenue (Smith, 1993).The Home Care Client Satisfaction Instrument is a consumer-focused quality management tool designed to measure overall satisfaction with care through a 15-question Likert scale instrument (Westra et al, 1995). Another consumer model yielding positive results using focus group feedback from clients and care givers was developed by the Visiting Nurses Association (VNA) of Cleveland (Stricklin, 1995). Data sets of clinical information, such as those developed through the Omaha System and the National Association of Home Care (NAHC) (Martin, Leak, and Aden, 1992; NAHC, 1994) are useful in measuring quality of care. "Report cards" of outcomes of health care agencies are becoming more readily available to consumers of health care. Finally, in the area of standards and guidelines, Maturan and Zander

(1993) discuss CareMaps developed by VNA First for use in their managed care system. Created to build on successive outcomes of each home health client encounter, CareMaps contain a care timeline, a problem index, a critical path, and a variance record. As mentioned previously, partnerships between public and private entities using multiple methods of ensuring quality are essential for adequate protection of the health of communities (see the Research Brief).

Using QA/QI in TQM/CQI

Although the methods differ, the objective of both TQM/CQI and QA/QI programs is quality outcomes for clients. QA/QI methods and tools help agencies conform to standards required by external accrediting agencies. QA/QI provides a way to identify examples of substandard care and improve that care when standards are not met (Harris, 1990). QA is focused on problem detection, whereas TQM/CQI is focused on problem prevention and continuous improvement. The total quality philosophy states that quality cannot be "inspected in"; it must be

RESEARCH *Brief*

Client satisfaction as an outcome measure is an important determinant of quality in health care organizations. In this study, the researchers measured client satisfaction with care received from baccalaureate undergraduate student nurses. These students worked in an academic nursing center (ANC) as part of a community health clinical rotation. This academic nursing center is committed to program evaluation, and one facet of their evaluation is client satisfaction. The ANC used the University of North Dakota Survey, a modification of the Group Health Association of American (GHAA) Consumer Satisfaction Survey. This Likert scale (5 = excellent, 1 = poor) survey contained 14 questions that reflected the services provided by the students. Surveys were mailed to 190 clients seen by these students. Clients were in either the child health program, the community health services program, or the expectant family program. Of the 190 clients, 101 responded (53%). Means on each question ranged from 3.9 to 4.7. Only one question resulted in a rating of less than very good to excellent. The overall ratings revealed a highly satisfied group of clients with no significant difference among programs. Significant themes revealed in written comments were satisfaction with the amount of time spent in teaching and the inclusion of families in the program.

Lindsey DL, Henly SJ, Tyree EA: Outcomes in an academic nursing center: client satisfaction with student services, *J Nurs Care Qual* 11(5):30, 1997.

"built in." According to Tindall and Stewart (1993), under QA/QI there is generally little attention paid to prevention of errors or problems and minimal ownership of quality issues. Furthermore the QA process may come to a halt until another problem is found. Kaluzny, McLaughlin, and Simpson (1992) point out differences in traditional management models that use performance standards versus those that use TQM/CQI (Table 22-1).

DID YOU KNOW? *TQM/CQI gives direction for managing a system of care, whereas QA/QI focuses on the care a client receives within the system.*

Since common ground exists between TQM/CQI and QA/QI, positive aspects of a known quality assurance program can be integrated into a total quality approach. Strengths of quality assurance include a history of expertise in development of evaluation of structures, identification of high-priority problems, and development of knowledge in quality assessment and information systems. These strengths can be used to advantage in a CQI effort.

TABLE 22-1 Traditional Management Compared with TQM Model

TRADITIONAL MODEL	TQM MODEL
Legal or professional authority	Collective or managerial responsibility
Specialized accountability	Process accountability
Administrative authority	Participation
Meeting standards	Meeting process and performance expectations
Longer planning horizon	Shorter planning horizon
Quality assurance	Continuous improvement

Traditional Quality Assurance

Traditional quality assurance programs can fit well with the CQI process. Because organizations may implement only parts of the TQM process, it is important to understand existing traditional quality assurance programs. The overall goal of specific quality assurance approaches is to monitor the process and outcomes of client care. The goals are as follows:

1. Identify problems between provider and client.
2. Intervene in problem cases.
3. Provide feedback regarding interactions between client and provider.
4. Provide documentation of interactions between client and provider.

The specific approaches often are implemented voluntarily by agencies and provider groups interested in the quality of interactions in their setting. However, state and federal governments require mandatory programs within public health agencies. For instance, periodic utilization review, peer reviews (audits), and other quality control measures are required in public health agencies that receive funds from state taxes, Medicaid, Medicare, and other public funding sources. Examples of specific approaches to quality control are agency staff review committees (peer review), utilization review committees, research studies, PRO monitoring, client satisfaction surveys, risk management, and malpractice litigation.

Staff review committee

Staff review committees are the most common specific approach to quality assurance in the United States. Staff committees are designed to monitor client-specific aspects of certain levels of care. The audit is the major tool used to evaluate quality of care.

According to LoGerfo and Brook (1984) the **audit process** (Fig. 22-3) consists of six steps:

1. Selection of a topic for study
2. Selection of explicit criteria for quality care
3. Review of records to determine whether criteria are met
4. Peer review of all cases that do not meet criteria

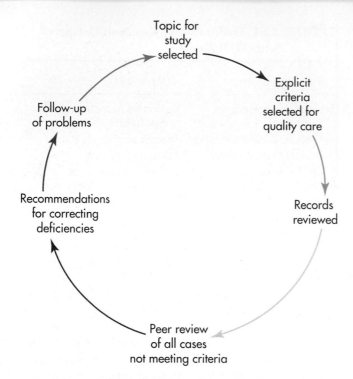

FIG. 22-3 The audit process.

5. Specific recommendations to correct problems
6. Follow-up to determine whether problems have been eliminated

Two types of audits are used in nursing peer review: concurrent and retrospective. The **concurrent audit** is a process audit that evaluates the quality of ongoing care by looking at the nursing process. Concurrent audit is used by Medicare and Medicaid to evaluate care being received by public health/home health clients. The advantages of this method are as follows:

• Identification of problems at the time care is given
• Provision of a mechanism for identifying and meeting client needs during care
• Implementation of measures to fulfill professional responsibilities
• Provision of a mechanism for communicating on behalf of the client

The disadvantages of the concurrent audit are as follows:

• It is time consuming.
• It is more costly to implement than the retrospective audit.
• Because care is ongoing, it does not present the total picture of care that the client ultimately will receive.

The **retrospective audit,** or outcome audit, evaluates quality of care through appraisal of the nursing process after the client's discharge from the health care system. The advantages of the retrospective audit are that it provides the following:

• Comparison of actual practice to standards of care
• Analysis of actual practice findings

• A total picture of care given
• More accurate data for planning corrective action

Disadvantages of the retrospective audit method are as follows:

• The focus of evaluation is directed away from ongoing care.
• Client problems are identified after discharge.

Thus corrective action can only be used to improve the care of future clients.

Utilization review

The purpose of **utilization review** is to ensure that care is needed and that the cost is appropriate (Davis, 1994). LoGerfo and Brook (1984) describe three types of utilization review:

1. *Prospective.* An assessment of the necessity of care before giving service
2. *Concurrent.* A review of the necessity of services while care is being given
3. *Retrospective.* An analysis of the necessity of the services received by the client after the care has been given

Each of these reviews assesses the appropriateness of the cost of care. Prospectively, care can be denied and money saved. Concurrently, services can be cut if they are not deemed essential. Retrospectively, payment can be denied to the provider if the care was not necessary.

Utilization review began in the middle part of the twentieth century out of concern for increasing health care costs. The first committees were developed by insurance companies and professional groups. Utilization review committees became mandatory under the 1965 Medicare law as a way to control hospital costs (Davis, 1994).

The utilization review process includes development of explicit criteria regarding the need for services and the length of service. Utilization review has been used primarily in hospitals to establish the need for client admission and to determine the length of hospital stay. In community and public health, especially home health care, utilization review establishes criteria for admission to agency service, the number of visits a client may receive, the eligibility for client services, such as a nursing aide or physical therapist, and discharge.

Utilization review has several advantages:

• Helps clients avoid unnecessary care
• May encourage the consideration of alternative care options, such as home health care rather than hospitalization
• Can provide guidelines for staff and program development
• Provides for agency accountability to the consumer

The major disadvantage of utilization review is that not all clients fit the classic picture presented by the "explicit criteria" used to determine approval or denial of care. For example, an elderly female client was admitted to a home health care agency for management after hospital discharge. The client was paraplegic as a result of a cerebrovascular accident. After several weeks of physical and speech therapy, the client showed little sign of progress. The utilization review committee considered the client's condition to be stable and did not recognize the continued need for management to prevent future complications; therefore Medicare payment was denied.

Appeal mechanisms have been built into the utilization review process used by Medicare and Medicaid. The appeal allows providers and clients to present additional data that may help to reverse the original decision to deny payment.

Risk management

Risk management committees often are a part of the QA/QI program of a community agency. **Risk management** seeks to reduce the agency's liability because of grievances brought against them. The risk management committee reviews all risks to which an agency is exposed. It reviews client and personnel safety policies and procedures and determines whether personnel are following the rules. Examples of problems reviewed by a risk management committee include administering incorrect vaccination dosage, pediatric client injury caused by a fall from an examining table, or injury to the nurse as a result of an accident while making a home visit. Incident reports are reviewed by the risk management committee for appropriate, accurate, and thorough documentation of any problem that occurs relating to clients or personnel. In addition, patterns are identified that may require changes in policy or staff development to correct the problem. As a part of risk management, grievance procedures are established for both clients and personnel.

Professional review organizations

The Professional Standards Review Organization (PSRO) was established in 1972 in an amendment to the Social Security Act (Public Law 92-603) as a publicly-mandated utilization and peer review program. This law provided that medical, hospital, and nursing home care under Medicare, Medicaid, and Title V Maternal and Child Health Programs would be reviewed for appropriateness and necessity and such care would be reimbursed accordingly.

In 1983 Congress passed the Peer Review Improvement Act (Public Law 97-248), creating PROs. PROs replaced PSROs and are directed by the federal government to reduce hospital admissions for procedures that can be performed safely and effectively in an ambulatory surgical setting on an outpatient basis and reduce inappropriate or unnecessary admissions or invasive procedures by specific practitioners or hospitals. Quality measures include reduction of unnecessary admissions caused by previous substandard care, avoidable complications and deaths, and unnecessary surgery or invasive procedures (Gremaldi and Micheletti, 1985).

Institutions contract with PROs for quality reviews. PROs are local (usually state) organizations that establish criteria for care based on local patterns of practice. They can be for-profit or not-for-profit organizations. They have access to physicians or may include physicians in their membership. PROs must define their operational objectives and are required to consult with nurses and other nonphysician health care providers when reviewing the activities of those professionals. PROs monitor access to care and cost of care. Professionals working under the regulation of PROs should develop accurate and complete documentation procedures to ensure compliance with the criteria of the PRO.

Debate has occurred over the limitations and benefits of the federally-mandated quality review process. Limitations include jeopardizing professional autonomy because decision making regarding care includes professionals, consumers, and government representatives. Another limitation of this process is the development of a costly control mechanism whereby client care activities may be determined by cost rather than by professional criteria. The benefit of the PSRO/PRO system has been the development of standards and the institution of peer review mechanisms to increase accountability for care provided (Greenberg and Lezzoni, 1995; Gremaldi and Micheletti, 1985; Lieski, 1985).

In 1985 PRO authority was expanded to include review of services offered by health maintenance organizations (HMOs) and competitive medical plans. In addition the Medicare Quality Assurance Act was passed to strengthen quality assurance programs and to improve access to posthospital care. This act required hospitals receiving Medicare payments to provide to Medicare beneficiaries written forms of discharge planning supervised by registered nurses and social workers.

Evaluative studies

Evaluative studies for quality health care increased during the twentieth century. Studies demonstrate the effect of nursing and health care interventions on client populations. Three key models have been used to evaluate quality: Donabedian's structure-process-outcome, the tracer, and the sentinel.

Donabedian's (1981, 1985, 1990) model introduced three major methods for evaluating quality care:
1. **Structure.** Evaluating the setting and instruments used to provide care. Examples of structure are facilities, equipment, characteristics of the administrative organization, client mix, and the qualifications of health providers.
2. **Process.** Evaluating activities as they relate to standards and expectations of health providers in the management of client care.
3. **Outcome.** The net change that occurs as a result of health care or the net result of health care.

The three methods may be used separately to evaluate a part of care. However, to get an overall picture of quality of care they should be used together.

The tracer method described by Kessner and Kalk (1973) is a measure of both process and outcome of care. This method is more effective in evaluating health care of groups than of individual clients. It is also more effective in evaluating care delivered by an institution than by an individual provider. Kessner and Kalk (1973) described the following essential characteristics for implementing the tracer method:

1. A tracer, or a problem, that has a definite impact on the client's level of functioning
2. Well-defined and easily diagnosed characteristics
3. Population prevalence high enough to permit adequate data collection
4. A known variation resulting from use of effective health care
5. Well-defined management techniques in either prevention, diagnosis, treatment, or rehabilitation
6. Understood (documented) effects of non-medical factors on the tracer.

Stevens (1985) provided a classification system for selecting client groups for tracer outcome studies in nursing:

1. A particular disease
2. Similar treatment
3. Similar needs
4. Similar community
5. Similar lifestyle
6. Similar illness stage

The tracer method provides nurses with data to show the differences in outcomes as a result of nursing care standards.

The sentinel method of quality evaluation is based on epidemiologic principles (Rutstein et al, 1976). This method is an outcome measure for examining specific instances of client care. The characteristics of this method are as follows:

- Cases of unnecessary disease, disability, complications, and death are counted.
- The circumstances surrounding the unnecessary event, or the sentinel, are examined in detail.
- A review of morbidity and mortality rates is used as an index to determine the critical increase in the untimely event, which may reflect changes in quality of care.
- Health status indicators, such as changes in social, economic, political, and environmental factors that may have an effect on health outcomes, are reviewed.

Changes in the sentinel indicate potential problems for others. For example, increases in encephalitis in certain communities may result from increases in mosquito populations.

Client satisfaction

Client satisfaction is another approach to measuring quality of care. Client satisfaction can be assessed using in-person or telephone interviews and mailed questionnaires. In nursing, satisfaction surveys are used to assess care received during a specific agency admission; the client's personal nursing care, or the total care that the client received from all services.

Satisfaction surveys may measure the interventions of client care, attitudes about the care received and the providers of care, and perceptions of the situation (environment) in which the care was received. Clients often are more critical of interpersonal and situational components of care than of the interventions of care.

Satisfaction surveys are an essential aspect of quality assessment. Survey data provide clues to reasons for client compliance or noncompliance with plans of care. The surveys also provide data about health-seeking behaviors, the probability of malpractice litigation, and the likelihood of continuing client-provider-agency relationships. The NLN (CHHA and CHS, 1988) provides an example of a client satisfaction survey (Discharged Patient Questionnaire) that can be used in a community health agency.

Malpractice litigation

Malpractice litigation is a specific approach to quality assurance imposed on the health care delivery system by the legal system. Malpractice litigation typically results from client dissatisfaction with the provider and with the content of the care received. Nursing is not immune from malpractice litigation. Nursing must continue to have a sound quality assurance program that ensures quality care. This will reduce the risk of quality control measures being imposed by an external source, such as the legal system.

MODEL QA/QI PROGRAM

The primary purpose of a QA/QI program is to ensure that the results of an organized activity are consistent with the expectations. All personnel affected by a quality assurance program should be involved in its development and implementation. Although administration and management are responsible for the quality of services, the key to that quality is the knowledge, skills, and attitudes of the personnel who deliver the service (Porter, 1988).

In 1977 the ANA introduced a model for a quality assurance program (ANA, 1977). Figure 22-4 depicts the model, which identifies seven basic components of a quality assurance program. According to Gottlieb (1988), quality assurance programs answer the following questions about health care services and nursing care:

1. What is being done now?
2. Why is it being done?
3. Is it being done well?
4. Can it be done better?
5. Should it be done at all?
6. Are there improved ways to deliver the service?
7. How much does it cost?
8. Should certain activities be abandoned and/or replaced?

The ANA model and Donabedian's framework for evaluating health care programs using the components of structure, process, and outcome can be used in developing a quality assurance program. Outcome is the most important ingredient of a program since it is the key to evaluation of providers and agencies by accrediting bodies, by insurance companies, and by Medicare and Medicaid through PROs and other accrediting agencies.

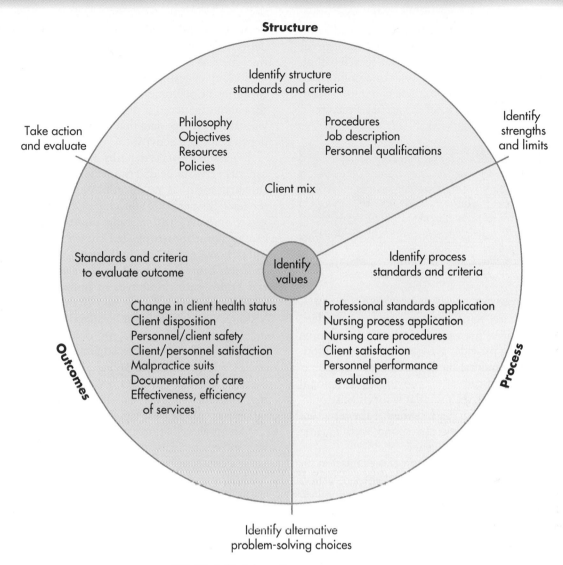

FIG. 22-4 Model quality assurance program.

Structure

The philosophy and objectives of an agency serve to define the structural standards of the agency. Evaluation of structure is a specific approach to quality appraisal. In evaluating the structure of an organization, the evaluator determines whether the agency is adhering to the stated philosophy and objectives. Is the agency providing services to populations across the life span? Are primary, secondary, and/or tertiary preventive services offered? Standards of structure are defined by the licensing or accrediting agency (e.g., the NLN standards for accrediting home health agencies) (CHHA/CHS, 1986).

Values identification, the first step in a quality assurance program, serves to define the beliefs of the agency about humanity, nursing, the community, and health. The beliefs of the community, the population to be served, and the providers of care are equally important to the agency beliefs, and all need to be considered to provide quality service.

Identification of standards and criteria for quality assurance begins with writing the philosophy and objectives of the organization. These program objectives, written in the 1990s, defined the intended results of nursing care, descriptions of client behaviors, and/or change in health status to be demonstrated on discharge (Rinke and Wilson, 1988).

Once objectives are formulated, the resources needed to accomplish the objectives should be identified. The personnel, supplies and equipment, facilities, and financial resources that are needed should be described. Once resources are determined, policies, procedures, and job descriptions should be formed to serve as behavioral guides to the employees of the agency. These documents should reflect the essential nursing and other health provider qualifications needed to implement the services of the agency.

Standards of structure are evaluated internally by a committee composed of administrative, management, and staff members for the purpose of doing a self-study. Standards of structure also are evaluated by a utilization review committee often composed of an external advisory group with community representatives for all services offered through an agency, such as a nurse, a physical therapist, a speech pathologist, a physician, a board member, and an administrator from a sister agency. The data from these committees identify the strengths and weaknesses of the agency structure.

> **NURSING TIP**
>
> *Know the standards of care for your agency. Keep your eyes open for recurring practices that are not up to the quality standards of your agency. For example, your clients complain daily about long waits for service. Chances are that these same practices may be occurring in other areas of the agency, and knowing this helps the agency improve quality.*

Process

The evaluation of process standards is a specific appraisal of the quality of care being given by agency providers, such as nurses. Agencies use various methods to determine criteria for evaluating provider activities: conceptual models, such as a developmental model or Neuman's Systems Model; the standards of care of the provider's professional organization, such as the ANA standards for nursing practice; or the nursing process. The activities of the nurse are evaluated to see whether they correspond with nursing care procedures defined by the agency.

The primary approaches used for process evaluation include the peer review committee and the client satisfaction survey. The techniques used for process evaluation are direct observation, questionnaire, interview, written audit, and videotape of client and provider encounters.

Although many audit instruments are available, Schmele has developed and tested an instrument based on the nursing process and applied this tool in the community. The Schmele Instrument to Measure the Process of Nursing Practice in Community Nursing Service is a three-part instrument that includes data from direct observation, from the record audit, and from the client by means of a survey questionnaire. Each technique involves evaluation of the four steps of the nursing process (Schmele, 1985; Meisenheimer, 1989). Schmele developed a second instrument, the SIMP-H, to measure the process of nursing practice in home health (see Appendix C.4).

Once data are collected to evaluate nursing process standards, the peer review committee reviews the data to identify strengths and weaknesses in the quality of care delivered. The peer review committee usually is an internal committee composed of representatives of the nursing staff who are trained to administer audit instruments and conduct client interviews.

Outcome

The evaluation of outcome standards, or the result of nursing care, is one of the more difficult tasks facing nursing today. The ability to identify changes in the client's health status as a result of nursing care provides nursing data that

demonstrate the contribution of nursing to the health care delivery system. Research studies using the tracer or sentinel method to identify client outcomes and client satisfaction surveys can be used to measure outcome standards. Measures of outcome standards include client admission data about the level of dependence or the acuity of problems and discharge data that may show changes in levels of dependence and activity.

From these data, strengths and weaknesses in nursing care delivery can be determined. The most common measurement methods are direct physical observations and interviews. Rissner (1975) developed a client satisfaction survey to evaluate client attitudes and the content of nursing care in a primary setting. The survey has been adapted for use in home health care by Reeder (Meisenheimer, 1989).

Instruments also have been developed to measure general health status indicators in home health (Choi et al, 1987; Gould, 1985; Padilla and Grant, 1987). The Omaha Visiting Nurses Association Problem Classification System includes nursing diagnosis, protocols of care, and a problem rating scale to measure nursing care outcomes (Martin et al, 1993). (See Chapter 10 for a discussion of the Omaha System.) Nursing has been involved primarily in evaluating program outcomes to justify program expenditures rather than in evaluating client outcomes.

Outcome evaluation assumes that health care has a positive effect on client status. The major problem with outcome evaluation is determining which nursing care activities are primarily responsible for causing changes in client status (Chernin and Ayer, 1990; Rapheal, 1991). In nursing there are multiple uncontrolled factors in the field, such as environment and family relationships, that have an effect on client status. Often it is difficult to determine whether these factors are the cause of changes in client status or whether nursing interventions have the most effect. The NLN has published useful guides for developing outcome criteria (Rinke and Wilson, 1988).

Types of problems studied in a quality assurance program include reasons for the following:
- Client death
- Client injury
- Personnel and client safety
- Agency liability
- Increased costs
- Denied reimbursement by third-party payers
- Client complaints
- Inefficient service
- Staff noncompliance with standards of structure
- Lack of resources
- Unnecessary staff work and overtime
- Documentation of care
- Client health status

Table 22-2 summarizes quality assurance measures.

Evaluation, Interpretation, and Action

Interpreting the findings of a quality care evaluation is an essential component of the process. It allows for the identification of discrepancies between the quality care standards of the agency and the actual practice of the nurse or other health providers. These patterns reflect the total agency's functioning over time and generate information for decisions to be made about the strengths and limitations of the agency. Regular intervals for evaluation should be established within the agency, and periodic reports should be written so that the combined results of structure, process, and outcome efforts can be analyzed and health care delivery patterns and problems can be identified. These reports should be used to establish an ongoing picture of changes that occur within an agency to justify community nursing services.

Identification and choices of possible courses of action to correct the weaknesses within the agency should involve both the administration and the staff. The courses of action chosen should be based on their significance, economic benefit, and timeliness. For example, if there is a nursing problem in the recording of client health education, the agency administration and staff may analyze the problem to see why it is occurring. Reasons for recording inadequacies given by the nurses include a lack of time to do paperwork properly, case overloads that reduce the amount of time spent with clients, and lack of available resources for health education. If such reasons are given, it would not be appropriate for management to deal with the problem by providing a staff development program on the importance of doing and recording health education. It would be more important to assess how to provide the time and resources necessary for the nurses to offer health education to the clients. Economically, it may be more beneficial to provide dictating equipment and clerical assistance so that nurses can dictate notes and other paperwork, thereby providing more client contact time, or it may be more beneficial economically to employ an additional nurse and reduce caseloads.

TABLE 22-2 Quality Assurance Measures

STRUCTURE	PROCESS	OUTCOME
INTERNAL AGENCY	**PEER REVIEW COMMITTEES**	**INTERNAL AGENCY COMMITTEES**
Self-study	Prospective audit	Evaluative studies
Review agency documents	Concurrent audit	Survey health status
	Retrospective audit	
EXTERNAL AGENCY	**CLIENT**	**CLIENT**
Regulatory audit	Satisfaction survey	Malpractice suits
Utilization review	Satisfaction survey	

Taking action is the final step in the QA/QI model. Once the alternative courses of action are chosen to correct problems, actions must be implemented for change to occur in the overall operation of the agency. Follow-up and evaluation of actions taken must occur for improvement in quality of care to occur. Although health provider evaluation will continue to be included in a quality improvement effort, the focus of a CQI effort emphasizes the process and not the person. The assumption here is that health care professionals and other employees customarily want to do the best job possible for the client, and problems or variations in a process should not be automatically attributed to their behavior (Laffel and Blumenthal, 1993). Although frequent feedback should be given to all employees, the hallmark of quality improvement is continuous learning. Staff development must be ongoing for all employees.

Documentation is essential to the evaluation of quality care in any organization. The following section focuses on the kinds of documentation that normally occur in a community health agency.

RECORDS
Purposes

Records are an integral part of the communication structure of the health care organization. Accurate and complete records are required by law and must be kept by all government and nongovernment agencies. In most states, the state departments of health stipulate the kind and content requirements of records for community health agencies.

Records provide complete information about the client, indicate the extent and quality of services being rendered, resolve legal issues in malpractice suits, and provide information for education and research.

Community and Public Health Agency Records

Within the community or public health agency many types of records are kept and used to predict population trends in a community, to identify health needs and problems, to prepare and justify budgets, and to make administrative decisions. The kinds of records kept by the agency may include reports of accidents, births, census, chronic disease, communicable disease, mortality rates, life expectancy, morbidity rates, child and spouse abuse, occupational illness and injury, and environmental health.

Other types of records kept within the agency are those used to maintain administrative contact and control of the organization. Three types of records make up this category: clinical, service, and financial. The clinical record is the client health record. The provider service records include information about the number of clinic clients seen daily, the immunizations given, home visits made daily, transportation and mileage, the provider's time spent with the client, and the amount and kinds of supplies used. The service record is completed on a daily basis by each provider and is summarized monthly and annually to indicate trends in health care activities and costs relative to personnel time, transportation, maintenance, and supplies. The provider service records are used to correlate with the agency's financial records of salaries, overhead, and transportation costs, and they serve as the basis for the cost accounting system (Pickett and Hanlon, 1990). These records are basic to peer review and audit.

Three additional kinds of service records seen in the community health agency are the central index system, the annual implementation plan, and the annual summary of agency activities. The central index system is a data-filing system that indicates the services requested, services offered, active and inactive clients of the agency, and a profile of the agency's clients.

The annual implementation plan is developed at the beginning of each fiscal year to define the short-term and long-term goals of the agency. The annual implementation plan serves as the basis for the agency's annual summary. The annual summary reflects the success of the agency in meeting the annual objectives, changes in population trends and health status during the year, the actual versus the projected budget requirements, the number of services offered, the number of clients served, and the plans and changes recommended for the future. This plan serves as the basis for the evaluation of agency structure.

As an outgrowth of quality assurance efforts in the health care system, comprehensive methods are being designed to document and measure client progress and client outcome from agency admission through discharge. An example of such a method is the client classification system developed at the Visiting Nurses Association of Omaha, Nebraska (Martin, 1982, Martin, Scheet, and Stegman, 1993). This comprehensive method for evaluating client care has several components: a classification system for assessing and categorizing client problems, a database, a nursing problem list, and anticipated outcome criteria for the classified problem. Such schemes are viewed as having the potential to improve the delivery of nursing care, documentation, and the descriptions of client care. Briefly, implementation of comprehensive documentation methods enhances nursing assessment, planning, implementation and evaluation of client care, and it allows for the organization of pertinent client information for more effective and efficient nurse productivity and communication.

clinical application

Margaret, a community health nursing student, has been asked to be a member of the health care team designated to monitor the quality of service provided to the clients and community of the health care agency. As a member of this committee, she wants to identify the current system used to monitor quality.

To prepare for her role in planning and implementing a QA/QI program, she reads the federal and state regulations to identify those elements that, by law, must be included in the QA/QI program. She finds that Medicare now has specific tools to measure outcomes of client care. She learns that when the Medicare evaluator visits the agency, Margaret will be making home visits with the evaluator to directly observe the physical appearance of the client.

At the first meeting, the student is interested in the relationship between philosophy and objectives of the agency. Does the philosophy reflect beliefs about the clients to be served by the agency, the type of nursing care and services to be delivered, the population or the community to be served, and beliefs about health care versus illness care? Do the objectives of the agency reflect the stated beliefs in the philosophy? For example, does the philosophy indicate beliefs about client education or research? If so, are there agency objectives that address providing health education or enhancing research related to better client care?

Once the committee establishes from the philosophy and objectives that the agency's goal is to deliver primary health care services to the total population of the community, Margaret is interested in the standards of care used to deliver quality health care. In nursing, are the ANA standards for nursing practice used to evaluate nursing care given? Are the nurses employed by the agency qualified to fulfill their job descriptions through education, experience, or both?

Then the committee looks at the employment criteria of the agency. Do the criteria reflect the beliefs of the agency about nursing and the agency goals? Do the agency's policies and procedures assist the nurse in meeting the stated standards of care.

Given the structure of the agency, how is the process of care evaluated? Does the agency use prospective, concurrent, or retrospective audits to evaluate the process of care given? Are the audits designed to measure the standards of care used by the agency? How is the data used after it is collected? Is there any evidence that the evaluation makes a difference? Has the process of care changed as a result of the evaluation?

After the structure and process elements are identified, the committee members and the student turn their attention to the outcome elements. What questions should be asked about outcome?

A. How is health outcome defined by the agency: client satisfaction, change in health status, number of malpractice suits, or number of Medicare payments received?

B. How is the data used to make a difference in future quality outcomes?

Answers are in the back of the book.

KEY POINTS

- The health care delivery system is the largest employing industry in the United States; society is demanding increased efficiency and effectiveness from the system.

- Quality control is the tool used to ensure effectiveness and efficiency.
- The managed care industry is changing the face of the American health care delivery system and how quality is defined and measured.
- Objective and systematic evaluation of nursing care has become a priority within the profession for several reasons, including the effects of cost on health care accessibility, consumer demands for better quality care, and increasing involvement of nurses in public and health agency policy formulation.
- Total Quality Management/Continuous Quality Improvement (TQM/CQI) is a management philosophy new to the health care arena. It is prevention oriented and process focused. Its primary focus is to deliver quality health care. *Quality* is defined as customer satisfaction.
- Public and private sectors are forming partnerships to monitor performance of all players in health care delivery to improve the health of communities.
- Quality assurance/quality improvement (QA/QI) is the monitoring of client care activities to determine the degree of excellence attained in implementation of the activities.
- Quality assurance has been a concern of the profession since the 1860s, when Florence Nightingale called for a uniform format to gather and disseminate hospital statistics.
- Licensure has been a major issue in nursing since 1892.
- Two major categories of approaches exist in QA/QI today: general and specific.
- Accreditation is an approach to quality control used for institutions, whereas licensure is used primarily for individuals.
- Certification combines features of both licensing and accreditation.
- Three major models have been used to evaluate quality: Donabedian's structure-process-outcome model, the sentinel model, and the tracer model.
- Seven basic components of a quality assurance program are 1) identifying values; 2) identifying structure, process, and outcome standards and criteria; 3) selecting measurement techniques; 4) interpreting the strengths and weaknesses of the care given; 5) identifying alternative courses of action; 6) choosing specific courses of action; and 7) taking action.

- Records are an integral part of the communication structure of a health care organization. Accurate and complete records are by law required of all agencies, whether governmental or nongovernmental.
- QA/QI mechanisms in health care delivery are the mechanisms for controlling the system and requesting accountability from individual providers within the system. Records help establish a total picture of the contribution of the agency to the client community.

critical thinking activities

1. Write your own definition of TQM/CQI; compare your definition with the one given in the text. Are they the same or different? Give justification for your answer.
2. How does traditional QA/QI fit into the TQM/CQI effort. Explain the relative importance of a continuing QA/QI effort.
3. Interview a nurse who is a coordinator of or is responsible for QA/QI in a local health agency. Ask the following questions and add others you may wish to have answered.
   a. Does the agency subscribe to the TQM/CQI approach to management?
   b. If not, is the agency incorporating elements of the TQM/CQI process as outlined by Deming in his 14 points?
   c. Is a traditional method of quality assurance used to ensure quality?
   d. Describe the components of the QA/QI program.
   e. How are records used in your QA/QI effort.
   f. Discuss the approaches and techniques that are used to implement the QA/QI program.
   g. How has the QA/QI program changed in the health agency over the past 20 years?
   h. What influence has the QA/QI program had on decreasing problems attributable to process? To provider accountability?
   i. List and describe the types of records usually kept in a community health agency. Explain the purpose of each type of record.
4. Conduct an assessment of your community. Identify partnerships necessary to ensure quality health outcomes for your community from the data gathered.

Bibliography

Al-Assaf AF: Historical evolution of managed care quality. In Al Assaf AF, editor: *Managed care quality: a practical guide,* New York, 1998, CRC Press.

Al-Assaf AF: Data management for total quality. In Al-Assaf AF, Schmele JA, editors: *The textbook of total quality in healthcare,* Delray Beach, Fla, 1993, St Lucie Press.

American Nurses Association: *Quality model: a plan for implementation of the standards of nursing practice,* Kansas City, Mo, 1977, the Association.

American Nurses Association: *A conceptual model of community health nursing,* Kansas City, Mo, 1982, the Association.

American Public Health Association: *Healthy communities 2000: model standards, guidelines for community attainment of the year 2000 national health objectives,* ed 3, Washington, DC, 1991, the Association.

American Public Health Association: *The definition and role of public health nursing: a statement of the public health nursing section on the delivery of health care,* Washington, DC, 1996, the Association.

Association of Community Health Nursing Educators: *Essential components of master's level practice in community health nursing,* Lexington, Ky, 1991a, the Association.

Association of Community Health Nursing Educators: *Essentials of baccalaureate education,* Louisville, Ky, 1991b, the Association.

Association of Community Health Nursing Educators: *Perspectives on doctoral education in community health nursing,* Lexington, Ky, 1993, the Association.

Berwick DM: Continuous improvement as an ideal in healthcare, *N Engl J Med* 320:53, 1989.

Bushy A: Empowering initiatives to improve a community's health status, *J Nurs Care Qual* 11(4):32, 1997.

Cary A: Credentialing: opportunities and responsibilities in nursing. In Lambert C, Lambert V: *Perspectives in nursing,* Norwalk, Conn, 1989, Appleton & Lange.

Continued

Bibliography—cont'd

Chernin S, Ayer T: The outcome audit: assuring quality care, *Caring* 9(2):8, 1990.

Choi T et al: Health specific family coping index for noninstitutional care. In Rinke L, editor: *Outcome measures in home care,* vol 1, New York, 1987, NLN.

Council of Home Health Agencies and Community Health Services: *Accreditation of home health agencies and community nursing services: criteria and guide for preparing reports,* New York, 1986, NLN.

Council of Home Health Agencies and Community Health Services: *Administrator's handbook for the structure, operation, and expansion of home health agencies,* New York, 1988, NLN.

Davis ER: *Total quality management for homecare,* Gaithersburg, Md, 1994, Aspen.

Deming WE: *Out of the crisis,* Cambridge, Mass, 1986, MIT, Center for Advanced Engineering Study.

Donabedian A: *Exploration in quality assessment and monitoring, vol 2,* Ann Arbor, Mich, 1981, Health Administration Press.

Donabedian A: *Explorations in quality assessment and monitoring, vol 3,* Ann Arbor, Mich, 1985, Health Administration Press.

Donabedian A: The seven pillars of quality, *Arch Pathol Lab Med* 114:1115, 1990.

Durch JS, Bailey LA, Stoto MA, editors: *Improving health in the community,* Washington, DC, 1997, National Academy Press.

Gottlieb H: Quality assurance: a blueprint for improved patient care and service, *Home Healthcare Nurs* 6(3):11, 1988.

Gould J: Standardized home health nursing plans: a quality assurance look, *Qual Rev Bull* 11(11):334, 1985.

Greenberg LG, Lezzoni LI: Quality. In Calkins D, Fernandopulle RJ, Marino BS: *Health care policy,* Cambridge, Mass, 1995, Blackwell Science.

Gremaldi PL, Micheletti JA: PRO objectives and quality criteria, *Hospitals* 59:64, 1985.

Halverson PK, Kaluzny AD, McLaughlin CP: *Managed care and public health,* Gaithersburg, Md, 1998, Aspen.

Harris JS: The bridge for quality assurance to quality improvement, *J Occ Med* 17:1175, 1990.

Hart C: *Handout Northern Telecom,* Research Park Triangle, NC, 1993, University Quality Forum.

Jennison B, Young G, Brown S: *Licensing, accreditation and certification,* Boston, 1993, Little, Brown & Co.

Joint Council Committee on Quality in Public Health: *Promoting quality care for communities: the role of health departments in an era of managed care,* Washington, DC, 1996, National Association of City and County Health Officials.

Jonas S: Measurement and control of the quality of health care. In Kooner AR, editor: *Health care delivery in the United States,* New York, 1986, Springer.

Jost TS: Oversight of the quality of medical care: regulation, management or the market? *Arizona Law Rev* 37:825, 1995.

Juran JM: *Juran's quality handbook,* New York, 1998, McGraw-Hill.

Kaluzny AD, McLaughlin CP, Simpson K: Applying total quality management concepts in public health organizations, *Public Health Rep* 107(3):257, 1992.

Kessner DM, Kalk CE: Assessing health quality-the case for tracers, *N Engl J Med* 288:189, 1973.

Kinney ED, Freedman JA, Cook CA: Quality improvement in community-based, long-term care: theory and reality, *Am J Law Med* 20(1-2):59, 1994.

Kovner A, Jonas S, editors: *Jonas and Kovner's health care delivery in the United States,* New York, 1998, Springer.

Laffel G, Blumenthal D: The case for using industrial quality management science in health care organizations. In Al-Assaf AF, Schmele JA, editors: *The textbook of total quality in healthcare,* Delray Beach, Fla, 1993, St Lucie Press.

Lalonde B: Assuring the quality home care via the assessment of client outcomes, *Caring* 7(1):20, 1988.

Lasker RD et al: *Medicine and public health: the power of collaboration,* New York, 1997, The New York Academy of Medicine.

Lieski AM: Standards: the basis of a quality assurance program. In Meisenheimer CG, editor: *A complete guide to effective programs,* Rockville, Md, 1985, Aspen.

Lindsey DL, Henly SJ, Tyree EA: Outcomes in an academic nursing center: client satisfaction with student services, *J Nurs Care Qual* 11(5):30, 1997.

LoGerfo J, Brook R: Evaluation of health services and quality of care. In Williams S, Torrens P, editors: *Introduction to health services,* New York, 1984, John Wiley & Sons.

Lohr KN, editor: *Medicare: a strategy for quality assurance,* vol 1, Washington, DC, 1990, National Academy Press.

Maibusch RM: Evolution of quality assurance for nursing in hospitals. In Schrolder PS, Maibusch RM, editors: *Nursing quality assurance,* Rockville, Md, 1984, Aspen.

Martin KS, Scheet NJ, Stegman MR: Home health clients: characteristics, outcomes of care, and nursing interventions, *Am J Public Health* 83(12):1730, 1993.

Martin K, Leak G, Aden C: The Omaha system: a research based model for decision making, *J Nurs Admin* 22:47, 1992.

Martin K: A client classification system adaptable for computerization, *Nurs Outlook* 30:515, 1982.

Maturan VL, Zander K: Outcomes management in a prospective pay system, *Caring* 12(6):46, 1993.

McLaughlin CP, Kaluzny AD: Defining total quality management/continuous quality improvement. In McLaughlin CP, Kaluzny AD, editors: *Continuous quality improvement in healthcare: theory, implementation and applications,* Gaithersburg, Md, 1994, Aspen.

Meisenheimer C: *Quality assurance for home health care,* Rockville, Md, 1989, Aspen.

National Association of Home Care: Draft uniform data set for home care and hospice, *Caring* 13(6):10, 1994

National Association of City and County Health Officials: *APEXPH in practice,* Washington, DC, 1995, NACCHO.

National Association of County Health Officials: *APEXPH: assessment protocol for assessment in public health,* Washington, DC, 1991, NACHO.

National Association for Healthcare Quality: *Risk management: NAHQ guide to quality management,* Skokie, Ill, 1993, NAHQ Press.

Padilla G, Grant M: Quality of life as a cancer nursing outcome variable. In Rinke L, editor: *Outcome Measures in Home Care* 1:169, 1987.

Phaneuf M: A nursing audit method, *Nurs Outlook* 5:42, 1965.

Pickett G, Hanlon J: *Public health administration and practice,* St Louis, 1990, Mosby.

Porter A: Assuring quality through staff nurse performance, *Nurs Clin North Am* 23(3):649, 1988.

Rapheal C: Response to: Quality assurance mechanisms in home care: measurement of quality and outcomes in home health care. In National League for Nursing: *Mechanisms of quality in long-term care: service and clinical outcomes* (Pub No 41-2382), New York, 1991, NLN.

Rinke L, Wilson A: Client oriented project objectives, *Caring* 7(1):25, 1988.

Rissner N: Development of an instrument to measure patient satisfaction with nurses and nursing care in primary care settings, *Nurs Res* 24(1):45, 1975.

Rutstein DD et al: Measuring the quality of medical care: a clinical method, *N Engl J Med* 294:582, 1976.

Schmele JA: Research and total quality. In Al-Assaf AF, Schmele JA, editors: *The textbook of total quality management,* Delray Beach, Fla, 1993, St Lucie Press.

Schmele J: A method for evaluating nursing practice in a community setting, *Qual Rev Bull* 11(4):115, 1985.

Smith BA: A TQM model for home care coordination and provider partnering, *Caring* 12(9):54, 1993.

Stevens-Barnum B, Kerfoot K: *The nurse as executive,* Gaithersburg, Md, 1995, Aspen.

Stevens B: *The nurse as executive,* Lincolnwood, Ill, 1985, Contemporary Publishing.

Stricklin MLV: Home care consumers speak out on quality, *Home Healthcare Nurse* 11(6):10, 1995.

Tindall BS, Stewart DW: Integration of total quality and quality assurance. In Al-Assaf AF, Schmele JA, editors: *The textbook of total quality in healthcare,* Delray Beach, Fla, 1993, St Lucie Press.

US Public Health Service: *Essentials of public health nursing practice and education consensus conference,* Washington, DC, 1984, US Government Printing Office.

Verhey M: Quality management in home care: models for today's practice, *Home Care Provider* 1(4):180, 1996.

Weiss M: The quality evolution in managed care organizations: shifting the focus to community health, *J Nurs Care Qual* 11(4):27, 1997.

Weitzman B: The quality of care: assessment and assurance. In Kovner A, editor: *Health care delivery in the United States,* New York, 1990, Springer.

Westra BL et al: Development of the home care client satisfaction instrument, *Public Health Nurs* 12:393, 1995.

Williams S, Torrens P, editors: *Introduction to health services,* New York, 1998, Delmar.

Young G: The privatization of quality assurance in health care. In Halverson PK, Kaluzny AD, McLaughlin CP: *Managed care and public health,* Gaithersburg, Md, 1998, Aspen.

CHAPTER 23

Group Approaches in Community Health

PEGGYE GUESS LASSITER

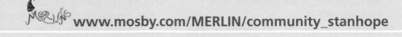

OBJECTIVES

After reading this chapter, the student should be able to do the following:

- Describe member interaction and group purpose as the major elements of a group.
- Analyze the effect of cohesion on group effectiveness.
- Identify the influence of group norms on group members.

- Explain the usefulness of groups in promoting individual health.
- Evaluate nursing behaviors that assist groups in promoting health for individuals.
- Identify the groups constituting a community and illustrate links between them.
- Describe the role of the nurse working with established groups toward community health goals.

KEY TERMS

cohesion	group culture	maintenance norms	selected membership
communication structure	group purpose	member interaction	groups
conflict	group structure	norms	task function
established groups	informal groups	reality norms	task norm
formal groups	leadership	role structure	
group	maintenance functions		*See Glossary for definitions*

CHAPTER OUTLINE

Group Concepts
    Group Definition
    Group Purpose
    Cohesion
    Norms
    Leadership
    Group Structure

Promoting the Health of Individuals Through Group Work
    Choosing Groups for Health Change
    Beginning Interactions
    Conflict
    Strategies for Change

Evaluation of Group Progress
Building Effective Work Teams
Community Groups and Their Contribution to Community Life
Working with Groups Toward Community Health Goals

www.mosby.com/MERLIN/community_stanhope

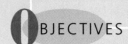

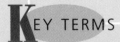

Working with groups is an important community nursing skill. Groups are an effective and powerful way to initiate and implement changes for individuals, families, organizations, and the community. People naturally form groups in the home setting; in turn, smaller groups in the community dramatically influence the community's health. Nurses who work with groups understand group concepts and group process. Groups form for various reasons. They may form for a clearly stated purpose or goal, or they may form naturally as individuals are attracted to each other by shared values, interests, activities, or personal characteristics.

Community groups represent the collective interests, needs, and values of individuals; they provide a link between the individual and the larger social system. Individual attitudes are developed in families and friendships. Throughout life, membership in other groups influences thoughts, choices, behaviors, and values as people socialize and interact. Through groups, people may express personal views and relate them to the views of others. Groups serve as communication networks and may be viewed as an organization of community parts.

Groups can bring about changes to improve the health and well-being of individuals and communities. Some individual changes for health are difficult or impossible to achieve without group support and encouragement.

All nurses have group experience. In daily practice, nurses routinely plan and use health-focused action with clients, other nurses, and other health care workers. Nurses often participate in groups in which they observe their own responses to members and leaders. Such study and experience aid nurses in applying group concepts in a variety of settings.

As discussed in Chapter 13, groups can be used to communicate health information in a cost-effective way to a number of clients who meet together, rather than repeating the information several times to individuals. During a time of decreasing resources, groups are an increasingly popular format for nursing intervention.

Understanding the community and assessing its health begin by identifying groups and their goals, member characteristics, and their place in the community structure. Through community groups, nurses help people identify priority health needs and capabilities and make valuable community changes.

GROUP CONCEPTS

The basic group concepts described in this section may be used in nursing practice to identify community groups and their contributions to community life and to assist groups work toward community and individual health goals.

Group Definition

A **group** is a collection of interacting individuals who have a common purpose or purposes. Each member influences and is in turn influenced by every other member to some extent. Key elements in this definition of group are **member interaction** and **group purpose.** The following examples illustrate member interaction and group purposes. Families are a unique and familiar example of community groups. Family purposes are numerous, including providing psychological support and socialization for their members. Usually, families share kinship bonds, living space, and economic resources. Interactions are diverse and frequent.

A second example is groups formed in response to particular community needs, problems, or opportunities. For example, in one community, residents banded together to form a neighborhood association to protect their health and welfare. This neighborhood of upper middle-class homes was located in an unincorporated area. For 3 years the residents were threatened with multiple environmental hazards, including a forest fire (fire hydrants had been overlooked in developing part of the area), establishment of a small airport near the homes, and construction of an interstate highway adjacent to the homes. To protect their interests, residents formed a neighborhood association and elected officers to represent their interests in a constructive manner.

Other groups in the community occur spontaneously because of mutual attraction between individuals and obvious and keenly felt personal needs. Young and single adults sharing similar desires for socialization and recreation may form loosely structured groups. Through parties and other social meetings, the young adults establish new ways of behaving and relating. They select partners, test ideas and attitudes, and establish their identity within a group of people with similar developmental needs. Their unstated purpose is to test and become familiar with adult roles.

A fourth example is health-promoting groups, which are formed as people meet in the community and health care settings and discover common challenges to their physical and emotional well-being. The purposes of health-promoting groups are to improve members' health and deal with specific threats to health. Chapters of Alcoholics Anonymous, Parents Without Partners, and La Leche League illustrate health-promoting groups. Members both give and receive personal support and participate in group problem solving and education. These groups may be one of two types: established groups or selected membership groups. Both types of groups are discussed later in this chapter.

> **NURSING TIP**
>
> *When the purpose for a group is clearly stated and agreed upon, the groups becomes increasingly attractive for members.*

How do purpose and interaction vary in these four examples? Some groups, such as the neighborhood association and La Leche League, have an obvious purpose that can be easily stated by members. For families, social groupings, and many spontaneously formed groups, the purposes are unstated. However, the purpose can be determined by studying their activities as a group over time. Purpose and member interaction are important components of all groups.

Group Purpose

When the need for a particular health change is identified and group work is selected as the most effective way to make it happen, a clear statement and presentation of the proposed group's purpose are essential. A clear purpose helps in establishing criteria for member selection.

A clear statement of purpose proved valuable in forming a new group in one city's housing development. The local department of social services had received numerous reports of child abuse and neglect. Routine home visits for well-child care documented high stress between parents and their offspring, and some parents requested guidance from the nurse in child discipline. The nurse proposed that a parent group address this community need. Nurses selected the following purpose for the group: dealing with kids for child and parent satisfaction. The purpose indicated both the process (to help parents deal with children) and the desired outcome (satisfaction for parents and children). As potential members were approached, this statement of purpose for the group helped the individuals decide whether they wanted to join.

When a group makes a public appeal for members and accepts everyone who wants to join, the membership is self-selected, based on the stated group purpose. In this type of recruitment, publicity must reach those in need of particular health changes. Prospective members often want to discuss the purpose with leaders or clarify questions concerning the purpose at the first group meeting. Their commitment to group health is partly based on individual goals and how well the group goal satisfies personal objectives.

Cohesion

Cohesion is the amount of attraction between individual members and between each member and the group. Individuals in a highly cohesive group identify themselves as a unit, work toward common goals, endure frustration for the sake of the group, and defend the group against outside criticism. Attraction increases when members feel accepted and liked by others, see similar qualities in one another, and share similar attitudes and values (Fig. 23-1). Members' traits that increase group cohesion and productivity include the following:
- Compatible personal and group goals
- Attraction to group goals
- Attraction to other selected members
- Appropriate mix of leading and following skills
- Good problem-solving skills.

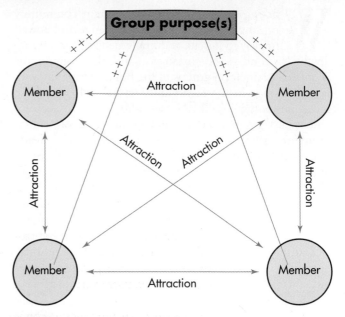

FIG. 23-1 Cohesion is the measure of attraction between members and member attraction to group purpose(s).

A **task function** is anything a member does that deliberately contributes to the group's purpose. Members with task-directed abilities become more attractive to the group. These traits include strong problem-solving skills, access to material resources, and skills in directing. Of equal importance are abilities to affirm and support individuals in the group. These functions are called **maintenance functions** because they help other members stay with the group and feel accepted. The ability to help people resolve conflicts and ensure social and environmental comfort is also a maintenance function. Both task and maintenance functions are necessary for group progress. Naturally, those members who supply such group requirements are attractive, and an abundance of such traits within the membership tends to increase group cohesion.

Other group members' traits may decrease cohesion and productivity. These include the following:
1. Conflicts between personal and group goals
2. Lack of interest in group goals and activities
3. Poor problem-solving and communication abilities
4. Lack of leadership skills
5. Disagreement about types of leadership
6. Aversion to other members
7. Behaviors and attributes that are poorly understood by others

See the Research Brief on group cohesion effects.

Usually, the more alike group members are, the stronger a group's attraction, whereas differences tend to decrease attractiveness. Members' perceptions of differences can create marked competition and jealousy. At the same time, personal differences can increase group cohesion if they support complementary functioning or provide contrast-

RESEARCH *Brief*

Two Canadian studies, one with university aerobics classes and a second with participants in private exercise clubs, report a significant relationship between member perception of group cohesion and individual attraction to group task and to social interaction. Adherence was measured by attendance in the exercise programs of more than 4 weeks.

In both studies, adherents were discriminated from drop-outs by measures of group cohesion perception. For university groups, measures of task cohesion were more discriminating, whereas for private fitness club groups, measures of social cohesion were more discriminating. Findings of the studies support the following views:

- Perceptions of cohesiveness operate in exercise groups.
- Perceptions of cohesiveness in exercise classes play an important role in the adherence behavior of individual participants.
- Task and social factors of cohesion vary by setting and moderate the cohesion-adherence relationship.
- A team-building approach may enhance cohesiveness and adherence among group participants in different programs for health behavior change.

Spink KS, Carson AV: Group cohesion effects in exercise class, *Small Group Res* 25(1): 26, 1994.

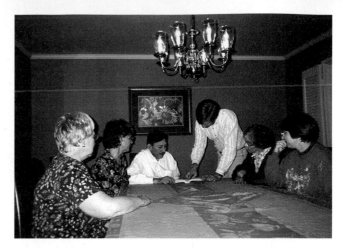

Cohesive community groups can support and help one another.

ing viewpoints necessary for decision making. This only reinforces the idea that cohesion factors are complex; many factors influence member attraction to each other and to the group's goal. In either case, group productivity and member satisfaction are positively affected by high group cohesion. Two examples illustrate factors that influence group cohesion.

A nurse initiated and provided beginning leadership for a group of clients who had been treated for burns. Ten residents, all from one town, had been discharged after 3 months in the local burn unit. The stated purpose for the group was to assist members in the difficult transition from hospital to home. Each individual had been treated for extensive burns in an intensive care treatment center; each had relied heavily on health workers for physical, social, and emotional rehabilitation; and each had faced the challenge of resuming work and family roles. Individuals shared some similar experiences and hopes for the future but varied in the amount of trauma and stress experienced. They also differed widely in psychological readiness for return to ordinary daily routines. One woman in the group was able to return quickly to her job as cashier in a large supermarket. The strength of her determination to overcome public reaction to her scars, coupled with an ability to "use the right words" and an empathy for others, distinguished her from others in the group. These differences

proved attractive to other members, inspiring them to work toward a return to their own roles in life. Other members saw her differences as attainable.

The cohesion for this group was provided by the members' attraction to the common purpose of returning to successful life patterns and managing relationships with others. Each member also believed that interaction with others with similar burn experiences could help them reach that goal. This example shows that certain member experiences, such as crises or traumas, may help individuals identify with each other and may increase member attraction.

Being different from the general population and similar to the other group members is, for some, a compelling force for membership in the group. Others are repelled by the group because they do not want to be identified by an aversive characteristic, such as disfigurement. Empathy for another's pain, learned only through mutual experience, may provide each individual with a required perspective for problem solving or affirming another's view. The nurse in this example helped members use common experiences and learn from their differences. The group was effective.

Differences created tension in one self-help group for victims of spouse abuse; in this group, nurses met a severe challenge stemming from the differences they presented as nonvictims. The nurses had been invited by professional staff to assist the group in its process toward the goal of "learning to manage: safety, health, and independence." Victim members of the group believed that the nurses could not truly understand the intensely personal and devastating injury each had experienced and told the nurses so. They isolated the nurses from membership but tolerated their presence. Attraction of the group diminished, and attendance at meetings fell. Discussion of superficial issues occupied group time as the victim members avoided topics of member safety and violence in general. Differences between the nurses and victims hampered group cohesion; the group was not effectively addressing its goal, and members felt isolated.

In response to this deterioration, the nurses encouraged all members to describe experiences seen as threatening to self-respect in their family and work roles. The nurses revealed some of their own struggles for responsible self-direction and control. Revealing their vulnerability made the nurses more attractive to the group. The members were able to accept the nurses, whom they now saw as more similar to themselves. They promptly refocused their efforts on the purpose of the group.

Group members supported one another to assert individual rights for safety, to locate employment, to make necessary living arrangements for independence from the abuser, and to identify needs for personal interactional changes. The clear purpose of maintaining member safety, combined with the new, broader common goal of asserting one's self-respect, contributed to successful group work.

Members' attraction to the group also depends on the nature of the group. Factors include the group programs, size, type of organization, and position in the community. When goals are perceived clearly by individuals and group activities are believed to be effective, attraction to the group is increased.

The concept of cohesion helps to explain group productivity. Some cohesion is necessary for people to remain with a group and accomplish the set goals. Attractiveness positively influences members' motivation and commitment to work on the group task. Cohesion for groups may be increased as members better understand the experiences of others and are able to identify common ideas and reactions to various issues. Nurses facilitate this process by pointing out similarities, contrasting supportive differences, or helping members redefine differences in ways that make those dissimilarities compatible.

Norms

Norms are standards that guide, control, and regulate individuals and communities. Group norms set the standards for group members' behaviors, attitudes, and perceptions. All groups have norms and mechanisms whereby conformity is accomplished (Sampson and Marthas, 1990). Group norms serve three functions:
1. Ensure movement toward the group's purpose or tasks
2. Maintain the group through various supports to members
3. Influence members' perceptions and interpretations of reality

Even though certain norms keep the group focused on its task, a certain amount of diversion is permitted as long as members respect central goals and feel committed to return to them. This commitment to return to the central goals is the **task norm;** its strength determines the group's keeping to its work.

Maintenance norms create group pressures to affirm members and maintain their comfort. Individuals in groups seem most productive and at ease when psychological and social well-being is nurtured. Maintenance behaviors include identifying the social and psychological tensions of members and taking steps to support those members at high-stress times. Health supportive maintenance norms may direct the group's attention to conditions such as temperature, space, and seating to ensure the physical comfort of the group during meeting times. This attention to arrangements may include meeting in places that are easily accessible and comfortable to the participants, providing refreshments, and scheduling meetings at convenient times.

WHAT DO YOU THINK? *Why might seniors finding haven at the senior center wish to avoid topics about conflict and declining health?*

A third and equally important function of group norms relates to members' perceptions of reality. Daily behavior is largely based on the way each aspect of life is understood. Through socialization, individuals learn how to gather information, assign meaning, and react to situations in a way that satisfies needs. Decision-making and action-taking processes are influenced by the meanings ascribed by a group's **reality norms.** Individuals look to others to reinforce or to challenge and correct their ideas of what is real. Groups serve to examine the life situations confronting individuals. As individuals gather information, attempt to understand that information, make decisions, and consider the facts and their implications, they can take responsible action, not only in relation to themselves and their group, but also for the community (see the Research Brief about a senior citizen center).

Group (task, maintenance, and reality) norms combine to form a **group culture.** Although working with a group does not mean dictating its norms, the nurse can support helpful rules, attitudes, and behaviors. Norms form when these rules, attitudes, and behaviors become part of the life of the group, independent of the nurse.

Figure 23-2 shows that reality norms influence members to see relevant situations in the same way as other members see them. They may feel strong normative pressures to support members who are considering change. Benne (1976), describing how small groups contribute to planned changes, points out that people develop their values by internalizing their particular small groups' norms, especially their families' norms. "Changes in value orientations of individuals may be accomplished by seeking and finding significant membership in a small group with norms that are different in some respects from the normative orientation these individuals bring to a group" (Benne, 1976, p. 76).

To illustrate, suppose a group of individuals with diabetes defines an uncontrollable diet as harmful; members

RESEARCH Brief

Engaging with others, working toward common goals, and belonging to a group were very strong values for seniors in a Philadelphia senior citizen center. At this center and surrounding neighborhood over a 3-year period, ethnographic data were collected through observation. Data showed the importance of finding social relationships with others in a safe place for seniors in an inner city neighborhood. The seniors negotiated dangerous streets, where violent assaults and drug dealing were common, to come together with familiar persons similar to themselves in age and in socioeconomic and ethnic backgrounds. They came for caring, friendly relationships and to fit into a social order within the haven of the senior center. Seniors in the study attempted to avoid conflict and discussing topics of declining health and social discrimination. They tried to maintain vitality and youth and upheld norms for propriety and trust. For those who live in dangerous public places, especially for the vulnerable elderly, finding a haven to avoid social isolation is a means of maintaining health.

Kaufmann KS: Center as haven: findings of an urban ethnography, *Nurs Res* 44(4):231, 1995

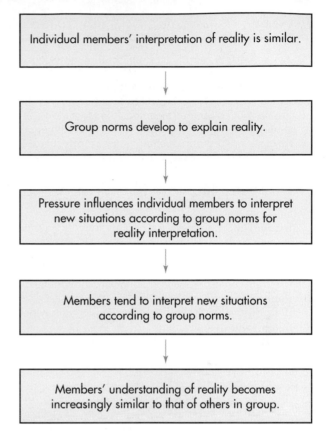

FIG. 23-2 Influence of group reality norms on individual members.

may try to influence one another to maintain diet control. The role of the nurse in this group is to provide accurate information about diet and the disease process, including cause and effect between food intake and disease. The nurse also continually displays a belief that health through diet control is attainable and desirable.

When members of any group have similar backgrounds, their scope of knowledge may be limited. For example, female members in a spouse abuse group may believe that men are exploitive and harmful based on common childhood and marriage experiences. Such a stereotypical view of men could be reinforced by similar perceptions in other members; this might lead to continuing anger, fear of interactions with men, and a hostile or helpless approach to family affairs. Nurses or group members who have known men in loving, helpful, and collaborative ways can describe their different and positive perceptions of men, thereby adding information and challenging beliefs. Thus the group functions to influence members' perceptions and interpretations of reality. The health and condition of the individual improves as members' perceptions of reality become based on a full range of data and as cause-and-effect factors are understood. Nurses bring an important perspective to groups in which similar backgrounds limit the understanding and interpretation of personal concerns.

Leadership

Leadership is a complex concept. It consists of behaviors that guide or direct members and determine and influence group action. Positive leadership defines or negotiates the group's purpose, selects and helps implement tasks that accomplish the purpose, maintains an environment that affirms and supports members, and balances efforts between task and maintenance. An effective leader attends to member communications and interactions as they unfold in the here-and-now. Attention to both spoken words and body language provides leaders and members continuous feedback, alerting members to changing group needs and encouraging them to take responsibility and pride in their own involvement.

Leadership is essential for effective groups. Leading may be concentrated in one or a few persons or may be shared by many. Generally, shared leadership increases productivity, cohesion, and satisfying interactions among members. A democratic approach to leading is most effective when there are many alternatives, much information is needed, and issues of values and ethics are involved (Sampson and Marthas, 1990).

After initiating or establishing a group, nurses may facilitate leadership within and among members, frequently relinquishing central control and encouraging members to determine the ultimate leadership pattern for their group. Of course, nurses differ widely in preference for leadership style. In some settings and circumstances, a single authority seems necessary (e.g., when members have limited skills

BOX 23-1 Examples of Leadership Behaviors

- *Advising.* Introducing direction based on knowledgeable opinion
- *Analyzing.* Reviewing what has occurred as encouragement to examine behavior and its meaning
- *Clarifying.* Checking out meanings of interaction and communication through questions and restatement
- *Confronting.* Presenting behavior and its effects to the individual and group to challenge existing perceptions
- *Evaluating.* Analyzing the effect or outcome of action or the worth of an idea according to some standard
- *Initiating.* Introducing topics, beginning work, or changing the focus of a group
- *Questioning.* Bringing about analysis of a view or views by questions that support examination
- *Reflecting behavior.* Giving feedback on how behavior appears to others
- *Reflecting feelings.* Naming the feelings that may be behind what is said or done
- *Suggesting.* Proposing or bringing an idea to a group
- *Summarizing.* Restating discussion or group action in brief form, highlighting important points
- *Supporting.* Giving the kind of emotionally comforting feedback that helps a person or group continue ongoing actions

or limited time or when groups claim discomfort with shared responsibility for leading).

Experiences with committees, work teams, and client groups promote self-confidence and increase appreciation of the leading capabilities of others. Practice teaches that getting selected tasks done is only one group outcome. A second, equally valuable result is watching members become more competent and able to share more responsibility. Shared leadership limits power seekers and supports group wholeness, flexibility, and freedom.

Leadership behaviors and definitions are listed in Box 23-1. Sources of leader influence are knowledge, ability, access to needed resources, personal attractiveness, status or position in the community or organization, and ability to control sanctions for others.

Leadership is typically described as patriarchal, paternal, or democratic; each of these styles has a particular effect on members' interaction, satisfaction, and productivity. Groups may reflect one or a combination of styles.

When one person has the final authority for group direction and movement, the leadership style is patriarchal or paternal. Patriarchal leadership may control members through rewards and threats, often keeping them in the dark about the goals and rationale behind prescribed actions. Paternal leadership wins the respect and dependence of its followers by parental-like devotion to members' needs. The leader controls group movement and progress through interpersonal power. Patriarchal and paternal styles of leadership are authoritarian. These styles are effective for groups such as a disaster team, in which the immediate task accomplishment or high productivity is the goal. However, group morale and cohesiveness are typically low under these styles of leadership, and members may fail to learn how to function independently. In addition, issues of authority and control may disrupt productivity if the group members challenge the power of the leader.

Paternal leadership was effective in the following situation. Mary Jones, a nurse, called her neighbors together to alert them to the threat of drug traffic in the neighborhood. The residents agreed with Mary that several recent drug-related arrests in the area signaled a need for community concern. No one knew what to do, but all believed that quick action was necessary. Mary had experience in organizing people, knew of local resources, and thought that information, education, and residents' collaboration with police could substantially control the local drug traffic problem. She organized the neighborhood group, assigned and monitored their tasks, and praised them as they made progress toward the goal of keeping the area free of drug sales.

Democratic leadership is cooperative in nature and promotes and supports members' involvement in all aspects of decision making and planning. Members influence each other as they explore goals, plan steps toward the goals, implement those steps, and evaluate progress.

A more common experience for nurses is illustrated in the following example. A committee of nurses for a small community health organization met weekly to improve nursing services. Tom initiated a revision of the written standards. Several members of the group felt threatened by Tom's idea. They feared that their daily work would change and that a resulting evaluation using new standards would find them inferior or necessitate that they alter familiar procedures. Jane supported updating the standards. She also recognized the necessity of continuing support and affirmation of each nurse's worth on the committee. While Tom pushed the committee toward revising the standards, she often interrupted to ask members to respond and to make suggestions, noting to the group the excellent contributions that were made. Sara provided a touch of humor whenever group tension became high. Amber provided a critical, questioning support to the decision-making process and encouraged the members to evaluate each step. In these and other ways, group members shared leadership tasks. Some served predominantly to push the group toward its objective, whereas others facilitated that movement by maintaining member involvement through support. For this group, the chairperson served as convener but did not dominate. The members were able to write and implement an audit for new nursing standards in a democratic leadership style.

> ### BOX 23-2 Examples of Group Role Behaviors
>
> - *Follower.* Seeks and accepts the authority or direction of others
> - *Gatekeeper.* Controls outsiders' access to the group
> - *Leader.* Guides and directs group activity
> - *Maintenance specialist.* Provides physical and psychological support for group members, thereby holding the group together
> - *Peacemaker.* Attempts to reconcile conflict between members or takes action in response to influences that disrupt the group process and threaten its existence
> - *Task specialist.* Focuses or directs movement toward the main work of the group

Group Structure

Structure describes the particular arrangement of group parts as they combine to make up the group as a whole. A **communication structure** identifies message pathways and member participation in sending and receiving messages. People who are active in receiving and sending messages and who serve as channels for messages are important in the structure. These "central" individuals influence the group because of their access to and interpretive control over communication flow. Communication and role structures are interrelated.

Role structure describes the expected behaviors of members in relation to each other as the group interacts. The role assumed by each member serves a purpose in the life of that group. Examples of roles are leader, follower, task specialist, maintenance specialist, evaluator, peacemaker, and gatekeeper (Box 23-2). Members' roles in the group may be described by their predominant actions. Identification of communication patterns helps to determine roles because people occupying particular roles characteristically use certain kinds of communication.

Group structure emerges from various member influences, including the members' understanding and support of the group purpose. Nurses assess the group structure as it relates to goal accomplishment. Many groups also consider their own structure, assess its usefulness in relation to member comfort and productivity, and then plan for a different division of tasks that is agreeable to the whole.

In the earlier example of nurses working on standards of nursing service, Tom served as task specialist, Jane as maintenance specialist, and Amber as evaluator. They consistently occupied particular roles and were expected by others to maintain their behavior to serve the group purposes.

A person occupying a gatekeeper's role controls outsiders' access to the group. Gatekeepers either facilitate or block communication between outsiders and group members. Identification of those in gatekeeper roles is crucial when established groups are used for community health.

The gatekeeper usually confronts the nurse after beginning contacts are attempted. An invitation to communicate further with group members is extended only after the nurse and gatekeeper determine mutual benefits and possible risks from continued contact between the nurse and the group.

PROMOTING THE HEALTH OF INDIVIDUALS THROUGH GROUP WORK

Health behavior is influenced greatly by the groups to which people belong. Individuals live within a social structure of significant others such as family members, friends, coworkers, and acquaintances. The patterns and directions of everyday activities are learned in a family, and these are later reinforced or challenged by new groups. These groups constitute the context in which values, beliefs, and attitudes are formed; individuals usually consider the responses of others in all types of decisions regarding personal welfare.

The following example illustrates the effects of a person's social network on health behavior. Mary Berton was worried about a lump she had recently discovered in her breast. She first asked her husband, Lew, to confirm its presence, which he did. He agreed that she should arrange for a diagnostic evaluation, and an appointment was arranged. Mary talked with Lew about the possible consequences of malignancy, and she noted Lew's concern for her safety. She was fearful of radical surgery and its effects on her relationship with Lew, but she did not discuss that with him. Mary telephoned two close friends from her workplace and asked them to meet her for coffee. Although they thought it was premature to fret about the lump being malignant, they discussed all they knew about treatment for breast cancer, including the trials, defeats, and successes of three mutual friends who had had surgery for breast cancer. Each of the friends had reacted differently to her own situation, and Mary's friends retold familiar details. The retelling seemed important to understanding the current situation and helping Mary sort out her feelings. The outcome for Mary of retelling was her improved understanding of the situation and her own response to it. She was assisted in facing the reality of risk, recognizing the need to follow through with diagnostic procedures, selecting able medical sources, and managing her emotional stress.

Mary's friends' and her husband's responses to her situation influenced her assessment, decision making, and subsequent behavior. The work done by Mary and her social network in response to her health need was important. It illustrates a common mechanism among individuals and the groups to which they belong. The groups described in this example are Mary's family group, which includes Mary and Lew, and Mary's friendship group, of which those who met for coffee are a subset.

Groups who will support an individual's health changes are unavailable to some people because of their social or emotional isolation. Isolated individuals may have low self-esteem, be mentally ill, or occupy positions of low status in their family or community. They may be disadvantaged, gifted, or deviant, or they may simply live in a rural area or be engaged in solitary work. These individuals benefit greatly through newly organized groups established for specific purposes.

Although social support is basic to health, the absence of negative social interactions is of equal importance to well-being. Groups sometimes oppose health. Friends who use addictive drugs are a clear example of such a group. It may be impossible for an individual to quit drug use while associating with such friends. To effect a lasting behavior change, an addicted individual needs support and new friends who do not abuse drugs. In such circumstances the individual must leave his or her group of associates, even if he or she must move from the neighborhood where they gather.

As nurses increase their knowledge of group concepts, develop skills in working with varied groups, and learn to employ the power in groups for individual changes, they will become available, visible, and sought for group work.

Choosing Groups for Health Change

Nurses frequently use groups to help individuals within a community after studying the overall needs of the community and its people. Such a study is based on client contacts, expressed concerns from various community spokespersons, health statistics for the area, available health resources, and the community's general well-being. These data point to the community's strengths and critical needs. Just as other nursing interventions are based on the assessment of needs and knowledge of effective treatment, group formation is determined by the assessment of priority community needs for individual health change.

At times nurses work with existing groups, and at other times they form new groups. Initiation of change and recruitment of a nurse may come not just from the nurse, but from individuals, the affected groups, or a related organization. A decision about whether to work in established groups or to begin new ones is based on the clients' needs, the purpose of existing groups, and the membership ties in existing groups.

Established groups

There are advantages to using **established groups** for individual health change. Membership ties already exist, and the structure already in place can be used. It is not necessary to find new members because compatible individuals already form a working group. Established groups usually have operating methods that have already proved successful; an approach for a new goal is built on this history. Members are aware of each other's strengths, limitations, and preferred styles of interaction. Members' comfort levels, stemming from their experience together, facilitate their focus on the new goal.

Established groups have a strong potential for influencing members. Ties between members have been enhanced through successful group endeavors. Their bonds are usually multidimensional because of the length of time they have spent together. Such rich ties support group change efforts for individuals' health.

Before deciding to work with particular established groups, the nurse must judge whether introducing a new focus is compatible with existing group purposes. In some cases, individual health goals will enhance existing group purposes, and the nurse is an important resource for bringing information for health, behavior, and group process.

How can the nurse enter existing groups and direct their attention to individual health needs? One nurse employed by an industrial firm noted the harmful effect of managerial stress on several individuals. They had elevated blood pressure, stomach pain, and emotional tension. The nurse learned that the employees with stress were all members of a jogging team that met weekly for conversation in addition to regular workouts. The other joggers readily accepted the offer to work together on individual stress management, recognizing that their fellow members were facing high-stress circumstances and the accompanying danger to health. High-level health had been a value shared by all team members, and although jogging was seen as an enjoyable and health-promoting activity, they had never talked about a shared purpose for improved health. In this circumstance the nurse saw a need for stress reduction, thought that the individuals at risk could achieve stress reduction if supported through a group process from valued friends, and proposed that a new purpose be added to the jogging team's activities.

Selected membership groups

In some situations, using existing groups is undesirable or impossible. The nurse then begins a selection process and brings a new group into existence. Nurses are familiar with group work in which members are selected because of their health. For instance, individuals with diabetes are brought together to consider diet management and physical care and to share in problem-solving remedies; community residents are brought together for social support and rehabilitation after treatment for mental illness; or isolated elderly persons are brought together for socialization and hot meals.

Members' attributes are an important consideration in composing a new group. Members are attracted to others from similar backgrounds, with similar experiences, and with common interests and abilities. Selecting members so that common ties or interests balance out dissimilar traits is therefore an important consideration.

Membership ties are influential; even in newly formed groups, people bring emotional and social ties from previous and parallel group memberships. People are influenced by the interaction in the newly formed group and by their alliance with other important groups to which they belong. Memory serves to keep the norms and role expectations from one group present in a person as he or she moves from one group to another. Individual behavior is then influenced not only by the membership, purpose, attraction, norms, leadership, and structure of the group, but also by those processes remembered from other valued group memberships. Consideration of the multiple influences on members helps to determine an appropriate grouping for each situation and its particular dimensions.

When the nurse is able to arrange it, the membership for **selected membership groups** should contain one or more individuals with expressive and problem-solving skills and others who are comfortable in supportive roles. Many people demonstrate abilities in task and maintenance functions, and others have undeveloped potential for such functions. Support and training for group effectiveness within the unit build cohesion. As members perform increasingly valuable functions for the group, they become more attracted to it and more attractive to others.

WHAT DO YOU THINK? *Will a group of similar individuals work together better than a group of dissimilar individuals? List similarities between individuals that increase their attraction to each other.*

The size of the group influences effectiveness; generally 8 to 12 people are considered a good number for group work focused on individual health changes. Groups of up to 25 members may be effective when their focus is on community needs, such as the group discussed previously who formed a neighborhood association. Large groups often divide and assign tasks to the smaller subgroups, with the original large groups meeting less frequently for reporting and evaluation.

Recruitment and selection of the most appropriate members for any group can be facilitated by setting member criteria. The criteria usually suggest a mixture of member traits, allowing for balance for the processes of decision making and growth.

Beginning Interactions

Once a group forms, work begins on the stated purpose. Early meetings require further clarification of both individual and group goals. Members with varying degrees of openness present themselves and their backgrounds. They begin to interact with each other by seeking and giving information about themselves and their circumstances and simultaneously demonstrating their capabilities in problem solving and group participation. The nurse assists by supporting ideas and feelings, inviting participation, giving information, seeking and providing clarification, and suggesting structure. Subsequent steps are then planned not only according to the nurse's skill and preference but also according to the group composition and the skills brought by members.

Nurses in the beginning groups should place the priority on helping members interact with a degree of satisfaction. This requires close attention to maintenance tasks of attending, eliciting information, clarifying, and recognizing contributions of members. Attending includes simple responses to people, such as listening carefully to their speech and noting their mood, dress, and informal conversation as they enter the meeting. Attending behavior communicates recognition and acceptance of the person and his or her presentations to the group.

A beginning format that focuses on whatever brought each member to the group provides recognition and helps the individual acknowledge similar and different perspectives. Members may be asked to describe what each hopes to accomplish in the group and what experiences each has previously had in groups. Member-to-member exchanges are encouraged; individuals are recognized and supported as they take on leadership functions.

Even in these beginning sessions, roles and a structure for the new group begin to take shape. Members try out familiar roles and test their individual abilities. Those approaches to member support, leadership, and decision making that are comfortable and productive become normative ways for the group to work. The nurse helps by creatively evaluating the appropriateness of style and productivity of roles. The work of the group is begun even as the goals for health change are examined carefully and are realistically accepted. During this early period, members' attractions to one another and to the group begin to develop. How to initiate and conduct group work in the community setting, using the example of addressing disease prevention through a community agency, is presented in the How To box.

HOW TO *Initiate and Conduct Group Work in the Community Setting*

Example: Group work to address disease prevention through a community agency
Purposes for group members:
1. *To increase awareness of common risks to health.*
2. *To improve health through problem solving.*
3. *To foster health promotion behaviors.*
   Planning and implementation steps:
1. *Seek consultation from community agency staff about priority health concerns and interests of the population which the agency serves.*
2. *Determine times when members can meet, when meetings may be held, and standards and procedures related to working within the agency.*
3. *Select a health-focused topic of interest. Develop a teaching plan; submit plan to designated agency contact for information and approval.*
4. *Market group teaching through a variety of strategies. Make the purpose, benefits to members, length of meeting, place, and time clear in the recruitment. Group members may volunteer, be referred, or be selected through leaders' interviews. Number should be limited to ten to fifteen per group.*
5. *Meet with group at designated times. Stick to teaching plan; submit needed revision to agency contact.*

Continued

6. *Record and evaluate process and outcome of group teaching. Keep a meeting journal.*
7. *Keep agency staff up-to-date on progress throughout the group meeting block of time.*
8. *Meet with agency staff for a summary report of the group project making recommendations for continued teaching and/or other health focused follow-up for members.*
9. *Write summary report.*

Conflict

Although **conflict** occurs normally in all human relations, people generally see conflict as the opposite of harmony, a state of interference to guard against. This view is an unfortunate one because the tensions of difference and potential conflict actually help groups work toward their purposes. Understanding common causes of conflict, conflict management approaches, and conflict resolution models is especially important in this decade of challenges to health and health care systems and increasingly violent expressions of community conflict.

Conflict arises whenever individuals perceive that their concerns have been or are about to be frustrated (Sitkin and Bies, 1993). Conflict signals that antagonistic points of view must be considered and that one must reexamine beliefs and assumptions underlying relationships. Some sources of concern for people are security, control of self and others, respect between parties, and access to limited resources; in groups, members express frustrations about trust, closeness and separation, and dependence and independence. These themes of interpersonal conflict operate to some extent in all interactions; they are not unique to groups. Within a group, because of members' regular and committed associations toward a common purpose, such issues are key; responding to them appropriately encourages personal growth and the facing of frustrations in the group.

Thomas (1992) differentiates between two potentially positive dimensions of response to conflict: assertiveness (attempting to satisfy one's own concerns) and cooperativeness (attempting to satisfy the concerns of others). Behaviors that reflect either assertiveness or cooperativeness and also hold the potential to satisfy the frustrated parties include confrontation, competition, compromise, reconciliation, and collaboration. Avoidance, forcing with power, capitulation, and excluding a member are conflict responses that fail to satisfy the concerns of frustrated parties.

Resolving conflict within groups depends on open communication among all parties, diffusion of negative feelings and perceptions, focusing on the issues, fair procedures, and a structured approach to process. Steps of conflict resolution in a group are listed in the following How To box, presenting a sequence of behaviors that support and encourage participants to acknowledge and resolve conflicts.

1. *Give a full description of concerns and divergent views.*
2. *Clarify assumptions on the conflict issue.*
3. *Specify underlying factors, including beliefs, individual desires, and expectations.*
4. *Identify the real issue or issues.*
5. *Jointly search for a collaborative resolution through a problem-solving approach.*
6. *Finalize resolution agreement (either a full agreement or a compromise in which each party is satisfied on important points).*

Conflict can be overwhelming, especially when members believe that the expression of controversy is unacceptable or unresolvable. Conflict suppressed over time tends to build up and finally explode out of proportion to the current frustration. A group that repeatedly avoids expressing conflict becomes fragile, unable to adapt to growth within the group, and helpless to face challenges. Conflict may be destructive if contentious parties fail to respect the rights and beliefs of others.

WHAT DO YOU THINK? *Collaboration is the most effective approach to conflict resolution.*

Conflict-acknowledging and problem-solving approaches that respect others and represent self-concerns are first learned in families and other small groups. These lessons teach people to embrace conflict as a natural occurrence that supports growth and change. Other individuals learn to avoid conflict or to disregard others in the promotion of self. Individuals may evaluate conflict management styles and refine skills in collaborative groups that support expression and resolution of conflict. Examination of conflict and resolution in supportive groups results in enhanced working relationships, stress reduction, and better coping.

Conflict management theory proposes that collaboration produces superior outcomes in conflict resolution; full participation of concerned parties, respecting the concerns of each and working toward full consensus, is useful. Some writers suggest that collaboration is impractical, requiring a long-term commitment to change at the individual, group, and institutional levels. Hindrances to collaboration are seen as competitive incentives, individuals having insufficient problem-solving skills, shortness of time, and lack of trust between parties (Thomas, 1992). Management strategies considered more practical than full collaboration include restructuring of settings, helping concerned parties reframe frustration as less stressful, and increasing competitive incentives. Although some circumstances undoubtedly warrant these less visionary responses to conflict, collaboration more completely resolves frustration and differences.

The following example illustrates conflict resolution through collaboration. A small church in a rural town initiated a project for youth recreation because fast driving around the countryside was the primary form of recreation for the teens. A roadway was frequently used as a speedway by the restless youth. The church enlisted the high-school principal and the nurse to work with a project group. All supported the development of a local youth center and worked energetically toward the goal.

After 2 months of steady cooperation, arguments began to erupt at meetings. Conflict about the supervision of the proposed center, the site for the physical plant, and numerous smaller concerns dominated planning time. The group consisted of active, aggressive members; four individuals dominated the discussions and resisted argument resolution. After several frustrating meetings, the nurse asked the group to explore each person's concerns and individual views on the direction and interaction of their work together. Welcoming an opportunity to relieve tension, members described their hopes, misgivings, and frustrated expectations related to the project. Each person elaborated on his or her assumptions about who would do what and how work should proceed. From this full discussion, the real issue became clear to all: disagreement related to members' functions in the project. The four dominant individuals expressed personal wishes to direct the planning and displayed aggravation when these attempts were thwarted. Other members described supportive and task functions but did not seek dominance in leadership functions. The open analysis of role structure made it clear to the members that arguments grew out of competition for directing roles rather than from true disagreements about the recreation project. Members searched for a collaborative resolution to the issue. They reached agreement to divide the work into several task areas to be led by separate area directors. Members expressed relief that basic agreement about the purpose remained intact, and they were able to modify their role expectations to accommodate all members. They joked together about being a collection of bosses and renewed their productive work.

Strategies for Change

Nurses can help goups to meet established health goals through their knowledge of health and health risks for individuals, groups, and communities. Skill in problem solving for change is key to accomplishing health goals.

Change, whether welcome or not, is disruptive to the client. Even though moving from a familiar way of being and interacting with others is uncomfortable (and resisted), all human systems do change over time because of development within the system and adaptation to outside stimuli. A change for one person in a group has effects on every other member. The disruption of growth, new opportunities, and threats to security trigger a fertile period for reevaluating, selecting new directions, improving, and maturing. Change creates opportunity for learning that is more than mastery of new information and identification of appropriate adjustment resources.

As discussed throughout this chapter, healthful change requires knowledge, practice of new skills, examination of attitudes and values about the change, and adjustment of roles in one's personal group or network. Helping people accomplish needed changes is ideally done within the small group context.

Basic teaching helps members understand the known association among environment, body response, wellness, and pathological states that are pertinent to desired changes. Together, group members focus on the reality of the problems and ways to understand them. A group reaches its full potential for effecting individual change when members work actively and directly through discussion and other approaches to problem solving. Such group work produces individual outcomes for healthful change.

Expectant-parent groups illustrate a type of community group in which teaching is an appropriate method. Participants need to understand facts concerning pregnancy, labor and delivery, self-care, infant care, parenting, and adjusting to change. They also need to practice the skills required in anticipated tasks and to explore their attitudes and emotional responses to the anticipated family changes. Specific learning activities in the group might include demonstration and practice for baby baths and situation enactment of family activity after the baby comes home. Such experiential learning activities, which require interaction among members and involve topics highly relevant to the goal of change, are useful.

One approach for improved health involves analyzing both supportive and interfering forces that affect movement toward the particular change proposed for improved health, including sources such as important individuals within the family, work, and community groups. These forces are identified during group meetings when group members learn from one another and the nurse how to help overcome interferences and promote facilitative factors.

DID YOU KNOW? *Most of the* Healthy People 2000 *priorities may be effectively addressed in health promotion and disease prevention groups. In groups, individuals may learn healthier behaviors, they may examine attitudes and values that are barriers to changing risk related behaviors, and they can gain support from others in changing from high-risk to healthy lifestyle choices. For example, groups may support physical activity and fitness, sound nutrition, and safe sexual practices. Through group support, individuals may conquer smoking, drug abuse, or abusive relationships. They may identify and reduce exposure to environmental hazards and promote safer physical settings for all. For a review of* Healthy People 2000 *priorities, see the* Healthy People 2000 Review *of the National Center for Health Studies (1995).*

With the support of a group, people often make needed changes for health that they are unable to accomplish on their own or with the help of just one individual. Skillful use of group methods can help the client analyze the problem, help sustain motivation for change, support the client during vulnerable periods, and provide quick interpersonal feedback for success and failure. The discomfort associated with change is greatly mitigated through the relationships with others in beneficial groups.

Evaluation of Group Progress

Evaluation of individual and group progress toward health goals is important. (A Guide for Evaluation of Group Effectiveness is shown in Appendix E.3). Action steps toward the goal are identified early in the planning stage. These small steps may be responses to learning objectives (listed action steps designed to support facilitative forces and deal with resistive forces), or they may reflect the group's problem-solving plan. These action steps and the indicators of achievement are discussed and written in a group record. Celebration is built into the group's evaluation system to help individuals recognize and reinforce each step toward the health goal. Celebration may include concrete rewards such as special foods and drinks, or it may be the personal expression of joy and member-to-member approval. Celebration for group accomplishments marks progress, rewards members, and motivates each person to continue.

Building Effective Work Teams

Team work is essential for nursing in all health care settings. In community work the team often includes workers from other health care disciplines and community residents. Team members' satisfaction and work team effectiveness depends on several key factors, including behavioral traits of team members, their expertise for producing the work product, the leader's and members' skill at team building, and their knowledge of group process. Group process concepts such as cohesion, purpose, task function, maintenance function, leadership, and conflict resolution guide nurses in effective team functioning.

: NURSING TIP

Help-group members recognize traits and interests that they have in common and how some differences in skills among individuals help to complement the main group purpose.

Effective teams begin with selection of members who have the specialized knowledge and skill to produce the desired product. Nurses who want effective teams become part of the hiring and personnel selection process. Training for skills can occur after hiring for some if most members come with relevant education and experience for the work. Good teams need a balance of member behavior types including those who are self-reliant and task oriented, those who are enthusiastic and people oriented, those that are loyal and close in interpersonal relationships, and those that are factual and evaluative in style (Clark, 1994). Once

a core team is selected, the leader and team members should evaluate the mix of member behavior types and target recruitment for persons exhibiting personal styles needed by the team.

Cohesiveness in the team, as for other groups, is increased by the connections among members. Cohesion and member attraction is built through regular contacts and interactions that strengthen team identity. For example, identity is enhanced by pointing out cooperation and success in meeting goals. Members are asked to share their experiences and expertise. They are encouraged to work together on parts of the work assignments. Negative approaches such as identifying a common enemy or competing with other teams should be used sparingly because they set up win-lose situations (Clark, 1994).

Often the issue that divides team coworkers is the purpose or perceived reason for conducting work. Purposes of team work must be clearly stated. If there is a disagreement about the guiding goal and secondary objectives, members will function at cross purposes and find tension in interaction. As in other groups, team leaders must clearly define and negotiate purposes, objectives, and member roles.

Work projects are divided into the tasks that must be undertaken. Responsibilities of each team member should relate directly to the purpose of the unit's function. The most important criteria in assigning and delegating responsibility are the ability of the team member to carry out the task and fairness of the assignment. As tasks are assigned or negotiated among members, differences in interpretation of work purpose will be identified. Sometimes the guiding purpose is rightfully redefined; more often team members refine their understanding of the work goal and adjust role expectations accordingly.

A successful team attends to the maintenance needs of members by observing for physical, social, and emotional comfort. Members' comfort includes satisfaction with progress toward work purpose and their perception of others' affirmation of their part in accomplishment of work. Support from others and the leader leads to strong team identification with the work unit. Clear leadership in work teams is essential as it is for all groups. Although leadership and decision making may be concentrated in one person or more equally shared among all, the pattern and legitimacy of leading should be firmly established and agreed upon by the team. Leading patterns may change over the life of the group; at each pattern change the team adjusts expectations on lines of direction, responsibility, and evaluation. Clear communication holds top priority among effective team members. Messages are quickly clarified when they seem vague or contradictory.

Differences expressed as conflicts are also addressed quickly by a successful team. Members are alert to the factors within and from outside that facilitate their performance. Barriers to accomplishing purpose are acknowledged, and the group makes decisions on how to deal with such barriers. Work is monitored by evaluating the group process in attaining purposes and by evaluating outcomes as they relate to the stated team purpose. From time to time the team reassesses its purposes, effectiveness in work together, and levels of member satisfaction.

Sometimes teams are ineffective because of the common and chronic problem of inadequate staffing. Effective nursing teams must confront the problem when it occurs. A strong team will point out inadequacies and its consequences on health care, public relations, and inability to expand programs. When administration does not respond, the team my go public with the problem to make the public and regulatory agencies aware of the issue. Such steps require strong team members who support one another and do not back off from pressure (Clark, 1994). Strong and effective teams are able to effect organizational change for improved health care.

COMMUNITY GROUPS AND THEIR CONTRIBUTION TO COMMUNITY LIFE

An understanding of group concepts provides a starting point for identifying community groups and how they function as components of the community. Because individuals develop, refine, and change their ideas within the context of the groups to which they belong, groups are vital to community well-being. Groups help identify community problems and are key in the management of interactions within the community and between the community and larger society.

Community groups may be informal (e.g., social networks, friendships, neighborhood groups) or formal (e.g., school, church, business groups). **Formal groups** have a defined membership and specific purpose. They may or may not have an official place in the community's organization. In **informal groups,** the ties between members are multiple, and the purposes are unwritten yet understood by members. Informal groups can be identified through interviews with key spokespersons. Information about when and why they gather is learned through interviews or observing gatherings to which the nurse is invited. Informal groups often are featured in the news when they are distinguished for community action or service. Formal groups usually can be identified in a variety of community media with meetings announced and business reported publicly. Membership lists, goals, and mission statements are usually written and available to interested persons.

Typically, residents willingly describe the informal and formal groups in their communities after they learn the nurse's purpose for entering and studying their community.

Group communication and member interactions across groups influence the overall harmony and free exchange in the community. Many communities encourage cooperation among groups through interagency councils, and many naturally occurring links among groups exist through family, friendships, and other relationships. Local extended-family groups, club relationships, work, and other acquaintance networks may influence the activities of seemingly separate groups in the larger community.

The nurse discerns goals for the community and for various groups through media reports, from community informants, and from local archives. These goals tell of resources and visions for change as perceived by the people living and working in the local community. Data may be organized according to the opinions and behaviors of the groups identified. Such information about community groups and assessment data are used with community representatives to plan desired interventions. Groups are both units of community analysis and vehicles for change.

Small groups can influence and change the larger social community of which they are a part. The social system depends on groups for governing, making policy, determining community needs, taking steps to alleviate those needs, and evaluating program outcomes. The small group is a mechanism for interrelatedness between community subsystems, certain subsystems and their counterparts in the larger social structure, and factions within subsystems. Change in the composition and function of strategic small groups may produce change for the wider social system that depends on small groups for direction and guidance (Benne, 1976).

WORKING WITH GROUPS TOWARD COMMUNITY HEALTH GOALS

Nurses use their understanding of group principles to work with community groups to make needed health changes. The groupings appropriate for this work include both established, community-sanctioned groups and groups for which nurses select members representing diverse community sectors.

Existing community groups formed for community-wide purposes such as elected executive groups, health-planning groups, better-business clubs, women's action groups, school boards, and neighborhood councils are excellent resources for community health assessment because part of their ongoing purpose is to determine and respond to community needs. In addition, they are already established as part of the community structure. When a group representing one community sector is selected for community health intervention, the total community structure is studied. Data about family ties, experiences with resource centers, and lifelong contacts to other sector groups are evaluated. Groups reflect existing community values, strengths, and normative forces.

How might nurses help established groups to work toward community goals? The same interventions recommended for groups formed for individual health change are beneficial to community health-focused groups. Such interventions include the following:
- Building cohesion through clarifying goals and individual attraction to groups
- Building member commitment and participation
- Keeping the group focused on the goal

- Maintaining members through recognition and encouragement
- Maintaining member self-esteem during conflict and confrontation
- Analyzing forces affecting movement toward the goal
- Evaluating progress

When nurses enter established groups, they need to assess the leadership, communications, and normative structures. This facilitates group planning, problem solving, intervention, and evaluation. The steps for community health changes parallel those of decision making and problem solving in other methodologies.

One nurse, Mrs. Winter, was asked to meet with a neighborhood council to help them study and "do something about" the number of homeless living on the streets. Mrs. Winter was known to residents from a local clinic, and they knew she also consulted at a shelter for the homeless in an adjacent community. When the council invited her, they stated that "our intent is to be part of the solution rather than part of the problem." Mrs. Winter accepted the invitation to visit. She learned that the neighborhood council had addressed concerns of the neighborhood for 20 years protecting zoning guidelines, setting up a recreational program for teens, organizing an after-school program for latch-key children, and generally representing the homeowners of the area. The neighborhood was composed of low-income families who took great pride in their homes. After meeting with the council and listening to their description of the situation, Mrs. Winter agreed to help and she joined the council.

As the first step in addressing the problem, the council conducted a comprehensive problem analysis on the homeless situation. All known causes and outcomes of homeless persons on the street were identified, and the relationships between each factor and the problem were documented from literature and from the local history. Mrs. Winter lent her expertise in health planning and her knowledge of the homeless and health risks. She suggested negotiation between the council and the local coalition for the homeless, recognizing that planning would be most relevant if homeless individuals participated. The council was cohesive and committed to the purpose, had developed working operations, and did not need help with group process. They made adjustments in their usual group operation to use the knowledge and health-planning skills of Mrs. Winter.

Interventions for the homeless included establishment of temporary shelters at homes on a rotating basis, provision of daily meals through the city council or churches, and joining the area coalition for the homeless. This example shows how an established, competent group addressed a new goal successfully by building on existing strengths in partnership with the nurse. Community groupings, because of their interactive roles, seem to be logical and natural ways for people who work together for community health change. As the decision-making and problem-solving capabilities of community groups are strengthened, the groups become more able representatives for the whole community. Nurses improve the community's health by working with groups toward that goal.

clinical application

Two case scenarios are listed in this Clinical Application. The first explores a situation when conflict within a group is ignored. The second presents effective group work.

Four nursing students in Chicago decided to work with parents at a drop-in family resource center as part of their undergraduate field experience. Parents at the center wanted to learn how to provide nutritious low-cost meals at home. The four students recruited three of the center parents who used the drop-in center's programs regularly. The group of students and parents decided to teach economical food planning and preparation through cooking and serving simple meals and explaining how to plan, select, and prepare them. The meals were planned for three consecutive Mondays at the center.

On the first scheduled Monday, everyone in the group worked together successfully. Eight parents attended the class, enjoyed a good economical meal, and were interested in learning how to plan and prepare it. At the close of the evening, three of the students announced that they would be unable to come the following Monday. The parents and remaining student on the teaching team felt abandoned and resentful but carried on planning for the next session. They did not talk about their resentment to the offending students even though they were left unfairly "holding the bag."

A. What went wrong in this example?

Two nurses worked with a group of 12 high school juniors as part of a health education course in an inner city neighborhood. The class met weekly in 90-minute sessions for 6 weeks. Faculty members for the class from the high school selected participants, shared their existing curriculum, and supported the purpose of the group. That purpose was to address issues that students identified as the most troublesome in their lives through group process.

As the class began, students asked for a review of sexually transmitted diseases, how to identify symptoms, and how to avoid risky behaviors. The leaders responded to requests with complete descriptions of prevention approaches and treatment. Discussion moved to teen relationships and communication. It became clear that verbal and physical violence were of even more importance to the teens than their concern about STDs.

The teens said that they were comfortable with the nurses who identified themselves as helpers who cared about students and their daily challenges. Students described how violence played an important part in everyday interactions. They described a culture in which a person must fight to be honorable, one in which fighting often occurred before irritations and provocations were carefully considered. One would fight first, in this culture, and ask questions later. Some felt safe in the neighborhood only when armed with a gun or knife. Both girls and boys were expected to fight for self and friends. The norm for fighting was clearly named. The teens were at risk for harm and death related to beliefs that problems are best solved through violent means.

With this knowledge the group members refocused on conflict resolution through other means than violence. The group lent support as members described recent deaths of friends from fierce acts. Because of their fears, students were willing to consider peaceful ways to solve problems in spite of the norms that were held about fighting. Students questioned their own attitudes and beliefs. They realized that friends greatly influenced how they thought they should behave. They began to change some of their ideas. Initiated by the class group, a nonviolent support club was established with the full sponsorship of the high school. It was one means to encourage continuing change for nonviolent resolution of conflict.

B. Can individuals develop healthy attitudes and change risk behaviors even when their peer culture values run counter to these changes?

Answers are in the back of the book.

KEY POINTS

- Working with groups is an important skill for nurses. Groups are an effective and powerful vehicle for initiating and implementing healthful changes.
- A group is a collection of interacting individuals with a common purpose. Each member influences and is influenced by other group members to varying degrees.
- Group cohesion is enhanced by commonly shared characteristics among members and diminished by differences among members.
- Cohesion is the measure of attraction between members and the group. Cohesion or the lack of it affects the group's function.
- Norms are standards that guide and regulate individuals and communities. These norms are unwritten and often unspoken and serve to ensure group movement to a goal, to maintain the group, and to influence group members' perceptions and interpretations of reality.

- Some diversity of member backgrounds is usually a positive influence on a group.
- Leadership is an important and complex group concept. Leadership is described as patriarchal, paternal, or democratic.
- Group structure emerges from various member influences, including members' understanding and support of the group purpose.
- Conflicts in groups may develop from competition for roles or member disagreement about the roles ascribed to them.
- Health behavior is greatly influenced by the groups to which people belong and for which they value membership.
- An understanding of group concepts provides a basis for identifying community groups and their goals, characteristics, and norms. Nurses use their understanding of group principles to work with community groups toward needed health changes.

critical thinking activities

1. Consider three groups of which you are a member. What is the stated purpose of each one? Are you aware of unstated but clearly understood purposes? What is the nature of member interaction in each group? How do purpose and interaction differ in the three groups?
2. Observe two working groups in session from the community, a health care agency, or a school. Notice the attractiveness of each group through the eyes of its members.
3. List actions that nurses may take to assist groups in various aspects of their work, such as member selection, purpose clarification, arrangements for comfort in participation, and group problem solving.
4. Observe a nurse working with a health promotion group. Does he or she function in the way you anticipated? What nursing behavior facilitated the group process? List the areas of skill and knowledge most likely to be expected of the nurse by the community residents' groups.
5. Identify areas of conflict in a work group to which you belong. Describe how one of these expressed or potential conflicts could be managed. Use the steps for conflict resolution outlined in the How To Resolve Conflicts in Groups feature presented in the chapter. What role would you take? Practice conflict-acknowledging and problem-solving behaviors in the next conflict you encounter.

Bibliography

Benne KD: The current state of planned changing in persons, groups, communities, and societies. In Bennis WG et al, editors: *The planning of change,* New York, 1976, Holt, Rinehart, & Winston.

Brown L: Normative conflict management theories: past, present and future, *J Organizational Behav* 13(3):303, 1992.

Clark CC: *The nurse as group leader,* ed 3, New York, 1994, Springer.

Kaufmann KS: Center as haven: findings of an urban ethnography, *Nurs Res* 44(4)231, 1995.

National Center for Health Statistics: *Healthy people 2000 review, 1994,* Hyattsville, Md, 1995, US Public Health Service.

Sampson EE, Marthas M: *Group process for the health professions,* ed 3, Albany, NY, 1990, Delmar.

Sitkin SB, Bies RJ: Social accounts in conflict situations: using explanations to manage conflict, *Hum Relations* 46(3):349, 1993.

Spink KS, Carson AV: Group cohesion effects in exercise class, *Small Group Res* 25(1):26, 1994.

Thomas KW: Conflict and conflict management: reflections and update, *J Organizational Behav* 13(3):265, 1992.

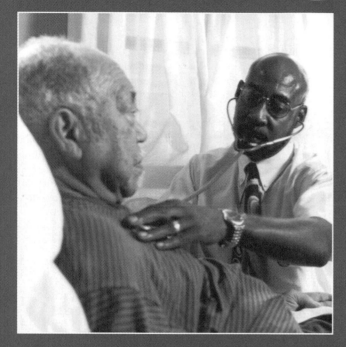

PART Five

Issues and Approaches in Family and Individual Health Care

The family is a major influence on the individual's concept of health and illness. It is within the family that a person's sense of self-esteem and personal competence is developed. The action taken by or for the person with a health problem depends on this sense of self-worth and the family's definition of illness. Environmental, social, cultural, and economic factors, as well as the resources of the community to meet health needs, influence the family's health risks and reaction to health. The goals of the nation for the Year 2000 name the individual as the primary target for changing the overall health of the nation, whereas the goals for the Year 2010 will focus more on the community as the primary target. Through family support the individual may develop the responsibility to participate in activities that will lead to a healthier lifestyle.

Major health problems of individuals can be identified and related to their developmental phase. This factor becomes evident when age-specific morbidity data are reviewed. Community health nurses can influence the actions and reactions to health of all individuals in the community from birth through senescence. The community health nurse can influence the health of children by introducing healthy parenting behaviors, risk factor appraisal, and age appropriate interventions.

Women and men are faced with many life changes and challenges, some of which are gender specific. Previous lifestyles and increases in stress from social, environmental, and economic constraints often result in risk for major health problems during adulthood.

The community health nurse's primary function with persons of all ages should be to promote quality and quantity of life. As the elderly segment of the population continues to grow, the health care delivery system and nurses must address and plan strategies to cope with increasing longevity, chronic health problems, and technological advances, as well as twenty-first century economic, social, and health issues.

Chapters 24 and 25 discuss family development, assessment, and health risks. Chapters 26 through 29 explore the major developmental tasks, health needs, risk factors, and issues for individuals from birth through senescence. Chapter 30 focuses attention on the needs of a special population, the physically compromised. Community health nursing interventions must be refined to assist this group in meeting their health care needs. Public health nurses assess the risk of age-related issues in populations, promote the development of programs and policies that will promote initiatives to enhance population health status, and ensure that such programs are available to address the health risks.

Family Development and Family Nursing Assessment

SHIRLEY M.H. HANSON & JOANNA ROWE KAAKINEN

OBJECTIVES

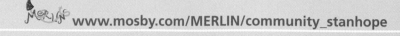
www.mosby.com/MERLIN/community_stanhope

After reading this chapter, the student should be able to do the following:

- Explain the importance of family nursing in the community setting.
- Describe family demographic trends.
- Predict how demographic changes affect health of families
- Define family, family nursing, family health, and healthy/nonhealthy families.
- Analyze changes in family function and structure.
- Name the three sources for emerging family nursing theories.
- Compare and contrast the four family social science theoretical frameworks
- Explain the various steps of the family nursing process.

- Summarize the importance of the assessment to the intervention outcomes.
- Compare and contrast the four ways to view family nursing.
- Compare and contrast two different models and approaches that can be used for family assessment and intervention.
- Explain one assessment model and approach in detail.
- Summarize how the genogram and ecomap can be used for family assessment.
- Describe the various barriers to family nursing.
- Share the implications for family policy.
- Explore issues of families in the future.

KEY TERMS

barriers to family nursing
cohabitation
dual-career marriages
dysfunctional families
ecomap
family

family demographics
family functions
family health
family nursing
family nursing assessment
family nursing diagnosis

family nursing process
family nursing prognosis
family nursing theory
family structure
Family Systems, Stressor,
 Strength Inventory (FS³I)

Friedman Family
 Assessment Model
functional families
genogram

See Glossary for definitions

CHAPTER OUTLINE

Family nursing is practiced in all settings. The trend in the delivery of health care has been to move health care to community settings; thus family nursing is very pertinent to public and community health nurses. **Family nursing** is a specialty area that has a strong theory base and is more than just "common sense" or viewing the family as the context for individual health care. Family nursing consists of nurses and families working together to ensure the success of the family and its members in adapting to responses of health and illness. The purpose of this chapter is to present a current overview of families and family nursing, theoretical frameworks, and strategies to assess and intervene with families in the community.

FAMILY NURSING IN THE COMMUNITY

As the basic social unit of society, within the family is where health care decisions are made. Families are responsible for providing or managing the care of family members. In the current health care system, families are significant members of health care teams since they are the everpresent force over the lifetime of care. In the current health care delivery system, families are more responsible than ever for assisting in the health care of ill family members. Health care occurs in families who are in the larger community and society.

Nurses are responsible for helping families promote their health, meet family health needs, and cope with health problems within the context of the existing family structure and community resources. To collaborate with families and develop useful interventions, nurses must be knowledgeable about family structures, functions, processes, and roles. In addition, nurses must be aware of and understand their own values and attitudes pertaining to their own families as well as being open to different family structures and cultures.

FAMILY DEMOGRAPHICS

Family demographics is the study of the structure of families and households and the events that alter the structure (Teachman, Polonko, and Scanizoni, 1987). Changes in the family and household structures can be explained by the events that alter status or position within the structure. The changes noted in family structure, values, and forms since 1950 are believed to stem from a weakening in the following American ideals: "a) to marry, b) to remain married, c) to have children, d) to restrict intimate relations to marriage, and e) to maintain separate roles for males and females" (Thornton, 1989, p. 873).

An important use of family demography by nurses is to forecast and predict stresses and developmental changes experienced by families and to identify possible solutions to family problems. It is important to note that families have changed over time in structure. The speed of the changes that occurred at the close of the twentieth century, its implications for family relationships, and the ability of

families to meet the changing needs of their members are all critical.

Marriage/Remarriage

Marriage remains a popular American ideal. At the present time, more than 90% of Americans marry during their lifetime. In 1995, 78% of the population over 18 years of age were married, which represents an increase from 61% in 1991 (US Census Bureau, 1992, 1995a). What is significant is not the number who get married but the fact that people are delaying marriage until they are older and the significantly higher divorce rate for young couples who marry before 24 years of age.

The median age for both genders at the time of first marriage has increased steadily since the beginning of the twentieth century. In 1995, the median age of first marriage for women was 24.5 years and 26.9 years for men (US Census Bureau, 1995b). Factors associated with age differences at the time of marriage are education, labor force participation, income, and premarital fertility. Education and job aspirations tend to influence the postponing of marriage, whereas dating or early heterosexual involvement and sexual experimentation may lead to early marriages for both males and females. Many early marriages are preceded by a premarital pregnancy, although willingness to have an abortion or to experience a premarital birth may delay marriage (NCHS, 1994).

A trend that is significant for the twentieth century is the increasing number of interracial marriages. McCray (1994) stresses the importance of multiculturalism and the changing dynamics of cultural diversity with the following predictions for 2010 (Davidson and Moore, 1996, p. 17).

- Hispanics will replace African-Americans as the nation's largest minority group.
- Caucasians will represent a bare majority.
- Asian Americans, who will remain the fastest growing minority, will triple their birthrate.
- The Native American population will double.
- The total U.S. population will increase 52% from 258 million to 392 million.

Interracial marriages, although infrequent, have steadily increased from 1.4% of all marriages in 1980 to 2.4% in 1995 (US Census Bureau, 1995b). One important point to consider from this statistic is the number of children born to interracial couples. Between 1970 to 1988 there were an estimated 1 to 2 million children born to interracial couples (O'Hare, 1992), indicating that families are becoming more diverse.

Until 1920 most of the people who remarried were widowed; now most people who remarry are divorced (Cherlin 1992). Most divorced people (75%) remarry, although it is more likely for men than for women (Eshlemann, 1997). It is estimated that three-fourths of the women who divorce in their forties will never remarry (Bumpasss, Sweet, and Martin, 1990). One-half of divorced and one-half of widowed men remarry within 2.2 years of the date that their last marriage ended. The median interval of remarriage for divorced women is 2.5 years and 4.6 years for widows (NCHS, 1994). There is greater diversity among couples who remarry than among those marrying for the first time. Men and women who remarry tend to differ in 1) age by a greater margin than men and women in their first marriages, 2) religious background, and 3) educational level (Davidson and Moore, 1996).

Dual-career marriages, or marriages where both partners work, have risen as more women enter the labor force. Family issues that are central to this demographic change are childcare, role overload (especially for women), and lack of shared household responsibilities among the couple. The cost of childcare places an additional financial burden on dual career families. It is estimated that the financial advantage over single earners drops by 68% when childcare is a family issue in dual-career marriages (Hanson and Ooms, 1991). The number of non-day shifts worked is higher in dual-career families so that one parent can be home with the children at all times, which has implications for family structures and functions.

Divorce

Each year in the United States, more than 2 million couples divorce, and more than 1 million children are affected by the divorce. Nearly 10 million children under 18 years of age lived with a biological parent and a stepparent or with two parents who were remarried. About 70% of these children lived with their biological mother and stepfather, and 30% lived with both natural parents (born after the mother remarried). Nearly one-half of all the children from divorced families have not seen one of their biological parents, usually the father, in the previous 5 years. Only one child in six whose parents were separated or divorced interacted with the outside biological parent about once a week (Furstenberg and Spannier, 1984).

Divorce has steadily increased since 1860 (Cherlin, 1992). The most concerning aspect of the increasing divorce rate was the rapid increase in the 1960s and 1970s, with its peak in 1979 (Levinson, 1995). High divorce rates have been related to the increase in the number of women in the work force and a more social acceptance of divorce. Davidson and Moore (1996) summarize the following effects on the divorced family:

- Adjustment depends on a supportive positive response from parents and married friends.
- Men experience more severe initial responses after divorce, but women have a longer recovery period.
- Divorce is more devastating and lasts longer for the children than the parents.
- Female children appear to be less vulnerable to divorce, but they actually internalize their stress as evidenced by lowered self-esteem and depression later.
- Many courts base custody on the best interests of the child.
- Both parents are responsible for child support.

In 1988 the median length of a marriage for divorcing couples was 7 years (NCHS, 1994). Approximately one-third of the divorces occurred before the fourth year of marriage. Some of the premarital factors associated with marital disruption are as follows (Davidson and Moore, 1996; Teachman, Polonko, and Scanzioni, 1987):

1. Less than a high school education
2. A premarital birth or premarital pregnancy
3. Marrying during the teen years or in the early twenties
4. Husband's frequent unemployment
5. Cohabitation

Postmarital factors leading to divorce are spousal behavior, inability to manage conflict, sexual incompatibility, and poor quality of marriage (Davidson and Moore, 1996).

The characteristics of people who divorce vary by age, race, religion, socioeconomic level, and the number of remarriages. Divorce rates are higher for people who get married in their early twenties or younger. The divorce rate for African-Americans is higher than for Caucasians. Protestants have a higher divorce rate than Catholics. People with a higher education and income level have lower divorce rates than less educated and lower income levels. Remarriages are less stable than first marriages since 75% of remarriages end in divorce (Hanson and Boyd, 1996a; Eshleman, 1997).

Cohabitation

One of the most dramatic changes in family structure has been **cohabitation,** or living together before marriage. Davidson and Moore (1996) suggest that the reasons for this shift are new sex norms and more tolerant parental attitudes regarding cohabitation. People who cohabitate are more likely to be over the age of 25, nonreligious, and less educated; to live in urban areas; and to never have been married (Davidson and Moore, 1996). Individuals who marry after they cohabitate have higher divorce rates than those who do not (Eshleman, 1997).

The number of unmarried couples living together rose from 523,000 in 1970 to 2.9 million in 1990 (US Census Bureau, 1991). In addition, the number of children of cohabiting couples rose from 53,000 in 1970 to 3.6 million in 1995 (US Census Bureau, 1995b).

WHAT DO YOU THINK? *Cohabitation before marriage does not increase or decrease the probability of divorce.*

Births

Birthrates in the United States vary by year and by state. In the United States there has been a trend to delay the birth of the first child and to have fewer children. There was an 884% increase in the number of children born to unmarried women between 1950 and 1992 (Eshleman, 1997), and this number continues to rise. In 1950 the ratio of children born to unmarried women was 1 in 205 births;

in 1970 it was 1 in 10 births; in 1980 it was 1 in 5 births; in 1990 it was 1 in 4 births; and in 1992 it rose to 1 in 3 births (Eshleman, 1997). The significant increase in births is not for mothers in the teenage years but for women 25 years of age or older.

Single-Parent Families

The number of children spending part of their childhood with one parent has resulted from the increased number of divorces and children being born outside of marriage (Bianchi, 1995). It is projected that approximately one-half to three-fourths of all children will spend some time living in a single-parent family (Levinson, 1995).

In 1990 there were over 7 million single-mother households and approximately 2 million single-father households (US Census Bureau, 1994b). It is predicted that by the age of 17, 80% of Caucasian children and 94% of African-American children born in 1980 will have spent at least some time in homes with only one parent (Espenshade, 1987). In 1995, 18.9 million children under 18 years of age lived with only one parent.

The number of single-parent households varies widely by ethnicity. In 1995, 21% of the children living with one parent were Caucasian, 68% were African-American, and 33% were Hispanic (US Census Bureau, 1995b). Although the most significant increase in the number of single-parent families involves single-mother households, between 1980 and 1995 the percentage of single-father households rose from 1.6% to 3.4% for Caucasians, from 2% to 4% for African-Americans, and 1.5% to 4% for Hispanics.

One of the major outcomes in single-mother households is the dramatic increase of children living in poverty (Bowen, Desimore, and McKay, 1995; Lino, 1995). About 46% of single-mother households fall below the poverty level (NCHS, 1994, 1995). In 1993 there were 12.3%, or 8.4 million families, living under the poverty level. The numbers vary by ethnicity; 9.4% of these families were Caucasian, 31.3% were African-American, and 27.3% were Hispanic.

Grandparent Households

The number of children who live with a grandparent has increased by 79% from 2.7 million in 1970 to 4 million in 1995. Of the 4 million, 57% live with a grandparent without either of their parents present in the household (US Census Bureau, 1995b). This change has altered the traditional supportive role of grandparenting to that of primary child rearing.

It is important for nurses to keep themselves informed and up-to-date regarding demographic trends pertaining to children and families. There are many family types other than those presented in this chapter, such as single households with no children, child-free couples, gay and lesbian couples, and intergenerational households.

Such knowledge is essential so that nurses can identify high-risk populations such as children living in poverty,

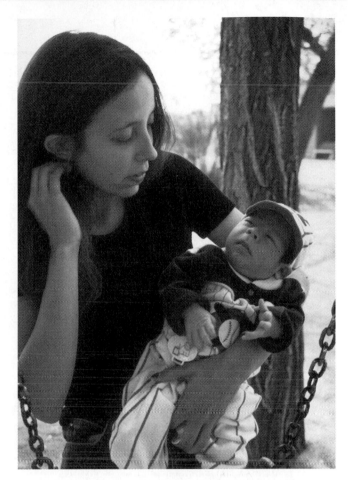

A young single mother with her infant son.

children of working mothers who care for themselves (latch key children), and elderly women living alone. Changing demographics have implications for planning health, developing community resources, and becoming politically active so that scarce funds and resources can be made available for health services needed by the growing, diverse population.

DEFINITION OF FAMILY

The definition of family is critical to the practice of nursing. Family has traditionally been defined using the legal concepts of relationships such as biologic/genetic blood ties, adoption, guardianship, or marriage. Since the 1980s a broader definition of family has been used that moved beyond the traditional blood, marriage, and legal constrictions.

Family refers to two or more individuals who depend on one another for emotional, physical, and/or financial support. The members of the family are self-defined (Hanson and Boyd, 1996a)

Nurses working with families should ask people who they consider to be their family and then include those members in health care planning. The family may range from traditional notions of the nuclear and extended fam-

Families in Canada

Karon Foster, Toronto Public Health and Ryerson Polytechnical University

TYPES OF FAMILIES

Most Canadians live in some type of family setting. There has been over a 45% increase in the number of families since 1971; in 1996 there were 7.8 million families (Statistics Canada, 1998). Married-couple families are still the most common form of family. In 1996, 73% of all families were married-couple families. The traditional nuclear family, composed of two parents and children, makes up 45% of all families. Empty nesters (parents whose children are grown and not living with the parents) are the fastest growing family type, and in 1996 37% of families were this type. There has been a 4% increase in the number of common-law families over a 10-year period. In 1996, common-law couples headed 12% of all families, for a total of over 2 million common-law families (Statistics Canada, 1998). Common-law families without children are the most frequent type of common-law relationship. The province of Quebec has the highest number of common-law families.

Single-parent families account for 15% of all families. In 1996, there were 1.1 million single-parent families, an increase of 33% since 1986 (Statistics Canada, 1998). Women head more than 80% of these single-parent families. This large percentage is due to changes in the divorce laws that have resulted in an increased number of divorces and the custody of children being awarded to mothers. Quebec has the highest number of single parents. Another change in single-parent families is the increasing number of single parents who have never been married. In 1996, the parent of 22% of single-parent families was never married (Statistics Canada, 1998). Approximately, 24% of families consist of only one person (Statistics Canada, 1998). Elderly women and men are the individuals most likely to live on their own. Another rising trend is the number of married couples remaining childless. In 1991, 41% of families without children were childless couples (Novara, 1993).

BIRTHRATES

Canadian families are also smaller than they were 20 years ago. Since 1991, the average number of persons per family has been 3.1. Most of the change in family size occurred before the mid-1980s. A declining birthrate has contributed to the smaller size of families. Married-couple families have the largest number of children per family as compared with common-law or single-parent families. Canada's birthrate has decreased considerably over the past 40 years, from a rate of over 25 births per 1000 people. In 1996, the birthrate was 12.5 births per 1000 people (Statistics Canada, 1997). Many women now marry at a later age and delay having children until they are older and established in their careers. In 1994, the average age of women having their first child was 28.2 years compared with 23 years in the 1960s (Almey, 1995; Statistics Canada, 1996). Birthrates have risen significantly for women over 30. Women 30 to 34 years of age now have higher birthrates than women 20 to 24 years of age.

MARRIAGE AND DIVORCE RATES

Changes in the marriage and divorce rates have influenced the structure of the Canadian family. Marriages still outnumber divorces, with 157,000 marriages and 71,000 divorces in 1996 (Statistics Canada, 1998). The marriage rate has stopped falling, and there was a slight increase in the number of marriages from 1987 to 1990. In 1996, the marriage rate was 5.3 marriages per 1000 people (Statistics Canada, 1997). Most first-time couples are delaying marriage until their late twenties. In 1995, the average age of brides was 27 years and for grooms was 29 years (Statistics Canada, 1998). The number of remarriages continues to increase; one-quarter of all marriages has a partner who has been previously married. In 1996, 1 in 5 people who remarried was a divorcee compared with 1 in 10 remarried people in 1974 (Statistics Canada, 1998). The divorce rate has dropped since 1985 when the divorce laws changed. The divorce rate in 1995 was 2.6 divorces per 1000 people (Statistics Canada, 1997). Divorce rates are highest among young adults in their late twenties.

LOW INCOME FAMILIES

A major concern for health professionals is the number of families who exist on low incomes. Statistics Canada defines low income as spending 55% or more of a total income on food, shelter, and clothing (1998). In 1995, 5.5 million Canadians had low incomes (Statistics Canada, 1998). Single mothers have the lowest incomes. Approximately 62% of female single-parent families have low incomes (Stephens et al, 1994). About 1 in 6 children under the age of 12 lives in a single-mother family (Stephens et al, 1994). Statistics Canada reports that 28.3% of families with children under the age of 18 are low income (1998). Childhood poverty in Canada has become a serious issue.

WORKING MOTHERS

Another trend that is changing family life is the increasing number of mothers who are employed outside of the home. In 1994, 77% of women with children between 7 and 17 years of age were employed while 63% of women with preschoolers were employed (Scott, 1996). Working mothers must juggle the responsibilities of family and a job, which affects family life. More than half of working mothers identify difficulties in managing family life. Affordable and accessible childcare is an issue that working families face.

GOVERNMENT BENEFITS FOR FAMILIES

In Canada, there are some benefits to assist families. Under the Employment Insurance Act, maternity and parental ben-

Families in Canada—cont'd

efits are available to eligible parents. Natural mothers can receive a maximum of 15 weeks of maternity benefits surrounding the birth of the baby. Natural and adoptive parents are eligible for a maximum of 10 weeks of parental leave from the child's birth or from the child's arrival in the home. Revenue Canada allows families with children to claim certain income tax deductions. Parents who are employed or who are enrolled in an educational program are allowed to claim childcare expenses as a deduction. For families with children under the age of 7, there is a child tax-benefit supplement.

In summary, the shape of Canadian families continues to change. Empty nesters, single-parent families, and common-law families continue to increase in number. Issues such as affordable and accessible childcare and poverty continue to affect some Canadian families.

Bibliography
Almey M: *Women in Canada: a statistical report*, ed 3, Ottawa, 1995, Statistics Canada.

Human Resources Development Canada: *Employment insurance: maternity, parental and sickness benefits*, Hull, 1998, Author.

Novara P: *A portrait of families in Canada: target groups project*, Ottawa, 1993, Statistics Canada, Housing, Family, and Social Statistics Division.

Scott K: *The progress of Canada's children 1996*, Toronto, 1996, Canadian Council on Social Development.

Statistics Canada: Social indicators, *Canadian Social Trends*, p 31, Winter 1997

Statistics Canada: *Morality: summary of causes 1994*, Ottawa, 1996, Statistics Canada, Health Statistics Division

Statistics Canada: Household and family life. In Wood J, editor: *Canada year book 1999*, Ottawa, 1998, Statistics Canada, Dissemination Division.

Stephens T et al: *Health and the Canadian family*, Ottawa, 1994, Minister of Supply and Services.

Canadian spelling is used.

---

ily to such "post-modern" family structures as single-parent, step, and same-gender families.

DID YOU KNOW? *Most nursing students tend to view family narrowly and based only on their own family of origin. Therefore it is important to study family nursing to broaden your understanding of other family variations.*

FAMILY FUNCTIONS

Throughout history, a number of functions have traditionally been performed by families (Hanson and Boyd, 1996a). Six of these **family functions** are summarized:

1. Families exist to achieve financial survival. Families are economic units to which all members contribute and from which all family members benefit.
2. Families exist to reproduce the species.
3. Families provide protection from hostile forces.
4. Passing along the culture, including religious faith, is an important function for families.
5. Families educate (socialize) their young.
6. Families confer status in society.

Historically, families that performed all of these six functions were considered healthy and good.

In contemporary times, the traditional functions of families have been modified and new functions have been added. For example, the financial function of families has changed so that family members do not need each other to stay financially healthy as much as they did in the past. Many married couples are electing to be child-free rather than to reproduce. Families depend on other agencies to provide safety such as law enforcement while other agencies are involved in the passing of the religious faith (e.g., churches or synagogues). Education (socialization function) is relegated to the schools. Family names are no longer needed to confer status.

Several new functions are more prominent in modern families. The relationship function has become important in contemporary families, thus putting a great deal of pressure on how people get along and their level of satisfaction. The health function has become more evident because it is the basis of a lifetime of physical and mental health or the lack thereof. The functions that served families have evolved and changed over time. Some have become more important and others less so.

FAMILY STRUCTURE

Family structure refers to the characteristics and demographics (gender, age, number) of individual members who make up family units. More specifically, the structure of a family defines the roles and the positions of family members (Box 24-1).

Family structures have changed over time. The great speed at which changes in family structure, values, and relationships are happening makes working with families at the beginning of the twenty-first century exciting and challenging. As social norms have become more tolerant of a range of choices in relation to managing one's life, there is no longer a general consensus that the traditional nuclear family model is the only "right" model. There is no "typical family" model. As a consequence, there is a growing number of family and household types. There is an increasing awareness that more variety exists within and among particular family structures. For example, the single-mother household may be represented by the un-married, teenage mother with an infant (unplanned pregnancy), the divorced mother with one or more children; or the career-oriented woman in her late thirties who elects to have a baby and remain single.

An individual may participate in a number of family life-course experiences over a lifetime (Fig. 24-1). For example, a child may spend the early, formative years in the family of origin (mother, father, sibling); experience some years in a single-parent family because of divorce; and participate in a stepfamily relationship when the single parent who has custody remarries. This same child as an adult may experience several additional family types.

As an adult, the individual may cohabitate while completing a desired education, marry and have a commuter-type marriage while developing a career, subsequently divorce, and become the custodial parent. The adult may eventually cohabitate with another partner and finally marry another partner who also has children. As this couple ages they will address issues of the aging family, and subsequently the woman will be an elderly single widow. Nurses will work with families representing various structures and living arrangements.

BOX 24-1 Family and Household Structures

MARRIED FAMILY
Traditional nuclear family
Dual-career family
  Spouses reside in same household
  Commuter marriage
Husband/father away from family
Stepfamily
  Stepmother family
  Stepfather family
Adoptive family
Foster family
Voluntary childlessness

SINGLE-PARENT FAMILY
Never married
  Voluntary singlehood (with children, biological or
  adopted)
  Involuntary singlehood (with children)

Formerly married
  Widow (with children)
  Divorced (with children)
    Custodial parent
    Joint custody of children
    Binuclear family

MULTIADULT HOUSEHOLD (WITH OR WITHOUT CHILDREN)
Cohabiting couple
Communes
Affiliated family
Extended family
New extended family
Home-sharing individuals
Same-sex partners
Fictive kin

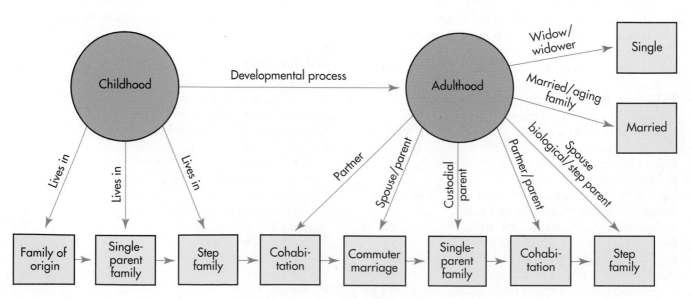

FIG. 24-1 Family career of an individual.

Prospects for families for the twenty-first century are numerous. New family structures that currently are experimental will emerge as everyday "natural" families (e.g., families in which the members are not related by blood or marriage, but who provide the services, caring, love, intimacy and interaction needed by all persons to experience a quality life).

FAMILY HEALTH

Despite the focus on **family health** within nursing, the meaning of family health lacks consensus and is not precise. The term *family health* is often used interchangeably with the concepts of family functioning, healthy families, or familial health. Hanson and Boyd (1996a) define family health as "a dynamic changing relative state of well-being which includes the biological, psychological, sociological, cultural, and spiritual factors of the family system."

This bio/psycho/socio/cultural/spiritual approach refers to individual members as well as the family unit as a whole. An individual's health (wellness and illness continuum) affects the entire family's functioning, and in turn the family's functioning affects the health of individuals. Thus assessment of family health involves simultaneous assessment of individual family members and the family system as a whole.

Healthy/Nonhealthy Families

Terms related to healthy versus nonhealthy families have varied in the literature. Health professionals have tended to classify clients and their families into two groups: "good families" and "bad families" in need of psychosocial evaluation and intervention (Satariano and Briggs, 1993). The term *family health* implies mental health rather than physical health. Recently the popular term for non-healthy families is **dysfunctional families,** also called noncompliant, resistant, or unmotivated, phrases that denote families who are not functioning well with each other or the world. The label "dysfunctional family" does not allow for family change and intervention and needs to be dropped from the nursing language. Families are neither all good nor all bad; therefore nurses need to view family behavior on a continuum of need for intervention when the family comes in contact with the health care system.

Family with strengths, or **functional families,** are terms often used to refer to healthy families. There has been research about healthy families, but it is clear that they all fall into the category of relational needs. This means that in healthy families, the basic survival needs are met. The traits ascribed to healthy families are based on attachment and are affectionate in nature (Carter and McGoldrick, 1988).

Curran (1983, 1985) reported traits of healthy families as well as family stressors that are useful for nurses to include in their assessment. Box 24-2 shows characteristics of families who are healthy and functioning well in society.

FOUR APPROACHES TO FAMILY NURSING

Central to the practice of family nursing is conceptualizing and approaching the family from four perspectives. All have legitimate implications for nursing assessment and intervention (Figs. 24-2 and 24-3). The approach that nurses use is determined by many factors, including the health care setting, family circumstances, and nurse resources.

1. *Family as the context,* or structure, has a traditional focus that places the individual first and the family second. The family as context serves as either a resource or a stressor to individual health and illness. A nurse using this focus might ask an individual client, "How has your diagnosis of insulin-dependent diabetes affected your family?" or "Will your need for medication at night be a problem for your family?"

2. *Family as the client.* The family is first and individuals are second. The family is seen as the sum of individual family members. The focus is concentrated on each individual as he or she affects the family as a whole. From this perspective, a nurse might say to a family member who has just become ill, "Tell me about what has been going on with your own health and how you perceive each family member responding to your mother's recent diagnosis of liver cancer."

3. *Family as a system.* The focus is on the family as client, and the family is viewed as an interactional system in which the whole is more than the sum of its parts. This approach simultaneously focuses on individual members and the family as a whole at the same time. The interactions between family members become the target for nursing interventions (e.g., the direct interactions between the parents, or the indirect interaction between the parents and the child). The systems approach to family always implies that when something

---

BOX 24-2 Characteristics of Healthy Families

1. The family tends to communicate well and listen to all members.
2. The family affirms and supports all of its members.
3. Teaching respect for others is valued by the family.
4. The family members have a sense of trust.
5. The family plays together, and humor is present.
6. All members interact with each other, and a balance in the interactions is noted among the members.
7. The family shares leisure time together.
8. The family has a shared sense of responsibility.
9. The family has traditions and rituals.
10. The family shares a religious core.
11. Privacy of members is honored by the family.
12. The family opens its boundaries to admit and seek help with problems.

Adapted from Curran D: *Traits of a healthy family,* Minneapolis, 1983, Winston Press (Harper & Row).

Family As Context

Individual as foreground
Family as background

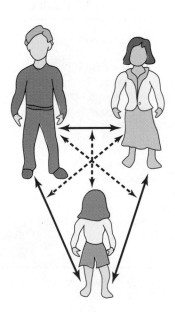

Family As Client

Family as foreground
Individual as background

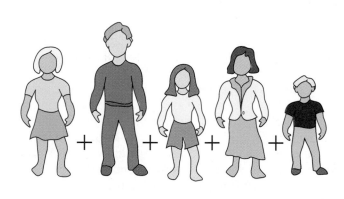

Family As System

Interactional family

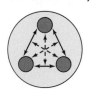

Family As Component
of Society

Legal

Education

Family

Health

Religion

Social

Financial

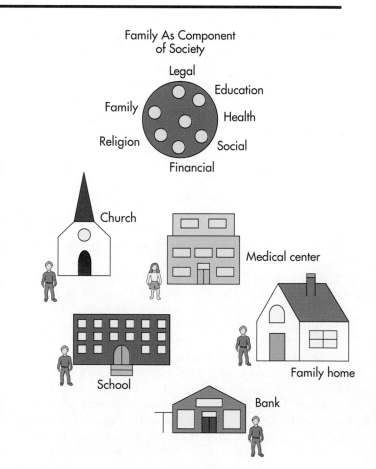

Church

Medical center

School

Family home

Bank

FIG. 24-2 Approaches to family nursing. (From Hanson SMH, Boyd ST: *Family health care nursing: theory, practice, and research,* Philadelphia, 1996, FA Davis.)

happens to one family member, the other members of the family system are affected. Questions nurses ask when approaching a family as system are, "What has changed between you and your spouse since your child's head injury?" or "How do you feel about the fact that your son's long-term rehabilitation will affect the ways in which the members of your family is functioning and getting along with one another?"

WHAT DO YOU THINK? *All families have secrets. Some information gleaned from families may be overexaggerated, minimized, or withheld.*

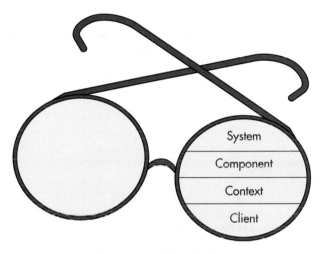

FIG. 24-3 Four views of family through a lens.

4. *Family as a component of society.* The family is seen as one of many institutions in society, along with health, education, religious, or financial institutions. The family is a basic or primary unit of society, as are all the other units, and they are all a part of the larger system of society. The family as a whole interacts with other institutions to receive, exchange, or give services and communicate. Nurses have drawn many of their tenets from this perspective as they focus on the interface between families and community agencies.

THEORETICAL FRAMEWORKS FOR FAMILY NURSING

Family nursing theory is an evolving synthesis of the scholarship from three different traditions: family social science, family therapy, and nursing (Fig. 24-4). In this chapter, only family social science theories are reviewed in depth. A more in-depth presentation of family theory development can be found elsewhere (Hanson, Kaakinen, and Friedman, 1998).

The first and oldest tradition that contributed to the model of family nursing theory came from the *family social science tradition.* These theories were developed from various family social science disciplines (largely sociology and psychology) (Jones and Dimond, 1982). Four conceptual approaches have dominated the field of marriage and family within the family social science tradition: structural-functional theory, systems theory, developmental theory, and interactionist theory (Klein and White, 1996; Nye and Berardo, 1981). These approaches are constantly evolving, which makes the knowledge base more user friendly.

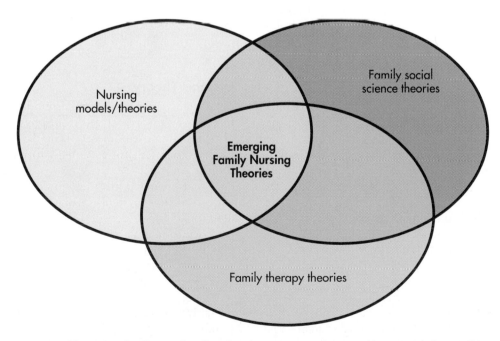

FIG. 24-4 Emerging family nursing theories. (From Hanson SMH, Kaakinen JR, Friedman MM: In Friedman MM: *Family nursing: research, theory, and practice,* Stamford, Conn, 1998, Appleton & Lange.)

The second tradition that followed the family social science theories was in the field of *marriage and family therapy*. Early theorists drew from existing social science theories to understand explanations of family events and to develop approaches for family treatment. Over time, family therapy theories have been classified in a variety of ways by various theorists (psychoanalytic, experiential, communication, strategic, behavioral, cognitive, structural, narrative, and solution-focused approaches) (Becvar and Becvar, 1996; Gladding, 1995).

The third and most recent tradition comes from the practice of nursing itself. The development of *nursing models and theories* over the last three decades profoundly influenced the practice of nursing. This nursing theories tradition influenced nursing theorists such as Nightingale, Peplau, Levine, Johnson, Neuman, Roy, King, Rogers, Orem, and Watson. The current state of the art of family nursing theory is a blend of the family social theories, family therapy theories, and nursing theories. Nurses are challenged to view current diverse families through this multi-conceptual lens and develop creative unique solutions to family needs.

The following is a summary of the four major family social theories and what they have contributed to family nursing theory.

Structure-Functional Theory

The structure-functional framework from a social science perspective defines families as social systems. Families are examined in terms of their relationship with other major social structures (institutions) such as health care, religion, education, government, and/or the economy. This perspective looks at the arrangement of members within the family, relationships between the members, and the roles and relationships of the members to the whole family (Artinian, 1994; Friedman, 1998). The primary focus is to determine how family patterns are related to other institutions in society and to consider the family in the overall structure of society. Emphasis is placed on the basic functions of families. With family structure as the focus, the major concern is how well the structure performs its functions. Individuals or family units receive little attention in this approach. Families are studied from the status-role perspective. Family theorists use this approach to understand the social or family system and its relationship to the overall social system. This approach describes the family as open to outside influences, yet at the same time the family maintains its boundaries. The family is seen as passive on adapting to the system rather than an agent of change. The framework emphasizes a static society structure and neglects change as a structural dynamic. Assumptions of this perspective include the following:

- A family is a social system with functional requirements.
- A family is a small group that has basic features common to all small groups.

- Social systems, such as families, accomplish functions that serve the individuals in addition to those that serve society.
- Individuals act within a set of internal norms and values that are learned primarily in the family through socialization.

Nurses refer to this model when they talk about the structure, forms, or type of family such as single-parent families, step-families, nuclear families, or extended families. Other structural dimensions of families include role structure, value system, communication patterns, power structure, or support networks (Friedman, 1998). This perspective is a useful framework for assessing families and health. Illness of a family member results in alteration of the family structure and function. If a single mother is ill, she cannot carry out her various roles, so grandparents or siblings may have to assume child-care responsibilities. Family power structures and communication patterns are affected with an illness of parents. The family assessment includes determining if changes resulting from the illness influence the family's ability to carry out its functions. Sample assessment questions are "How did the death alter the family structure?" and "What family roles were changed with the onset of the chronic illness?" Interventions become necessary when a change in the family structure alters the family's ability to function. Examples of interventions using this model include helping families use existing support structures and helping families modify the way they are organized so that role responsibilities can be distributed.

The major strength of the structure-functional theory to family nursing is its comprehensive approach that views families in the broader community in which they live. The major weakness of this approach is the static picture of family, which does not allow for dynamic change over time.

Systems Theory

The systems approach to understanding families was influenced by theory derived from physics and biology. A system is composed of a set of interacting elements; each system can be identified and is distinct from the environment in which it exists. An open system exchanges energy and matter with the environment (negentropy), whereas a closed system is isolated from its environment (entropy). Systems depend on both positive and negative feedback to maintain a steady state (homeostasis). Seeking therapy when the marital relationship is strained is an example of using negative feedback to maintain a steady state. Assumptions of the systems perspective include the following:

- Family systems are greater than and different from the sum of their parts.
- There are many hierarchies within family systems and logical relationships between subsystems (e.g., mother-child, family-community).

- There are boundaries in the family system that can be open, closed, or random.
- Family systems increase in complexity over time, evolving to allow greater adaptability, tolerance to change, and growth by differentiation.
- Family systems change constantly in response to stresses and strains from within and from outside environments. There are structural similarities in different family systems (isomorphism).
- Change in one part of family systems affects the total system.
- Causality is modified by feedback; therefore causality never exists in the real world.
- Family systems patterns are circular rather than linear; change must be directed toward the cycle.
- Family systems are an organized whole; therefore individuals within the family are interdependent.
- Family systems have homeostasis features to maintain stable patterns that can be adaptive or maladaptive.

The family system perspective encourages nurses to view clients as participating members of a family. Nurses using this perspective determine the effects of illness or injury upon the entire family system. Emphasis is on the whole rather than on individuals. Nursing assessment of family systems includes assessment of individual members, subsystems, boundaries, openness, inputs and outputs, family interactions, family processing, and adaptation or change abilities. Assessment questions include "Who is in the family system?" and "How has one member's critical illness affected the entire family system?" Interventions need to assist individual, subsystem, and whole family functioning. Some nursing strategies using this approach include establishing a mechanism for providing families with information about their family members on a regular basis and discussing ways to provide for a normal family life for family members after someone has become ill.

The major strength of the systems framework is that it views families from both a subsystem and suprasystem approach. That is, it views the interactions within and between family subsystems as well as the interaction between families and the larger supersystems, such as community, world, and universe. The major weakness of the systems framework is that the focus is on the interaction of the family with other systems rather than on the individual, which is sometimes more important.

Developmental Theory

Individual developmental theory has been core to nursing of people across the life span. This approach looks at the family system over time through different phases that can be predicted and known family transitions based on norms.

Evelyn Duvall (1977) in her classic book, *Family Development*, presents a synthesis of developmental concepts. In essence, she takes the principles of individual develop-

ment and applies them to the family as a unit. Her stages of family development are based on the age of the eldest child. Overall family tasks are identified that need to be accomplished for each stage of family development. Developmental concepts include moving to a different level of functioning, implying progress in a single direction. Family disequilibrium and conflicts are described as occurring during transition periods from one stage to another. The family has a predictable natural history designated by stages, beginning with the simple husband-wife pair. The group becomes more complex with the addition of each new child over time. The group again becomes simple and less complex as the younger generation leaves home. Finally the group comes full circle to the original husband-wife pair. At each family life-cycle stage, there are developmental needs of the family and tasks that must be performed. These concepts are further refined by Duvall and Miller (1985).

Developmental theory is an attempt to integrate the small scale (interactive framework) and large scale (structural framework) analyses of the other two approaches while viewing the family as an open system in relation to structures in society (Jones and Dimond, 1982). Developmental theory explains and predicts the changes that occur to humans or groups over time. Achievement of family developmental tasks helps individual members to accomplish their tasks. This framework assists nurses in anticipating clinical problems in families and in identifying family strengths. The framework serves as a guide in assessing the family's developmental stage, the extent to which families are fulfilling the tasks associated with their respective stage, the family's developmental history, and the availability of resources essential for performing developmental tasks.

In conducting an assessment of families using the developmental model, there are several questions that can be asked: Where does this family place on the continuum of the family life cycle? What are the developmental tasks that are not being accomplished? Typical kinds of nursing intervention strategies using this perspective help families understand individual and family growth and development stages and help families deal with the normal transition periods between developmental periods (e.g., tasks of the school-age family member versus tasks of the adolescent family member).

Family nurses must recognize that in every family there are both individual and family developmental tasks that need to be accomplished for every stage of the individual/family life cycle that are unique to that particular group.

Other basic assumptions of systems theory include:
- Families change and develop in different ways because of internal and environmental stimulation.
- Developmental tasks are goals worked toward rather than specific jobs completed at once.
- Each family is unique in its composition and complexity of age-role expectations and positions.

- Individuals and families are a function of their history as well as the current social structure.
- Families have enough in common despite the way they develop over the family life span.
- Families may arrive at similar developmental levels through different processes.

The major strength of this approach is that it provides a basis for forecasting what a family will be experiencing at any period in the family life cycle (e.g., role transitions and family structure changes). The major weakness is the fact that the model was developed at a time when the traditional nuclear family was emphasized. However, Friedman (1998) explores family life-cycle or career stages in divorced families, stepparent families, and domestic-partner relationships. The perfect progress of families from marriage through death is not a current reality. What happens to the stages of the individual/family life cycle when there is a divorce, death, adoption, and the other multiple forms that we now call family?

Interactionist Theory

Interactionist theory views families as units of interacting personalities and examines the symbolic communications by which family members relate to one another. Within the family, each member occupies a positions to which a number of roles are assigned. Members define their role expectations in each situation through their perceptions of the role demands. Members judge their own behavior by assessing and interpreting the actions of others toward them. The responses of others in the family serve to challenge or reinforce family members' perceptions of the norms of role expectations (Bomar, 1996). Central to the interaction approach is the process of role taking. Every role exists in relation to some other role, and interaction represents a dynamic process of testing perceptions about one another's roles (Stanhope, 1996). The ability to predict other family members' expectations for one's role enables each member to have some knowledge of how to react in the role and indicates how other members will react to performing the role.

George Herbert Mead (1934) is credited with synthesizing previous work to bring together mind, self, and society as major concepts in the school known as "symbolic interactionism." He describes the human mind's capacity to organize and control responses by selecting one option over another (reflection) and to derive meaning from symbols and gestures in interacting with others. The self emerges from these interactions with others and is a symbolic object in the mind's eye, apart from the body or from other objects or persons. A person derives the symbolic self from his or her social group and setting. Changes made in the social order mandate earlier changes in self. For example, family violence cannot be abolished until the "selves" making up society see these practices as criminal acts that violate individuals and families.

Some of the major assumptions of this framework are as follows:
- Complex sets of symbols having common meanings are acquired through living in a symbolic environment.
- Individuals distinguish, evaluate, and assign meaning to symbols.
- Behavior is influenced by meanings of symbols or ideas rather than by instincts, needs, or drives; therefore the meaning an individual assigns to symbols is important to understanding behavior.
- The self continues to change and evolve over time through introspection caused by experience and activity.
- The evolving self has several dimensions: the physical body and characteristics and a complex social self. The "me" is a conventional, habitual self that consists of learned, repetitious responses. The "I" is spontaneous to the individual.
- Individuals are actors as well as reactors; they select and interpret the environment to which they respond.
- Individuals are born into a dynamic society.
- The nature of the infant is determined by the environment and responses to the infant rather than by a predisposition to act in a certain way (this is now being challenged).
- Individuals learn from the culture and become the society.
- Individuals' behavior is a product of their history, which is continually being modified by new information.

Assessment of families using the interaction framework emphasizes interaction between and among family members and family communication patterns about health and illness behaviors appropriate for different roles. Nurses intervene by strategies focused on the following (Bomar, 1996):
1. Effectiveness of communications among members
2. Ability to establish communication between nurses and families
3. Clear and concise messages between members
4. Similarities between verbal and nonverbal communication patterns
5. Directions of the interaction

Nurses can center their attention on how family members interact with one another, so this approach is useful in explaining family communication, roles, decision making, and problem solving (Friedman, 1998).

The major strength of this approach is the focus on internal processes within families such as roles, conflict, status, communication, responses to stress, decision-making, and socialization. Processes rather than end products of social interactions are the major focus; thus this framework has been used by many nurse scholars. The major weakness is the broadness and lack of agreement about concepts and assumptions of the theory, which has made it difficult to refine. Interactionalists consider families to be comparatively closed units with little relation to the outside society.

Conclusions Regarding Family Nursing Theory

Currently there is no singular theory or conceptual framework from nursing, family social science, or family therapy that fully describes the relationships and dynamics for family life and family nursing theory. Thus an integrated approach is necessary for the theory, practice, research, and education of family nursing. One theoretical perspective does not give nurses a sufficiently broad knowledge upon which to assess and intervene with families. Therefore nurses must draw upon multiple theories to work effectively with families.

Of the three categories of theory, the family social science theories are the most well developed and informative with respect to how families function, the environment-family interchange, interactions within the family, how the family changes over time, and the family's reaction to health and illness. One striking limitation in using family social science theories as a basis for assessment and intervention in family nursing is that their clinical application is limited, although recent work has made some strides in this direction (Berkey and Hanson, 1991; Danielson, Hamel-Bissell, and Winstead-Fry, 1993; Friedman, 1998; Hanson and Boyd, 1996a; Vaughan-Cole et al,

1998; Wright and Leahey, 1995). Family therapy theories are the next most developed theories and come from a professional/practice background rather than an academic discipline such as family social science. More family nursing theory, practice, and research is drawing from family therapy theories as the specialty grows more sophisticated. Of all three, theory basis nursing models are the least developed. The major drawback to the nursing models is that they originated using the individual as the focus, and only a few evolved to fit a family or group focus (Berkey and Hanson, 1991) (see the Research Brief).

FAMILY NURSING PROCESS

The **family nursing process** is a dynamic organized method of critically thinking about the family. It is problem solving with the family to help the family successfully adapt to identified health care needs (Ross, 1996). The family nursing process is the application of the basic nursing process and is grounded in knowledge of family nursing and family theory (Hanson and Boyd, 1996a).

The family nursing process consists of the following steps adapted specifically with family as the focus group (Carnevali and Thomas, 1993):

1. *Collection of a family nursing database (general or focused).* Data collection is focused on both identification of problem areas and strengths of the family. Often this and the following step of diagnostic reasoning become

RESEARCH *Brief*

There are many issues pertaining to family nursing assessment and intervention that need to be studied. Although family social science has been around for the last 25 years, the field focused its previous work on the theoretical foundations of family and just recently looked at family health and the application of theory to practice. Concurrently, nursing research is also about 25 years old and has focused largely on individuals rather than on the family as a unit. The merger of family social science and family therapy into nursing to form a new specialty called *family nursing* has only received attention in the last 7 years. Much work needs to be done by family nursing researchers. Considerations for research include the following.

1. Development of additional family nursing assessment models. Currently there are three major models, Hanson and Mischke (1996), Friedman (1998), and Wright and Leahey (1994), all of which have a very different focus and yield different data.
2. Field test the existing family nursing assessment models. The existing three models mentioned previously have received very little field testing for clinical or research utility.

3. Develop measurement instruments that are psychometrically tested specifically for nursing of families. Little measurement instrumentation has been developed by and for nurses for use with families as a unit.
4. Field test existing family measurement instruments for their adaptability to family nursing and family health. There are hundreds of instruments purportedly developed for use in family social science, but they have not been adapted for clinical use in health care.
5. Further work needs to be done on diagnostic taxonomies that focus on families as a unit of analysis/care. Presently the health care model is driven by individual diagnostic taxonomies, which influence the kind of care nurses give families.
6. There is a need for a paradigm shift from individual health care to family health care. Most students of nursing are not educated in family assessment. Nursing educators need to find more effective ways of teaching family concepts to nursing students of all levels.

Boyd ST, Hanson SMH: Theoretical and research foundations. In Hanson SMH, Boyd ST, editors: *Family health care nursing theory, practice and research*, Philadelphia, 1996, F.A. Davis.

integrated so that assessment and analysis of the data collected occurs concurrently. Nurses make inferences and draw conclusions about the data they collect, which in turn directs more data collection or defines the problem areas.

2. *Diagnostic reasoning and generation of specific family nursing diagnosis.* In this step, nurses make clinical judgments about which problems can be solved by nursing intervention, which problems need to be referred to other professionals, and areas of concern to which the family is successfully adapting on its own without intervention. The problems that require nursing intervention are specifically stated as family nursing diagnoses. The family nursing diagnosis provides direction for the collaboration of the nurse and the family in designing a plan of action. Diagnostic statements for the family as a whole can be derived from any of the common taxonomies that contain statements related to families, such as the North American Nursing Diagnosis Association (NANDA; Gordon, 1997-1998), *Diagnostic and Statistical Manual of Mental Disorders* (DSM-IV; APA, 1994), *International Classification of Disease* (ICD; AMA, 1997), or the Omaha System (Martin and Scheet, 1992).

3. *Collection of nursing and medical data and generating of data-supported nursing prognosis for each family nursing diagnosis.* The nursing prognosis is a nursing judgment, based on the holistic view of the family and its members, that predicts the probability of the family's ability to respond to the current situation. The predictive, or statement, outlines the most successful course of action on which to focus the interventions.

4. *Treatment planning based on both family nursing diagnosis and prognosis, plus additional data on daily living and family resources and deficiencies, should influence planned nursing actions.* The nurse and family work in a partnership to design and contract for a plan of action based on identified family strengths. The goal of the plan of action is to have the family successfully manage its health care concerns.

5. *Implementation of family negotiated plans of action.* The specific family and nursing interventions are carried out by the identified party, family member or provider, to achieve the goals upon which they agreed.

6. *Evaluation of family/family members' responses to plans of action, effects of family diagnosis, prognosis, and previous treatment.* The evaluation phase is based on the family outcomes, not on the effectiveness of the interventions. Modification of family nursing diagnosis and plans occurs as necessary based on an on-going evaluation.

7. *Termination of the nurse-family partnership is included in the plan of action and is implemented based on the evaluation.* A more detailed discussion of the family nursing process occurs in the following sections demonstrating how to implement the process.

NURSING TIP

Assessment is interactive. As you are evaluating families, they are evaluating you.

Collection of Data

The first step in the traditional nursing process is assessment, which is a comprehensive data-collection process. The assessment process is one of the most critical steps in the nursing process because it directs the whole problem-solving process. The selection of the appropriate assessment tool is made by the nurse based on areas of concern identified by the referring source (e.g., the physician) and the theoretical framework the nurse is using. Two family assessment tools are discussed in detail later in this chapter.

Purpose of the family interview

The purpose of the initial family interview is to identify the health concerns of the family. The central issues often are not the same as the problem for which the family was referred. See the following case study:

The Raggs family is referred to the home health clinic by a physician for medication management after Sam, the 73-year-old husband, was discharged from the hospital with the diagnosis of insulin-dependent diabetes mellitus (NIDDM), which he has had for 13 years. The potential area of concern that prompted the referral was the actual administration of insulin. After the initial interview the nurse finds that administration of the medication is not the central issue for Sam and his wife, Rose, but how to manage his nutrition. The inference of the referral source was that the family knew how to manage the dietary aspects of diabetes because Sam had NIDDM for 13 years. In this particular case, the focus needs to be on the nutritional management rather than medication administration.

HOW TO *Plan for the Assessment Process*

Assessment of families requires an organized plan before you see the family. This planning includes the following:

1. *Why are you seeing the family?*
2. *Who will be present during the interview?*
3. *Where will you see the family and how will the space be arranged?*
4. *What are you going to be assessing?*
5. *How are you going to collect this data?*
6. *What are you going to do with the information you find?*

Identification of a potential problem area

Data collection begins with the identification of a potential problem area identified by a variety of sources, which include the family, the physician, a school nurse, or a case worker. The identification of a problem, actual or potential, triggers the nurse to establish contact with a family. Several examples follow:

1. A family is referred to the home health agency because of the birth of the newest family member. In

that district, all births are automatically followed up with a home visit.

2. A family calls the Visiting Nurse Association to request assistance in providing care to a family member who has a terminal health care problem.
3. The school nurse is asked to conduct a family assessment by a teacher who noticed that a student has frequent absences and has had significant behavior changes in the classroom.
4. A physician requests a family assessment with a child who has failure to thrive.

The initial source of referral has identified an actual or potential family health care problem. The specific problem or the central issue may not have been identified at this point. One of the most important pieces of information provided by the referral source is the focus or the cluster of cues, or symptoms, that lead someone to believe that a problem might exist. The cluster of cues helps to focus the assessment process and selection of the appropriate family assessment tools.

As soon as the referral occurs, the nurse begins the assessment process and data collection. Sources of preencounter data collected before the family interview by the nurse include the following:

- *Referral source.* The information collected from the referral source includes the cues that lead them to identify that a problem area exists for this family. Demographic information may be obtained from the referral source. Both subjective and objective information is helpful in the assessment process.
- *Family.* A family may identify a health care concern and seek help. During the initial intake or screening procedure, valuable information can be collected that provides the focus for the assessment interview between the nurse and the family. Information is collected by the nurse during the interaction with the family member on the phone while making arrangements for the initial appointment. This information might include family members' views of the problem, surprise that the referral was made, reluctance to set up the meeting, avoiding setting up the interview, or recognizing that a referral was made or that a probable health care concern exists.
- *Previous records.* Previous records may be available for review before the first meeting between the nurse and the family. Often a record release for information is necessary to obtain family or individual records.

Setting up the meeting with the family

Before contacting the family to arrange for the initial appointment, the nurse decides the best place to conduct the interview. Often this decision is dictated by the type of agency with which the nurse works (e.g., home health is conducted in the home), or the mental health agency may choose to have the family meet in the neighborhood clinic office.

There are several advantages to conducting the interview in the family home. The everyday environment of the family can be viewed by the nurse during the visit. An important reason to conduct home interviews is to emphasize that the problem is the responsibility of the whole family and not one family member. The family members are likely to feel more relaxed and demonstrate typical family interactions in their own environment. The convenience of conducting the interview in the home may increase the probability of having more family members present. Two important disadvantages of conducting the interview in the home are that 1) the home may be the only sanctuary or safe place for the family or its members to be away from the scrutiny of others, and 2) to conduct an interview in the personal space of the family requires skilled communication ability on the part of the nurse.

Conducting the family interview in the office or clinic allows for easier access to consult with other health care providers about the problem. An advantage of using the clinic may be that the family situation is so intense that a more formal, less personal setting may be necessary for the family to begin discussion of emotionally charged issues. A disadvantage of conducting the family interview in the office is that it may reinforce a possible culture gap between the family, since the nurse does not see the everyday family environment.

HOW TO *Set an Appointment with the Family*

The assessment process starts immediately upon referral to the nurse. The following are suggestions that will make the process of arranging a meeting with the family easier:

1. *Remember that the assessment is reciprocal and the family will be making judgments about you when you call to make the appointment.*
2. *Introduce yourself and the purpose for the contact.*
3. *Do not apologize for contacting the family. Be clear, direct, and specific about the need for an appointment.*
4. *Arrange a time that is convenient for all parties that gets the most family members present.*
5. *Confirm place, time, date, and directions.*

After the decision is made regarding the place of the family interview, the appointment needs to be arranged with the family. The nurse needs to be confident and organized when making the initial contact. After the introduction, the nurse concisely states the reason for requesting the family visit. All family members are encouraged to attend the interview. Several possible times for the appointment can be offered, which allows the family to select the most convenient time for all members to be present. Often this occurs in the late afternoon or evening.

Family Nursing Diagnosis

The family nursing diagnosis is based on the nurse determining the central issue of concern with the family. It is important for the nurse to state the specific family nursing diagnosis because it provides the framework for the remaining steps in the family nursing process. The **family nursing diagnosis** is a public statement of the problem and the specific reason that brings the nurse and family together to solve a family health care need (Ross, 1996). If the family nursing diagnosis is not properly identified, the family and the nurse will collect data, design interventions, and implement plans of care that do not meet the family's needs. A key factor to identifying the correct family nursing diagnosis is asking broad-based questions that allow for data collection in multiple ways concurrently. The importance of identifying the central issue of concern and accurately making the family nursing diagnosis is demonstrated by comparing the following two scenarios:

Scenario #1: The hypothesized central issue for the Raggs family was identified by the referral source: Is insulin being administered correctly by the Raggs family? Based on this central issue, evidence was collected and the family nursing diagnosis identified was the following: Lack of family knowledge related to the administration of insulin secondary to new diagnosis of insulin-dependent diabetes as evidenced by 1) verbal statements of concern about giving the injection, 2) difficulty drawing up the accurate amount of insulin, and 3) questions about the storage of insulin. This nursing diagnosis focuses further data collection and plan for interventions on 1) the psychomotor skills of family members necessary to give the insulin injection, 2) the correct amount of insulin to give according to blood glucose level, and 3) the correct storage and handling of the medication and the equipment.

Based on this family nursing diagnosis, the nurse concluded that the most important area to concentrate on was the ability of the family to administer medication. The data collection process and the nurse's thinking were focused on a single problem, not the whole effect of this health issue on the family. The identification of other family health care needs may occur, but the identification will be delayed, which may cause potential harm.

Scenario #2: The real central issue for the Raggs family identified by the nurse conducting the assessment is as follows: What is the best way to ensure that the Raggs family understands the relationship of insulin-dependent diabetes and the administration of medication? After collecting evidence, the family nursing diagnosis was the following: Lack of family knowledge related to health care management of a family member who has been newly diagnosed with insulin-dependent diabetes.

Asking a broader-based question allows the nurse to view the whole picture of the family dealing with this specific health concern and directs the data-collection process. More evidence was collected in this case scenario because more options for possible interventions were considered concurrently in the data-collection process. Areas of data collection for this nursing diagnosis were 1) administration of medication, 2) nutritional management, 3) blood glucose monitoring, 4) activity exercise, and 5) knowledge of pathophysiology of diabetes. The nurse was able to collect data looking at the family in a more holistic fashion. The central issue for the family centered around nutritional management, which ultimately affects the administration of medication.

The major difference between the two scenarios presented above was the way in which the nurse framed the question. In the first scenario the nurse asked a question that allowed for only one aspect of the family and the health care concern to be considered at a time. This type of step-by-step problem-solving process is tedious, time consuming, and will likely cause error in the identification of the most pressing family nursing diagnosis. In the second scenario, the nurse asked a question that allowed for critical thinking about several options concurrently.

An important part of defining the family nursing process is continuous reflective questioning, which helps to keep the central issue in focus and allows for modification of the family nursing diagnosis (Alfaro-Lefevre, 1994). The following are helpful reflective questions:

- Am I continuing to focus on the central issue?
- Am I sure that I am understanding the information correctly?
- Is everyone involved focused on the central issue?
- Have I collected enough information to be drawing inferences or conclusions?
- Have I made any assumptions that might not be true or valid?

The family nursing diagnoses should not be limited to the few that are endorsed by the NANDA (Gordon, 1997-1998). The taxonomies presented previously are other useful tools for coming up with family nursing diagnoses. After the family nursing diagnosis has been identified and verified with the family, the next step is the family nursing prognosis.

Family Nursing Prognosis

The **family nursing prognosis** is a realistic statement about the ability of the family to successfully adapt to the nursing diagnosis given the strengths of the family, the pattern of family response in similar situations, and the direction of the family health care problem. The prognosis statement represents the nurse's judgment of the evidence presented in the family assessment process. Family nursing prognosis "is a prediction of the possible or probable course of events and outcomes associated with a particular family health status or family situation under various circumstances, treatment options or lack of treatment" (Carnevali and Thomas, 1993, p. 80).

The family prognosis contains information about "areas where changes can occur, types of outcomes and direction of change" (Carnevali and Thomas, 1993, p. 80). The treatment plan is based on predicting the areas in which the family can change to achieve successful adaptation.

The areas of change may be focused on the family's response to the situation, the family system process, and the family function most affected or family components, such as roles, communication, decision making, or stress and coping. The nurse can predict the course of events or the pattern of change expected to occur given information known about the family. The types of outcomes that the nurse considers are as follows:

- Preventing a potential problem
- Minimizing the problem

- Stabilizing of the problem
- A deteriorating problem.

A case example showing the importance of the prognosis statement follows:

Scenario #3: The home hospice nurse has been working with the Brush family for three weeks. The Brush family consists of the following members, who all live in the home:
- Dylan (father)
- Myra (mother)
- William (10-year-old son)
- Jessica (7-year-old daughter)
- Beatrice (grandmother, Myra's mother)

Beatrice was diagnosed with terminal liver cancer 4 weeks ago. The Brush family all agreed that Beatrice should live with them and be cared for until her death in their home. Beatrice has other children who live in the same city. The hospice nurse in collaboration with the Brush family identified several family nursing diagnoses, but the following family nursing diagnosis is of major importance because it affects the lives of all family members: Family role conflict related to the maternal grandmother moving into her daughter's home after being diagnosed with terminal liver cancer. The daughter showed her role conflict by stating, "Sometimes I do not know who I am—daughter, nurse, mother, or wife."

The prognosis for resolving the role conflict experienced by Myra can be minimized for success by working with the family to spread the caregiver role among the extended family members, to negotiate certain tasks and who performs them, and by providing for respite care. One of the strengths of the family is agreement that caring for the dying grandmother in the home is the "right" ethical choice for them. The disruption to the family and their expected roles will be short term because the grandmother will probably not live for more than 4 months. Home hospice has been contacted and is involved in the care management. The family has a strong internal and external support system. The extended family is willing to be involved in the care of Beatrice.

The prognosis is critical because it serves as the foundation for the interventions or strategies of action that the family and nurse design in response to the identified family nursing diagnosis. The area of change in the case study is family roles and the expected behaviors of each family member. The course of events is short term, but Myra's role conflict may increase as her caregiver role becomes more intense as her mother gets worse. The type of outcome is to mobilize resources to minimize Myra's role conflict.

Planning, Implementing, and Evaluating

After the prognosis statement is made, it is important for the nurse to determine if the family responses to the problem require nursing intervention or if should they be referred to a different professional. The planning phase is a form of contracting with families. The contract, or plan of action, includes establishing goals, plans of action, determining who does what in the plan, and building the evaluation steps. The written plan of care 1) ensures involvement

of each person, 2) involves people in their own care, and 3) increases autonomy and self-esteem of the family members.

Once the nurse determines that the identified central issues are appropriate for nursing, the planning and intervening aspects of the family nursing process help the family members be part of the solution. The degree of involvement of each family member varies and needs to be negotiated among the family members with the help of the nurse. The types of plans and the implementing and evaluating processes are specific to the family and the family nursing diagnosis. The plan, implementation, and evaluation are designed based on the evidence collected in the assessment and the prognosis statement.

During the planning stage, it is important for the nurse to recognize that the family has the right to make its own health decisions. The role of the nurse is to offer guidance to the family, provide information, and assist in the planning process. An important part of the planning phase is to determine who does what. The nurse may assist the family by 1) providing direct care, which the family cannot; 2) removing barriers to needed services, which helps the family to function; and 3) improving the capacity of the family to act on its own behalf and assume responsibility (Friedman, 1998).

In the reflective critical thinking process, the nurse should ask the following questions while assisting the family in designing the plan of action (Freidman, 1998):

1. Is this plan being developed in collaboration with the family?
2. Will the proposed approaches enhance family strengths and increase family member independence?
3. Is this action within the information and skill level of the family members or their own resources?
4. On a scale of one to ten (with ten being the highest), how committed and motivated are family members to adhere to the plan?
5. Are there adequate resources available to carry out the plan?
6. How would family members respond to these questions?
7. Will this action diminish or strengthen the coping ability of the family?

Building the plan of action for the family on family strengths increases the liklihood that the family will achieve the desired outcome. Once the plan has been developed and all individuals involved have approved or committed to the plan, the plan is put into effect. Data collection continues throughout the implementation phase and is part of the formative evaluation process. When a plan is not working well, the nurse and the family should work together to determine the barriers of implementation. Family apathy and indecision are known to be barriers to implementation (Friedman 1998). Friedman (1998) identified the following nurse-related barriers to implementation: 1) imposing ideas, 2) negative labeling, 3) overlooking strengths, and 4) neglecting cultural or gender implications. Family apathy may occur because of value differences between the nurse and the family; the family may be overcome with a sense of hopelessness, the family may view the problems as too overwhelming; or the family may have a fear of failure. Additional factors to be considered are that the family may be indecisive because they cannot determine which course of action is better, the family may have an unexpressed fear or concern; or the family has a pattern of decision making only when faced with a crisis.

The evaluation process contains both formative (ongoing) and summative (ending) evaluation components. The evaluation is based on the family outcomes and response to the plan, not the success of the interventions. An important part of the plan is the termination of the relationship between the nurse and the family.

NURSING TIP

Too much disclosure during the early contacts between the family and nurse may scare the family away. Slow the process down and take time to build trust.

Termination of the Nurse-Family Relationship

Termination is phasing out the nurse from family involvement. When termination is built into the plan, the family benefits from a smooth transition process. The family is given credit for the outcomes of the plan that they helped design. Strategies often used in the termination component are decreasing the sessions with the nurse, extending invitations to the family for follow-up, and making referrals when appropriate. The termination should include a summative evaluation meeting where the nurse and family put a formal closure to their relationship.

When termination occurs suddenly, it is important for the nurse to determine the forces bringing about the closure. The family may be initiating the termination prematurely, which requires a renegotiating process. The insurance or agency requirements may be placing a financial constraint on the amount of time the nurse can work with a family. Regardless of how termination comes about, it is an important aspect in the family nursing process.

The family nursing process summarized in this section represents a critical thinking approach to working with families. The assessment aspect of the nursing process is a crucial component to successful intervention and is described in detail in the next section.

BARRIERS TO PRACTICING FAMILY NURSING

Many barriers exist that affect the practice of family nursing in a community setting. Two significant **barriers to family nursing** are the narrow definition of family used by health care providers and social policy makers and the lack of consensus of what is a healthy family. Other barriers are summarized by Hanson and Boyd (1996a) and Gillis (1993):

- Until the last decade, most practicing nurses had little exposure to family concepts during their undergraduate education and have continued to practice using the individual focus. Family nursing was viewed as "common sense" and not a theory-based nursing approach.
- There has been a lack of good comprehensive family assessment models, instruments, and strategies in nursing.
- Nursing has strong historical ties with the medical model, which views families as structure and not central to individual health care.
- The traditional charting system in health care has been oriented to the individual.
- The medical and nursing diagnosis systems used in health care are disease centered, and diseases are focused on individuals.
- Insurance carriers have traditionally based reimbursement and coverage on an individual basis, not as a family unit.
- The hours during which health care systems provide services to families are at times of day when family members cannot accompany one another.

These and other obstacles to family nursing practice are slowly shifting. Nurses must continue to lobby for changes that are more conducive to caring for the family as a whole.

FAMILY NURSING ASSESSMENT

Family nursing assessment is the cornerstone for family nursing interventions. By using a systematic process, family problem areas are identified and family strengths are emphasized as the building blocks for interventions. Building the interventions with family-identified problems and strengths allows for equal family and provider commitment to the solutions and ensures more successful interventions. Two family assessment models and approaches are presented: the Family Assessment Intervention Model and the Family Systems, Stressor, Strength Inventory (FS³I) (Hanson and Mischke, 1996; Hanson and Boyd, 1996a; Hanson and Kaakinen, 1996) and the Friedman Family Assessment Model and Short Form (Friedman, 1998). Genograms and ecomaps are presented as strategies to assess families that provide a clear, concise picture of intergenerational patterns and social supports or direction of family stress. Nurses are encouraged to select the model and strategy that provides the best fit to their particular philosophy and practice, or nurses can use a combination of both (see the Case Study in Appendix I.4).

Family Assessment Intervention Model and Family Systems, Stressor, Strength Inventory (FS³I)

The Family Assessment Intervention Model is based on an extension of Betty Neuman's Health Care Systems Model and uses a family-as-client approach (Hanson and Mischke, 1996; Neuman, 1989; Reed, 1993). This model reflects a systems approach.

In this model, families are subject to the tensions produced when stressors (see arrows in Fig. 24-5), in the form

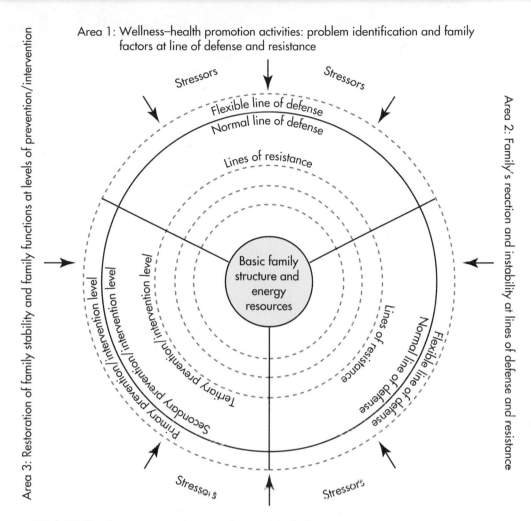

Area 1: Wellness–health promotion activities: problem identification and family factors at line of defense and resistance

Stressors   Stressors

Flexible line of defense
Normal line of defense

Lines of resistance

Basic family structure and energy resources

Area 2: Family's reaction and instability at lines of defense and resistance

Area 3: Restoration of family stability and family functions at levels of prevention/intervention

Primary prevention/intervention level
Secondary prevention/intervention level
Tertiary prevention/intervention level

Lines of resistance
Normal line of defense
Flexible line of defense

Stressors   Stressors

FIG. 24-5 Family assessment intervention model. (From Hanson SMH, Mischke KM: Family health assessment and intervention. In Bomar PJ, editor: *Nurses and family health promotion: concepts, assessment, and interventions,* Philadelphia, 1996, WB Saunders. Adapted from the Neuman Health Care Systems Model.)

of problems, penetrate their defense system. The family's reaction depends on how deeply the stressor penetrates the family unit and how capable the family is of adapting to maintain its stability. The lines of resistance protect the family's basic structure, which includes the family's functions and energy resources. The core contains the patterns of family interactions and unit strengths. The basic family structure must be protected at all costs or the family will cease to exist. Reconstitution or adaptation is the work the family undertakes to preserve or restore impaired family stability after stressors penetrate the family lines of defense, altering usual family functions. The model addresses three areas:

1. Health promotion, wellness activities, problem identification, and family factors at lines of defense and resistance
2. Family reaction and stability at lines of defense and resistance
3. Restoration of family stability and family functioning at levels of prevention

The basic assumptions for this family-focused model are listed in Box 24-3.

An assessment instrument based on this model was developed and named the **Family Systems, Stressor, Strength Inventory (FS³I)** (Hanson and Mischke, 1996). The FS³I is a family health assessment/measurement instrument that provides for quantitative and qualitative input by all family members and the nurse. It focuses on identifying stressful situations occurring in families and the strengths families use to maintain health functioning despite their problems. The FS³I is divided into three sections: 1) Family Systems Stressors: General, 2) Family Stressors: Specific, and 3) Family System Strengths. See Appendix I.2 for the forms.

The data collected by this instrument determine the level of prevention/intervention needed: primary, secondary, and tertiary (Pender et al, 1992). The primary prevention mode focuses on movement of the individual and family toward a positively balanced state of increased health or health promotion activities. Primary interventions include providing families with information about their strengths, supporting their coping and functioning abilities, and encouraging attempts toward wellness through family education. Secondary prevention modes address actions necessary to attain system stability after the family system has been invaded by stressors or problems. Secondary interventions include helping the family members handle their problems, helping them find and use appropriate treatment, and intervening in crises. The tertiary prevention mode includes those actions instituted to maintain systems stability. Tertiary intervention strategies are initiated after treatment has been completed and may include coordination of care after discharge from the hospital or rehabilitation services.

In summary, the FS³I focuses on two concepts of family health: family stressors and family strengths. It provides nurses with entry into the family system to gather data useful for nursing intervention.

Friedman Family Assessment Model

The **Friedman Family Assessment Model** (Friedman, 1998) draws heavily on the structural-functional framework and on developmental and systems theory. The model takes a broad approach to family assessment, which views families as a subsystem of society. The family is viewed as an open social system. The family's structure (organization) and functions (activities and purposes) and the family's relationship to other social systems are the focus of this approach.

This assessment approach is important for family nurses because it enables them to assess the family system as a whole, as part of the whole of society, and as an interaction system. The general assumptions for this model are contained in Box 24-4.

The guidelines for the Friedman Assessment Model consist of six broad categories of interview questions:
1. Identifying data
2. Developmental family stage and history
3. Environmental data
4. Family structure, including communication, power structures, role structures, and family values
5. Family functions, including affective, socialization, and health care
6. Family coping

Each category has several subcategories. There are both long and short forms of this assessment tool. See Appendix I.3 for the short form.

In summary, this approach was developed to provide guidelines for family nurses who are interviewing a family

---

BOX 24-3 Basic Assumptions for Family Assessment and Intervention Model

1. Although each family as a family system is unique, each system is a composite of common, known factors or innate characteristics within a normal, given range of response contained within a basic structure.
2. Many known, unknown, and universal environmental stressors exist. Each differs in its potential for disturbing a family's usual stability level, or normal line of defense. The particular interrelationships of family variables—physiological, psychological, sociocultural, developmental, and spiritual—at any time can affect the degree to which a family is protected by the flexible line of defense against possible reaction to one or more stressors.
3. Over time, each family/family system has evolved a normal range of response to the environment, referred to as a *normal line of defense*, or usual wellness/stability state.
4. When the cushioning, accordion-like effect of the flexible line of defense is no longer capable of protecting the family/family system against an environmental stressor, the stressor breaks through the normal line of defense. The interrelationships of physiological, psychological, sociocultural, developmental, and spiritual variables determine the nature and degree of the system reaction or possible reaction to the stressor.
5. The family, whether in a state of wellness or illness, is a dynamic composite of the interrelationships of

physiological, psychological, sociocultural, developmental, and spiritual variables. Wellness is on a continuum of available energy to support the system in its optimal state.
6. Implicit within each family system is a set of internal resistance factors, known as *lines of resistance*, which function to stabilize and return the family to the usual wellness state (normal line of defense), or possibly to a higher level of stability, after an environmental stressor reaction.
7. Primary prevention relates to general knowledge that is applied in family assessment and intervention in identification and mitigation of risk factors associated with environmental stressors to prevent possible reaction.
8. Secondary prevention relates to symptomatology after reaction to stressors, appropriate ranking of intervention priorities, and treatment to reduce their noxious effects.
9. Tertiary prevention relates to the adjustive processes taking place as reconstitution begins and maintenance factors move the client back in a circular manner toward primary prevention.
10. The family is in dynamic, constant energy exchange with the environment.

Based on data from Berkey KM, Hanson SMH: *Pocket guide to family assessment and intervention*, St Louis, 1991, Mosby; Neuman B: *The Neuman systems model*, ed 2, Norwalk, Conn, 1989, Appleton & Lange to gain an overall view of what is going on in the family. The questions are extensive, and it may not be possible to collect all the data at one visit. All the categories may not be pertinent for every family.

Summary of Family Assessment Models

Each family nursing assessment model and approach is unique and creates a different database upon which to plan interventions. The Family Assessment Intervention Model and the Family Systems Stressor Strength Inventory (FS^{3}I) measure very specific dimensions and give a microscopic view of family health. The Friedman Family Assessment Model is more broad and general. It is particularly useful for viewing families in their communities. Examples of completed family assessment tools are in the Case Study presented in Appendix I.4.

Genograms and Ecomaps

The genogram and ecomap are essential components of any family assessment, which should be used concurrently with either one or both of the assessment approaches just described.

BOX 24-4 Assumptions Underlying Friedman's Family Assessment Model

1. The family is a social system with functional requirements.
2. A family is a small group possessing certain generic features common to all small groups.
3. The family as a social system accomplishes functions that serve the individual and society.
4. Individuals act in accordance with a set of internalized norms and values that are learned primarily in the family through socialization.

From Friedman MM: *Family nursing: theory and practice*, ed 4, Norwalk, Conn, 1998, Appleton & Lange.

Genogram

The **genogram** displays pertinent family information in a family tree format that shows family members and their relationships over at least three generations (McGoldrick and Gerson, 1985). The genogram shows family history and patterns of health-related information, which is a rich source of information from which to plan interventions. The identified patient (IP) and his or her family are highlighted on the genogram. Genograms enhance nurses' abilities to make clinical judgements and connect them to family structure and history.

A form that can be used for developing genograms is depicted in Figure 24-6, and the genogram symbols most often used in a genogram are shown in Figure 24-7. An outline for a brief genogram interview is presented in Box 24-5 with genogram interpretive categories in Box 24-6. A sample of a three-generation genogram is depicted and discussed in the Case Study in Appendix I.4. The health history for all family members (morbidity, mortality, onset of illness) is important information for family nurses and can be the focus of analysis of the family genogram. Most families are cooperative and interested in completing the genogram. A genogram does not have to be completed in one sitting and becomes a part of the ongoing health care record.

Ecomap

The **ecomap** is a visual picture of the family unit in relation to the community. The ecomap serves as a tool to organize and present factual information and thus allows the nurse to have a more holistic and integrated perception of the family situation. The ecomap shows the nature of the relationships among family members and between family members and the community; it is "an overview of the family in their situation, picturing both the important nurturing and stress-producing connections between the family and the world" (Ross and Cobb, 1990, p. 176). The nurse starts with a blank ecomap, which consists of a large

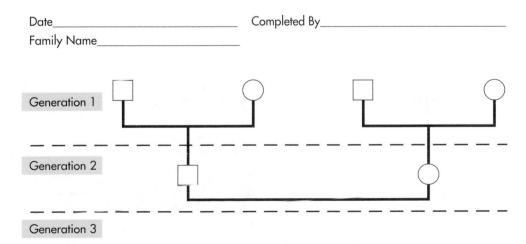

Date_____ Completed By_____

Family Name_____

Generation 1

Generation 2

Generation 3

FIG. 24-6 Genogram form. (Adapted from McGoldrick M, Gerson R: *Genograms in family assessment*, New York, 1985, WW Norton.)

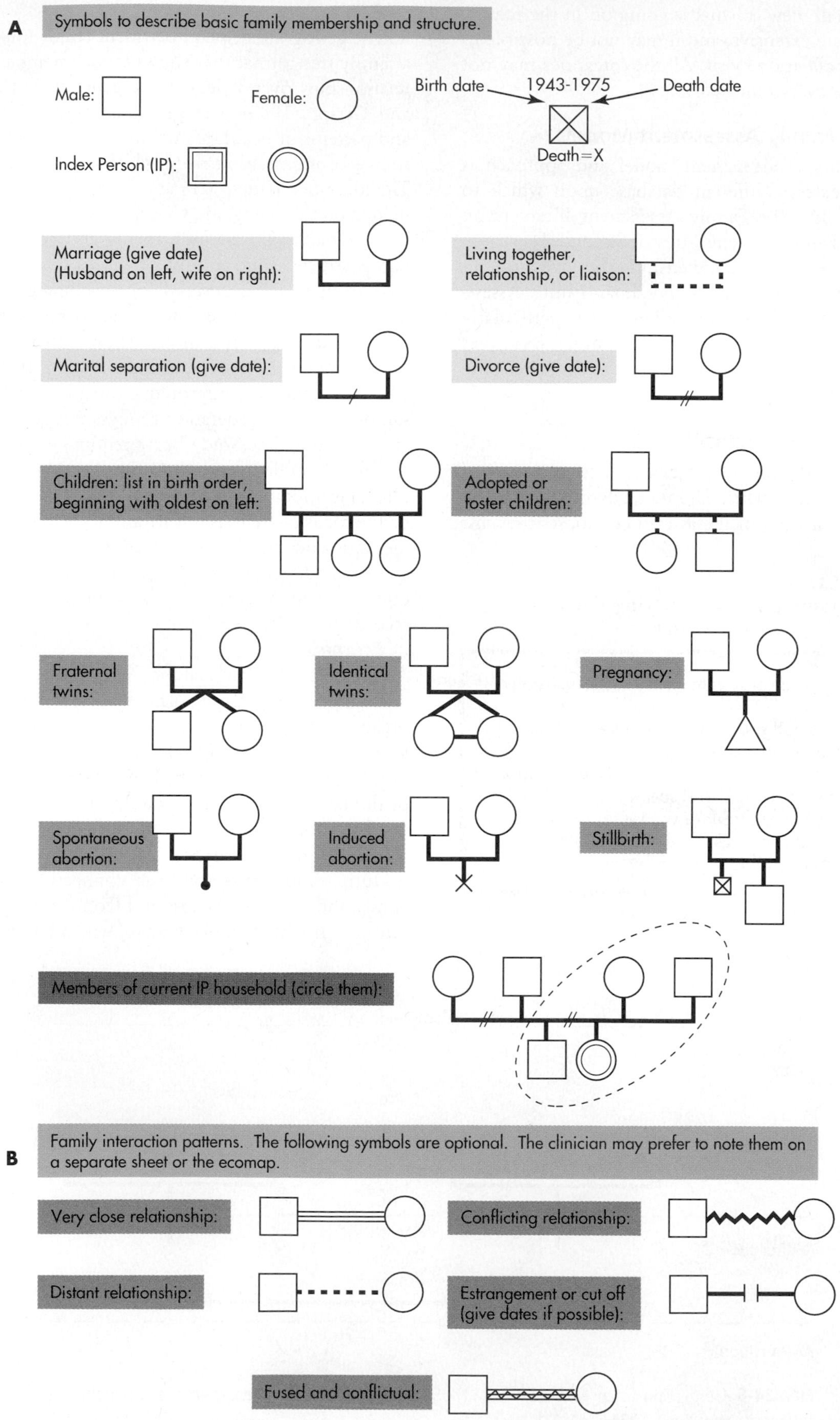

A Symbols to describe basic family membership and structure.

Male: □   Female: ○

Index Person (IP): ▣   ◎

Birth date → 1943-1975 ← Death date

Death=X

Marriage (give date) (Husband on left, wife on right):

Living together, relationship, or liaison:

Marital separation (give date):

Divorce (give date):

Children: list in birth order, beginning with oldest on left:

Adopted or foster children:

Fraternal twins:

Identical twins:

Pregnancy:

Spontaneous abortion:

Induced abortion:

Stillbirth:

Members of current IP household (circle them):

B Family interaction patterns. The following symbols are optional. The clinician may prefer to note them on a separate sheet or the ecomap.

Very close relationship:

Conflicting relationship:

Distant relationship:

Estrangement or cut off (give dates if possible):

Fused and conflictual:

FIG. 24-7 Genogram symbols. (Adapted from McGoldrick M, Gerson R: *Genograms in family assessment,* New York, 1985, WW Norton.)

Continued

C Medical history. Since the genogram is meant to be an orienting map of the family, there is room to indicate only the most important factors, such as major or chronic illnesses and problems. Include dates in parentheses where possible. Use diagnostic labels where available (e.g., cancer, stroke, schizophrenia).

D Other family information of special importance may also be noted:

1. Ethnic background and migration date
2. Religion or religious change
3. Education
4. Occupation or unemployment
5. Military service
6. Retirement
7. Trouble with law
8. Physical abuse or incest
9. Obesity
10. Chemical use (smoking, alcohol, marijuana, etc.)
11. Dates when family members left home (e.g., LH '74)
12. Current location of family members

It is useful to have a space at the bottom of the genogram for notes on *other key information*. This would include date of original genogram, critical events, changes in the family structure since the genogram was made, hypotheses, and other notations of major family issues or changes. Notations should always be dated and kept to a minimum since every extra piece of information on a genogram complicates it and therefore diminishes its readability.

FIG. 24-7, Cont'd For legend see previous page.

BOX 24-5 Outline for a Genogram Interview

For each person on the genogram, the following information may be included. The nurse should determine which of the following information is relevant to include on the genogram depending on the issues that the family is concerned about.
- First name
- Age
- Date of birth
- Occupation
- Health problems
- Cause of death
- Dates of marriages, divorces, separations, commitments, cohabitation, and remarriages
- Education level
- Ethnic or religious background

Adapted from McGoldrick M, Gerson R: *Genograms in family assessment*, New York, 1985, W.W. Norton.

BOX 24-6 Genogram Interpretive Categories

The following areas are important to observe in the family genogram:
1. *Family structure:* nuclear, blended, single-parent household, gay-lesbian relationship, cohabitation, divorces, separations
2. *Sibling subsystem group:* birth order, gender, distance between age of children
3. *Pattern of repetition:* look for patterns of repetition across the generations relative to family structure, family behaviors, family health problems, patterns of relationships, family violence, abuse issues, and poverty
4. *Life events:* look for similar types of events across generations, family transitions, family traumas

Adapted from McGoldrick M, Gerson R: *Genograms in family assessment*, New York, 1985, W.W. Norton.

---

circle with smaller circles around it (Fig. 24-8). The identified client and his or her family are placed in the center of the large circle in a genogram format. The outer smaller circles around the family unit represent "significant people, agencies, or institutions in the family's environment" (Wright and Leahey, 1994, p. 55) that interact with the different family members. The nature, quality of the relationships, and direction of energy flow between the family members and the subsystems are shown by different connecting lines.

The ecomap serves as a tool to organize and present information, allowing the nurse to have a more holistic and integrated perception of the family situation. Not only does it portray the present situation, but it also can be used to set goals for the future by encouraging connection and exchange with individuals and agencies in the community.

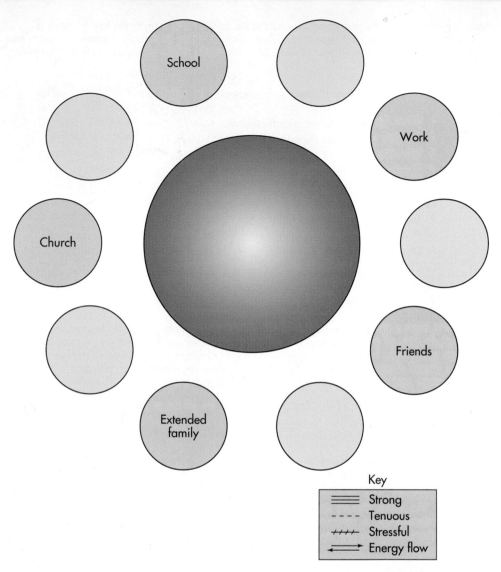

FIG. 24-8 Ecomap form. (Adapted from Friedman MM: *Family nursing: research and practice,* Norwalk, Conn, 1998, Appleton & Lange.)

A more detailed discussion of ecomapping can be found in Hanson (1996), Hartman (1978), McGoldrick and Gerson (1985), and Ross and Cobb (1990). An example of a completed ecomap is shown in the Case Study in Appendix I.4.

FUTURE IMPLICATIONS

Future Implications for Family Nursing

Family nursing practice is an evolving area of nursing (Kirschling, 1994) and will continue to be a significant aspect of health care in the future, especially with the current focus of health care reform in the United States. The barriers confronting the practice of family nursing need to be integral aspects addressed in new health care delivery systems.

Most nursing research has focused on the individual, not family health care (Boyd and Hanson, 1996a). Research pertaining to family and mental health is further advanced

than family and physical health. Recently nursing has awakened to the connection between family dynamics and health and illness. More family-centered research needs to be conducted by family nurses.

Future Implications for Family Policy

As professionals, nursing is accountable for participating in the development of legislation and family policy. Government actions that have a direct or indirect effect on families is called *family policy.* All government actions, whether at the local, county, state, or national level, affect the family either directly or indirectly. The range of social policy decisions that affect families is vast, such as health care access and coverage, low-income housing, social security, welfare, food stamps, pension plans, affirmative action, and education. "Although all government polices affect families, in both negative and positive ways, the

United States has no overall, official explicit family policy" (Zimmerman, 1992, p. 4).

Most government policy indirectly affects families. Much debate has taken place within government regarding the definition of family. An argument often cited for the lack of more explicit family policies is related to the financial burden that would occur if the definition of family was too broad.

The national health promotion and disease prevention objectives outlined in both *Healthy People 2000* (USDHHS, 1990) and *Healthy Communities 2000* (APHA, 1991) have direct and indirect consequences and outcomes that affect families. The Family Leave legislation passed in the 1990s by the U.S. Congress is an example of a type of family policy that has been positive for families. A family member may take a defined amount of leave for family events (e.g., births, deaths) without fear of losing his or her job. Equally important today is the role that families will be assigned in health care reform. Since families are a primary source for health care beliefs and delivery, it is important that the issues of families and their place in health care reform be obvious. "All policies affect families, strengthening or diminishing their ability to sustain themselves and to prepare the next generation" (Elliott, 1993, p. ii).

At the beginning of the twenty-first century, it is natural and wise to look forward and speculate on the future of family nursing, families, and what this might mean for family social policy. A brief discussion is provided for students to ponder and realize that we all have an opportunity to write the script for this new century.

Future of Families

Each family is an unexplored mystery, unique in the ways in which they meet the needs of their members and society. Healthy and vital families are essential to the world's future because each family member is affected by what their families have invested in them or failed to provide for their growth and well-being. Families will continue to survive and serve as the basic social unit of society.

The following projections and trends for the future of families provide an important lens to view the future:

- Marriage rates remain high in the United States and are among the highest of all developed nations in the world. However, there has been a slight decline in the rate of marriage since World War II, largely because of the trend to postpone marriage and the increase in the rates of cohabitation. Nevertheless, marriages continue to dissolve as a result of abandonment, separation, divorce, or death of a spouse.
- Divorce rates during the 1970s and 1980s increased rapidly. More than 60% of all marriages end in divorce. In recent years, there has been a slight trend downward, possible resulting from the increase in age at first marriage, which lowers the risk of divorce. According to Gelles (1995), divorce will continue to be the typical way that the majority of marriages end.

- Children will increasingly live in below-poverty-level, single-mother households because of lack of support from fathers.
- Birthrates appear to be generally down since the baby boom. Children's overall share of the population has declined since 1970 and will continue to decline in the foreseeable future as fertility rates stay low and baby boomers age. Delays in first marriage often means that couples delay having their first child. The birthrate among women who have never married is rising and will likely continue; unmarried motherhood currently accounts for almost one-third of all births in the United States. Fertility rates will likely stay below replacement for the general population, although there is a significant variation in fertility rates across socioeconomic, racial, and ethnic groups.
- The proportion of married women (with or without children) employed in the workforce has increased rapidly in the past 40 years, with the greatest growth among married women with preschool children. The combined effects of the economy and women's movement will continue the upward trend in maternal employment. Mothers in two-parent households carry increasing economic responsibilities.
- The future of families is one of diversity of family forms and structures. There is little evidence that any of the forces will move families back toward the "idyllic nuclear family of the 1950s" (Gelles, 1995). Families and intimate relationships will continue to evolve. For example, continued development exists in single-parent families, gay and lesbian relationships, interracial marriages, and multigenerational families (new extended family). Diversity includes both cohabitation and living as single.
- The future of families will call for increased and changing marital roles. Twenty years ago, it was predicted by many that household equality was quickly approaching. However, it appears that working women simply added a second "shift" to their lifestyles. The home and child care are still considered the province and responsibility of women. Although more men are involved in housework and child care, more men also have abandoned their families and failed to provide court-ordered child support after divorce. There is reason to predict that role options in families will continue to become more flexible. There is also reason to believe that families will always have a gender-based division of labor.
- Parents face growing concerns about caring for children through more years of education (and living at home) at the same time that their own longer-living parents survive. Middle-age adults find themselves in the "sandwich generation" between prolonged dependency of adult children remaining or returning to the home of origin and elderly parents and grandparents entering into their homes on a somewhat permanent basis. It is estimated that 20% of American children will be raised

by their grandparents (Burton, Dilworth-Anderson, and Merriwether-deVries, 1995).

- Families will have more complicated family histories and kinship relationships resulting from divorce, remarriage, and serial relationships. Society will need to come up with a whole new vocabulary on how to relate to the complexity of relationships in modern families.
- The increase in the number of elderly persons accompanied by the decline in the fertility rate and decreased mortality rate has a direct effect on families. The fastest growing population group includes individuals older than 85 years of age who are more likely to be frail, dependent, and have multiple health needs. The availability of kin to provide family care becomes a major issue for families. Families will be managing care of family members from a distance, via phone, e-mail, and fax technology (Kaakinen, in press; Kinsella, 1996). In the future the old will be cared for by their children in their eighties or grandchildren in their sixties (Dreman, 1997; Kaakinen, in press).
- Although controversial, genetic technology will be a part of the future. Today there is rapid movement toward a future when knowledge of genetic makeup and its implications for individual futures will radically transform the world. There are social, legal, political and ethical issues arising for the future from recent discoveries made in genetic research.

Gelles (1995, p. 508) believes that the two major threats and unknowns to families in the future are the following:

1. *AIDS.* "The cloud that hangs over the family and intimate relations is not divorce, cohabitation, working mothers, or alternative lifestyles. Today's cloud is AIDS (acquired immunodeficiency syndrome)." The disease was barely recognized 10 years ago and today it has moved way beyond its original gay male culture.
2. *Status of American children.* The status of children in families has changed, and the changes have not all been to the advantage of the children. Although some argue that the key change is the absence of fathers, the major structural change is the poverty that affects children in single-parent homes. There is a signifcant increase in the percentage of children in the United States who live in poverty. The major problems that children face do not come from cohabitation, day care, or the fact that their mothers work. Families are not declining because of divorce, working mothers, and lower fertility. The family is declining because American society continues to ignore the needs of a substantial portion of its children. Many children do not get immunizations, are not fed or clothed, do not get health care, and live in dangerous environments.

clinical application

The idealized family portrayed in the media during the twentieth century consists of a working father, a mother that stays home, and their children. Many families today compare their turbulent, hectic lives with those of the fictionalized past and find their situations wanting.

A. Did the idealized version of the traditional family ever really exist?
B. Some people believe that American families are in decline while others believe that families are healthy. What do you think?
C. What do you think is happening with American families and what do you think the future will bring?
D. What are the implications for the practice of family community nursing?

Answers are in the back of the book.

KEY POINTS

- Families are the context within which health care decisions are made. Nurses are responsible for assisting families in meeting health care needs.
- Family nursing is practiced in all settings
- Family nursing is a specialty area that has a strong theoretical base and is more than just common sense.
- Family demographics is the study of structures of families and households as well as events that alter the family, such as marriage, divorce, births, cohabitation, and dual careers.
- Demographic trends affecting the family include the age of individuals when he or she marries, increase in intraracial marriages with children, most divorced people remarrying, increase in dual-career marriages, increased number of children from maritally disrupted families, high divorce rate, dramatic increase in cohabitation, increased number of children who spend time in a single-parent family, delay of childbirth, increased number of children born to women who are single or who have never married, and increased number of children who live with grandparents.
- Traditionally, families have been defined as a nuclear family: mother, father, and young children. There is a variety of family definitions, such as a group of two or more, a unique social group, and two or more persons joined together by emotional bonds.
- The six functions performed by families are economic survival, reproduction, protection, cultural heritage, socialization of young, and conferring status.
- Family structure refers to the characteristics, gender, age, and number of the individual members who make up the family unit.
- Family health is difficult to define, but it includes the biological, psychological, sociological, cultural, and spiritual factors of the family system.
- There are four approaches to viewing families: family as context, family as client, family as a system, and family as a component of society.
- Structural functional frameworks view the family as a social system with members who have specific roles and functions.
- Systems theory describes families as a unit of the whole composed of members whose interactional patterns are the focus of attention.
- Family development is one theoretical framework used to study families. This approach emphasizes how families change over time and focuses on interactions and relationships among family members.

- Interactional framework focuses on the family as a unit of interacting personalities and examines the communication processes by which family members relate to one another.
- Nurses should ask clients whom they consider to be family and then include those members in the nurse's health care plan.
- The family nursing process is a dynamic, systematic, organized method of critically thinking about the family.
- The purpose of the initial family interview is to identify the health concerns of the family.
- The family nursing diagnosis is based on the nurse determining the actual issues of concern within the family.
- An important part of defining the family nursing process is continuous reflective questioning.
- The family prognosis is a realistic statement about the ability of the family to successfully adapt to the nursing diagnosis.
- It is essential in the beginning of the planning step to determine if the family's response to the problem requires nursing intervention or should be referred to a different professional.
- It is important for the nurse to recognize that the family has the right to make its own health decisions.
- The nurse, in working with families, must evaluate the family outcomes and response to the plan, not the success of the interventions.
- Two family assessment models and approaches are the Family Assessment Intervention Model and the Family Systems Stressor Strength Inventory (FS³I).
- The Friedman Family Assessment Model takes a macroscopic approach to family assessment, which views the family as a subsystem of society.
- The FS³I measures very specific dimensions and gives a microscopic view of health.
- The whole family picture is enhanced by merging data from both assessment tools.
- Genograms and ecomaps are essential components of any family assessment.
- The future of family, health care, and nursing is not an exact science. However, all areas are under change and there are many challenges to be understood and overcome in the new century.

critical thinking activities

1. Select six or more health professionals and ask them to define family. Analyze the responses for commonalities and differences. Write your definition of family.
2. Define *family nursing*.
3. Discuss how family fits into nursing.
4. Form small groups and discuss the implications of family demography and demographic trends for nursing.
5. Develop a typology of the different family structures and household arrangements representative of the community. This information may be available from various sources, such as the health department, schools, other social and welfare agencies, and census data.
6. Identify five barriers to practicing family nursing in a community setting.
7. Describe how a family assessment is different than an individual client assessment.
8. Discuss the importance of family nursing diagnosis and prognosis related to developing a plan of action with a family.
9. Explain why family assessment is the most critical aspect of the family nursing process.
10. What kind of difficulties could you experience when arranging for a family assessment interview?
11. Discuss factors to be considered when determining the place to conduct a family assessment interview. Include pros and cons.
12. How would you select which family assessment tool to use?
13. Describe and compare the Family Systems Stressor Strength Inventory (FS³I) assessment tool and the Friedman Family Assessment Model.
14. Draw your own family genogram and ecomap. Discuss how they are used in family nursing.
15. Discuss the role of nursing related to family policy.
16. Summarize and contrast the four family social science theories.
17. Break into small groups and have students discuss the family from the four family social science theories.

Bibliography

Alfaro-LeFevre R: *Applying nursing process: a step-by-step process,* ed 3, Philadelphia, 1994, J.B. Lippincott.

American Medical Association: *International classification of diseases: clinical modifications* (ICD-9-CM), Vol 1 and 2, 9th revision, Dover, Delaware, 1997, AMA.

American Psychiatric Association: *Diagnostic and statistical manual of mental disorders,* ed 4, Washington, DC, 1994, the Association.

American Public Health Association: *Healthy communities 2000: model standards: guidelines for community attainment of year 2000 national health objectives,* Washington, DC, 1991, the Association.

Artinian NT: Selecting model to guide family assessment, *Dimens Crit Care Nurs* 14(1):4, 1994.

Becvar DS, Becvar RJ: *Family therapy: a systemic integration,* Boston, 1996, Allyn & Bacon.

Bender DL, Leone B: *The family in America: opposing viewpoints,* San Diego, 1991, Greenhaven Press.

Berkey KM, Hanson SMH: *Pocket guide to family assessment and intervention,* St Louis, 1991, Mosby.

Bianchi SM: The changing demographic and socioeconomic characteristics of single parent families. In Hanson SMH et al, editors: *Single parent families,* New York, 1995, Haworth Press.

Bomar P: *Nurses and family health promotion: concepts, assessment, and interventions,* ed 2, Philadelphia, 1996, W.B. Saunders.

Boss PG et al: *Sourcebook of family theories and methods: a contextual approach,* New York, 1993, Plenum.

Bowen G, Desimore L, McKay J: Poverty and the single mother family: a macroeconomic perspective. In Hanson SMH et al, editors: *Single parent families,* New York, 1995, Haworth Press.

Boyd ST, Hanson SMH: Theoretical and research foundations. In Hanson SMH, Boyd ST, editors: *Family health care nursing theory, practice and research,* Philadelphia, 1996a, F.A. Davis.

Boyd ST, Hanson SMH: Family nursing practice in the 21st century. In Hanson SMH, Boyd ST: *Family health care nursing: theory, practice and research,* Philadelphia, 1996b, F.A. Davis.

Broderick CB: Beyond the five conceptual frameworks: a decade of development in family theory, *J Marriage Fam* 33:129, 1971.

Continued

Bibliography—cont'd

Bumpass LL, Sweet JA, Martin TC: Changing patterns of remarriage, *J Marriage Fam* 52:747, 1990.

Burton LM, Dilworth-Anderson P, Merriwether-deVries C: Context and surrogate parenting among contemporary grandparents. In Hanson SMH et al, editors: *Single-parent families: diversity, myths, and realities*, New York, 1995, the Haworth Press.

Carnevali D, Thomas M: *Diagnostic reasoning and treatment decision making in nursing*, Philadelphia, 1993, J.B. Lippincott.

Carter E, McGoldrick M: The family life cycle and family therapy: an overview. In Carter E, McGoldrick M, editors: *The changing family life cycle: a framework for family therapists*, New York, 1988, Gardner Press.

Cherlin AJ: *Marriage, divorce, remarriage,* Cambridge, 1992, Harvard University Press.

Curran D: *Traits of a healthy family,* Minneapolis, 1983, Winston Press (Harper & Row).

Curran D: *Stress and the healthy family,* Minneapolis, 1985, Winston Press (Harper & Row).

Danielson CB, Hamel-Bissell B, Winstead-Fry P: *Families, health and illness: perspectives on coping and intervention,* St Louis, 1993, Mosby.

Davidson JK, Moore NB: *Marriage and family: change and continuity,* Boston, 1996, Allyn & Bacon.

Dreman S, editor: *The family on the threshold of the 21st century,* Mahwah, NJ, 1997, Lawrence Erlbaum Associates.

Duvall EM: *Marriage and family development,* ed 5, Philadelphia, 1977, J.B. Lippincott.

Duvall EM, Miller BL: *Marriage and family development,* ed 6, New York, 1985, Harper & Row.

Elliott B: *Vision 2010: families and health care,* Minneapolis, 1993, National Council on Family Relations.

Epenshade TJ: Marital careers of American women: a cohort life table analysis. In Bongaarts J, Burch TK, Wachter KW, editors: *Family demography: methods and their application,* New York, 1987, Oxford University Press.

Eshleman JR: *The family,* ed 8, Boston, 1997, Allyn & Bacon.

Fawcett J: *Analysis and evaluation of conceptual models of nursing,* ed 3, Philadelphia, 1995, F.A. Davis.

Friedemann ML: *The framework of systemic organization: a conceptual approach to families and nursing,* Thousand Oaks, 1995, Sage.

Friedman MM: *Family nursing: research, theory and practice,* ed 4, Norwalk, Conn, 1998, Appleton & Lange.

Furstenberg FF, Spannier GB: *Recycling the family: remarriage after divorce,* Beverly Hills, Calif, 1984, Sage.

Gelles RJ: *Sociology: an introduction,* ed 5, New York, 1995, McGraw Hill.

Gillis CL: Family nursing research, theory and practice. In Wegner GD, Alexander RJ: *Readings in family nursing,* Philadelphia, 1993, J.B. Lippincott.

Gladding ST: *Family therapy: history, theory, and practice,* Englewood Cliffs, NJ, 1995, Prentice Hall.

Gordon M: *Manual of nursing diagnosis,* New York, 1997-1998, McGraw-Hill.

Hanson SL, Ooms T: The economic costs and rewards of two-earner, two-parent families, *J Marriage Fam* 51:622, 1991.

Hanson SMH: Family assessment and intervention. In Hanson SMH, Boyd S: *Family health care nursing: theory, practice and research,* Philadelphia, 1996, F.A. Davis.

Hanson SMH, Boyd ST: Family nursing: an overview. In Hanson SMH, Boyd ST: *Family health care nursing: theory, practice and research,* Philadelphia, 1996a, F.A. Davis.

Hanson SMH, Boyd ST: *Family health care nursing: theory, practice and research,* Philadelphia, 1996b, F.A. Davis.

Hanson SMH, Heims ML: Family nursing curricula in U.S. schools of nursing, *Family Relations* 31(7):303, 1993.

Hanson SMH, Heims ML, Julian DJ: Education for family health care professionals: nursing as a paradigm, *Family Relations* 41:49, 1992.

Hanson SMH, Kaakinen J: Family nursing assessment. In Stanhope M, Lancaster J, editors: *Community health nursing: promoting health of aggregates, families, and individuals,* ed 4, St Louis, 1996, Mosby.

Hanson SMH, Kaakinen JR, Friedman MM: Theoretical approaches to family nursing. In Friedman MM: *Family nursing: theory and practice,* ed 4, Norwalk, Conn, 1998, Appleton & Lange.

Hanson SMH, Mischke K: Family health assessment and intervention. In Bomar P, editor: *Nurses and family health promotion: concepts, assessments and interventions,* ed 2, Philadelphia, 1996, W.B. Saunders.

Hartman A: Diagrammatic assessment of family relationships, *Social Casework* 59:465, 1978.

Jones SL, Dimond SL: Family theory and family therapy models: comparative review with implications for nursing practice, *J Psychosoc Nurs Ment Health Serv* 20(10):12, 1982.

Kaakinen J: An ecological view of elders and their families: needs for the 21st century. In Dempsey C, Butkus R, editors: *All creation is groaning,* Collegeville, Minn, in press, Liturgical Press.

Kinsella K: Aging and the family: present and future demographic issues. In Blieszner T, Bedford V, editors: *Aging and the family: theory and research,* Westport, Conn, 1996, Praeger.

Kirschling JM: "Success" in family nursing: experts describe phenomena, *Nurs Health Care* 15:186, 1994.

Klein DM, White JM: *Family theories: an introduction,* Thousand Oaks, Calif, 1996, Sage.

Levinson D, editor: *Encyclopedia of marriage and the family,* vol 1, New York, 1995, Simon & Schuster Macmillan..

Lino M: The economics of single parenthood: past research and future directions. In Hanson SMH et al, editors: *Single parent families,* New York, 1995, Haworth Press.

Lueckenotte A: *Gerontologic nursing,* St Louis, 1996, Mosby.

Macklin ED: Nontraditional family forms. In Sussman MB, Steinmetz SK, editors: *Handbook of marriage and the family,* New York, 1988, Plenum.

Martin K, Scheet M: *The Omaha system: application for community health nursing,* Philadelphia, 1992, W.B. Saunders.

McCray JW: Multicultural diversity and ethical considerations in research design, *J Home Econ* 86(2):41, 1994.

McGoldrick M, Gerson R: *Genograms in family assessment,* New York, 1985, W.W. Norton.

Mead G: *Mind, self and society,* Chicago, 1934, University of Chicago Press.

National Center for Health Statistics: Births, marriages, divorces, and deaths for 1993, *Mon Vital Stat Rep* 42(12), 1994.

National Center for Health Statistics: *Health: United States, 1993,* DHHS Pub No (PHS) 94-1232, Hyattsville, Md, 1994, US Public Health Service.

National Center for Health Statistics: *Health: United States, 1994,* DHHS Pub No (PHS) 95-1232, Hyattsville, Md, 1995, US Public Health Service.

Neuman B, editor: *The Neuman systems model,* ed 2, Norwalk, Conn, 1989, Appleton & Lange.

Nye FI, Berardo F, editors: *Emerging conceptual frameworks in family analysis,* New York, 1981, Praeger.

O'Hare WP: America's minorities: the demographics of diversity, *Population Bulletin* 47(4):1992

Pender N et al: Health promotion and disease prevention: toward excellence in nursing practice and education, *Nurs Outlook,* 40:106 1992.

Reed KS: *Betty Neuman: the Neuman systems model,* Newbury Park, Calif, 1993, Sage.

Ross BJ: Nursing process and family health care. In Hanson SMH, Boyd S: *Family health care nursing: theory, practice and research,* Philadelphia, 1996, F.A. Davis

Ross BJ, Cobb KL: *Family nursing: a nursing process approach,* Redwood City, Calif, 1990, Addison-Wesley.

Satariano HJ, Briggs NJ: The good family syndrome. In Wegner GD, Alexander RJ: *Readings in family nursing,* Philadelphia, 1993, J.B. Lippincott.

Settles BH: A perspective on tomorrow's families. In Sussman MB, Steinmetz SK, editors: *Handbook of marriage and the family,* New York, 1987, Plenum.

Stanhope M: Family theories and development. In Stanhope M, Lancaster J, editors: *Community health nursing: promoting health of aggregates, families, and individuals,* ed 4, St Louis, 1996, Mosby.

Sussman MB, Steinmetz SK, editors: *Handbook of marriage and the family,* New York, 1987, Plenum.

Teachman JD, Polonko KA, Scanzioni J: Demography of the family. In Sussman MB, Steinmetz SK, editors: *Handbook of marriage and the family,* New York, 1987, Plenum.

Thornton A: Changing attitudes toward family issues in the United States, *J Marriage Fam* 51: 873, 1989.

US Census Bureau: *Current population reports, Series p-20-477 and p-20-478,* Washington, DC, 1994a, US Government Printing Office.

US Census Bureau, Rawlings SW, Saluter A: *Household and family characteristics: March 1994,* Current population reports, Series p-20, No. 483, Washington, DC, 1994b, US Government Printing Office.

US Census Bureau: *Marital status and living arrangements: March 1990,* Current population reports, Series p-20, No. 450, Washington, DC, 1991, US Government Printing Office.

US Census Bureau, Saluter A: *Marital status and living arrangements: March 1995,* PPL-52, 1995b.

US Census Bureau: *Marriage, divorce, and remarriage in the 1990's,* Current population reports, Series p-23, No 180, Washington, DC, 1992, US Government Printing Office.

US Census Bureau: *Statistical abstract of the United States, 1995,* Current population reports, Series p-60, No 184, Washington DC, 1995a, US Government Printing Office.

US Census Bureau: *Statistical abstract of the United States,* ed 115, Washington, DC, 1995c, US Government Printing Office.

US Department of Health and Human Services: *Healthy people 2000: national health promotion and disease prevention objectives,* Washington, DC, 1990, USDHHS.

US Department of Health and Human Services: *International classification of diseases,* ed 4, Washington, DC, 1991, USDHHS.

Vaughan-Cole B et al: *Family nursing practice,* Philadelphia, 1998, W.B. Saunders.

Whall AL: *Family therapy theory for nursing: four approaches,* Norwalk, Conn, 1986, Appleton-Century-Crofts.

Wright LM, Leahey M: *Nurses and families: a guide to family assessment and intervention,* ed 2, Philadelphia, 1994, F.A. Davis.

Zimmerman S: *Family policies and family wellbeing: the role of political culture,* Newbury Park, Calif, 1992, Sage International.

CHAPTER 25

Family Health Risks

CAROL LOVELAND-CHERRY

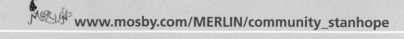 www.mosby.com/MERLIN/community_stanhope

OBJECTIVES

After reading this chapter, the student should be able to do the following:

- Analyze the various approaches to defining and conceptualizing family health.
- Analyze the major risks to family health.
- Analyze the interrelationship among individual health, family health, and community health.

- Explain the relevance of knowledge about family structures, roles, and functions for the family-focused community health nursing process.
- Explain the application of the nursing process (assessment, planning, implementation, evaluation) for reducing family health risks and promoting family health.

KEY TERMS

adaptive model	family crisis	initiation phase	social risks
biologic risk	family health	life-event risk	termination phase
clinical model	health risk appraisal	lifestyle risk	transitions
contracting	health risk reduction	postvisit phase	
economic risk	health risks	previsit phase	
empowerment	home visits	risk	
eudaimonistic model	in-home phase	role-performance model	*See Glossary for definitions*

CHAPTER OUTLINE

Early Approaches to Family
  Health Risks
    Health of Families
    Health of the Nation
Concepts in Family Health Risk
    Family Health
    Health Risk
    Health Risk Appraisal
    Health Risk Reduction

Life Events
    Family Crisis
Major Family Health Risks
    Biologic Risk
    Social Risk
    Economic Risk
    Lifestyle Risk
    Life-Event Risk

Community Health Nursing
  Approaches to Family Health
  Risk Reduction
    Family Health Risk Appraisal
    Home Visits
    Contracting with Families
    Enabling and Empowering
      Families
Community Resources

506

The importance of the family in promoting the health of individuals and communities is well established (Bomar, 1996; Feetham et al, 1992; Gilliss et al, 1989; Nightingale et al, 1978). Acknowledgment of the family as a client unit has been a basic assumption underlying the practice of community health nursing, but how does family health fit into the larger health care picture, such as *Healthy People 2000*? Do families have a contribution to make? Are the broader health goals sensitive to the needs of the family?

In establishing health objectives for the nation, an emphasis has been placed on both health promotion and risk reduction. Reducing the risks to segments of the population is a direct way of improving the health of the general population. Specific risks have been identified and related to specific objectives. Although none of the objectives directly address families, the family is both an important environment affecting the health of individuals and a unit whose health is basic to that of the community and larger population. It is within the family that health behavior, including health values, health habits, and health risk perceptions, are developed, organized, and performed. Individuals' health behaviors are affected by and acted out within the family environment, larger community, and society. In turn, the larger community and society are made up of and depend upon the functioning of individuals for continued well-being. For example, traditional indices of morbidity and mortality rates are computed on the basis of grouped data about individuals (see Chapter 11).

To intervene effectively and appropriately with families to reduce their health risk and thereby promote their health, it is necessary to understand family structure and functioning, family theory, nursing theory, and models of health risk (see Chapters 10, 14, and 24). However, it is necessary to go beyond the individual and the family and understand the complex environment in which the family exists. Increasing evidence of the effect of social, biological, economic, and life events on health requires a broader approach to addressing health risks for families. Pender (1996) identifies six categories of risk factors: genetics, age, biologic characteristics, personal health habits, lifestyle, and environment.

In this chapter, health risks in these six categories for families are identified and analyzed, and approaches to reducing these risks are discussed. Options for structuring nursing interventions with families to decrease health risks and to promote health and well-being are explored.

EARLY APPROACHES TO FAMILY HEALTH RISKS
Health of Families

Early consideration of the family in health and illness focused on three major areas: 1) the effect of illness on families, 2) the role of the family in the cause of disease, and 3) the role of the family in use of services. In his classic review of the family as an important unit, Litman (1974) points out the important role that the family plays in health and illness as a primary unit of health care and emphasizes that the relationship among health, health behavior, and family "is a highly dynamic one in which each may have a dramatic effect on the other" (Litman, 1974, p. 495). Mauksch (1974) proposes the idea of distinguishing family health from individual health. Pratt's (1976) examination of the role of the family in health and illness expanded the literature to include the role of family health in promoting behavior. Pratt proposes the "energized family" as being an ideal family type most effective in meeting health needs. The energized family is characterized by promoting freedom and change, a variety and active contact with other groups and organizations, flexible role relationships, equal power structure, and a high degree of autonomy in family members. Doherty and McCubbin (1985) propose a family health and illness cycle with six phases:
1. Family health promotion and risk reduction
2. Family vulnerability and illness onset
3. Family illness appraisal
4. Family acute response
5. Family and health care system interaction
6. Family adaptation to illness

Health of the Nation

Paralleling the focus in family studies on health, increased attention was being given to ways to improve the health of everyone in the United States. As the result of major public health and scientific advances, the leading causes of morbidity and mortality shifted from infectious diseases to chronic diseases, accidents, and violence, all of which have strong lifestyle and environmental components. A population-focused study in Alameda County, California (Belloc and Breslow, 1972) demonstrated relationships between seven lifestyle habits and morbidity and mortality. These habits were 1) sleeping 7 to 8 hours daily, 2) eating breakfast almost every day, 3) never or rarely eating between meals, 4) being at or near recommended height-adjusted weight, 5) never smoking cigarettes, 6) moderate or no use of alcohol, and 7) regular physical activity.

A growing body of literature supported the notion that lifestyle and the environment interact with hereditary tendencies for disease. In response to these findings and the limited effect of medical interventions on the growing incidence and prevalence of injuries and chronic disease, the government launched a major effort to address the health status of the population. Part of this effort was a report by the Division of Health Promotion and Disease Prevention of the Institute of Medicine (IOM) that examined the critical components of the physical, socioeconomic, and family environments related to decreasing risk and promoting health (Nightengale et al, 1978). The *Surgeon General's Report on Health Promotion and Disease Prevention* (Califano, 1979) described the risks to good health. Health objectives for the nation were established and then evaluated and restated for the year 2000 (USDHHS, 1991).

Within this context, the notion of **risk,** a factor predisposing or increasing the likelihood of ill health, took on increased importance. Specific attention was paid to those "environmental and behavioral influences capable of provoking ill health with or without previous predisposition" (Califano, 1979, p. 13). The reduction of health risks is a major approach to improving the health of the nation. Although the family is considered an important environment related to achieving important health objectives, limited attention and research have been given to family health risk.

CONCEPTS IN FAMILY HEALTH RISK

Individuals participate in behaviors for two motivations. One of these underlying forces is health promotion, "behaviors directed toward increasing the level of well-being and actualizing the health potential of individuals, families, communities and society" (Pender, 1996, p. 4). In contrast, health protecting behaviors are those "directed toward decreasing the probability of specific illness or dysfunction in individuals, families, and communities, including active protection against unnecessary stressors" (Pender, 1996, p. 4). The same behavior may be undertaken from either of the two perspectives. Health risk is conceptually consistent with the notion of health protecting behaviors.

Understanding family health risk requires an examination of several related concepts: family health, family health risk, risk appraisal, risk reduction, life events, lifestyle, and family crisis. Although health is a vague term that can be defined from a number of perspectives, it usually is defined by the individual within his or her own culture and value system. Similarly, illness is the experience of a disease process.

Family Health

Family theorists refer to healthy families but generally do not define family health. Based on the various family theoretical perspectives (see Chapters 10, 14, and 24) definitions of healthy families can be derived within the guidelines of any one of the frameworks. For example, within the perspective of the developmental framework, **family health** can be defined as possessing the abilities and resources to accomplish family developmental tasks. Thus the accomplishment of stage-specific tasks is one indicator of family health.

From the perspective of Neuman's model (1989), family health would be defined in terms of system stability as characterized by five interacting sets of factors: physiological, psychological, sociocultural, developmental, and spiritual.

Another dimension of family health can be identified using Smith's (1983) four models of health, which are listed in Table 25-1: clinical model, role-performance model, adaptive model, and eudaimonistic model.

The following clinical example applies these models to one family's situation:

The Harris family consists of Mr. and Mrs. Harris, 12-year-old Kevin, and 6-year-old Leisha. Kevin was recently diagnosed with insulin-dependent diabetes mellitus (IDDM), and the family was referred by the endocrinology clinic for community health nursing service to work with the family in adjusting to the diagnosis.

The focus in a **clinical model** approach might be to identify realistic perceptions of health risks for Kevin and to teach the parents how to recognize and deal with symptoms of complications. Assessment would include completing a family health/illness history, determining Mr. and Mrs. Harris' perceptions and knowledge of diabetes mellitus, identifying the family's health care resources, and recognizing their concerns about caring for a child with a chronic disease.

Assessment in the **role-performance model** includes exploring with the family their feelings about their abilities and resources to accomplish developmental tasks. This family is in the developmental stage of families with school-age children based on the age of the oldest child. Developmental tasks for families in this stage include the following (Duvall and Miller, 1985, p. 217):
1. Providing suitable housing and health care for the family
2. Meeting family costs and making adjustments when the wife/mother works
3. Allocating and monitoring responsibilities for maintaining the home
4. Continuing socialization through wider community participation
5. Encouraging husband-wife, parent-child, and child-child communication
6. Rearing children with appropriate parenting skills in two-parent, one-parent, or reconstituted family households
7. Demonstrating interest in children's schooling and in their acquisition of basic skills and knowledge
8. Recognizing achievement and growth of individual family members and building solid values and morals in the family

Assessment in the **adaptive model** focuses on identifying with the family the kinds of changes that have occurred since Kevin's diagnosis and the different or new demands that have resulted. The nurse would work with the family members to help them adapt to having a child with a chronic illness and to repattern their lives to deal with the related increased and different demands on the family. By pointing out the knowledge and skills that the family already has and the ways to adapt them to the changes in the family system, the nurse builds on family competencies. Another potential intervention would be to identify appropriate services in the community, such as support groups and summer camps for children with diabetes mellitus.

In the **eudaimonistic model,** the nurse could work with the family in reassessing family goals and ways to meet them. The diagnosis of a family member with a chronic condition indicates assessment of family values and goals, such as socializing and educating children, family recreation, and patterns of interacting. It might be ap-

TABLE 25-1 Smith's Four Models of Health

MODEL	VIEW OF HEALTH	ASSESSMENT	NURSING GOALS
Clinical	*Individual:* The absence of disease *Family:* The absence of disease or dysfunction	Includes family health/illness history; family's definition of health and illness; family's value of health; family's knowledge of health promotion and illness prevention/treatment; family practices related to nutrition, sleep/rest, exercise, and recreation; use of alcohol, tobacco, drugs; family processes for determining illness and whether and how professional care will be sought	To promote family's physical, mental, and social health; to provide comfort in the family; to prevent deterioration of family system
Role performance	*Individual:* Effective performance of roles *Family:* Effective meeting of family functions and developmental tasks	Includes family's current developmental stage/history; family's role structure, socialization patterns, resources for meeting functions and developmental tasks; family's perceptions of family functioning	To promote effective performance of family functions; to promote achievement of developmental tasks; to assist in identifying and mobilizing support systems and resources
Adaptive	*Individual:* Condition of the whole person engaged in effective interaction with physical/social environment *Family:* Condition of the whole family engaged in effective interaction with physical/social environment; family/environment fit	Includes the identification of family coping patterns, social networks, and support systems; family's perceptions of their environment; family's flexibility in altering behaviors, roles, rules, and perceptions when needed	To promote the family's adaptation and health-directed patterning with the environment
Eudaimonistic	*Individual:* Complete development of individual's potential for general well being and self-realization *Family:* Development of family's well-being and maximum potential	Includes family's values and goals; family interaction patterns of recreation and relaxation; family cohesion; family promotion of autonomy	To clarify family's values; to assist in identifying and prioritizing family's goals; to assist family in implementing plans to meet goals

Adapted from Smith JA: *The idea of health: implications for the nursing professional,* New York, 1983, Teachers College Press, Columbia University.

propriate to inform the family about how they could offer support to other families in similar circumstances. Based on the assessment, the nurse can assist the family in identifying areas of strength and areas where external community resources may be necessary.

Health Risk

Several factors contribute to the experience of healthy/unhealthy outcomes. Clearly, not everyone exposed to the same event will have the same outcome. The factors that determine or influence whether disease or other unhealthy results occur are called **health risks.** This notion of controlling health risks is central to disease prevention and health promotion (Califano, 1979). Health risks can be classified into general categories. Califano (1979) identifies four major categories: inherited biological risk, environmental risk, behavioral risk, and age-related risk. Each of these categories of risk is discussed in terms of family health risk in the following section. Although risk factors can singly influence outcomes, the cumulated risks can work in combination with one another. Their combined effect is more than the sum of the individual effects. For example, a family history of cardiovascular disease is a single risk factor that is effected by smoking, a behavioral risk. This combination of risks is greater for males than females (up to a certain age). Thus the combined effect of a family history, smoking, and being male is greater than merely considering each of the three individual risk factors.

Health Risk Appraisal

Health risk appraisal refers to the process of assessing the presence of specific factors within each of the categories that have been identified as being associated with an increased likelihood of an illness, such as cancer, or an unhealthy event, such as an automobile accident. Several techniques have been developed to accomplish health risk appraisal, including computer software programs and paper and pencil instruments. The general approach is to determine whether a risk factor is present and to what degree. Based on scientific evidence, each factor is weighted and a total sum score is derived.

Health Risk Reduction

Health risk reduction is based on the assumption that decreasing the number of risks or the magnitude of risk will result in a lower probability of the undesired event (e.g., substance abuse in adolescents). Reduction of health risks can be accomplished through a variety of approaches, usually specific to the theory and research knowledge related to the particular risk. In considering health risk reduction, it is important to note that the characteristics of the specific risk influence individuals' and families' tolerance of the risk (Pender, 1996). Pender (1996) provides examples of the effects of the nature of risks:

1. Voluntarily assumed risks are tolerated better than those imposed by others.
2. Risks over which scientists debate and are uncertain are more feared than risks on which scientists agree.
3. Risks of natural origin are often considered less threatening than those created by humans.

Thus risk reduction is a complex process that requires knowledge of the specific risk and families' perceptions of the nature of the risk.

Life Events

Life events can increase the risk for illness and disability. These events can be categorized as either normative or nonnormative. Normative events are those that generally are expected to occur at a particular stage of development or of the lifespan.

Normative events can be identified from the Family Developmental Framework. Examples of normative events are a child leaving home to go to college, retirement from work, and starting a first job. Nonnormative events, in contrast, are those that are not anticipated to occur with any ability to predict (e.g., loss of a job). Furthermore, life events and the accumulation of such events can, under certain conditions, result in a family crisis.

> **WHAT DO YOU THINK?** *Government priority to funding health risk reduction and health promotion programs, including assistance programs, would have greater benefit to the population's health than funding for illness activities.*

Family Crisis

A crisis exists when the family is not able to cope with the event and becomes disorganized or dysfunctional. When the demands of the situation exceed the resources of the family, a **family crisis** exists. When families experience a crisis or crisis-producing event, they attempt to gather their resources to deal with the demands created by the situation. Burr and colleagues (1994) differentiate between family resources and family coping strategies. The former are the resources that a family has available to them. The latter are the "active processes and behaviors families actually try to do to help them manage, adapt, or deal with the stressful situation" (Burr et al, 1994, p. 129). Thus if a family were to experience an unexpected illness in the main wage earner, family resources might include financial assistance from relatives or emotional support. Family coping strategies, in contrast, would include whether the family asked a relative to loan them emergency funds or talked with relatives about the worries they were experiencing. Based on the existing literature, Burr and colleagues developed a three-level classification of coping strategies with seven major categories, 20 subcategories, and 41 sub-subcategories. Although the last level is too extensive to present here, the seven major categories and 20 subcategories are listed in Table 25-2.

MAJOR FAMILY HEALTH RISKS

Risks to families' health arise in several major areas: biologic risk, social risk, economic risk, lifestyle risk, and life events leading to crisis. In most instances, no one of these five areas is sufficient to be a single threat to family health; rather a combination of risks from two or more categories is more usual. For example, there may be a family history of cardiovascular disease, but often the health risk is compounded by an unhealthy lifestyle. An understanding of each of these categories provides the basis for a comprehensive perspective on family health risk assessment and intervention.

Beginning with the Surgeon General's report (Califano, 1979), an emphasis in health promotion and disease prevention has focused on these lifestyle patterns. *Healthy People 2000* targets areas in health promotion, health protection, preventive services, and surveillance and data systems to describe age-related objectives (USDHHS, 1991). Included in the area of health promotion are physical activity and fitness, nutrition, tobacco use, use of alcohol and other drugs, family planning, mental health and mental disorders, and violent and abusive behavior. Health protection activities include issues related to unintentional injuries, occupational safety and health, environmental health, food and drug safety, and oral health. Preventive services relate to reducing risk related to illness and include maternal and infant health, heart disease and stroke, cancer, diabetes and chronic disabling conditions, HIV infection, sexually transmitted diseases, immunization and infectious diseases, and clinical preventive services. The interrelationships among the various groups of risk are clear when the objectives for the nation are considered.

TABLE 25-2 Burr and Klein's Conceptual Framework of Coping Strategies

HIGHLY ABSTRACT STATEGIES	MODERATELY ABSTRACT STRATEGIES
1. Cognitive	1. Be accepting of the situation and others 2. Gain useful knowledge 3. Change how the situation is viewed or defined (reframe the situation)
2. Emotional	4. Express feelings and affection 5. Avoid or resolve negative feelings and disabling expressions of emotion 6. Be sensitive to others' emotional needs
3. Relationships	7. Increase cohesion (togetherness) 8. Increase adaptability 9. Develop increased trust 10. Increase cooperation 11. Increase tolerance of one another
4. Communication	12. Be open and honest 13. Listen to one another 14. Be sensitive to nonverbal communication
5. Community	15. Seek help and support from others 16. Fulfill expectations in organizations
6. Spiritual	17. Be more involved in religious activities 18. Increase faith or seek help from God
7. Individual development	19. Develop autonomy, independence, and self-sufficiency 20. Keep active in hobbies

From Burr WR et al: *Reexamining family stress: new theory and research*, Thousand Oaks, Calif, 1994, Sage.

Biologic Risk

The family plays an important role both in the development and in the management of a disease or condition. Several illnesses have a familial component that can be accounted for either from a genetic basis or established lifestyle patterns. These formulated factors contribute to the **biologic risk** for certain conditions. Patterns of cardiovascular disease, for example, often can be traced through many generations of families. Such families are said to be at risk for cardiovascular disease. How or whether cardiovascular disease is found in a family is often influenced by the lifestyle of the family. Consistent research evidence supports the positive mediating effects of diet, exercise, and stress management on preventing or delaying cardiovascular disease. An inclination for hypertension can be managed by following a low-sodium diet, maintaining a normal weight, regular exercise, and effective stress management techniques, such as meditation. Diabetes mellitus is another disease with a strong genetic pattern, and the family plays a major role in the management of the condition. Family patterns of obesity increase the risk in individuals for a number of conditions, including coronary heart disease, hypertension, diabetes, some types of cancer, and gallbladder disease (USDHHS, 1991).

Another form of biologic risk experienced by families is being susceptible to certain illnesses. Generally, if a family maintains a level of general health, individual members are less at risk for contracting certain infectious diseases. This protection can be extended by maintaining health practices, such as current immunizations, adequate nutrition, and adequate rest (see Chapter 38).

Social Risk

The importance of **social risks** to families' health is gaining increased recognition (see Chapters 7 and 8). Living in high-crime neighborhoods, communities without adequate recreational or health resources, communities that have major chemical noise or other contaminants, or other high-stress environments increases a family's health risk. One social stress is discrimination, whether racial, cultural, or other. The psychological burden resulting from discrimination is a stressor in and of itself and also adds to the effects of other stressors. The implication of these examples of risky social situations is that they contribute to the stressors experienced by the families. If adequate resources and coping processes are not available, breakdowns in health can occur.

Economic Risk

The poor are at greater risk for health problems (see Chapter 32). **Economic risk** is determined by the relationship between family financial resources and demands on those resources. Having adequate financial resources means that a family is able to purchase the necessary commodities related to health. These include adequate housing, clothing, food, education, and health/illness care. The amount of money that a family has available needs to be considered relative to spending and to social factors. A family may have an income well above the poverty level, but because of a devastating illness in a family member, the family may not be able to meet financial demands. Likewise, families from ethnic populations frequently experience discrimination in finding housing; even if they find housing, they may not be welcome and may be harassed, resulting in increased stress.

Unfortunately, not all families have access to health care insurance. For families at the poverty level, programs like Medicaid are available to pay for health and illness care; families in the upper income brackets can either afford to pay for health care out-of-pocket, purchase health insurance, or are in employment situations that have health care benefits. An increasing number of families have major wage earners in jobs that do not have health benefits, do not have a sufficient income to purchase health care, and earn too much money to qualify for public assistance programs. Consequently, many families have financial resources that allow them to maintain a subsistence level but that limit the quality of their purchasing power. Illness care may be available but not preventive care; food high in fat and calories may be affordable, while fresh fruit and vegetables are not. A U.S. Department of Agriculture (USDA) study found that for "every $1.00 spent on a pregnant woman in its Women, Infants and Children (WIC) program, $1.77 to $3.13 is saved in Medicaid costs during her child's first 60 days of life" (Greer, 1995, p. 6).

Lifestyle Risk

Personal health habits continue to contribute to the major causes of morbidity and mortality in the United States (see Chapter 14). The pattern of personal health habits and risk behaviors defines individual and family **lifestyle risk.** The family is the basic unit within which health behavior, including health values, health habits, and health risk perceptions, is developed, organized, and performed. Families maintain major responsibility for determining what food is purchased and prepared, setting sleep patterns, planning family activities, setting and monitoring norms about health and health risk behaviors, determining when a family member is ill, determining when health care should be obtained, and carrying out treatment regimens. Diet has been identified as an element in 5 of the 10 leading causes of death in the United States (USDHHS, 1991). General guidelines from the USDHHS and the USDA include eating a variety of foods; maintaining healthy weight; choosing a diet low in fat and cholesterol, including plenty of vegetables, fruits, and grain products; moderate use of sugars, salt, and sodium; and alcohol consumption only in moderation.

DID YOU KNOW? *Adolescents from families that have close, supportive interactions, clearly set and enforced rules, and parents who are involved with their children have decreased risk for alcohol use or misuse. These family patterns can be enhanced through family-focused intervention sessions in the home.*

Multiple health benefits of regular physical activity have been identified; regular physical exercise is effective in health promotion, disease prevention, and health maintenance. Among the benefits of regular physical activity are increased muscle strength, endurance, and flexibility; management of weight; prevention of colon cancer, stroke, and back injury; and prevention and management of coronary heart disease, hypertension, diabetes, osteoporosis, and depression (USDHHS, 1991). Families structure time and activities and can be helped to select between those that are sedentary and those that provide moderate, regular physical activity.

Substance use is a major contributor to morbidity and mortality in the United States. Tobacco use has been identified as the single most preventable cause of death; it has been associated with several types of cancer, coronary heart disease, low birth weight, prematurity, sudden infant death syndrome, and chronic obstructive pulmonary disease. Furthermore, passive smoking has been linked to disease in nonsmokers and children. Drug use, including alcohol, is a major social and health problem. Alcohol use is a factor in approximately 50% of homicides, suicides, and motor vehicle deaths (USDHHS, 1991). Drug use is associated with transmission of HIV, fetal alcohol syndrome, liver disease, unwanted pregnancy, delinquency, school failure, violence, and crime. The literature consistently identifies the effects of family factors, such as family closeness, families doing activities together, and behavior modeled in the family as decreasing the risk of children for substance use.

Although violence and abusive behavior are not limited to families, the amount of intrafamilial violence is thought to be underestimated. The obvious difficulties in collecting sensitive data from families make it difficult to obtain accurate statistics on family violence. Evidence supports the intergenerational nature of violence and abuse; abusers were often abused as children.

Life-Event Risk

Transitions, movement from one stage or condition to another, are times of potential risk for families. Transitions present new situations and demands for families. These experiences often require that families change behaviors, schedules, and patterns of communication; make new decisions; reallocate family roles; learn new skills; and identify and learn to use new resources. The demands that transitions place on families have implications for the health of the family unit and individual family members and can be considered as **life-event risk.** How well prepared families are to deal with transitions is affected by the nature of the event. If the event is a normative, or anticipated, event, then it is possible for families to identify needed resources, make plans, learn new skills, or otherwise prepare for the event and its consequences. This kind of anticipatory preparation can increase the family's coping processes and lessen stress and negative outcomes. If, on the other hand, the event is nonnormative, or unexpected, families have little or no time to prepare and the outcome can be increased stress, crisis, or even dysfunction. Table 25-3 lists family stages and the developmental tasks associated with each stage.

Several normative events have been identified for families. The developmental family framework organizes these events within a staged model and identifies important transition points. The developmental model provides a useful framework for identifying normative events and preparing families to cope successfully with related demands. The developmental tasks associated with each stage define the types of skills families need to acquire. The kinds of normative events families experience usually are related to the addition or loss of a family member, such as the birth or adoption of a child, the death of a grandparent, a child moving out of the home to go to school or take a job, or the marriage of a child. There are health-related responsibilities associated with each of these tasks. For example, the birth or adoption of a child requires that families learn about human growth and development, parenting, immunizations, management of childhood illnesses, normal childhood nutrition, and safety issues.

Nonnormative events present different kinds of issues for families. The nature of unexpected events can be either positive or negative. A job promotion or inheriting a substantial sum of money may be unexpected but are usually positive events. More often nonnormative events are unpleasant, such as a major illness, divorce, the death of a child, or loss of the main family income.

Regardless of whether a life event is normative or nonnormative, it is often a source of stress for families. Several theoretical frameworks have been developed to examine the processes of family stress and coping. Perhaps the most widely used and developed is the ABC-X model and its evolution over time. The model was originally developed by Hill (1949) and was based on work with families separated by war. Within the model, crisis (X) was proposed to be a product of the nature of the event (A), the family's definition of the event (B), and the resources available to the family (C). McCubbin extended the model to the Double ABC-X Model to encompass the period after the initial crisis and introduced the idea of a pile-up of stressors. Adaptation or maladaptation by the family is proposed to be predicted by the pile up of stressors (Aa), the family's perception of the crisis (Bb), and new resources and coping strategies (Cc).

TABLE 25-3 Family Developmental Tasks

FAMILY STAGES	DEVELOPMENTAL TASKS
Beginning family	Establishing a marriage Relating to kin network Family planning
Early childbearing family	Stabilizing the family unit Reconciling family members' conflicting developmental tasks Facilitating developmental needs of mother, father, and infant
Family with preschool child(ren)	Nurturing and socializing children Maintaining a stable marriage
Family with school-age child(ren)	Socializing children Promoting school achievement Maintaining satisfactory marital relationship
Family with teenager(s)	Balancing teenage freedom and responsibility Maintaining open parent-child communication Maintaining a stable marital relationship Building a foundation for future family stages
Launching family	Releasing children as young adults Readjusting the marriage Assisting aging parents
Middle-age family	Strengthening the marital relationship Sustaining relationships with parents and children Providing a healthy environment Cultivating leisure-time activities
Aging family	Adjusting to retirement Maintaining satisfactory living arrangement Adjusting to reduced income Adjusting to health problems Adjusting to death of spouse

Adapted from Friedman MM: *Family nursing; theory and assessment*, East Norwalk, Conn 1992, Appleton & Lange.

Burr and colleagues (1994) recently challenged this linear view of families and stress and coping. They advocate a more systems-oriented conceptualization of family stress. They point out that families develop a series of processes to manage or transform inputs to the system (e.g., energy, time) to outputs (e.g., cohesion, growth, love) known as "rules of transformation." Over time, families develop these patterns in sufficient quantity and variety to handle most changes and challenges; this is referred to as "requisite variety of rules of transformation." It is when families do not have an adequate variety of rules to allow them to respond to an event that the event then becomes stressful. Rather than proceeding to deal with the situation, they fall into a pattern of trying to figure out what it is they need to do and the usual tasks of the family are not adequately addressed. Rules that were implicit in the family are now reconsidered and redefined.

Furthermore, the reformulation of family stress theory proposes three levels of stress: Level I is change "in the fairly specific patterns of behavior and transformation processes" (e.g., change in who does which household chores); Level II is change "in processes that are at a higher level of abstraction" (e.g., change in what are defined as family chores); and Level III are changes in highly abstract processes (e.g., family values) (Burr et al, 1994, pp. 44-45). There are coping strategies identified to address each level of stress that families go through in sequence, if necessary (see the Research Brief about the Neuman Systems Model).

COMMUNITY HEALTH NURSING APPROACHES TO FAMILY HEALTH RISK REDUCTION
Family Health Risk Appraisal

Assessment of family health risk requires multiple approaches to address the many components of risk. As in any assessment, the first and most important task is to get to know the family, their strengths, and their needs (see Chapter 24). This section focuses on appraisal of family health risks within biologic, social, economic, lifestyle, and life events risk.

Biologic health risk

One of the most effective techniques for assessing the patterns of health and illness in families is the use of the family genogram (Bahr, 1990). See Chapter 24 for further discussion and example of a genogram.

A genogram is a schematic representation of a family that depicts the family unit of immediate interest and includes several generations using a series of circles, squares, and connecting lines. Basic information on composition of the family, relationships in the family, and patterns of health and illness can be obtained by completing the genogram with the family. As shown in Figure 25-1, a square indicates a male, a circle indicates a female, and an "x" through either a square or a circle indicates a death. Marriage is indicated by a solid horizontal line and offspring/children by a solid vertical line. A broken horizontal line indicates a divorce or

RESEARCH *Brief*

Based on results of a study of 50 families who had experienced a variety of stressors, Burr and colleagues (1994) examined the changes experienced under stress in nine areas of family life: marital satisfaction, family rituals and celebrations, quality of communication, family cohesion, functional quality of the executive subsystem, quality of the emotional atmosphere, management of daily routines and chores, contention, and normal family development versus changed or arrested development. The results of the study support that families did use the proposed strategies, both the helpful ones and the harmful ones, with significant differences between men and women on 10 of the 80 strategies. Women tended to use a wider range of strategies, and men tended to use more of the harmful strategies. The results supported the sequencing and developmental nature of families' use of strategies in acute stressor situations but not in chronic stressor situations. Thus the pattern was evident in stresses, such as bankruptcy, but not in families with a child with a chronic condition.

Results of this work provide direction for community health nursing intervention with families over the lifespan. The three levels share similarities with Neuman's (1989) flexible lines of defense (Level I change), normal line of defense (Level II change), and lines of resistance (Level III change). Based on Neuman's model, primary prevention strategies (e.g., parenting classes) would be appropriate for dealing with Level I change; secondary prevention strategies (e.g., crisis intervention) for dealing with Level II change; and tertiary prevention strategies (e.g., family therapy) for dealing with Level III change.

Burr WR et al: *Reexaming family stress: new theory and research*, Thousand Oaks, Calif, 1994, Sage; Neuman B: *The Neuman systems model*, ed 2, Norwalk, Conn, 1989, Appleton & Lange.

separation. Dates of birth, marriage, death, and other important events can be indicated where appropriate. Major illness or conditions can be listed for each individual.

The genogram in Figure 25-1 was completed for the Graham family. Some of the interesting patterns that can be seen from the genogram are the repeated recurrence of hypertension, adult onset diabetes, cancer, and hypercholesterolemia. Completion of a genogram requires interviews with the family members. Bahr suggests that a family chronology, a time-line of family events over three generations, be completed to extend the genogram.

A more intensive and quantitative assessment of a family's biologic risk can be achieved through the use of a standardized family risk assessment. Because such assess-

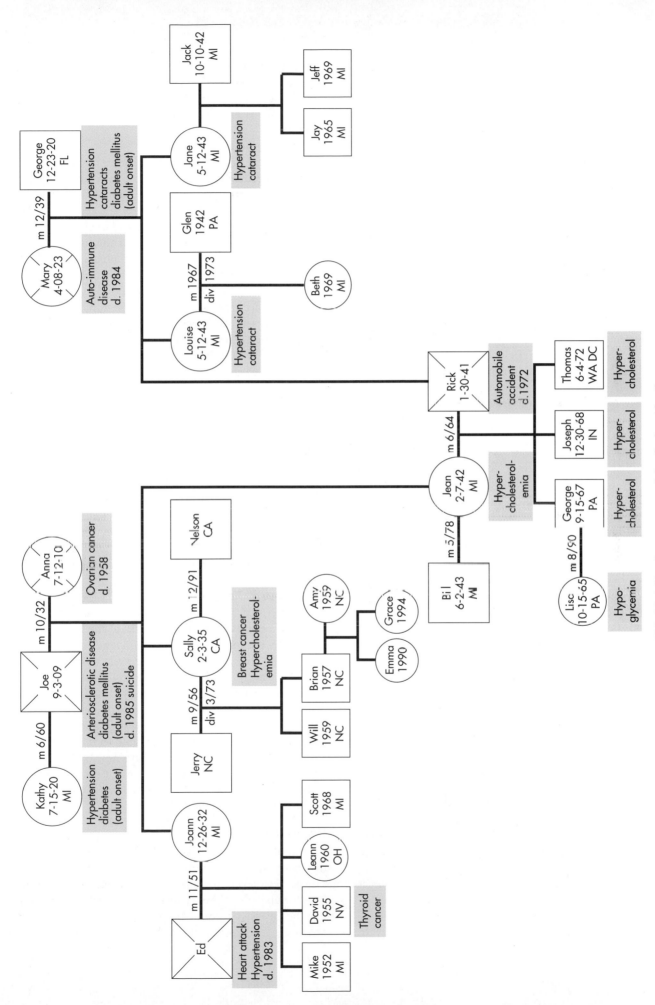

FIG. 25-1 Family genogram of the Graham family.

ments involve other areas in addition to biologic risk, one will be described later in this section after the description of assessment of other types of risk.

Social health risk

Assessment of social health risk is less well defined and developed. Information on relationships that the family has with others such as relatives and neighbors; their connections with other social units, church, school, work, clubs, and organizations; and the flow of energy, positive or negative, can be assessed through the use of an ecomap (see Chapter 24 for further discussion and an example of an ecomap).

An ecomap is merely a visual representation of the family's interactions with other groups and organizations, accomplished using a series of circles and lines. The family of interest is represented by a circle in the middle of a page; other groups and organizations are then indicated by other circles; lines, representing the flow of energy, are drawn between the family circle and the circles representing other groups and organizations. An arrowhead at the end of each line indicates the direction of the flow of energy (into or out of the family), and the boldness/darkness of the line indicates the intensity of the energy. Thus an ecomap drawn for the Graham family (Fig. 25-2) indicates that much of the family energy goes into work (also a source of stress) for the parents. In contrast, major sources of energy for the Grahams are their immediate and extended families and friends.

Other aspects of social risk include characteristics of the neighborhood and community where the family lives. If the nurse has worked in the general geographic area, he or she already may have done a community assessment (see Chapter 15) and have a working knowledge of the neighborhood and community. It is important, however, for information to be obtained from the family in order to understand their perceptions.

Information about the origins of the family is useful to understand other social resources and stressors. Information about how long the family has lived in their current location and the origin and immigration patterns of their family and ancestors provides insight into the pressures they experience.

Economic health risk

Financial information often is considered private by families. It is not necessary to know actual family income except in certain instances when it is necessary to determine whether families are eligible for programs or benefits. It is useful to know whether the family's resources are adequate to meet the demands. In terms of health risk, it is important to understand the resources that families have to obtain health/illness care; adequate shelter, clothing, and food; and access to recreation. Families with limited resources may qualify for programs such as Medicaid, Aid to Dependent Families, WIC, or Maternal Support Systems/Infant Support Systems. Families with wage earners with health/medical benefits and those with sufficient income usually are able to afford adequate health care. Unfortunately, there is a growing number of families whose main wage earner is employed but receives no health/medical benefits.

Lifestyle health risk

Families are the major source of factors that can promote or inhibit positive lifestyles. They regulate time and energy and the boundaries of the system. A number of tools exist for assessing individuals' lifestyle risks, but few are available for assessing family lifestyle patterns. Although assessment of individual lifestyle contributes to determining the lifestyle risk of a family, it is important to look at risks for the family as a unit. One approach is to identify family patterns for each of the lifestyle components included in *Healthy People 2000*. Within the areas of health promotion, health protection, and preventive services, lifestyle can be assessed on several dimensions. Based on the literature in health behavior research, the critical dimensions include the following:

- Value placed on the behavior
- Knowledge of the behavior and its consequences
- Effect of the behavior on the family
- Effect of the behavior on the individual
- Barriers to performing the behavior
- Benefits of the behavior

In terms of specific behaviors, it is important to assess the frequency, intensity, and regularity of the behavior. It also is important to evaluate the resources available to the family for implementing the behavior. Thus items for assessment of physical activity include the value that a family places on physical activity, the hours that a family spends in exercise, the kinds of exercise the family does, and resources available for exercise.

Life-event health risk

As discussed previously, both normative and nonnormative life events pose potential risks to the health of families. Even events that generally are viewed as being positive require changes and can place stress on a family. The normative event of the birth of a child, for instance, requires considerable changes in family structures and roles. Furthermore, family functions are expanded from previous levels, requiring families to add new skills and establish additional resources. These changes in turn can result in strain and, if adequate resources are not available, stress. Therefore to adequately assess the risks associated with life risks, both normative and nonnormative events occurring in the family need to be considered.

Home Visits

Community health nurses work with families in a variety of settings including clinics, schools, support groups, and offices. However, an important aspect of community health nursing's role in reducing health risks and promoting the health of populations has been the tradition of providing services to individual families in their homes.

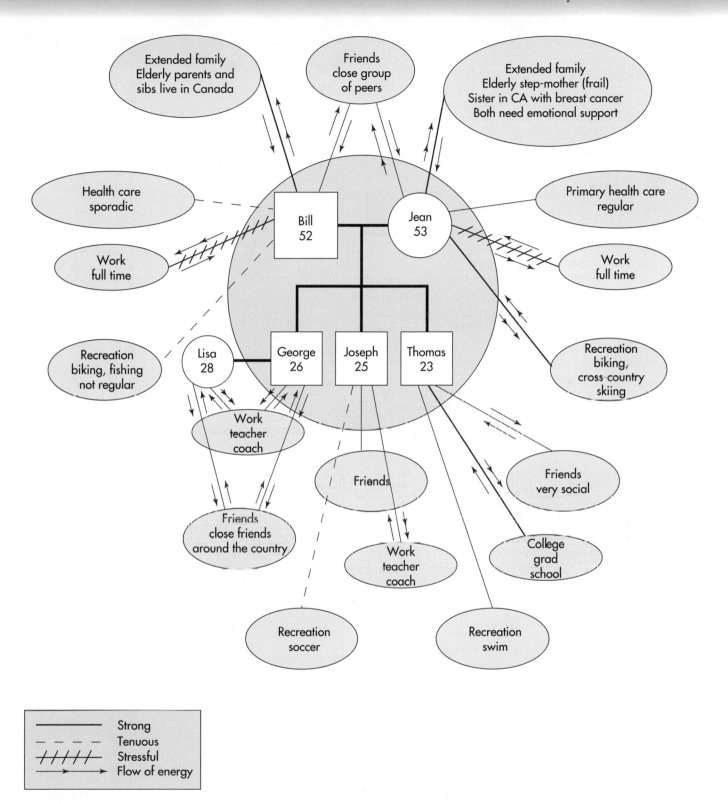

FIG. 25-2 Ecomap of the Graham family.

Purpose

Home visits give a more accurate assessment of the family structure, the natural or home environment, and behavior in that environment. Home visits also provide opportunities to identify both barriers and supports for reaching family health promotion goals. The nurse can work with the client first hand to adapt interventions to meet realistic resources. Meeting the family on their home ground also may contribute to the family's sense of control and active participation in meeting their health needs.

The majority of the studies evaluating the home have focused on the maternal-child population (Bradley and Martin, 1994; Kang et al, 1995; Olds and Kitzman, 1993).

Home visiting programs are receiving increased attention and are used to provide a broad range of services to achieve a variety of health-related goals. If the home visit is to be a valuable and effective intervention, careful and systematic planning must occur.

> **NURSING TIP**
>
> *A home visit is more than just an alternative setting for service; it is an intervention.*

Advantages and disadvantages

Recently, the effectiveness of providing large portions of health promotion services in this mode has been critically reexamined by agencies such as health departments and visiting nurses associations (VNAs) (Barnes-Boyd, Norr, and Nacion, 1998; Olds and Kitzman, 1993). Advantages include convenience for the client, client control of the setting, provision of an option for those clients unwilling or unable to travel, the ability to individualize services, and a natural, relaxed environment for the discussion of concerns and needs. Costs are a major disadvantage. The cost of previsit preparation, travel to and from the home, time spent with one client, and postvisit preparation is high. Many agencies have actively explored alternative modes of providing service to families, particularly group interventions (see Chapter 23). The important issue is determining which families would most benefit from them and how home visits can most effectively be structured and scheduled. With increasing demands for home health care, the home visit is again becoming a prominent mode for delivery of nursing services (see the Research Brief about the article by Kang and colleagues).

Building a trusting relationship with the client is the cornerstone of successful home visits. There are five basic helping skills that are fundamental to effective home visits: observing, listening, questioning, probing, and prompting. The need for these skills is evident in all phases of the home visit process.

Process

The components of a home visit are summarized in Table 25-4 and are discussed in the following sections.

Initiation phase. Usually, a home visit is initiated as the result of a referral from a health or social agency. However, a family may request services or the nurse may initiate the home visit as a result of case-finding activities. The **initiation phase** is the first contact between the nurse and the family. This provides the foundation for an effective therapeutic relationship. Subsequent home visits should be based on need and mutual agreement between the nurse and the family. Frequently, nurses are not sure of the reason for the visit. This carries with it the potential for

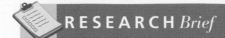

RESEARCH *Brief*

The purpose of this multisite field experiment was to test the efficacy of hospital and home visit interventions to improve interaction between mothers and preterm infants. The outcomes of a hospital intervention, State Modulation (focused on teaching mothers to read the behavior cues and modulate the states of consciousness of preterm infants during feedings), and the home visit intervention, Nursing Systems for Effective Parenting-Preterm (NSTEP-P), were compared with a hospital program on car seats and standard public health nursing home visits. The sample of 327 mothers and their preterm infants (less than 36 weeks gestational age at discharge) were randomly assigned to intervention groups based on their education. Highly educated mothers (equal to or more than 13 years of education) were assigned to hospital programs and the less-educated mothers (equal to or less than 12 years of education) were assigned to combinations of hospital and home visit programs. The outcomes were evaluated at 40, 46, and 60 weeks conceptual age.

The results supported suggest that State Modulation treatment and NSTEP-P are cost-effective treatments for families with healthy preterm infants. State Modulation treatment alone is a powerful intervention for well-educated mothers. State Modulation treatment in combination with NSTEP-P is most effective for mothers with limited formal education. The cost of the two programs, $100 for State Modulation and $550 for combined State Modulation and nine visit NSTEP-P, were proposed to be cost-effective approaches for promoting positive developmental outcomes for preterm infants via improved mother-infant interactions. The results also support consideration of the use of these interventions by public health nurses with vulnerable populations in the changing health care environment.

Kang R et al: Preterm infant follow-up project: a multi-site field experiment of hospital and home intervention programs for mothers and preterm infants, *Public Health Nurs* 12(3):171, 1995.

the visit to be compromised and to come aimlessly or abruptly to a premature halt. Regardless of the reason for making a home visit, it is necessary that the nurse be clear about the purpose for the visit and that this perception or understanding be shared with the family.

Previsit phase. The **previsit phase** has several components. For the most part, these are best accomplished in order, as presented in the How To box.

The possibility exists that the family may refuse a home visit. Less-experienced nurses or students may interpret this as a personal rejection when it is not. Families make

TABLE 25-4 Phases and Activities of a Home Visit

PHASE	ACTIVITY
I. Initiation phase	Clarify source of referral for visit
	Clarify purpose for home visit
	Share information on reason and purpose of home visit with family
II. Previsit phase	Initiate contact with family
	Establish shared perception of purpose with family
	Determine family's willingness for home visit
	Schedule home visit
	Review referral and/or family record
III. In-home phase	Introduce self and professional identity
	Interact socially to establish rapport
	Establish nurse-client relationship
	Implement nursing process
IV. Termination phase	Review visit with family
	Plan for future visits
V. Postvisit phase	Record visit
	Plan for next visit

HOW TO *Prepare for the Home Visit: Previsit Phase*

- *First, if at all possible, the nurse should contact the family by telephone before the home visit to introduce oneself, to identify the reason for the contact, and to schedule the home visit. A first telephone contact should be a maximum of 15 minutes. The nurse should give name and professional identity, for example, "This is Karen Smith. I'm a community health nurse from the Middle County Health Department").*

- *The family should be informed of how they came to the attention of the community health nurse, for example, as the result of a referral or a contact from observations or records in the school setting. If a referral has been received, it is important and useful to ascertain whether the family is aware of the referral. This will show a valuing of the client's input and involvement in care.*

- *A brief summary of the nurse's given information allows the family to know the extent of the nurse's knowledge about the family. For example, the nurse might say, "I understand that your baby was discharged from the hospital yesterday and that you requested some assistance with caring for the child at home."*

- *A visit that is appropriate for the nurse and the family should be scheduled for as soon as possible. Letting the family know agency hours available for visits, the approximate length of the visit, and the purpose of the visit are helpful to the family in determining when to set the visit. Although the length of the visit may vary, depending on circumstances, approximately 30 minutes to 1 hour is usual depending on the reason for the visit.*

- *If possible, the visit should be arranged when as many as possible of the family members will be available for the entire visit. It is also important for the nurse to tell the client about any fee for the visit and subsequent visits and possible methods for payment.*

- *The telephone call can terminate with a review by the nurse of the time, place, and purpose for the visit and a means for the family to contact the nurse in case they need to verify or change the time for the visit or to ask questions. If the family does not have a telephone, another method for setting up the visit can be used. The most obvious is dropping off a note at the family home or sending a letter or postcard informing the family of when and why the home visit will occur with a means for the family to contact the nurse if necessary.*

decisions about when and which outsiders are allowed entry into their home. The nurse needs to explore the reasons for the refusal; there may be a misunderstanding about the reason for a visit or there may be a lack of information about services. The contact may be terminated as requested if the nurse determines that either the situation has been resolved or services have been obtained from another source, and if the family understands that services are available and how to contact the agency if desired. However, the nurse should leave open the possibility of future contact. There are instances when the nurse will be mandated to persist in requesting a home visit because of legal obligations, such as follow-up of certain communicable diseases.

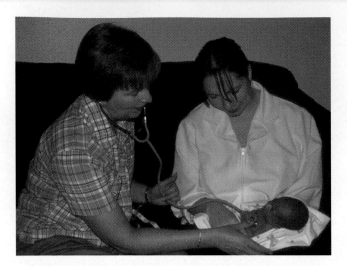

A nurse conducts a physical assessment of an infant during a home visit to the mother and her new baby.

Before visiting the family, it can be useful for the nurse to review the referral or, if not a first visit, the family record. If there is a time lapse between the contact and the visit, a brief telephone call to confirm the time often prevents the nurse from finding no one at home for the visit.

In-home phase. The actual visit to the home constitutes the **in-home phase** and affords the nurse the opportunity to assess the family's neighborhood. An issue that may arise either in approaching the family home or once the family has opened the door to the nurse is that of personal safety. Nurses need to examine personal fears and objective threats to determine if safety is indeed an issue. Certain precautions can be taken in known high-risk situations. Agencies may provide escorts for nurses or have them visit in pairs, readily identifiable uniforms may be required, or a sign-out process indicating timing and location of home visits may be used routinely. The nurse needs to use caution; if a reasonable question about the safety of making the visit exists, the visit should not be made.

The nurse needs to be aware that families may feel that they are being "checked up on," are seen as being inadequate or dysfunctional, or that their privacy is being impinged upon. Nursing services, especially those from health departments, have been identified by the public as being "public services" for needy families or those with insufficient funds to pay for care. These potential areas of concern underlie the needs for sensitivity on the part of the nurse, the need for clarity in information regarding the reason for visits, and the need to establish collaborative, trusting relationships with the family.

Another factor that may affect the nature of the home visit is whether the visit is viewed as "voluntary" or "required" (Byrd, 1995). A "voluntary" home visit (need for a visit by the client) is characterized by easier entry for the nurse, client-controlled interaction, an informal tone, and mutual discussion of frequency of future visits. In con-

trast, the client has little felt need for "required" home visits (often legally mandated), entry is difficult for the nurse; the interaction is nurse controlled; there is a more formal, investigatory tone to the visit with distorted nurse-client communication; and there is no mutual discussion of frequency of future visits.

The changing nature of the American family can make it difficult to schedule visits during what have been traditional agency hours. The number of working single-parent or dual-income, two-parent families is increasing, which means that families are busy with more demands on their time. Even if one parent is at home during the usual work day, the ideal is to work with the entire family unit. This often is not possible because of conflict between agency hours and school or work schedules. It may be possible to schedule a visit at the beginning or end of a day to meet with working or school-age members. In some parts of the country, agencies are reconsidering traditional hours and Monday through Friday visits.

Families may or may not be able to control interruptions during the visit. Telephones ring, pets join in the visit, people come and go, and televisions are left on. The nurse can ask that for a limited time televisions be turned off or other disruptive activities be limited. Families may be so used to the background noises and routine activities that they do not recognize them as being potentially disruptive.

The actual home visit includes several components. Once at the family home, the nurse needs to again provide personal and professional identification. It is important to tell the client the location of the agency if not known. This is part of the introductory phase. Then there should be a brief social period to allow the client to assess the nurse and to establish rapport. The next step is a description by the nurse of his or her role, responsibilities, and limitations. Another important component of the home visit is to determine what the client's expectations are for the home visit.

The major portion of the home visit is concerned with establishing the relationship and implementing the nursing process. Assessment, intervention, and evaluation are ongoing. What actually occurs in the home visit is largely determined by the reason or focus for the visit. Some reasons for visits are listed in Box 25-1.

It is important that the nurse be realistic about what can be accomplished in a home visit. In some situations, one visit may be all that is possible or appropriate. In this instance, needs and resources for meeting needs are explored with the family and it is determined whether further services are desired or indicated. If further services are indicated and the current agency is not appropriate, the nurse can assist the family in identifying other services available in the community and can help in initiating any referrals. Although it is not unusual to have only one home visit with a family, often multiple visits are made. The frequency and intensity of home visits vary with not only the needs of the family but also whether the family is eligible

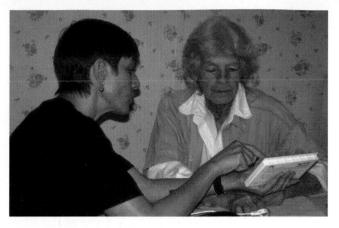

A nurse explains medication procedures to a client during a home visit.

for services and agency policies and priorities. It is realistic to expect initial assessment and at least the beginning of building a relationship to occur on a first visit.

Termination phase. When the purpose of the visit has been accomplished, the nurse reviews with the family what has occurred and what has been accomplished as the major focus of the **termination phase.** This provides a basis for planning further home visits. Ideally, termination of the visit and, ultimately, termination of service begins at the first contact with the establishment of a goal or purpose. If communication has been clear to this point, the family and nurse can now plan for future visits, specifically the next visit. Planning for future visits is part of another issue: setting goals and planning service. Contracting is a constructive approach to working with clients and is receiving increasing attention by health professionals. The purpose and components of contracting with clients are discussed in the next section.

Postvisit phase. Even though the nurse has now concluded the home visit and left the client's home, responsibility for the visit is not complete until the interaction has been recorded. A major task of the **postvisit phase** is documenting the visit and services provided. Agencies may or may not organize their records by families. That is, the basic record may be a "family" folder or record with all members included in one record, or each family member receiving services has a separate record with other family members' records cross-referenced. In reality the concept of a family-focused record often does not occur. History and background usually are given to some extent for the family, but often the focus shifts to individual health histories. Consequently, nursing diagnoses, goals, and interventions are directed towards individual family members rather than the family unit. Record systems and formats vary from agency to agency. The nurse needs to become familiar with the particular system used in the agency. All systems should include a database; a nursing diagnosis and problem list; a plan, including specific goals; actual actions and interventions; and evaluation. These are the basic elements needed for legal and clinical purposes. The format may consist of narratives; flow sheets, problem-oriented medical records (POMR); subjective, objective, assessment plan (SOAP); or a combination of formats. It is important that recording be current, dated, and signed.

Be sure to use theoretical frameworks that are appropriate to the family-centered nursing process. For example, a nursing diagnosis of "ineffective mothering skill related to lack of knowledge of normal growth and development" is an individual-focused nursing diagnosis. "Inability for family to accomplish stage-appropriate task of providing safe environment for preschooler related to lack of knowledge and resources" is a family-focused nursing diagnosis based on knowledge of the developmental approach to families. At times it may be necessary to present information for a specific family member. However, the emphasis should be on the individual as a member of, and within the structure of, the family.

Contracting with Families

Increasingly, health professionals look at working with clients in a more interactive, collaborative style. This approach is consistent with a more knowledgeable public and the recent self-care movement. **Contracting,** which is an agreement between two or more parties, involves a shift in responsibility and control to a shared effort by client and professional versus that of the professional alone. The ANA's *Standards of Community Health Nursing Practice* (1986) explicitly states the rights of clients to participate actively in planning their own health care; these same standards designate that "in partnership with the family and individual" the community health nurse collects, interprets, and analyzes data; formulates and validates diagnoses; formulates plans and implements interventions; and evaluates process and revision of the plan. This active involvement of the client is reflected in several of the existing nursing models, with Orem as an example (1995). Contracting is one strategy aimed at promoting a collaborative working relationship (in this instance, one specifically focused on health risk reduction and health promotion).

Contracting is one way of formally involving the family in the nursing process and explaining their roles. Some nurses are reluctant to use the term "contracting" but discuss it in terms of mutual goal setting. Some of this reluctance may be related to the potential legal terms of a contract, whether formal or informal. There may be concern about possible liability in terms of services agreed upon versus those received and the agreed-upon outcomes. In some cases, the connection between contracting and compliance may be contrary to a philosophy of an interactive partnership between nurse and client.

Thus an important issue is the purpose and/or philosophy that underlies the nurse's use of contracting with families. If contracting is viewed only as another approach to increasing compliance, the basic premises of the concept are violated. Contracting should address the issue of control by client versus control by the professional.

Purposes

The purpose of the agreement is to enhance and support the clients' active role in health care by defining clients' and professionals' roles in accomplishing health-related goals. The nursing contract is a working agreement that is continuously renegotiable and may or may not be written. A nursing contract may be either a contingency or a noncontingency contract. A contingency contract states a specific reward for the client after completion of the client's portion of the contract; a noncontingency contract does not specify rewards. The implied rewards are the positive consequences of reaching the goals specified in the contract.

In the instance of family health risk reduction, it is essential that the contract be made with all responsible and appropriate members of the family. Involving only one individual is invalid if the goal is family health risk reduction, which requires a total family system effort and change. Scheduling a visit with all family members present may require extra effort; if meeting with the entire family is not possible, each family member can review a contract, give input, and sign it. This allows for active participation by all family members without the necessity of finding a time when everyone involved can be present.

Process of contracting

Contracting is a learned skill on the part of both the nurse and the family. All parties involved need to know the purpose and process of contracting. There are three general phases: beginning, working, and termination. The three phases can be further specified into seven sets of activities. The phases and activities are summarized in Table 25-5.

TABLE 25-5 Phases and Activities in Contracting

PHASE	ACTIVITY
I. Beginning phase	Mutual data collection and exploration of needs and problems Mutual establishing of goals Mutual development of a plan
II. Working phase	Mutual division of responsibilities Mutual setting of time limits Mutual implementation of plan Mutual evaluation and renegotiation
III. Termination phase	Mutual termination of contract

The first activity involves both the family and the nurse in data collection and analysis of the data. An important aspect of this step is obtaining the family's view of the situation and its needs and problems. The nurse can present his or her observations and validate them with the family and also obtain the family's view.

It is important that goals be mutually set and realistic. A pitfall for nurses and clients who are new to contracting is to set overly ambitious goals. The nurse should recognize that there may be discrepancies between professional priorities and those of the client and determine whether negotiation is required. Because contracting is a process characterized by renegotiation, the goals are not static.

Throughout the process, the nurse and family need to continually learn and recognize what each can contribute to meeting health needs. This exploration of resources allows both parties to become aware of their own and others' strengths and requires a review of the nurse's skills and knowledge, family support systems, and community resources.

Developing a plan to meet the goals involves specifying activities, prioritizing goals, and selecting a starting point. Next the nurse and the family need to decide who will be responsible for which activities. Structuring time limits involves deciding on a deadline for accomplishing or evaluating progress towards accomplishing a goal and the frequency of contacts. At the agreed-upon time, the nurse and family together evaluate the progress to date in both process and outcome. Based on the evaluation, the contract can be modified, renegotiated, or terminated.

Advantages and disadvantages of contracting

Contracting takes time and effort and may require the family and nurse to reorient their roles. Increased control on the part of the family also means increased responsibility. Some nurses may have difficulty relinquishing the role of the controlling expert professional. Contracts will not always be successful and contracting is neither appropriate nor possible in some cases. Some clients do not want to have this kind of involvement; they prefer to defer to the "authority" of the professional. Included in this group are individuals with minimal cognitive skills, those who are involved in an emergency situation, those who are unwilling to be more active in their care, and those who do not see control or authority for health concerns within their domain. Some of these clients may learn to contract; some never will.

The use of the nursing process does not necessarily provide an active role for the family as a client; it assumes that needs exist based only on professional judgment and that changes can and should be made within the family unit. Contracting is one alternative approach that depends on the value of input from the nurse and the family, competency of the family, responsibility on the part of the family, and the dynamic nature of the process, which not only allows for but also requires continual renegotiation. Although it may not be appropriate in all situations or with all families, contracting can give direction and structure to health risk reduction and health promotion in families.

Enabling and Empowering Families

Help-giving interventions do not always have positive outcomes for clients. If families do not perceive a situation as a problem or need, offers of help may cause resentment. Help giving also may have negative consequences if there is not a match between what is expected and what is offered. Nurses' failure to recognize families' competencies and to define an active role for families can lead to dependency and lack of growth for families. This can be frustrating for both the nurse and the family. For families to become active participants, they need to feel a sense of personal competence and a desire for and willingness to take action. Recently, approaches for helping individuals and families assume an active role in their health care have focused on empowerment (Rodwell, 1996). Definitions of **empowerment** reflect three characteristics of the empowered family seeking help:

- Access and control over needed resources
- Decision-making and problem-solving abilities
- Ability to communicate and obtain needed resources

The last characteristic refers to the fact that families may need to learn how to identify sources of help, how to contact agencies, how to ask critical questions, and how to negotiate with agencies to have family needs met. These characteristics generally reflect a process by which people (individuals, families, organizations, or communities) take control of their own lives. The outcomes of empowerment are positive self-esteem, the ability to set and reach goals, a sense of control over life and change processes, and a sense of hope for the future (Rodwell, 1996).

Empowerment requires a viewpoint that often conflicts with the views of many helping professions, including nursing. Empowerment's underlying assumption is one of a partnership between the professional and the client versus one in which the professional is dominant. First, families are assumed to be either competent or capable of becoming competent. This implies that the professional is not an unchallengeable authority who is in control. Second, an environment that creates opportunities for competencies

to be used is necessary. Finally, families need to identify that their actions result in behavior change. A community health nursing intervention that incorporates the principles of empowerment would be directed toward the building of nurse-family partnerships that emphasize health risk reduction and health promotion. The nurse's approach to the family should be positive and focused on competencies rather than on problems or deficits. The interventions need to be consistent with family cultural norms and the family's perception of the problem. Rather than making decisions for the family, the nurse would support the family in primary decision-making and bolster their self-esteem by recognizing and using family strengths and support networks. Interventions promoting family behaviors increase family competency and decrease the need for outside help, resulting in families seeing themselves as being actively responsible for bringing about desired changes. The goal of an empowering approach is to create a partnership between the nurse and the family characterized by cooperation and shared responsibility.

COMMUNITY RESOURCES

Families have varied and complex needs and problems. The community health nurse often mobilizes several resources in order to effectively and appropriately meet family health promotion needs. Although the specific resources vary from community to community, general types can be identified. Government resources such as Medicare, Medicaid, Aid to Families of Dependent Children, Supplementary Security Income, Food Stamps, and WIC are available in most communities. These programs primarily provide support for basic needs (e.g., illness/health care, nutritional needs, funds for housing and clothing), and funds are based on the meeting of eligibility criteria.

In addition to government agencies providing health-related services to families, most communities have voluntary (nongovernmental) programs. Local chapters of such organizations as the Cancer Society, Heart Association, Lung Association, and Muscular Dystrophy Association provide educational and support services and some direct services to individuals and families regarding specific conditions. These agencies provide primary prevention and health promotion services, as well as screening programs and assistance, once the disease or condition is diagnosed. Local social service agencies, such as Catholic Social Services, provide direct services, such as counseling to families. Other voluntary organizations provide direct service (e.g., shelters for the homeless or battered individuals, substance abuse counseling and treatment, Meals on Wheels, transportation, clothing, food, furniture).

Health resources in the community may be proprietary, voluntary, or public. In addition to private health care providers, community health nurses should be aware of voluntary and public clinics, screening programs, and health promotion programs.

Identifying resources in a community requires time and effort. One obvious and valuable source is the telephone book. Often community service organizations, such as the Chamber of Commerce and the local health department, publish community resource listings. Regardless of how the resource is identified, the community health nurse must be familiar with the type of service offered and any requirements or costs involved. If this information is not available, the community health nurse can contact the resource.

Locating and using these systems often requires skills and patience that many families lack. Community health nurses work with families to identify community resources and as a client advocate in helping families learn to use resources. This may involve sharing information with families, rehearsing with families what questions to ask, preparing required materials, making the initial contact, and arranging transportation. The appropriateness and effectiveness of resources should be evaluated with families after referrals.

clinical application

The initial referral for community health nursing service to a family provides limited information, and the situation that develops may be much more complex than anticipated. The following example, based on an actual case, illustrates the issues and approaches outlined in this chapter.

A referral was received at the Middle County Health Department indicating that Amy Cress, age 16, had been referred by the school counselor at the local high school for prenatal supervision. Amy was 4 months pregnant, in apparently good health, in the tenth grade, and living at home with her mother, stepfather, and younger sister. The family lived in a rural area outside of a small farming community. The father of the baby also lived in the community and continued to see Amy on a regular basis. The referral information provided the community health nurse with a beginning, but limited, assessment of the family situation.

A. What would you do first as the community health nurse assigned to this family?
B. How would you help this family empower themselves to take responsibility for this situation?
C. After initial contact, how would you extend the assessment to the entire family system?
D. Would you contract with this family? How? On what terms?

Answers are in the back of the book.

KEY POINTS

- The importance of the family as a major client system for community health nursing in reducing health risks and promoting health of individuals and populations is well documented; the family system is a basic unit within which health behavior, including health values, health habits, and health risk perceptions, is developed, organized, and performed.

- Knowledge of family structure and functioning, family theory, nursing theory, and models of health behavior are fundamental to implementing the nursing process with families in the community. However, community health nurses need to go beyond the individual and family and understand the complex environment in which the family functions to be effective in reducing family health risks. Categories of risk factors that are important to family health are biologic risk, lifestyle risk, social risk, life-event risk, and economic risk.

- Several factors contribute to the experience of healthy/unhealthy outcomes. Not everyone exposed to the same event will have the same outcome. The factors that influence whether disease or other unhealthy results occur are called *health risks*. The cumulated risks are synergistic; their combined effect is more than the sum of the individual effects.

- An important aspect of community health nursing's role in reducing health risk and promoting the health of populations has been the tradition of providing services to individual families in their homes.

- Home visits afford the opportunity to gain a more accurate assessment of the family structure and behavior in the natural environment. Home visits also provide opportunities to make observations of the home environment and to identify both barriers and supports to reducing health risks and for reaching family health goals.

- Increasingly, health professionals have come to look toward working with clients in a more interactive, collaborative style.

- Contracting, which is an agreement between two or more parties, involves a shift in responsibility and control to a shared effort by client and professional versus that of professional alone.

- Families have varied and complex needs and problems. The community health nurse often mobilizes several resources to effectively and appropriately meet family health needs.

critical thinking activities

1. Select one of the year 2000 objectives and identify how biologic risk, social risk, economic risk, lifestyle risk, and life-event risk contribute to family health risk for that objective.
2. Select three to four families (hypothetically or from actual situations) representative of different ethnic and socioeconomic backgrounds. Complete a family genogram and ecomap for each family, and identify and compare major health risks.
3. Select one or more agencies in which community health nurses work, and examine the agency's and community health nursing's philosophies and objectives with emphasis on individual care, family care, illness care, risk reduction, and health promotion.
4. Identify three community health problems in your community, and discuss the implications of these problems for the health of families. Identify three health problems common to families in your community, and discuss the implications of the problems for the health and/or health care resources of the community.

Bibliography

American Nurses Association, Council of Community Health Nurses: *Standards of community health nursing practice,* Kansas City, Mo, 1986, American Nurses Association.

Bahr KS: Student responses to genogram and family chronology, *Family Relations* 39(3):243, 1990.

Barnes-Boyd C, Norr KF, Nacion KW: Evaluation of an interagency home visiting program to reduce postneonatal mortality in disadvantaged communities, *Public Health Nurs* 13(3):201, 1998

Belloc NB, Breslow L: Relationship of physical health in a general population survey, *Am J Epidemiol* 93:329, 1972.

Bomar PJ, editor: *Nurses and family health promotion: concepts, assessment, and interventions,* Baltimore, 1996, Williams & Wilkins.

Bradley PJ, Martin J: The impact of home visits on enrollment patterns in pregnancy-related services among low-income women, *Public Health Nurs* 11(6):392, 1994.

Burr WR et al: *Reexamining family stress: new theory and research,* Thousand Oaks, Calif, 1994, Sage.

Byrd ME: The home visiting process in the contexts of the voluntary vs. required visit: examples from fieldwork, *Public Health Nurs* 12(3):196, 1995.

Califano JA Jr: *Healthy people: the Surgeon General's report on health promotion and disease prevention,* Washington, DC, 1979, US Government Printing Office.

Doherty WJ, McCubbin HI: Family and health care: an emerging arena of theory, research and clinical intervention, *Family Relations* 34(1):5, 1985.

Duvall EM, Miller BC: *Marriage and family development,* ed 6, New York, 1984, Addison and Wesley.

Feetham SL et al, editors: *The nursing in families: theory/research/education/practice,* Thousand Oaks, Calif, 1992, Sage.

Gilliss C et al, editors: *Toward a science of family nursing,* Menlo Park, Calif, 1989, Addison-Wesley.

Greer C: Something is robbing our children of their future, *Parade Magazine,* pp 4-6, March 5, 1995.

Hill R: *Families under stress,* New York, 1949, Harper.

Kang R et al: Preterm infant follow up project: a multi-site field experiment of hospital and home intervention programs for mothers and preterm infants, *Public Health Nurs* 12(3):171, 1995.

Keller LO et al: Population-based public health nursing interventions: a model from practice, *Public Health Nurs* 15(3):207, 1998.

Litman TJ: The family as a basic unit in health and medical care: a social behavioral overview, *Soc Sci Med* 8:495, 1974.

Mauksch HO: A social science basis for conceptualizing family health, *Soc Sci Med* 8:521, 1974.

Neuman B: *The Neuman systems model,* ed 2, Norwalk, Conn, 1989, Appleton & Lange.

Nightingale EO et al: *Perspectives on health promotion and disease prevention in the United States,* Washington, DC, 1978, Institute of Medicine, National Academy of Sciences.

Olds DL, Kitzman H: Review of research on home visiting for pregnant women and parents of young children, *The Future of Children: Home Visiting* 3(3):53, 1993.

Orem DE: *Nursing: concepts of practice,* ed 5, St Louis, 1995, Mosby.

Pender NJ: *Health promotion in nursing practice,* ed 3, Stamford, Conn, 1996, Appleton & Lange.

Pratt L: *Family structure and effective health behavior,* Boston, 1976, Houghton-Mifflin.

Pyen CW: Wide disparity exists in poverty guidelines for property tax breaks, *The Ann Arbor News,* pp C1, C2, March 19, 1995.

Rodwell CM: An analysis of the concept of empowerment, *J Adv Nurs* 23:305, 1996

Smith JA: *The idea of health: implications for the nursing professional,* New York, 1983, Teachers College Press, Columbia University

US Department of Health and Human Services: *Healthy people 2000: national health promotion and disease prevention objectives,* Washington, DC, 1991, USDHHS, Public Health Service.

US General Accounting Office: *Home visiting: a promising early intervention strategy for at-risk families,* Washington, DC, 1990, United States General Accounting Office.

Child and Adolescent Health

MARCIA K. COWAN

OBJECTIVES

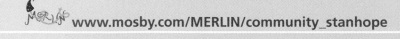

www.mosby.com/MERLIN/community_stanhope

After reading this chapter, the student should be able to do the following:

- Describe significant physical and psychosocial developmental factors characteristic of the child and adolescent population.
- Examine the role of the nurse and discuss appropriate nursing interventions that promote and maintain the health of children and adolescents.

- Discuss major health problems of children and adolescents.
- Evaluate the role of the community health nurse with specific at risk populations in the community.
- Describe ways to promote child and adolescent health within the community.

KEY TERMS

accommodation
adolescent period
assimilation
attention deficit disorder (ADD)
cognitive development

development
growth
homeless child syndrome
immunization
infancy
neonatal period

preschool period
psychosocial development
puberty
secondhand smoke
scheme
school-age period

sudden infant death syndrome (SIDS)
toddler period

See Glossary for definitions

CHAPTER OUTLINE

The future of the United States depends on how the children are cared for. Focusing on the health needs of children increases the chances of future adults who value and practice healthy lifestyles. Community-oriented nurses have two major roles in the area of child and adolescent health:

1. The nurse provides direct services to children and their families: assessment, management of care, education, and counseling.
2. Nurses are involved in the assessment of the community and the establishment of programs to ensure a healthy environment for its children.

The roles of the nurse offer the opportunity to teach healthy lifestyles to children and caregivers and to provide family-centered care in the ambulatory setting. This chapter provides information on the assessment of children and adolescents and activities to promote health. The content includes principles of growth and development from birth through adolescence and major health problems seen in this population. *Healthy People 2000* and *Healthy People 2010* objectives are used as a framework for focusing on needs of children in the community. Several programs are presented to show the various ways that nurses work with children and families.

STATUS OF CHILDREN

There were 69 million children in the United States in 1996, representing one fourth of the population. One in five of these children were living in poverty. This number increases to one in four children under 6 years of age. In 1994, one in three families with children had inadequate housing or could not afford their housing. One in three children lived in single parent households. This number increases to one out of two minority children. Children who are living with unmarried mothers are more likely to be poor than children living with married partners (NCHS, 1998). To combat this problem, the U.S. Congress passed the Child Health Insurance Program (CHIPS) legislation in 1999 to cover children for basic preventive services and episodic illness services for unserved children.

In 1994, one in seven children had no health insurance. This includes 1.3 million teenagers. By 2000, the number of uninsured children is estimated to reach 12.6 million (NCHS, 1998).

DID YOU KNOW? *One third of the uninsured children in the United States are eligible for Medicaid programs.*

In 1994, 3.1 million children were reported to be abused or neglected, with 2000 deaths. This is a number that is often underreported since it is difficult to prove. Abuse occurs in all income, racial, and ethnic groups. The number of cases is increasing significantly (Children's Defense Fund, 1996). At either end of the age spectrum, children are at great risk. Although infant mortality rates are decreasing, 7.9 out of 1000 babies die in the first year of life. The mortality rate for minority infants is twice that of Caucasian infants (NCHS, 1998).

In 1996, 800,000 teenagers became pregnant, most unintentionally (see Chapter 33). Sexually transmitted diseases and genital carcinomas are increasing among teens. Each year, 500,000 to 1.5 million teenagers run away or are forced out of their homes. More than one half are 15 to 16 years of age. About 1 out of 20 teenagers leaves high school before graduation. One out of eleven 16 to 19 year olds is detached, not in school or working. One fourth of violent crimes are committed by juveniles 12 to 17 years of age. Of all violent crimes, teenagers are most often the victims (NCHS, 1998) The status of children and teenagers in the United States compares poorly with other industrialized nations of the world.

CHILD DEVELOPMENT

Physical Growth and Development: Neonate to School Age

Growth is the measurable aspect of the individual's size; **development** involves the observable changes in the individual. A unique feature of the pediatric population is the ongoing process of growth and development, resulting in physical, cognitive, and emotional changes. Health visits or well-child checkups are scheduled at key ages to monitor these processes. Nursing assessments include growth and health status, developmental level, and the quality of the parent-child relationship. Table 26-1 identifies recommendations for schedules and components of well-child assessments as recommended by the American Academy of Pediatrics (AAP) and the Guide to Clinical Preventive Services (see Appendix A.2). The nurse needs to be aware of issues of concern at each age.

Assessment strategies and tools, common concerns and problems, and specific interventions for each age group are further discussed in Appendixes E.4 to E.8.

Focus of assessment

Neonates. The **neonatal period** extends from birth to 1 month of age. It is a time of transition. Organ systems undergo changes that allow extrauterine existence. Cardiopulmonary shunts close to enable lung function. Pulmonary pressures change, reflecting changes in circulation and air expansion of the lungs. The liver and kidneys increase regulatory functions. The gastrointestinal system matures as it processes nutrients. Sensory stimulation bombards the baby. Physiologic stabilizing and rapid growth highlight this time. Weight gain averages $\frac{1}{2}$ to 1 ounce per day. The nurse assesses the stability of the neonate by physical examination, including vital signs and weight (see Appendixes E.4 and F.2).

The parents are learning how to meet the needs of the baby. The nurse assesses his or her ability to respond to the neonate's needs. Feeding, elimination, and sleep patterns are frequently issues of concern. Nurses provide information to help families understand the temperament and be-

TABLE 26-1 Guidelines for Well Child Care

| | AGE | | | | | | | | | | | |
| | MONTHS | | | | | | | YEARS | | | | |
	2	4	6	9	12	15	18	2	3	4-6	7-9	10-13	14-21
Physical exam	*	*	*	*	*	*	*	*	*	*	*	*	*
Height, weight	*	*	*	*	*	*	*	*	*	*	*	*	*
Head circumference	*	*	*	*	*	*	*	*	*				
Blood pressure									*	*	*	*	*
Vision	s	s	s	s	s	s	s	s	*	*	*	*	*
Hearing	s	s	s	s	s	s	s	s	s	*	*	*	*
Developmental	*	*	*	*	*	*	*	*	*	*	*	*	*
LABORATORY TESTS													
Hct/Hb				*						*		*	
Urinalysis										*		*	
Cholesterol screen								c		c		c	c
Lead level					*					*			
Pap smear													
Sexually transmitted diseases screening												^	^
TB skin test +					*					*		*	
ANTICIPATORY GUIDANCE													
Feeding/nutrition	*	*	*	*	*	*	*	*	*	*	*	*	*
Growth/development	*	*	*	*	*	*	*	*	*	*	*	*	*
Behavior	*	*	*	*	*	*	*	*	*	*	*	*	*
Safety/poisons/injury	*	*	*	*	*	*	*	*	*	*	*	*	*
Sexual behaviors											a	a	a
Substance abuse											a	a	a
Physical activity										a	a	a	a

s, subjectively determined by behavioral observations; formal assessment as determined by history; *a*, as appropriate for age; *b*, evoked otoacoustic emissions testing within the first 3 months, preferably before discharge from the nursery; +, recommendations will vary according to state guidelines and individual risk; *c*, based on assessment of family risk factors; ^, annually if sexually active.
Modified from American Academy of Pediatrics: *Guidelines for health supervision III: American Academy of Pediatrics guide to clinical preventive services*, Elk Grove Village, Ill, 1997, Author.

havior of neonates. The goal of care is to support the family as they increase their caregiving skills.

Early discharge from the hospital at 24 hours of age often gives the community health nurse responsibility to assess physical status, monitor family coping, refer to community resources as needed, and teach infant care (Table 26-2). The nurse should be aware of factors that place the infant at risk (Box 26-1) and danger signs indicating need for referral.

Infants. Infancy extends from 1 month to 1 year. During this time, rapid growth continues. Infants usually double the birth weight by 6 months and triple the birth weight by 1 year. Length usually increases by 10 to 12 inches (25 to 30 cm). Nurses identify and intervene in situations when the infant is at risk because of health or socioeconomic problems. Nursing interventions include monitoring of growth and development with particular attention to areas of feeding, sleeping, elimination, development, and safety (Table 26-3).

Feeding and elimination dominate many of the parent's concerns. Increasing stomach capacity and growth needs may cause overfeeding and spitting up. Gastrointestinal reflux is fairly common in infancy. Stool patterns change in early infancy, which may confuse parents.

DID YOU KNOW? *Many parents think that their child should be potty trained by 2 years of age. Only 4% of children are actually potty trained by age 2; 22% by age 2½; 60% by age 3; and 80% by age 3 ⅓.*

Sleep is another area of concern. Parents often have unrealistic ideas about infant sleep. By 4 to 6 months of age, infants can sustain longer sleep periods without night feedings. New developmental skills, such as pulling up or walk-

TABLE 26-2 Assessing the Neonate

ASSESSMENT	FOCAL POINTS	NURSING IMPLICATIONS

Physical	Assess stabilization of transition
	Assess vital signs:
	    Temperature: 98.6° to 99.5° F (37° to 37.5° C) rectally
	    Heart rate: 120 to 140 beats/min
	    Respiratory rate: 40 to 60 breaths/min
	Assess for growth:
	    Weight gain 1/2 to 1 ounce/day (15 to 30 g)
	    Length 1/2 to 1 inch/month (1.2 to 2.5 cm)
	    Head circumference: 0.6 inch/month (1.5cm)
	Assess for normal variations and minor abnormalities (see Appendix E.4)
	Screening (generally performed before nursery discharge): PKU, hypothyroid, sickle cell, galactosemia, hearing
		Identify deviations and refer as needed
		Teach cord care, circumcision care, bathing, diaper area and skin care, temperature-taking techniques, normal variations of color, activity patterns, and variations in respiratory patterns
		Teach signs of illness and how to contact health care provider

Nutrition	Assess feeding behaviors and parent comfort with feeding technique Assess adequacy of caloric intake based on weight gain and output	Teach feeding techniques including breastfeeding, formula preparation, burping, and positioning Identify concerns related to getting enough to eat, spitting up, gas, and colic
Elimination	Urine output: at least 6 to 8 wet diapers/day Stool patterns may vary from several times per day to every 3 to 4 days. Loose to firm consistency is normal Straining with bowel movements is common	Educate and reassure parents regarding normal elimination patterns
Sleep	Assess sleep patterns noting high variability between active and quiet babies. Average 16 hours per day	Encourage supine sleep position Offer strategies to encourage night sleep
Development	Observe responses to tactile, auditory, taste, and visual stimuli Note ability to self quiet, reflex responses, habituate, and state transition	Identify behaviors showing individuality, competence, consolability, and responsiveness Adapt caregiving stategies to match temperament
Safety	Dependency on caregiver for safety	Offer anticipatory guidance for well child care and immunizations Discuss falls, carseat, water temperature, and fire safety in the home

ing, may interfere with night sleep. Illnesses and teething may also cause infants to resume night wakening. Parents may want to help the infant learn self-comforting skills to go back to sleep.

The second half of infancy brings major accomplishments in gross motor activities. Rolling, sitting, pulling up, and walking bring safety concerns. Parents should be given anticipatory guidance in these areas (see Appendix E.5).

Toddlers and preschoolers. The **toddler period** consists of the second and third years of life. The **preschool period** encompasses ages 3 to 5 years. Slowing and stabilization of growth are hallmarks of this period as reflected by changes in appetite and eating patterns. Increased physical ability and independence forces parents to deal with discipline issues. The number of acute illnesses increases.

Children will test limits, seeking rules and trying to make sense of the world. Negativism and aggressive behaviors upset parents and caregivers but are often a result of the child's frustrations. Discipline is important method of teaching self-control. It is not punishment, it is a training process to help children deal with their emotions. Parents are role models for behavior.

Physical punishment by adults teaches aggressive behavior and lack of self control. Outbreaks should be avoided. If the child is tired, avoid going to the grocery store at that time. Distraction may prevent tantrums. Parents need to reward behaviors that are positive and ignore negative behaviors. Short time-outs may be useful to remove children from the situation. Alternatively a "big hug" may help restrain an out-of-control child until calm is restored. Often

---

BOX 26-1 Identification of "At Risk" Newborns

History. Family history of major disease; gestational or delivery complications

General appearance. Congenital malformations; birth trauma

Head. Bulging or sunken fontanel; macrocephaly; microcephaly

Heart. Rapid, slow, or irregular rate; heart murmur

Respiratory. Rapid, noisy, or difficult respirations; persistant cough

Temperature. Hypothermia; fever

Growth. Macrosomia; intrauterine growth retardation

Neurologic. Hypertonia; hypotonia; lethargy; jitery; irritability, seizures; abnormal cry

Color. Cyanosis; jaundice; pallor

Skin. Petechiae; purpura; bleeding sites

Gastrointestinal. Vomiting; diarrhea; poor feeding; abdominal distention

Output. Abnormal voiding; delayed stooling; hematochezia

Adapted from Watterberg K, Gallaher KJ: Signs and symptoms of neonatal illness. In Hoekelman R et al, editors: *Primary pediatric care,* ed 3, St Louis, 1997, Mosby.

---

the tantrum is an attempt to get attention. Explanations should be brief and succinct. Long lectures are poorly understood and often teach that "out-of-control" behavior gets attention.

Toddlers and preschoolers are often around other children (e.g., daycare centers), increasing exposure to viruses and bacteria. There may be more episodes of acute illnesses, including upper respiratory infections, otitis media, and stomach viruses. Allergies may influence health. Children of this age are often suffer from "runny, drippy" noses. Children average one acute illness per month.

NURSING TIP

Examination of infants through preschoolers is easiest if the child is being held by the parent. It helps to offer the child a piece of examining equipment to handle. Showing the child how the equipment is used before using it on the child helps to alleviate fears. Describing what is happening may increase the child's confidence.

Nurses monitor growth and development and offer anticipatory guidance about behavior and acute illness (Table 26-4) (see also Appendix E.6).

School-age children. The **school-age period** begins at school entry and continues until the beginning of puberty, usually around 10 years of age. Although this has been considered a time of latency for children, it is not uneventful. Physical growth is typically slow and steady. The focus shifts from family to peers as school fills more of the day. This is a time of competition. The child compares himself or herself with others in school performance, sports, and appearance. Opportunities for success and positive feedback are critical for the child's feeling of accomplishment (see Appendix E.7).

Actively involve the child in the assessment and education process. Encouraging participation models taking responsibilty for making healthy lifestyle choices. Acute illnesses decrease during this time. School adjustment, peer relations, and learning problems are issues to explore. Nurses assess growth and sexual development, dental health, sleep and eating patterns, immunization status, hearing, and vision (Table 26-5).

Sports physicals are a common reason for seeking health care. Guidelines for sports safety should be discussed (Box 26-2). Another important issue involves television viewing. Television time is inactivity. Program content may be inappropriate. Parents need to limit the time spent watching, select programs carefully, view programs with children, and discuss content (see Appendix E.7).

WHAT DO YOU THINK? *On Saturday morning television there are an average of 20 to 25 violent acts per hour during cartoons. During the first hour of prime-time network television, 75% of the shows include sexual talk or behavior. Should the government become involved in what is shown or in the development of ratings systems?*

Health assessment tools

Growth charts. Height, weight, and head circumference (until 3 years of age) are noted at each health visit to record the rate of growth. Measurements are plotted on standard growth curves and compared with normals for the age (see a pediatric text for examples). The child's pattern of growth is more important rather than a single measurement. Most healthy children will follow the same growth percentile over time.

Developmental assessment. Children follow predictable patterns of development. Developmental standards have been established based on age levels at which children master key motor, language, adaptive, and social behaviors. Developmental screening tests compare an individual child with the average standard and are used to identify children requiring further evaluation and intervention. Table 26-6 on p. 534 provides an overview of frequently used tools (see also Appendixes F.5 and F.7). See Box 26-2 for guidelines for children involved in sports.

Temperament and behavioral assessments. Behavioral characteristics or temperament have an important role in how a child interacts with others and the environment. Nurses use information about temperament and behavior to help parents understand the child'sneeds, which may have a positive influence on the parent-child relationship. Table 26-6 lists tools to assess these characteristics.

TABLE 26-3 Assessing the Infant

ASSESSMENT	FOCAL POINTS	NURSING IMPLICATIONS

Physical	Continued assessment of stabilization of organ systems
	Vital signs:
	  Heart rate: 115 to 130 beats/min
	  Respiratory rate: 20 to 40 breaths/min
	Growth:
	  Weight gain:
	    First 6 months: 6 to 8 oz/wk (180 to 240 g)
	    Second 6 months: 3 to 4 oz/wk (90 to 120 g)
	  Length increase:
	    First 6 months: 1 inch/month (2.5 cm)
	    Second 6 months: ½ inch/month (1.25 cm)
	Tooth eruption begins at average of 6 months
	Primary series of immunizations
	Hearing: turns to sounds, babbles
	Vision: increased tracking of objects
		Anticipatory guidance regarding acute illness; risk factors include daycare, smoke exposure, and poor handwashing
		Discuss risk/benefits of immunizations
		Refer abnormal physical findings

Nutrition	Assess feeding patterns and techniques Identify parent concerns Addition of solids at 6 months of age Breastfeeding or formula throughout the first year of life with weaning to a cup around 12 months Fluoride source identified	Introduction of new foods with progression from spoon feeding to soft finger foods Introduction of cup
Elimination	Urine output continues to be at least 6 to 8 wet diapers/day Stools are soft to firm; easily passed; varying from daily to every few days	Educate and reassure parents regarding normal elimination patterns
Sleep	3 months: 70% sleep 8 hours at night with two naps during the day 6 months: 80% sleep 8 hours at night with variable naps during the day 12 months: 90% sleep 8 to 12 hours at night with average of one 2-hour nap during the day	Teaching strategies to promote falling asleep independently, self comfort techniques, and bedtime routines
Development	Development proceeds in cephalocaudal progression Behaviors progress from reflexive and involuntary to purposeful and voluntary Reaching, holding, mouthing activities of the hands predominate during early infancy Rolling and sitting occur during middle infancy, with more shaking and banging of objects Pulling up, crawling, and walking occur during late infancy	Anticipatory guidance includes education regarding attachment, stranger awareness, separation anxiety, and night wakening Encourage ways to play with the infant to encourage development
Safety	Increasing gross and fine motor skill increase safety Environmental risks include lead exposure	Education regarding risks for falls, choking, aspiration, poison prevention, use of car seat, burn prevention Screen for lead toxicity if appropriate Offer anticipatory guidance for well child care and immunizations

Physical Growth and Development: Adolescence

The **adolescent period** refers to ages 11 through 21. **Puberty** refers to the biologic changes that occur during this time, including the growth spurt and the development of secondary sexual characteristics. The growth spurt is mediated by both growth hormone and sex steroids. The duration of the growth spurt averages 24 to 36 months, ending with epiphyseal closure. The onset varies with the individual and includes increases in both height and weight. The development of secondary sex characteristics is measured on a scale developed by Tanner (see Appendix F.6). Breast bud is the first sign of sexual development for a majority of females. Testicular enlargement is the first for a majority of males.

TABLE 26-4 Assessing Toddlers and Preschool Children

ASSESSMENT	FOCAL POINTS	NURSING IMPLICATIONS

Physical	Assessment of organ systems: increased frequency of upper respiratory illness, otitis media, allergy symptoms, gastrointestinal illness
	Vital signs:
	    Heart rate: 100 to110 beats/min
	    Respiratory rate: 20 to 40 breaths/min
	    Blood pressure: average 98/60 mm Hg
	Growth rate markedly decreased
	Weight gain averages 5 lb/year (2.27 kg)
	Height increases 3 to 4 inches/year (7.6 to 10 cm)
	Dental: 20 primary teeth by age 2
	Anterior fontanel closes by 18 months
	Normal progression from bowlegs (12 to 18 months) to knock knees (18 to 24 months)
		Anticipatory guidance regarding acute illness; risk factors include daycare, smoke exposure, and poor handwashing
		Management of upper respiratory illness, gastrointestinal viruses, otitis media, allergies
		Education regarding when to contact health care provider
		Refer abnormal physical findings
		Discuss risks/benefits of immunizations
		Cleaning and flossing of teeth/dental referral
		Vision screening age 3 and preschool
		Audiometry age 3 to 4; sooner if concerns

Nutrition	Slowing of growth results in decreased caloric needs and diminished appetite Obtain dietary history; food preferences and food jags are common Self feeding skills increase	Reassure with information related to growth needs and intake Encourage offering small, nutritious snacks frequently
Elimination	Most children demonstrate readiness for toilet training between the ages of 2 and 3 Inappropriate emphasis on defecation may result in constipation	Anticipatory guidance on cues for readiness, strategies to toilet train, and ways to discourage constipation or retention problems
Sleep	By age 3, most children sleep 8 to 12 hours at night, with an afternoon nap until age 3 to 5 Nightmares and night terrors may interrupt patterns of night sleep	Provide guidance regarding routine and common problems Encourage bedtime routine

Development	Toddler period:
	    Increasing motor skills
	    Increasing autonomy and independence, with resulting periods of ambivalance
	    May show negativism and aggression when frustrated
	    Parallel play with peers
	Preschool period:
	    Increasing verbal skills
	    Increasing initiative, but with difficulty with impulse control
	    Interacts more with peers but can lead to conflicts
		Developmental screening using standardized assessment tools, history, and observation
		Discipline strategies: effective use of time-out, ignoring negative behaviors, rewarding positive behaviors, avoiding conflict by distraction or timing of activities

Safety	Increasing gross and fine motor skills, imitation, and independence increase risks for injury	Provide anticipatory guidance related to climbing, falls, outdoor supervision, poison prevention, drownings, burns, guns, sunburn, and car seat

Emotional and cognitive changes also occur during this progression toward maturity and independence. These processes may start before physical changes and may last beyond the end of growth. Emotional growth is as varible as biologic growth and occurs with periods of development and regression. The process of change may involve a great deal of stress for families, although most adolescents cope well with the conflicts (Neinstein, 1996) (Fig. 26-1). Some topics for parents to consider in the overall health of their adolescent are listed in Box 26-3.

Early adolescence (ages 10 to 13) includes the onset of puberty and many physical changes. The adolescent is concerned with appearance and sex characteristcs and compares his or her body with those of others. Conflicts with family may begin. Impulse control may be limited.

By middle adolescence (ages 14 to 16), the majority of pubertal changes have occurred. Appearance is still a focus, but there is a growing acceptance and comfort with the body. Risk taking is fueled by a sense of invulnerability. Peer values become the standards for behavior.

TABLE 26-5 Assessing School-Age Children

ASSESSMENT	FOCAL POINTS	NURSING IMPLICATIONS

Physical	Decreasing number of acute illnesses
	Vital signs:
	  Heart rate: 60 to 100 beats/min
	  Respiratory rate: 18 to 30 breaths/min
	  Blood pressure range: 90/60 to 108/66 mm Hg
	Growth rate stable
	Weight gain: 5 to 7 pounds/yr (2.27 to 3 kg)
	Height increase: 2.5 inches/yr (6 cm)
	Loss of primary teeth
	Vision 20/20
	Skeletal growth: lengthening of legs and trunk, widening of thighs and shoulders
		Provides anticipatory guidance regarding normal growth patterns
		Identification of deviant growth patterns
		Inspect number and condition of teeth, noting loss of deciduous teeth and eruption of permanent teeth
		Provides education on preventive dental care
		Identification of dental problems

Nutrition	Caloric needs increase with periods of increased growth Average requirements: 2400 to 2800 kcal/day Capable of selecting and preparing own meals Vulnerable to advertising Tends to have strong food preferences Tends to snack frequently	Obtain diet history Provide education regarding balanced diet, healthful snacks, need for breakfast, and exercise needs Identify eating disorders
Sleep	Obtain history of sleep requirements Ideal sleep: 9 hr/night with regularity of schedule	Identification of deviant sleep patterns Provide counseling on meeting sleep requirements
Development	Increasing coordination of fine and gross motor skills, including eye-hand coordination Increasing intellectual competency with transition from concrete to abstract conceptualization Moving from egocentrism Time of intense competition between peers in school and activities Needs successful experiences	Involve child in discussions Provide anticipatory guidance regarding safety, independence, peer pressure, and conformity Assessment of school performance Identify need to provide opportunities for successful experiences
Safety	Involve child in education	Sports safety, including protective equipment. Bicycle safety: helmets, road rules Seat belts

Late adolescents (ages 17 to 21) have completed growth and can focus on values and personal identity. Vocational goals and financial responsibilites are topics of concern. The ability to compromise and set limits improves.

Physical illness declines during adolescence. Injury and violence are the leading causes of morbidity and mortality. Studies of early and middle adolescents report increasing sexual activity, multiple sex partners, pregnancy, and sexually transmitted diseases (CDC, 1996). Experimentation with alcohol, smoking, and drugs occurs at younger ages. Screening and education may prevent health problems during this period. The Guidelines for Adolescent Preventative Services (GAPS), released by the American Medical Association (GAPS Executive Committee, Department of Adolescent Health, 1995), recommend yearly visits between ages 11 and 21 to identify adolescents who have considered or begun risky behaviors (Box 26-4). The goals of nursing care include early detection of physical, emotional, and behav-

BOX 26-2 Guide to Sports Safety

- Children should be grouped according to weight, size, maturation, and skill level.
- Qualified and competent persons should be available for supervision during games and practices.
- Adequate and appropriate sized equipment should be available.
- Goals should be developmentally and physically appropriate for the child.

ioral problems. Nurses promote healthy lifestyle choices and update immunizations (Table 26-7). Strategies to increase communication with adolescents are identified in the How To box. GAPS also recommends parent guidance visits during early and middle adolescence.

TABLE 26-6 Assessment Tools

TEST	FOCUS	AGES	SUMMARY
Denver II	Developmental screen	0-6 yr	Screening of gross motor, fine motor, adaptive/language, and personal/social skills
Revised Denver Prescreening Developmental Questionnaire	Developmental screen	3 mo-6 yr	Parent questionnaire Short form of the Denver to identify children who need further testing
Developmental Profile II	Developmental screen	0-9 yr	Structured interview with parent Screens physical/motor, self-help, social, academic, and communication skills
Preschool Readiness Experimental Screening Scale	Preschool readiness	4-5 yr	Addresses school-related skills and maturation
Early Language Milestone Scale	Speech and language screening	0-36 mo	Screening tool for general speech/language development Includes visual, auditory receptive, and auditory expressive areas Combines history, direct testing, and observation
Denver Articulation Screening Examination	Speech and language screening	2-6	Word imitation to screen articulation and intelligibility of speech
	Infant behavior, state, and temperament patterns	0-1 mo	Assessment of reflexes and behavioral responses. Tests for state and individual characteristics to identify abnormalities and for parent education.
Infant Temperament Questionnaire	Temperament	1-12 mo	Child's temperamental characteristics identified based on parental responses
Toddler Development Scale		1-3 yr	Assess the following aspects of temperament: activity, rhythmicity, adaptability, approach, sensory threshold, intensity, mood, distractibility, and persistence
Behavioral Style Questionnaire		3-7 yr	
Middle Childhood Questionnaire		8-12 yr	

HOW TO *Communicate with Adolescents*

- *Identify what issues remain confidential.*
- *Move from less personal to more personal topics.*
- *Use open-ended questions.*
- *Use matter-of-fact style.*
- *Acknowledge that discussion of sensitve subjects may cause uncomfortable feelings.*
- *Talk in terms that adolescents will understand.*
- *Use nonjudgmental responses.*
- *Listen.*
- *Obtain information from the adolescent directly; plan on time with the adolescent without the parent for interview.*
- *Depersonalize questions (e.g., "Many teenagers go to parties where drugs are used. Do you?").*

Psychosocial Development

The child's growth process includes **psychosocial development.** The work of Erik Erikson focuses on the interaction of emotional, cultural, and social forces on personality development. Personality development culminates in the achievement of ego identity, which involves accepting oneself and having the skills for healthy functioning in society. Erikson believed that development is a continual process that occurs in distinct stages. At each stage, a developmental crisis requires resolution. Although a child never completely finishes all the developmental tasks in a given stage, some degree of mastery and comfort must be achieved before proceeding successfully to the next stage. As internal conflicts are resolved, there is new orientation to self and society. This sets the stage for the next conflict. Each crisis emerges from the mastery of the previous stage. All new development is rooted in prior experiences. Difficulty with resolution of the crisis will cause problems progressing through the subsequent stages.

The first five stages of Erikson's model deal with the tasks of childhood and adolescence; the last three stages deal with adulthood.

1. *Trust versus mistrust* involves the period of infancy. The infant learns to trust both self and the environment based on how consistently needs are met. If needs are met inconsistently, the infant feels a sense of confu-

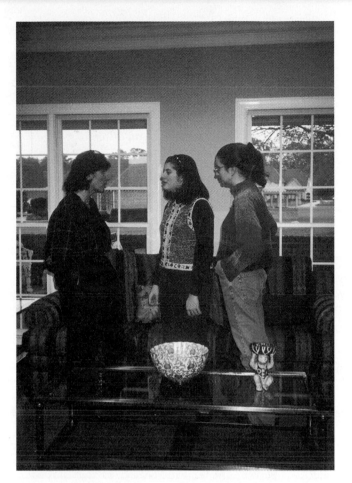

FIG. 26-1 Conflict between parents and teenagers is normal as teenagers experience physical and emotional growth processes.

sion and mistrust. Resolution, or moving through this stage to the next, depends on the quality of interaction and attachment between the parent and infant.

2. *Autonomy versus shame and doubt* encompasses early childhood and involves the child's developing physical and mental skills. Resolution is supported as parents allow increasing independence and acquiring of skills. When parents have appropriate expectations and encourage autonomy, the child develops a sense of control over self and environment. The child feels inadequate if not allowed the opportunity for mastery.

3. *Initiative versus guilt* occurs during preschool and early school-age years. The child achieves mastery through initiation of activity and asking questions. This stage also includes incorporation of adult standards and learning to take responsibility for one's own actions. Restriction may lead to a sense of guilt about thoughts and actions.

4. *Industry versus inferiority* occurs as the child moves from initiating to completing of projects. This occurs during middle and late childhood. Competition and peer involvement increase during this time. The child uses expanding cognitive skills to become a productive member of a group. The status in the group and self-esteem are challenged if the child feels that he or she is not "good enough."

5. *Identity versus identity diffusion* is the classic task of adolescence. The conflict is to achieve a sense of self and a set of values and a belief system. This is accomplished by "trying on" various roles and receiving responses from others. Identity diffusion results when the adolescent is unable to acquire a sense of self or direction or to find a way to "fit" into the surrounding world (Table 26-8) (Sahler and Wood, 1997).

Cognitive Development

The work of Jean Piaget is widely used to understand the process of **cognitive development.** According to Piaget, learning results from actively manipulating objects and information, followed by a mental processing of the event. As the child interacts with the environment, new objects and problems are discovered. The child creates mental schemes or thought patterns to understand the encounter. The **scheme** is the action pattern and the mental basis for the action. It permits the child to receive information from the world, make sense of it, and predict future events. Development occurs as the schemes increase in scope and complexity.

TABLE 26-7 Assessing Adolescents

Assessment	Focal Points	Nursing Implications

Physical	Decreasing number of acute illnesses
	Vital signs:
	    Heart rate: 55 to 110 beats/min
	    Respiratory rate: 16 to 20 breaths/min
	    Blood pressure range: 110/66 to 120/76 mm Hg
	Growth spurt may last 24 to 36 months and occurs for females between 9½ and 14 years of age for and males between 10½ and 16 years of age
	Weight gain varies:
	    Males: 12.5 to 29 lb (5.7 to 13.2 kg)
	    Females: 10 to 23 lb (4.6 to 10.6 kg)
	Height increases:
	    Males: 10 to 11 inches (26 to 28 cm)
	    Females: 9 to 11 inches (23 to 28 cm)
	Loss of primary teeth completed/addition of wisdom teeth
	Vision 20/20
	Growth of reproductive organs
	Skeletal growth: mass doubles
	Fat deposits and muscle mass increase
	Skin: increase of acne
	Hair growth: axillary and pubic; males: facial, chest, and extremities
	Development of secondary sexual characteristics (Tanner staging)
	    Females: menarche averages 121/4 years; Tanner stage 3 to 4
	    Males: ejaculation Tanner stage 3; fertility Tanner stage 4
		Provides anticipatory guidance regarding normal growth patterns
		Identification of deviant growth patterns
		Inspect number and condition of teeth, noting loss of deciduous teeth and eruption of permanent teeth
		Provides education on preventive dental care
		Identification of dental problems
		Address issues of sexuality, including abstinance: physical and emotional changes, peer pressure verses option to decline, responsiblility for sexual behaviors
		Provide information on preventing pregnancy and sexually transmitted diseases
		Teach breast and testicular self-examination
		Immunizations
		Screening for hypertension
		Screening adolescents at risk for hyperlipidemia

Nutrition	Caloric needs increase with periods of increased growth; average requirements:
	    Males 3000 kcal/day
	    Females 2100 kcal/day
	Capable of selecting and preparing own meals
	Increased occurrence of eating disorders: anorexia, bullemia, pica, obesity
		Obtain diet history
		Provides education regarding balanced diet, healthful snacks, need for breakfast, and exercise needs
		Identifies eating disorders, obesity, and problems with body image
		Refers as appropriate

Sleep patterns	Obtain history of sleep requirements Ideal sleep: 9 hr/night with regularity of schedule	Identification of deviant sleep patterns Provide counseling on meeting sleep requirements
Development	Early adolescence (10-13 yr): focus on body changes and comparison to peers; beginning separation from parents and challenging authority Middle adolescence (14-17 yr): increasing involvement with peers and independence from family; sexual exploration Late adolescence (18-21 yr): concern with future plans; likely to be involved in committed intimate relationship	Discuss school performance. Identify plans for future including school, work, relationships with family and peers, life skills. Strategies to improve communication skills. Strategies for anger management and conflict resolution without violence. Strategies for handling independence.
Safety	Injury and accidents are the leading cause of morbidity and mortality in this age group Risk-taking behaviors result from feelings of invincibility, challenging authority, and seeking peer approval.	Education regarding tobacco and substance abuse, including alcohol, steroids, and over-the-counter substances; driving; sports safety, including protective equipment, seat belts, firearms

Base on data from Neinstein L: *Adolescent health care; a practical guide,* ed 3, Philadelphia, 1996, Williams & Wilkins; Millonig VL: *The pediatric nurse practitioner certification review guide,* Potomac Md, 1990, Health Leadership Associates.

TABLE 26-8 Erikson's Stages of Ego Development

Age	Psychosocial Conflict	Resolution
0-1 yr	Trust/mistrust	Sense of hope
2-3 yr	Autonomy/ shame or doubt	Self-confidence and self-control
4-5 yr	Initiative/guilt	Independence
6-11 yr	Industry/inferiority	Competence
12-18 yr	Identity/identity diffusion	Sense of self/ loyalty

Assimilation is the process of integrating new experiences into existing schemes. When new information cannot fit into the existing schemes, the child must modify schemes or develop new schemes. This process is **accommodation.** The general thought process or mental activity is an operation.

Piaget identified four stages of cognitive development that represent increasing problem-solving ability (Table 26-9). A transition period with combinations of behaviors exists between each of the stages. The nurse must understand characteristics of cognitive ability at each stage to work effectively with the child and family.

1. The *sensorimotor period* from birth to 2 years of age involves the operation of object permanence, causality, and symbolism. The infant moves through progressive stages from an inability to remember objects not seen to an ability to locate an object if only a part of it is visible. The toddler later learns to locate a totally hidden object. At first the toddler cannot find a hidden object if it is moved to another location unless he sees it moved. The toddler can then locate the object after a series of moves without actually seeing the moves to achieve object permanence. By similar progressions, the concept of cause and effect emerges. The infant moves from simply recreating accidentally discovered effects (such as kicking movements) to moving a toy, to increasingly complex behaviors to cause events (such as winding up a toy to make it move). Symbolic representation involves a progression from using the same actions on all objects to using an object to represent another correctly (e.g., offering a doll a drink from a toy cup).

2. During the *preoperational stage* from ages 2 to 7 years, children are magical thinkers. They are unable to separate stories and fantasy from reality. This stage is divided into two periods. The first period, the preconceptual stage from 2 to 4 years of age, is characterized by increasing symbolism in play and language. The child is unable to take the perspective of another or imagine how another might feel or think. The second period is the intuitive phase from 4 to 7 years of age.

The child is very literal in understanding of words and is apt to confuse coincidental occurrences with causation. During this phase the child can only deal with one aspect of an object at a time, enabling very simple classification or grouping.

3. The *concrete operations* stage from 7 to 11 years of age enables new skills but only with directly perceived information. The child is unable to perform mental operations requiring abstract thinking. The understanding of the concept of relations is evidenced by the ability to classify objects by characteristics, order a series of objects, and understand that the properties of objects remain the same even if the appearance is altered.

4. *Formal operations,* beginning at approximately 11 years of age, enable the child to work with abstract ideas and use inductive and deductive reasoning to solve problems. With this stage comes the ability to construct new thoughts and ideas from previously obtained information and to form hypotheses. Development of formal operations continues through adolescence and into adulthood, although some people never completely progress through this stage (Sahler and Wood, 1997).

An understanding of cognitive abilities of the child enables the nurse to plan appropriate teaching strategies. A teaching session on nutrition, including superheroes and incorporating imitation as a strategy to choose healthful food, would be appropriate for a 4-year-old child who is in the preoperational stage. An 8-year-old child has the ability to understand food groups and composition of a healthy diet; these skills would guide the content and approach used to offer nutrition information. Concrete thinkers need visual methods of teaching, such as pictures and diagrams, and would benefit from "hands on" experiences. Those with formal operation abilities would be able to form and test hypotheses.

Piaget's theory offers information to help parents understand and cope with the child's behavior. Parents are often distressed because the infant cries with separation and is afraid of strangers between 7 and 9 months of age. Offering information about the development of object permanence and the ability to handle several pieces of information at the same time is reassuring. Separation anxiety or protest results from the infant's ability to remember that the parent exists even though not seen, which is a newly emerging skill at this age. Stranger anxiety or awareness occurs because the infant is able to compare two sets of information simultaneously: familiar and unfamiliar people. It is helpful for parents to understand the behavior as a normal part of cognitive development (Brazelton, 1994).

NUTRITION

Promoting good nutrition and dietary habits is one of the most important parts of maintaining child health. The first 6 years are the most important for developing sound life-

TABLE 26-9 Piaget's Stages of Cognitive Development

STAGE	AGE	CHARACTERISTICS	EXAMPLE
Sensorimotor	0-8 mo	Reflex behaviors become purposeful	Moves fist while grasping rattle; repeats action to shake rattle for the sound it makes
	8-18 mo	Object permanence: objects and people exist when not present	Looks for hidden toy or cries for mother when she leaves
	18-24 mo	Symbolism: objects can represent other objects; words can represent objects; beginning of mental representation: think before doing action	Gets an object from another room; knows mentally what object is even if not seen and can think about getting it before acting
Preoperation	2-7 yr	Self awareness: aware of self as separate from events in environment; development of a sense of vulnerability	Questions to learn about environment
		Egocentric: inability to take other's view	Develops fears as unable to separate reality from things seen on television or heard
		Symbolism: language is literal; blending of real world and fantasy; increasing complexity of symbolic play	Learns from imitation
		Irreversibility: cannot reverse an action or situation	Nightmares seem "real"
		Finalism: every event has direct cause and every question has direct answer	Cannot retrace steps of situation to look for lost thing
		Centration: only focuses on one aspect of situation	Changing shape changes toy: rolling out a ball of clay makes it bigger
		Magical thinking: not a clear sense of what is real; confuses coincidence with causation	Fascination with monsters and superheroes to cope with sense of vulnerability
Concrete operation	7-11 yr	Learns by manipulation of objects	Has better understanding of time, place, number
		Classification: orders objects by characteristics	Enjoys collections because of the ability to group and classify
		Conservation: understands that properties of objects remain the same despite change of appearance	Ability to understand beyond the literal meanings of words
		Egocentricity: considers other view point	Increasing use of humor, riddles, and jokes
		Internal regulation: able to send messages to self	Participates in group games; peer relationships important
			Increasing ability to apply relationships, build upon previous experiences and make inferences as long as the ideas involve concrete or physical objects
Formal operation	11-19 yr	Hypothesizes: uses propositonal thinking, which does not require experience with the problem	Ability to perform scientific process
		Considers alternative explanation for same phenomenon	Follows train of thought to a logical conclusion
		Considers alternate frames of reference	Idealism may interfere with reality
		Tests hypothesis with deductive reasoning	Begins to form personal rules and values
		Synthesizes and integrates concepts to other schemes	
		Works with abstract ideas	
		Reflective, futuristic thinking	

TABLE 26-10 Daily Dietary Guidelines: Childhood and Adolescence

	1 TO 3 YEARS		4 TO 6 YEARS		7 TO 12 YEARS		ADOLESCENCE	
	SERVINGS/ DAY	SERVING SIZE	SERVINGS/ DAY	SERVING SIZE	SERVINGS/ DAY	SERVING SIZE	SERVINGS/ DAY	SERVING SIZE
MILK/DAIRY 1/2 c milk = 1 oz cheese or 1/2 c yogurt or 1/2 c pudding	2	1/2c	2	3/4 c	2-3	1 c	2-3	1 c
PROTEIN 1 oz lean meat = 1 egg or 1 oz cheese or 2 T peanut butter or 1/4 c cottage cheese or 1/2 c dried peas or beans	2	1 oz	2	2 oz	2	2 oz	2-3	2 oz
VEGETABLES/FRUITS 1 small fruit = 1/2 c juice or 1/2 cut fruit	4-5	3-4 T (1/4 c)	4-5	4-6 T (1/2 c)	At least 5	1/3-1/2 c	At least 5	1/2c
BREADS/CEREALS 1 slice – 1/2 c cereal or 1 oz cold cereal or 1/2 c pasta or 2-3 crackers	3-4	1/2 slice	4	1/2 slice	6-11	1 slice	6-11	1 slice

Adapted from American Academy of Pediatrics Committee on Nutrition: *Pediatric nutrition handbook*, ed. 4, Elk Grove Village, Ill, 1998, Author.
c, Cup; T, tablespoon.

time eating habits. The quality of nutrition has been widely accepted as an important influence on growth and development. It is now becoming recognized for an important role in disease prevention.

Atherosclerosis begins during childhood. Other diseases, such as obesity, diabetes, osteoporosis, and cancer, may have early beginnings also (Forbes, 1997). *Healthy People 2000* objectives include reducing obesity, improving the quality of the diet, and increasing cardiovascular fitness. Educating children and their families is an appropriate way to accomplish these objectives (USDHHS, 1991).

Factors Influencing Nutrition

The child and family both provide a range of variables that influence nutritional habits. Ethnic, racial, cultural, and socioeconomic factors influence what the parents eat and how they feed their children. The child brings individual issues to the nutritional arena, such as slow eating, picky patterns, food preferences, allergies, acute or chronic health problems, and changes with acceleration and decel-

eration of growth. Parents often have unrealistic expectations of what children should eat. Table 26-10 offers guidelines to daily requirements for all ages.

Nutritional Assessment

Physical growth serves as an excellent measure of adequacy of the diet. Height, weight, and head circumference, if younger than 3 years old, plotted on appropriate growth curves at regular intervals allow assessment of growth patterns. Good nutritional intake supports physical growth at a steady rate (Fig. 26-2).

A 24-hour diet recall by the parent is a helpful screening tool to assess the amount and variety of food intake. If the recall is fairly typical for the child, the nurse can compare the intake with basic recommendations for the child's age. It is important to ask about the family's and child's concerns regarding diet. It is also helpful to look at the family's meal patterns. A key area of nutrition assessment includes the child's and family's exercise. Behavior problems that occur during meals may also be an issue.

Nutrition During Infancy

The first year of life is critical for growth of all major organ systems of the body. Most of the brain growth that occurs during the life span occurs during infancy. The digestive and renal systems are immature at birth and during early infancy. Certain nutrients are not handled well. Energy needs are high. Nutrition during this time influences how an infant will grow and thrive.

Types of infant feeding

Breast milk is the preferred method of infant feeding. Breast milk provides appropriate nutrients and antibodies for the infant. Breastfed infants have fewer illnesses and allergies. If breastfeeding is not chosen, commercially prepared formulas are an acceptable alternative. Although evaporated milk with added sugar has been used in the past as a low-cost alternative to breast milk, it is now discouraged. Errors in mixing and the lack of vitamins and minerals have been common problems.

The method of feeding is a choice that parents should make with guidance and education. The advantages and disadvantages of breast, formula, and combination feeding should be discussed with the parents.

Nurses should be prepared to instruct and support parents in the feeding method of their choice. For breastfeeding, teaching topics include comfortable position, appropriate techniques, feeding frequency, the let-down reflex, care of breasts, and length of feedings. The mother's feelings about nursing her infant and the presence or absence of family support are important to success. For bottle feeding, parents need instruction about preparation and care of equipment and formula, position, frequency, and amount of feeding. Parents may need to discuss feelings about the method of feeding.

Supplements

Current recommendations from the American Academy of Pediatrics indicate that the iron in breast milk is highly available to the infant. Breastfed infants do not require iron supplementation. Infants who are not breastfed should be given a commercial formula that is fortified with iron. Addition of iron to formula has reduced the incidence of anemia and does not cause stomach symptoms. After 4 to 6 months of age, iron needs are further met by the introduction of iron fortified cereals.

Fluoride at 0.25 mg/day is recommended for infants who drink ready-to-feed formula or formula mixed with water from a supply containing less than 0.3 ppm of fluoride. Fluoride is currently started at 6 months of age and maintained until 16 years of age. Fluoride is not recommended for breastfed infants whose mothers have a fluoridated water supply (AAP Committee on Nutrition, 1998)

Introduction of solid foods

Current trends include the introduction of solids between 4 and 6 months of age. There is no nutritional, developmental, or psychological advantage to starting earlier. Studies have not shown that cereal helps a baby sleep longer. Parents need to know the risks of feeding solids too early:

- The incidence of constipation is greater when solid food intake is too high.
- Early introduction of solids may lead to overfeeding and obesity.
- There is a greater possibility of food allergy because immunoglobulin A (IgA) production is insufficient for solid foods until closer to 6 months.
- If the infant lowers milk intake because of filling on solids, there may be an imbalance of nutrients.

Once parents have decided to start solids, nurses can help them plan a schedule for starting appropriate foods. Dry cereal fortified with iron is a useful starter food because of the ease of digestion (see Appendix E.9).

At 1 year of age, the infant may be changed from formula to whole milk. Skim, lowfat, and 2% milk are not recommended for babies less than 2 years of age because of insufficient fat and caloric content (AAP Committee on Nutrition, 1998).

Nutrition During Childhood

The skill and desire to self-feed begins at approximately 1 year of age. The parental role begins to shift at this time to providing a balanced, healthy range of foods as the child assumes more independence. Growth rate and caloric needs decrease during this time. Nurses can best assist parents by offering information on daily needs and healthy food choices. Suggestions for children might include the following:

- Frequent, small meals may be better accepted.
- Offer a balanced diet incorporating variety and foods that the child likes.
- Limit milk intake to the recommendations for age.
- Consider the child's development and safety; avoid nuts, popcorn, grapes, and similar foods to decrease risk of aspiration in young children.

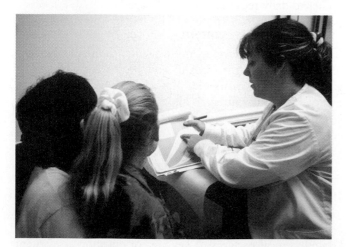

FIG. 26-2 A nurse explains the growth patterns on a growth chart to a child and her mother.

- Encourage children to help with food selection and preparation based on developmental skills.
- Generally, vitamin and iron supplements are not necessary.
- Avoid using food as a punishment or reward.

Fat content in the diet should be restricted to less than 30% beginning at 2 years of age, with no more than 10% of the total calories coming from saturated fats. Studies show that children as young as 2 to 6 years of age have diets higher in total fats and in saturated fats than recommended. In general, the family diet does not contain enough fiber-rich foods or fruits and vegetables. Diets of school-age children have been shown to be low in calcium. Children also need regular physical activity. Observations of children indicate that they are too sedentary. The entire family may benefit from suggestions to modify the diet:

- Choose low-fat protein sources: plant proteins, such as beans, peas, and wholegrain products or lean cuts of meat, chicken, or fish, trimming visible fat.
- Broil, bake, stir-fry, or poach foods rather than fry.
- Use polyunsaturated and monosaturated fats found in nuts, seeds, nut butters, wheat germ, and vegetable oils.
- Decrease salt, sugar, and fats.
- Increase complex carbohydrates: breads, grains, cereals.
- Increase fruits and vegetables to at least 5 serving/day, especially green and orange vegetables and citrus fruits.
- Use low-fat dairy products.
- Increase calcium intake through low-fat dairy products, calcium-fortified products, and supplements, if necessary.
- Maintain regular activity (e.g., exercise, sports, household chores) and limit television viewing.

Remind parents that they are teaching children lifelong strategies to prevent illness and promote good health (AAP Committee on Nutrition, 1998).

Adolescent Nutritional Needs

The preadolescent and adolescent years are a time of increased growth that is accompanied by increases in appetite and nutritional requirements. Caloric and protein requirements increase for boys 11 to 18 years of age. Girls have an increased protein need but a decreased caloric need during the same age span. The iron needed by the adolescent is nearly double that needed by adults.

Adolescent nutritional needs are influenced by physical alterations and psychosocial adjustments. Teenagers are often free to eat when and where they choose. Eating habits acquired from the family are dropped. Food away from home is a major souce of nutrition. Fad foods and diets are prominent. Accelerated growth and poor eating habits make the adolescent at risk for poor nutritional health. Adolescents have the most unsatisfactory nutritional status of all age groups. Deficiencies in iron, vitamins, calcium, riboflavin, and thiamine are most common (Neinstein and Schack, 1996).

Nurses initiate activities that promote improved nutritional status. Such activities include the following:

- Provision of information on good nutrition in individual or group sessions
- Diet assessment
- Educational activities that focus on effects of fad foods and diets
- Supplying of "at risk" nutrients
- Provision of a daily food guide (see Table 26-10)
- Suggested snacks and "on the run" foods that supply essential nutrients
- Relationship of good nutrition to healthy appearance

IMMUNIZATIONS

Routine **immunization** of children has been very successful in the prevention of selected diseases. The ultimate challenge is making sure that children receive immunizations (Fig. 26-3). Cost and convience are two critical issues in determining whether children are immunized. Successful programs combine low-cost or free immunizations provided at convient times and locations. It is important to urge parents to obtain immunizations for their children, focusing on the issue at every opportunity.

The goal of immunization is to protect by using immunizing agents to stimulate antibody formation (see Chapter 38 for types of immunity). Immunizing agents for active immunity are in the form of toxoids and vaccines. Toxoid is a bacterial toxin (e.g., tetanus, diphtheria) that has been heated or chemically treated to decrease the virulence but not the antibody-producing ability. Vaccines are suspensions of attenuated (live) or inactivated (killed) microorganisms. Examples include pertussis (inactivated bacteria); measles, mumps, and rubella and oral polio (live attenuated virus); and hepatitis B (inactivated virus).

The neonate receives placental transfer of maternal antibodies. This natural passive immunity lasts for about 2

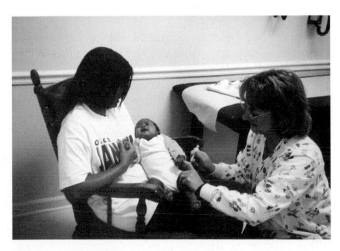

FIG. 26-3 An infant receives a regularly scheduled immunization.

TABLE 26-11 Recommended Immunization Schedules for Children Not Immunized in First Year of Life

TIME INTERVAL/AGE	IMMUNIZATION	COMMENT
YOUNGER THAN 7 YEARS		
First visit	DTaP or DTP, Hib, HBV, MMR, OPV or IPV	MMR if child is 12 mo; TB testing may be done at the same visit; Hib is not indicated if the child is >60 mo.
Interval After First Visit		
1 mo	DTaP or DTP, HBV, Var	
2 mo	DTaP or DTP, Hib, OPV or IPV	Second dose of Hib is not indicated if >15 mo when first dose was given.
at least 8 mo	DTaP or DTP, HBV, OPV or IPV	
4-6 yr	DTaP or DTP, OPV or IPV, MMR #2	DPT or DaTP not necessary if the fourth dose was given after 4 yr; OPV not necessary if the third dose was given after 4 yr.
11-12 yr	Td	Repeat every 10 years throughout life
7 YEARS AND OLDER		
First visit	HBV, OPV or IPV, MMR, Var, Td	Var: susceptible children 13 yr or older receive 2 doses at least 1 month apart.
Interval After First Visit		
2 mo	HBV, OPV or IPV, MMR#2, Td	Minimal interval between doses of MMR, HBV, IPV is 1 mo.
8-14 mo	HBV, OPV or IPV, Td	
10 years after last Td	Td	Repeat every 10 years throughout life.

HBV, Hepatitis B virus; *DTP*, diphtheria-tetanus toxoid-pertussis; *DTaP*, diphtheria-tetanus toxoid-acellular pertussis; *Hib*, *Haemophilus influenzae* type b conjugate vaccine; *IPV*, inactivated polio vaccine; *OPV*, oral polio vaccine; *MMR*, measles-mumps-rubella; *Td*, adult tetanus-diphtheria toxoid (used after age 7); *Var*, varicella.
Adapted from American Academy of Pediatrics: *1997 Red book: report of the committee on infectious diseases*, ed 24, Elk Grove Village, Ill, 1997, Author.

months. Protection is temporary and is only to diseases to which the mother has sufficient antibodies. The immune system of both term and preterm infants is capable of adequate antibody response to immunizations by 2 months of age. Generally, this is the recommended age to start immunizations. (Exception: the hepatitis B series may begin at birth.)

The interval between immunizations is important to the immune response. After the first injection, antibodies are produced slowly and in small concentrations (primary response). Subsequent injections with the same antigen are recognized by the body, and antibodies are produced much faster and in higher concentration (secondary response). Because of this secondary response, once an initial immunization series has been started, it does not need to be restarted if interrupted, regardless of the length of time elapsed. Once the initial series is completed, boosters are required at the appropriate intervals to maintain an adequate concentration of antibodies.

Recommendations

Immunization recommendations rapidly change as new information and products are available. Two major organizations are responsible for guidelines: the American Acad-

emy of Pediatrics (AAP) and the U.S. Public Health Service's Advisory Committee on Immunization Practices (ACIP). Table 26-11 and Table 26-12 list current recommendations. The main goal of the guidelines is to provide flexibility to ensure that the largest number of children will be immunized. All health care providers are urged to access immunization status at every encounter with children and to update immunizations whenever possible. See Appendix D.3 for immunizing agents, contraindications, and side effects.

Contraindications

There are relatively few contraindications to giving immunizations. Minor acute illness is not a contraindication. Immunizations should be defered with moderate or acute febrile illnesses because the reactions may mask the symptoms of the illness or the side effects of the immunization may be accentuated by the illness.

People with the following conditions are not routinely immunized and require medical consultation: pregnancy, generalized malignancy, immunosuppressive therapy or immunodeficiency disease, sensitivity to components of the agent, or recent immune serum globulin, plasma, or blood administration.

TABLE 26-12 Immunization Schedule: Range of Ages for Routine Immunizations

VACCINE	BIRTH	2 MO	4 MO	6 MO	12 MO	15 MO	18 MO	4-6 YR	11-12 YR	14-16 YR
HBV	HBV #1 →	HBV #2 →		HBV #3 →						
DTP		DTP #1*	DTP #2*	DTP #3*	DTP #4*^	or DTaP+ →		DTP #5 or DtaP	Td →	
Hib		Hib #1*	Hib #2*	Hib #3*	Hib #4*					
OPV		OPV #1	OPV #2	OPV #3 →				OPV #4		
MMR				MMR #1 →				MMR #2 →		

Vaccine abbreviations *HBV*, Hepatitis B virus; *DTP*, diphtheria-tetanus toxoid-pertussis; *DtaP*, diphtheria-tetanus toxoid-acellular pertussis; *Hib*, Haemophilus influenzae type b conjugate vaccine; *IPV*, inactivated polio vaccine; *OPV*, oral polio vaccine; *MMR*, measles-mumps-rubella; *Td*, adult tetanus-diphtheria toxoid (used after age 7) *Var*, varicella
*DTP and Hib combination vaccine may be given when DTP and Hib are administered simultaneously
+Dtap #4 or DTP #4 may be given as early as 12 months if 6 months have elapsed since DTP #3
‡if not given previously; may begin the series at any visit
§ACIP recommends 2 doses of IPV at 2 and 4 months, followed by 2 doses of OPV at 6 to 18 months and 4 to 6 years
‖susceptible children 13 years or over should receive 2 doses at least 1 month apart
¶MMR#2 may be administered at any visit provided 1 month has elapsed since dose #1 and both given after 12 months of age.
Adapted from American Academy of Pediatrics; *Recommended childhood immunization schedule*, United States, January 1999, ed 24, Elk Grove Village, Ill, 1997, American Academy of Pediatrics

Legislation

The National Childhood Vaccine Injury Act became effective in 1988. It requires providers to advise parents and clients about the risks and benefits of the immunizing agent as well as possible side effects. Informed consent is recommended. Vaccine Information Statements (VIS) are used for this purpose. Provisions for reporting specific compensable adverse reactions to specific vaccines are also covered in this act (AAP, 1997). This program allows compensation for vaccine-related events. Since enactment lawsuits have been reduced, drug manufacturers have had less of a liability burden (AAP, 1997).

Vaccines for Children (VFC), an entitlement program enacted in 1995, is designed to provide free vaccines to eligible children. This program includes children on Medicaid, children without health insurance, Native Americans, and those whose health insurance does not cover immunizations. Although this program is limited in scope, it reflects a commitment to child health and a beginning to an expanding focus on prevention.

MAJOR HEALTH PROBLEMS
Injuries and Accidents

Injuries and accidents are the most important cause of disease, disability, and death among children. Injuries cause one-half of all childhood and three-fourths of all adolescent deaths in the United States. Each year, 20% to 25% of all children will have a serious problem related to accidents or injuries. Most are preventable. The key to changing behaviors is teaching age-appropriate safety.

Motor vehicle accidents are the leading cause of death among children and teenagers. One-fourth of those deaths involved drunk drivers. Two-thirds of the children who are killed in motor vehicle accidents are unrestrained. Surveys show that 20% of infants and 40% of children and teens are unrestrained in cars (Fig. 26-4). As many as 80% of children who are using seat belts or carseats are restrained incorrectly (National Center for Injury, 1998). Motor vehicle accidents not only include automobile collision but also pedestrian injury. Drowning and burns account for most of the other deaths; poisons and falls also contribute heavily. Development is an important issue in identifying risks to children. Table 26-13 lists the three leading injury causes of death by age.

Infants

Infants have the second highest injury rate of all groups of children. Small size contributes to the type of injury. The small airway may be easily occluded. The small body fits through places where the head may be entrapped. Infants are handled on high surfaces for the convenience of the caregiver, placing them at great risk for falls. In motor vehicle accidents, small size is a great disadvantage and increases the risk for crushing or being propelled into surfaces. Immature motor skills do not allow for escape from injury, placing them at risk for drowning, suffocation, and burns.

Toddlers and preschoolers

This population experiences a large number of falls and poisonings, as well as motor vehicle accidents. They are active, and their increasing motor skills make supervision difficult. They are inquisitive and have relatively immature logic abilities.

School-age children

The school age group has the lowest injury death rate. At this age, it is difficult to judge speed and distance, placing them at risk for pedestrian and bicycle accidents. Universal use of bicycle helmets would prevent 135 to 155 deaths and 39,000 to 45,000 head injuries per year. Peer pressure often inhibits the use of protective devices such as helmets and limb pads. Sports and athletic injuries are increased in this age group (National Center for Injury Prevention and Control, 1998).

Adolescents

Injury accounts for 75% of all deaths during adolescence. Risk-taking becomes more conscious at this time, especially among males. The death and serious injury rates for males are three times higher than for females. Adoles-

cents are at the highest risk of any age group for motor vehicle deaths, drowning, and intentional injuries. Use of weapons and drug and alcohol abuse play an important role in injuries in this age group (Neinstein, 1996). Youth gangs are more violent and seem to be increasing in prevalence. Suicide is the second leading cause of death among youth between the ages of 15 and 24 (National Center for Injury Prevention and Control, 1998). Poor social adjustment, psychiatric problems, and family disorganization increase the risk for suicide.

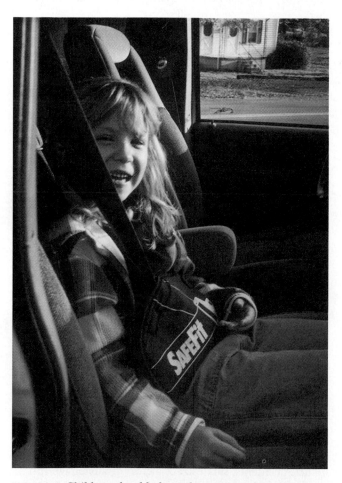

FIG. 26-4 Children should always be restrained while riding in a vehicle.

WHAT DO YOU THINK? *Most states have enacted laws allowing health care providers to treat adolescents in certain situations without parental consent. These include emergency care, substance abuse, pregnancy, and birth control. All 50 states recognize the mature minors doctrine. This allows youths 15 years of age and older to give informed medical consent if it is apparent that they are capable of understanding the risks and benefits and if the procedure is medically indicated.*

If a minor can give consent, is there also an obligation to maintain confidentiality when providing health care? Health care providers are guided by three premises. It is thought that adolescents may not seek health care if they believe that their parents will be notified. Many providers note that the client is the adolescent, not the parent. Federal and state statutes and professional ethical standards support confidentiality for adolescents. In most situations, it is important to provide confidentiality. At certain times, release of information should occur despite the adolescent's desire for confidentiality. These include legal situations (e.g., physical abuse) or if the minor poses a danger to self or others (English, 1996).

Sandy, a 15 year old, has revealed to the nurse that she has become sexually active with her boyfriend. She has no interest in any form of birth control. The nurse wants to involve her parents, but Sandy does not want them to know. What are the issues? What are Sandy's rights? What strategies could the nurse use in this situation?

Injury and accident prevention

The nurse has a responsibility in the prevention of accidents and injuries. The nurse is responsible for identification of risk factors by assessing the characteristics of

TABLE 26-13 Types of Injury Causing Death By Age Group (yr) *

<1	1 TO 4	5 TO 14	15 TO 20
Aspiration	Fires/burns	Pedestrian	Motor vehicle accident
Homicide	Drowning	Motor vehicle accident	Suicide
Motor vehicle accident	Motor vehicle accident	Drowning	Homicide

*Listed in order of frequency.
Based on data from Baker SP et al: *The injury fact book*, ed 2, New York, 1992, Oxford Press.

the child, family, and the environment. Interventions include anticipatory guidance, environmental modification, and safety education. Education should focus on age-appropriate interventions based on knowledge of leading causes of death and risk factors.

Topics to consider are listed in Box 26-5 (see also Appendix E.11). The Research Brief about the Niffenegger article discusses a study involving handwashing practices.

Acute Illness

Infection is the most significant cause of illness in infants and children. Infectious diseases, whether bacterial or viral in origin, are usually associated with a variety of symptoms: fever, upper respiratory symptoms, generalized discomfort and malaise, loss of appetite, rash, vomiting, and diarrhea. Most are self-limited and can be handled by the family at home with interventions to prevent complications. The nurse may need to identify whether the child can be managed at home based on the severity of symptoms and the family's abilty to provide care. The nurse may be involved in developing a home care plan. Also the nurse teaches the family about the illness and prevention of its spread. Nursing interventions for home care of a child with a gastrointestinal virus are shown in Box 26-6.

Infectious diseases may be more serious in younger children and infants. Neonates, because of immunologic immaturity, are more susceptible to bacterial illness with spread to multiple organ systems, called *sepsis*. Children of all ages are at risk for invasion of the spinal fluid, or meningitis. The morbidity and mortality rates of these forms of infection vary with the age of the child, causative organism, severity of the illness, and the onset of treatment. The nursing role includes early identification and referral (see a pediatric text for signs and symptoms of sepsis and meningitis), supporting the family during the treatment phase, and follow-up care as indicated. Preventive measures include family education in hygiene and identification of environmental sources of infection (see Appendix E.8).

Sudden Infant Death Syndrome

Sudden death may occur in infants with a specific disorder such as meningitis or a chronic illness. When no specific cause of death can be determined, the death is labeled **sudden infant death syndrome (SIDS)**. Each year, over 5000 infants die of SIDS in the United States, making it the most common cause of death during the first year of life. Few factors can be used to predict the occurrence. Most deaths occur between 1 and 5 months of age, although it may occur up to 1 year of age. Only a small number of infants who died of SIDS experienced a previous episode of cyanosis or apnea. Cardiorespiratory monitoring has not

---

BOX 26-5 Injury Prevention Topics

Car restraints, seat belts, air bag safety
Preventing fires, burns
Poison prevention
Preventing falls
Preventing drowning, water safety
Bicycle safety
Safe driving practices
Sports safety
Pedestrian safety
Gun control
Decreasing gang activities
Substance abuse prevention

RESEARCH *Brief*

Data were gathered to determine if an instructional program for child care could significantly reduce the spread of infectious diseases in the test center. In a test group of 3 to 5 year olds and their teachers, classes were held on germs and handwashing. A similar control group maintained their usual handwashing practices. During 21 weeks, including cold and flu season, the test group had significantly fewer colds than the control group.

Past reasearch suggests that children in center care are 18 more times as likely to become ill than children who stay at home. This study demonstrates a way to improve those statistics. Nurses who are in a position to consult schools and daycare centers can develop educational strategies that are age appropriate and may make a difference in illness in their community.

Niffenegger JP: Proper handwashing promotes wellnes in child care, *J Pediatr Health Care* 11:1, 1997.

BOX 26-6 Nursing Guide: Home Management of Gastrointestinal Virus (GEV) in Children

- Education regarding expected course of the illness: GEV is usually self-limited with vomiting lasting 1 to 2 days and diarrhea lasting up to 7 to 10 days.
- Progressive diet management: NPO for 3 to 4 hours; sips of oral electrolye solution every 5 to 10 minutes for 2 hours; clear liquids (primarily oral electrolyte solution) for the rest of the day; bland, easily digested foods (BRAT diet: banana, rice, applesauce, toast) for the next 24 to 48 hours.
- Fever management with antipyretic agent if needed (avoid aspirin).
- Monitor for signs of dehydration and intructions on seeking further care: urinates less than usual; parched, dry mouth and mucus membranes; poor skin turgor; sunken eyes with no tears; irritability; lethargy.
- Prevention of spread: instructions on handwashing technique.

been shown to decrease the incidence. SIDS occurs more often in preterm and low-birth-weight infants and possibly in infants with upper respiratory tract infections. SIDS also occurs more often in male infants and in low socio-economic groups. Maternal cigarette smoking increases the risk 3 to 4 times. The risk to siblings is unclear at present. Studies show that the prone sleeping position and tight swaddling may increase the risk. The incidence has de-creased 38% since the supine sleep position has been pro-moted. There is no test to identify infants who may die, making this a frustrating clinical problem (Brooks, 1997).

When an infant dies, the family requires tremendous support. The nurse provides empathetic support and as-sists the family as they progress through the grief process and deal with siblings and other family members. Referral to support groups may be helpful.

Nursing interventions for SIDS include teaching of the following prevention strategies:
- Supine position for healthy infants
- No parental smoking
- Improved access to prenatal and postnatal health care
- Teaching and providing close follow-up care for high-risk groups
- Improved use of baby monitors for selected infants

Chronic Health Problems

Improved medical technology has increased the number of children surviving with chronic health problems. Exam-ples include Down syndrome, spina bifida, cerebral palsy, asthma, diabetes, congenital heart disease, cancer, hemo-philia, bronchopulmonary dysplasia, and acquired im-munodeficiency syndrome (AIDS). Despite the differences in the specific diagnoses, the families have complex needs and similar problems. Several variables exist to assess for each child and family:
- Is the condition stable or life threatening?
- What is the actual health status?
- What is the degree of impairment to the child's ability to develop?
- What type and what is the frequency of treatments and therapy required?
- How often are health care visits and hospitalizations re-quired?
- To what degree are the family routines disrupted?

The common issues of chronic health problems include the following:
- All children and adolescents with chronic health prob-lems need routine health care. The same issues of pedi-atric health promotion and health care need to be ad-dressed with this group.
- Ongoing medical care specific to the health problem needs to be provided. Examples include monitoring for complications of the health problem, specific medica-tions, dietary adjustments, and therapies such as speech, physical, or occupational therapy. Ongoing evaluation of the effectiveness of treatment protocols is critical.

- Care is often provided by multiple specialists. There is a need for coordinating the scheduling of visits, tests, or procedures and the treatment regimen.
- Skilled care procedures are often required and may in-clude suctioning, positioning, medications, feeding techniques, breathing treatments, physical therapy, and use of appliances.
- Equipment needs are often complex and may include monitors, oxygen, ventilators, positioning or ambula-tion devices, infusion pumps, and suction machines.
- Educational needs are often complex. Communication between the family and team of health care providers and teachers is essential to meet the child's health and educational needs.
- Safe transportation to health care services and school must be available. Several barriers exist, including fam-ily resources, location, ability to be fitted appropriately in car restraint systems, and the amount and size of supportive equipment.
- Financial resources may not be adequate to meet the needs.
- Behavioral issues include the effect of the condition on the child's behavior as well as other family members. Chronic health problems may cause stress on relation-ships.

Nursing interventions in the primary care setting with a child diagnosed with insulin-dependent diabetes mellitus serve as a model for pediatric chronic health problems. Box 26-7 lists nursing care for diabetic children.

Alterations in Behavior

Behavioral problems in the child and adolescent are highly variable and may include eating disorders, attention prob-lems, substance abuse, elimination problems, conduct dis-orders and delinquency, sleep disorders, and school mal-adaptation. A healthy self-concept is supported by positive interactions with others. Problem behaviors may provide negative feedback, which may generate low self-esteem. A child's coping mechanisms are influenced by the individ-ual developmental level, temperament, previous stress ex-periences, role models, and support of parents and peers. Maladaptive coping mechanisms present as problem be-haviors. Inappropriate behaviors may lead to further phys-ical or developmental problems.

The common areas of behavior problems are as follows:
- Interplay of self-concept and self-esteem
- Need for a family-centered approach to management
- Multidisciplinary teams often involved in care

Attention deficit disorder (ADD) interventions are presented as a model for nursing management of a behav-ior problem (Box 26-8). ADD is a combination of inatten-tion and impulsiveness, and it may include hyperactivity not appropriate for age. ADD frequently includes low self-esteem, labile mood, low frustration tolerance, temper out-bursts, and poor academic skills. The evaluation is based on symptoms. Diagnosis is made by excluding other dis-

BOX 26-7 Nursing Guide: Insulin-Dependent Diabetes Mellitus in Children

- Follow-up care to evaluate child for disease control and to ensure that the family is coping well with management of care
- Family teaching including the following:
  Disease process, complications, insulin action
  Insulin therapy: technique; storage; dose adjustment
  Glucose monitoring: technique; frequency of readings; interpretation of results
  Diet regulation: diet developed to consider family diet, food preferences, and schedules: diet plan; timing meals and snacks; allowing for occasional treats and modifications for "special times"
  Exercise planning: type; intensity; duration; monitoring; relationship of diet and insulin to exercise; coordination with family patterns and school activity
  Smoking prevention: additive effects to vascular disease
  Skin care and hygiene to prevent infections
  Emergency management of hypoglycemia and hyperglycemia
- Coordination of specialty services: eye care, endocrinology, nutritionist, primary care provider
- Referral to support groups, camps for psychosocial needs
- Referral for qualification for state or federal programs (e.g., Children's Specialty Services)

BOX 26-8 Nursing Guide: Attention Deficit Disorder

- *Assessment.* History, physical, parent/family assessment, learning and psychoeducational evaluations.
- *Behavioral modifications.* Home and school: teaching families techniques to support clear expectations, consistent routines, positive reinforcement for appropriate behavior, and time out for negative behaviors.
- *Classroom modifications.* Consult with family and teachers to meet individual needs for remediation or alternate instruction methods if necessary; structuring activities to respond to the child's needs.
- *Support:* Referral to family therapy, support groups, or mental health services to assist development of positive coping behaviors.
- *Medications.* Consult with physician to monitor for therapeutic and adverse effects.
- *Follow-up.* Assess at 3- to 6-month intervals when stable. Dynamic process affected by relationships with others. Behaviors will change with age; problem may persist through adulthood.

Modified from Miller KJ, Costellanos FX: Attention deficit/ hyperactivity disorders, *Pediatr Rev* 19:11, 1998.

orders. Symptoms vary with severity of the problem, and interventions range from simple to complex. A familial tendency exists; several members of a family may be affected. Treatment involves a family focus and includes health professionals and educators (Miller and Castellanos, 1998).

PROGRESS TOWARD CHILD HEALTH: NATIONAL HEALTH OBJECTIVES

Healthy People is a national effort to improve the health of the population. In 1979, the Public Health Service set out objectives for improved health status and prevention to be achieved by 1990. The year 2000 health objectives expanded the focus from avoiding premature death to prevention of illness and disability. The 2010 health objectives will expand the efforts further based on data gathered. Three themes prevail: 1) prevent illness and disability, 2) reduce disparities in health among populations, 3) and increase accessibility of health services.

WHAT DO YOU THINK? *The number of children with health insurance is decreasing. Should insurance companies be required to sell "children only" policies for families who cannot afford the cost of premiums for the entire family?*

States, cities, and communities throughout the country are using *Healthy People* objectives to develop health promotion programs and services. The focus is the families, neighborhoods, schools, and workplaces, which are the environments where change can occur. Race, ethnic group, gender, and economic status influence the level of health.

The Centers for Disease Control and Prevention (CDC) estimated that over one half of the 2.1 million premature deaths in the nation are preventable with changes in individual behavior and improved access to health care. *Healthy People 2000* goals embrace strategies to improve prevention efforts in sources of premature death, which are listed in Table 26-14. All areas apply directly to the child and adolescent population. Progress toward objectives in specific child and adolescent areas are reviewed in Table 26-15 (USDHHS, 1991).

NEEDS OF CHILDREN WITHIN THE COMMUNITY

Nursing, through developing and coordinating community services and through formation of public policies, promotes the well-being of children within the community. Assessments are made to identify the needs and target populations at risk. Programs based on the needs of specific at-risk populations are developed for the delivery of health care.

Strategies for Health Care in the Community

Nurses are in a position to work with groups of families or children through programs targeting the health care needs of those at risk. Three strategies for common pediatric concerns are identified to model nursing interventions in the

TABLE 26-14 Sources Of Premature Death

TARGET AREA	NUMBER OF DEATHS ANNUALLY
Tobacco use	400,000
Inappropriate diet and exercise patterns	300,000
Underage drinking	100,000
Under immunization	63,000
Firearms	35,000
Sexually transmitted diseases	30,000
Poor access to health care services	290,000
Total number of preventable deaths/yr	**1,218,000**

Adapted from US Department of Health and Human Services: *Healthy people 2000: midcourse review and 1995 revisions*, Washington, DC, 1991, USDHHS.

TABLE 26-15 Progress of *Healthy People 2000* Objectives: Pediatric Applications

OBJECTIVE	MOVING TOWARD GOAL	MOVING AWAY FROM GOAL
Fewer people overweight		X
More people exercising regularly	X	
Fewer youth beginning to smoke	X	
Decreased alcohol and drug use in those 12 to 17 years of age	X	
Fewer teen pregnancies		X
Fewer homicides and assault injuries		X
Fewer unintentional injuries and deaths	X	
Increased use of car safety restraints	X	
No children with elevated blood lead	X	
Fewer children with dental caries	X	
Fewer newborns of low birth weight		X
Fewer sexually transmitted diseases	X	
Higher immunization levels	X	
No barriers to preventive services		X

Adapted from US Department of Health and Human Services: *Healthy people 2000: midcourse review and 1995 revisions*, Washington, DC, 1991, USDHHS.

community. Strategies include programs based in the home, targeted at the needs of homeless persons, or centered in daycare or school settings.

Home-based service programs

Home-based service programs vary in goals and target populations. In general, home visiting programs increase use of available community resources by bringing the services into the home or neighborhood or by promoting awareness of resources (Box 26-9). By working on problems within the home setting, families can strengthen problem-solving abilities. Home visitor programs may offer the following services based on needs of the community:

- Monitoring the health status of vulnerable populations
- Childrearing education
- Counseling services
- Social support
- Clinical services
- Safety instruction

Programs may consist of professional and trained lay people forming a team to provide services. Home-based programs have been shown to decrease preterm and low-birth-weight deliveries, improve parenting capabilities, enhance the development of disabled children, promote early hospital discharge, and decrease health care costs (Olds, 1991). Specific programs might include home visiting programs to support the transition from hospital to home for preterm infants or programs to prevent home accidents and injury.

Interventions are based on assessment of the needs of the child and family (see Appendix I.1). Areas to be assessed include interactions and relationships, environment, and developmental appropriateness (Box 26-10).

Programs for homeless families

Actual numbers of homeless children and adolescents are difficult to determine. Estimates vary from 200,000 to 800,000 children and adolescents. Families comprise the fastest growing segment of the homeless population; 25% to 40% of homeless are families, often a single mother with 2 or 3 children (NCHS, 1998). The longer the duration and the amount of disruption of support systems determine the effects of homelessness on health. Children in homeless situations are often not immunized and suffer from poor nutrition. There is limited or no access to health care. Often there is increased exposure to environmental hazards, violence, and substance abuse. The combination of health problems, environmental dangers, and stress is referred to as the **homeless child syndrome** (Redlener, 1991).

Children experience chronic illness, such as tuberculosis, asthma, anemia, and chronic otitis media. Hospitalizations are more frequent in this population. Behavioral problems may exist, such as sleep disorders, withdrawal, aggression, or depression. School performance problems may arise from lack of regular attendance. Many of the children demonstrate developmental delays as a re-

BOX 26-9 **Community Resources for Children's Health Care**

Children's service clinics
Well child clinics
Immunization clinics
Infectious disease clinics
Children's Specialty Services
Family violence/child abuse centers
School health programs
Head Start
Parents Anonymous
Crisis hotlines
Community education classes
Early Intervention/Developmental Services
Childbirth education classes
Breastfeeding support groups
Parent support groups
Family planning clinics
Women, Infant's, and Children (WIC) programs
Medicaid
Youth employment/training programs

BOX 26-10 **Components of the Home Assessment**

INTERACTIONS AND RELATIONSHIPS
Interaction with home visitor
Ease of family members
Accurate representation of the normal relationships

Interaction/relationships Observed Between Family Members
Express positive responses to the child
Family members talk to child and respond to child
Age-appropriate discipline and restriction

ENVIRONMENT
Age/type of building
Adequate sanitation facilities: waste disposal, washing facilities
Adequate refrigeration
Type of heating and cooling systems/routinely maintained
Adequate space
Safety:
    Fire/burns: smoke detector; fire extinquisher; hot water temperature plan established; limit exposure to sources of burns (fireplaces, heating units)
    Falls/injury: hazards identified and limited (e.g., stairs, windows); firearms absent or secured; toys and furniture safe
    Poison prevention: hazards identified and limited; Ipecac; emergency procedure

DEVELOPMENTAL OPPORTUNITES
Toys, games, books appropriate for age
Controlled use of television and radio
Family expectations of child appropriate
Child given age-appropriate responsibilities
Family encourages and supports activies to develop skills

sult of the lack of an appropriate environment to foster development.

The nurse may be involved in outreach programs combining health care workers and community members to take the health care services to the homeless (see Box 26-11). Identifying a consistent team to provide continuity of care on a regular basis is important. The family is often removed from its network of neighbors, friends, relatives, and the usual health care providers. Emphasis should be placed on preventive and follow-up care and immediate problems. Services include physical examinations, behavioral and developmental assessments, nutritional support, screening tests, and immunizations (Redlener, 1991).

Daycare and school

Daycare centers and schools provide an environmental framework for the child and adolescent population. Over 7 million children under 6 years of age are enrolled in daycare. Studies have shown that these children are 18 times more likely to acquire infectious diseases than children who are not in daycare (Brunell, 1994). Most of these diseases for the older child and adolescent originate in school. The nurse can establish programs and serve as a resource to daycare centers and schools.

Nurses can provide information regarding illness and injury prevention for child care providers and teachers to improve health and safety. Centers and schools may need assistance in developing standards for hygiene, sanitation, and disinfection to prevent the spread of disease. This may include handwashing, food preparation, and cleaning of toys and equipment. Requirements for immunizations of both children and staff may need to be established. Guidelines for care of sick children should be developed. Staff members may benefit from educational programs on top-

ics such as infectious diseases, cardiopulmonary resuscitation (CPR), behavior management and discipline, or other concerns that they may have.

Health education should be incorporated into the school curriculum for older children and adolescents. The students should be encouraged to participate in identifying the content and presentation of the material. Topics may include sports participation, self-care, and health-related topics, such as prevention of disease.

Education for families of the children may focus on coping strategies, such as division of responsibilities, identification of frustrations, and dealing with behaviors that signify stress and tension. Nurses are in a key position to consult with these populations and serve as a resource for program development.

Service Programs for Children in the Community

Types of services offered based on the priorities from *Healthy People 2000* objectives include health promotion, health protection, and preventive services. Many of the

---

BOX 26-11 Healthy People 2000 Priorities: Examples of Child and Adolescent Focus

- *Health promotion.* Breastfeeding support programs, parenting skills classes, prevention of tobacco use, parent support groups, screening for families at risk for child abuse/neglect, nutrition education programs
- *Health protection.* Injury prevention counseling, toy safety seminars, playground safety, sports physicals and safety instruction, dental screenings, fluoride supplementation, car seat loan programs
- *Preventive services.* WIC programs, family planning services, immunization programs, lead screening, hearing and vision screening

---

RESEARCH *Brief*

America's youth are engaged in risky health behaviors. Those who smoke cigarettes are the most likely to have many poor health habits. An NCHS survey of randomly selected youths 12 to 21 years of age documented an association between smoking and other unhealthy behaviors. Current smokers were 3 to 17 times more likely to have used other substances, such as alcohol and marijuana. Almost 50% of the smokers drank alcohol and were more likely to binge drink than nonsmokers. Almost 40% have engaged in physical fighting and carrying weapons, including guns and knives. Other behaviors occurred at a higher rate among smokers: 60% engaged in sexual intercourse, 66% failed to use a seat belt, 50% failed to exercise regularly, and 87% reported a diet lacking in fruits and vegetables.

The survey focused on the adolescent period when many life-long habits and attitudes are set. This information helps nurses understand the scope and connections between risky behaviors. Nurses can use this information to educate families, preadolescents, and adolescents as a prevention strategy.

National Center for Health Statistics: *Relationship between cigarette smoking and other unhealthy behaviors among our nation's youth,* Advance Data No. 263, NCHS office of public affairs, April 24, 1995.

---

health care needs of children and adolescents fall within these priorities. Box 26-11 lists examples. To address these priorities, the nurse may be involved in community assessment, political action, and establishment of programs. Three program ideas with strong implications regarding the health of children are presented as models.

Smoking prevention

Smoking has been identified as the most important preventable cause of morbidity and mortality in the United States, yet 50 million Americans smoke. Smoking is associated with cardiovascular disease, cancer, and lung disease. Parents often do not understand or believe the effects of smoking on children. Children exposed to **secondhand smoke** experience increased episodes of ear and upper respiratory tract infections. Children of smokers are more likely to smoke. Teenagers who become smokers are rarely able to quit (Rasco, 1992).

The number of teenagers smoking has not decreased since 1980, with the age of onset of smoking becoming younger. Statistics show that as many as 6 million teenagers and 100,000 preteens smoke on a daily basis. Tobacco industry advertising has increased through use of advertisements, billboards, and sponsorship of sporting events. Cigarette advertisements appear in "teen" magazines, and companies offer logo products that appeal to children. More than 80% of a group of 6-year-old children were able to associate a picture of Joe Camel with cigarettes. Although 46 states have laws prohibiting the sale of cigarettes to minors, restrictions are not enforced. Minors are able to purchase tobacco products 46% to 88% of the time (MacKenzie, Bartecchi, and Schrier, 1994). See the Research Brief about cigarette smoking.

Interventions to discourage smoking focus on the parent, the child or adolescent, and public policy. Parents should be offered educational programs dealing with the negative effects of smoking on children, interventions to stop smoking, and ways to create a "smoke-free" environment. Behavior modification techniques should be incorporated.

Anti-smoking programs directed toward children and teenagers are more successful if the focus is on short-term effects rather than long-term effects. Developmentally, children and teenagers cannot visualize the future to imagine the consequences of smoking. The immediate health risks and the cosmetic effects should be emphasized. Teaching should include how advertising puts pressure on people to smoke. Music, sports, and other activities, including stress reduction techniques, should be encouraged. Teaching social skills to resist peer pressure is critical.

Nurses should become politically active in the area of smoking. Banning tobacco advertising, enforcing restrictions of sale to minors, increasing funds for anti-smoking education, and restriction of public smoking may reduce the incidence of smoking.

WHAT DO YOU THINK? *Taxes should be increased on tobacco products to provide funding for health care programs and to discourage young people from smoking.*

Reduction of gun violence

Each day in the United States, 13 children are killed and 30 are wounded in gun-related accidents, suicides, and homicides. Often with each event, other children are affected by witnessing gun violence or knowing the victims.

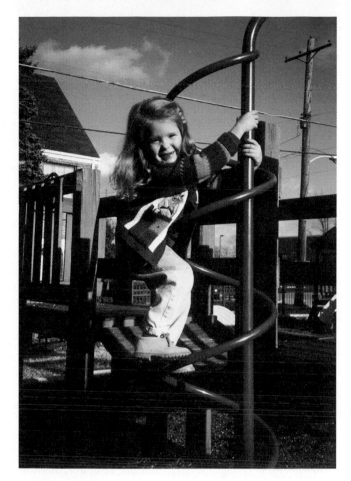

FIG. 26-5 Playground injuries are frequent among young children.

More than 135,000 children are carrying guns to school, many obtained in their own homes. At least 50% of the families in this country report owning guns, many of which are stored loaded. In a national survey, one-third of teens and preteens reported that they could obtain a gun (Havens and Zink, 1994).

Consequences of gun violence are serious. Permanent, debilitating physical injuries are sustained. Little is known about the emotional effects of being a victim of or witnessing acts of violence, but it has been proposed that the effects are long lasting. The financial burden of treatment and rehabilitaton is high and often not completely compensated.

Some of the factors associated with gun violence include access to firearms, substance abuse, poverty, and cultural acceptance of violent behavior. Interventions must begin early and address each of these factors.

Nurses can actively participate in efforts to reduce gun violence among young people. Numerous legislative actions have been proposed limiting the sale of handguns to minors and restricting possession of guns in schools. The Brady Bill authorized a waiting period for handgun purchases, raised licensing fees for gun dealers, and required

---

BOX 26-12 Guidelines for Playground Safety

- Playgrounds should be surrounded by a barrier to protect children from traffic.
- Activity centers should be distributed to avoid crowding in one area.
- Finishes should meet CPSC regulations for lead.
- Durable materials should be used.
- Sand, gravel, wood chips, and wood mulch are acceptable surfaces for limiting the shock of falls.
- Equipment should be inspected regularly for protrusions that could puncture skin or entangle clothes.
- Not recommended: multiple-occupancy swings, animal swings, rope swings, and trampolines.

Based on data from Swartz MK: Playground safety, *J Pediatric Health Care* 6(3):161, 1992.

police notification of multiple gun purchases. Nurses can urge legislators to support gun control legislation. Nurses can collaborate with schools to develop programs to discourage violence among children. Community programs focusing on gun storage, safety at school, and managing aggressive behavior need to be offered. Families may need support in supervising their children after school. Community efforts to enchance family stability and promote self-esteem are vital to decreasing violence (Havens and Zink, 1994).

Promoting safe playgrounds

Schools, daycare centers, and community groups often need guidance toward developing safe places for children to play. One child is injured on a playground every 2½ minutes. Each year over 66,000 children sustain severe injuries. The most frequent injuries are falls, with three-fourths involving head injuries (National Center for Injury Prevention, 1998) (Fig 26-5).

The U.S. Consumer Product Safety Commission has published guidelines for playground safety. Guidelines include structure, materials, surfaces, and maintenance of equipment. The developmental skills of specific ages are incorporated, as well as recommendations for physically challenged children. Nurses can use these guidelines to help the community establish standards for play areas. Box 26-12 summarizes these guidelines.

ROLE OF THE COMMUNITY HEALTH NURSE IN CHILDREN'S HEALTH

A major goal of the *Healthy People 2000* objectives is improving access to health care for children, specifically for preventive services and immunizations. The nurse is in a key position to bring about this goal. Nurses may practice in a variety of settings, including community health centers, school-based clinics, or home health programs. They may provide care through well child clinics, immunization programs, federally mandated programs such as the WIC program, or specific state-funded programs, such as Head

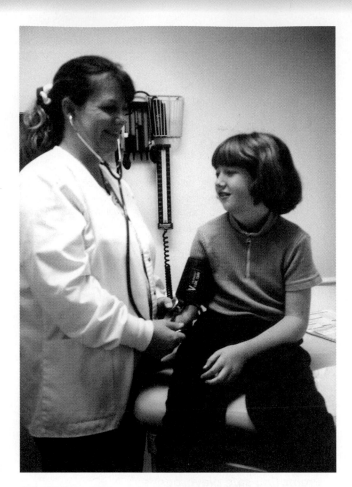

FIG. 26-6 A child gets her blood pressure taken during a well child care assessment.

Start (see Appendix A.1). Nurses provide health supervision and well child care. The nursing process and a knowledge base of the factors unique to this population provide a framework of care.

The nursing assessment includes a health history of health and illness patterns. A complete history is usually obtained at the first visit, with interim history obtained at subsequent visits. The nurse assesses the adequacy of growth, nutritional status, and concerns about diet. A physical examination is performed, the extent of which varies with the purpose of the visit. For well child care, a complete assessment, including vital signs; hearing, vision, and dental screening; and laboratory tests, is done (Fig. 26-6). Developmental and behavioral assessments enable early detection of problems and are an important component of health supervision. The nurse identifies psychosocial and emotional concerns of the child and family. Family assessment enables the nurse to identify problems that may interfere with parenting abilities (see Appendix I.1 and Box 26-10 on home assessment).

The nursing plan of care includes three major components. The first is the management of actual or potential health problems. The second involves both education and

antipatory guidance. This enables families to understand what to expect in the areas of growth and development as well as social, emotional, and cognitive changes. The nurse offers information to promote healthy life styles and to prevent health problems and accidents. A third role is case management or coordination of care. For example, the nurse serves to coordinate referrals to community agencies, other health care services or providers, or assistance programs. See Box 26-9 for a list of community resources.

Evaluation of care has always been a critical part of the nursing process. It is now a necessity in the current health care environment with health care payers requiring justification of the cost of health care services. Nurses identify and document positive outcomes from the interventions. This may include objectives such as increased knowledge or observable changes in behaviors.

clinical application

John D. is a 9 year old brought to the clinic by his mother for follow-up of an emergency department visit 5 nights ago for an episode of asthma. John has a history of recurrent episodes of wheezing and respiratory distress occurring on a regular basis since he was 4 years of age. Until 4 or 5 months ago, John has been under good control using a combination of bronchodilators and cromolyn sodium inhalers on a prescribed protocol, based on peak flow meter readings. Mrs. D reports that over the past few months, John has been uncooperative about his asthma. He refuses to use his flow meter and would not use his maintenance medication at school. During this episode, he even refuses to use his bronchodilator at school, even though he is still "sick." Mrs. D is very frustrated and states that she just "can't understand him at all." She reports no changes at home or at school. John is an excellent student, who gets along well with peers, participates in many activities and sports, and normally is very cooperative with both parents. He frequently "picks on" his sister, but his mother perceives this as appropriate. Mrs. D does admit that since the weather has been so rainy, she has smoked inside the house a few times.

The clinic nurse reviews this information with the nurse practitioner who is his health care provider. They review findings from his assessment. Physical examination is unremarkable except for evidence of an upper respiratory tract infection and peak flow readings in the clinic of 60% to 80% of his expected baseline. His medication orders from the emergency department are appropriate for his condition and include albuterol and cromolyn sodium inhalations tid to qid using a spacer device. John is fairly knowledgable about his asthma and treatment regimen, but he has "forgotten" some of the information he learned when he first started his treatment. He admits that he does not go to the office to use his inhalers at school but does not reveal why.

A. Which of the following actions would be the most appropiate for the nurse?
  1. Discuss the need to change medications with the nurse practitioner since John seems unable to stay well on the current regimen.
  2. Advise John and his mother that he must use his albuterol and cromolyn sodium inhalers. Review the pathophysiology of asthma, how the medications work, and orders for administration. Schedule a follow-up visit to see how well he is doing.
  3. Ask John what could be done to make it easier for him to use his medications. Set up a contract with John, allowing him a reward system for compliance with his asthma protocol. Review asthma information using hands-on activities and games.
  4. Refer John to an asthma specialist since he is having problems with control.
B. In talking with John's mother, the nurse should stress the importance of her smoking outside. In addition to the risks of second-hand smoke, Mrs. D. needs to know which of the following?
  1. John will sense that she does not love him if she smokes inside.
  2. John learns by observing role models. She models noncompliance with the treatment plan when she "breaks the rules."
  3. If she is to smoke inside, she should do it when John is asleep so he will not be aware of the problem.
  4. When the weather is bad, smoking is acceptable in the house as long as there is adequate ventilation.
C. The nurse refers the family to the regional asthma support program through the American Lung Association. He receives information about an asthma summer camp and names of children his age with asthma. Identify principles of development of school age children that support this intervention.
D. John's immunization record was reviewed. He has had: OPV #4, DTP #5, MMR#1, and a PPD (age 4). What immunizations, if any, does he need at this time?

Answers are in the back of the book.

KEY POINTS

- Physical growth and development is an ongoing process resulting in physical, cognitive, and emotional changes that affect health status.
- Good nutrition is essential for healthy growth and development and influences disease prevention in later life. The adolescent population is at greatest risk for poor nutritional health.
- Immunizations are successful in prevention of selected diseases. Barriers to immunizing children are cost and inconvenience.

- Pyschosocial development is subject to the interaction of emotional, cultural, and social forces. Resolution of crises at each stage of development is important for mastery of skills needed to accept oneself and to function in society.
- Cognitive development follows an orderly process of increasing complexity of thought and action patterns. Understanding the child's congnitive level is the basis of effective interventions.
- The family is critical to the growth and development of the child. Social support is one of the most powerful influences on successful parenting.
- Accidents and injuries are the major cause of health problems in the child and adolescent population. Most are preventable. Nurses have a major role in anticipatory guidance and prevention.
- Nurses are involved in strategies to meet the needs of the pediatric population in the community. Home based service programs have been successful in providing care for at risk populations. Children of homeless families are at risk for health problems, environmental dangers, and stress. Community programs to provide health care for the homeless may decrease those risks. Use daycare and school as a framework for offering education and services to groups of children, adolescents, and their families.
- Service programs aimed at decreasing smoking, reduction of gun violence, and community playground safety are important aspects of the *Healthy People 2000* initiative and help to ensure a safer future for children.

critical thinking activities

1. Develop a plan of immunization for a 5 1/2 year old who has had one DTP, Hib, and OPV.
2. Administer the Denver II or DDST-R to a 9-month-old infant. Develop a plan of anticipatory guidance.
3. Develop a plan of nursing care for a family who has experienced a SIDS death.
4. Develop a plan of nursing care for a family who has a 12-year-old child with spina bifida and a family with a 12-year-old child with leukemia. Note the commonalities.
5. Develop a nutritional program for a) mothers who are breastfeeding their infants, b) a group of 5 year olds in a kindergarten class, c) and a group of high school sophomores. What factors do these programs have in common? How do they differ?
6. Administer a safety survey (TIPP program from the American Academy of Pediatrics or develop your own) to assess the home environment of a 6 month old and a 5 year old. Develop a plan of education and anticipatory guidance for the family.

Bibliography

American Academy of Pediatrics: *1997 Red book: report of the committee on infectious diseases,* ed 24, Elk Grove Village, Ill, 1997, Author.

American Academy of Pediatrics Committee on Nutrition: *Pediatric nutrition handbook,* ed 4, Elk Grove Village, Ill, 1998, Author.

Brazelton TB: *Touchpoints,* New York, 1994, Addison-Wesley.

Brooks JG: Sudden infant death syndrome. In Hoekelman R et al, editors: *Primary pediatric care,* ed 3, St Louis, 1997, Mosby.

continued

Bibliography—cont'd

Brunell PA, editor: New CEC national program to improve quality of day care setting, *Infect Dis Watch* 4:1, 1994.

Centers for Disease Control and Prevention: Youth risk surveillance, 1995, *MMWR Morb Mortal Wkly Rep* 43, 1996.

Children's Defense Fund: *The state of America's children yearbook,* Washington, DC, 1996, Author.

English A: Understanding legal aspects of care. In Neinstein L: *Adolescent health care; a practical guide,* ed 3, Philadelphia, 1996, Williams & Wilkins.

Forbes GB: Nutrition. In Hoekelman R et al, editors: *Primary pediatric care,* ed 3, St Louis, 1997, Mosby.

GAPS Executive Committee, Department of Adolescent Health: *American Medical Association guidelines for adolescent preventative services, recommendations monograph,* Chicago, 1995, American Medical Association.

Havens DMH, Zink RL: A pediatric nurse practitioner call to arms: new solutions needed for nation's growing public health problem, *J Pediatr Health Care* 8:3, 1994.

MacKenzie TD, Bartecchi CE, Schrier MD: The human costs of tobacco use, *N Engl J Med* 330:14, 1994.

Miller KJ, Costellanos FX: Attention deficit/hyperactivity disorders, *Pediatr Rev* 19:11, 1998.

Millonig VL: *The pediatric nurse practitioner certification review guide,* Potomac Md, 1990, Health Leadership Associates.

National Center for Health Statistics: *FASTATS,* Washington, DC, 1998, US Government Printing Office.

National Center for Injury Prevention and Control: *Fact sheet* [on-line], Nov, 1998. Available: www.cdc.gov/ncipc/duip

Neinstein L: *Adolescent health care: a practical guide,* ed 3, Philadelphia, 1996, Williams & Wilkins.

Neinstein LS, Schack LE: Nutrition. In Neinstein L: *Adolescent health care; a practical guide,* ed 3, Philadelphia, 1996, Williams & Wilkins.

Olds DL: Nonphysician home visits. In Green M, Haggerty RJ, editors: *Ambulatory pediatrics,* ed 4, Philadelphia, 1991, W.B. Saunders.

Physicians desk reference, Montvale, NJ, 1998, Medical Economics Company.

Rasco C: Discouraging smoking: interventions for pediatric nurse practitioners, *J Peditric Health Care* 6(4):200, 1992.

Redlener I: Health care for homeless children: special circumstances. In Green M, Haggerty RJ, editors: *Ambulatory pediatrics,* ed 4, Philadelphia, 1991, W.B. Saunders.

Sahler OJZ, Wood BL: Theories and concepts of development as they relate to pediatric practice. In Hoekelman R et al, editors: *Primary pediatric care,* ed 3, St Louis, 1997, Mosby.

Swartz MK: Playground safety, *J Pediatric Health Care* 6(3):161, 1992.

US Department of Health and Human Services: *Healthy people 2000: midcourse review and 1995 revisions,* Washington, DC, 1991, USDHHS.

Watterberg K, Gallaher KJ: Signs and symptoms of neonatal illness. In Hoekelman R et al, editors: *Primary pediatric care,* ed 3, St Louis, 1997, Mosby.

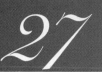

Women's Health

SHIRLEEN LEWIS-TRABEAUX & DEMETRIUS J. PORCHE

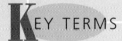 www.mosby.com/MERLIN/community_stanhope

OBJECTIVES

After reading this chapter, the student should be able to:

- Define the term *women's health.*
- Describe the women's health movement in the United States.
- Describe the health status of women in the United States.
- Discuss the development of women.

- Examine issues of young adult women, women in midlife, and older women.
- Discuss the major health alterations of women.
- Identify the health needs of special populations of women.
- Explain the term *the cost of caregiving.*
- Analyze health policy and legislation that influences women's health.

KEY TERMS

anorexia
anovulatory
bulimia
caregiver burden

estrogen replacement
   therapy
hormone replacement
   therapy (HRT)
liposuction

menopause
osteoporosis
perimenopausal
preconceptional
   counseling

urinary incontinence
women's health
women's health
   movement
See Glossary for definitions

CHAPTER OUTLINE

The authors would like to acknowledge the contributions of Dr. Linda Corson Jones who died in 1997.

This chapter examines the health status of women in the United States and worldwide. The history of the women's health movement is presented. The relatively new but growing body of literature that documents the distinctive nature of women's development is explored. Major health issues of women, such as heart disease, cancer, HIV, reproductive health, depression, midlife, and aging, are presented. The issue of abuse against women is covered in Chapter 37. Strategies in which community health nurses can help women meet health needs throughout the life span are emphasized. The pivotal role of women in ensuring the family's and community's health is highlighted in the discussion of programs for women's health services. Factors influencing women's access to health services, including unequal services, financial and employment issues, gender-power issues, family considerations, health behaviors of women, and health care providers' attitudes, are considered. Health policy, including major legislation affecting women's health services and future directions for women's health, is discussed.

DEFINITIONS

To understand women's health issues, one must first understand the term **women's health.** The American Academy of Nursing's 1996 Expert Panel on Women's Health says that women's health includes their entire life span and involves health promotion, maintenance, and restoration. This term, women's health, recognizes that the health of women is related to the biological, social, and cultural dimensions of women's lives. Moreover, women's normal life events or rites of passage, such as menstruation, childbirth, and menopause, are considered part of normal female development, rather than syndromes or diseases requiring medical treatment only. This broad emphasis on women's health is in contrast to the view of women in terms of their reproductive health or their role in parenting children.

HISTORY OF THE WOMEN'S HEALTH MOVEMENT

The **women's health movement** has its origin in the feminist movement. The first wave of feminism began in the United States in the mid-nineteenth century. Industrialization created changes in the social and family structure of women's lives. The burden of women's work at home decreased and large numbers of women left the workforce. During this time birth rates decreased and life expectancy increased. Women were then free to achieve more education and to spend more energy on social reform.

The second wave of feminism in the 1960s and 1970s gave birth to the women's health movement. At this time, fertility continued to decrease, and women continued to earn higher education. Women's health was considered within the domain of the obstetrician and gynecologist. In the 1960s Congress passed Title VII, which banned sexual discrimination in the workplace, and civil rights for women became an important issue.

Women's health issues focused on their bodies throughout the 1970s. A women's health conference was held in Boston in 1969 to discuss "Women and Their Bodies." In 1973, the Supreme Court reviewed the case of Roe v. Wade and the decision of the court resulted in legalized abortion. This was viewed by many as a great success in establishing women's health. The first Feminist Women's Health Center was founded in Los Angeles, California. This center served as a prototype for other women's health centers and focused on self-determination and the need to change the power relationships within medicine.

The medicalization of childbirth began to change in 1972 with the formation of the International Childbirth Education Association (ICEA). The ICEA created changes in childbirth such as rooming in, having husbands present during delivery, natural childbirth, and birthing centers, and it promoted increased use of midwives.

A National Women's Health Network (NWHW), established in 1974 to monitor national health care policy, functions as a clearinghouse and advocates for women's health. In 1986, the National Institutes of Health (NIH) developed a health care policy that called for the inclusion of women in clinical research. In 1990, the Office of Research on Women's Health within the NIH was formed. This office has the responsibility to address women's health issues (Geary, 1995).

The women's health movement that was initiated at the grassroots level has now become a national movement. Although the importance of women's health began gaining national recognition during the last two decades, issues related to women's health continue to exist. For example, the rate of breast cancer deaths has increased, yet no one knows why (Cooper et al, 1998). Heart disease is a major killer of women, but until recently the majority of research has been conducted on men. Women are the fastest-growing high-risk group for developing human immunodeficiency virus (HIV), yet only in the last few years have national HIV treatment studies included women. Most types of depression are twice as common in women as they are in men. Domestic violence, including sexual, physical, and psychological abuse, remain significant health problems for women (discussed in Chapter 37).

NURSING TIP

Women should be actively involved in the planning of women's health programs. Include women who are representative of the target population to serve as formal or informal leaders, gatekeepers, or role models.

HEALTH STATUS OF WOMEN

Unfortunately, millions of people, particularly women, do not have access to basic resources to attain a state of health. In most countries women live longer than men, but women are generally less healthy. This difference in health is related to poverty. Although women compose half of the world's population, they represent 70% of the people in the world who live in poverty (Craft, 1997a). In the United States, two thirds of all poor adults are women. Of those individuals living below the poverty level, most are single mothers with children.

In the last half of the twentieth century, the number of women working outside of the home increased by 170% (NWHIC, 1998a). Projections are that by the year 2005 nearly 50% of the work force will be women (Bureau of Labor Statistics, 1996). Although women have made progress in obtaining managerial and executive jobs, the majority of women continue to work in traditionally low-paying occupations such as teacher, clerical, cashier, manager, administrator, and registered nurse. Earning for women have improved significantly in the past 30 years; however, women still earn less than men do. For every dollar a man earns a woman earns about 75 cents. Even when women perform the same work as men, they may earn less. For example in nursing, a traditionally female occupation, female registered nurses earn less than their male counterparts (Bureau of Labor Statistics, 1996). Two thirds of all part-time workers are women (Bureau of Labor Statistics, 1995). Part-time workers are less likely to have job-sponsored medical benefits, such as medical leave and insurance, and are more likely to depend on assistance programs such as Medicaid and Medicare.

Although women have made some strides in their efforts to achieve financial equality during the last decade, progress has been slow. Worldwide the education of women is the single most important factor in the improvement of the health of women and their families. As women are educated, their socioeconomic status improves and mortality rates decline (Craft, 1997b). Because women's financial stability is closely linked to health outcomes, it is essential to promote policies that support the advancement of women. Nurses can play a vital role as key mobilizers in empowering women, empowering themselves, and working with communities to take control of women's health and ensure that resources are developed to benefit both genders equally (Conway-Welch et al, 1997).

DEVELOPMENTAL THEORIES

Major theories of human development are based on the work of men such as Erikson, Freud, Piaget, and Kohlberg. An inherent gender bias appears to exist in the work of these classic human developmental theorists because their research was based on males. Consequently, theories of men's development became the accepted normal adult development for all. When research findings do not easily apply to women, it is assumed that the problem is with the female gender and not with the research. For example, in Erikson's now-classic stages of psychological development, the stage of identity formation is identified as crucial in the development of a normal healthy adult. To achieve identity formation, an individual must separate and be-

come autonomous from others. As a result of Erikson's work, many developmental psychologists continue to define normal development in terms of autonomy, independence, and separation. A female's identity may not be found through independence and separation but instead in the relationships that she forms with others.

Until the 1960s the classic developmental theories, on which modern developmental psychology is based, were unchallenged. Three factors led women to challenge the male-dominated human development theories. First, in the 1960s the feminist movement pushed women's issues to the front. Second, the number of women psychologists increased significantly in the 1970s. Finally, female psychologists began to conduct research with women.

As the evolution of women's developmental theory advances, more will be learned about qualities important to women's development, such as nurturing and intimacy. To effectively support women, nurses need to understand the importance of relationships and responsibilities to women.

HEALTH PROMOTION AND LIFESTYLE ISSUES: WOMEN ACROSS THE LIFE SPAN

A life span approach to women's health recognizes that the health status of a woman in one phase of her life affects subsequent phases, as well as the lives of her children (Craft, 1997b). This section discusses adolescent and young adult women, women in midlife, and older women. Issues concerning special populations of women are examined, and reproductive health is discussed.

Adolescent and Young Adult Women

Adolescence, ages 12 through 18 or 21, is the gateway to adulthood and a time of major physical, emotional, and social changes. Female identity develops during adolescence and early adulthood. In childhood many girls are socialized to be passive, and they are not expected or encouraged to achieve as much as boys. Because of this early female socialization, many adolescent and young adult women experience difficulties developing their sense of identity, self-esteem, and independence. Sadly, females who fail to develop self-worth are often underachievers and perform poorly in school.

Adolescence and early adulthood is also a time when young women make choices about diet, physical activity, tobacco and alcohol use, and sexual practices that can influence their health throughout life. Girls who enter adolescence with low self-worth are more vulnerable to choosing health-damaging behaviors (USDHHS, PHSOWH, 1998a).

Nurses can work with other health providers, parents, schools, and religious and community organizations to provide girls with positive messages, meaningful opportunities, and accurate information about their health. A national public education campaign called "Girl Power!" began in 1996. The campaign is designed to help 9- to 14-year-old girls empower themselves to build skills and self-confidence in academics, arts, and sports. The campaign also addresses issues such as tobacco, alcohol and other drugs, premature sexual activity, physical activity, nutrition, and mental health (USDHHS, PHSOWH, 1998b).

In adolescence and young adulthood, females are developing bone mass that will be critical to the prevention of osteoporosis. Consequently, it is very important for young females to establish a lifelong habit of regular weight-bearing physical activities such as walking, running, dancing, aerobics, soccer, and weight-lifting. Also, this age group needs adequate calcium in their diet to help build healthy bones. Regular physical activity also enhances psychological health and in turn increases self-esteem and reduces stress. Competitive team sports promote cooperation and assertiveness. These social skills can be useful to adolescents and young women throughout their lives (USDHHS, PHSOWH, 1998a). Suggestions for eating healthily and exercising regularly are listed below.

Women in Midlife

Ages 35 to 65 years are commonly referred to as *midlife*. This transition time represents the more mature years after young adulthood but before the senior years. Today it is expected that a woman will live one third of her life past menopause.

Midlife is a time of physiological, psychological, and social changes for women. **Menopause** is a biological transition in women's lives that has personal, social, and cultural significance (Woods, 1994). Although menopause is a universal life transition for women during midlife, women are poorly prepared for what to expect during this stage.

Natural menopause is a gradual process, with progressive changes in **anovulatory** cycles and eventual cessation of menses. In the 8 to 10 years preceding menopause, hormonal changes occur that eventually lead to amenorrhea. During the **perimenopausal** period, women may note a number of changes resulting from a reduced production of estrogen. The most common physical symptoms are bleeding pattern changes, hot flashes, genital and skin changes, weight gain, and cardiovascular and bone changes (Rousseau, 1998). Additionally, emotional symptoms include irritability, fatigue, tension, nervousness, depression, and inability to concentrate. Some of these changes are apparent (hot flashes), but others are silent (cardiovascular and bone changes), having no immediate signs or symptoms.

Hormone replacement therapy (HRT) is the most frequently prescribed therapy for symptoms related to menopause. In addition to reducing hot flashes, HRT appears to retard the development of osteoporosis, reduce urinary incontinence and vaginal dryness, prevent thinning of the skin, reduce the risk of heart disease, reduce the risk of Alzheimer's disease, and positively affect mood. Despite the number of health benefits that can be documented for HRT, great controversy still surrounds this form of therapy. Some women do not like the side effects of HRT, such as headaches, nausea and vomiting, bloating, weight gain, and irritation with contact lenses. HRT may also increase the likelihood of developing gallbladder disease, endometrial cancer, and breast cancer.

Increasingly, women want to be actively involved in selecting therapies for managing the effects of hot flashes and other symptoms that occur during midlife. Many women choose self-management approaches, including

---

HOW TO *Eat Healthy and Be Physically Active*

1. Set realistic personal goals that focus on personal health and well-being, not weight loss
2. Measure progress by changes in fitness and energy level, as well as improvements in blood pressure, glucose, and lipids
3. Make lifestyle changes that are internally motivated (for self) rather than externally motivated (for spouse, family, or friends)
4. Do not go on a diet; gradually make healthy dietary and lifestyle choices
5. Identify weaknesses in dietary practices and physical activity habits and plan strategies for dealing with them
6. Develop good long-term eating practices such as the following:
   a. Include the daily servings from each food group in the food guide pyramid
   b. Choose to eat more whole grains, cereals, beans, soy products, as well as five fruits and vegetables a day
   c. Avoid one of the pitfalls of overeating by not skipping meals or getting hungry
   d. Always eat breakfast
   e. Always have healthy foods available for snacking
7. Realize that regular physical activity is an absolute requirement to maintain a healthy body weight
8. Participate in regular physical activity that is enjoyable, convenient, and inexpensive
9. Find an exercise partner or exercise classmates to help motivation
10. Find a sport you enjoy and do it regularly
11. Consider walking, running, dancing, aerobics, soccer, or weight-lifting
12. Take a break from physical activity at least one day per week

Adapted from Manore M: Running on empty: health consequences of chronic dieting in active women, American College of Sport's Medicine (ACSM) *Health and Fitness Journal* 2(2):24, 1998.

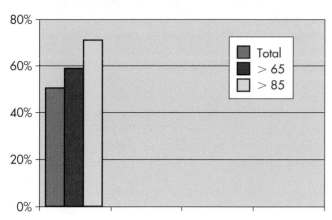

FIG. 27-1 Female population in the United States. (From Administration on Aging: *Profile of older Americans: 1997* [on-line], 1997. Available: www.aoa.dhhs.gov)

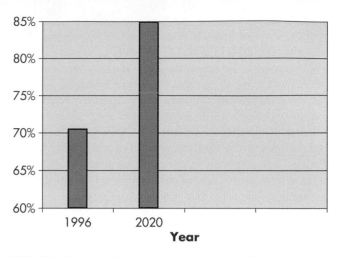

FIG. 27-2 Projected increase in the number of women aged over 85 years. (From Administration on Aging: *Profile of older Americans: 1997* [on-line], 1997. Available: www.aoa.dhhs.gov)

self-help groups, relaxation techniques, biofeedback, imagery, exercise, and herb and vitamin therapies.

Self-management of hot flashes includes an awareness of patterns and precipitating factors, such as particular foods or environmental temperatures to avoid. Spicy foods, alcohol, and caffeine may increase hot flashes. Many women find that their hot flashes are worse when environmental temperatures are highest. Some women elect to wear only cotton clothing because cotton does not trap heat and moisture like synthetic fabrics. Women may be able to reduce nighttime awakenings caused by hot flashes by sleeping in a cool bedroom. Some women find sleeping on cotton sheets helpful. Some research indicates that regular exercise may reduce the severity of hot flashes. Smoking reduces estrogen levels and may increase the risk of hot flashes.

Increasingly, women in midlife are known as the "sandwich generation." Many of these women are raising children while caring for aging parents or in-laws or assisting in the parenting of their grandchildren. Many are juggling parenting, employment, and caring for aging parents. The nurse should be knowledgeable about community services to assist these women. For example, the AARP has information and guidance for caregivers.

Older Women

Most older Americans are women. Women make up 51% of the total U.S. population, 59% of the over-65 population and 71% of Americans over age 85 (USPHSOWH, 1996) (Fig. 27-1). The fastest-growing segment of the population is Americans over the age of 85. By the year 2020, older women will account for 85% of persons aged 85 and over who live alone (Administration on Aging, 1997) (Fig. 27-2). The life expectancy for women is 79.3 years, versus 72.5 years for men. Projections for the year 2050 show the

life expectancy for women and men to increase to 85 years and 80 years, respectively (U.S. Census Bureau, 1996a).

For many women, the years past retirement are a time of enrichment and personal growth. After years of working and caring for their families, they may finally have time for themselves. Some women discover creativity within them that they were not aware existed or previously did not have time to foster. Some become writers and artists for the first time at 60 or 70 years old. Women also enjoy their older years traveling, reading, studying, gardening, and spending time with family. Unfortunately, for some of these women and many others, growing older also means facing a series of hardships and losses.

The longer women live, the poorer they become as a result of such factors as death of spouse, limited fixed incomes, and higher cost of living, including out-of-pocket health care cost. Almost three-fourths of the nation's elderly poor are women (USDHHS, PHSOWH, 1998c). Social Security benefits are the primary source of income for older women today. Older women are only half as likely as older men to be receiving pension income. The median income of older persons in 1995 was $16,684 for males and $9,626 for females (Administration on Aging, 1997).

Because women have a greater life expectancy than men do, they are more susceptible to disabilities associated with aging. It is estimated that half the additional life expectancy of women is spent in a state of disability. As the need for health care services increases with age, many elderly women are propelled further into poverty. Most women age 65 and over have Medicare coverage. Unfortunately, Medicare covers only about half of the medical cost. Medicaid is a supplemental insurance available to low-income persons. Older women spend up to 25% of their meager disposable income on out-of-pocket health care expenses (Administration on Aging, 1997). Sadly, two thirds of older women do not seek preventive services such as mammograms because of cost and problems with transportation (USDHHS, PHSOWH,1998c).

Caregiving has defined the lives of many women. This continues as women age and care for ill husbands. The demands of caregiving for a spouse are often the most difficult for women because of their own age, fading health, and lack of resources. For almost 1.3 million children, the grandmother is the primary caregiver. Community health services should be diverse enough to meet the needs of older women in a variety of circumstances (Administration on Aging, 1997).

Women are three times more likely than men to be widowed. Over half of elderly widows now living in poverty were not poor before their husbands died. Poverty increases with age and is more prevalent among older women of color who live alone (Administration on Aging, 1997). Widowed women are at increased risk for social isolation, depression, poverty, and substance abuse. As women age and become more frail they may limit their activities outside the home because of fear of crime, further isolating them.

When elderly women require care, it is frequently middle age daughters who assume responsibility for their mothers. Thus the cycle of caregiving is complete for one woman and continues for another. For those women who live beyond 85 years old, there may be no loved ones to care for them. They may die alone and neglected.

Special Populations

Four groups of women warrant special consideration because of the uniqueness of their lives. In this section, minority women, single mothers, lesbians, and women in prison are discussed. Adolescent pregnancy is discussed in Chapter 33 .

Minority women

About 26% of the female population in the United States are members of racial and ethnic minority groups. The largest minority population is African-American women, followed by Hispanics, Asian/Pacific Islanders, and American Indian/Alaska Natives. The fastest growing minority group is Asian/Pacific Islanders, followed by Hispanics.

The life expectancy for minority women is lower than that for Caucasian women. African-American women have a life expectancy of 73.5 years, compared to 79 years for Caucasian women. Income and education influence the health status of minority women. Most minority women have less formal education, earn less, are poorer, and use fewer health services than Caucasian women.

Certain diseases are more prevalent among some groups of minority women. The risk of heart disease among minority women is higher because the incidences of obesity and cigarette smoking are greater. Certain cancers have higher incidences in some groups than in others. Among Vietnamese women the rate of cervical cancer is three times

higher than that of the second-highest group. Stomach cancer is more common among Japanese and Korean women, the incidence of lung and colorectal cancer are higher among Alaska Native women, and American Indian women have a high incidence of cancer of the gallbladder. Regardless of the health problem, the outcome for poor minority women is worse than for Caucasian women. For example, although the incidence of breast cancer is higher for Caucasian women, African American women are more likely to die from the disease (NCHS, 1996).

Nurses should be sensitive to the needs of minority women. Nurses can collaborate with other health disciplines to assure that the special needs of minority women are met. Minority women require culturally sensitive health care services. Translators or bilingual nurses should be available for non–English-speaking women. Minority nurses or nurses trained in minority women's health issues should provide community-oriented prevention and treatment programs in the neighborhoods where minority women live and work (USDHHS, PHSOWH, 1998d).

Single mothers

In 1996, women were responsible for three of every ten households (U.S. Census Bureau, 1996b). Single mothers are six times as likely as single fathers to be raising children. The poverty rate for families supported by single women is higher than for married couples, and nonpayment of child support is a major factor that contributes to the financial decline of many female-headed families. In 1998, only 50% of women due to receive child support payment received the full amount awarded by the courts. The average amount of child support received in 1991 was $3011 dollars per year (U.S. Census Bureau, 1995).

Although adolescent pregnancy is an important issue, there are some women who choose to be single mothers. In 1997, 41% of single mothers had never married (U.S. Census Bureau, 1997). Some plan their pregnancy, and others choose to become single parents when they learn they are pregnant. Adolescent and minority single mothers may choose to remain single because of the decline in the number of males available to marry. A growing profile of a single mother by choice is a woman who is older, well educated, and financially able. Women who elect to become pregnant outside of marriage arrange for purposeful intercourse or artificial insemination, whereas others choose single-parent adoption.

Most single mothers do the work of two parents with the resources of one. The combined effect of the multiple responsibilities of home and a job can lead to depression and stress. Single mothers often feel lonely and isolated. A solid social network of family and friends can contribute to the well-being and satisfaction of single mothers.

Lesbians

It is difficult to determine the actual number of lesbians because they often do not reveal their sexual preferences and remain an unrecognized population. It is estimated that 2% to 10% of the female population are lesbians.

Women's Health in Canada

Karon Foster, Toronto Public Health and Ryerson Polytechnical University

LIFE EXPECTANCY AND CAUSES OF DEATH

Canadian women have seen their life expectancy improve over the past 40 years. Today, a female child can expect to live to age 81, except Aboriginal girls who can expect to live to age 75. In 1994, there were 99,335 female deaths with a death rate of 5.3 per 1,000 population (Statistics Canada, 1996). Heart disease, cancer, and motor vehicle accidents are the leading causes of death for women. For women age 20 to 44, motor vehicle accidents followed by breast cancer and suicides are the three leading causes of death. For women 45 to 64 years, cancer and circulatory diseases account for 74% of all deaths (Health Reports, 1995). For women 65 years and older, the leading causes of death are ischemic heart disease, cerebrovascular disease, and cancer, followed by pneumonia and influenza. Falls among the elderly are also a significant cause of death. Female mortality statistics for 1994 indicated 38,688 deaths due to circulatory disease, 26,310 cancer deaths, 8,255 deaths due to respiratory diseases, and 4,150 deaths due to accidental injuries (Statistics Canada, 1996). Lung and breast cancers account for most of the cancer deaths, with deaths from lung cancer now exceeding those of breast cancer.

CHRONIC CONDITIONS AND INJURIES

The National Population Health Survey Overview 1996/97 (NPHS) showed the chronic diseases with the highest incidence for women were nonarthritic back problems, arthritis/rheumatism, migraine, and hypertension (Statistics Canada, 1998). Other health problems include asthma, cataracts, heart disease, urinary incontinence, ulcers, cancer, diabetes, sexually transmitted diseases, and HIV infections. Women 65 years and older have higher incidence rates of arthritis/rheumatism, heart disease, and cancer. Younger women report migraines and allergies as common health problems. This survey also showed that repetitive strain injuries (RSI) and other injuries were also a health concern. In 1995, approximately 2 million Canadians over the age of 12 had experienced a RSI (Statistics Canada, 1998). Women most commonly reported injuries to the wrist, hand, or fingers with most of these injuries occurring at work or school. Fifty-one per cent of women reported accidental falls resulting in sprains, strains, or broken bones.

HEALTH CARE PRACTICES

How frequently do women seek health care and what preventive health practices do they participate in? Surveys show that most women report visiting a health care professional at least once per year (NPHS 98). Women over 65 years visited health professionals more frequently than younger women. General practitioners and dentists were the health professionals most commonly seen. The Canadian Cancer Society recommends that women over 50 have mammogram screening done every 2 years and that all women do breast self-examination (BSE) monthly. In the Health Population Survey, 80% of women in this age group reported having a mammogram done within 2 years (Statistics Canada, 1998). The proportion of women practising BSE has dropped since 1985. In 1990, 28% of women had never done BSE, 27% did BSE on a monthly basis, 19% did BSE every 2 to 3 months, and 27% did it even less frequently (Normand 1995). Only one third of women in the high-risk group report performing monthly BSE (Normand, 1995). The National Workshop on Screening for Cancer of the Cervix recommends that all sexually active women be regularly screened with a Pap smear every 3 years until age 70. Although, this recommendation was initially made 10 years ago, recent findings indicate that 1 in 6 Canadian women over 18 have never had a Pap test (Lee, Parsons, & Gentleman, 1998). Also, 1 in 4 women in the targeted group had not been screened according to the guidelines. Clearly, health professionals need to increase women's awareness of these screening procedures and encourage women to participate in these preventive health practises.

LIFESTYLE PRACTICES

Lifestyle factors such as smoking, alcohol use, diet, and physical activity also influence the health of women. Cigarette smoking is a risk factor for heart disease, stroke, and cancer. The percentage of Canadian women who smoke has declined in the past 15 years. In 1994, 28 % of women over the age of 15 were current smokers, while 34 % had never smoked, and 28% had stopped smoking (Normand, 1995). Women 20 to 24 years are the most likely to smoke. Smoking among teenage girls increased from 21% in 1990 to 29% in 1994.

Alcohol consumption is associated with injuries and many diseases. In 1993, 45 % of women 15 years and older reported having consumed an alcoholic beverage at least once a month. Twenty to twenty-four year olds have the highest incidence of alcoholic consumption.

Physical activity is promoted as a behaviour to prevent disease and maintain health. Forty-six per cent of women surveyed were moderately active (Normand, 1995). Older women are less active than young women are, and women with chronic health problems are more sedentary. Women are less physically active than men are; this can be attributed to women's responsibilities in caregiving and housework.

Obesity is a factor in heart disease and diabetes and has been linked with endometrial and breast cancer in women. The Heart Health Survey 92 found 27% of women have a Body Mass Index over 27 (Shah, 1994). Diet is a major factor in diseases such as cancer, heart disease, and osteoporosis. Most deaths for cardiovascular disease occur in individuals with elevated blood cholesterol. Elevated blood cholesterol levels have been noted in 43% of Canadian women (Shah, 1994).

Continued

Women's Health in Canada—cont'd

In summary, women's life expectancy has improved in Canada; however, cancer and heart disease pose major threats to the health of women. Preventive health practices, lifestyle changes, and a variety of health promotion strategies need to be use in order to address these threats.

Bibliography

Lee J, Parsons G, Gentleman J: Falling short of PAP testing guidelines, *Health Rep* 10(1):9, 1998.

Normand J: *Women in Canada: a statistical report*, ed 3, Ottawa,1995, Statistics Canada.

Shah CP, Shah S, Shah R: *Determinants of health and disease: public health and preventive medicine in Canada*, ed 3, Toronto, 1994, University of Toronto Press.

Statistics Canada: *Mortality: summary list of causes of death 1994*, Ottawa, 1996, Statistics Canada Health Statistics Division.

Statistics Canada: *National population health survey overview 1996/97*. Ottawa, 1998, Statistics Canada Health Statistics Division.

Wilkins K: Causes of death: how the sexes differ, *Health Rep* 7(2)33, 1995.

Canadian spelling is used.

There are lesbian women in all races, classes, and ethnic groups. Lesbians are both similar to and different from heterosexual women. Many lesbian women hide their sexual preference from neighbors, family, co-workers, and health care providers out of fear of discrimination and reprisal. Although the American Psychiatric Association recognized lesbianism as a normal sexual choice in 1972, heterosexism and homophobia contribute to the prejudice, fear, and discrimination that lesbian women endure. Many lesbians are denied jobs, housing, and custody of their children on the basis of their sexual orientation. Sometimes, prejudice and fear are acted out in the form of violence against lesbian women. The decision to live openly as a lesbian is a difficult one. The term *coming out* refers to the decision to disclose one's sexual identity rather than hiding it (APA, 1998). Many women report knowing as teenagers that they were attracted to females but denying their feelings out of fear. Many marry, have children, and only later in life acknowledge their sexual preference. Divorced lesbians with children are often denied custody of their children on the basis of their sexual preference.

The health needs of lesbians have not been well studied. Although many of the health care needs of lesbian women are the same as those of heterosexual women, some special considerations exist. For example, risk factors for breast cancer such as nulliparity, obesity, and high alcohol intake are more prevalent in the lesbian population; therefore they may be at higher risk for breast cancer. There is also a misconception among lesbians, as well as among health care professionals, that lesbians are at low risk for sexually transmitted diseases. Studies have found that bacterial vaginosis, trichomonas, and monilial vaginitis are very common among lesbian women (Roberts and Sorensoen, 1995). Lesbians should be advised to avoid contact with vaginal secretions and menstrual blood. To avoid unprotected oral sex, lesbians can use latex barriers, such as a dental dams. Lesbians need to also know the importance of regular pelvic examinations, Pap screening, and screening for genital infections (Levinson and White, 1995).

▌WHAT DO YOU THINK? *Courts of law have questioned the suitability of lesbians as parents. The courts have expressed concern that children of lesbian parents will suffer psychologically as a result of their upbringing. There is a fear that these children will experience impaired social relations and have sexual identity crises.*

Overall, the results of research to date suggest that home environments provided by lesbian parents are as likely as those provided by heterosexual parents to support and enable children's psychological growth. Additionally, children of lesbian mothers develop patterns of gender-role behavior that are much like those of other children. Also, children of lesbian parents have normal relationships with peers and their relationships with adults of both sexes are also satisfactory. On the basis of existing research findings, fears about children of lesbians being sexually abused by adults, ostracized by peers, or isolated in single-sex lesbian or gay communities are unfounded (Patterson, 1998).

Nurses should be aware of the parenting and reproductive needs of lesbians (Roberts and Sorenson, 1995). The issue of lesbian parents is controversial. The 1980s are known as the "lesbian baby boom" because the number of lesbian couples who choose to have children increased (Zeidenstein, 1990).

Many lesbians delay health care to avoid an encounter with a health care provider. Lesbian women complain of health care providers assuming their heterosexuality with questions such as, "What method of birth control do you use?" Because nurses tend to reflect the dominant culture, they may have a lack of knowledge about lesbian lifestyles and health concerns. Lesbian women are more likely to reveal their true selves to nurses who are open and nonjudgmental. If a woman can feel comfortable enough to disclose her lesbianism, the quality of health care that she receives is improved. Nurses can create a nonthreatening environment by asking questions such as, "Are you in a committed relationship?" "Are you single-partnered or married?" "Is your partner a man or a woman?" (Levinson and White, 1995).

Unfortunately, many lesbian women experience increased stress and depression because of social isolation, prejudice, and discrimination. The prevalence of substance use and abuse is greater among lesbians. Mental health counseling is recommended for depression. Alcoholics Anonymous or Narcotics Anonymous groups are active throughout the country. Many communities have active lesbian women's support groups.

Women in prison

Although women represent only a small percentage (5.2%) of the total state prison population, this number has increased significantly. Between 1986 and 1991 the number of women in state prisons grew by 75%. The upsurge in the female prison population is directly attributed to drugs and drug-related crimes. Over 75% of all women in prison have children, and two thirds have children under age 18. Many women in prison are poor, minority, and single mothers. The majority of women in prison report that their children's grandparents are the primary care givers (Bureau of Justice Statistics, 1994).

The problems of incarcerated women are not unlike those of women everywhere. About 6% of inmates enter prison pregnant (Bureau of Justice Statistics, 1994). Pregnant women in prison are more likely than women in the general population to be chemically dependent and enter prenatal care late. The stress of being in prison is worsened by pregnancy. Nursing interventions must be aimed at intensive health education related to childbirth and childcare. Inmates should be encouraged to discuss their concerns in self-help groups. Also, group counseling sessions for inmates and their families are suggested, as well as instruction in stress management and self-esteem enhancement (Fogel, 1993).

Reproductive Health

Women often enter the health care system because of reproductive issues or problems. It is not surprising that nurses provide a range of services in the area of reproductive health. *Healthy People 2000* identifies several objectives for improving maternal and infant health during the childbearing years, including increasing prenatal care, reducing complications of pregnancy, and decreasing low birth weight and infant mortality. In addition, improvement in preconceptional counseling and prenatal and newborn screening is sought.

U.S. women have a wide array of effective contraceptives from which to choose. Nurses need to take an active role in discussing contraception use with all women of childbearing age. Much of the literature focuses on the problem of unintended pregnancy among adolescents. Lit-

tle attention has been paid to the contraceptive concerns of adult women. Health care providers erroneously assume that adult women are fully informed about contraception, use their method correctly and consistently, and are highly satisfied (NWHIC, 1998a).

Effective contraceptive counseling requires not only accurate knowledge of current contraceptive choices but also a nonjudgmental approach. Women should be encouraged to talk about intimate family and individual issues. The goal of contraceptive counseling is to ensure that women receive appropriate instruction in order to make informed reproductive choices.

Assessment should include questions about sexual behavior; medical history; health habits, including smoking; past contraceptive methods; contraceptive failures; and motivation. Choice of method depends on compliance and motivation. Critical questions must be addressed such as, Is the woman able to take daily pills or insert a diaphragm before each act of intercourse? Does the woman want to practice the minimal compliance with contraception required by the intrauterine device (IUD), Norplant, or Depo-Provera? Contraception instruction should include discussion of all the options available. Women may put themselves at risk for unintended pregnancy through their choices if not appropriately informed. Many women seek contraceptive services with a specific contraception method in mind. Research has documented, however, that many women have wrong information regarding risks of various contraceptive methods. For example, women often overestimate the cancer risks of oral contraceptives.

A comprehensive presentation of contraception options is also important because women use many different methods and change methods often. An outline of contraceptive methods is presented in Table 27-1. Many times they never fill a prescription or purchase the over-the-counter methods. Sometimes women change contraception methods between health care visits. Women who had previously selected a highly effective pregnancy prevention option (e.g., oral contraceptives) may switch to a method that is much less effective (e.g., condoms or withdrawal) without discussing this change with a health care professional (USDHHS, PHSOWH, 1998b). Careful discussion of all the contraceptive options may prevent some of these problems.

In recent years a movement to expand the concept of prenatal care to include **preconceptional counseling** has gained momentum (Earls, 1998; Kogan et al, 1998). Preconceptional counseling includes education, assessment, diagnosis, and interventions to address risks before conception. The goal of preconceptional care is to reduce or eliminate risks for both the woman and the infant. Preconceptional care provides the nurse with an opportunity to initiate reproductive health promotion strategies. Enthusiasm for preconceptional care has increased as the rates for low birth weight, infant mortality, and congenital malformations have remained the same. Increasingly, it is

TABLE 27-1 Contraceptive Methods: Advantages and Disadvantages

CONTRACEPTIVE METHOD	ADVANTAGES	DISADVANTAGES
Spermicides	50% to 95% effective Inexpensive Convenient and easily accessible Provides some STD protection Few side effects	Local irritation
Male latex condom	97% effective Inexpensive Fairly easy to use Reduces risk of STDs	May decrease sensation Allergies Some lubricant products destroy latex
Female condom	95% effective Provides protection from STDs Provides control to women	Expense
Diaphragms	95% effective May insert up to 6 hours before sex Reduce risk of cervical cancer	Increase frequency of urinary tract infections Associated with toxic shock syndrome Can remain in place no longer than 24 hours Avoid during menses Device should be fitted by health care provider
Cervical caps	75% to 90% effective Provides contraception for 48 hours	Must be removed after 48 hours Risk for toxic shock syndrome Odor problems may be experienced Device must be fitted by health care provider
Intrauterine devices	98% to 99% effective No systemic effects Immediately reversible	Risk of uterine perforation Increase in spontaneous abortions Ectopic pregnancy risk may be increased Uterine bleeding and pain Pelvic infection
Combination oral contraceptives	99% effective Convenient and easy to use Rapidly reversible Provides women with control Prevention of fibrocystic disease	Must have daily adherence No STD protection Expensive Possible systemic side effects
Norplant	99% effective Needs little motivation from client to adhere Rapid reversibility Avoids risk of estrogen	Difficult removal Disrupts menstrual bleeding pattern
Depo-Provera	99% effective Easy to use Decreased menstrual flow	Unpredictable uterine bleeding Changes in lipids
Emergency postcoital contraception	75% effective Provides late protection Used in cases of abuse/rape	Must be started soon Systemic side effects such as nausea

From Uphold C, Graham M: *Clinical guidelines in family practice*, ed 3, Gainesville, Fla, 1998, Barmarrae Books.

recognized that many risks can be identified and corrected before conception. For example, research has linked inadequate intake of folic acid with the development of neural tube defects. Additional folic acid during the first 6 weeks of pregnancy may protect against neural tube defects. Thus the U.S. Public Health Service (1996) recommends that all women of childbearing age who are capable of becoming pregnant should consume 0.4 mg of folic acid per day.

Preconception assessment provides an opportunity to discuss a woman's family, medical, reproductive, nutri-

tional, and social history. For example, exposure to tobacco and alcohol may be detected. Education about the effects of these on the fetus can be explored, and efforts aimed at decreasing exposure can be taken.

Prenatal care is strongly associated with improved birth outcomes. A number of barriers exist for women seeking prenatal care. Many times women are hesitant to seek early prenatal care because of the cost. Some women lack transportation and must travel great distances to seek care, especially in rural areas. Women may face a bureaucratic system that is understaffed and underfinanced. Some physicians will not treat Medicaid clients or those with little insurance (Roberts et al, 1998). Often clinics are crowded; the waiting time is long. Moreover, most clinics do not offer childcare services.

Pregnant women cite a number of factors that increase their motivation to seek prenatal care, including transportation, telephone or mailed reminders, childcare, cash payments, layette gifts, and posters. U.S. social policy provides few supports for childbearing families. This is in direct contrast to most other industrialized countries. European countries, with infant mortality rates lower than the U.S. rate, provide all mothers with early adequate prenatal care. Many countries offer additional support for pregnant women. Pregnant Japanese women can ride free on city buses. In England, health visitors (public health nurses) visit all new mothers. France has developed an elaborate cash payment program for women engaged in prenatal care. Most industrialized countries have established policies that protect not only the mother and infant but also the family as well. Among these countries, only the United States and South Africa do not have a charter that states that the health and well-being of families is a national priority. The United States is also one of the few industrialized countries without a central administrative office to coordinate policies and initiatives for maternal-child health.

In addition to lack of prenatal care, lifestyle problems such as inadequate nutrition, smoking, substance use, poor maternal health, psychological distress, and violence are important contributors to high infant mortality. Promoting healthy lifestyle behaviors and reducing risk factors should provide the core of prenatal care. Nurses should also address areas such as taking vitamin or mineral supplements, stress management, gaining an appropriate amount of weight, seeking social support, and parent education.

WOMEN'S HEALTH PROBLEMS: ACUTE AND CHRONIC

Heart Disease

Heart disease is the leading cause of death among women over 50 and the second leading cause of death among women ages 35 to 39 years (NWHIC, 1998a). Although women are less likely to have heart attacks than men , they are more likely to die from heart attacks. After menopause and by age 75, the incidence of heart disease in women exceeds that of men (Arnstein, Buselli, and Rankin, 1996).

Although a number of researchers are now studying women and heart disease, the traditional knowledge base (including diagnosis and therapeutics) is based on studies using men. The presentation of heart disease in women is different from men. Men with heart disease initially experience an acute myocardial infarction with few warning signs. Women with heart disease are more likely to report chest pain and other symptoms before experiencing a myocardial infarction. Nearly 90% of women with a myocar-

dial infarction report chest pain. Additionally, women are more likely to present with upper abdominal pain, dyspnea, nausea, and fatigue (Hill and Geraci, 1998; Manson et al, 1997). Women may delay seeking treatment, expecting that a heart attack involves much more pain than they are experiencing. In addition, women's complaints may not be taken seriously by health care providers, who may attribute symptoms to stress. Thus women may be misdiagnosed until their condition warrants emergency surgery (Hill and Geraci, 1998).

Cessation of smoking is the most important factor in decreasing the morbidity and mortality of heart disease in women. Women who are heavy smokers are at two to four times higher risk of coronary artery disease than women who do not smoke (Flack, O'Connor, and Wei, 1998). Women over 35 years old who smoke cigarettes and take oral contraceptives are at the greatest risk of developing heart disease (Gallagher et al, 1996).

As a preventive measure, nurses should inform women who smoke of other contraceptive methods available to them. Nurses should develop community-focused programs about how to modify risk factors of heart disease such as smoking, obesity, alcohol consumption, diet, stress management, and activity level. Community-level primary prevention should include increasing women's awareness and knowledge level of heart disease. It is important for the nurse to teach clients about symptoms of heart disease. Angina may be manifested as chest pain radiating down one or both arms or it may be experienced as pressure, chest fullness lasting several minutes, a choking sensation, lightheadedness, fainting, and shortness of breath (Hill and Geraci, 1998).

Secondary community-level interventions should focus on screening for risk factors that can be modified, such as cholesterol, hypertension, glucose, and weight screening programs (Ahmed, Clasen, and Donnelly, 1998). Other standard diagnostic tests not typically used for routine screening purposes, such as treadmill exercises and thallium scan, were developed for men. Therefore they may not be as reliable or as sensitive for women and are typically used in secondary prevention for acute illness. Drugs typically prescribed for the treatment of women with heart disease, such as beta blockers, nitrates, and calcium channel blockers, were not originally tested with women. Therefore the nurse should be alert that women may not respond to these drugs in the same manner as men.

Postmenopausal women are at risk for heart disease because of decreased levels of estrogen. Hormone replacement therapy (HRT) reduces the risk of death from heart disease (Gallagher et al, 1998). HRT is the hormone combination of estrogen and progesterone. Hormone replacement therapy is used for women who have not had a hysterectomy. **Estrogen replacement therapy** is use of the single hormone estrogen. Estrogen replacement therapy is used in women who have had a hysterectomy (Gallagher et al, 1998). The U.S. Preventive Services Task Force (1996) recommends that all women be counseled about HRT. Estrogen replacement therapy is contraindicated for some women. The nurse should be aware of the benefits and contraindications of this therapy. Contraindications include unexplained vaginal bleeding, active liver disease, chronic impaired liver functions, recent vascular thrombosis, and breast or endometrial cancer.

Women may also react to cardiac surgery differently than men. Because coronary artery disease develops 10 to 20 years later in women than men, women who require cardiac surgery are much older than their male counterparts. This may be one of the reasons that women have higher mortality rates during surgery than men. One study found that whereas men viewed surgery as a major event in their lives, women viewed the surgery as a part of growing old. These differences in perceptions influence postsurgical recovery. Postoperatively, more men participated in cardiac rehabilitation than women. Women were less likely to follow discharge instructions; they allowed family responsibility and level of fatigue to guide their postoperative activity (Hawthorne, 1994).

Cancer

Cancer is the second leading cause of death for women. The most common types of cancer in women are lung, breast, colorectal, ovarian, cervical, and pancreatic. Lung cancer is the leading cause of cancer deaths among women, surpassing breast and colorectal cancer (Baldini and Strauss, 1997; NWHIC, 1998a). Most lung cancer is preventable by modifying lifestyle, such as through smoking cessation.

More women between ages 25 and 35 smoke than any other age group. African-American women in this age group are more likely to smoke than Caucasian women (Baldini and Strauss, 1997). The smoking cessation rate for African-American smokers is significantly less than for Caucasians.

The U.S. Preventive Services Task Force (1996) does not recommend screening asymptomatic individuals without symptoms for lung cancer. The task force recommends that all individuals should be counseled about the use of tobacco products and encouraged to initiate a smoking cessation program. To be effective, smoking cessation programs for young women need to consider some of the powerful forces that encourage young women to initiate and continue smoking. For a number of years, cigarette advertisements have promoted smoking in women through an emphasis on slimness (e.g., Virginia Slims). This has resulted in many young women associating smoking with maintaining an acceptable body weight.

Nurses need to target young African-American women for education about the dangers of smoking. Oakley (1994) described smoking as "increasingly a marker for poverty" that is a powerful "strategy for calming the nerves and coping with stress" (p. 432). Findings from research studies focusing on African-American women's attitudes and practices regarding smoking offer insights that are important in planning smoking cessation programs (NWHIC, 1998a; Shervington, 1994). Many women identified only a few risks of smoking. Barriers to smoking cessation were closely linked to their difficult life situations. Barriers include living in highly stressful environments; feeling isolated and without social support; and choosing smoking as an affordable, legal pleasure given limited financial resources. Women stated that a comprehensive smoking cessation program that has other purposes meaningful to their lives, such as dealing with disappointments, handling stress, and obtaining resources, would be more effective.

Breast cancer is the second most common cancer in women (Catalano and Satariano, 1998). Carcinoma of the breast accounts for 32% of female cancers (Kuter, 1996). Although earlier detection and better reporting may account for some of the increase in incidence, other causes of this are increased life span, earlier menarche, and increased commitment to careers that result in delayed childbearing. The mortality rate from breast cancer has changed little since 1930. The 5-year survival among women with localized breast cancer has improved since the 1940s (Press, 1998). Therefore early detection of breast cancer is the most important strategy to increase breast cancer survival.

Risk factors that have been identified for breast cancer are listed in Box 27-1. It has been estimated that many cases of breast cancer cannot be explained by these established risk factors. Approximately 75% of the women with breast cancer do not have a high-risk profile (Kuter, 1996). Moreover, most risk factors cannot be reduced by lifestyle modifications. The major risk factor is advancing age; breast cancer increases significantly for women over 50 years old.

Although breast cancer occurs most frequently in women of higher socioeconomic status, financially disadvantaged women have the highest mortality rate. The high mortality rate among these women may be related to lack of information about the disease and inadequate health care, which often results in late-stage diagnosis and delayed

---

BOX 27-1 Risk Factors Associated with Breast Cancer

Over 50 years of age
Family history (mother, sister, daughter)
Genetic predisposition
Previous breast cancer
First pregnancy after 30 years of age
Nulliparity
Menarche before 12 years of age
Menopause after 55 years of age
Proliferative atypical breast hyperplasia
History of ovarian or endometrial cancer
Obesity after menopause
High socioeconomic status

treatment. Financially disadvantaged women are much less likely to have regular mammograms. Financial concerns such as fear of job loss and making ends meet leave little time for health promotion efforts such as breast self examination (Catalano and Satariano, 1998; McCance and Jorde, 1998).

Early detection remains the primary factor in survival for women with breast cancer. All women should receive age-appropriate periodic screening and education. This includes a combination of mammography, clinical breast examination, and breast self-examination (BSE) teaching. An objective of *Healthy People 2000* is to increase to at least 80% the proportion of women 40 years and over who have ever had a clinical breast examination and a mammogram.

The American Cancer Society (ACS) guidelines for mammography are the most widely accepted. ACS recommends that annual mammography begin by age 40 years and consist of annual clinical examination, with a screening mammography performed at 1- to 2-year intervals. States with high rates of mammography screening have demonstrated reduced breast cancer fatality rates, presumably as a result of diagnosing breast cancer at an earlier stage (Cooper et al, 1998).

Despite mass media publicity about the high rates of breast cancer and the importance of early detection, many women do not follow to recommended screening guidelines for BSE, clinical breast examination, and mammography. During the 1990 National Health Survey, only about two thirds of women aged 50 to 59 reported ever having had a mammogram (NCHS, 1993). In 1994 the Agency for Health Care Policy and Research (AHCPR) released a comprehensive review of research surrounding clinical breast examination and mammography and excellent recommendations for health care providers. The report recognizes that women may lack information or harbor fears of embarrassment and pain about being examined. A nurse's recommendation to seek breast cancer screening can be a very powerful motivator. A number of studies report that more than 90% of women had a mammography after their health care provider recommended it (Breen and Kessler, 1994).

Nurses will find the AHCPR practice guidelines helpful in counseling women about mammography. Nurses need to inform women that mammography is the most sensitive and specific screening test for breast cancer currently available. Women need to understand the difference between screening and diagnostic mammography. Women with breast signs or symptoms such as a mass, skin changes, and nipple discharge should request diagnostic rather than screening mammography. Women need to be informed that the procedure can be uncomfortable or painful. If possible, women should schedule mammography when they are not experiencing cyclical breast tenderness or have conditions that increase breast density. Women's privacy should be respected. Women should not be required to walk or wait in a public area while wearing an examination gown.

Older women have been identified as a group that is less likely to participate in breast cancer screening. They are less likely to perform BSE, to obtain clinical breast examinations, and to seek mammograms. Elderly women giving reasons for not participating in screening cite lack of knowledge about cancer, particularly the fact that risk of cancer increases with age. Messages on breast cancer frequently do not acknowledge the older woman's degree of risks. This is evidenced by the breast cancer educational information portraying younger women in photography and artwork. Thus this message may be creating a myth that older women are not vulnerable to this disease. Nurses need to target older women for breast cancer teaching and screening. Nurses should implement strategies that decrease the financial barriers to screening and social marketing programs that improve the public's acceptance of screening programs. Educational initiatives should be culturally sensitive. In addition, pictures and written materials should be designed for all ages.

The incidence of reproductive cancers increases with age. Women over 40 years old are at increased risk for cervical, uterine, and ovarian cancer (Wertheim, Soto-Wright, and Goodman, 1996). Ovarian cancer causes more deaths than all other forms of gynecological cancer combined. Overall, 1 in 70 women will develop ovarian cancer during their lifetime. The incidence of ovarian cancer increases with age, from 1.4 per 100,000 women younger than 40 years of age to 38 per 100,000 women older than 60 years of age with a peak incidence at 59 years of age (Wertheim, Soto-Wright, and Goodman, 1996). Symptoms of ovarian cancer usually do not occur until the disease has progressed to an advanced stage. Consequently, most women with ovarian cancer are first diagnosed during an advanced stage. A major risk factor for ovarian cancer is family history of breast or ovarian cancer. Other risk factors for ovarian cancer include nulliparity, late first pregnancy, infertility, late menopause, high-fat diet, higher socioeconomic status, a family history of ovarian cancer, and occupational exposure to talc and asbestos. The periodic pelvic examination is the only reliable screening test available.

About one third of gynecological cancers include uterine cancers (cervical and endometrial). Endometrial cancer is the most common malignant disease of the female genital tract. Endometrial cancer occurs most often in postmenopausal women, with the average age at diagnosis of 61 years. A woman's lifetime risk of developing endometrial cancer is 2% to 3% (Wertheim, Soto-Wright, and Goodman, 1996). Risk factors include nulliparity, late menopause, early menarche, anovulation, obesity, liver disease, high socioeconomic status, and a family history of breast cancer. Symptoms of endometrial cancer include abnormal vaginal bleeding and an enlarged uterus. The Papanicolaou (Pap) test is a poor screening test for endometrial cancer; endometrial biopsy is an accurate diagnostic method for endometrial cancer. There are not enough data, however, to justify screening of the general population of postmenopausal women with endometrial biopsies (Press, 1998).

With early detection, appropriate treatment, and adequate follow-up, cervical cancer is one of the most preventable diseases. Major risk factors for cervical cancer include cigarette smoking, low socioeconomic status, a history of multiple sexual partners, early onset of sexual activity, and use of oral contraceptives. Moreover, sexually transmitted viral diseases such as herpes and human papilloma have recently been recognized as playing a possible role in the development of cervical cancer (Wertheim, Soto-Wright, and Goodman, 1996).

Early symptoms of cervical cancer can include vaginal bleeding or discharge, symptoms often associated with douching and sexual intercourse. The principal screening test for cervical cancer is the Pap test. It is responsible for a dramatic reduction of cervical cancer during the last two decades. All women should be educated about the importance of having regular gynecological examinations. Only 50% of women 18 years and over report having an annual Pap test (NCHS, 1993). Over 30% of poor women over age 65 have never had a Pap smear (Chapman, 1997). An objective of *Healthy People 2000* is to increase to at least 95% the proportion of women 18 years and over who have ever had a Pap test and to at least 85% those who have received a Pap test in the preceding 1 to 3 years. The U.S. Preventive Services Task Force (1996) recommendations call for Pap tests to begin when the female first engages in sexual intercourse or by age 18 years. The test should be performed every 1 to 3 years on females who have been or are sexually active. The American College of Obstetricians and Gynecologists recommends a yearly Pap test. Some women may experience financial barriers to receiving the appropriate Pap test as recommended (US Preventive Services Task Force, 1996). Nurses should refer such women to available community resources that provide these services for financially challenged women or develop programs for these women.

Human Immunodeficiency Virus

HIV is a major health problem and cause of death among women. Women represent the fastest growing groups of individuals with acquired immunodeficiency syndrome (AIDS) in the United States. By the year 2000, it is projected that more women than men will have AIDS in this country.

DID YOU KNOW? *Perinatal transmission of HIV can be significantly reduced if an HIV-infected women is placed on antiretroviral prophylaxis after the first trimester and during labor and delivery, and the infant receives prophylactic antiretroviral therapy for 6 weeks after birth.*

Many women are at risk because they are not aware of the modes of HIV transmission and do not acknowledge their risk behaviors (Soet, DiIorio, and Dudley, 1998). The highest HIV seroprevalence rates in women are found in women of childbearing age. Injection drug use or being the sexual partner of an injecting drug user are the main risk factors for women (Kazanjian and Eisenstat, 1996).

More than 70% of women with HIV are African-American or Hispanic. Although membership in an ethnic group is not a risk factor, the overrepresentation is linked to the disproportionate numbers of minority members engaged in high-risk behaviors, such as multiple sexual exposures. Most HIV-infected women are clustered within urban areas where poverty and drug abuse are prevalent.

Research findings point to several distinctions about women with HIV. Generally, women with HIV have many more coexisting problems than men, including malnutrition, other sexually transmitted diseases (STDs), substance abuse, lack of social support, and poor access to health care (Minkoff, DeHovitz, and Duerr, 1995). The disease progression of HIV differs between women and men. For example, *Pneumocystis carinii* pneumonia and Kaposi's sarcoma are often seen as AIDS-defining illnesses in men with AIDS. The occurrence of these illnesses are less among women. Vaginal fungal infections, especially those caused by *Candida albicans,* are frequently the presenting illness in women with AIDS (Minkoff, DeHovitz, and Duerr, 1995). Women with HIV are also prone to cervical neoplasias and pelvic inflammatory disease. Gender differences in the clinical symptoms of AIDS may contribute to women receiving a later diagnosis or a misdiagnosis. The problem of early recognition of HIV infection in women may result in insufficient or incorrect health care treatment. The nurse should know gender differences in the symptoms of HIV infection and educate their clients about these symptoms.

Since women of childbearing age are the largest at-risk group for becoming infected with HIV, attention to issues of perinatal HIV transmission are important. Perinatal transmission is the most common route of HIV infection in children (Minkoff, DeHovitz, and Duerr, 1995). The rate of perinatal HIV transmission can be reduced to as low as 8.3% with prophylactic zidovudine therapy during pregnancy, delivery, and in the infant (Minkoff, DeHovitz, and Duerr, 1995).

DID YOU KNOW? *Women are experiencing an alarming increase in the number of HIV/AIDS cases. The increase in HIV/AIDS cases in women of childbearing age will directly affect the number of HIV/AIDS cases in the pediatric population.*

The nurse should discuss a number of issues with HIV-seropositive women, including the possibility of perinatal transmission to the fetus and the unknown effect of the pregnancy on their own HIV disease state. It is recommended that all HIV-seropositive pregnant women receive counseling about HIV testing and fetal risk with all options explored including abortion and sterilization procedures. HIV-seropositive status, however, may not be a decisive factor for a woman deciding to continue or terminate her pregnancy. In fact, a number of surveys have found that most women choose to continue their pregnancy despite their HIV status (Minkoff, DeHovitz, and Duerr, 1995). Complex social, cultural, and psychological factors often determine whether a woman becomes pregnant and influences the commitment she has to the pregnancy. Nurses need to recognize the powerful cultural dynamics that surround the life choices that HIV-seropositive women make for themselves, their children, and their families. They must be prepared to assist and support women's decisions.

HIV is often a family illness, resulting in extraordinary needs that embrace several domains: physical, psychosocial, spiritual, and economic. The lives of these families are frequently complicated by the death of one or more parents and a child because of HIV illness. In addition, the same circumstances that may have led the mother to become infected with HIV may undermine her ability to provide care for her HIV-infected infant and her other children. Many of these families have other problems: poverty, isolation, poor education, unemployment, inadequate housing, and drug use. Health care that demonstrates appreciation and respect for HIV-infected families is a challenge.

Women and Weight Control

Americans, particularly women, spend a great deal of time, money, and effort in pursuit of the slender body. For women, obesity is a stigma in U.S. culture. Research has consistently documented that more women than men are dissatisfied with their bodies. Often, women of normal weight and even underweight women view their bodies as too large. Moreover, females begin developing a fear of obesity in childhood.

In the dominant American culture, thinness symbolizes competence, success, control, power, and sexual attractiveness. This culture's preoccupation with thinness and shape of women can be seen in the popular media "waif" models. People may associate obesity with laziness and a lack of willpower.

Obesity is defined as an increase in body weight of 20% or more above the desirable body weight. The number of overweight women in the United States is increasing. The prevalence of overweight women ages 20 to 74 increased from 27% to 37% between 1976 and 1994. The *Healthy People 2000* objective is a decrease to 20%. African-American women increased from 44% to 52%, and the *2000* objective is a decrease to 30%. Among Mexican-American women the incidence increased from 39% to 50%, and the *2000* objective is 25% (USDHHS, PHS, 1998) (Fig. 27-3). The prevalence of obesity and the associated risks of obesity in the development of diabetes, hypertension, cardiovascular disease, and other medical problems make obesity

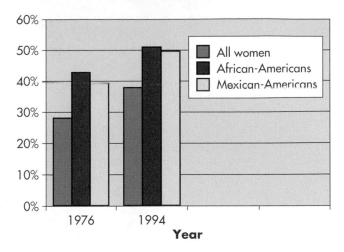

FIG. 27-3 *Healthy People 2000* rates of obesity among women of different ethnicities in two different years. (From U.S. Department of Health and Human Services, Public Health Service: *Healthy people: progress review women's health* [online], 1998. Available: odphp.osophs.dhhs.gov/pubs/hp2000/PROGRVW/women/women.htm)

a major health problem among women. The nurse can provide education regarding weight and obesity's risks to health.

Because obesity in women is such a stigma in western culture, women are at highest risk for suffering adverse social and psychological consequences of obesity. These consequences can include social and financial discrimination. More women enter weight treatment programs for their perceived loss of attractiveness rather than for health concerns. Recently, a nondieting approach to increasing self-esteem in obese women was demonstrated to be beneficial to the emotional health of these women (Ciliska, 1998).

In the last 20 years, reports of disordered eating have noticeably increased. Many girls and women are dissatisfied with their current shape and weight, but only a small number of these actually develop serious eating disorders. The most common eating disorders seen in women are anorexia nervosa and bulimia. **Anorexia** is defined as fear of gaining weight and disturbances in perception of the body. Excessive weight loss is the most noticeable clue. Individuals with anorexia rarely complain of weight loss because they view themselves as normal or overweight. Many of these women struggle with psychological problems, including depression, obsessive symptoms, and social phobias. **Bulimia** is characterized by persistent concern with body shape and weight, recurrent episodes of binge eating, a loss of control during these binges, and use of extreme methods to prevent weight gain, such as purging, strict dieting, fasting, or vigorous exercise. Unlike anorexia, bulimia is observed across all weight categories, with most women being within a normal weight range. Although bulimia is considered less dangerous medically than anorexia, electrolyte imbalance and dehydration can create serious physical complications, such as cardiac dysrhythmias.

Nurses are in a prime position to include assessment for eating disorders and referral for treatment into their routine clinical practices. The goal of the nurse is to identify not only those women with eating disorders, but also those women at risk for developing eating problems. See the Research Brief for a discussion of a study about overeating. Through a thorough physical and psychosocial assessment, as well as a history of dietary practice, the

---

RESEARCH *Brief*

The purpose of this study was to compare eating patterns of women who experience episodes of weight cycling with women of normal weight. A subject was identified as a weight cycler if she reported two cycles of weight loss and regain greater than 10 pounds in the last 2 years.

Semistructured interviews were conducted on 15 women with normal weight and 30 women who were in a previous study of motivational states associated with overeating episodes. The women were between the ages of 21 and 53 years of age, with a weight grouping of normal, overweight, or obese.

This study identified four common themes that emerged from the semistructured interviews: planned overeating; power/control; relationships with others; and unpleasant feelings. All of the women reported planning to overeat. The overweight women planned to overeat when alone, whereas the obese women overate with others present. The normal-weight women overate when celebrating special occasions. Personal power or control over their eating was felt by 73% of normal-weight women, 30% of overweight women, and 50% of obese women. Unpleasant feelings related to overeating included anxiety, tension, stress, boredom, tiredness, and loneliness. Obese women reported more boredom, tiredness, and loneliness than overweight and normal-weight women when overeating.

Nurses can use these study findings to plan health promotion strategies for women who have experienced overeating or to prevent women from experiencing feelings that pose the risk for overeating. Reducing overweight and obesity in women will accomplish the reduction or elimination of a major risk factor for several acute and chronic illnesses. Nurses planning women's health programs should include strategies such as group counseling, peer support programs, encourage expression of unpleasant feelings, planned activities to reduce fatigue and occupy their time, and stress management programs to reduce feelings of anxiety, tension, and stress.

Popkess-Vawter S, Brandau M, Straub J: Triggers of overeating and related intervention strategies for women who weight cycle, *Appl Nurs Res* 11(2):69, 1998.

---

nurse may be able to identify women with eating disorders and provide appropriate referrals. Community health nurses should promote healthy eating habits and regular physical activity as a weight control strategy.

Cosmetic Surgery

Many women today will go to great lengths in search of the perfect body. Beauty-enhancing procedures such as **liposuction** operations, breast enlargements, eyelid lifts, facelifts and aesthetic dentistry are now available to women. The most popular form of cosmetic surgery is liposuction, which involves surgical removal of excess fatty tissue through the insertion of suction tubes in specific areas. Between 1992 and 1997 the number of liposuctions increased 215% and the number of breast augmentations increased by 275% (National Clearinghouse of Plastic Surgery Statistics, 1997). The field of cosmetic surgery is one of the largest money-makers in medicine. Cosmetic surgery is an unregulated field, and the risk of complications are rising as record numbers of physicians compete for a share of the market. Also, new procedures and instruments are being rushed to the market without clinical trials. For example, in 1996 the ultrasonic liposuction machine was introduced in the United States. Later it was discovered that it can cause internal tissue damage and scarring if used incorrectly, and many physicians were not properly trained in the proper use. The nurse should inform women of the risk associated with beauty enhancement procedures. Women who want to have cosmetic surgery should be advised to carefully select a qualified physician (Gilbert, 1998).

Some experts believe that, in the future, gender differences in mortality will not be as great between men and women. A decline in cardiovascular mortality rates among males is expected to result in an increased life expectancy for men. It is also forecast that the life expectancy among women will decline as they assume many of the poor health habits traditionally associated with men, such as cigarette smoking and alcohol use. In addition, as women become more integrated into the labor force, they will be increasingly exposed to occupational hazards and job stresses.

Although women may live longer than men, they experience more morbidity and use health services at higher rates than men. The three major chronic conditions women experience are heart conditions, arthritis, and hypertension. The three major causes of mortality in women are heart disease, cancer, and cerebrovascular disease.

Arthritis

Arthritis is the most prevalent chronic condition experienced by women; it is three times as common in women than men (Ross, 1997). In general, the majority of the clients with rheumatoid arthritis are women (Grisso, Ness, and Hendrix, 1997). The rate of arthritis increases significantly with age. Many arthritic diseases exist; the most common form of arthritis is degenerative joint disease, or osteoarthritis. About 25% of women with arthritis experience some limitations in activity because of their condition. Women with arthritis often suffer from chronic, often debilitating, pain. The monetary cost of managing this pain can be devastating to an older woman's limited income (Kington and Smith, 1997; Tindall, 1997). Other areas of concern include obtaining adequate sleep, dealing with medications, maintaining energy, and experiencing depression/anxiety. Nurses can encourage women to prevent progression of osteoarthritis through education on the relationship between obesity and increased "wear and tear" on joints. In addition, women should be cautioned to protect their joints from repeated trauma. Physical therapy may be helpful in reducing pain and disability.

Osteoporosis

Osteoporosis is a major health problem for postmenopausal and elderly women. Osteoporosis causes between 1.3 and 1.5 million spinal, hip, and forearm fractures annually (Whitmore, 1998). The most common fracture associated with osteoporosis is compression fracture of the vertebrae. These fractures may result in curvature of the spine and reduced thoracic volume, leading to a compromised respiratory system. Hip fractures are the second most common fractures associated with osteoporosis. The incidence of this type of fracture increases with age. In 1996 the incidence of hip fractures among Caucasian women 85 years of age and over was 2804 per 100,000. The *Healthy People 2000* objective is to reduce the number of hip fractures to 2177 per 100,000 (USDHHS, PHS, 1998).

The health consequences of osteoporosis are tremendous. Individuals may face pain, surgery, hospitalization, loss of independence, and decreased quality of life. Hip fracture is the leading cause of loss of independent living for women. Of the women who survive a hip fracture, over 50% will never be able to walk without aid, and some women will be forced into long-term care (Whitmore, 1998; Woodhead and Moss, 1998). Among medically ill and functionally impaired clients with hip fractures, mortality is increased (Magaziner et al, 1997). Women experience a gradual increase in their risk of mortality for 5 years postfracture.

Two groups of variables contribute to the risk of developing osteoporosis. The first group includes factors that women cannot modify: 50 years and over, being Caucasian or Asian, having a petite or slim bone structure, being menopausal or having experienced an early menopause, and having a family history of osteoporosis (Whitmore, 1998; Woodhead and Moss, 1998). The second group consists of variables that women can modify: inadequate intake of calcium, limited exercise, smoking, and excessive alcohol use. Prevention of osteoporosis includes maintaining a desirable weight; maintaining an adequate intake of dietary calcium, phosphorus, and vitamin D; and participating in regular weight-bearing exercise. Re-

searchers have found that women begin experiencing significant bone loss as early as 35 years old. Therefore premenopausal women should be encouraged to take 1000 mg of calcium daily; postmenopausal women need calcium supplementation of 1500 mg a day and a vitamin D supplement. Weight-bearing exercises and estrogen replacement therapy are also recommended (Woodhead and Moss, 1998).

Prevention efforts for osteoporosis should be targeted at young girls as they develop health promotion behaviors. It is believed that women increase bone mass through their twenties, and women with higher bone mass in early adulthood may be able to resist the effects of age-related bone loss (Whitmore, 1998; Woodhead and Moss, 1998). Anorexia and exercise to the point of amenorrhea may be hazardous to women's bones (McGee, 1997). Athletic women should be counseled about preserving bone density. Nursing interventions for adult women include eliciting a careful family, social, and dietary history and teaching preventive behaviors.

For postmenopausal women, nurses should obtain yearly height measures and observe for clinical features of osteoporosis (kyphosis). Nurses can also teach women how to prevent or slow the progression of osteoporosis. Women often consume less than half the recommended daily calcium intake which predisposes them to osteoporosis (NWHIC, 1998b). The researchers found women lacked knowledge about the importance of calcium, exercise, and estrogen replacement therapy to prevent osteoporosis. Moreover, for many women, a low income created an economic barrier to obtaining adequate calcium.

Urinary Incontinence

Urinary incontinence (UI) is a major women's health issue. **Urinary incontinence** is defined as a condition in which involuntary loss of urine occurs. Urinary incontinence creates a social or hygienic problems for women (Jay and Staskin, 1998). The prevalence of UI in women ranges from 10% to 25% (Jay and Staskin, 1998). Of the people over 65 years of age, 20% are incontinent. It is believed that the incidence of UI is greatly underreported, since many women believe that losing continence is just the normal result of childbearing or growing older. Urine loss may vary from small infrequent amounts to large, frequent amounts.

The consequences of UI can be devastating. UI creates a financial burden to individuals. As a nation the direct cost of urinary incontinence exceeds $10.5 billion annually (Gallo, Fallon, and Staskin, 1997). Individuals typically experience a loss in self-esteem, a sense of guilt, and isolation. UI in elderly persons is the major factor contributing to the family's decision to seek institutional care. In elderly persons, skin breakdown can contribute to the development of pressure ulcers.

As seen by the advertising and brisk sales of perineal pads or diapers, many women attempt to manage the problem without seeking professional help. Some studies have estimated that fewer than 50% of individuals with severe incontinence seek professional help. Individuals may wait between 7 and 9 years to seek help (Jay and Staskin, 1998). The vast majority of women are never asked questions about UI during a routine physical examination. An objective of *Healthy People 2000* is to increase to at least 60% the proportion of providers of primary care for older adults who routinely evaluate people aged 65 years and older for UI. UI is not, however, restricted just to the older population. Evidence is mounting that young, healthy, nulliparous females often experience UI, especially during exercise. Activities that provoke the highest degree of UI involve jumping, high-impact landings, and running. Women who participate in gymnastics, basketball, and running typically experience some UI.

Because so many women will not initiate discussion about problems with UI, introducing the topic and taking a urinary history to determine if a woman has urinary control difficulties are important. Simple questions may invite a woman to begin sharing, such as, "Are you having any problems with urination or bladder control?" or "Do you ever unintentionally lose urine?" Women often restrict fluids because of urge incontinence. Restricting fluids may actually worsen incontinence because the bladder does not fill to its normal capacity. Fluids help to distend the bladder to its normal capacity, which maintains bladder tone. Decreased fluid intake can also lead to dehydration, cystitis, and constipation. Highly concentrated urine can irritate the bladder mucosa and increase the urge to urinate.

Nurses can encourage a number of behaviors that can prevent or minimize UI. Women should be encouraged to maintain adequate hydration (2000 to 3000 ml a day). Constipation can exacerbate incontinence by putting pressure on the bladder and obstructing the urethra. Some fluids increase the urge to urinate; caffeine beverages and citrus juices should be avoided. Obesity can contribute to incontinence; therefore weight reduction may reduce UI. Low estrogen levels can lead to flaccid muscle tissue, causing stress incontinence. Perimenopausal and postmenopausal women can be counseled about HRT. Strengthening the sphincter and supporting structures of the bladder (Kegel exercises) should be promoted. Pelvic muscle assessment should become as much a part of preventive health care of women as annual Pap tests and regular mammography. Although several surgical interventions exist for UI, the success rate varies greatly. Comprehensive behavioral and medical management of UI is recommended before referral for surgery (Jay and Staskin, 1998).

Depression

Mental illness patterns vary for women and men. Findings from epidemiology through community-based surveys indicate that women are more likely to experience major depression and phobias. It is possible that one in 10 women in a primary care setting may be experiencing major depression (Landau and Milan, 1996). Men have higher rates of antisocial personality disorder and alcohol abuse.

A number of factors that may contribute to the development of depression in women have been identified, including unhappy intimate relationships, history of sexual and physical abuse, reproductive events, multiple roles, ethnic minority status, low self-esteem, poverty, and unemployment. Nursing research has also documented the importance of women's social networks in protecting them from depression and enhancing their self-esteem (Woods et al, 1994). Women may derive great satisfaction from interpersonal relationships, but they are also at greater risk for depression when conflict in these relationships occur.

Research is beginning to document that older women are a high-risk group for depression. Causes of depression in older women are loss of physical health, loss of a spouse from death or divorce, and financial problems.

Nurses should be aware of the signs and symptoms of depression. Depression may be identified in the workplace, adversely affecting the woman's work satisfaction and performance. Prompt referral for professional mental health services should be made if depression is suspected. Women may also benefit from a group support that focuses on developing coping skills for dealing with difficult relationships and role conflict.

NATIONAL HEALTH OBJECTIVES FOR WOMEN

Over 60 of the national *Healthy People 2000* objectives specifically target the health of women (Box 27-2). A progress review of the *Healthy People 2000* objectives found a number of improvements in women's health. There was a decline in the rate of females that smoke cigarettes (Fig. 27-4). The rate of unintended pregnancy has also declined. The number of live births among females ages 15 to 17 years old declined (Fig. 27-5). The percentage of female receiving prenatal care increased. The females age 50 and over receiving a clinical breast examination and a mammogram increased (Fig. 27-6).

Unfortunately, there were increases in the incidence of hip fractures among white women 85 years and over (Fig. 27-7). Also, the prevalence of overweight females increased (see Fig. 27-3) (USDHHS, PHS, 1998). The nurse can improve the outcome of women's health by providing culturally sensitive comprehensive services. Ways to provide quality women's health services are listed in the How To box on p. 574.

PROGRAMS AND SERVICES FOR WOMEN

Changes in the health care delivery system have a profound effect on women. Women are the gatekeepers of their families' health care. They make three fourths of the health care decisions in American households. Additionally, women make over 61% of physician visits and purchase 59% of prescription drugs (Smith Barney Research, 1997). Because of women's greater involvement with health services, they can play a major role in family health promotion.

BOX 27-2 National Health Objectives for Women

The following are *Healthy People 2000* objectives that focus on women's health issues:

- Reduce overweight to a prevalence of no more than 30% among African-American women age 20 and older
- Reduce overweight to a prevalence of no more than 25% among Hispanic women age 20 and older
- Reduce overweight to a prevalence of no more than 41% among women with high blood pressure
- Increase calcium intake so at least 50% of youth ages 12 to 24 and 50% of pregnant and lactating women consume three or more servings daily of foods rich in calcium, and at least 50% of people ages 25 and older consume two or more servings daily
- Reduce iron deficiency to less than 3% among children ages 1 through 4 and among women of childbearing age
- Increase to at least 75% the proportion of mothers who breastfed their babies in the early postpartum period and to at least 50% the proportion who continue breastfeeding until their babies are 5 to 6 months
- Reduce cigarette smoking to a prevalence of no more than 12% among women of reproductive age
- Reduce cigarette smoking to a prevalence of no more than 10% among pregnant women
- Reduce pregnancies among girls ages 17 and younger to no more than 50 per 1000 adolescents
- Reduce to no more than 30% the proportion of all pregnancies that are unintended
- Reduce the prevalence of infertility to no more than 6.5%
- Reduce the maternal mortality rate to no more than 3.3 per 100,000 live births
- Reduce breast cancer deaths to no more than 20.6 per 100,000 women
- Reduce deaths from cancer of the uterine cervix to no more than 1.3 per 100,000 women

From USDHHS: *Healthy people 2000: national health promotion and disease prevention objectives*, Washington, DC, 1992, Author.

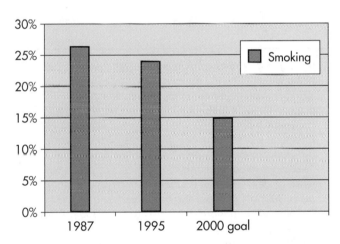

FIG. 27-4 *Healthy People 2000* progress for the percentage of women who smoke. (From U.S. Department of Health and Human Services, Public Health Service: *Healthy people: progress review women's health* [on-line], 1998. Available: odphp.osophs.dhhs.gov/pubs/hp2000/PROGRVW/women/women.htm)

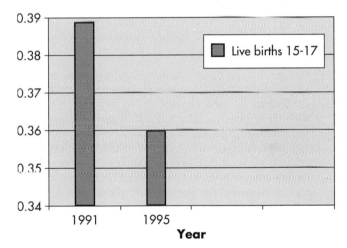

FIG. 27-5 *Healthy People 2000* progress for the number of live births amoung females ages 15 to 17. (From U.S. Department of Health and Human Services, Public Health Service: *Healthy people: progress review women's health* [on-line], 1998. Available: odphp.osophs.dhhs.gov/pubs/hp2000/PROGRVW/women/women.htm)

A visit with a health provider can be an opportunity for women to share issues of concern in their lives and receive information to make informed decisions about their family's health. Women must be provided with the information that they need to make informed decisions. Nurses should encourage women to make use of all health visits to get health advice for themselves and their families.

Traditional centers of care for women like Planned Parenthood, feminist women's health centers, and local community health centers can serve as models for women-centered health care delivery. Unfortunately such centers are not included in large managed care organizations (MCO). The women's health service providers authorized by MCOs do not copy these traditional women's health care models. Subsequently, women suffer from the loss of women's centered care (Taylor and Woods, 1996).

As a female-dominated profession, nurses have personal insight into women's health issues. Nurses should be

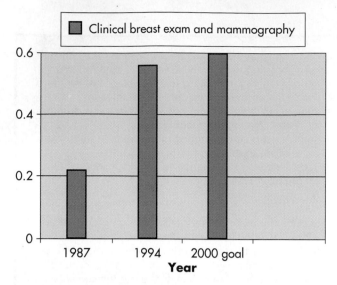

FIG. 27-6 *Healthy People 2000* progress for women receiving a clinical breast examination and a mammogram. (From U.S. Department of Health and Human Services, Public Health Service: *Healthy people: progress review women's health* [on-line], 1998. Available: odphp.osophs.dhhs.gov/pubs/hp2000/PROGRVW/women/women.htm)

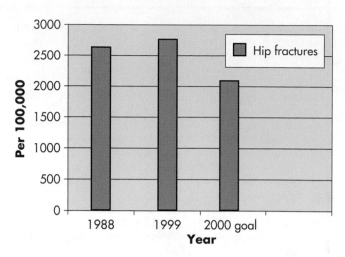

FIG. 27-7 Incidence of hip fractures in Caucasian women 85 years and older. (From U.S. Department of Health and Human Services, Public Health Service: *Healthy people: progress review women's health* [on-line], 1998. Available: odphp.osophs.dhhs.gov/pubs/hp2000/PROGRVW/women/women.htm)

▤ HOW TO *Provide Quality Women's Health Services*

- *Include women of various ages, ethnic groups, and socioeconomic status when planning women's health programs.*
- *Identify the specific health needs of targeted communities before planning programs .*
- *Provide comprehensive women's services, minimally including gynecological and reproductive services, health education programs, general medical services, shelter resources for women and children, transportation, translation , multicultural counseling, and referral network.*
- *Learn about women's unique response to health issues.*
- *Provide culturally relevant outreach to inform women about the magnitude of threats to health from smoking, poor diet, and lack of exercise.*
- *Improve your cultural and linguistic competence through continuing education, travel, and working with diverse cultural groups.*
- *Develop new and effective ways to influence girls and women to engage in physical activity throughout life.*
- *Participate in partnerships and community coalitions to develop women's health services in nontraditional*

- *setting, e.g., churches, schools, workplaces, and beautician shops.*
- *Affiliate with other community-based organizations to provide services such as: childcare and educational completion programs.*
- *Integrate women's service programs with childcare programs to develop family health services.*
- *Seek ways to control and diminish the rising prevalence of depression in women, e.g., stress management, support groups, and assertiveness training.*
- *Strive to expand women's access to HIV/AIDS prevention counseiing and treatment programs.*
- *Participate in the development of data collection strategies for population groups that have not been adequately monitored, such as lesbians and poor and less educated women.*
- *Ensure that all health-related programs take into account women's needs, particularly single mothers, minorities, lesbians, and women in prison.*

Adapted from US Department of Health and Human Services, Public Health Service: *Healthy people: progress review women's health* [on-line], 1998. Available: odphp.osophs.dhhs.gov/pubs/hp2000/PROGRVW/women/women.htm

involved in the planning and evaluation of women's health services. Effective women's health programs recognize and respect the diversity of color, age, ethnicity and culture among women across their life span. More focus must be on social issues that directly affect women's health such as racism, sexism, ageism, violence against women, gender roles, poverty and health belief systems. (Taylor and Woods, 1996). Refer to the previous How To box for suggestions for providing quality women's health services.

BOX 27-3 U.S. Preventive Health Service Recommendations

PRIMARY PREVENTION STRATEGIES FOR WOMEN

- Regular dental examinations
- Regular physical examinations, including Pap test and mammography
- Adequate calcium intake
- Regular physical activity; including weight-bearing activities
- Diet with less than 30% fat; limit cholesterol intake; increase intake of high-fiber foods
- Limit alcohol and tobacco use; encourage smoking cessation programs
- Hormone replacement therapy for perimenopausal and postmenopausal women
- Family planning and contraceptive counseling
- Home smoke detectors and security systems
- Daily dental care: floss and brush with fluoride toothpaste
- Set home water temperature at 120° to 130° F
- Appropriate immunizations: pneumococal, influenza, and tetanus-diphtheria boosters
- Use of lap/shoulder belts
- Sexually transmitted disease prevention: use barrier protection consistently and correctly

From U.S. Preventive Services Task Force: *Guide to clinical preventive services: report of the U.S. Preventive Services Task Force*, Washington, DC, Philadelphia, 1996, Williams & Wilkins.

BOX 27-4 Possible Components of a Comprehensive Women's Health Program

- Comprehensive reproductive and gynecological services, including screenings for breast and cervical cancer and sexually transmitted diseases, preconceptual counseling, and abortion counseling and referral, as well as services for fertility or infertility, late pregnancy, and menopause for women at midlife
- Health promotion that focuses on physical fitness and nutrition; avoidance of cigarettes, alcohol, and other substances; stress management; violence prevention; occupational exposure, including injury prevention; self-image and self-esteem for adolescents and young adult women
- Parenting classes for young mothers
- Immunizations
- Screening, counseling and referral for mood disorders, depression, caregiver role strain and stress-related illnesses, violence and abuse
- Close monitoring of women at midlife and older for early detection of heart disease; breast, cervical, and colon cancer; diabetes; lung disease; arthritis; and other chronic illnesses

Based on data from Taylor D, Woods N: Changing women's health, changing nursing practice, *JOGGN* 25(9):791, 1996.

There is a national initiative to provide quality women's health services. In 1996 the Department of Health and Human Services (USDHHS) established six national centers of excellence in women's health. The centers will use a one-stop shopping approach to providing a comprehensive array of women's health services. The centers will also conduct women's health research and provide educational programs and materials on women's health. The USDHHS anticipates that these women's health centers will serve as a model to be duplicated throughout the country (USDHHS, 1996). U.S. Preventive Health Service Recommendations for primary prevention strategies for women are listed in Box 27-3. Nurses can work together with other health care professionals to provide comprehensive women's health services. Suggested components of a comprehensive women's health program are listed in Box 27-4.

ISSUES, TRENDS, AND POLICY AFFECTING WOMEN'S HEALTH
The Cost of Caregiving

Caregiving is a major role of women throughout their life span. Today, 72% of unpaid family caregivers are women, the majority of whom are midlife daughters or daughters-in-law (Robinson, 1997). For many women, caring for family members is informal care that they provide in addition to paid employment outside the home. Mothers assume the primary responsibility for the health and illness of their young families, wives often care for their aging and ill husbands, and daughters and daughters-in-law care for aging parents or in-laws. Unfortunately, in today's society the role of caregiver is devalued. Most women today are juggling the roles of wife, employee, and caregiver to children, parents, and in-laws with little assistance from spouses, employers, and government.

The wages lost by women to fulfill their role as caretaker of the family's health are immeasurable. It is estimated that 9% of family caregivers leave the work force to provide care, 29.4% adjust their work schedule, and 18.1% take time off without pay. In a family with three or more children women spend about 90 hours a week in paid and unpaid work, while men typically spend only 60 hours (APA, 1998). It has been estimated that women who provide uncompensated care for elderly family members spend an average of 28 to 40 hours a week (Robinson, 1997).

The added responsibility and financial strain of the caregiver role can lead to **caregiver burden** and increased stress. When a young mother must take time off of work to keep a health care provider appointment or to care for a sick child, she loses wages. When a daughter who is caring for an elderly relative at home is forced to quit her job or work part time, the interruption in employment can mean a decline in family income and loss of insurance coverage and retirement contributions.

As the health care industry continues cost containment, services once provided in hospitals and other health care settings are now being provided by women (Robinson, 1997; Taylor and Woods, 1996). Who will care for today's caregivers? The next generation is smaller and the number of caregivers are fewer. They may not be able to provide the amount of informal kin care provided today. The ability of these women to finance their own care in the future may be limited by their caregiving activities today (Robinson, 1997).

Access to medical care is linked to health insurance. Women are twice as likely as men to be underinsured. Women lack health insurance for various reasons. Many women work part-time or are employed in low-paying jobs that do not provide insurance coverage (USDHHS, PH-SOHW, 1998c). For example, of the three million women who are childcare workers, most earn incomes at or below poverty level, and few have health insurance.

Despite women's central role in providing care, very few women participate in public decisions regarding health care. A powerful minority of male physicians, legislators, and health care administrators control decisions regarding research, public policy, and health care (Quimby, 1994). In recent years this has begun to change. More women are entering traditionally male-dominated fields of medicine, research, and health care administration. More women are in Congress now than at any other time in U.S. history. As more women participate in the decision-making process, more women's health issues are addressed.

Health Policy and Legislation

Two pieces of legislation, the Women's Health Equity Act (WHEA) of 1990 and the Family and Medical Leave Act of 1993 (FMLA), address many of the needs specific to women. The Women's Health Equity Act (WHEA) was passed in response to the gross inequities in research between men and women's health issues. As a result of WHEA, women's health has emerged as a field of discussion, study, and research in many schools of nursing and medicine. The Women's Health Initiative is a $625-million, 14-year study of diseases in women that began in 1993. It is the largest study of diseases in women ever conducted (Geary, 1995). This initiative has begun to identify the unique women's health issues.

The FMLA provides job protection and continuous health benefits (if applicable) to eligible employees who need extended unpaid leave. Eligible employees can take 12 weeks annually for serious personal or family health conditions or for the birth or adoption of a child. Family is defined as the employee's child, spouse, or parents (National Partnership of Women and Families, 1998). The FMLA is particularly beneficial to women who work outside of the home and are family caregivers. Before this legislation, many women had to quit or were terminated from their jobs in order to care for a newborn or an ill family member. The loss of employment benefits created financial hardship for many women and served to punish female caregivers. The FMLA may be of little benefit for low-income women, since 12 weeks without pay is financially ruinous.

Although the FMLA has provided much-needed assistance to families caring for aging family members, much work still needs to be done. Currently, elderly married couples are required to spend much of their assets in order for Medicare to pay for the cost of nursing home care. Because wives typically live longer than their husbands, it is often the wife who must place her husband in a nursing home and as a consequence live in poverty (National Partnership for Women and Families, 1998).

Another piece of legislation that has a major impact on poor women is The Personal Responsibility and Work Opportunity Reconciliation Act, commonly known as the welfare reform law, which was passed in 1996. The law provides the states with block grants called Temporary Assistance for Needy Families (TANF). The law, which requires welfare recipients to work, provides transportation, childcare and housing assistance for families on welfare. Families on welfare are also able to retain their Medicaid benefits. The new law also requires states to initiate child support enforcement (CSE) efforts (USDHHS Administration for Children and Families, 1998) The full impact of this piece of legislation is not yet known. For some women it is an opportunity to improve the quality of life for themselves and their families. For other women and their children the law is certain to have a devastating effect.

Although women's issues are at the front of public policy today, much work still needs to be done. Those most vulnerable populations in a society are the very young and the very old. Because women are the primary family caregivers at both ends of the age continuum, a national child care policy and a policy on aging are of particular concern. The United States is the only country in the industrialized world that does not have a national childcare policy. In Europe, parents pay much less for childcare that is rated better than that in the United States. Whereas parents in Europe typically pay 5% to 15% of the cost of their children's childcare, their U.S. counterparts pay more than 90%. It is estimated that the average parent pays $2600 for childcare annually. It is further estimated that in order to provide good childcare, the cost would be $5000 annually. In Europe the cost is $7000 to $10,000 per child per year. The added cost goes to fund the salary and benefits of European childcare workers. A national policy on childcare similar to that in European countries would not only provide assistance to parents but would also lift millions of childcare workers out of poverty (Scarr et al, 1993).

The nurse must advocate for legislation of public policies that support issues important to the lives of all women and their families. Policies should address women's physical, mental, and social well-being. It is also important that the nurse promote self-advocacy among women.

clinical application

The following situation involves the needs and health problems of a middle-age woman and her family.

Mrs. Johnson is a 50-year-old African-American woman who works as a nursing assistant at a long-term care facility for elderly persons. She is a widow with two adult children. Her third child, Michael, was murdered 2 years ago while walking home one night. He was 18 years old. Her daughters Vicky, age 32, and Jackie, age 30, live in the neighborhood. She has four grandchildren: Jamil, age 14; Shandra, age 12; Chrystal, age 8; and Shaquil, age 6. Mrs. Johnson's 70-year-old mother, Mrs. Smith, now lives with her since she suffered a mild stroke 2 months ago and can no longer manage alone. The community health nurse visits three times a week to monitor Mrs. Smith's blood pressure and cardiovascular status.

Mrs. Johnson rises early to prepare breakfast for her mother and help her dress. She also prepares her mother's lunch before she leaves for work. Mrs. Smith can ambulate around the house with the aid of a walker and is independent in most of her activities of daily living.

When Mrs. Johnson returns home in the evening, she prepares dinner and helps her mother prepare for bed. She shops, cleans her house, and does laundry on Saturdays. She relies on public transportation. Vicky and Jackie provide assistance when they can, although both women work full time and have children.

Since her son's death, Mrs. Johnson has become active in community organizing efforts to stop the violence in her neighborhood. She attends weekly meetings at her church. The neighborhood has changed in the 30 years that she has lived there. It is now a dangerous place to live. She knows that there is drug dealing, and sometimes at night she hears the sound of gunfire. She worries about the safety of her grandchildren, especially Jamil. On Sundays she attends church and cooks dinner. Her daughters and grandchildren often come for Sunday dinner.

One day when the nurse visits Mrs. Smith, Mrs. Johnson is home. Mrs. Johnson mentions to the nurse that she has a history of hypertension that is controlled with medication and diet. However, she has not taken her Aldomet for 2 days. She will not be able to fill her prescription until Friday when she is paid. The nurse takes her blood pressure, which is 190/100 mm Hg.

The nurse recommends that Mrs. Johnson go to the public health clinic and see the nurse practitioner. At the clinic the nurse completes a health history and learns that Mrs. Johnson has smoked 15 to 20 cigarettes a day for the past 30 years. She has not had a Pap test in 5 years. She has no health insurance and no sick leave. A 24-hour dietary recall reveals that Mrs. Johnson had eggs, bacon, and juice for breakfast; hamburger and french fries for lunch; and red beans with sausage for dinner. She had potato chips and a coke for an afternoon snack and cookies and

milk at bedtime. Her blood pressure remains high at 190/96 mm Hg.

A. What additional information should be collected about Mrs. Johnson?
B. What are your nursing diagnoses?
C. What factors must be considered when developing a plan of care?
D. What are the continued health risks for Mrs. Johnson and her family?
E. Identify women's health issues from the chapter that apply to Mrs. Johnson's life.
F. Identify community resources that might be of assistance to Mrs. Johnson and her mother.

Answers are in the back of the book.

KEY POINTS

- The women's health movement was pivotal in bringing national recognition to women's health issues.
- Women have a longer life expectancy than men. However, women are more likely to have acute and chronic conditions that require them to use health services more than men.
- Relationships are crucial to the development of female identity.
- A life span approach to women's health recognizes that the health status of a woman in one phase of her life affects subsequent phases, as well as the lives of her children.
- Women are known as the gatekeepers of health. Women make three fourths of the health care decisions in American households.
- Women of color are more likely to have poor health outcomes because of a poor understanding of health, lack of access to health care, and lifestyle practices
- Smoking is a risk factor for a number of major health problems, including lung cancer, heart disease, osteoporosis, and poor reproductive outcomes
- Caregiving is a major role of women throughout their life span. The added responsibility and financial strain of the caregiver role can lead to caregiver burden.
- The failure to include women in medical research has resulted in a lack of understanding about the distinctive issues surrounding the diagnosis and treatment of the major diseases for women
- Heart disease is the leading cause of death among women over 50 and the second leading cause of death among women ages 35 to 39.
- Cancer is the second leading cause of death for women.
- In responses to the past lack of equality in health-related research and the provision of clinical care, there is now a major national focus on women's health issues.

critical thinking activities

1. Design a teaching plan for a middle-age woman that reflects a maximum level of health promotion.

critical thinking activities—cont'd

2. Analyze mortality and morbidity data in your county and rank the order of the 10 most prevalent health problems for women. Compare these to men's health problems.

3. Interview three women (young, middle age, and older). Compare and contrast their major health concerns.

4. Using a telephone book or community resources directory, list and evaluate health promotion and illness prevention services available for women. Include fees, location, and range of services.

Bibliography

Administration on Aging: *Profile of older Americans: 1997* [on-line], 1997. Available: www.aoa.dhhs.gov

Ahmed S, Clasen M, Donnelly J: Management of dyslipidemia in adults, *Am Fam Phys,* 57(9):2192, 1998.

American Psychological Association: *Working mothers: happy or haggard?* [on-line], 1998. Available: www.apa.org/psychnet

Arnstein P, Buselli E, Rankin S: Women and heart attacks: prevention, diagnosis and care, *Nurse Pract* 21(5):57, 1996.

Baldini E, Strauss G: Women and lung cancer: waiting to exhale, *Chest* 112(4):229, 1997.

Breen N, Kessler L: *Changes in the use of screening mammography: evidence from the 1987 and 1990 National Health Interview Surveys, Am J Public Health* 84:62, 1994.

Bureau of Justice Statistics Bulletin: *Women in prison* [on-line], 1994. Available: www.fed stats.gov

Bureau of Labor Statistics: *Employment and earnings, January 1996* [on-line], 1996. Available: stats.bls.gov

Bureau of Labor Statistics: Unpublished data, annual averages 1995 [on-line], 1995. Available: stats.bls.gov/

Catalano R, Satariano W: Unemployment and the likelihood of detecting early-stage breast cancer, *Am J Public Health* 88(4):586, 1998.

Chapman G: Patterns of cervical carcinoma in women of advanced age. *JAMA,* 89(12):801, 1997.

Ciliska D: Evaluation of two nondieting intervention for obese women, *Western J Nurs Res* 20(1):119, 1998.

Conway-Welch C et al: Women's health and women's health care: recommendations of the 1996 AAN expert panel on women's health, *Nurs Outlook,* 45(1):7, 1997.

Cooper G et al: An ecological study of the effectiveness of mammography in reducing breast cancer mortality, *Am J Public Health* 88(2):281, 1998.

Craft N: Women's health: a global issue, *Br Med J* 315(7116):1154, 1997a.

Craft N: Life span: conception to adolescence (women's health, part 2*), Br Med J* 315(7117):1227, 1997b.

Earls F: Positive effects of prenatal and early childhood interventions, *JAMA* 14:1271, 1998.

Flack J, O'Connor C, Wei J: Four commonly seen cardiovascular diseases, *Patient Care* 32(9):98, 1998.

Fogel CI: Pregnant inmates: risk factors and pregnancy outcome, *J Obstet Gynecol Neonat Nurs* 22(1):33, 1993.

Gallagher J et al: Why HRT makes sense, *Patient Care* 30:166, 1996.

Gallo M, Fallon P, Staskin D: Urinary incontinence: steps to evaluation, diagnosis, and treatment, *Nurse Pract* 22(2):21, 1997.

Geary M: An analysis of the women's health movement and its impact on the delivery of health care within the United States, *Nurse Pract* 20(11):24, 1995.

Gilbert S: Gauging the risk factors in search of a perfect face, *The New York Times* [on-line], 1998. Available: www.nyt.com

Grisso J, Ness R, Hendrix S: Update in women's health, *Ann Intern Med* 127(11):1006, 1997.

Hawthorne M: Gender differences in recovery after coronary artery surgery, *Image J Nurs Sch* 26(1):75, 1994.

Hill B, Geraci S: A diagnostic approach to chest pain based on history and ancillary evaluation, *Nurse Pract* 23(4):20, 1998.

Jay J, Staskin D: Urinary incontinence, *Adv Nurse Pract* 6(10):32, 1998.

Kazanjian P, Eisenstat S: Human immunodeficiency virus. In Noble J, editor: *Textbook of primary care medicine,* ed 2, St Louis, 1996, Mosby.

Kington R, Smith J: Socioeconomic status and racial and ethnic differences in functional status associated with chronic diseases, *Am J Public Health* 87(5):805, 1997.

Kogan M: The changing pattern of prenatal care utilization in the United States 1981-1995, using different prenatal care indeces, *JAMA* 279(20):1661, 1998.

Kuter I: Breast cancer. In Noble J, editor: *Textbook of primary care medicine,* ed 2, St Louis, 1996, Mosby.

Landau C, Milan F: Depression. In Noble J, editor: *Textbook of primary care medicine,* ed 2, St Louis, 1996, Mosby.

Levinson W, White J: Lesbians: what a primary care physician needs to know, *Western J Med* 62(5):463, 1995.

Magaziner J et al: Excess mortality attributable to hip fracture in white women aged 70 years and older, *Am J Public Health* 87(10):1630, 1997.

Manore M: Running on empty: health consequences of chronic dieting in active women, American College of Sports Medicine (ACSM) *Health and Fitness Journal* 2(2):24, 1998.

Manson M et al: Cardiovascular disease in women: a statement for health care professionals from the American Heart Association, *Circulation* 96:2468, 1997.

McCance K, Jorde L: Evaluating the genetic risk of breast cancer, *Nurse Pract* 23(8):14, 1998.

McGee C: Secondary amenorrhea leading to osteoporosis: incidence and prevention, *Nurse Pract* 22(5):38, 1997.

Minkoff H, DeHovitz J, Duerr A: *HIV infection in women,* New York, 1995, Raven Press.

National Center for Health Statistics: *Health promotion and disease prevention: United States, 1990,* Series 10, No163, USDHHS Pub No185, Hyattsville, Md, 1993, USD-HHS.

National Center for Health Statistics: [on-line], 1996. Available: www.cdc.gov/nch-swww/nchshome.htm

National Clearinghouse of Plastic Surgery Statistics: [on-line], 1997. Available: www.plastic surgery.org

National Partnership for Women and Families: *Guide to the family and medical leave act: questions and answers* [on-line], 1998. Available: www.nationalpartnership.org/index.html

National Women's Health Information Center: *Priority women's health issues* [on-line], 1998a. Available www.4women.org/owh/pub/womhelahtis-sues/whipriority.htm

National Women's Health Information Center: *Osterporsis overview* [on-line], 1998b. Available: www.4women.org/nwhic

National Women's Health Information Center: *HHS issues first comprehensive survey of working women's health* [on-line], 1998c. Available: www.4women.org/nwhic

Oakley A: Who cares for health? social relations, gender and the public health, *J Epidemiol Community Health* 48:427, 1994.

Patterson C: *Lesbian and gay parenting: a summary of resource findings* [on-line], 1998. Available: www.apa.org/psychnet.

Popkess-Vawter S, Brandau M, Straub J: Triggers of overeating and related intervention strategies for women who weight cycle, *Appl Nurs Res* 11(2):69, 1998.

Press M: Gynecologic cancers, *Cancer* 83(8):1751, 1998.

Quimby CH: Women and the family of the future, *J Obstet Gynecol Neonat Nurs* 23(2):113, 1994.

Roberts R et al: Barriers to prenatal care: factors associated with initiation of care in a middle-class midwestern community, *J Fam Practice* 47(1):53, 1998.

Roberts SJ, Sorenson L: Lesbian health care: a review and recommendations for health promotion in primary care settings, *Nurse Practitioner* 20(6):42, 1995.

Robinson KM: Family care giving: who provides the care, and at what cost? *Nurs Econ* 15(2):243, 1997.

Ross C: A comparison of osteoarthritis and rheumatoid arthritis: diagnosis and treatment, *Nurse Pract* 22(9):20, 1997.

Rousseau ME: Women's midlife health: reframing menopause, *J Nurse-Midwifery* 43(3):208, 1998.

Scarr S et al: Quality of child care as an aspect of family and child care policy in the United States, *Pediatrics* 91(1):182, 1993.

Shervington DO: Attitudes and practices of African-American women regarding cigarette smoking: implications for interventions, *J Natl Med Assoc* 86(5):337, 1994.

Smith Barney Research: *The new women's movement: women's healthcare,* April, 1997.

Soet J, DiIorio C, Dudley W: Women's self-reported condom use: intra and interpersonal factors, *Women Health* 27(4):19, 1998.

Taylor D, Woods N: Changing women's health, changing nursing practice, *JOGGN* 25(9):791, 1996.

Tindall W: When joints—and cost—become inflamed, *Business and Health* 15(12):47, 1997.

US Census Bureau, Economic and Statistics Administration: *Household and family characteristics* [on-line], 1996a. Available: www.census.gov/population/www/socdemo/hh-fam.html

US Census Bureau, Economic and Statistics Administration: *Household and family characteristics* [on-line], 1997. Available: www.census.gov/population/www/socdemo/hh-fam.html

US Census Bureau, Economic and Statistics Administration: *Who receives child support?* [on-line], 1995. Available: www.census.gov/socdemo/www/chld-supp.html

US Census Bureau: *Life expectancy at birth, age 65, and age 85, by sex and race/Hispanic origin: 1995 and 2050* [on-line], 1996b. Available: www.census.gov/statab/www

US Department of Health and Human Services: *Healthy people 2000: national health promotion and disease prevention objectives,* Sudbury, Mass, 1992, Jones & Bartlett.

US Department of Health and Human Services: *HHS launches "centers of excellence in women's health"* [on-line], 1996. Available: www.hhs.gov

US Department of Health and Human Services, Administration for Children and Families: *Welfare reform* [on-line], 1998. Available: www.acf.dhhs.gov/news/welfare

US Department of Health and Human Services, Public Health Service: *Healthy people: progress review women's health* [on-line], 1998. Available: odphp.osophs.dhhs.gov/pubs/hp2000/PROGRVW/women/women.htm

US Department of Health and Human Services, Public Health Service Office on Women's Health: *PHSOWH fact sheet: adolescent and young adult women's health* [on-line], 1998a. Available: phs.os.dhhs.gov/progorg/ophs

US Department of Health and Human Services, Public Health Service Office on Women's Health: *PHSOWH fact sheet: HHS girl power! campaign* [on-line], 1998b. Available: www.health.org/power

US Department of Health and Human Services, Public Health Service Office on Women's Health: *PHSOWH fact sheet: older women's health* [on-line], 1998c. Available: phs.os.dhhs.gov/progorg/ophs

US Department of Health and Human Services, Public Health Service Office on Women's Health: *PHSOWH fact sheet: the health of minority women* [on-line], 1998d. Available: phs.os.dhhs.gov/progorg/ophs

US Department of Labor: *Women's bureau: facts on working women* [on-line], 1996. Available: stats.bls.gov

US Preventive Services Task Force: *Guide to clinical preventive services: report of the U.S. Preventive Services Task Force, Washington, DC, 1996,* Philadelphia, 1996, Williams & Wilkins.

US Public Health Service, Office on Women's Health: *Women's health issues* [on-line], 1996. Available: www.4women.org/owh/pub/womhealth

Wertheim I, Soto-Wright V, Goodman H: Gynecologic cancers. In Noble J, editor: *Textbook of primary care medicine,* ed 2, St Louis, 1996, Mosby.

Whitmore S: Rebuilding bone, *Adv Nurse Pract* 6(9):30, 1998.

Woodhead G, Moss M: Osteoporosis: diagnosis and prevention, *Nurse Pract* 23(11):18, 1998.

Woods NF: Menopause—challenges for future research, *Exp Gerontol* 29(3/4):237, 1994.

Woods NF et al: Depressed mood and self esteem in young Asian, black and white women in America, *Health Care Women Int* 15:243, 1994.

Zeidenstein L: Gynecological and childbearing needs of lesbians, *J Nurse Midwifery* 35(1):10, 1990.

CHAPTER 28
Men's Health

THOMAS KIPPENBROCK

OBJECTIVES

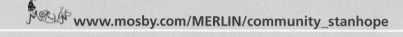

www.mosby.com/MERLIN/community_stanhope

After reading this chapter, the student should be able to do the following:

- Identify legislation affecting men's health.
- Explain the unique aspects of developmental stages and tasks that affect young and middle-age men.
- Discuss risk factors and their consequences on men's health.

- Understand how the lifestyles that men lead affect their health.
- Identify legislation affecting men's health.
- Describe the nurse's role in maintaining and promoting men's health.
- Describe the advance practice nurse's role in men's health.

KEY TERMS

assaultive violence
body maintenance
development
digital rectal examination (DRE)

generativity versus stagnation
intimacy versus isolation
men's health nurse practitioner (MHNP)

men/women death ratio
moral development
prostate cancer
psychosocial development
testicular cancer

testicular self-examination (TSE)

*See **Glossary** for definitions*

CHAPTER OUTLINE

How Men Define Health
Health Status of Men in the United States
Male Development
    Psychosocial
    Moral
Men's Health and Mortality
Gender Differences
Cultural Differences
Leading Causes of Men's Deaths

Heart and Cardiovascular Diseases
Cancer
Accidents
Pulmonary Diseases
Human Immunodeficiency Virus and Acquired Immunodeficiency Syndrome
Suicide
Homicide

Alcohol-Induced Disorders
Men's Health Practices in Everyday Life
Nurse's Role in Men's Health
    Educator
    Client Advocate
    Case Manager
    Men's Health Nurse Practitioner

Males are physiologically more vulnerable than females. More male infants die at birth. More males die of cardiovascular, liver, and chronic pulmonary diseases, as well as cancers and suicide. Males have a shorter predicted life span. Many explanations exist for such differences in gender health outcomes: genetics, risk-taking behaviors, stressors, ignoring warning signs, and many others. This chapter discusses men's health by reviewing developmental stages of men, identifying men's health problems and needs, and exploring the nurse's role in maintaining and promoting men's health in the community.

Men's health, as a separate and distinct practice of care, is at an early developmental level. Men's health goes beyond care of the prostate, genitalia, sexual dysfunction, and associated diseases. Today's focus is on the entire person, requiring a holistic approach.

This chapter also addresses the goals of *Healthy People 2000* (USDHHS, 1991) of increasing the healthy life span of Americans, reducing health disparities among Americans, and helping people achieve access to preventive services by focusing on the unique health needs of men. Health promotion strategies are described to help men deal effectively with the leading causes of death affecting them. In addition, nursing interventions are discussed that are designed to help men take advantage of preventive services that they tend to overlook to a greater extent than do women. The strategies described in this chapter illustrate the many ways in which the *Healthy People 2000* goals and objectives can be applied to men.

HOW MEN DEFINE HEALTH

Although men and women have similar ideas about health, there are some distinct differences. Most people view health as being closely associated with well-being. Both men and women define health comprehensively and refer to it as a state or condition of well-being, and they often relate this condition to capacity, performance, and function.

Health is related to a sense of self and the physical body, and both are tied to past and future actions. When men are asked about health, they look at physical, mental, and emotional well-being. Also, they believe the state of self has the potential to affect the state of others. Many men believe health is individual. This means one person's idea of health and well-being may differ from another's thoughts of being healthy. Men frequently refer to healthiness as "keeping" or "being in control" and "minding" one's body. Men seem to imagine themselves as having "power over" their relationship to their bodies. Men speak about their bodies as though they "belong" to them in the same way an object belongs to them (Saltonstall, 1993).

The times are changing from focusing on diseases and treatments to a new health care focus on identifying health needs and preventing health problems. This preventive focus is a wise one: men have been identified as a high-risk group. They frequently engage in compensatory, aggressive, and risk-taking behavior predisposing them to illness, injury, and even death.

Men tend to avoid medical help as long as possible, leading to serious health problems. With the exception of orthopedics and pediatrics, females use medical specialties more often than men. "Many men simply don't seek medical advice, or take action in preventive health care, unless it's absolutely necessary" (Rafuse, 1993, p. 329).

Men need to openly express their health care concerns. Health care professionals can help men examine their concerns by encouraging them to discuss nonhealth problems, as well as health care problems, and by promoting preventive health care. Although some men are apprehensive about intimate interaction with professionals, strategies can be used to reduce men's anxiety. Nurses should remove physical barriers separating themselves from the client, use handouts and other written information to support verbal instructions, and show a genuine interest in men's needs.

HEALTH STATUS OF MEN IN THE UNITED STATES

As described in Chapter 3, the 1990s have seen considerable attention focused on health reform, with finances playing a key role. Both men and women will be affected by changes in health care. Review of past health care legislation affecting men may provide clues to where future legislation is going. Rules and regulations on elder care, work-related injuries, and veterans' services have affected men's health.

Most Americans turning 65 years old are eligible for Medicare, Part A, consisting of hospital insurance, skilled nursing facilities, home health care, and hospice care. Disabled men are also eligible for these benefits. Currently, millions of men participate in this government-operated insurance plan. Medicare, Part B, which requires subscribers to pay a monthly fee, provides 80% coverage on other medical-related expenses such as physician costs. As described in Chapter 5, to hold down the spiraling cost of Medicare, a prospective payment system was established. This system allows pretreatment diagnosis billing categories for almost all U.S. hospitals reimbursed by Medicare.

The Worker's Compensation Act (WCA) and Americans with Disabilities Act (ADA) are two significant laws affecting men's health because of the high occupational accident rate. The WCA required all industrial employers to carry worker's compensation for their employees in cases of job-related injuries; however, some nonprofit organizations are exempt. Worker's compensation insurance pays for an employee's partial lost wages and medical costs encountered. If the employee is permanently disabled, the worker is entitled to additional money.

The ADA was designed to protect people from being discriminated against in the workplace; this means employers are prohibited from discriminating against quali-

---

BOX 28-1 **Tasks of the Young Adult Male**

- Develops an intimate relationship with another
- Chooses a mate
- Establishes a husband or father role or both
- Manages a household independent of his parents' home and care
- Develops a career or vocation
- Continues development of a social structure
- Develops a community role focusing on citizenship
- Develops a lifestyle suitable to his philosophy on life

BOX 28-2 **Tasks of the Middle-Age Adult Male**

- Promotes a deep relationship with the spouse
- Nurtures and shares in the growth of children and the next generation
- Adjusts to physical changes
- Reassesses self and career goals
- Achieves desired goals in life and career
- Builds acceptable leisure activities
- Copes with the empty nest syndrome

---

fied disabled individuals in hiring, promotion, job assignment, discharge, pay, and all other "terms, conditions, and privileges" of employment. An ADA-qualified individual is defined as a person with a disability who meets the skill, experience, education, and other job-related requirements of a position held or desired and who, with or without reasonable changes in the work environment, can perform the essential functions of a job. If a person is injured on the job, the employer has to look at all circumstances and evaluate how the employee may be taken care of after the injury.

With more men taking on parenting and elder caregiver roles, the Family and Medical Leave Act offers opportunities to meet family responsibilities. An eligible employee is entitled to a maximum of 12 weeks for the birth of a child, to care for an ill child or spouse, to adopt or accept a foster or an adoptive child, and, last, for his recovery from a serious health condition. When the person's leave is over, he is entitled to return to work in the same or an equivalent position with the same or equivalent pay scale and benefits. During the leave, the employer is not required to pay the employee, although vacation time, personal time off (PTO), or sick leave can be used. Other benefits such as life insurance and health insurance will continue; however, the employer is only required to pay for the employee.

The effects of war have influenced men's health care legislation. Until the Vietnam era, most American veterans were men. Since the mid-1970s women have entered the armed forces and are eligible for veterans' benefits. Nevertheless, the majority of veterans are men. Health-related veterans' benefits include hospital and nursing home care, counseling for sexual trauma, alcohol and drug treatments, prosthetic services, outpatient pharmacy services, and dental services. Other entitlements include a pension program.

MALE DEVELOPMENT

Development is a process by which humans change in structure, thoughts, or behaviors as a consequence of biological or environmental factors. Usually these changes are progressive and cumulative; they are not as rapid in adults as they are in children. Because adult men and women follow similar developmental patterns, developmental theorists have not typically separated the genders.

Psychosocial

Erikson (1968) explained the **psychosocial development** of adults as stages in which a person's abilities or experiences dictate major life adjustments in his or her social environment or self. The following is an overview of psychosocial development focusing on men during their young and middle adulthood.

Young adulthood (20 to 45 years of age)
Erickson labels this stage **intimacy versus isolation.** Each person must establish a secure personal identity. Once this task is accomplished, the person is able to form intimate and loving relationships. The young adult male begins to focus on developing close relationships with others and eventually choosing a mate. Box 28-1 provides a summary of tasks. These relationships lead to forming his own family and pursuing a career. Around 30 years of age and again at 40 years, there is a time of reevaluation during which the person closely examines himself regarding goals and accomplishments. This may be a crisis period for men, and they may decide to make changes in their lives.

Middle adulthood (40 to 65 years of age)
Erickson labels middle adulthood as **generativity versus stagnation.** This stage focuses on contributions to the next generation. Men are involved in sharing, nurturing, and contributing to the growth of others. Box 28-2 lists tasks for this stage. Middle adulthood has been typically defined as being a period of stability, yet many men undergo a transition period equal to or greater than the one they experienced in adolescence. Jung (1933) noted a gradual personality change in which men search their inner selves for a greater meaning in their lives. At this time, men may begin to acknowledge "tender feelings" and are more expressive. Marriage and the spousal relationship are the best predictors of male midlife satisfaction and perceived stress reduction. Thus a redefinition of husband and father roles may occur. Men also must cope with the physical changes that occur during this time.

Moral

Over time, society has changed from hunting and gathering to farming, manufacturing, and service. In prehistoric times, humans' need to hunt and kill game was essential for survival; however, with the discovery of machines, en-

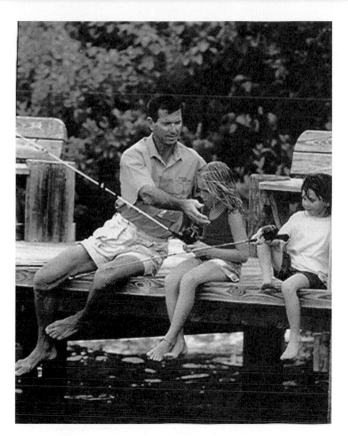

During the young adulthood stage, men generally focus on marriage and family issues.

ergy, and agriculture, the need to kill should cease. Yet humans continue to kill and commit crimes against humanity. Questions about human moral development can be explained by reviewing related theory. This chapter further explores why some men resort to violence.

Kohlberg (1984) focused on the **moral development** of the individual. As a person reasons and thinks about moral issues and problems, the individual should become motivated to develop new and broader viewpoints. People do not lose the insight they have gained earlier but instead build on it. Kohlberg divided moral development into stages or levels of reasoning. Box 28-3 summarizes these stages, which are hierarchical. Progression usually occurs with advancement from one stage to the next; however, individuals may regress to a previous stage. Stage advancement does not depend on physical maturity. The typical movement through stages is an orderly process from a focus on self to the larger society and universal principles.

MEN'S HEALTH AND MORTALITY

In the United States, men's life expectancy for all ages is one of the lowest in developed countries and much lower than women. At birth a male born in the United States can expect to live until 73.8 years of age, compared to 79.6 years for women. Canadian men's life expectancy is 75.6 years, as compared to 81.4 years for Canadian women (see the Canadian box). The European counties of France (73.8 years), Netherlands (74.1 years), and Norway (74.2 years) have higher life expectancy than American men, and similarly the women outlive the European men (82.4, 80.3, and 80.3 years, respectively). Japanese men outlive U.S. men by almost 4 years (76.4 years), but once again Japanese women outlive the men (82.4) (Statistical yearbook, 1997).

For American adolescents (15 to 24 years of age) and young adult men (25 to 34 years of age), death rates are more than twice those of men in Japan and the Netherlands. In addition, American men ages 45 to 54 years rank second-highest in death rates among the 13 developed countries; but, interestingly enough, mortality has significantly declined for American men ages 45 to 54 years. The least progress toward decline in death rates is in the men's age group of 25 to 34 years. Accidents, homicides and other violence, cancers, circulatory system diseases, and infectious and parasitic diseases account for most deaths in developed countries. American men rank high in all areas except the last one. The good news is that there has been a decline in men's ischemic heart disease in the United States; however, American men's and women's heart disease mortalities are still among the highest in the world (US Congress, Office of Technology Assessment, 1993).

GENDER DIFFERENCES

Gender differences start at birth. U.S. male neonate, postneonate, and infant death rates are higher than those of females. For example, Caucasian males babies' death rates are 450 neonate, 249 postneonate, and 699 infants, compared to Caucasian females rates of 364, 194, and 555 per 100,000 live births for the same group. African-American male babies are considerably higher (1063, 571, and 1634) compared to

Men's Health in Canada

Karon Foster, Toronto Public Health and Ryerson Polytechnical University

LIFE EXPECTANCY AND CAUSES OF DEATH

Canadian men have seen their life expectancy improve over the past 40 years. Today, a male child can expect to live to age 75. In 1994, there were 109,742 male deaths, which is a death rate of 8.7 deaths per 1,000 population (Statistics Canada, 1996). The major killers of men are heart disease, cancer, and respiratory diseases. In men ages 20 to 44, the leading causes of death are suicide and injuries from motor vehicle accidents, followed by HIV and cancer. For men ages 45 to 64 the leading causes of death are cancer, circulatory disease, and suicide. Lung cancer and ischemic heart disease are the major threats to men of this age. For men over 65, the order is reversed, with circulatory disease killing more men than cancer. Ischemic heart disease, lung cancer, and stroke are the main causes of death for this age group. Suicide and falls are also significant causes of death for those over 65 years.

Mortality statistics for males in 1994 showed there were 31,014 deaths due to cancer and 39,885 deaths due to circulatory diseases. Deaths due to respiratory disease ranked third with 10,087 and included pneumonia, influenza, asthma, bronchitis, and obstructive airway disease (Statistics Canada, 1996). In the same year there were 2,969 deaths due to suicide (Statistics Canada, 1996). The most common cancer deaths in men are due to tracheal, bronchus, and lung cancers, followed by prostate and intestinal cancers. The mortality rate due to prostate cancer has increased in the last 15 years, and it is estimated there will be 7,800 deaths by 2016 (Ellison et al, 1998). Ischemic heart disease and cerebrovascular diseases are the leading causes of circulatory deaths.

CHRONIC CONDITIONS AND INJURIES

The National Population Health Survey Overview 1996/97 (NPHS) showed the chronic diseases with the highest incidence for men were non-arthritic back problems, arthritis/rheumatism, hypertension, and heart disease, followed by cataracts, asthma, migraine, bronchitis, diabetes, and cancer (Statistics Canada, 1998). Other health problems include skin cancer and a rising incidence of prostate cancer. With the current rise in prostate cancer it is estimated that 1 in 11 men will develop prostate cancer. Men 65 years and older have higher incidence rates of arthritis/rheumatism, heart disease, and cancer. The incidence rates for these diseases were higher in men in low-income levels. Testicular cancer is the leading cancer in men between 15 and 34 years of age. This survey also showed that repetitive strain injuries (RSI) and other injuries were also a health concern. In 1995, approximately 2 million Canadians over the age of 12 had experienced a RSI (98). Men most commonly reported injuries to the back and spine, with the highest percentage of these injuries occurring at work or school followed closely by sports and leisure activities. Thirty-nine percent of men reported accidental falls resulting in sprains, strains, or broken bones. Twenty-five percent of men reported an injury in both the 1994/95 and 1996/97 surveys.

HEALTH CARE PRACTICES

How frequently do men seek health care and what preventive health practices do they participate in? Most men report visiting a health care professional at least once per year (NPHS 98). Males over 65 years visited health professionals more frequently than younger men. General practitioners and dentists were the health professionals most commonly seen, whereas chiropractors were the most common alternative health care service provider consulted. Hypertension is one of the major chronic illness reported in men, and it is also a risk factor for cardiovascular disease. Regular blood pressure (BP) screening is an important factor in monitoring hypertension. The NPHS survey of 1996/97 showed 68% of people over the age of 12 had a yearly BP screening. The frequency of BP screening, however, is lower in men. To detect testicular cancer, the Canadian Cancer Society recommends that men examine their testicles once a month. With the current increase in prostate cancer, early screening is important to control the disease. The Task Force on Periodic Health Examination recommends a yearly digital rectal examination for men over 40 years. At this point the serum prostate specific antigen test is not routinely recommended for all men because of controversy over its use as a screening method.

LIFESTYLE PRACTICES

Lifestyle factors such as smoking, alcohol use, diet, and physical activity also influence the health of men. Cigarette smoking is a risk factor for heart disease, stroke, and cancer. The percentage of Canadian men who smoke has declined sharply in the past 15 years. In 1994, 33% of men over the age of 15 were current smokers (Millar and Beaudet, 1996). Men 20 to 44 years are the most likely to smoke. Smoking behaviour was higher in men who consumed alcohol on a regular basis.

Alcohol consumption is associated with injuries and many diseases. The 1994 NPHS showed 69% of men consumed alcohol at least once a month (Millar and Beaudet, 1996). Men ages 25 to 29 had the highest incidence of alcohol use.

Physical activity is promoted as a behaviour to prevent disease and maintain health. Men are more physically active in their leisure time than women are. Canadian men have gradually become more physically active. In 1994, 20% of men were physically active (Millar and Beaudet, 1996).

In 1991, 30% of men were considered overweight, an increase from 1985 data (Millar and Stephens, 1993). The 1992 Heart Health Survey found that 35% of men had a

Men's Health in Canada—cont'd

Body Mass Index over 27 (Shah, 1994). Most deaths for cardiovascular disease occur in individuals with elevated blood cholesterol. Forty-eight percent of Canadian men have elevated blood cholesterol levels (Shah, 1994). There has been an increase in the elevated blood cholesterol levels for men ages 18 to 44 years.

OCCUPATIONAL HEALTH

Men experience risks to their health from exposure to hazardous materials in their work and from work-related injuries. Occupational health is a provincial responsibility, and government monitoring of health and safety is carried out by different agencies in each province. Employers are required to provide information about substances in the workplace that are hazardous to a worker's health through the Workplace Hazards Management Information System (WHMIS) program. Compensation for injuries that occur during employment is provided through Workman's Compensation.

In summary, men's life expectancy has improved in Canada. However, cancer, heart disease, and respiratory disease pose major threats to the health of men. Health professionals need to encourage men to make lifestyle changes and incorporate a variety of health promotion strategies into their practise in order to address these health threats.

Bibliography

Ellison L, et al: Monograph series on aging-related diseases: X prostate cancer. Ottawa, Health Canada, *Laboratory Center for Disease Control* 19(1):1, 1998, [on-line]. Available: www.hc-sc.gc.ca/hph/lcdc/bcrdd/hdsc/s7_e.html#16

Millar W, Beaudet M: Health facts from the 1994 National Population Health Survey, *Canadian Social Trends* 40:24, 1996.

Millar W, Stephens T: Social status and health risks in Canadian adults, *Health Rep* 5(2):147, 1993.

Shah CP, Shah S, Shah R: Determinants of health and disease. In *Public health and preventive medicine in Canada*, ed 3, Toronto, 1994, University of Toronto Press.

Statistics Canada: *National population health survey overview 1996/97*, Ottawa, 1998, Statistics Canada Health Statistics Division.

Statistics Canada: *Mortality: summary list of causes of death 1994*, Ottawa, 1996, Statistics Canada Health Statistics Division.

Wilkins K: Causes of death: how the sexes differ, *Health Rep* 7(2):33, 1995.

Canadian spelling is used.

African-American female babies (905, 481, 1386) for each of the groups (Report of final mortality statistics, 1997).

On the other end of the life span, men have a shorter life expectancy than women. Government data revealed that the U.S. life expectancy for men at birth was a record in 1995 but men still live considerably fewer years than women. African-American and Caucasian men can expect to live 66.1 and 73.8 years, compared with 74.2 and 79.6 years for African-American and Caucasian women. The gender differences is 8.1 years for African-Americans and 5.8 years for Caucasians (Report of final mortality statistics, 1997). In 1991 the age-adjusted death rate for men of all races was 1.7 times higher than that of women. The **men/women death ratio** has fluctuated somewhat over the past years. The recent low was 1.5 in 1950, compared with 1.8 in 1970.

Men engage in more risk-taking behaviors than women. This is particularly true with behaviors involving physical challenges or illegal behavior. Men drink more alcohol than women, which may explain men's higher mortality from accidents, liver cirrhosis, and some types of cancer. Men's jobs are more hazardous, resulting in more job-related accidents. Men are also exposed to more industrial carcinogens. Other areas contributing to gender differences in morbidity or mortality may include stress responses, genetics, physiological differences, environmental factors, and preventive behavior. Often, differences are related to several combined factors.

Similarities and differences exist as to the leading causes of death among men and women (Table 28-1). Heart disease and cancer are by far the leading causes of mortality for both genders. The most prominent gender death rate differences are for pulmonary diseases, human immune virus (HIV), suicides, homicides, accidents, and alcoholism-related diseases. For example, HIV deaths are almost five times higher in men than in women; suicides are more than four and one-half times higher; homicides are more than three times higher; and accidents and liver diseases are more than two times higher. Even though cerebrovascular disease, pneumonia, diabetes, are leading causes of men's deaths, they will not be discussed because women have similar death rates.

CULTURAL DIFFERENCES

Men's health status differ among the various cultures and races. In the general population, mortality is higher for African-Americans than for Caucasian populations. For example, there was a 1.6 times higher age-adjusted death rate for both sexes in the African-American population compared to Caucasians. Likewise, the age-adjusted death rate was higher (1.7) for African-American males than for Caucasian males. When analyzing the leading causes of death, African-American male death rates exceed Caucasian male rates in the top seven leading causes (heart disease, cancers, HIV, cerebrovascular disease, accidents, homicides, and diabetes mellitus). The African-American male life expectancy at birth is 66.1, compared to 73.8 for Caucasian males. Life expectancy for Caucasian males was 7.7 years higher than for African-American males in 1995. Disease such as HIV infections, heart disease, homicide, cancer, and perinatal conditions accounted for the differences.

Within the Hispanic population, the age-adjusted death rate for males was 1.9 times higher than that of females, compared to 1.6 for non-Hispanic Caucasians. When ana-

lyzing age groups, Hispanic males experienced 3 to 4 times higher death rates than Hispanic females for the ages 15 to 44 (Report of final mortality statistics, 1997).

LEADING CAUSES OF MEN'S DEATHS
Heart and Cardiovascular Diseases

For men, heart disease is the leading cause of death. The age-adjusted men's death rate in 1995 was 226 per 100,000 population, accounting for 31% of all of men's causes of mortality. This health statistic is unquestionably significant in young and middle-age men. For young men (25 to 44 years), heart disease is 2.6 times higher than for females; for middle-age men (45 to 64 years), it is 2.5 times higher (Table 28-2) (Report of final mortality statistics, 1997).

Coronary heart disease (CHD) is the leading cause of morbidity and mortality in the United States despite the decline during the last three decades. Over 700,000 people were hospitalized with acute myocardial infarctions (MI) in 1997. About 400,000 people die annually from CHD, accounting for one third of all deaths (Hunink et al, 1997). Table 28-3 describes differences in the types of chest pain.

Gaziano (1998) identified two factors contributing to future heart disease in the United States. One factor is the anticipated aged population, who will have more incidents of cardiovascular disease. Several physiological changes occur as a person ages, including an increase in the size of the heart. The biggest changes take place on the left side of the heart, or the pumping side. Heart mass increases 1 to 1.5 g/yr between ages 30 and 90 years. However, the heart may atrophy if the person has an extended illness. Aging results in valve and vascular changes, and systolic blood pressure rises because of less compliant blood vessels.

TABLE 28-1 **Leading Causes of Death, Age-Adjusted Death Rate, and Death Ratio (as Compared with Those Among Women)**

CAUSE OF DEATH	DEATH RATE: MALES	DEATH RATE: FEMALES	DEATH RATIO
Heart	226.6	132.9	1.7
Cancer	156.8	110.4	1.4
Cerebrovascular disease	28.9	24.8	1.2
Accidents	44.1	17.5	2.5
Motor vehicle	22.7	10.07	2.3
Other	21.4	7.5	2.9
Chronic obstructive pulmonary disease	26.3	17.1	1.5
Pneumonia	16.5	10.4	1.6
HIV	26.2	5.2	5.0
Diabetes	14.4	12.4	1.2
Suicide	18.6	4.1	4.5
Homicide	14.7	4.0	3.7
Chronic liver	11.0	4.6	2.4

From Report of final mortality statistics, 1995, *Monthly Vital Statistics Rep* 45(2; suppl), 1997.

TABLE 28-2 **Heart and Vascular Disease Death Rates and Death Ratios of Young and Middle-Age Men and Women**

CAUSE	DEATH RATE: 25-44 YEARS OF AGE			DEATH RATE: 45-64 YEARS OF AGE		
	MEN	WOMEN	DEATH RATIO	MEN	WOMEN	DEATH RATIO
Heart	29.6	11.5	2.6	286.8	112.7	2.5
CV disease	4.5	3.9	1.1	33.2	25.4	1.3

From Report of final mortality statistics, 1995, *Monthly Vital Statistics Rep* 45(2; suppl), 1997. *CV*, Cardiovascular.

TABLE 28-3 **Assessing Chest Pain**

	ANGINA	MYOCARDIAL INFARCTION
Onset	Sudden or gradual	Sudden
Duration	Usually >15 min	30 to 120 min
Location	Substernal or anterior chest; however, not sharply localized	Same as for angina
Radiation	Back, neck, arms, jaw, abdomen, or fingers	Jaws, neck, back, shoulder, and one or both arms
Quality and intensity	Mild to moderate as tightness, pressure described squeezing, and crushing	Persistent and severe pressure similarly described as angina pain

The other factor influencing more heart disease is found in the very young. Evidence from the Bogalusa Heart Study showed that children and young adults had traditional risk factors related to atherosclerosis in the aorta and coronary arteries. In an autopsy of 86 Caucasian males, 52 African-American males, and 66 females, researchers found the extent of aortic and coronary artery vessels with fatty steaks and fibrous plaques increasing with age among chilren and young adults. Among the cardiovascular risk factors found on the dead subjects: body mass index, systolic and diasystolic blood pressure, serum concentrations of total cholestrol, triglycerides, low-density lipoproteins cholesterol, and high-density lipoprotein cholesterol were strongly associated with the extent of lessions in the aorta and conoray arteries. In addition, cigarette smokers had more lessions than nonsmokers (Berenson et al, 1998). See the Research Brief about the article by Marciniak and colleagues.

The decline in the age-adjusted rates of CHD and strokes have been attributed to improved treatment and primary and secondary prevention among middle-age and older populations. Efforts against smoking, screening for hypertension and high cholestrol blood levels, and improved treatments of acute MI have had direct results in recent CHD declines. Hunink et al (1997) estimated that 25% of the CHD mortality decline was owned to primary prevention. Also, much of the decline was explained by improved CHD client management through risk factor reduction and treatments. Interventions to decrease lipoproteins explained one third of the CHD mortality. This effect is explained by diet or lipid-lowering medications.

RESEARCH *Brief*

Preintervention and postintervention acute myocardial infarction (AMI) sample from a four-state region was studied. The research goal was to improve the quality of care for AMI clients. Samples were studied at two time periods in the regional sample, as well as indicator comparisons made with a random sample from across the county. Morality comparisons involving all AMI clients nationwide were collected. The results revealed the quality of care was better in the four-state region. Treatments such as administration of aspirin during hospitalization, prescription of beta-blockers at discharge, and smoking cessation counseling lead to improved health outcomes. Mortality at 30 days decreased from 19% to 17%, the length of stays decreased from 8 to 6 days, and the postinfarction 1-year mortality was significantly reduced.

Marciniak TA et al: Improving the quality of care for medicare patients with acute myocardial infarction: results from the cooperative cardiovascular project, *JAMA* 279(17):1351, 1998.

Cancer

Malignant neoplasms are the second leading cause of death for men of all ages. The age-adjusted death rate is 157 per 100,000 population, accounting for 24% of all men's deaths in the United States (Report on Final Mortality Statistics, 1995, 1997). A discussion of the most significant cancers affecting men will be addressed: prostate, testicular, and skin.

Prostate cancer

The second most common cancer among U.S. men, next to pulmonary neoplasms, with a reported age-adjusted death rate of 13.1 cases per 100,000 per population, is **prostate cancer** (Report on final mortality statistics, 1997). The risk for prostate cancer increases with each decade after 50 years of age and is highest among men 75 years and older. In reviewing race and ethnic data, African-American men have the highest reported death percentages (9.4%), followed by Caucasian men, 6.2%; Hispanic men, 6.1%; American Indian men, 5.4%; and Asian men the lowest at 3.7% (Landis et al, 1998). See the Research Brief about the Albertsen et al article about prostate cancer.

The exact cause of prostate cancer is unknown. Genetics, hormones, diet, environment, and viruses have all been implicated as risk factors. Early diagnosis is essential because treatment is usually unsuccessful unless it is done in the early stages of the disease. One diagnostic problem is the lack of symptoms; thus the cancer may be advanced before detection.

The two most commonly used early diagnosis methods are an annual **digital rectal examination (DRE)** and the serum prostate-specific antigen (PSA). DRE can detect palpable masses. The presence of asymmetry, induration, or a firm nodule is a sign of cancer. Men identify the examination as painful and avoid the procedure; however, the test is inexpensive and results are quick. PSA is a serum protease used to detect nonpalpable and recurrent prostrate lesions. Serial measurements increase over time and are more important than an elevated one-time result (Pobursky, 1995). Other forms of testing include transrectal ultrasounds, x-ray assessment, computerized tomography and magnetic resonance imaging (MRI), and biopsy.

More frequent examinations are recommended for men who are considered at risk. Two factors considered to indicate risk are (1) men with continuing urinary symptoms and a history of blood relatives with prostatic cancer, and (2) men with benign prostatic hypertrophy or a partial prostatectomy.

The most frequent treatment option includes a wait-and-monitor period. Continued assessment of urine, DRE, and PSA assessment is used in the early cancer stage. More intense treatment may include one or a combination of the following: radiation therapy, hormonal therapy, pharmacological management, or surgical management. Even though survival rates have improved, it is still necessary to continue to educate men concerning the risks and the need for regular examinations. The 5-year survival rate for Caucasian men is 90%; for African-American men it is 75% (Landis et al, 1998).

Closely related and a precursor to prostate cancer is benign prostatic hyperplasia (BPH). Aging is the major risk factor for BPH. By 60 years of age, more than 50% of men will experience BPH. This rate increases to 90% by 85 years of age. In fact, one in four U.S. men will require treatment of symptomatic BPH by 80 years (Treating your enlarged prostate, 1994). Symptoms may include frequency of urination, nocturia, urgency, straining to urinate, hesitancy in urination, weak or intermittent stream, and feeling of incomplete emptying. Prostate enlargement does not necessarily correlate with the severity of the symptoms or the amount of restriction to urine flow. Complications may include urinary retention, renal insufficiency, urinary tract infections, hematuria, or bladder stones.

Symptom assessment may be done using a self-administered questionnaire called the International Prostate Symptom Scores (I-PSS). This questionnaire consists of six symptom-related questions and one quality-of-life question. The symptoms include most of those discussed above: incomplete emptying, frequency, intermittency, urgency, weak stream, and straining. Symptoms are scored from 0 (not at all) to 5 (almost always). The total score can range from 0 (asymptomatic) to 35 (symptomatic). The quality-of-life question has six possible responses ranging from delighted to terrible. Additional diagnostic tests are also used to reach a diagnosis. These include uroflometry, postvoid residual urine, pressure flow studies, and urethrocystoscopy.

Testicular cancer

Testicular cancer is a commonly found solid-tumor malignancy in men 15 to 35 years of age. The etiology of this cancer, testicular germ cell, is unknown. Many possible explanations exist, such as age, endocrine and genetic disorders, or socioeconomic and occupational factors.

The most common presenting symptom is a painless, firm scrotal mass or swelling accidentally discovered. Low back pain may result with retroperitoneal lymph node involvement. It is unfortunate that most men do not practice risk appraisal strategies to detect this cancer. Walker (1993) found 83% of men do not perform **testicular self-examination (TSE).**

Modeling and guided practice should be components of a comprehensive testicular educational program. Instructions are on how to perform a month TSE are provided below and in Figure 28-1. A program may consist of audiovisual aids and pamphlets followed by step-by-step procedures and return demonstrations. These approaches lead to increased frequency of TSE and enhanced comfort levels of the men performing the procedure (Walker, 1993). If tumors are found, the most common form of management is retroperitoneal lymph node dissection and chemotherapy for metastases larger than 3 cm.

Skin cancer

The three main types of skin cancers are basal and squamous cell carcinoma and malignant melanomas. When these are combined, skin cancers ranked as the fifth highest new reported cancers among men, with 67, 600 cases (Landis et al, 1998). Men's death rate (3.3/100,000 population) was much higher than women's death rate in 1995

RESEARCH *Brief*

A total of 767 men with localized prostate cancer diagnosed between 1971 to 1984, 55 to 74 years old at the time of diagnosis, and either not treated with or treated with immediate or delayed hormone therapy were studied 10 to 20 years after first being diagnosed. The research goal was to estimate survival rates based on the type of treatments. The researchers found men with well-differentiated prostate disease identified by prostate biopsy faced a minimal risk of death from the tumor within 15 years after diagnosis. Conversely, men with poorly differentiated disease faced a high death risk when treated conservatively. Men with moderately differentiated disease faced a modest death risk that increased slowly after 15 years. Unclear to the researchers is whether the moderately differentiated group would actually benefit from more aggressive treatments.

Albertsen PC et al: Competing risk analysis of men aged 55 to 74 years at diagnosis managed conservatively for clinical localized prostate cancer, *JAMA* 280:975, 1998.

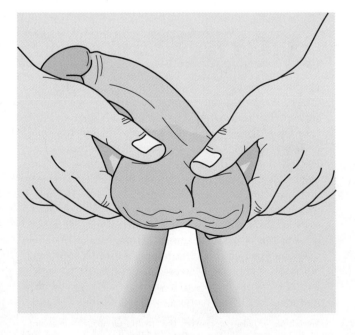

TSE

FIG. 28-1 Performing a testicular self-examination.

(1.9/100,000 population) (Report of final mortality statistics, 1997).

Prolonged sun exposure and high ultraviolet B cause skin cancer. Red-, blond-, or light brown-haired men with light complexions or freckles are the most susceptible. Also, men with a history of long-term occupational or recreational sun exposure such as farmers, construction workers, sailors, swimmers, surfers, and sunbathers are at high risk.

HOW TO *Perform a Step-by-Step Monthly Testicular Self-Examination (TSE)*

1. Perform the TSE during a warm bath or shower.
2. Roll each testicle between your thumb and fingers using warm hands. Testicles should be egg shaped, 4 cm, oblong, similar in size, and have a rubbery texture; the left dangles lower than the right.
3. Check the epididymis for softness and slight tenderness.
4. Check the spermatic cord for firm, smooth tubular structure.

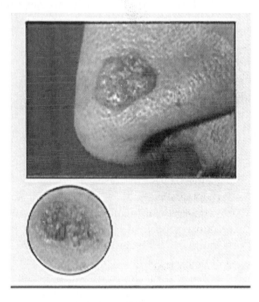

FIG. 28-2 Skin cancer.

Malignant melanoma is the deadliest form of skin cancer and the incidence is rising worldwide (Fig. 28-2). This cancer can metastasize to the brain, lungs, bones, liver, and other areas of the skin with generally fatal results. With early screening, the 5-year relative survival rate for Caucasians is 88% and 67% for African-Americans (Landis et al, 1998).

Prevention includes decreasing exposure to direct sunlight, especially between the peak hours of 10 AM and 3 PM. Men should wear protective clothing and use a sunblock of at least SPF 15 or higher when outside. Regular skin inspection and assessment are also important. Early diagnosis and treatment increase the chances of recovery.

Accidents

The fourth leading cause of men's death for all ages, accounting for age-adjusted death rates of 44 per 100,000 population, is accidental death. The death rate data are highly significant in men 15 to 24 years old (56 per 100,000 population) and 25 to 44 years old (51 per 100,000 population) (Report of final mortality statistics, 1997).

Fatal accidents

Men are at higher risk for fatal occupational injuries than women. In 1992 men accounted for about 90% of all fatally injured workers. This is high, since men accounted for approximately 55% of the workforce. A breakdown of occupational fatalities by gender is listed in Table 28-4.

The most recent data reveal that transportation and assault/violent acts were the two leading fatal occupational injuries, accounting for 58% of men's deaths in this category. Other leading fatal injuries were contact with objects and equipment, falls, exposure to harmful substances or environment, and fires. The men/women occupational death ratios differed greatly. For example, the men's death rate resulting from contact with objects and equipment was 46 times greater than in women, 42 times greater for fire and exposure, 33 times greater for harmful substances and environmental exposure, 19 times greater for falls, 14 times greater for transportation, and 6 times greater for assaults and violent acts (Toscango and Windau, 1994).

TABLE 28-4 Number and Percent Distribution of Fatal Occupational Injuries By Gender

	MEN (N=5657)		WOMEN (N=426)	
	NUMBER	PERCENT	NUMBER	PERCENT
Transportation	2263	40	162	38
Assaults and violent acts	1018	18	183	43
Contact with objects and equipment	962	17	21	5
Falls	566	10	30	7
Exposure to harmful substances or environment	566	10	17	4
Fire and exposure	170	3	4	1

From Toscano G, Windau J: *Fatal work injuries: results from 1992 national census*, Report 870, Washington, DC, 1994, US Department of Labor, Bureau of Labor Statistics.

Nonfatal accidents

Sprains and strains accounted for approximately 1 million of the total 2.3 million work-related injuries in 1992. About one fifth of the nonfatal injuries occurred to the back, caused by overexertion from lifting, pulling, or pushing objects or persons. Again, men accounted for nearly two thirds of these cases. Occupations with the highest back injuries were nonconstruction laborers, truck drivers, and nursing aides or orderlies (U.S. Department of Labor, 1994).

Pulmonary Diseases

Chronic obstructive pulmonary disease is the fifth leading cause of age-adjusted death among men. Men have a 1.5 times greater chance of dying from chronic pulmonary problems than women. It should be noted that the incidence of emphysema and respiratory system cancer death rates are higher in men than in women (Report of final mortality statistics, 1997).

Smoking is a definite pulmonary disease risk factor. Traditionally, men have used tobacco more than women; however, this trend is changing. Early studies found that men were more likely than women to become regular smokers. More recent data indicate women are more likely than men to have tried smoking. In recent decades the public, and especially men, have received education concerning the dangers of smoking. This has resulted in a decrease in the prevalence of smoking, chiefly in men. Evidence indicates men's cessation rates were higher than women's in middle-age and older smokers during the 1960s and 1970s. In the United States, education is an important factor concerning gender differences in smoking. Men in two categories—ages 19 to 24 years old, and those who had attended college—are less likely than females to become smokers.

WHAT DO YOU THINK? *It is clear that tobacco use in any form has detrimental effects on personal health. Current legislation has limited or banned smoking in public places. These policies have been criticized by smokers who cite the "common courtesy approach" as being effective.*

Human Immunodeficiency Virus and Acquired Immunodeficiency Syndrome

Acquired immunodeficiency syndrome (AIDS) is a major health concern in the world and United States. AIDS is the leading cause of death in the United States for men ages 25 to 44, fourth for the 45 to 64 age group, sixth for the 15 to 24 age group, and it is the seventh leading cause of death for men of all age groups. There is a wide difference in death rates between men and women. For all ages and all races, the age-adjusted men's death rate from AIDS is 26 per 100,000 population, compared with women's 5.7 per 100,000 population. Evaluating race and gender, the African-American male death rate is highest at 82, followed by Caucasian males at 28, compared with African-American females at 25 and Caucasian females at 5 per 100,000 (Report of final mortality statistics, 1997).

The incidence of HIV in the United States during the 1990s had fallen to a level below the peak of the mid-1980s (Karon et al, 1996), but much of the decline reflects trends in Caucasian homosexual men older than 30 years. There is some evidence that the rate is once again increasing. Teenagers and young adults engaging in high-risk sexual behaviors, and drug use is the reason the epidemic continues in this age group. Among the 38 million persons born between 1965 and 1974, 42,240 persons had developed AIDS starting in 1996. African-American men had the highest incidence of AIDS with 124 per 100,000, followed by Hispanic men with 56 per 100,000, and Caucasian men 23 per 100,000, respectively. Homosexual contract was the leading exposure category for young Caucasian, African-American, and Hispanic men with AIDS. In 1995, the incidents of AIDS attributed to homosexual contact was 4 times higher in African-American men and 2 times higher in Hispanic men than in Caucasian men. Injection drug use was the second leading exposure category, followed by heterosexual contact third (Rosenberg and Biggar, 1998).

AIDS spreads by direct contact with infected blood or body fluids, including vaginal secretions, semen, and breast milk. High-risk groups include sexually active men with multiple partners and intravenous drug users. The risk of HIV and AIDS being introduced through blood and blood products has been greatly reduced. All blood donated in the United States has been tested for the HIV antibody since 1985. Individuals who donate are also screened as to health history and risk behaviors.

The signs and symptoms of AIDS vary from person to person but may include diarrhea, night sweats, fever, weight loss, fatigue, persistent cough, and memory problems. A person may be asymptomatic or have any one or a combination of symptoms. Treatment is directed at symptom relief, and two drugs are used to slow the progression of the disease: azidothymidine (AZT) and dideoxyinosine (ddI).

The occurrence of this disease has created both ethical and financial questions. The cost for care and treatment of AIDS continues to grow, and many male AIDS clients find insurance companies refusing to pay as costs soar. Men have been fired from their jobs, refused medical treatment, and driven out of their communities. Although such discrimination is against the law, it still occurs. Ethical standards of confidentiality, privacy, and treatment have been challenged. The result is that men with HIV and AIDS remain silent about their disease. Many persons in high-risk groups decline to be tested out of fear of potential results. Healthcare workers both in acute care and community health must maintain confidentiality and demonstrate high ethical standards.

DID YOU KNOW? *If a person with HIV or AIDS knowingly infects another person, it may be considered a criminal offense.*

Suicide

Some of the most significant gender health differences occur in the mental health domain. The age-adjusted suicide death rate in men is 19 per 100,000 population, compared with 4 for women, representing nearly a five-fold gender difference. In addition, suicide is the ninth leading cause of death overall for men; high-risk groups are men 15 to 24 years old (the third leading cause) and men 25 to 44 years old (the fourth leading cause) (Report of final mortality statistics, 1997).

Suicide is a significant problem in men, since they are more likely to make a serious attempt to kill themselves rather than to use a suicide attempt as a cry for help. Elderly persons are more likely to use violent and lethal means, and they communicate their intentions less frequently.

Suicide is tragic, since it can often be prevented and such a loss causes grief for family members and friends. Nurses in community health often can identify men at risk for suicide. Table 28-5 shows selected suicidal risk factors. A study by Canetto (1994) found the two major reasons for the high male suicide rate was maladaptive coping to external stressors and socially reinforced behaviors.

Despite the widespread use of telephone crisis lines, school-based intervention programs, and antidepressive medications, high rates of suicide continue. All suicide attempts should be taken seriously. The nurse's goal is to detect risk factors, promote safety, prevent self-harm, make appropriate referrals, and help people back to health.

Homicide

Men are also prone to engage in dangerous and risky behavior, such as carrying weapons and fighting. The age-adjusted homicide death rate for men is 15 per 100,000 population, compared with 4 for women. Homicides are the tenth leading cause of death in men of all ages. More significantly, for 15- to 24-year-old men, all races, the death rate is 34 per 100,000 population and the second leading cause of death (Report of final mortality statistics, 1997).

Assaultive violence is defined as "nonfatal and fatal interpersonal violence where physical force or other means is used by a person with intent of causing harm, injury, or death to another" (Rosenberg and Mercy, 1991, p. 14). Specifically, a national poll found that 34% of U.S. adults have witnessed a man beating his wife or girlfriend. Also, the violent nature of men is exemplified by research that found that 14% of all women have had a violent action committed against them by a man at some time (EDK Associates, 1993). These statistics continue to increase (see Chapter 37).

Multiple causes are attributed to violent behavior. For example, brain dysfunction is associated with irregularities in the limbic system, the part of the brain that regulates emotions and motivation and is associated with violence. Other causes of dysfunction include organic brain disease, psychosis, depression, mental retardation, and brain tumors.

Violence is associated with social, economic, cultural, and environmental factors that especially contribute to assaults among African-American youth (Hammond and Yung, 1993). Poverty and inner-city residency also have been shown to be strongly associated with violent victimization among all adolescents. For African-American males 15 to 24 years, homicide is the leading cause of death at 132 per 100,000 population. Further, for African-American males 25 to 44 years, the death rate is 78 per 100,000 population, making it the second leading death cause in their age bracket (Report of final mortality statistics, 1997).

The Justice Department estimates half the households in the United States have a gun (Maguire and Pastore, 1994). One example of health-related problems of gun ownership is workplace homicides. Gunshot wounds account for more than 80% of workplace homicides, and male workers make up 83% of the victims (Windau and Toscano, 1994).

Little is known about the long-term effects men experience following sexual assaults. Nurses need to understand violent crimes and develop prevention and educational programs for assisting the male victim. For now nurses

TABLE 28-5 Suicide Risk Factors

FACTORS	CONDITIONS
Gender	Men use more violent means and have a higher completed suicide rate.
Marital status	Unmarried men have a greater risk than married men.
Employment	Unemployed men are at greater risk.
Previous attempts	Men with more than one attempt have a much higher chance of attempting it again. One quarter to one half of deaths are by people who have made previous attempts.
Family history	A positive family history increases the risk of suicides.
Medical illness	Men suffering from terminal illness or other medical conditions are at high risk.

must continue to support and provide counseling for the male victim who demonstrates emotional distress.

Violence is a public health emergency. Solutions are complex but are believed to be reachable. First, nurses need to identify signs and symptoms of violent behavior. The practitioner should be concerned about a man who is excessively restless and agitated; he may pace up and down or start pounding on walls, doors, furniture, and other objects. He may appear angry and tense by clenching his teeth, jaw, and fists. His voice may become loud, and he may use profanity. He may become argumentative by refusing to follow directions and making threats. Another sign to watch for includes impulsive behaviors. Alcohol and drug abuse and psychiatric disorders are highly associated with violent behavior. Finally, the most predictive indicator of violence is a history of aggressive behavior and family violence.

Alcohol-Induced Disorders

In 1991 the National Council on Alcoholism and Drug Dependence (1991) estimated 10.5 million U.S. adults showed symptoms of alcoholism. In addition, 7.2 million showed continued heavy drinking patterns with impaired health or social functioning. An evaluation of gender differences reveals the men's age-adjusted death rate for alcohol-induced causes is 10.8 per 100,000 population compared with 3.0 for women (Report of final mortality statistics, 1997).

Chronic liver disease and cirrhosis represent a health hazard associated with alcohol abuse. Age-adjusted gender death rates from alcohol abuse demonstrate striking differences: 11.0 for men compared with women at 4.6 per 100,000. Furthermore, African-American men have an even higher death rate of 14.7, compared to 6.0 for African-American women. Age-related data demonstrate some interesting comparisons. The death rate for men 25 to 44 years old was 7.5 per 100,000 population, making it the seventh leading cause of death, and for men ages 45 to 64 years it was 30.0, making it the sixth leading cause of death (Report of final mortality statistics, 1997).

Patterns of alcohol, tobacco, and drug usage established during the teen years often persist into adulthood, contributing to a leading cause of mortality and morbidity. Alcohol is closely associated with several negative aspects of society: suicide, violent crime, birth defects, and domestic and sexual abuse. Rivara et al (1997) found alcohol and illicit drug use were associated with increased risk of violent deaths in the home. Males drinking and using drugs accounted for the majority of the homicide (63%) and suicide (72%) victims.

Alcohol is the major cause of all fatal and nonfatal motor vehicle accidents among teenage drivers. Bachman et al (1991) described the highest drinking rates in teens among Caucasian, American-Indian, and Hispanic males in their senior year of high school. Among high school seniors, males drink more (binge drinking) than females in all ethnic groups. In addition to alcohol-related injuries, illnesses, and deaths, drinking can have negative consequences on family, friends, and employment.

Alcohol leads to dependence associated with one's inability to cut down on drinking, including morning drinking, memory losses, and other related medical problems. Almost 50% of separated and divorced men under 45 years of age have been exposed to alcoholism in the family. Also, separated and divorced men are three times more likely than married men to say they have been married to an alcoholic or problem drinker (National Council on Alcoholism and Drug Dependence, 1991).

Society must remember that alcohol consumption is a major drug problem. Nurses must start educating the younger population about the effects of alcohol. One focal point is the message to "stop underage drinking." Even though alcohol use by persons under 21 years of age is illegal in most states, alcohol is easily accessible. Education is the best prevention at this time and should begin in elementary schools.

MEN'S HEALTH PRACTICES IN EVERYDAY LIFE

Men and women both have unquestionable biological and physiological needs for rest, exercise, and food consumption to maintain health. When asked, men and women differ on the most important needs to maintain health. Women listed food first, then exercise, and then rest. Men rate exercise first, then sleep, and food last. Men emphasized the nutrient quality of food; women focused on the food's calories rather than its nutrient quality. Men perceived body maintenance activities as essential to producing health for oneself and emphasized sports and outdoor activities as influencing better body maintenance. Further, men viewed the body as a medium of action; function and capacity were of major importance (Saltonstall, 1993).

The concept of **body maintenance** images has two components: inner and outer. *Inner* refers to optimal functioning, performance, and capacity to do things. *Outer* refers to appearance, movement within social space, and having the potential to be heard and touched. Men discern the inner phenomenon as a function and capacity more than the outer body phenomenon of appearance. Men would rather look at how they went through the day, what they accomplished, and what kind of physical shape they are in so they can perform their tasks and life activities. Less attention is given to having good color and skin tones.

Bird and Fremont (1991) compared men's and women's social roles related to time use and health. Even though men reported poorer health than women, men spend more time in paid work hours with higher wages associated with better health. Women, on the other hand, spend more time doing housework, have a slightly lower educational level, and have less paid work hours and lower wages, all of which are associated with poorer health. Neither gender was shown to spend much time helping others, which has been shown to improve health. Gender differences favor men's health and their perception of health. Men do benefit from the role of being the family's primary breadwinner.

Men need to take an individual conscious look at themselves and develop a plan to stay healthy and free of illness by becoming knowledgeable about health and their own individual bodies. Along with knowledge comes desire to be healthy. In addition, men need to set health-related goals and develop an action plan. With the support of the nursing profession, men can take responsibility in changing and maintaining healthier lifestyles. Table 28-6 summarizes men's biological and psychosocial health care needs.

TABLE 28-6 Men's Health Care Needs

	BIOLOGICAL	PSYCHOSOCIAL	COMBINATION
Expression		Desire to communicate with others about health care concerns	
Support		Support from others about certain sex roles and lifestyles that influence their physical and mental health	
Respect and dignity			Attention from professionals regarding factors that may cause illness or affect a man's expression of illness, including occupational factors, leisure patterns, and interpersonal relationships
Health-seeking knowledge and behaviors	Information about their body's functions, what is normal and abnormal, what action to take, and the contributions of proper nutrition and exercise. Self-care instruction including testicular and genital self examinations Physical examination and historytaking that include sexual and reproductive health and illness across the life span		
Holistic medical care and availability		Adjustment of health care system to men's occupational constraints regarding time and location of source of health care	Treatment for problems of couples, including interpersonal problems, infertility, family planning, sexual concerns, and sexually transmitted diseases
Parental guidance		Help with fathering (e.g., being included as a parent in care of children) Help with fathering as a single parent, in particular, with a child of the opposite sex, in addressing the child's sexual development and concerns	
Coping		Recognition that feelings of confusion and uncertainty in a time of rapid social change are normal and may mark onset of healthy adaptation to change	
Fiduciary		Financial ways to obtain the above	

NURSE'S ROLE IN MEN'S HEALTH

Nurses in community health have knowledge and skills enabling them to assess, diagnose, plan, implement, and evaluate the care of men. Nurses, using a range of skills and in a variety of roles, work with men in diverse communities ranging from isolated agricultural regions to densely populated cities. The roles of educator, client advocate, case manager, and men's health nurse practitioner are discussed.

Educator

The goal of client education is to provide knowledge and skills for learning new behaviors or changes affecting health-related behaviors. The educator's goal is to improve or maintain the health status of men. When the nurse encounters men in the clinics, health departments, or their homes, a teaching opportunity exists. The myth about men not being receptive to health information is not substantiated. Glasser (1990) reported men were willing to use health departments to receive health care information and products. Survey findings indicated men used family planning services at a Midwestern county public health department. The authors reported that men not only accompanied their female partners in the family planning process and provided emotional support to their partners, but also took an active part in the family planning process. Also, other men received birth control products distributed by the department.

Client Advocate

The goal of client advocacy is to ensure that men's long-term health care needs are met. The goal for the advocacy role is to inform and support men in their health care decisions. The nurse needs to become knowledgeable about the health care options and to support the client in his decisions. For example, a male client who has had a myocardial infarction needs to be informed about his treatment options (i.e., diet, exercise, drugs, therapy, stress reduction, and surgical interventions). The nurse should help the man make his decisions in the most effective and cost-conscious manner.

> **NURSING TIP**
>
> *Use therapeutic communication skill of empathy and respect when gathering information from men about their health.*

Case Manager

Being a case manager of men's health means more than just coordinating client services. The role involves problem solving and managing men's health care services in a supportive, effective, and efficient manner. The American Nurses Association (1988) described the nursing care manager's role as "a health care delivery process whose goals are to provide quality health care, decrease fragmentation, enhance the client's quality of life, and contain cost." The

actual role of the case manager is structured to the client's needs (see Chapter 19).

Men's Health Nurse Practitioner

Typically, men choose not to communicate their health concerns to physicians. In the office and clinics, pleasantries and shallow comments are exchanged, with critical health care concerns avoided. Physicians rarely give their male clients adequate time for reflective discussion and thoughtful communications about their health needs. Further, physicians focus on pathologic findings and "cure" treatments. Prevention and health promotion activities are not high priorities.

A **men's health nurse practitioner (MHNP)** would alleviate some of these concerns. This advance practice role would deliver comprehensive men's health care. The provider would assess and manage minor health problems, as well as manage acute and chronic conditions. Conducting histories and physical examinations, ordering and interpreting diagnostic studies, prescribing medications and treatments, providing health maintenance care, promoting positive health behaviors and self-care, and collaborating with physicians and other health professionals are some of the MHNP's functions and roles. Effective interpersonal skills and empathetic listening are important communication skills the nurse practitioner would use to facilitate men discussing their health concerns. The nurse in community health can work with the MHNP by assessing the needs of the population served by the MHNP and developing health promotion and disease prevention programs and group activities to increase the health status of men in the community.

clinical application

Using the concepts in this chapter, analyze the following case. Focus on the issues of how men define health, developmental patterns, the health practices of men, and a nursing care plan.

John, a 29-year-old Caucasian man with a wife and three children, was employed as a sales representative in a small, rural community. John's health was excellent except for injuries sustained in a car accident several years ago that required three blood transfusions. After the accident, John returned to work, thinking he was fully recovered. His business success continued, and he was well respected by employers, coworkers, and community leaders.

Years after the accident, John became ill with pneumonia requiring hospitalization. While he was hospitalized, a blood test discovered HIV. A series of devastating events followed. John and his family decided to keep his condition confidential so he could live the rest of his life as normally as possible.

When John returned to work from the hospital, his coworkers seemed distant and they avoided him. He began to receive threatening telephone calls telling him to leave town, and his car was spray-painted with derogatory words. Clearly, there had been a breach of confidentiality. John later discovered his hospital file was marked "AIDS" in large red letters. Further, he learned nurses refused to care for him while he was hospitalized and he was the dinner conversation focus throughout the hospital.

John's circumstances worsened, and he felt isolated and rejected. He eventually was fired from work, thereby losing health insurance for himself and his family. His wife divorced him. All his accumulated wealth was depleted. He could not pay his hospital bills; his financial state was compounded by filing for bankruptcy. John was now homeless. His symptoms gradually progressed. He had a fever, tachypnea, lymphadenopathy, night sweats, and diarrhea. A friend suggested he visit the clinic. Further, John is reluctant to speak about his disease. He is extremely fatigued and whispers softly. He refuses any government services; however, you are able to convince him to enter the homeless shelter across the street for the night. You ask him to return to the clinic in the morning.

Imagine you are the nurse in the public health clinic.

A. What information do you want to collect?
B. What nursing diagnoses are relevant based on the collected data?
C. What short-term goals are appropriate for the first clinic visit?
D. What long-term goal do you want to plan with John?
E. What social and health agencies would you consult in planning for John's care?
F. What outcome criteria should you use to evaluate the effectiveness of your plans and interventions?

Answers are in the back of the book.

KEY POINTS

- Men are physiologically the more vulnerable gender, demonstrated by shorter lifespans and a higher infant mortality.
- Men's psychosocial and moral development continues through young and middle adulthood.
- Life expectancy of men in the United States is one of the lowest in developed countries.
- Men engage in more risk-taking behaviors, such as physical challenges and illegal behaviors, than do women.
- The most significant death rate differences between men and women are AIDS, suicides, homicides, and accidents.

- Men tend to avoid diagnosis and treatment of illnesses that may result in serious health problems.
- Legislation has been enacted that is helpful to men in the areas of elder care, worker's compensation, Americans with disabilities, family and medical leaves, and veterans.
- The men's health nurse practitioner is an advance practice role focusing on the comprehensive health needs of men.

critical thinking activities

1. Interview six men ranging in age from 21 to 70 years and ask them to list what they believe are health risk factors for them, what activities they regularly engage in that promote health, and what changes they believe they should make to promote their own health and reduce any existing risk factors.
2. Using the information gathered in activity 1, design a plan for health promotion for each man who is interviewed, using the man's lifestyle, occupation, interest in social and recreational activities, income level, health risks, limitations in activities, and medical conditions. Review this plan with the man and determine how effectively the plan fits his perception of what he might do to ensure a healthier state.
3. Using the information gathered from the interviews and from the design of the health plan, determine at which developmental level the man is functioning. Is the level consistent with the age of the man?
4. Because morbidity and mortality data indicate that women live longer than men in the United States, Interview 10 women ranging in age from 21 to 70 years and compare their health status, health risks, and participation in health-promoting behaviors with those of the 10 men who were interviewed to see what differences exist that might explain this differing life expectancy.
5. Using the leading causes of death described in this chapter that affect men, design a diet for men from two different cultural groups in the United States that would promote health and reduce the risks from the leading causes of death among men.
6. Because violence, suicide, and accidents are major causes of mortality for men in the United States, look at your community and describe the leading risk factors for violence, suicide, and accidents. Do each category separately. Use statistical data to document incidence. What agencies exist in the community to help prevent death or disability from these three risk factors?

Bibliography

Albertsen PC, et al: Competing risk analysis of men aged 55 to 74 years at diagnosis managed conservatively for clinical localized prostate cancer, *JAMA* 280:975, 1988.

American Nurses Association: *Nursing care management*, Kansas City, Mo, 1988, American Nurses Association.

Bachman JG et al: Racial/ethnic differences in smoking, drinking, and illicit drug use among American high school seniors, *Am J Pub Health* 81(3):372, 1991.

Berenson GS, Sathanur R: Association between multiple cardiovascular risk factors and atherosclerosis in children and young adults, *N Engl J Med* 338(23):1650, 1998.

Bird C, Fremont A: Gender, time use, and health, *J Health Soc Behav* 32:114, 1991.

Canetto SS: Gender issues in the treatment of suicidal individual, *Death Studies* 18:513, 1994.

EDK Associates: *Men beating women: ending domestic violence: a qualitative and quantitive study of public attitudes on violence against women*, New York, 1993, Author.

Continued

Bibliography—cont'd

Erikson E: *Identity: youth and crisis,* New York, 1968, WW Norton.

Gaziano JM: When should heart disease prevention begin? *N Engl J Med* 338:(23)1690, 1998.

Glasser M: Males use of public health departments' family planning services, *Am J Pub Health* 80:611, 1990.

Hammond W, Yung B: Psychology's role in public health response to assaultive violence among young African-American men, *Am Psychologist* 48:142, 1993.

Hunink GM et al: The recent declines in mortality from coronary heart disease, 1980-1990: the effect of secular trends in risk factors and treatment, *JAMA* 277(7):535, 1997.

Jung CG: *Modern man in search of a soul,* New York, 1933, Harcourt Brace Jovanovich.

Karon J et al: Prevalence of HIV infections in the united states, 1984 to 1992, *JAMA* 276:126, 1996.

Kohlberg L: *Psychology of moral development: the nature and validity of moral stages,* San Francisco, 1984, Harper.

Landis S: Cancer statistics, 1998, *CA Cancer J Clin* 48:6, 1998.

Maguire K, Pastore A: *Sourcebook of criminal justice statistics, 1993,* Washington, DC, 1994, US Department of Justice, Bureau of Justice Statistics.

Marciniak TA et al: Improving the quality of care for medicare patients with acute myocardial infarction: results from the cooperative cardiovascular project, *JAMA* 279(17):1351, 1998.

National Council on Alcoholism and Drug Dependence: *Alcoholism in the family,* Hyattsville, Md, 1991, NCHS.

Pobursky J: Prostrate cancer: detection and treatment options, *Today's OR Nurse* 17:5, 1995.

Rafuse J: Men's attitudes about seeking healthcare may put them at risk, conference told, *J Can Med Assoc* 149:329, 1993.

Report of final mortality statistics, 1995, *Monthly Vital Statistics Rep* 45, 2;(Suppl), 1997.

Rivara F et al: Alcohol and illicit drug abuse and the risk of violent death in the home, *JAMA* 278:569, 1997.

Rosenberg P, Biggar R: Trends in HIV incidence among young adults in the united states, *JAMA* 279:1894, 1998.

Rosenberg M, Mercy J: Assaultive violence. In Rosenberg M, Mercy J, editors: *Violence in America: a public health approach,* New York, 1991, Oxford University Press.

Saltonstall R: Healthy bodies, social bodies: men's and women's concepts and practices of health in everyday life, *Soc Sci Med* 36:7, 1993.

Statistical yearbook, 1995, New York, 1997, United Nations.

Toscano G, Windau J: *Fatal work injuries: results from 1992 national census,* Report 870, Washington, DC, 1994, US Department of Labor, Bureau of Labor Statistics.

Treating your enlarged prostate. AHCPR Pub No 94-0583, Rockville, Md, 1994, Public Health Service, Agency for Health Care Policy and Research.

US Congress, Office of Technology Assessment: *International health statistics: what the numbers mean for the United States: background paper,* Pub No OTA-BP-H-116, Washington, DC, 1993, US Government Printing Office.

USDHHS: *Healthy people 2000: national health promotion and disease prevention objectives,* Washington, DC, 1991, USDHHS, Public Health Service.

US Department of Labor: *Work injuries and illnesses by selected characteristics,* Pub No USDL-94-213, Washington, DC, 1994, Bureau of Labor Statistics.

Walker R: Modeling and guided practice as components within a comprehensive testicular self-examination educational program for high school males, *J Health Educ* 24:162, 1993.

Windau J, Toscano G: *Workplace homicides in 1992,* Report 870, Washington DC, 1994, US Department of Labor, Bureau of Labor Statistics.

Elder Health

KATHLEEN FLETCHER & CYNTHIA J. WESTLEY

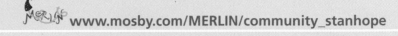

OBJECTIVES

After reading this chapter, the student should be able to do the following:

- Describe the changing demography of elders in the United States
- Define terms commonly used to refer to elders
- Discuss various biological, psychosocial, and developmental theories of aging
- Identify the multidimensional influences on aging and how these affect the health status of an elder

- Detail the components of a comprehensive health assessment of an elder
- List chronic health problems often experienced by elders
- Describe several community-based models for gerontology nursing practice
- Examine role opportunities in gerontological nursing for nurses in community health

KEY TERMS

advance directives	durable power of	gerontology	neglect
ageism	attorney	gerontological nursing	Patient Self-Determina-
aging	ego-integrity versus	instrumental activities of	tion Act
basic activities of daily	despair	daily living	respite care
living	elder abuse	life review	three Ds
chronic illness	five Is	living will	wellness
	geriatrics	long-term care	*See Glossary for definitions*

CHAPTER OUTLINE

The authors would like to acknowledge the contribution of Delois Skipwith and Patricia Birchfield to this chapter in previous editions.

The growth of the population ages 65 and older in the United States has steadily increased since the turn of the century. In 1900 approximately 4% of the population was over age 65; today elders account for nearly 13% of the U.S. population. In the year 2030 the percentage of individuals over age 65 is projected to be about 25%. The effect this demographic shift has on nursing practice in all settings is considerable. Estimates are that two thirds of a nurse's career today is spent working with elders (Simmons et al, 1998). Since most health care for elders is delivered outside of the acute care setting, nurses in community health in particular have been providing nursing care to an increased proportion of elders, which calls for specialized knowledge, skills, and abilities in gerontology.

This chapter begins by describing the demographic profile of elders living in the United States and giving some introductory terminology. The multidimensional influences of aging and disease are then presented, followed by a detailed description of the gerontological assessment skills needed by the nurse. The chapter concludes with a discussion of role opportunities for practicing gerontology in the community.

DEMOGRAPHICS

An individual born in 1900 could expect to live to be about 47 years of age. A newborn in 1996 could expect to live to be about 76 years of age. The older population numbered 34 million in 1996, about one in every eight Americans (AARP, 1996). The oldest old (those over age 85) are the fastest growing subgroup of elders. The longer an individual lives, the more likely that person will live even longer. Persons reaching age 65 have an average life expectancy of an additional 18 years. Future growth projections reveal that by the year 2030, when the baby boom generation reaches age 65, there will be about 70 million elders. That number represents more than twice the number of elders in society today.

A closer look at the demographics of elders today reveals a sex ratio of 145 women for every 100 men. Women outlive men by about 7 years, an advantage that is suspected to be biological. Minority populations today represent about 15% of all elders, with projections that the minority composition will double by the year 2030. Geographical location of elders does not reflect equal distribution across states; in fact, in 1996 half of all persons over age 65 lived in nine states (Box 29-1).

Most older adults live in a noninstitutional community setting, and a majority (67%) of them live with someone else. About 4% of the elderly live in a nursing home, a likelihood that increases significantly as one ages. For example, for persons in the 65 to 74 age group the percentage of individuals in a nursing home is 1%; it increases to 5% for persons ages 75 to 84, and to 15% for those elders over age 85. Elders as a whole are not an affluent group. For those reporting income to the IRS in 1996, 40% reported an annual income of less than $10,000. Chronological age is an arbitrary way to project health care needs since among elders there is a wide difference in the health state. The age of 65 has been used as a benchmark since 1935, when Franklin Delano Roosevelt used this age in eligibility criteria for Social Security. This seemed to be a reasonable criteria at the time since most individuals did not live long enough to collect Social Security. As life expectancy has grown, consideration has been given to increasing the age at which one might be eligible for Social Security. Although chronological age is limiting, some projections in the area of physical function and prevalence of chronic illness can be made. More than half of elders report having difficulty in carrying out **basic activities of daily living** (ADLs such as bathing, dressing, eating) and **instrumental activities of daily living** (IADLs such as preparing meals, taking medications, managing money), with a disproportionate share of individuals with disability in the higher age group (Fig. 29-1).

The last few years of an elder's life are often spent in declining physical functioning. A goal for nurses is to help

---

BOX 29-1 Geographic Distribution of Elders: Top 9 States

California	Ohio
Florida	Illinois
New York	Michigan
Texas	New Jersey
Pennsylvania	

Based on data from American Association of Retired Persons: *A profile of older Americans: 1995*, Washington, DC, 1995, the Association.

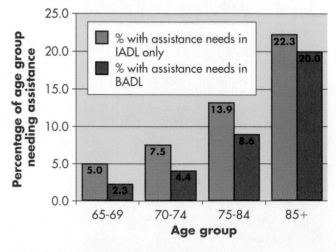

FIG. 29-1 Percentage needing assistance with activities of daily living by age: 1992. (From American Association of Retired Persons: *A profile of older Americans: 1995*, Washington, DC, 1996, the Association.)

elders maximize functional status and minimize functional decline. Health promotion and disease prevention strategies must be emphasized in the elderly.

WHAT DO YOU THINK? *Surveys documenting the functional status rating of an individual by the nurse, the caregiver, and the clients themselves often differs. What factors cause the different perspectives in measuring and noting functional status?*

DEFINITIONS

Aging, if defined purely from a physiological perspective, has been described as a process of deterioration of body systems. This definition is obviously inadequate to describe the multidimensional aging process in elders. **Aging** can be more appropriately defined as the sum total of all changes that occur in a person with the passing of time. Influences on how one ages come from several domains that include the physiological processes, as well as psychological, sociological, and spiritual processes. The physiological declines associated with aging have been easier to understand than aging as a process of growth and development.

Myths associated with aging have evolved over time. Some of the common myths involve the perception that all elders are infirm, senile, cannot adapt to change, and cannot learn new behaviors or skills. These myths are easily debunked by elders who run marathons, learn to use the internet, and are vibrant members of society. **Ageism** is the term used for prejudice about older people. Prejudice may be obvious or subtle. Ageism fosters a stereotype of elders that does not allow them to be viewed realistically.

Changing demographics have facilitated the recognition of the special needs for elders and the expansion of knowledge about the aging process. **Gerontology** is the specialized study of the processes of growing old. **Geriatrics** is the study of disease in old age. The American Nurses Association (ANA) encourages the use of the broader term *gerontological nursing* to refer to specialized nursing of elders that encompasses a health, as well as an illness, perspective. **Gerontological nursing** is the specialty of nursing concerned with assessment of the health and functional status of older adults, planning and implementing health care and services to meet the identified needs, and evaluating the effectiveness of such care (Lueckenotte, 1996).

THEORIES OF AGING

There is no one definition of aging; however, circadian rhythms and metabolic clocks suggest that metabolic age is a more accurate measure of status than chronological age. Aging begins with conception and occurs continuously over time. Lack of a clear definition of aging leads to many theories that attempt to explain a variety of influences on what we know as a complex process. Although it is inevitable that all persons will age, each individual organism ages at different rates.

Hayflick (1994) noted that "Aging is not merely the passage of time. It is the obvious biological events that occur over a span of time. There is no perfect definition of aging, but, as with love and beauty, most of us know it when we experience it or see it." No one theory or definition can explain the process of aging. Thus, biological, psychosocial, and developmental theories of aging have been developed.

Biological Theories

These theories have a central theme of change. They are explained on molecular, cellular and systemic levels. Genetics effects occur at all levels. Great strides are being made in understanding changes in aging; however, many questions remain unanswered. An individual theory may not totally answer the questions of aging but may attempt to explain the forces within the body that affect the aging process. Table 29-1 summarizes biological theories of aging.

Other biological influences such as environment and nutrition need consideration as well. The daily ingestion of many substances can produce unhealthy changes. These include smoke and other air pollutants, mercury, lead, arsenic, and pesticides. What is eaten also can have a significant influence on aging. Too many, too few, or too poor in quality nutrients can negatively influence aging. A lot of notice has been given to the influence of nutritional supplements on the aging process. It is important for nurses to keep an open mind to clients' desire for information. It is important that information is grounded in objective research and that clients are educated to be careful consumers.

Psychosocial Theories

Psychologists study personality, development, heredity, environmental influences, intelligence, memory, and psychogenic disorders. Sociologists study attitudes, family structures, economic influences, cultural differences, and political influences. In the study of aging they come together to address the effect of behavior of the elderly on aging.

Disengagement theory (Cuming and Henry, 1961) states that society and individuals disengage in mutual withdrawal, allowing the individual to become more self-focused and balanced. This is contrasted to the activity theory. Activity theory states that it is important to maintain regular roles and activities that are both social and solitary and to develop new roles to substitute for lost roles. Most normal elders do make choices, influenced by past experiences, to maintain a high level of activity.

Continuity theory focuses on the relationship between continued, consistent activity; coping abilities; and life satisfaction. Past experiences, decisions, and behaviors determine the predisposition to make present and future choices. Four patterns of personality and coping have been identified that are developed in early adulthood and con-

TABLE 29-1 Summary of Biological Theories of Aging

THEORY	DYNAMICS	RETARDANTS
STOCHASTIC THEORIES		
Error	Faulty synthesis of DNA and/or RNA	
Somatic	Alteration in RNA/DNA; protein or enzyme synthesis causes defective structure of function	
Transcription	Failure of transcription or translation between cells; malfunctions of RNA or related enzymes	
Free radical	Oxidation of fats, proteins, carbohydrates, and elements creates free electrons that attach to other molecules, altering cellular function	Improve environmental monitoring; decrease intake of free radical–stimulating foods; increase vitamin A and C intake (mercaptans; increase vitamin E; use of coenzyme Q10)
Cross-link	Lipids, proteins, carbohydrates, and nucleic acid react with chemicals or radiation to form bonds that cause an increase in cell rigidity and instability	
Clinker	Mix of somatic, free radical, and cross-link theories	
Wear and tear	Repeated injury or overuse of cells, tissue, organs, or systems	
NONSTOCHASTIC THEORIES		
Programmed	Biological clock triggers specific cell behavior at specific time	Hypothermia and diet can delay cell division but not number of divisions
Run-out-of-program	Organism capable of specific number of cell divisions and specific life span	
Neuroendocrine	Control mechanism (pituitary and hypothalamus) regulate interplay between various organs and tissues; efficiency of signals between mechanism is altered or lost	Treatment with potent hormones such as DHEA (dehydroepiandrosterone) and RU486
Immunological/autoimmune	Alteration of B and T cells leads to loss of capacity for self-regulation; normal or age-related cells recognized as foreign matter; system reacts by forming antibodies to destroy these cells	Immunoengineering, selective alteration, and replacement or rejuvenation of immune system

From Ebersole P, Hess P: *Toward health aging: human needs and nursing response*, ed 5, St Louis, 1998, Mosby.

tinue into later life as an individual adapts to life changes (Havighurst et al, 1969):

- Integrated personalities: mature and happy, with varied activity levels
- Defended personalities: distressed, trying to maintain middle-age values and norms
- Passive-dependent personalities: apathetic, with high dependency needs
- Unintegrated personalities: exhibiting mental illness

Humanistic theorists, such as Carl Rogers and Abraham Maslow, give a holistic view of development that tries to account for different human experiences. Humanistic theory views people as unique, self-determined, worthy of respect, and guided by a variety of basic human needs. Rogers believed that the process of becoming a fully functioning adult is aided throughout life by important relationships that provide unconditional positive regard (Berger, 1994). Maslow thought that an individual's behavior was motivated by universal needs that range from the most basic (food, sleep, safety) to the highest need for self-actualization (Maslow, 1968).

There is a complex interaction between culture, health status, socioeconomic status, and personality influences on aging. When performing an assessment the nurse must consider the client's current situation and social network, as well as past history of coping behavior, and must try to not make assumptions about the individual's chronological age.

Developmental Theories

Aging is a process, and all individuals must perform certain developmental tasks at different stages of life. Clark

TABLE 29-2 Physiological Aging Changes in Body Systems

	AGE-RELATED CHANGE	IMPLICATION FOR NURSING
Skin	Skin thins	Prone to skin breakdown and injury
	Atrophy of sweat glands	Increased risk of heat stroke
	Decrease in vascularity	Frequent pruritus
		Dry skin
Respiratory	Decreased elasticity of lung tissue	Reduced efficiency of ventilation
	Decreased respiratory muscle strength	Prone to alelectasis and infection
Cardiovascular	Decrease in baroreceptor sensitivity	Prone to orthostatic hypotension and falls
	Decrease in number of pacemaker cells	Increased prevalence of dysrhythmias
Gastrointestinal	Dental enamel thins	Peridontal disease common
	Gums recede	Prone to swallowing dysfunction
	Delay in esophageal emptying	Prone to constipation
	Decreased muscle tone	
	Altered peristalsis	
Genitourinary	Decreased number functioning nephrons	Modifications in drug dosing may be required
	Reduced bladder tone and capacity	Incontinence more common
	Prostate enlargement	May compromise urinary function
Neuromuscular	Decrease in muscle mass	Decrease in muscle strength
	Decrease in bone mass	Osteoporosis increases risk of fracture
	Loss of neurons/nerve fibers	Altered sensitivity to pain
		Delayed reaction time
Sensory	Decreased visual acuity, depth perception; adaptation to light changes	May pose safety issue
	Loss of auditory neurons	Hearing loss may cause limitation in activities
	Altered taste sensation	May change food preferences and intake
Immune	Decrease in T cell function	Increased incidence of infection
	Appearance of autoantibodies	Increased prevalence of autoimmune disorders

and Anderson (1967) characterized developmental tasks as an internal change process. They refer to adaptive tasks as the externalization of that internal process. Their theory demonstrates that while aging has positive and negative consequences, individuals continue to adjust and adapt by the following:

- Recognition of aging and definition of limitations
- Redefinition of physical and social life space
- Substitution of alternate sources of need satisfaction
- Reassessment of criteria for evaluation of the self
- Reintegration of values and life goals

Erik Erickson's (1959) stages of development are widely cited as a way of viewing development across the life span. His eighth stage, **ego-integrity versus despair,** describes the process of examining one's own life in relation to humanity and the world. A sense of failure can lead to despair, depression, and fear of death rather than acceptance and satisfaction.

The process of **life review** involves recalling past life experiences in attempt to believe that one's life has had meaning and to prepare for death without fear. Reminiscence can help maintain self-esteem and reaffirms a sense of identity (Burnside and Haight, 1994). Eagan (1996) developed a Reminiscing Game to help players share their life philosophy and early memories. Nurses can use tools like this and can employ active listening techniques to help clients validate their lives, resolve conflicts, and complete the tasks of aging.

Numerous predictable and unpredictable events occur in an individual's life. Even as we acknowledge the complexity and individuality of aging, we seek to compartmentalize and organize the process through theories. Theories can provide a useful framework as long as the nurse maintains an appreciation of the differences of the individual elders he or she encounters.

MULTIDIMENSIONAL INFLUENCES ON AGING

The elder experiences aging in many ways: physiologically, psychologically, sociologically, and spiritually. Physiologic changes occur in all body systems with the passing of time. There is considerable variation in how and when these processes occur between individuals, as well as the degree of aging within the various body systems in the same individual. Table 29-2 highlights physiological changes with the aging of body systems and the nursing implications of these changes. The effect of these physiological changes overall result in a diminished physiological reserve, decrease in homeostatic mechanisms, and a decline in immunological response.

No known intrinsic psychological changes occur with aging. The personality and developmental theories noted above imply certain expectations and behaviors assigned

Men

Women

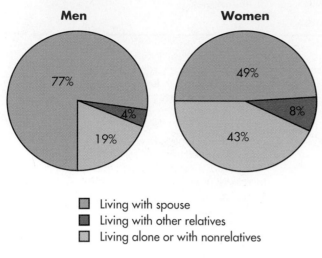

- ☐ Living with spouse
- ☐ Living with other relatives
- ☐ Living alone or with nonrelatives

FIG. 29-2 Living arrangements of persons 65+: 1995. (Data from US Census Bureau: *Statistical abstract of the United States,* ed 113, Washington, DC, 1993, US Government Printing Office.)

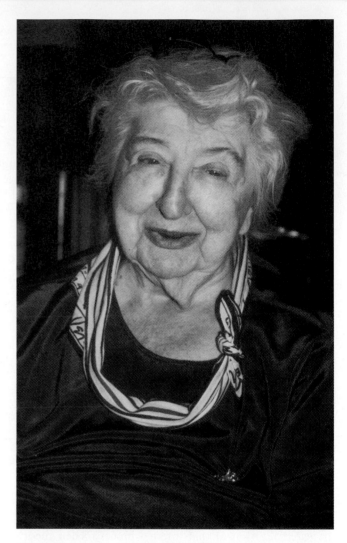

Although now in a wheelchair, this 88-year-old former operating room nurse still enjoys each day to its fullest.

to later life; however, these are not specific or discrete. The influences of the environment and culture on personal development and maturation are substantial and further limit the ability of the nurse to predict how an individual psychologically ages.

Some known and some disputed changes in brain function over time may influence cognition and behavior. Reaction speed and psychomotor response is somewhat slower, which can be related to the neurological changes with aging. This is demonstrated particularly during timed tests of performance where speed is an influencing variable. It has also been demonstrated in simulated tests of driving skills where speed of response, perception, and attention slow with age. Typically older individuals can learn and perform as well as younger individuals, though they may be slower and it may take them longer to accomplish a specific task.

Intellectual capacity does not decline with age as was previously thought. An age-associated memory impairment, benign senescent forgetfulness, involves very minor memory loss. This is not progressive and does not cause dysfunction in daily living. Reassurance is important for the older adult and families since anxiety often exacerbates the problem of mild memory impairment. Memory aides (e.g., mnemonics, signs, notes) may help the elder compensate for this type of impairment.

There are many external influences on mental health and aging, particularly those associated with loss and change. Adapting and coping responses of even the most resilient individuals will be challenged when successive losses and changes occur within a relatively short period.

The later years for many elders mark a period of changing social dynamics. Social networks provide the structure for social support. Demographics of marital status and living arrangements of elders reveal the magnitude of social change. Half of all older women in 1995 were widows.

There were five times as many widows (8.6 million) as widowers (1.7 million) in 1995 (AARP, 1996). Although women are more likely to live alone than men (Fig. 29-2), they frequently have more extensive social networks than men, who rely more dominantly on the spousal support.

Higher socioeconomic status, income, and education tend to be reflected in large and differing social networks (Ebersole and Hess, 1999). Families typically remain involved with aging parents, with estimates that over 5 million are involved in some type of parent care. Not all individuals do remain in their own home or in the home of another. A relatively small percentage (4%) of the 65+ population lived in nursing homes in 1995, with the likelihood of nursing home residency increasing with advanced age. As one ages, social role and status may change, and elders are more vulnerable to social isolation.

Though most of the multidimensional influences of aging are marked by decline and loss, some have suggested that there is an increased spiritual awareness and consciousness as one ages and that religion is a powerful cul-

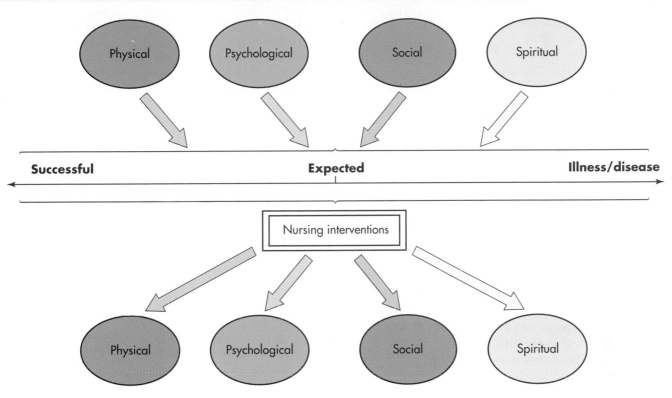

FIG. 29-3 Elder health comprehensive assessment model.

tural force in the lives of older clients. *Spirituality* refers to the need to transcend physical, psychological, and social identities to experience love, hope, and meaning in life. Religious affiliations and religious rituals are one aspect of spirituality that can include other activities and relationships. Caring for pets and plants or experiencing nature through a walk in the woods can also foster spiritual growth. Physical and functional impairments and fear of death may challenge one's spiritual integrity. Having a strong sense of spirituality enables individuals who are physically and functionally dependant on others to avoid despair by appreciating that they are still capable of giving and deserving of receiving love, respect, and dignity.

COMPONENTS OF A COMPREHENSIVE HEALTH ASSESSMENT

Assessing the health status of the elder poses challenges because of the wide variability of health in elders. It is important to look at the many dimensions of health on a continuum, as shown by the elder health comprehensive assessment model in Figure 29-3.

If one were to look at physiological, psychological, sociological, and spiritual domains, the elder may be at various points on this continuum. For example, an individual may demonstrate successful psychological aging through adaptating and coping while experiencing a physiologically terminal disease or significant functional impairments. The nurse intervenes appropriately in each of these domains to help the elder age successfully in each of these domains.

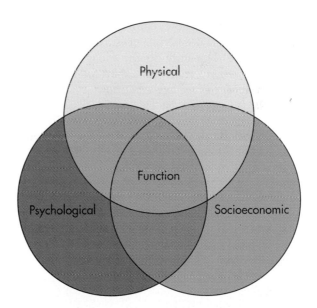

FIG. 29-4 Kane's conceptualization of central function. (From Kane RL, Ouslander JG, Abrass IB: *Essentials of clinical geriatrics*, ed 3, New York, 1994, McGraw-Hill.)

Effective care of elders by the nurse requires an accurate assessment of their health status. The goal of this care is to optimize health status and function and to minimize health decline and functional deterioration. Central to the comprehensive assessment of an elder is a functional assessment (Fig. 29-4).

Finding a good assessment instrument that reflects all of these domains and that is reasonable in terms of length is important. The Multidimensional Functional Assessment of the Older American Resources and Services (OARS) organization is a lengthy and comprehensive tool designed to evaluate most of the domains mentioned above. The tool is designed to evaluate ability, disability, and the capacity level at which the elder is able to function. Five dimensions are considered for assessment: social resources, economic resources, physical health, mental health, and activities of daily living. Each component uses a quantitative rating scale. At the conclusion of the assessment a cumulative impairment score (CIS) is established. Once problems are assessed through a multidimensional process, the nurse uses the nursing process to diagnose and intervene (see Chapter 15).

CHRONIC HEALTH CONCERNS OF ELDERS IN THE COMMUNITY

Chronic illnesses occur over a long period with occasional acute exacerbations and remissions. They can affect multiple systems and be expensive and discouraging. The prevalence of chronic disease rises with lengthening of life span and highly technical medical care. Until the late 1930s illnesses were generally caused by bacteria or parasites. With antibiotics, immunizations, and public health measures these diseases have decreased in western nations with other conditions becoming more common health problems. Table 29-3 shows the prevalence of chronic conditions for men and women. Not only do chronic conditions cause disability and activity restriction, they often require frequent hospitalizations for exacerbations.

TABLE 29-3 Rank Order Prevalence of Chronic Conditions by Gender per 1000 People Ages 65 and Older (1990)

CONDITION	RATE
MEN	
Hearing impairment	830
Arthritis	750
Heart disease	680
Hypertension	589
Vision impairment	382
Orthopedic impairment	273
WOMEN	
Arthritis	1100
Hypertension	853
Hearing impairment	564
Vision impairment	546
Heart disease	534
Orthopedic impairment	501

From US Census Bureau: *Statistical abstract of the United States,* ed 113, Washington, DC, 1993, US Government Printing Office.

Health care in general is oriented toward acute illness. In **chronic illness,** cure is not expected, so nursing activities need to be more holistic, addressing function, wellness, and psychosocial issues. With chronic illness the focus is on healing (a unique process resulting in a shift in the body/mind/spirit system) rather than curing (elimination of the signs and symptoms of disease). Eliopoulos (1997) lists the following goals for chronic care:
- Maintain or improve self-care capacity
- Manage the disease effectively
- Boost the body's healing abilities
- Prevent complications
- Delay deterioration and decline
- Achieve highest possible quality of life
- Die with comfort, peace, and dignity

The trajectory model of chronic illness (Corbin and Cherry, 1997) traces a course of illness through phases upward, downward, or plateaued.

HOW TO *Evaluate the Phases of Chronic Illness Using the Trajectory Model*

The chronic illness may include the following:
- *A pretrajectory phase, noting which factors put an individual at risk*
- *A trajectory phase where symptoms become noticeable*
- *Stable and/or unstable phases as the symptoms vary from controlled to reactivated*
- *Acute and/or phases where symptoms or the development of the illness became more serious or life threatening*
- *A comeback phase of gradual return to an acceptable level of function*
- *A downward course of decline, deterioration, and an inability to control symptoms, to dying or a shutting down of body processes*

Attention is paid to the client's self-concept and self-esteem, as well as the resources that are needed to manage the disease outside the medical system. Goals for care are structured to help clients adjust their day-to-day choices to maintain the highest level of functional ability possible within the limits of their conditions. The motivation to make lifestyle choices necessary to cope with chronic illness stems from the fear of death; disability; pain; and negative effects on work, family, or activity. Redeker (1988) developed the Health Belief Model to explain how individuals decide whether a choice is worth taking action. According to this model, knowledge of a medical condition does not affect compliance as much as personal thoughts and feelings and a therapeutic alliance with health care providers.

Tierney et al (1994) outlines chronic conditions that can adversely affect the aging experience. These include intellectual impairment, immobility, instability, incontinence, and iatrogenic drug reactions, called the **five Is,** and

HOW TO *Assess Environmental Factors Affecting Risks of Falling in the Home*

Environmental Area or Factor	Objective and Recommendation
All areas: lighting	Absence of glare and shadows; accessible switches at room entrance; night light in bedroom, hall, bathroom
Floors	Nonskid backing for throw rugs; carpet edges tacked down; carpets with shallow pile; nonskid wax on floors; cords out of the walking path; small objects (e.g., clothes, shoes) off floor
Stairs	Lighting sufficient, with switches at top and bottom of stairs; securely fastened bilateral handrails that stand out from wall; top and bottom steps marked with bright, contrasting tape; stair rises of no more than 6 inches; steps in good repair; no objects stored on steps
Kitchen	Items stored so that reaching up and bending over are not necessary; secure step stool available if climbing is necessary; firm, nonmovable table
Bathroom	Grab bars for tub, shower, toilet; nonskid decals or rubber mat in tub or shower; shower chair with handheld shower; nonskid rugs; raised toilet seat; door locks removed to ensure access in an emergency
Yard and entrances	Repair of cracks in pavement, holes in lawn; removal of rocks, tools, other tripping hazards; well-lit walkways, free of ice and wet leaves; stairs and steps as above
Institutions	All the above; bed at proper height (not too high or low); spills on floor cleaned up promptly; appropriate use of walking aids and wheelchairs
Footwear	Shoes with firm, nonskid soles; low heels (unless person is accustomed to high heels); avoidance of walking in stocking feet or loose slippers

From Tinetti ME, Speechley M: Prevention of falls among the elderly, *N Engl J Med* 320:1055, 1989.

the **three Ds** of intellectual impairment: dementia (progressive intellectual impairment), depression (mood disorder), and delirium (acute confusion).

Immobility is most often caused by degenerative joint disease and results in pain, stiffness, loss of balance, and psychological problems. Fear of falling is a major cause of immobility. This is related to instability, which results in falls in 30% of elders each year.

Urinary incontinence often contributes to institutional care and social isolation. For that reason it is difficult to estimate the numbers of individuals and cost of incontinence. It is important to address continence routinely in the assessment process, identify the type of incontinence, and intervene appropriately.

Iatrogenic drug reactions result from changes in the older individual's absorption, metabolism, and excretion process that lead to altered responses to drugs. Many elderly take numerous medicines, increasing the chance of drug reactions.

WHAT DO YOU THINK? *The average older adult in the community has eleven different prescriptions filled each year. What are some of the hazards of this situation?*

One often overlooked concern of elders is that of abuse. **Elder abuse** encompasses physical, psychological, financial, and social abuse or violation of an individual's rights (McKenna, 1997). Abuse consists of the following:
• The willful infliction of physical pain or injury
• Debilitating mental anguish and fear

• Theft or mismanagement of money or resources, and/or
• Unreasonable confinement or the depriving of services

Neglect refers to a lack of services that are necessary for the physical and mental health of an individual by the individual or a caregiver. Elderly persons can make independent choices with which others may disagree. Their right to self-determination can be taken from them if they are declared incompetent. Exploitation is the illegal or improper use of a person or their resources for another's profit or advantage. During the assessment process, nurses need to be aware of conflicts between injuries and explanation of cause, dependency issues between client and caregiver, and substance abuse by the caregiver. Nearly all 50 states have enacted mandatory reporting laws and have instituted protective service programs. The local social services agency or area agency on aging can help with information on reporting requirements.

The **Patient Self-Determination Act** of 1991 requires those providers receiving Medicare and Medicaid funds to give clients written information regarding their legal options for treatment choices if they become incapacitated. A routine discussion of advance medical directives can help ease the difficult discussions faced by health care professionals, family, and clients. The nurse can assist an individual to complete a values history instrument. These instruments ask questions about specific wishes regarding different medical situations. This clarifying process then leads to completion of **advance directives** to document these preferences in writing. There are two parts to the advance directives. The **living will** allows the client to express wishes regarding the use of medical treatments in the event of a terminal illness. A **durable power of attorney** is the legal way for the client to designate someone else to make health care decisions when he or she is unable to do so. A Do Not Resuscitate order (DNR) is a specific order from a physician not to use cardiopulmonary resuscitation. State laws vary widely regarding the implementing of these tools, so it is important to consult a knowledgeable source of information. It is also important to involve the family, and especially the designated decision maker or agent, in these discussions so that everyone is clear about the client's choices.

> **DID YOU KNOW?** *OBRA spells out the rights of the elderly as the right to the following:*
> - *Individualized care*
> - *Be free from discrimination*
> - *Privacy*
> - *Freedom from neglect and abuse*
> - *Control one's own funds*
> - *Sue*
> - *Freedom from physical and chemical restraint*
> - *Involvement in decision making*
> - *Vote*
> - *Have access to community services*
> - *Raise grievances*
> - *Obtain a will*
> - *Enter into contracts*
> - *Practice the religion of one's choice*
> - *Dispose of one's own personal property*

Family Caregiving

Eighty-five percent of all elderly live in homes alone, with spouses, or other family or friends. Female spouses represent the largest group of family caregivers of the. *Stress, strain, burden,* and *burnout* are words that are used to reflect the negative effects of family caregiving. Issues involve the work itself, past and present relationships, effect on others, and the caregivers' lifestyle and well-being. It is estimated that at least 5 million adults are providing direct care to an elderly relative at any given time, with another 44 to 45 million assuming some type of responsibility for an elder relative. For many families the caregiving experience is a positive, rewarding, and fulfilling one. Nursing intervention can facilitate good health for older persons and their caregivers, and contribute to meaningful family relationships during this period. Eliopoulos (1997) uses the acronym "TLC" to represent these interventions:

- T = training in care techniques, safe medication use, recognition of abnormalities, available resources
- L = leaving the care situation periodically to obtain respite and relaxation and maintain their normal living needs
- C = care for themselves (the caregiver) through adequate sleep, rest, exercise, nutrition, socialization, solitude, support, financial aid, and health management

> **NURSING TIP**
>
> *Older adults are at increased risk for infection. Prevention in the community includes encouraging routine hand-washing and adapting universal precautions specifically to the practice setting.*

COMMUNITY-BASED MODELS FOR GERONTOLOGICAL NURSING

Nursing Roles

Communities are where people live, work, and socialize. Often older people can remain in the setting of their choice by modifying the environment and providing of support services. Community health settings include public health departments, nurse-managed health centers, ambulatory care clinics, and home health agencies. The cultural values of the community shape lifestyle and influence health status. Legislation that affects the health care system is a product of that culture. Dramatic changes have occurred since the Social Security Act was enacted in 1935 (Table 29-4). The demographic changes in this country mean that there is an ever-growing population of older adults. Most of these individuals wish to stay in their own homes and communities and will be frequent consumers of health and other services. Nurses are involved in direct care, providing self-care information, supervision of paraprofessionals, or collaborating with other disciplines to provide the most appropriate, high-quality, cost-effective care at the most appropriate level and location. Service opportunities are located on a continuum detailed in Box 29-2.

A knowledge of community resources is a fundamental part of caring for the elderly in any community. The nurse assesses the need for and helps develop the resources. Most communities have an information and referral system, as well as a public directory of services available. Every community has an area agency on aging that coordinates planning and delivery of needed services and can be a good resource for the nurse.

Community Care Settings

Senior centers

Senior centers were developed in the early 1940s to provide social and recreational activities. Now many centers are multipurpose, offering recreation, education, counseling, therapies, hot meals, and case management, as well as health screening and education. Some even offer primary care services. Nurses have a unique opportunity to provide services to a group of elderly who wish to remain independent in the community.

Adult day health

Adult day health is for individuals whose mental and/or physical function requires them to need more health care and supervision. It serves as more of a medical model than the senior center and often individuals return home to their caregivers at night. Some settings offer **respite care**

TABLE 29-4 Health Care–Related Political Events Relevant to Elder Health

Date	Event	Impact
1935	Social Security Act signed	Increases financial security
1948	Hospital Construction and Facilities Act (Hill-Burton)	Provides funds for construction of long-term care facilities
1950	First National Conference on Aging in Washington, DC	Beginning of federal policy and national attention to problems of aged
1963	Kennedy formed President's Council on Aging; designated May as Older American's Month	
1965	Older American's Act	Mandates comprehensive services by states
	Social Security Act Amendments	
	Medicare (Title XVIII)	National medical insurance for all older adults
	Medicaid (Title XIX)	Federal/state program to increase medical services for poor and disabled; more nursing homes and federal regulations
	Title XX	In-home services for indigent through Social Services
1972	Medicare reform	Professional Standards Review Organizations to review hospital services for overuse
		Intermediate care facilities reimbursed
		New regulations
1973	Older Americans Act	Establishes area agencies on aging to coordinate amendment's services
		Increases public transportation to rural areas, concentrating on elderly and disabled
		Establishes National Clearing House for Aging
1976	Title V of Older Americans Act	Funds appropriated for multipurpose Senior Centers
1981	Omnibus Reconciliation Act (OBRA)	Provides funds for community, preventive programs leading to growth in home health services
1982	Tax Equity and Fiscal Responsibility (TEFRA)	Introduces idea of prospective payment for Medicare instead of fee-for-service
1983	Diagnostic Related Groups (DRGs)	Hospital prospective payment plan to control Medicare costs
1987	New OBRA laws	Increases standards of care in nursing homes
		Established ombudsman programs
1990	Americans with Disabilities Act	Prohibits discrimination against disabled individuals
1991	Patient Self Determination Act	Increases importance of advance directives
1996	Health Insurance Portability and Accountability Act	Safeguards health coverage for people who change jobs
		Establishes medical savings accounts for medical and long- term expenses
1997	Balanced Budget Act	Establishes Medicare +Choice program to expand plan choices through managed care companies
		Changes reimbursement for long- term care and home health to prospective payment
		Increases preventive services offered

for short-term overnight relief for caregivers. This provides caregivers the opportunity to work or have personal time during the day. Oftentimes support groups for caregivers are offered by nurses.

Home health

Home health can be provided by working in multidisciplinary teams. Nurses provide individual and environmental assessments, direct skilled care and treatment, and short term guidance and instruction. Nurses often function independently in the home and must rely on their own resources and knowledge to improvise and adapt care to meet the client's unique physical and social circumstances. They work closely with the family and other caregivers to provide necessary communication and continuity of care.

Hospice

Hospice represents a philosophy of caring for and supporting life to its fullest until death occurs. The hospice team encourages the client and family to jointly make decisions to meet physical, emotional, spiritual, and comfort needs.

Assisted living

Assisted living covers a wide variety of choices from a single shared room to opulent independent living accommodations in a full-service, life care community. The differences are related to the contract signed for the type and extent of the amenities provided. The role of the nurse varies depending on the philosophy and leadership of the management of the facility. The nurse generally provides

BOX 29-2 Continuum of Care for Elderly

IN-HOME

Home safety assessment and equipment
Meals on Wheels
Homemaker and chore services
Telephone reassurance/friendly visitor
Personal emergency response system
Pharmacies/grocers that deliver
Area Agency of Aging services
State health, legal, social service departments
Adult protective services—city social services
Home health aide
Home health nurses and therapists
Hospice

COMMUNITY-BASED

Specialized transportation for disabled
Multipurpose senior centers
Health screenings/health fairs
Congregate meal sites
Community mental health clubhouses
Adult day health care
Respite care
Community nursing clinics
Comprehensive geriatric medical service
Medicare and Medicaid HMOs
Caregiver or disease-focused support groups
Case/disease management
Health promotion/self-care classes

HOUSING

Elder Cottage Housing Opportunity (ECHO)
Home sharing
Accessory apartments
Foster home
Group home
Assisted living facility
Life care community
Retirement village
Intermediate care facility
Skilled nursing facility
Rehabilitation hospital
Subacute unit/hospital
Acute care hospital
State mental hospital

RESEARCH *Brief*

The Mobile Health Unit was implemented to increase access to nursing services, to improve and/or maintain functional status and health status, and to increase health promotion behaviors of rural elderly residents experiencing difficulty obtaining health care because of illness, transportation problems, or financial factors. For 222 project participants, 1773 encounters were completed, with a mean number of visits per individual of 7.9. Participants in the project demonstrated increased breast and cervical cancer screenings; increased immunization rates for influenza, pneumonia, and tetanus; and decreased use of the emergency room. This project represents an alternative model of health care delivery in a rural area with limited resources and health care providers.

Alexy BB, Elnitsky CL: Rural mobile health unit: outcomes, *Public Health Nurs* 15(1):3, 1998.

assessment and interventions, medication review, education, and advocacy.

Nursing homes

Nursing homes, or **long-term care** facilities as they are often called, house only 5% of the elderly population at a given time; however, 25% of those over 65 years old will spend some time in a nursing home. Nursing homes provide a safe environment, special diets and activities, routine personal care, and the treatment and management of health care needs for those needing rehabilitation, as well as those needing a permanent supportive residence. Nursing homes are moving more towards the prospective payment model of the hospital and will be based on the nursing assessment.

Creative models for nurses have been established in the various settings described. The Visiting Nurse Association of Springfield, Massachusetts uses the Geriatric Resource Nurse model (Francis, 1998). Originally developed in the acute care setting, the VNA tailored this model to home care. The VNA prepared nurses interested in geriatrics with the knowledge, skills, and abilities necessary to become resource nurses to the home care staff. The Research Brief describes a Mobile Health Unit for nursing services.

Senior nutrition sites have begun to expand services to include primary care. The Geriatric Assessment and Intervention Team (GAIT) Initiative is an example of a community-sponsored program that seeks and visits vulnerable elderly persons (JABA, 1998). The GAIT Initiative is an example of a community-sponsored program that seeks out and goes to vulnerable elderly. The team consists of a nurse practitioner, case manager, and geriatric social worker who use the rural nutrition site as a home base. Their goal is to improve access to appropriate health care with an emphasis on health promotion and disease prevention.

Nursing homes are increasingly contracting with physician/nurse practitioner teams who have gerontological expertise to provide primary care to the nursing home residents. Examples of effective models include Evercare (Ryan, 1999) and the Fallon Health Systems (Burl, 1998). The advanced practice gerontological nurse practitioner, in addition to providing primary care, also frequently educates the nursing staff on gerontological issues.

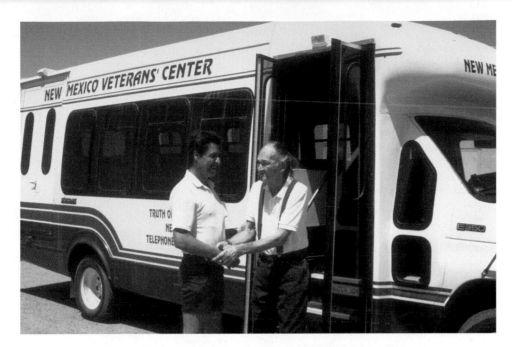

This elderly man lives in a residential center for veterans.

ROLE OPPORTUNITIES FOR NURSES: HEALTH PROMOTION, DISEASE PREVENTION, AND WELLNESS

Nurses in community health focus on the prevention of disease and the promotion and maintenance of health. To achieve these goals, nurses are involved in client and community education, counseling, advocacy, and care management. The overall goal is improving the individual's and the community's health through collaborative practice with other members of the health care team. Achieving this goal involves the nurse in all three levels of prevention. Examples of preventive activities for the elderly in the community include the following:

- Primary: preventing heatstroke, managing stress, reducing the risk of cancer through diet, offering free flu shots
- Secondary: screening for blood pressure, cholesterol, glaucoma, blood glucose
- Tertiary: teaching diabetics how to identify and prevent foot complications, or a support group for dialysis clients.

The nurse should be familiar with the guidelines for screening preventive services for individuals 65 years of age and older (see Appendix A.2) recommended by the U.S. Guide to Clinical Preventive Services.

Healthy People 2000 (USDHHS, 1991) offers direction through measures for reducing and preventing unnecessary disease, disability, and death across the life span. The goals are increasing the span of healthy life of Americans, reducing health disparity among Americans, and achieving access to preventive services for all Americans through health promotion protection, and preventive services. Box 29-3 summarizes the *Healthy People 2000* objectives for adults ages 65 and older. Health promotion activities involve behaviors that positively affect a person's health status. The Put Prevention into Practice program is designed to help health care professionals structure their preventive activities. Although many older adults enjoy good health, many live with chronic conditions and need support to maximize their strengths.

The term **wellness** was coined by Travis (1977) to help bring to mind the idea of health as holistic rather than merely the absence of disease or illness. It includes the physical, emotional, mental, and spiritual components of a person. With this approach in chronic illness it is possible for individuals to maintain their own individual optimal level of wellness along a continuum shown in Figure 29-5 (Ebersole and Hess, 1998). The traditional way of looking at health as either present or absent is less helpful for the elderly. More appropriate is the positive approach of addressing risk factors that affect the experience of chronic illness. Travis outlines five dimensions of wellness:

1. Self-responsibility: The core of wellness, encouraging self-help strategies, taking control of health and life choices, and partnering with health care providers rather than abdicating control.
2. Nutritional awareness: Learning about the selection and preparation of food and developing eating habits leading to a more balanced, nutritionally appropriate diet.
3. Physical fitness: Involving aerobic capacity, body structure, body composition, balance, muscle flexibility, and muscle strength.
4. Stress management: Developing new attitudes and ways to cope with events in life that seem beyond control and that cause negative physical and mental problems.

29-3 *Healthy People 2000* **Selected National Objectives for Adults Ages 65 and Older**

HEALTH PROMOTION
Reduce

- Suicide among white males
- Death by motor vehicle accidents (age 70+)
- Death from falls and fall-related injury, particularly age 85+
- Death from residential fires
- Hip fractures
- Number of persons who have difficulty performing two or more personal care activities so as to enhance independence
- Significant visual impairment
- Epidemic-related days of restricted activity

Increase

- Years of healthy life to at least 65 for African-Americans and Hispanics

RISK REDUCTION
Increase

- The percentage of individuals who regularly participate in light-to-moderate activity for at least 30 minutes a day
- Immunization levels for pneumococcal influenza among the chronically ill older population
- The percentage of older persons who receive, within appropriate intervals, screening and immunization services and at least one counseling service

SERVICES AND PROTECTION
Increase

- Percentage of recipients of home food services
- Percentage of older adults who have the opportunity to participate yearly in at least one organized health promotion program through senior centers, life care facilities, or community-based settings serving the older adult
- Percentage of states in the United States that have design standards for signs, signals, markings and lighting, and other roadway environmental improvements to enhance visual stimuli and protect the safety of older drivers and pedestrians
- The proportion of primary care providers who routinely review with their clients prescribed and over-the-counter medications each time a new medication is prescribed
- The usage of the oral care system
- The proportion who receive clinical breast examinations and mammograms
- The number of women age 70+ with uterine cervix who receive Pap tests

Extend

- Long-term institutional facilities, the requirement for oral examinations, and service provided to new admissions no later than 90 days after entering a facility.

From USDHHS: *Healthy people 2000*, Pub No (PHS) 91-50212, Washington, DC, 1991, US Government Printing Office.

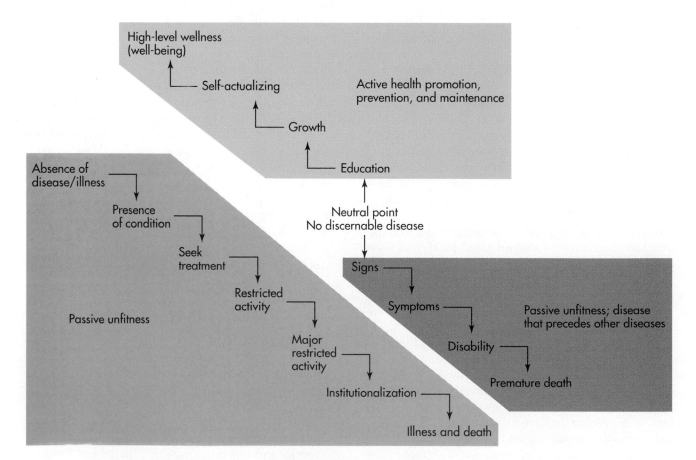

FIG. 29-5 Comparison of a wellness/health continuum with the traditional medical continuum. (From Ebersole P, Hess P: *Toward health aging: human needs and nursing response,* ed 5, St Louis, 1998, Mosby.)

5. Environmental sensitivity: Influencing one's personal room/home space; physical earth issues of conservation and pollution; and social components of government, economics, and culture.

While persons do slow down and are more susceptible to disease as aging occurs, it is the advances in prevention and wellness measures that delay the onset of debilitating disease and functional decline and expand the years of quality life. Nurses can provide health education and screening and other wellness programs for individuals and groups in all settings. Another important role for nurses is participating in research related to the outcomes of care and cost effectiveness of different health promotion programs.

The aging population is creating a major shift in the health care needs of the present and future. Controlling national health care expenditures is a major issue. New directions in the health care for older adults means significant changes in social, political, and economic policies and structures (Corbin and Cherry, 1997). Nurses are in a position to influence these changes. Since no one holds a crystal ball about where these changes will lead having knowledge, being involved, flexible, and creative will help. It is to nurses that older adults turn for advice and counseling about the confusing array of services and choices available. Nurses must be role models for positive attitudes toward and advocates for the unique needs of older adults in different community settings.

clinical application

Mrs. Eldridge, a 79-year-old widow, was reported by neighbors and the administrator of the senior high-rise where she lived to the nurse who visited residents of the high-rise. Mrs. Eldridge lives alone, and no one had been observed coming or going from her apartment recently. When Mrs. Eldridge has been seen by her neighbors, she appears self-neglected and does not appear to recognize her neighbors.

The nurse made a visit to Mrs. Eldridge's apartment and validated the unkempt appearance of both. Mrs. Eldridge answered the door and was pleasant but unkempt with an odor of stale urine. Even though Mrs. Eldridge was hesitant and unsure in her answers, the history revealed medical problems. A son and daughter-in-law lived in the next county and phoned at least once a week; their number was taped to the table by the phone. Several pill bottles were observed on the kitchen counter with the names of a local physician and pharmacist.

The nurse, while at Mrs. Eldridge's home, noted that both she and her clothes were dirty and that she moved without aids and appeared steady on her feet. The kitchen was littered with unwashed dishes and empty frozen-food boxes, which Mrs. Eldridge could not recall being bought or delivered. An open billfold with several bills was lying open on the kitchen counter, as well as an uncashed Social Security check.

What should the nurse do about the situation as she found it?

A. Call adult protective services and get an emergency order to put Mrs. Eldridge in a nursing home.
B. Call Mrs. Eldridge's son and see if his mother can move in with him since she cannot take care of herself.
C. Complete a physical and mental examination to first determine the cause of Mrs. Eldridge's situation.
D. Call Mrs. Eldridge's pharmacist to see what medications she is taking.
E. Call Mrs. Eldridge's son to discuss the situation with him and to make plans with him and his mother for her future.

Answers are in the back of the book.

KEY POINTS

- The growth of the population 65 and older in the United States is steadily growing, accompanied by an increase in chronic conditions, greater demand for services, and strained health care budgets.
- Most older adults live in the community. The last few years of life often represent functional decline. Nurses strive to help the person maximize functional status and minimize costs through direct care and appropriate referral to community resources.
- Nurses address the chronic health concerns of elders with a focus on maintaining or improving self-care and preventing complications to maintain the highest possible quality of life.
- Assessing the elder incorporates physical, psychological, social, and spiritual domains. Individual and community-focused interventions involve all three levels of prevention through collaborative practice.

critical thinking activities

1. Describe your impression of a typical elder and compare it with the demographic information on elders given in this chapter.
2. From the previous clinical application, identify an example of a theory of aging and an example of ageism, and write at least two nursing diagnoses.
3. From television portrayals, identify both positive and negative ways in which elders are portrayed.
4. Interview an elder within your family, and ask him or her to list any health problems, how your relative would rate his or her health on a scale of 1 to 10 (with 10 being the highest), and what is included in a typical day's activities. Also, ask the elder to keep a 24-hour dietary recall.
5. From the information in activity 4:
   a. Devise screening recommendations for your relative.
   b. Derive at least one nursing diagnosis.
   c. What theory of aging best fits your relative?

continued

critical thinking activities—cont'd

6. Interview a peer to determine what myths of aging they perceive about elders.
7. Describe what you can do to aid in overcoming the myths and examples of ageism that are pervasive in society.

8. Discuss the perceptions of nurses who work in long-term care institutions.

Bibliography

Alexy BB, Elnitsky C: Rural mobile health unit: outcomes, *Public Health Nurs* 15(1):3, 1998.

American Association of Retired Persons: *A profile of older Americans: 1995,* Washington, DC, 1996, the Association.

Berger KS: *The developing person through the lifespan,* ed 3, New York, 1994, Worth.

Burl JB et al: Geriatric nurse practitioners in long-term care: demonstration of effectiveness in managed care, *J Am Geriatr Soc* 46:506, 1998.

Burnside I, Haight B: Reminiscence and life review: therapeutic interventions for older people, *Nurse Pract: Am J Primary Health Care,* 19(4):55, 1994.

Clark M, Anderson PB: *Culture and aging: an anthropological study of older Americans,* Springfield, Ill, 1967, C.C. Thomas.

Corbin J, Cherry J: Caring for the aged in the community. In Swanson E, Tripp-Reimer T, editors: *Chronic illness and the older adult,* New York, 1997, Springer.

Cumming E, Henry H: *Growing old: the process of disengagement,* New York, 1961, Basic Books.

Ebersole P, Hess P: *Toward health aging: human needs and nursing response,* ed 5, St Louis, 1998, Mosby.

Egan DE: The reminiscing game, *Pennsylvania Nurse* 50(2):22, 1996.

Eliopoulos C: *Gerontological nursing,* ed 4, Philadelphia, 1994, J.B. Lippincott.

Erickson EH: *Identity and the lifecycle,* New York, 1959, International Press.

Francis D, Fletcher K, Simon L: The geriatric resource nurse model of care: a vision for the future, *Nurs Clin North Am* 33(3)481, 1998.

Havighurst RL, Neugarten BL, Tobin SS: Disengagement and patterns of aging. In Neugarten BL, editor: *Middle age and aging.* Chicago, 1968, University of Chicago.

Hayflick L: *How and why we age,* New York, 1994, Ballantine Books.

Jefferson Area Board for Aging: *Your pathway to health: senior wellness network and a geriatric assessment intervention team* (brochure), Charlottesville, Va, 1998, Author.

Kane RL, Ouslander JG, Abrass IB: *Essentials of clinical geriatrics,* ed 3, New York, 1994, McGraw-Hill.

Lueckenotte A: *Gerontological nursing,* St Louis, 1996, Mosby.

Maslow A: *Toward a psychology of being,* ed 2, Princeton, NJ, 1968, Van Nostrand.

Matteson MA, McConnell ES, Linton AD: *Gerontological nursing: concepts and practice,* ed 2, Philadelphia, 1997, W.B. Saunders.

McKenna LS: Elder abuse: preparing to identify and intervene in health care, *Home Care Provider* 2(1):30, 1997.

Redeker N: Health beliefs and adherence in chronic illness, *Image J Nurs Sch* 29(1):31, 1988.

Ryan J: Collaboration between the nurse practitioner and physician in long-term care. In Fletcher K, editor: The nurse practitioner in long-term care, *Lippincott's Primary Care Practice,* April/May, 1999.

Simon L, Fletcher K, Francis D: The geriatric resource model of care: a vision for the future. In Abraham I, Fulmer T, Milisen K, editors: Advances in geriatric nursing, *Nurs Clin North Am* 33(3):481, 1998.

Stackhouse JC: *Into the community: nursing in ambulatory and home care,* Philadelphia, 1998, Lippincott-Raven.

Tierney LM, McPhee SJ, Papadakis MA: *Current medical diagnosis and treatment,* ed 35, East Norwalk, Conn, 1996, Appleton & Lange.

Travis J: *Wellness workbook: a guide to high level wellness,* Mill Valley, Calif, 1977, Wellness Resource Center.

US Census Bureau: *Statistical abstract of the United States,* ed 113, Washington, DC, 1993, US Government Printing Office.

US Department of Health and Human Services: *Healthy people 2000,* Washington, DC, 1991, US Government Printing Office.

CHAPTER 30

The Physically Compromised

MARY ANN MCCLELLAN

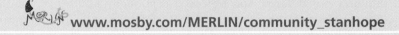

OBJECTIVES

After reading this chapter, the student should be able to do the following:

- Define selected terms related to the concept of physically compromised
- Discuss implications of definitions of developmentally disabled, handicapped, disabled, impaired, and chronically ill.
- List six types of conditions that may cause a person to become physically compromised.
- Compare the effects of being physically compromised on the individual, the family, and the community.

- Describe the implications of being physically compromised for selected populations (rural, low income, work site populations).
- Examine selected issues for those who are physically compromised (abuse, health promotion).
- Discuss relationships between being physically compromised and the objectives of both *Healthy People 2000* and *Healthy Communities 2000.*
- Examine the nurse's role in caring for people who are physically compromised.

KEY TERMS

Americans with
 Disabilities Act
chronic disease
developmental disability

disability
disorder
functional limitations

handicap
impairment
physically compromised

severe chronic disability
work disability

See Glossary for definitions

CHAPTER OUTLINE

Definitions and Concepts
Scope of the Problem
Effects of Being Physically Compromised
   Effects on the Individual
   Effects on the Family
   Effects on the Community

Special Populations
   Rural Populations
   Low-Income Populations
   Occupation and Worksite
Selected Issues
   Abuse
   Health Promotion

Healthy People 2000 Objectives
Healthy Cities
Role of the Nurse
Legislation

Early public health nursing emphasized home care of the sick and the poor, prevention of communicable diseases, and conditions of hygiene in the home and the community. Federal funding in the 1960s allowed for state and local health departments to expand services to include the following: secondary prevention through early detection of selected chronic diseases (e.g., cancer, glaucoma), family planning services to improve the health of mothers and children, and expanded community health nursing services to those who were mentally handicapped. Home health care through the Medicare program increased at about the same time. These changes, along with laws affecting handicapped and developmentally disabled people and many of the objectives of *Healthy People 2000* and the Healthy Cities movement (see Chapter 17), have led to more opportunities for nurses to work with families and other community groups that have members who are physically compromised in some manner.

This chapter defines several terms related to being physically compromised, discusses the scope of the problem, and describes the effects of disabling conditions on individuals, families, and communities. It discusses the relationships between these problems, *Healthy People 2000* and *Healthy Communities 2000* specific objectives, and the concepts of Healthy Cities. Of special importance is the nurse's role and interventions with individuals, families, and communities in dealing with or preventing these health problems.

DEFINITIONS AND CONCEPTS

This chapter's topic, community members who, at some point across the life span, are physically compromised, is so broad that definitions of several related terms are necessary.

The term **developmental disability** relates to the functioning of a person and comes from the Rehabilitation, Comprehensive Services, and Developmental Disabilities Amendments of 1978 (Public Law 95-602): A **severe, chronic disability** of a person is a condition with the following characteristics:

- Relates to a mental or physical impairment or a combination of mental and physical impairments
- Occurs before the person reaches age 22
- Is likely to continue indefinitely
- Results in substantial functional limits in three or more areas of major life activity
- Reflects the person's need for a combining and sequencing of special interdisciplinary or basic care, treatment, or other services that are of lifelong or extended duration and are individually planned and coordinated

: NURSING TIP

Major life activities refer to self-care, receptive and expressive language, learning, mobility, self-direction, capacity for independent living, and financial sufficiency.

A **disability** "is any restriction or lack (resulting from an impairment) of ability to perform an activity in the manner or within the range considered normal for a human being" (Badley, 1993) "at that chronological age" (Heerkens et al, 1994). The medical model has dominated the definition of a disability. Other models and definitions include such areas as interactions and relationships among the individual, society, and the environment (Imrie, 1997; Orr and Schkade, 1997; Peters, 1996). In addition, culture has been considered (Banja, 1996). An **impairment** "is any loss or abnormality of psychological, physiological or anatomical structure or function. 'Impairment' is more inclusive than '**disorder**' in that it covers losses, e.g., the loss of a leg is an impairment, but not a disorder" (Badley, 1993, p. 162).

Functional limitations are essentially descriptions of functions such as hearing, seeing, grasping, moving, climbing, and reading. Emphasis is placed on the level of func-

BOX 30-1 Conditions Related to Disability in Persons 15 Years Old or Older

AIDS or AIDS-related condition
Alcohol- or drug-related problem or disorder
Arthritis or rheumatism
Back or spine problems (including chronic stiffness or deformity of the back or spine)
Blindness or other visual impairment (difficulty seeing well enough, even with glasses, to read a newspaper)
Broken bone/fracture
Cancer
Cerebral palsy
Deafness or serious trouble hearing
Diabetes
Epilepsy
Head or spinal cord injury
Heart trouble (including coronary heart disease and arteriosclerosis)
Hernia or rupture
High blood pressure (hypertension)
Kidney stones or chronic kidney trouble
Learning disability
Lung or respiratory trouble (asthma, bronchitis, emphysema, respiratory allergies, tuberculosis, or other lung trouble)
Mental retardation
Missing legs, feet, arms, hands, or fingers
Paralysis of any kind
Senility/dementia/Alzheimer's disease
Speech disorder
Stiffness or deformity of the foot, leg, arm, or hand
Stomach trouble (including ulcers, gall bladder, or liver conditions)
Stroke
Thyroid trouble or goiter
Tumor, cyst, or growth
Other

From Centers for Disease Control and Prevention: Prevalence of disabilities and associated health conditions, United States, 1991-1992, *MMWR Morb Mortal Wkly Rep* 43(40):730, 1994.

tion rather than the purpose of the activity so that functional limitation can be associated with the disability. For example, an impairment in the strength or range of motion of the arm could lead to functional limitations in grasping or reaching. These in turn could give rise to disabilities, for example, inability to reach up to high shelves, get dressed, perform hair care, or cook (Badley, 1993, p. 165).

Handicap refers to social implications for a person who is impaired or disabled. A **handicap** is a disadvantage for a given individual with an impairment or a disability that limits or prevents the fulfillment of a role that is normal for that individual. Handicap reflects the value attached to an individual's situation or experience by others when it departs from the norm, and the individual's performance or status and the expectations of the individual himself or of the particular group of which he is a member (Badley, 1993).

Chronic disease, or illness, refers to any long-lasting condition or illness. Disease processes (e.g., diabetes mellitus, cancer, tuberculosis) or a congenital or an acquired condition (e.g., Down syndrome, severe burns, amputation of a limb), are examples of chronic diseases. Therefore concepts related to disabilities, handicaps, impairments,

and functional limitations may apply to individuals with a chronic disease or other conditions. For nurses working with those with a chronic disease, the onset, course, outcome, and degree of limits are important factors to assess in deciding the meaning of the disease to individuals and the families.

A person who is **physically compromised** may have any or all the conditions listed in Box 30-1.

SCOPE OF THE PROBLEM

There are nursing implications for individuals who are physically compromised, for their families, for the populations and subpopulations which they make up, and for the communities in which they live. The nurse must remember that some clients prefer to be regarded as being physically challenged or physically compromised, while others may think such terms minimize the importance of the needs and problems of people who are disabled. See Appendixes H.2, I.5, and J.6 for a thorough review of assessment tools for use with people who are physically compromised.

People may be physically compromised from many different causes. Three major categories of such causes summarized in Figure 30-1 are injuries, developmental disabil-

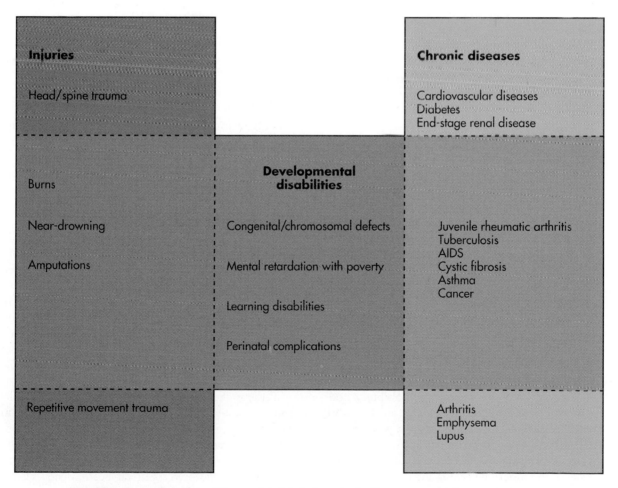

FIG. 30-1 Examples of conditions related to being physically compromised.

ities, and chronic diseases. As Figure 30-1 indicates, some of these conditions may occur at different ages and stages of development of the individual. Therefore the effects on the person's life are influenced by the timing as well as by the severity of the condition. Several specific conditions and inherited problems can cause disability. These include genetic disorders, acute and chronic illnesses, violence, to-bacco use, lack of access to health care, or failure to eat correctly, exercise regularly, or manage stress effectively. Other causes include perinatal complications, injuries, substance abuse, environmental problems, and unsanitary living conditions. One example includes both tobacco use and environmental problems. In 1996, cigarette smoking prevalence was added to the nationally notifiable health problems to be reported to the Centers for Disease Control and Prevention (CDC) by states. Approximately 15 million children and adolescents were exposed to cigarette smoke in their homes in 1996 (CDC, 1997). Appendix B lists selected national organizations, including those with information about disabilities.

By definition, developmental disabilities start before age 22 and continue throughout the person's lifetime. There are no specific statistics on total numbers of children's developmental disabilities in this country. However, the CDC's Survey of Income and Program Participation (SIPPS), 1991-1992, estimated that about 3.8 million (7.9%) persons under 17 years of age had a disability at that time (McNeil, 1995). In addition, usually about 10% to 15% of children in the United States have some type of special health care needs. About 1% to 2% of all children have conditions severe enough to limit daily functioning (Francis, 1995). Nearly 6.2% (almost 2 million) of adolescents ages 10 to 18 years, live with some limits on their activities due to chronic conditions.

Data about disabilities among adults are also inadequate. However there has been a continued decline between 1982 and 1994 in the prevalence of disability in those over 65, from 24.9% to 21.3% (Manton, Corder, and Stallard, 1997). The National Long-Term Care Surveys of the 1980s showed widening differences in disability between African-American and Caucasian elderly populations. Institutional care for the same groups was about the same (Clark, 1997). Liao et al (1999) found that those with higher income had less illness and disability and a better quality of life in their last years.

Work disability, the inability to perform work for 6 months or more due to a mental, physical, or other health condition (CDC, 1993), costs billions of dollars each year in lost wages and direct and indirect medical costs in this country. In 1990 an estimated 12.8 million people ages 16 to 64 years were believed to have a work disability. About half of these were severe (CDC, 1993). The greatest work disability in the South occurred among those who were of female, rural, elderly, less educated, African-American, and below poverty level (Holzer et al, 1996). The effects of personal income on the functional status and early retirement

of those with chronic diseases is significant (Kingston and Smith, 1997).

EFFECTS OF BEING PHYSICALLY COMPROMISED

The extent to which the physically compromised individual may need extra support, care, and services from the family unit and the community is shown in Box 30-2. Understanding the relationships of these three is best grasped by starting with the stresses placed on the individual.

Effects on the Individual

Health care tends to be organized around medical diagnoses rather than an individual's degree and kind of functional strengths and limitations. However, the effects of being physically compromised vary with the cause of the disability, the person's resilience, the severity of limitations, and other factors (Turner-Henson and Holaday, 1995). Because it is not possible to discuss here every cause of being physically compromised, some of their effects will be discussed, instead, from a life span perspective.

Children: infancy through adolescence

Perhaps the wide variety of effects, as they relate to cause, is best shown by looking at some specific examples. For instance, infants and children, even those whose parents have accepted their need for gastrostomies, usually have poor growth and development. Better nutrition often improves the children's general health. They seem more

---

BOX 30-2 **Potential Effects of Being Physically Compromised Related to Individuals, Families, and Communities**

PERSON
Related health problems (e.g., nutrition, oral health, hygiene, limited activity and stamina)
↓ Self-concept/self esteem
↓ Life expectancy and ↑ risk for infection and secondary injury
Developmental tasks; change in role expectations

FAMILY
Stress on family unit
Need for ↑ use of external resources in role expectations
↓ options in use of any discretionary income
Social stigma

COMMUNITY
Need/demand to reallocate resources
Discomfort or fear due to lack of knowledge of disability
Need to comply with legislation
Services provided by health department, health care providers
↑ need for other services beyond medical diagnosis (e.g., transportation, etc.)

↑ Increased; ↓, decreased.

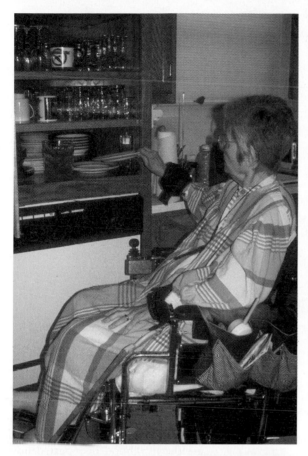
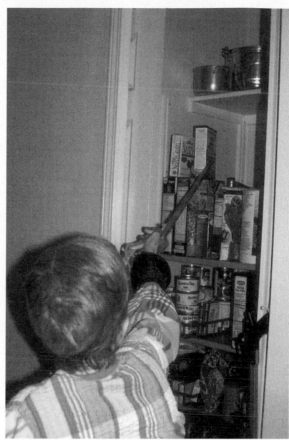
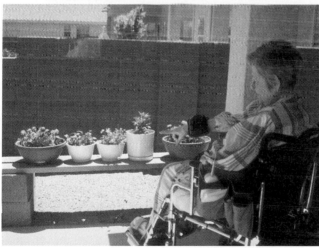
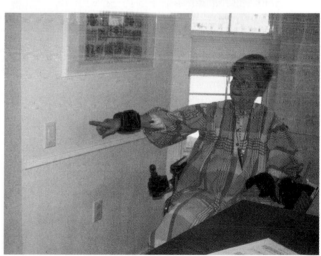

This disabled woman is able to live in and maintain her own home, including growing plants and flowers, with the help of easy-access devices and lower light fixtures and cabinets.

alert and responsive. However, past negative experiences with oral feedings may result in continued facial defensiveness. For example, they may turn away from parents' kisses (Thorne, Radford, and McCormick, 1997). In addition, children with significant sensory deficits (e.g., hearing or vision impairments) are at risk for social isolation, cognitive and neuropsychological impairment, and developmental delays (Schilling and DeJesus, 1993; Trüster and Brambring, 1992).

Social implications for children who are chronically ill are important. School-age children who are chronically ill may be discriminated against in their school systems, peer groups, communities, and government institutions. A study by Cole, Roberts, and McNeal (1996) looked at school children's perceptions of imaginary chronically ill peers with diabetes mellitus, asthma, AIDS, or cystic fibrosis. The fourth-, fifth-, and sixth-grade students thought all of the diseases were contagious and had difficulty accepting them as peers. Such results showed a need for early education for children about those with chronic diseases.

The effects on adolescents' development may vary with the time of onset of the physical problem. The effect seems to be less when the onset occurs in early adolescence rather than in middle or late adolescence. Children with chronic diseases diagnosed earlier may be seen as regressing in development during adolescence. However, their behavior may simply mean a change in already-achieved tasks that will permit chronically ill adolescents to express themselves in new ways (Weekes, 1995). Remember that adolescence is often a time when behaviors seem to regress. Adolescents who are physically compromised may be like their healthier peers in many ways. For example, adolescents who are developmentally delayed vary in employment rates. Adolescents' sociodemographic characteristics are often more important in successful employment than are their disabilities (Rimmerman et al, 1996). Adolescents who have chronic health problems are found to be as sexually active as their well peers. The visibility of the chronic conditions does not seem to affect the adolescents' sexual behavior (Suris et al, 1996).

Transitions. Predictable transition points in a child's development can be difficult for those with disabilities and for their families. Children's first words, first steps, and first days at school are important events. These may highlight the differences between what is "normal" and what children's true abilities are (Mallory, 1996).

Of special concern is the change to adulthood by adolescents with disabilities. Parents often begin worrying about this issue when their children are between 5 and 10 years old. That is the age range in which the permanence of their disability is clearer. Many students with disabilities do not complete high school, have poor success in college settings, and are unemployed (Brown and Nourse, 1997). There is likely to be variation in success rates depending on such factors as the types of children's disabilities and

the socioeconomic levels of their families. Some of the barriers faced by these adolescents include the following ones: they are often seen as "permanent children" by their parents; others have very low expectations of those with disabilities; and parents and children are seldom involved in early planning for work and independent living (Wagner and Blackorby, 1996).

Adults

Chronic diseases may have major effects on adults. One recent report of disability in adults showed the interaction of selected conditions in select populations. Table 30-1 summarizes some of these (Kington and Smith, 1997; Pablos-Möndez, Blustein, and Kirsch, 1997; Picavet and van den Bos, 1997; Wilkins and Park, 1996; Wray, 1996).

Other conditions known to have major effects on the adult population include injuries that may lead to early death. Costs of low back pain (LBP), possibly resulting from repeated microtrauma, are estimated to be about $85 billion a year in this country. Effects of LBP vary from minor inconvenience to major disability and psychosocial dysfunction in the person and his family (Simmonds, Kumar, and Lechelt, 1997). Ongoing communication problems in adults with traumatic brain injury (TBI) have associated hearing and/or speech problems and comorbid disabilities of agility and mobility (Labinski, Moscato, and Willer, 1997). Older adults with fragility fractures are much more likely to die in the 6 months postfracture. Hip fractures also increase the likelihood of repeated hospitalizations, needed help for activities of daily living (ADL), and the need to enter a nursing home for the first time. The effects of fragility fractures are worsened by the presence of preexisting chronic diseases (Cooper, 1997; Wolinsky, Fitzgerald, and Stump, 1997).

External factors that affect chronic illness on adults include previous problem-solving skills and management of tasks related to their conditions and to development. Alcohol and drug use, living arrangements, insurance, prescription drug spending, the physical environment, the use of assistive equipment, and sexuality are all factors that affect adult responses to chronic illness (Abstracts of the International Seminar on Women and Disability, 1997; Hub-

TABLE 30-1 Selected Conditions in Various Populations

POPULATION	CONDITIONS
Hispanic	Diabetes mellitus and tuberculosis comorbidity; ↑ hypertension rates
African-American (preretirement age)	Disability and work experience
Dutch	Mobility disability with musculoskeletal disorders, lung diseases, neurological disorders, heart diseases, diabetes, and cancer
Canadian (55 years + living in a community)	Disability with epilepsy, stroke, arthritis/rheumatism, back problems, and cataracts
African-American adults (generally)	↑ hypertension, diabetes mellitus, and arthritis

↑, Increased.

bard et al, 1996; Kochhar and Scott, 1997; Mueller et al, 1997; Satariano, 1997; Verbrugge et al, 1997). When considering the effects of disability among the elderly on activities of daily living, the progression of the loss of abilities was first walking, followed by bathing, transferring, dressing, toileting, and feeding. Women outlive men, just as in the well population, but were disabled for a significantly longer time (Dunlop, Hughes, and Manheim, 1997).

Effects on the Family

Most people who are physically compromised are cared for at home by one or more family members. As many as one of every seven adults in this country may be caring for relatives or friends. More than one in five of these care-givers is usually a woman aged 35 to 64. About one third of this care may be given to people who are elderly (Marks, 1996). Figure 30-2 depicts some of the issues and concerns that occur when a family member is disabled and the effect of the disability on the family unit. Clearly, the entire family system is affected in families with members who are disabled (Garlow and Turnbull, 1993).

Children: infancy through adolescence

Many children with chronic illnesses or defects are surviving conditions that would have been fatal 20 years ago.

Children's disability may have long-term effects on the primary caregiver, usually the mother, and on the marital relationship. Mothers of severely brain-injured children describe these children and themselves as "different people" after the accidents (Guerrieve and McKeever, 1997). Mothers' perceptions of the effect of their chronically ill children has on their families directly affects maternal mental health (Ireys and Silver, 1996). The family's response to a child's disability may also affect the child. If the family and mother have a positive psychological adjustment, so will the child. An area of conflict for parents of children with disabilities may be in the school setting. One study reports differences in parent and teacher ratings of adaptive behavior in children with disabilities. The teachers' ratings were higher than those of the parents (Voelke et al, 1997). There is a need for a greater array of community and support services for children with disabilities who have behavior problems (Floyd and Gallagher, 1997).

Effects on siblings may vary with the particular disorder of the disabled children. If the disorder is emotional or communicative rather than physical, the sibling may have difficulty adjusting (Fisman et al, 1996). Williams (1997), in a recent review of more than 40 studies on the effects of chronically ill children on their siblings, found that about 60% reported an increased risk of adjustment for siblings;

FIG. 30-2 Factors influencing a family unit when a member is physically compromised.

RESEARCH *Brief*

This article describes the need for and development of the TIMDAC. No previous tool existed for measuring death anxiety of child with HIV/AIDS and that was culturally sensitive to African-American and Hispanic (Latino) populations. The test uses projective technique with four colored pictures to interview children. The child tells a story about each picture. Death anxiety-related (DAR) and non–death anxiety–related (NDAR) responses are totaled. A death anxiety profile is created from this process. Interrater reliability in the final study was .80. However, the authors pointed out that studying the construct validity of an instrument is ongoing, especially with projective techniques.

Implications for nurses include the following:

1. Children with life-threatening illnesses have less psychological damage when the family communicates openly about the disease. Therefore nurses need to support family openness in discussing the meaning of his or her illness with the child.

2. Emotional needs of HIV-infected and AIDS-diagnosed children should be investigated clinically. Nurses need to listen to these children's anxiety about and perceptions of death.

Ireland M, Malgady RG: Thematic Instrument for Measuring Death Anxiety in Children (TIMDAC), *J Pediatr Nurs* 14(1):28, 1999.

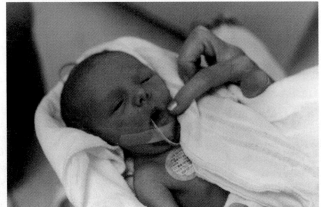

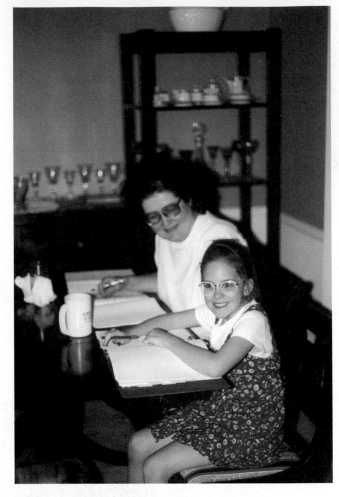

A, An at-risk infant girl who was one month premature and delivered by stat C-section due to abruption. Apgars were 1[1] and 5[3]. **B,** The same child at 10 years of age. She is profoundly hearing impaired. Her parents' commitment has helped her to be mainstreamed successfully, and she is able to do her own homework.

30% reported no risk. About 10% showed both positive and negative effects of having a disabled sibling.

Families with an infant who needs technologically assisted care at home may have home health nurses present 12 to 18 hours each day. The presence of these nonfamily members may add stress to the family (Murphy, 1997). Going through such life-threatening, prolonged illnesses as leukemia in a child is very stressful for the whole family. Some of these children may show such problems as posttraumatic stress, depression, anxiety, and learning problems. The parents of such children seem to be affected even more (Stuber, 1996) (see the Research Brief about the article by Ireland and Malgady).

Adults

The situation of adults who are physically compromised produces a variety of effects on their family unit. For example, the financial effect of having a disabled family member may be worse if that person has been the main source of family income.

Other concerns related to children living in a home with one or more disabled adults are risks for accidental in-

juries and the potential for behavioral problems (Gates and Lackey, 1997). Another issue involves the developmentally delayed adults. Parents are often very concerned about the future of these adult children as the parents themselves age (Mengel, Marcus, and Dunkle, 1996).

Family members who are caregivers for physically compromised adults are most likely to be spouses or daughters of the affected individuals. Family caregivers are often poorly trained and at risk for injury (Brown and Mulley, 1997).

Pruchno, Patrick, and Burant (1997) confirmed that African-American mothers of adult children with disabilities experience greater caregiver burden and caregiver satisfaction than do Caucasian mothers. The meaning to a family of a member's disability is affected by that family's cultural background. Cultural implications and differences are found in the following areas (McCallion et al, 1997):

• How disability is perceived
• Who are "family"
• Who provides care
• How the family makes decisions

- What family members think of each other
- What support families receive from friends and community
- Why the family moved
- Cultural values important to family members
- Family willingness to accept services from outside the family
- The family's first language
- Families' concerns about service providers

Effects on the Community

The presence of physically compromised people and their families in a community may have far-reaching effects on all aspects of community life. The community may be called upon to respond in new ways to these citizens, especially as a result of federal laws affecting those who are disabled.

Children: infancy through adolescence

The inclusion of children with complex medical problems in the New York City school system has created the need for skilled services of at least 150 nurses. A special curriculum to insure these skills was developed by the school system (Lipper et al, 1997).

Children who are chronically ill or disabled and who enter school for mainstream education need more support from the community. Properly modified regular education can meet the learning needs of many students with disabilities (Terman et al, 1996). However, increased resources and support for regular classrooms, increased teacher training, and committed local school systems are requirements to successfully include children with disabilities.

Public schools must evaluate their effectiveness with students who are disabled, which adds to the cost of educating children. Education of local pediatricians and nurses helps to attain supportive and knowledgeable collaboration for the development of early intervention programs in the schools.

Transition points in children's lives require the investment of additional community resources. Parents will feel highly involved in decisions about their disabled children in inclusive school environments. Teachers are generally positive about parent involvement. Both groups will learn to value the need for shared commitment among all these involved (Bennett, Deluca, and Bruns, 1997). Contact, books about disabled children, and discussions about attitudes can help preschool-age children develop positive attitudes and acceptance of people with disabilities (Favazza and Odom, 1997).

Adults

One of the most visible ways in which those with disabilities affect their communities is through the changes that become necessary to accommodate access to buildings. The effects of facilities at hotels and motels on those with disabilities has been varied. Upscale lodgings are more likely to be accessible; however, some economy chains are recognized as having consistently accessible facilities (England, 1996). Increasing awareness of needs of library patrons with disabilities had changed some services. One area of limitation has been use of adaptive technology that permits disabled users to search a library's online catalog and databases (Nelson, 1996).

The managed care system has seemingly failed to recognize basic characteristics of chronic disease and disability and the services needed to care for these clients. Persons with chronic conditions are the fastest-growing, costliest, and most complex group receiving health care (Bringewatt, 1997). Sources of costs for chronic health problems include poor psychosocial adjustment and increased demands for screening of communicable diseases (Watt et al, 1997).

Tuberculosis is an example of a communicable disease that is also a chronic health problem of varying severity. At least one major health department has had many increased demands on its tuberculosis (TB) control program for screening of low- or no-risk people and information by the general public.

Those with disabilities have had effects on the Medicaid and Medicare systems (Davis and O'Brien, 1996). Medicare data show that persons with disabilities have more functional limitations, poorer health status, lower incomes, and experience more barriers to health care than aged Medicare beneficiaries. Information from Medicaid shows that significant increase in the Medicaid disabled population has led to the young disabled outnumbering the Medicaid-eligible elderly. Medicaid serves an increasingly younger disabled population.

One way in which people with developmental disabilities may affect their communities can be influenced by possible changes in Medicaid. For example, the number of persons with developmental disabilities projected to lose Medicaid long-term care services in the year 2002 is about 21% of those served in 1992. This change will increase the burden of care on the communities in which these people live.

SPECIAL POPULATIONS
Rural Populations

There is disagreement among policymakers at all government levels about the definition of the word "rural." The two most common definitions are those of the Census Bureau and the Office of Management and Budget (OMB). The Census Bureau classifies people based on the population size and residential population density of the places they live. The OMB classifies counties as either metropolitan or nonmetropolitan depending on whether the county has a large city and suburbs (Johnson-Webb, Baer, and Gesler, 1997).

As mentioned in Chapter 16, rural dwellers may be at greater risk for disability than urbanites, in particular from agricultural-related injuries and chronic illness. Table 30-2 summarizes some of the hazards and their potentially disabling effects. During the last 40 years, death rates in agriculture have declined 24%. In the same period death and injury rates in mining and construction, the other most hazardous industries, have fallen 75% (Schulman et al, 1997).

TABLE 30-2 Agricultural Industry and Disabling Conditions

ORGAN SYSTEM OR DISORDER	PRINCIPAL EXPOSURES	POSSIBLE DISABILITY MANIFESTATIONS
Lungs	Organic dust, microbes, molds, fungi, endotoxins, allergens	Chronic bronchitis, asthma, hypersensitivity pneumonitis, organic dust, toxic syndrome
Cancer	Herbicides, insecticides, fungicides, fumes, sunlight, diet, unknown	Non-Hodgkin's lymphoma; Hodgkin's disease, multiple myeloma, soft-tissue sarcoma, leukemias, skin cancer, prostate cancer, stomach, pancreas, testicle, glioma
Neurological disorders	Herbicides, insecticides, fungicides, solvents, fumigants	Acute intoxication, Parkinson's disease, peripheral neuritis, Alzheimer's disease, acute and chronic encephalopathy
Accidents	Tractor rollovers, machine injuries, animal injuries, farmyard injuries	Suffocation, crushing, amputations, eye injuries
Hearing loss	Motor noise, animal noise	Deafness
Skin	Pesticides, fuels, fungi, sun	Dermatitis, cancer
Stress and well-being	Isolation, intergenerational problems, violence, substance abuse, incest	Depression, suicide, poor coping, physical disability resulting from inadequate attention to health.

From Zejda TE, McDuffie HH, Dosman JA: *West J Med* 158(1):56, 1993.

Children who work in agriculture have over 23,000 injuries and 300 deaths on American farms every year. One article describes a study that found adolescents were being exposed to serious safety hazards on North Carolina farms. Most were exposed to injury by tractors, large animals, all-terrain vehicles, farm trucks, and rotary mowers. Over 30% were exposed to pesticides and tobacco harvesters. Common injuries included insect stings, cuts, burns, and falls (Schulman, Evenson, Runyan, Cohen, and Dunn, 1997).

Parents also allow children ages 9 to 14 years to do high-risk chores under two circumstances: when the families feel pushed for money or when the labor force is inadequate. The economic benefit of safety behavior is an area that needs to be stressed by nurses. Such an approach would more likely encourage teaching by parents and the role modeling of safety (Kidd et al, 1997).

On family farms, even though most parents are aware of high-risk activities, they allow children to take part in hazardous work. Fathers' attitudes most strongly account for their willingness to let children drive a tractor, to be an extra rider on a tractor, or to be near the hind legs of a dairy cow. These attitudes relate to a desire for children to gain work experience, to develop a work ethic and self-confidence, to save time and money, and the fathers' wishes to spend time with and supervise the children (Lee et al, 1997).

Those who have had a previous injury that limited their ability to work the farm are at increased risk for another farm-related injury. Such repeat injuries increase the likelihood of ongoing disabilities among older farmers (Browning et al, 1998). Non-Hodgkin's lymphoma (NHL), another problem for farmers in the central United States,

is associated with exposures to infectious microorganisms and pesticides (Keller-Byne, Khuder, Schaub, and McFee, 1997).

In addition to health problems peculiar to their lifestyle, people who live in rural areas can also have some of the same health problems as urban dwellers with fewer options for dealing with these problems, both for informal and formal sources of care and support. Rural residents generally experience barriers to access to primary care. However, these problems are greater for persons with disabilities (Lishner, Richardson, Levine, and Patrick, 1996). Main barriers to use of preventive services includes problems with ability to pay, perception of need, service availability, accessibility of services, and perception of racism (Schoenberg and Coward, 1998; Strickland and Strickland, 1996). It is important for the nurse to maintain current knowledge about services available at the local, county, and state levels.

Aging and disability are concerns of rural nurses. Older adults from nonmetropolitan areas are more likely to be able to perform functional activities of daily living and self-care activities both with and without disability. It is possible that rural older adults may discount the significance of decreasing functional ability and to what has to be done in a day's work. Such "normalizing" of aging may affect ways in which aging rural populations use primary care and long-term care services (Rabiner et al, 1997).

Low-Income Populations

Physically compromised individuals often experience poverty, as do other special population groups: single parents and their children, the aged, the unemployed, and members of racial and ethnic minorities. Persons with low income have less access to health care throughout their lives and are less likely to participate in all levels of prevention. Therefore they are at greater risk for the onset of disabling conditions and for more rapid progression of disease processes. Those in poverty are also at greater risk for disabling conditions resulting from lifestyle, such as injuries, tobacco abuse, and inadequate nutrition.

Those who are disabled and in poverty are less likely to be able to provide for their special needs from their own resources. Those who are physically compromised are often unemployed, including those who are able to work and who seek jobs. Employers may be reluctant to hire personnel whose conditions may increase health insurance costs. Therefore lack of insurance through the work setting further limits access to health care by those who are physically compromised.

The prevalence of chronic illness among U.S. youth is a significant public health concern. The lack of transition services for these youth fosters major delays in further education, vocational rehabilitation, and employment. For these and other reasons, many youth with chronic health problems must cope with the additional burden of poverty (Ireys, Salkeyer, Kolodner, and Bijur, 1996). Other factors that affect low-income, physically comprised clients' access to needed services are inadequate transportation, lack of coordination of care, and limited locally available services for those who cannot pay for them. Figure 30-3 provides an illustration of the relationship between poverty and disabilities.

Occupation and Worksite

Several issues related to occupation and disability are of concern to nurses. Many chronic diseases can result from or be created by worksite hazards (Bowden and McDiarmid, 1994; Stellman, 1994). In addition, work-related injuries and the severity and length of disability are believed to be seriously underreported (Oleinick et al, 1994). Some recent studies have increased available information in this area. Work-related injuries include the following:

- Head injuries
- Carpal tunnel syndrome
- Obesity-related hip and knee pain
- Hip pain related to heavy lifting
- Low back pain
- Functional limitations related to falls (Blanc et al, 1996; Gillen et al, 1997; Menard, 1996; Sobti et al, 1997)

The more severe the injury, the greater number of days lost from work.

Ponzer et al (1997) studied the level of disability caused by injury to working-age women. These women were injured seriously enough that they were admitted to the hospital. They found that injury recovery was associated with injury severity; frequency of previous injury, or trauma recurrence; and self-assessed mental and physical health during hospitalization. They recommended that psychiatric, psychological, and social support be offered to all injured clients as part of the medical care provided to them. One

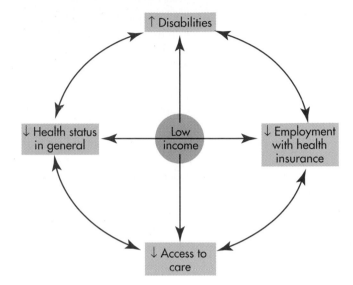

FIG. 30-3 Relationships of poverty and disability.

option to monitor these needs would be follow-up by a nurse.

Other family members' disability status may be caused by worksite conditions (Bowden and McDiarmid, 1994). For example, a positive association has been identified between mental retardation in 10-year-old children and their mothers' employment in textile and garment industries (Decouflé et al, 1993).

Blatter and others (1997) found statistically significant associations between certain paternal occupational exposures and the occurrence of spina bifida in their children. These occupational risks were low exposure to welding fumes and to UV radiation during welding. There were suggestive findings of an association between spina bifida and moderate or high exposure to cleaning agents, moderate to high pesticide exposure, and stainless steel dust.

One of the most common problems in the work setting is chronic pain, a costly work problem. It is usually started by an injury or disease process and is seldom cured. The goal of the nurse working with such clients is to help them learn to manage the pain, rather than letting pain control them. One recommendation is that the health care system and industry work together to conduct studies toward the development of effective chronic pain treatment protocols (Hart, 1997).

Children are at particular risk for work-related disability. The U.S. Department of Labor estimates that over 4 million children are legally employed in this country. The department also estimates that another 1 to 2 million are employed illegally. Working in agriculture and delivering the newspaper are the most hazardous areas of employment for children and adolescents. However, other types of employment also present threats to children's health. Poverty, massive immigration, and reduced enforcement of federal child labor laws are principally responsible for the resurgence of child labor in the U.S. in the last 20 years (Landrigan and McCammon , 1997) .

The **Americans with Disabilities Act** of 1990 includes provisions for certain employers to make "reasonable accommodations" in the work environment in order to facilitate employment of those who are physically compromised. However, there are many continuing questions in interpreting and carrying out the requirements of the law. For example, an elevator may have a control panel with Braille printing, may be at wheelchair level, and may have "buttons" to press that are sensitive to warmth for those with inadequate strength to press them. What is the employer's responsibility to an employee who has bilateral amputation of both arms below the shoulder and whose prostheses includes a type of hook that prevents his readily pressing elevator buttons?

In one example of accommodation, Daly and Bound (1996) analyzed data from a health and retirement study. They found that many workers who suffered from health limits were directly accommodated by their employers. Those who did not receive such accommodation often adapted to their limits by changing their job demands or by changing jobs entirely.

Vocational assessment and evaluation play a significant part in optimizing rehabilitation outcomes of people with disabilities. The focus is the individual's current employability (functional) level using an asset approach. This describes the client's strengths and limitations and identifies services required to achieve vocational rehabilitation goals for the individual. Disability affects a company's profits, regardless of how or where the disability occurred. A comprehensive disability management program must be developed and implemented in order to reduce losses secondary to disability. Primary prevention to reduce disability through lifestyle changes should also be a part of such a program (Chan et al, 1997; Lukes and Wachs, 1996).

SELECTED ISSUES

Abuse

Most of the literature on abuse of those who are physically disabled concerns children and the elderly. However, nurses must be knowledgeable about state laws related to reporting suspected abuse of those of any age who are disabled.

For adults, abuse associated with physical disability has been identified as occurring after the disability. In children, physical disability may result from abuse or neglect, or abuse may occur after the onset of disability. A form of child abuse, Munchausen by proxy syndrome, may present as a developmental disability or with neurological symptoms, especially seizure activity. Several studies have shown that adults and children who are developmentally delayed are at higher risk for sexual abuse than the general public.

Much has been written about characteristics of abusers and the children and elderly adults who are abused. The interaction among the environment, the victim, and the abuser seems to be most important. Figure 30-4 includes several factors to consider. For example, those who are physically compromised and who are in group residences or who must travel long distances in buses may be at risk for abuse from a variety of possible predators. Such potential victims seem to be especially at risk if they cannot communicate (Porter et al, 1995). Children with cerebral palsy or other conditions affecting their appearance, gait, and mobility are a vulnerable group. They are more likely to be victimized by their peers. Therefore they need special support and protection at school and in other settings with groups of children (Dawkins, 1996). See the Research Brief about the article by Kotch et al on p. 626.

Breakdowns in parent/child interactions often result from the lack of maternal/caregivers knowledge of the young children's cues or of the limited capacity of some children with disabilities to stimulate their caregivers. Nurses might need to facilitate caregiver-child interactions by interpreting the child's cues, for example (Hadadian, 1996).

Of special interest to nurses is the concern that the services developed to help children with disabilities may contribute to their increased risk for abuse. For example, depersonalizing potential victims is a critical factor in making violence toward them acceptable. One study found that nurses used the term "baby" with parents of term healthy newborns. The same nurses used the more distancing term "infant" with parents whose newborns had disabilities (Sobsey, 1997).

Children's disabilities are unlikely to be identified if the child must enter the child protection system with a state, another way to depersonalize the child. Such limits could mean that children may not receive all the care that they need; or, in many cases, a consideration is given only to the living situation's ability to protect and care for them, while the abused or neglected children's special education needs are not taken into account. Often, routine lack of compliance with special education on the part of the involved school system is a major problem to be overcome (Bonner et al, 1997; Weinberg, 1997).

Research on abuse of those who are physically compromised, as well as the many effects on the abused person, is not currently well developed. Nevertheless, the nurse's comprehensive approach to health problems promotes his or her ability to consider multiple factors in these situations.

Health Promotion

Health promotion usually focuses on the primary prevention of conditions that may lead to disability (e.g., smoking cessation to prevent lung cancer). Physically compromised clients also need information and counseling for health promoting behaviors, since such behavior may slow the progress of a condition or prevent added pathology. For example, a child with a serious congenital heart defect does not need the added insult of increased respiratory infections from exposure to second-hand cigarette smoke.

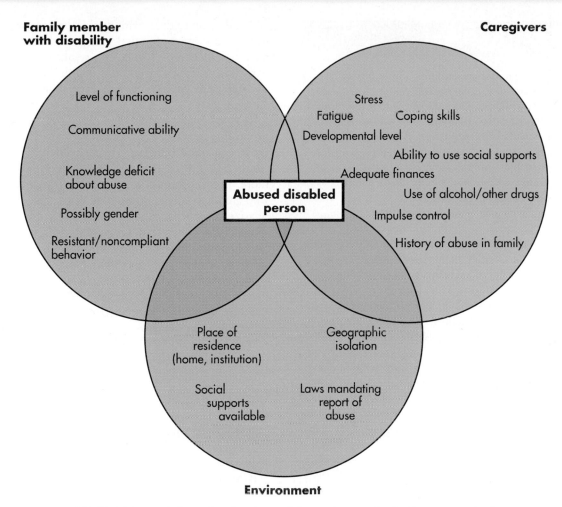

FIG. 30-4 Factors influencing the abuse of those who are physically compromised.

Health promotion is a multidimensional concept that applies to all individuals regardless of disability. Strategies are needed to expand the knowledge base of health promotion for those who are physically compromised. Research, partnerships, and communication with those with disabilities and among health care professionals are recommended (Fowler, 1997). Persons with chronic disability have frequently defined themselves in terms of their physical problems and sick role. Davidhizar and Shearer (1997) believed that a client may be diagnosed with a physical illness, a chronic illness, or a disability. However, such clients might still work to attain high-level wellness by functioning in an integrated way with the environment.

Health within illness is beginning to gain recognition in nursing. Little research has been done in this area. In one study, however, several themes were used to describe participants' experiences of health with illness, including honoring oneself, seeking and connecting with others, creating opportunities, celebrating life, transcending self, and acquiring a state of grace (Lindsey, 1996).

Many health promotion and disease prevention needs are similar across the life span; these include exercise, diet, avoidance of excess substance use, and injury prevention. However, specific problems and interventions to deal with these needs may vary according to such factors as age, specific disabling condition, and developmental status. For example, nutritional needs of premature infants may focus on adequate energy, protein, fat, vitamins and minerals. An older adult with Type II diabetes mellitus may be concerned primarily with reducing his or her risk of experiencing a myocardial infarction.

Because one of the most important needs of those with disabilities is that of appropriate nutrition, nurses may consult with dietetics professionals or refer clients to them for assistance. For example, a client with Down syndrome may need a lower caloric intake than nondisabled persons his age. A dietitian could provide information or counseling about managing this need (Cloud, 1997).

DID YOU KNOW? *Mexican Americans 65 years and older with type 2 diabetes mellitus have a greater prevalence and health burden from the disease than do non-Hispanic and African-American of the same age group. This is especially true among elderly men (Black, Ray, and Markides, 1999).*

RESEARCH *Brief*

Mothers of 708 mainly at-risk infants were interviewed in their homes soon after their babies' discharge from the hospital. These children were at risk due to low birthweight, congenital defects, maternal age <14 to 17 years, or other medical/social problems. The interview included items thought to be related to the ecological model of child maltreatment from behavior domains of the child, family, social, and parent. State (North Carolina) child abuse and neglect central registry data were tracked every 6 months until these children became 4 years old.

Some of the predisposing risk factors found soon after birth would still predict child maltreatment reports through 4 years of age. Generally, families with low levels of support had a higher risk of being reported for child maltreatment. Those families with higher levels of mothers' being depressed and/or with life event stress and low social support had up to 4 times the risk of being reported for child maltreatment.

Implications for nursing practice include the following:
1. Nurses need to include assessment of social support for the mother and family, especially when caring for high-risk children.
2. Ongoing, periodic monitoring and support by community health nurses can identify developing problems, reinforce effective parental behavior and problem solving, and help access formal or informal community support services.

Kotch JB: Predicting child maltreatment in the first 4 years of life from characteristics assessed in the neonatal period, *Child Abuse Neglect* 23(4):305, 1999.

Traditional rehabilitation of clients with developmental disabilities who are in residential facilities is enhanced by involvement of a dietitian (Hogan and Evers,1997). Families and professionals can work together to meet the nutritional needs of children with disabilities and chronic health care problems. Doing so before a child becomes severely malnourished or a family becomes dysfunctional is possible with such an approach (Secrist-Mertz et al, 1997).

A large body of research about exercise science has been published in the last 30 years. However, little information is available on the activity patterns and physiological responses to exercise in people with disabilities. The availability of such information will be helpful to nurses in counseling those with disabilities.

A variety of smoking cessation treatments are effective with the disabled as with well populations. These treatments can be used with groups of smokers who have chronic illnesses (Wewers and Ahijevych, 1996).

In addition to those with disability, caregivers also need health promotion. Spousal caregivers are especially vulnerable to health problems. This results from the relentless demands of caregiving combined with the grief process associated with changes in role expectations (Jackson and Cleary, 1995).

It is especially important to establish lifelong, health-promoting behaviors in children who are disabled. Unfortunately, parents may be so overwhelmed by care for such children that this aspect of care is not considered. Furthermore, health promotion and disease protection for those who are physically compromised often have not been emphasized in primary care or in rehabilitation. Table 30-3 summarizes issues that limit access to health care and health promotion for those who are physically compromised (Gans et al, 1993; Nosek, 1992).

Access to physicians' offices can be improved in the following areas (Jones and Tamari, 1997):
- Transportation and entrance to the facility
- Entrance to the office
- Waiting rooms
- Restrooms
- Examination rooms
- General building features

> **WHAT DO YOU THINK?** *Nurses should participate in analyzing various types of data, e.g., traffic accident patterns, to identify problems that could be improved with public health approaches/interventions.*

HEALTHY PEOPLE 2000 OBJECTIVES

Appendix A.1 summarizes the *Healthy People 2000* objectives. Clearly many of the national health goals that apply to people without disabling conditions also apply to people who are physically compromised. For example, Objective 17 deals with diabetes mellitus and the resulting disabling complications. Other objectives with clear relevance to the disabled person include those that deal with physical activity and fitness, nutrition, educational and community-based programs, unintentional injuries, occupational safety and health, environmental health, oral health, maternal and infant health, immunization and infectious diseases, and clinical preventive services. Sexually transmitted diseases, Objective 19, may also be seen to apply to the infants who are congenitally infected (USDHHS, 1991).

When the *Healthy People 2000* project started, those involved in developing the objectives recognized the limited data available for many health problems. Therefore Objective 22, concerned with surveillance and data systems, was included. As a result, CDC has obtained and provided more useful data on conditions that lead to disability in this country.

Examples of recent reports on surveillance results, with implications for disability prevention or management, include those on the incidence of birth defects in the United

TABLE 30-3 Impediments to Primary Health Care of the Physically Compromised

ISSUES	EXAMPLES
Transportation	May not be able to drive; limited flexibility in public/private transporation; may need specially equipped van
Access to clinic/office	Entrances, halls, restrooms may all be inadequate. Examination tables, scales, life equipment unavailable or inappropriate. Increased time needed for disabled client's visit.
Inadequate care from primary care providers	Limited or no training in primary care needs/health promotion of those with disabilities; lack of understanding reasons that those with disabilities often delay treatment until at crisis levels; limited ability to distinguish between progress in a disability and different, new health problems.
Information given to clients	Often unavailable or available only to few specialists; may not have been given basic health information in school; most have never received comprehensive rehabilitation.
Finances	Health maintenance/health promotion costly: good food, someone to obtain and prepare it; exercise: transporation, fees of facilities and assistant with exercise.
Personal assistance	Needed by some with disabilities for most basic health activities, hygiene, laundry, etc.

Base on data from Gans BM: *Arch Phys Med Rehabil* 74(12-S):S15, 1993; Nosek MA: *J Womens Health* 1(4), 1992

States and toy-related injuries among U.S. children and teenagers. Surveillance activities include identifying children with fetal alcohol syndrome (FAS) and those who were seriously hearing impaired (CDC, 1997). Preventive-care practices are crucial in reducing the complications and disability from chronic disease. Such information can be useful for nurses working with clients.

HEALTHY CITIES

Healthy Communities 2000 (APHA, 1991) gives communities a way to establish local goals to achieve the objectives of *Healthy People 2000*. One of the subsystems within a community that is identified as a committee is Population Groups (Flynn et al, 1993). These committees should include, in addition to "able-bodied people," those who are physically compromised or their representatives if they are unable to participate. It would also be useful if those who are physically compromised could participate on other committees (e.g., Education, Employment, Planning and Housing). Such involvement can aid people with disabilities to enhance their leadership skills, specifically interpersonal and decision-making skills. These improved skills can lead to empowerment of those in this population (Walker and Doherty, 1994).

Families are grounded in the communities in which they live. Informal support networks, or systems, are key factors in assisting families. When such supports are inadequate, such formal helping systems as social/psychological services, provided by a healthy community, might be key (Patterson and Blum, 1996).

Requirements for a health city include the following:
1. The ability to meet developmental needs (food, clothing, shelter), functional and aesthetic needs, communication and networks, ecological considerations, and attention to competing priorities for creation of a stable infrastructure.
2. The flexibility to cope with change or crisis.
3. The competence that makes it possible for individuals or groups to use the city.
4. The ability to perform its educational role, which is defined as learning that permits questions; is free from prejudiced opinions; and is open to the possibility that there are different ways of viewing a problem.

These requirements apply to all citizens, including those who are physically compromised. One of the major elements of the Healthy Cities project as described in Chapter 17 is the understanding that the health of communities and people who live in them are dependent upon the environment. *Healthy People 2000* (USDHHS, 1991) environmental health objectives include those for control of asthma and lead poisoning from environmental conditions. Asthma is a relatively common reason for being physically compromised. Lead poisoning may result in a developmental disability in learning. Tobacco use may also be regarded as having significance for the environmental effects on health. Objective 3.5 deals with reducing the beginning of smoking by children and youth, which is influenced by imitation of others and by advertisement. Also, Objective 3.5 recognizes the importance of second-hand smoke on children's health.

Healthy cities may support some of the needs of those with disabilities by encouraging participation in sports. Participation in athletic competition is beneficial to most individuals who wish to take part (Rothner, 1996). Athletes with disabilities demonstrate the same percentage of injury as the athlete without disability in similar sports activities. As with athletes with no disabilities, preparation and supervision of the disabled can prevent many injuries.

Another example of a healthy city is that almost all states have developed initiatives to provide families with developmentally disabled children a variety of supportive goods and services. Much of this has been provided at local levels. Healthy communities explore ways to include people of all ages with disabilities in their communities. Services promote collaboration and integration of the individual into the community and decision-making occurs at the local level (Agosta and Melda, 1996).

The greatest obstacles faced by people with disabilities are often attitudinal ones. Programs that place responsibility for rehabilitation and integration within the community can foster a better understanding of the issues. Until significant progress is made in this area, problems of access in communities that serve to ignore those with disabilities will continue (Peat, 1997).

In a recent report, the Institute of Medicine (1996) recommended that government public health agencies develop the capacity to identify and work in partnership with all the agencies that influence a community's health. This approach may emphasize the involvement of such established institutions and agencies as local hospitals and health departments (Burger, McMahon, Sellaro, and Stefanak, 1998). The nurse working with individuals or populations who are physically compromised can be a member of the partnership.

ROLE OF THE NURSE

Many factors influence the role of the nurse who works with those who are physically compromised. These factors include, of course, the community's awareness of those who are disabled and its commitment to their health needs. But of particular influence is the agency in which

the nurse works. The structure and priorities of an agency determine whether a nurse will carry a general caseload or focus on service to a special population. If funding sources are dedicated to particular programs (e.g., tuberculosis control, maternal-child health services), care for those who are physically compromised may be dispersed throughout several program areas and may be difficult to identify.

In dealing with those who are physically compromised, the nurse's role may further change as the focus varies from the levels of individuals, families, groups, or entire communities. For instance, the nurse may be a caregiver and apply the nursing process and principles of epidemiology at any of the above listed levels. This may include, among other things, assessing, implementing, and evaluating technical care for a ventilator-dependent client at home.

A second role, long associated with community health nurses, is that of *educator*, that is, one who provides clients at any level with sufficient knowledge to enable them to decide on the most appropriate behavior for their own needs. The nurse may provide an entire community with information about reducing disability by decreasing a specific cause, such as spinal cord injury. The closely-related *counseling* role of the community health nurse is of value in that clients learn to improve their problem-solving skills as the community health nurse guides them.

The community health nurse's role as an *advocate* for individuals and families or groups of those who are physically compromised is especially important. An advocate is

---

HOW TO *Promote Appropriate Use of Asthma Medications by Children*

A. Collaborate/coordinate efforts with health care provider managing child's asthma.
  1. Personnel in all areas in which child uses drugs need to be informed of regimen
  2. Be aware of factors that could affect adherence to regimen:
     a. Prolonged therapy
     b. Medications used prophylactically
     c. Delayed consequences of nonadherence
     d. Drugs expensive, hard to use
     e. Family concerns about side effects
     f. Adherence less likely with mild or severe asthma; most likely with moderate asthma
     g. Child with cognitive or emotional problems
     h. Poorly functioning family
     i. Strong alternative health beliefs
     j. Multiple caregivers
B. Assess child's adherence to regimen
  1. Count pills; float test for remaining amount in inhalers (gross estimate)
  2. Ask child, "In an average week, how many puffs of your inhaler do you actually get?"
  3. Refill history from pharmacist (information can be obtained from child's health care provider)

C. Interventions
  1. Educate child, parents, and other caregivers
  2. Encourage adaptation of regimen to family's needs
     a. Health care provider may need additional information about family situation
     b. Signed, dated, written permission to exchange information with such a provider is needed
  3. Encourage consideration of acceptability of medication to child, family
  4. Be encouraging, caring, supportive, and willing to work with family
  5. Follow-up and monitor progress closely, including school attendance, etc. when appropriate
  6. Consider home visits, e.g., to assess/manage environmental triggers
  7. Identify an "asthma partner," another adult besides parents when they do not reliably monitor child
  8. Use a contract for adherence
  9. In extreme cases, especially with young and/or ill children, consider reporting family to Child Protective Services for medical neglect

someone who speaks on behalf of others who are unable to speak for themselves. One of the potential problems with this role is that the nurse may unintentionally foster excessive dependence by individuals, families, or other groups. The nurse focuses on using advocacy to support those who need this service. At the same time, the chance to observe the nurse's data-collecting and negotiating skills can be of use as a model for clients who are capable of using such knowledge. For example, the nurse might advocate a school environment that is adapted to the specific needs of children who are wheelchair mobile but who do not necessarily have to be limited to their chairs, without explicitly telling the children what they should do about the use of their wheelchairs. The nurse may help a family caregiver of a disabled individual by validating that the caregiver's own basic needs are being sacrificed and by identifying ways that this problem can be moderated.

As a *referral agent,* the nurse maintains current information about agencies whose services are of potential use to those who are disabled. Referral, one of the most important functions of the nurse, is the process of directing clients to the resources that can meet their needs. For self-directed clients and families, information about an agency's services, phone number, and address may be adequate. For a family with little understanding of how systems work for a developmentally delayed child, more specific guidance and case conferences with the local school may be necessary to coordinate the child's health-related and educational needs.

As a *primary care provider,* one who gives essential care universally accessible to all, the nurse may be the most logical person to ensure that primary prevention for other health problems (e.g., communicable diseases), and information about health promotion are made available to clients who are physically compromised. On a more individualized basis, the *case manager* role means meeting the needs of clients by developing a plan of care to reach that goal. The nurse may also see that others carry out the plan and is responsible for evaluating the plan's effectiveness. For example, a client who has been disabled through complications of diabetes mellitus may have several complex needs related to dealing with immediate problems such as adjusting to the amputation of one or more limbs, learning strategies for better management and compliance to slow progress of other complications. The nurse or case manager will, with the client and family, develop a plan to meet those needs and establish a time frame to evaluate specific outcomes.

In the role of *coordinator,* the nurse is not responsible for developing the overall plan of client care. Instead, responsibilities include assisting clients and families by organizing and integrating the resources of other agencies or care providers to meet clients' needs most efficiently. For example, with the family's agreement, the nurse may arrange for a family to see a social worker on the same day that they bring their child to be followed up in a pediatric cardiology clinic.

The nurse performs the functions of a *collaborator* by taking part in joint decision making with clients, families, groups, and communities. Collaboration may, of course, be part of the community health nurse's role with other care providers, too. This role is of particular importance as the nurse seeks to involve those who are physically disabled in community-level decisions that affect their lives. An example is working with agencies or groups who make decisions about community housing for those who are physically compromised.

The role of the nurse as *casefinder* is historically a basic part of public health nursing. Nurses identify individuals with disabilities who need services they are not currently receiving. Developmental, vision, and hearing screening of young children by the nurse are examples of ways in which this role is carried out. It is important to bear in mind that, although the nurse's efforts are for a particular client, the focus of casefinding is on monitoring the health status of entire groups or communities. Casefinding in tuberculosis may indicate the increase in a population of this chronic disease, which is also a communicable disease. The nurse may also identify those who are members of vulnerable populations and who are not yet physically compromised. Such people may have limited or no access to health promotion or disease prevention services or may be unaware of those for which they are eligible.

The nurse may function as a change agent at all levels, including the health care delivery system. A *change agent* is one who originates and creates change. This process includes identifying a need for change, enlightening and motivating others as to this need, and starting and directing the proposed change. The nurse may function in the role by helping to obtain more appropriate health care services for those who are physically compromised.

LEGISLATION

A nurse who works with clients who are physically compromised may have a general caseload of clients of all ages while another, such as a school nurse, may see clients in a specific age group. A nurse's need to know about laws related to specific groups will vary with the population that is the nurse's focus of care. Box 30-3 summarizes categories of historically significant federal legislation designed to benefit those who are disabled. For in-depth information about federal laws in each category since 1914, consult the National Information Center for Children and Youth with Disabilities (1991) and Reed (1992).

Rehabilitation services were originally developed through legislation for veterans of World War I. In time, others who were physically compromised were regarded less as sources of embarrassment to their families and more as citizens who should participate as fully as possible in all aspects of society. This change in attitudes is reflected in major laws being passed. Most recently, the Americans with Disabilities Act of 1990, PL 101-336, with subsequent amendments has had far-reaching effects on the civil rights of those in the community

EDUCATION
Early childhood special education
Elementary and Secondary Education Act and Amendments
Vocational education for those who are disabled

REHABILITATION
Vocational
Medical, including Medicare and Medicaid
Rehabilitation

SERVICES
Economic assistance
Facility construction and architectural design
Deinstitutionalization and independent living
Civil Rights and Advocacy

Based on data from National Information Center for Children and Youth with Disabilities: *NICHCY News Digest* 1(1):12, 1991.

who are physically compromised. Significantly, this act includes all of the following:

• Persons who have a physical or mental impairment that substantially limits one or more of the major life activities of such an individual
• Persons who have a record of such an impairment
• Persons who are perceived or regarded as having a disability

Examples include someone with a condition that is not presently disabling (e.g., hypertension or a mild congenital special deformity) .

Herr (1997) describes the Individuals with Disabilities Education Act of 1990 as one of those rare pieces of landmark legislation. Everyone concerned needs to maintain the effectiveness of such legislation so that school systems will be fair and provide administrative equity to all. Actions can include the following:

1. Promoting the fundamental principle that "all means all" because all children with disabilities must be educated
2. Leveling the "playing field" by retaining the balance of due process safeguards to prevent abuses and infringements of rights
3. Respecting partnerships and the orderly process that the Act promotes now
4. Understanding the interrelated role of advocacy and monitoring to ensure compliance with the law
5. Strengthening the Act to help children with disabilities and their families to live productive lives.

Nurses are in positions to provide advocacy for these children by supporting such actions.

For older adults, the ADA and the adoption of living wills and related protections by various states are impor-

tant recent legislative changes. These support the legal rights of older and disabled people in attempting to live as normal lives as possible and to make their own decisions about serious or terminal illnesses (Slavitt and LaBant, 1996).

In addition, most states and many large cities and counties have their own laws prohibiting discrimination on the basis of disability. Such laws sometimes offer greater protection to employees by extending coverage to smaller employers, by using more expansive definitions of disability than those used under the ADA, and by expanding the duty to accommodate to require that employers assist employees with disabilities to move to new positions for which they are qualified. As such, it is important to be familiar with state law in the area in which nurses practice and how it may affect employer obligations to employees with disabilities (Pennell, 1997). Considering the potential significance of major legislation for nurses' practice, it may be necessary to provide or obtain continuing education on the topic.

The human immunodeficiency virus (HIV) epidemic, with the consequent disability and death by acquired immunodeficiency syndrome (AIDS), has been viewed as a condition in which those with HIV infection should be protected by law under disability rights. However, the recent use of new drugs implies to many that this is becoming a chronic but not disabling disorder. Parmet and Jackson (1997) believe that no longer considering HIV infection as a disability is dangerous. They fear that such an attitude will threaten legal protection of people with this condition.

The ADA has been an effective means of addressing allegations of employment discrimination brought forward by people with seizure disorders. However, it has not increased the number of people with disabilities who are employed. In combination with employer education and rehabilitation counseling, legislative protection can help those with epilepsy to be more successful in pursuing employment opportunities (Troxell, 1997).

The Federal Rehabilitation Act of 1973 and the Americans with Disabilities Act have given physically impaired athletes the legal means to challenge medical sports participation decisions. Health care providers who work with physically compromised individuals must recognize the potential conflict between medical safety recommendations and the expanded legal rights of these individuals. Prospective athletes, after being fully informed about risks of participation in sports, have greater responsibility in the decision-making process (Nichols, 1996).

There have been recent changes in the types of legal ways to correct violations that inhibit a student's right to free appropriate public education (FAPE). There has been increased use of compensating education, i.e., the awareness of additional educational services to a student. These have often been in the form of educational services beyond the age of eligibility for past violations to a student's right to an appropriate education. In addition, courts have increasingly considered monetary damages for "mental distress" or "pain and suffering" as potential remedies for people with disabilities who are judged to have been denied FAPE (Katsiyannis and Maag, 1997). Nurses may be in positions to emphasize to school systems and to parents of children with disabilities that compliance with the Individuals with Disabilities Education Act (IDEA) and other related laws is more cost effective in the long run.

In 1986 Part H was added to IDEA, expanding coverage to include infants and toddlers from birth to age two. Many of these children have multiple, serious health problems. Early intervention specialists, including nurses, are being faced with Do Not Resuscitate (DNR) orders. However, there is no specific legal guidance on implementing DNR orders in community settings (Brown and Valluzzi, 1995). All children with special health care needs should have clear emergency procedures and guidelines within their Individual Family Service Plan (IFSP) at school. All involved staff should be informed of the program's policies for emergency procedures, including DNR orders, and should be trained in appropriate interventions.

Assisted suicide of people with disabilities is an area with many ethical, legal, and practice considerations for health care providers. Part of the discussion focuses on whether physician-assisted suicide (PAS) should be considered as part of a medical treatment continuum. Another consideration is the possibility that viewing assisted suicide as a public health issue may provide insight into preventive measures to lower risk factors. This can also improve the lives of members of the community who are disabled (Blanck, Kirschner, and Bienen, 1997).

Both federal and state legislation and rules and regulations have implications for the nurse working with those who are disabled. The nurse must remember that other state and federal laws and rules and regulations are applicable for all citizens. For example, some states have wrongful death laws that specify who must be consulted and who can make decisions about the type of resuscitation to be used and under what circumstances.

🌱 clinical application

A referral was made to a public health department from a nearby regional level III neonatal intensive care unit (NICU) regarding discharge plans for a developmentally delayed infant. The infant, Joel, was born at 27 weeks of gestation and had remained in intensive care for 7 months. His hospital course was complicated by hyaline membrane disease, bronchopulmonary dysplasia, and intraventricular hemorrhage. At the time of discharge, Joel was receiving neither supplemental oxygen nor medications and was taking all of his feedings orally. There were strong indications of spastic diplegia, and he was diagnosed as having severe retinopathy of prematurity with the expectation of eventual

blindness. Family financial resources were extremely limited. Although Medicaid coverage was available for subsequent needs, the family owed over $100,000 to the hospital. Joel's grandmother would babysit while Mary, Joel's mother, finished high school. Joel's father, who was also 17 years old and unemployed, had not been active with Mary and her mother in the hospital discharge planning program. His involvement with Mary and Joel was expected to be minimal. The hospital was seeking a home evaluation before discharge.

What would you consider to be the first step in completing the home evaluation?

Answer is in the back of the book.

🅚EY POINTS

- The community health nurse has numerous opportunities to influence the development of disabling conditions through health promotion, especially health education for parents who might be high risks for having a disabled child, for children at risk for accidents and injuries, and for adults with chronic illnesses who might prevent disability through careful health practices.
- The majority of the objectives identified in *Healthy People 2000* apply to physically compromised individuals, their families, and communities.
- Physically compromised people need to participate in health promotion to prevent the onset of a new health disruption, to strengthen their well-functioning aspects, and to prevent further deterioration of their health problem.
- Nursing interventions for physically compromised clients requires attention to their health, as well as to the environment in which they live.
- Nurses influence policy decisions that affect the health and well-being of physically compromised individuals.
- Nurses must know both federal and state laws pertaining to disabilities to most effectively assist clients and their families.

🔍 critical thinking activities

1. Divide either the class or clinical group into two teams and debate: Children with developmental disabilities should (should not) be mainstreamed into classrooms with nondisabled children.
2. During a home visit to an adult (and then to a child) who has a chronic illness that leaves them physically compromised, answer the following questions:
   a. Could this disability have been prevented? If so, what steps much the nurse have taken to provide health promotion activities to prevent the occurrence of the disability condition?
   b. What role, if any, does the environment play in the onset of this compromising health condition?
   c. What preventive activities are currently needed to assure the highest possible quality of life for this person?

critical thinking activities—cont'd

3. For the next week look at each building that you enter :
   a. What accommodations have been made to allow physically compromised people to enter this building?
   b. What accommodations should still be made?
   c. Who should pay for these architectural accommodations?

4. Spend one day following your usual schedule using either crutches or a wheelchair, so you can understand better what it means to be physically compromised.
5. Using a telephone book or community resource directory for your town, identify all agencies whose scope of work would be devoted to assisting physically compromised individuals and their families

Bibliography

Abstracts of the International Seminar on Women and Disability, *Sexual Disabil* 15(1):11, 1997.

Agosta J, Melda K: Supporting families who provide care at home for children with disabilities, *Exceptional Children* 62(3):271, 1996.

Anke AGW et al: Long-term prevalence of impairments and disabilities after multiple trauma, *J Trauma: Injury Infect Crit Care* 42(1):54, 1997.

American Public Health Association: *Healthy communities 2000: model standards,* ed 3, Washington, DC, 1991, the Association.

Badley EM: An introduction to the concepts and classifications of the international classification of impairments, disabilities, and handicaps, *Disabil Rehabil* 15(4):161, 1993.

Banja JD: Ethics, values, and world culture: the impact on rehabilitation, *Disabil Rehabil* 18(6):279, 1996.

Bennett T, DeLuca D, Bruns D: Putting inclusion into practice: perspectives of teachers and parents, *Exceptional Children* 64(1):115, 1997.

Betz CL: A systems approach to adolescent tansitions: an opportunity for nurses, *J Pediatr Nurs* 11(5):271, 1996.

Black SA, Ray LA, Markides KS: The prevalence and health burden of self-reported diabetes in older Mexican Americans: findings from the Hispanic established populations for epidemiological studies of the elderly, *Am J Public Health* 89(4):546, 1999.

Blanc PD: Self-reported carpal tunnel syndrome: predictors of work disability from the National Health Interview Survey Occupational Health Supplement, *Am J Indust Med* 30(3):362, 1996.

Blanck P, Kirschner K, Bienen L: Socially assisted dying and people with disabilities: some emerging legal, medical, and policy implications, *Ment Phys Disabil Law Rep* 21(4):538, 1977.

Blatter BM: Paternal occupational exposure around conception and spina bifida in offspring, *Am J Indust Med* 32(3):283, 1997.

Bockenek WL: Primary care for persons with disabilities, *Am J Phys Med Rehabil* 76(3;suppl):S43, 1997.

Bonner BL, Crow SM, Hensley LD: State efforts to identify maltreated children with disabilities: a follow-up study, *Child Maltreatment* 2(1):52, 1997.

Boult C: Decreasing disability in the 21st century: the future effects of controlling six fatal and nonfatal conditions, *Am J Public Health* 86(10):1388, 1996.

Bowden KM, McDiarmid MA: Occupationally acquired tuberculosis: what's known, *J Occup Med* 36(3):320, 1994.

Braddock B: Medicaid and persons with developmental disabilities, *Ment Retard* 34(5):331, 1996.

Branch LG: Research on disability: where is it leading? *J Gerontol* 51B(4):S171, 1996.

Bringewatt RJ: Integrating care for people with chronic conditions, *Creative Nurs* 2(2):7, 1996.

Brown AR, Mulley GP: Injuries sustained by caregivers of disabled elderly people, *Age Aging* 26(1):21, 1997.

Brown P, Nourse SW: Moving from school to adult life, *Phys Med Rehabil Clin North Am* 8(2):359, 1997.

Brown SE, Valluzzi JL: Do not resuscitate orders in early intervention settings: who should make the decision? *Infants Young Children,* 7(3):13, 1995.

Browning SR: Agricultural injuries among older Kentucky farmers: the farm family health and hazard surveillance study, *Am J Indust Med* 33(4):341, 1998.

Buchanan RJ: Compliance with tuberculosis drug regimens: incentives and enablers offered by public health departments, *Am J Public Health* 87(12):2014, 1997.

Burger A: Healthy valley 2000, *Am J Public Health* 88(5):821, 1998.

Centers for Disease Control and Prevention: Prevalence of work disability, United States, 1990, *MMWR* 42(39):757, 1993.

Centers for Disease Control and Prevention: Prevalence of selected risk factors for chronic disease by education level in racial/ethnic populations, United States, 1991-1992, *MMWR* 43(48):894, 1994a.

Centers for Disease Control and Prevention: Prevalence of disabilities and associated health conditions, United States, 1991-92, *MMWR* 43(40):730, 1994b.

Centers for Disease Control and Prevention: Diabetes-specific preventive-care practices among adults in a managed-care population–Colorado, Behavioral Risk Factor Surveillance System, 1995, *MMWR* 46(43):1018, 1997a.

Centers for Disease Control and Prevention: Preventive-care knowledge and practices among persons with diabetes mellitus–North Carolina, Behavioral Risk Factor Surveillance System, 1994-1995, *MMWR* 46(43):1023, 1997b.

Centers for Disease Control and Prevention: Serious hearing impairment among children aged 3-10 years–Atlanta, Georgia, 1991-1993, *MMWR* 46(45):1073, 1997c.

Centers for Disease Control and Prevention: State-specific prevalence of cigarette smoking among adults, and children's and adolescents' exposure to environmental tobacco smoke, *MMWR* 46(44):1038, 1997d.

Centers for Disease Control and Prevention: Surveillance for fetal alcohol syndrome using multiple sources–Atlanta, Georgia, 1981-1989, *MMWR* 46(47):1118, 1997e.

Centers for Disease Control and Prevention: Temporal trends in the incidence of birth defects, *MMWR* 46(49):1171, 1997f.

Centers for Disease Control and Prevention: Toy-related injuries among children and teenagers–United States, 1996, *MMWR* 46(50):1185, 1997g.

Centers for Disease Control and Prevention: Trends in the prevalence and incidence of self-reported diabetes mellitus–United States, 1980-1994, *MMWR* 46(43):1014, 1997h.

Chan F et al: Vocational assessment and evaluation of people with disabilities, *Phys Med Rehabil Clin North Am* 8(2):311, 1997.

Chapman LJ et al: Agricultural safety efforts by county health departments in Wisconsin, *Public Health Rep* 111(5):437, 1996.

Clark DO: US trends in disability and institutionalization among older blacks and whites, *Am J Public Health* 87(3):328, 1997.

Clawson JA: A child with chronic illness and the process of family adaptation, *J Pediatr Nurs* 11(1):52, 1996.

Cloud HH: Expanding roles for dietitians working with persons with developmental disabilities, *J Am Dietet Assoc* 97(2):129, 1997.

Cole KL, Roberts MC, McNeal RE: Children's perceptions of ill peers: effects of disease, grade, and impact variables, *Children's Health Care* 25(2):107, 1996.

Cooper C: The crippling consequences of fractures and their impact on quality of life, *Am J Med* 103(2A):12S, 1997.

Daly MC, Bound J: Worker adaptation and employer accommodation following the onset of a health impairment, *J Gerontol* 51B(2):S53, 1996.

Davidhizar R, Shearer R: Helping the client with chronic disability achieve high-level wellness, *Rehabil Nurs* 22(3):131, 1997.

Davies M, Howlin P, Udwin O: Independence and adaptive behavior in adults with Williams Syndrome, *Am J Med Genetics* 70(2):188, 1997.

Davis MH, O'Brien E: Profile of persons with disabilities in Medicare and Medicaid, *Health Care Financ Rev* 17(4):179, 1996.

Dawkins JL: Bullying, physical disability and the pediatric patient, *Development Med Child Neurol* 38(7):603, 1996.

Decouflé P et al: Mental retardation in ten-year-old children in relation to their mothers' employment during pregnancy, *Am J Ind Med* 24(5):567, 1993.

Dickson IIG: Problems with the ICIDH definition of impairment, *Disabil Rehabil* 18(1):52, 1996.

Dokken DL, Syndnor-Greenberg N: Helping families mobilize their personal resources, *Pediatr Nurs* 24(1):66, 1998.

Drotar D: Relating parent and family functioning to the psychological adjustment of children with chronic health conditions: what have we learned? what do we need to know? *J Pediatr Psychol* 22(2):149, 1997.

Dunlop DD, Hughes SL, Manheim LM: Disabilities in activities of daily living: patterns of change and a hierarchy of disability, *Am J Public Health* 87(3):387, 1997.

Ehrlich GE, Wolfe F: On the difficulties of disability and its determination, *Rheumat Dis Clin North Am* 22(3):613, 1996.

Eliopoulos C: Chronic care coaches: helping people to help people, *Home Healthcare Nurse* 15(3):185, 1997.

England D: Accessibly inn correct, *Accent on Living* 41(3):26, 1996.

Favazza PC, Odom SL: Promoting positive attitudes of kindergarten-age children toward people with disabilities, *Exceptional Children* 63(3):405, 1997.

Ferrara MS, Buckley WE: Athletes with disabilities injury registry, *Adapted Phys Activ Q* 13(1):50, 1996.

Fisman S et al: Risk and protective factors affecting the adjustment of siblings of children with chronic disabilities, *J Am Acad Child Adolesc Psychiatry* 35(11):1532, 1996.

Floyd FJ, Gallagher EM: Parental stress, care demands, and use of support services for school-age children with disabilities and behavior problems, *Fam Relat* 46(4):359, 1997.

Flynn BC: Healthy cities: the future of public health, *Health Trends Transit* 4(3):12, 1993.

Fontana SA et al: The delivery of preventive services in primary care practices according to chronic disease status, *Am J Public Health* 87(7):1190, 1997.

Fowler SB: Health promotion in chronically ill older adults, *J Neurosci Nurs* 29(1):39, 1997.

Francis S: Disability and chronic illness. In Johnson BS: *Child, adolescent and family psychiatric nursing*, Philadelphia, 1995, J.B. Lippincott.

Gabor LM, Farnham R: The impact of children with chronic illness and/or developmental disabilities on low-income, single-parent families, *Infant-Toddler Interven* 6(2):167, 1996.

Gans BM, Mann NR, Becker BE: Delivery of primary care to the physically challenged, *Arch Phys Med Rehabil* 74(12-S):S-15, 1993.

Garlow JE, Turnbull HR III: Families and disability, *Vision 2010* 1(1):26, 1993.

Gates MF, Lackey NR: Youngsters caring for adults with cancer, *Image J Nurs Scholar* 30(1):11, 1998.

Gillen M et al: Insury severity associated with nonfatal construction falls, *Am J Indust Med* 32(6):647, 1997.

Guerriere D, McKeever P: Mothering children who survive brain injuries: playing the hand you're dealt, *J Soc Pediatr Nurses* 2(3):105, 1997.

Hadadian A: Attachment relationships and its significance for young children with disabilities, *Infant-Toddler Interven* 6(1):1, 1996.

Hart BG: Chronic pain management in the workplace, *AAOHN J* 45(9):451, 1997.

Heerkens YF et al: Impairments and disabilities—the difference: proposal for adjustment of the international classification of impairments, disabilities, and handicaps, *Phys Ther* 74(5):430, 1994.

Herr SS: Reauthorization of the Individuals with Disabilities Education Act, *Ment Retard* 35(2):131, 1997.

Hogan SE, Evers SE: A nutritional rehabilitation program for persons with severe physical and developmental disabilities, *J Am Dietet Assoc* 97(2):162, 1997.

Holzer CE et al: The demographics of disability in the south, *Comm Ment Health J* 32(5):431, 1996.

Hubbard JR, Everett AS, Khan MA: Alcohol and drug abuse in patients with physical disabilities. *Am J Drug Alcohol Abuse* 22(2):215, 1996.

Imrie R: Rethinking the relationships between disability, rehabilitation, and society, *Disabil Rehabil* 19(7):263, 1997.

Institute of Medicine: *Healthy communities: new partnerships for the future of public health*, Washington, DC, 1996, National Academy Press.

Ireys HT, Silver EJ: Perception of the impact of child's chronic illness: does it predict maternal mental health? *Development Behav Pediatr* 17(2):77, 1996.

Ireys HT et al: Schooling, employment, and idleness in young adults with serious physical health conditions: effects of age, disability status, and parental education, *J Adolesc Health* 19(1):25, 1996.

Johnson-Webb KD, Baer LD, Gesler WM: What is rural? issues and considerations, *J Rural Health* 13(3):253, 1997.

Jones KE, Tamari IE: Making our offices universally accessible: guidelines for physicians, *Canad Med Assoc J* 156(5):647, 1997.

Katsiyannis A, Maag JW: Ensuring appropriate education: emerging remedies, litigation, compensation, and other legal considerations, *Exceptional Children* 64(4):451, 1997.

Kawaga-Singer M et al: Panel III: behavioral risk factors related to chronic diseases in ethnic minorities, *Health Psychol* 14(7):613, 1995.

Keller-Byrne JE et al: A meta-analysis of non-Hodgkin's lymphoma among farmers in the central United States, *Am J Industr Med* 31(4):442, 1997.

Kidd P et al: The process of chore teaching: implications for farm youth injury, *Fam Comm Health* 19(4):78, 1997.

Kington RS, Smith JP: Socioeconomic status and racial and ethnic differences in functional status associated with chronic diseases, *Am J Public Health* 87(5):805, 1997.

Kochhar S, Scott CG: Living arrangements of SSI recipients, *Soc Sec Bull* 60(1):18, 1997.

Landrigan PJ, McCammon JB: Child labor—still with us, *Publ Health Rep* 112(6):466, 1997.

Lawrence RH, Jette AM: Disentangling the disablement process, *J Gerontol* 51B(4):S173, 1996.

Lee BC, Jenkins LS, Westaby JD: Factors influencing exposure of children to major hazards on family farms, *J Rural Health* 13(3):206, 1997.

Lefley HP: Synthesizing the family caregiving studies: implications for service plan-

Continued

Bibliography—cont'd

ning, social policy, and further research, *Fam Relations* 46(4):443, 1997.

Liao Y et al: Socioeconomic status and morbidity in the last years of life, *Am J Public Health* 89(4):569, 1999.

Lindsey E: Health within illness: experiences of chronically ill/disabled people, *J Adv Nurs* 24(3):465, 1996.

Lipper EG et al: Partnerships in school care: meeting the needs of New York City schoolchildren with complex medical conditions, *Am J Public Health* 87(2):291, 1997.

Lishner DM et al: Access to primary health care among persons with disabilities in rural areas: a summary of the literature, *J Rural Health* 12(1):45, 1996.

Lubinski R, Moscato BS, Willer BS: Prevalence of speaking and hearing disabilities among adults with traumatic brain injury from a national household survey, *Brain Injury* 11(2):103, 1997.

Lukes E, Wachs JE: Keys to disability management: a guide for the occupational health nurse, *Am Assoc Occupat Health Nurses J* 44(3):141, 1996.

Mallory BL: The role of social policy in life-cycle transitions, *Exceptional Children* 62(3):213, 1996.

Mansell S, Sobsey D, Moskal R: Clinical findings among sexually abused children with and without developmental disabilities, *Ment Retard* 36(1):12, 1998.

Manton KG, Corder L, Stallard E: Chronic disability trends in elderly United States populations: 1982-1994. *Proc Nat Acad Sci USA* 94(6):2593, 1997.

Marks NF: Caregiving across the life span, *Fam Relat* 45(1):27, 1996.

McCallion P, Janicki M, Grant-Griffin L: Exploring the impact of culture and acculturation on older families caregiving for persons with developmental disabilities, *Fam Relat* 46(4):347, 1997.

McNeil JM: Disabilities among children aged 17-years–United States, 1991-1992, *JAMA* 274(14):1112, 1995.

Menard MR: Comparison of disability behavior after different sites and types of injury in a workers' compensation population, *J Occupat Environment Med* 38(11):1161, 1996.

Mengel MH, Marcus DB, Dunkle RE: "What will happen to my child when I'm gone?" a support and education group for aging parents as caregivers, *Gerontolog* 36(6):816, 1996.

Mueller C, Schur C, O'Connell J: Prescription drug spending: the impact of age and chronic disease status, *Am J Public Health* 87(10):1626, 1997.

Murphy KE: Parenting a technology assisted infant: coping with occupational stress, *Social Work Health Care* 24(3-4):113, 1997.

National Information Center for Children and Youth with Disabilities: Selected, key federal statutes affecting the education and civil rights of children and youth with disabilities, *NICHCY News Digest* 1(1):12, 1991.

Nelson PP: Library services for people with disabilities: results of a survey, *Bull Med Librar Assoc* 84(3):397, 1996.

Newby NM: Chronic illness and the family life-cycle, *J Adv Nurs* 23(4):786, 1996.

Nichols AW: Sports medicine and the Americans with Disabilities Act, *Clin J Sport Med* 6(3):190, 1996.

Nolan CM: Topics for our times: the increasing demand for tuberculosis services–a new encumbrance on tuberculosis control programs, *Am J Public Health* 87(4):551, 1997.

Nosek MA: Primary care issues for women with severe disabilities, *J Womens Health* 1(4):245, 1992.

Orr C, Schkade J: The impact of the classroom environment on defining function in school-based practice, *Am J Occupat Ther* 51(1):64, 1997.

Pablos-Mèndez A, Blustein J, Knirsch CA: The role of diabetes mellitus in the higher prevalence of tuberculosis among Hispanics, *Am J Public Health* 87(4):574, 1997.

Parmet WE, Jackson DJ: No longer disabled: the legal impact of the new social construction of HIV, *Am J Law Med* 23(1):7, 1997.

Patterson J, Blum RW: Risk and resilience among children and youth with disabilities, *Arch Pediatr Adolesc Med* 150(7):692, 1996.

Peat M: Attitudes and access: advancing the rights of people with disabilities, *Can Med Assoc J* 156(5):657, 1997.

Pennell FE, Johnson J: Legal and civil rights aspects of vocational rehabilitation, *Phys Med Rehabil Clin North Am* 8(2):245, 1997.

Peters DJ: Disablement observed, addressed, and experienced: integrating subjective experience into disablement models, *Disabil Rehabil* 18(12):593, 1996.

Peterson JW, Sterling YM, Weekes DP: Access to health care: perspectives of African American families with chronically ill children, *Fam Comm Health* 19(4):64, 1997.

Picavet HSJ, van den Bos GAM: The contributions of six chronic conditions to the total burden of mobility disability in the Dutch population, *Am J Public Health* 87(10):1680, 1997.

Ponzer S et al: Women and injuries–factors influencing recovery, *Women & Health* 25(3):47, 1997.

Porter S, Yuille JC, Bent A: A comparison of the eyewitness accounts of deaf and hearing children, *Child Abuse Negl* 19(1):51, 1995.

Pruchno R, Patrick JH, Burant CJ: African American and white mothers of adults with chronic disabilities: caregiving burden and satisfaction, *Fam Relat* 46(4):335, 1997.

Rabiner DJ et al: Metropolitan versus non-metropolitan differences in functional status and self-care practice: findings from a national sample of community-dwelling older adults, *J Rural Health* 13(1):14, 1997.

Reed KL: History of federal legislation for persons with disabilities, *Am J Occup Ther* 46(5):397, 1992.

Reiss J et al: Enhancing the role public health nurses play in serving children with special health needs: an interactive video conference on Public Law 99-457 Part H, *Public Health Nurs* 13(5):345, 1996.

Reynolds MC, Heistad D: 20/20 analysis: estimating school effective-ness in serving students at the margins, *Exceptional Children* 63(4):439, 1997.

Richardson M: Addressing barriers: disabled rights and the implications for nursing of the social construct of disability, *J Adv Nurs* 25(6):1269, 1997.

Richmond TS: An explanatory model of variables influencing postinjury disability, *Nurs Res* 46(5):262, 1997.

Rimmer JH, Braddock D, Pitetti KH: Research on physical activity and disability: an emerging national priority, *Med Sci Sports Exercise* 28(11):1366, 1996.

Rimmerman A et al: Job placement of urban youth with developmental disabilities: research and implications, *J Rehabil* 62(1):56, 1996.

Rothner AD: Sports participation in children and adolescents with neurological impairments, *Va Med Q* 123(2):94, 1996.

Satariano WA: The disabilities of aging: looking to the physical environment, *Am J Public Health* 87(3):331, 1997.

Schilling LS, DeJesus E: Developmental issues in deaf children, *J Pediatr Health Care* 7(4):161, 1993.

Schoenberg NE, Coward RT: Residential differences in attitudes about barriers to using community-based services among older adults, *J Rural Health* 14(6):295, 1998.

Schulman MD et al: Farm work is dangerous for teens: agricultural hazards and injuries among North Carolina teens, *J Rural Health* 13(4):295, 1997.

Secrist-Mertz C et al: Helping families meet the nutritional needs of children with disabilities: an integrated model, *Children's Health Care* 26(3):151, 1997.

Simmonds MJ, Kumar S, Lechelt E: Psychosocial factors in disabling low back pain: causes or consequences? *Disabil Rehabil* 18(4):161, 1996.

Slavitt EB, LaBant TM: Living and leaving life on one's own terms: certain legal rights of older adults and persons with disabilities, *Topics Stroke Rehabil* 2(4):44, 1996.

Sobsey D: Letter to editor, *Child Abuse Neglect* 21(9):819, 1997.

Sobti A et al: Occupational physical activity and long-term risk of musculoskeletal symptoms: a national survey of post office pensioners, *Am J Industr Med* 32(1):76, 1997.

Stellman JM: Where women work and the hazards they may face on the job, *J Occup Health* 36(8):814, 1994.

Sterling YM, Peterson J, Weekes DP: African-American families with chronically ill children: oversights and insights, *J Pediatr Nurs* 12(5):292, 1997.

Strickland J, Strickland DL: Barriers to preventive health services for minority households in the rural South, *J Rural Health* 12(3):206, 1996.

Stuber ML: Psychiatric sequelae in seriously ill children and their families, *Psychiatr Clin North Am* 19(3):481, 1996.

Suris JC et al: Sexual behavior of adolescents with chronic disease and disability, *J Adolesc Health* 19(2):124, 1996.

Taanila A, Kokken J, Jörvelin M-J: The long-term effects of children's early-onset disability on marital relationships, *Development Med Child Neurol* 38(7):567, 1996.

Terman DL et al: Special education for students with disabilities: analysis and recommendations, *Future Children* 6(1):4, 1996.

Thorne S, McCormick J, Carty E: Deconstructing the gender neutrality of chronic illness and disability, *Health Care Women Internat* 18(1):1, 1997.

Thorne SE, Radford MJ, McCormick J: The multiple meanings of long-term gastrostomy in children with severe disability, *J Pediatr Nurs* 12(2), 89, 1997.

Troxell J: Epilepsy and employment: the Americans with Disabilities Act and its protections against employment discrimination, *Med Law* 16(2):375, 1997.

Trüster H, Brambring M: Early social-emotional development in blind infants, *Child Care Dev* 18(4):207, 1992.

Turner-Henson A, Holaday B: Daily life experiences for the chronically ill: a life-span perspective, *Fam Comm Health* 17(4):1, 1995.

Turner-Stokes L: Secondary safety of car adaptations for disabled motorists, *Disabil Rehabil* 18(6):317, 1996.

US Department of Health and Human Services: *Healthy people 2000: national health promotion and disease prevention objectives.* Washington, DC, 1991, USDHHS, Public Health Service.

US Office of Special Education and Rehabilitation Services: *Fifth annual report to Congress on the implementation of P.L. 94-142,* Washington, DC, 1983, US Government Printing Office.

Verbrugge LM, Rennert C, Madans JH: The great efficacy of personal and equipment assistance in reducing disability, *Am J Public Health* 87(3):384, 1997.

Voelke S: Discrepancies in parent and teacher ratings of adaptive behavior of children with multiple disabilities, *Ment Retard* 35(1):10, 1997.

Wagner MM, Blackorby J: Transition from high school to work or college: how special education students fare, *Future Children* 6(1):103, 1996.

Walker MB, Doherty AA: Healthy cities: empowering vulnerable populations for health through partnerships, *Fam Comm Health* 17(2):77, 1994.

Watt S et al: Age, adjustment and costs: a study of chronic illnesses, *Soc Sci Med* 44(10):1483, 1997.

Weekes DP: Adolescents growing up chronically ill: a life-span developmental view, *Fam Comm Health* 17(4):22, 1995.

Weinberg LA: Problems in educating abused and neglected children with disabilities, *Child Abuse Neglect* 21(9):889, 1997.

Wewers ME, Ahijevych KL: Smoking cessation interventions in chronic illness, *Annu Rev Nurs Res* 14:75, 1996.

Wilkins K, Park E: Chronic conditions, physical limitations and dependency among seniors living in the community, *Health Rep* 8(3):7, 1996.

Williams PD: Siblings and pediatric chronic illness: a review of the literature, *Internat J Nurs Stud* 34(4):312, 1997.

Winstead P, Bishop KK: Nurses and Public Law 102-119: a family-centered continuing education program, *J Contin Educ Nurs* 28(1):26, 1997.

Wolinsky FD, Fitzgerald JF, Stump TE: The effect of hip fracture on mortality, hospitalization, and functional status: a prospective study, *Am J Public Health* 87(3):398, 1997.

Wray LA: The role of ethnicity in the disability and work experience of preretirement-age Americans, *Gerontologist* 36(3):287, 1996.

Wright R: Physical disability: the long-term effects of child sexual abuse, *Sexual Disabil* 14(2):93, 1996

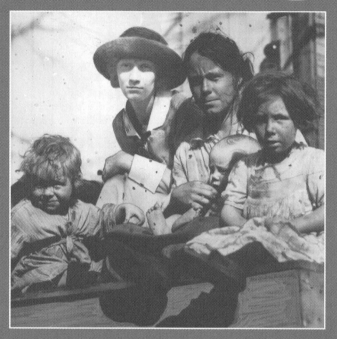

PART Six

Vulnerability:
Community-
Oriented
Nursing Issues
for the Twenty-
First Century

As the twenty-first century begins and the complexity of health and social problems increases, community health problems remain more a societal problem than an individual problem. Solutions will require an integrated social and health care approach that begins with a commitment to primary health care. Primary health care involves a partnership between public health and primary care to address the problems of the society as well as the individual.

Communities increasingly experience significant problems as a result of conditions that are often expensive and hard to treat: violence against people and property, unresolved mental health illnesses, abuse of substances among people of all groups, teen pregnancy, and an increasing number of people disenfranchised from society, whose personal resources and access to health and social services are limited. This section presents a discussion of the most common problems seen in our communities.

Chapter 31 sets the stage for this section by discussing the concept of vulnerability and the implications for communities of the growing number of vulnerable people. Chapter 32 describes poverty and homelessness as two conditions having profound effects on the health of individuals, families, and communities. Chapter 33 examines the growing community health problems arising from increased rates of teen pregnancy. Chapter 34 looks at the community health implications of the growing migrant population in cities and rural areas across the country. Mental health issues, substance abuse, and violence and human abuse are discussed in chapters 35, 36, and 37 respectively. The final two chapters, 38 and 39, discuss communicable diseases and HIV, hepatitis, and sexually transmitted diseases, problems that are on the increase.

Vulnerability and Vulnerable Populations: An Overview

JULIANN G. SEBASTIAN

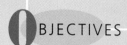 www.mosby.com/MERLIN/community_stanhope

OBJECTIVES

After reading this chapter, the student should be able to do the following:

- Define *vulnerability*.
- Describe vulnerable population groups.
- Analyze trends that have influenced the development of vulnerability among certain population groups and social attitudes toward vulnerability.
- Analyze the effects of public policies on vulnerable populations.
- Evaluate the usefulness and validity of a conceptual model of vulnerability.

- Explain how socioeconomic status, age, health status, and life experiences can predispose people to vulnerability.
- Describe outcomes of vulnerability from the individual, group, and societal perspectives.
- Identify assessment issues related to vulnerable population groups.
- Give examples of the nurse's role in planning and implementing care for vulnerable population groups.
- Explain how to evaluate outcomes of nursing interventions with vulnerable population groups.

KEY TERMS

1115 waiver
barriers to access
brokering health services
case finding
case management
chronically homeless
comprehensive services
culturally sensitive health
 education strategies
cumulative risks

cycle of vulnerability
differential vulnerability
 hypothesis
disadvantaged
disenfranchisement
distribution effects
empowerment
enabling
episodically homeless
federal poverty level

health field concept
hidden homeless
homeless
human capital
iterative assessment
 process
locus of control
market model
outreach
recidivism

resilience
risk
social Darwinism
social isolation
vulnerable population
 group
wrap-around services

See Glossary for definitions

CHAPTER OUTLINE

This chapter introduces the concept of vulnerability and the nursing roles for meeting the health needs of vulnerable population groups. Selected special population groups that are vulnerable to poorer health outcomes than others are described. Public policies that have influenced vulnerable groups and the effects of these policies are explored. The nature of vulnerability is analyzed, and factors that predispose people to vulnerability, outcomes of vulnerability, and the cycle of vulnerability are described. Community and public health nursing interventions are designed to help break the cycle of vulnerability. Numerous interventions are possible at the individual, family, group, and community level. This chapter details the nurse's use of the nursing process with vulnerable population groups and presents case examples throughout and at the end to clarify these ideas.

PERSPECTIVES ON VULNERABILITY

Definition

"Vulnerable populations are defined as social groups who have an increased relative risk or susceptibility to adverse health outcomes" (Flaskerud and Winslow, 1998, p. 69). In the context of health care, **risk** is an epidemiological term that means that some people have a higher probability of illness than others. In the familiar concept of the epidemiological triangle, the agent, host, and environment interact to produce illness or poor health. The natural history of disease model explains how certain aspects of physiology and the environment, including personal habits, social environment, and physical environment, make it more likely that one will develop particular health problems (Valanis, 1992). For example, a smoker is at risk of developing lung cancer because cellular changes occur with smoking. However, not everyone who is at risk develops health problems. Some individuals are more likely than others to develop those health problems for which they are at risk. These people are more vulnerable than others. The web of causation model better explains what happens in these situations. A **vulnerable population group** is a subgroup of the population that is more likely to develop health problems as a result of exposure to risk or to have worse outcomes from these health problems than the population as a whole. Vulnerability is an international concern, with different populations being most vulnerable in different countries.

According to the web of causation model of health and illness (Valanis, 1992), the interaction between numerous causal variables creates a more potent combination of factors predisposing an individual to illness (see Chapter 11 for more information on epidemiology). One way of thinking about this is that not only are more independent variables present (causal factors), but these variables interact, resulting in a higher probability of illness. This means that the relative risk of illness or poor health outcomes is greater for vulnerable populations (Aday, 1997). Members of vulnerable groups frequently have **cumulative risks,** or

combinations of risk factors (Nichols et al, 1986) that make them more sensitive to the adverse effects of individual risk factors that others might be able to overcome. Vulnerability, therefore, implies that certain people are more sensitive to risk factors than others (O'Connor, 1994).

Those who are at risk, but who are not as likely to develop the health problem are more resilient than their more vulnerable counterparts. Being at risk for a certain health problem is therefore necessary for development of that problem, but it is not sufficient. It also seems to be necessary to possess other characteristics that increase one's vulnerability before the health problem actually develops. For example, vulnerable population groups are those who are not only particularly sensitive to risk factors but also possess multiple, cumulative risk factors. This is referred to as the **differential vulnerability hypothesis** (Aday, 1993).

Health care professionals focus on the needs of special population groups. Special population groups are defined as low-income groups, minority groups, and people with disabilities in *Healthy People 2000* (USDHHS, 1991).

Vulnerable individuals and families often belong to more than one of these groups. For example, nurses work with pregnant adolescents who are poor, have been abused, and are substance abusers. Nurses also work with substance abusers who are HIV-positive and HBV-positive, as well as those who are severely mentally ill. Box 31-1 lists vulnerable population groups.

Nurses, other public health professionals, and policy makers are targeting health care interventions toward vulnerable population groups because these groups suffer from disparities in access to care, uneven quality of care, and the poorest health outcomes. Both *Healthy People 2000* and *Healthy Communities 2000* (APHA, 1991) highlight vulnerable population groups and illness prevention and health promotion objectives for them. Because of the continuing disparity in health status between certain special population groups and Americans as a whole, a major effort was begun to improve selected areas of health among African-Americans, Hispanics, American Indians, Alaska Natives, and Pacific Islanders (Hamburg, 1998). This will

---

BOX 31-1 Vulnerable Population Groups of Special Concern to Nurses

Poor and homeless persons
Pregnant adolescents
Migrant workers
Severely mentally ill individuals
Substance abusers
Abused individuals
Persons with communicable disease and those at risk
Persons who are HIV positive or have hepatitis B virus and sexually transmitted disease

be a major part of *Healthy People 2010*, which will be published in the year 2000. The areas targeted for improvement are as follows:

- Infant mortality
- Cancer screening and management
- Cardiovascular disease
- Diabetes
- HIV infection and AIDS
- Immunization rates

The following discussion points out some of the problems that each of the vulnerable populations just described has with access to care, quality and appropriateness of care, and health outcomes. Chapters 32 to 39 describe these vulnerable populations in more detail.

Description of Vulnerable Population Groups

Poor and homeless persons

Economic status is strongly related to health (Adler et al, 1997; USDHHS, 1998). People who are poor are more likely to live in hazardous environments that are overcrowded and have inadequate sanitation, work at high-risk jobs, eat less nutritious diets, and have multiple stressors, because they do not have the extra resources to manage unexpected crises and may not even have adequate resources to manage daily life (de la Barra, 1998; Erickson, 1996; Pappas, 1994). Poverty often reduces an individual's access to health care. In the developed countries of the world, this is more likely to be a problem for those just above the poverty line who are not eligible for public support, while in developing countries poverty is correlated with decreased access to health care. Children who are raised in poverty may be less able to develop resilience and more likely to be depressed later in life (Adler et al, 1997).

Although race is itself an important predictor of poor health outcomes, poverty seems to be a key causal factor for minority populations. In a study of the widening gap in life expectancy between African-Americans and Caucasians in the United States, researchers concluded that the causes of the differences were related to low socioeconomic status rather than race (Kochanek et al, 1994). It may also be that race and economic status interact in some situations, and that relationships between race and economic status vary by disease (Adler et al, 1997).

Poverty is more likely to affect women, children and the elderly, with over 80% of those in poverty being among these groups (Erickson, 1996; Ropers, 1991). These populations are already vulnerable to poor health outcomes, and adding the stressors associated with poverty increases the effect of vulnerability.

The gap between the rich and the poor has increased throughout the latter part of the twentieth century in the United States, corresponding with a decrease in federal assistance for the poor (Erickson, 1996). In 1979, 11.4% of the U.S. population lived in poverty, while in 1989, 31.5% of the population were poor (Shugars, O'Neill, and Bader, 1991). Poverty is a global problem. The gap between rich and poor countries, as well as between social strata within the developing countries in particular, has widened during this century (de la Barra, 1998). "The concentration of wealth has increased annually since 1991" (de la Barra, 1998, p. 47). This depletes human potential worldwide and creates economic, political, and cultural instability that all influence health. For example, children in the poorest sections of Accra, Ghana have three times the risk of infectious disease mortality and twice the risk of respiratory mortality as children in wealthier sections. Children under the age of 5 who live in poor sections of Sao Paulo, Brazil have mortality rates from infectious and respiratory diseases that are four times higher than those living in wealthier sections (de la Barra, 1998).

Poverty may be categorized as the following:

1. Acute poverty, which occurs suddenly after a crisis such as job loss or illness
2. Chronic poverty, which persists over many years
3. Absolute poverty, which indicates a lack of food, shelter, and clothing
4. Relative poverty, which indicates less-than-average resources
5. Administrative poverty, which refers to having met a governmentally determined standard for poverty (e.g., the federal poverty level)
6. Subjective poverty, in which the individual has inadequate income for basic necessities within a particular area (Erickson, 1996).

The interaction among multiple socioeconomic stressors makes people more susceptible to risks than others with more financial resources who may cope more effectively. For example, Felicia's situation illustrates how living environment and practical problems such as transportation and cost interact to make people who are poor particularly vulnerable to health problems.

Felicia is a 22-year-old single mother of three children whose primary source of income is Aid to Families with Dependent Children. She is worried about the future because she will no longer be eligible for welfare by the end of the year. She has been unable to find a job that will pay enough for her to afford child care. Her friend, Maria, said Felicia and her children could stay in Maria's trailer for a short time, but Felicia is afraid that her only choice after that will be a shelter.

Felicia recently took all three children with her to the health department because 15-month-old Hector needed immunizations. Felicia was also concerned about 5-year-old Martina, who had a fever of 100° to 101° F on and off for the past month. Felicia and her friends in the trailer park think that some type of hazardous waste from the chemical plant next door to the park is making their children sick. Now that Martina was not feeling well, Felicia was particularly concerned. However, the health department nurse told her that no appointments were available that day and that she would need to bring Martina back to the clinic on the next day. Felicia left discouraged because it was so difficult for her to get all three children ready and on the bus to go to the health department, not to mention the expense. She thought maybe Martina just had a cold and she would wait a little longer before bringing her back. However, she wanted to take care of Martina's problem before losing her medical card. Felicia is desperate to find a way to manage her money problems and take care of her children.

Extreme poverty, in the form of homelessness, affects women, children, and minorities more often than others (Erickson, 1996). Thirty percent of the homeless in the United States are families, and "85% of those families are headed by women of whom the majority are minorities" (Erickson, 1996, p. 165; Berne et al, 1990). Those who are homeless or marginally housed have even fewer resources than poor people who have adequate housing. Homeless and marginally housed people must struggle with heavy demands as they try to manage daily life. These individuals and families do not have the advantage of shelter and must cope with finding a place to sleep at night and to stay during the day, as well as finding food, before even thinking about health care. In fact, many of the health care needs of homeless individuals are related to their regular search for shelter and food. For example, homeless individuals often have foot problems from constant walking, hypothermia from exposure to the cold, and exacerbations of chronic health problems because they have no place to store their medications, cannot always find nutritious meals, and cannot maintain a healthy balance of rest and activity because of vagrancy laws that prohibit loitering in one place for a prolonged time (Sebastian, 1985).

Ferenchick (1992) compared the medical problems of homeless clients who were seen in a community health clinic with those of clients who had stable housing and those with unstable housing arrangements. He found that homeless clients were significantly more likely to have injuries, fractures, and dental problems than clients with housing. Homeless persons experience problems ranging from violence and trauma associated with life in the streets, to difficulty managing dental care because they have no place to store toothbrushes, toothpaste, and other dental supplies. Clinicians at the Montefiore Health Care Outreach Team for the Homeless (Plescia et al, 1997), located in the Bronx in New York City, found that the most common diagnoses from 1992 to 1995 were well-child and well-adult care, need for immunizations, chemical dependence, and upper respiratory infections. They also found a heavy emphasis on social issues. In a study of homeless shelters for women in Chicago, Barge and Norr (1991) found that the most common health problems of women in their childbearing years were hypertension, mental illness, and injuries, with infections, abuse, and STDs also reported but less often.

Pregnant adolescents

Adolescent pregnancy is a key contributing factor to familial cycles of poverty. Teenagers from poor families, or who are homeless or runaway, are more likely to get pregnant (Fullerton et al, 1997). Adolescents who choose to keep and raise their infants are more likely to remain poor

themselves. With increased social acceptability of out-of-wedlock pregnancy (Pierre and Cox, 1997), a large proportion of teenage mothers do choose to keep and raise their children (Yoos, 1987). This often results in interrupted education for one or both of the parents, limited job opportunities, additional expenses associated with child rearing, and a long-term cycle of economic problems that affect both the parents and their children. The teenage mother is often a single parent, with even more economic consequences. Economic problems are worsened by the many health problems associated with adolescent pregnancy.

Adolescent females (especially those under 14 years of age) are more likely to deliver low birth weight infants than are women in their twenties and thirties (Maynard, 1996; USDHHS, 1997). This is thought to result from the combined interaction of physiological variables (Yoos, 1987) and socioeconomic conditions (Trussell, 1988). Being unable to afford prenatal care, not knowing the importance of such care and how to obtain it, and often beginning prenatal care later in pregnancy than older mothers all contribute to the poor pregnancy outcomes of adolescents. Pregnant adolescents may also experience toxemia, pregnancy-induced hypertension, and anemia.

Migrant workers

With the growing number of legal and illegal immigrants in the United States throughout the 1990s (San Francisco Chronicle, 1998), the number of migrant workers in this country has also increased. Migrant workers face a wide variety of risk factors, including occupational risks associated with hazardous work and poor working conditions and socioeconomic risks from poverty and homelessness. The nature of occupational risks varies depending on the type of work. Many are employed on farms, planting and harvesting agricultural products. Others are employed in other types of seasonal labor, such as those who travel the horse racing circuit, working at race tracks and on horse farms (Ireson and Weaver, 1992). In addition to occupational risks, migrant workers are at high risk for tuberculosis (Ciesielski et al, 1994). Crowded living conditions, traveling to work in crowded buses, and malnutrition are risk factors to which migrant workers are exposed.

Migrant workers are **episodically homeless.** "Episodically homeless people are those who frequently go in and out of homelessness" (Institute of Medicine, 1988, p. 23). Because migrant workers obtain shelter in migrant camps while they are working but may not have a reliable place to live at other times, they are among the **hidden homeless.** These distinctions are important to consider when planning health services, since it is easy to forget that migrant workers have many of the same problems as those who are **chronically homeless** (Institute of Medicine, 1988).

Migrant workers also have serious problems with access to health care (Ciesielski et al, 1994). Some, but not all, migrant workers do not have citizenship status. Those who are illegal immigrants may have no legal access to health services, depending on the laws in a particular state. As the number of immigrants without access to public education, health care, and economic subsidies increases, the United States is developing a seriously underserved class of people with numerous health and social problems (San Francisco Chronicle, 1998).

Increasingly, migrant workers are settling in the communities in which they have worked, adding to the diversity of those communities. Public misunderstanding may lead to a reluctance to accept certain strategies for meeting needs. For example, in one community, an increasing proportion of Hispanic migrant workers who chose to stay in the community led to establishment of an Hispanic Neighborhood Center to meet their needs. However, neighbors objected, leading to community-wide debate about ways to help this special population.

Severely mentally ill individuals

Severely mentally ill (SMI) individuals, defined as those people with a major psychosis such as schizophrenia or bipolar disorder, also cope with a combination of health and socioeconomic problems. These disorders often manifest themselves during adolescence or young adulthood, at the very time when people are trying to establish themselves financially. Untreated severe mental illness interferes with a person's ability to function on a daily basis and thus makes it difficult to maintain a job. SMI individuals need multiple health and social services, such as antipsychotic medications, counseling and sometimes group therapy, and vocational assistance (Steinwachs et al, 1992).

Throughout the nineteenth and much of the twentieth centuries, SMI individuals in the United States were treated primarily by hospitalization for long periods. State mental hospitals were originally developed in the nineteenth century as restful places where a comprehensive, healing environment could be created (Grob, 1973). In fact, the original term *asylum* was intended to connote this idea of rest and refuge from the stresses of daily living. State mental hospitals were never supposed to become long-term care facilities for SMI individuals. However, the lack of adequate community resources for these people resulted in increasing reliance on them and, eventually, on the abuses and dysfunctions that were documented by Clifford Beers, who had himself been a patient in a state mental hospital (Grob, 1983). Eventually, public concern about mental hospitals led to the passage of the 1963 Community Mental Health Centers Act, which intended to deinstitutionalize the SMI population and create **comprehensive services** for them in their own communities.

Unfortunately, comprehensive service networks did not develop in every community, and many SMI individuals were left with fewer and more fragmented services than they needed to function. In many cases, people who had lived in mental hospitals for many years had no idea how to manage on their own in the community. Community agencies often work together to provide the individualized

care that many SMI people need to help them function and achieve a high quality of life in their communities (Steinwachs et al, 1992). It appears that the most effective approach to integrating community services for severely mentally ill individuals is through a single core provider agency that coordinates services provided by others within the community (Provan, 1997). Early work also suggests that the links between agencies must be consistent in order for clients to benefit from integration (Provan and Sebastian, 1998). For example, clients benefit more when agencies that coordinate care also participate in some way in the referral process, rather than having two groups of agencies performing these functions separately.

Behavioral managed care organizations currently provide much of the care for SMI individuals, especially as state Medicaid programs are contracting with such groups to provide SMI care (Mechanic, Schlesinger, and McAlpine, 1995). Some people believe that quality of care suffers as the managed care organizations limit services to reduce cost (Wells et al, 1995). One study (Nicholson et al, 1996) found that a mental health managed care company that aimed to reduce hospitalizations of children and adolescents was able to do so, resulting in part from clinicians' decisions to use hospitalization primarily for acute stabilization purposes and to refer more clients to outpatient crisis services. This study did not examine clinical outcomes of these decisions. Questions remain about whether such decisions shift costs to family members (Mechanic et al, 1995) and result in higher rates of **recidivism** (i.e., more frequent hospital admissions) (Callahan et al, 1995). Mentally ill individuals often do not have the resources to challenge eligibility rules and may suffer poorer health outcomes from service limitations that do not meet their needs. Young chronically mentally ill individuals without adequate access to care may be incarcerated for behaviors resulting from their mental health problems. Further, severely mentally ill individuals may lack routine preventive health care such as screening for common illnesses, and education and support for health prevention and illness promotion.

Substance abusers

Substance abuse is a growing problem in the United States. It includes abuse of legal and illegal substances, such as alcohol, tobacco, narcotic pain medications, and street drugs (e.g., cocaine, heroin, marijuana). Substance abuse creates both health and socioeconomic problems. For example, people who use cocaine may have heart problems and develop nasal and sinus pathology. Neurological problems may result from marijuana use. Alcohol abuse damages the liver and is a risk factor for certain forms of cancer. Alcoholic persons who are HIV-positive are at a higher risk of developing hepatitis (Anastasi and Rivera, 1994). Substance abusers have serious socioeconomic problems, including financial strain from the cost of the drugs, criminal convictions from illegal activities used to obtain the drugs, communicable diseases from sharing drug paraphernalia (from sexual activity such as prostitution to earn money for drugs), and from decreased inhibitions caused by the drugs themselves. There is also frequent family breakdown. Substance abusers may be reluctant to seek health care for fear of being "turned in" to criminal authorities.

Family and community violence

Violence within families and communities is a growing social and health problem (Erickson, 1996), affecting all age groups. Physical, emotional, and sexual abuse are issues, as well as neglect. Adult domestic violence of all types occurs more often than any other crime. Chez (1994, p. 33) says that "the term 'domestic violence' refers to a pattern of regularly occurring abuse and violence, or the threat of violence, in an intimate (though not necessarily cohabitating) relationship." Domestic violence occurs in one of five forms: physical, sexual, psychological, emotional, and economic (Chez, 1994). The incidence of child abuse has risen, with 2.9 million suspected cases reported in 1992 (Devlin and Reynolds, 1994).

Child neglect is the most common form of child abuse, followed by physical abuse and then sexual abuse (Finklehor, 1994). Child sexual abuse is a particular problem not only because of its long-term consequences for affected children, including posttraumatic symptoms, emotional problems, and addictive behaviors (Briere and Elliott, 1994), but also because the reported cases of child sexual abuse are rising faster than those for neglect and physical abuse (Finklehor, 1994). Abusive behavior seems to be related to a combination of problems, including mental health problems, substance abuse, and socioeconomic stressors such as family dysfunction and financial strain. Stressed families and those who are abusing substances are at high risk for child abuse (Devlin and Reynolds, 1994). Low income single mothers who lack social resources and have a history of childhood abuse, and in particular sexual abuse, are at especially high risk for abusive parenting (Hall, Sachs, and Rayens, 1998).

Factors such as gang membership, having friends or family members who belong to gangs, and having the support of peers for violent behavior are all related to a propensity for violence among vulnerable inner-city youth (Powell, 1997). It appears that the involvement of a positive adult role model outside the family and religion may serve as protective factors for youth who are at high risk for violent behavior.

Persons with communicable diseases and those at risk

Vulnerable populations are at a particularly high risk of contracting communicable diseases. The incidence of communicable and infectious diseases is increasing in the United States, partly because not all children are fully immunized, so the level of "herd immunity" for childhood diseases has dropped in some communities. Also, as more strains of multidrug-resistant bacteria develop, the incidence of communicable diseases increases. The measles outbreak in the United States in the early 1990s is one example of increased incidence from inadequate levels of herd immunity. Increases in numbers of people infected with dangerous strains of drug-resistant *Staphylococcus aureus* have been seen in recent years (Shovein and Young, 1992). The incidence of tuberculosis (TB) increased throughout the 1980s and 1990s, partly because of the decreased resistance of HIV-infected people to opportunistic infections (O'Brien and Bartlett, 1992). Persons who live or work in homeless shelters or drug treatment centers and substance abusers have a higher risk of becoming infected with TB than the rest of the population (Avey, 1993). New infectious syndromes are occurring, such as *Mycobacterium avium* complex (MAC) (Anastasi and Rivera, 1994; Benenson, 1990), which affects people who are HIV-positive. Crack cocaine users risk TB infection, partly because of the crowding and high traffic in crack houses and because of the coughing caused by smoking cocaine (Leonhardt et al, 1994).

Old and new sexually transmitted disease prevalence has risen throughout the century (Erickson, 1996), leading in many cases to long-term health, social, and economic consequences. Communicable diseases are a global issue, because international travel has made disease transmission so easy and rapid.

Questions have been raised in recent years about the safety of food and water supplies. For example, epidemics of staphylococcal food poisoning have occurred in the United States related to both political and economic problems. These outbreaks were traced to a chain of fast-food hamburger restaurants. Investigation revealed that standards for detecting potentially harmful levels of bacterial contaminants in raw meat were inadequate. Public health officials advised restaurants to cook meat to a high enough temperature to kill the bacteria, but this was not always done. As a result, large numbers of people became ill and two young children died. People who are the most likely to contract communicable and infectious diseases are those with compromised immune systems, such as people with HIV, acquired immunodeficiency syndrome (AIDS), and cancer, as well as very young and very old persons. Communicable disease prevalence can influence the social and economic health of a community because the greater the number of people who are sick, the fewer people who are available to do the work necessary to sustain other community functions.

Persons who are HIV-positive or have hepatitis and other sexually transmitted diseases

Persons who are HIV-positive or have HBV and other STDs are susceptible to further health and socioeconomic risks. They are more likely to develop other infectious diseases and certain forms of cancer. For example, persons who are HIV-positive risk developing opportunistic infections such as TB and cancers such as Kaposi's sarcoma. People who have certain STDs, such as herpes simplex type 2 infection, also risk cancer. Socioeconomic problems result from interference with work and family, and lifestyle disruptions. These problems are compounded if the individual loses his or her insurance. This can happen as a result of changing jobs and being refused coverage because of a preexisting condition, because the insurance rates for someone with a preexisting condition were high, or because the insurance company dropped that person's coverage altogether. Social, psychological, and emotional problems associated with these illnesses can be the most disruptive aspects.

 RESEARCH *Brief*

Providing care to children with HIV/AIDS can be an emotionally demanding and complex task. Caring for a child with HIV/AIDS may result in feelings of guilt, anxiety, stress, uncertainty, isolation and grief. Previous research has shown that social support interventions are effective strategies for mitigating stress. This study aimed to test the effectiveness of a social support boosting intervention on caregivers of children with HIV/AIDS.

Seventy caregivers participated in this two-group, repeated measures experimental study. Caregivers were divided into experimental and control groups. Within both groups, caregivers were stratified based on whether they were seropositive for HIV/AIDS (biological parents) or seronegative (blood relatives or foster parents). The experimental group received a social support boosting intervention, which was a form of modified case management. The intervention consisted of case managers helping participants identify sources of social support in the areas of emotional support, cognitive support, and instrumental support. Participants in the control group received standard care, which consisted of multidisciplinary health care for the child and respite and social services for the caregiver. Data were collected at entry into the study, 6 months after entry, and 12 months after entry.

The researchers found that seronegative caregivers reported significantly higher levels of perceived social support following the intervention, whereas the seropositive caregivers did not exhibit this outcome. The researchers hypothesized that the needs of caregivers who themselves had HIV/AIDS were more complex than those of caregivers who were not also concerned with the effects of HIV/AIDS on themselves. They recommended that nurses include social support boosting interventions for caregivers of children with HIV/AIDS and recognize the need for more individualized and complex nursing interventions with caregivers who are also seropositive for the virus.

Hansell PS: The effect of a social support boosting intervention on stress, coping, and social support in caregivers of children with HIV/AIDS, *Nurs Res* 47(2):79, 1998.

"HIV infection disproportionately affects racial and ethnic minorities and families with complex problems such as addiction. Eighty-one percent of the AIDS cases diagnosed in children under 13 years of age through June, 1996 were either African American or Hispanic" (Caliandro and Hughes, 1998, p. 107). Since many of these children lose their mothers to AIDS, grandmothers often rear them. African-American and Hispanic grandmothers who are caring for a child with AIDS are committed to the value of family, generally find joy and meaning in parenting and caring for these children, and focus much of their energies on managing both personal (e.g., emotional and physical health) and physical resources (e.g., finances and home and neighborhood safety) (Caliandro and Hughes, 1998). A major issue for people who are HIV-positive is the effects on family and social dynamics. Caregivers, family members, and life partners are affected by their loved ones' HIV disease and can benefit from nursing interventions such as social support. However, it appears that caregivers who are themselves HIV-positive require different types of social support than those caregivers who are not coping with personal disease while also caring for an HIV-positive child (Hansell et al, 1998) (see the Research Brief).

Racial and ethnic minority groups

In 1998, President Clinton initiated a program to decrease health disparities in six areas for members of racial and ethnic minority populations. The Presidential Initiative on Race recognizes that while the health of Americans has improved overall throughout the 1990s, certain racial and ethnic minority populations continue to experience a higher than average burden from poor health. The groups that are targeted in this initiative are African Americans, Hispanics, American Indians, Alaska Natives, and Pacific Islanders. These groups are expected to "grow as a proportion of the total U.S. population; therefore, the future health of America as a whole will be influenced substantially by success in improving the health of these racial and ethnic minorities" (Hamburg, 1998, p. 372).

Two examples of health disparities across population groups are in the areas of infant mortality and childhood immunization rates. In 1995, African-Americans had an infant mortality rate of 14.6 per 1000 live births, compared with 6.3 for Caucasians, and 5.3 for Asian Americans or Pacific Islanders. Each of the target populations in President Clinton's Initiative had lower childhood immunization rates than Caucasians in 1996. This initiative will direct funds toward research to learn more about the causes of these disparities and demonstration projects to test innovative care delivery models to reduce health disparities.

Special population groups differ in other countries. In Canada, Aboriginal Indians and people who live in remote rural areas in northern Canada need special attention to reduce health disparities. The infant mortality rate for Canada as a whole was 6.1 per 1000 live births in 1995. By comparison, the infant mortality rates for the Yukon and the Northwest Territories in Canada were 12.8 and 13.0 per 1000 live births (Statistics Canada, 1998).

Trends Related to Caring for Vulnerable Populations

During colonial times, persons with chronic physical or mental conditions were cared for in their own communities. Later, the social reforms of the nineteenth century led to institutional care for many of these individuals. At the beginning of the twenty-first century, there is a renewed emphasis on caring for vulnerable population groups in the community through partnerships between groups such as public health, managed care, and community groups. This has been referred to as "community-oriented managed care" (Aday, 1997, p. 16).

Many of the vulnerable population groups described in this chapter and Chapters 32 to 39 have less access to health services than other groups. The trend is toward more outreach and **case finding** to make access easier (AAN, 1992). A related trend is to develop culturally appropriate forms of outreach and care delivery in order to more effectively promote the health of these populations (AAN, 1992). For example, in many African-American communities, one of the most effective locations for outreach and community education is the neighborhood church or mosque. The American Cancer Society program, "Sister to Sister" involves African-American women going door to door in African-American neighborhoods providing individualized education about the importance of breast cancer screening.

There is also a trend toward providing more comprehensive, family-centered services when treating vulnerable population groups. Felicia Delacorte's situation, described previously, is a good example of the importance of providing comprehensive, family-centered, "one-stop" services. If Felicia had been able to have Martina checked while she was in for Hector's immunizations, Martina's health problem would have been treated at an earlier stage. Furthermore, if social and economic assistance were also provided and included in interdisciplinary treatment plans, the services would have been even more responsive to the combined effects of social and economic stressors on the health of special population groups. This situation is sometimes referred to as providing **wrap-around services,** in which comprehensive health services are available and social and economic services are "wrapped around" these services.

Finally, the trend is toward providing more of these comprehensive services in locations where people live and work, including schools, churches, neighborhoods, and workplaces. Nurses are beginning to develop mobile outreach clinics and take them to migrant camps, schools, and local communities. The shift away from hospital-based care includes a renewed commitment to the public health services that vulnerable populations need to prevent illness and promote health (Baker et al, 1994; Fielding and Halfon, 1994), such as reduction of environmental hazards and violence and assurance of safe food and water.

A major shift in providing care for certain vulnerable populations in the United States is the increasing reliance on private managed care by Medicaid and Medicare. Many states now have *1115 waivers* from the Health Care Financing Administration (HCFA) that permit them to test innovative approaches to organizing care for Medicaid beneficiaries (Epstein, 1997). An **1115 waiver** is a situation in which HCFA has given a particular state permission to waive certain usual Medicaid requirements in order to test unique approaches to providing health care in specific local areas. These waivers have been used in most cases to develop varied forms of managed care arrangements for all or part of the Medicaid beneficiaries in a state. An advantage of the waivers is they allow states to develop strategies that work best in their local communities, rather than mandating that all states use the same model.

Some vulnerable populations are such high financial risks and have such unique needs that their care is contracted to specialty groups. For example, mental health and substance abuse services are often contracted out to behavioral managed care firms. These contracts are referred to as "carve outs" because the care for a specific population has been carved out of an overall managed care plan for all other clinical populations. Other groups whose care may be "carved out" are the elderly, disabled populations, and children with special health care needs. Care also may be "carved out" as part of a block grant, in which funds are given in a block to a local area that focuses on a broad area, such as maternal and child health. Block grants are intended to enable local areas to have more control deciding how to spend the funds in order to respond to local needs and conditions. In one city, funds from a block grant broadly focused on energy and home heating were used to help support a homeless shelter.

The situation in Canada differs because control of local health care decisions rests largely at the level of provincial governments, rather than at the federal level. This permits responsiveness to local conditions and needs. A major challenge in today's health care environment is developing flexible new care delivery strategies for high-risk populations that are responsive to local cultural mores and social context, and that result in improved clinical outcomes at an affordable cost.

A disadvantage of mandated managed care for Medicaid enrollees is that studies to date have shown that the majority of beneficiaries remain on Medicaid less than a year (Carrasquillo et al, 1998), severely limiting the continuity of care that is available to them. One of the primary reasons for leaving Medicaid is a change in work status. While this has important benefits, if the individual chooses a managed care plan at a new place of employment, the likelihood is that he or she will also be required to select a new primary care provider from that particular company's panel of providers.

A second and related set of disadvantages relates to cultural variations across groups who normally receive Medicaid. American Indians may find that policies associated with Medicaid managed care plans require them to choose primary care providers who are not part of the Indian Health Service (Wellever, Hill, and Casey, 1998). These providers may be far from the individual's home and may not allow for the culturally appropriate practices that are accepted within the Indian Health Service. American Indians are likely also to believe that having their care managed by a group outside of the Indian Health Service interferes with their tribal authority. These problems can be handled by customizing requirements for the needs of the special population group (Wellever, Hill, and Casey, 1998).

PUBLIC POLICIES AFFECTING VULNERABLE POPULATIONS

Landmark Legislation

Public policy is shaped by legislation that specifies the general directions for government bodies to take. Even though laws may only relate to a certain proportion of the population, they tend to have a ripple effect and result in other groups following the general intent of the law. As seen in Box 31-2, various pieces of landmark legislation have affected vulnerable population groups throughout the twentieth century.

Three of these pieces of legislation provided for direct and indirect financial subsidies to certain vulnerable groups. The Social Security Act created the largest federal support program for elderly and poor Americans in history. This act sought direct payments to eligible individuals to ensure a minimal level of support for people at risk of problems resulting from inadequate financial resources. Later, the Medicare and Medicaid amendments to the Social Security Act of 1965 provided for the health care needs of elderly, poor, and disabled people who might be vulnerable to impoverishment resulting from high medical bills or to poor health status from inadequate access to health care. These acts created third-party health care payers at the federal and state levels. Title XXI of the Social Security Act, enacted in 1998, provides for the State Child Health Insurance Program (CHIP) to provide funds to insure currently uninsured children. In addition to CHIP, new outreach and casefinding efforts will enroll eligible children in Medicaid. "Taken together, these two approaches will seek to provide health insurance for at least half of the 10 million uninsured children in this country" (Hamburg, 1998, p. 375).

Three of the other laws created financial support for building health facilities, thereby improving access to health services for vulnerable groups. The Hill-Burton Act of 1946 provided financial support to build hospitals that would provide care to indigent people. The Community Mental Health Centers Act of 1963 funded construction of community mental health centers and training of mental health professionals who provided community-based care for the severely mentally ill individuals discharged from state mental hospitals. This overall policy of deinstitutionalization from mental hospitals was also included in the act and is similar to the current trend to treat more people in their communities and homes rather than in institutions. A policy that encourages more community-based care also requires that the community-based services that people need are developed and implemented. Finally, the Stewart B. McKinney Homeless Assistance Act of 1988 resulted in money for clinics and a wide variety of educational and social services for homeless individuals and families.

The other three pieces of legislation, the National Health Planning and Resource Development Act of 1974, the Tax Equity and Fiscal Responsibility Act of 1982, and the Balanced Budget Act of 1997, influenced the use of resources for providing health services. The National Health Planning and Resource Development Act was intended to provide local mechanisms for planning which types of health services and facilities were really needed so that duplication of expensive facilities and services would be avoided. The goal was to reduce the increasing cost of health services; this would indirectly influence access for vulnerable population groups by making health services more affordable. Also, part of the planning process included community health needs assessment, with the goal of providing balanced services so all would have access to the care they needed. The Tax Equity and Fiscal Responsibility Act (TEFRA) of 1982 focused on the cost of health services but did so in a very different way. This act was de-

---

BOX 31-2 Legislation That Has Affected Vulnerable Population Groups in the United States

LEGISLATION THAT PROVIDED FOR DIRECT AND INDIRECT FINANCIAL SUBSIDIES TO CERTAIN VULNERABLE POPULATION GROUPS

Social Security Act of 1935
Medicare and Medicaid Social Security Act amendments of 1965
State Child Health Insurance Program amendment, 1998

LEGISLATION THAT PROVIDED FINANCIAL SUPPORT FOR BUILDING HEALTH CARE FACILITIES

Hill-Burton Act of 1946
Community Mental Health Centers Act of 1963
Stewart B. McKinney Homeless Assistance Act of 1988

LEGISLATION THAT AFFECTED HOW HEALTH CARE RESOURCES WERE USED

National Health Planning and Resources Development Act of 1974
Tax Equity and Fiscal Responsibility Act of 1982
Federal Balanced Budget Act of 1997

signed to limit the rapid increase in health care costs, but it did not focus on community planning. Instead, TEFRA mandated that payment for hospital services for all Medicare patients would no longer be done on a retrospective cost basis; that is, the HCFA would no longer simply pay the bills that were submitted to them for Medicare enrollees. Now, the HCFA would pay for services on a prospective basis. The agency did so by developing a list of common medical diagnoses (diagnosis-related groups, or DRGs) and determining what they would pay for the care of people with these diagnoses. If hospitals provided services that cost more than the amount indicated on the list, those hospitals lost money. The effect was an increased emphasis on shorter hospital stays, more emphasis on identifying cost-effective treatments, and more emphasis on community-based care and care in the home. This was difficult for certain vulnerable groups, such as the homeless, who did not have the same level of resources and support to continue with the care necessary after discharge.

A similar shift in payment occurred with the stipulations related to home health in the Balanced Budget Act of 1997. In an attempt to curb the rapid growth in spending on home health and financial fraud in that industry, the HCFA moved toward prospective payment for home health services. More stringent regulations about which services would be reimbursed and for how long, may also limit access to care for certain vulnerable groups, such as frail elderly, chronically ill individuals whose care is largely home-based, and people who are HIV positive. The goal is to ensure that care is appropriate, rather than limiting access. Nurses and other health care providers must work even more closely with families to determine the kinds of services needed to foster self-care, and the optimal timing of these services. The Balanced Budget Act of 1997 also reduced payments for services for Medicare beneficiaries such that some providers have chosen to no longer treat Medicare beneficiaries. This means that those whose health needs may be high (some chronically ill and the elderly) may have limited access to care.

Implementation Issues

Once a law is passed, it must be put into place before it will have a substantial effect on the public. Often, unanticipated problems occur during the implementation phase. These problems sometimes mean that the "letter of the law" is followed but that the intentions of the law are not met. For example, the Community Mental Health Centers Act intended to move treatment of severely mentally ill people into the communities so they would have better outcomes. However, the community supports necessary to help this population were not always adequate, so many eventually lost contact with families and jobs and became homeless (Institute of Medicine, 1988). Another example of an unanticipated outcome is the effects that increasingly strict immigration and border control policies

have had on the flow of illegal immigrants into the United States. Mexican immigrants, in particular, have chosen to cross southern U.S. borders at increasingly risky locations, arriving in the country sick and injured. Another effect of policies that reduced benefits to legal immigrants was to create a new underserved population without equal access to public health and welfare services (San Francisco Chronicle, Oct. 13, 1998).

Implementation problems also occur because the law has unintended effects on other groups that lawmakers do not anticipate. These are called **distribution effects.** Distribution effects are seen in the criticisms that mental hospitals do not discharge people quickly because the administrators and staff had much to lose. Staff lost jobs and administrators lost perquisites such as homes and their own personal staff as censuses dropped (Torrey et al, 1990).

Even though laws such as Medicaid and the McKinney Act were passed to support care for vulnerable groups, some vulnerable individuals and families still do not have adequate access to care. Friedman (1994) argues that nonfinancial **barriers to access** include subtle and often unintentional discrimination. Subconscious discrimination can result in an inadequate number of providers who are willing to treat certain racial groups and people with certain diagnoses, such as HIV. Discrimination against certain diagnoses can influence which conditions insurers are willing to pay for. Other nonfinancial barriers include having inadequate providers in rural areas and certain sections in urban areas, and cultural barriers such as the inability of many vulnerable groups to manage the health care system (Friedman, 1994). One study (Gifford and Bettenhausen, 1997) found that receptionists in physician offices responded differently over the telephone to young women on Medicaid, thereby subtly creating barriers to access. Thus, even though laws have been passed to increase access to health services by vulnerable groups, inequities still exist for these populations because of attitudes.

Effects of Managed Care on Health Care for Vulnerable Populations

In many areas, the growth of public managed care (i.e., Medicaid and Medicare managed care options) has reduced the personal health services for individuals (e.g., primary care clinics in health departments). The competition for clients in heavy managed care markets has made it more attractive to private clinics and physicians' offices to provide the personal care services that some public health departments formerly provided because they can obtain payment for these services. Some public health departments have eliminated these services and focus on providing population-focused services only, such as communicable disease control, environmental services, and managing public food and water supplies (Aiken and Salmon, 1994). In this way, many public health departments are refocusing on the core functions of public health (i.e., assessment, policy, and assurance).

However, not all private health agencies choose to provide vulnerable populations with services, and many are concerned that disparities in health care access and outcomes could grow even greater. Aiken and Salmon (1994) explain that vulnerable populations are more expensive to treat, since they possess multiple, cumulative risks and require special service delivery considerations (e.g., to help overcome transportation problems or provide culturally competent care). Managed care organizations possess strong incentives to control costs by keeping their enrollees healthy. These groups may prefer to care for the healthiest people rather than those who are most vulnerable and, in fact, may find it necessary in order to remain financially solvent. As noted earlier, one approach that is used to manage care for high-risk populations is to contract their care to specialty organizations (referred to as "carve outs"). These specialty organizations often develop innovative approaches to caring for these high-risk populations.

For example, one school of nursing contracted with its regional Medicaid office to provide a new care delivery program for families with medically fragile children. This is a family program that aims to strengthen families who rear children with high-risk health problems. Nurse practitioners and a clinical nurse specialist provide primary care, urgent care, health education, health coaching, family counseling and support, and **case management** for families in the program. Most care is provided in the home, although the program staff also works with clients in hospitals, clinics, and physicians' offices in order to facilitate seamless care delivery.

Many argue that fundamental changes are needed in the way that health services are delivered (Baker et al, 1994). The American Nurses Association's proposal for health care reform (ANA, 1991) specifically focused on the need for special programs for vulnerable groups. This document proposed that special programs and outreach activities be developed for these groups. Nursing's plan for health care reform was noteworthy in its emphasis on both health services and broader social change. "National health reform must also consider the interrelationships between health and such factors as education, behavior, income, housing and sanitation, social support networks, and attitudes about health. Better health cannot be the nation's only goal when hunger, crime, drugs, and other social problems remain" (ANA, 1991, p. 14). Nurses should focus efforts on precursors to health to address the multidimensional nature of vulnerability.

CONCEPTUAL BASES OF VULNERABILITY

Vulnerability results from the combined effects of limited resources. Figure 31-1 shows the interactions between lim-

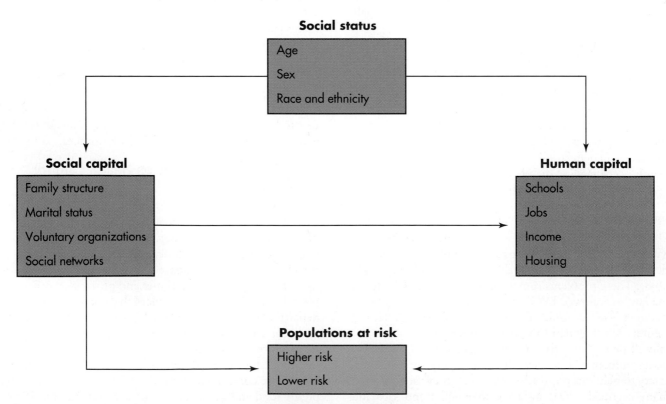

FIG. 31-1 Predictors of populations at risk. (From Aday LA: *At risk in America: The health and health care needs of vulnerable populations in the United States,* San Francisco, 1993, Jossey-Bass.)

itations in physical and environmental resources, personal resources (or human capital), and biopsychosocial resources (e.g., presence of illness and genetic predispositions) (Aday, 1993). Poverty, limited social support, and working in a hazardous environment are examples of limitations in physical and environmental resources. People with preexisting illnesses, such as those with communicable or infectious diseases, or those with chronic illnesses such as cancer, heart disease, or chronic airway disease, have less physical ability to cope with stressors than those without such physical problems. **Human capital** refers to all of the strengths, knowledge, and skills that give each individual potential to live a productive, happy life. People with little education have less human capital because their choices are more limited than those with higher levels of education.

Vulnerability is multidimensional; that is, multiple concepts are needed to understand what vulnerability means to those who experience it. Disempowerment, limited control, victimization, disadvantaged status, disenfranchisement, and health risks are the dimensions emphasized in this chapter. Figure 31-2 illustrates the dynamic interactions among these dimensions. It is important to emphasize,

however, that vulnerability is not simply a state of "deficiency." Rather, it is dynamic and can be counteracted by acquiring the resources necessary to function more easily in contemporary society and by fostering **resilience.** Nursing interventions should focus on the connections between these types of resources. Figure 31-3 shows one model for targeting interventions for vulnerable population groups. In this model, interventions such as case finding, health education, policy-making related to improving health for vulnerable populations are all appropriate interventions for nurses.

Disempowerment

Moccia and Mason (1986) stated that poverty is a power issue because it involves a lack of control over critical resources needed to function effectively in society. In contemporary American society, money is one of the most critical resources; insufficient financial means put individuals in dependent positions and further removes control over choices between available options. In addition, insufficient financial resources limit the degree of participation many have in making decisions that will affect them, thus limiting their potential to influence even the kinds of op-

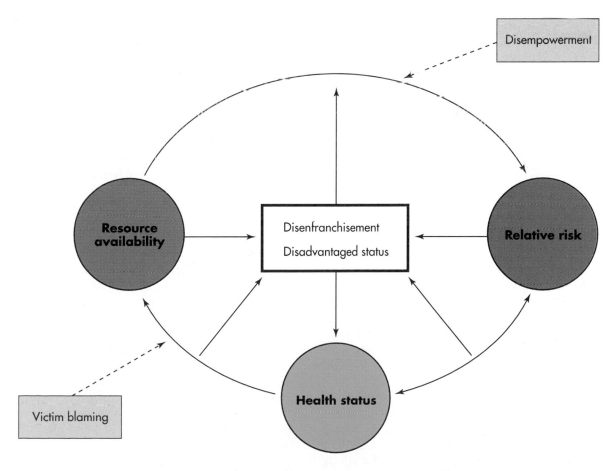

FIG. 31-2 Vulnerable population: social dynamics and outcomes. (Adapted from Flaskerud JA, Winslow BJ: Conceptualizing vulnerable populations health-related research, *Nurs Res* 47(2):70, 1998.)

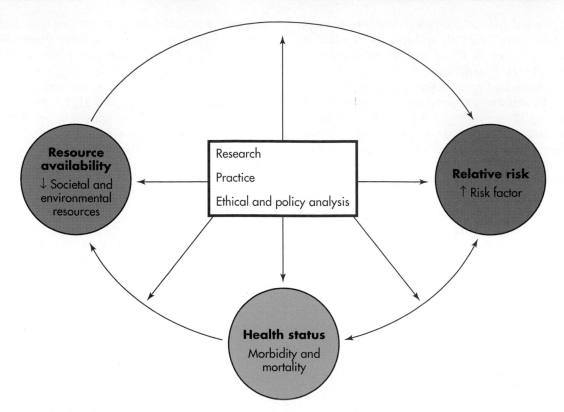

FIG. 31-3 Vulnerable Populations conceptual model for research and practice. (Adapted from Flaskerud JA, Winslow BJ: Conceptualizing vulnerable populations health-related research, *Nurs Res* 47(2):70, 1998.)

tions available to them. In the past, community health planning was often unintentionally patriarchal. Health professionals thought they knew better than lay people which health needs were most important and the best ways to provide services to meet those needs. This belief is changing because community health professionals emphasize empowering vulnerable groups and working as partners with them.

The **health field concept** explains how limited control over one's own health is part of vulnerability. This concept was developed by LaFramboise (1973, cited in Dever et al, 1988, p. 26) and expanded by Lalonde (1974, cited in Dever et al, 1988, p. 26). Individual control of health is only one factor in a comprehensive model of health in which biology, environment, and the health care system make up the remaining three foci. According to the health field concept, individuals share control and responsibility for their health status with society as a whole.

Individuals largely determine the behaviors they engage in that are health promoting or potentially health damaging. Although individuals do not control their biological heritage, they share some responsibility for the heritage they pass on to their offspring (e.g., through the effects that prenatal health and maternal lifestyle have on infant health). Society determines the types of health services and the types of reimbursement mechanisms available. Also,

society is responsible for many environmental hazards. Thus the health field concept explains how health status is affected by both individual factors (individual and biology) and broader societal factors (environment and health care system). The ongoing health of people with AIDS, for example, is affected not only by their own health behaviors, but also by the fact that they may lose access to medications and laboratory tests when their insurance policies are cancelled.

In many cases, aspects of the physical and social environment that adversely affect the health status of vulnerable populations are beyond their control and are the responsibility of society. For example, communities sometimes find it difficult to locate group homes for severely mentally ill clients in residential neighborhoods despite the emphasis on providing care for these individuals in more normal environments. Neighbors may fear mentally ill people, or they may worry that their property values will drop. If group homes are located in poor neighborhoods, residents are more likely to be victims of crime, to be exposed to environmental hazards such as air pollutants, and to feel ostracized.

Victim Blaming

Limited individual control over behavior is not the only issue related to health status and vulnerability. Dever et al

(1988) express concern that the current emphasis on individual control of health through lifestyle choices may result in blaming the victim for areas outside individual control. In the extreme, victim blaming relieves society from assuming responsibility for environmental issues and health service delivery issues.

Rosner (1982) concluded that victim blaming has become part of the outlook on care for the poor in American society. In the early days of the United States, the public believed that poverty was temporary and could be overcome. People felt a sense of responsibility to help the "truly needy" and believed that poor people were worthy of help. The thought that poverty might be permanent was in opposition to the developing American ideas of self-sufficiency and individual achievement.

Later, during the Industrial Revolution and the early part of the twentieth century, social attitudes shifted, and people thought that poor and dependent members of society somehow deserved their situations. This attitude justified limitations on social welfare that were actually caused by financial constraints on service availability. Ultimately, affluence was seen as a sign of morality, as the just reward for clever and hard-working members of society, and poverty was viewed as the outcome of immorality and slothfulness. Americans eventually adopted an attitude of ambivalence toward poor and dependent persons; those who were seen as temporarily poor were considered worthy of help, and those for whom poverty was considered a permanent state were not considered worthy of help (Rosner, 1982). Ambivalent attitudes toward vulnerable populations are common; for example, the public sometimes objects to spending tax dollars for treatment of HIV and substance abuse because some still think that people create these problems for themselves.

Such ambivalence seems to have increased in the last decade. Strict eligibility criteria are becoming more common for health and social services. Policy makers are concerned about welfare reform. Public sentiment seems to favor not providing financial entitlements for those who do not want to help themselves. Also, ambivalence toward the poor may have resulted partly from professional opinions regarding enabling behavior. The concept of **enabling** comes from the literature on addictions and refers to the behavior of people in the dependent person's environment that makes it possible for the addiction to continue, such as covering up and "making things right." Some think that the presence of loose eligibility criteria for health and social services enables individuals to maintain patterns of dependency. Rosner (1982) argued that attitudes favoring strict eligibility criteria are more likely during times of severely limited economic resources and that certain functions are served by blaming the victims of poverty and dependency.

These functions include the maintenance of a class system and the opportunity for middle-class and upper-class groups to practice charity and benevolence toward poor and dependent persons (Rosner, 1982). Curtin (1986) pointed out that contributing to these persons' needs gives people an opportunity for tax deductions and feelings of self-satisfaction from helping the less fortunate. The functions served by having lower-class groups in society are therefore both financial and psychological. Further division of the health care system into a two-tiered system of care based inherently on victim blaming of those at the lower level has resulted in part from a shift in the focus of health care from client care to a consumer commodity (Curtin, 1986). The emphasis on cost containment resulted in policies designed to limit those eligible for free or government-financed care, as opposed to earlier efforts to expand accessibility of services (Grau, 1987; Rosner, 1982), although health system reform may reverse this.

Disenfranchisement

Disenfranchisement refers to a feeling of separation from mainstream society in which the individual does not have an emotional connection with any group in particular or the larger social fabric in general. In addition to perceived disenfranchisement, certain groups such as the poor, the homeless, and migrant workers may essentially be "invisible" to society as a whole and forgotten in health and social planning. Disenfranchisement suggests that vulnerable groups do not have the social supports necessary to manage effectively an emotionally and physically healthy lifestyle. Many vulnerable individuals have limited formal support networks because they do not have well-established linkages with formal organizations in their communities, such as churches and schools. They may also have few informal sources of support, such as family, friends, and neighbors. For example, homeless individuals are often isolated and have few people that they can call on for assistance. It is not true, however, that all vulnerable groups have no sources of social support. Nurses should remember that although disenfranchisement is part of being vulnerable for many, strong support from churches, family, and neighbors may be advantages that some vulnerable individuals can draw upon, even though they may feel disenfranchised from society as a whole.

Disadvantaged Status

Thus, in many ways, vulnerable groups have limited control over potential and actual health needs. Since these groups are in the minority, they are more **disadvantaged** than others because typical health planning focuses on the majority. Ironically, the traditional public health emphasis on the utilitarian value of "the greatest good for the greatest number" places vulnerable populations at a disadvantage. Disadvantage also results from lack of resources that others may take for granted. Vulnerable groups have limited social and economic resources with which to manage their health care. The Family Resiliency Model predicts that families who have access to adequate resources can more effectively withstand stressors (McCubbin and McCubbin, 1991). For example, women sometimes choose to tolerate domestic violence rather than risk losing a place for themselves and their children to live. Women who are among the working poor are more likely to become homeless when they leave an abusive partner. They may not have adequate financial resources to pay for a place to live when they lose their partners' income. In their epidemiological study of the effects of undesirable life events, McLeod and Kessler (1990) found that lower socioeconomic status resulted in ". . . pervasive disadvantages inherent in the lives of persons who occupy lower-status positions" (p. 169).

Health Risk

Vulnerable populations not only experience multiple, cumulative risks, but they also seem to be particularly sensitive to the effects of those risks. Risks may originate in environmental hazards (e.g., lead exposure from peeling, lead-based paint) or social hazards (e.g., crime and violence), in personal behavior (e.g., diet and exercise habits), or from biological or genetic makeup (e.g., congenital addiction or compromised immune status). Members of vulnerable populations often have comorbidities, or multiple illnesses, with each affecting the other. These elements of multiple risk factors, cumulative effects of risk factors, and low thresholds for risk must be addressed when assessing the needs of vulnerable populations and designing services for them.

PREDISPOSING FACTORS

Socioeconomic Status

Social and economic factors predispose people to vulnerability. Poverty, a primary cause of vulnerability, is a growing problem in the United States (Northam, 1996; Pesznecker, 1984). Poverty is a relative state. The federal definition of poverty is used to develop eligibility criteria for entitlement and other programs. According to *Healthy People 2000* (USDHHS, 1991, p. 29) "Nearly 1 of every 8 Americans lives in a family with an income below the Federal poverty level." In 1998, the **federal poverty level** for a family of four was $16,450 for all states except Hawaii, Alaska, and the District of Columbia (Superintendent of Documents, 1998). However, many people who earn just a little more than the federal poverty level are unable to manage their living expenses, yet are ineligible for assistance programs. Poverty causes vulnerability by making it more difficult for people to function in society. It is often difficult for a young family with an employed father in the home to obtain financial support from social services, even if the father is earning less money than the family needs. This family is considered *near poor;* sometimes, in these situations, families decide they would be better off financially if the fathers were absent because they become eligible for welfare. Vulnerability results from families' efforts to do what is necessary to manage, even though it is disruptive to the family system.

Persons who do not have the financial resources to pay for medical care are considered medically indigent. They may be self-employed or work in small businesses and are unable to afford health benefits. Some people have inadequate health insurance coverage. This may be because either their deductibles and copayments are so high they have to pay for most expenses out-of-pocket or because few conditions or services are covered. In these situations, poverty in its relative sense causes vulnerability because uninsured and underinsured people are less likely to seek preventive health services because of the expense and are more likely to suffer the consequences of preventable illnesses.

Currently, health care reimbursement policies are based more on a market model than on a human service model. This type of model perpetuates inequities in service availability and accessibility. The **market model** assumes that people who have the resources to purchase services are the ones entitled to those services. Further, a market model assumes that consumers have the information and opportunity to make free choices about where to purchase services. Individuals unable to purchase services must somehow not be "fit" to receive services. Moccia and Mason (1986) observed that **social Darwinism** is a subtle social value in the United States. Social Darwinism refers to the idea of survival of the fittest in relation to the ability to purchase goods and services. Social Darwinism conflicts with the belief that at least some basic level of health care is a right and should be provided regardless of ability to pay. The two perspectives reflect the controversy in health care reform over how involved the government should be in providing health and social services to vulnerable groups.

One of the problems that results from this idea, whether intentional or not, is that policies that reflect this posture reinforce a cycle that may be almost impossible for disenfranchised individuals and groups to break out of (Curtin, 1986). For example, groups who are unable to afford adequate preventive services are likely to develop more chronic diseases, which further deplete the human potential in those groups. This is referred to as a drain on human capital, where *human capital* means that the potential of all people in the community is a valuable resource. Depletion of health status results in decreased human capital and limits the abilities of group members to obtain employment, seek advanced education, or behave in ways that improve their situations. Poor health leads to reduced human capital and to reduction in human capital that leads to higher overall levels of health risks (Aday, 1993). Ultimately the whole community suffers if the potential of its members is limited.

Like economic status, **social isolation** is strongly related to vulnerability. A study of gay men with AIDS (Rabkin et al, 1993) found that the men were optimistic, did not deny the severity of their illnesses, and displayed high levels of psychological resilience. The researchers attributed this to the fact that almost all the men reported having confidants, or "someone who was 'there' for them" (p. 167). Similarly, Hogan and DeSantis (1994) reported that adolescents who had experienced the death of a sibling were helped when they felt that their friends were "there for them."

Age-Related Causes

Vulnerable groups may share certain physiological and developmental characteristics that predispose them to unique risks. Among these, age is probably the most central variable. It has long been known that clients at the extreme ends of the age continuum are less able physiologically to adapt to stressors. For example, infants of substance-abusing mothers risk being born addicted and having severe physiological problems and developmental delays. Elderly individuals are more likely to develop active infections from communicable diseases such as TB and generally have more difficulty recovering from infectious processes than younger people because of their less effective immune systems. Chapter 36 discusses substance abuse, and Chapter 38 describes communicable disease risk.

Certain individuals are vulnerable at particular ages because of the interaction between crucial developmental characteristics and socioeconomic tensions. For example, adolescent females (especially those under age 14 years) are more likely to deliver low birth weight infants than women in their twenties (Simpson et al, 1997), probably because of physiological variables (Yoos, 1987), although socioeconomic conditions may play an equally important role (Trussell, 1988). An inability to afford prenatal care, lack of awareness of the existence of or importance of prenatal care, and a tendency to seek such care later in pregnancy than older mothers also contribute to poor pregnancy outcomes of adolescent females. Chapter 33 describes adolescent pregnancy in more detail.

Health-Related Causes

Changes in normal physiological status predisposes individuals to vulnerability. This may result from disease processes, such as in someone with one or more chronic diseases. Infection with HIV is a good example of a pathophysiological situation that increases vulnerability to opportunistic infections such as MAC because of immunodeficiency. Chapter 39 describes HIV, hepatitis, and STDs in detail. Physiological alterations may also result from accidents, injuries, or congenital problems leading to mental or physiological disability. Elderly individuals often exhibit vulnerability resulting both from age and from multiple chronic illnesses. Both factors result in limitations in functional status for many elderly persons, thereby leading to vulnerability to safety hazards and to loss of independence. Chapter 29 discusses elder health. Physically compromised individuals are another example of a vulnerable group, as discussed in Chapter 30.

Life Experiences

One's life experiences, especially experiences early in life, influence development of psychological vulnerability or resilience. For example, children who survive disasters may experience difficulties in later life if they do not receive adequate counseling (Yule, 1992). Internal **locus of control** appears to protect children (particularly adolescents) from the negative effects of disaster (Kimchi and Schaffner,

1990; Yule, 1992). Vulnerable population groups often develop an external locus of control. They may believe that events are outside their control and result from bad luck or fate. An external locus of control makes it more difficult for people to initiate action or to seek care for health problems. Such a point of view may make a person believe that health promotion and illness prevention activities are unimportant or ineffective because they do not believe they have much personal control over their own health status. Extroversion and flexibility are other personality characteristics that appear to be protective factors against early adversity (Yule, 1992). People who have been abused or those who have experienced chronic stressors throughout life may have depleted the reserves that others would normally have for coping with new stressors (Nurius et al, 1992).

OUTCOMES OF VULNERABILITY

Outcomes of vulnerability may be negative, such as lower health status than the rest of the population, or they may be positive with effective interventions. For example, culturally competent, family-focused community health nursing interventions may improve vulnerable populations' health status and empower such groups to promote their own health.

Poor Health Outcomes

Vulnerable populations often have worse health outcomes than others in terms of morbidity and mortality. These groups have high prevalence of chronic illnesses, such as hypertension, and high levels of communicable diseases, such as TB, HBV, STDs, and upper respiratory illnesses, including influenza. They have high mortality rates from crime and violence, including domestic violence. Other types of health outcomes that deserve further study include functional status, overall perception of physical and emotional well-being, quality of life, and satisfaction with health services.

Chronic Stress

Poor health creates stress as individuals and families try to manage health problems with inadequate resources. For example, if someone with AIDS develops one or more opportunistic infections and is either uninsured or underinsured, that person and the family and caregivers will have more difficulty managing than if the individual had adequate insurance. Vulnerable populations cope with multiple stressors, so managing multiple stressors creates a sort of "domino effect," with chronic stress likely to result. This can lead to feelings of hopelessness.

Hopelessness

Hopelessness results from an overwhelming sense of powerlessness and social isolation. For example, substance abusers who feel powerless over their addiction and who have isolated themselves from the people they care about may believe that no way exists to change their situation.

Feelings of hopelessness contribute to a continuing **cycle of vulnerability.**

Cycle of Vulnerability

The factors that predispose people to vulnerability and the outcomes of vulnerability create a cycle in which the outcomes reinforce the predisposing factors, leading to more negative outcomes. Unless the cycle is broken, it is difficult for vulnerable populations to change their health status. Nurses identify areas where they can work with vulnerable populations to break the cycle. The nursing process guides nurses in assessing vulnerable individuals, families, groups, and communities; developing nursing diagnoses of their strengths and needs; planning and implementing appropriate therapeutic nursing interventions in partnership with vulnerable clients; and evaluating the effectiveness of interventions.

ASSESSMENT ISSUES

Box 31-3 lists guidelines for assessing members of vulnerable population groups, whether individual or families. The following discussion expands on the points listed in that box.

Nursing Conceptual Approaches

Nursing assessment of vulnerable populations may be organized around any nursing conceptual framework that takes into account the multiple stressors experienced by these groups and the particular difficulties they have managing their health. Neuman, Roy, and Orem are particularly appropriate to use with vulnerable populations. Neuman's focus on identifying stressors and lines of resistance is a useful framework for organizing a nursing assessment because vulnerable populations experience multiple, overlapping stressors. Roy's emphasis on health-promoting modes of adaptation helps the nurse emphasize client strengths that are resources for coping with stressors. Orem's self-care approach directs the nurse to assess the client's self-care needs and abilities so therapeutic nursing interventions can target self-care deficits. These three nursing models are consistent with Pesznecker's (1984) adaptational model of poverty, which states that poor persons

---

BOX 31-3 Guidelines for Assessing Members of Vulnerable Population Groups

SETTING THE STAGE

- Create a comfortable, nonthreatening environment.
- Learn as much as you can about the culture of the clients you work with so that you will understand cultural practices and values that may influence their health care practices.
- Provide culturally competent assessment by understanding the meaning of language and nonverbal behavior in the client's culture.
- Be sensitive to the fact that the individual or family you are assessing may have other priorities that are more important to them. These might include financial or legal problems. You may need to give them some tangible help with their most pressing priority before you will be able to address issues that are more traditionally thought of as health concerns.
- Collaborate with others as appropriate; you should not provide financial or legal advice. However, you should make sure to connect your client with someone who can and will help them.

NURSING HISTORY OF AN INDIVIDUAL OR FAMILY

- You may have only one opportunity to work with a vulnerable person or family. Try to complete a history that will provide all the essential information you need to help the individual or family on that day. This means that you will have to organize in your mind exactly what you need to ask, and no more, and why the data are necessary.
- It will help to use a comprehensive assessment form that has been modified to focus on the special needs of the vulnerable population group with whom you work. However, be flexible. With some clients, it will be both impractical and unethical to cover all questions on a

comprehensive form. If you know that you are likely to see the client again, ask the less pressing questions at the next visit.
- Be sure to include questions about social support, economic status, resources for health care, developmental issues, current health problems, medications, and how the person or family manages their health status. Your goal is to obtain information that will enable you to provide family-centered care.
- Does the individual have any condition that compromises his or her immune status, such as AIDS, or is the individual undergoing therapy that would result in immunodeficiency, such as cancer chemotherapy?

PHYSICAL EXAMINATION OR HOME ASSESSMENT

- Again, complete as thorough a physical examination (on an individual) or home assessment as you can. Keep in mind that you should only collect data for which you have a use.
- Be alert for indications of physical abuse, substance use (e.g., needle marks, nasal abnormalities), or neglect (e.g., underweight, being inadequately clothed).
- You can assess a family's living environment using good observational skills. Does the family live in an insect- or rat-infested environment? Do they have running water, functioning plumbing, electricity, and a telephone?
- Is perishable food (e.g., mayonnaise) left sitting out on tables and countertops? Are bed linens reasonably clean? Is paint peeling on the walls and ceilings? Is ventilation adequate? Is the temperature of the home adequate? Is the family exposed to raw sewage or animal waste? Is the home adjacent to a busy highway, possibly exposing the family to high noise levels and automobile exhaust?

possess both individual and group factors, past experiences, and coping skills that, when combined with environmental factors such as stressors and stigma, lead to either healthy or unhealthy adaptive responses. Mediating factors such as public policy and social support can influence whether health-promoting or health-damaging adaptive responses are more likely. Pesznecker's model is particularly relevant to vulnerable populations, so nurses should consider using nursing conceptual frameworks that expand on this model as the basis for client assessment.

Because members of vulnerable populations often experience multiple stressors, nursing assessment must balance the need to be comprehensive and yet focus only on information that the nurse has a need for and that the client is willing to provide. The discussion that follows focuses on assessment of individual clients and families and on assessment of entire vulnerable population groups. With individuals and families, assessment can be intrusive and tiring, so it is important that the nurse have a reason for obtaining the data before asking the client. This means that assessing becomes an **iterative assessment process,** involving progressively more depth as the nurse refines his or her hypotheses about the nursing diagnose

Socioeconomic Considerations

Vulnerable populations typically have limited socioeconomic resources. Assessment should include questions about the clients' perceptions of socioeconomic resources, including identifying people who can provide support and financial resources. Support from other people may include information, caregiving, emotional support, and help with instrumental activities of daily living, such as transportation, shopping, and babysitting. Financial resources may include the extent to which the client can pay for health services and medications, as well as questions about eligibility for third-party payment. The nurse should ask the client about the perceived adequacy of both formal and informal support networks.

Physical Health Issues

Often, nurses see individual clients in clinic settings. These clients may be concerned about specific problems, which should be the initial priority. However, because vulnerable populations often find it difficult to seek routine health promotion and illness prevention services, nurses should take the opportunity to explain to clients the value of preventive assessment. If clients agree, nursing assessment should include evaluation of clients' preventive health needs, including age-appropriate screening tests, such as immunization status, blood pressure, weight, serum cholesterol, Papanicolaou smears, breast examinations, mammograms, prostate examinations, glaucoma screening, and dental evaluations. It may be necessary to make referrals to have some of these tests done for clients. Assessment should also include preventive screening for physical health problems for which certain vulnerable groups are at

a particularly high risk. For example, persons who are HIV-positive should be evaluated regularly for their T4 cell counts and for common opportunistic infections, including TB and pneumonia. Intravenous (IV) drug users should be evaluated for HBV, including liver palpation and serum antigen tests as necessary. Alcoholic clients should also be asked about symptoms of liver disease and should be evaluated for jaundice and liver enlargement. Severely mentally ill clients should be assessed for the presence of tardive dyskinesia, indicating possible toxicity from their antipsychotic medications. Chapters 32 to 39 provide more specific details about physical health assessment for vulnerable groups.

Biological Issues

Vulnerable populations should be assessed for congenital and genetic predisposition to illness and either receive education and counseling as appropriate or be referred to other health professionals as necessary. For example, pregnant adolescents who are substance abusers should be referred to programs to help them quit using addictive substances during their pregnancies and ideally after delivery of their infants as well. Pregnant women over age 35 should receive amniocentesis testing to determine if genetic abnormalities exist in the fetus. Specialized counseling about treatment and anticipatory guidance regarding the infant's needs can be provided by an advanced practice nurse or physician.

Psychological Issues

Vulnerable family groups should be assessed for the extent of stress the family may be experiencing and the presence of healthy or dysfunctional family dynamics. The nurse should also evaluate these families for effective communication patterns, caregiving capabilities, and the extent to which family developmental tasks are being met. Vulnerable individuals should be assessed for the presence of stressors, their usual coping styles, levels of self-efficacy (or the belief that one is capable of meeting life's challenges), their overall sense of well-being and level of self-esteem, and the presence of depression and anxiety (Berne et al, 1991; Pesznecker, 1984).

Lifestyle Issues

Nurses should assess lifestyle factors of vulnerable individuals, families, and groups that may predispose them to further health problems. Lifestyle factors include usual dietary patterns, exercise, rest, and the use of drugs, alcohol, and caffeine. For example, many homeless individuals eat their meals either at shelters or at fast-food restaurants. Because of the unpredictability of meals and food availability, it is often difficult for them to eat a diet that is low in fat, cholesterol, and sodium, and it is particularly difficult to eat the recommended five servings of fruit and vegetables per day. Cultural preferences may also influence lifestyle.

Environmental Issues

Vulnerable groups are more likely to be exposed to environmental hazards than other groups. Nurses should assess the living environment and neighborhood surroundings of vulnerable families and groups for environmental hazards such as lead-based paint, asbestos, water and air quality, industrial wastes, and the incidence of crime. Nurses must often establish partnerships with vulnerable groups to put changes into place, such as persuading a local industry to reduce the levels of effluents from their plants or working with local government and law enforcement to develop crime prevention programs.

PLANNING AND IMPLEMENTING CARE FOR VULNERABLE POPULATIONS

Planning and implementing care for members of vulnerable populations involves partnership between nurse and client. If the nurse directs and controls the client's care, the nurse will not be able to establish a trusting relationship and may inadvertently foster a cycle of dependency and lack of personal health control. In fact, the most important initial step is for the nurse to establish that he or she is trustworthy and dependable. For example, if the nurse works in a community clinic for substance abusers, he or she must overcome any suspicion that clients may have of the nurse and eliminate any fears that the nurse will manipulate them with "games."

Roles of the Nurse

Nurses working with vulnerable populations may fill numerous roles, including those listed in Box 31-4. They identify vulnerable individuals and families through **outreach** and case finding. They encourage vulnerable groups to obtain health services and develop programs that respond to their needs. Nurses teach vulnerable individuals, families, and groups strategies to prevent illness and promote health. They counsel clients about ways to increase their sense of personal power and help them identify strengths and resources (Chez, 1994). They provide direct care to clients and families in a variety of settings, including storefront clinics (Aiken and Salmon, 1994), mobile clinics, shelters (Mayo et al, 1996), homes, neighborhoods (Jenkins and Torrisi, 1997), work sites, churches, and schools (Hacker, 1996). For example, a nurse in a mobile migrant clinic might administer a tetanus booster to a client who has been injured by a piece of farm machinery and may also check that client's blood pressure and cholesterol level during the same visit. A home health nurse seeing a family referred by the courts for child abuse may weigh the child, conduct a nutritional assessment, and help the family learn how to manage anger and disciplinary problems. A nurse working in a school-based clinic may lead a support group for pregnant adolescents and conduct a birthing class. Nurses working with people being treated for TB monitor drug treatment compliance to ensure that they complete their full course of therapy

BOX 31-4 Nursing Roles When Working With Vulnerable Population Groups
Case finder Health teacher Counselor Direct care provider Monitor and evaluator of care Case manager Advocate Health program planner Participant in developing health policies

(Frieden, 1994). Nurses often function as case managers for vulnerable clients, making referrals and linking them with community services, and serve as advocates. The nurse functions as an advocate when referring clients to other agencies, working with others to develop health programs, and influencing legislation and health policies that affect vulnerable populations.

DID YOU KNOW? *Referring clients to community agencies involves much more than simply picking up the phone and making a call or completing a form. You should be certain that the agency to which you are referring a client is the right one to meet that client's needs. Nurses can do more harm than good by referring a stressed, discouraged client to an agency from which the client is not really eligible to receive services. Be sure to help the client learn how to get the most from the referral.*

The nature of nurses' roles varies depending on whether the client is a single person, a family, or a group. For example, a nurse might teach an HIV-positive client about the need for prevention of opportunistic infections, or may help a family with an HIV-positive member understand myths about transmission of HIV, or may work with a community group concerned about HIV transmission among students in the schools. In each case, the nurse teaches how to prevent infectious and communicable diseases, and the size of the group and the teaching methodologies vary. Box 31-5 lists principles for intervening with vulnerable populations.

Client Empowerment

Nurses should help all vulnerable groups achieve a greater sense of personal **empowerment,** since one of the core dimensions of vulnerability is a perception of powerlessness that can lead to hopelessness. Clients who feel empowered are more likely to be able to make autonomous decisions about their health care and improve their own health status. Nurses empower clients by helping them acquire the skills needed for healthy living and for being an effective

BOX 31-5 Principles for Intervening with Vulnerable Populations

GOALS

- Set reasonable goals that are based on the baseline data you collected. Focus on reducing disparities in health status among vulnerable populations and include the six target areas in the Presidential Initiative on Race and Ethnicity.
- Work toward setting manageable goals with the client. Goals that seem unattainable may be discouraging.
- Set goals collaboratively with the client as a first step toward client empowerment.
- Set family-centered, culturally sensitive goals.

INTERVENTIONS

- Set up outreach and casefinding programs to help increase access to health services by vulnerable populations.
- Try to minimize the "hassle factor" connected with your interventions. Vulnerable groups do not have the extra energy, money, or time to cope with unnecessary waits, complicated treatment plans, or confusion. As your client's advocate, identify what hassles may occur and develop ways to avoid them. This may include providing comprehensive services during a single encounter, rather than asking the client to return for multiple visits. Multiple visits for more specialized aspects of the client's needs, whether individual or family, reinforce a

perception that health care is fragmented and organized for the professional's convenience rather than the client's.
- Work with clients to ensure that interventions are culturally sensitive and competent.
- Focus on teaching clients skills in health promotion and disease prevention. Also, teach them how to be effective health care consumers. For example, role play, asking questions in a physician's office with a client.
- Help clients learn what to do if they cannot keep an appointment with a health care or social service professional.

EVALUATING OUTCOMES

- It is often difficult for vulnerable clients to return for follow-up care. Help your client develop self-care strategies for evaluating outcomes. For example, teach homeless individuals how to read their own TB skin test and give them a self-addressed, stamped card they can return by mail with the results.
- Remember to evaluate outcomes in terms of the goals you have mutually agreed on with the client. For example, one outcome for a homeless person receiving isoniazid therapy for TB might be that the person returned to the clinic daily for direct observation of the compliance with the drug therapy.

health care consumer. For example, one of the first steps in helping abused individuals is to empower them so they can begin to help themselves. Nurses can do this through active listening, by letting clients know that what is happening to them is illegal and that all people have the right to be safe, and by reassuring them that their fears and concerns are normal (Chez, 1994). Chez also suggests assisting the client to make independent decisions and helping clients recognize the strengths they can draw on to change the situation. Some examples of actions that abused women can decide to take include seeking help, seeking shelter, moving out of the house, notifying authorities, and separating or divorcing (Nurius et al, 1992).

One way to foster empowerment is to ensure that health-promoting strategies are culturally appropriate. For instance, culturally sensitive health education strategies ensure that information is provided in language that is meaningful to the group (semantic approach to cultural sensitivity) and that the cultural context is taken into account (instrumental approach to cultural sensitivity) as the educational program is designed (Bayer, 1994). **Culturally sensitive health education strategies** are based on respect for cultural diversity and demonstrate that the culture of the participants is respected. For example, when working with the homeless, it is important to build on the survival skills they have developed and to ensure that health programs reflect the fact that their first priority is usually sur-

vival. The culture of homelessness is oriented to the present, so a wide range of services should be available in a single location—"one-stop shopping" (Davis, 1996, p. 182).

NURSING TIP

Nurses demonstrate respect to clients of different cultural backgrounds by learning about the cultural norms, values and traditions of the groups within a particular community. It is particularly helpful to be fluent in a second language; e.g., nurses who work in communities with a large Hispanic population will find it useful to be fluent in Spanish. Similarly, nurses who work with people who are deaf should consider learning sign language.

WHAT DO YOU THINK? *Bayer (1994) says that public health professionals should not worry about being culturally sensitive when the values of a population subgroup threaten that group's health. According to the principled approach to cultural sensitivity, health professionals should not attempt to change cultural barriers to healthy behaviors because that would amount to imposing the values of the dominant group on the minority group (Bayer, 1994). Is this an example of the dominant culture being paternalistic and not respecting cultural diversity, or is it necessary to ignore cultural barriers to health when the public health at large is likely to be affected?*

HOW TO *Provide Comprehensive Care for Vulnerable Populations*

When working with vulnerable populations, try to have as many services as possible available in a single location and at convenient times. This "one-stop shopping" approach to care delivery is helpful for populations having multiple social, economic, and health- related stressors. While it may seem costly to provide comprehensive services in one location, it may save money in the long run by preventing illness.

Sometimes, the first step in empowering clients is functioning as an advocate for them, especially in the policy arena, where vulnerable populations may not always be represented. For example, in one community a nursing student learned that a social service agency had restrictive policies toward serving homeless alcoholic men. This was the primary agency that could provide shelter for these men, but their restrictive policies made it difficult for the men to obtain shelter as often as necessary. After advocating for the needs of this vulnerable population and persuading the agency to relax their policies, this nurse participated on the board of the agency to ensure that their policies continued to meet the needs. Providing shelter made it more likely that the men could get adequate rest, bathe, and dress in clean clothes so they could look for jobs and become more self-sufficient.

Levels of Prevention

Healthy People 2000 objectives emphasize preventing illness and promoting health. One way to do this is for vulnerable individuals to have a primary care provider who both coordinates health services for them and provides their preventive services. This primary care provider may be an advanced practice nurse or a primary care physician (e.g., a family practice physician). Another approach is for a nurse to serve as a case manager for vulnerable clients and, again, coordinate services and provide illness prevention and health promotion services.

HOW TO *Coordinate Services for Members of Vulnerable Populations*

Nurses who work with vulnerable populations often need to coordinate services across multiple agencies for members of these groups. It is helpful to have a strong professional network with people who work in other agencies. Effective professional networks make it easier to coordinate care smoothly and in ways that do not add to clients' stress. Nurses can develop strong networks by participating in community coalitions and attending professional meetings. When making referrals to other agencies, a phone call can be a helpful way to obtain information that the client will need about the visit. When possible, having an interdisciplinary, interagency team plan care for clients at high risk of health problems can be quite effective. It is crucial to obtain the clients' written and informed consent before engaging in this kind of planning due to confidentiality issues.

One example of primary prevention recommended for certain vulnerable groups is provision of prophylactic antituberculosis drug therapy for HIV-positive individuals who live in homeless shelters. Anastasi and Rivera (1994) explain that prophylactic drug treatment for persons who are HIV-positive may be either primary or secondary. The goal of primary drug treatment is to "prevent or delay the onset of symptoms of reactivated as well as newly acquired infections. The goal of secondary prophylaxis is to prevent or delay recurrent episodes of symptomatic infection. Both are intended to reduce the number of episodes of infection over a person's lifetime" (Anastasi and Rivera, 1994, p. 37). Another example of primary prevention is administering influenza vaccinations to vulnerable populations who are immunocompromised unless contraindicated. An example of secondary prevention is conducting screening clinics for vulnerable populations. For example, nurses who work in homeless shelters, prisons, migrant camps, and substance abuse treatment facilities should know that these groups are at a high risk for acquiring communicable diseases. Both clients and staff need routine screening for TB (Box 31-6). An example of tertiary prevention is conducting a therapy group with the residents of a group home for severely mentally ill adults. Nurses who work with abused women to help them enhance their levels of self-esteem are also providing tertiary preventive activities.

Strategies for Promoting Healthy Lifestyles

Helping vulnerable persons develop healthy lifestyle behaviors requires great sensitivity by nurses. They should focus on identifying clients' priorities and helping them meet these priorities. For example, discussing exercise with a homeless person requires empathy and creativity. Often, vulnerable individuals and families are coping with crises, so the nurse must begin by using crisis intervention strate-

---

BOX 31-6 Primary and Secondary Prevention for Populations at Risk for Communicable Diseases

People who spend time in homeless shelters, substance abuse treatment facilities, and prisons risk acquiring communicable diseases such as influenza and TB. Nurses who work in these facilities should plan regular influenza vaccination clinics and TB screening clinics. When planning these clinics, nurses should work with local physicians to develop signed protocols and should plan ahead for problems related to the transient nature of the population. For example, nurses should develop a way for homeless individuals to read their TB skin test if necessary and transfer the results back to the facility where the skin test was administered. It is helpful to develop a portable immunization chart, such as a wallet card, that mobile population groups such as the homeless and migrant workers can carry with them.

gies. After the crisis has been managed, a trusting relationship is likely to exist between the nurse and client, which forms the basis for health promotion interventions. Nurses must be sensitive to the lifestyles of their vulnerable clients and must develop methods of health promotion that recognize these lifestyle factors. For instance, Brennan's ComputerLink program for people with AIDS provides personal computers in the homes of people with AIDS and enables them to obtain information about ways to maintain a high quality of life in the privacy of their homes (Brennan and Ripich, 1994). Another example is a program that was designed to encourage inner-city Latino families to increase their intake of low-fat milk (Wechsler and Wernick, 1992). This successful program included providing money-off coupons for low-fat milk, making it less costly for families to purchase the milk.

Healthy People 2000 Objectives and *Healthy Communities 2000* Standards

The *Healthy People 2000* objectives emphasize illness prevention and health promotion. Objectives have been developed for health promotion, health protection, preventive services, and surveillance and data systems. Objectives that are relevant for vulnerable populations may be found in several areas. Within the health promotion category are objectives related to alcohol and other drugs, mental health and mental disorders, and violent and abusive behavior. The preventive services category contains objectives targeting maternal and infant health, HIV infection, STDs, and immunization and infectious diseases. Specific age-related objectives are outlined, as are objectives for special populations. The special population category for low-income persons is directly related to the vulnerable populations described in this chapter. The other special population categories are African-Americans, Hispanics, Asians and Pacific Islanders, American Indians and Native Americans, and persons with disabilities. These categories overlap with many of the vulnerable populations described in this chapter, although it would not be accurate to say that all members of any one of these groups are vulnerable. However, many minority populations are disproportionately represented in vulnerable groups, so nurses should focus special attention on the health objectives for the special populations identified in *Healthy People 2000*. This will help achieve the targeted goals for special populations in the Presidential Initiative on Race and Ethnic Disparities in Health (Hamburg, 1998).

The *Healthy People 2000* (USDHHS, 1991) objectives include targets for improvement over baseline incidence and prevalence statistics on illness and health problems. Many objectives include unique targets for special population subgroups with incidence and prevalence statistics that are much higher than for the population as a whole. For example, one of the physical activity objectives for lower-income adults is to "increase to at least 12% the proportion of people who engage in vigorous physical activity that promotes the development and maintenance of cardiorespiratory fitness 3 or more days per week." The target proportion for the population as a whole is 20% and is higher because their baseline level of 12% is higher than the baseline level of 7% for low-income adults. These targets are designed to be realistic improvements over the baseline levels. Communities should determine local incidence and prevalence statistics and establish realistic targets for improvement. For example, it would be unrealistic to establish the same goals for reducing the incidence of HIV infection for IV drug users as for the general population because the baseline rates are so much higher for IV drug users and because their risks are so much greater. Rather, nurses should work with local groups to establish goals and objectives that are substantially better than baseline rates but are potentially achievable. Later goals will use the new baselines, and the health status of the vulnerable population group should continuously improve.

The *Healthy People 2000 Midcourse Review* (USDHHS, 1995) shows that while progress has been made in achieving the objectives, wide disparities still exist between the health of special populations and the country as a whole. For example, between 1990 and 1992, the age-adjusted years of potential life lost (YPPL) before age 75 for the population as a whole was 8384 per 100,000. "For blacks and American Indians/Alaskan Natives in Indian Health Service areas (HIS) the rate are considerably higher, 15,468 and 11,875 respectively" (USDHHS, 1995, pp. 7-8). This reflects wide disparities in mortality from a number of causes, including infant mortality, accidents, violence, and early death from chronic illness.

A group of public health professionals representing several different agencies, including the American Public Health Association and the Centers for Disease Control and Prevention, developed a guide to help individual communities meet the *Healthy People 2000* national health objectives in their own areas. This guide, entitled *Healthy Communities 2000: Model Standards* (APHA, 1991), describes ways that communities can establish health objectives that are consistent with national health objectives but realistic for local communities. It also suggests activities to achieve local health objectives and ways to determine the capacity of the local health department to implement the activities and emphasizes developing partnerships with other agencies.

Comprehensive Services

In general, more agencies are needed that provide comprehensive services with nonrestrictive eligibility requirements. Communities often have many agencies that restrict eligibility for their services to people most likely to benefit from those services, or they limit eligibility to make it possible for more people to receive services. For example, shelters may prohibit people who have been drinking alcohol from staying overnight and sometimes limit the number of sequential nights a person can stay. Food banks usually limit the number of times a person can receive free food. Agencies are frequently very specialized as well. For vulnerable individuals and families, this means

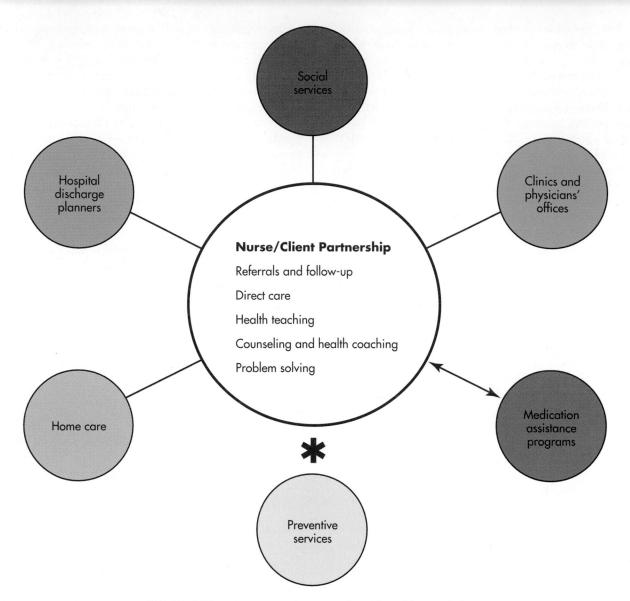

FIG. 31-4 The nurse as case manager for vulnerable populations

that they must go to many agencies to find services for which they qualify and that meet their needs. This is so tiring and discouraging that people are sometimes willing to forego help because it is just too difficult to obtain it. In their study of admission policies in homeless shelters for women in Chicago, Barge and Norr (1991) found that most shelters limited the numbers of pregnant women, women with children, and especially women with teenage boys. It is very difficult to help these clients achieve health promotion and illness prevention objectives if they have difficulty meeting basic needs for shelter.

Resources for Vulnerable Populations

Nurses should be thoroughly familiar with community agencies that offer a wide variety of health and social ser-

vices for vulnerable populations. Nurses should also follow up with the client after the referral if at all possible to ensure that the desired outcomes were achieved. Sometimes, excellent community resources may be available but impractical for clients because of transportation or reimbursement problems. Nurses should identify if these problems will interfere with clients following through with referrals and work with other team members to make the referral as convenient and realistic as possible. Although clients with social problems such as financial needs should be referred to social workers, nurses should understand the close connections between health and social problems and know how to work effectively with other professionals. A list of community resources can often be found in the telephone book, and many communities have publications that list community resources. Examples of agency resources found in most communities are as follows:

- Health departments
- Community mental health centers
- American Red Cross and other voluntary organizations
- Food and clothing banks
- Missions and shelters
- Nurse-managed neighborhood clinics
- Social service agencies such as Travelers' Aid and Salvation Army
- Church-sponsored health and social service assistance

Two other very important categories of resources for vulnerable populations are their own personal coping skills and social supports (McLeod and Kessler, 1990). These groups must often be quite resourceful and creative to manage in the face of multiple stressors. Nurses should work with clients to help them identify their own personal strengths and draw on those strengths when managing their health needs. Also, clients may be able to depend on informal support networks. Even though social isolation is a problem for many vulnerable clients, nurses should not assume that clients have no one who can help them.

Case Management

Case management involves linking client with services and providing direct nursing services to clients, such as teaching, counseling, screening, and immunizing (Bower, 1992). Lillian Wald was the first nurse case manager, linking vulnerable families with the wide variety of services needed to help them stay healthy (Buhler-Wilkerson, 1993). Aiken and Salmon (1994, p. 327) explain that "public health nurses represent the interface between personal health services and population-based health promotion." Linking, or **brokering health services,** is accomplished by making appropriate referrals and by following up with clients to ensure that the desired outcomes from the referral were achieved. Nurses have been effective case managers in community nursing clinics, in health departments, and in case management programs where the focus included both community and hospital care. Nurse case managers emphasize health promotion and illness prevention with vulnerable clients and focus on helping them avoid unnecessary hospitalization. Figure 31-4 illustrates the coordination and brokering aspect of the nurse's role as case manager for vulnerable populations.

EVALUATION OF NURSING INTERVENTIONS WITH VULNERABLE POPULATIONS

Evaluation of therapeutic nursing interventions begins with client goals and objectives and focuses on the extent to which client health outcomes were achieved. Nurses may evaluate individual client goal achievement, the extent to which a vulnerable family achieved goals developed in partnership with the nurse, or the extent to which a nursing program achieved its objectives. Evaluation takes place while providing care and gives the nurse a basis for

revising therapeutic interventions to make them more effective. Evaluation also takes place when a case is closed or when a program is completed and gives nurses data to use in providing care to similar clients or programs in the future. The types of client outcomes that may be evaluated include improved quality of life, improved indicators of physical health status (e.g., blood pressure, skin integrity, mobility), reduced depression or anxiety, improved functional status, increased levels of knowledge about health behaviors, and satisfaction with care. Nurses use a variety of scales to evaluate these outcome indicators; they sometimes interview clients or administer short questionnaires; and they use laboratory reports and results of health assessments to help evaluate goal achievement with individuals and clients. Incidence and prevalence data, survey data, and service utilization data are used to evaluate health programs for vulnerable populations.

 clinical application

Assume that you are a nurse working in a migrant health clinic. Use the ideas presented in the chapter to plan nursing interventions for Dorothy Green. Ms. Green, a 46 year old farm worker pregnant with her fifth child, came in requesting treatment for swollen ankles. During your assessment, you learned that she had seen the nurse practitioner at the local health department 2 months ago. The NP gave her some sample vitamins, but Ms. Green lost them. She has not received regular prenatal care and has no plans to do so. Her previous pregnancies were essentially normal, although she said she was "toxic" with her last child. She also said that her middle child was "not quite right". He is in the seventh grade at age 15 but seems to manage adequately. Ms. Green is 5'2", weighs 180 pounds, and has a blood pressure of 160/90 with pitting edema of the ankles and a mild headache.

Ms. Green says that she usually takes chlorpromazine hydrochloride (Thorazine) but has run out of it and cannot afford to have her prescription refilled. She says that she has been in several mental hospitals over the last few years and describes her behavior as getting more agitated and having problems managing her daily activities. As her agitation grows, she says that she usually hears voices and this really makes her aggressive.

None of her children live with her, and she has no plans for taking care of the infant. She thinks she will ask the child's father, a racetrack worker, to help her since she usually travels around the country with him.

A. What additional information do you need to help you adequately assess Ms. Green's health status and current needs?

B. What nursing diagnoses are suggested by the brief historical, physical, and socioeconomic data presented?

Answers are in the back of the book.

KEY POINTS

- Vulnerable populations are more likely to develop health problems as a result of exposure to risk or to have worse outcomes from those health problems than the population as a whole. Vulnerable populations are more sensitive to risk factors than those who are more resilient and are more often exposed to cumulative risk factors. These populations include poor or homeless persons, pregnant adolescents, migrant workers, severely mentally ill individuals, substance abusers, abused individuals, persons with communicable diseases, and persons with sexually transmitted diseases, including HIV and HBV.
- All countries have these special population groups that are more vulnerable to poor health than others. The specific groups vary across countries, depending on local political, economic, cultural, and demographic characteristics.
- Health care is increasingly moving into the community. This began with deinstitutionalization of the severely mentally ill population and is continuing today as hospitals reduce inpatient stays. Vulnerable populations need a wide variety of services, and because these are often provided by multiple community agencies, nurses coordinate and manage the service needs of vulnerable groups.
- Public policies sometimes provide financial assistance for vulnerable populations and sometimes provide money to build health facilities and train professionals to work with vulnerable groups. Unanticipated implementation problems often further disadvantage vulnerable populations. Health care reform policies are focused on controlling costs and may have the unintended effect of limiting services to vulnerable populations.
- The health field concept suggests that both individuals and society are responsible for health status. Individuals and groups may be vulnerable to social and health problems both as a result of their own actions and the policies and decisions made at the societal level. There are many dimensions to vulnerability, including limited control over one's own health, victimization, disenfranchisement, disadvantaged status, powerlessness, and cumulative health risks.
- Socioeconomic problems, including poverty and social isolation, physiological and developmental aspects of age, poor health status, and highly stressful life experiences, predispose people to vulnerability. Vulnerability can become a cycle, where the predisposing factors lead to poor health outcomes, chronic stress, and hopelessness. These outcomes increase vulnerability.
- Nurses assess vulnerable individuals, families, and groups to determine which socioeconomic, physical, biological, psychological, and environmental factors are problematic for clients. They work as partners with vulnerable clients to identify client strengths and needs and develop intervention strategies designed to break the cycle of vulnerability.
- Community health nursing roles when working with vulnerable populations include health teacher, counselor, direct care provider, case manager, advocate, health program planner, and participant in developing health policies. Nurses focus on empowering clients to prevent illness and promote health, and they work to achieve the *Healthy People 2000* national health objectives with vulnerable populations. Nurses link clients with resources in the community and monitor client outcomes to ensure that community referrals are effective.
- Evaluation of therapeutic nursing interventions with vulnerable populations occurs both during and after service delivery. Results of evaluations are used to make revisions in nursing care, with the ultimate goal of improving client outcomes.

critical thinking activities

1. Vulnerability implies that certain populations have both a higher relative risk of illness due to the presence of multiple risk factors and a greater sensitivity to the effects of individual risk factors. Identify populations in your community that you think are more vulnerable to poor health than others. List the risk factors members of these populations are more likely to have, and identify the prevalence of these risk factors in your community. Discuss with your classmates or a nurse in a clinical agency the effect you believe these risk factors are having on the health of vulnerable populations in your community. Analyze whether members of these special populations seem to be more sensitive to the effect of the risk factors than the population as a whole.

2. Examine health statistics and demographic data in your geographical area to determine which vulnerable groups predominate in your area. Look through your phone book for examples of agencies that you think provide services to these vulnerable groups. Make appointments with key individuals in several of these agencies to discuss the nature of their target population, the types of services provided, and the reimbursement mechanisms for these services. Various class members should visit different agencies and then share their results during class. Based on your findings, identify gaps or overlaps in services provided to vulnerable groups in your community. What might be some ways to manage these gaps and overlaps to help clients receive the services they need?

3. Debate with your class the nature and extent of services that you believe should be made available to the homeless. Defend your position regarding "enabling" and "worthiness."

4. Health care spending accounts for about 15% of the gross domestic product (GDP). Most people do not want to spend any more of the GDP on health care. Assuming then that the amount of money available to spend on health care is fixed at any point in time, explain what proportion of that money you think the federal government should spend on prevention and treatment of AIDS, substance abuse, severe mental illness, and breast cancer. What criteria did you use to arrive at your conclusions?

5. To what extent do you think economic issues and social values play a role in the way that health services are offered to vulnerable population groups? Explain why you think the population as a whole should or should

not pay for care for vulnerable groups. Read the article by Grey (1994) in the reference list on the development of health services for migrant workers for an example of this debate.

6. Discuss the types of assistance you might provide to the following clients:
   a. A chronically homeless, pregnant, 33-year-old, mildly mentally retarded woman and her unemployed boyfriend
   b. A 14-year-old runaway girl who is earning money through prostitution and has a drug habit
   c. A 22-year-old woman with four children who is receiving welfare and whose boyfriend smokes crack cocaine
   d. An HIV-positive woman with no family and few friends who is trying to make plans for someone to care for her three children after her death
   e. A 56-year-old alcoholic male migrant farm worker whose TB skin test just came back positive

What kinds of nursing needs do these clients have in common? Analyze the dimensions of vulnerability described in this chapter in terms of how these clients may possess these characteristics and how you, as a nurse, can help them break out of the cycle of vulnerability.

7. Examine the pros and cons of school-based clinics for adolescents. Do you think reproductive services should be included in such clinics? What are the ethical issues involved in providing reproductive information to adolescents, with or without parental consent and involvement?

8. Interview nurses at a health department to identify which personal care services they provide to vulnerable populations and which population-based services they provide. Discuss their opinions about whether personal care services should only be provided by private agencies.

Bibliography

AAN Expert Panel Report: Culturally competent health care, *Nurs Outlook* 40(6):277, 1992.

Aday LA: *At risk in America: the health and health care needs of vulnerable populations in the United States,* San Francisco, 1993, Jossey Bass.

Aday LA: Vulnerable populations: a community-oriented perspective, *Fam Community Health* 19(1):1, 1997.

Adler NE et al: Socioeconomic inequalities in health: no easy solution. In Lee PR, Estes CL, editors: *The nations' health,* ed 5, Sudbury, Mass, 1997, Jones & Bartlett.

Aiken LH, Salmon ME: Health care workforce priorities: what nursing should do now, *Inquiry* 31(3):318, 1994.

American Nurses Association: *Nursing's agenda for health care reform,* Kansas City, Mo, 1991, the Association.

American Public Health Association: *Healthy communities 2000: model standards,* ed 3, Washington, DC, 1991, the Association.

Anastasi JK, Rivera J: Understanding prophylactic therapy for HIV infections, *Am J Nurs* 94(2):36, 1994.

Avey MA: TB skin testing: how to do it right, *Am J Nurs* 93(9):42, 1993.

Baker EL et al: Health reform and the health of the public: forging community health partnerships, *JAMA* 272(16):1276, 1994.

Barge FC, Norr KF: Homeless shelter policies for women in an urban environment, *Image J Nurs Sch* 23(3):145, 1991.

Bayer R: AIDS prevention and cultural sensitivity: are they compatible? *Am J Public Health* 84(6):895, 1994.

Benenson AS: *Control of communicable diseases in man,* ed 15, Washington, DC, 1990, American Public Health Association.

Berne AS et al: A nursing model for addressing the health needs of homeless families, *Image J Nurs Sch* 22(1):8, 1991.

Bower KA: *Case management by nurses,* Kansas City, Mo, 1992, American Nurses Association.

Brennan PF, Ripich S: Use of a home-care computer network by persons with AIDS, *Int J Technol Assess Health Care* 10(2):258, 1994.

Briere JN, Elliott DM: Immediate and long-term impacts of child sexual abuse, *Future Child Sex Abuse Child* 4(2):54, 1994.

Buhler-Wilkerson K: Bringing care to the people: Lillian Wald's legacy to public health nursing, *Am J Public Health* 83(12):1778, 1993.

Caliandro G, Hughes C: The experience of being a grandmother who is the primary caregiver for her HIV-positive grandchild, *Nurs Res* 47(2):107, 1998.

Callahan JJ et al: Mental health/substance abuse treatment in managed care: the Massachusetts Medicaid experience, *Health Affairs* 14(3):173, 1995.

Carrasquillo O et al: Can Medicaid managed care provide continuity of care to new Medicaid enrollees: an analysis of tenure on Medicaid, *Am J Public Health* 88(3):464, 1988.

Chez N: Helping the victim of domestic violence, *Am J Nurs* 94(7):32, 1994.

Ciesielski S et al: The incidence of tuberculosis among North Carolina migrant farmworkers, 1991, *Am J Public Health* 84(11):1836, 1994.

Curtin L: Throwaway people? *Nurs Manage* 17(12):7, 1986.

Davis RE: Tapping into the culture of homelessness, *J Prof Nurs* 12(3):176, 1996.

De la Barra X: Poverty: the main cause of ill health in urban children, *Health Educ Behav* 25(1):46, 1998.

Dever GEA, Sciegaj M, Wade TE: Creation of a social vulnerability index for justice in health planning, *Fam Comm Health* 10(4):23, 1998.

Devlin BK, Reynolds E: Child abuse: how to recognize it, how to intervene, *Am J Nurs* 94(3):26, 1994.

Epstein AM: Medicaid managed care and high quality: can we have both? *JAMA* 278(19):1617, 1997.

Erickson GP: To pauperize or empower: public health nursing at the turn of the 20th and 21st centuries, *Public Health Nurs* 13(3):163, 1996.

Ferenchick GS: The medical problems of homeless clinic patients: a comparative study, *J Gen Intern Med* 7:294, 1992.

Fielding J, Halfon N: Where is the health in health system reform? *JAMA* 272(16):1292, 1994.

Finklehor D: Current information on the scope and nature of child sexual abuse, *Future Child Sex Abuse Child* 4(2):31, 1994.

Flaskerud JH, Winslow BJ: Conceptualizing vulnerable populations health-related research, *Nurs Res* 47(2):69, 1998.

Freedberg L, McLeod RG: The other side of the law: despite all efforts to curb it, immigration is rising, *San Francisco Chronicle,* Oct 13, 1998.

Frieden TR: Tuberculosis control and social change, *Am J Public Health* 84(11):1721, 1994.

Friedman E: Money isn't everything: nonfinancial barriers to access, *JAMA* 271(19):1535, 1994.

Fullerton D et al: Preventing untended teenage pregnancies and reducing their

Continued

Bibliography—cont'd

adverse effects, *Quality in Health Care* 6(2):102, 1997.

Gifford BD, Bettenhausen KL: Physicians' receptiveness to teen Medicaid recipients seeking office-based prenatal care, *Fam Comm Health* 20(2):70, 1997.

Grau L: Illness-engendered poverty among the elderly, *Women Health* 12(3/4), 1987.

Grey MR: The medical care programs of the Farm Security Administration, 1932 through 1947: a rehearsal for national health insurance? *Am J Public Health* 84(10):1678, 1994.

Grob G: *Mental institutions in America: social policy to 1875*, New York, 1973, Free Press of Glencoe.

Grob G: *Mental illness and American society: 1875-1940*, Princeton, NJ, 1983, Princeton University Press.

Hacker K: Integrating school-based health centers into managed care in Massachusetts, *J School Health* 66(9):317, 1996.

Hall LA, Sachs B, Rayens MK: Mothers' potential for child abuse: the roles of childhood abuse and social resources, *Nurs Res* 47(2):87, 1998.

Hamburg M: Eliminating racial and ethnic disparities in health: response to the Presidential initiative on race, *Public Health Rep* 113(July/August):372, 1998.

Hansell PS et al: The effect of a social support boosting intervention on stress, coping, and social support in caregivers of children with AIDS, *Nurs Res* 47(2):79, 1998.

Hogan NS, DeSantis L: Things that help and hinder adolescent sibling bereavement, *West J Nurs Res* 16(2):132, 1994.

Institute of Medicine: *Homelessness, health, and human needs*, Washington, DC, 1988, National Academy Press.

Ireson C, Weaver D: Marketing nursing beyond the walls, *J Nurs Adm* 22(1):57, 1992.

Jenkins M, Torrisi D: Community partnership primary care case study: Abbottsford Community Health Center, *Nurse Practitioner Forum* 8(1):21, 1997.

Kimchi J, Schaffner B: Childhood protective factors and stress risks. In Arnold LE, editor: *Childhood stress*, New York, 1990, Wiley.

Kochanek KD, Maurer JD, Rosenberg HM: Why did black life expectancy decline from 1984 through 1989 in the United States? *Am J Public Health* 84(6):938, 1994.

Leonhardt KK et al: A cluster of tuberculosis among crack house contacts in San Mateo County, California, *Am J Public Health* 84(11):1834, 1994.

Maynard R, editor: *Kids having kids: a Robin Hood Foundation special report on the cost of adolescent childbearing*, New York, 1996, Robin Hood Foundation.

Mayo K: Community collaboration: prevention and control of tuberculosis in a homeless shelter, *Public Health Nurs* 13(2):120, 1996.

McCubbin MA, McCubbin HI: Family stress theory and assessment: the resiliency model of family stress, adjustment, and adaptation. In McCubbin HI, Thompson AI, editors: *Family assessment inventories for research and practice*, Madison, Wisconsin, 1991, University of Wisconsin.

McLeod JD, Kessler RC: Socioeconomic status differences in vulnerability to undesirable life events, *J Health Soc Behav* 31:162, 1990.

Mechanic D, Schlesinger M, McAlpine DD: Management of mental health and substance abuse services: state of the art and early results, *Milbank Q* 73:19, 1995.

Moccia P, Mason DJ: Poverty trends: implications for nursing, *Nurs Outlook* 34(1):20, 1986.

Nichols J, Wright LK, Murphy JF: A proposal for tracking health care for the homeless, *J Comm Health* 11(3):204, 1986.

Nicholson J et al: Impact of Medicaid managed care on child and adolescent emergency mental health screening in Massachusetts, *Psychiatric Services* 47(12):1344, 1996.

Northam S: Access to health promotion, protection, and disease prevention among mpoverished individuals, *Public Health Nurs* 13(5):353, 1996.

Nurius PS, Furrey J, Berliner L: Coping capacity among women with abusive partners, *Violence Vict* 7(3):229, 1992.

O'Brien LM, Bartlett KA: TB plus HIV spells trouble, *Am J Nurs* 92(5):28, 1992.

O'Connor FW: A vulnerability-stress framework for evaluating clinical interventions in schizophrenia, *Image J Nurs Sch* 26(3):231, 1994.

Pappas G: Elucidating the relationships between race, socioeconomic status, and health, *Am J Public Health* 84(6):892, 1994.

Pesznecker B: The poor: a population at risk, *Public Health Nurs* 4(1):237, 1984.

Pierre N, Cox J: Teenage pregnancy and prevention programs, *Curr Op Pediatr* 9(4):310, 1997.

Plescia M et al: A multidisciplinary health care outreach team to the homeless: the 10-year experience of the Montefiore Care for the Homeless Team, *Fam Comm Health* 20(2):58, 1997.

Powell KB: Correlates of violent and nonviolent behavior among vulnerable inner city youths, *Fam Comm Health* 20(2):38, 1997.

Provan KG: Services integration for vulnerable populations: lessons from community mental health, *Fam Comm Health* 19(4):19, 1997.

Provan KG, Sebastian JG: Networks within networks: interoganizational delivery systems in community mental health, *Acad Manage J*, Aug, 1998.

Rabkin JG et al: Resilience in adversity among long-term survivors of AIDS, *Hosp Comm Psychiatry* 44(2):162, 1993.

Ropers RH: *Persistent poverty*, New York, 1991, Plenum Press.

Rosner D: Health care for the "truly needy": nineteenth-century origins of the concept, *Milbank Mem Fund Q* 60(3):355, 1982.

Sebastian JB: Homelessness: a state of vulnerability, *Fam Comm Health* 8(3):11, 1985.

Shovein J, Young MS: MRSA: Pandora's box for hospitals, *Am J Nurs* 92(2):48, 1992.

Shugars DA, O'Neill EH, Bader JD, editors: *Healthy America: practitioners for 2005, an agenda for U.S. health professional schools*, Durham, NC, 1991, Pew Health Professions Commission.

Simpson CC et al: Preventing pregnancy in early adolescence: identifying risks, *ADVANCE Nurse Practit* 5(4):22, 1997.

Statistics Canada: infant mortality rates, 1998. Available online [www.statcan.ca/english/Pgdb/people/Health/health21.htm] Dec 8, 1998.

Steinwachs DM et al: Service systems research, *Schizophr Bull* 18:627, 1992.

Superintendent of Documents: *Federal Register 63(36)*, Washington, DC, 1998, US Government Printing Office.

Torrey EF et al: *Care of the seriously mentally ill: a rating of state programs*, ed 3, Washington, DC, 1990, Public Health Citizen Health Research Group and the National Alliance for the Mentally Ill.

Trussell J: Teenage pregnancy in the United States, *Fam Plann Perspect* 20(6):262, 1988.

US Department of Health and Human Services: *Healthy people 2000: midcourse review.* Washington, DC, 1995, US Government Printing Office.

US Department of Health and Human Services: *Healthy people 2000: national health promotion and disease prevention objectives.* Washington, DC, 1991, Government Printing Office.

US Department of Health and Human Services: Secretary Shalala launches new national strategy to prevent teen pregnancy: new state-by-state data show decline in teen birth rates, *Health and Human Services News*, 1, 1997.

US Department of Health and Human Services, Public Health Service: *Health, United States*, Washington, DC, 1998, US Government Printing Office.

Valanis B: *Epidemiology in nursing and health care,* ed 2, East Norwalk, Conn, 1992, Appleton & Lange.

Wechsler H, Wernick SM: A social marketing campaign to promote low-fat milk consumption in an inner-city Latino community, *Public Health Rep* 107(2):202, 1992.

Wellever A, Hill G, Casey M: Medicaid reform issues affecting the Indian Health Care System, *Am J Public Health* 88(2):193, 1998.

Wells KB et al: Issues and approaches in evaluating managed mental health care, *Milbank Q* 73:57, 1995.

Will MB: Referral: a process, not a form, *Nursing '77* 7:44, 1977.

Yoos L: Perspectives on adolescent parenting: effect of adolescent egocentrism on the maternal-child interaction, *J Pediatr Nurs* 2(3):193, 1987.

Yule W: Resilience and vulnerability in child survivors of disasters. In Tizard B, Varma V, editors: *Vulnerability and resilience in human development,* London, 1992, Kingsley.

CHAPTER

32

Poverty and Homelessness

CHRISTINE DIMARTILE BOLLA

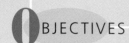

OBJECTIVES

After reading this chapter, the student should be able to do the following:

- Analyze the concept of poverty.
- Discuss nurses' perceptions about poverty and health.
- Describe the social, political, cultural, and environmental factors that influence poverty.
- Discuss the effects of poverty on the health and well-being of individuals, families, and communities.

- Analyze the concept of homelessness.
- Discuss nurses' perceptions about homelessness and health.
- Describe the social, political, cultural, and environmental factors that influence homelessness.
- Discuss the effects of homelessness on the health and well-being of individuals, families, and communities.
- Discuss nursing interventions for poor and homeless individuals.

KEY TERMS

Consumer Price Index (CPI)
crisis poverty
cultural attitudes
deinstitutionalization
Elizabethan poor laws
federal income guidelines
gentrification

historical factors
homelessness
Interagency Council on the Homeless (ICH)
knowledge
media discourses
near poor

neighborhood poverty
persistent poverty
personal beliefs
poverty
poverty thresholds
Stewart B. McKinney Assistance Act

Temporary Assistance to Needy Families (TANF)
values
Women, Infants, and Children (WIC)

See Glossary for definitions

CHAPTER OUTLINE

Concept of Poverty
    Personal Beliefs, Values, and Knowledge
    Cultural Attitudes, Media Discourses, and Historical Factors
Defining and Understanding Poverty
    Social Definitions of Poverty
    Political Dimensions
    Cultural Perspectives
    Environmental Perspectives

Poverty and Health: Effects Across the Life Span
    Childbearing Women and Poverty
    Children and Poverty
    Older Adults and Poverty
    The Community and Poverty
Understanding the Concept of Homelessness
    Personal Beliefs, Values, and Knowledge

Clients' Perceptions of Homelessness
Homelessness in the United States
Causes of Homelessness
Effects of Homelessness on Health
    Homelessness and At-Risk Populations
    Federal Programs for the Homeless
Role of the Nurse

The author wishes to acknowledge the contributions of Teresa Acquaviva and Jeanette Lancaster to the content of this chapter.

merican cultural values are based on self-reliance, responsibility and accountability. Therefore interventions aimed at improving the plight of the poor and homeless are constrained by issues of power, politics, and arguments concerning social versus individual responsibility.

Nurses encounter poor persons, families, and aggregates in a variety of settings, such as private homes, congregate living situations, schools, churches, clinics, and meal sites. To provide effective care for individuals, families, and aggregates living in poverty, nurses must develop concepts of poverty and homelessness that include historical, social, political, economic, biological, psychological, and spiritual factors. To appreciate the concepts of poverty and homelessness, one must begin with self-examination of personal beliefs, values, and knowledge about poverty and homelessness. Next, one must develop an understanding of the history of public responses to poor and homeless persons, and the relationship of this history to public and personal responses today that influence perceptions of poor and homeless persons. The nurse must identify health care needs, barriers to care, and essential nursing services for poor and homeless individuals, families, and aggregates. To provide effective nursing interventions, the nurse must understand the epidemiology, health problems, and risk factors associated with poverty (Carney, 1992).

This chapter describes the many ways in which poverty and homelessness affect the health status of individuals, families, and communities. It also suggests nursing intervention strategies with poor and homeless aggregates.

CONCEPT OF POVERTY

Individual perceptions of poverty and poor persons are rooted in social, political, cultural, and environmental factors. Personal beliefs, social values, personal knowledge of poverty, cultural attitudes, media views, and historical factors influence a person's understanding of poverty.

Personal Beliefs, Values, and Knowledge

To be effective, nurses must recognize and acknowledge the personal beliefs, values, and knowledge that form their own world views and influence the way they practice. **Personal beliefs** are ideas about the world that an individual believes to be true. Personal opinions concerning individuals on public assistance are examples of personal beliefs. Societal **values** are attitudes, customs, and ways of behaving that members of a society regard as either appropriate or inappropriate. Perceptions of individual versus social responsibility for health and well-being are rooted in society's values. **Knowledge** is information thought to be true by an individual, group or society. Perceptions of the differences between truth and nontruth influence what is considered legitimate knowledge by an individual, family, group, or the greater society.

Cultural Attitudes, Media Discourses, and Historical Factors

Cultural attitudes are the beliefs and perspectives that a society values. Perspectives regarding individual responsibility for health and well-being in the United States are influenced in part by prevailing cultural attitudes. **Media discourses,** or views, involve communication of thoughts and attitudes through literature, film, art, TV, and newspapers. Media images of persons on welfare influence, and are influenced by, cultural attitudes and values. **Historical factors** include acts, ideas, and events that have shaped current attitudes. **Elizabethan poor laws** and colonial settlement laws, for example, specified who should be given assistance and who should not. The history of society's responses to poverty and poor persons has influenced the way poverty is understood and responded to today (Katz, 1989).

HOW TO *Test Values and Beliefs About Poverty*

Nurses should ask themselves the following questions about poverty and persons living in poverty:

1. *What do I believe to be true about being poor?*
2. *What do I personally know about poverty?*
3. *How have family and friends influenced my ideas about being poor?*
4. *Have I ever personally been poor?*
5. *How have media images of poor persons helped to shape our images of poverty and poor persons?*
6. *What do I feel when I see a hungry child? A hungry adult?*
7. *Do I believe that people are poor because they just don't want to work? Or do I believe that society has a significant influence on one's becoming poor?*
8. *What really causes poverty?*

The questions listed above may seem abstract, but nurses are often faced with concrete questions that test their values and beliefs. Nurses may more comprehensively evaluate their beliefs, values, and knowledge regarding poverty by considering the following clinical situations:

- You are conducting health screening at a homeless shelter and one of the clients asks you for money for bus fare. Do you give it to her?
- You are in the home of an elderly client whose kitchen is covered with roaches. What are your obligations in terms of the client's home environment? Where do you sit if he offers you a chair?
- You are making a visit to an especially unclean home. What do you do if the client offers you some food?
- How would you target interventions for an aggregate of poor and/or homeless families in a local shelter?
- How could you effectively advocate for a group of medically indigent men?

There are no easy answers to these questions. However, nurses' behaviors in these situations influence their relationships with clients who are poor.

In addition to personal beliefs, values, and knowledge, nurses should consider how nursing theories and theories from other disciplines influence the care they provide to persons living in poverty (Carney, 1992). Many nursing theories are based on the assumption that human beings have inherent dignity and worth. Some theories view the human being as a system in continuous interaction with the environment. Other theories suggest that the human being is continuous with, and inseparable from, the environment. In community oriented nursing, the concepts of person, health, environment and nursing are reconceptualized to encompass a population focus. The concept of environment, for example, can be reconceptualized to include economics, power, class, race, politics, sexual orientation, and access to health care (Stevens, 1989).

Nursing is based on valuing individuals, promoting health, and respecting the dignity and quality of life (Roy and Andrews, 1991). Conflicts in values, beliefs, and perceptions often arise when nurses work with persons from different social, cultural, and economic backgrounds. A lack of agreement between the professional's and the client's perception of need can lead to conflict. As a result of this conflict, clients may fail to follow the prescribed treatment protocol; the nurse may then inaccurately interpret the client's behavior as resistance, lack of cooperation, or noncompliance.

Nurses should evaluate clients and aggregates in the context of environment to develop effective nursing interventions. Treating medical problems alone is inadequate. Instead, care must be multidimensional and include biological, psychological, social, environmental, economic, and spiritual factors.

DEFINING AND UNDERSTANDING POVERTY

More than 40 million persons have incomes below the federal poverty level (National Coalition for the Homeless, 1998), and 20.5% of America's young children live in poverty. Persons living in poverty, however, are not a homogenous group. It is essential to listen closely to clients in order to individualize their care and to avoid making inappropriate assumptions concerning their needs. In addition, the fears and misconceptions of health care providers related to poverty can create barriers that prevent them from fully engaging in relationships with those who come from different socioeconomic and cultural backgrounds. By taking the time to know clients by name and to listen to the stories of their lives, nurses begin the process of breaking down the barriers of fear, isolation, uncertainty, and the unknown.

Social Definitions of Poverty

Social definitions of poverty vary. Raspberry (1994) states that one of the difficulties of dealing with poverty and welfare reform is the lack of a common language and a common view. According to Sebastian (2000), poverty refers to having insufficient financial resources to meet basic living

expenses. These expenses include costs of food, shelter, clothing, transportation, and medical care. People who are poor are more likely to live in dangerous environments, to work at high-risk jobs, to eat less nutritious foods, and to have multiple stressors. They often lack the tangible and emotional resources to manage expected crises because, for them, managing their daily lives is a serious challenge (Pappas, 1994).

For years, income level has been used as the criterion that determines whether or not someone is poor. While income continues to be the measurement of choice, the federal poverty guidelines have been renamed "federal income guidelines." Income is also a qualifying factor for a variety of programs, such as federal housing subsidies; Temporary Assistance to Needy Families (TANF, formerly called AFDC); medical assistance; food stamps; **Women, Infants, and Children (WIC)**; and Head Start.

Poverty is a power issue, according to some authors, because it involves a lack of control over critical resources needed to function effectively in society. The federal government uses two terms to discuss poverty: poverty thresholds and poverty guidelines. The **poverty thresholds** are issued by the U.S. Census Bureau and are used primarily for statistical purposes. The **federal income guidelines** are issued by the U.S. Department of Health and Human Services (USDHHS) and are used to determine whether a person or family is financially eligible for assistance or services under a particular federal program. The federal income guidelines are updated annually to be consistent with the Consumer Price Index. The **Consumer Price Index (CPI)** is a measure of the average change over time in the prices paid by urban consumers for a fixed market basket of consumer goods and services (Gibson, 1998).

Many people who earn slightly more than the government-defined income levels (listed in Table 32-1) are unable to meet living expenses and are not eligible for government assistance programs. In a family of four, for

TABLE 32-1 Poverty Thresholds in 1997, by Size of Family and Number of Related Children Under 18 Years of Age

SIZE OF FAMILY UNIT	INCOME GUIDELINE ($)
1	8350
2	10,473
3	12,802
4	16,400
5	19,380
6	21,886
7	24,802
8	27,590

From US Census Bureau: *Current population survey*, Washington, DC, 1998, US Government Printing Office.

example, whose annual income is considered above the defined income level of $16,400, the adult family members would not qualify for Medicaid in some states. Persons and families whose income is above the federal income guidelines but insufficient to meet living expenses are often called the **near poor** (Sebastian, 2000). **Poverty** can also be defined as a variety of conditions involving differences in home and environment, material possessions, educational and occupational resources, and financial resources (Carney, 1992).

Social scientists often use terms describing types of poverty, such as persistent poverty and neighborhood poverty. **Persistent poverty** refers to individuals and families who remain poor for long periods and who pass poverty on to their descendants. **Neighborhood poverty** refers to geographically defined areas of high poverty characterized by dilapidated housing and high levels of unemployment. Raspberry (1994) states that poverty embraces a wide range of conditions: "The poverty of the working poor, for instance, is quite different from the poverty of teenage mothers. The poverty of those idled by plant closings or similar economic events is different from the poverty of those who lack marketable skills, and different yet from the poverty of those who can't hold a job or who don't want one" (p. A25).

While the social definitions used to describe and identify various types of poverty are interesting, they are not sufficient. For nurses, the most significant factor is her/his ability to accept and respect clients and attempt to understand how their life situations influence their health and well-being. Being poor is one variable that must be measured against the presence of other variables that may increase or decrease the negative effects of poverty.

Political Dimensions

A historical review reveals that poverty in the United States was not recognized as a social problem before the Civil War. The prevalent attitude during that time was that poverty was an individual's problem, and poor individuals had only themselves to blame. Generally, society did not assume responsibility for alleviating the plight of the poor. However, the post-Civil War industrialized society changed this attitude. Widespread unemployment, undesirable working conditions, insufficient wages, and substandard housing forced a rethinking of public responsibility for the poor (Wilson, 1987). Many laws concerning public health and housing were passed. This social reform movement led to an early interest in urban poverty research (Bremner, 1956; Miller, 1966). Despite influences of the depression of the 1930s and national discussion of New Deal legislation, such as the Social Security Act of 1935, the public's interest in the plight of the poor was not sustained (Wilson, 1987).

A resurgence of political activity on behalf of disadvantaged groups occurred during the late 1950s and early 1960s. In 1959 the Kerr-Mills Act increased funds for health care for aged persons (Plotnick and Skidmore,

1975). In 1961 President Kennedy approved a pilot food program in response to the hunger he observed on the campaign trail (Price, 1994). In 1963 President Kennedy instructed his administration to develop a major policy effort to combat poverty. After Kennedy's assassination, President Johnson sustained the interest in the antipoverty campaign. Johnson established the War on Poverty in 1964, which emphasized job-training programs and community organization and involvement (Plotnick and Skidmore 1975; Wilson, 1987). In 1964 the Social Security Administration established the income level of the official poverty line. Individuals and families with incomes below the federal poverty line were considered to be living in poverty. In 1965 the Medicare amendments to the Social Security Act were passed. After 1965 considerable research focused on poverty as it related to education, health, housing, the law, and public welfare (Wilson, 1987).

Policy changes during the 1980s led to an emphasis on defense spending, rather than social programs. Jargowsky and Bane (1990) noted that a series of events in the 1980s, such as the visibility of the homeless and the media attention on the "underclass," rekindled public interest in issues of poverty.

During the 1990s interest grew in reforms in health care and the welfare system. In 1994 a record 14.3 million people received welfare benefits, representing a 31% increase since 1989 (DeParle, 1994). In 1996, a bill creating the **Temporary Assistance for Needy Families (TANF)** program was enacted. This welfare reform legislation replaced the Aid to Families with Dependent Children (AFDC) program with a program of temporary welfare benefits called Temporary Assistance to Needy Families. Under TANF recipients of benefits are provided with benefits for a limited time and are required to find jobs and/or to enroll in job training programs. The economic and social effects of the TANF program are not currently known.

WHAT DO YOU THINK? *Opinions and beliefs about welfare differ among recipients, taxpayers, politicians, economists, health care providers, and others. Some people believe that welfare benefits are inadequate, whereas others argue that welfare breeds dependency and illegitimacy. Families receiving welfare benefits also have differing views.*

The political debate in the 1990s has been whether to abolish or to reform welfare. Aid to Families with Dependent Children (AFDC) has been replaced with the Temporary Assistance to Needy Families (TANF) program. What is the relationship between welfare reform and health? What implications does welfare reform have on nurse working in the community? How would you have redesigned the welfare system?

Cultural Perspectives

Writing about the concept of poverty, Carney (1992) states that the meaning of poverty differs greatly among cultures.

Poverty and Homelessness in Canada

Lianne Jeffs, Registered Nurses Association of Ontario and University of Toronto

POVERTY

Poverty is a major health and social issue and is one of the most important determinants affecting the health and well-being of a nation. In Canada, many people are just a paycheque, divorce, or illness away from being poor. There is no official poverty line in Canada. The poverty threshold level used by Statistics Canada is Low Income Cut-off (LICO), which is based on a sustenance concept of poverty and calculated on expenditure patterns. Currently, an individual is considered poor if 55% of his or her income is spent on food, shelter, and clothing. Most of the individuals living in poverty in Canada are children, women, elderly, and the Aboriginal population.

Since 1989 the rate of child poverty has increased by 46%, as currently 1 in 5 children in Canada are poor (Campaign 2000, 1998). Although the United Nations (UN) Human Development Index rates Canada as one of the best countries to live in, the UN Human Poverty Index ranks Canada only tenth in its treatment of the poor. In fact, the gap between the privileged and disadvantaged children in Canada is among the most marked in the industrialised world. Between 1989 and 1994, the child poverty rate rose and fell with the unemployment rate whereas in 1994 and 1995, the child poverty rate continued to increase despite the decline in the unemployment rate (the jobs that were created were largely part-time and consequently did not provide the same economic benefit as full-time employment) (Campaign 2000, 1998). Poverty in children is strongly associated with lower health status and other health and social issues (Canadian Institute of Child Health, 1994). Being poor has severe consequences for a child's emotional development. Living in substandard housing, not having enough to eat or adequate clothing, and not having access to play and recreation facilities all influence a child's emotional well-being. Increased incidence of family dysfunction, child abuse and neglect, and child and parental depression are also effects of poverty.

In Canada, women are at a higher risk for poverty than men are as the poverty rate for women has been at least 4% to 5% higher than men. In 1994, 20% of women as compared to 15% of men were poor, and women represented almost 60% of all poor Canadians (Statistics Canada, 1995). Over the last 15 years, the overall poverty rate for senior citizens in Canada has decreased, falling to 17.2% in 1994 (National Council of Welfare, 1996). Social programs such as the federal Old Age Security, the Guaranteed Income Supplement, the Spouse's Allowance, and the Canada/Quebec Pension Plan and income supplements provided by five provinces and territories are strongly associated with decreasing the poverty rate in the elderly population (Canadian Public Health Association, 1997a). There is concern, however, for women over the age of 75, since 40% of these women live alone, are poor, and are too frail to look after themselves. Health effects associated with poverty in the elderly population include activity limitations and exacerbations of chronic illness and disease.

The Aboriginal population is the most economically disadvantaged in Canada, and poverty is widespread within this group. The Aboriginal population includes status and non-status Indians living on and off reserves, as well as the Metis and the Inuit peoples. The poverty rate for those Indian families living on the reserves is 47.2%, which is three times the overall poverty rate for Canada (Oberle, 1993). In 1990, more than half of adult Aboriginal people reported annual incomes below $10,000, whereas only 6% reported annual incomes of $40,000 or more. The Aboriginal people have a lower health status, lower life expectancy, and increased morbidity and mortality rates (including infant mortality rate) than the overall Canadian population (Canadian Public Health Association, 1997a).

HOMELESSNESS

Homelessness, whether a cause or a consequence of ill health, has emerged as a fundamental health issue for Canadians. The causes of homelessness have been linked to poverty, changes in the housing market, and changes in the delivery of mental health services. Similar to the United States, the shift of mental health services from institutions to the community (deinstitutionalization) in the Canadian health care system is a significant cause of homelessness. Among the homeless of Canada are adolescents (street youth), persons living with mental illness, and Aboriginal people. The most alarming demographic change noted among homeless is the rapid growth in the number of homeless women and children (Canadian Public Health Association, 1997b). In 1986, it was estimated that between 130,000 to 250,000 people living in Canada did not have homes or lived in grossly inadequate housing conditions. Although there has been no recent report on the national state of homelessness, regional reports, research studies, and community agency reports have provided compelling evidence that there has been a substantial growth in homelessness across Canada (Canadian Public Health Association, 1997b). The most common health issues associated with homelessness are communicable diseases such as tuberculosis, HIV/AIDS and other sexually transmitted diseases, severe infections, musculoskeletal disease, dental problems, assault, mental health and suicide, increased drug and substance use, and decreased access to health services.

POVERTY AND HOMELESSNESS INITIATIVES

Over the years there have been substantial cuts to social services and programs in Canada. Employment insurance and

Economic Delivery of Health Care in Canada–cont'd

welfare programs have been cut, and public health services and social housing services have been shifted to municipalities. Cash transfers from the federal government (Canada Health and Social Transfer) have been reduced from $18.5 billion to $12.5 billion since 1995. As a result of these cuts, hundreds of community agencies and social programs have closed, and there is limited funding for existing programs and agencies in Canada. The growth of poverty and homelessness has prompted many local municipalities and community agencies to develop new programs and strengthen existing programs. Examples of these programs are food banks, healthy children programs, and interventions for the homeless such as street patrols, cold weather alert systems and mobile health units. A recent initiative in Toronto saw a coalition of individuals and agencies form the Toronto Disaster Relief Committee, which is calling on all levels of government to declare homelessness a national disaster requiring humanitarian relief. This committee, co-founded by Cathy Crowe, a registered nurse who has worked for years with the homeless population, is also urging the development of a National Homelessness Relief and Prevention Strategy that will provide homeless people with immediate health protection and housing and prevent further homelessness.

Canada signed the International Covenant on Economic, Social, and Cultural Rights, which guarantees every individual's right to an adequate standard of living, including adequate food, clothing, and housing. In this context the government needs to ensure that future social policy initiatives address the growing social disparities in Canada to improve upon the minimal efforts currently being directed towards improving living standards or advancing economic policies.

Bibliography

Campaign 2000: *Child poverty in Canada report card 1998*, Toronto, 1998, Author.

Canadian Institute of Child Health: *The health of Canada's children: a CICH profile*, ed 2, Ottawa, 1994, Author.

Canadian Public Health Association: *Health impacts of social and economic conditions: implications for public policy*, Ottawa, 1997a, the Association.

Canadian Public Health Association: *1997 position paper on homelessness and health*, Ottawa, 1997b, the Association.

National Council of Welfare: *Poverty profile 1994*, Ottawa, 1996, Author.

Oberle P: *The incidence of family poverty on Canadian Indian reserves*, Ottawa, 1993, Indian and Northern Affairs.

Statistics Canada: *Women in Canada: a statistical report*, ed 3, Ottawa, 1995, Statistics Canada Target Groups Project.

Canadian spelling is used.

For example, in India and Japan the poor have been respected because of the political and religious systems that give meaning to their lives. Western cultures, however, tend to view most aspects of poverty as negative.

Environmental Perspectives

The causes of poverty are complex and interrelated. In recent decades the number of adult and elderly Americans living in poverty has decreased, while the number of women and children living in poverty has increased. The following reasons affect the growing number of poor persons in the United States:
- Decreased earnings
- Increased unemployment rates
- Changes in the labor force
- Increase in female-headed households
- Inadequate education and job skills
- Inadequate antipoverty programs
- Inadequate welfare benefits
- Weak enforcement of child support statutes
- Dwindling Social Security payments to children
- Increased numbers of children born to single women

As the fiscal characteristics of most industrialized nations have changed from industrial economies to service economies, job opportunities have increasingly excluded workers who do not have, as a minimum, a high school education. Many manufacturing jobs do not pay sufficient salary to support a family. Also, many jobs at the lower end of the pay scale do not include health care or retirement benefits.

POVERTY AND HEALTH: EFFECTS ACROSS THE LIFE SPAN

The number of persons living in poverty in the United States increased by almost 26% from 25.4 million to 31.9 million between 1970 and 1988. By 1996, 36.5 million Americans lived in poverty (Dalaker et al, 1998). In addition to the increase in the numbers of persons living in poverty, there has been a significant increase in the number of Americans living in extreme poverty, an increase of 500,000 persons from 1995. In 1996, for example, 14.4 million people—nearly 40% of all poor persons—had incomes of less than half the poverty level (National Coalition for the Homeless, 1998).

Poverty directly affects health and well-being. Persons living in poverty and near-poverty have higher rates of chronic illness, higher infant morbidity and mortality, shorter life expectancy, more complex health problems, and more significant complications and physical limitations resulting from chronic disease. These poor health outcomes are often secondary to barriers that impede access to health care, such as inability to pay for health care, lack of insurance, geographical location, language, maldistribution of providers, transportation difficulties, inconvenient clinic hours, and negative attitudes of health care providers toward poor clients. Hospitalization rates for poor persons are three times those for persons with higher incomes (Ensign and Santelli, 1998). Some health problems having a higher incidence among poor persons include asthma, diabetes, and hypertension.

Childbearing Women and Poverty

Poverty, while presenting a significant obstacle to health across the life span, has an especially negative effect on women of childbearing age. Women living in poverty demonstrate lower levels of physical functioning, as well as higher reported levels of bodily discomfort than women in higher socioeconomic groups. Prevalence rates for ulcer disease, asthma and anemia are significantly higher among women living in poverty. Poor women also report significantly more HIV risk behaviors than more affluent women (Weinreb et al, 1998a).

Poverty has significant effects on poor teenaged women. Poor teens are four times more likely than nonpoor teens to have below-average academic skills. Regardless of their race, poor teens are nearly three times as likely to drop out of school as their nonpoor counterparts. Teenage women who are poor and who have below-average skills are more likely to have children than nonpoor teenage women. Poor pregnant women are more likely than other women to receive late or no prenatal care and to deliver low birth weight babies, premature babies, or babies with birth defects (Johnson et al, 1991).

Welfare reform will likely affect the health and well-being of childbearing women and their families. For example, the Personal Responsibility and Work Opportunity Reconciliation Act of 1996 requires more families to work to receive assistance. This requirement will force legislators to target funding for childcare subsidies for families going from welfare to work but will decrease the amount of funding available for other working poor women and their children. Changes in welfare policy are generally propelled by the goals of adults. Unfortunately, two thirds of those receiving cash benefits are children (National Center for Children and Poverty, 1998a).

Children and Poverty

Many of the children of the United States are members of the 5H Club. They are hungry, homeless, hugless, hopeless, and without health care (Elders, 1994). The 1996 poverty rate of 20.5% for children is almost twice as high as the poverty rate for any other age group. Forty percent of persons living in poverty are children (National Coalition for the Homeless, 1998). Moreover, poverty among young children (ages 0 to 5) has increased across all racial and ethnic groups, as well as in all urban, suburban, and rural geographical areas. In 1997, 24% of young children in the United States lived in poverty (National Center for Children in Poverty, 1999).

> ■ **DID YOU KNOW?**
> - *The majority (64%) of all poor children under the age of 6 live with at least one working parent.*
> - *The young child poverty rate in the United States is 33% to 66% higher than that of other Western industrialized countries.*
> - *Eleven percent of children under the age of 6 in the United States live in extreme poverty (less than 50% of the poverty level).*
> - *Forty-four percent of children in the United States live in or near poverty (below 185% of the poverty level) (National Center for Children in Poverty, 1997a).*

Changes in welfare policy will affect family income, parenting behaviors, and children's access to services (National Center for Children and Poverty, 1998b). Decreases in family income may result in an increase in the number of children living in extreme poverty, and will increase parental stress. Increased parental stress can have a negative effect on the well-being of children. Welfare changes that deny social and health services to the poor have negative effects on the health and well-being of poor children.

Young children (0 to 5 years of age) are at highest risk for the most harmful effects of poverty. Shore (1997a) examined the effects of inadequate nutrition on brain development. According to Shore, sound nutrition during the first years of life is crucial for emotional and intellectual development. Unfortunately, many children live in poverty during the early childhood years. Nearly 1 in 4 children in the United States lived in poverty in 1995. Poor children face several factors that increase their risk for impaired brain development. According to recent research, the time period encompassing the prenatal period through early childhood represents a critical period during which the brain is directly affected by environmental stimulation (National Center for Children in Poverty, 1997b). Several risk factors appear to impede brain development in young children, including inadequate nutrition (Brown and Pollitt, 1996); maternal substance abuse (Mayes, 1996); maternal depression (Belle, 1990); exposure to environmental toxins (National Health/Education Consortium, 1991); trauma and abuse (Brooks-Gunn et al, 1995); and quality of daily care (Burchinal, Lee, and Ramey, 1996). Unfortunately, poor children have greater exposure to these identified risk factors (National Center for Children in Poverty, 1997b).

The document *Healthy People 2010* (USDHHS, 1997) acknowledges the effect of low income and low educational and occupational levels on infant mortality, prematurity, low birth weight, birth defects, and infant deaths. Other effects are listed in Box 32-1. Poverty also increases the likelihood of chronic disease, injuries, traumatic death,

BOX 32-1 The Effects of Poverty on the Health of Children

Higher rates of prematurity, low birth weight, and birth defects
Higher infant mortality rates
Increased incidence of chronic disease
Increased incidence of traumatic death and injuries
Increased incidence of nutritional deficits
Increased incidence of growth retardation and developmental delays
Increased incidence of iron deficiency anemia
Increased incidence of elevated lead levels
Increased incidence of infections
Increased risk for homelessness
Decreased opportunities for education, income, and occupation

NURSING TIP

A client's advice to nurses caring for the poor:
- Treat the poor like everyone else.
- Do not be condescending.
- Do not make it obvious that someone is poor.
- Do not prejudge; ask if someone wants to pay on their bill.
- Remember that people can't always pay for their medicine
- Suggest programs that might help, such as food banks, churches, and clothing centers.
- Poor people need a lot of support.
- Many poor people need help to learn how to promote their own health given a paucity of resources.

developmental delays, poor nutrition, inadequate immunization levels, iron deficiency anemia, and elevated blood lead levels. Furthermore, children of poverty are more likely than nonpoor children to be hungry and suffer from fatigue, dizziness, irritability, headaches, ear infections, frequent colds, weight loss, inability to concentrate, and increased school absenteeism (Brown and Pollitt, 1996; U.S. Department of Commerce, 1996).

Older Adults and Poverty

In 1993, an estimated 12% of older adults (65 years and over) lived in poverty (U.S. Department of Commerce, 1996). This figure represents a decrease in the poverty rate for this age group. The decrease is a consequence of improvements in Social Security and the Supplemental Security Income Program. Certain elderly groups, however, continue to be vulnerable to the effects of poverty. Older African-Americans, for example, are at significantly greater risk for chronic and nutritionally related diseases than older Caucasian adults (Schoenberg and Gilbert, 1998).

Older adults living in poverty have a disproportionately greater likelihood of poor health outcomes than their more affluent counterparts. Studies comparing selected characteristics of persons residing in geographical areas of concentrated affluence with those of persons living in areas of concentrated poverty have demonstrated that affluence has a significant protective effect on the health of older adults (Waitzman and Smith, 1998). Prevalence rates for chronic illness and chronic illness complications, general morbidity, poor dental health, and overall mortality are significantly greater among poor older adults (Persson et al, 1998; Waitzman and Smith, 1998). Moreover, poor older adults are more likely to seek acute crisis care rather than preventive health care. Older adults are particularly at risk because they may be alone and are unable to manage their personal affairs. Many older adults are eligible for benefits but do not know how to access them.

The Community and Poverty

Poverty can affect both urban and rural communities. A number of characteristics describe poor communities. For example, poorer neighborhoods have a greater number of minority residents and single-parent families, higher rates of unemployment, and lower wage rates. Residents of poor neighborhoods also are more likely to be victims of crime, substance abuse, racial discrimination, and police brutality. Differences in quality and level of education also exist. Health care is less available to residents of poor neighborhoods. Housing conditions in some areas are deplorable, with many families living in run-down shacks or condemned apartment buildings. Residents are often exposed to environmental hazards, such as inadequate heating and cooling, exposure to rain and snow, inadequate water and plumbing, and the presence of pests and other vermin (Jargowsky and Band, 1990).

Since being poor affects the health and well-being of individuals, families, and communities, nurses need to acknowledge that poverty exists and influences health. Poverty is a part of the picture, not the whole picture. Being poor is a health risk factor that should be assessed; however, nurses need to examine individual and community strengths, resources, and sources of support.

UNDERSTANDING THE CONCEPT OF HOMELESSNESS

Understanding the concept of homelessness similarly requires considerable reflection and analysis. A number of variables, such as personal beliefs, personal/society's values, cultural norms, political debate, and personal knowledge/ experience influence the nurse's perception of the phenomenon of homelessness. The life stories of homeless clients can help nurses understand this significant public health problem.

Personal Beliefs, Values, and Knowledge

Poverty can lead to homelessness. **Homelessness,** like poverty, is a complex concept. The questions in the How To box on p. 674 prompt self-evaluation about homelessness.

:HOW TO *Evaluate the Concept of Homelessness*

- *What is it like to live on the streets?*
- *What issues might confront a young mother and her children inside a homeless shelter?*
- *How is it that people are so poor that they have no place to go?*
- *What really causes homelessness?*
- *How do you respond to the person on the street asking for money to buy a sandwich or catch a bus?*
- *How is your response different (or not) when a young mother with children asks you for money?*
- *How do you react to the smell of urine in a stairwell or elevator?*

Although people who have never been homeless cannot truly understand what it means to be homeless, nurses can explore their personal beliefs, values, and knowledge of homelessness in order to increase their sensitivity regarding homeless clients and aggregates.

Clients' Perceptions of Homelessness

People who live on the street are the poorest of the poor. Often, however, they become faceless, nameless, invisible, and inaudible (Cangialosi, 1994). As nurses begin to work with homeless groups and to know their clients by name, they engage in therapeutic relationships. The homeless want a place of their own, stability, and relationships. Baumann (1993) discussed the personal meaning of homelessness with 15 homeless mothers. The Research Brief describes the following themes: boundaries (social physical, symbolic), connections, fatigue/despair, lack of self-respect, lack of self-determination, and lack of privacy.

Homelessness in the United States

According to the Stewart B. McKinney Act of 1994, a person is considered homeless who "lacks a fixed, regular, and adequate night-time residence and; ... has a primary night time residency that is: (A) a supervised publicly or privately operated shelter designed to provide temporary living accommodations; (B) an institution that provides a temporary residence for individuals intended to be institutionalized; or (C) a public or private place not designed for, or ordinarily used as, a regular sleeping accommodation for human beings" (National Coalition for the Homeless, 1998, p.1). This definition generally refers to persons who are homeless on the streets, in shelters, or who face eviction within one week.

Current estimates of homelessness in the United States indicate that the homeless population grows by nearly 5% per year. During 1996, an estimated 1.2 to 2 million persons experienced homelessness (National Coalition for the Homeless, 1998). It is difficult to report accurately the number of homeless persons in any community. Counts of visible homeless persons are used to generate statistics related to homelessness in the United States.. For example, people living in homeless shelters, eating in soup kitchens,

RESEARCH *Brief*

What does it mean to be homeless? Data from interviews with 15 respondents provided the themes mentioned previously.

- Three types of boundaries were identified: physical, social, and symbolic.
- The women felt vulnerable because they lacked physical boundaries.
- The women said that they used a lot of energy to maintain connections.
- The homeless women experienced fatigue and despair.
- Being displaced was part of the homeless experience that threatened the women's self-respect.
- The women were frustrated with the effort needed to determine the course of their lives.
- Privacy, as needed for individual and family integrity, was hard to find.
- Participants moved frequently.

This study describes how it feels to be homeless and to have responsibilities for children for whom one cannot fully provide.

Baumann S: The meaning of being homeless, *Scholarly Inq Nurs Pract* 7(1):59, 1993.

or sleeping on sidewalks and in parks are part of the estimates of homeless people at any given period of time. Precise calculation of the number of homeless persons at a point in time is complicated by several factors (Link et al, 1994):

- Homeless persons are often hard to locate because many sleep in boxcars, on roofs of buildings, in doorways, under freeways. Others stay temporarily with relatives. Figures given by statisticians fail to include these invisible persons.
- Once located, many homeless persons refuse to be interviewed or deliberately hide the fact that they are homeless.
- Some persons experience short intervals of homelessness or may have intermittent homeless episodes. They are more hard to identify at any specific point in time.
- It is hard to generalize from one location to another. For example, the numbers and patterns of homelessness are different in large versus small cities or in urban versus rural areas.

Link and colleagues (1994) conducted a comprehensive study of homeless using different methods from most previous studies and found a much higher reported rate of homelessness. They conducted surveys of 1507 residents of the continental United States in a 4-month period to determine if the persons had ever been homeless and if they had been homeless in the last 5 years. They found that 13.5 million adults (or 7.4% of the U.S. population)

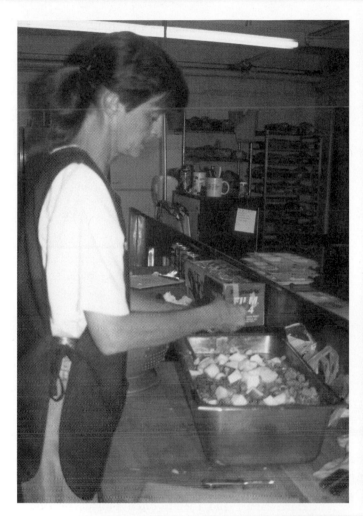

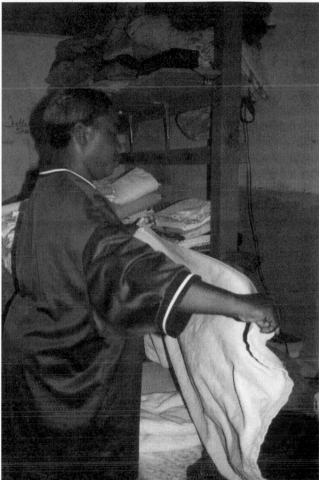

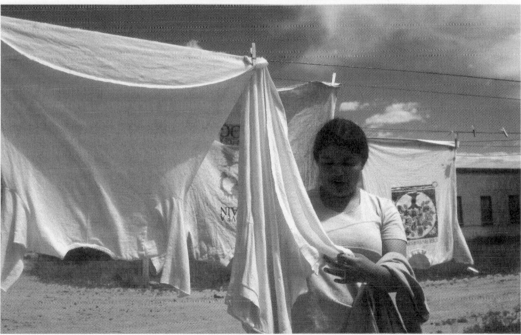

Increasingly women, many with children, are becoming part of the homeless population. Each of these women is a resident in a homeless shelter where residents help with the cooking, laundry, and other chores.

had been homeless in the last 5 years. Because they had such a large number of reported instances of homelessness, the researchers examined possible causes for the differences. One factor may have been that no definition of homelessness was used, so persons surveyed may have interpreted the term differently. Also, participants may be more willing to say that they have been homeless, since the data were being gathered retrospectively (or after the homeless period occurred). Also, the study only included persons with telephones at the time of data collection. However, despite the unique features of the study, it appears that homelessness may be much more widespread than statistics generally indicate and that the homeless population changed dramatically in the 1990s. Previously, people thought of the homeless as middle-age alcoholic men who lived on the streets. Families, children, single women, recently unemployed persons, substance abusers, adolescent runaways, and mentally ill individuals have now joined this traditional population.

The concept of homelessness includes two rather broad categories. The first category encompasses persons living in crisis poverty. These are people whose lives are generally marked by hardship and struggle. For them, homelessness is often transient or episodic. Persons living in **crisis poverty** often resort to brief stays in shelters or other temporary accommodations. Their homelessness may result from lack of employment opportunities, lack of education, obsolete job skills, or domestic violence. Such issues lead to persistent poverty and need to be addressed along with efforts to find stable housing.

Persons in the second category (persistent poverty) are homeless men and women with chronic mental or physical disabilities, and they are the group that is most frequently identified with homelessness in the United States. Physical and mental disabilities in this group often coexist with alcohol and other drug abuse, severe mental illness, other chronic health problems, and/or chronic family difficulties. They lack money and family support, often end up living on the streets, and their homelessness is often persistent. Members of this group need economic assistance, rehabilitation, and ongoing support.

Many of today's homeless are people who in previous decades had homes and managed to survive on limited incomes. Today the homeless population includes people of every age, sex, ethnic group, and family type (Vredevoe et al, 1992). Surprisingly, the single homeless tend to be younger and better educated than stereotypes would suggest. Many are longstanding residents of their communities and have some history of job success (Vladek, 1990). Box 32-2 summarizes the characteristics of America's homeless.

Homeless people are found in both rural and urban areas. Many sleep at night in shelters but are asked to vacate these shelters during the day. This means that during the day, they sit or stand on the street, in parks, alleys, shop-

---

BOX 32-2 Who Are America's Homeless?

Families
Children
Single women
Female heads of household
Adults who are unemployed, earn low wages, or are migrant workers
People who abuse alcohol or other substances
Abandoned children
Adolescent runaways
Elderly persons with no place to go and no one to care for them
Persons who are mentally ill
Vietnam-era veterans

From *Health: United States, 1998*, DHHS Pub No (PHS) 08-1232, Washington, DC, 1998, U.S. Government Printing Office.

---

ping centers, libraries, and in places such as trash bins, cardboard boxes, or under loading docks at industrial sites. They may also seek shelter in public buildings, such as train and bus stations. Those who do not sleep in shelters may sleep in single-room occupancy hotels, all-night movie theaters, abandoned buildings, and vehicles (Vredevoe et al, 1992).

Rural communities, despite their peaceful images, are not immune to homelessness. The extent of the problem is more often disguised than in the urban areas because rural people are often more likely to help one another. Therefore, family and friends often provide temporary housing to their neighbors who have no place to live (Dahl et al, 1993).

Causes of Homelessness

Most people move into homelessness gradually. Once they give up their own dwellings, they move in with family or friends. Only when all other options are exhausted do people go to shelters or seek refuge on the streets. Many factors contribute to the increasing numbers of homeless persons, including a growing number of people living in poverty, a decrease in the number of affordable housing units, emergency demands on income, gentrification of neighborhoods, alcohol and drug addiction, and a decrease in the number of transitional treatment facilities for deinstitutionalized mentally ill individuals (Arno et al, 1996; Culhane et al, 1997; de la Barra, 1998; National Coalition for the Homeless, 1998).

As noted previously, the percentage of people living below the poverty level has increased. Changes in the housing market have also had a profound negative effect on many persons who were marginally meeting their financial obligations. The move to upgrade urban housing, or **gentrification,** began with a positive intent that unfortunately led to negative consequences for many of the former residents of urban areas. During the 1980s, the supply of low-income housing dropped by about 2.5 million units; simultaneously, a large increase occurred in the need for low-income housing units. Historically, urban neighborhoods provided homes for older adults and poor persons. As neighborhoods were modernized, former residents were often unable to afford either to use existing housing in the old neighborhoods or to locate new housing elsewhere. In many older neighborhoods, people who are now homeless previously lived in SRO (single-room occupancy) buildings where they rented rooms on a long-term basis. Urban renewal eliminated many of the SROs and left a more attractive, better maintained neighborhood that became unaffordable for its former residents. A poignant example of the effects urban gentrification on the poor recently occurred in Oakland, California, where the condemnation and closure of the Hotel Royal, combined with decreased availability of other similarly priced SRO hotels, forced the majority of its residents to become homeless (Fagan, 1998). One of the tenants said, "I hate those fleas, I hate the cold, I hate that they haven't fixed up this disgusting place I have to live in. But even more, I hate how they are just tossing us on the street without hardly any notice; this isn't what you'd call great, but at least it was home. Until now" (p. A20).

Deinstitutionalization of chronically mentally ill individuals from public psychiatric hospitals increased the number of homeless persons. Deinstitutionalization intended to replace large state psychiatric hospitals with community-based treatment centers. The goal was for clients to have shorter stays in mental health facilities and move into appropriately designed and readily available community-based care. Unfortunately, those hospitals were often either downsized or closed, and federal and state governments failed to allocate the needed funds to provide community-based services. Indeed, fewer than 800 of the intended community mental health centers were ever built (Jackson and McSwane, 1992). According to statistics from the National Coalition for the Homeless (1998), 38% of single homeless adults suffer from a significant mental illness.

EFFECTS OF HOMELESSNESS ON HEALTH

Homelessness is correlated with poor health outcomes. Homeless individuals suffer significantly greater incidences of acute and chronic illness, AIDS, and trauma (Busen and Beech, 1997). Even though they are at higher risk of physiological problems, homeless persons have greater difficulty accessing health care services (Gillis and Singer, 1997). Health care is usually crisis oriented and sought in emergency departments, and those who access health care have a hard time following prescribed regimens (Gelberg et al, 1996). An insulin-dependent diabetic man who lives on the street may sleep in a shelter. His ability to get adequate rest, exercise, take insulin on a schedule,

eat regular meals, or follow a prescribed diet is virtually impossible. How does one purchase an antibiotic without money? How is a child treated for scabies and lice when there are no bathing facilities? How does an elderly man with peripheral vascular disease elevate his legs when he must be out of the shelter at 7 AM and on the streets all day? In addition to these challenges related to self-care, health promotion and maintenance is most often given lower priority than obtaining food and shelter. Homeless people spend most of their time trying to survive. Just getting money to buy food is a major chore. While some homeless persons are eligible for entitlement programs, such as TANF, WIC, or Social Security, others must beg for money, sell plasma or blood products, steal, sell drugs, or engage in prostitution.

Some of the specific health problems accompanying homelessness include hypothermia, infestations, peripheral vascular disease, hypertension, respiratory infections, tuberculosis, AIDS, trauma, and mental illness (White et al, 1997)). Disorders caused by exposure include hypothermia and heat-related illnesses, such as heat stroke. The prevalence of diabetes, poor skin integrity, chronic disease, nutritional deficits, trauma, and use and abuse of alcohol and illicit drugs compounds the effects of exposure. In addition to promoting decreased sensitivity to hot and cold, the use of street drugs can lead to hyperthermia or hypothermia (Brickner et al, 1996).

Cardiovascular and respiratory diseases in the homeless population include peripheral vascular disease, hypertension, tuberculosis, pneumonia, and chronic obstructive pulmonary diseases. Homeless persons spend many hours on their feet and often sleep in positions that compromise their peripheral circulation. Hypertension is exacerbated by high rates of alcohol abuse and high sodium content of foods served in fast-food restaurants, shelters, and other meal sites. Crowded living conditions put homeless persons at risk for exposure to viruses and bacteria that cause pneumonia and tuberculosis. In addition, high rates of tobacco, alcohol and illicit drug use diminish immune response and contribute to increased prevalence of chronic obstructive pulmonary disease in homeless persons (White et al, 1997).

AIDS is also a growing concern among the homeless population. The seroprevalence of the human immunodeficiency virus (HIV) infection in the homeless is estimated to be at least double that found in the general population. The use of intravenous drugs and sexual assault are other risk factors. Homeless persons with AIDS tend to develop more virulent forms of infectious diseases, have longer hospitalizations, and less access to treatment (Fournier, 1998; Gelberg et al, 1996).

Trauma is a significant cause of death and disability in the homeless population. Major trauma includes gunshot wounds, stab wounds, head trauma, suicide attempts, and fractures. Minor trauma includes bruises, abrasions, concussions, sprains, puncture wounds, eye injuries, and cellulitis (Heffron et al, 1997).

As discussed previously, deinstitutionalization has contributed to the growing number of homeless persons who suffer from mental illnesses, including schizophrenia and affective disorders. The prevalence of alcohol and substance abuse compounds the effects of mental illness. Many homeless persons were mentally ill before becoming homeless, whereas others develop acute mental distress as a result of being homeless. While treatment modalities may exist, homeless persons are often unable to gain access to mental health treatment facilities. Barriers to treatment include lack of awareness of treatment options, lack of available space in treatment facilities, inability to pay for treatment, lack of transportation, and nonsupportive attitudes of service providers (Hilfiker, 1994).

In addition to the physiological effect on health, homelessness also influences psychological, social, and spiritual well-being. Becoming homeless means more than losing a home, or a regular place to sleep and eat; it also means losing friends, personal possessions, and similar surroundings. Homeless persons live in chaos, confusion, and fear.

Homelessness and At-Risk Populations

Being homeless affects good health across the life span. Imagine the effect of homelessness on pregnancy, childhood, adolescence, or older adulthood; each group has different needs. Nurses must be aware of the unique needs of homeless clients across the life span.

Homeless pregnant women are at high risk for complex health problems. Pregnancy outcomes for homeless pregnant women are significantly poorer than for pregnant women in the general population. Pregnant homeless women present several challenges. They have higher rates of sexually transmitted diseases and higher incidences of addiction to drugs and alcohol, poorer nutritional status, and a higher incidence of poor birth outcomes (i.e., lower birth weight and lower Apgar scores). Although homeless women who are pregnant are at increased risk for pregnancy complications, they have less access to prenatal care (Beal and Redlener, 1995).

The health problems of homeless children, although similar to those of poor children, often have more serious consequences. Homeless children have poorer health than children in the general population. In addition, homeless children experience more symptoms of acute illness, such as fever, ear infection, diarrhea, and asthma than their housed counterparts (Weinreb et al, 1998b). Homeless children living on the streets in urban areas are at greatest risk of poor health (de la Barra, 1998). Menke and Wagner (1998) compared mental health, physical health, and healthcare practices of homeless, previously homeless, and nonhomeless school-age children, and found that homeless children demonstrated higher levels of anxiety, were significantly more depressed, and were at higher risk for physical

and mental health problems than poor children who were not homeless. Homeless children are at greater risk for inadequate nutrition, which can lead to delayed growth and development, failure to thrive, or obesity. Homeless children also experience higher rates of school absenteeism, academic failure, and emotional and behavioral maladjustments. The stress of homelessness can be manifested in behaviors such as withdrawal, depression, anxiety, aggression, regression, or self-mutilation (Davidhizar and Frank, 1992).

More than 2 million adolescents are homeless. Homeless adolescents living on the streets exhibit greater risk taking behaviors, poorer health status, and decreased access to health care than teens in the general population (Ensign and Santelli, 1997). In addition, homeless adolescents are at high risk of contracting serious communicable diseases, such as AIDS and hepatitis B, and more likely to use alcohol and illicit substances. They often have histories of runaway behavior, physical abuse and sexual abuse (Busen and Beech, 1997). Once on the streets, many homeless adolescents exchange sex for food, clothing, and shelter. In addition to the increased risk of STDs and other serious communicable diseases, homeless adolescent girls who exchange sex for survival are at high risk for unintended pregnancy (Rew, 1996). A study comparing homeless adolescents with domiciled teens found that homeless youth initiated sexual activity at an earlier age, were less likely to use contraception at first sexual experience, were twice as likely to have been pregnant, had more sex partners, and were twice as likely to have visited an emergency room in the past 12 months (Ensign and Santelli, 1998). Homeless youth have higher rates of depression, lower self-esteem, more suicidal ideation, and poorer overall health than their domiciled counterparts (Unger et al, 1997).

Homeless older adults are the most vulnerable of the impoverished elderly population. They have lived in longstanding poverty, have fewer supportive relationships, and are likely to become homeless as a result of catastrophic events. Life expectancy for homeless older adults is about 20 years less than for middle-class older adults (Hilfiker, 1994). Permanent physical deformities, often secondary to poor or absent medical care, are common among homeless older adults. Homeless older adults suffer from untreated chronic conditions, tuberculosis, hypertension, arthritis, cardiovascular disease, injuries, malnutrition, poor oral health, and hypothermia (Hilfiker, 1994; Schoenberg and Gilbert, 1998). As with younger homeless persons, older adults who are homeless must focus their energy on survival.

Federal Programs for the Homeless

A tremendous need exists for comprehensive, affordable, and accessible care for the nation's homeless population. The federal government officially became involved with meeting the needs of the homeless in 1987 with the passage of the **Stewart B McKinney Assistance Act** (P.L. 100-77). Title 11 of the McKinney Act provided funding for outpatient health services; however, the monies for these services were not large, and many needs go unmet. The act grants homeless children the same access to education as permanently housed children. This act also created the **Interagency Council on the Homeless (ICH)** to coordinate and direct federal homeless activities (Velsor-Friedrich, 1993a, 1993b).

The ICH is made up of the heads of 16 federal agencies that have programs or activities for the homeless. The general goals of the ICH are to improve federal programs for the homeless through better coordination and linkages, decreasing the amount of documentation required to qualify for benefits. By targeting the most vulnerable segments of the homeless population, the ICH intends to influence the problem of homelessness. Children are a priority for the ICH (Velsor-Friedrich, 1993a).

Homeless families with children are eligible to receive shelter and nutrition assistance from the U.S. Department of Agriculture WIC program. Persons receiving WIC benefits receive vouchers entitling them to free nutritious foods and infant formulas from local grocers. The Temporary Assistance to Needy Families (TANF) program can be a key source of income for homeless families.

Unfortunately, health care for homeless persons tends to be fragmented and limited in scope. Some of the most useful health care programs for the homeless begin with grants from private funding agencies, such as the Robert Wood Johnson Foundation and the Pew Charitable Trusts. Projects funded by these agencies have followed sound public health principles by encouraging community involvement, public/private partnerships, and commitment to outreach. Most of these projects rely heavily on nurse practitioners and physician assistants to deliver care in collaboration with physicians, nurses, and social workers. In recent years, many schools of nursing have received funding from the Division of Nursing in the USDHHS to establish nurse-managed centers for the homeless. Both faculty and students provide a range of services in these centers.

ROLE OF THE NURSE

Nurses have a critical role in the delivery of health care to poor or homeless people. To be effective, nurses need strong assessment skills, current knowledge of available resources, and an ability to convey respect, dignity, and value to each person. Nurses need to be able to work with poor and homeless clients to promote, maintain, and/or restore health. Nurses must be prepared to look at the whole picture: the person, the family, or the community interacting with the environment.

- *Create a trusting environment.* Trust is essential to the development of a therapeutic relationship with poor or homeless persons. Many clients and families have been disappointed by their interactions with health care and social systems and are mistrustful and see little hope

for change. By following through and doing what they say they will do, nurses can establish trusting relationships with clients. If the answer to a question is unknown, an appropriate response might be, "I don't know the answer, but I will try to find out. Let me make a few phone calls and I will let you know Friday." Reliability helps to build the foundation for a trusting relationship.

- *Show respect, compassion, and concern.* Poor and homeless clients are defeated so often by life's circumstances that they may feel that they do not deserve attention. Listen carefully and empathize with clients so that they believe that they are worthy of care. Too often, poor and homeless persons are not treated with respect and dignity by health and social services workers. Since clients respond well to nursing interactions that demonstrate respect, it is helpful to use reflective statements that convey acceptance and understanding of their situation.
- *Do not make assumptions.* A comprehensive and holistic assessment is crucial to identifying underlying needs. Just because a young mother with three preschool children misses a clinic appointment does not mean that she does not care about the health of her children. She may not have transportation, one child may be sick, or she may be sick. Find out the reason for the absence and help solve the problem.
- *Coordinate a network of services and providers.* The multiple and complex needs of poor and homeless people make working with them exceedingly challenging. Many services exist, but often the people who could benefit are unaware of their existence. Developing a coordinated network of providers involves conducting a thorough assessment of the service area to identify federal, state, and local services available for poor and homeless clients. Where are the food banks? Where can you get clothing? What programs are available in the local churches and schools? How do people access these services? What are the eligibility requirements? How helpful are the people who work at the service agencies? What service is provided to eligible individuals and families? Nurses can identify these services and help link families with appropriate resources. In addition, a thorough assessment of available services for homeless persons in a nurse's service area can identify significant gaps in essential services. Once these gaps are identified, nurses serving as case managers can work with other health care providers and with community members to advocate for necessary services for homeless clients.

NURSING TIP

Case management is an intervention strategy that can be used by nurses working with families who are poor or homeless (Wagner and Menke, 1992).

HOW TO *Apply Case Management Strategies to Working With the Homeless*

- *Determine available services and resources.*
- *Determine missing resources and develop creative solutions for service deficiencies.*
- *Integrate and use clinical skills.*
- *Establish long-term therapeutic relationships with families.*
- *Enhance the family's personal coping skills, survival skills, and resourcefulness.*
- *Facilitate service delivery on behalf of the family.*
- *Guide the family toward the use of appropriate community resources.*
- *Communicate and collaborate with professionals from multiple service systems.*
- *Advocate for the development of creative solutions.*
- *Participate in policy analysis and political activism.*
- *Manipulate and modify the environment as needed.*
- *Connect with local, state, and federal legislators.*

- *Advocate for accessible health care services.* Poverty and homelessness create a number of barriers that prevent access to health care services. Nurses can advocate for accessible and convenient locations of health care services. Neighborhood clinics, mobile vans, and home visits can bring health care to people unable to access care. Coordinating services at a central location often improves client compliance since it reduces the stress of getting to multiple places. Many homeless shelters and transition housing units have clinics on site. These multi-service centers provide health care, social services, day care, drug and alcohol recovery programs, and comprehensive case management. Multiservice models are usually multidisciplinary. For example, mid-level practitioners (NPs and PAs), public health nurses, social workers, psychologists, child psychologists, and administrative personnel might provide a network of support for clients in shelters and low-income housing facilities.
- *Focus on prevention.* Nurses can use every opportunity to provide preventive care and health teaching. Important health promotion (primary prevention) topics include child and adult immunization, and education regarding sound nutrition, foot care, safe sex, contraception, and prevention of chronic illness. Screening for health problems such as tuberculosis, diabetes, hypertension, foot problems, and anemia is an important form of secondary prevention. Know what other screening and health promotion services are available in the target area, such as nutrition programs, job training programs, educational programs, housing programs, and legal services. All these services may be included in a comprehensive plan of care.
- *Know when to walk beside the client and when to encourage the client to walk ahead.* This area is often difficult for the nurse to implement. Nursing interventions range from extensive care activities to minimal support. At times

nursing actions include providing encouragement and support, or providing information. At other times, nurses may actually call a pediatrician to set up an appointment for a sick child and may call again to see that the appointment was kept. Nurses assess for the presence of strengths, problem-solving, and coping ability of an individual or family while providing information on where and how to gain access to services.

For example, a local hospital may provide free mammograms for uninsured women. Women who qualify for this free service may not take advantage of it because they are afraid that they may have breast cancer. Nurses can find out about this important service, inform the women of the service, teach them about the importance of preventive care, and assess and deal with fear and anxiety. The challenge for the nurse becomes choosing whether to schedule the appointments for the women or providing them with a referral sheet, knowing that many will not follow through. The choice is not clear, but the goal is to make available a needed screening intervention without taking away the woman's right to decide what to do for herself.

- *Develop a network of support for yourself.* Caring for poor and homeless persons is challenging, rewarding, and at times exhausting. It is important to find a source of personal strength, renewal, and hope. The people you encounter are often looking to you to maintain hope and provide encouragement. Discover for yourself what restores and encourages you. For some nurses it is poetry, music, painting, or weaving. For others it is a walk in a peaceful place, a weekend retreat, a good run, a workout at the gym, or meeting with other nurses who are engaged in the same work. Be attentive to your own needs, and create the time and space to restore your spirit.

clinical application

Tonya, a single mother with AIDS, lives in an apartment with seven other family members and her children, who are HIV-positive. Tonya does not often keep her children's numerous appointments at the immunology clinic. How do you respond?

- **A.** Make an unsolicited telephone call or visit to Tonya and her family to let them know they are important and that the nurse is thinking about them.
- **B.** Call child protective services to report her failure to keep her children's appointments because she is noncompliant and neglectful of her children.
- **C.** Do a more thorough assessment to determine why appointments are missed.

Answer is in the back of the book.

KEY POINTS

- Health care in this country is comprised of a personal care system and a public health system, with overlap between the two systems.
- To understand the concepts of poverty and homelessness, consider your personal beliefs and attitudes, clients' perceptions of their condition, and the social, political, cultural, and environmental factors that influence poverty and homelessness.
- The definition of poverty varies depending on what source is consulted. The federal government defines poverty based on income, family size, age of the head of household, and number of children under 18 years of age. Those who are poor insist that poverty has less to do with income and more to do with a lack of family, friends, love, and support.
- Factors leading to the growing number of poor persons in the United States include decreased earnings, diminishing availability of low-cost housing, increases in the number of households headed by women (women's incomes are traditionally lower than men's), inadequate education, lack of marketable job skills, welfare reform, and reduced Social Security payments to children.
- Poverty has a direct effect on health and well-being across the life span. Poor persons have higher rates of chronic illness, higher infant morbidity and mortality, shorter life expectancy, and more complex health problems.
- Child poverty rates remain twice as high as those for adults. Children in single-parent homes are twice as likely to be poor as those who live in homes with two parents. Younger children (0 to 5) are at highest risk for developmental delays and damage caused by inadequate nutrition and/or lack of health care.
- Poverty affects both urban and rural communities. The poorer the neighborhood the greater is the proportion of residents who are members of minority groups.
- At present, the following groups often constitute the homeless in both rural and urban areas: families, single mothers, single women, recently unemployed persons, substance abusers, adolescent runaways, mentally ill individuals, and single men.
- Factors contributing to homelessness include an increase in the number of persons living in poverty, diminishing availability of low-cost housing, increased unemployment, substance abuse, lack of treatment facilities for mentally ill persons, domestic violence, and family situations causing children to run away.
- The complex health problems of homeless persons include inability to get adequate rest, exercise, and nutrition; exposure; infectious diseases; acute and chronic illness; infestations; trauma; and mental health problems.
- Nurses have a critical role in the delivery of care to persons who are poor and homeless. Nurses bring to each client encounter the ability to assess the client in context, and to intervene in ways that restore, maintain, or promote health.
- In addition to interactions with individuals who are poor or homeless, nurses use the nursing process to assess, diagnose, plan, implement, and evaluate population-focused interventions.

critical thinking activities

1. Examine health statistics and demographic data to identify the rate of poverty and homelessness in your geographical area. What resources and agencies are available in your area to support homeless persons? What services are available from federal, state, and local sources? Identify a specific geographical region and assess this target area in terms of services for poor and homeless persons. Do a literature search to identify recommended state-of-the-art interventions for poor and homeless persons. Compare the recommended programs and interventions with those available in your target area. How does your area measure up? What do you recommend to fill the gaps?
2. Examine the specific programs identified in the assessment above. How do those who need services access them? Working with other students, make appointments with key persons in the agencies identified above to find out what each agency offers, which particular aggregate is served, how clients access the services, who is eligible, how the agency receives funding, and what methods are used to evaluate the agency's ability to meet the needs of its targeted aggregates.
3. Identify nurses in your community who work with the homeless or with other vulnerable groups. Invite these nurses to come to a class meeting to share their experiences. What constitutes a typical workday? What are the rewards and challenges of working with vulnerable populations? How do they deal with the frustrations and challenges of their work? What advice might they offer to students working with vulnerable aggregates? What programs do they recommend? How are they involved in political advocacy activities related to vulnerable aggregates?
4. Imagine yourself as a nurse working in a homeless shelter or making a home visit to a family in an impoverished neighborhood. How have your life experiences and education prepared you (or not) for these situations? What are your expectations? Write down your fears, anxieties, and apprehensions? Discuss your writings with classmates.
5. Discuss welfare reform with other students. How does our welfare system work? Who receives welfare? Who is eligible for benefits? How do people apply for welfare? What are the strengths and weaknesses of welfare reform in America? What are the financial and personal costs of welfare reform? Identify federal and state senators and representatives in your districts. Where do they stand on the issue of welfare reform? How would you restructure our welfare system?

Bibliography

Arno PS et al: The impact of housing status on health care utilization of persons with HIV disease, *J Health Care Poor Underserved* 7(1):36, 1996.

Baumann S: The meaning of being homeless, *Scholarly Inq Nurs Pract* 7(1):59, 1993.

Beal AC, Redlener I: Enhancing perinatal outcome in homeless women: the challenge of providing comprehensive health care, *Semin Perinatol* 19(4):307, 1995.

Bremner RH: *From the depths: the discovery of poverty in the United States,* New York, 1956, University Press.

Brickner PW et al: *Health care of homeless people,* New York, 1996, Springer.

Brooks-Gunn J et al: Toward an understanding of the effects of poverty upon children. In Fitzgerald HB, Lester BM, Zuckerman B, editors: *Children of poverty: research, health and policy issues,* New York, 1995, Garland Publishing.

Brown L, Pollitt E: Malnutrition, poverty and intellectual development, *Scientific Am* 274(2):38, 1996.

Burchinal M, Lee M, Ramey C: Type of day care and preschool intellectual development in disadvantaged children, *Child Develop* 60(1):128, 1996.

Busen NH, Beech B: A collaborative model for community-based health care screening of homeless adolescents, *J Prof Nurs* 13(5):316, 1997.

Busen NH, Beech BL: A collaborative model for community-based health car4e screening of homeless adolescents, *J Prof Nurs* 13(5):316, 1997.

Cangialosi G: *A kairos winter,* Washington, DC, 1994, Servant Leadership School Publication.

Carney P: The concept of poverty, *Public Health Nurs* 9(2):74, 1992.

Clarke PN et al: Health and life problems of homeless men and women in the southeast, *J Comm Health Nurs* 12(2):101, 1995.

Culhane DP, Averyt JM, Hadley TR: The rate of public shelter admission among Medicaid-reimbursed users of behavioral health services, *Psychiatric Service* 48(3):390, 1997.

Dahl S, Gustafson C, McCullagh M: Collaborating to develop a community-based health service for rural homeless persons, *J Nurs Admin* 23(4):41, 1993.

Davidhizar R, Frank B: Understanding the physical and psychosocial stressors of the child who is homeless, *Pediatr Nurs* 18(6):559, 1992.

de la Barra X: Poverty: the main cause of ill health in urban children, *Health Educ Behav* 25(1)46, 1998.

Dalaker J, Naifeh M: *U.S. Bureau of the Census, Current Population Reports,* Series P60-201, Poverty in the United States, Wash-ington, DC, 1998, US Government Printing Office.

DeParle J: Welfare as we've known it, *New York Times,* p. E4, June 19, 1994

Efron D et al: Children in homeless families in Melbourne: health status and use of health services, *Med J Austr* 165(11-12): 640, 1996.

Elders J: *An urban health crisis,* Keynote address presented at Mothers and Children 1994, Washington, DC, 1994.

Ensign J, Santelli J: Health status and service use: comparison of adolescents at a school-based health clinic with homeless adolescents, *Arch Pediatr Adolesc Med* 152(1):20, 1998.

Ensign J, Santelli J: Shelter-based homeless youth: health and access to care, *Arch Pediatr Adolesc Med* 151(8):817, 1997.

Fagan K: Resident hotel's 60 tenants evicted: Oakland calls Hotel Royal a health hazard, *San Francisco Chronicle,* p. A20, May 14, 1998.

Flynn L: The health practices of homeless women: a causal model, *Nurs Res* 46(2):72, 1997.

Fournier AM, Carmichael C: Socioeconomic influences on the transmission of human immunodeficiency virus infection: the hidden risk, *Arch Fam Med* 7(3):214, 1998.

Gelberg L, Doblin BH: Ambulatory health services provided to low-income an homeless adult patients in a major community health center, *J Gen Intern Med* 11(3):156, 1996.

Gibson S: *Understanding the consumer price index: answers to some questions,* Washington, DC, 1998, Bureau of Labor Statistics.

Gillis LM, Singer J: Breaking through the barriers: healthcare for the homeless, *J Nurs Admin* 27(6):30, 1997.

Hatton DC: Managing health problems among homeless women with children in a transitional shelter, *Image J Nurs Sch* 29(1):33, 1997.

Heffron WA, Skipper BJ, Lambert L: Health and lifestyle issues as risk factors for homelessness, *J Am Board Fam Pract* 10(1):6, 1997.

Hilfiker D: *Not all of us are saints: a doctor's journey with the poor,* New York, 1994, Hill & Wang.

Hunter JK et al: Factors limiting evaluation of health care programs for the homeless, *Nurs Outlook* 45(5):224, 1997.

Jackson MPO, McSwane DA: Homelessness as a determinant of health, *Public Health Nurs* 9(3):185, 1992.

Jargowsky MP, Band MJ: Ghetto poverty: basic questions. In Lynn KE, McGeary M, editors: *Inner city poverty in the United States,* Washington, DC, 1990, National Academy Press.

Jezewski MA: Staying connected: the role of facilitating health care for homeless persons, *Public Health Nurs* 12(3):P203, 1995.

Johnson D et al: *Child poverty in America,* Washington, DC, 1991, Children's Defense Fund.

Katz MB: *The undeserving poor: from the war on poverty to the war on welfare,* New York, 1989, Pantheon Books.

Killion CM: Special health care needs of homeless pregnant women, *Adv Nurs Sci* 18(2):44, 1995.

Kitazawa S: Tuberculosis health education: needs in homeless shelters, *Public Health Nurs* 12(6):409, 1995.

Kleinman LC et al: Homing in on the homeless: assessing the physical health of homeless adults in Los Angeles County using an original method to obtain physical examination data in a survey, *Health Serv Res* 31(5):533, 1996.

Kreider B, Nicholson S: Health insurance and the homeless, *Health Econ* 6(1):31, 1997.

Link BG et al: Lifetime and five year prevalence of homeless in the United States, *Am J Public Health* 84(12):1907, 1994.

Mayes L: *Early experience and the developing brain: the model of prenatal cocaine exposure.* Paper presented at the invitational conference: "Brain development in young children: new frontiers for research, policy and practice," Chicago, June 12, 1996, University of Chicago.

McGee D et al: Use of a mobile health van by a vulnerable population: homeless sheltered women, *Health Care Women Internat* 16(5):451, 1995.

Menke EM, Wagner JD: A comparative study of homeless, previously homeless, and never homeless school-aged children's health, *Iss Comprehen Pediatr Nurs* 20(3):153, 1998.

Miller HP: *Poverty American style,* Calif, 1966, Wadsworth.

National Center for Children and Poverty: *Anticipating the effects of federal and state welfare changes on systems that serve children,* New York, 1998a, Columbia University.

National Center for Children and Poverty: *How welfare reform can help or hurt children,* New York, 1998b, Columbia University.

National Center for Children in Poverty: *Poverty and brain development in early childhood,* New York, 1997b, Columbia University.

National Center for Children in Poverty: *Young children in poverty fact sheet,* New York, 1997a, Columbia University.

National Coalition for the Homeless: *How many people experience homelessness? Fact sheet #3,* Washington DC, 1998a, Author.

National Coalition for the Homeless: *Why are people homeless? Fact Sheet #1,* Washington DC, 1998b, Author.

National Health/Education Consortium: Healthy brain development, *The National Health/Education Consortium Report,* 1991.

Nyamathi A, Flaskerud J, Leake B: HIV-risk behaviors and mental health characteristics among homeless or drug-recovering women and their closest sources of social support, *Nurs Res* 46(3):133, 1997.

Pappas G: Elucidating the relationships between race, socio-economic status and health, *Am J Public Health* 84(6):892, 1994.

Persson RE et al: Oral health and medical status in dentate low-income older adults, *Specialty Care Dentistry* 18(2):70, 1998.

Plotnick R, Skidmore F: *Progress against poverty: a review of the 1974-1974 decade,* New York, 1975, Academic Press.

Price J: More mouths, more money, *Washington Times,* p. A6, April 19, 1994.

Raspberry W: Several kinds of poverty, *Washington Post,* p. A25, May 27, 1994.

Rew S: Health risks of homeless adolescents: implications for holistic nursing, *J Holistic Nurs* 14(4):348, 1996.

Robertson MJ, Winkleby MA: Mental health problems of homeless women and differences across subgroups, *Annu Rev Public Health* 17:311, 1996.

Roy C, Andrews H: *The Roy adaptation model: the definitive statement,* East Norwalk, Conn, 1991, Appleton and Lange.

Schoenberg NE, Gilbert GH: Dietary implications of oral health decrements among African-American and white older adults, *Ethnic Health* 3(1-2):59, 1998.

Sebastian J: Vulnerable populations in the community. In Stanhope M, Lancaster J, editors: *Community and public health nursing: process and practice for promoting health,* ed 5, St Louis, 2000, Mosby.

Shore R: *Rethinking the brain: new insights into early development,* New York, 1997, Families and Work Institute.

Stein JA, Gelberg L: Comparability and representativeness of clinical homeless, community homeless, and domiciled clinic samples: physical and mental health, substance use, and health services utilization, *Health Psychol* 16(2):155, 1997.

Unger JB et al: Homeless youths and young adults in Los Angeles: prevalence of mental health problems and the relationship between mental health and substance abuse disorders, *Am J Psychol* 25(3):371, 1997.

US Department of Commerce: *Dynamics of economic well-being: who stays poor? who doesn't? current population reports: household economic studies,* Washington, DC, 1996, Author.

US Department of Health and Human Services: *Leading indicators for Healthy People 2010: a report from the HHS group on sentinel objectives,* Washington, DC, 1998, USDHHS, Public Health Service.

Velsor-Friedrich B: Homeless children and their families: Part I, the changing picture, *J Pediatr Nurs* 8(2):122, 1993a.

Velsor-Friedrich B: Homeless children and their families: Part II, Federal programs and health care delivery systems, *J Pediatr Nurs* 8(3):190, 1993b.

Vladek BC: Health care and the homeless: a political parable for our time, *J Health Polit Policy Law* 15(2):305, 1990.

Vredevoe J, Menke E, Woo J: The homeless population, *Western J Nurs Res* 14(6):731, 1992.

Wagner JD, Menke EM, Ciccone JK: What is known about the health of rural homeless families? *Public Health Nurs* 12(6):400, 1995.

Waitzman NJ, Smith KR: *Separate but unequal: the effects of economic segregation on mortality in metropolitan America,* Washington, DC, 1997, US Census Bureau, US Government Printing Office.

Weinreb L et al: Health characteristics and medical service use patterns of sheltered homeless and low-income housed mothers, *J Gen Intern Med* 13(6):389, 1998a.

Weinreb L et al: Determinants of health and service use patterns in homeless and low-income housed children, *Pediatrics* 102(3 Pt 1):554, 1998b.

White MC et al: Association between time homeless and perceived health status among the homeless in San Francisco, *J Comm Health* 22(4):271, 1997.

Wilson WJ: *The truly disadvantaged: the inner city, the underclass, an public policy,* Chicago, 1987, University of Chicago Press.

Zima BT et al: Mental health problems among homeless mothers: relationship to service use and child mental health problems, *Arch Gen Psychiatry* 53(4):332, 1996.

CHAPTER

33 Teen Pregnancy

DYAN ARETAKIS

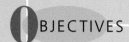 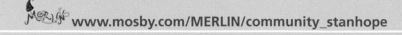

OBJECTIVES

After reading this chapter, the student should be able to do the following:

- Discuss approaches that could be used in working with the adolescent client.
- Identify trends in adolescent pregnancy, births, abortions, and adoption in the United States.
- Discuss reasons that may affect whether a teenager becomes pregnant.

- Explain some of the deterrents to the establishment of paternity among young fathers.
- Develop nursing interventions for the prevention of pregnancy problems that adolescents are at risk of experiencing.
- Identify nursing activities that may contribute to the prevention of adolescent pregnancy.

KEY TERMS

abortion	gynecological age	prematurity	sexual victimization
adoption	low birth weight	prenatal care	statutory rape
birth control	paternity	repeat pregnancy	weight gain
coercive sex	peer pressure	sexual debut	*See Glossary for definitions*

CHAPTER OUTLINE

Adolescent Health Care in the United States
Adolescent Client
Trends in Adolescent Sexual Behavior and Pregnancy
Background Factors
  Sexual Activity and Use of Birth Control
  Peer Pressure and Partner Pressure

Other Factors
Young Men and Paternity
Early Identification of the Pregnant Teen
Special Issues in Caring for the Pregnant Teen
  Violence
  Initiation of Prenatal Care
  Low-Birth-Weight Infants and Preterm Delivery

Nutrition
Infant Care
Repeat Pregnancy
Schooling and Educational Needs
Teen Pregnancy and the Nurse
  Home-Based Interventions
  Community-Based Interventions

Teen pregnancy is an area of great public concern because of the significant impact on communities. Resources to support the special needs of pregnant teenagers are decreasing, and the costs of sustaining young families over time is prohibitive. Many teenagers who become pregnant are caught in a cycle of poverty, school failure, and limited life options. Other teens will face these issues after a pregnancy occurs. Even under the ideal circumstances of adequate finances, loving and supportive families, and good birth outcomes, a teen parent must circumvent her own necessary developmental tasks to raise her child.

There is neither a uniform reason that teens become pregnant nor a universally acceptable solution. The causes of teen pregnancy are diverse and affected by changing moral attitudes, sexual codes, and economic circumstances. The strain that teen pregnancy places on the health care and social service systems is enormous. Social concern also is raised about the lost potential for young parents when pregnancy occurs and the academic and economic disadvantages that their children will experience. Nurses are in a key position to understand how teen pregnancy affects both the individual and the community. This chapter presents a variety of issues associated with teen pregnancy and proposes nursing interventions to promote healthy outcomes for individuals and communities.

DID YOU KNOW? *States spend more on the costs of supporting teen parents and their children than on preventing teen pregnancy. For example, in the Southern states only a penny is invested in the primary prevention of pregnancy for every dollar spent on public programs to support families begun by teenagers.*

ADOLESCENT HEALTH CARE IN THE UNITED STATES

Adolescents are generally a healthy age group. When they seek health care services it is for reasons quite different than those of adults or young children. The greatest causes of teen mortality result from high-risk behaviors: motor vehicle accidents (usually including alcohol), homicide, suicide, and accidental injuries (such as falls, fires, or drowning). Teens often engage in behaviors that put them at risk for life-threatening diseases. For example, each year one quarter of both new HIV infections and newly identified sexually transmitted diseases occur among adolescents. It is during the teen years that other behaviors are initiated (e.g., smoking, decreased activity, and poor nutrition) that can ultimately lead to poor health during the adult years. Working with teens requires that the nurse provide health education and also influence behavior change that can significantly alter a young person's life.

Several national surveys have assessed health issues facing adolescents. Seventh- to twelfth-graders have high rates of alcohol use (17% in the past month); cigarettes (25% are current smokers); marijuana use (25% had ever tried); victim violence (24%); and weapon possession (12% carried a weapon in the previous month) (Resnick et al, 1997). Mental health issues are strongly associated with girls during the adolescent years: 18% of high school girls reported eating disorders of binging and purging, 20% had been victims of childhood physical and sexual abuse, and 25% experienced depression. Boys experienced similar mental health concerns but at slightly lower rates (Commonwealth Fund, 1997). Suicide was considered by 10% of girls and 7.5% of boys and attempted by 5% and 2%, respectively (Resnick et al, 1997).

Most adolescents do not seek care for the problems described above. First, access to health care may be hindered because of a limited number of professionals who have expertise in dealing with teenagers. Second, costs of care or availability of insurance may limit services. Third, adolescents need to believe that their visits are confidential before they will honestly reveal information. Finally, health care professionals must be able to discuss sensitive topics in a nonjudgmental and supportive manner. They need to demonstrate a desire to work with youth. A knowledge of adolescent behaviors, health risks, and the social context in which an adolescent lives assist the nurse in the promotion of health by providing anticipatory guidance about **peer pressure,** assertiveness, and future planning. Involvement and education of the parents about youth culture and development serves to promote positive and supportive parenting of teens.

ADOLESCENT CLIENT

Adolescents have limited experience independently seeking health care. When they do seek care, it is often to discuss concerns about a possible pregnancy or to find a **birth control** method. These teens also may need assistance negotiating complex health care systems. Special approaches in both the client interview and subsequent client education are often warranted. The behavior of adolescents toward the nurse can range from mature and competent during one visit to hostile, rude, or distant at other times because behavior often reflects intense anxiety over what the teen is experiencing.

Because client interviews usually begin with evaluation of a chief complaint, teens need to know that their concerns are heard. Health care providers may have their own opinions about what teenagers need and may fail to take the chief complaint seriously. For example, when a teen expresses a desire to become pregnant, this should be discussed in depth even though the nurse may feel uncomfortable providing information to a teen about how to conceive. During the interview the nurse can provide preconception counseling and emphasize the need to achieve good health and to establish a health-promoting lifestyle before pregnancy. Health risks to the mother, as well as to fetal development, can be discussed. Not only does information presented this way demonstrate that

BOX 33-1 **Sexually Transmitted Diseases and Teen Pregnancy**

Sexually transmitted diseases (STDs) affect 25% of sexually experienced teenagers each year. STDs are more easily transmitted to women than men and can be more difficult to detect. STD infections among women can contribute to infertility, cancer, and ectopic pregnancy. When a young women is pregnant, these infections can cause premature rupture of membranes, premature labor, and postpartum infection. Also, the baby can be affected by all STDs in several ways: prematurity and low birth weight, febrile infection after delivery, long-term infection, and even death (e.g., exposure to viral infections such as HPV, HSV, HBV, and HIV).

The pregnant adolescent is at high risk for acquiring an STD because she may not be using contraceptives such as condoms. During the pregnancy, she will require periodic STD screening. STD education and counseling should accompany this screening. Information given should include ways to reduce one's risk such as maintaining a mutually monogamous relationship and using latex condoms.

BOX 33-2 **Reproductive Health Care and Adolescents' Rights**

No federal regulation requires a young person to have parents involved in decisions on contraception services provided by federal programs. States cannot prohibit an adolescent access to contraception. Several Supreme Court decisions protect this access:
- 1965: *Griswold v. Connecticut*—the right to prevent pregnancy through the use of contraceptives is protected by the right to privacy.
- 1972: *Eisenstad v. Baird*—the right to privacy in contraceptive use is extended to unmarried individuals.
- 1977: *Carey v. Population Services International*—the right to privacy is specifically extended to minors.

Modified from Center for Population Options: *Adolescent abortion and mandated parental involvement: the impact of back alley laws on young women*, Washington, DC, 1993, Author.

the nurse has heard what the teen is saying, but it also allows the nurse to provide useful health information that may encourage the teen to examine her plans carefully, seriously, and maturely.

It is important to pay attention to what the teen fails to verbalize. Knowledge of adolescent health care issues is valuable so that the nurse can anticipate other health concerns and provide an environment in which the adolescent feels safe in raising other concerns. By creating a caring and understanding atmosphere, the nurse can encourage the young person to discuss concerns about family violence, drugs, alcohol, or dating.

Discussing reproductive health care is a sensitive matter for both teens and many adults. Teens may have difficulty expressing themselves because of a limited sexual vocabulary or embarrassment due to their lack of knowledge. The nurse must recognize this potential deficit and embarrassment and assist teens by anticipating concerns. It is also important to allow teens to express themselves in their own language, which may include crude or offensive words. Nurses must learn about common slang expressions and common misconceptions so they do not miss important concerns that a teenager might have. The nurse can offer more appropriate terms once trust is established.

Teens may have difficulty discussing topics that provoke a judgmental reaction, such as discussing sexually transmitted diseases (STDs) (Box 33-1). It is important for the nurse to choose neutral words to elicit symptoms (e.g., "Has there been a change in your typical vaginal discharge?"). This approach also gives the nurse a chance to educate the young client about normal anatomy and physiology.

Considerable debate exists over whether adolescents should make reproductive health care decisions without

their parents' knowledge. As seen in Box 33-2 the adolescent's right to privacy, and thus her right to contraceptive treatment, is federally protected. Obstacles to services do exist, however, and this may result in a teen not receiving contraceptive information and treatment. Obstacles can include lack of transportation to a health care facility, money to pay for services, or permission to leave school early to attend an appointment.

Abortion services for adolescents are not clearly defined. No federal protection is extended to adolescents requesting abortion services, and the adolescent's right to privacy and ability to give consent varies by state, as seen in Box 33-3. Confidential care to teenagers may mean the difference between preventing an unwanted pregnancy, an abortion, or a birth. This care can influence whether prenatal visits begin in the first trimester versus the second or third trimester. Teens have varied reasons for pursuing confidential care, including seeking independence as well as serious and well-founded concerns about a parent's potential reaction (i.e., abuse of the teen). Once nurses recognize the reason for confidential care they can work with teens to discuss reproductive health care needs with the family. To do so, first clarify family values about sexuality and family communication styles with the teen. In a dysfunctional family, referral to community agencies (e.g., child protective services, Al-Anon) may be necessary. However, the nurse may need to honor the adolescent's need for confidentiality for an unknown period and proceed with the usual interventions, such as pregnancy testing, options counseling, and referral for clinical care.

TRENDS IN ADOLESCENT SEXUAL BEHAVIOR AND PREGNANCY

Approximately 1 million teens become pregnant each year, and more than half go on to have babies. Births to teenagers make up 12% of all births in the United States (ACOG, 1998). The numbers of teens who become preg-

BOX 33-3 Abortion and Adolescent Rights

- *Parental consent laws:* The parents of a young woman who is under 18 years of age seeking an abortion must give permission to the abortion provider before the abortion is performed. These laws are enforced in 16 states: Alabama, Indiana, Kentucky, Louisiana, Maine, Massachusetts, Michigan, Mississippi, Missouri, North Carolina, North Dakota, Pennsylvania, Rhode Island, South Carolina, Wisconsin, and Wyoming.
- *Parental notification laws:* One or both parents of a young woman seeking an abortion must be notified by the abortion provider before the abortion is performed. These laws are enforced in 14 states: Arkansas, Delaware, Georgia, Idaho, Iowa, Kansas, Maryland, Minnesota, Nebraska, Ohio, South Dakota, Utah, Virginia and West Virginia.
- *Judicial bypass:* In a 1979 Supreme Court decision, it was ruled that any mandatory parental consent law must allow the young woman an opportunity to be granted an exception or waiver to the law. A young woman could appeal directly to a judge, who would decide either that she was mature enough to make this decision or that the abortion would be in her best interest.

Data from the Center for Population Options: *Adolescent abortion and mandated parental involvement: the impact of back alley laws on young women*, Washington, DC, 1993, Author; National Abortion and Reproductive Rights Action League Foundation: *Who decides? a state by state review of abortion and reproductive rights*, Washington, DC, 1998, NARAL.

BOX 33-4 Healthy People 2000 Objectives Related to Adolescent Reproductive Health

1. Reduce pregnancies among girls ages 17 and younger; special population targets are African-American and Hispanic girls ages 15 to 19.
2. Reduce rape and attempted rape of young women.
3. Increase calcium intake to three or more servings daily of foods rich in calcium for youth aged 12 to 24 and for pregnant and lactating women.
4. Reduce the proportion of adolescents who have engaged in sexual intercourse.
5. Increase abstinence from sexual activity for the previous 3 months among sexually active adolescents ages 17 and younger.
6. Increase contraceptive use, especially those methods that prevent pregnancy and provide barrier protection against disease, among sexually active young people ages 19 and younger.
7. Increase the proportion of sexually active unmarried young women whose partner used a condom at last intercourse.
8. Increase the proportion of sexually active unmarried young men ages 15 to 19 who used a condom at last intercourse.
9. Increase the proportion of persons ages 10 to 18 who have discussed human sexuality, including values surrounding sexuality, with their parents and/or have received information through another parentally endorsed source, such as youth, school, or religious programs.
10. Increase the proportion of primary care providers who provide age-appropriate preconception care and counseling.
11. Increase discussions among persons ages 10 and older with family members on topics related to nutrition, physical activity, sexual behavior, tobacco, alcohol, other drugs, or safety.

Modified from USDHHS: *Healthy People 2000: national health promotion and disease prevention objectives*, Washington, DC, 1991, USDHHS, Public Health Service.

nant are generally identified in the following way: by age group (younger than 15, ages 15 to 17, ages 18 to 19); by pregnancy outcomes (birth, induced abortion, or spontaneous abortion); by rates (number of pregnancies, births, and abortions per 1000 young women); and by race/ethnicity (black, white, Hispanic/Latino). Teen birth rates increase by age, with the highest rates occurring among 19-year-olds. Pregnancy and birth rates increased steadily among teens of all ages from 1986 to 1991 and declined among teens of all ages and ethnicity from 1991 to 1996 (CDC, 1997). Decreases from 25% to 22% were also noted in the repeat teen birth rate from 1991 to 1996. These decreases are attributed to stabilization of the numbers of teens becoming sexually active and increased condom use (CDC, 1997). Over the last 36 years, rates and numbers of births to teens have fluctuated widely. The highest rates occurred in the 1960s and 1970s, followed by a drop to the lowest point in 1986 and since rising and falling again (Moore et al, 1997).

Hispanic/Latino teens currently have the highest rate of births at 107/1000. This is more than double the rate of white teens (39/1000) (Moore et al, 1997). Black teens have the next highest rate (99/1000). Decreases in birth rates occurred among all ethnic/racial groups from 1991 to 1995.

The greatest decrease was of births to black teens. Seventy-six percent of teens are unmarried at the time of their child's birth, a number that has quadrupled since 1960 (Moore et al, 1997). *Healthy People 2000* (USDHHS, 1991) has identified goals to reduce teen pregnancy and birth rates (Box 33-4).

In 1994, 35% of pregnancies to teenagers were ended by elective abortion (ACOG, 1998) Elective abortion rates for teenagers increased from the time of legalization in 1973 until 1986. From 1986 to 1994, there was a 21% decrease in abortions to teens (Moore et al, 1997). This decrease is due in part to decreases in the pregnancy rate but may also result from laws that have required parental notification for minors requesting abortion services in some states. Black and white teens choose abortion at similar rates. Adolescents who terminate their pregnancies by abortion differ from those who give birth in the following ways: they are more likely to complete high school, are more successful in school, have higher educational aspirations, and are more likely to come from a family of a higher socioeconomic status (Alexander and Guyer, 1993).

The United States leads the developed world in rates of teenage pregnancy, teen births, and teen abortions. Teens in Sweden have the highest rate of sexual activity (the United States is second), but they experience fewer pregnancies, births, and abortions. If these same comparisons are made with only white teens, the United States still leads in the number of pregnancies, births, and abortions. Comparisons with statistics in other countries suggests that much of this difference is caused by the limited use of contraceptives among teens, as well as a general ambivalence about providing comprehensive sexuality education at home and at school for children and adolescents in the United States (Hatcher et al, 1998).

BACKGROUND FACTORS

Many adults have difficulty understanding why young people would jeopardize their careers and personal potential by becoming pregnant during the teen years. Adolescents, however, view the world differently than do adults. Teens often feel invincible and therefore do not anticipate any risk for the consequences related to their behaviors. That is, they may not believe that sexual activity will lead to pregnancy. When teens become pregnant, they do not think that the negative outcomes they are advised of could come true. Many teens believe that they are unique and different and that everything will work out fine. The developmental circumstances of adolescence, coupled with potential background disadvantages, can magnify the problems facing the pregnant and parenting teen. Pregnant teens often express the unrealistic attitude that they can do it all: school, work, parenting, and socializing (Fig. 33-1).

The characteristics of the teens who are giving birth is changing. A disproportionate number of teens who give birth are poor (more than three quarters), have limited educational achievements, and see few advantages in delaying pregnancy since they do not expect that their circumstances will improve at a later time (Nord et al, 1992). Most teens report that their pregnancy was unplanned. They typically say they think a pregnancy should be delayed until people are older, have completed their education, and are employed and married (Hatcher et al, 1998). Their behaviors, however, do not support the opinions they express. In fact, some teens actually seem ambitious about becoming pregnant. Several of the factors that often contribute to pregnancy are discussed next.

Sexual Activity and Use of Birth Control

The **sexual debut,** or first experience, with intercourse for a teen will have a significant impact on pregnancy risk. Although the percentage of sexually active teens today is much greater than it was in the 1970s, decreases over the last five years have been noted. In the ninth grade 37% of students are sexually active; 48% by tenth grade; 58% in the eleventh grade and 66% by the twelfth grade. Male students (12%) and black students (24%) were more likely than white, Hispanic/Latino, or female students to initiate sexual activity before age 13. Black students (73%) are more likely to report a history of sexual activity, followed by Hispanic/Latino (57%) and white students (48%) (CDC, 1996).

> **DID YOU KNOW?** *In 1996 Congress passed the Personal Responsibility and Work Opportunity Reconciliation Act. This welfare reform package strives to discourage teen pregnancy and other nonmarital births in a variety of ways. Emphasis is on the primary prevention of pregnancy through abstinence education and discouraging sex before marriage. Further, benefits may be withdrawn if adolescent parents do not live in an adult-supervised home and attend school.*

The *Healthy People 2000* goal is to reducce to no more than 15% by age 15 and no more than 40% by age 17 the number of adolescents who have engaged in sexual inter-

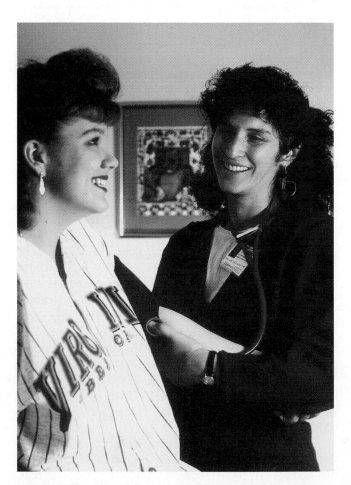

FIG. 33-1 The United States leads the developed world in the rates of teen pregnancy.

course (baseline of 27% girls and 33% boys by age 15; 50% girls and 66% boys by age 17, reported in 1988).

Although more teens have begun using birth control in the past 10 years, there still is progress to be made; 78% of adolescent girls (Moore et al, 1998) report use of birth control at first voluntary coitus. Teen males use condoms with increasing frequency (99% reported using condoms at some time during the past year) but not consistently. Overall, 44% of teen males use condoms consistently, with the greatest use reported by black teen males and the lowest use reported by Hispanic/Latino teen males (Moore et al, 1998). Half of all first-time pregnancies occur within 6 months of initiating intercourse (Hatcher et al, 1998). Teens harbor many myths that contribute to poor use of birth control, such as believing you cannot get pregnant the first time, or they may have erroneous knowledge about a woman's fertile time. Failure to use birth control by teens can also reflect their embarrassment in discussing this practice with partners, friends, parents, and health care providers and the obstacles they encounter finding facilities that provide confidential and affordable birth control (Hatcher et al, 1998).

The earlier the sexual debut, the less likely a birth control method will be used, since younger teens have less knowledge and skill related to sexuality and birth control. School-based sex education can come too late or not at all. Birth control is usually discussed in the secondary-school curriculum, but this could be eighth grade in one school district and tenth in another; school curricula are not standardized. Younger teens may falsely believe that they are too young to purchase birth control methods such as condoms. Confidential reproductive health care services may be available for teens, but problems are still associated with transportation, school absences, and costs of care that ultimately restrict access to these services.

Inconsistent use of birth control can reflect teens' willingness to take risks, their dissatisfactions with available birth control methods, and their ambivalence about becoming pregnant. Real and perceived side effects of birth control methods can discourage use. Hormonal methods such as Depo-Provera (an intramuscular injection every 3 months) and Norplant (a 5-year implant) appeal to some women because the method is less directly tied to coitus. These newer methods may have nuisance-type side effects (e.g., irregular bleeding) that are unappealing to many women. Table 33-1 describes hormonal birth control methods.

The use of alcohol and other substances is common among adolescents and can contribute to unplanned pregnancy. Mood-altering effects may reduce inhibitions about engaging in intercourse and interfere with the proper use of a chosen birth control method.

Peer Pressure and Partner Pressure

Peer pressure among teens is not a new phenomenon, but many of the influences have become more serious. Influence has expanded from fashion and language to cigarettes, substance abuse, sexuality, and pregnancy. Teens are more likely to be sexually active if their friends are sexually active (Perkins, 1991). Peers reinforce teen parenting by exaggerating birth control risks, discouraging abortion and **adoption,** and glamorizing the impending birth of the child.

Both young men and women may think that allowing a pregnancy to happen verifies one's love and commitment for the other. In addition, young men from socioeconomically disadvantaged backgrounds may be more likely to say that fathering a child would make them feel more manly and are less likely to use an effective contraceptive (Marsiglio, 1993).

TABLE 33-1 Hormonal Birth Control Methods

METHOD	PERCENTAGE PREGNANT WITH PERFECT USE	PERCENTAGE PREGNANT WITH TYPICAL USE	PATTERN OF USE	PERCENTAGE OF CONTINUATION AT 1 YEAR	PERCENTAGE OF TEENS USING METHOD	COMONLY REPORTED REPORTED SIDE EFFECTS
Norplant	0.05	0.05	Insert every 5 years	88	2.2	Menstrual irregularities; hirsutism, acne, scalp hair loss, weight gain, headache, mood changes
Depo-Provera	0.3	0.3	Inject every 3 months	70	7.9	Menstrual irregularities; weight gain
Birth control pills	0.1	5	Take a pill daily	71	35.4	Nausea; menstrual irregularities; breast tenderness; weight gain

Data from Hatcher RA et al: *Contraceptive technology*, New York, 1998, Ardent Media; Emans SJ, Laufer MR, Goldstein DP: *Pediatric and adolescent gynecology*, ed 4, Philadelphia, 1998, Lippincott-Raven.

Other Factors

Other factors influencing teen pregnancy are a history of **sexual victimization,** family structure, and parental influences. Pregnant teenagers may have a greater likelihood of having been sexually abused during their lifetime, with rates recorded as high as 62% (Stock et al, 1997). Adolescent females with a history of sexual abuse are at risk for earlier initiation of voluntary sexual intercourse, are less likely to use birth control, are more likely to use drugs and alcohol at first intercourse, and are more likely to have older sexual partners (Boyer and Fine, 1992). The youngest women are more likely to experience **coercive sex** (74% of women who had intercourse before age 14 reported that it was involuntary) (Moore et al, 1998). Young women may also become pregnant as a result of forced sexual intercourse. A history of sexual victimization will influence a young woman's ability to exert control over future sexual experiences, which will affect the use or nonuse of birth control and rejection of unwanted sexual experiences. Parker and colleagues have found that 21% of pregnant adolescents reported violence during the pregnancy, a rate greater than that reported by adult women (Covington et al, 1997). In addition, young women who have experienced a lifetime of economic, social, and psychological deprivation may think that a baby will bring joy into an otherwise bleak existence. Some mistakenly think that a baby can provide the love and attention that her family has not provided.

> **WHAT DO YOU THINK?** *In response to federal welfare reform recommendations, there has been a recent trend toward the enforcement of statutory rape laws by individual states. These laws make it a crime to have sexual contact with a person before the age of consent is reached (which varies among states). Supporters of this action think that this will discourage adult men from relationships with minors and consequently reduce teen pregnancy. Opponents believe that this strategy does not take into account the complex issues involved in teen pregnancy (such as poverty and limited opportunities for young women) and think it may do more to distance a father from involvement in his child's life.*

Family structure can influence adolescent sexual behavior and pregnancy. Adolescents raised in single-parent families may be more likely to have intercourse and to give birth than those raised in two-parent families. This difference is striking: sexual activity will occur among 22% of girls from two-parent families and 44% of girls from other family situations. A similar difference is also seen in the likelihood of giving birth by age 20 (Moore et al, 1998). The age of a young woman when the family structure changes is also important. The most vulnerable age for a family change to occur is 14 (Hollander, 1993).

Parenting styles can influence a young woman's risk for early sexual experiences and pregnancy. Parents who are extremely demanding and controlling or neglectful and who have low expectations are least successful in instilling parental values in their children. Parents who have high demands for their children to act maturely and who offer warmth and understanding with parental rules have children more likely to exhibit appropriate social behavior and to delay early sexual experiences and pregnancy. Children of parents who are neglectful are the most sexually experienced, followed by children of parents who are very strict. Further, parents who discuss birth control, sexuality, and pregnancy with their children can positively influence delay of sexual initiation and effective birth control use. Parents who do not communicate about sexuality with their teens may find them more at risk for sexual permissiveness and pregnancy (East and Felice, 1992).

YOUNG MEN AND PATERNITY

One in 15 males becomes a father during the teen years. While one third of the fathers of babies born to teens are teens themselves, more than half the fathers are between ages 20 and 24. Most fathers of babies born to adolescent mothers are 2 to 3 years older than the mother (Robinson, 1988). Teen fathers face special challenges because of concomitant social problems and limited future plans or ability to provide support. There also may be an overlap between young fatherhood and delinquency. Young fathers who demonstrate law-breaking behaviors, alcohol or substance use, school problems, and aggressive behaviors may have difficulty developing a positive fathering role (Stouthaner-Loeber and Wei, 1998).

Paternity, or fatherhood, is legally established at the time of the birth for a teen who is married. However, it is more difficult to establish paternity among nonmarried couples. Some of the difficulty lies in the complexity of the specific state system for young men to acknowledge paternity. In some states, a young man may have to work with the judicial system outside of the hospital after the birth, and if he is under age 18, he may need to involve his parents.

Some young couples do not attempt to establish paternity and prefer a verbal promise of assistance for the teen mother and child. Although a verbal commitment may be acceptable when the child is born, the mother may become more inclined to pursue the establishment of paternity later when the relationship ends or for reasons related to financial, social, or emotional needs of the child. Young women who receive state or federal assistance (e.g., Aid for Dependent Children, Medicaid) may be asked to name the child's father so the judicial process can be used to establish paternity.

Young men react differently when they learn that their partner is pregnant. The reaction often depends on the nature of the relationship before the pregnancy. Many young men will accompany the young woman to a health care center for pregnancy diagnosis and counseling. A large percentage of young men will continue to accompany the young woman to some prenatal visits and may even attend the delivery (Robinson, 1988). These young men may also

Teen Pregnancy in Canada

Karen Wade, Toronto Public Health and University of Toronto

ADOLESCENT SEXUAL BEHAVIOUR IN CANADA

The Canada, Youth, and AIDS Study (1988) surveyed 38,000 Canadian adolescents in Grades 7, 9, 11, and first year college or university to explore their sexual behaviours. Results revealed that 31% of Grade 9 boys and 21% of Grade 9 girls had engaged in sexual intercourse. By the time they reached Grade 11, 49% of boys and 46% of girls had been sexually active. In Canada, as in the United States, unprotected sexual activity is commonplace among youth and poses serious health threats, including sexually transmitted diseases, HIV infection, and unplanned pregnancy. Many sexually active teens do not use condoms or use them inconsistently (Health Canada, 1997; King et al, 1988; Richardson and Beazley, 1997; Svenson et al, 1992; Thomas, DiCenso, and Griffith, 1998). Among Canadian females, adolescents 15 to 19 years old have the highest rates of chlamydia and gonorrhoea of all age groups (Health Canada, 1997) and the number of people in their twenties with AIDS is increasing, indicating infection in the teen years (Frank, 1996).

TRENDS IN ADOLESCENT PREGNANCY IN CANADA

Wadhera and Millar (1997) reviewed data related to teenage pregnancy in Canada from 1974 to 1994. The teenage pregnancy rate (live births, therapeutic abortions [including those performed in free-standing clinics], miscarriages, and stillbirths per 1000 female population) in Canada dropped overall from 1974 to 1994 from 53.7 to 48.8 per 1000. However, since 1987 the rate has increased almost every year (Wadhera and Millar, 1997). This rate may be an underestimate of the true rate for several reasons. Nonhospitalized miscarriages and illegal abortions in Canada have been estimated to be as high as 17%, which is above the annual rate of 3% to 7% that Wadhera and Millar (1997) used in their calculations. The rates reflect the year in which the pregnancies end, so they do not include pregnancies that began at age 19 and ended at age 20 (Wadhera and Millar, 1997).

In 1974 the majority (66%) of teenage pregnancies in Canada ended in a live birth, while 26% of teens had therapeutic abortions and 8% had stillbirths or miscarriages. By 1994, although the majority of teenage pregnancies ended in a live birth, almost as many (45%) ended in a therapeutic abortion. In 1994, the teen abortion rate in Canada was 22 abortions per 1000 women ages 15 to 19, accounting for almost 20% of all abortions performed in 1994, compared with only 6% of live births in 1994 (Wadhera and Millar, 1997).

Although the trends in pregnancy rates of younger and older teens reflect a similar pattern as the trends in overall adolescent pregnancy rates, there are marked differences in the adolescent pregnancy rates of younger and older Canadian teens. In 1994, the pregnancy rate of 15- to 17-year-olds was 30.2 per 1000 population, which, although lower than the rate of 33.8 in 1974, has been rising since 1987. Pregnancy rates of 18- to 19-year-olds are more than double those of 15- to 17-year-olds. The pregnancy rate of 18- to 19-year-olds fell from 83.7 per 1000 in 1974 to 61.8% in 1984 and then climbed to 76.2 in 1994 (Wadhera and Millar, 1997).

In 1994, teenage pregnancy rates varied substantially among Canadian provinces and territories from a low of 31.5 per 1000 in Prince Edward Island to a high of 136.7 per 1000 in the North West Territories. Wadhera and Millar (1997) note that these rates do not include abortions performed in clinics because these data do not always include the woman's age or province/ territory of residence.

In 1988, the most recent year for which figures are available to compare Canada's teenage pregnancy rate (excluding stillbirths/miscarriages) to other major countries, Canada's rate was 40 pregnancies per 1000 women ages 15 to 19. This rate was higher than that of Sweden, Finland, Denmark, the Netherlands, and Japan but lower than the rates in Czechoslovakia, Hungary, New Zealand, England, Wales, Iceland, and the United States. Of the countries for which data were available, the United States had the highest adolescent pregnancy rate, at almost 100 per 1000, as well as the highest teen abortion rate at 44 legal abortions per 1000. In 1988, Canada's teen birth rate of 24 live births per 1000 was significantly lower than the U.S. rate of 53 per 1000 (Allan Guttmacher Institute, 1994, as cited in Wadhera and Millar, 1997). Wadhera and Millar (1997) cite data from The Allan Guttmacher Institute (1996), as well as the United States Monthly Vital Statistics Reports (1996), which show that although U.S. pregnancy, birth, and abortion rates continue to exceed those of Canada, slow steady declines have been evident since the early 1990s, in contrast with increases in Canadian rates during the same time period.

Bibliography

Frank J: 15 years of AIDS in Canada, *Canadian Social Trends* 41:4, 1996.

Health Canada: *Sexual risk behaviours of Canadians*, Ottawa, 1997, Bureau of HIV/AIDS and STD Epi Update Series, Laboratory Center for Disease Control.

King AJC et al: *Canada, youth, and AIDS study*, Ottawa, 1988, Health Canada, Federal Centre for AIDS.

Richardson HRL, Beazley RP: Factors influencing condom use among students attending high school in Nova Scotia, *Can J Human Sexuality* 6(3):185, 1997.

Svenson LW et al: Rural high school students' knowledge, attitudes, and behaviours related to sexually transmitted diseases, *Can J Public Health* 83(4):260, 1992.

Thomas BH, DiCenso A, Griffith L: Adolescent sexual behaviour: results from an Ontario sample. Part II: Adolescent use of protection, *Can J Public Health* 89(2):94, 1998.

Wadhera S, Millar WJ: Teenage pregnancies, 1974 to 1994, *Health Reports* (Statistics Canada, Catalogue 82 003 XPB), 9(3):9, 1997.

Canadian spelling is used.

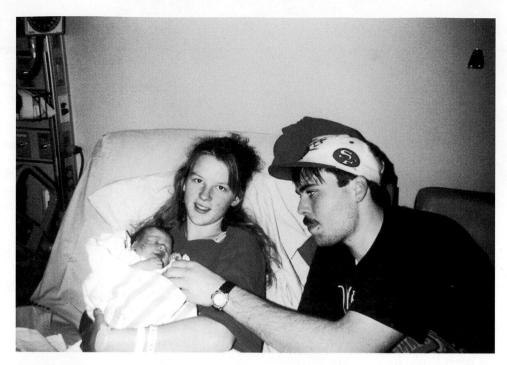

FIG. 33-2 It is important to include both the teen mother and father in teaching about child development.

want to and need to be involved with their children regardless of changes in their relationships with the teen mother. It is not unusual for a young man to be excluded or even rejected by the young woman's family (usually her mother). He may then begin to act as though he is disinterested when he may really feel that he cannot provide resources for his child or know how to take care of him or her (Rhein et al, 1997) (Fig 33-2).

Nurses can acknowledge and support the young man as he develops in the role of father. His involvement can positively affect his child's development and provide greater personal satisfaction for himself and greater role satisfaction for the young mother (Rhein et al, 1997). The immediate concerns revolve around his financial responsibility, living arrangements, relationship issues, school, and work. Establishing an opportunity to meet with the young man and both families is helpful to clarify these issues and identify roles and responsibilities.

Young men who grow up in poor families are more likely to believe that fathering a child can make them feel manly, and they are more likely to be pleased with a pregnancy than their affluent counterparts. These young men are also less likely to use or to discuss birth control with a partner. Young men who had previously impregnated a young woman are more likely to feel and act this way (Marsiglio, 1993).

EARLY IDENTIFICATION OF THE PREGNANT TEEN

Some teens delay seeking pregnancy services because they fail to recognize signs such as breast tenderness and a late period because they are experiencing a variety of other pubertal changes. Most young women, however, suspect pregnancy as soon as a period is late. These young women may still delay seeking care since they falsely hope that the pregnancy will just go away. A teen also may delay seeking care to keep the pregnancy a secret from family members, who may pressure her to terminate the pregnancy, or because of fears about gynecological examinations (Cartwright et al, 1993).

Nurses must be sensitive to subtle cues that a teenager may offer about sexuality and pregnancy concerns. Such cues include questions about one's fertile period or requests for confirmation that one need not miss a period to be pregnant. Once the nurse identifies the specific concern, information can be provided about how and when to obtain pregnancy testing. The nurse should determine how a teenager would react to the possible pregnancy before completing the test. If the test is negative, the nurse should take the opportunity to assess whether the young woman would consider counseling to prevent pregnancy. A follow-up visit is important after a negative test to determine if retesting is necessary or if another problem exists.

> **NURSING TIP**
>
> *An important counseling opportunity presents itself when a teen has a pregnancy test that is negative. Use this time to clarify a desire or disinterest in pregnancy and help empower her to influence her reproductive future.*

A young woman with a positive pregnancy test requires a physical examination and pregnancy counseling. It is advantageous to offer these at the same time so that the counseling is consistent with the findings of the examination. The purpose of the examination is to assess the duration and well-being of the pregnancy, as well as to test for sexually transmitted infection. The pregnancy counseling should include the following: information on adoption, abortion, and child-rearing; an opportunity for assessment of support systems for the young woman; and identification of the immediate concerns she might have.

The availability of affordable abortion services up to 13 weeks' gestation varies from community to community. Similarly, second-trimester services may be available locally or involve extensive travel and cost. The nurse should be knowledgeable about abortion services and provide information or refer the pregnant teenager to a pregnancy counseling service that can assist.

The pregnant teenager needs information about adoption, such as current policies among agencies that allow for continued contact with the adopting family. Also, church organizations, private attorneys, and social service agencies provide a variety of adoption services with which the nurse should be familiar. Box 33-5 lists guidelines for adoption counseling. *Healthy People 2000* objectives include efforts to increase to 90% the proportion of pregnancy counselors who offer positive, accurate information about adoption to their unmarried clients with unintended pregnancies (baseline: 60% of pregnancy counselors in 1984). At this time, 8% of adolescent women age 17 and under relinquish custody of their infants (ACOG, 1998).

Pregnancy counseling requires that the nurse and young woman explore strengths and weaknesses for personal care and responsibility during a pregnancy and parenting. Young women vary in their interest in including the partner or their parents in this discussion. Issues to raise include education and career plans, family finances and qualifications for outside assistance, and personal values about pregnancy and parenting at this time in their life. Often it is difficult to focus on counseling in any depth at the time of the initial pregnancy testing results. A follow-up visit is usually more productive and should be arranged as soon as possible.

As decisions are made about the course of the pregnancy, the nurse is instrumental in referral to appropriate programs such as WIC (Supplemental Food Program for Women, Infants, and Children), Medicaid, and prenatal services. The young woman and her family also need to know about expected costs of care and, if there is a family insurance policy, whether it will cover the pregnancy-related expenses of a dependent child. For those without insurance, the family can apply for Medicaid or determine whether local facilities offer indigent care programs (e.g., Hill-Burton programs for assistance with hospital expenses). The nurse can also begin prenatal education and

counseling on nutrition, substance abuse and use, exercise, and special medical concerns.

SPECIAL ISSUES IN CARING FOR THE PREGNANT TEEN

Pregnant teenagers are considered high-risk obstetrical clients. Many of the complications of their pregnancy result from poverty, late entry into **prenatal care,** and limited knowledge about self-care during pregnancy. Nursing interventions through education and early identification of problems may dramatically alter the course of the pregnancy and birth outcome.

Violence

Teens are more likely to experience violence during their pregnancies than adult women. Age may be a factor in their greater vulnerability to potential perpetrators that include partners, family members, and other acquaintances. Violence in pregnancy has been associated with an in-

---

BOX 33-5 Guidelines for Adoption Counseling

1. Assess your own thoughts and feelings on adoption. Do not impose your opinion on the decision-making process of teen mothers.
2. Be knowledgeable about state laws, local resources, and various types of adoption services.
3. Choose language sensitively. For example:
   a. Avoid saying "giving away a child" or "putting up for adoption." It is more appropriate and positive to say "releasing a child for adoption," "placing for adoption," or "making an adoption plan."
   b. Avoid saying "unwanted child" or "unwanted pregnancy." A more appropriate term may be "unplanned pregnancy."
   c. Avoid saying "natural parents" or "natural child," since the adopted parents would then seem to be "unnatural." The terms "biological parents" and "adopted parents" are more appropriate.
4. Assess when a discussion of adoption is appropriate. It can be helpful to begin with information on adoption, then explore feelings and concerns over time. Individuals will vary in how much they may have already considered adoption, and this will influence the counseling session.
5. Assess the relationship between the pregnant teen and her partner and what role she expects him to play. Discuss the reality of this.
6. It may be helpful for a pregnant teen to talk with other teens who have been pregnant, are raising a child, have released a child for adoption, or have been adopted themselves.
7. A young woman can be encouraged to begin writing letters to her baby. These can be saved or given to the child when released to the adoptive family.

Adapted from Brandsen CK: *A case for adoption*, Grand Rapids, Michigan, 1991, Bethany.

creased risk of substance abuse, poor compliance with prenatal care, and poor birth outcomes. In the case of partner violence, young women may be protective of their partners due to fear or helplessness. Eliciting this history from an adolescent does not happen easily. The nurse must inquire about violence at every visit. Frequent routine assessments are more revealing than inquiries at just the first prenatal visit (Covington et al, 1997). The nurse must also observe for physical signs of abuse, as well as for controlling or intrusive partner behavior (see the Research Brief).

Initiation of Prenatal Care

Pregnant adolescents differ remarkably from pregnant adults in initiation and compliance with prenatal care. Inadequate prenatal care has been negatively associated with health risks to both the mother and the fetus. Half of all pregnant teens delay entering prenatal care until after the first trimester, whereas one quarter of women of all ages delay until after the first trimester (Children's Defense Fund, 1994; VanWinter and Simmons, 1990). Teens report that the greatest barrier to care is real or perceived cost (Cartwright et al, 1993). Other barriers include denial of the pregnancy, fear of telling parents, transportation, dislike of providers' care, and offensive attitudes among clinic staff toward pregnant teens (Cartoof et al, 1991; VanWinter and Simmons, 1990).

Once a teen is enrolled in prenatal care, the nurse becomes an important liaison between personnel at the clinical site and the young woman. Confusion and misunderstandings easily occur when teens do not understand what a health care provider says to them. Often these misunderstandings are based on lack of knowledge about basic anatomy and physiology. For example, a teen may be told as she gets close to term that the head of the baby is down and it can be felt. This is an alarming piece of information for a young woman who imagines the entire baby could just pop out any time!

Cooperation between the nurse and the clinical staff can also maximize the client's compliance with special health or nutritional needs. For example, a teen who has premature contractions may be placed on bed rest and instructed to increase fluids. The nurse who makes home visits can provide additional assessment of the teen's condition and can solve problems about self-care, hygiene, meals, and school.

Low-Birth-Weight Infants and Preterm Delivery

Teens are more likely than adult women to deliver infants weighing less than 5½ pounds or to deliver before 37 weeks' gestation. The risk of **low birth weight** or **prematurity** is greater for younger teens and for a second birth to a teen, especially if it is within 1 year of the first. These low-birth-weight and premature infants are at greater risk for death in the first year of life and are more at risk for long-term physical, emotional, and cognitive problems (Nord et al, 1992). For example, low-birth-weight and pre-

RESEARCH *Brief*

This study looked at the incidence of abuse by developmental age and the relation it might have to pregnancy planning, high school participation, substance use during pregnancy, pregnancy complications, and infant birth weight.

The 559 ethnically diverse study participants were between the ages of 13 and 19 and receiving prenatal care at clinics in the Northwest. The teens were interviewed one time during their pregnancy. Abuse was measured by the Abuse Assessment Screen, which has reported validity and reliability. Substance abuse was identified by confidential self-reporting and information about pregnancy complications was determined from the medical records.

In this study 37% of adolescents reported abuse in the past year and 14% during the pregnancy. The highest rates of abuse occurred during middle adolescence (ages 16 to 17) and dropped significantly by age 18. Although this study did not identify the perpetrator, it was assumed that in some cases it was a family member. The authors speculate that some abuse may decline at age 18 when some young women moved away from the family home. Deleterious pregnancy outcomes, such as low birth weight, were not increased among those reporting the greatest abuse. Overall, rates of abuse among pregnant teens were not as high as those reported by other studies. The authors conclude that more abuse will be reported by teens if screening is done multiple times throughout the pregnancy.

Curry MA, Doyle BA, Gilhooley J: Abuse among pregnant adolescents: differences by developmental age, *MCN* 23(3):144, 1998.

mature infants can be more difficult to feed and soothe. This challenges the limited skills of the young mother and can further strain relations with other members of the household, who may not know how to offer support or assistance.

The risk of low-birth-weight and premature births can be averted by the teen's early initiation into prenatal care. Although such births still occur, it is important to work closely with the teen mother as soon as she is identified as pregnant to try to promote compliance with prenatal care visits and self-care during the pregnancy. After the pregnancy, these infants and their mothers will benefit from frequent nursing supervision to ensure that their care is appropriate and that everyone in the home is coping adequately with the strain of a small infant.

Nutrition

The nutritional needs of a pregnant teenager are especially important. First, the teen lifestyle does not lend itself to overall good nutrition. Fast foods, frequent snacking, and

TABLE 33-2 Adolescent Nutritional Needs During Pregnancy

NUTRIENT	DAILY REQUIREMENT DURING PREGNANCY*	FOOD SOURCE
Calcium	1200-1500 mg	Macaroni and cheese; Taco Bell Chili Cheese burrito; pizza; McDonald's Big Mac; puddings, milk; yogurt
Iron	30 mg (adolescents should take 30-60 mg elemental iron a day as a supplement)	Meats, dried beans and peas, dark green leafy vegetables, whole grains, fortified cereal
Zinc	15 mg	Seafood, meats, eggs
Folate (folic acid)	0.4 mg (prenatal vitamins contain 0.4 to 1.0 mg of folic acid)	Green leafy vegetables, liver, breakfast cereals.
Vitamin A	800 RE	Dark yellow and green vegetables, fruits
Vitamin B_6	2.2 mg	Chicken, fish, liver, pork, eggs
Vitamin C	70 mg	Green and red peppers, collard greens, broccoli, spinach, tomatoes, potatoes, strawberries, citrus fruits

*Higher ranges are especially important for the younger pregnant teen

hectic social schedules limit nutritious food choices. Snacks, which account for approximately a third of a teen's daily caloric intake, tend to be high in fat, sugar, and sodium and limited in essential vitamins and minerals. Second, the nutritive needs of both pregnancy and the concurrent adolescent growth spurt require the adolescent to change her diet substantially. The growing teen must increase caloric nutrients to meet individual growth needs as well as allow for adequate fetal growth. Third, poor eating patterns of the teen and her current growth requirement may leave her with limited reserves of essential vitamins and minerals when the pregnancy begins. The nurse can assess the pregnant teenager's current eating pattern and provide creative guidance. For example, protein can be increased at fast-food establishments by ordering milkshakes instead of soft drinks and cheeseburgers or broiled chicken sandwiches instead of hamburgers. Snack foods can be purchased for eating on the way to school in the morning and for midmorning snacks (Story, 1990).

The recommended nutritional needs of the adolescent may depend on the **gynecological age** of the teen, that is, the number of years between her chronological age and her age at menarche, as well as her chronological age. Young women with a gynecological age of 2 or less years or under the age of 16 may have increased nutrient requirements because of their own growth. Further, the younger and still-growing teen may compete nutritionally with the fetus. Fetuses may show evidence of slower growth in young women ages 10 to 16 years (Scholl et al, 1997; Story, 1990). The nurse, in collaboration with the WIC nutritionist, can determine the nutritional needs of the pregnant teenager to tailor education appropriately. Table 33-2 describes adolescent nutritional needs in pregnancy.

Weight gain during pregnancy is one of the strongest predictors of infant birth weight. Although precise weight gain goals in adolescence are controversial, pregnant adolescents who gain 26 to 35 pounds have the lowest incidence of low-birth-weight babies (Story, 1990). Younger

TABLE 33-3 Gestational Weight Gain Recommendations for Adolescents*

PREPREGNANT WEIGHT CATEGORIES†	RECOMMENDED TOTAL GAIN	
	KG	LB
Underweight (BMI 19.8)	12.5-18	28-40
Normal weight (BMI 19.9-26)	11.5-16	25-35
Overweight (BMI 26-29)	7.0-11.5	15-25
Very overweight (BMI 29)	7.0-9.1	15-20

*Very young adolescents (14 years of age or younger or less than 2 years postmenarche) should strive for gains at the upper end of the range.

†BMI (body mass index) is calculated as weight (kg)/height squared (m).

From Gutierrez Y, King JC: Nutrition during teenage pregnancy, *Pediatr Ann* 22(2):99, 1993.

teen mothers (ages 13 to 16), because of their own growth demands, may need to gain more weight then older teen mothers (ages 17 and over) to have the same-birth-weight baby. Differentiating the still-growing teen from the grown teen may not be possible in the clinic setting, so encouraging teens to gain at the upper end of their weight goals may be the best approach (Lederman, 1997). Teenagers who begin the pregnancy at a normal weight should be counseled to begin weight gain in the first trimester and average gains of 1 pound per week for the second and third trimesters (Gutierrez and King, 1993). Table 33-3 shows the recommendations established by the Institute for Medicine for adolescent gestational weight gain by prepregnant weight categories.

It is important for the nurse to assess the attitudes of the pregnant teen about weight gain and to follow her progress. Studies indicate that most teenagers view prenatal weight gain positively. However, teens who are overweight before pregnancy may have negative attitudes about weight gain (Story, 1997). Family support of the pregnant teen can be a strong influence in adequate weight gain and good nutrition during the pregnancy (Stevens-Simon et al, 1993). Nutrition education should emphasize what accounts for weight gain and how fetal growth will benefit.

Iron deficiency is the most common nutritional problem among both pregnant and nonpregnant adolescent females (Story, 1997). The adolescent may begin a pregnancy with low or absent iron stores because of heavy menstrual periods, a previous pregnancy, growth demands, poor iron intake, or substance abuse. The increased maternal plasma volume and increased fetal demands for iron (especially in the third trimester) can further compromise the adolescent. Iron deficiency in pregnancy may contribute to increased prematurity, low birth weight, postpartum hemorrhage, maternal headaches, dizziness, shortness of breath, and so on (Story, 1990). The nurse can reinforce the need for the teen to take prenatal vitamins during pregnancy and after the baby's birth. Vitamins should contain 30 to 60 mg elemental iron daily. The nurse should educate about iron-rich foods and foods that promote iron absorption, such as those containing vitamin C.

Infant Care

Many adolescents have cared for babies and small children and feel confident and competent. Few teens are ever prepared, however, for the reality of 24-hour care of an infant. The nurse can help prepare the teen for the transition to motherhood while she is still pregnant. The trend toward early discharge from the hospital has made prenatal preparation even more important. The nurse can enlist the support of the teen's parents in education about infant care and stimulation. Young fathers-to-be would benefit from this education as well. Family values, practices, and beliefs about child care may be deeply embedded and require the nurse to work gently and persuasively to challenge any that may be detrimental to an infant (Wayland and Rawlins, 1997). For example, a family may believe that corporal punishment is a necessary component of child-rearing.

Adolescents often lack the self-confidence and knowledge required to positively interact with their infants (Diehl, 1997). They may also have unrealistic expectations about their children's development; for example, they may expect their children to feed themselves at an early age (Castiglia, 1990a). Teen parents often lack knowledge about infant growth and development, as seen in their limited verbal communication with their children, limited eye contact, and the tendency to display frustration and ambivalence as mothers (Koniak-Griffin and Verzemnieks, 1991). Over time, adolescents can improve their ability to foster their children's emotional and social growth. Children of adolescent mothers have also been found to be at risk for academic and behavior problems in late childhood and adolescence (Diehl, 1997). These risks can be reduced

when the teen mother receives professional intervention and supervision in the area of infant cognitive development (Ruff, 1990).

Abusive parenting is more likely to occur when the parents have limited knowledge about normal child development. It may also be more likely to occur among parents who cannot adequately empathize with a child's needs. Younger teens are particularly at risk for being unable to understand what their infant or child needs. This frustration may be exhibited as abusive behavior toward the child (Diehl, 1997).

After the birth of the baby, the nurse should observe how the mother responds to infant cues for basic needs and distress. Specific techniques that the new mother can be instructed to use in early child care are listed below. It is important to begin parenting education as early as possible. Adolescents who feel competent as parents have enhanced self-esteem, which in turn positively influences their relationship with their child (Diehl, 1997). Recognizing these good parenting skills and providing positive feedback help a young mother gain confidence in her role.

HOW TO *Promote Teen Mother/Newborn Interactions*

1. Make eye contact with your baby. Position your face 8 to 10 inches from your baby's face and smile.
2. Talk to your baby often. Use simple sentences, but try to avoid baby talk. Allow time for your baby to "answer." This will help your baby acquire language and communication skills.
3. Babies often enjoy when you sing to them, and this may help soothe them during a difficult time or help them fall asleep. Experiment with different songs and melodies to see which your baby seems to like.
4. Babies at this age cannot be spoiled. Instead, when babies are held and cuddled, they feel secure and loved.
5. Babies cry for many reasons and for no reason at all. If your baby has a clean diaper, has recently been fed and is safe and secure, he or she may just need to cry for a few minutes. What works to calm your baby may be different from other babies you have known. You can try rocking, gentle reassuring words, soft music, or quiet.
6. Make feeding times pleasant for both of you. Do not prop the bottle in your baby's mouth. Instead, you should sit comfortably, hold your baby in your arms, and offer the bottle or breast.
7. When babies are awake, they love to play. They enjoy taking walks and looking at brightly colored objects or pictures and toys that make noises, such as rattles and musical toys.

Repeat Pregnancy

Teen mothers who experience a closely spaced second pregnancy, or **repeat pregnancy,** have poorer educational and economic outcomes. Twenty-four percent of teens will have a second birth within 24 months, and the younger the teen, the greater the risk of an early second pregnancy (Kalmuss and Namerov, 1994). Nurses should recognize the risk factors for a second teen pregnancy: teens from disadvantaged backgrounds, teens from large families, those who are married, and those who had discontinued their education after the delivery of the first child. Also, teens who reported a planned first pregnancy are more likely to have a second pregnancy within 24 months to complete their family. Parenting adolescents who return to school after the birth of their first child, regardless of prior school performance, are least likely to repeat a pregnancy and more likely to use birth control (Kalmuss and Namerov, 1994).

Discussions about family planning should be initiated during the third trimester of the current pregnancy. Contraceptive options should be reviewed, and the young woman should begin identifying the methods she is most likely to use. It is helpful to determine at this time the methods she has used in the past, her satisfaction or dissatisfaction, and reasons for use or nonuse. Many teens express unrealistic goals, such as "I am never going to have sex again" or "I need a break from guys," and they may erroneously believe that they are unable to conceive for some time after the delivery. After delivery, the nurse should follow up on the young woman's plan. Obstacles to obtaining contraceptives may exist, and the nurse can identify these and help problem solve with the new mother.

Schooling and Educational Needs

Adolescents who become parents may have had limited school success before the pregnancy. As noted previously, the potential for a closely spaced second birth may be delayed by return to school. Federal legislation passed in 1972 prohibits schools from excluding students because they are pregnant. Greater emphasis is placed on keeping the pregnant adolescent in school during the pregnancy and returning as soon as possible after the birth. Several factors may positively influence a young woman's return to school. These include her parents' level of education and their marital stability, small family size, whether there have been reading materials at home, whether her mother is employed, and whether the young woman is African-American (Ahn, 1994; Klerman, 1993). A practical challenge for young parents is locating and affording quality child care; difficulties with this may prevent the highly motivated teenager from returning to school. In the past 30 years, the percentage of parenting teens who return to school and graduate has improved significantly (Nord et al, 1992).

Young women who have pregnancy complications may seek home instruction. This decision is made according to regulations issued by the state boards of education. Some young women have difficulty attending school because of the normal discomforts of pregnancy or because of social and emotional conflicts associated with the pregnancy. Teens who leave school without parental or medical excuses may face legal problems because of truancy. This increases the potential for them to become school dropouts. The nurse can determine if this has happened and try to coordinate with the school personnel (and school nurse if one exists) to tailor efforts for a particular pregnant teen to keep her in school. Specific needs to address include: (1) using the bathroom frequently, (2) carrying and drinking more fluids or snacks to relieve nausea, (3) climbing stairs and carrying heavy bookbags, and (4) fitting comfortably behind stationary desks. Schools that are committed to keeping students enrolled are generally helpful and will assist in accommodating special needs.

TEEN PREGNANCY AND THE NURSE

The nurse can influence teen pregnancy through appropriate interventions at home and in the community.

Home-Based Interventions

Young women at risk for pregnancy can be identified in families currently receiving services by the nurse. Younger sisters of pregnant teens are at a twofold-increased risk for becoming pregnant themselves (East and Felice, 1992). Anticipatory guidance that addresses sexuality issues can be offered to the parents of all preteens and teens during home visits to increase their knowledge and awareness.

Visiting the pregnant teen in her home allows the nurse to obtain an assessment of the facilities available at home for management of her pregnancy needs and suitability of the environment for her child. Some specific areas to assess are adequacy of heating and cooling, a source of water, cleanliness of the home, cooking facilities, and food storage. The nurse may find it more convenient for parents and other family members to participate in education and counseling sessions in their own home. Also, the need for financial assistance and other social service support may be more easily identified. It has been demonstrated that home visiting by nurses during a young woman's pregnancy is positively associated with increases in birth weight and increased use of prenatal care and support services (Deal, 1994) (Fig 33-3).

When a teen pregnancy occurs, the family dynamics can shift. Families may go through stages of reactions. First, a crisis stage may occur, characterized by many emotions and conflict. By the third trimester, a honeymoon stage may occur, with greater acceptance and understanding of the teen and the impending birth. Finally, after the infant's birth, reorganization may occur, during which conflict may emerge again over issues of child care and the young woman's role. The nurse can facilitate family coping and resolution of these stages by treating the family as client and assessing each person's role and strengths. Ultimately, family support for a teen parent can positively influence both mother and infant (Ruchala and James, 1997; Wilkerson, 1991).

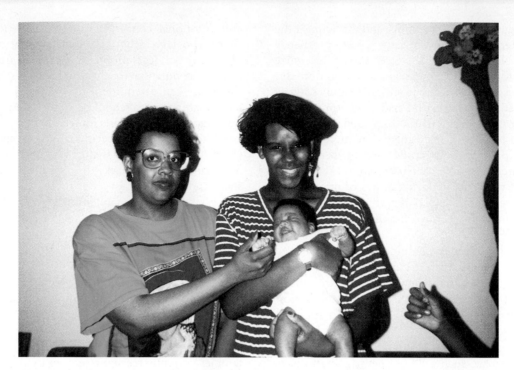

FIG. 33-3 Both the teen mother and the teen's own mother can be included in health teaching.

Community-Based Interventions

Broad-based coalitions and planning councils are forming in many areas to facilitate a comprehensive approach to teen pregnancy. These groups usually include health care professionals, social workers, clergy, school personnel, businessmen, legislators, and members of other youth-serving agencies. The nurse can have a significant role on this team by participating in or organizing community assessments, public awareness campaigns, group education (for professionals, parents, and youth), and interdisciplinary programs for high-risk youths. Community acceptance is more likely when there is a broad base of support for activities directed at the reduction of teen pregnancy or reduction of consequences.

Healthy Communities 2000: Model Standards use the objectives of *Healthy People 2000* and allow for modification of programs to tailor them to each community. These model standards can be used by a broad-based coalition or by a lead agency, such as the public health department. Initially an assessment of need is done, followed by a determination of local priorities. Goals for the individual community can then be established and a plan of action developed. Efforts should be evaluated on a regular basis.

The nurse can also be a valuable asset to schools. Family life education programs are strongly recommended or mandated in 46 states, and all 50 states recommend or mandate AIDS education (Kirby et al, 1994). Health teachers may call on nurses for educational materials or assistance with classroom instruction, especially in the areas of family planning, STDs, and pregnancy. Schools that do not have nurses may arrange to have the nurse available for health consultations with students during school hours. Schools may also request that nurses participate on their health advisory boards.

School-based clinics are operating in more than 400 middle and high schools in the United States. The services offered may include counseling, referrals, general health evaluations, and family planning. Some of these programs have been found to delay the onset of intercourse and increase the use of contraception (Kirby et al, 1994). The nurse can assist school systems to design these programs and can also refer young women in need of reproductive health care services.

Nurses bring their knowledge about youth and reproductive behavior to any organization or group that has teens, their parents, or other professionals working with teens. Churches are becoming increasingly interested in addressing the needs of their youth, especially since teen sexual activity, pregnancy, and parenting are affecting more of their members.

DID YOU KNOW? *Emergency contraception can reduce the risk of pregnancy by 75% when used within 72 hours after unprotected intercourse. Although this is an effective and safe method, a regularly used birth control provides greater protection.*

Community coalitions can look to the *Healthy People 2000* for planning and the *Healthy Communities 2000* standards for modifying these goals to meet the needs of individual communities.

clinical application

Kristen is a nurse in a small southern city. In her assessment of the community she identifies large numbers of pregnant and parenting teenagers enrolled at the local high school. In response to this she develops a school-based young mother's educational program. The program is endorsed by school administrators who recognize that this program will encourage teens to remain in school, as well as provide good physical and social support from a knowledgeable professional

As a trusting relationship evolves between the nurse and the students, their special needs become apparent. The nurse uses her knowledge of community resources and makes referrals to various agencies and organizations. Examples of referrals are a church-based program for maternity clothing and baby equipment; the family stress clinic for one young woman and her parents; the health department for WIC registration and home visiting; the pediatric specialty clinic for one student's asthma symptoms, which have been exacerbated by the pregnancy.

One student, a tenth-grader, is withdrawn. She does not talk with the other students, nor does she reveal information about herself. The nurse is concerned and arranges to spend extra time with this student. Eventually the young woman explains that her boyfriend has begun hitting her when they argue.

Which of the following steps should Kristin, the nurse, take?

A. Notify the school officials and contact the police.
B. Encourage the student to develop a safety plan and include her parents or other adults in her care.
C. Follow the state laws for reporting domestic violence or child abuse.
D. Lead a group discussion on partner violence.

Answer is in the back of the book.

KEY POINTS

- The provision of reproductive health care services to adolescents requires sensitivity to the special needs of this age group. This includes being knowledgeable about state laws regarding confidentiality and services for birth control, pregnancy, abortion, and adoption.
- Pregnant teenagers have a substantial percentage of the first births in the United States. They are more likely to deliver prematurely and have a baby of low birth weight. This risk can be reduced by early initiation of prenatal care and good nutrition.
- Factors that can influence whether a young woman becomes pregnant include a history of sexual victimization, family dysfunction, substance use, and failure to use birth control. Several factors may overlap.

- Nutritional needs during pregnancy can be challenged if the teenager has unhealthy eating habits and begins the pregnancy with limited reserves of vitamins and minerals. With education, the adolescent can make good food choices while still snacking or eating fast foods. Weight gain during pregnancy is a significant marker for a normal-weight baby.
- Young men need special attention and preparation as they become fathers. The interventions include information about pregnancy and delivery, declaration of paternity, care of infants and children, and psychosocial support in this role.
- The pregnant teen will need support during her pregnancy and in child-rearing. Families may provide most of this support. However, many communities have a variety of services available for adolescents. These services include financial assistance for medical care, nutritional programs, and school-based support groups.
- Adolescent parents have unrealistic expectations about their children and consequently do not know how to stimulate emotional, social, and cognitive development. The children born to adolescents are at risk of academic and behavioral problems as they become older. Teens who receive education on normal development and child care will be more likely to avert these problems with their children.
- During a pregnancy, teenagers are expected to attend school. Homebound instruction is reserved for those with medical complications. Teen mothers who return to school and complete their education after the birth of their child are less likely to have a repeat pregnancy. Problems finding child care and the need to have an income can create an obstacle to school return.
- Community coalitions, which include nurses, can have a significant impact on teen pregnancy. These coalitions generally have diverse representation from the community, and therefore their activities meet with more community support.

critical thinking activities

1. Become familiar with statistics on teen pregnancy, births, miscarriages, and abortions in your area. Collect information also on utilization of prenatal care, low-birth-weight and premature deliveries, high school completion, and repeat pregnancies.
2. Call or visit local schools and interview the school nurse or guidance counselors about teen pregnancy. Determine what resources are available through the schools for pregnancy prevention. Assess the family life education curriculum, and identify a teaching project for nursing students.
3. Design and offer a childbirth preparation class for pregnant teens and their support persons. Include a plan for identifying potential participants, select a site that is accessible, and develop an evaluation method.
4. Assess reproductive health care services to young men in your community. Design an awareness campaign targeting young men on paternity issues and the prevention of pregnancy.

Bibliography

Ahn N: Teenage childbearing and high school completion, *Fam Plann Perspect* 26(1):17, 1994.

Alan Guttmacher Institute: *Sex and America's teenagers,* New York, 1994, Author.

Alderman EM, Fleischman AR: Should adolescents make their own health care choices? *Contemp Pediatr,* January 1993, p 65.

Alexander CS, Guyer B: Adolescent pregnancy: occurrence and consequences, *Pediatr Ann* 22(2):85, 1993.

American College of Obstetricians and Gynecologists (ACOG): *Adolescent pregnancy fact sheet,* Washington DC, 1998, ACOG

American Public Health Association: *Healthy Communities 2000: model standards,* ed 3, Washington, DC, 1991, the Association.

Boyer D, Fine D: Sexual abuse as a factor in adolescent pregnancy and child maltreatment, *Fam Plann Perspect* 24(1):4, 1992.

Brandsen CK: *A case for adoption,* Michigan, 1991, Bethany.

Cartoof VG, Klerman LV, Zazveta VD: The effect of source of prenatal care on care-seeking behavior and pregnancy outcomes among adolescents, *J Adolesc Health* 12:124, 1991.

Cartwright PS et al: Teenagers' perceptions of barriers to prenatal care, *South Med J* 86(7):737, 1993.

Castiglia PT: Adolescent mothers, *J Pediatr Health Care* 4(5):262, 1990a.

Castiglia PT: Adolescent fathers, *J Pediatr Health Care* 4(6):311, 1990b.

Centers for Disease Control and Prevention: Youth Risk Behavior Surveillance–United States, 1995, *MMWR* 45(SS-4):1, 1996.

Centers for Disease Control and Prevention: State-specific birth rates for teenagers–United States, 1990-1996, *MMWR* 46(36):837, 1997.

Children's Defense Fund: *The state of America's children yearbook,* Washington, DC, 1994, Author.

Commonwealth Fund: *The commonwealth fund survey of the health of adolescent girls,* New York, 1997, Author.

Covington DL et al: Improving detection of violence among pregnant adolescents, *J Adolesc Health* 21(1):18, 1997

Curry MA, Doyle BA, Gilhooley J: Abuse among pregnant adolescents: differences by developmental age, *MCN* 23(3):144, 1998.

Deal LW: The effectiveness of community health nursing interventions: a literature review, *Public Health Nurs* 11(5):315, 1994.

Diehl K: Adolescent mothers: what produces positive mother-infant interaction, *MCH* 22(2):89, 1997

Donovan P: Can statutory rape laws be effective in preventing adolescent pregnancy, *Fam Plann Perspect* 29(1):30, 1997

East PL, Felice ME: Pregnancy risk among the younger sisters of pregnant and childbearing adolescents, *J Dev Behav Pediatr* 13(2):128, 1992.

Emans SJ, Laufer MR, Goldstein DP: *Pediatric and adolescent gynecology,* ed 4, Philadelphia, 1998, Lippincott-Raven.

Fiscella K et al: Does child abuse predict adolescent pregnancy? *Pediatrics* 101(4 Pt 1):620, 1998.

Gutierrez Y, King JC: Nutrition during teenage pregnancy, *Pediatr Ann* 22(2):99, 1993.

Hamberger LK, Ambuel, B: Dating Violence, *Pediatr Clin N Amer* 45(2):381, 1998.

Hatcher RA et al: *Contraceptive technology,* New York, 1998, Ardent Media.

Hollander D: Family instability, stress heighten adolescents' risk of premarital birth, *Fam Plann Perspect* 25(6):284, 1993.

Kalmuss DS, Namerow PB: Subsequent childbearing among teenage mothers: the determinant of a closely spaced second birth, *Fam Plann Perspect* 26(4):149, 1994.

Kirby D et al: School-based programs to reduce sexual risk behaviors: a review of effectiveness, *Public Health Rep* 109(3):339, 1994.

Klerman LV: Adolescent pregnancy and parenting: controversies of the past and lessons for the future, *J Adolesc Health* 14:553, 1993.

Koniak-Griffin D, Verzemnieks I: Effects of nursing intervention on adolescents' maternal role attainment, *Issues Compr Pediatr Nurs* 14(2):121, 1991.

Kreutzer, TA: *Expenditures and investments: adolescent pregnancy in the south,* vol II, Washington, DC, 1997, Southern Regional Project on Infant Mortality.

Lederman SA: Nutritional support for the pregnant adolescent. In Adolescent nutritional disorders prevention and treatment, *Ann NY Acad Sci* 817:304, 1997.

Marsiglio W: Adolescent males' orientation toward paternity and contraception, *Fam Plann Perspect* 25(1):22, 1993.

Moore KA, Driscoll AK, Lindberg LD: *A statistical portrait of adolescent sex, contraception and childbearing,* Washington DC, 1998, National Campaign to Prevent Teen Pregnancy.

Moore KA et al: *Facts at a glance.* Sponsored by the Charles Stewart Mott Foundation, Flint, Mich, Washington DC, 1997, Child Trends.

National Abortion and Reproductive Rights Action League Foundation: *Who decides? a state by state review of abortion and reproductive rights,* Washington DC, 1998, NARAL.

National Campaign to Prevent Teen Pregnancy: *Whatever happened to childhood? the problem of teen pregnancy in the U.S.,* Washington DC, 1997, Author

Nord CW et al: Consequences of teenage parenting, *J Sch Health* 62(7):310, 1992.

Perkins JL: Primary prevention of adolescent pregnancy, *Birth Defects* 27(1):33, 1991.

Resnick MD et al: Protecting adolescents from harm, *JAMA* 278(10):823, 1997.

Rhein LM et al: Teen father participation in child rearing: family perspectives, *J Adolesc Health* 21(4):244, 1997.

Robinson B: *Teenage fathers,* Lexington, Mass, 1988, Heath.

Ruchala PL, James DC: Social support, knowledge of infant development and maternal confidence among adolescent and adult mothers, *JOGGN* 26(6):685, 1997.

Ruff CC: Adolescent mothering: assessing their parenting capabilities and their health education needs, *J Natl Black Nurses Assoc* 4(1):55, 1990.

Scholl TO, Hediger ML, Schall JI: Maternal growth and fetal growth: pregnancy course and outcome in the Camden study in Adolescent Nutritional Disorders Prevention and Treatment, *Ann NY Acad Sci* 817:292, 1997.

Stevens-Simon C, Nakashima I, Andrews D: Weight gain attitudes among pregnant adolescents, *J Adolesc Health* 14(5):369, 1993.

Stock JL et al: Adolescent pregnancy and sexual risk taking among sexually abused girls, *Fam Plann Perspect* 29(5):200, 1997.

Story M, editor: *Nutrition management of the pregnant adolescent,* Washington, DC, 1990, National Clearinghouse.

Story M: Promoting healthy eating and ensuring adequate weight gain in pregnant adolescents: issues and strategies, in Adolescent Nutritional Disorders Prevention and Treatment, *Ann NY Acad Sci* 817:321, 1997.

Stouthamer-Loeber M, Wei EH: The precursors of young fatherhood and its effect on delinquency of teenage males, *J Adol Health* 22(1):56, 1998.

USDHHS: *Healthy People 2000: national health promotion and disease prevention objectives,* Washington, DC, 1991, USDHHS, Public Health Service.

VanWinter JT, Simmons PS: A proposal for obstetric and pediatric management of adolescent pregnancy, *Mayo Clin Proc* 65:1061, 1990.

Wayland J, Rawlins R: African American teen mothers' perceptions of parenting, *J Pediatr Nurs* 12(1):13, 1997

Wilkerson NN: Family focused secondary prevention, *Birth Defects* 27(1):33, 1991.

Migrant Health Issues

KIM DUPREE JONES, CHERYL PANDOLF SCHENK, & MARIE NAPOLITANO

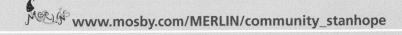

www.mosby.com/MERLIN/community_stanhope

OBJECTIVES

After reading this chapter, the student should be able to do the following:

- Define the term *migrant farm worker* and discuss the difficulty in determining the definition.
- Describe common health problems of the migrant farm worker and farm worker families.
- Examine the barriers to migrant farm workers and their families in securing health care.
- Evaluate successful programs that encourage health promotion among migrant farm workers and their families.

- Analyze the role of the nurse in planning and providing care to migrant farm workers and their families.
- Evaluate legislation that has assisted in the provision of health care services for these groups.
- Discuss proposed health reform legislation and the effects of the provision of health care services on migrant farm workers and their families.
- Describe the cultural needs of migrant farm workers and their families, and list methods of providing culturally based nursing care through assessment, planning, intervention, and evaluation.

KEY TERMS

cultural differences
machismo
migrant farm worker

Migrant Health Act
migration

National Advisory Council
  on Migrant Health
personalismo

pesticide exposure
working conditions
See Glossary for definitions

CHAPTER OUTLINE

Definition of Migrant
Migrant Health Problems
  Health and Health Care
  Work Conditions
  Pesticide Exposure
  Housing
  Women

Children and Youth
Barriers to Migrant Health Care
Social and Cultural Considerations
  in Migrant Health Care
  Work Ethic and Gender Roles
  Family
  Health Values

Interactive Styles
Health Promotion and Illness Prevention
Role of the Nurse
Legislative Issues

Imagine yourself working in the tobacco fields 14 hours a day in temperatures over 100° F with no drinkable water or bathrooms. After work, you come home to a two-bedroom trailer shared with 15 other workers. Your home has no indoor plumbing or air conditioning. You expect to have a stiff back and aching knees from your day's labor but are fearful that the constant skin rashes and eye irritation are from pesticides sprayed in the fields. Although a neighboring county has a health care facility for migrant farm workers, transportation is a problem, and the luxury of a paid sick day does not apply to you. What would you do?

Migrant farm workers and their families are one example of a vulnerable population. Vulnerable populations are characterized by unique social, economic, and health risks that lead to disenfranchisement, victimization, and helplessness. *Healthy People 2000* (USDHHS, 1991), a document containing national strategies to promote health and prevent disease, does not specifically address migrant farm workers. However, the objective for clinical preventive services (number 21.5) is to "assure that at least 90 percent of people for whom primary care services are provided directly by publicly funded programs are offered, at a minimum, the screening, counseling, and immunization services recommended by the U.S. Preventive Task Force" (USDHHS, 1991, p. 539). Community and migrant health centers are an example of publicly funded primary care centers that provide some services to migrant farm workers and their families. Other *Healthy People 2000* objectives that could be expanded to include migrant farm workers involve the health of Hispanic individuals, lower-income individuals, and farm and agricultural workers as an extension of occupational safety and health.

DEFINITION OF MIGRANT

The Office of Migrant Health defines a **migrant farm worker** as an individual "whose principal employment is in agriculture on a seasonal basis, who has been so employed within the last 24 months and who establishes for the purpose of such employment a temporary abode" (p. 8). For the purposes of this chapter, only the migrant farm worker is discussed. Also, this text refers to migrant workers of Mexican heritage unless otherwise noted.

Although migrant farm workers have been a vital link in putting food on the dinner table for decades, little is known about them. For example, much debate surrounds the actual number of migrant workers due to differences in definitions, divergent methodologies for estimating numbers of workers, and whether dependents are included. The Office of Migrant Health indicates there are an estimated 4.2 million persons in migrant and seasonal farm work, of which only approximately 12% to 15% are served by federally supported migrant health centers (USDHHS, 1993). Crawford (1994) demonstrates major flaws in the manner in which migrant workers have traditionally been counted

and tracked, particularly in the Hispanic Health and Nutrition Examination Survey (HHANES), the only existing comprehensive study of the health of Mexican-Americans in the United States.

Migrant farm workers traditionally have followed one of three migratory streams (Eastern, originating in southern Florida; Midwestern, originating in southern Texas; and Western, originating in southern California). However, as workers increasingly travel throughout the country seeking employment, these streams are becoming less distinct. There is also a growing trend toward importing workers to Canada on temporary work visas from the Caribbean Islands.

MIGRANT HEALTH PROBLEMS

At a 1993 farm worker hearing before the National Advisory Council on Migrant Health, past and present migrant farm workers indicated that the problems that most concern them involve health and health care, work conditions, pesticide exposure, housing, women, and children and youth. Some of their actual testimonies, first names, and states of residence are given in Box 34-1.

Health and Health Care

Although migrant farm workers are concerned about specific illnesses, the themes of fundamental economic, societal, vulnerability and political conditions that lead to poor health are more often discussed. Migrant farm workers experience limited access to health care. Financial, cultural, transportation, mobility, language, and occupational factors are frequently cited as the major barriers that limit access to health care for farm workers. Furthermore access to dental, mental health, and pharmacy services are even more problematic (Adam, 1994; Mobed, Gold and Schenker, 1992).

The National Migrant Resource Program, Inc. (1990, p. 2), reports that in the United States, "Migrant farm workers' infant mortality rate is 25% greater than the national average; their life expectancy is 49 rather than 75 years; the rate of parasitic infection among some sets of farm workers approaches 50 times that of the total population." Also, migrant farm workers are 300 times more likely to contract hepatitis. Studies reporting the frequency and severity of health problems for which migrant workers and their families seek care include the following, in descending order: skin infections, muscle strain/sprain and upper respiratory infection (Johnsrud et al, 1998). Other leading causes of morbidity and mortality among migrants include infectious diseases such as tuberculosis (TB) and human immunodeficiency virus (HIV) disease. Although traditional health care services perceive problems concerning TB tracking and medication compliance to be important, migrant families are often unable to complete treatment because of extreme poverty, frequent moves, and cultural norms that encourage use of medication only for pain.

BOX 34-1 What Migrants Say About . . .

HEALTH AND HEALTH CARE

"What we have to do is reeducate our people and let them know that we have many rights to live and work and to educate and to have health care. And without health care, we cannot have the other three." Unidentified Male Farm Worker, California

WORK CONDITIONS

"We're used to working. We don't want to be given things. We just want to be respected and to be paid the salaries." Teresa, California

"Right now, because I'm here today (testifying at hearing on work conditions), I may not have my job. Possibly I may not have my job tomorrow." Jose, California

PESTICIDE EXPOSURE

"You go to the fields and you think that it's a foggy day because it's so pretty and it's white, but it's actually the chemicals that have been sprayed." Adelaide, California

"Pesticides presently occupy us tremendously during our work. We wear rubber gloves and that in itself creates a problem because it takes flesh, pieces of flesh from our hands." Guadalupe, California

HOUSING

"My slogan is, there must be a way to build houses. I believe we have the right to live in a decent way. We are the labor force. It's like we are foreigners—I am a U.S. citizen.

Farmworkers come here with hope, but go home worse off than before." Unidentified Male Farmworker, Colorado

"We have no coolers in the summer and no heaters in the winter. Temperatures range up to 100 degrees in the summer and 30 degrees in the winter. We work out in the open for 12 or more hours and after working there for more than 12 hours, we have no place to rest. This creates a tremendous amount of frustration, not being able to provide the children with the minimum for comfort." Margarita, California

"The foremen even charged (the farmworkers) for sleeping under the trees." Teresa, California

WOMEN

". . . Another thing I would like to mention is the way we are treated as women. As women we are discriminated with our co-workers because they see us as insignificant beings. The men think that they are superior." Maria, California

CHILDREN AND YOUTH

". . . (the children) go out to the fields. They lay under the trees and there is a residue falling on the children. They are picking grapes, what happens? The sprayers are there with the residue falling on the children." Irma, Oregon

"We have worked in the fields! Well, I'm not very young but I've left some of my youth in the work." Juliana, Washington

From Calarneau C, editor: *Under the weather: farm worker health*, Austin, Texas, 1993, National Advisory Council on Migrant Health, Bureau of Primary Health Care, USDHHS.

Work Conditions

Much is heard about unsafe **working conditions** in agriculture, especially involving migrant farm workers. Migrant farm workers are faced with questionable farmer payment practices, inadequate record keeping, below–minimum wage salary, and lack of enforcement regarding legislation for field sanitation and safety regulations. The vast number of farms covered by a single government inspector make upholding the standards for workers' safety and for fairness virtually impossible.

The work of migrant farm workers exposes these individuals to numerous health problems. Injuries are reported as the leading cause of mortality and morbidity among agricultural workers (Ciesiclski, Hall, and Sweeney, 1991). Lack of a comprehensive surveillance system makes it difficult to know the extent of injuries within the migrant population. Reported injuries have included fractures or sprains from falls from ladders or equipment; strains and sprains from prolonged stooping, heavy lifting, and carrying; amputations, deaths, and crush injuries from tractors, trucks, or other machinery; pesticide poisoning; electrical injuries; and drowning in ditches.

The physical demands of harvesting crops 12 to 14 hours a day take their toll on the musculoskeletal system. For example, a worker using improper body mechanics to stoop over with straight legs and pull up weeds or produce will inevitably suffer back pain, whereas the worker who lifts 50-pound crates of produce onto a truck bed all day may complain of shoulder and wrist pain. Naturally occurring chemicals or applied poisons can cause irritation to the skin (contact dermatitis) or to the eyes (allergic or chemical conjunctivitis).

Because such luxuries as paid vacation and sick time or workers' compensation do not exist for most migrants, they often work in pain. Simply stated, if they do not work, they do not make money. It is understandable, therefore, why they fear to leave the fields to seek health care during working hours. In a sample of 287 migrant farm workers who sustained significant on-the-job injuries, only 35% received medical care (Ciesiclski et al, 1991). Furthermore, people who live with chronic pain typically do not sleep well and are more likely to make mental mistakes in the fields that further endanger their health. Working with automated machinery is especially risky under these circumstances.

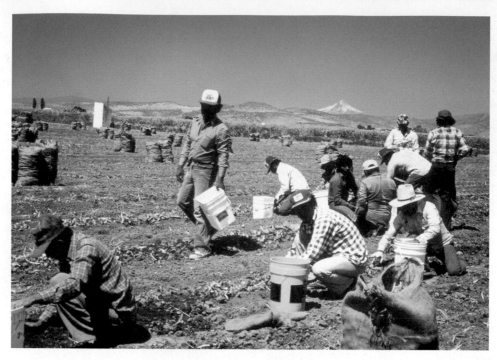

Migrant farm workers working in fields.

Pesticide Exposure

The vast majority of the North American food supply is treated with pesticides. Organophosphate anticholinesterase pesticides make up the largest group of pesticides in current use. These pesticides are known to affect normal neuromuscular functioning. Farm workers are exposed not only to the immediate effects of working in fields that are foggy or wet with pesticides, but also to the unknown long-term effects of chronic exposure to pesticides. The migrant farm worker's dwelling also can be a major source of contamination for the worker and his family. Acute health effects of **pesticide exposure** include mild psychological and behavioral deficits such as memory loss, difficulty with concentration, mood changes, abdominal pain, nausea, vomiting, diarrhea, headache, malaise, skin rashes, and eye irritation. Acute severe pesticide poisoning can result in death. More chronic exposure may lead to cancer, blindness, Parkinson's disease, infertility or sterility, liver damage, and polyneuropathy and neurobehavioral problems. Although legislation is in effect to minimize pesticide risk, migrant farm worker families remain at high risk for exposure. Lack of resources for monitoring, culturally inappropriate educational methods, fear of losing one's job or day's wage, and language differences are just a few barriers that hinder a safer pesticide environment for migrant farm workers.

Housing

Housing for migrant farm workers and their families is a problem of both quality and quantity. When migrant farm workers were asked by members of the National Advisory Council on Migrant Health where they had lived since working in the United States, they listed the following sites: in trailers, dirt-floor houses, cabins, labor camps, garages, cars, caves, boxes, ditch banks, tents, chicken coops; under trees, bridges, or tarps; in orchards, parks, fields, yards, streets; and next to highways and railroad tracks.

Cost of housing and cramped living conditions are also problematic. The weekly rent for a trailer may be $150. The farm worker may only make $25 a day. Therefore it is not unusual to find 10 to 15 people living in a single dwelling designed to accommodate three or four.

For migrant farm workers, housing is usually tied to the worker's job. Therefore, when a job is completed, the worker becomes simultaneously homeless and unemployed. This forced **migration** leaves little time or energy to seek out higher-quality housing.

Women

Hispanic women, as with most women throughout the world, are subject to oppression through both the expectations of their own families and communities and policies in various countries. Migrant women who work in the fields report harm from personal violence. They are concerned about working with pesticides that may cause birth defects and miscarriage. Furthermore, whether women work in the fields or at the camps at home, childcare is their responsibility.

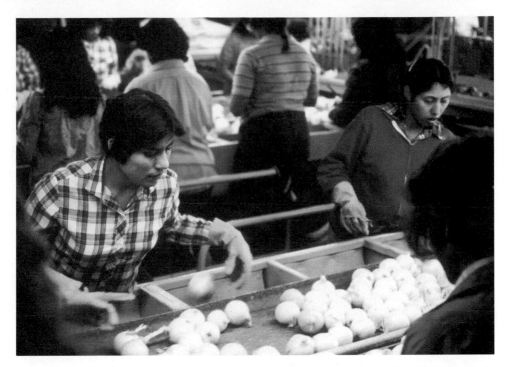

Many women have to work in fields or do related food-processing tasks. In addition to their farm work, they are also responsible for all child-rearing duties.

Some women describe taking infants and small children into the fields and tell horror stories about children being maimed or killed by farm equipment. Migrant Head Start is an option for children 6 months to 5 years old. However, inadequate funding results in lack of services for all migrant children. State and nationally sponsored summer school programs for farm workers' children over 3 years of age are in place in some areas of the United States.

Some women stay at the camp and care for several children whose parents are in the fields. These women suffer from isolation, depression, and anxiety. Many report being forbidden to leave the children except for 1 hour once a week, which they must spend buying food and other supplies for their family. A small number of programs have been funded to educate the migrant women to become lay health care workers. These women serve as a link between existing health care agencies and the migrant farm worker families. For example, in Oregon, La Familia Sana have educated migrant farm worker families regarding pesticide exposure and intervened with families regarding childhood immunizations and domestic violence.

Children and Youth

Migrant farm worker parents want a better future for their children. In fact, this strong desire was the catalyst for many farm workers to leave their country of origin. These children often appear to the outsider as happy, outgoing, and inquisitive. On the surface, they may look like children in any other aggregate. However, these children often suffer from health care deficits including malnutrition (vi-tamin A, iron), infectious diseases (upper respiratory infection, gastroenteritis), dental caries (due to prolonged use of the bottle, bottle propping, limited access to fluoride), inadequate immunization status, pesticide exposure, accidents, and limited access to drug and alcohol prevention and rehabilitation programs.

Children of migrant farm workers may need to work for the family's economic survival. Many work in the fields while others care for the children left at home and face special challenges in education, including having to be fluent in two languages and competent in two cultures. This is especially difficult for children who may change schools several times in a year or who miss several days because of travel. In fact, the child of a migrant farm worker is likely to attend an average of 24 different schools by fifth grade (National Farmworker Health Conference, 1998). Some federally funded summer programs offer supplemental schooling for children of migrant farm workers.

BARRIERS TO MIGRANT HEALTH CARE

"Farm workers' unmet needs for basic health care is not only a national disgrace, but also a national challenge" (USDHHS, p. 20 [1993 Recommendations]).

The **Migrant Health Act** funds more than 100 migrant health projects in the United States that have 364 actual clinic sites serving more than 500,000 farm workers and their families located in 40 states and in Puerto Rico. Surveys indicate that only 12% to 15% of eligible migrants use clinic services (Decker and Knight, 1990; Galarneau, 1993; Helsinki Commission, 1993; USDHHS, 1993). Fac-

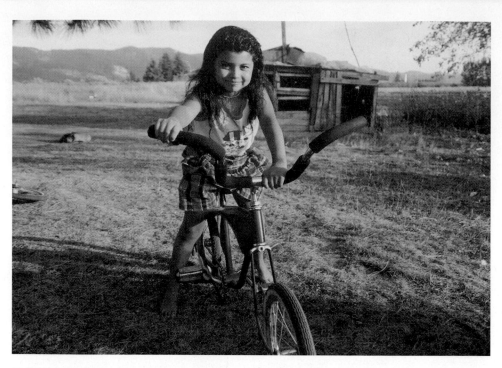

Children of migrant farm workers experience many hardships. They may have to help with the agricultural work while trying to maintain their schoolwork and to fit into two different cultures. These can be difficult efforts, especially if the children have to move a lot or are sick very much.

tors that limit adequate provision of health care services include:
- *Lack of knowledge.* Many migrant farm workers and their families live in a clustered environment close to work. Minimal outreach by bicultural/bilingual workers to this community is a frequently cited reason for the limited knowledge about the services that are available.
- *Lack of income.* The average reported farm worker income in the United States is about $7500 per year based on hourly wages or by amount of produce harvested each day (National Agricultural Workers Survey, 1997). Earning potential may be compromised by broken machinery, drought or rain, and lack of transportation to the next work site. Also, crew leaders are often paid by the farmer and expected to distribute wages to the workers. It is reported that some crew leaders keep a portion of workers' salaries for themselves and that some farm owners deduct Social Security monies, which may or may not be submitted to the government. All these inequities create a vicious cycle of poverty for the farm worker. Studies contend that two thirds of farm workers can live on the money they earn, but they have no money for health care and emergencies (Caudle, 1993; Helsinki Commission, 1993).

WHAT DO YOU THINK? *Substandard wages paid to migrant farm workers allow Americans to pay less for their fruits and vegetables.*

- *Availability of services.* The Welfare Reform legislation of 1996 changed the availability of federal services accessible to certain immigrants to this country (National Housing Law Project, 1996). Immigrants are treated differently depending on whether they were in the United States before August 22, 1996 and the category of immigrant to which they are designated. As a result of this legislation, each state determined whether to fill any or part of the services gap to immigrants. Many legal immigrants and undocumented immigrants are ineligible for services such as Supplemental Security Income (SSI) and food stamps. Furthermore, workers may not remain in a geographical area long enough to be considered for benefits or may lose benefits when they relocate to a state with different eligibility standards. Federal funding for Migrant Health Services ($70.6 million in 1998) has not kept pace with escalating costs and is equivalent to $100 per user per year, which is inadequate to meet minimal health needs. Finally, less than 20% of the total farmworker population is reached by public health funds (Helsinki Commission, 1993; Medicaid, 1991; Mines et al, 1997; National Farmworker Health Conference, 1998).

DID YOU KNOW? *In many states, workers' compensation benefits are not available to migrant farm workers for on-the-job injuries (Mines et al, 1997).*

- *Location of services.* Health care services may be located a great distance from work or home with no transportation to and from sites. Privacy is compromised when migrant workers depend on employers to provide transportation to clinics (Casseta, 1994; Caudle, 1993; USDHHS, 1993).

- *Hours.* Many health services are available during work hours and inconvenient to workers, who are only paid when picking; therefore seeking health care reduces earnings (Bishop and Harrison, 1987).
- *Child care.* Lack of affordable and accessible childcare for all migrant children compromises safety. Infants and small children may be left with older children or taken to the fields where overheating and death can occur. Also, health care services for adults and children are less readily obtained without available childcare.
- *Mobility and tracking.* Although families move from job to job, their health care records do not typically go with them, thereby leading to fragmented services in such areas as tuberculosis treatment and immunizations. For example, health departments are known to dispense tuberculosis (TB) medications on a monthly basis. Treatment for TB requires 6 to 12 months of medication for adequate treatment. When the migrant farm worker relocates, he or she must independently seek out new health services to continue medications. Furthermore, fear of immigration authorities deters clients with TB from seeking continued health care (Asch, Leake and Gerberg, 1994).
- *Discrimination.* Although migrant farm workers and their families bring revenue in to the community, they are often perceived as poor, uneducated, transient, ethnically distinct, and shiftless. In the authors' experience, even children experience discrimination when they are told to sit in the back of the school bus. Interviews with migrant families reveal a hesitancy to secure care when they interpret treatment by health care staff as not accepting of them (Decker and Knight, 1990; Helsinki Commission, 1993; USDHHS, 1993).

> **DID YOU KNOW?** *Farm worker children are excluded from the protection of the 1938 Child Labor act. Children as young as 10 can work in the fields. Annually, 300 children die in work-related injuries, and 25,000 are injured (Helsinki Commission, 1993).*

- *Documentation.* Many farm workers and their families are legal residents of the United States. However, some workers are "illegal" and not in compliance with Immigration and Naturalization Service regulations. Some illegal workers fear that securing services in a federally funded or state-funded clinic may lead to discovery and deportation.
- *Lack of bicultural/bilingual health care staff.* The recruitment and retention of bicultural/bilingual health care provider staff is a priority of the National Advisory Council on Migrant Health (1998). Many sources and interviews with migrant workers and their families indicate that lack of culturally competent staffing is a factor in using services.

> **NURSING TIP**
> *If you regularly work with Hispanic migrant workers, you can be more helpful if you learn some key Spanish words and phrases.*

SOCIAL AND CULTURAL CONSIDERATIONS IN MIGRANT HEALTH CARE

Recognition of societal norms and respecting **cultural differences** are central to succeeding and thriving in one's environment. This may be evidenced by gaining employment, accessing education, and receiving health care. Nurses must acknowledge the unique culture and values of migrant farm workers and their families in planning and providing care for this aggregate.

Work Ethic and Gender Roles

Males in the Hispanic culture may identify with the concept of **machismo,** the quality of dominance and chauvinism. Machismo may be further defined as courage, strength, honor, virility, pride, and dignity (de la Rosa, 1989; Decker and Knight, 1990). Because the workers may identify with machismo, a situation that may compromise or threaten this quality may undermine self-concept. Examples of this might be if a worker is ill and cannot support his family or if women seek health care without the consent of the male head of the family.

The wife/mother often decides when health care services are needed. She still maintains the traditional role of childcare giver with meal, shopping, and household responsibilities. The male head of the family is in charge of finances and transportation and makes the final decision about whether to secure health care services.

Family

The male head of the family approves decisions, and family needs, or familialism, are a priority over individual needs. Illness or disability of a family member is a family issue, and the family decides whether to seek care. At times, an illness or other problems may be kept solely within the family. For example, substance abuse is often considered a moral illness and a family responsibility rather than an illness to be discussed with non–family members.

Love of their children, rather than concern for their own health, may encourage migrant parents to adopt healthier lifestyles. One example is when the parents of a child with asthma choose to stop smoking (Marin, 1990). Health care may not be sought if there is a question of pride or a concern that seeking care is seen as a weakness or irresponsibility on the part of the family and the patriarch. Approval of an intervention by the family, and especially the male head of the family, will more likely lead to compliance (Caudle, 1993; Smith, 1988).

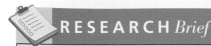

RESEARCH *Brief*

This master's research project evaluated data from the Virginia Garcia Migrant Clinic's mobile van program to migrant labor camps in 1997. The purpose of the project was to describe the population seen; the types of health needs; and the diagnoses, interventions, and referrals made by the van personnel. Of the 847 clients seen, 79% were male and 21% were female, with the average age 26 years. Forty-five percent of the clients were evaluated by a primary care provider, while the remaining 55% received preventive services such as blood pressure screening and tetanus vaccine. The top three diagnoses were skin infection, muscle strain/sprain, and upper respiratory infection. Medications and education were the major primary care interventions identified. Analgesics, antifungals, antibiotics, and antacids were the most common medications dispensed. Eighty-three clients were referred from the van, with 68 of those being referred in to the main clinic. Other referrals were made to dental and eye clinics.

Johnsrud P et al: *Migrant outreach van evaluation,* Oregon Health Sciences University, School of Nursing, 1998. Unpublished masters thesis.

Health Values

Although certain health beliefs and practices have been identified with Latino cultures, the nurse must remember that beliefs and practices differ between countries, regions, and individuals. Health is seen as a harmonious relationship between the social and spiritual sides of being. Illness occurs when this relationship is disrupted or a break occurs with cultural norms. Although some traditional health care practices are acknowledged and accepted, farm worker families also believe in seeking treatment from family members and from folk healers or, if from Mexico, curanderas (Caudle, 1993; Smith, 1988). Folk remedies may be tried first and may remain a mainstay of therapy even if traditional care is sought later. Prayer is extremely important, since most families are Roman Catholic and healing is considered a gift from God.

Interactive Styles

In seeking a health care provider, clients prefer **personalismo,** a provider with a similar background, culture, and language as themselves. Emotionality of the language and the nuances of slang are difficult to translate and may be limited if the services of an interpreter are used. Culturally, Hispanics prefer polite, respectful, nonconfrontational relationships with others, or simpatia. At times, because of simpatia, families may appear to understand what is being said to them when they do not. That is, the nurse may be providing information that is too complex for the client and the family yet they believe it would be rude to tell the

nurse that his or her information is unclear to them. During the visit to the clinic, family and friends (collectivism) may want to witness the examination and discuss the treatment plan (Caudle, 1993; Marin, 1990).

WHAT DO YOU THINK? *Assume you are examining a 16-year-old girl who was cut on the knee while working in the fields. Her mother, father, and aunt want to join you while you examine the girl. Should you allow them to come into the treatment room or tactfully point them toward the waiting room?*

HEALTH PROMOTION AND ILLNESS PREVENTION

Most farm workers do not view illness as a problem unless the condition prevents them from working. If health care is sought, the expectation (and need) is that a quick and complete recovery with no delay in resuming work will result. Health promotion and disease prevention are difficult concepts for migrant workers to embrace because of limited education, lack of future orientation, and their compromised access to health care. The authors saw this issue repeatedly in several situations:

- A farm worker with peptic ulcer disease and blood in his stools wanted relief from pain but would not admit or accept that cigarette smoking and alcohol consumption aggravated his condition.
- A young worker who was nauseated and vomiting while working with tobacco wanted relief from vomiting; however, he did not welcome the information that nicotine poisoning might be causing his illness.
- A worker had heat exhaustion because of refusing to drink water during the course of a 12-hour day in 90° temperatures. If she was hydrated, she would earn less money because of time away from the fields to void. Her lack of fluids put her at risk for cystitis and pyelonephritis.

Health promotion begins by informing the farm worker family about the resources available. Several migrant health programs have recruited migrant workers to serve as outreach workers and lay camp aides to assist in outreach and health education of the workers. Outreach, as defined by the Migrant Health Program, should "improve utilization of health services, improve effectiveness of health services, provide comprehensive health services, be accessible, be acceptable, and be appropriate to the population served" (USDHHS, 1993, p. 54). Outreach programs succeed because they recognize the diversity of this group and the need for flexibility in the provision of services. Because these outreach workers are members of the migrant community, they are trusted and know the culture and the language (Larson and Watkins, 1990; Watkins and Larson, 1991).

The Department of Maternal and Child Health of the School of Public Health at the University of North Carolina at Chapel Hill initiated an outreach program with the Tri-County Community Health Center, a federally

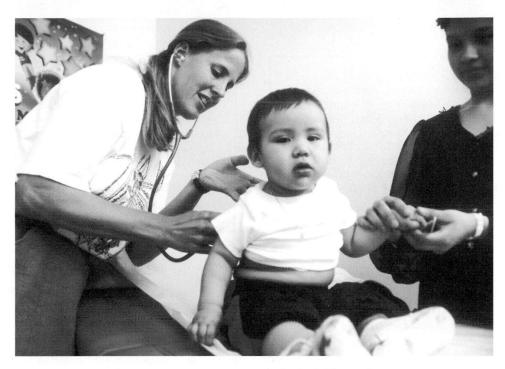

A nurse examines a migrant worker's child at a clinic.

funded migrant health clinic. Lay health advisors from the farm workers' camps educated workers and their families in the camps and helped to determine those in need of health services. Women were recruited who had leadership ability, respect, caring, and interest in learning about health issues and the importance of sharing that knowledge (Larson and Watkins, 1990). With some training on child health needs, environmental concerns, and resources available, they became ready resources within the camp. Lay workers reported several contacts each week with farm workers who sought out information on health care and resources. While actual statistical data showed no change in specific disease rates in camps, some anecdotal evidence suggests that their presence had a positive impact on health. Information would be further disseminated as women moved from camp to camp. The women who participated reported an increased sense of self-esteem and empowerment (Watkins and Larson, 1991). A similar program is sponsored by the Midwest Migrant Health Information Office in conjunction with the Catholic Consortium for Migrant Health Funding.

Education sessions taught by camp aides at the Salud Clinic Outreach program in Oregon focused on concepts of hygiene to prevent the spread of gastrointestinal problems. Farm worker women involved in these sessions were willing to learn these concepts because they were unaware that hygiene and the spread of disease were related (Bishop and Harrison, 1987). La Clinica del Carino in Hood River, Oregon, recruited farm worker women and developed a culturally competent mental health and substance abuse education program for women and adolescents. The Family Health/La Clinica in Washington State developed "Las

Comadres," a support network for farm worker women who had been removed from the feminine support network they had at home. Camp health aides and lay health advisors remain identified with their culture, promote preventive health care, and encourage their neighbors to learn about and take responsibility for their health care (Larson and Watkins, 1990).

ROLE OF THE NURSE

The health status of all people is a function of their ecology, or all that "touches" them. The nurse keeps a finger on the pulse of the community by remaining active in those political, social, religious, and employment areas that involve the client. Acting as a community educator, knowledgeable about how to obtain the latest information and resources, the nurse can work to assess the infrastructure of the community. These nursing actions sound straightforward but several barriers must be overcome. For example, in rural communities where most persons are well known to one other, where farmers hold the community "purse strings," and where migrant workers often are exploited, discriminated against, and ostracized, how can nurses make a difference in the health of migrant farm workers and their families?

The nurse can be a catalyst for change using the nursing process to assess farm worker needs continually, directing members in search of health care services, and evaluating the success of their efforts. For example, the nurse may analyze a community and determine that health care should be offered to farm worker families from 6 PM to 9 PM weekdays. Box 34-2 presents one migrant community care analysis. The nurse would then work with other health care

> ## BOX 34-2 Example of Assessment with Migrant Workers
>
> Faculty members and health nursing and family nurse practitioner students relocated to a rural southeastern U.S. county to provide health care to migrant farm workers. During the 2-week experience, the authors noted that migrant workers were most receptive to obtaining health services after 4 PM. The authors also realized that a mobile health van located in the camps where the workers lived was used more often than a better-equipped migrant health care facility located farther away.

> ## BOX 34-3 Resources for the Nurse Working with Migrant Farm Workers
>
> **FILMS AND VIDEOS**
>
> "Health of America's Harvesters: The Migrant Health Program." Produced by Alan McGill, 1990. (Contact the National Migrant Resource Program.)
> "Frontline: New Harvest, Old Shame." Produced by Hector Galan, PBS, 1990. (Contact your public or university library.)
>
> **WRITTEN MATERIALS**
>
> Johnston HL: *Health for the nation's harvesters: a history of the migrant health program in its economic and social setting,* Farmington Hills, Mich, 1985, National Migrant Worker Council.
> National Advisory Council on Migrant Health: *1993 recommendations of the National Advisory Council on Migrant Health,* Rockville, Md, 1993, Author.
> Rust GS: Health status of migrant farmworkers: a literature review and commentary, *Am J Public Health* 80(10):1213, 1990.
> Wilk VA: *The occupational health of migrant and seasonal farmworkers in the United States,* ed 2, Washington, DC, 1986, Farmworker Justice Fund.
>
> **ORGANIZATIONS**
>
> Bureau of Primary Health Care
> Migrant Health Program
> 4350 East West Highway, 7th Floor
> Bethesda, MD 20814
> (301) 594-4303
>
> National Migrant Resource Program, Inc.
> and/or Migrant Clinicians Network, Inc.
> 1515 Capital of Texas Hwy. South, Suite 220
> Austin, TX 78746
> (512) 328-7682

See this book's website at www.mosby.com/MERLIN for additional resources.

agencies to write grants and hire culturally competent personnel to provide these services. Services could include minor acute care and stable chronic care. The needs assessment might also indicate inadequate child and adult immunizations, which may best be provided in the fields, camps, and schools. The nurse may create an immunization tracking system to share information with other counties and states as the farm workers migrate. Culturally specific health promotion and disease prevention materials would be provided, as well as information about referral sources. Box 34-3 lists selected resources for the nurse working with migrant farm workers.

LEGISLATIVE ISSUES

In the late 1930s and 1940s, the Farm Security Act (later part of the U.S. Department of Agriculture) constructed migrant farm worker housing and provided basic health services. In 1946, this program provided health care services to more than 100,000 workers and worker families. This program dissolved in 1947 with all other war relief programs. Farm worker services were without any federal regulations until September 1962, when President John F. Kennedy signed the Migrant Health Act, funded under Section 329 of the Public Health Service Act, which provided primary and supplemental health services to migrant workers and their families. This act provides for professional and lay health workers, outreach, transportation, and environmental services, although not all services are provided at all clinic sites.

During 1992, more than 535,000 migrant farm workers and their families received services. The act was funded at $57.3 million in 1993. Average funding is equivalent to $100 per user per year. As mentioned earlier, this act funds more than 100 migrant health projects that support 364 sites located in 40 states and Puerto Rico. The act encourages cooperative agreements with state agencies and state and regional primary care associations to augment health care services and delivery. Partnerships are promoted between migrant health centers and state and local health departments, area health education centers, hospitals, specialty and social service providers, and residency programs. The migrant health centers are part of the Bureau of Primary Health Care, Health Resources and Services Administration, Public Health Service in the Department of Health and Human Services.

The **National Advisory Council on Migrant Health** meets three times a year to advise, consult with, and make recommendations concerning the organization, operation, selection, and funding of migrant centers. Recommendations for 1993 were as follows (USDHHS, 1993):

- *Housing.* The council advocated appropriate and safe housing for migrant farm workers and their families, with no less than 10,000 units per year over the next 10 years. As a result of this recommendation, a work group called the National Hispanic Housing Council was formed and developed criteria and recommendations addressing the needs of worker housing. This recommendation urged that Section 8 HUD funds for housing be available to migrant farm workers.

- *Appropriations and reauthorization.* The council recommended an annual appropriation of $100 million for the Migrant Health program and perinatal services. Current funding provides for only 12% to 15% of those who are eligible use the migrant program services.
- *Mental health.* The council urged full integration of mental health services into migrant health programs. Note: 1994 recommendations urged that $5 million in funding for mental health services be allocated.
- *Family issues.* The council recommended that all special projects take into consideration the farm worker family. Specific issues revolve around adequate schooling for children, lack of prenatal care for women, domestic violence, child abuse, and day-care needs. Note: As a result of this recommendation, there has been an interagency Memorandum of Agreement between the Migrant Health Program and the Migrant Head Start Program to allow interaction when planning direct service delivery.
- *Health reform.* The council urged that all migrant farm workers and their families, regardless of immigration status, should be serviced by any reform. Benefits would be portable, and there would be state-by-state reciprocity for Medicaid. Note: Additional information published in a 1998 update to the recommendations stated a reinforced need for portable benefits, no limitations on out-of-area coverage in that this may directly limit benefits to the highly migratory migrant farm worker, a definition of employer that could be used by the migrant farm worker, and mandatory coverage for the undocumented worker (USDHHS, 1994).
- *Outreach.* The council recommended increased resources for outreach programs and urged that all new federal initiatives include a migrant component and a special allocation for this population.
- *Occupational and environmental health.* The council recommended the establishment of an interagency group with the Department of Labor, OSHA, and the Social Security Administration to address the enforcement of regulations and laws protecting the farm workers' health and safety. (Note: full implementation of the Environmental Protection Agency's Worker Protection Standards was instituted on Jan. 1, 1995.) These standards include (USDHHS, 1994):
  - A "right to know" section so that information on pesticides will be available to the farm worker
  - Strict rules on field reentry after pesticide use
  - Readily available decontamination facilities for the farm worker
- *Health professions.* The council recommended incentives to increase the recruitment and supply of health care workers, with emphasis on bicultural/bilingual providers.

- *Research.* The council recommended the accumulation of hard data on the population and basic health status indicators of migrant farm workers, with cooperative efforts from other state and federal agencies.
- *Oral health.* The council recommended the inclusion of oral health care into Section 329 of the Public Health Service Act, as well as oral health being listed as a Medicaid benefit (USDHHS, 1994).

 clinical application

Louisa is 17 years old and has spent most of her life as a migrant farmworker. Her family, her father and two other siblings, work most of the year traveling the East Coast of the United States picking crops in season. She is presently picking tobacco in the southeastern United States. One evening after finishing her work she asks to speak with Joan, the nurse, who is with the medical van parked outside the trailer camp where Louisa and her family live. She is most concerned about a rash on her hands, arms, and chest. Joan also notes that Louisa's eyes are red and she occasionally coughs. She asks Joan for something for her rash. She wants treatment quickly, so the rash will go away and she will be able to work without scratching. Louisa seems to be in a great hurry and says she does not want her father to know she stopped by the van because he would be angry. While waiting for the nurse practitioner, Joan, who speaks fluent Spanish, asks if Louisa has any other problems. Initially hesitant, Louisa says she wishes she should go to school on a regular basis. She is most concerned about her brother and sister, age 8 and 10, who work in the fields as well. She says they constantly cough and have been having breathing trouble, especially when her father smokes, the wind blows dust around their trailer, or when picking crops soon after pesticides have been sprayed.

A. Determine the additional information needed to complete an assessment of Louisa and her family. Recognizing the specific cultural concerns, how would you obtain this information?
B. List community resources that might be available for Louisa and her family.
C. Discuss potential barriers that may prevent access to health care and other services.

Answers are in the back of the book.

KEY POINTS

- A migrant farm worker is a laborer whose principal employment involves moving from farm to farm planting or harvesting agricultural products and attaining temporary housing.

KEY POINTS—Cont'd

- An estimated 3 to 5 million migrant farm workers are in the United States. These numbers are controversial because of the inconsistency in defining farm workers and limitations in obtaining data.
- The life expectancy of the migrant farm worker is 49 years, compared with 75 years for other U.S. residents.
- Health problems of migrant farm workers are linked to their work environment, limited access to health services and education, and lack of economic opportunities.
- Migrant farm workers are faced with questionable farmer payment practices, inadequate record keeping, below–minimum wage standards, and lack of enforcement regarding legislation for field sanitation and safety regulations.
- Farm workers are exposed not only to the immediate effects in the fields (foggy or wet with pesticides), but also to unknown long-term effects of chronic exposure to pesticides.
- When harvesting is completed, the farm worker becomes simultaneously homeless and unemployed. Forced migration to find employment leaves little time or energy to seek out and improve living standards.
- Hispanic women are subject to oppression through both expectations of their own families and communities and policy decisions that work against them.
- Children of migrant farm workers may need to work for the family's economic survival.

critical thinking activities

1. Interview health care workers such as nurses, physicians, dentists, mental health providers, social workers, and registered dietitians and determine their definition of migrant farm worker. Ask them to describe their experiences working with migrant farm workers. Compare and contrast their definitions and experiences.
2. Interview community leaders to determine the presence of migrant farm workers in your area. Compare and contrast information about migrant farm workers by interviewing teachers, clergy, and politicians versus migrant outreach workers, Wage and Hour personnel, Department of Labor personnel, and Migrant Head Start program employees.
3. In some areas of the United States, placement agencies specialize in helping businesses hire migrant workers. Determine whether an agency of this type exists in your area. If yes, interview a key person and ask questions that would enable you to access such things as: how they recruit workers; how long workers typically stay in one location; what health screening they do? Who provides health services to the workers they place?
4. Determine eligibility for Medicaid and Aid to Families with Dependent Children services. You may consult the county health department and the state office. Do migrant workers in your state qualify?
5. Design a clinic to provide health care to migrant workers in your area. What services would you provide? What hours would you operate? How would you staff the clinic?

Bibliography

Adam V: Health status of vulnerable populations, *Ann Public Health* 15:487, 1994.

Asch S, Leake B, Gerberg L: Does fear of immigration authorities deter tuberculosis patients from seeking care? *West J Med* 161(4):373, 1994.

Bishop M, Harrison M: *Farm labor camp outreach project: a step toward meeting the health care needs of the Hispanic farm worker in Oregon.* Unpublished report, 1987.

Cassetta R: Needs of migrant health workers challenge RNs, *Am Nurse* 6(6):34, 1994.

Caudle P: Providing culturally sensitive health care to Hispanic clients, *Nurse Pract* 18(12):40, 1993.

Ciesiclski S, Hall SP, Sweeney M: Occupational health injuries among North Carolina migrant farm workers, *Am J Public Health* 81(7):926, 1991.

Crawford LH: *Linkages between the health care system and Mexican-American migrant farm workers.* Unpublished doctoral dissertation, Atlanta, 1994, Georgia State University.

de la Rosa M: Health care needs of Hispanic Americans and the responsiveness of the health care system, *Health Soc Work* 14:105, 1989.

Decker S, Knight L: Functional health assessment: a seasonal migrant farm worker community, *J Community Health Nurs* 7(3):141, 1990.

Duggar B: *Access of migrant and seasonal farm workers to Medicaid covered health care services.* Unpublished paper, 1990.

Galarneau C, editor: *Under the weather: farm worker health,* Austin, Texas, 1993, National Advisory Council on Migrant Health, Bureau of Primary Health Care, USDHHS.

Helsinki Commission: *Migrant farm workers in the United States: briefings of the Commission on Security and Cooperation in Europe,* Washington, DC, 1993, US Government Printing Office.

Johnsrud P et al: *Migrant outreach van evaluation,* Oregon Health Sciences University, School of Nursing, Unpublished masters thesis, 1997.

Larson K, Watkins E: *Migrant and lay health programs: their role and impact,* Chapel Hill, NC, 1990, University of North Carolina at Chapel Hill Press.

Marin B: AIDS prevention for non Puerto Rican Hispanics. In Leukefeld C, Batjes R, Amsel Z, editors: *AIDS and intravenous drug use: community interventions and prevention,* New York, 1990, Hemisphere.

Medicaid and migrant farm worker families: analysis of barriers and recommendations for change, Washington, DC, 1991, National Association of Community Health Centers.

Mines R, Gabbard S, Steinman A: *A profile of U.S. farm workers, demographics, household composition, income and use of services,* U.S. Department of Labor, Office of the Assistant Secretary for Policy, Commission on Immigration Reform, April, 1997.

Mobed IK, Gold E, Schenker M: Occupational health problems among migrant and seasonal farmworkers, *West J Med* 157(3):367, 1992.

National Agricultural Worker's Survey, 1997, US Department of Labor, Office of the Assistant Secretary for Policy.

National Farmworker Health Conference, National Advisory Council on Migrant Health. May 13-17, 1998, Houston, Tex.

National Housing Law Project, US Department of Labor, Office of the Assistant Secretary for Policy: Washington, DC, 1996, US Government Printing Office.

National Migrant Resource Program: *Migrant and seasonal farm worker health objectives for the year 2000,* Austin, Tex, 1990, Author.

Smith LS: Ethnic differences in knowledge of sexually transmitted diseases in North American blacks and Mexican American migrant farm workers, *Res Nurs Health* 11:51, 1988.

US Department of Health and Human Services: *1993 recommendations of the National Advisory Council on Migrant Health,* Austin, Texas, 1993, National Advisory Council on Migrant Health, National Migrant Resource Program.

US Department of Health and Human Services: *1994 update to the recommendations of the National Advisory Council on Migrant Health,* Austin, Texas, 1994, National Advisory Council on Migrant Health, National Migrant Resource Program.

US Department of Health and Human Services: *1998 update to the recommendations of the National Advisory Council on Migrant Health,* Austin, Texas, 1998. National Migrant Resource Program.

US Department of Health and Human Services: *Healthy People 2000: national health promotion and disease prevention objectives,* Washington, DC, 1991, USDHHS, Public Health Service.

Watkins E, Larson K: *Migrant lay health advisors: a strategy for health promotion, a final report,* Chapel Hill, NC, 1991, University of North Carolina at Chapel Hill.

Mental Health Issues

PATRICIA B. HOWARD

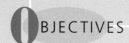BJECTIVES

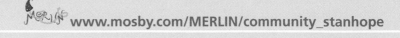www.mosby.com/MERLIN/community_stanhope

After reading this chapter, the student should be able to do the following:

- Describe the history of community mental health and make predictions about the future.
- Discuss essential mental health services and corresponding national objectives for healthier people.
- Analyze the status of the population who have mental illness in the United States.
- Evaluate standards, models, concepts, and research findings for use in community mental health nursing practice.

- Describe the role of the community mental health nurse with people and groups at risk for psychiatric mental health problems.
- Apply the nursing process in community work with clients diagnosed with psychiatric disorders, families at risk for mental health problems, and populations at risk.
- Examine ways to improve the mental health of people who are at risk in a complex society.

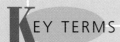EY TERMS

Americans with Disabilities Act (ADA)
community mental health
community mental health centers (CMHCs)

Community Support Program (CSP)
consumer
consumer advocacy
deinstitutionalization
institutionalization

mental health problems
National Alliance for the Mentally Ill (NAMI)
National Institute of Mental Health (NIMH)
pharmacokinetics

relapse management
severe mental disorders
systems theory

See Glossary for definitions

CHAPTER OUTLINE

Providing adequate care to mentally ill people is complex and influenced by many individual and community factors. Some of these factors are 1) the scope and chronicity of mental illness, 2) the uncertainty about specific cause, cure, and treatment for most severe mental disorders, and 3) the severe disabling nature of some mental disorders. Limited resources compound the problems and present challenges in community mental health work.

Cultural beliefs and economics influence the amount and types of services and treatment available in countries. However, two universal truths exist: services for people with mental disorders are inadequate in all countries, and the impact of mental illness on families, communities, and nations is profound. Therefore specialized knowledge and skills about severe mental illness and mental health problems are necessary for effective community and public health nursing practice. It is helpful to understand both the organization of mental health services from a historical perspective and trends in current health care demands and delivery. Knowledge about populations at risk for psychiatric mental health problems and understanding illness outcomes in terms of biopsychosocial consequences are even more important. Finally, it is necessary to refine and broaden nursing process skills in treatment planning to include the impact of mental illness on families and the community.

This chapter focuses on the development of community mental health services, current health objectives for mental health and mental disorders, and the role of the nurse in community settings. Frameworks and concepts useful in community mental health nursing practice are also presented. Because other chapters in this book are devoted to high-risk groups such as the homeless population and those with substance abuse problems, this chapter focuses on populations who have long-term, severe mental disorders and groups who are vulnerable to mental health problems. **Severe mental disorders** are determined by diagnosis and criteria that include degree of functional disability (APA, 1994). **Mental health problems** are difficulties related to an individual's inability to negotiate the daily challenges of life without experiencing undue social isolation, emotional distress, or behavioral incapacity (USDHHS, 1991).

STATUS OF THE MENTALLY ILL IN THE UNITED STATES

Persons with mental illness have numerous problems. Many lack access to adequate health services and others have inadequate housing. Even so, advances have been made in the treatment of mental illness. These advances have been influenced by two major movements: consumer advocacy, and better understanding of the neurobiology of mental illness (Center for Mental Health Services [CMHS], 1996; Keltner et al, 1998; Levin and Petrila, 1996). A third movement, managed care, has influenced

changes in the treatment of the mentally ill, and it is unclear whether these changes will be positive or negative.

Consumer Advocacy

Similar to other advocacy movements, those for people with mental illness came about to fulfill unmet needs. Specifically, the **National Alliance for the Mentally Ill (NAMI)** was the first group to advocate for better services. This **consumer advocacy** group worked to establish education and self-help services for individuals and families with mental illness (Lefley, 1996). Efforts of NAMI gained momentum in the early 1980s. Subsequently, political groups and legislative bodies responded with direct support. One example of direct support was funding for the **Community Support Program (CSP)** by the **National Institute of Mental Health (NIMH)**. The CSP provides grant monies to states to develop comprehensive services for persons discharged from psychiatric institutions (Lefley, 1996). These and similar efforts have helped bring consumers, families, and professionals together to work toward improvement in the treatment and care of persons with mental illness.

Neurobiology of Mental Illness

Although the brain-mind-soul continuum remains unclear (Keltner et al, 1998), more is now known about the neuroanatomic functions of the brain than at any time in history. For example, neuroradiology techniques aid diagnosis and treatment of people with psychiatric disorders. Also, angiography is used to screen for abnormalities of the vascular system like atherosclerosis or brain tumors that can result in behavior changes. Diagnosis is also improved by using non-invasive scanning of the brain. For example, computed axial tomography (CAT) scans provide a cross-sectional view of the brain, whereas nuclear magnetic resonance (NMR) offers the advantage of imaging the brain from different planes. Still other techniques like positron emission tomography (PET) and single photon emission computed tomography (SPECT) provide information about cerebral blood flow and brain metabolism. Information like this can lead to better understanding about illnesses like dementia.

Discoveries in psychopharmacology have also revolutionized treatment of mental illness (Fawcett and Barkin, 1998; Honigfeld et al, 1998; Keltner and Folks, 1997). The new atypical antipsychotic drugs used in the treatment of schizophrenia have led to improved quality of life for many. Moreover, there is less risk for side effects with these new medications. Additionally, selective serotonin reuptake inhibitors (SSRI) are considered the first choice in the treatment of depression because they lead to good responses with fewer side effects.

Managed Care

Managed care is "the practice of making informed judgments of what patients need, and then managing the treatment to insure that patients get necessary and appropriate care" (CMHS, 1996, p. 3). Managed mental health care is growing rapidly yet, despite its size and importance, little is known about it. Indeed, information from evaluation research in managed care systems about consumer outcomes like health status, quality of life, functioning, and satisfaction will not be readily available until after the year 2000 (Leff and Woocher, 1998). Since one purpose of managed care is to control costs, oftentimes by substituting less costly services for more costly ones (CMHS, 1996), the findings about consumer outcomes are critical. For example, community care is less costly than hospital care. However, the services must fit the needs of the consumer, and research can help guide care decisions about the fit. Currently, many changes are taking place in the managed care arena. These changes present challenges for nurses who need to make judgments about the positive and negative outcomes of these changes on the people they care for even before research findings that can be generalized to the population are readily available.

EVOLUTION OF COMMUNITY MENTAL HEALTH CARE

In the United States today, **community mental health** is the primary model of care for people with mental illness. Components of the model include team care, case management, outreach, and prevention. In most states the model is implemented through comprehensive **community mental health centers (CMHCs),** yet neither the model and its components nor the CMHCs are refined processes and systems of care. Rather, the model continues to evolve in this era of health care reform as the CMHCs react to societal, political, and fiscal pressures.

The community mental health model of care is also used in many other western countries, and the trend is evolving in many eastern countries. For example in Korea, Kim (1998) is developing a community-based program where psychiatric nursing care is given to people with long-term psychiatric problems. In Hong Kong—a major financial and trade city—mental health services were largely based in hospitals until the early 1990s; now community mental health nurses provide care in day and residential centers (Pang et al, 1997; Yip, 1998). Historically, both in the United States and abroad, reform movements influenced the development of mental health services and models of care whether they were located in hospital or community settings.

Historical Perspectives

Before the eighteenth century, treatment of people with mental disorders was based on superstitions or beliefs that mentally ill people were possessed by demons, and both cause and cure were attributed to witches and magicians. Near the end of the eighteenth century, in a movement influenced by Philippe Pinel (1759 to 1820) in France and Benjamin Rush (1745 to 1813) in America, the revolution

in mental health care known as humanitarian reform took place (Donahue, 1985; Taylor, 1994). Humanitarian reform led to hospital expansion and the community mental health movements.

Humanitarian reform

Before the humanitarian reform movement, persons with mental illness were often housed in jails because health and social services had not been developed. Even after the development of hospitals as a site of treatment following the reform movement, persons with mental disorders were neglected and mistreated. For example, the first psychiatric hospital in the United States was built in Williamsburg, Virginia in 1773, but approximately 50 years passed before widespread construction of facilities in other states took place (Taylor, 1994; Worley, 1997). One person in particular, Dorothea Dix, led reform efforts to correct types of practices that were inhumane (Worley, 1997).

Dorothea Lynde Dix (1802 to 1887) focused attention on three populations: criminals, those with mental disorders, and victims of the Civil War (Donahue, 1985; Worley, 1997). She said that people with mental disorders needed health and social services, and her efforts resulted in improved organization of mental health services. Moreover, her work led to the development of hospitals as the primary site of care where she influenced standards for hospital administration and nursing care. Because of her lifetime efforts, often through political action, treatment for mentally infirm persons was altered on both the North American and European continents.

Hospital expansion, institutionalization, and the mental hygiene movement

Psychiatric hospitals constructed during the expansion era were located in rural areas. They were intended for small numbers of clients. However, they soon became overcrowded with people who had severe mental disorders, the elderly, and immigrants who were poor and unable to speak English (Donahue, 1985; Taylor, 1994; Worley, 1997). Similar conditions for the same era have been reported about treatment in other countries (Yip, 1998). Clients were essentially separated from the community and isolated from their families. Many were institutionalized for the rest of their lives, largely in response to a continued fear of persons with mental disorders. **Institutionalization** of large numbers of people, combined with minimal information about cause, cure, and care, resulted in overcrowded conditions and exploitation of clients.

At the turn of the twentieth century, institutional conditions were reported publicly in the United States by Clifford Beers, who knew about psychiatric hospital treatment from personal experiences (Lefley, 1996). Beers urged reform and influenced the founding of the National Committee for Mental Hygiene. During the mental hygiene movement, attention shifted to ideas about prevention, early intervention, and the influence of social and environmental factors on mental illness. These ideas about treatment also influenced the development of multidisciplinary approaches to treatment. The mental hygiene and community mental health movements increased understanding about mental illness. Understanding about the scope of mental illness became even more evident during World War II during the conscription process for the armed services.

Many of the persons screened for military service during World War II were found to have neurological and psychiatric mental health disorders. Even more military personnel required treatment for mental health problems associated with social and environmental stress during and after the war, not only in the United States but also in Europe, Russia, and Pacific Rim countries (Grob, 1991; Yip, 1998). At the same time the community mental health model continued to expand slowly while populations consisting of individuals with severe mental disorders and elderly persons with dementia grew larger in the state hospitals. Demands for mental health services in communities, combined with concerns about conditions of state psychiatric hospitals, prompted federal legislation that influenced development of the community mental health concept.

Federal Legislation for Mental Health Services

The first major piece of legislation to influence mental health services in the United States was the Social Security Act in 1935. The Social Security Act, in response to economic and social problems of the era, shifted the responsibility of care for ill people from the state to the federal government. The federal government's role expanded when the demand for mental health services increased during World War II. Key points of legislation that influenced the development of community mental health services are summarized in Table 35-1.

In 1946, the National Mental Health Act was passed and the NIMH administered its programs (Taylor, 1994; Worley, 1997). Objectives included development of education and research programs for community mental health treatment approaches. The Act also included financial incentives for training grants to increase the number of professional workers, including nurses, in mental health services. Education and research programs materialized readily, along with advances in science and technology and the development of psychotropic medications (Keltner and Folks, 1997; Worley, 1997).

In 1955 the Mental Health Study Act was passed and the Joint Commission on Mental Illness and Health was established by the NIMH (Taylor, 1994). Members of the commission studied national mental health needs and submitted a report entitled Action for Mental Health to Congress. Recommendations of the report included continued development of research and education programs, early and intensive treatment for acute mental illness, and shifting the care of severely mentally ill persons away from the large hospitals to psychiatric wards in general hospitals and to community mental health clinics. Community services were to include aftercare services after hospitalization for individuals with major mental illness (Grob, 1991). The shift in the locus of care from state hospitals to community systems was begun.

The Community Mental Health Centers Act (CMHC) was passed in 1963, and the CMHC concept was formalized. Federal funds were designated to match state funds to construct CMHCs and start programs. CMHCs offered short-term and partial hospitalization, aftercare, emergency services, outpatient treatment, rehabilitation, and vocational counseling. However, many CMHCs, especially

TABLE 35-1 Legislation That Influenced Community Mental Health Services

YEAR	LEGISLATION	FOCUS
1955	Mental Health Study Act	Resulted in Joint Commission on Mental Illness and Health that recommended transformation of state hospital systems and establishment of community mental health clinics
1963	Community Mental Health Centers Act	Marked beginning of community mental health centers concept and led to deinstitutionalization of large psychiatric hospitals
1975	Developmental Disabilities Act	Addressed the rights and treatment of people with developmental disabilities and provided foundation for similar action for individuals with mental disorders
1977	President's Commission on Mental Health	Reinforced importance of community-based services, protection of human rights, and national health insurance for mentally ill persons
1978	Omnibus Reconciliation Act	Rescinded much of the 1977 commission's provisions and shifted funds for all health programs from federal to state governments
1986	Protection and Advocacy for Mentally Ill Individuals Act	Legislated advocacy programs for mentally ill persons
1990	Americans with Disabilities Act	Prohibited discrimination and promoted employment opportunities for persons with disabilities, including mental disorders

those in poor and rural areas, were unable to generate adequate money for continuing their start-up programs. The deinstitutionalization of persons with severe mental disorders was well underway before some of these shortcomings were recognized.

Deinstitutionalization

Deinstitutionalization involved moving large numbers of people out of the state psychiatric hospitals. The cost of institutional care was perhaps the main reason for the movement; other influences included discovery of psychotropic medications and civil rights activism (Grob, 1991; Keltner and Folks, 1997; Worley, 1997). The goal of deinstitutionalization was to improve the quality of life for people with mental disorders by providing services in the communities where they lived rather than in large institutions. To change the locus of care, large hospital wards were closed and persons with severe mental disorders were returned to the community to live. Many were discharged to the care of family members; others went to nursing homes. Still others were placed in apartments or other types of adult housing; some of these were supervised settings, and others were not.

Not surprisingly, as with any abrupt, dramatic change, problems related to unexpected service gaps between the hospitals and CMHCs led to continuity-of-care problems. For example, although families were not prepared for the treatment responsibilities they had to assume, few mental health systems offered them education and support programs. Also, although many elderly clients were admitted to nursing homes and personal care settings, education programs were seldom available for staff, who often lacked the skills necessary to treat persons with mental disorders. And finally, some clients found themselves in independent settings such as rooming houses and single-room occupancy hotels with little or no supervision. Clients, families, communities, and the nation suffered as poor living and social conditions were associated with mental disorders (Grob, 1991). These types of issues prompted additional legislation and advocacy efforts.

Civil rights legislation for persons with mental disorders

The development of CMHCs was based on the principle that persons with mental disorders had a right to treatment in the least restrictive environment (Perlin, 1994). Although CMHCs did prove less restrictive than institutions, they lacked necessary services. For example, people with severe mental disorders require daily monitoring or hospitalization during acute episodes of illness. Even though hospital services were available, many individuals expressed their rights to refuse treatment and resisted admission. Also, transitional care following discharge for those persons who were admitted to hospitals was not available in most communities (Grob, 1991). In addition to the right to refuse treatment, advocates for mentally ill individuals focused on such civil rights issues as segregated services, inhumane practices in psychiatric hospitals, and

failure to include clients in treatment planning. Activism for minorities and handicapped persons also influenced civil rights legislation for persons with mental disorders. In particular, during the 1970s institutional conditions of persons with developmental handicaps prompted the Developmental Disabilities Assistance Act and Bill of Rights Act (Wasserbauer, 1996). Other legislation shifted funding from the federal to the state level.

State systems of mental health services developed in diverse ways and were often inadequate. In general, individuals with severe mental disorders were vulnerable and neglected and either lacked or were unable to access health and social services. In an effort to offset these problems, in 1986 the federal Protection and Advocacy for Mentally Ill Individuals Act was legislated. Advocacy programs for mentally ill persons became part of the same state advocacy systems developed earlier under the Developmental Disability Act (Wilk, 1993). In spite of advocacy efforts and legislation, the CMHCs were unable to meet the increased and diverse demands for mental health services in their communities. The lack of services combined with concerns about discrimination against all people with disabilities led to additional legislation.

Americans with Disabilities Act of 1990

In 1990 the **Americans with Disabilities Act (ADA)** was passed. The ADA mandated that individuals with mental and physical disabilities be brought into the mainstream of American life (Perlin, 1994; Wasserbauer, 1996). To promote the mainstreaming process, the ADA addressed three major issues: (1) employment; (2) public services, programs, and activities; and (3) public accommodations (Brazelon Center for Mental Health Law, 1994; Perlin, 1994). For example, the ADA seeks to end discrimination against persons with mental impairment or other disabilities in areas of employment, including job application, hiring, advancement, and discharge practices. Also, the ADA mandates that state and local governments administer services in ways that are integrated and applicable for specific populations, including persons with psychiatric mental health disorders. Violations of the ADA are considered similar to violations of the Equal Protection Clause of the Constitution (Perlin, 1994).

DID YOU KNOW? *The Americans with Disabilities Act (ADA) of 1990 prohibits employment discrimination against people with mental disabilities. Since the ADA went into effect, many persons with mental disorders have filed discrimination charges. Employers need assistance in understanding functional limitations commonly associated with mental disorders. Limitations include difficulty concentrating and dealing with stress.*

Even so, implementing the law may not be a smooth process (Wilk, 1993), and many health care providers, including nurses (Wasserbauer, 1996), do not know about provisions of the ADA. History reveals that past legislation promoted the rights of persons with mental disorders, but litigation was also responsible for the lack of growth, if not decline, in community mental health services (Perlin, 1994; Wilk, 1993). The community mental health nurse can advocate for clients to ensure equality in access to health services, housing, and employment.

Advocacy efforts

In this discussion the **consumer** refers to persons who are current or former recipients of mental health services. As in all areas of health care, the rights and wishes of consumers are important in planning and delivering services. However, consumers of mental health services have traditionally had difficulty advocating for themselves. For example, in the past, treatment programs fostered passivity in clients and excluded them from the treatment planning process. In addition, family members were responsible for

---

BOX 35-1 Advocacy and Self-Help Organizations

- Community Support Program (CSP): A program of the U.S. Department of Health and Human Services (USDHHS), Substance Abuse and Mental Health Administration (SAMSHA), Center for Mental Health Services (CMHS), that developed plans for a model continuum of care, offers grants for demonstration programs including community rehabilitation projects, and provided money to states for development of consumer and family services and advocacy efforts.
- Consumer/Survivor Mental Health Research and Policy Work Group: An endeavor sponsored by the Mental Health Statistics Improvement Program of the CMHS to initiate consumer representation in activities of the National Association of State Mental Health Program Directors (NASMHPD).
- Judge David L. Bazelon Center for Mental Health Law Project (MHL): An organization of attorneys and mental health professionals who advocate for consumers on legal and policy matters.
- National Alliance for the Mentally Ill (NAMI): A family organization that promotes family support groups, education programs, public campaigns to reduce stigma, and advocacy for mental health policy and services at local and national levels.
- NAMI Consumers Council: A consumer advocacy group that advocates for improved and effective psychiatric services and consumer empowerment.
- National Association of Psychiatric Survivors (NAPS): A consumer organization that advocates for such things as involuntary treatment and some forms of treatment like electroconvulsive therapy.
- National Mental Health Association (NMHA): An organization aimed at improving mental health in the population at large emphasizing prevention.
- National Mental Health Consumers' Association (NMHCA): A consumer organization that advocates for improvements in the mental health system.

See this book's website at *~~* www.mosby.com/MERLIN for more information about these organizations.

---

care in the home, but they lacked resources and even information about treatment (Lefley, 1996). Like consumers, family members suffered from the stigma of mental illness and public attitudes that contributed to self-advocacy problems. In contrast, self-advocacy and involvement in treatment planning foster self-confidence, promote participation in service, and may influence policy decisions. Consumer and family groups foster these objectives.

Family members led self-advocacy efforts in the 1970s when small groups organized to challenge and change mental health services. These early efforts resulted in the formation of the National Alliance for the Mentally Ill (NAMI), which today has both state and local affiliates. Soon, consumer groups formed to advocate for better services, changes in mental health policy, self-help programs in treatment, and empowerment. Several advocacy groups that support these consumer efforts are summarized in Box 35-1. In their assessment of resources, nurses can identify community advocacy and support groups.

CURRENT AND FUTURE PERSPECTIVES IN MENTAL HEALTH CARE

Agreement is widespread that health care services are lacking both nationally and internationally. In the United States, large segments of the population do not have basic health care services or insurance to cover both expected and unexpected illnesses (ANA, 1991; CMHS, 1996; Feingold, 1994; Navarro, 1994). Also, consumers, family members, and health care providers are concerned about issues of basic treatment, continuity of care, housing, and costs for acute and long-term mental health services (CMHS, 1996; Krauss, 1993, 1994; Leff and Woocher, 1998; Worley, 1997). Therefore health care reform is currently a major political, social, and economic issue.

If changes occur, they will take time because they will involve alterations in the current health care delivery system. In the meantime, nurses working in communities must understand the model of care called managed care, the scope of mental illness, and the national health objectives designed to promote the health and welfare of persons with mental health problems.

Era of Managed Care

Managed care is an approach to the delivery of health services that emphasizes cost control and appropriate utilization of services to offset more costly treatments (CMHS, 1996; Leff and Woocher, 1998; Manderscheid and Henderson, 1995). Managed care seeks to reduce hospital stays and increase community care, since care tends to cost more in hospitals than in community settings. Nurses conduct comprehensive client histories to determine health problems and interventions that improve quality of care and cost effectiveness. In home health settings, nurses screen for ineffective coping techniques such as use of alcohol or other substances to offset the stress of traumatic life events, thereby preventing further problems and costly care. They also screen for signs of psychiatric disorders in primary care and community health care settings. These types of nursing assessments and subsequent interventions may offset costly treatment in hospital settings.

: DID YOU KNOW? *Managed cared programs tend to reduce coverage for inpatient hospital stays for mental illness. However, community survival for people with serious mental illness requires a broad range of well-coordinated services including mental and physical health, housing assistance, substance abuse treatment for some, and social and vocational rehabilitation.*

Providing the range of community services necessary for persistent mental illness is difficult without sufficient funds for health and social services (CMHS, 1996). Clearly, managed care has changed the mental health field and more changes are anticipated. Nurses need to be informed about changes in the health care system and how these changes affect persons with mental illness. Such information enables nurses to advocate for adequate services to meet the needs of individuals with severe and persistent mental illness. The services must include access to mental health services in work and school settings.

National Objectives for Mental Health Services

Goals of the community mental health movement are consistent with health promotion and disease prevention objectives outlined in *Healthy People 2000* and those forthcoming in *Healthy People 2010* (USDHHS, 1991). These objectives emphasize the importance of personal responsibility in developing patterns of healthy living. They also address health issues of vulnerable populations, including people with mental disorders. Table 35-2 gives target populations and problems. Objectives focus on all age groups, identify specific target populations, and highlight the grave nature of problems associated with mental illness.

Model standards for implementing national objectives

Useful guidelines for implementing *Healthy People 2000* objectives are available in *Healthy Communities 2000: Model Standards* (APHA, 1991). The standards cover the priority areas and populations identified in the *Healthy People 2000* objectives, and they are recommended for use in determining needs at state and community levels. Overall, the goal for mental health and mental disorders emphasizes prevention, maintenance, or restoration of mental health and independent functioning. Another goal is to decrease disparities in health among population segments, including those listed in Table 35-2. However, as previously mentioned, individuals with mental health problems have historically lacked adequate services and frequently lack accessible services today. Also, preventive mental health programs are essentially nonexistent today (Krauss, 1993), although they were recommended as early as the mental hygiene movement. The model standards can be used to slow or reverse these trends. For example, nurses can (1) promote use of the standards in the agencies where they are employed, (2) use the standards in community assessment activities, and (3) introduce information about the

TABLE 35-2 Problems and Populations Targeted in National Health Objectives for Mental Health

PROBLEM	TARGET POPULATION
Persistent mental disorders	Children Adolescents Adults
Adverse health effects from stress	Adults
Injurious suicide attempts	Adolescents
Suicide	Adolescents Adult and elderly men Native Americans and Alaska natives in reservation states
Maltreatment	Children and youth age 18 yr and younger
Assault injuries	Children age 12 yr and older Adults
Physical abuse	Women
Rape and attempted rape	Women and adolescents age 12 yr and older
Homicide	Children age 3 yr and younger Spouses African-American men and women Hispanic-American men Native Americans and Alaska natives in reservation states

Modified from USDHHS: *Healthy People 2000: national health promotion and disease prevention objectives*, Washington, DC, 1991, USDHHS, Public Health Service.

standards to other groups and agencies, including local consumer and family organizations. Other ways to use the standards with specific populations are included in the discussion about the scope of mental illness.

Scope of Mental Illness

Mental illness is prevalent in all segments of societies. For discussion, the scope of mental illness may be broken into two useful classifications: severe mental disorders and mental health problems.

Severe mental disorders

Severe mental disorders strike at the human qualities of thought and behavior. Because of limitations in existing databases, it is difficult to explain prevalence rates of mental illness. However, reports available from the CMHS (1996) indicate there are at least 10 million people age 18 years or older in the United States with severe mental illness. The estimated prevalence rate of serious emotional disturbance in children age 9 to 17 years is 9% to 13%; prevalence rates for children less than 9 years cannot be estimated because of inadequate databases (CMHS, 1996). Severe mental disorders are persistent, disabling, and affect persons of all ages, races, and socioeconomic levels. Severe mental illness in adults is more common among women, those with less than $20,000 family income, and those with less than a college education. Severe mental illnesses include mood disorders and depression, anxiety and phobic disorders, antisocial personality disorders, schizophrenia and schizoaffective disorders, and organic brain syndrome. Although these conditions are often defined in terms of serious disability and long-term duration, treatment emphasizes care in the least restrictive setting and mainstreaming individuals into community life.

Many adults with severe mental illness seek treatment in the general medical sector, including primary care settings and emergency rooms. Children living in poverty are an especially vulnerable population. Schools, social service agencies, and the juvenile justice system are common sites for mental health services for this age group (CMHS, 1996).

At present, many people with severe mental disorders live in poverty because they lack the ability to earn or maintain a suitable standard of living. For example, as many as one third to one half of the homeless population, which averages 600,000 persons daily, are affected with a severe mental disorder (NIMH, 1991; Krauss, 1993). Thus nursing care can be provided in shelters, soup kitchens, and other places where people seek food and protection. For example, depression affects more than 11 million people in the United States, many of whom are homeless (Isaacs, 1998). Specific assessment skills with depressed people include empathy and adequate time to establish a therapeutic relationship. Nursing interventions include 1) referral to a community based agency that provides shelters, if indicated; 2) counseling, and 3) referral for antidepressant therapy.

Even those persons who live with family caregivers or who are in supervised housing are at risk for inadequate services since the long-term care they require frequently depletes human and fiscal resources. Indeed, even caregivers may be at risk for mental health problems (Biegel et al, 1991; Howard, 1994, 1998). In addition to counseling, supportive listening, and stress management education, the nurse can refer family caregivers to the local Alliance for the Mentally Ill for group support services. Other important community resources include crisis intervention services, intensive care services for those who are a danger to themselves or others, rehabilitation services, and follow-up or continuing care in clinics and home settings (APHA, 1991). In addition to local crisis and mental health service centers, there are national organizations designed for groups with specific problems. Box 35-2 lists examples. Many of these organizations have local chapters or information can be accessed from the Internet.

Mental health problems of high-risk populations

As indicated in the definitions at the beginning of this chapter, mental health is a dynamic process that enables and promotes the individual's physical, cognitive, affective, and social functioning. In contrast, threats to mental health create stress that undermines functional, interpersonal, and intrapersonal interactions and diminishes the individual's ability to pursue and achieve life's goals. Both internal and external factors influence an individual's mental health status. Internal factors include the biopsychosocial makeup or personality characteristics of the individual. External factors involve socioenvironmental forces, including the values, beliefs, and material assets of communities. Values and beliefs influence the allocation of resources for neighborhoods and schools and can contribute to or undermine the mental health of people in communities.

BOX 35-2 Examples of Sources of Information and Help for People with Mental Illness and Mental Health Problems

Alcoholics Anonymous
Al-Anon
American Anorexia/Bulimia Association
American Association of Suicidology
Anxiety Disorders Association of America
Attention Deficit Information Network
Children and Adults with Attention Deficit Disorder
Depressive/Manic Depressive Association
Gamblers Anonymous
National Center for Post-Traumatic Stress Disorder
National Center for Learning Disabilities
Obsessive-Compulsive Foundation, Inc.
Overeaters Anonymous
Schizophrenics Anonymous

See this book's website at www.mosby.com/MERLIN for more information about these organizations.

Mental health problems are manifested in many ways. Untoward incidents or even anticipated life events can diminish physical, cognitive, affective, and social functioning. For example, in most situations, either anticipated or unexpected death of a family member results in grief that may temporarily interrupt functional activities of surviving family members. Loss of appetite, sadness, difficulty making decisions, and disturbed sleep patterns are common during bereavement. Given adequate support and adaptation, most persons resume their lifestyles following the death of a loved one in spite of the sadness that they are likely to experience. When people do not have adequate resources, or when bereavement is complicated because of the conditions of the situation, there is an increased risk for threats to the mental health of surviving family members. Some may experience chronic sorrow that may be a normal response to loss (Eakes, Burke, and Hainsworth, 1998). Important interventions with individuals experiencing sorrow and grief are to encourage roles and activities that promote comfort and reduce isolation. For example, cause of death and age of survivors are two conditions that place people at risk during this particular life event. When the cause of death is suicide, family members may experience bereavement complications from reactions such as guilt or they may experience chronic sorrow. If the death is due to acquired immunodeficiency syndrome (AIDS), bereavement complications may be associated with a stigma that increases stress and slows adaptation of surviving family members. Death of a family member can affect survivors of different ages in various ways. Infants and youth may be deprived of significant nurturing and care that will result in long-term emotional deficits, whereas adults are at increased risk for stress related to role changes, and elderly persons are vulnerable to social isolation as relatives and friends die. In any of these situations, individual or group therapy may be indicated not only for the immediate situation but also for prevention of longer-term problems.

However, bereavement is not the only cause of diminished mental health. Other causes include but are not limited to physical health problems, disabilities resulting from trauma, exposure to violence in the neighborhood, job loss and unstable employment, and unanticipated environmental disasters that result in loss. Since multiple threats to mental health exist, it is useful to organize the study of problems according to risk. Populations are at risk at all ages along life's continuum.

Children and adolescents. Some children are at risk for acute or chronic mental health problems from neglect, and still others develop problems even in the presence of positive parenting. For example, risks during the prenatal period may be a result of exposure to maternal health deficits such as inadequate nutrition or poor physical health. Children may develop depression associated with loss following divorce even though both parents may provide nurturing and attention.

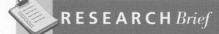

RESEARCH *Brief*

A critical review of research studies on the identification and treatment of children's mental health by primary care providers was conducted. The authors examined methods and findings of studies published on the topic from 1979 to 1994. They found that primary care providers underidentified mental health problems among children and adolescents unless impairments were severe. Based on study findings, these authors concluded that large numbers of children with mental health problems are not identified or are not treated. Recommendations include the importance of well-child care and continuity of care to promote recognition and treatment of child and adolescent mental health problems.

Richardson LA et al: Identification and treatment of children's mental health problems by primary care providers: a critical review of research, *Arch Psych Nurs* 10(5):293, 1996.

Types of mental health problems typically diagnosed during childhood are depression, anxiety, and attention deficit disorder. Examples of chronic disorders commonly seen are mental retardation, Down syndrome, and autism. Children are also at increased risk for acute and chronic mental health problems resulting from situations in their environment. Examples of environmental factors include crowded living conditions, violence, separation from parents, and lack of consistent caregivers. These problems affect growth and development and influence mental health during adolescence.

The incidence of suicide suggests that many problems during adolescence are so profound that these adolescents see no alternative but death. Studies reveal a steady increase in the number of suicides during adolescence (USDHHS, 1991). Among males between the ages of 15 and 19 years, it is the second leading cause of death (Krauss, 1993). Among adolescent girls, anxiety and phobia are not uncommon, and suicidal behavior, if not actual suicide, is associated with depression. Serious public health problems associated with violence in society and in families also take their toll on adolescents. Teenagers are among those who are most likely to be victims of homicide or experience mental health problems related to intrafamilial violence (USDHHS, 1991). Target populations for health and human service objectives related to reducing rape and attempted rape include female children 12 years and older, those pertaining to assault injuries include both males and females over 12 years of age, and those designed to interrupt the intergenerational cycle of abuse are directed at children of both genders regardless of age (USDHHS, 1991). Other common problems during adolescence include conduct disorders, eating disorders, and substance abuse. It is important for nurses to assess, intervene, and refer for all these conditions and risk factors in schools, day care centers, and other places where children and adolescents spend time. See the Research Brief about identification and treatment of mental health problems in children.

Children and adolescents require a variety of mental health services, including crisis intervention and both short- and long-term counseling. Nurses working in community settings, well-child clinics, and home health can help to offset this problem through prevention, education, and including parents in program planning. When conditions are identified, early intervention and continuity of care can promote optimal functioning and may offset chronic conditions. Since many children and adolescents lack services or access to them, community mental health assessment activities are essential. Assessment activities include identifying types of programs available or lacking in places where children and adolescents spend time. In addition to schools and homes of clients served in programs, assessment should be done in day-care centers, churches, and organizations that plan and guide age-specific play and entertainment programs. The model standards also emphasize access to preschool programs, school health education, and health promotion in postsecondary institutions to reduce the risk of mental health problems (APHA, 1991). Assessment data are essential for planning and developing programs that address mental health problems prevalent from the prenatal period through adolescence. Preventing problems during these developmental periods can reduce mental health problems in adulthood.

Adults. In addition to severe disorders such as major depression and schizophrenia, adults suffer from multiple sources of stress that contribute to their mental health status. Sources of stress include multiple role responsibilities, job insecurity, and unstable relationships. These and other conditions can undermine mental health and contribute to domestic violence and substance abuse in all populations regardless of income or culture. Other mental health problems during adulthood are caused by factors similar to those of childhood.

For example, environmental and intrafamilial violence threatens the lives of adults. As described in chapter 37, homicide, suicide, and domestic violence rates are high in the United States. Recent research suggests that domestic violence can lead to posttraumatic stress disorder (PTSD) and major depression among women (Breslaw et al, 1997). A study of Vietnam veterans with severe combat PTSD also revealed many subjects had been abused as children (Johnson, Rosenheck, Fontana et al, 1996). Other mental health problems of adults include eating disorders, panic disorder, and psychosocial problems related to AIDS and other medical conditions. These and other disabling conditions affect family members. See the Research Brief about caregiving for children with schizophrenia.

Most family caregivers are women who care for a spouse, aging parent, or child with a long-term disabling

RESEARCH *Brief*

Mothers and fathers were the subjects of these studies about caregiving for adult children with schizophrenia. In both studies, subjects were middle-age and older adults. Cross-sectional data in the form of in-depth interviews were based on naturalistic inquiry. Findings of the first study with maternal caregivers led to a description of the stages and concepts of lifelong learning about how to live with a child who had schizophrenia. Findings of the second study indicated that fathers too were engaged in a prolonged caregiving event. Three themes explained the extent to which these fathers engaged in caregiving: involvement in care, unresolved issues, and severity of the event.

Implications for nursing practice are as follows:
1. Home care services and transition programs from the hospital to community services are important for families with relatives who have severe mental disorders.
2. Interventions with families should include education, respite services, and stress management.

Howard PB: Lifelong maternal caregiving for children with schizophrenia, *Arch Psych Nurs* 8(2):107, 1994; Howard PB: The experience of fathers of adult children with schizophrenia, *Issues Ment Health Nurs* 19(2):399, 1998.

---

illness (Biegel et al, 1991). These caregivers are also at risk for health disruption. Specifically, mothers and fathers caring for adult children with schizophrenia are at risk for increased threats to mental health during their own adult years and into old age (Howard, 1994, 1998). Caregivers of persons with severely disabling mental disorders often have their mental health threatened by guilt (Natale and Barron, 1994), lack of social support (Norbeck et al, 1991), and chronic strain (Reinhard, 1994). Other chronic conditions that threaten the mental health status of caregivers are Alzheimer's disease and human immunodeficiency virus (HIV)/AIDS. Specifically, caregivers of older relatives with Alzheimer's are at increased risk for strain and burden (Kuhlman et al, 1991; Pallett, 1990), and those who care for loved ones with HIV/AIDS have high levels of distress (McShane, Bumbalo, and Patsdaughter, 1994) and heightened anxiety and depression (Wiener et al, 1994). During stressful life events such as these, it is important for caregivers to know how to manage the many competing demands in their lives.

Activities to improve the mental health status of adults include public education programs, prevention approaches, and providing mental health services in primary care. Specific approaches include use of community support groups, education about lifestyle management to reduce stress, and work site programs aimed at reducing employee stress (APHA, 1991). Nevertheless, most programs currently available for adults with mental health problems primarily monitor or restore health rather than prevent problems. Barriers to preventive services include inadequate financing for mental health services and fragmented care (Krauss, 1993; Leff and Woocher, 1998).

Older adults. In the United States the population over 65 years of age has steadily increased since the turn of this century. Today persons who reach 65 years can expect to live into their 80s. Moreover, the segment of the older adult population that is growing most rapidly in the United States today are those persons age 85 years and older (USDHHS, 1991; Krauss, 1993). Although many older people maintain highly functional lives, others have mental health deficits because of normal sensory losses related to aging, failing physical health, difficulty performing activities of daily living, and social deprivation or isolation. Life changes related to work roles and retirement often result in reduced social contacts and support. Other previously described losses are associated with the death of a spouse, other family members, or friends. Reduced social networks and contacts brought about by these life events can influence mood and contribute to serious states of depression.

Depression affects functional independence and contributes to suicide. In the United States, men between age 65 and 74 years are in the highest risk category for suicide (USDHHS, 1991). Another factor linked to suicide in this age group is chronic illness. Common physical problems of older adults include terminal illnesses associated with cancer and chronic conditions such as arthritis, osteoporosis, and cardiovascular and respiratory disease. Brain disorders such as Alzheimer's disease, dementia, and stroke are also common among older adults. All these conditions have an effect on the mental health status of individuals and their family caregivers.

Healthy aging activities such as physical activity and establishing social networks improve the mental health of older adults. Because older adults, like younger people, are victims of violence in the environment and in their homes, the national health objectives refer to reducing the incidence of abuse (USDHHS, 1991). Strategies that address the problem of elder abuse include early screening for risk factors in all primary care settings and organizing health promotion programs through senior centers or other community-based settings (APHA, 1991). Home health care nurses can assess and intervene to offset those at risk for abuse. For example, stress management for caregivers and respite day-care programs for an elderly family member can reduce stress and prevent abuse.

Low-income, ethnic, and minority groups. Although all socioeconomic and cultural groups have mental health problems, low-income groups are at greater risk because they often lack minimal resources for meeting basic physical and mental health needs. Ethnic and minority groups also are at risk since they may lack supportive reference groups and access to adequate, culturally sensitive services (Baker et al, 1993; Lantican, 1998; Sandhaus, 1998).

People who live in poverty often have low incomes and live in substandard, overcrowded conditions that contribute to stress in activities of daily living. In single-parent families, a subgroup of the low-income population, depression is not uncommon. One study found that more than half (59.6%) of a sample of low-income single mothers (N = 255) had high depressive symptoms. In addition, depression was associated with fewer social resources and greater everyday stressors and was a predictor of parenting attitudes (Hall et al, 1991). Beck (1998) studied the effects of postpartum depression on the development of children. She found that postpartum depression had a moderate to large adverse effect on infants' behavior, although it weakened as the child grew older. Predictors of postpartum depression are prenatal depression and lack of social support (Beck, 1998). Single-parent families are at risk. Interventions include individual or group therapy with women and enhancing the roles of those who provide social support, such as the child's father.

Substandard living conditions also compromise children. For example, children in low-income families often have elevated blood lead levels that can result in serious mental and physical impairments. Even more serious, these children are more vulnerable to death from fire and drowning, and all age groups in low-income families are at risk because of violence in their neighborhoods (USDHHS, 1991).

Physical illness, infectious disease, and hazards in the environment also contribute to the mental health status of any individual or group. Nonetheless, individuals in low-income groups are at increased risk for serious illness and infectious disease, including tuberculosis and HIV infections (USDHHS, 1991; Sandhaus, 1998). Homeless mentally ill persons who live in poverty are at increased risk for tuberculosis and HIV infections because of their self-care and cognitive deficits combined with overcrowded, unsanitary living conditions (Colson, Susser, and Valencia, 1994).

Members of minority groups are likely to have low-income groups with earnings at or below the poverty line (USDHHS, 1991; Krauss, 1994; Sandhaus, 1998). In addition, these groups are at increased risk for mental health problems because they lack access to mental health services (Padgett et al, 1994; Sandhaus, 1998).

The predominant minority populations in the United States are African-Americans, Hispanics, Asian- and Pacific Islander-Americans, native Americans, and Alaska natives (USDHHS, 1991). Within each of these groups are subgroups with unique cultural differences that have been shaped by social, political, and historical factors (Lantican, 1998; Sandhaus, 1998). Therefore it is important to avoid simplification and overgeneralization in discussions about the characteristics and problems of minorities. Rather, it is critical to conduct community assessments to determine unique characteristics and factors that contribute to mental health deficits within specific aggregates of the population (APHA, 1991). The information presented here is intended to stimulate thinking and awareness for developing nursing process activities in individual communities.

Today, African-Americans make up the largest minority group in the United States. African-Americans live in all regions of the United States and are represented in all socioeconomic groups, yet one third live in poverty and one half are exposed to the high stress of inner-city conditions (USDHHS, 1991; Padgett et al, 1994). Among the many subgroups of the African-American population, African-American elders (aged 65 years and older) represent a unique reference group when it comes to health care. This group had few health care facilities available to them before and during desegregation. This experience and other complex socioenvironmental issues shaped their health beliefs and influenced their awareness about services that may be available for their quality of life and mental well-being (Baker, et al, 1993).

Factors affecting the mental health status of a significant number of African-Americans are similar to those described for low-income families. Still others are exposed to urban problems such as violence. As noted in Table 35-2, ethnic groups are target populations for both homicide and suicide. These conditions suggest that violence, stress, despondency, and other severe emotional conditions are influenced by environmental conditions. Similar problems threaten the mental health status of the second largest minority group in the United States.

Hispanic-Americans are the second largest and fastest growing minority group in America with 87% living in urban areas (the largest concentrations are in western states, Florida, and New York [Grothaus, 1996; USDHHS, 1991]). Migrant farm workers are also an important subpopulation among Hispanics. As discussed in Chapter 34, migratory living patterns marked by low income, poor education, and lack of health services contribute to stressful living conditions. Nurses and nurse practitioners are the primary health care providers for migrant laborers and their roles include case management and interagency collaboration (Sandhaus, 1998). Interagency collaboration includes networking and referral to community mental health agencies and advanced practice psychiatric nurses when drug and alcohol abuse or mental illness are the primary health problems. Hispanic-Americans living in low-income urban areas are subject to many of the conditions described for low-income and disadvantaged African-American families. Outcomes of these living conditions are also similar. For example, the high rates of unintentional injuries and homicide among young Hispanic men (USDHHS, 1991) not only reveal serious stressful living conditions but also suggest strain, loss, and potential bereavement complications for family members.

Nurses working with Mexican-American families must understand their cultural and family dynamics to provide health services. The first step in establishing the therapeutic relationship is to establish an environment "where the family feels heard, understood, and accepted" (Grothaus, 1996, p. 37). The Mexican-American population is predicted to rise significantly; therefore nurses need knowledge and skill in cross-cultural therapies. Nurses also need to include the consumer perspective in planning and evaluating mental health service delivery (Lantican, 1998), including access to care.

Eleven million Asian- and Pacific Islander-Americans who speak over 30 different languages and have diverse cultures make up the third largest minority group in the United States (USDHHS, 1991). Approximately three quarters are from Southeast Asia, and many are refugees. The largest number of this population lives in California. Whereas Asian- and Pacific Islander-Americans, like other minority groups, are represented in all socioeconomic strata, many are in the lower-income groups. The lower-income groups include refugees and recent immigrants who are dealing with the displacement issues of loss, adjustment, and adaptation. Losses often involve forfeiture of family, traditions, and lifestyles for cultures that may seem alien. Adjustments and adaptations include those basic to daily living: learning new languages, laws, and monetary systems and locating support systems. Finding support systems includes acquainting oneself with the health care delivery system. Assessment, planning, and interventions with members of this population and those with diverse languages, customs, and beliefs must include information about their health beliefs and an understanding of the health care system in the United States and of the services that are available to them. Nurses must look at the leadership in other countries when making recommendations or developing programs. For example, Kim, (1998), a professor of nursing in South Korea reported on a community-based care approach for mentally ill clients and their families. A psychosocial rehabilitation model emphasizing client and family education and restructuring the clients' environment is used. Restructuring the clients' environment includes using day care as a place to practice social skills (Kim, 1998). Considering the culture of the population is a key component in any program.

Diversity also characterizes the numerous tribes that make up the native American and Alaska native population. These descendants of the original North American residents number approximately 1.6 million and are currently the fourth largest minority group in the United States. About one third of native Americans live on reservations or historic trust lands, whereas approximately 50% live in urban areas (USDHHS, 1991). Approximately 25% of this minority group live below the poverty line and have threats to mental health that are similar to those described for all low-income groups. Other problems are similar to those described for other minority groups. For example, suicide, homicide, and unintentional injuries are common (see Table 35-2). These problems suggest serious mental health deficits that are important to address when working in communities. More detailed information is available from the Indian Health Service. Community assessments that include data about specific populations from organized agencies such as the Indian Health Service are important, since assessment data guide role activities during all steps of the nursing process.

ROLE OF THE NURSE IN COMMUNITY MENTAL HEALTH

The role of the nurse in community mental health was shaped by the evolution of services and the work of nursing pioneers. Development of a knowledge base for the nursing discipline and changes in practice settings prompted recent redefinitions of the scope of psychiatric mental health clinical practice (ANA, 1994). The practice standards reflect the values of the profession, describe the responsibilities of nurses, and provide direction for the delivery and evaluation of nursing care with specific populations. Target populations are consistent with those identified in national health objectives. The statement also describes the roles of nurses in both advanced and basic level practice.

Advanced practice psychiatric nurses have graduate education. They provide primary, secondary, and tertiary care to individuals, groups, families, adults, children, and adolescents. Depending on state laws, some prescribe medications and have hospital admission privileges (Talley and Caverly, 1994). Recently, the psychiatric nurse practitioner title and role have been described (Caverly, 1996), as well as models for practitioner programs that blend psychiatric and primary care skills (Dyer et al, 1997). The blended nurse practitioner role has been a response to some shifts in the health care system away from specialization towards comprehensive services that address both physical and mental health problems.

Nurses prepared at the undergraduate level provide basic primary, secondary, and tertiary services that are equally valuable. Specific roles and functions of nurses at the basic level listed in Box 35-3 are based on clinical nursing practice and standards (ANA, 1994). The functions suggest the overlapping roles of practitioner, educator, and coordinator.

Practitioner

Objectives of the practitioner role are to help the client maintain or regain coping abilities that promote functioning. This involves using the nursing process to guide the diagnosis and treatment of human responses to actual or potential mental health problems (ANA, 1994). Role functions at the basic practitioner level include case management, counseling, milieu therapy, and psychobiological interventions with individuals and with groups. Practitioner skills are used in a variety of settings including the home and often with large groups of people in specific neighborhoods, schools, and public health districts.

For example, many clients who have schizophrenia live in personal care homes. These clients require biopsy-

---

BOX 35-3 Roles and Functions in Psychiatric-Mental Health Nursing Practice

ROLES
Practitioner
Educator
Coordinator

FUNCTIONS
Advocacy
Case-finding and referral
Case management
Community action
Counseling
Crisis intervention
Health maintenance
Health promotion
Health teaching
Home visits
Intake screening and evaluation
Milieu therapy
Psychobiological interventions
Self-care activities

Adapted from American Nurses Association: *A statement on psychiatric-mental health clinical nursing practice and standards of psychiatric-mental health clinical nursing practice*, Washington, DC, 1994, American Nurses Publishing.

---

chosocial interventions related to medication management, milieu management for improved social interaction, and assistance with self-care activities for community living such as use of public transportation (Liberman et al, 1993; Murphy and Moller, 1993). Also, the practitioner increasingly coordinates these activities with staff members in community settings. Therefore coordination of care is often the means for promoting treatment plan outcomes and enhancing quality of life for clients. These activities can support positive outcomes for others in the community at large.

For example, family members are a primary support system for individuals with schizophrenia. Whether the client lives in a personal care home, family residence, or another setting, counseling family members and the client about the illness may offset the stressors of caregiving. Moreover, educating the public may reduce the stigma and offset social isolation for both clients and families. For the community, implications of these basic-level functions may include public support for needed services and decreased costs of health care resulting from reduced hospitalization. As suggested in these examples, practitioner and educator roles overlap.

Educator

The educator role uses teaching-learning principles to increase understanding about mental illness and mental health. The educator role is foundational to health maintenance, health promotion, and community action. Teaching clients about illness symptoms and the benefits of medications promotes health maintenance and may reduce the risk for illness relapse (Murphy and Moller, 1993; Moller and Murphy, 1997). Similar education programs for family members increase their ability to monitor illness symptoms and identify events that lead to relapse (Murphy and Moller, 1993; Moller and Murphy, 1997).

At the community level, both formal and informal teaching is important. One important objective for health promotion is to teach positive coping skills. An example of an ineffective coping skill among individuals is overmedicating. Even when medications are properly used in treatment, the nurse requires specialized knowledge about drug interactions and pharmacokinetics. **Pharmacokinetics** refers to the absorption, distribution, metabolism and elimination of drugs in the body (Keltner and Folks, 1997). Factors that influence pharmacokinetics include anatomic and physiological changes that occur with aging or with coexisting mental and physical conditions. Even use of nonprescription medication (i.e., over-the-counter drugs) can influence pharmacokinetics.

NURSING TIP

Nurses need to teach individuals and groups about the consequences of medication use and misuse.

WHAT DO YOU THINK? *Although psychopharmacology, which began in the 1950s, has dramatically improved the lives of people with severe mental illness, controversies exist about medication side effects and the cost of monitoring some of the more serious side effects. For example, side effects of antipsychotic drugs can cause central and peripheral nervous system manifestations.*

Peripheral nervous system effects include hypotension, urinary retention, sedation, and weight gain. Central nervous system side effects include parkinsonian symptoms such as tremors and rigidity and even more serious manifestations: tardive dyskinesia and neuroleptic malignant syndrome. Do the benefits offered by these medications justify their side effects?

Coordinator

Coordination of care is a basic principle of the multidisciplinary team approach in community mental health services. Yet homelessness suggests there is lack of coordination as well as limited services in most communities. Therefore, at minimum, the role of coordinator must include case-finding, referral, and follow-up to evaluate system breakdown and deficits. Because of current system deficits, nurses in community mental health function as coordinators who carry out intake screening, crisis intervention, and home visits. The coordinator role also tries to improve the client's health and well-being by promoting independence and self-care in the least restrictive environ-

ment. These functions are consistent with descriptions of case management that emphasize continuity of care for individuals who need complex services (Bachrach, 1994).

HOW TO *Assess the Mental Health Needs of Homeless People*

Because of the temporary relationships between homeless people and health care providers, it is difficult to accurately assess their needs. Walker, 1998, suggests the following. Work to create a climate of credibility and trust. This may require "hanging out" in a series of unscheduled visits with homeless people and offering them a sandwich or a cup of coffee, listening to their worries and concerns, or handling obvious physical needs like open sores or head lice. Information may be gathered through seemingly casual encounters in alleys, soup kitchens, shelters, or on the sidewalk.

To achieve these objectives and improve services, the nurse must work with a variety of professionals, including advanced practice nurses, social workers, physicians, psychologists, occupational and vocational therapists, and rehabilitation counselors. Since nonlicensed paraprofessionals are frequently involved in direct care activities, their services must be directed, coordinated, and evaluated within the context of treatment planning. Finally, coordination also involves work with individuals who may not have formal preparation but who are essential for positive treatment outcomes. These individuals include family members, shelter volunteers, consumer support groups, and community leaders who can influence development of services. The coordinator role clearly offers nurses an opportunity to identify health system effectiveness and ineffectiveness.

Frameworks

A basic principle of the community mental health movement was that people had a right to mental health services; another principle asserted that those with disorders had a right to services in the least restrictive environment. Prevention has been emphasized since the inception of the movement. Theories and concepts that help to explain relationships or the dynamics of mental illness provide useful frameworks for fostering these objectives.

Systems theory

Systems theory is a useful framework for community mental health practice because it emphasizes the relationship of the elements of a unit to the whole. To understand either the element or the whole, one must examine the interactions and relationships that exist between them. A holistic view of system and subsystems can be applied in a variety of ways in community mental health practice. One example of subsystems in a community are its cultural groups. Subsystems of the cultural groups are families; subsystems of the families are individuals. Using systems theory to explore the background, conditions, and context of situations will reveal information about the positive and negative forces that either promote or undermine the well-being of any unit in the system.

Other useful theories to enhance understanding of the multidimensional aspects of community mental health nursing are those that explain biological systems, personality, life span development, and family dynamics.

Prevention

Health promotion and illness prevention are fundamental to community mental health practice as well as national objectives previously described (APHA, 1991; USDHHS, 1991). Therefore the concepts of primary, secondary, and tertiary levels of prevention are useful in practice.

Primary prevention refers to the reduction of health risks. It involves the identification of conditions that have the potential of causing stress and illness. Most functions of the educator role are aimed at primary prevention. Examples include giving education and lifestyle management classes for caregivers of individuals with severe mental disorders.

Secondary prevention refers to activities aimed at reducing the prevalence or pathological nature of a condition. Many functions of the practitioner role are aimed at secondary prevention. Providing individual and group psychotherapy, case referral, and follow-up to determine the need for additional services and coordinating services following crisis intervention are all examples of secondary prevention.

Tertiary prevention refers to restoration and enhancement of functioning. Many practitioner and coordinator role activities are aimed at tertiary prevention. They include monitoring illness symptoms and treatment responses, coordinating transition from the hospital to the community, and identifying respite care options for caregivers.

Vulnerability-stress model

The vulnerability-stress-coping-competence model of major mental disorders was designed for use in the rehabilitation of individuals with severe mental illness (Liberman et al, 1993). Within the context of biological, environmental, and behavioral factors, the model explains the onset, course, and outcome of severe mental illness, emphasizing the importance of social skills development necessary for community living.

Liberman et al (1993) explained that individuals with severe mental disorders have psychobiological vulnerabilities because of the interplay between genetic brain impairments, not yet fully understood, and stressful life events. According to the theory, biological vulnerability inhibits social skills development during the early years of life. Also, social skills deficits combined with stressful life events can overwhelm the individual's coping ability and result in illness symptoms. Protective factors, another concept of the theory, are important moderators of vulnerability and stress (Liberman et al, 1993). Coping and competence are viewed as essential protective factors. Moreover, coping and competence are "exercised" by "families," "natural support systems," and "professional treatment" as well as the individual who is ill (Liberman et al, 1993). Other protective

factors are rehabilitation programs, housing programs, and case management. Relapse management is central to many of the programs and activities that enhance coping skills and competence.

Relapse management

As a case manager it is important for the community mental health nurse to foster coping and competency aimed at managing illness symptoms with consumers, family members, and other caregivers. The aim of managing illness symptoms is to offset relapse. Since **relapse management** is a major goal of interventions in community mental health nursing, the Moller-Murphy Symptom Management Assessment Tool (MM-SMAT) (Murphy and Moller, 1993) may be especially useful during nursing process activities.

The MM-SMAT was developed to provide consumers, family members, and professionals with a common framework for managing neurobiological disorders such as schizophrenia, bipolar disorder, and major depression (Murphy and Moller, 1993), and it is compatible with vulnerability-stress models of mental illness. Categories of the MM-SMAT focus on the frequency, intensity, and duration of symptoms for the purpose of identifying health, environmental, and behavioral triggers that may lead to illness relapse. Examples of triggers are poor nutrition, poor social skills, hopelessness, and poor symptom management. Once triggers are identified, interventions aimed at fostering effective coping skills can be introduced to offset relapse of symptoms. For example, an intervention that may promote effective coping to offset social isolation is guiding the client to organized consumer group activities available in the community. Another is to promote consumer and family efforts at job training through community vocational agencies. Still another is to promote competency in family members by coordinating services that enhance their understanding of the illness, provide social support, and include respite when needed. Finally, medication management is an important intervention for offsetting relapse.

Scientific advances that led to the use of lithium in the treatment of mania, chlorpromazine (Thorazine) in the treatment of schizophrenia, and imipramine (Tofranil) in antidepressant therapy revolutionized mental health care and services (Keltner and Folks, 1997). More recently in the United States, risperidone (Land and Salzman, 1994) and clozapine (Keltner and Folks, 1997; Clarke and Yaeger, 1994) were introduced for treatment of clients who experienced severe side effects or who did not respond to more traditional antipsychotic drugs (Breier et al, 1993). New antidepressant agents referred to as selective serotonin reuptake inhibitors (SSRIs) have also been introduced. Although these new drugs have dramatically improved the lives of many people with mental disorders, they are not without controversy. Perhaps the greatest controversy is to prescribe medications without incorporating other relapse management approaches. In the nursing process, psychopharmacology should be used with social, behavioral, and psychotherapeutic interventions that take into consideration the cultural dimensions of the client (Keltner and Folks, 1997; Clarke and Yaeger, 1994).

clinical application

Mary, a 62-year-old grandmother, and John, her 66-year-old husband, live in a four-room house in a rural area not far from a large city. Their 28-year-old daughter Ann and her 6-year-old son Jason live with Mary and John. Ann was diagnosed with schizophrenia when she was 20 years old, divorced a short time later when Jason was an infant, and moved home to live with her parents. Ann has been hospitalized frequently for treatment of her psychiatric disorder. Most of the time, she was hospitalized because symptoms of her illness recurred after she quit keeping appointments at the CMHC and refused to take her antipsychotic medications. Other patterns of behavior included leaving home unannounced, seeking rides with strangers, and going into the city, where she lived on the streets for days at a time. Because of these problems, Ann was incarcerated in the legal system and declared mentally incompetent when Jason was 2 years old. At that time, Mary and John legally adopted Jason.

Although there have been few changes in Ann's course of illness during the time since the court ruling, some recent self-care activities suggested that she was more accepting of her illness and treatment plan, including medications. A community mental health nurse from a home health agency was assigned case management activities during Ann's last hospitalization. During the hospitalization, infectious diseases, including HIV, were ruled out, but Ann was identified as being at risk because of her lifestyle. The nurse established rapport with Ann during hospitalization and began home visits during the week of discharge. Case management activities were to include education and family support. Following in-depth assessment activities in the home, including use of the MM-SMAT with Ann and her parents, the nurse developed a comprehensive treatment plan incorporating levels of prevention for members of the family.

With Ann, tertiary prevention activities included a plan to help her to identify situations and behaviors that put her at risk for illness relapse, monitoring of medications, teaching about risks for infectious disease including HIV, and exploring options for psychosocial rehabilitation. Tertiary prevention activities for Mary and John included referral to the local NAMI affiliate for supportive services and encouragement of continued work with teachers at Jason's school. The comprehensive plan also revealed the importance of secondary and primary prevention measures.

Because of her multiple roles and limited support outside the family, Mary was at increased risk for continued stress. She also had early signs of depression that included tearfulness, sleep disturbance, loss of appetite, and inability to concentrate. Therefore the nurse arranged for immediate intake and assessment for services at the CMHC. With encouragement, John took over more of the child care activities with Jason. In time, these tertiary and secondary activities resulted in a more stable environment for the family, and since all family members were in agreement, the nurse began to explore supervised housing options for Ann. John and Mary became more active in the local NAMI affiliate. The nurse provided primary prevention activities with the NAMI group by giving a talk about lifestyle management and by recommending an advanced psychiatric nurse consultant for more comprehensive program development.

A. Where do many caregivers find social support networks?
B. If Jason shows signs of behavioral problems, who can give assessment information?
C. In addition to education, what other case management activities are important in Ann's care?
D. If Mary's depression is managed with medications, what nursing care activities are important?

Answers are in the back of the book.

KEY POINTS

- Reform movements and subsequent federal legislation influenced the development of the current community mental health model that includes team care, case management, prevention, and rehabilitation components of service.
- During this current decade, federal legislation in the United States focused on mainstreaming persons with mental disabilities into American life by legislating access to employment, services, and housing.
- People are at risk for threats to mental health at all ages across the life span. Low-income and minority groups are often at increased risk because they lack access to services and because programs may lack cultural sensitivity.
- Homelessness and substandard living conditions contribute to psychosocial problems related to social isolation and also increases the risk for infectious diseases, including tuberculosis (TB) and HIV, among persons with severe mental disorders.
- National health objectives to promote health and services for persons who have mental health problems and severe mental disorders illustrate the scope of mental illness and provide direction for community mental health practice.
- Guidelines for attaining national health objectives were designed to help individuals at regional and local levels establish health priorities that include those for mental illness.
- Recent redefinitions of ANA standards provide a framework for the roles and functions of community mental health nurses.
- Frameworks that are useful in community mental health nursing include primary, secondary, and tertiary levels of prevention, vulnerability-stress models, and relapse management.

critical thinking activities

1. For 1 week, keep a list of incidents related to mental health problems that you read about in local newspapers or hear about on the radio and television. Categorize the incidents according to age, gender, socioeconomic, and ethnic or minority status.
2. Visit a local shelter or organization that offers temporary protection for persons with mental disorders. Determine services that are available or lacking for children, women, and men.
3. Visit with representatives of your local self-help organizations for consumers to determine types of problems they have and adequacy of resources for people with severe mental disorders and their caregivers to determine gaps in services. Develop a list of the agencies in your community that provide direct or indirect services for those with mental illness and their families.
4. Interview a school nurse, an occupational health nurse, an emergency room nurse, or a hospice nurse in your community to discuss types of mental health problems they deal with in their practice settings. Determine resources that are available or lacking for primary, secondary, and tertiary prevention.
5. Interview a nurse working in a local community mental health agency to discuss roles, functions, programs, and resources available or lacking for primary, secondary, and tertiary prevention. Compare findings about prevention programs with information obtained from the preceding interview.
6. As a class activity, arrange for a panel of speakers representing the minority populations described in this chapter. Discuss their views about the way culture shapes thinking about mental illness and determine types of culturally sensitive services that are available or lacking in your community.
7. Review articles in at least four research journals to determine current research findings about severe mental disorders and mental health problems, and to compare nursing care in the United States with that of other countries.

Bibliography

American Nurses Association: *Nursing's agenda for health care reform,* Pub No PR 3 220M, Washington, DC, 1991, American Nurses Publishing.

American Nurses Association: *A statement on psychiatric-mental health clinical nursing practice and standards of psychiatric-mental health clinical nursing practice,* Washington, DC, 1994, American Nurses Publishing.

American Psychiatric Association: *Diagnostic and statistical manual of mental disorders,* ed 4, Washington, DC, 1994, the Association.

American Public Health Association: *Healthy communities 2000: model standards, guidelines for community attainment of the year 2000 national health objectives,* ed 3, Washington, DC, 1991, the Association.

Bachrach LL: The Carter commission's contributions to mental health service planning, *Hosp Community Psych* 45(6):527, 1994.

Baker FM, Lavizzo-Mourey R, Jones BE: Acute care of the African-American elder, *J Geriatr Psych Neurol* 6:66, 1993.

Beck CT: The effects of postpartum depression on child development: A meta-analysis, *Arch Psych Nurs* 12(1):12, 1998.

Brazelon Center for Mental Health Law: Mental disability law in 1993, *Clearinghouse Review,* p 1322, March 1994.

Biegel DE, Sales E, Schulz R: *Family caregiving in chronic illness,* Newbury Park, Calif, 1991, Sage.

Breier A et al: Clozapine treatment of outpatients with schizophrenia: outcome and long-term response patterns, *Hosp Community Psych* 44(12):1145, 1993.

Breslaw N et al: Psychiatric sequelae of post-traumatic stress disorder in women, *Arch Gen Psych* 54:81, 1997.

Caverly SE: The role of the psychiatric nurse practitioner, *Nurs Clin North Am* 31(3):449, 1996.

Center for Mental Health Services: *Mental health, United States, 1996.* In Manderscheid RW, Sonnenschein MA, editors: DHHS Pub No (SMA) 96-3098. Washington, DC, 1996, Supt of Docs, US Government Printing Office.

Clarke DE, Yaeger SF: Addressing emerging social needs of patients treated with new neuroleptics, *J Psychosoc Nurs* 32(11):19, 1994.

Colson P, Susser E, Valencia E: HIV and TB among people who are homeless and mentally ill, *Psychosoc Rehab J* 17(4):157, 1994.

Donahue MP: *Nursing: the finest art,* St Louis, 1985, Mosby.

Dyer JG et al: The psychiatric-primary care nurse practitioners: a futuristic model for advanced practice, *Arch Psych Nurs* 11(1):2, 1997.

Eakes GG, Burke ML, Hainsworth MA: Middle-range theory of chronic sorrow, *Image J Nurs Sch* 30(2):179, 1998.

Fawcett J, Barkin RL: A meta-analysis of eight randomized double-blind, controlled clinical trials of Mirtaziapine for the treatment of patients with major depression and symptoms of anxiety, *J Clin Psychiatry* 59:123, 1998.

Feingold E: Health care reform: More than cost containment and universal access, *Am J Pub Health* 84(5):727, 1994.

Grob GN: *From asylum to community,* Princeton, NJ, 1991, Princeton University Press.

Grothaus KL: Family dynamics and family therapy with Mexican Americans, *J Psychosoc Nurs* 34(2):31, 1996.

Hall LA et al: Psychosocial predictors of maternal depressive symptoms, parenting attitudes, and child behavior in single-parent families, *Nurs Res* 40(4):214, 1991.

Honigfeld G et al: Reducing clozapine-related morbidity and mortality: 5 years of experience with the Clozaril National Registry, *J Clin Psychiatry* 59(supp 3):3, 1998.

Howard PB: Lifelong maternal caregiving for children with schizophrenia, *Arch Psych Nurs* 8(2):107, 1994.

Howard PB: The experience of fathers of adult children with schizophrenia, *Issues Ment Health Nurs* 19:399, 1998.

Isaacs A: Depression and your patient, *AJN* 98(7):26, 1998.

Johnson DR et al: Outcome of intensive inpatient treatment for combat-related post-traumatic stress disorder, *Am J Psych* 153:771, 1996.

Keltner NL, Folks GD: *Psychotropic drugs,* ed 2, St Louis, 1997, Mosby.

Keltner NL et al: *Psychobiological foundations of psychiatric care,* St, Louis, 1998, Mosby.

Kim S: Out of darkness, *Reflections* 24(3):8-12, 1998.

Krauss J: *Health care reform: essential mental health services,* Washington, DC, 1993, American Nurses Publishing.

Krauss J: The mental status of health care reform, *Arch Psych Nurs* 8(1):1, 1994.

Kuhlman GJ et al: Alzheimer's disease and family caregiving: critical synthesis of the literature and research agenda, *Nurs Res* 40(6):331, 1991.

Land W, Salzman C: risperidone: a novel antipsychotic medication, *J Hosp Community Psychiatry* 45(5):434, 1994.

Lantican L: Mexican American clients' perceptions of services in an outpatient mental health facility in a border city, *Issues Ment Health Nurs* 19:125, 1998.

Leff HS, Woocher LS: Trends in the evaluation of managed mental health care, *Harvard Rev Psychiatry* 5:344, 1998.

Lefley HP: Impact of consumer and family advocacy movements on mental health services. In Levin B, Petrila J, editors: *Mental health services: a public health perspective,* New York, 1996, Oxford University Press.

Liberman RP et al: Innovations in skills training for the seriously mentally ill: the UCLA social and independent living skills modules, *Innovations Res* 2(2):43, 1993.

Manderscheid RW, Henderson MJ: *Federal and state legislative and program directions for managed care: Implications for case management,* Rockville, Md, 1995, USDHHS, Substance Abuse and Mental Health Services Administration, Center for Mental Health Services.

McShane RE, Bumbalo JA, Patsdaughter CA: Psychological distress in family members living with Human Immunodeficiency Virus/Acquired Immune Deficiency Syndrome, *Arch Psych Nurs* 8(1):53, 1994.

Moller M, Murphy M: The three R's rehabilitation program: a prevention approach for the management of relapse symptoms associated with psychiatric diagnosis, *Psych Rehab J* 20(3):42, 1997.

Murphy MF, Moller MD: Relapse management in neurobiological disorders: the Moller-Murphy Symptom Management Assessment Tool, *Arch Psych Nurs* 7(4):226, 1993.

Natale A, Barron C: Mothers' causal explanations for their sons' schizophrenia: relationship to depression and guilt, *Arch Psych Nurs* 8(4):228, 1994.

National Institute of Mental Health: *Caring for people with severe mental disorders: a national plan of research to improve services* (DHHS publication no. ADM91-1762), Washington, DC, 1991, US Government Printing Office.

Navarro V: The future of public health in health care reform, *Am J Pub Health* 84(5):729, 1994.

Norbeck JS et al: Social support needs of family caregivers of psychiatric patients from three age groups, *Nurs Res* 40(4):208, 1991.

Padgett DK et al: Ethnicity and the use of outpatient mental health services in a national insured population, *Am J Pub Health* 84(2):222, 1994.

Pallett PJ: A conceptual framework for studying family caregiver burden in Alzheimer's-type dementia, *Image J Nurs Sch* 22(1):52, 1990.

Pang A et al: Community psychiatry in Hong Kong, *Int J Soc Psychiatry* 43(3):213, 1997.

Perlin ML: Law and the delivery of mental health services in the community, *Am J Orthopsych* 64(2):194, 1994.

Reinhard SC: Perspectives on the family's caregiving experience in mental illness, *Image J Nurs Sch* 26(1):70, 1994.

Richardson LA et al: Identification and treatment of children's mental health problems by primary care providers: a critical review of research, *Arch Psych Nurs* 10(5):293, 1996.

Sandhaus S: Migrant health: a harvest of poverty, *AJN* 98(9):52, 1998.

Talley S, Caverly S: Advanced practice psychiatric nursing and health care reform, *Hosp Commun Psych* 45(6):545, 1994.

Taylor CM: *Essentials of psychiatric nursing,* ed 14, St Louis, 1994, Mosby.

US Department of Health and Human Services: *Healthy People 2000: national health promotion and disease prevention objectives,* Washington, DC, 1991, USDHHS, Public Health Service.

Walker C: Homeless people and mental health: a nursing concern, *AJN* 98(11):26, 1998.

Wasserbauer LI: Psychiatric nurses' knowledge of the Americans with Disabilities Act, *Arch Psych Nurs* 10(6):324, 1996.

Wiener L et al: The HIV-infected child: parental responses and psychosocial implications, *Am J Orthopsych* 64(3):485, 1994.

Wilk RJ: Federal legislation for rights of persons with mental illness: obstacles to implementation, *Am J Orthopsych* 63(4):518, 1993.

Worley NK: *Mental health nursing in the community,* St. Louis, 1997, Mosby.

Yip KS: A historical review of mental health services in Hong Kong (1841 to 1995), *International Journal of Social Psychiatry* 44(1):46, 1998.

Alcohol, Tobacco, and Other Drug Problems in the Community

MARY LYNN MATHRE

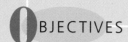 www.mosby.com/MERLIN/community_stanhope

OBJECTIVES

After reading this chapter, the student should be able to do the following:

- Analyze personal attitudes toward alcohol, tobacco, and other drug problems.
- Differentiate among the terms *substance use, abuse, dependence,* and *addiction.*
- Examine the differences among the major psychoactive drug categories.

- Explain the role of the nurse in primary, secondary, and tertiary prevention of alcohol, tobacco, and other drug problems as it relates to individual clients and their families.
- Evaluate the role of the nurse in primary, secondary, and tertiary prevention of alcohol, tobacco, and other drug problems as it relates to the community and national policies.

KEY TERMS

addiction treatment
Alcoholics Anonymous
 (AA)
alcoholism
antiprohibitionists
blood alcohol concentra-
 tion (BAC)
brief interventions
codependency

cross-tolerance
denial
depressants
detoxification
drug addiction
drug dependence
enabling
fetal alcohol syndrome
 (FAS)

hallucinogens
harm reduction
inhalants
injection drug users
mainstream smoke
neurotransmitters
polysubstance use or
 abuse
prohibition

psychoactive drugs
set
setting
sidestream smoke
stimulants
substance abuse
tolerance
withdrawal
See Glossary for definitions

CHAPTER OUTLINE

Substance abuse is a national health problem that is linked to numerous forms of morbidity and mortality. Between 25% and 40% of all general hospital admissions are related to the effects of alcohol abuse (Institute for Health Policy, Brandeis University, 1993), and one in five dollars of Medicaid is spent on substance abuse (Merrill et al, 1993). More deaths and disabilities annually are attributed to substance abuse than to any other preventable cause. Of the 2 million U.S. deaths each year, one quarter are attributed to tobacco, alcohol, and illicit drug use (Institute for Health Policy, Brandeis University, 1993). The National Household Survey on Drug Abuse estimates that 12.8 million Americans (6.1% of the population age 12 or older) currently use illicit drugs, while 32 million Americans (15.8% of the population) had engaged in binge or heavy drinking (Substance Abuse and Mental Health Services Administration, 1996). The substance abuser is not only at risk for personal health problems but may be a threat to the health and safety of family members, coworkers, and other members of the community.

Substance abuse and addiction affect all ages, races, sexes, and segments of society. As seen in Appendix A.1, *Healthy People 2000* (USDHHS, 1991) lists "tobacco" as the third priority area and "alcohol and other drugs" as the fourth priority area, with a total of 46 objectives, as well as related objectives in other priority areas. The newer phrase of *alcohol, tobacco, and other drug (ATOD) problems* rather than *substance abuse* reminds us that alcohol and tobacco represent the major drugs of abuse when discussing substance abuse, drug addiction, or chemical dependency.

This chapter begins by providing a broad perspective of ATOD problems to clarify the relevant issues. A historical overview of ATOD problems and attitudes towards ATOD users and addicts are examined to differentiate drug problems from those created by lack of information, the war on drugs, and unfounded fears. Relevant terms are defined to decrease the confusion caused by frequent misuse of terms. The major drug categories are described, including information on commonly used substances and current ATOD use trends. The remainder of the chapter examines the role of the nurse in primary, secondary and tertiary prevention and how the nurse can improve the outcomes for individuals, families and communities with ATOD problems when using a harm reduction model. The reader is encouraged to consider possible nursing strategies to operationalize the *Healthy People 2000* objectives for substance abuse problems.

ATOD PROBLEMS IN PERSPECTIVE

ATOD abuse and addiction can cause multiple health problems for individuals. Heavy ATOD use has been associated with many problems, including neonates with low birth weight and congenital abnormalities; accidents, homicides, and suicides; chronic diseases, such as cardiovascular diseases, cancer, and lung disease; violence; and family disruption. Factors that contribute to the substance abuse problem include lack of knowledge about the use of drugs; the labeling of certain drugs (alcohol, nicotine, and caffeine) as nondrugs; lack of quality control of illegal drugs; and drug laws that label certain drug users as criminals.

Historical Overview

Psychoactive drug use has been part of most cultures since the beginning of humanity. Often a culture encourages use of some drugs while discouraging the use of others. Caffeine, alcohol, and tobacco are socially acceptable drugs in the United States and Canada, whereas other cultures prohibit their use. Conversely, marijuana, cocaine, and heroin use are not accepted in mainstream U.S. society, although these substances are considered sacred or beneficial and their use is accepted in various other cultures.

The United States' primary solution to various "drug problems" has been prohibition. During alcohol **prohibition** from 1920 to 1933, the United States experienced a sharp increase in violent crime and corruption among law officials secondary to the illicit marketing of alcohol. Distilled beverages were pushed because of the higher profit margin per bottle of liquor than for beer or wine. The high alcohol content in illicit moonshine caused severe health problems. The alcohol prohibition was eventually recognized as a failure and repealed (Rose, 1996).

Similar problems are occurring with the current *War on Drugs* and the newer prohibition on marijuana, cocaine, and other drugs. An increase in violent crime and corruption among law officials as a result of the illicit market is becoming a major national problem. Stronger drugs are pushed because of their greater profits. In the past two decades, the U.S. war on drugs has escalated. New laws have created mandatory sentences for drug offenders, are destroying civil liberties, and are putting most resources into law enforcement rather than drug education and treatment (Baum, 1997; Davis, 1998; Heather et al, 1993; Vallance, 1993) (Fig. 36-1).

From 1993 to 1997, 50% of the drug treatment centers closed, and from 1991 to 1997, 60% of the adolescent treatment centers closed because insurance companies cut back on coverage for addiction treatment (Moyers, 1998). A recently formed group, Physician Leadership on National Drug Policy, has found that drug addiction can be treated with as much success as illnesses such as diabetes, hypertension, and asthma and that treatment is much more cost-effective than putting addicts in prison (Marwick, 1998) (Fig. 36-2). A comparison of two nationwide treatment studies (one from 1979 to 1981 and the other from 1991 to 1993) confirmed the effectiveness of drug abuse treatment, but identified an "alarming drop over time" in support services which address medical, psychological, family, legal, vocational, and financial problems (Mueller and Wyman, 1997).

Attitudes and Myths

Attitudes are developed through cultural learning and personal experiences. Attitudes toward ATOD problems are

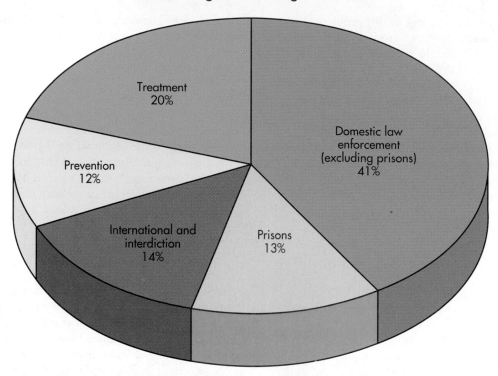

FIG. 36-1 Federal drug control budget for 1998.

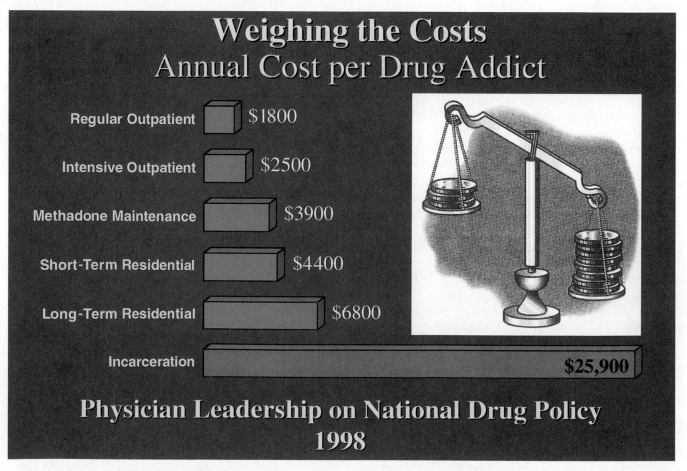

FIG. 36-2 Weighing the costs—annual cost per drug addict. (Prepared by Physician Leadership on National Drug Policy [PLNDP] National Project Office, Brown University Center for Alcohol and Addiction Studies, Providence, Rhode Island, 1998.)

influenced by the way society categorizes drugs as either "good" or "bad." In the United States, good drugs are over-the-counter (OTC) or those prescribed by a health care provider, yet this makes them no less problematic or addictive. Bad drugs are the illegal drugs, and persons who use these drugs are considered criminals regardless of whether the drug has caused any problems.

Americans rely heavily on prescription and OTC drugs to relieve (or mask) anxiety, tension, fatigue, and physical or emotional pain. Rather than learning nonmedicinal methods of coping, many people choose the "quick fix" and take pills to deal with their problems or negative feelings.

Addicts are often viewed as immoral, weak-willed, or irresponsible persons who should try harder to help themselves. Although alcoholism was recognized as a disease by the American Medical Association in 1954 and drug addiction was recognized as a disease some years later, much of the public and many health care professionals have failed to change their attitudes and accept alcoholics and addicts as ill persons in need of health care.

Nurses must examine their attitudes toward ATOD use, abuse, and addiction before working with this health problem. To be therapeutic, the nurse must develop a trusting, nonjudgmental relationship with the client. Systematic assessment for ATOD problems is based on an awareness that there may be problems with legal drugs as well as illegal drugs. If the nurse's attitude toward a client with a drug abuse problem is negative or punitive, the issue may never be directly addressed or the client may be avoided. If the client senses the negative attitude of the health care provider, either by words or tone of voice, communication may cease and information withheld (Tweed, 1989). To develop a therapeutic attitude, the nurse must realize that any drug can be abused, that anyone may develop drug dependence, and that drug addiction can be successfully treated.

Myths develop over years, and if myths are not questioned, many attitudes may be formed based solely on fiction rather than fact. Some common myths are as follows: "An alcoholic is a skid row bum"—less than 5% of persons with addictions fit this description. "If you teach people about drugs, they will abuse them"—although it is true that people may choose to use drugs if they have knowledge about them, it is more likely that people without knowledge about them will abuse them. "Addiction is a sin or moral failing"—addiction is recognized as a health problem involving biopsychosocial factors, and persons who use drugs do not do so with the intent to become addicted.

Paradigm Shift

Hopefully the new millennium will see a major shift in how the United States conceptualizes ATOD problems. The old criminal justice model is based on stereotypes, misinformation, and punishment and uses war tactics to fight the drug users, addicts, and suppliers (fellow citizens). Campaigns have been launched using the slogans "zero tolerance" for drug users, "just say no" to drugs, and striving for a "drug free America"—all of which vilify the drug user or drug addict. This punitive approach to illicit drug use hinders open communication between the health care professional and the drug user. Those who are abusing drugs, experiencing secondary health problems, or possibly becoming addicted may not seek help for fear of being arrested or confined.

The American Public Health Association is currently reviewing the **harm reduction** model, an approach used in Great Britain, the Netherlands, and Australia (Des Jarlais, 1995). This new public health model is based on understanding that addiction is a disease, that any psychoactive drug can be abused, that accurate information can help persons make responsible decisions about drug use, and that persons who have ATOD problems can be helped. This approach accepts the reality that psychoactive drug use is endemic, and subsequently the focus is on pragmatic interventions, especially education to reduce the adverse consequences of drug use and treatment for addicts. The United States has already taken a harm reduction approach with tobacco and alcohol. Educational campaigns are used to inform the public about the health risks of tobacco use. Warnings have appeared on tobacco product labels since 1967 as a result of the Surgeon General's 1966 report on the dangers of smoking. In 1971 a ban on television and radio cigarette advertising was imposed. Cigarette smoking has decreased from 42% of the population in 1965 to 29%, or about 62 million Americans, in 1996 (National Institute on Drug Abuse, 1998c).

Education is beginning to address the dangers of alcohol abuse and establish guidelines for safe alcohol use. Alcohol consumers are choosing lower alcohol-content products such as beer and wine coolers rather than distilled products (Kinney and Leaton, 1995). Nurses have a responsibility to seek the underlying roots of various health problems and plan action that is realistic, nonjudgmental, holistic, and positive, and a harm reduction model for ATOD problems facilitates such an approach.

Definitions

The terms *drug use* and *drug abuse* have virtually lost their usefulness because the public and government have narrowed the term drug to include only illegal drugs, rather than including prescription, over-the-counter (OTC), and legal recreational drugs. The current phrase *alcohol, tobacco, and other drugs (ATOD)* is a reminder that the leading drug problems are with alcohol and tobacco. The term *substance* broadens the scope to include alcohol, tobacco, legal drugs, and even foods. **Substance abuse** is the use of any substance that threatens a person's health or impairs his or her social or economic functioning. This definition is more objective and universal than the government's definition of drug abuse, which is the use of a drug without a prescription or any use of an illegal drug. Although any drug or food can be abused, this chapter focuses on **psy-**

choactive drugs: drugs that affect mood, perception, and thought.

Drug dependence and drug addiction are frequently used interchangeably, but they are not synonymous. **Drug dependence** is a state of neuroadaptation (a physiological change in the central nervous system [CNS]) caused by the chronic, regular administration of a drug in which continued use of the drug becomes necessary to prevent withdrawal symptoms (O'Brien, 1996). This happens when persons are given an opiate such as morphine on a regular basis for pain management. To prevent withdrawal symptoms, the morphine should be gradually tapered rather than abruptly stopped.

Drug addiction is a pattern of abuse characterized by an overwhelming preoccupation with the use (compulsive use) of a drug, securing its supply, and a high tendency to relapse if the drug is removed. Frequently, addicts are physically dependent on a drug, but there also appears to be an added psychological component that causes the intense cravings and subsequent relapse. In general, anyone can develop a drug dependence caused by regular administration of drugs that alter the CNS; however, only 7% to 15% of the drug-using population will develop a drug addiction. The reason some people develop a drug addiction and others do not is not completely understood and continues to be an area of much research.

Alcoholism is addiction to the drug called alcohol. Alcoholism and drug addiction are recognized as illnesses under a biopsychosocial model. Simply stated, the disease concept of addiction and alcoholism identifies them as chronic and progressive diseases in which a person's use of a drug or drugs continues despite problems it causes in any area of life—physical, emotional, social, economical, or spiritual.

PSYCHOACTIVE DRUGS

Although any drug can be abused, ATOD abuse and addiction problems generally involve the psychoactive drugs. Because they can alter emotions, these drugs are used for enjoyment in social and recreational settings and for personal use to self-medicate physical or emotional discomfort. Psychoactive drugs are divided into categories according to their effect on the CNS and the general feelings or experiences the drugs may induce. A pharmacology text will provide detailed information on these drug categories (e.g., depressants, stimulants, and hallucinogens). Often if persons cannot obtain their drug of choice, another drug from the same category will be substituted. For example, a person who cannot drink alcohol may begin using a benzodiazepine as an alternative because both are CNS depressants. Table 36-1 ranks commonly used drugs regarding the severity of withdrawal, the reinforcement potential, degree of tolerance, dependence (addiction) potential, and level of intoxication.

Depressants

Depressants lower the body's overall energy level, reduce sensitivity to outside stimulation, and, in high doses, induce sleep. Low doses of depressants may produce a feeling of stimulation caused by initial sedation of the inhibitory centers in the brain. In general, depressants decrease heart rate, respiration rate, muscular coordination, and energy and dull the senses. Higher doses lead to coma and, if the vital functions shut down, death. Major

TABLE 36-1 Ranking* of Risks of Six Commonly Used Drugs

	WITHDRAWAL		REINFORCEMENT		TOLERANCE		DEPENDENCE		INTOXICATION*	
	NIDA	UCSF	NIDA	UCSF	NIDA	UCSF	NIDA	UCSF	NIDA	UCSF
Nicotine	3	3	4	4	2	4	1	1	5	6
Heroin	2	2	2	2	1	2	2	2	2	2
Cocaine	4	3	1	1	4	1	3	3	3	3
Alcohol	1	1	3	3	3	4	4	4	1	1
Caffeine	5	4	6	5	5	3	5	5	6	5
Marijuana	6	5	5	6	6	5	6	6	4	4

Ranking Scale: 1 = most serious; 6 = least serious.

Ranking by Dr. Jack E. Henningfield of the National Institute on Drug Abuse (NIDA) and Dr. Neal L. Benowitz of the University of California at San Francisco (UCSF).

*Explanation of terms: *withdrawal*, presence and severity of characteristic withdrawal symptoms; *reinforcement*, substance's ability, in human and animal tests, to get users to take it repeatedly and instead of other substances; *tolerance*, amount of substance needed to satisfy increasing cravings and level of plateau that is eventually reached; *dependence (addiction)*, difficulty in ending use of substance, the relapse rate, the percentage of people who become addicted, addict's self-reporting of degree of need for substance and continued use in face of evidence that it causes harm; intoxication-level of intoxication associated with addiction, personal and social damage that substance causes.

From Hilts PJ: Is nicotine addictive? depends on whose criteria you use, *New York Times*, C3, August 2, 1994.

categories include alcohol, barbiturates, benzodiazepines, and the opioids.

Alcohol

Alcohol (ethyl alcohol or ethanol) is the oldest and most widely used psychoactive drug in the world. Approximately 65% of Americans age 18 and older consume alcohol, and approximately 5.2% are alcohol dependent, 8% are problem drinkers, and 9.4% are at-risk drinkers (exceed the recommended guidelines) (Manwell et al, 1997). Alcohol abuse ranks third following coronary diseases and cancer as the major cause of death in the United States. The life expectancy of a person with alcoholism is reduced by 15 years, and mortality is $2\frac{1}{2}$ times greater than that of persons without alcoholism (Kinney and Leaton, 1995).

Alcohol abuse costs billions of dollars in lost productivity, property damage, medical expenses from alcohol-related illnesses and accidents, family disruptions, alcohol-related violence, and neglect and abuse of children. Chronic alcohol abuse exerts profound metabolic and physiological effects on all organ systems. Gastrointestinal (GI) disturbances include inflammation of the GI tract, malabsorption, ulcers, liver problems, and cancers. Cardiovascular disturbances include cardiac dysrhythmias, cardiomyopathy, hypertension, atherosclerosis, and blood dyscrasias. CNS problems include depression, sleep disturbances, memory loss, organic brain syndrome, Wernicke-Korsakoff syndrome, and alcohol withdrawal syndrome. Neuromuscular problems include myopathy and peripheral neuropathy. Males may experience testicular atrophy, sterility, impotence, or gynecomastia, and females who consume alcohol during pregnancy may reproduce neonates with fetal alcohol syndrome (FAS) or fetal alcohol effects (FAE). Some of the metabolic disturbances include hypokalemia, hypomagnesemia, and ketoacidosis. Also, endocrine disturbances may result in pancreatitis or diabetes (National Institute on Alcohol Abuse and Alcoholism, 1997).

The concentration of alcohol in the blood is determined by the concentration of alcohol in the drink, the rate of drinking, the rate of absorption (slower in the presence of food), the rate of metabolism, and a person's weight and gender. The amount of alcohol the liver can metabolize per hour is equal to about $\frac{3}{4}$ ounce of whiskey, 4 ounces of wine, or 12 ounces of beer. Figure 36-3 shows the effects on the CNS as the **blood alcohol concentration (BAC)** increases. However, with chronic consumption, tolerance will develop and a person can reach a high BAC with minimal CNS effects.

Gender affects the BAC because females have less alcohol dehydrogenase activity than men (except for males with chronic alcoholism). Because this enzyme detoxifies alcohol, a deficiency results in a higher bioavailability of alcohol. Consequently, females suffer the long-term effects of alcohol intake at much lower doses in a shorter time span (Frezza et al, 1990; Talashek et al, 1994).

Alcohol use in moderation may provide health benefits by providing mild relaxation and lowering the serum cholesterol (Coate, 1993). *Moderate Drinking* (Kishline, 1994) provides guidelines for achieving the health benefits and reducing the harmful effects.

> **NURSING TIP**
>
> *The National Institute on Alcohol Abuse and Alcoholism recommends the following limitations for persons who drink: For men—no more than two drinks per day. For women—no more than one drink per day. For persons over age 65—no more than one drink per day (1995).*

Barbiturates

Since barbituric acid was discovered in 1864, hundreds of derivatives have been developed. These drugs are generally known as sleeping pills or "downers." High doses help people sleep, and low doses have a calming effect.

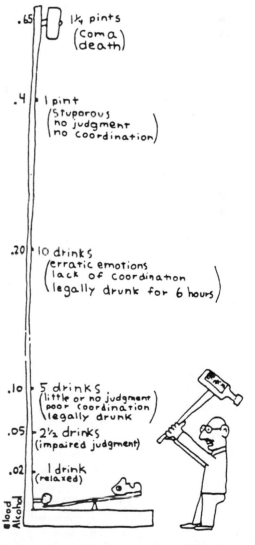

FIG. 36-3 Blood alcohol level and related CNS effects of a normal drinker (160-lb male) according to the number of drinks consumed in 1 hour. (From Kinney J, Leaton G: *Loosening the grip,* ed 5, St Louis, 1995, Mosby.)

The short-acting barbiturates, similar to alcohol in their effects, are frequently abused. These drugs are not as toxic to the body's organ systems as alcohol; however, the tolerance that develops is more dangerous. **Tolerance** (the need for a higher dose to yield the same effect) to the effects on mood develop faster than the physical tolerance to the lethal dose, resulting in a greater risk of accidental overdose. When barbiturates are used in combination with alcohol, a synergistic reaction occurs and the risk of overdose is greatly increased.

Benzodiazepines

Benzodiazepines were introduced in the 1960s and marketed to housewives as the cure for everyday stress. In 1994, more than 80 million benzodiazepine prescriptions were filled, with 1 in 10 Americans reporting use of a benzodiazepine once a year or more for a medical reason other than insomnia (Gold et al, 1995). At one time, diazepam (Valium) and chlordiazepoxide (Librium) were marketed for the treatment of alcoholism, but it soon became apparent that these drugs produced an alcohol-like effect and that persons with alcoholism became addicted to these drugs.

These drugs continue to be misprescribed for long-term therapy rather than treating the underlying stress. The benzodiazepines have a relatively safe therapeutic index (difficult to overdose), but withdrawal can be life threatening.

Opioids

Opiates include the natural drugs found in the opium poppy, namely, opium, morphine, and codeine. Opioids are synthetic drugs, such as heroin (semisynthetic), meperidine, methadone, oxycodone, and propoxyphene, that mimic the effects of the natural opiates. Opiates are by far the most effective drugs for pain relief. Opioid addicts (approximately 0.1 percent of opioid users) take prescription opioid analgesics obtained legally (present with false or exaggerated complaints of pain) or illegally (forged prescriptions or diversion).

The United States has approximately 750,000 to 1 million heroin addicts, and more than 2 million people who have tried it (O'Brien, 1996). The typical heroin addict is male, is from a poor socioeconomic background, and began use between 16 and 19 years of age (Foley, 1993).

Tolerance develops quite readily with opioids and can reach striking levels. Tolerance to one opioid extends to other opioids, and thus **cross-tolerance** can occur. Physical dependence also develops quite quickly; less than 2 weeks of continuous use can cause withdrawal symptoms if not tapered. Chronic abuse of the opioids causes few physiological problems except for constipation. The negative consequences primarily result from their illegal status. Heroin is usually consumed intranasally, subcutaneously, intravenously, or by inhalation and costs $10 to $100 per bag. A "bag" varies in amount and purity, but the purity has increased in the 1990s to 45% or greater, which makes it strong enough to inhale. This encourages some persons to try it who would never inject (O'Brien, 1996).

Stimulants

People use **stimulants** to feel more alert or energetic by activating or exciting the nervous system. An increase in alertness and energy results as the stimulant causes the nerve fibers to release noradrenaline and other stimulating **neurotransmitters.** However, these drugs do not simply give the person more energy; they only make the body expend its own energy sooner and in greater quantities than it normally would.

If used carefully, stimulants are useful and have few negative health effects. The body must be allowed time to replenish itself after use of a stimulant. The "cost" for the "high" is the "down" state following the use of a stimulant: a feeling of sleepiness, laziness, mental fatigue, and possibly depression. Many persons abusing stimulants soon begin a vicious cycle of avoiding the down feeling by taking another dose and can become physically dependent on the stimulant to function. Common stimulants include nicotine, cocaine, caffeine, and amphetamines.

Nicotine

One in five deaths in the United States is attributed to cigarettes (Institute for Health Policy, Brandeis University, 1993). The Centers for Disease Control and Prevention (CDC) estimates more than 430,000 deaths per year are caused by complications of cigarette smoking, including 30% of all heart disease deaths, 90% of all lung cancer victims, and about 90% of all chronic obstructive pulmonary disease deaths (Fiore, 1993; Leshner, 1998). See Fig. 36-4 for cigarette smoking mortality. The *Morbidity and Mortality Weekly Report (*MMWR, July 8, 1994) estimated 1993 smoking-related medical costs at $50 billion. In an analysis of 1987 data, the *Report* found that more than 40% of the total annual medical care expenditures were attributable to smoking. Cancer mortality could be reduced by approximately 25% if smoking were eliminated.

Nicotine, the active ingredient in the tobacco plant, is a particularly toxic drug. To protect itself, the body quickly develops tolerance to the nicotine. If a person smokes regularly, tolerance to nicotine develops within hours, compared with days with heroin or months with alcohol. Pipes and cigars are less hazardous than cigarettes because the harsher smoke discourages deep inhalation. However, pipes and cigars increase the risk of cancer of the lips, mouth, and throat.

Smoke can be inhaled directly by the smoker (**mainstream smoke**), or it can enter the atmosphere from the lighted end of the cigarette and be inhaled by others in the vicinity (**sidestream smoke**). Sidestream smoke contains greater concentrations of toxic and carcinogenic compounds than mainstream smoke. Diseases and conditions associated with smoking include cancer, cardiovascular and pulmonary problems, and perinatal effects. Smoking bans are being adopted with the intent to reduce the discomfort and health hazards among nonsmokers. See the Research Brief about nicotine metabolism and intake.

Nicotine is also used as chewing tobacco or snuff. Marketed as "smokeless tobacco," a wad is put in the mouth

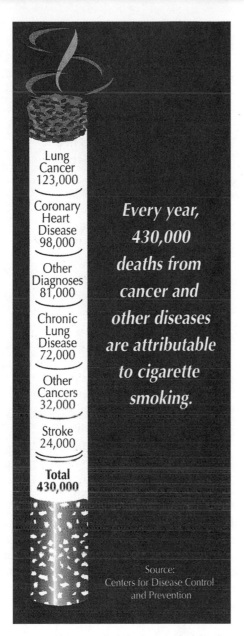

FIG. 36-4 Cigarette smoking mortality. (From Centers for Disease Control and Prevention, Atlanta, Georgia).

RESEARCH *Brief*

Using a sample of 40 black and 39 white smokers, cotinine, a metabolite of nicotine, and nicotine were measured in the urine of smokers after given infusions of deuterium-labeled nicotine and continuing their regular smoking patterns. Both groups were matched by age (mean, 32.5 and 32.3), body weight, and number of cigarettes smoked daily (mean, 14 and 14.7). The total and nonrenal clearance of nicotine was not significantly different in comparing the two groups. The total and nonrenal clearance of cotinine was significantly lower in blacks than in whites. The intake of nicotine per cigarette smoked was estimated to be 30% higher in blacks than in whites based on cotinine levels during smoking and clearance results. Additional testing showed that cotinine half-life was longer, but not significantly, in blacks than in whites indicating varying nicotine metabolism rates.

Blacks in this study had both a slower clearance of cotinine and a higher intake of nicotine per cigarette. Previous studies have shown that a genetic trait that may protect an individual from nicotine addiction may be missing in blacks. These results may help explain why blacks are at higher risk of lung cancer and have higher rates of relapse with smoking cessation strategies.

Perez-Stable EJ et al: Nicotine metabolism and intake in black and white smokers, *JAMA* 280:152, 1998.

could be dissolved in water and used intravenously or orally when mixed in soft drinks. By the early 1900s the common route of administration of the white powder was intranasal "snorting" (Weil and Rosen, 1993).

In the 1970s "freebasing" was introduced. This involved making the hydrochloride salt a more volatile substance using highly flammable substances such as ether to convert the powder to a crystal that could then be smoked in a pipe. By the early 1980s another form of smokeable cocaine was introduced. Cocaine was dissolved in water, mixed with baking soda, and then heated to form rocks, or "crack." Approximately 90% of cocaine users have snorted cocaine, 33% have smoked it, and 10% have injected it (Warner, 1993). Intranasal cocaine has been a popular recreational drug among the rich and famous, but the cheaper crack form, sold in small quantities at $2 to $20, has become popular, particularly among inner-city black populations.

WHAT DO YOU THINK? *More than 400,000 whites use cocaine, compared to 200,000 Hispanics and 48,000 African-Americans (Marwick, 1998). However, 99% of the drug-trafficking defendants in the United States between 1985 and 1987 were African-American (Baum, 1997).*

and the nicotine is absorbed sublingually. Higher doses of nicotine are delivered in the smokeless forms because the nicotine is not destroyed by heat. Nevertheless, this form is less addictive because nicotine enters the bloodstream less directly.

Cocaine

Cocaine comes from the coca shrub found on the eastern slopes of the Andes mountains and has been cultivated by South American Indians for thousands of years. The Indians chew a mixture of the coca leaf and lime to get a mild stimulant effect similar to coffee. By 1860 cocaine was isolated from the plant as a hydrochloride salt. It

Cocaine produces a feeling of intense euphoria, increased confidence, and a willingness to work for long periods. Smoking cocaine gives intense effects because the drug quickly reaches the brain through the blood vessels in the lungs.

Cocaine's interaction with dopamine seems to be the basis for the addictive patterns. The extreme euphoria is believed to be caused by cocaine's effect of dopaminergic stimulation. Chronic administration can lead to neurotransmitter depletion (especially of dopamine), which results in an extreme dysphoria characterized by apathy, sadness, and anhedonia (lack of joy). Thus a cocaine user can get caught up in a dangerous cycle of gaining an extreme high followed by an extreme low and avoiding that low by consuming more cocaine. Crack addiction develops rapidly and is expensive, with addicts needing between $100 and $1000 per day. Addicts soon learn that their ill health and drug use are related, but, overwhelmed by cravings, they may resort to criminal activities (theft or prostitution) to get the drug.

Street cocaine ranges in purity from 5% to 60% and may be cut with other drugs, such as procaine or amphetamine, or any white powder, such as sugar or baby powder. The incidence of cocaine-related emergency room visits increased twelvefold from 1985 to 1992. Some of this increase results from poor quality control; however, most is the result of the use of crack (Weiss et al, 1994). High doses can cause extreme agitation, hyperthermia, hallucinations, cardiac dysrhythmias, pulmonary complications, convulsions, and possibly death (Das and Laddu, 1993; Warner, 1993).

Caffeine

Caffeine is one of the most widely used psychoactive drugs in the world, with a U.S. daily per capita consumption of 211 mg. Caffeine in soft drinks and cold coffee drinks is becoming the drug of choice for American youth. New names such as Surge, Zapped, Jolt, and Outburst and slogans such as "slammin a Dew" (for Mountain Dew) reflect the marketing strategy for "power" drinks aimed at teens (Cordes, 1998).

Caffeine is found in coffee, tea, chocolate, soft drinks, and various medications (Table 36-2). Moderate doses of caffeine from 100 to 300 mg per day increase mental alertness and probably have little negative effect on health. Higher doses can lead to insomnia, irritability, tremulousness, anxiety, cardiac dysrhythmias, and headaches. Regular use of high doses can lead to physical dependence, and the withdrawal symptoms may include headaches, slowness, and occasional depression (Strain et al, 1994). Treating afternoon headaches with analgesics containing caffeine may in reality be preventing a withdrawal symptom from heavy morning coffee consumption.

Amphetamines

Amphetamines are a class of stimulants similar to cocaine, but the effects last longer and the drugs are cheaper. Amphetamines have a chemical structure similar to adrenaline and noradrenaline and are generally used to decrease fatigue, increase mental alertness, suppress appetite, and create a sense of well-being. Amphetamines were issued to American soldiers during World War II to decrease fatigue and increase mental alertness. They are currently popular among truck drivers and college students.

These drugs are taken orally, intranasally, by injection, or they are smoked. When taken intravenously, they quickly induce an intense euphoric feeling (a "rush"). The user may speed for several days (go on a "speed run") and then fall into a deep sleep for 18 or more hours ("crash"). "Ice," a smokeable form of crystallized methamphetamine, was introduced in the late 1980s as an alternative to crack because it can be easily manufactured and the effects last up to 24 hours. Methamphetamine use first appeared in Honolulu and western areas of the continental United States. Use increased in the 1990s in both rural and urban areas of the South and Midwest (National Institute on Drug Abuse, 1998a).

Other drugs containing caffeine, ephedrine, or phenylpropanolamine (singly or in combination), referred to as "look-alikes," gained market attention after access to amphetamines was controlled by prescription. These chemicals are often found in OTC cold remedies as a nasal decongestant and in diet pills (e.g., Dexatrim).

TABLE 36-2 Caffeine Content in Commonly Consumed Substances

SUBSTANCE	CAFFEINE CONTENT (MG)
Coffee (5 oz)	
Brewed	60-180
Instant	30-120
Decaffeinated	1-5
Chocolate	
Cocoa (5 oz)	2-20
Semisweet (1 oz)	5-35
Tea (5 oz)	
Brewed	20-90
Iced	67-76
Soft drink (12 oz)	
Colas	40-45
Mountain Dew	53
Orange, ginger ale, root beer	0
Prescription drugs	
propoxyphene (Darvene)	32.4
Fiorinal	40
ergotamine (Cafergot)	100
Over-the-counter drugs	
Aqua-ban	100
Anacin	32
Excedrin	65
No Doz	100
Vivarin	200

Marijuana

Marijuana (*Cannabis sativa* or *Cannabis indica*) is the most widely used illicit drug in the United States. Estimates of regular users range from 20 to 30 million Americans, and as many as 60% of those between the ages of 18 and 25 years have tried marijuana at some time. Use peaked among high school seniors in the late 1970s, when about 60% reported having used marijuana and nearly 11% reported daily use. By 1997, just under 50% reported having used marijuana, and 5.8% were daily users (Cargo, 1998).

Compared with the other psychoactive drugs, marijuana has little toxicity and is one of the safest therapeutic agents known (Petro, 1997). However, because of its illegal status, there is no quality control and a user may consume contaminated marijuana. Users enjoy a mild euphoria, a relaxed feeling, and an intensity of sensory perceptions. Side effects include dry and reddened eyes, increased appetite, dry mouth, drowsiness, and mild tachycardia. Adverse reactions include anxiety, disorientation, and paranoia.

The greatest physical concern for chronic users is possible damage to the respiratory tract. Tolerance can develop as well as physical dependence; however, the withdrawal symptoms are benign. Addiction can occur for some chronic users and is difficult to treat because the progression tends to be subtle.

Before the *Marihuana Tax Act of 1937*, tincture of cannabis was listed in the *U.S. Pharmacopoeia* through 1941 for such ailments as migraines, spasticity, and dysmenorrhea and in the treatment of heroin or cocaine addiction. In 1970 marijuana was placed in the Schedule I category of drugs by the passage of the *Controlled Substances Act* and has not been available for medicinal use. The only legal access to this medicine has been through the U.S. Food and Drug Administration's (FDA's) Compassionate Investigational New Drug Program. In 1992 this program was closed, and there are only eight remaining legal clients (Mathre, 1997). In response to this complete prohibition, some health care organizations support access to this medication through formal resolutions, including eight state nurses' associations (Arkansas, California, Colorado, Mississippi, North Carolina, New Mexico, New York, and Virginia as of 1998), the National Nurses Society on Addictions (Access to Therapeutic Cannabis, 1995), and the American Public Health Association (Access to Therapeutic Marijuana/Cannabis, 1996).

DID YOU KNOW? *Marijuana contains a group of compounds called cannabinoids. A synthetic oral preparation (dronabinol) of the primary psychoactive cannabinoid, delta-9-tetrahydrocannabinol (THC), is available by prescription as a Schedule II drug. However, new research shows that other non-psychoactive cannabinoids are believed to have more therapeutic value (Mathre, 1997).*

DID YOU KNOW? *Before the marijuana prohibition, cannabis was a popular plant grown for its fiber (hemp), seed (popular birdseed), oil, and medicinal as well as psychoactive properties. During World War II, the hemp fiber was so valuable that farmers were required to grow marijuana to ensure a supply. Hemp fiber and seeds do not contain enough active THC to produce any psychoactive effects and these products are becoming available in the United States.*

Hallucinogens

Also called *psychedelics* (mind vision), **hallucinogens** can produce hallucinations. Many of these drugs have been used for centuries in religious ceremonies and healing rituals and used by many cultures to produce euphoria and as aphrodisiacs. For these drugs, the user's mood, basic emotional makeup, and expectations (set) along with the immediate surroundings (setting) influence the mental effects experienced by the user. The physical effects are more constant and produce CNS stimulation.

The two broad chemical families of hallucinogens are the indole hallucinogens and those that resemble adrenalin and amphetamines. The indoles are related to hormones (serotonin) made in the brain by the pineal gland and include such drugs as lysergic acid diethylamide (LSD), psilocybin, mushrooms, and morning glory seeds. The second group lacks the chemical structure called the indole ring and includes peyote, mescaline and MDMA (Ecstasy). Phencyclidine (PCP) is in a class by itself. LSD and PCP will be discussed.

Lysergic acid diethylamide

LSD is the most well-known drug in the hallucinogen category. It is one of the most potent drugs known, over 3000 times more potent than mescaline (O'Brien, 1996). It is administered orally in small tablets, in gelatin chips ("window panes"), or on pieces of paper soaked with the drug or stamped with ink containing LSD. The effects from a dose of 25 to 300 micrograms can last up to 10 to 12 hours (Weil and Rosen, 1993).

The desired effects include euphoria, a heightened sense of awareness, distorted perceptions, and synesthesia (a mixing of senses, i.e., sounds appearing as visual images). Adverse reactions to LSD include depersonalization, hypertension, panic, and psychosis. Another adverse reaction may be a flashback, or a recurrence of the "trip" weeks or months after the LSD is ingested. Flashbacks can be frightening, especially because of their unpredictability, but will decrease in frequency over time.

Phencyclidine

Phencyclidine (PCP) is a potent anesthetic and analgesic with CNS depressant, stimulant, and hallucinogenic properties. A high incidence of PCP use was seen in the early 1980s primarily in the metropolitan areas of Los Angeles, Washington, D.C., and New York City (Brust, 1993). PCP comes in pill or powder form and has often been sold as mescaline, psilocybin, THC, or other drugs. "Angel dust" is PCP sprinkled on a marijuana joint.

The mental effects vary but often include a feeling of disconnection from the body and reality, apathy, disorganized thinking, a drunk-like state, and distortions of time and space perception. Adverse reactions include combative behavior, inability to talk, a rigid robotic attitude, confusion, paranoid thinking, catatonia, coma, and convulsions. Unlike the other hallucinogens, phencyclidine can be addicting.

Inhalants

Initiation of inhalant use generally occurs during adolescence and from 1990 to 1995, the largest incidence was seen in 14- and 15-year-olds. Currently there are no significant differences between sexes. Forty-three percent of those who reported using in the 1990 to 1995 surveys used inhalants on multiple occasions (Neumark et al, 1998). In the United Kingdom approximately 5% of teenage deaths result from volatile substance abuse, with up to one third of these deaths occurring among first-time users (Ramsey et al, 1995).

The **inhalants** do not fit neatly into other categories but include gases and solvents. The three main types of inhalants are organic solvents, volatile nitrites, and nitrous oxide. These substances are inhaled ("huffed") from bottles, aerosol cans, or soaked cloth or put into bags or balloons to increase the concentration of the inhaled fumes and decrease the inhalation of other substances in the vapor (e.g., paint particles).

Organic solvents include rubber cement, model airplane glue, paint thinner, and aerosol products such as spray paint, deodorant, and hair spray. The effects are similar to alcohol but have a rapid onset and last a short time. The user initially feels stimulated as inhibitions are depressed; then a drunk-like state is experienced and possibly hallucinations. Users may also experience headache, tinnitus, diplopia, abdominal pain, nausea, or vomiting. "Sudden sniffing death" may occur, which appears to be related to acute cardiac dysrhythmia (Dinwiddie, 1994). These drugs are inexpensive and easy to obtain by youth.

Amyl nitrite is the most common of the volatile nitrites and is most often used by urban male homosexuals. It is frequently used during sexual activity to intensify the experience and prolong orgasm. This yellow liquid is packaged in cloth-covered glass capsules that have to be popped (hence the common name of "poppers") to release the drug for inhalation.

Often referred to as laughing gas, nitrous oxide is widely used in dentistry and minor surgery as a tranquilizer to sedate and create an analgesic effect by changing the client's mood and interpretation of pain. Nitrous oxide is also found in whipping cream aerosol cans ("whippets") and is released by spraying the can upside down. Dangers with administration increase when inhaling directly from pressurized tanks because the gas is very cold and can cause frostbite to the nose, lips, and vocal cords. Also, if nitrous oxide is not mixed with oxygen, the user may die from asphyxiation (Espeland, 1993).

PREDISPOSING/CONTRIBUTING FACTORS

In addition to the specific drug being used, two other major variables influence the particular drug experience: set and setting (Weil and Rosen, 1993). To understand various patterns of drug use and abuse by individuals, all three factors (drug, set, and setting) should be considered.

Set

Set refers to the individual using the drug, as well as that individual's expectations, including unconscious expectations, about the drug being used. A person's current health may alter a drug's effects from one day to the next. Some people are genetically predisposed to alcoholism or other drug addiction, and their chemical makeup is such that the disease process is triggered simply by consuming the drug. Persons with underlying mood disorders or other mental illness may try to self-medicate with psychoactive drugs. Sometimes their choice of drug may exacerbate their symptoms, as with a depressed person consuming alcohol and becoming more depressed.

With psychoactive drugs the user may not notice any mind-altering effects with medicinal use. This may happen to a child with cancer using marijuana to stop the nausea and vomiting secondary to the chemotherapy. However, an older person using marijuana for the same reason, who believes the stories that marijuana causes insanity, may experience an exacerbation of the sensory effects secondary to their expectations.

Setting

Setting is the influence of the physical, social, and cultural environment within which the use occurs. Social conditions influence the use of drugs. The fast pace of life, competition at school or in the workplace, and the pressure to accumulate material possessions are daily stressors. Pharmaceutical, alcohol, and tobacco companies are continuously bombarding the public with enticing advertisements pushing their products as a means of feeling better, sleeping better, having more energy, or just as a "treat." People grow up believing that most of life's problems can be solved quickly and easily through the use of a drug.

For persons of a lower socioeconomic background and with minimal education or employment possibilities, many of life's opportunities may seem out of reach. For these people, psychoactive drug use may offer a way to numb the pain or escape from their hopeless reality. These people rarely seek relief through a physician's prescription or other therapeutic measures. Instead, they rely on alcohol or illicit drugs, which are more readily available. For some, illicit drug dealing may appear to be the only way out of the poverty and unemployment path.

Biopsychosocial Model of Addiction

Many theories exist on the etiological factors of addiction, and no consensus exists on specific causes. The underlying etiological factors include the belief that addiction is a disease, a moral failing, a psychological disturbance, a personality disorder, a social problem, a dysbehaviorism, or a maladaptive coping mechanism. Different people develop addiction in different ways. For example, some alcoholics say, "I knew I was an alcoholic from my first drink; I drank differently than others." Others have no family history of addiction, but when stressed (chronic pain, significant losses, or abusive relationships resulting in low self-esteem) they find that drugs may temporarily relieve their stress. Over time, heavy use of one or more drugs to cope with the stress may lead to addiction. Current research is focusing on the neurochemistry of addiction, which shows actual brain chemistry changes among addicts. The biopsychosocial model provides a framework to understand addiction as the result of the interaction of multiple factors.

PRIMARY PREVENTION AND THE ROLE OF THE NURSE

The harm reduction approach to substance abuse puts the focus on health promotion and disease prevention. Primary prevention for ATOD problems includes 1) the promotion of healthy lifestyles and resiliency factors and 2) education about drugs and guidelines for use. Nurses are ideally prepared to use health promotion strategies such as promoting and facilitating healthy alternatives to indiscriminate, careless, and often dangerous drug use practices and providing education about drugs to decrease harm from irresponsible or unsafe drug use.

Promotion of Healthy Lifestyles and Resiliency Factors

Assisting clients to achieve optimal health includes identifying interventions other than or in addition to the use of drugs whenever possible. Teaching assertiveness and decision-making skills helps clients increase self-responsibility for health and increase their awareness of the various options.

Nagging health problems such as difficulty sleeping, muscle tension, lack of energy, chronic stress, and mood swings are common reasons people turn to medications, especially the psychoactive drugs. Nurses can help clients understand that medications mask problems rather than solving them. Stress reduction and relaxation techniques along with a balanced lifestyle can address these problems more directly than medications (Dodge, 1991; Rassool and Winnington, 1993). Lack of sleep, improper diet, and lack of exercise contribute to many health complaints. Assisting clients to balance their rest, nutrition, and exercise on a daily basis can reduce these complaints. Nurses can provide useful information to groups, assisting the develop-

ment of community recreational resources, or facilitating stress reduction, relaxation, or exercise groups. Nurses can help persons increase their awareness of drug-free community activities. Listed below are community-based activities in which the nurse may become involved.

DID YOU KNOW? *The National Nurses Society on Addictions (NNSA), through a grant by the U.S. Center for Substance Abuse Prevention (CSAP), offers primary prevention workshops for nurses and has an independent-study program available for purchase (Jack and Snow, 1994). The workshops and independent study highlight community involvement and cultural diversity issues.*

HOW TO *Set Up Community-Based Activities Aimed at Substance Abuse Prevention*

- *Increase involvement and pride in school activities*
- *Organize student assistant programs (students helping students)*
- *Organize a Students Against Drunk Driving (SADD) chapter*
- *Mobilize parent awareness and action groups (e.g., MADD)*
- *Increase availability of recreation facilities*
- *Encourage parental commitment to nondrinking parties*
- *Encourage religious institutions to convey nonuse messages and provide activities associated with nonuse*
- *Curtail media messages that glamorize drug and alcohol use*
- *Support and reinforce antidrug use peer pressure skills*
- *Provide general health screenings, including ATOD use*
- *Collaborate among community leaders to solve problems related to crime, housing, jobs, and access to health care*

Lack of educational opportunities, job training, or both can contribute to socioeconomic stress and poor self-esteem, which can lead to drug use to escape the situation. Nurses can help clients identify community resources and solve problems to meet basic needs rather than avoid them.

In addition to decreasing risk factors associated with ATOD problems, it is important to increase protective or resiliency factors. Children from high-risk environments who survive successfully have more resiliency factors than do those who do not survive (Kumpfer and Hopkins, 1993). Prevention guidelines to teach parents and teachers how to increase resiliency in youth include the following strategies:

- Empower them to develop an increased sense of responsibility for their own success
- Help them to identify their talents

- Motivate them to dedicate their lives to helping society rather than believing that their only purpose in life is to be consumers
- Provide realistic appraisals and feedback; stress multicultural competence; encourage and value education and skills training
- Increase cooperative solutions to problems rather than competitive or aggressive solutions.

Drug Education

ATOD problems include more than abuse of psychoactive drugs. Today more than 450,000 different drugs and drug combinations are available, and prescription drugs are involved in almost 60% of all drug-related emergency room visits and 70% of all drug-related deaths. Approximately 25% of elderly hospital admissions result from problems related to noncompliance and drug reactions (Larrat et al, 1990).

Nurses are experts in medication administration and understand the potential dangers of indiscriminant drug use and the inherent inability of drugs to "cure" all problems. Nurses can influence the health of clients by destroying the myth of good drugs versus bad drugs. This means teaching clients that no drug is completely safe and that any drug can be abused and helping persons learn how to make informed decisions about their drug use to minimize the potential harm.

Drug technology is growing, yet the public receives little information about how to safely use this technology. Harm reduction as a goal recognizes that people consume drugs and that they need to know about the use of drugs and risks involved in order to make responsible decisions about their drug use. Drug education should begin on an individual basis by reviewing the client's prescription medications. Because a physician or nurse practitioner has prescribed the medication, clients often presume there is little risk involved.

Is the client aware of any untoward interactions this drug may have with other drugs being used or with food? A common occurrence with drug users is the use of drugs from different categories used together or at different times to regulate how they feel, known as **polysubstance use or abuse.** For example, a person may drink alcohol when snorting cocaine to "take the edge off"; or some intravenous drug users combine cocaine with heroin (speedball) for similar reasons. Polysubstance use can cause drug interactions that can have additive, synergistic, or antagonistic effects. Indiscriminant polysubstance abuse may lead to serious physiological consequences and can be complicated for the health care professional to assess and treat.

People need to know what questions to ask regarding their personal drug use and should be encouraged to seek the answers to these questions before using any drug. Encouraging clients to ask questions regarding their drug use can increase their responsibility for personal health as well as increase their awareness that drugs will alter their body chemistry. Below are seven questions that can assist clients in obtaining the essential information necessary to decrease the possible harm from unsafe medication consumption.

HOW TO *Determine the Relative Safety of a Drug for Personal or Client Use*

Before using a drug/medication always determine:
- *The chemical being taken*
- *How and where the drug works in the body*
- *The correct dosage*
- *Whether there will be drug interactions*
- *If there are allergic reactions*
- *If there will be drug tolerance*
- *If the drug will produce physical dependence**

*Caution: Approximately 10% of the population may suffer from the disease of addiction. For them, responsible use of psychoactive drugs is limited secondary to their disease. They need to notify their physician of the addiction if use of psychoactive medicines is being considered in treatment.

From Miller M: *Drug consumer safety rules*, Mosier, Ore, 1994, Mothers Against Misuse and Abuse.

Nurses can identify various references and community resources available to provide the necessary information, and they can clarify the information. User-friendly reference texts are available that offer information about drug interactions among medications, other drugs (including alcohol, tobacco, marijuana, and cocaine), and other substances (food and beverages), and serve as an excellent guide for the nurse as well as for the client's personal and family use (Griffith, 1998; Rybacki and Long, 1999).

As people learn to ask questions about their prescription medications, the nurse can encourage them to ask the same questions regarding self-administration of OTC and recreational drugs. This does not mean that nurses should encourage other drug use but rather that the potential harm from self-medication can be reduced if clients have the necessary information to make more informed decisions.

As parents learn to seek information regarding their use of medications, they begin to act as role models for their children. It can be confusing for children and adolescents to be told to "just say no" to drugs while they see their parents or drug advertisements try to "quick fix" every health complaint with a medication.

The simple "just say no" approach does not help young people for several reasons. First, children are naturally curious, and drug experimentation is often a part of normal development (Shedler and Block, 1990). Second, children from dysfunctional homes often use drugs to obtain attention or to escape an intolerable environment. And finally, the "just say no" approach does not address the powerful influence of peer pressure (Donaldson et al, 1994).

Drug education has moved into the school curriculum, with Project DARE (Drug Abuse Resistance Education) the most widely used school-based drug-use prevention

BOX 36-1 The Evolution of Prevention

Prevention approaches have evolved since the 1960s, when there was a high level of illegal drug use. The first response was to use scare tactics. Drugs were shown as harmful, and the information was often exaggerated or inaccurate. Information from peers often invalidated these scare tactics and caused distrust of the "experts." During the early 1970s, some professionals began using the strategy of giving accurate information to young people. This strategy may have increased usage rates, creating educated drug users. By the late 1970s, the focus was on teaching young people life skills, which included personal self-awareness, independent living, job skills, and communication skills. In the early 1980s, healthy alternatives to ATOD use looked at natural highs through recreational experiences. Also in the 1980s, emphasis was placed on changing policies to decrease drug use. These policy changes centered around legislative and law enforcement efforts. By the late 1980s community involvement, which attempted to bring societal pressure to bear on the problem, was begun. The strategy for the 1990s was a comprehensive approach that combined all of the previous approaches with the exception of scare tactics.

From Nurse Training Course, "Prevention of Alcohol, Tobacco, and Other Drugs," developed by the National Nurses Society on Addictions, Macro International Inc, and J & E Associates, under contract by the Center for Substance Abuse Prevention, 1994.

program in the United States. This program uses law enforcement officers to teach the material, but recent studies find that it is less effective than other interactive prevention programs and may even result in increased drug use (Ennett et al, 1994). Basic ATOD prevention programs for young people should combine efforts to increase resiliency factors with drug education. Nurses can serve as educators or as advisors to the school systems or community groups to ensure all of these areas are addressed. Role-playing is useful in teaching many of these skills. Box 36-1 provides an historical overview of the prevention approaches.

SECONDARY PREVENTION AND THE ROLE OF THE NURSE

To identify substance abuse and plan appropriate interventions, nurses must assess each client individually. When drug abuse, dependence, or addiction is identified, nurses must assist clients to understand the connection between their drug use patterns and the negative consequences on their health, their families, and the community.

Assessing for ATOD Problems

Assessing for substance abuse problems should be included in health assessments. An assessment of self-medication practices as well as recreational drug use should be done at the time of the medication history. This puts all relevant drug use history together and aids in the assessment of drug use patterns. When working with a client over time, periodic assessment of drug use patterns will alert the nurse to any changes requiring intervention.

After obtaining a medication history, follow-up questions can determine if problems exist. For prescription drug use, is the client following the directions correctly? Nurses should inquire about any prescribed psychoactive drug use: How long has the client been taking the drug? Has the client increased the dosage or frequency above the prescription?

When assessing self-medication and recreational or social drug use patterns, nurses should determine the reason for use. Some underlying health problems (e.g., pain, stress, weight, or insomnia) may be alleviated by nonpharmaceutical interventions. Nurses should ask about the amount, frequency, duration of use, and route of administration of each drug. Nursing tip: Think of "the 4 Hs" to remember what to ask when assessing drug use patterns: How taken (route), How much, How often, and How long.

To establish the presence of a substance abuse problem, determine if the drug use is causing any negative health consequences or problems with relationships, employment, finances, or the legal system. Below are examples of questions to ask to determine the presence of socioeconomical problems that are often secondary to substance abuse.

HOW TO *Assess Socioeconomical Problems Secondary to Substance Abuse*

If the client admits to use of alcohol, tobacco or other drugs, ask the following questions:
1. *Do your spouse, parents, or friends worry or complain about your drinking or using drugs?*
2. *Has a family member gone for help about your drinking or using drugs?*
3. *Have you neglected family obligations secondary to drinking or using drugs?*
4. *Have you missed work because of your drinking or using drugs?*
5. *Does your boss complain about your drinking or using drugs?*
6. *Do you drink or use drugs before or during work?*
7. *Have you ever been fired or quit secondary to drinking or using drugs?*
8. *Have you ever been charged with driving under the influence (DUI) or drunk in public (DIP)?*
9. *Have you ever had any other legal problems related to drinking and using drugs, such as assault and battery, breaking and entering, or theft?*
10. *Have you had any accidents while intoxicated, such as falls, burns, or motor vehicle accidents?*
11. *Have you spent your money on alcohol or other drugs instead of paying your bills (telephone, electricity, rent, etc.)?*

If there is a pattern of chronic, regular, and frequent use of a drug, nurses should assess for a history of withdrawal symptoms to determine if there is physical dependence on

Use of Alcohol, Tobacco and Other Drugs in Canada

Pat Sanagan, Toronto Public Health
Maureen Cava, Toronto Public Health and University of Toronto

The Canadian approach to substance abuse prevention builds on the desire to provide a balance among prevention, intervention, treatment, and legislation. Canada recognizes that drug use needs to acknowledge multiple realities: that poverty, racism, homelessness, and other systemic issues play a large role in drug-related problems and that developing appropriate prevention and treatment programs is needed. This is balanced with the concerns around supply and a legislative framework to reduce drug trafficking.

Health Canada's *Drug Strategy* (1998) acknowledges the complexity of drug use and has a long-term goal to reduce the harm associated with alcohol and other drugs to individuals, families, and communities.

CANADIAN STATISTICS

The most recent statistics about Canadian drug use contained in *Canada's Alcohol and Other Drugs Survey* (Health Canada, 1995) indicate an overall drop in substance use between 1984 and 1994, with some areas to watch, one being cannabis use and another being injecting behaviour. Tobacco use had declined significantly until 1989, when rates stabilised. At least one province has noted increased rates in use by young people of 5% to 7% since 1991 (Ontario Tobacco Research Unit, 1998). Several provinces survey student drug use every two years. The most recent reports from Ontario and Nova Scotia (Adlaf, Ivis, and Smart, 1997; Government of Nova Scotia, 1998) indicate that, while previous surveys showed an increase in cannabis use, this had slowed, while binge-drinking and some hallucinogen use among young people had increased.

CANADIAN COSTS

The Canadian Centre on Substance Abuse (1996) estimates that substance abuse costs more than $18.45 billion annually in Canada, representing $649 per capita. Tobacco and alcohol account for the greatest percentage of these costs, with tobacco costs estimated at $9,559.8 million, alcohol at $7,522.1 million, and illicit drugs at $1,371.0 million in 1992.

CANADIAN RESPONSE

Canadian community health nurses are involved in health promotion and disease prevention related to substance use at the individual, family, aggregate, and community level.

Strategies are targeted at primary, secondary, and tertiary prevention. Primary prevention includes development of programs and policies dealing with the effect of advertising, taxation, and labeling on tobacco, alcohol, over-the-counter medication, and herbal use. Strategies for secondary prevention include working with at-risk groups, developing appropriate and effective harm reduction programs, and assessment and referral interventions. Tertiary prevention initiatives include collaboration with treatment centres to ensure comprehensive client aftercare, and advocacy to provide treatment options to recognize a range of needs.

EMERGING SUBSTANCE USE ISSUES FOR CANADIAN COMMUNITY HEALTH NURSES

Three key substance use issues are emerging that Canadian nurses should focus on:
1. The development of "Low-risk Drinking Guidelines" for groups at risk (Walsh, Bondy, and Rehm, 1998).
2. The increase in HIV/AIDS and Hepatitis B and C in drug users in communities across Canada, but particularly in Vancouver, Ottawa, and Montreal (Armstrong, 1998).
3. The relationship between poverty, homelessness, mental illness, and addiction (Golden, 1999).

Bibliography
Adlaf E, Ivis F, Smart R: *Ontario student drug use survey 1977-1997*, Ontario, 1997, Centre for Addiction and Mental Health, ARF Division Document Series No. 136.
Armstrong R: Searching for bargains and doing more with less, *Canadian AIDS News* 10(2):2, 1998.
Golden A: *Taking responsibility for homelessness: an action plan for Toronto*, Toronto, 1999, City of Toronto.
Government of Nova Scotia: *Nova Scotia student drug use survey*, Halifax, Nova Scotia, 1998, Author.
Health Canada: *Canada's alcohol and other drugs survey*, Ottawa, 1995, Author.
Health Canada: *Canada's drug strategy*. Ottawa, 1998, The Office of Alcohol Drugs and Dependency Issues.
Ontario Tobacco Research Unit: *Monitoring the Ontario tobacco strategy: progress toward our goals*, Fourth Annual Monitoring Report, Toronto, 1998, Ontario Tobacco Research Unit.
Single E et al: *The costs of substance abuse in Canada: a cost estimation study*, Toronto, 1996, Canadian Centre on Substance Abuse and the Centre for Addiction and Mental Health (ARF Division).
Walsh G, Bondy S, Rehm J: Review of Canadian low-risk drinking guidelines and their effectiveness, *Canadian Journal of Public Health*, 89(4):241, 1998.

Canadian spelling is used.

the drug. A progression in drug use patterns and related problems warns about the possibility of addiction.

Denial is a primary symptom of addiction. Methods of denial include lying about use, minimizing use patterns, blaming or rationalizing, intellectualizing, changing the subject, using anger or humor, and "going with the flow" (agreeing there is a problem, stating behavior will change, but not demonstrating any behavior changes). Suspect a problem if the client becomes defensive or exhibits other behavior indicating denial when asked about alcohol or other drug use.

Drug Testing

During the 1980s preemployment or random drug testing in the workplace gained popularity. Drug testing can be done by examining a person's urine, blood, saliva, breath (alcohol), or hair. The most common method of drug screening is urine testing. Urine testing only indicates past use of certain drugs, not intoxication. Thus persons can be identified as having used a certain drug in the recent past, but the degree of intoxication and extent of performance impairment cannot be determined with urine testing. Also, most drug-related problems in the workplace are due to alcohol, and alcohol is not always included in a urine drug screen. Other problems with urine testing include using it as a tool of intimidation, false positives, invasion of privacy, and not being cost effective.

When is drug testing appropriate? Drug testing secondary to documented impairment may help to substantiate the cause of the impairment and serve as a backup rather than the primary screening method. It is also useful for recovering addicts. Part of their treatment is to abstain from psychoactive drug use; therefore a urine test yielding positive results for a drug indicates a relapse.

Blood, breath, and saliva drug tests can indicate current use and amount. Any of these tests can help to determine alcohol intoxication, and they often are used to substantiate suspected impairment. A serum drug screen can be useful when overdose is suspected to determine the specific drug ingested. The testing of hair is gaining attention because the results can provide a long history of drug use patterns.

Employee assistance programs (EAPs) are being established in work settings, with at least 30% of U.S. workers having access to an EAP. Roughly 86% of work sites with 5000 or more employees have EAPs (Callery, 1994). These programs can identify health problems among employees and offer counseling or referral to other health care providers as necessary. EAPs provide early identification of and intervention for substance abuse problems; they also offer services to employees to reduce stress and provide health care or counseling so that they may prevent substance abuse problems from developing. Nurses frequently develop and run these programs.

High-Risk Groups

Identifying high-risk groups helps nurses design programs to meet specific needs and to mobilize community resources.

Adolescents

The younger a person is when beginning intensive experimentation with drugs, the more likely dependence will develop. Heavy drug use during adolescence can interfere with normal development. Note that *Healthy People 2000* Objectives 3.5 and 4.5 refer to delay of the initiation of use of tobacco, alcohol, and marijuana.

Reports from annual high school drug surveys monitor the national trends among youth, including data on lifetime use, recent use, and daily use. Regarding lifetime use from the 1997 survey, by the eighth grade 53.8% have tried alcohol, 47.3% smoked cigarettes, 22.6% tried marijuana,

and 4.4% tried cocaine. By twelfth grade, about 81.7% have used alcohol, 65.4% smoked cigarettes, 49.6% used marijuana, and 8.7% tried cocaine (National Institute on Drug Abuse, 1998b). These figures are probably low in that they do not include high-school dropouts.

Family-related factors (genetics, family stress, parenting styles, child victimization) appear to be the greatest variable which influences substance abuse among adolescents. The co-occurrence with psychiatric disorders (especially mood disorders) and behavioral problems are also associated with substance abuse among adolescents, leaving peer pressure as a lesser influential factor. Research suggests that successful social influence-based prevention programs may be driven by their ability to foster social norms that reduce an adolescent's social motivation to begin using ATOD. The most effective treatment approach for adolescents appears to be the use of family-oriented therapy (Weinberg et al, 1998).

Elderly persons

Elderly persons (65 years of age and older) represent 13% of the U.S. population and are the fastest growing segment of U.S. society, expected to represent 21% by the year 2030. They consume more prescribed and over-the-counter medications than any other age group. Approximately 27% of all tranquilizer prescriptions and 38% of hypnotic prescriptions in 1991 were written for older adults. Alcohol and prescription drug misuse affects as many as 17% of adults age 60 and older. Problems with alcohol consumption, including interactions with prescribed and over-the-counter drugs, far outnumber any other substance abuse problem among the elderly (Center for Substance Abuse Treatment, 1998).

The increased use of prescription drugs and alcohol by elderly persons may be related to coping problems. Problems of relocation, possible loss of independence, retirement, illness, death of friends, and lower levels of achievement contribute to feelings of sadness, boredom, anxiety, and loneliness. Factors such as slowed metabolic turnover of drugs, age-related organ changes, enhanced drug sensitivities, a tendency to use drugs over long periods, and a more frequent use of multiple drugs all contribute to greater negative consequences from drug use among the elderly population.

Often alcohol abuse is not identified because its effects on cognitive abilities may mimic changes associated with normal aging or degenerative brain disease. Also, depression may simply be attributed to the more frequent losses rather than the depressant effects of alcohol, and the elderly person may subsequently receive medical treatment for depression rather than alcoholism.

IV drug users

In addition to the problem of addiction, intravenous (IV) drug users are at risk for other health complications. IV administration of drugs always carries a greater risk of overdose because the drug goes directly into the bloodstream. With illicit drugs the danger is increased because the exact dosage is unknown. In addition, the drug may be contaminated with other chemicals that can cause negative consequences. Often IV drug users make their own solution for IV administration and any particles present can result in complications from emboli.

The sharing of needles has been a common practice among addicts. The spread of human immunodeficiency virus (HIV) through needle sharing is a public health risk. Hepatitis and other bloodborne diseases can also be transmitted through contaminated needles. Infections and abscesses may develop secondary to dirty needles or poor administration techniques.

Injection drug users (those who self-administer intravenously or subcutaneously) represent the most rapidly growing source of new AIDS cases and are at the greatest risk for spread of the virus in the heterosexual community. Primarily because of this trend, emphasis is being placed on reducing the transmission of this disease through contaminated needles. Abstinence is ideal but unrealistic for many addicts. Using the harm reduction model, the nurse should provide education on use of bleach to clean needles between use and needle exchange programs to decrease the spread of the virus. Studies indicate that needle exchange programs have not increased injection drug abuse but have, in fact, increased the number of people entering treatment programs (Schwartz, 1993).

Drug use during pregnancy

Most drugs can negatively affect a fetus. Thus the use of any drug during pregnancy should be discouraged unless medically necessary. *Healthy People 2000* Objectives 14.4 and 14.10 address this issue. **Fetal alcohol syndrome (FAS)** has been identified as the third leading cause of birth defects and the leading cause of mental retardation in the United States (Cordero et al, 1994; Peterson and Lowe, 1992). Although it appears an epidemic of drug use (other than alcohol) occurred among pregnant women during the 1980s, with a leveling off between 1988 and 1990, both the size and severity of the epidemic have been overstated. The National Hospital Discharge Survey found that about half (53%) of the discharged infants of drug-using parturient women were drug-affected newborns (Dicker and Leighton, 1994). See the Research Brief about use of illicit drugs by pregnant women.

Despite the increased focus on drug abuse interventions, many pregnant women with drug problems do not receive the help they need. This may be a result of ignorance, poverty, lack of concern for the fetus, lack of available services, and fear of the consequences. The fear of criminal prosecution may push addicted women farther away from the health care system, cause them to conceal their drug use from medical providers, and cause them to deliver their babies in out-of-hospital settings, thus further jeopardizing the pregnancy outcome (Chavkin and Kandall, 1990; Fiesta, 1991; Hutchings, 1993; Kain et al, 1993).

WHAT DO YOU THINK? *In some states, pregnant women who are using illicit drugs are reported to child protective services because of the potential harm to the fetus. Will this practice do more harm than good? What about women who drink alcohol or smoke cigarettes?*

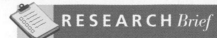

RESEARCH *Brief*

The purpose of the study was to identify infant and maternal outcomes associated with self-reported illicit drug use during pregnancy and to determine whether illicit polydrug use before pregnancy caused added risk to the mother or infant. Participants were identified from newborn referrals to the local visiting nurses association and unrestricted birth certificates over a 3-month study period in a city outside of Boston. Of 360 mothers contacted, 284 (78.9%) agreed to participate. Data were collected using an interview schedule designed for this study and were analyzed using descriptive statistics and logistic regression. Of the subjects, 26.8% reported using any illicit drug, 22.5% reported marijuana use, and 10.6% reported cocaine use during pregnancy.

Pregnant users of illicit drugs had a 120% greater risk of experiencing premature birth, precipitous labor, low weight gain, placental abruption, and/or vaginal bleeding than nonusers. Infants of the drug users had a 180% greater risk of being small for gestational age, having low birth weight, having early gestational age, and/or being shaky or jittery. The use of drugs before pregnancy but not during pregnancy was not associated with any negative maternal or fetal outcome.

Nurses can identify women who are illicit drug users and provide outreach and treatment to ensure future low-risk pregnancies. This study describes specific implications for home health nurses.

Mahoney DL: Infant and maternal outcomes associated with self-reported illicit drug use during pregnancy, *J Addictions Nurs* 10(3):115, 1998.

Use of illicit drugs

The solution of "just say no" is both simplistic and misleading. Indiscriminant use of "good" drugs has caused more health problems from side effects, adverse reactions, drug interactions, dependence, addiction, and overdoses than use of "bad" drugs. However, the war on drugs focuses on illicit drugs and punishes illicit drug users. The black market associated with illicit drug use puts otherwise law-abiding citizens in close contact with criminals, prevents any quality control of the drugs, increases the risk of acquired immunodeficiency syndrome (AIDS) and hepatitis secondary to needle sharing, and hinders health care professionals' accessibility to the abuser or addict.

Lack of quality control (unknown strength and purity) can cause unexpected overdoses or secondary effects of the impurities. A synthetic analog of fentanyl (3-methylfentanyl) marketed as "heroin" is 6000 times as potent as morphine. Unsafe administration (contaminated needles) lead to local and systemic infections. The high cost on the black market leads to crime to support the addiction.

WHAT DO YOU THINK? *Antiprohibitionists believe that the prohibiton of drugs causes greater societal problems than the use of those drugs and that the government has no right to forbid adults from what they choose to ingest. Although antiprohibitionists are often called "legalizers," this label is misleading because it implies that by "legalizing" a drug, the government is condoning its use. Do you understand the difference between the terms? If some drugs should be prohibited, who should decide which drugs to prohibit? Should persons be incarcerated because they have consumed a prohibited drug?*

Codependency and Family Involvement

Drug addiction is often referred to as a family disease, with one in four Americans experiencing family problems related to alcohol abuse. A recent study shows that 52.9% of Americans age 18 and older have a family history of alcoholism among first- or second-degree relatives (Dawson and Grant, 1998). People in a close relationship with the addict often develop unhealthy coping mechanisms to continue the relationship. This behavior is known as **codependency,** a stress-induced preoccupation with the addicted person's life, leading to extreme dependence and excessive concern with the addict (Talashek et al, 1994).

Strict rules typically develop in a codependent family to maintain the relationships: don't talk, don't feel, don't trust, don't lose control, and don't seek help from outside the family. Codependents try to meet the addict's needs at the expense of their own. Codependency may underlie many of the medical complaints and emotional stress seen by health care providers such as ulcers, skin disorders, migraine headaches, chronic colds, and backaches.

When the addicted person refuses to admit the problem, the family continues to adapt to emotionally survive the stress of the addict's irrational, inconsistent, and unpredictable behavior. Members of the family will consequently develop various roles that tend to be gross exaggerations of normal family roles. Members cling irrationally to these roles, even when they are no longer functional.

One of the most significant roles a family member may assume is that of an enabler. **Enabling** is the act of shielding or preventing the addict from experiencing the consequences of the addiction. As a result the addict does not always understand the cost of the addiction and thus is "enabled" to continue to use.

Although codependency and enabling are closely related, a person does not have to be codependent to enable. Anyone can be an enabler: a police officer, a boss or coworker, and even a drug treatment counselor. Nurses who do not address the negative health consequences of the drug use with the addicted person are enablers.

The nurse can assist families to recognize the problem of addiction and help them confront the addicted member in a caring manner. Whether or not the addicted family

BOX 36-2 Brief Interventions Using the FRAMES Acronym

- *Feedback.* Provide the client direct feedback about the potential or actual personal risk or impairment related to drug use.
- *Responsibility.* Emphasize personal responsibility for change.
- *Advice.* Provide clear advice to change risky behavior.
- *Menu.* Provide a menu of options or choices for changing behavior.
- *Empathy.* Provide a warm, reflective, empathetic, and understanding approach.
- *Self-efficacy.* Provide encouragement and belief in the client's ability to change.

Adapted from Bien TH, Miller WR, Tonigan JS: Brief interventions for alcohol problems: a review, *Addictions* 88:315, 1993.

member is agreeable to treatment, the family members should be given some guidance about the literature and services that are available to help them cope more effectively. The nurse can help identify treatment options, counseling assistance, financial assistance, support services, and (if necessary) legal services for the family members. Children of ATOD abusers or addicts are themselves at a greater risk for developing addiction and must be targeted for primary prevention.

TERTIARY PREVENTION AND THE ROLE OF THE NURSE

The nurse is in a pivotal position to help the addict and the addict's family. The nurse's knowledge of community resources and how to mobilize them can significantly influence the quality of care clients receive.

Many people with alcoholism and drug addiction become lost in the health care system. If satisfactory care is not provided in one agency or the waiting list is months long, the person may give up rather than seek alternative sources of care. The nurse who knows the client's history, environment, support systems, and the local treatment programs can offer guidance to the most effective treatment modality. **Brief interventions** by health care professionals who are not treatment experts are effective in helping ATOD abusers and addicts reduce their consumption or follow through with treatment referrals (Bien et al, 1993; Center for Substance Abuse Treatment, 1997; Minicucci, 1994). Box 36-2 describes six elements commonly included in brief interventions using the acronym FRAMES.

Strategies used with clients may vary depending on their readiness for change. Understanding the stages of change listed in Box 36-3 and recognizing which stage a client is in are important factors in determining which interventions and programs may be most helpful to the client (Center for Substance Abuse Treatment, 1997; Prochaska et al, 1992).

BOX 36-3 Stages of Change

PRECONTEMPLATION

At this stage the person does not intend to change in the foreseeable future. The person is often unaware of any problem. Resistance to recognizing or modifying a problem is the hallmark of precontemplation.

CONTEMPLATION

At this stage the individual is aware that a problem exists and is seriously thinking about overcoming it but has not yet made a commitment to take action. The nurse can encourage the individual to weigh the pros and cons of the problem and the solution to the problem.

PREPARATION

Preparation was originally referred to as decision making. At this stage the individual is prepared for action and may reduce the problem behavior but has not yet taken effective action (e.g., cuts down amount of smoking but does not abstain).

ACTION

At this stage the individual modifies his or her behavior, experiences, or environment to overcome the problem. The action requires considerable time and energy. Modification of the target behavior to an acceptable criterion and significant overt efforts to change are the hallmarks of action.

MAINTENANCE

In this stage the individual works to prevent relapse and consolidate the gains attained during action. Stabilizing behavior change and avoiding relapse are the hallmarks of maintenance.

Adapted from Prochaska JO, DiClemente CC, Norcross JC: In search of how people change: applications to addictive behaviors, *Am Psychologist* 47(9):1102, 1992.

After the client has received treatment, the nurse can coordinate aftercare referrals and follow up on the client's progress. The nurse can provide additional support in the home as the client and family adjust to changing roles and the stress involved with such changes. The nurse can support addicted persons who have relapsed by reminding them that relapses may well occur, yet encouraging them and their families to continue to work toward recovery and an improved quality of life.

Detoxification

Detoxification is the clearing of one or more drugs from the person's body and managing the **withdrawal** symptoms. Depending on the particular drug and the degree of dependence, the time period may range from a few days to several weeks. Because withdrawal symptoms vary (depending on the drug used) and range from uncomfortable to life threatening, the setting for and management of withdrawal depend on the drug used.

Drugs such as stimulants or opiates may produce withdrawal symptoms that are uncomfortable but not life threatening. Detoxification from these drugs does not require direct medical supervision, but medical management of the withdrawal symptoms increases the comfort level. On the other hand, drugs such as alcohol, benzodiazepines, and barbiturates can produce life-threatening withdrawal symptoms. These clients should be under close medical supervision during detoxification and should receive medical management of the withdrawal symptoms to ensure a safe withdrawal. For those who develop delirium tremens, 15% may not survive despite medical management; therefore close medical management is initiated as the blood alcohol level begins to fall.

A general rule in detoxification management is to wean the person off the drug by gradually reducing the dosage and frequency of administration. Thus a person with chronic alcoholism could be safely detoxified by a gradual reduction in alcohol consumption. In practice, however, the switch to another drug, usually a benzodiazepine, often offers a safer withdrawal from alcohol as well as an abrupt end to the intoxication from the drug of choice. For example, chlordiazepam (Librium) is commonly used for alcohol detoxification.

DID YOU KNOW? *Because of cost-containment efforts, more primary care providers and drug treatment programs use outpatient or home detoxification for persons requiring medical detoxification for alcohol withdrawal. Nurses can provide the necessary monitoring and evaluation of the client's health status in the home environment to reduce the risk of medical complications related to alcohol withdrawal, as well as to provide encouragement and support for the client to complete the detoxification.*

DID YOU KNOW? *Auricular acupuncture (needles inserted in the ear) can be effective in treating withdrawal symptoms from various drugs and as an aid during substance abuse treatment and relapse prevention. It is a specific acupuncture technique that is quick, inexpensive, and safe. In some states nurses who are trained in this technique can be certified to use it to help with substance abuse detoxification and treatment (Moner, 1996).*

Addiction Treatment

Addiction treatment differs from the management of negative health consequences of chronic drug abuse, overdose, and withdrawal. **Addiction treatment** focuses on the addiction process: helping clients view addiction as a chronic disease and assisting them to make lifestyle changes to halt the progression of the disease. According to the disease theory, addicts are not responsible for the symptoms of their disease; they are, however, responsible for treating their disease. On any given day, more than 800,000 persons receive addiction treatment in specialized programs. In 1991 most clients (82%) were outpatients (Institute for Health Policy, Brandeis University, 1993).

Most treatment facilities are multidisciplinary because the intervention strategies require a wide range of approaches. Their programs involve interactions among the addict, family, culture, and community. Strategies include medical management, education, counseling, vocational rehabilitation, stress management, and support services. In general, there are two basic approaches to addiction treatment: 1) medical management or controlled use and 2) total abstinence. The key to effective treatment is to match individual clients with the interventions most appropriate for them.

Controlled use and medical management

For those addicted individuals unwilling or unable to completely abstain from psychoactive drugs, other drugs can assist them in abstaining from their drug of choice. Up to the early 1900s, U.S. physicians sometimes prescribed morphine for alcoholic persons because of the extensive physical damage or aggressive behavior caused by the alcohol. The person with alcoholism would instead become addicted to morphine but would not suffer most of the negative physical or behavioral consequences related to alcoholism (Brecher, 1972).

A similar philosophy is applied today with the methadone maintenance program for treatment of heroin addiction. Methadone, when administered in moderate or high daily doses, produces a cross-tolerance to other narcotics, thereby blocking their effects and decreasing the craving for heroin. The advantages of methadone are that it is long acting, effective orally, and inexpensive and has few known side effects. The oral use of methadone offers a solution to the danger of the spread of AIDS and other bloodborne infections that commonly occur among needle-sharing addicts. More recently, trends indicate that many persons with IV heroin addiction are also "shooting" (taking intravenously) cocaine, and since methadone does not affect the cocaine cravings, a polysubstance-addicted individual on a methadone maintenance program may still continue with IV drug use. Although not recognized as a cure for heroin (or other opiate) addiction, methadone maintenance reduces deviant behavior and introduces addicted persons to the health care system. This may ultimately lead to total abstinence.

For some persons, medical treatment is used to negate the high from their drug of choice or deter use by negative interactions. Naltrexone (Trexan) can be used with opiate addiction. It is a pure opiate antagonist that blocks the effects of all opium-derived compounds. This can help the client by preventing the psychological and physical reinforcements of opiates if a person should slip and use an opiate. More recently, naltrexone also has been effectively used to block the pleasure produced by alcohol (Volpicelli et al, 1995).

Total abstinence

Total abstinence is the most recommended treatment for ATOD addiction. People who are addicted to a particular drug (e.g., cocaine) are advised to abstain from the use of all psychoactive substances. The use of another drug may simply reinforce the craving for the original drug and cause relapse. More commonly, the addiction merely transfers to the replacement substance.

Treatment may be on an inpatient or outpatient basis. In general, the more advanced the disease is, the greater the need for inpatient treatment. Inpatient treatment programs usually last 28 days, although they may range from less than 1 week to 90 days. Once a person has completed detoxification (considered the first phase of the treatment process), the programs use counseling and group interaction to help him or her stay clean long enough for the body chemistry to rebalance. This is often a difficult time for persons recovering from addictions because they may experience mood swings and difficulty sleeping and dealing with emotions.

The educational segment of the program focuses on providing information about the disease concept and how drugs affect a person physically and psychologically. Clients are informed of the various lifestyle changes that are recommended and learn about tools to assist them in making these changes. Discharge planning continues throughout treatment as clients build the support systems that they will need when they leave the controlled environment of a treatment center and face pressures and temptations (triggers) that may lead to relapse.

Long-term residential programs, also called halfway houses, have been developed to ease the person recovering from an addiction back into society. These facilities provide continued support and counseling in a structured environment for persons needing long-term assistance in adjusting to a drug-free lifestyle. The residents are expected to secure employment and take responsibility in managing their financial obligations.

Outpatient programs are similar in the education and counseling offered, but they allow the clients to live at home and continue to work while undergoing treatment. This method is very effective for persons in the earlier stages of addiction who feel confident that they can abstain from drug use and have established a strong support network.

Most programs have incorporated family counseling and education. In addition, specific programs are being developed to address the needs of various populations such as adolescents, women during pregnancy, specific ethnic groups, and health care professionals.

Recovery from addiction involves a lifetime commitment and may include periods of relapse. The addicted person must realize that modern medicine has not found a cure for addiction; therefore returning to drug use may ultimately reactivate the disease process.

Smoking cessation programs

A goal of *Healthy People 2000* is to decrease the incidence of smoking to 15% of the population. The 1987 baseline for males was 31% and by 1994 it was 28%. The baseline for females was 27% and by 1994 it has decreased to 23%

BOX 36-4 Smoking Cessation Resources

American Cancer Society
777 3rd Ave
New York, NY 10017
"Smart Move" (video and literature)
"Fresh Start" smoking cessation program

American Heart Association
7272 Greenville Ave.
Dallas, TX 75231
(214) 373-6300
"In Control: Freedom from Smoking" program

American Lung Association
1740 Broadway
New York, NY 10019
"Freedom From Smoking for You and Your Family"

Americans for Nonsmokers Rights
2054 University Ave. #500
Berkley, CA 94704

Anti-Tobacco Initiative
American Public Health Association
1015 Fifteenth St., N.W.
Washington, DC 20005

ASH (Action on Smoking and Health)
2013 H St. N.W.
Washington, DC 20006

Five Day Plan to Stop Smoking (general headquarters)
Seventh Day Adventist Church
Narcotics Education Division
6840 Eastern Ave. N.W.
Washington, DC 20012

National Interagency Council on Smoking and Health
Room 1005, 291 Broadway
2BB:New York, NY 10007

Office of Cancer Communications
National Cancer Institute
National Institutes of Health
Bethesda, MD 20205
(800) 638-6694
(800) 492-6600 in Maryland

Office on Smoking and Health
U.S. Department of Health and Human Services
Room 1-58
5600 Fishers Lane
Rockville, MD 20857
(800) 232-1311
"Action Guide to Second-hand Smoke"
"African American Quitting Guide"

SmokEnders
Memorial Parkway
Phillipsburg, NJ 08864
(908) 454-4357

STAT (Stop Teenage Addiction to Tobacco)
511 East Columbus Ave.
Springfield, MA 01105
(413) 732-7828

For more information, see the WebLinks on this book's website at www.mosby.com/MERLIN.

(National Center for Health Statistics, 1997). Nurses can not only become active in smoking prevention programs, but also in community efforts to assist persons to quit smoking.

Nearly 35 million Americans try to quit smoking each year. Less than 10% of those who try to quit on their own are able to stop for a year. Studies show that significantly greater cessation rates occur for smokers receiving interventions compared to those smokers who do not receive interventions. Interventions that involve medications and behavioral treatments appear most promising (Leshner, 1998).

Nicotine replacement therapy can be used to help smokers to withdraw from nicotine while focusing their efforts on breaking the psychological craving/habit. Four types of nicotine replacement products are available: nicotine gum and skin patches are available over the counter, and nicotine nasal spray and inhalers are available by prescription. These products are about equally effective and can almost double the chances of successfully quitting.

Other treatments include smoking cessation clinics, hypnosis, and acupuncture. The most effective way to get people to stop smoking and prevent relapse involves multiple interventions and continuous reinforcement since most smokers require several attempts at cessation until they are successful. Many resources are available on smoking cessation programs and support groups, including those listed in Box 36-4. Helping the client develop a plan to stop smoking can increase the likelihood of success. *Nursing Care of the Patient Who Smokes* by Rienzo (1993) provides further information on how to quit smoking.

WHAT DO YOU THINK? *Research has shown that antidepressants can help persons stop smoking. Glaxo-Wellcome has developed a specific drug, bupropion hydrochloride, for persons to use to help them stop smoking. Insurance companies do not pay for the use of this medicine.*

Support Groups

The founding of **Alcoholics Anonymous (AA)** in 1935 began a strong movement that recognized the important role of peer support in the treatment of a chronic illness. AA groups have developed throughout the world, and their success has led to the development of other support groups such as Narcotics Anonymous (NA) for persons with narcotic addictions and Pills Anonymous for persons with polydrug addictions. Similar programs have been developed for process addictions, such as Overeaters Anonymous and Gamblers Anonymous.

AA and NA help addicted people develop a daily program of recovery and reinforce the recovery process. The fellowship, support, and encouragement among AA members provide a vital social network for the person recovering from an addiction.

Al-Anon and Alateen are similar self-help programs for spouses, parents, children, or others involved in a painful relationship with an alcoholic (Nar-Anon for those in relationships with persons with narcotic addictions). Al-Anon family groups are available to anyone who has been affected by their involvement with an alcoholic person. The purposes of Alateen include providing a forum for adolescents to discuss family stressors, learn coping skills from one another, and gain support and encouragement from knowledgeable peers. Adult Children of Alcoholics (ACOA) groups are also available in most areas to address the recovery of adults who grew up in alcoholic homes and are still carrying the scars and retaining dysfunctional behaviors.

For some persons the AA program places too much emphasis on a higher power or focuses too much on the negative consequences of past drinking. Women for Sobriety focuses on rebuilding self-esteem, a core issue for many women with alcoholic problems (Kaskutas, 1994). Rational Recovery has a cognitive orientation and is premised on the assumption that ATOD addiction is caused by irrational beliefs that can be understood and overcome (Galanter et al, 1993).

Outcomes

Health promotion and risk reduction are basic concepts in community and public health nursing. Promoting a healthy environment in the home and local community provide individuals and families a nurturing environment to achieve optimal health. Individuals with high self-esteem, access to health care, and information about the health risks related to drug use can be responsible for their personal health and make informed decisions about drug use. Nurses can assess the health of the community and its citizens, prioritize the needs, and identify local resources to collaborate with others to develop strategies that will improve the underlying health of the community.

Early identification and intervention for persons with ATOD problems can prevent many of the harmful physical, emotional and social consequences that may occur if abuse continues and may also prevent abuse patterns from developing into addiction. The nurse must assess individual and community ATOD problems and can then target at risk groups to develop strategies to increase assessment and provide appropriate interventions. Review the national health objectives for the tobacco and substance abuse areas and note how many can be achieved with secondary prevention strategies.

A study of California drug treatment centers found that for every dollar spent on treatment, the public saves 7 dollars in health care and crime costs (National Opinion Resource Center, 1994). Besides monetary savings, treatment helps addicted individuals and their families recover from the devastating effects of addiction. Addicts and their families often become hopeless and helpless while actively addicted. The nurse can offer hope in affirming the addict's self worth and be the bridge to community resources to assist in treatment and recovery.

Many of these expected outcomes for ATOD problems have been slighted because of a lack of funding with the federal strategies focused on law enforcement and punishment rather than education and treatment. The greatest challenge for nurses is to influence policy makers to put the emphasis on health care for this major health problem.

clinical application

Jane Doe, RN, is a home health case manager in a large low-income housing area in her local community. She designs care plans and coordinates health care services for clients who need health care at home. She makes the initial visits to determine the level and frequency of care and acts as supervisor of the volunteers and nurses' aids who perform most of the day-to-day care. Single parent families are the norm, and drug dealing is commonplace in this housing area.

Jane made a home visit to Anne, a 26-year-old mother of three, who is taking care of her 62-year-old maternal grandfather, Mr. Jones, who is recovering from cardiac bypass surgery. He has a smoking history of 2 packs per day for almost 40 years and had decreased to 1 ppd since his surgery, but refuses to quit. He had a history of alcohol dependence, reportedly consuming up to a fifth of liquor a day, and a history of withdrawal seizures. Four years ago he went through an alcohol detoxification but refused to stay at the facility for continued treatment, stating he could stay sober on his own. Since that time he has had several binge episodes, but Anne reports that he has not been drinking since the surgery. A widower for 5 years, Mr. Jones now lives with Anne.

Anne is a widow and has two sons, ages 3 and 9, and a daughter, age 5. The oldest son's father is an alcoholic who is currently incarcerated for manslaughter while driving under the influence of alcohol, and the father of her two youngest children was killed by a stray bullet in a cocaine

Continued

clinical application—cont'd

bust 3 years ago. Years earlier, Anne and her husband had smoked crack cocaine for several months but both stopped when she became pregnant with their youngest child and had remained cocaine free. Anne was still angry at the system and frightened of police officers since the drug raid in which her husband was killed. Other residents had been hurt, and less than $500 worth of cocaine was found three apartments away from hers.

Anne doesn't consume alcohol, but smokes 1 to 2 packs per day. She quit smoking during her pregnancies, but restarted soon after each birth.

A. What type of interventions can Jane provide for Mr. Jones regarding his smoking?
B. How can Jane help Anne cope with the potential risk of Mr. Jones continuing to drink when he progresses to more independence?
C. How can Jane help Anne with her cigarette smoking?
D. Knowing there is a genetic link to alcoholism and the high rate of drug problems in the housing area, how can Jane help prevent Anne and her children from developing substance abuse problems?
E. What problems seem greater because of the drug laws, and what can Jane do to help make the environment safer and more nurturing?

Answers are in the back of the book.

KEY POINTS

- Substance abuse is a national health problem linked to numerous forms of morbidity and mortality.
- Harm reduction is a new approach to ATOD problem that deals with substance abuse primarily as a health problem rather than a criminal problem.
- All persons have attitudes about the use of drugs that influence their actions.
- Social conditions such as a fast-paced life, excessive stress, and the availability of drugs influence the incidence of substance abuse.
- Important terms to understand when working with individuals, groups, or communities for whom substance abuse is prevalent are *drug dependence, drug addiction, alcoholism, psychoactive drugs, depressants, stimulants, marijuana, hallucinogens,* and *inhalants.*
- Primary prevention for substance abuse includes education about drugs and guidelines for use, as well as the promotion of healthy alternatives to drug use for either recreation or to relieve stress.
- Nurses can play a key role in developing community prevention programs.

- Secondary prevention depends heavily on careful assessment of the client's use of drugs. Such assessment should be part of all basic health assessments.
- High-risk groups include pregnant women, young people, elderly persons, intravenous drug users, and illicit drug users.
- Drug addiction is often a family, not merely an individual, problem.
- Codependency describes a companion illness to the addiction of one person in which the codependent member is addicted to the addicted person.
- Brief interventions by nurse can be as effective as treatment.
- Nurses are in ideal roles to assist with tertiary prevention for both the addicted person and the family.

critical thinking activities

1. Read your local newspaper for 4 days and select stories that illustrate the effect of substance abuse on individuals, families, and the community.
2. For each of the stories in the newspaper related to substance abuse, describe preventive strategies that a nurse might have tried before the problem reached such a dire state.
3. Looking at your local community resources directory (or the telephone book), identify agencies that might serve as referral sources for individuals or families for whom substance abuse is a problem.
4. In groups of three to five students, discuss your personal attitudes toward drinking, smoking, and drug abuse. Discuss each category of substance abuse separately. Consider the following areas: sex, age, amount, time, occasion, place where substance abuse occurs, companions, motivation, and incentives.
5. Review popular magazine and television advertisements for alcohol, tobacco, and other medicines (e.g., sleepers, analgesics, laxatives, stimulants). In small groups discuss the messages conveyed in the advertisements and what the implications would be for client education to reduce possible harm from misuse and abuse of these substances.
6. Attend an open AA or NA meeting and an Al-Anon meeting. Go alone if possible or with an alcoholic or a drug-addicted friend. As the members introduce themselves, give your first name and state, "I am a visitor." Plan to listen and do not attempt to take notes. Respect the anonymity of the persons present. Discuss your experiences later in a group.
7. In groups of four or five, review the national health objectives in *Healthy People 2000* (see Appendix A.1) under "Tobacco" and "Alcohol and Other Drugs." Pick an objective from each section, and brainstorm about possible community efforts a nurse could initiate to reach that objective.

Bibliography

American Public Health Association: Access to therapeutic marijuana/cannabis #9513, *Am J Pub Health* 36(3):441, 1996.

Baum D: *Smoke and mirrors: the war on drugs and the politics of failure,* Boston, 1997, Little, Brown, and Company.

Bien TH, Miller WR, Tonigan JS: Brief interventions for alcohol problems: a review, *Addiction* 88:315, 1993.

Brecher EM: *Licit and illicit drugs,* Boston, 1972, Little, Brown and Company.

Brust JCM: Other agents: phencyclidine, marijuana, hallucinogens, inhalants, and anticholinergics, *Neurol Clinics* 11(3):555, 1993.

Callery YC: Chemical abuse rehabilitation for hospital employees, *AAOHNJ* 42(4):67, 1994.

Cargo S: Increases in teen drug use appear to level off, *NIDA Notes* 13(2):10, 1998.

Center for Substance Abuse Treatment: *A guide to substance abuse services for primary care clinicians,* Treatment Improvement Protocol (TIP) Series, Number 24. DHHS Pub. No. (SMA) 97-3139. Washington, DC, 1997, US Government Printing Office.

Center for Substance Abuse Treatment: *Substance abuse among older adults,* Treatment Improvement Protocol (TIP) Series, Number 26. DHHS Pub. No. (SMA) 98-3179. Washington, DC, 1998, US Government Printing Office.

Chavkin W, Kandall SR: Between a "rock" and a hard place: perinatal drug abuse, *Pediatrics* 85(2):223, 1990.

Coate D: Moderate drinking and coronary heart disease mortality: evidence from NHANES I and the NHANES I follow-up, *Am J Pub Health* 83(6):888, 1993.

Cordero JF, Floyd RL, Martin ML, et al: Tracking the prevalence of FAS, *Alcohol Health Res World* 18(1):82, 1994.

Cordes H: Generation wired: caffeine is the new drug of choice for kids, *The Nation* 266(15):11, 1998.

Das G, Laddu A: Cocaine: friend or foe? *Intern J Clin Pharmacol Ther Toxicol* 31(9):449, 1993.

Davis AY: Masked racism: reflections on the prison industrial complex, *ColorLines* 1(1):1, 1998.

Dawson DA, Grant BF: Family history and gender: their combined effects on DSM-IV alcohol dependence and major depression, *J Stud Alcohol* 59(1):97, 1998.

Des Jarlais DC: Editorial: harm reduction—a framework for incorporating science into drug policy, *Am J Pub Health* 85(1):10, 1995.

Dicker M, Leighton EA: Trends in the US prevalence of drug-using parturient women and drug-affected newborns, 1979 through 1990, *Am J Pub Health* 84(9):1433, 1994.

Dinwiddie SH: Abuse of inhalants: a review, *Addiction* 89(8):925, 1994.

Dodge VH: Relaxation training: a nursing intervention for substance abusers, *Arch Psychiatr Nurs* 5(2):99, 1991.

Donaldson SI, Graham JW, Hansen WB: Testing the generalizability of intervening mechanism theories: understanding the effects of adolescent drug use prevention interventions, *J Behav Med* 17(2):195, 1994.

Ennett ST et al: How effective is drug abuse resistance education? a meta-analysis of Project DARE outcome evaluation, *Am J Pub Health* 84(9):1394, 1994.

Espeland K: Inhalant abuse: assessment guidelines, *J Psychosoc Nurs Ment Health Serv* 31(3):11, 1993.

Fiesta J: Mother vs child: a legal controversy, *Nurs Management* 22(10):14, 1991.

Fiore MC: Treatment options for smoking in the '90s, *J Clin Pharmacol* 34(3):195, 1993.

Foley KM: Opioids, *Neurol Clinics* 11(3):503, 1993.

Frezza M et al: High blood alcohol levels in women: the role of decreased gastric alcohol dehydrogenase activity and first-pass metabolism, *N Engl J Med* N 322(2):95, 1990.

Galanter M, Egelko S, Edwards H: Rational recovery: alternative to AA for addiction? *Am J Drug Alcohol Abuse* 19(4):499, 1993.

Gold MS et al: Epidemiology of benzodiazepine use and dependence, *Psychiatric Annals* 25(3):146, 1995.

Griffith WH: *Complete guide to prescription and nonprescription drugs,* New York, 1998, The Body Press/Perigee.

Heather N et al, editors: *Psychoactive drugs and harm reduction: from faith to science,* London, 1993, Whurr.

Hilts PJ: *Is nicotine addictive? Depends on whose criteria you use.* New York Times, August 2, 1994, p C3.

Hutchings DE: The puzzle of cocaine's effects following maternal use during pregnancy: are there reconcilable differences, *Neurotoxicol Teratol* 15:281, 1993.

Institute for Health Policy, Brandeis University: *Substance abuse: the nation's number one health problem, key indicators for policy,* Princeton, NJ, 1993, The Robert Wood Johnson Foundation.

Jack L, Snow D: *Prevention of alcohol, tobacco, and other drug problems: an independent study for nurses,* Raleigh, NC, 1994, US Center for Substance Abuse Prevention and the National Nurses Society on Addictions.

Kain ZN, Rimar S, Barash PG: Cocaine abuse and the parturient and effects on the fetus and neonate, *Anesth Analg* 77(4):835, 1993.

Kaskutas LA: What do women get out of self-help? their reasons for attending Women for Sobriety and Alcoholics Anonymous. *J Subst Abuse Treat* 11(3):185, 1994.

Kinney J, Leaton G: *Loosening the grip,* ed 5, St Louis, 1995, Mosby.

Kishline A: *Moderate drinking,* NY, 1994, Crown Trade Paperbacks.

Kumpfer KL, Hopkins R: Prevention: current research and trends, *Psychiatr Clin North Am* 16(1).11, 1993.

Larrat EP, Taubman AH, Willey C: Compliance-related problems in the ambulatory populations, *Am Pharmacy NS* 30(2):18, 1990.

Leshner AI: Addiction research can provide scientific solutions to the problem of cigarette smoking, *NIDA Notes,* 13(3):3, 1998.

Mahoney DL: Infant and maternal outcomes associated with self-reported illicit drug use during pregnancy, *J Addictions Nurs* 10(3):115, 1998.

Manwell L et al: Tobacco, alcohol, and drug use in a primary care sample: 90 day prevalence and associated factors, *J Addict Dis* 17(1):67, 1997.

Marwick C: Physician leadership on national drug policy finds addiction treatment works, *JAMA* 279(15):1149, 1998.

Mathre ML, editor: *Cannabis in medical practice: a legal, historical, and pharmacological overview of the therapeutic use of marijuana,* Jefferson, NC, 1997, McFarland & Company.

Medical-care expenditures attributable to cigarette smoking—US, 1993, *MMWR* 43(26):469, 1994.

Merrill J, Fox K, Chang H: *The cost of substance abuse to America's health care system: report 1: Medicaid hospital costs,* New York, 1993, Center on Addictions and Substance Abuse at Columbia University.

Miller M: *Drug consumer safety rules,* Mosier, Ore, 1994, Mothers Against Misuse and Abuse.

Minicucci DS: The challenge of change: rethinking alcohol abuse, *Arch Psychiatr Nurs* 8(6):373, 1994.

Moner SE: Acupuncture and addiction treatment, *J of Addictive Diseases* 15(3):79, 1996.

Moyers BD, Casiato T, Hughes K: Moyers on addiction: close to home (5-part video series), Princeton, NJ, 1998, Films for the Humanities and Sciences.

Mueller MD, Wyman JR: Study sheds new light on the state of drug abuse treatment nationwide, *NIDA Notes* 12(5):1, 1997.

National Center for Health Statistics: *Healthy people 2000 review,* 1997, Hyattsville, Md, 1997, Public Health Service.

National Institute on Alcohol Abuse and Alcoholism: *The physician's guide to helping patients with alcohol problemsi,* Rockville, Md, 1995, Author.

National Institute on Alcohol Abuse and Alcoholism: Alcohol's effect on organ function, *Alcohol Res World* 21(1):3, 1997.

National Institute on Drug Abuse: Comparing methamphetamine and cocaine, *NIDA Notes,* 13(1):15, 1998a.

National Institute on Drug Abuse: Trends in drug use among 8th, 10th, and 12th graders, *NIDA Notes* 13(2):15, 1998b.

National Institute on Drug Abuse: Facts about nicotine and tobacco products, *NIDA Notes,* 13(3):15, 1998c.

National Nurses Society on Addictions: Access to therapeutic cannabis, *J Addictions Nurs* 8(1):18, 1996.

National Opinion Research Center: *Evaluating recovery services: the California drug and alcohol treatment assessment,* Chicago, 1994, Author.

continued

Bibliography—cont'd

Neumark YD, Delva J, Anthony JC: The epidemiology of adolescent inhalant drug involvement, *Arch Pediatr Adolesc Med* 152:781, 1998.

O'Brien CP: Drug abuse and drug addiction. In Hardman JG, Limbird LE, editors: *Goodman & Gilman's the pharmacological basis of therapeutics,* ed 9, New York, 1996, McGraw-Hill.

Perez-Stable EJ et al: Nicotine metabolism and intake in black and white smokers. *JAMA* 280(2): 152, 1998.

Peterson PL, Lowe JB: Preventing fetal alcohol exposure: a cognitive behavioral approach. *Int J Addict* 27(5):613, 1992.

Petro DJ: Pharmacology and toxicity of cannabis. In Mathre ML, editor: *Cannabis in medical practice: a legal, historical and pharmacological overview of the therapeutic use of marijuana,* Jefferson, NC, 1997, McFarland & Company.

Prochaska JO, DiClemente CC, Norcross JC: In search of how people change: applications to addictive behaviors, *Am J Psychol* 47(9):1102, 1992.

Ramsey J et al: Volatile substance abuse in the United Kingdom. In Kozel N, Sloboda Z, De La Rosa M, editors: *Epidemiology of inhalant abuse: an international perspective,* Rockville, Md, 1995, National Institute on Drug Abuse, NIDA Research Monograph 148; NIH publication 95-3831.

Rassool GH, Winnington J: Using psychoactive drugs, *Nurs Times* 89(47):38, 1993.

Rienzo PG: *Nursing care of the patient who smokes,* New York, 1993, Springer.

Rose KD: *American women and the repeal of prohibition,* New York, 1996, New York University Press.

Rybacki JJ, Long JW: *The essential guide to prescription drugs.* New York, 1999, Harper Perennial.

Schwartz RH: Syringe and needle exchange programs worldwide, *South Med J* 86(3):323, 1993.

Shedler J, Block J: Adolescent drug use and psychological health: a longitudinal inquiry, *Am Psychol* 45(5):612, 1990.

Strain EC et al: Caffeine dependence syndrome: evidence from case histories and experimental evaluation, *JAMA* 272(13):1043, 1994.

Substance Abuse and Mental Health Services Administration: *National household survey on drug abuse advance report No. 18,* Rockville, Md, 1996, SAMHSA.

Talashek ML, Gerace LM, Starr KL: The substance abuse pandemic: determinants to guide interventions, *Pub Health Nurs* 11(2):131, 1994.

Tweed SH: Identifying the alcoholic client, *Nurs Clin North Am* 24(1):13, 1989.

US Department of Health and Human Services: *Healthy People 2000: national health promotion and disease prevention objectives,* Washington, DC, 1991, USDHHS, Public Health Service.

US Department of Health and Human Services: *Reducing the health consequences of smoking: 25 years of progress. A report of the Surgeon General,* Washington, DC, 1989, US Government Printing Office.

Vallance TR: *Prohibition's second failure: the quest for a rational and humane drug policy,* Wesport, Conn, 1993, Greenwood Publishing Group.

Volpicelli JR et al: Effect of naltrexone on alcohol "high" in alcoholics, *Am J Psychiatry* 152(4):613, 1995.

Warner EA: Cocaine abuse, *Ann Intern Med* 119(3):226, 1993.

Weil A, Rosen W: *Chocolate to morphine: understanding mind-active drugs,* Boston, 1993, Houghton Mifflin.

Weinberg NZ et al: Adolescent substance abuse: a review of the past 10 years, *J Am Acad Child Adolesc Psychiatry* 37(3):252, 1998.

Weiss RD, Mirin SM, Bartel RL: *Cocaine,* ed 2, Washington, DC, 1994, American Psychiatric Press.

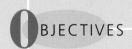
Violence and Human Abuse

JACQUELYN C. CAMPBELL & KÄREN M. LANDENBURGER

OBJECTIVES

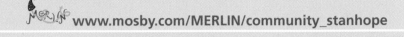

www.mosby.com/MERLIN/community_stanhope

After reading this chapter, the student should be able to do the following:

- Discuss the scope of the problem of violence in American communities.
- Examine at least three factors existing in most communities that influence violence and human abuse.
- Identify at least three types of community facilities that can help prevent violence.
- Identify typically noticed indicators of child abuse.
- Define the four general types of child abuse: neglect, physical, emotional, and sexual.
- Discuss abuse of elderly persons as a growing community health problem.

- Evaluate the role that nurses can assume with rape victims.
- Analyze primary preventive nursing interventions for community violence.
- Evaluate the different responses that a nurse would expect to see in a battered woman from the beginning of the abuse until after the relationship has ended.
- Discuss the principles of nursing intervention with violent families.
- Describe specific nursing interventions with battered women.

KEY TERMS

assault	emotional neglect	physical abuse	suicide
battered child syndrome	empowerment	physical neglect	survivors
child neglect	forensic	rape	violence
elder abuse	homicide	sexual abuse	wife abuse
emotional abuse	incest	spouse abuse	*See Glossary for definitions*

CHAPTER OUTLINE

Social and Community Factors
  Influencing Violence
    Work
    Education
    Media
    Organized Religion
    Population
    Community Facilities

Violence against Individuals or
  Oneself
    Homicide
    Assault
    Rape
    Suicide
  Family Violence and Abuse
    Development of Abusive
      Patterns

Types of Family Violence
Nursing Interventions
  Primary Prevention
  Secondary Prevention
  Tertiary Prevention:
    Therapeutic Intervention with
    Abusive Families
Clinical Forensic Nursing

The word "violence" comes from the Latin *violare*, meaning to violate, injure, or rape. Indeed, violence is a violation, with both emotional and physical effects. Unfortunately the United States has the fifth highest homicide rate in the world. Newspaper headlines and television reports are filled with news of violence. Although considerable progress has been made in decreasing rates of death from all other causes since 1940, the risk of assault and homicide in the United States has increased (USDHHS, 1991). The violence in our streets and in our homes threatens the health and well-being of our entire population.

It is not clear from research if violence stems from an innate aggressive drive or is primarily learned behavior. Clearly, all human beings have the capability for violence, yet some entire societies are basically nonviolent (Counts et al, 1992). Therefore it is important to understand under what conditions aggression and violence are increased and, conversely, what keeps them in check and promotes nonviolent conflict resolution.

Violence is a community health nursing concern. Significant mortality and morbidity result from violence. Communities across the United States are voicing anger and fear about rising crime and violence rates. Medical, nursing, psychology, and social service professionals have been slow in developing a response to violence that is integral to their daily professional lives. As a result, the estimated 4 million victims of violence annually may not receive the best care possible. In addition, the extent of their pain that could have been avoided by community health prevention efforts is unknown.

Violence is generally defined as those nonaccidental acts, interpersonal or intrapersonal, that result in physical or psychological injury to one or more persons. Violent behavior is predictable and thus preventable (Rosenberg and Fenley, 1991), especially with community action. Violence is a major cause of premature mortality and lifelong disability and violence-related morbidity is a significant factor in health care costs. Violence is the twelfth leading cause of death in the United States and the sixth leading cause of premature mortality (USDHHS, 1991). A section of the National Objectives for the Year 2000 is devoted to violence, providing official recognition of the need for health professionals to address this issue (see Appendix A.1).

This chapter examines violence as a public health problem and discusses how nurses can help individuals, families, groups, and communities cope with and reduce violence and abuse. Nurses have access to clients in a wide variety of settings, including the home. Since they are in key positions to detect and intervene in community and family violence, nurses need to understand how community-level influences can affect all types of violence.

SOCIAL AND COMMUNITY FACTORS INFLUENCING VIOLENCE

Many factors in a community can support or minimize violence. Changing social conditions, multiple demands on people, economic conditions, and institutions that make up a given society or community influence the level of violence and human abuse. The following discussion of selected contemporary social conditions helps to explain factors that influence violent behavior.

Work

Productive and paid work is an expectation in mainstream American society, especially for men. Work can be fulfilling and contribute to a sense of well-being; it can also be frustrating and unfulfilling, contributing to stress that may lead to aggression and violence. Unemployment is also associated with violence both within and outside the home.

When jobs are repetitive, boring, and lacking in stimulation, frustration mounts. Some work environments discourage creativity and reward conformity and "following the rules." In many work settings people try to get ahead regardless of the cost to others. Workers often go home feeling physically and psychologically drained. They may have worked at a back-breaking pace all day only to be yelled at by the boss for what seemed like a trivial oversight. It is hard to separate feelings generated at work from those in the home environment.

For example, a father arrives home feeling tired, angry, and generally inadequate because of a series of reprimands from his boss. Soon after he sits down, his 4-year-old son runs through the house pretending to fly a wooden airplane. After about three loud trips past his father, who keeps shouting for the child to be quiet and go outside, the airplane hits the father in the head. The father may strike out in frustration and anger.

During economic downturns, people may be afraid to give up jobs that are frustrating, are boring, or create stress. Family needs may necessitate that they keep the hated job. They feel trapped and may resent those who depend on them. This frustration and resentment may lead to violence.

Unemployment may precipitate aggressive outbursts. The inability to secure or maintain a job may lead to feelings of inadequacy, guilt, boredom, dissatisfaction, and frustration. Unemployment does not fit the image of the ideal man in American society, and these men are more likely to be violent both within and outside the family (Tolman and Bennett, 1990).

Young, minority males have the highest rates of unemployment in the United States, even in times of prosperity ranging upwards to 50%. This group also has the highest rate of violence. They live in a world of oppression, with lack of opportunity and enormous anger. They feel that they are pushed out of mainstream society and are on the receiving end of the fallout of policies that ignore their dilemmas and give them no stake in mainstream America. Most analyses conclude that the differential rates of violence between African-Americans and whites in the United States have more to do with economic realities, such as poverty, unemployment, and overcrowding, than with race (Hawkins, 1993; Reiss and Roth, 1994).

Education

In recent years schools have assumed many responsibilities traditionally assigned to the family. Schools teach sexual development, discipline children, and often serve as a place to "dump" children who have no other place to go. Large classes often mean that teachers spend more time and energy monitoring and disciplining children than challenging and stimulating them to learn. In large classes, children who do not conform to norms of expected behavior are often isolated. The nonconforming child is simply removed from the classroom because time is not available to help the child learn alternative ways of behavior.

It is ironic that parents often punish children for hitting or biting other children by spanking them. Corporal punishment is also still used in many U.S. schools. Such punishment only reinforces the child's tendency to strike out at others. Schools are often places where the stressors and frustrations that can contribute to violence are rampant, and violence is learned rather than discouraged; yet school can be a powerful contributor to nonviolence. Classes can help adolescents learn peaceful conflict resolution and the issues of date rape and help young children deal with the threat of sexual abuse (Gelles and Conte, 1990; Webster, 1993). Parents can be advised of the availability of these kinds of programs, and school boards should be urged to adopt them into the curriculum.

Media

The media can be instrumental in campaigns against violence. Recent television programs, both documentaries and dramatizations, and print articles have heightened public awareness about family violence. Abused women and rape victims have especially benefited from media attention, which tends to lessen the stigma of such victimization. The media are also useful in publicizing services. However, the media have often served as a source of frustration to poor persons in U.S. society, as a cause of public apathy, and as a model of violence to be emulated.

Television, movies, newspapers, and magazines show happy, fun-loving people. Television parades all the wonders money can provide; yet for many Americans, the hope of buying many of these nonessentials seems unrealistic. Such polarization between what is available and what is possible provides fertile ground for the development of abusive patterns. Frustration, unfilled dreams, and unmet wishes are often handled through hurting someone who cannot fight back.

The media cater to children by advertising products to buy and things to do. Parents may get angry when their children request the foods, toys, and clothes they see on television, in magazines, or in newspapers or hear advertised on the radio. In addition, many toys and video games encourage violence through play.

Too often the media portray the world as a violent place. When the public is convinced that violence is rampant, there are two possible results. People may become blasé about violence and no longer feel outraged and galvanized to action when terrible things happen in their community. On the other hand, some become frightened of their neighbors, isolate themselves, and refuse to become involved when someone needs help. Neither response is useful in any community-action program.

Hitting, kicking, stabbing, and shooting are seen daily as ways to handle anger and frustration. By the age of 18 years, the average child has seen 1800 murders and countless acts of nonfatal violence on television. Often in these acts of violence, the good guys conquer the bad ones. Thus violence is often seen as justified when the perpetrator views the cause to be worthy. Frequent violent television viewing by children has been associated with aggressive behavior in longitudinal research (Campbell and Humphreys, 1993). On the other hand, the media can be a powerful force for increasing public awareness of various forms of violence and what can be done to address them (Kline et al, 1998).

Organized Religion

Three human needs (stimulation, a sense of worth or power, and some degree of closeness and intimacy) are often provided by the church (Prince, 1980). Religion may encourage nonviolent conflict resolution, and the church, clergy, and church groups often provide positive role models and reinforcement for peaceful behavior.

Historically, a seemingly contradictory relationship exists between abuse and religion. For example, many religious groups uphold the philosophy of "spare the rod, spoil the child." Also, some faiths uphold the victimization of people with their disapproval of divorce. Family members may stay together, although they are at emotional or physical war with one another, because of religious commitments (Prince, 1980).

Although controversial, guilt can be a form of victimization. Some religious bodies seem more concerned about using religious beliefs to keep members "in line" than offering suggestions and encouragement for behavior. Rigid guidelines complete with predictions of dire spiritual consequences can produce guilt and lowered self-esteem.

Population

A community's population can influence the potential for violence. Density, poverty, and diversity, particularly racial tension and overt racism, contribute to violence (Evans and Taylor, 1995; Hampton and Yung, 1996).

High-population-density communities can positively or negatively influence violence. Those with a sense of cohesiveness may have a lower crime rate than areas of similar size that lack social and cultural groups to support unity among members. Bonds formed among church groups, clubs, and professional organizations may promote harmony among members. Such groups provide members an opportunity to talk about stressors rather than to respond through violence. For example, residents of public housing often form neighborhood associations to deal with situations common to many or all residents. Tension can often be released in a productive way through projects carried out by the association.

Some high-population areas experience a community feeling of powerlessness and helplessness rather than one of cohesiveness. Lack of jobs and low paying jobs result in feelings of inadequacy, despair, and social alienation. Social alienation and exclusion from opportunities can lead to decreased social cohesion and increased violence (Moore and Harrisson, 1995; Wilkinson, 1997). Fear and apathy may cause community residents to withdraw from social contact. Withdrawal can foster crime because many residents assume someone else will report suspicious behavior, or they fear reprisals for such reports.

Youths often attempt to deal with feelings of powerlessness by forming gangs. Poverty and lack of education appear to be the overriding risk factors. A number of these young adults have attempted to deal with their feelings by turning to crime against people and property to release frustration. In many cities these gangs have been highly destructive. Unfortunately many programs have focused on family functioning based on secondary prevention through intervention with families rather than focusing on primary prevention and the primary issues leading to gang membership (Winfree, Esbensen, and Osgood, 1996).

Other high-population areas may be characterized by a *sense of confusion,* resulting in disintegration and disorganization. These areas often have transient populations who have limited physical or emotional investment in the community. Lack of community concern allows crime and violence to go unchecked and may become a norm for the area. Also, as crime increases, residents who are able to move leave the area. This increases community disintegration because the residents who leave are often the most capable members of the population.

The potential for violence also tends to increase among highly diverse populations. Differences in age, socioeconomic status, ethnicity, religion, or other cultural characteristics may disrupt community stability. Highly divergent groups may not communicate effectively and neither accept nor understand one another. Many such groups become hostile and antagonistic toward one another. Each group may see the other as different and not belonging. The alienated group may become the focal point for the others' frustrations, anger, and fears. Racism, classism, and heterosexism are examples of major causes of community disintegration resulting in a vicious cycle of dishonesty, distrust, and hate.

Community Facilities

Communities differ in the resources and facilities they provide to residents. Some are more desirable places to live, work, and raise families and have facilities that can reduce the potential for crime and violence. Recreational facilities such as playgrounds, parks, swimming pools, movie theaters, and tennis courts provide socially acceptable outlets for a variety of feelings, including aggression.

Spectator sports, such as football or hockey, also allow members of the community to express feelings of anger and frustration. However, viewing sports can encourage a sense of violence as participants hit or shove one another.

Although the absence of such facilities can increase the likelihood of violence, their presence alone does not prevent violence or crime. These facilities are adjuncts and resources that residents can use for pleasure, personal enrichment, and group development.

Familiarity with factors contributing to a community's violence or potential for violence enables nurses to recognize them and intervene accordingly. It is the nurse's responsibility to work with the citizens and agencies of the community to correct or improve deficits.

VIOLENCE AGAINST INDIVIDUALS OR ONESELF

The potential for violence against individuals (e.g., murder, robbery, rape, and assault) or oneself (e.g., suicide) is directly related to the level of violence in the community. Persons living in areas with high rates of crime and violence are more likely to become victims than those in more peaceful areas. The major categories of violence addressed in this chapter are described in terms of the scope of the problem in the United States and underlying dynamics.

Homicide

Homicide is the eleventh leading cause of death for all Americans, and the number one cause of death for young (age 15 to 34 years) African-American men and women (U.S. Public Health Service, 1990). However, the African-American homicide rate has decreased significantly since 1970, whereas the white homicide rate has increased (U.S. Public Health Service, 1990; Bureau of Justice Statistics, 1997). Although the data are not adequate, it also appears that Hispanic-American males have a much higher rate of homicide than non–Hispanic-American whites. Homicide is increasing the most among adolescents, but even among very young children in the United States, homicide occurs at an alarming rate. As many as 4.2 per 100,000 children age 3 years and younger were killed by another person, usually a family member (U.S. Public Health Service, 1990). Only 13% to 15% of all homicides in the United States are caused by strangers (Riedel, 1998). When strangers are involved, many of these homicides are related to the illegal substance–abuse network.

The majority of homicides, however, are perpetrated by a friend, acquaintance, or family member during an argument. Therefore prevention of homicide is at least as much an issue for the public health system as for the criminal justice system (Rosenberg and Fenley, 1991).

Homicide within families

At least 13% of the homicides in the United States occur within families (Bachman, 1994), and half of these occur between spouses. These numbers, however, do not include unmarried couples who are living together or those who are either divorced or estranged, a group at higher risk. Husbands comprised about 60% of perpetrators in spousal homicides, and self-defense is involved approximately seven times as often when wives kill their husbands than vice versa (Campbell, 1995; Bachman, 1994).

An alarming aspect of family homicide is that small children often witness the murder or find the body of a family member. No automatic follow-up or counseling of these children occurs through the criminal justice or mental health system in most communities. These children are at great risk for emotional turmoil and for becoming involved in violence themselves.

The underlying dynamics of homicide within families vary greatly from those of other murders. Homicide within families is most often preceded by abuse of a family member (Campbell, 1991). Thus prevention of family homicide involves working with abusive families. The chance of eventual homicide must always be kept in mind when working with these families. Nurses have a "duty to warn" family members of the possibility of homicide when severe abuse is present, just as they warn of the hazards of smoking (Campbell, 1995). Other nursing care issues are discussed further in the section on family violence.

Assault

The death toll from violence is indeed staggering, yet the physical injuries and emotional costs of **assault** are equally important issues in terms of the acute health care system and both public health nursing and home health care. At least 100 nonfatal assaults occur for each homicide that occurs in the United States (US Public Health Service, 1990). Of all simple and aggravated assaults, 33% resulted in injury (Reiss and Roth, 1993). The greatest risk factor for an individual's victimization through violence is age, with youth at significantly higher risk. Whereas more males than females are victims of homicide and assault, women are more likely to be victimized by a relative, especially a male partner (Bachman, 1994). Sometimes the difference between a homicide and an assault is only the response time and quality of emergency transport and treatment facilities. Whatever community measures are used to address homicide are also useful to combat assault. In addition, nurses find that assaulted persons are often seen in home health care with long-term health problems such as head injuries, spinal cord injuries, and stomas from abdominal gunshot wounds. In addition to physical care, nurses must also address the emotional trauma resulting from a violent attack by helping victims talk through their traumatic experience to try to make some sense of the violence, and by referring them for further counseling if anxiety, sleeping problems, or depression persists after the assault.

Rape

Currently **rape** is one of the most underreported forms of human abuse in the United States. Although the number of rapes reported to law enforcement agencies has decreased since 1993, only a third of victims or survivors report rape/sexual assault to a law enforcement agency. The rates of completed and attempted rape are equivalent (Reiss and Roth, 1993). In 1992 there were 84 rapes per 100,000 women, the lowest since 1976 (US Department of Justice, 1997). Victim reporting of rape has improved. Hospital, emergency personnel, and police have better protocols for victims of rape. Although the collection of information leading to prosecution is emphasized, the protocols try to ensure respectful and supportive treatment for victims. Another important factor is the recognition of date and marital rape. Official recognition of rape regardless of a victim's relationship to the perpetrator has led to an increased number of women reporting rape. Rape also happens to men, especially boys and young men, but the statistics on the incidence of male rape vary. A major problem in obtaining statistics is that the definition of rape adopted by the Federal Bureau of Investigation for compiling the Uniformed Crime Reports is limited to penile-vaginal penetration only (Koss and Harvey, 1991). It appears that the emotional trauma to a male rape victim is at least as serious as that for a woman.

For reported rapes, cities constitute higher risk areas than do rural areas, and the hours between 8 PM and 2 AM, weekends, and the summer are the most critical times. In about half of rapes the victim and the offender meet on the street, whereas in other cases the rapist either enters the victim's home or somehow entices or forces the victim to accompany him.

Prevention of rape, as in other forms of human abuse, requires a broad-based community focus for educating both the community as a whole and key groups such as police, health providers, educators, and social workers. Rape rates and community-level variables such as community approval and legitimization of violence (e.g., violent network television viewing and permitting corporal punishment in schools) appear related and underscore the need for community-level intervention (Donat and D'Emilio, 1997).

Attitudes

The first priority is to change attitudes about rape and about victims or survivors. Rape is a crime of violence, not a crime of passion. The underlying issues are hostility, power, and control rather than sexual desire. The defining issue is lack of consent of the victim. When a woman or man refuses any sexual activity, that refusal means "no." People have the right to change their mind, even when they seemed initially acquiescent. Pressure in the form of physical contact, threats, or deliberate inducement of drug or alcohol intoxication is a violation of the law. There must also be an end to the myths that women say "no" to sex when they really mean "yes" and that the victims of rape are culpable because of the way they dress or act. On college campuses, negative attitudes toward acquaintance or date rape are slow to change. Women on college campuses underreport allegations of rape because of issues of confidentiality and fear of being discredited (Koss and Cook , 1998).

Pornography

It is unclear whether a relationship exists between the viewing of pornographic material showing violence against women and aggressive sexual behavior (Cottle et al, 1997; Kimmel, 1996; Russell, 1995a). However, there is enough evidence to recommend keeping violent pornography illegal, especially for minors. Prevention also involves providing information to women about self-protection, including self-defense procedures, avoiding high-risk locations, and safeguarding one's home against unwanted entry.

Victim or survivor

During the act of rape, survivors are often hit, kicked, stabbed, and severely beaten. It is this violence that most traumatizes the person because of the fear for her life and her helplessness, lack of control, and vulnerability.

People react to rape differently, depending on their personality, past experiences, background, and support received after the trauma. Some cry, shout, or discuss the experience. Others withdraw and fear discussing the attack. During the immediate as well as the follow-up stages, victims tend to blame themselves for what has happened. It is important while working with rape victims that nurses help them identify the issues behind self-blame. Although fault should not be placed on survivors, they should be taught to take control, learn assertiveness, and therefore believe that they can take certain actions to prevent future rapes. Survivors need to talk about what happened and to express their feelings and fears in a nonjudgmental atmosphere. Nonjudgmental listening is important.

In any psychological trauma, the right to privacy and confidentiality is of the utmost importance. Victims should be given privacy, respect, and assurance of confidentiality. They also should be told about health care procedures conducted immediately after the rape and should be linked with proper resources for ease of reporting. Nurses often provide continuous care once the victim enters the health care system. Because many victims deny the event once the initial crisis is past, a single-session debriefing should be completed during the initial examination. The physical assessment, examination, and debriefing should be carried out by specially trained providers (Aiken and Speck, 1995).

In several states nurses perform the physical examination in the emergency department to gather evidence (e.g., hair samples and skin fragments beneath the victim's fingernails) for criminal prosecution (Ledray and Simmelink, 1997). This is an important intervention since physicians may be impatient with the time required for this procedure; nurses can take advantage of this opportunity to provide therapeutic communication. Nurses can be trained to conduct the examination easily, and their evidence is credible and effective in resultant court proceedings (Ledray and Simmelink, 1997). Nurses can lobby for changes in hospital policies and state laws to make this strategy a reality in all states.

Rape is a situational crisis for which advance preparation is rarely possible. Therefore nursing efforts are directed toward helping victims cope with the stress and disruption of their lives caused by the attack. Counseling focuses on the crisis and the concomitant fears, feelings, and issues involved. Nurses can help survivors problem-solve to develop ways to regroup personal forces. If posttraumatic stress disorder has developed, professional psychological or psychiatric treatment is indicated.

Many rape victims need follow-up mental health services to help them cope with the short- and long-term effects of the crisis. The time after a rape is one of disequilibrium, psychological breakdown, and reorganization of attitudes about the safety of the world. Common, everyday tasks often tax an individual's resources. Many individuals forget or fail to keep appointments. Therefore nurses can make appropriate referrals and obtain permission from the victim to remain in contact through telephone conversations. In this manner the ongoing needs of the victim can be assessed and support, encouragement, and resources can be offered as needed (Koss and Harvey, 1991).

DID YOU KNOW? *Forty to forty-five percent of physically abused women are also being forced into sex. This has implications for the prevention of unintended and adolescent pregnancies, human immune virus (HIV), acquired immunodeficiency syndrome (AIDS), and repeat sexually transmitted diseases (STDs), as well as for women's healthy sexuality and self-esteem.*

Suicide

In 1994, suicides were committed by 31,142 people in the United States. This is a rate of 12 per 100,000 people. Rates are higher for males, the elderly, non-Hispanic whites, and American Indians/Alaskan Natives (CDC, 1997). The risk for death by **suicide** is greater than for death by homicide (Reiss and Roth, 1993). Approximately 11.6 suicides per 100,000 people occur in the United States (US Public Health Service, 1990). The incidence of suicide increases with age, reaching a high of 40 per 100,000 among persons over 75 years of age.

Among adolescents the incidence of actual suicide is equally alarming. According to the National Institute of Mental Health, more than 6000 adolescents kill themselves each year. This figure means that every 90 minutes an adolescent commits suicide; in addition, it is estimated that every day 1000 more will attempt it (Oliphant, 1986). Leading risk factors for adolescent suicide are low self-esteem, chronic depression, incest, and extrafamilial sexual and physical abuse (Eggert et al, 1994; Hernandez et al, 1993).

Males commit suicide three times more often than females, although females attempt suicide more often. The number one risk factor for actual and attempted suicide in adult women is spousal abuse (Stark and Flitcraft, 1991). Suicide is four times more frequent among whites than among African-Americans. Affluent and educated people have higher rates of suicide than do the economically and educationally disadvantaged.

Nursing care must focus on family members and friends of suicide victims. **Survivors** often feel angry toward the dead person, yet frequently turn the anger inward. Likewise, survivors frequently question their own liability for the death. The impact of suicide can affect family, friends, co-workers, and the community. Survivors may have difficulty dealing with their feelings toward the dead person. They may have difficulty concentrating and may limit their social activities because it is often difficult for both survivors and their friends to talk about the suicide. Nurses can help survivors cope with the trauma of the loss and make referrals to a counselor or support groups.

FAMILY VIOLENCE AND ABUSE

Family violence, including **sexual abuse, emotional abuse,** and **physical abuse,** causes significant injury and death. These three forms tend to occur together as part of a system of coercive control. Generally, violence within families is perpetrated by the most powerful against the least powerful. Thus approximately 90% of all "spouse abuse" is directed primarily toward wives (although they may physically fight back), whereas approximately 7% to 8% is mutual violence, and 2% to 3% is husband abuse (Campbell and Humphreys, 1993).

Recognizing the battered child or spouse in the emergency room is relatively simple after the fact. It is unfortunate that, by the time medical care is sought, serious physical and emotional damage may have been done. Nurses are in a key position to predict and deal with abusive tendencies. By understanding factors contributing to the development of abusive behaviors, nurses can identify abuse-prone families.

Development of Abusive Patterns

Factors that characterize people who become involved in family violence include upbringing, living conditions, and increased stress. Understanding how these factors influence the development of abusive behavior can help the nurse deal with abusive families.

Upbringing

Of all the factors that characterize the background of abusers, the most predictably present is previous exposure to some form of violence (Straus and Gelles, 1990). As children, abusers were often beaten themselves or witnessed the beating of siblings or a parent. Children raised in this way may abhor the use of violence, but they have had no experience with other models of family relationships.

Physical punishment of children appears to be associated with future abuse of both children and spouses, especially when used frequently and severely (Straus and Gelles, 1990). Childhood physical punishment teaches children to use violent conflict resolution as an adult. A child may learn to associate love with violence because a parent is usually the first person to hit a child. Children may think that those who love them also are those who hit them. The moral rightness of hitting other family members thus may be established when physical punishment is used to train children, especially when it is used more than occasionally. These experiences predispose children ultimately to use violence with their own children.

As well as having a history of child abuse themselves, people who become abusers tend to have hostile personality styles and be verbally aggressive. They have often learned these characteristics from their own childhood experiences. Their parents may have set unrealistic goals, and when the children failed to perform accordingly, they were criticized, demeaned, punished, and denied affection. These children may have been told how to act, what to do, and how to feel, thereby discouraging the development of normal attachment, autonomy, problem-solving skills, and creativity (Briere et al, 1996). Children raised in this way grow up feeling unloved and worthless. They may want a child of their own so that they will feel assured of someone's love.

To protect themselves from feelings of worthlessness and fear of rejection, abused children form a protective shell and grow increasingly hostile and distrustful of others. The behavior of potential abusers reflects a low tolerance for frustration, emotional instability, and the onset of aggressive feelings with minimal provocation. Because of their emotional insecurity, they often depend on a child or spouse to meet their needs of feeling valued and secure. When their needs are not met by others, they become overly critical. Critical, resentful behavior and unrealistic expectations of others lead to a vicious cycle. The more critical these people become, the more they are rejected and alienated from others. Abusive individuals tend to perceive that the target of their hostility is "out to get them." These distorted perceptions can be detected when parents talk about an infant crying or keeping them up at night "on purpose" (Briere et al, 1996; Campbell and Humphreys, 1993).

Increased stress

A perceived or actual crisis may precede an abusive incident. Because crisis reinforces feelings of inadequacy and low self-esteem, a number of events often occur in a short time to precipitate abusive patterns. Unemployment, strains in the marriage, or an unplanned pregnancy may set off violence.

The daily hassles of raising young children, especially in an economically strained household, intensify an already stressed atmosphere for which an unexpected and difficult event provides a catalyst for violence. Straus and Gelles (1990) found associations among stressful life events, poverty, the number of small children, and family violence.

Crowded living conditions may also precipitate abuse. The presence of several people in a small space heightens tensions and reduces privacy. Tempers flare because of the constant stimulation from others.

Social isolation is associated with abuse in families (Briere et al, 1996; Straus and Gelles, 1990). Such isolation reduces social support, decreasing a family's ability to deal with stressors. The problem may be intensified if a violent family member tries to keep the family isolated to escape detection. Therefore when a family misses clinic or home visit appointments, nurses need to keep in mind that abuse may be present. Nurses can encourage involvement in community activities and can help neighbors reach out to neighbors to help prevent abuse.

Frequent moves disrupt social support systems, are associated with an overall increased stress level, and tend to isolate people, at least briefly. Mobility can have a serious negative effect on the abuse-prone family. These families do not readily initiate new relationships. They rely on the family for support. Resources may be unfamiliar or inaccessible to them. Because frequent moving may be both a risk factor for abuse and a sign of an abusive family trying to avoid detection, nurses should assess such families carefully for abuse.

Types of Family Violence

Since various forms of family violence and violence outside the home often occur together, nurses who detect child abuse should also suspect other forms of family violence. When elderly parents report that their (now adult) child was abused or has a history of violence toward others, the nurse should recognize the potential for elder abuse. Physical abuse of women is frequently accompanied by sexual abuse both inside and outside marital rela-

tionships. Severe wife abusers may have a history of other acts of violence. Families who are verbally aggressive in conflict resolution (e.g., using name calling, belittling, screaming, and yelling) are more likely to be physically abusive. Although the various forms of family violence are discussed separately, they should not be thought of as totally separate phenomenon.

No member of the family is guaranteed immunity from abuse and neglect. Spouse abuse, child abuse, abuse of elderly persons, serious violence among siblings, and mutual abuse by members all occur. Although these examples are not inclusive, they demonstrate the scope of family violence.

Child abuse

The most recent published national survey projected that nearly 1.5 million children and adolescents are subjected to abusive physical violence each year (Straus and Gelles, 1990). This is probably a conservative figure, since only the most severe cases are reported. In addition a greater number of children each year witness domestic violence (Campbell and Humphreys, 1993; Peled, 1996). Child maltreatment was rarely discussed in medical literature until Henry Kempe et al published their classic article in 1962, which coined the term **battered child syndrome.**

Kempe and his associates (1962) generated public and professional concern over child maltreatment. Their work led to the passage in 1974 of the Child Abuse Prevention and Treatment Act, which mandated reporting by professionals of child maltreatment.

The presence of child abuse signifies ineffective family functioning. Abusive parents who recognize their problem are often reluctant to seek assistance because of the stigma attached to being considered a child abuser.

Children are frequent victims of abuse because they are small and relatively powerless. In many families only one child is abused. Parents may identify with this particular child and be especially critical of the child's behavior. In

---

HOW TO *Identify Potentially Abusive Parents*

The following characteristics in couples expecting a child constitute warning signs of actual or potential abuse.

1. *Denial of the reality of the pregnancy, as seen in a refusal to talk about the impending birth or to think of a name for the child*
2. *An obvious concern or fear that the baby will not meet some predetermined standard: sex, hair color, temperament, or resemblance to family members*
3. *Failure to follow through on the desire for or seeking of an abortion*
4. *An initial decision to place the child for adoption and a change of mind*
5. *Rejection of the mother by the father of the baby*
6. *Family experiencing stress and numerous crises so that the birth of a child may be the "straw that broke the camel's back"*

7. *Initial and unresolved negative feelings about having a child*
8. *Lack of support for the new parents*
9. *Isolation from friends, neighbors, or family*
10. *Parental evidence of poor impulse control or fear of losing control*
11. *Contradictory history*
12. *Appearance of detachment*
13. *Appearance of misusing drugs or alcohol*
14. *Shopping for hospitals or health care providers*
15. *Unrealistic expectations of the child*
16. *Abuse of mother by father, especially during pregnancy*
17. *Child is not biological offspring of male stepfather or mother's current boyfriend*

some cases the child may have certain qualities such as looking like a relative, being handicapped, or being particularly bright and capable, that provoke the parent.

Abusive parents tend to be very controlling of their children's behavior and insensitive to their needs (Humphreys and Ramsey, 1993). They often have unrealistic expectations of the child's developmental abilities. The nurse must not only teach them what is normal but also address their underlying emotional needs. These parents often experience pain and poor emotional stability and need intervention as much as their children. Below are some of the behavioral indicator of potentially abusive parents.

Foster care. When child abuse is discovered, the child is often placed in a foster home. It is unfortunate that there is not enough good foster care for all abused children, and many foster care situations are also abusive. Abused children generally want to return to their parents, and the goal of most agencies is to keep natural families together as long as it is safe for the child. However, a family preservation approach is not always effective in keeping children safe (Chalk and King 1998). Many times the nurse's role involves helping to monitor a family in which a formerly abused child is returned after a time in foster care. Keen judgment and close collaboration with social services are necessary in these situations. The nurse must ensure the safety of the child, while working *with* the parents in an empathetic way. The nurse's goal is to enhance their parenting skills, not to be viewed as yet another watchdog.

Another point to keep in mind about abusive parents is that the wish to replace a child who has been removed by the courts because of abuse is a normal response to the grief of losing a child. Rather than regarding another pregnancy as a sign of continued poor judgment or pathological behavior, the pregnancy can be perceived by the nurse as an opportunity for intensive intervention to prevent the abuse of the expected child. Generally, the parents are equally eager to avoid further problems if enlisted as partners in the project.

Indicators of child abuse. It is essential that nurses recognize the physical and behavioral indicators of abuse and neglect. Child abuse ranges from violent physical attacks to passive neglect. Violence such as beating, burning, kicking, or shaking may lead to severe physical injury. Passive neglect may result in insidious malnutrition or other problems. Abuse is not limited to physical maltreatment but includes emotional abuse such as yelling at or continually demeaning and criticizing the child.

Emotional abuse involves extreme debasement of feelings and may result in the child feeling inadequate, inept, uncared for, and worthless. Victims of emotional abuse learn to hide their feelings to avoid incurring additional scorn. They may act out by performing poorly in school, becoming truant, and being hostile and aggressive. Children who are abused or who witness domestic violence can

suffer developmentally (Wolak and Finkelhor, 1998). Often adolescents run away from home as a direct result of domestic violence (Nadon, Koverola, and Schludermann, 1998).

HOW TO *Recognize Actual or Potential Abuse*

1. An unexplained injury
   a. Skin: burns, old or recent scars, ecchymosis, soft tissue swelling, human bites
   b. Fractures: recent or ones that have healed
   c. Subdural hematomas
   d. Trauma to genitalia
   e. Whiplash (caused by shaking small children)
2. Dehydration or malnourishment without obvious cause
3. Provision of inappropriate food or drugs (alcohol, tobacco, medication prescribed for someone else, foods not appropriate for the child's age)
4. Evidence of general poor care: poor hygiene, dirty clothes, unkempt hair, dirty nails
5. Unusually fearful of nurse and others
6. Considered to be a "bad" child
7. Inappropriately dressed for the season or weather conditions
8. Reports or shows evidence of sexual abuse
9. Injuries not mentioned in history
10. Seems to need to take care of the parent and speak for the parent
11. Maternal depression
12. Maladjustment of older siblings

Physical symptoms of physical, sexual, or emotional stress may include hyperactivity, withdrawal, overeating, dermatological problems, vague physical complaints, stuttering, enuresis (bladder incontinence), and encopresis (bowel incontinence). It is ironic that bed-wetting is often a trigger for further abuse, which makes for a particularly vicious cycle. When a child displays physical symptoms without clear physiological origin, ruling out the possibilty of abuse should be part of the nurse's assessment process.

Child neglect. The two categories of **child neglect** are physical and emotional. **Physical neglect** is defined as failure to provide adequate food, proper clothing, shelter, hygiene, or necessary medical care (Campbell and Humphreys, 1993). Physical neglect is most often associated with extreme poverty.

In contrast, **emotional neglect** is the omission of basic nurturing, acceptance, and caring essential for healthy personal development. These children are largely ignored or in many cases treated as nonpersons. Such neglect usually affects the development of self-esteem. It is difficult for a neglected child to feel a great deal of self-worth because the parents have not demonstrated that they value the child.

Neglect is more difficult to assess and evaluate than abuse because it is subtle and may go unnoticed. Astute observations of children, their homes, and the way in which they relate to their caregivers can provide clues of neglect.

Sexual abuse. Child abuse also includes sexual abuse. Approximately one of four female children and one of ten males in the United States will be subject to some form of sexual abuse by the time they reach 18 years of age. The exact prevalence is difficult to obtain because not all children have the cognitive ability to describe these experiences (Kendall-Tackett and Marshall, 1998). This abuse ranges from unwanted sexual touching to intercourse. The majority of childhood sexual abuse is perpetrated by someone the child knows. Between one half and one third of all sexual abuse involves a family member (Russell, 1995b). Although sexual abuse is perpetrated across caregivers, a child's risk for abuse is higher with stepparents or nonrelated caregivers (Gelles, 1998). The long-term effects of sexual abuse are depression, sexual disturbances, and substance abuse (Carlson et al, 1997).

Research has shown that many of the characteristics of physically abusive and sexually abusive parents, such as unhappiness, loneliness, and rigidity, are shared by both groups (Milner and Robertson, 1990). However, sexually abusive parents report fewer family problems and a more positive view of the child than do physically abusive parents.

Father-daughter incest is the type of **incest** most often reported (Herman and Hirschman, 1993). Many cases of parental incest go unreported because victims fear punishment, abandonment, rejection, or family disruption if they acknowledge the problem. Incest occurs in all races, religious groups, and socioeconomic classes. Incest is receiving greater attention because of mandatory reporting laws, yet all too often its incidence remains a family secret.

Because nurses are often involved in helping women deal with the aftermath of incest, it is crucial to understand the typical patterns and the long-term implications. A typical pattern is as follows. The daughter involved in paternal incest is usually about 9 years of age at the onset and is often the oldest or only daughter. The father seldom uses physical force. He most likely relies on threats, bribes, intimidation, or misrepresentation of moral standards or exploits the daughter's need for human affection (Herman and Hirschman, 1993).

Nurses must be aware of the incidence, signs and symptoms, and psychological and physical trauma of incest. Green (1996) identified clusters of affective symptoms, including low self-esteem, depression, and intrusive imagery. Somatic symptoms include headaches, eating and sleeping disorders, menstrual problems, and gastrointestinal distress. Other symptoms include difficulties in social situations, especially in forming and maintaining close relationships with men, and behavioral symptoms such as substance abuse and sexual dysfunction.

Adolescents may display inappropriate sexual activity or truancy or may run away from home. Running away is usually considered a sign of delinquency; however, an adolescent who runs away may be using a healthy response to a violent family situation. Therefore the assessment should ask about sexual and physical abuse at home and plan appropriate intervention.

Houck and King (1989) say that the effects of any kind of child maltreatment can be lessened if the child has a nonoffending parent, another relative, or an adult outside the family to provide stable, ongoing support and emotional nurturance. Even so, adult survivors of sexual abuse often have significant health problems that need to be addressed in terms of the ongoing effects of their adult experiences (Draucker, 1993).

Abuse of female partners

Although women do abuse men, by far the greatest proportion of what is often discussed as spouse abuse or domestic violence is actually wife abuse. At least 1.8 million women are battered by their husbands each year in the United States (Straus and Gelles, 1990). Neither the term **wife abuse** nor **spouse abuse** takes into account violence in dating or cohabiting relationships or violence in same sex-relationships. *Spousal or partner violence* is a more inclusive term to refer to all kinds of violence between partners, and all adults should be assessed for violence in their primary intimate relationships. Though there are no prevalence studies on violence in same sex-relationships, the incidence is considered to be that same as in heterosexual relationships. The abuse of female partners has the most serious community health ramifications because of the greater prevalence, the greater potential for homicide (Campbell, 1995), the effects on the children in the household, and the more serious long-term emotional and physical consequences.

Victims of child abuse and individuals who saw their mothers being battered are at risk of using violence toward an intimate partner, whether one is male or female (Straus and Gelles, 1990). However, using evidence of a violent childhood to identify women at risk of abuse is less useful since abuse cannot be predicted based on characteristics of the individual woman. It is the violent background of an abusive male, combined with his tendencies to be possessive, controlling, and extremely jealous, that is most predictive of abuse. Substance abuse is also associated with battering, although it cannot be said to "cause" the violence.

Signs of abuse. Battered women often have bruises and lacerations of the face, head, and trunk of the body. Attacks are often carefully inflicted on parts of the body that can easily be disguised by clothing. This pattern of proximal location of injuries (breasts, abdomen, upper thighs, and back) rather than distal is characteristic of abuse (Campbell and Sheridan, 1989). When a woman has a black eye or bruises about the mouth, the nurse should ask, "Who hit you?" rather than, "What happened to you?" The latter implies that the nurse is neither knowledgeable nor comfortable with violence, and this may prompt the woman to fabricate a more acceptable cause of her injury.

Once abused, women tend to exhibit low self-esteem and depression (Campbell et al, 1997). They have more physical symptoms of stress than women in troubled relationships and also frequently complain of chronic pain. Both of these symptoms may be related to repeated injuries, as well as to the intense stress of a violent relationship (Campbell and Humphreys, 1993).

Abuse as a process. Research by both Landenburger (1989) and Campbell et al (1994) suggests that there is a process of response to battering over time wherein the woman's emotional and behavioral reactions change. At first there is a great need to minimize the seriousness of the situation. The violence usually starts with a slight shove in the middle of a heated argument. All couples fight, and if there is any physical aggression, both the man and woman tend to blame the incident on something external such as a particularly stressful day at work or drinking too much. The male partner usually apologizes for the incident and, as with any problem in a relationship, the couple tries various strategies to improve the situation. Although marital counseling may be useful at this early stage, it is generally contraindicated at all other stages because of the risk to the woman's safety. Unfortunately, abuse tends to escalate in frequency and severity over time, and the man's remorse tends to lessen (Campbell and Humphreys, 1993).

Because women have often been taught to take responsibility for the success of a relationship, they usually go through a period in which they tend to change their behavior to end the violence. They may even blame themselves for infuriating their spouse. Women who blame themselves for provoking the abuse are more likely to have low self-esteem and be depressed than those who do not blame themselves. The majority of battered women do not blame themselves for provoking the abuse, and any self-blame tends to decrease over time (Campbell, 1989a). Women find that no matter what they do, the violence continues. During this period the woman tries to hide the violence because of the stigma attached. She tries to placate her spouse and feels she is losing her sense of self (Landenburger, 1998; Ulrich, 1989). The woman is also typically concerned about her children whether she leaves or stays.

Some abuse escalates to the point that the woman is kept in terror, similar to a prisoner of war (Okun, 1986). She is constantly subjected to emotional degradation, absolute financial dependency, sadistic physical and sexual violence, and control of all her activities. She is in terror that her partner will try to kill her, her children, or both if she attempts to leave. This fear is, in fact, often justified. Clinically, she may experience learned helplessness, traumatic stress syndrome, or both and will need intensive therapy. She may kill herself or her abuser to escape because she sees no other way out (Campbell, 1992). A nurse encountering an abusive situation such as this needs to consider the safety of the woman and her children as the

priority. The woman will need an order of protection, a legal document specifically designed to keep the woman's abuser away from her. She will also need help in getting to a safe place, such as a wife abuse shelter. At the very least, the woman must design a carefully thought-out plan for escape and arrange for a neighbor or an adolescent child to call the police when there is another violent episode.

The more frequently encountered battered woman is one who has tried several times to leave. She will eventually successfully do so or otherwise manage to end the violence (Campbell et al, 1994). Each attempt to leave is a gathering of resources, a trial of her children's ability to survive without a father, and a testing of her partner's promises to reform. When and if it becomes clear that he is not going to change and she has the emotional support and the financial resources to do so, she will end the relationship. Often this will involve using a shelter for abused women or individual advocacy and support groups and/or the criminal justice system.

An alternative to ending the relationship is the male partner's attendance at programs for batterers. These programs have been shown to be most effective if they are court mandated and if the man's underlying values about women are addressed, as well as his violence (Dutton, 1995; Edleson and Tolman 1992). Abused women need affirmation, support, reassurances of the normalcy of their responses, accurate information about shelters and legal resources, and brainstorming about possible solutions. These needs can be met by other women in similar situations and by professionals such as nurses (Campbell 1998). Women should not be pushed into actions they are not ready to take.

After the abuse has ended, a period of recovery ensues. This includes a normal grief response for the relationship that has ended and a search for meaning in the experience (Landenburger, 1989; Landenburger, 1998). Thus a formerly battered woman who is feeling depressed and lonely after the relationship has ended is exhibiting a normal response for which support is needed.

Intimate partner sexual abuse. Because 40% to 45% of battered women are also sexually abused (Campbell, 1989b), the nurse must carefully assess for this form of violence in women in ongoing relationships. In fact, between 10% and 14% of all American women have been raped within a marriage. This sexual abuse is not always accompanied by physical abuse.

The notion that men have a right to force their wives to have sex comes from traditional English law that stated that a woman gave irrevocable and perpetual consent to her husband on marriage to have sex whenever and however he wanted. This legal tradition was reflected in the laws of 47 states in the United States as recently as 1980 as a marital rape exemption. In other words, a man could not be charged with rape if the victim was his wife. By 1994 only 7 states still retained this provision, but the fact that it is still legal for a man to rape his wife in any state is alarming. Serious physical and emotional damage has been documented from marital rape (Campbell and Alford, 1989). There is also an alarming incidence of date rape, the dynamics of which may parallel marital rape.

To assess for sexual assault, the question of "Have you ever been forced into sex you did not wish to participate in?" should be used in all nursing assessments to see if marital rape, date rape, or rape of a male has occurred.

Abuse during pregnancy. Battering during pregnancy has serious implications for the health of both women and their children. Approximately one of six pregnant women is physically battered during pregnancy, with a larger proportion (20%) of adolescents abused during pregnancy than adult women. Although abuse during pregnancy occurs across ethnic groups, white women experience a significantly higher severity of abuse than African-American or Hispanic women (McFarlane and Parker, 1994). These women are at risk for spontaneous abortion, premature delivery, low-birth-weight infants, substance abuse during pregnancy, and depression (Campbell et al, 1992; McFarlane, Parker, and Soeken, 1994). Abuse before pregnancy often precedes abuse during pregnancy. See the Research Brief.

Generally, the same dynamics of coercive control operate when a woman is battered during pregnancy. The largest group of one sample of 76 battered women were subject to the same abuse whether or not they were pregnant. About 20% escaped abuse during pregnancy, although they were abused again after the baby was born. Another 35% indicated that their perception of the reason for abuse during pregnancy was that their partner was jealous of or angry at the baby (Campbell et al, 1993). It could be anticipated that this group of infants would be at particularly high risk of child abuse after they are born. The main difference found between women who were battered during pregnancy and those who were not was that those women battered during pregnancy had been battered more frequently and severely previous to their pregnancy (Campbell et al, 1993). The clear implication is that all pregnant women should be assessed for abuse at each prenatal care visit, and postpartum home visits should include assessment for child abuse and partner abuse. In as many as 77% of families where there is severe wife abuse, there is also child abuse (Straus and Gelles, 1990).

Abuse of elderly persons

Elder abuse is a form of family violence that is becoming more apparent. About 4% of senior citizens suffer from some form of abuse, neglect, or exploitation (Weith, 1994). Similar to spouse abuse and child abuse, most cases of elder abuse go unreported. As with other forms of human abuse, elder maltreatment includes emotional, sexual, and physical neglect, as well as physical and sexual violence, with financial abuse and violation of rights particular issues for elders (Weiner, 1991). In addition, similar to spouse abuse, alcohol abuse is used as an excuse (Anetzberger et al, 1994).

Types of elder abuse. The elderly are neglected when others fail to provide adequate food, clothing, shelter, and physical care and to meet physiological, emotional, and safety needs. Elder neglect either through lack of care or improper care can be considered criminal neglect.

Roughness in handling elderly people can lead to bruises and bleeding into body tissues because of the fragility of their skin and vascular systems. It is often difficult to determine if the injuries of elderly persons result from abuse, falls, or other natural causes. Careful assessment both through observation and discussion can help in determining the cause of injuries. Other ways in which elderly persons are physically abused occur when caregivers impose unrealistic toileting demands and when the special needs and previous living patterns of the person are ignored.

Elderly persons can also be abused with regard to nutrition. They may be given food that they cannot chew or swallow or that is contraindicated because of dietary restrictions. Caregivers may overlook food preferences or social or cultural beliefs and patterns about food. Elderly people may become undernourished if they can neither prepare their own food nor eat the food that is prepared for them.

Caregivers occasionally give elderly people medication to induce confusion or drowsiness so that they will be less troublesome, will need less care, or will allow others to gain control of their financial and personal resources. Once medicated, elderly persons have few ways to act on their own behalf.

The most common form of psychological abuse is rejection or simply ignoring elderly people. This kind of treatment conveys that they are worthless and useless to others. Elderly persons may subsequently regress and become increasingly dependent on others, who tend to re-

---

RESEARCH *Brief*

Nursing researchers evaluated the safety behaviors of equal numbers of Hispanic, African-American, and white women abused during pregnancy (N = 132) who received a 10-minute nursing intervention for domestic violence three times during pregnancy. There was a significant increase in each of the 15 safety behaviors (such as hiding money and car keys, asking neighbors to call the police, removing weapons) over time with the largest increase after the first intervention (outcomes were measured twice during pregnancy and three times in the year post partum). Since one out of six women is abused during pregnancy, nurses need to provide this tested intervention to increase safety for them and their infants.

McFarlane J et al: Safety behaviors of abused women after an intervention during pregnancy. *JOGNN* 27(1):64, 1998.

sent the imposition and demands on their time and lifestyles. The pattern becomes cyclical: the more regressed the person becomes, the greater the dependence. Further, the elderly people's past accomplishments and present abilities are not consistently acknowledged, causing them to feel even less capable. Indicators of actual or potential elder abuse are listed below.

HOW TO *Identify Potential or Actual Elder Abuse*

- *Unexplained or repeated injury*
- *Fear of the caregiver*
- *Untreated sores or other skin injuries, such as decubitus ulcers, excoriated perineum, burns*
- *Overall poor care (e.g., unclean, given inappropriate food)*
- *Withdrawal and passivity*
- *Periods of time when the elderly person is unsupervised*
- *Failure to seek appropriate medical care*
- *Contractures resulting from immobility or restraint*
- *Unwillingness or inability of caregiver to meet elderly person's needs*
- *Improper home repair*
- *Unsafe home situation (e.g., poor heating, ventilation, dangerous clutter)*

Adapted from Phillips LR: Abuse/neglect of the frail elderly at home: an exploration of theoretical relationships, *J Adv Nurs* 8:379, 1983; Fulmer T: Mistreatment of elders, assessment, diagnosis, and intervention, *Nurs Clin North Am* 24(3):707, 1989.

Precipitating factors for elder abuse. Caregivers abuse elderly people for a variety of reasons. Elderly family members may impose a physical, emotional, or financial burden on the caregiver, leading to frustration and resentment. The abuser may reverse earlier family patterns, whereby the abuser was previously abused by the elderly person (Anetzberger et al, 1994).

Many people tend to think of abused elderly individuals as dependent on others for their care. A factor that increases the risk of elder abuse is the dependency of a significant other on the elderly person (Lang, 1993). Spouses who batter continue to abuse as they age. Additionally, children who have lived in abusive households learn that behavior (Baron and Welty, 1996). Also, many female abused elderly persons are battered women who have become old. Thus, although it is important to assess for elder abuse when the elderly person is in need of care from family members, all elderly persons should be assessed for abuse.

Confused and frail elderly persons are a high-risk group for abuse. Large numbers of frail elderly people, many with serious physical or mental impairments, live in the community and are cared for by their families. Also, those with Alzheimer's disease and other dementias have a greater risk for physical abuse than elderly persons with other illnesses. These illnesses place a high burden on the caregiver and subsequent depression of the caregiver

(Coyne et al, 1993). Living with and providing care to a confused elderly person are difficult, round-the-clock tasks that often exhaust family members. Family stress increases as members must work harder to fulfill their other responsibilities in addition to the needs of the elderly person.

Prevention strategies. Fulmer (1989) suggested the following prevention strategies for communities:

1. Develop new ways to provide assistance to caregiving families, including helping them decide about discontinuing caregiving at home
2. Publicize existing supports for caregiving families
3. Involve all community organizations in developing new supports and training, such as Neighborhood Watch programs for families with elderly persons.

In addition, nurses must help families who plan to take care of an elderly member at home to fully evaluate that decision and prepare for the stressors that will be involved. A plan for regular respite care for the elderly person is absolutely necessary. Strategies for the primary and secondary prevention of abuse of elderly persons include victim support groups, senior advocacy volunteer programs, and training for providers working with elderly persons (Wolf et al, 1994).

Elderly people need to retain as much autonomy and decision-making ability as possible. Nurses have many ways to detect abuse among elderly persons and the skills and responsibility for discovering abuse, giving treatment, and making referrals. Many families who care for elderly members exhaust their resources and coping ability. Nurses can help them find new sources of support and aid.

NURSING INTERVENTIONS
Primary Prevention

To prevent violence and human abuse, a community approach is essential. First, the community can take a stand against violence and make sure their elected officials and the local media consider nonviolence a priority. Nurses as community advocates can help with this process. In the legislative arena, laws are needed to outlaw physical punishment in schools and marital rape. State laws can enforce mandatory arrest for abusers, which has been shown to decrease repeat offenses, at least for men who are employed and well connected in their communities (Edleson and Tolman, 1992).

Strong community sanctions against violence in the home can reduce abuse levels (Counts et al, 1992; Levinson, 1989). Neighbors keeping an eye out and working together to address problems in other families is not an invasion of privacy but a sign of community cohesiveness. Nurses can work with advocate groups to make sure police deal with assault within marriage as swiftly, surely, and severely as assault between strangers. Nurses can encourage others to interfere when they see children beaten in a grocery store, notice that an elderly person is not being properly cared for, see a neighborhood bully beat up his classmates, or hear a neighbor hitting his wife.

Second, persons can take measures to reduce their vulnerability to violence by improving the physical security of their homes and learning personal defense measures. Nurses can encourage people to keep windows and doors locked, trim shrubs around their homes, and keep lights on during high-crime periods. Many neighborhoods organize crime watch programs and post signs to that effect. Other signs indicate that certain homes will assist children who need help; these homes are identified by the sign of a hand, usually posted in a window. Other neighbors informally agree to monitor one another's property and safety. Also, many law enforcement agencies evaluate homes for security and teach individual or neighborhood safety programs. Individuals install home security systems, participate in personal defense programs such as judo or karate, and purchase firearms for their protection.

Unfortunately, handguns are far more likely to kill family members than intruders (Kellerman and Reay, 1986). Accidental firearm death is a leading cause of death for young children, and handguns kept in the home are unfortunately easy to use in moments of extreme anger with other family members or extreme depression. The majority of homicides between family members and most suicides involve a handgun. Nursing assessments should include a question about guns kept in the home. The family should be made aware of the risk that a handgun holds for family members. If the family thinks that keeping a gun is necessary, safety measures should be taught, such as keeping the gun unloaded and in a locked compartment, keeping the ammunition separate from the gun and also locked away, and instructing children about the dangers of firearms. Lobbying for handgun-control laws is a primary prevention effort that can significantly decrease the rate of death and serious injury caused by handguns in the United States.

Assessment for risk factors

Identification of risk factors is an important part of primary prevention. Although abuse cannot be predicted with certainty, several factors influence the onset and support the continuation of abusive patterns. Nurses can identify potential victims of abuse because they see clients in a variety of settings. Factors to include in an assessment of an individual or family's potential for violence are categorized by Logan and Dawkins (1986) as illustrated in Fig. 37-1.

The nurse must also be able to identify "red-flag" antisocial behaviors that might lead to abusive patterns. According to Klingbeil (1986), high-risk categories of behavior include the following:

1. Psychiatric diagnosis such as depression
2. Pattern of substance abuse
3. Loss and grief after death of a loved one
4. Isolation
5. Lack of support system
6. Homelessness

7. Previous history of assaultive or suicidal behavior
8. Chronic unemployment
9. Presence or use of weapons; previous arrests
10. History of runaways
11. Single-car auto accidents
12. Psychosomatic complaints

WHAT DO YOU THINK? *Most experts on violence agree that all women entering the health care system should be asked about domestic violence and sexual assault experience; yet men are also victimized by violence, even though little is known about their responses to such experiences. Some experts think that health care professionals should ask men if they are perpetrators of violence as a secondary prevention activity, reasoning that if identified early, such behavior may be more amenable to interventions. Others are concerned that since it is not certain what health care system interventions are most effective for male perpetrators or victims of violence, it is premature to do routine screening. There is also some concern that perpetrators of domestic violence or child abuse may become angry if asked about their violent behavior and retaliate against the family member.*

Individual and family strategies for primary prevention

Primary prevention of abuse includes strengthening individuals and families so they can cope more effectively with multiple life stressors and demands and reducing the destructive elements in the community that support and encourage violence. In their work in schools, community groups, employee groups, day-care centers, and other community institutions, nurses can foster healthy developmental patterns and identify signs of potential abuse.

Providing support and psychological enrichment to at-risk individuals and families often prevents the onset of health disruption. For example, nurses can strengthen and teach parenting abilities. Basic skills such as diapering, feeding, quieting, and even holding and rocking a baby can be the focus of a class or home or clinic visit. Parents also need to learn acceptable and workable ways to discipline children so that limits are maintained without causing the child emotional or physical harm.

Mutual support groups are valuable for new parents, families with special children, or abused people themselves. Such groups have variable formats and can provide information, support, and encouragement. Nurses can help begin such groups or can actually serve as group leaders. Chapter 23 describes the role of the nurse in working with community groups.

Secondary Prevention

When abuse occurs, nurses can initiate measures to reduce or terminate further abuse. Both developmental and situa-

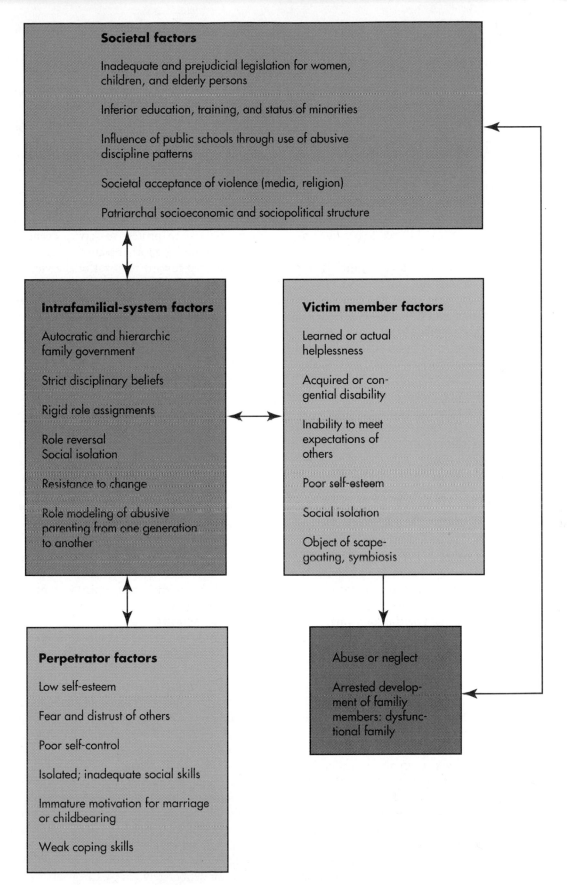

FIG. 37-1 Factors to include when assessing an individual's or family's potential for violence.

tional crises present opportunities for abusive situations to develop. Violence is a family crisis and should be handled using crisis intervention strategies.

Nursing intervention can help participants discuss the problem and seek ways to deal with the tension that led to the abusive situation. Injured persons must be temporarily or permanently placed in a safe location. Secondary preventive measures are most useful when potential abusers recognize their tendency to be abusive and seek help. For children, there is often a need for 24-hour child protection services or caregivers who can take care of the child until the acute family or individual crisis is resolved. Respite care is extremely important in families with frail elderly members. Telephone crisis lines can be used to provide immediate emergency assistance to families.

Effective communication with abusive families is important. Typically, these families do not want to discuss their problems and many are embarrassed to be involved in an abusive situation. Often a lot of guilt is involved. Effective communication must be preceded by an attitude of acceptance. It is often difficult for nurses to value the worth of an individual who willfully abuses another. The behavior, not the person, must be condemned.

Additionally, families do not always know how to have fun. Nurses can assess how much recreation is integrated into the family's lifestyle. Through community assessment, nurses know what resources and facilities are available and how much they cost. Families may need counseling about the value of recreation and play in reducing tension and appropriately channeling aggressive impulses.

Tertiary Prevention: Therapeutic Intervention with Abusive Families

Although it may be hard to form a trusting relationship with abusive families, nurses are often in key positions to act as case manager, coordinating the other agencies and activities involved. Principles of giving care to families who are experiencing violence include the following:
- Intolerance for violence
- Respect and caring for all family members
- Safety as the first priority
- Absolute honesty
- **Empowerment**

Nurses must clearly indicate that any further violence, degradation, and exploitation of family members will not be tolerated, but that all family members are respected, valued human beings. However, everyone must understand that the safety of every family member is the first priority.

Abusers often fear they will be condemned for their actions, so it is often difficult to make and maintain contact with abusive families. Although nurses convey an attitude of caring and concern for them, families may doubt the sincerity of this concern. They may avoid being home at the scheduled visit time out of fear of the consequences of the visit or an inability to believe that anyone really wants

to help them. If the victim is a child, parents may fear that the nurse will try to remove the child.

Nurses are mandatory reporters of child abuse, even when only suspected, in all states. They are also mandatory reporters of elder abuse and abuse of other physically and cognitively dependent adults as well as of felony assaults of anyone in most states. The mandatory reporting laws also protect reporters from legal action on cases that are never substantiated. Even so, physicians and nurses are sometimes reluctant to report abuse. They may be more willing to report abuse in a poor family than in a middle-class one, or they may think that an elderly person or child is better off at home than in a nursing home or foster home. Referral to protective service agencies should be viewed as enlisting another source of help, rather than an automatic step toward removal of the victim or criminal justice action. This same attitude can be communicated to families so that reporting is done with families rather than without their knowledge and prior input. Absolute honesty about what will be reported to officials, what the family can expect, what the nurse is entering into records, and what the nurse is feeling is essential.

To further empower the family, the nurse needs to recognize and capitalize on the violent family's strengths, as well as to assess and deal with its problems. The nurse must use a nurse-family partnership rather than a paternalistic or authoritarian approach. The family is generally capable of generating many of its own solutions, which will be much more culturally appropriate and individualized than those the nurse may generate. Victims of direct attack need information about their options and resources and reassurance that abuse is unfortunately rather common and that they are not alone in their dilemma. They also need reassurance that their responses are normal and that they do not deserve to be abused. Continued support for their decisions must be coupled with nursing actions to ensure their safety.

Nursing actions

The nurse can meet the family's therapeutic needs in a variety of ways. Besides referral to appropriate community agencies, nurses can act as role models for the family. During clinic and home visits, nurses can demonstrate constructive adult-child interactions. Nurses often teach mothers child-care skills such as proper feeding, calming a fretful child, effective discipline, and constructive communication.

Nurses can demonstrate good communication skills and discipline by teaching both parents and children in a calm, respectful, and informative manner. Caregivers, especially those caring for children, handicapped people, or elderly persons, may need to learn age-appropriate expectations. It is unreasonable to expect a 14-month-old infant to differentiate between right and wrong. Children at this age do not deliberately annoy caregivers by breaking delicate pieces of china. Likewise, a person with poor sphincter control does not willingly soil clothes or bedding.

Role modeling can be used with abuse victims of all ages. When providing nursing care to abused spouses or to elderly persons, nurses can demonstrate communication skills, conflict resolution, and skill training. For example, adult children often become abusive toward their parents when they become frustrated in trying to care for the elderly person. During home visits, nurses can show them how to physically and psychologically care for the relative. The nurse can work with caregivers to help them develop approaches that are acceptable to the individual elderly person. Assessment, creativity, and critical thinking help the nurse, family, and client learn how to meet client and family needs without causing undue stress and frustration.

The emotional investment and sheer drain of energy required to effectively work with abusers and victims of abuse cannot be disregarded. Abusers present difficult clinical challenges because of their reluctance to seek help or to remain actively involved in the helping process.

Referral is an important component of tertiary prevention. Nurses should know about available community resources for abuse victims and perpetrators. Some of these resources are listed in Box 37-1. If attitudes and resources are inadequate, it is often helpful to work with local radio and television stations and newspapers to provide information about the nature and extent of human abuse as a community health problem. This also helps to acquaint people with available services and resources. Frequently, people do not seek services early in an abusive situation because they simply do not know what is available to them. Ideally, a program or plan for abused people begins with a needs assessment to identify potential clients and to determine how to effectively serve this group. Nurses can help to get programs started and provide public education.

Nursing interventions specific to female partner abuse

Women in abusive relationships most often seek care for injuries in an emergency setting, a physician's office, or a prenatal clinic. Generally, these women are seeking assistance for injuries sustained during physically abusive episodes (Tilden and Shepard, 1987). Despite the overall incidence of battering and its resultant physical and emotional health problems for women, health professionals, even those in emergency departments, often fail to identify abused women, and are often seen as paternalistic, judgmental, insensitive, and less effective and helpful than they could be.

Because of the stigma involved, women and health care providers may hesitate to initiate discussion about abuse. However, the majority of battered women say they would have liked to talk about the issue with a health care professional if they were asked (Campbell and Humphreys, 1993). Because abuse develops slowly, starting with minor psychological abuse and building to more severe physical incidents, it often goes unrecognized by victims and health care providers alike until a severe episode occurs.

The quality of health care that a battered woman receives often determines whether she follows through with referrals to legal, social service, and health care agencies. In emergency departments, at least 15% of adult women patients have been physically or sexually abused by a partner or ex-partner (Dearwater et al, 1998). Care in the emergency department is often fragmented and necessarily oriented toward life and death situations. Therefore women may not be adequately assessed and often receive little or no specific emotional support or intervention. A cycle persists in which women seek care and receive either no interventions or ineffective interventions. This cycle perpetuates feelings of anger and inadequacy within health care providers, resulting in blame placed on women for their lack of compliance to remedies offered.

Managed care and clinic settings may be the best places to routinely screen for domestic violence. Between 10% and 25% of adult women in these primary care settings have been physically abused within the last year (Campbell, 1998). Hopefully if battered women are identified in those settings, effective interventions can be provided that will prevent the kind of serious injury resulting in later emergency department visits (see the Research Brief earlier in the chapter).

However, many battered women hesitate to identify themselves as victims of domestic violence for several reasons. They may fear that revelation will further jeopardize their safety, increase their sense of shame and humiliation, and minimize the repetitive or serious nature of the violence. This hesitation to speak out often makes it difficult for health care professionals to identify the battered woman. In addition, the very nature of the systems in which victims of violence introduce themselves can be barriers. Emergency departments, clinics, managed care settings and health departments are busy places. Staff members work hard to maintain the functioning of these facilities. Sometimes it is difficult in such chaotic settings for staff members to realize that they may be the first or only health provider to recognize violence in their clients' lives and that women need them to take the time to deal with this issue (Senter, 1993).

BOX 37-1 Common Community Services

Child protective services
Child abuse prevention programs
Adult protective services
Parents Anonymous
Wife abuse shelter
  Program for children of battered women
  Community support group
  24-hour hotline
  Legal advocacy or information
State coalition against domestic violence
Batterer treatment
Victim assistance programs
Sexual assault programs

Studies have found that only a small percentage of battered women in emergency departments and other health care settings were identified as such and treated for the abuse, despite the significant prevalence (Campbell and Sheridan, 1989; Dearwater et al, 1998). Battered women present for treatment in a number of ways, including physical complaints (such as not being able to sleep or chronic pain) related to the chronic stress of living in an abusive situation or old injuries. They may be unaware of the relationship of their symptoms to the violence in their lives. For the battered woman and the staff to begin to make the connection between her life situation and the presenting complaints, the nurse needs to ask direct questions in a supportive, open, and concerned manner (King and Ryan, 1989).

Assessment. Assessment for all forms of violence against women should take place for all women entering the health care system. The assessment should be ongoing and confidential. A thorough assessment gathers information on physical, emotional, and sexual trauma from violence, risk for future abuse, cultural background and beliefs, perceptions of the woman's relationships with others, and stated needs. The assessment should be conducted in private. Other adults who are present should be directed to the waiting area and told that it is policy that initially women are seen alone. Women should be asked directly if they were in an abusive relationship as a child or are currently in an abusive relationship as an adult. They should also be asked if they have ever been forced into sex that they did not wish to participate in. Shame and fear often make disclosure difficult. Verbal acknowledgment of the situation and emotional and physical support assist women in talking about past or current circumstances.

Women can be categorized into three groups: no, low, or moderate to high risk. Women with no signs of current or past abuse are considered at no risk. At the initial assessment a woman may hesitate to speak of concerns she has. Future visits should include questioning a woman about whether there have been any changes in her life or whether she has additional information or questions about topics discussed at previous visits.

Women at low risk show no evidence of recent or current abuse. Education that helps a woman gain perspective on her situation and her needs should be discussed. Resource materials including group and individual formats can be suggested. The risk level should be recorded, and preventive measures and teaching should be documented.

Assessment of moderate to high risk includes evaluation of a woman's fear for both psychological and physical abuse. Lethality potential should be assessed (Campbell, 1995). Risk factors for lethality include behaviors such as stalking or frequent harassment, threats or an escalation of threats, use of weapons or threats with weapons, excessive control and jealousy, and public use of violence. Statements from an abuser such as "If I can't have you, no one

can" should be taken seriously. In all cases a history of abuse and alcohol and drug use should be collected and carefully documented. The determined risk level should also be documented along with any past or present physical evidence of abuse from prior or current assault; this evidence should be photographed, shown on a body map, or described narratively. It is important that the assailant be identified in the record; this can take the form of either quotes from the woman or subjective information. These records can be very important for women in future assault or child custody cases, even if the woman is not ready to make a police report at the present time.

Immediate care for a woman in a potentially harmful or present abusive situation involves the development of a safety plan. A woman can be assisted to look at the options available to her. Shelter information, access to counseling, and legal resources should be discussed. If a woman wants to return to her partner, she can be helped in the development of plans that can be carried out if the abuse continues or becomes more serious.

Whenever there is evidence of sexual assault within the prior 24 to 48 hours, a rape kit examination should be performed. Lists of resources such as rape crises clinics and support groups for survivors of physical and emotional abuse should be made available.

Prevention. Prevention, public policy, and social attitudes are intertwined. Our society has taken a major step toward the secondary prevention of abuse through the establishment of programs that encourage women and children to speak about their experiences. Nurses need to support these programs further by believing the experiences they are told. In the development of laws that punish child and woman abuse, society has given some support to the victims of abuse. Often, however, the victims are again victimized by disbelief of their experiences, a devaluing of the effects of these assaults, and a focus on assisting the perpetrators of the crimes. Primary prevention includes a social attitudinal change. Both girls and boys need to be taught human values of interdependence, respect for human life, and a commitment to empathy and strength in the development of the human species regardless of gender, race, or socioeconomic status. We must urge continued progress toward eliminating the feminization of poverty and ensuring gender parity in economic resources. In addition, local communities must make it clear that violence against women is not tolerated by eliminating pornography, mandating arrests of abusers, and creating a general climate of nonviolence.

Abused women need assistance in making decisions and taking control of their lives. Community health, prenatal, planned parenthood, primary care, and emergency department nurses are involved with women at key times when they can be screened for the presence or absence of abuse. Mechanisms for screening women who are either abused or at risk for abuse are available (McFarlane et al,

1991). To intervene effectively, nurses must understand abuse as a cumulative process that must be examined as a continuum within the context of a relationship (Landenburger, 1989). During this process the abuse, the relationship, and a woman's view of self-change require time-specific interventions. Women are often blamed and held responsible for the abuse inflicted on them by their male partners (Landenburger, 1998). Subsequently women are either assisted in a way that discounts their feelings and further devalues them, or the abuse is ignored.

Strategies addressing education for health professionals. A variety of strategies have been reported that address the knowledge deficit of health practitioners on abuse issues. The National March of Dimes Birth Defects Foundation has sponsored a variety of training sessions for health professionals and produced an excellent training manual that addresses violence against women and battering during pregnancy (McFarlane and Parker, 1994). The nursing intervention recommended was tested experimentally with battered women receiving the intervention significantly increasing their safety behaviors throughout the pregnancy and one-year postpartum (McFarlane et al 1998).

Helton et al (1987a and b) report that 6 months after receiving 20 hours (2 1/2 days) of training, 75% of the 841 health professionals who participated in the March of Dimes course were routinely assessing for battering during pregnancy or were in the process of developing an assessment protocol within their practices. Tilden and Shepard (1987) instituted a battered women identification training program for emergency department (ED) personnel in a large urban medical center and reported that the incidence of recorded positive histories of adult family violence rose from 9.72% before training to 22.97% after the education program and implementation of an interview protocol.

After inception of a hospital-based family violence program housed in an urban ED, Sheridan (1998) demonstrated that the number of positive and probable battered women rose from 242 in 1986 to 337 in 1987, approximately a 40% increase in identification. The program included ongoing in-service training of all emergency department personnel including nonmedical support staff (i.e., unit secretaries, housekeepers, and security guards), as well as daily chart audits and telephone follow-up calls.

CLINICAL FORENSIC NURSING

Clinical forensic nursing is a relatively new specialty that has an interesting history and pattern for development. This field is defined as the "application of clinical and scientific knowledge to questions of law and the civil or criminal investigation of survivors of traumatic injury and/or patient treatment involving court-related issues" (Lynch, 1993, p. 8). John Butts, chief medical examiner for Alberta, Canada, in 1975 established a program using registered nurses as medical examiner investigators. He did this because he saw that nurses had a good education in medical

terminology, pharmacology, and the ability to be sensitive and communicate effectively with grieving families. As has been well established in this chapter, trauma as a result of violence is a growing public health problem. There are many people who survive trauma and are considered to be "living forensic patients" in contrast to earlier descriptions of forensics that dealt primarily with death.

Simply defined, **forensic** means "pertaining to the law." Currently, forensic specialists evaluate and assess victims of rape, drug and alcohol addiction, domestic violence, assaults, automobile or pedestrian accidents, incest, medical malpractice, and the injuries associated with food and drug tampering (Lynch, 1995). While much of the work in forensic nursing occurs in the emergency department, there is clearly a public health nursing role in primary prevention as well as in follow up if the events listed above do not occur.

When a client is admitted to a hospital with traumatic injuries he or she should be evaluated as to the forensic nature of the injuries. The nurse most often comes in contact with police, victims and perpetrators of violence or crime in the emergency department. The nurse provides a vital link between the investigative process, health care and the court (Lynch, 1995). There are specific actions that nurses should take when they come in contact with victims. It is important that evidence be collected in such a way that the collection itself protects rather than destroys or alters the evidence. For example, when cutting a shirt off a victim who has been shot in the chest, be sure to not cut through the bullet hole in the shirt. Rather cut to the side of the hole to protect the point of origin of the bullet for later criminal investigation.

The most common types of evidence are clothing, bullets, blood stains, hairs, fibers, and small pieces of material such as fragments of metal, glass, paint and wood. Lynch (1995) provides detailed guidelines about how to process clothing that includes what to look for, how to document what is found, how to remove the clothes and preserve them, and how to determine who should have custody of the clothes. She also describes what is called the "chain of custody," which means who gets control of items that may provide evidence about what happened. She describes in-depth wound characteristics and how they should be handled.

According to Lynch (1995, pp. 496-497) implementation of the clinical forensic nursing role includes the ability to do the following:
- Develop the appropriate forensic protocols in compliance with accreditation standards
- Triage clients at risk for forensic injuries
- Report to proper legal agencies
- Document, collect and preserve evidence
- Secure evidence and maintain the chain of custody and
- Serve as liaison between the health care institution, law enforcement agencies, and medical examiner/coroner

and make referrals when medical treatment and/or crisis intervention is required.

Maintaining an index of suspicion is important. Community and public health nurses, like their colleagues in the emergency department, have many opportunities to observe for signs of violence and to determine if the injuries occurred from natural or unnatural causes. Prevention is a key antiviolence strategy. Nurses should observe for injuries, listen for conversation that would suggest that violence is present in the family or the potential for violence is great, and be aware of the risk factors and compare known risk factors to the characteristics of the people with whom they work. It is believed that violence is underreported, and this may be particularly true for rape. For this reason, assessment, observation, and evaluation must always be present.

clinical application

Mrs. Smith, a 75-year-old bedridden woman, consistently became rude and combative when her daughter, Mary, attempted to bathe her and change her clothes each morning. During a home visit, Mary told the nurse, Mrs. Jones, that she had gotten so frustrated with her mother on the previous morning that she had hit her. Mary felt terrible about her behavior. She stressed that her mother's incontinence made it essential that she be kept clean; her clothes had to be changed every day for her own safety and physical well-being.

A. How should Mrs. Jones respond to this disclosure?
B. What specific nursing actions should be taken?
C. What ongoing services does the nurse need to provide?

Answers are in the back of the book.

KEY POINTS

- Violence and human abuse are not new phenomena, but they have increasingly become community health concerns.
- Communities throughout the United States are angry and frustrated about increasing levels of violence.
- Nurses can evaluate and intervene in incidents of community and family violence; to intervene effectively, the nurse must understand the dynamics of violence and human abuse.
- Factors influencing social and community violence include changing social conditions, economic conditions, population density, community facilities, and institutions within a community, such as organized religion, education, the mass communication media, and work.
- The potential for violence against individuals or against oneself is directly related to the level of violence in the community. Identification and correction of factors affecting the level of violence in the community constitute one way of reducing violence against family members and other individuals.

- Violence and abuse of family members can happen to any family member: spouse, elderly person, child, or developmentally disabled person.
- People who abuse family members were often themselves abused and react poorly to real or perceived crises. Other factors that characterize the abuser are the way the person was raised and the unique character of that person.
- Child abuse can be physical, emotional, or sexual. Incest is a common and particularly destructive form of child abuse.
- Spouse abuse is usually wife abuse. It involves physical, emotional, and, frequently, sexual abuse within a context of coercive control. It usually increases in severity and frequency and can escalate to homicide of either partner.
- Nurses are in an excellent position to identify potential victims of family abuse because they see clients in a variety of settings, such as schools, businesses, homes, and clinics. Treatment of family abuse includes primary, secondary, and tertiary prevention and therapeutic intervention.

critical thinking activities

1. For 1 week keep a log or diary related to violence.
   a. Make a note of each time you feel as though you are losing your temper. Consider what it might take to cause you to react in a violent way.
   b. Think back; when was the last time you had a violent outburst? What precipitated it? What were your thoughts? What were your feelings? How might you have handled the situation or those feelings without reacting in a violent way?
   c. During this same week make note of the episodes of violent behaviors you observe. For example, do parents hit children in the supermarket? What seems to precipitate such outbursts? What alternatives might exist for reacting in a less violent way?
2. If you learned, after a careful assessment of your community, that family violence is a significant community health problem, what plan of action might you take to intervene? Remember that the goal is to promote health; outline a plan of action with objectives, timetables, implementation strategies, and evaluation plans for intervening in family violence in your community.
3. Complete a partial community assessment to determine the actual incidence and types of violence in your community.
4. What resources are available in your community for victims of violence? Interview a person who works in an agency that seeks to aid victims of violence. What is the role of the agency? Do its services seem adequate? Who is eligible? Is there a waiting list? What is the fee scale?
5. Cut out all stories about violence in your local newspaper every day for 2 weeks. Note the patterns. Is the majority of the violence perpetrated by strangers or family members? How are the victims portrayed? What kinds of families are involved? What kinds of stories and families get front-page treatment rather than a few lines in the back of the paper?

Bibliography

Aiken MM, Speck PM: Sexual assault and multiple trauma: a sexual assault nurse examiner (SANE) challenge, *J Emerg Nurs* 21(5):466, 1995.

Anetzberger GJ, Korbin JE, Austin: Alcoholism and elder abuse, *J Interpersonal Violence* 9(2):184, 1994.

Bachman R: *Violence against women: a national crime victimization survey report*, Washington, DC, 1994, US Department of Justice, Office of Justice Programs, Bureau of Justice Statistics.

Baron S, Welty A: Elder abuse, *J Gerontol Soc Work* 25(1/2):33, 1996.

Behaviors related to unintentional and intentional injuries among high school students—United States, 1991, *MMWR* 41(41):760,1992.

Bowker LH: *Beating wife-beating*, Lexington, Mass, 1983, Lexington Books.

Briere J et al: *The APSAC handbook on child maltreatment*. Thousand Oaks, Calif, 1996, Sage.

Bureau of Justice Statistics: *Criminal Victimization 1996*, Washington, DC, 1997, US Department of Justice.

Campbell, JC: *Assessing dangerousness: potential for further violence of sexual offenders*, Newbury Park, Calif, 1995, Sage.

Campbell JC: A test of two explanatory models of women's responses to battering, *Nurs Res* 38(1):18, 1989a.

Campbell, JC: Battered woman syndrome: a critical review, *Violence Update* 1(4):1, 1990.

Campbell JC: *Empowering survivors of abuse: health care, battered women and their children*. Newbury Hills, Calif, 1998, Sage.

Campbell JC: "If I can't have you, no one can": homicide in intimate relationships. In Radford J, Russell DEH, editors: *Femicide: the politics of woman killing*, Boston, 1992, Twayne.

Campbell JC: Women's responses to sexual abuse in intimate relationships, *Health Care Women Int* 10:335, 1989b.

Campbell JC: In Sampselle CM, editor: *Violence against women: nursing research, education, and practice issues*, Washington, DC, 1991, Hemisphere Publishing.

Campbell JC, Alford P: The dark consequences of marital rape, *Am J Nurs* 89:946, 1989.

Campbell JC, Humphreys J: *Nursing care of survivors of family violence*, St Louis, 1993, Mosby.

Campbell JC, Oliver C, Bullock L: Why battering during pregnancy? *AWHONN's Clinical Issues in Perinatal and Women's Health Nursing*, 4(3):343, 1993.

Campbell JC, Sheridan DJ: Clinical articles: emergency nursing interventions with battered women, *J Emerg Nurs* 15(1):12, 1989.

Campbell JC et al: Correlates of battering during pregnancy, *Res Nurs and Health* 15:219, 1992.

Campbell JC et al: Nursing care of abused women. In Campbell J, Humphreys J editors: *Nursing care of survivors of family violence*, St. Louis, 1993, Mosby.

Campbell JC et al: Relationship status of battered women over time, *J Fam Viol* 9:99, 1994.

Carlson RB et al: A conceptual framework for the long term psychological effects of traumatic childhood abuse, *Child Maltreatment* 2(3):272, 1997.

Centers for Disease Control and Prevention: Regional variations in suicide rates—United States, 1990-1994, *MMWR* 46(34):789, 1997.

Chalk R, King PA: *Violence in families: assessing prevention and treatment programs*. Washington, DC, 1998, National Academy Press.

Cottle CE et al: Conflicting ideologies and the politics of pornography. In O'Toole LL, Schiffman JR, editors: *Gender violence: interdisciplinary perspectives*, New York, 1997, New York University Press.

Counts D, Brown J, Campbell J: *Sanctions and sanctuary*, Boulder, Col, 1992, Westview Press.

Coyne AC, Reichman WR, Berbig LJ: The relationship between dementia and elder abuse, *Am J Psychiatry* 150(4):643, 1993.

Dearwater S et al: Prevalence of domestic violence treated in a community hospital emergency department, *JAMA* 280(5):433, 1998.

Donat PL, D'Emilio N: A feminist redefinition of rape and sexual assault: historical foundations and change. In O'Toole LL, Schiffman JR, editors: *Gender violence: interdisciplinary perspectives*, New York, 1997, New York University Press.

Draucker CB: Childhood sexual abuse: sources of trauma, *Issues Ment Health Nurs* 14(3):249, 1993.

Dutton DG: *The domestic assault of women*, Newton, Mass, 1995, Allyn & Bacon.

Edleson JL, Tolman RM: *Intervention for men who batter*, Newbury Park, Calif, 1992, Sage.

Eggert LL et al: Prevention research program: reconnecting at-risk youth, *Issues Ment Health Nurs* 15(2):107, 1994.

Evans JP, Taylor J: Understanding violence in contemporary and earlier gangs: an exploratory application of the theory of reasoned action, *J Black Psychology*, 21(1):71, 1995.

Fulmer T: Mistreatment of elders, assessment, diagnosis, and intervention, *Nurs Clin North Am* 24(3):707, 1989.

Gelles RJ: The youngest victims: violence toward children. In Bergen RK, editor: *Issues in intimate violence*, Thousand Oaks, Calif, 1998, Sage.

Gelles R, Conte J: Domestic violence and sexual abuse of children: a review of research in the eighties, *J Marriage Fam* 52(4):1045, 1990.

Green AH: Overview of child sexual abuse. In Kaplan SJ, editor: *Family violence: a clinical and legal guide*, Washington, DC, 1996, American Psychiatric Press.

Hampton RL, Yung BR: Violence in communities of color: where we were, where we are, and where we need to be. In Hampton RL, Jenkins P, Gullotta TP, editors: *Preventing violence in America*, Thousand Oaks, Calif, 1996, Sage.

Hawkins DF: Inequality, culture, and interpersonal violence, *Health Affairs* 12(4):80, 1993.

Helton AS, McFarlane J, Anderson ET: Battered and pregnant: a prevalence study, *Am J Pub Health* 77(10):1337, 1987a.

Helton A, McFarlane J, Anderson E: Prevention of battering during pregnancy: focus on behavioral change, *Public Health Nurs* 4(3):166, 1987b.

Herman J, Hirschman L: Father daughter incest. In Bart PB, Moran EG, editors: *Violence against women: the bloody footprints*, Thousand Oaks, Calif, 1993, Sage.

Hernandez JT, Lodico M, DiClemente RJ: The effects of child abuse and race on risk taking in male adolescents, *J Natl Med Assoc* 85(8):593, 1993.

Houck GM, King MC: Child maltreatment: family characteristics and developmental consequences, *Issues Ment Health Nurs* 10:193, 1989.

Humphreys J, Ramsey AM: Child abuse. In Campbell J, Humphreys J, editors: *Nursing care of survivors of family violence*, St Louis, 1993, Mosby.

Kempe CH et al: The battered child syndrome, *JAMA* 181:17, 1962.

Kellermann AL, Reay DT: Protection or peril? an analysis of firearm-related deaths in the home, *N Engl J Med* 314(24):1557, 1986.

Kendall-Tackett K, Marshall R: Sexual victimization of children: incest and child sexual abuse. In Bergen RK, editor: *Issues in intimate violence*, Thousand Oaks, Calif, 1998, Sage.

Kimmel MS: Does censorship make a difference? an aggregate empirical analysis of pornography and rape, *J Psychol Human Sexuality* 8(3):1, 1996.

King M, Ryan J: Abused women: dispelling myths and encouraging intervention, *Nurse Pract* 14:47, 1989.

Klein E et al: *Ending domestic violence: changing public perceptions/halting the epidemic*, Newbury Parks, Calif, 1997, Sage.

Continued

Bibliography—cont'd

Klingbeil K: Interpersonal violence: a comprehensive model in a hospital setting—from policy to program. In *The Surgeon General's workshop on violence and public health report,* DHHS Pub No HRS-D-MC 86-1, Washington DC, 1986, Health Resources and Services Administration, USDHHS, Public Health Service.

Koss MP, Harvey MR: *The rape victim: clinical and community intervention,* ed 2, Newbury Park, Calif, 1991, Sage.

Koss MP, Cook SL: Facing the facts: date and acquaintance rape are significant problems for women. In Bergen RK, editor: *Issues in intimate violence,* Thousand Oaks, Calif, 1998, Sage.

Landenburger K: A process of entrapment in and recovery from an abusive relationship, *Issues Ment Health Nurs* 10:209, 1989.

Landenburger, K: *Exploration of women's identity: clinical approaches with abused women. Empowering survivors of abuse: Health care, battered women and their children,* Newbury Hills, Calif, 1998, Sage.

Lang SS: Finding refute traditional views on elder abuse, *Human Ecology Forum* 21(3):30, 1993.

Ledray LE, Simmelink K: Sexual assault: clinical issues:efficacy of SANE evidence collection: a Minnesota study, *J Emerg Nurs* 23(1):75, 1997.

Levinson D: *Family violence in cross-cultural perspective,* Newbury Park, Calif, 1989, Sage.

Logan BB, Dawkins CE: *Family-centered nursing in the community,* Menlo Park, Calif, 1986, Addison-Wesley.

Lynch VA: Forensic nursing: diversity in education and practice, *J Psychosoc Nurs* 31(11):7, 1993.

Lynch VA: Clinical forensic nursing: a new perspective in the management of crime victims from trauma to trial, *Crit Care Nurs Clin North Am* 7(3):489, 1995.

McFarlane J et al: Assessing for abuse: self-report versus nurse interview, *Public Health Nurs* 8: 245, 1991.

McFarlane J et al: Safety behaviors of abused women after an intervention during pregnancy, *JOGNN* 27(1):64, 1998.

McFarlane J, Parker B: *Abuse during pregnancy: a protocol for prevention and intervention,* White Plains, New York, 1994, March of Dimes Birth Defects Foundation.

McFarlane J, Parker B, Soeken K: Abuse during pregnancy: effects on maternal complications and birthright in adult and teenage women, *Obstet Gynecol* 84(3):323, 1994.

Milner JS, Robertson KR: Comparison of physical child abusers, intrafamilial sexual child abusers, and child neglecters, *J Interpersonal Violence* 5(1):37, 1990.

Moore R, Harrisson S: In poor health: socioeconomic status and health chances: a review of the literature, *Social Sciences in Health* 1(4):221, 1995.

Nadon SM, Koverola C, Schludermann EH: Antecedents to prostitution: childhood victimization, *J Interpersonal Violence* 13(2):206, 1998.

Okun LE: *Woman abuse: facts replacing myths,* Albany, NY, 1986, State University of New York Press.

Oliphant C, editor: *Health scene,* Pendleton, OR, 1986, Pendleton Community Hospital.

Peled E: Secondary victims no more: refocusing intervention with children. In Edleson JL, Eisikovits ZC, editors: *Future interventions with battered women and their families: visions for policy, practice, and research,* Thousand Oaks, Calif, 1996, Sage.

Phillips LR: Abuse/neglect of the frail elderly at home: an exploration of theoretical relationships, *J Adv Nurs* 8:379, 1983.

Pillemer K, Finkelhor D: The prevalence of elder abuse: a random sample survey, *Gerontologist* 28:51, 1988.

Prince J: A systems approach to spouse abuse. In Lancaster J: *Community mental health nursing: an ecological perspective.* St Louis, 1980, Mosby.

Public Health Improvement Plan, Olympia, Wash, 1994, Washington State Department of Health.

Reiss AJ, Roth JA, editors: *Understanding and preventing violence,* vol 1-4, Washington, DC, 1993/1994, National Academy Press.

Renzetti CM: Violence in lesbian and gay relationships. In O'Toole LL, Schiffman JR, editors: *Gender violence: interdisciplinary perspectives,* New York, 1997, New York University Press.

Riedel M. Counting stranger homicides, *Homicide studies* 2:206, 1998

Rosenberg ML, Fenley MA, editors: *Violence in America: a public health approach,* New York, 1991, Oxford.

Russell DEH: Pornography and rape: a causal model, *Prevention in Human Services* 12(2):45, 1995a.

Russell DEH: The prevalence, trauma, and sociocultural cause of incestuous abuse of females: a human rights issue. In Rolf K et al, editors: *Beyond trauma: cultural and societal dynamics,* New York, 1995b, Plenum.

Senter S: *Program planning manual for implementing a response to domestic violence in hospital emergency departments,* Seattle, Wash, 1993, Seattle-King County Department of Public Health.

Sheridan D: Health care based programs for domestic violence survivors. In Campbell J: *Empowering survivors of abuse: health care, battered women and their children.* Newbury Park, Calif, 1998, Sage.

Stark E, Fitzcraft A: Spouse abuse. In Rosenberg ML, Finley MA: *Violence in America,* New York, 1991, Oxford.

Straus MA, Gelles RJ: *Physical violence in American families: risk factors and adaptations to violence in 8,145 families.* New Brunswick, NJ, 1990, Transaction.

Tilden VP, Shepard P: Increasing the rate of identification of battered women in an emergency department: use of a nursing protocol, *Res Nurs Health* 10:209, 1987.

Tolman RM, Bennett LW: A review of research on men who batter, *J Interpersonal Violence* 5(1):87, 1990.

Ulrich YC: Cross-cultural perspective on violence against women, *Response Victimiz Women Child* 12(1):21, 1989.

US Department of Health and Human Services: *Healthy People 2000: national health promotion and disease prevention objectives,* Washington, DC, 1991, USDHHS, Public Health Service.

US Department of Justice: *Murder in families: violence against women,* Washington, DC, 1994, Bureau of Justice Statistics.

US Department of Justice: *Sex offenses and offenders: an analysis of data on rape and sexual assault,* Washington, DC, 1997, Bureau of Justice Statistics, NCJ-163392.

US Surgeon General: *Workshop on violence and public health report,* DDHS Pub No HRS-D-MC 86-1, Washington, DC, 1986, Health Resources and Services Administration, US Public Health Service, USDHHS.

Webster DW: The unconvincing case for school-based conflict resolution, *Health Affairs* 12(4):126, 1993.

Weiner A: A community based education model for identification and prevention of elder abuse, *J Gerontol Soc Work* 16(3-4):107, 1991.

Weith ME: Elder abuse: a national tragedy, *FBI Law Enforcement Bulletin* 63(2):24, 1994.

Wilkinson RG: Comment: Income, inequality, and social cohesion, *Am J Public Health* 87(9):1540, 1997.

Winfree LT, Esbensen F, Osgood DW: Evaluating a school-based gang-prevention program, *Evaluation Review* 20(2):181, 1996.

Wolak J, Finkelhor D: Children exposed to partner violence. In Jasinski JL, Williams LM, editors: *Partner violence: a comprehensive review of 20 years of research,* Thousand Oaks, Calif, 1998, Sage.

Wolf RS, Pillemer K, Wilson NL: What's new in elder abuse programming, *Gerontologist* 34(1):126, 1994.

Whyte W: Forensic nursing: A review of concepts and definitions, *Nursing Standard* 11(23) 46, 1997.

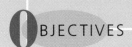

CHAPTER 38

Communicable Disease Risk and Prevention

FRANCISCO S. SY & SUSAN C. LONG-MARIN

OBJECTIVES

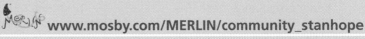

www.mosby.com/MERLIN/community_stanhope

After reading this chapter, the student should be able to do the following:

- Discuss the current impact and threats of infectious diseases on society.
- Explain the agent-host-environment triad and how these elements interact to cause infectious diseases.
- Evaluate the factors leading to the emergence or reemergence of infectious diseases.
- Define and discuss the implications of immunity in terms of active immunity, passive immunity, and herd immunity.
- Define surveillance and discuss the functions and elements of the surveillance system.

- Analyze why tuberculosis is once again considered an important public health problem and discuss diagnostic tools, treatment, prevention, and control measures.
- Describe the risk of foodborne illness and appropriate prevention measures, giving special attention to salmonella and *E. coli* 0157:H7.
- Examine the rise in parasitic infections, the population particularly at risk, and possible preventive measures.
- Apply the three levels of prevention and give appropriate examples of preventive interventions.
- Evaluate the multisystem approach to control of communicable diseases.

KEY TERMS

acquired immunity
active immunization
agent
common vehicle
communicable disease
communicable period
disease
elimination

emerging infections diseases
endemic
environment
epidemic
epidemiological triad
eradication
herd immunity

horizontal transmission
host
incubation period
infection
infectiousness
natural immunity
nosocomial infection
pandemic

passive immunization
resistance
surveillance
universal
vector
vertical transmission

See Glossary for definitions

CHAPTER OUTLINE

continued

CHAPTER OUTLINE—cont'd

The topic of communicable diseases includes the discussion of a wide and complex variety of organisms; the pathology they may cause; and their diagnosis, treatment, prevention, and control. This chapter presents an overview of the communicable diseases with which community and public health nurses deal most often. Diseases are grouped according to descriptive category (by mode of transmission or means of prevention) rather than by individual organism (*E. coli*) or taxonomic group (viral, parasitic). Detailed discussion of sexually transmitted diseases, HIV/AIDS and viral hepatitis is provided in Chapter 39. Although not all infectious diseases are directly communicable from person to person, the terms *infectious* diseases and *communicable* diseases are used interchangeably throughout this chapter.

HISTORICAL AND CURRENT PERSPECTIVES

In 1900, communicable diseases were the leading causes of death in the United States. By 2000, improved nutrition and sanitation, vaccines, and antibiotics have put an end to the epidemics that once ravaged entire populations. In 1900 tuberculosis was the second leading cause of death; in 1995 this disease killed less than 1400 people or was responsible for about 0.06% of all deaths in the United States (NCHS, 1996). As individuals live longer, chronic diseases—heart disease, cancer, and stroke—have replaced infectious diseases as the leading reasons for death. Infectious diseases, however, have not vanished. They are still the number one cause of death worldwide. Infectious diseases account for 25% of all physician visits each year, and antibiotics are the second most prescribed type of drugs in the United States (CDC, 1994a).

DID YOU KNOW? *During the past decade, as rates of infectious disease have increased, the use of antibiotic drugs has grown significantly. Antibiotics are now the second most prescribed group of drugs in the United States. With the introduction of new antibiotic drugs come new forms of antibiotic drug resistance, a problem that is further exacerbated by inappropriate use of antibiotics.*

New killers are emerging, and old familiar diseases are taking on different, more virulent characteristics. Consider the following recent developments. The advent of the AIDS epidemic in the 1980s reminds us of plagues from the past and challenges our ability to contain and control infection like no other disease in this century. AIDS and accidents are now the leading killers of persons 25 to 44 years of age. Legionnaire's disease and toxic shock syndrome, unknown at mid-century, have become part of common vocabulary. The identification of infectious agents causing Lyme disease and Ehrlichiosis has provided two new tickborne diseases to worry about. In the summer of 1993 in the southwestern United States, healthy young adults were stricken with a mysterious and unknown but often fatal respiratory disease that is now known as Hantavirus pulmonary syndrome. Methicillin-resistant *Staphylococcus aureus* is now resistant to all but one antibiotic, vancomycin. A severe, invasive strain of *Streptococcus pyogenes Group A* drew public attention in 1994, referred to by the press as the "flesh-eating" bacteria. Consumption of improperly cooked hamburgers and unpasteurized apple juice contaminated with a highly toxic strain of *E. coli* (*Escherichia coli 0157:H7*) caused illness and death in children across the county. In 1996, 10 states had outbreaks of diarrheal disease traced to imported fresh berries. The implicated organism in these outbreaks, *Cyclospora cayetanensis* (a coccidian parasite), was only diagnosed in humans in 1977; it had only been reported in American outbreaks three times before 1996 (CDC, 1996a). Also in 1996, the fear that "mad cow disease" (bovine spongiform encephalopathy) could be transferred to humans through beef consumption led to the slaughter of thousands of British cattle and a ban on the international sale of British beef. The highly fatal Ebola virus, unknown to most people 20 years ago, is now the subject of movies and best-selling books.

It is estimated that in the United States 90,000 people per year die from microbial causes separate from AIDS-associated illnesses (McGinnis and Foege, 1993). The eco-

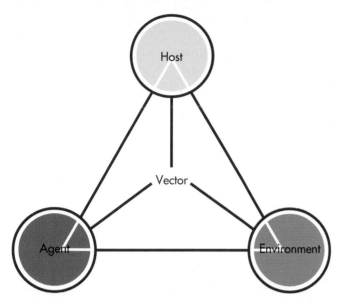

FIG. 38-1 The epidemiological triad of a disease. (From Gordis L: *Epidemiology*, Philadelphia, 1996, W.B. Saunders.)

nomic burden of infectious diseases is staggering. The annual combined direct cost and lost productivity due to intestinal infections is estimated at $30 billion, while the annual treatment cost for sexually transmitted diseases, excluding AIDS, is $5 billion. Annual direct medical cost due to nosocomial infections is $4.5 billion, and the combined medical cost and lost productivity for influenza is $17 billion per year. The yearly estimated cost of antimicrobial resistance is $4 billion (CDC, 1994a).

Because of the morbidity, mortality, and associated cost of infectious diseases, the national health promotion and disease prevention goals outlined in *Healthy People 2000* list a number of objectives for reducing the incidence of these illnesses. Examples of targeted areas for reduction are as follows:

- Indigenous cases of vaccine-preventable disease
- Epidemic-related pneumonia deaths among people aged 65 or older
- Viral hepatitis
- Tuberculosis
- Nosocomial infections
- Selected diseases of international travelers
- Bacterial meningitis
- Diarrheal diseases of children in day care
- Acute middle ear infections in young children
- Pneumonia-related days of restricted activity.

An objective for reducing salmonellosis and other foodborne infections is found in the section for food and drug safety. Although infectious diseases may not be the leading cause of death at the beginning of the twenty-first century, they continue to present varied, multiple and complex challenges to all health care providers. Nurses must know about these diseases in order to effectively participate in diagnosis, treatment, prevention, and control.

BOX 38-1 Six Characteristics of an Infectious Agent

- *Infectivity.* The ability to enter and multiply in the host.
- *Pathogenicity.* The ability to produce a specific clinical reaction after infection occurs.
- *Virulence.* The ability to produce a severe pathological reaction.
- *Toxicity.* The ability to produce a poisonous reaction.
- *Invasiveness.* The ability to penetrate and spread throughout a tissue.
- *Antigenicity.* The ability to stimulate an immunological response.

TRANSMISSION OF COMMUNICABLE DISEASES

Agent, Host, and Environment

The transmission of **communicable diseases** depends on the successful interaction of the infectious agent, host and environment. These three factors comprise the **epidemiological triad.** (Fig. 38-1). Changes in the characteristics of any of the factors may result in disease transmission (Benenson, 1995). Consider the following examples. Antibiotic therapy may not only eliminate a specific pathological agent but may also alter the balance of normally occurring organisms in the body. As a result, one of these agents overruns another, and disease, such as a yeast infection, occurs. HIV performs its deadly work not by directly poisoning the host but by destroying the host's immune reaction to other disease-producing agents. Individuals living in the temperate climate of the United States do not contract malaria at home, but they may become infected if they change their environment by traveling to a climate where malaria-carrying mosquitoes thrive. As these examples illustrate, the balance among agent, host, and environment is often precarious and may be unintentionally disrupted. Entering the twenty-first century, the potential results of such disruption requires attention as advances in science and technology, destruction of natural habitats, explosive population growth, political instability, and a worldwide transportation network combine to alter the balance among the environment, people, and the agents that produce disease.

Agent factor

Four main categories of infectious agents can cause infection or disease: bacteria, fungi, parasites, and viruses. The individual **agent** may be described by its ability to cause disease and the nature and the severity of the disease. Terms commonly used to characterize infectious agents are defined in Box 38-1.

Host factor

A human or animal **host** may harbor an infectious agent. The characteristics of the host that may influence the spread of disease are host resistance, immunity, herd immunity, and infectiousness of the host. **Resistance** is the ability of the host to withstand infection and may be due to natural or acquired immunity.

Natural immunity refers to species-determined innate resistance to an infectious agent. For example, opossums rarely contract rabies. **Acquired immunity** is the resistance acquired by a host due to previous natural exposure to an infectious agent. Having measles once protects against future infection. Acquired immunity may be induced by active or passive immunization. **Active immunization** refers to the immunization of an individual by administration of an antigen (infectious agent or vaccine) and is usually characterized by the presence of an antibody produced by the individual host. Vaccinating children against childhood diseases is an example of inducing active immunity. **Passive immunization** refers to immunization through the transfer of specific antibody from an immunized individual to a nonimmunized individual, such as the transference of antibody from mother to infant or by administration of an antibody-containing preparation (immune globulin or antiserum). Passive immunity from immune globulin is almost immediate but short-lived. It is often induced as a stop-gap measure until active immunity has time to develop after vaccination. Examples of commonly used immunoglobulins include those for hepatitis A, rabies, and tetanus.

Herd immunity refers to the immunity of a group or community. It is the resistance of a group of people to invasion and spread of an infectious agent. Herd immunity is based on the resistance of a high proportion of individual members of a group to infection. It is the basis for increasing immunization coverage for vaccine-preventable diseases. Higher immunization coverage will lead to greater herd immunity which in turn will block the further spread of the disease.

Infectiousness is a measure of the potential ability of an infected host to transmit the infection to other hosts. It is concerned with the relative ease with which the infectious agent is transmitted to others. Individuals with measles are extremely infectious; the virus spreads readily on airborne droplets. A person with Lyme disease cannot spread the disease to other people; the infected tick can.

Environment factor

The **environment** refers to all that is external to the human host including physical, biologic, social, and cultural factors. These environmental factors facilitate the transmission of an infectious agent from an infected host to other susceptible hosts. Reduction in communicable disease risk can be achieved by altering these environmental factors. Using mosquito nets and repellants to avoid bug bites, installing sewage systems to prevent fecal contamination of water supplies, and washing utensils after contact with raw meat to reduce bacterial contamination are all examples of altering the environment to prevent disease.

Modes of Transmission

Infectious diseases can be transmitted horizontally or vertically. **Vertical transmission** is the passing of the infection from parent to offspring via sperm, placenta, milk, or contact in the vaginal canal at birth. Examples of vertical transmission are transplacental transmission of HIV and syphilis. **Horizontal transmission** is the person-to-person spread of infection through one or more of the following four routes: direct/indirect contact, common vehicle, airborne, or vectorborne. Sexually transmitted diseases are spread by direct sexual contact. Enterobiasis or pinworm infection can be acquired through direct contact or indirect contact with contaminated objects such as toys, clothing, and bedding. **Common vehicle** refers to transportation of the infectious agent from an infected host to a susceptible host via water, food, milk, blood, serum, or plasma. Hepatitis A can be transmitted through contaminated food and water, hepatitis B through contaminated blood products. Legionellosis and tuberculosis are both spread via contaminated droplets in the air. Vectors can be arthropods such as ticks and mosquitoes or other invertebrates such as snails that can transmit the infectious agent by biting or depositing the infective material near the host.

Disease Development

Exposure to an infectious agent does not always lead to an infection. Similarly infection does not always lead to disease. Infection depends on the infective dose, infectivity of the infectious agent, and immunocompetence of the host. It is important to differentiate infection and disease as clearly illustrated by the HIV/AIDS epidemic. **Infection** refers to the entry, development, and multiplication of the infectious agent in the susceptible host. **Disease** is one of the possible outcomes of infection, and it may indicate a physiological dysfunction or pathological reaction. In an example from the sports world, compare the case of Magic Johnson with that of Greg Louganis. Both publicly announced that they had tested positive for HIV, but while Johnson was asymptomatic, Louganis had developed the clinical signs of AIDS. Or in other words, Johnson was infected but not diseased, Louganis was both infected and diseased.

DID YOU KNOW? *Only discovered in 1983, an infectious agent,* Helicobacter pylori, *is now recognized as the major factor in peptic ulcer disease.*

Incubation period and communicable period are not synonymous. **Incubation period** is the time interval between invasion by an infectious agent and the first appearance of signs and symptoms of the disease. The incubation periods of infectious diseases vary from 2 to 4 hours for staphylococcal food poisoning to 10 to 15 years for AIDS. **Communicable period** is the interval during which an infectious agent may be transferred directly or indirectly from an infected person to another person. The period of communicability for influenza is 3 to 5 days after the clinical onset of symptoms. Hepatitis B–infected persons are infectious many weeks before the onset of first symptoms and remain infective during the acute phase and chronic carrier state, which may persist for life.

Disease Spectrum

Persons with infectious diseases may exhibit a broad spectrum of disease that ranges from subclinical infection to severe and fatal disease. Those with subclinical or inapparent infections are important from the public health point of view since they are a source of infection and may not be cared for like those with clinical disease. They should be targeted for early diagnosis and treatment. Those with clinical disease may exhibit localized or systemic symptoms and mild to severe illness. The final outcome of a disease may be recovery, death, or something in between, including a carrier state, complications requiring extended hospital stay, or disability requiring rehabilitation. At the community level, the disease may occur in endemic, epidemic, or pandemic proportion. **Endemic** refers to the constant presence of a disease within a geographic area or a population. Pertussis is endemic in the United States. **Epidemic** refers to the occurrence of disease in a community or region in excess of normal expectancy. Although people tend to associate large numbers with epidemics, even one case can be termed epidemic if the disease is considered previously eliminated from that area. **Pandemic** refers to an epidemic occurring worldwide and affecting large populations. HIV/AIDS is both epidemic and pandemic since the number of cases is growing rapidly across various regions of the world as well as in the United States.

SURVEILLANCE OF COMMUNICABLE DISEASES

During the first half of the twentieth century, the weekly publication of national morbidity statistics by the U.S. Surgeon General's Office was accompanied by the statement, "No health department, state or local, can effectively prevent or control disease without knowledge of when, where, and under what conditions cases are occurring." (CDC, 1996a). **Surveillance** gathers the *who, when, where* and *what;* these elements are then used to answer *why.* A good surveillance system will systematically collect, organize, and analyze current, accurate, and complete data for a defined disease condition. Resulting information is promptly released to those who need it for effective planning, implementation, and evaluation of disease prevention and control programs.

Elements of Surveillance

The basic 10 elements of surveillance are the routine sources of data on disease occurrence, which include mortality registration, morbidity reporting, epidemic reporting, epidemic field investigation, laboratory reporting, individual case investigation, surveys, utilization of biologics and drugs, distribution of animal reservoirs and vectors, and demographic and environmental data.

Nurses may be involved at different levels of the surveillance system. They play important roles in collecting data, making diagnoses, reporting cases, and providing feedback information to the general public. Examples of possible activities include investigating sources and contacts in outbreaks of pertussis in school settings or shigellosis in day care; TB testing and contact tracing; collecting and reporting information pertaining to notifiable communicable diseases; and providing morbidity and mortality statistics to those who request them including the media, the public, those planning services, and those writing grants.

List of Reportable Diseases

Requirements for disease reporting in the United States are mandated by state rather than federal laws and regulations. The list of reportable diseases in each state varies. State health departments, on a voluntary basis, report cases of selected diseases to the Centers for Disease Control and Prevention (CDC) in Atlanta, Georgia. The 52 diseases presently included in the National Notifiable Diseases Surveillance System (NNDSS) at CDC are listed in Box 38-2. The NNDSS data are collated and published weekly in the *Morbidity and Mortality Weekly Report* (MMWR). Final reports are published annually in the *Summary of Notifiable Diseases* (CDC, 1996a).

EMERGING INFECTIOUS DISEASES

Emergence Factors

Emerging infectious diseases are those in which the incidence has actually increased in the past two decades or has the potential to increase in the near future. These emerging diseases may include new or known infectious diseases. Consider the following examples. Identified only in the past two decades when sporadic outbreaks occurred in Sudan and Zaire, Ebola virus is a mysterious new killer with a frightening mortality rate that sometimes reaches 90%, has no known treatment, and has no understood reservoir in nature. It appears to be transmitted through direct contact with bodily secretions and as such can potentially be contained once cases are identified. Why outbreaks occur is not understood. Ebola is an example of new viruses that may appear as civilization intrudes farther and farther into previously uninhabited natural environments changing the landscape and disturbing ecological balances that may have existed unaltered for hundreds of years.

Closer to home, Hantavirus was first detected in 1993 in the Four Corner area of Arizona and New Mexico when a mysterious and deadly respiratory disease appeared to target young, healthy Native Americans. The disease was soon discovered to be a variant of but to exhibit different pathology from a rodentborne virus previously known only in Europe and Asia. Transmission is thought to occur through aerosolization of rodent excrement. One explanation for the outbreak in the Southwest is that an unseasonably mild winter led to an unusual increase in the rodent population; more people than usual were exposed to a virus that had until that point gone unrecognized in this country. Infection in Native Americans first brought attention to Hantavirus because of a cluster of cases in a small geographical area, but no evidence suggests that any ethnic group is particularly susceptible to this disease. Hantavirus has now been diagnosed in sites across the United State. The best protection against this virus seems to be avoiding rodent-infested environments.

BOX 38-2 Nationally Notifiable Infectious Disease

1. AIDS	27. Malaria
2. Anthrax	28. Measles
3. Botulism	29. Meningococcal disease
4. Brucellosis	30. Mumps
5. Chancroid	31. Pertussis
6. *Chlamydia trachomatis,* genital infections	32. Plague
7. Cholera	33. Poliomyelitis
8. Coccidioidomycosis	34. Psittacosis
9. Cryptosporidiosis	35. Rabies, animal
10. Diphtheria	36. Rabies, human
11. Encephalitis, California	37. Rocky Mountain spotted fever
12. Encephalitis, eastern equine	38. Rubella
13. Encephalitis, St. Louis	39. Rubella, congenital syndrome
14. Encephalitis, western equine	40. Salmonellosis
15. *Escherichia coli* O157:H7	41. Shigellosis
16. Gonorrhea	42. Streptococcal disease, invasive, Group A
17. *Haemophilus influenzae,* invasive disease	43. *Streptococcus pneumoniae,* drug-resistant
18. Hansen disease (leprosy)	44. Streptococcal toxic-shock syndrome
19. Hantavirus pulmonary syndrome	45. Syphilis, congenital
20. Hemolytic uremic syndrome, postdiarrheal	46. Syphilis
21. Hepatitis A	47. Tetanus
22. Hepatitis B	48. Toxic-shock syndrome
23. Hepatitis, C/non A, non B	49. Trichinosis
24. HIV infection, pediatric	50. Tuberculosis
25. Legionellosis	51. Typhoid fever
26. Lyme disease	52. Yellow fever

NOTE: Although not a nationally notifiable disease, CSTE recommends reporting of cases of chickenpox via the NNDSS.
From Epidemiology Program Office: *National notifiable infectious diseases,* Atlanta, 1998, Centers for Disease Control and Prevention (www.cdc.gov/epo/dphsi/infdis.htm).

TABLE 38-1 Factors That May Influence the Emergence of New Infectious Diseases

CATEGORIES	SPECIFIC EXAMPLES
Societal events	Economic impoverishment; war or civil conflict; population growth and migration; urban decay
Health care	New medical devices; organ or tissue transplantation; drugs causing immunosuppression; widespreaduse of antibiotics
Food production	Globalization of food supplies; changes in food processing and packaging
Human behavior	Sexual behavior; drug use; travel; diet; outdoor recreation; use of child care facilities
Environmental changes	Deforestation/reforestation; changes in water ecosystems; flood/drought; famine; global warming
Public health infrastructure	Curtailment or reduction in prevention programs; inadequate communicable disease surveillance; lack of trained personnel (epidemiologists, laboratory scientists, vector and rodent control specialists)
Microbial adaptation and change	Changes in virulence and toxin production; development of drug resistance; microbes as cofactors in chronic diseases

From Centers for Disease Control and Prevention: *Addressing emerging infectious disease threats: a prevention strategy for the US,* Atlanta, 1994, CDC.

Not only is HIV/AIDS a relatively new disease, but the resultant immunocompromise is largely responsible for the rising numbers of previously rare opportunistic infections such as cryptosporidiosis, toxoplasmosis, and pneumocystis pneumonia. HIV may have existed in isolated parts of sub-Saharan Africa for years and emerged only recently into the rest of the world as the result of a combination of factors including new roads, increased commerce, and prostitutes. Tuberculosis is a familiar face turned newly aggressive. After years of decline, it has resurged as a result of drug resistance and infection secondary to HIV/AIDS.

Several factors, operating singly or in combination, can influence the emergence of these diseases as shown in Table 38-1 (CDC, 1994a). Except for microbial adapta-

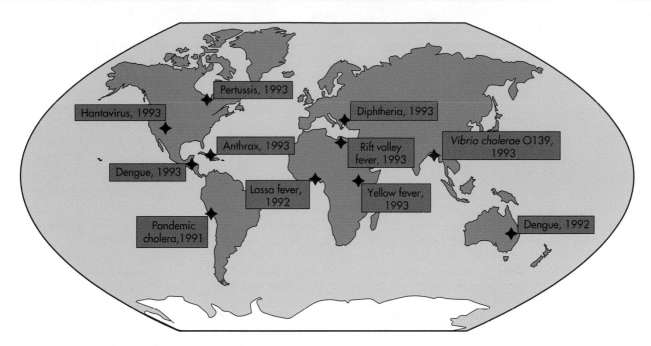

FIG. 38-2 Examples of emerging and resurgent infectious diseases in the 1990s. (From Centers for Disease Control and Prevention: *Addressing emerging infectious disease threats: a prevention strategy for the US,* Atlanta, 1994a, CDC.)

tion and changes made by the infectious agent such as those likely in the emergence of *Escherichia coli 0157:H7,* most of the emergence factors are consequences of activities and behavior of the human hosts, and environmental changes such as deforestation, urbanization, and industrialization. The rise in households with two working parents has increased the number of children in day care, and with this shift has come an increase in diarrheal diseases such as shigellosis. Changing sexual behavior and illegal drug use influence the spread of HIV/AIDS as well as other sexually transmitted diseases. Before the use of large air-conditioning systems with cooling towers, legionellosis was virtually unknown. Immigrants, legal and illegal, as well as travelers bring with them a variety of known and potentially unknown diseases. In order to prevent and control these emerging diseases, effective ways to educate people and change their behavior and to develop effective drugs and vaccines must be developed. Also, current surveillance systems should be strengthened and expanded to improve the detection and tracking of these diseases.

Examples of Emerging Infectious Diseases

Examples of emerging and resurgent infectious diseases around the world are shown in Fig. 38-2 (CDC, 1994a). Selected emerging infectious diseases, including a brief description of the diseases and symptoms they cause, their modes of transmission, and causes of emergence are listed in Table 38-2.

PREVENTION AND CONTROL OF COMMUNICABLE DISEASES

Communicable disease can be prevented and controlled. The goal of prevention and control programs is to reduce the prevalence of a disease to a level at which it no longer poses a major public health problem. In some cases, diseases may even be eliminated or eradicated. The goal of **elimination** is to remove a disease from a large geographical area such as a country or region of the world. **Eradication** is the irreversible termination of all transmission of infection by extermination of the infectious agents worldwide (CDC 1993b; Last, 1983). The World Health Organization (WHO) officially declared the global eradication of smallpox on May 8, 1980 (Evans, 1985). After the successful eradication of smallpox, the eradication of other communicable diseases became a realistic challenge. Polio appears to have been eliminated from the Americas (CDC, 1994d). No cases of indigenous polio caused by wild-type virus have been reported in the United States since 1979. The WHO has adopted a resolution for eradication of paralytic poliomyelitis and dracunculiasis (guinea worm infection) from the world by the year 2000.

Primary, Secondary, and Tertiary Prevention

Prevention of communicable diseases can be attained at three levels: primary, secondary, and tertiary (Last, 1983). Primary prevention seeks to reduce the incidence of disease through health promotion and education or, in other words, preventing disease before it happens. Examples include im-

TABLE 38-2 Examples of Emerging Infectious Diseases

INFECTIOUS AGENT	DISEASES/SYMPTOMS	MODE OF TRANSMISSION	CAUSES OF EMERGENCE
Borrelia burgdorferi	Lyme disease: rash, fever, arthritis, neurological and cardiac abnormalities	Bite of infective Ixodes tick	Increase in deer and human populations in wooded areas
Escherichia coli 0157:H7	Hemorrhagic colitis; thrombocytopenia; hemolytic uremic syndrome	Ingestion of contaminated food, especially undercooked beef and raw milk	Likely caused by a new pathogen
Ebola-Marburg Viruses	Fulminant, high mortality, hemorrhagic fever	Direct contact with infected blood, organs, secretions, and semen	Unknown
Legionella pneumophila	Legionnaires' disease: malaise, myalgia, fever, headache, respiratory illness	Air cooling systems, water supplies	Recognition in an epidemic situation
Hantaviruses	Hemorrhagic fever with renal syndrome; pulmonary syndrome	Inhalation of aerosolized rodent urine and feces	Human invasion of virus ecological niche
Human immuno-deficiency virus HIV-1	HIV infection; AIDS/HIV disease; severe immune dysfunction, opportunistic infections	Sexual contact with or exposure to blood or tissues of infected persons; perinatal	Urbanization; lifestyle changes; drug use; international travel; transfusions; transplant
Human papilloma-virus	Skin and mucous membrane lesions (warts); strongly linked to cancer of the cervix and penis	Direct sexual contact, contact with contaminated surfaces	Newly recognized; changes in sexual lifestyle
Cryptosporidium	Cryptosporidiosis; infection of epithelial cells in gastrointestinal and respiratory tracts	Fecal-oral, person-to-person, waterborne	Development near watershed areas; immunosuppression
Pneumocystis carinii	Acute pneumonia	Unknown; possibly airborne or reactivation of latent infection	Immunosuppression

Based on data from Ledeberg J, Shope RE, Oaks SC: Emerging infections: microbial threats to health in the US, Washington DC, 1992, National Academy Press; Centers for Disease Control and Prevention: *MMWR* 43(RR-7):1, 1994.

munization against communicable diseases, malaria chemoprophylaxis, the adoption of universal precautions by health care workers, the promotion of safer sex, and making water and the environment safe.

Secondary prevention targets the reduction of disease prevalence and disease morbidity through early diagnosis and treatment. Examples are skin testing for tuberculosis, serological screening for HIV, screening for sexually transmitted diseases (STDs), contact investigation in tuberculosis control programs, and partner notification in AIDS and STD programs.

WHAT DO YOU THINK? *Refusal of preventive health care to illegal immigrants may prove a threat to the public's health.*

Tertiary prevention works to reduce complications and disabilities related to disease through treatment and mental and physical rehabilitation. Two examples of tertiary prevention are *Pneumocystis carinii* pneumonia (PCP) chemoprophylaxis for people with AIDS and providing

footwear and gloves to leprosy clients to prevent trauma to their insensitive and deformed hands and feet.

Multisystem Approach to Control

Communicable diseases represent an imbalance in the harmonious relationship between the human host and the environment. This state of imbalance provides the infectious agent an opportunity to cause illness and death in the human population. Given the many factors that can disrupt the agent-host-environment relationship, a multisystem approach to control of communicable diseases, as presented in Table 38-3, must be developed (Wenzel, 1992).

NURSING TIP

When dealing with a communicable disease that has outbreak potential, include family members and close contacts as well as the sick person when developing a treatment and prevention plan.

TABLE 38-3 A Multisystem Approach to Communicable Disease Control

GOAL	EXAMPLE
Improve host resistance to infectious agents and other environmental hazards	Improved hygiene, nutrition, and physical fitness; increased immunization coverage; provision of chemoprophylaxis and chemotherapy; stress control and improved mental health
Improve safety of the environment	Improved sanitation, provision of safe water and clean air; proper cooking and storage of food; control of vectors and animal reservoir hosts
Improve public health systems	Increased access to health care; adequate health education; improved surveillance systems
Facilitate social and political changes to ensure better health for all people	Individual, organizational, and community action; legislation

Adapted from Wenzel RP: Control of communicable diseases. In Last JM, Wallace RB, editors: *Public health and preventive medicine*, ed 13, Norwalk, Conn, 1992, Appleton & Lange.

VACCINE-PREVENTABLE DISEASES

Vaccines are one of the most effective methods of preventing and controlling communicable diseases. The smallpox vaccine, which left distinctive scars on so many shoulders, is no longer in use because the smallpox virus has been declared totally eradicated from the world's population. Diseases such as polio, diphtheria, pertussis, and measles, which previously occurred in epidemic proportions, are now controlled by routine childhood immunization. They have not, however, been eradicated, so children need to be immunized against these diseases. In the United States, "No shots, no school" legislation has resulted in the immunization of most children by the time they enter school. However, many infants and toddlers, the group most vulnerable to these potentially severe diseases, do not receive scheduled immunizations despite the availability of free vaccines. Inner-city children from minority and ethnic groups are at risk for incomplete immunization.

The Childhood Immunization Initiative (CII), begun in 1993, set national goals for immunization and provided federal money for vaccines, immunization delivery programs, and immunization research. State governments and health departments across the country responded to this initiative, and by 1996 a total of 30 states and 14 urban areas had achieved all the CII vaccination coverage goals targeted to be attained by 1996 (CDC, 1997a) (see the Research Brief).

Since many children receive their immunizations at public health departments, nurses play a major role in the effort to increase immunization coverage of infants and toddlers. These nurses can track children known to be at risk for underimmunization and call or send reminders to their parents. They can help avoid missed immunization opportunities by checking the immunization status of every young child they encounter whether the clinic or home visit is immunization related or not. In addition, they can organize immunization outreach activities into the community that deliver immunization services; pro-

 RESEARCH *Brief*

A study of Los Angeles African-American newborns and their families was done to determine how effective parent education and case management might be in developing parent understanding of and demand for immunizations that in turn might influence providers to not miss opportunities to immunize during child health visits.

Newborns and their families were randomly assigned to a case management or a control group and observed through their first birthday. Families in the case management group were regularly visited and telephoned, educated on the importance and safety of immunizations, and encouraged to request immunizations from their providers. After children turned 1 year, their parents were interviewed and provider records were examined.

Missed opportunities occurred at more than 50% of the visits of all children whose records were examined. Home visits and parent education were only minimally associated with reducing missed opportunities. Missed opportunities occurred more often with private than public providers and at visits for acute illness than well-child visits. The implications for nursing practice from the study conclusions are:

1. Missed opportunities to immunize are primarily determined by factors controlled by the provider. Immunization history of every child presenting for a child health visit should be assessed and immunization considered if no appropriate contraindications are present.
2. Community health nurses who may contact families for a variety of reasons during and outside child health visits are in an excellent position to assess immunization status and encourage immunization when needed.

Wood D: Reducing missed opportunities to vaccinate during child health visits: how effective are parent education and case management, *Arch Pediatr Adolesc Med* 152(3):238, 1998.

Communicable Disease Risk and Prevention in Canada

Jann Houston, Toronto Public Health

CANADIAN NOTIFIABLE DISEASE LIST

In Canada, each province legislates its own list of reportable diseases. The following list indicates the diseases that are reported by each province to Health Canada.

- AIDS
- Amoebiasis
- Botulism
- Brucellosis
- Campylobacteriosis
- Chancroid
- Chickenpox
- Genital Chlamydia
- Cholera
- Diphtheria
- Giardiasis
- Gonococcal Infections
- Gonococcal Ophthalmia Neonatorum
- *Haemophilus influenzae* type b
- Hepatitis A
- Hepatitis B
- Hepatitis C
- Hepatitis Non-A, Non-B
- Legionellosis
- Leprosy
- Listeriosis (all types)
- Malaria
- Measles
- Meningitis, Pneumococcal
- Meningitis, Other Bacterial
- Meningitis, Viral
- Meningococcal Infections
- Mumps
- Paratyphoid
- Pertussis
- Plague
- Poliomyelitis
- Rabies
- Rubella
- Rubella, Congenital
- Salmonellosis
- Shigellosis
- Syphilis, Congenital
- Syphilis, Early Latent
- Syphilis, Early Symptomatic
- Syphilis, Other
- Tetanus
- Trichinosis
- Tuberculosis
- Typhoid
- Verotoxigenic *E. coli*
- Yellow Fever

INFECTIOUS DISEASES
Meningococcal Disease

In 1996 in Canada, there were 215 reported cases of meningococcal infections. Group B has been the most common cause of disease in the Americas. Community outbreaks of group C disease, affecting school and college-aged youths, have occurred with increasing frequency in Canada and the United States since 1990 (LCDC, 1999).

Tuberculosis (TB)

Although Canada has one of the lowest reported incidence rates of TB in the world, it is an important disease in certain high-risk populations, including Aboriginal peoples, foreign-born residents from countries with a high prevalence of TB, disadvantaged inner-city populations, and those with HIV infection. In 1996 there were 1849 reported cases of tuberculosis in Canada (LCDC, 1999). An important strategy that is now being implemented in certain jurisdictions is Direct Observed Therapy. This approach ensures that individuals take the prescribed course of therapy, and public health staff can also help to assist clients to obtain the health care and social support that they need.

VACCINE-PREVENTABLE DISEASES
Measles, Mumps, and Rubella

The National Advisory Committee on Immunization now recommends that children receive a first dose of measles vaccine at 12 months of age and a second dose at either 18 months or at 4 to 6 years of age (National Advisory Committee on Immunization [NACI], 1998). Since the introduction of this two-dose schedule in 1996, reported measles cases in Canada have dropped from 2361 in 1995 to 335 in 1996 (LCDC, 1999). There are approximately 500 cases of mumps reported in Canada each year (LCDC, 1999). The overall incidence of rubella in Canada has remained low; however, outbreaks continue to occur in certain geographic centres. In Canada, there were 302 reported cases of rubella in 1996 (LCDC, 1999).

Haemophilus influenzae type b (Hib)

In the early 1990s, Hib was the most common cause of bacterial meningitis in Canada. Since the introduction of a new vaccine in 1992, the number of cases in Canada has decreased by more than 70%. In 1996 there were 55 reported cases of Hib in Canada (LCDC, 1999).

Pertussis

Since the introduction of the vaccine in 1943, rates of pertussis have decreased over 90% in Canada. In 1996, Canada had 5408 reported cases of pertussis (LCDC, 1999). Canada has also introduced the new acellular pertussis vaccine. The use of whole cell pertussis is no longer recommended in Canada (NACI, 1998).

Communicable Disease Risk and Prevention in Canada—cont'd

Influenza

Influenza occurs in Canada every year, generally during the late fall and winter. Canada, like other countries, has been affected by major influenza pandemics (e.g., in 1889-1890, 1918-1919, 1957-1958, and 1968-1969). The National Advisory Committee on Immunization recommends that priority be given to ensuring annual vaccination of people at high risk since this is the single most important measure for reducing the impact of influenza (NACI, 1998).

IMMUNIZATION

In Canada, immunization cannot be made mandatory because of the Canadian Constitution. Only three provinces (out of 10 provinces and 3 territories) require proof of immunization for school entrance. The delivery of immunization services also varies in Canada, although immunization is provided free to all citizens. In some provinces and territories, the public health care system administers all childhood immunizations and in others private physicians provide the immunization with vaccine ordered from local public health units (LCDC, 1996). The National Advisory Committee on Immunization recommends the following Canadian Vaccination Schedule for Infants and Children (NACI, 1998):

Age	DtaP	IPV	Hib	MMR	Td	Hep B* 3 doses
2 months	X	X	X			Infancy
4 months	X	X	X			
6 months	X	X †	X			
12 months				X		
18 months	X	X	X	X ‡or		
4-6 years	X	X	X	X ‡		
14-16 years					X	Preadolescence (9-13 years)

DtaP, Diphtheria, tetanus, pertussis (acellular) vaccine; *Hib*, *Haemophilus influenzae* type b conjugate vaccine; *MMR*, Measles, mumps and rubella vaccine; *Td*, Tetanus and diphtheria toxoid "adult type"; *Hep B*, Hepatitis B vaccine.

*Hepatitis B vaccine can be routinely given to infants or preadolescents, depending on the provincial/territorial policy.

†This dose is not needed routinely, but can be included for convenience.

‡A second dose of MMR is recommended, at least 1 month after the first dose given. For convenience, options include giving it with the next scheduled vaccination at 18 months of age or with school entry (4 to 6 years) vaccinations (depending on the provincial/territorial policy), or at any intervening age that is practicable.

Bibliography

Health Protection Branch-Laboratory Centre for Disease Control: *Canadian national report on immunization*, Ottawa, 1996, Health Canada.

Health Protection Branch-Laboratory Centre for Disease Control: *Notifiable diseases on-line*, Ottawa, 1999, Health Canada.

National Advisory Committee on Immunization: *Canadian immunization guide*, ed 9, Ottawa, 1998, Canadian Medical Association.

Canadian spelling is used.

---

vide answers to parents' questions and concerns about immunization; and educate parents about why immunizations are needed, inappropriate contraindications to immunization, and the importance of completing the immunization schedule on time.

Routine Childhood Immunization Schedule

Children in the United States are routinely immunized against the following 10 diseases:

1. Hepatitis B
2. Diphtheria
3. Pertussis (whooping cough)
4. Tetanus
5. Paralytic poliomyelitis (polio)
6. *Haemophilus influenzae* type B (Hib)
7. Measles
8. Mumps
9. Rubella
10. *Varicella* (chickenpox)

To the undoubted relief of parents who feared days of work lost to caring for children miserable with chickenpox, the *Varicella* vaccine was licensed for general use in April 1995. Diphtheria, pertussis, and tetanus (DTP) are usually given in combination as are measles, mumps, and rubella (MMR). To achieve recommended immunization levels by 2 years of age, most of these immunizations should begin when an infant reaches 2 to 3 months of age. Live vaccines—measles, mumps, rubella (MMR), and polio—should be completed by 15 and 18 months, respectively. *Varicella* may be given at any visit after the first birthday. Table 26-12 in Chapter 26 provides the 1998 immunization schedule recommended by the Advisory Committee on Immunization Practices, American Academy of Pediatrics, and the American Academy of Family Physicians. Other vaccines available for use in special circumstances include those against hepatitis A, influenza, meningococcal meningitis, plague, pneumococcal pneumonia, rabies, and yellow fever.

Measles

Measles is an acute, highly contagious disease that is considered a childhood illness but is often seen in the United States in adolescents and young adults. Symptoms include fever, sneezing and coughing, conjunctivitis, small white spots on the inside of the cheek (Koplik spots), and a red, blotchy rash beginning several days after the respiratory signs. Measles is caused by the rubeola virus and is transmitted by inhalation of infected aerosol droplets, direct contact with infected nasal or throat secretions, or with articles freshly contaminated with the same nasal or throat secretions. Its very contagious nature, combined with the fact that people are most contagious before they are aware they are infected, makes measles a disease that can spread rapidly through the population. Infection with measles confers lifelong immunity (Benenson, 1995).

Measles and malnutrition form a deadly combination for many children in the developing world. Despite the introduction in 1963 of a live attenuated measles vaccine that is safe, effective, and widely available, measles still causes 10% of total deaths in children less than 5 years of age and is the eighth leading cause of death worldwide. Much of this mortality is preventable by immunizing all infants (CDC, 1997b).

Immunization has decreased the measles cases in the United States. Before 1963, 200,000 to 500,000 cases of measles were reported yearly, but by 1983 reported cases had fallen to an all-time low of less than 1500. Then in the late 1980s the incidence of measles began to climb again. In 1989 to 1991, more than 55,000 cases of measles were reported. This increase resulted from low immunization rates among preschool children and was countered with efforts to increase immunization rates and the routine use of two doses of measles vaccine for all children (CDC, 1997c).

With the exception of outbreaks in 1994 that occurred predominantly among high school– and college-age persons, many of whom had received only one previous dose of measles vaccine, reported measles cases have continued to drop since 1991. In 1997 only 138 cases were reported to CDC, the lowest number of cases reported since measles became a nationally reportable disease in 1912 and a 55% decrease from the previous record low of 309 cases reported in 1995 (CDC, 1998b).

As vaccine coverage of children ages 19 to 35 months improves (91% in 1996) and increasing numbers of schools require second-dose coverage, the pattern of infection is shifting from underimmunization of infants and school-age children to disease acquired from other countries. Of the 138 measles cases reported in 1997, 41% were documented as imported. The fact that these imported cases did not result in outbreaks suggests that vaccination efforts in this country have been successful in increasing herd immunity against measles. Groups who remain at greatest risk for measles are those who do not routinely accept immunization, such as those with religious or philosophical objections, students in schools that do not require two doses of vaccine, and infants in areas where immunization coverage is low. The exposure of these groups to an imported case could result in a major outbreak (CDC, 1998b).

Healthy People 2000 calls for the sustained elimination of indigenous measles in the United States and the Pan American Health Organization has called for the elimination of measles from the Western Hemisphere by the year 2000. Once considered an impossibility, the goal of global elimination is now being considered. Efforts to meet this goal will require 1) rapid detection of cases and implementation of appropriate outbreak control measures, 2) achievement and maintenance of high levels of vaccination coverage among preschool-age children in all geographical regions, 3) greater implementation and enforcement of the two-dose schedule among young adults, 4) the determination of the source of all outbreaks and sporadic infections, and 5) cooperation among countries in measles control efforts (CDC, 1997b). Nurses work to receive reports of cases, investigate and initiate control measures for outbreaks, and to use every opportunity to immunize adolescents and young adults who lack documentation of two doses of measles vaccine. Those who work in regions where illegal immigration is common and/or where groups obtain exemption from immunization on religious grounds need to be especially alert for cases and the need for prompt outbreak control among these particularly susceptible populations.

Rubella

The rubella (German measles) virus causes a mild febrile disease with enlarged lymph nodes and a fine, pink rash that is often difficult to distinguish from measles or scarlet fever. In contrast to measles, rubella is only a moderately contagious illness. Transmission is through inhalation of or direct contact with infected droplets from the respiratory secretions of infected persons. Children may show few or no constitutional symptoms, whereas adults usually experience several days of low-grade fever, headache, malaise, runny nose, and conjunctivitis before the rash appears. Many infections occur without a rash.

Although still primarily a childhood disease, rubella occurs more often in adolescents than do measles or chickenpox. When children are well immunized, infections in these older populations become more important with outbreaks in institutions, universities, and the military. Infection confers lifelong immunity. Rubella is most common in winter and spring (Benenson, 1995). Since 1991, cases have fallen to all time lows with an annual case average of 183 for 1992 to 1996. The percentage of cases among Hispanics increased from 19% in 1991 to 68% in 1996 (CDC, 1997d).

For many years, because it caused only a mild illness, rubella was considered to be of minor importance. Then, in 1941, the link between maternal rubella and certain congenital defects was recognized, and this disease suddenly assumed major public health significance. Congenital rubella syndrome (CRS) occurs in greater than 25% of infants born to women who are infected with rubella during the first trimester of pregnancy (Gershon, 1995). Rubella infection, in addition to intrauterine death and spontaneous abortion, may result in anomalies that can affect single or multiple organ systems. Defects include cataracts, congenital glaucoma, deafness, microcephaly, mental retardation, cardiac abnormalities and diabetes mellitus.

Healthy People 2000 calls for the sustained elimination of both indigenous rubella and CRS. Preventing rubella and CRS will require many of the same efforts discussed with measles, including achievement and maintenance of high rates of immunization among preschoolers, early detection and outbreak control, taking advantage of opportunities such as high school and college entrance to immunize susceptible adolescents, extending immunization opportunities to religious groups that traditionally do not seek health care, and targeting adolescent and young adults who are particularly susceptible because they come from or are exposed to persons from countries that do not routinely vaccinate against rubella. The increasing number of cases in persons of Hispanic background suggests a population to which immunization efforts should be specifically targeted.

Pertussis

Pertussis (whooping cough) begins as a mild upper respiratory infection that progresses to an irritating cough that within 1 to 2 weeks may become paroxysmal (a series of repeated violent coughs). The repeated coughs occur without intervening breaths and can be followed by a characteristic inspiratory "whoop." Pertussis is caused by the bacteria *Bordetella pertussis* and is transmitted via an airborne route through contact with infected droplets. It is highly contagious and considered endemic in the United States. Vaccination against pertussis is a part of the routine childhood immunization schedule. Treatment of infected individuals with antibiotics such as erythromycin may shorten the period of communicability but does not relieve symptoms unless given early in the course of the infection. A 2-week treatment with antibiotics is recommended for family members and close contacts of infected individuals, regardless of immunization status. (Benenson, 1995).

Before the development of a whole-cell vaccine in the 1940s, pertussis resulted in hundreds of thousands of cases and thousands of deaths per year, the majority of cases occurring in children under 5 years. Since vaccine licensure, the number of cases in the United States has steadily declined, hitting a record low in 1976 of just over 1000 cases. However, since the early 1980s, pertussis cases have shown cyclic increases every 3 to 4 years (CDC 1995a). In 1996 to 1997, over 13,000 cases were reported (CDC, 1998c).

While immunization coverage of U.S. children 19 to 35 months of age has been increasing throughout the 1990s, some parents have hesitated to vaccinate their children against pertussis. This hesitation is a result of the frequency of minor adverse reactions to the whole-cell pertussis vaccine, as well as publicity surrounding infrequent but serious adverse reactions and the inaccurate suggestion that pertussis vaccine could result in permanent neurological damage. The licensure in 1996 of an acellular vaccine associated with fewer adverse reactions that can be administered to very young infants may help improve acceptance of pertussis immunization (Marwick, 1996).

Although pertussis is still predominantly a disease of young children, the increasing number of cases in adolescents and young adults is a growing problem. Infants are the group most susceptible to pertussis and the most likely to suffer complications. An examination of 13,615 cases reported during 1992 to 1994 showed 41% in infants less than 1 year of age (the majority less than six months old); 20% in children 1 to 4 years olds, 11% in those 5 to 9 years old, and 28% in those age 10 years and older (CDC 1995a). In 1996, 44% of all reported pertussis cases occurred among persons age 10 years or older. Cases in very young children, especially those younger than 6 months, are attributed to not being fully immunized because of age. Cases in older children largely result from underimmunization and cases in adolescents and adults with histories of complete immunization are attributed to waning immunity. Although natural infection with pertussis results in permanent immunity, immunization through vaccination does not. Because pertussis in adolescents and adults may be a mild disease without the characteristic signs seen in children, it may go underdiagnosed and underreported in these age groups. These individuals then become an important reservoir for the disease, and because pertussis is highly contagious, are responsible for its spread to infants and children as well as other adults. Pertussis vaccines are not labeled for use in individuals older than 6 years; catching up children who are missing doses and boostering for waning immunity are not presently options for preventing outbreaks. The routine boostering of adults for pertussis is under discussion. Increasing physician awareness of pertussis in older children and adults to increase prompt detection and treatment may help curtail outbreaks (CDC, 1997e).

Nurses may expect periodic outbreaks of pertussis because of its cyclical nature. Working with the community to maintain the highest possible levels of immunization coverage can minimize these outbreaks. Because of the contagious nature of pertussis, nurses play a major role in limiting transmission during outbreaks by ensuring appropriate treatment of family members, classmates, and other close contacts.

Influenza

Influenza is a viral respiratory infection often indistinguishable from the common cold or other respiratory diseases. Transmission is airborne and through direct contact with infected droplets. Unlike many viruses that do not survive long in the environment, the "flu" virus is thought to survive for many hours in dried mucus. Outbreaks are common in the winter and early spring in areas where people gather indoors such as in schools and nursing homes. Gastrointestinal and respiratory symptoms are common. Because symptoms do not always follow a characteristic pattern, many viral diseases that are not influenza are often called "flu." The most important factors to note about influenza are its epidemic nature and the mortality that results from its pulmonary complications, especially in the elderly.

There are three types of influenza viruses: A, B, and C. Type A is usually responsible for large epidemics, whereas outbreaks from type B are more regionalized and those from type C are less common and usually only result in mild illness. Influenza viruses often change the nature of their surface appearance or alter their antigenic make-up. Types B and C are fairly stable viruses, but type A changes constantly. Minor antigenic changes are referred to as antigenic *drift* and cause yearly epidemics and regional outbreaks. Major changes such as the emergence of new subtypes are called antigenic *shift;* these only occur with type A viruses. Antigenic *shift* and *drift* leads to epidemic outbreaks every few years and pandemic outbreaks every 10 to 40 years. Mortality rates associated with epidemics may be higher than those in non-epidemic situations (Benenson, 1995).

In 1997 in Hong Kong, the first known cases of human illness associated with an avian influenza virus, A (H5N10), were reported. Referred to in the press as Hong Kong "Bird Flu," this virus appears to have been transmitted to people through contact with infected poultry. As a result of this association, Hong Kong officials ordered the slaughter of all chickens in and around Hong Kong, which appears to have stopped the spread of this disease. No cases have been reported outside Hong Kong. Although investigation of this disease did not rule out the possibility of human to human transmission, the fact that it did not spread more readily among a population essentially without antibodies to this virus suggests that it is not being efficiently transmitted among people (CDC, 1998d).

Influenza vaccines are prepared each year based on the best possible prediction of what type and variant of virus will be most prevalent that year. Because of the changing nature of the virus, immunization is necessary yearly and is given in the early fall before the flu season begins. Immunization is highly recommended for the elderly, individuals with chronic respiratory disease, or those with other chronic disease conditions that impair the immune system, as well as health-care workers and anyone involved in essential community services. Although immunization is recommended for the previously mentioned groups, any individual may benefit from this protection. Flu shots do not always prevent infection, but they do result in milder disease symptoms. Immunization of adults involves one injection. Children less than 12 years of age may initially receive two doses 1 to 2 weeks apart and subsequently one dose on a yearly basis. Sensitivity to eggs is a contraindication to immunization, and pregnant women should avoid immunization in the first trimester of pregnancy (Benenson, 1995).

Unlike the immunizations for childhood diseases, flu shots are largely targeted at an adult population. Over 80% to 90% of all influenza-associated deaths in the United States occur in people age 65 and older.

Since adults do not use health care services as regularly as children do, different approaches may be required to reach higher immunization coverage rates among adults. Public health nurses often spearhead influenza immunization campaigns that target adults such as by having nurses stationed at polling places during elections or in the parking lots of health departments, churches, and schools conducting "drive-up" clinics. As with children, nurses should check immunization history and encourage immunization for every adult encountered in a clinic or home visit.

FOODBORNE AND WATERBORNE DISEASES

Foodborne illness, or "food poisoning," is often categorized as food infection or food intoxication. Food infection results from bacterial, viral, or parasitic infection of food and includes salmonellosis, hepatitis A, and trichinosis. Food intoxication results from toxins produced by bacterial growth, chemical contaminants (heavy metals), and a variety of disease producing substances found naturally in certain foods such as mushrooms and some seafood. Examples of food intoxications are botulism, mercury poisoning, and paralytic shellfish poisoning. Table 38-4 presents some of the most common agents of food intoxication, their incubation period, source, symptoms, and pathology. Although not a hard and fast rule, food infections are associated with incubation periods of 12 hours to several days after ingestion of the infected food, whereas intoxications become obvious within minutes to hours after ingestion. Botulism is a clear exception to this rule with an incubation period of a week or more in adults. The expression "ptomaine poisoning" often used when discussing foodborne illness does not refer to a specific causal organism.

It is estimated that somewhere between 6.5 and 81 million cases of foodborne illness occur each year in the United States, cause 4000 to 9000 deaths, and result in as much as 8 to 23 billion dollars in medical costs and lost productivity (Stephenson, 1997). This range of estimates is so wide since there is no structured, national surveillance system and most cases are never reported. In an effort to more precisely determine the burden of foodborne diseases in the United States, the CDC in 1994 instigated the Foodborne Diseases Active Surveillance Network (FoodNet). This program monitors foodborne disease outbreaks in five sites and specifically tracks confirmed cases of disease resulting from seven agents that can cause foodborne disease: *Campylobacter, E.coli 0157:H7, Listeria, Salmonella, Shigella, Vibrio,* and *Yersinia.*

WHAT DO YOU THINK? *Food irradiation is one option being strongly considered to prevent outbreaks of foodborne disease.*

TABLE 38-4 Commonly Encountered Food Intoxications

CAUSAL AGENT	INCUBATION PERIOD	DURATION	CLINICAL PRESENTATION	ASSOCIATED FOOD
Staphylococcus aureus	30 min-7 hr	1-2 days	Sudden onset of nausea, cramps, vomiting, and prostration often accompanied by diarrhea; rarely fatal	All foods, especially those most likely to come into contact with foodhandlers' hands that may be contaminated by purulent discharges from infections of the eyes and skin
Clostridium perfringens (strain A)	6-24 hr	1 day or less	Sudden onset of colic and diarrhea, maybe nausea; vomiting and fever unusual; rarely fatal	Inadequately heated meats or stews; food contaminated by soil or feces becomes infective when improper storage or reheating allows multiplication of organism
Vibrio parahemolyticus	4-96 hr	1-7 days	Watery diarrhea and abdominal cramps; sometimes nausea, vomiting, fever, and headache; rarely fatal	Raw or inadequately cooked seafood; period of time at room temperature usually required for multiplication of organism
Clostridium botulinum	12-36 hr, sometimes days	Slow recovery, may be months	CNS signs; blurred vision, difficulty in swallowing and dry mouth followed by descending symmetrical flaccid paralysis of an alert person; "floppy baby" w/infant botulism; fatality <15% with antitoxin and respiratory support	Home-canned fruits and vegetables that have not been preserved with adequate heating; infants have become infected from ingesting honey

Based on data from Benenson AS, editor: *Control of communicable diseases in man*, ed 16, Washington, DC, 1995, American Public Health Association.

Recently, publicity has surrounded the deaths of children who ate undercooked fast-food hamburgers containing a virulent strain of *E. coli;* nationwide outbreaks of diarrheal disease from *Cyclospora* contaminated Guatemalan raspberries; outbreaks of hepatitis A in school children who consumed tainted frozen strawberries; and salmonella infections associated with uncooked poultry and eggs. While the very young, the very old, and the very debilitated are most susceptible, everyone can acquire foodborne illness regardless of socioeconomic status, race, sex, age, occupation, education or area of residence. However, a new, particularly susceptible population is emerging as a result of the increasing older population, the growing numbers of immunocompromised individuals (resulting from chemotherapy, immunosuppressive drugs and AIDS), and the larger numbers of children surviving debilitating illness. At the same time the centralized food production and processing system with its widespread distribution network increases the potential for any contamination to result in a large-scale foodborne disease outbreak. Public health officials think that the number of reported cases of foodborne illness vastly underestimates the true number of cases and that the number of foodborne outbreaks is likely to increase.

Ten Golden Rules for Safe Food Preparation

Protecting the nation's food supply from contamination by all virulent microbes is a complex issue that will be in-

credibly costly and time consuming to address. However, much foodborne illness, regardless of causal organism, can easily be prevented through simple changes in food preparation, handling, and storage to destroy or denature contaminants and prevent their further spread. Because these measures are so important in preventing foodborne disease, *Healthy People 2000* has included an objective directed toward them, and the World Health Organization (WHO) has developed the "Ten Golden Rules for Safe Food Preparation" presented in Box 38-3 (Benenson, 1995).

Salmonellosis

Salmonellosis is a bacterial disease characterized by sudden onset of headache, abdominal pain, diarrhea, nausea, sometimes vomiting, and almost always fever. Onset is typically within 48 hours of ingestion, but the clinical signs are impossible to distinguish from other causes of gastrointestinal distress. Diarrhea and lack of appetite may persist for several days, and dehydration may be severe. While morbidity can be significant, death is uncommon except among infants, the elderly and the debilitated. The rate of infection is highest among infants and small children. It is estimated that only a small proportion of cases are recognized clinically and that only 1% of clinical cases are reported. The number of salmonella infections yearly may actually number in the millions (Benenson, 1995).

BOX 38-3 Ten Golden Rules for Safe Food Preparation

1. Choose food processed for safety.
2. Cook food thoroughly.
3. Eat cooked food immediately.
4. Store cooked food carefully.
5. Reheat cooked foods thoroughly.
6. Avoid contact between raw foods and cooked foods.
7. Wash hands repeatedly.
8. Keep all kitchen surfaces meticulously clean.
9. Protect foods from insects, rodents, and other animals.
10. Use pure water.

From Benenson AS, editor: *Control of communicable diseases in man,* ed 15, Washington, DC, 1990, American Public Health Association.

Outbreaks occur commonly in restaurants, hospitals, nursing homes, and institutions for children. The transmission route is ingestion of food derived from an infected animal or contaminated by feces of an infected animal or person. Meat, poultry, and eggs are the foods most often associated with salmonellosis outbreaks. Animals are the common reservoir for the various *Salmonella* serotypes although infected humans may also fill this role. Animals are more likely to be chronic carriers. Reptiles such as iguanas have been implicated as salmonella carriers along with pet turtles, poultry, cattle, swine, rodents, dogs, and cats. Person-to-person transmission is an important consideration in day care and institutional settings.

Escherichia coli 0157:H7

Escherichia coli 0157:H7 belongs to the enterohemorrhagic category of *E. coli* serotypes that produce a strong cytotoxin that can cause a potentially fatal hemorrhagic colitis. This pathogen was first described in humans in 1992 following the investigation of two outbreaks of illness that were associated with consumption of hamburger from a fast-food restaurant chain. It is estimated that in this county up to 500 deaths a year may be caused by *E. coli* 0157:H7. Undercooked hamburger has been implicated in several outbreaks, as have roast beef, alfalfa sprouts, unpasteurized milk and apple cider, municipal water, and person-to-person transmission in day care centers (CDC, 1994 g). Infection with 0157:H7 causes bloody diarrhea, abdominal cramps, and infrequently fever. Children and the elderly are at highest risk for clinical disease and complications. Hemolytic uremic syndrome is seen in 5% to 10% of cases and may result in acute renal failure. The case-fatality rate is 3% to 5%.

Hamburger often appears to be involved in outbreaks because the grinding process exposes pathogens on the surface of the whole meat to the interior of the ground meat, effectively mixing the once-exterior bacteria thoroughly throughout the hamburger so that searing the surface is no longer sufficient to kill all the bacteria. Tracking the contamination is complicated by the fact that hamburger is often made of meat ground from several sources. The best protection against this pathogen, as with most foodborne pathogens, is to thoroughly cook food before eating it.

Waterborne Disease Outbreaks and Pathogens

Waterborne pathogens usually enter water supplies through animal or human fecal contamination and frequently cause enteric disease. They include viruses, bacteria, and protozoans. Hepatitis A virus is probably the most publicized waterborne viral agent, although other viruses may also be transmitted by this route (enteroviruses, rotaviruses, and paramyxoviruses). The most important waterborne bacterial diseases are cholera, typhoid fever, and bacillary dysentery. However, other *Salmonella* types, *Shigella, Vibrio,* and various coliform bacteria including *E. coli* 0157:H7 may be transmitted in the same manner. In the past, the most important waterborne protozoans have been *Entamoeba histolytica* (amebic dysentery) and *Giardia lamblia,* but recent outbreaks of cryptosporidiosis in municipal water like that which resulted in diarrheal outbreaks that crippled the city of Milwaukee in 1993 have pushed *Cryptosporidium* into the debate over how to best safeguard municipal water supplies. Protozoans do not respond to traditional chlorine treatment as do enteric and coliform bacteria.

The CDC defines an outbreak of waterborne disease as an incident in which two or more persons experience similar illness after consuming water that epidemiological evidence implicates as the source of that illness. Only a single incident is required in cases of chemical contamination. The CDC and the Environmental Protection Agency (EPA) maintain a collaborative surveillance program for collection and periodic reporting of data on the occurrence and causes of waterborne disease outbreaks.

VECTORBORNE DISEASES

Vectorborne diseases are transmitted by vectors, usually arthropods, either biologically or mechanically. With biologic transmission, the **vector** is necessary for the developmental stage of the infectious agent. An example would be mosquitoes that carry malaria. Mechanical transmission occurs when an insect simply contacts the infectious agent with its legs or mouth parts and carries it to the host. For example, flies and cockroaches may contaminate food or cooking utensils.

Vectorborne diseases commonly encountered in the United States are those associated with ticks such as Lyme disease (*Borrelia burgdoferi*), Ehrlichiosis (*Ehrlichia chafeensis*), and Rocky Mountain spotted fever (*Rickettsia rickettsii*). Nurses who work with large immigrant populations or with international travelers may encounter malaria and dengue fever, both carried by mosquitoes. Plague *(Yersinia pestis)* is carried by fleas of wild rodents. More rarely seen are babesiosis *(Babesia microti),* tularemia *(Francisella tularensis),* and Q fever *(Coxiella burnetii),* all associated with ticks.

Lyme Disease

Parents in Lyme, Connecticut, concerned about the unusual incidence of juvenile rheumatoid arthritis in their children, first brought attention to the tickborne infection that is now referred to as Lyme disease. Although first described in 1975, Lyme disease is now the most common vectorborne disease in the United States (CDC, 1997f). The causative agent, the spirochete *Borrelia burgdoferi*, was not identified until 1982. Lyme disease became a nationally notifiable disease in 1991. Lyme disease is transmitted by Ixodid ticks that are associated with white-tailed deer (*Odocoileus virginianus*) and the white-footed mouse (*Peromyscus leucopus*). Lyme disease has been reported throughout the United States with cases concentrated in rural and suburban areas of the northeast, mid-Atlantic states, north, upper central region, and Pacific coast states (Dennis, Fikrig, and Schaffner, 1999). This disease usually occurs in summer during tick season.

The clinical spectrum of Lyme disease can be divided into three stages. Stage I is characterized by erythema chronicum migrans, a distinctive skin lesion often called a bull's-eye lesion because it begins as a red area at the site of the tick attachment that spreads outward in a ring-like fashion as the center clears. About 50% to 70% of infected persons develop this lesion 3 to 30 days after a tick bite. The skin lesion may be accompanied or preceded by fever, fatigue, malaise, headache, muscle pains and a stiff neck, as well as tender and enlarged lymph nodes and migratory joint pain. Most clients diagnosed in this early stage respond well to 10 to 14 days of oral tetracycline or penicillin.

If not treated during this first stage, Lyme disease can progress to stage II, which may include additional skin lesions, headache, and neurological and cardiac abnormalities. Clients who progress to stage III have recurrent attacks of arthritis and arthralgia, especially in the knees, that may begin months to years after the initial lesion. The clinical diagnosis of classical Lyme disease with the distinctive skin lesion is straightforward. Illness without the lesion is more difficult to diagnose, since serological tests are more accurate in stages II and III than in stage I (Steere, 1995). A newly approved vaccine promises to curb the growth of this disease (Dennis, Fikrig, and Schaffner, 1999). It is suggested that the vaccine will be most appropriate for use in high-risk regions.

Rocky Mountain Spotted Fever

Contrary to its name, Rocky Mountain spotted fever (RMSF) is seldom seen in the Rocky Mountains and most commonly occurs in the Southeast, Oklahoma, Kansas, and Missouri. The infectious agent is *Rickettsia rickettsii*. The tick vector varies according to geographic regional. The dog tick, *Dermacentor variabilis*, is the vector in the eastern and southern United States RMSF is not transmitted from person to person. It is thought that one attack confers lifelong immunity.

Clinical signs include sudden onset of moderate to high fever, severe headache, chills, deep muscle pain, and malaise. About 50% of cases experience a rash on the extremities that spreads to most of the body. Many cases of what has been referred to as "spotless" RMSF may be caused by a newly identified tickborne organism, *Ehrlichia chafeensis*. RMSF responds readily to treatment with tetracycline. Definitive diagnosis can be made with paired serum titers. Since early treatment is important in decreasing morbidity and mortality, treatment should be started in response to clinical and epidemiological considerations rather than waiting for laboratory confirmation (Benenson, 1995).

Prevention and Control of Tickborne Diseases

Vaccines are not currently available for any tickborne diseases except tularemia; work is being done on a vaccine for Lyme disease. The best preventive measures are wearing protective clothing when outdoors and searching for ticks. Protective clothing includes long-sleeve shirts and long pants tucked into socks. Ticks require a prolonged period of attachment (6 to 48 hours) before they start blood feeding on the host; prompt tick discovery and removal can help prevent transmission of disease. Ticks should be removed with steady, gentle traction on tweezers applied to the head parts of the tick (Walker et al, 1995). The tick's body should not be squeezed during the removal process to avoid infection that could be transmitted from resultant tick feces and tissue juices. When outdoors, tick repellents containing diethytoluamide (DEET) can offer effective protection, but significant toxicity, including skin irritation, anaphylaxis, and seizures, has been reported in children.

DISEASES OF TRAVELERS

Individuals traveling outside of the United States need to be aware of and take precautions against potential diseases to which they may be exposed. Which diseases and what precautions will depend on the individual's health status, the particular travel destination, the reason for travel, and the length of travel. Persons who plan to travel in remote regions for an extended period may need to consider rare diseases and take special precautions that would not apply to the average traveler. Consultation with public health officials can provide specific health information and recommendations for a given situation.

Upon return from visiting exotic places, travelers may bring back with them an unplanned souvenir in the form of disease. Therefore, in a presenting client, a history of travel should always be closely considered. Even the apparently healthy returned traveler, especially if residing in a tropical country for some time, should undergo routine screening to rule out acquired infections. Likewise, refugees and immigrants may arrive with infectious health problems ranging from helminth infections to diseases of major public health significance such as tuberculosis, malaria, cholera, and hepatitis. Community health nurses may find themselves dealing with these diseases since refugees are often processed and treated through the public health system.

Malaria

Caused by the bloodborne parasite *Plasmodium*, malaria is a potentially fatal disease characterized by regular cycles of fever and chills. Transmission is through the bite of an infected *Anopheles* mosquito. The word *malaria* is based on an association between the illness and the bad air of the marshes where the mosquitoes breed. Malaria is an old disease that first appears in recorded history in 1700 BC China. Today malaria poses a major health risk since there is no vaccine available to protect against this disease that causes as many as 200 to 300 million cases and 1 to 2 million deaths per year.

Malaria prevention depends on protection against mosquitoes and appropriate chemoprophylaxis. Of the four types of human malaria, *Plasmodium ovale* and *Plasmodium vivax* can lead to relapsing malaria; more seriously, *Plasmodium falciparum,* is drug resistant. Thus decisions about antimalarial drugs must be tailored individually, based on the types of malaria in the specific area of the country to be visited, the purpose of the trip, and the length of the visit. The CDC and the World Health Organization publish guides to the status of malaria and recommendations for prophylaxis on a country-by-country basis. At this time, there is no one drug or drug combination known to be safe and efficacious in preventing all types of malaria. Antimalarials are generally started a week to several weeks before leaving the country and are continued for 4-6 weeks after returning. Despite appropriate prophylaxis, malaria may still be contracted. Travelers should be advised of this fact and urged to seek immediate medical care if they exhibit symptoms of cyclical fever and chills upon return home. Immigrants and visitors from areas where malaria is endemic may also become clinically ill after entering this country. Since the malaria parasite is bloodborne, blood donors should be questioned about a history of exposure to malaria.

Foodborne and Waterborne Diseases

As in this country, much foodborne disease abroad can be avoided if the traveler eats thoroughly cooked foods prepared with reasonable hygiene; eating foods from street vendors may not be a good idea. Trichinosis, tapeworms, and fluke infections, as well as bacterial infections, result from eating raw or undercooked meats. Raw vegetables may act as a source of bacterial, viral, helminth, or protozoal infection if they have been grown with or washed in contaminated water. Fruits that can be peeled immediately before eating such as bananas are less likely to be a source of infection. Dairy products should be pasteurized and appropriately refrigerated.

Water in many areas of the world is not potable (safe to drink), and drinking this water can lead to infection with a variety of protozoal, viral and bacterial agents including amoeba, *Giardia, Cryptosporidium,* hepatitis, cholera, and various coliform bacteria. Unless traveling in an area where the piped water is known to be safe, only boiled water (boiled for 1 minute), bottled water, or water purified with iodine or chlorine compounds should be consumed. Ice should be avoided since freezing does not inactivate these agents. If the water is questionable, choose coffee or tea made with boiled water, carbonated beverages without ice, beer, wine, or canned fruit juices.

Diarrheal Diseases

Travelers often suffer from diarrhea, so much so that colorful names such as "Montezuma's Revenge," "Turista," and "Colorado Quickstep," among a few, exist in our vocabulary to describe these bouts of intestinal upset. Some of these diarrheas do not have infectious causes and result from stress, fatigue, schedule changes, and eating unfamiliar foods. Acute infectious diarrheas are usually of viral or bacterial origin. *E. coli* probably causes more cases of traveler's diarrhea than all other infective agents combined (Mandell et al, 1995). Protozoan-induced diarrheas such as those resulting from *Entamoeba* and *Giardia* are less likely to be acute and more commonly to present once the traveler returns home. Travelers need to be careful about what they eat and drink.

ZOONOSES

A zoonosis is an infection transmitted from a vertebrate animal to a human under natural conditions. The agents that cause zoonoses do not need humans to maintain their life cycles; infected humans have simply somehow managed to get in their way. Means of transmission include animal bites, inhalation, ingestion, direct contact, and arthropod intermediates. This last transmission route means that some vectorborne diseases may also be zoonoses. Other than vectorborne diseases, some of the more common zoonoses in the United States include toxoplasmosis (*Toxoplasma gondii*), cat scratch disease (*Bartonella henselae*), brucellosis (*Brucella* species), listeriosis (*Listeria monocytogenes*), salmonellosis (*Salmonella* serotypes*),* and rabies (Family *Rhabdoviridae,* genus *Lyssavirus*).

Rabies (Hydrophobia)

One of the most feared of human diseases, rabies has the highest case fatality rate of any known human infection, essentially 100%. In the 1970s three cases of presumed rabies recovery were reported. All had received preexposure or postexposure prophylaxis. Since that time, despite the intensive medical care available in the United States, no survivors have been reported. A significant public health problem worldwide with an estimated 30,000 deaths a year, rabies in humans in the United States is a rare event due to the widespread vaccination of dogs begun in the 1950's. Today the major carriers of rabies in the United States are not dogs but wild animals—raccoons, skunks, foxes, and bats. Small rodents, rabbits and hares, and opossums rarely carry rabies. Epidemiological information should be consulted for information on the potential carriers for a given geographic region. The east coast of the United States is presently experiencing an epizootic (epidemic) of raccoon rabies.

Rabies is transmitted to humans by introducing virus-carrying saliva into the body usually via an animal bite or scratch. Transmission may also occur if infected saliva comes into contact with a fresh cut or intact mucus membranes. Rabies is found in neural tissue and is not transmitted via blood, urine, or feces. Airborne transmission has been documented in caves with infected bat colonies. Transmission from human to human is theoretically possible but has not been documented except for 6 cases of rabies acquired by receiving corneal transplants harvested from individuals who died of undiagnosed rabies (Fishbein, et al, 1995). Guidelines for organ donation now exist to prevent this possibility.

The best protection against rabies remains vaccinating domestic animals—dogs, cats, cattle, and horses. If an individual is bitten, the bite wound should be thoroughly cleaned with soap and water and a physician consulted immediately. Suspicion of rabies should exist if the bite is from a wild animal or an unprovoked attack from a domestic animal. Even when there is no suspicion of rabies, a physician should be contacted since tetanus or antibiotic prophylaxis may be indicated.

No successful treatment exists for rabies once symptoms appear, but if given promptly and as directed, postexposure prophylaxis (PEP) with human rabies immune globulin and rabies vaccine can prevent the development of the disease. Three products are licensed for use as rabies vaccine in the United States: human diploid cell vaccine (HDCV), rabies vaccine adsorbed (RVA), and purified chick embryo cell (PCEC) culture (RabAvert™)(CDC, 1998d). The vaccine is administered in a series of five 1-ml doses injected into the deltoid muscle. Reactions to the vaccine are fewer and less serious than with previously used vaccines. Individuals who deal frequently with animals such as zookeepers, lab workers, and veterinarians may choose to receive the vaccine as preexposure prophy-laxis. The decision to administer the vaccine to a bite victim depends on the circumstances of the bite and is made on an individual basis.

Recommendations for providing postexposure prophylaxis treatment are provided by the Advisory Committee for Recommendations on Immunization Practices available through local public health officials or the CDC. In general, cats and dogs that have bitten someone and have verified rabies vaccinations are confined for 10 days for observation. Treatment is initiated only if signs of rabies are observed during this period. If the animal is known to be or suspected to be rabid, treatment begins immediately. If the animal is unknown to the victim and escapes, then public health officials should be consulted for help in deciding whether treatment is indicated. With wild animal bites, treatment is begun immediately. With bites from livestock, rodents, and rabbits, treatment is considered on an individual basis. Decisions to treat become more complicated for possible nonbite exposure to saliva from known infected animals, and again public health officials are helpful in making these treatment decisions (CDC, 1991a).

PARASITIC DISEASES

Parasitic diseases are more prevalent in developing countries than the United States due to tropical climate and inadequate prevention and control measures. A lack of cheap and effective drugs, poor sanitation, and a scarcity of funding lead to high reinfection rates even when control programs are attempted. Parasites are classified into four groups: nematodes (roundworms), cestodes (tapeworms), trematodes (flukes), and protozoa (single celled animals). Nematodes, cestodes, and trematodes are all referred to as helminths. Table 38-5 presents examples of diseases caused by parasites from these groups.

TABLE 38-5 Selected Parasite Categories

CATEGORY	PARASITE AND DISEASE
Intestinal nematodes	*Ascaris lumbricoides* (roundworm) *Trichuris trichiura* (whipworm) *Ancylostoma, Necator* (hookworm) *Enterobius vermicularis* (pinworm)
Blood and tissue nematodes	*Wuchereria bancrofti* (filariasis) *Onchocerca volvulus* (river blindness)
Cestodes	*Taenia solium* (pork tapeworm) *Taenia saginata* (beef tapeworm)
Trematodes	*Schistosoma* species (schistosomiasis)
Protozoans	*Giardia lamblia* (giardiasis) *Entamoeba histolytica* (amebiasis) *Plasmodium* species (malaria) *Leishmania* species (leishmaniasis) *Trypanosoma* species (African sleeping sickness, Chagas' disease) *Toxoplasma gondii* (toxoplasmosis)

Based on data from Brown H, Neva FA: *Basic clinical parasitology*, ed 5, Norwalk, Conn, 1983, Appleton-Century-Crofts.

Nurses and other health professionals should be aware of the increasing detection of parasitic infections in the United States Several factors that have affected these recent developments include increases in each of the following:

- International travel
- Immigration of persons from developing countries
- Incidence of AIDS with secondary parasitic opportunistic infections such as *pneumocystis carinii* pneumonia, cryptosporidiosis, and toxoplasmosis
- Recognition of *Giardia* and *Cryptosporidium* as common infectious agents in day care centers and waterborne disease outbreaks
- Incidence and recognition of sexually transmitted parasitic enteric infections acquired through oral-anal sex
- Recognition of *Cryptosporidium* species as pathogens in immunocompetent individuals due to improvement in stool examination techniques (Kappus et al, 1994)

Intestinal Parasitic Infections

Enterobiasis (pinworm) is the most common helminth infection in the United States with an estimated 42 million cases a year. Pinworm infection is most common among children and most prevalent in crowded and institutional settings. Pinworms resemble small pieces of white thread and can be seen with the naked eye. Diagnosis is usually accomplished through pressing cellophane tape to the perianal region early in the morning. Treatment with oral vermicides results in a cure rate of 90% to 100%.

A study by state diagnostic laboratories found intestinal parasites in 20% of 216,275 stool specimens examined. The most commonly identified parasites were *Giardia lamblia*, *Entamoeba histolytica*, *Trichuris trichiura* (hookworm), and *Ascaris lumbricoides* (roundworm) (Kappus et al, 1994). The opportunities for widespread indigenous transmission of these intestinal parasites are limited because of improved sanitary conditions in this country. Effective drug treatment is available for these intestinal parasitic infections.

Parasitic Opportunistic Infections

Some of the common parasitic opportunistic infections in AIDS and other immunocompromised clients include *Pneumocystis carinii* pneumonia, cryptosporidiosis, microsporidiosis, and isosporiasis. *Pneumocystis carinii* pneumonia (PCP) occurs in 80% of AIDS clients. Airborne transmission is presumed. *P. carinii* is found in the lungs and causes severe pneumonia in immunocompromised clients. It does not cause infection in immunocompetent persons. Effective drugs for treatment and prophylaxis of PCP are available such as trimethoprim-sulfamethoxazole and pentamidine isethionate (Martinez, Suffredini, and Masur, 1992).

Cryptosporidium, *Microsporidium*, and *Isospora belli* are intestinal protozoans transmitted by the fecal-oral route that cause diarrheal disease. The AIDS epidemic has brought about an increased incidence of illness due to these organisms. Up to 15% to 20% of refractory unexplained diarrhea in AIDS clients may be due to microsporidiosis. An estimated 10% to 15% of AIDS clients in this country and as many a 30% to 50% around the world have developed chronic cryptosporidiosis. Infection with *I. belli* among AIDS clients is in the United States is rare (about 1%), but 15% to 20% of Haitian and African clients may be infected. There is currently no consistently effective and FDA approved drug treatment for cryptosporidiosis or microsporidiosis. Trimethoprim-sulfamethoxazole is effective for isosporiasis (DeVita, Hellman, and Rosenberg, 1997).

Control and Prevention of Parasitic Infections

Nurses and other health care workers can make a correct diagnosis and provide appropriate treatment and client education in an effort to prevent and control parasitic infections. Diagnosis of parasitic diseases is based on history of travel, characteristic clinical signs and symptoms, and the use of appropriate laboratory tests to confirm the clinical diagnosis. Knowing what specimens to collect, how and when to collect these specimens, and what laboratory techniques to use are all important in interpreting laboratory results. Effective drug treatment is available for most parasitic diseases. High drug cost and drug resistance and toxicity are some of the common therapeutic problems. Measures for prevention and control of parasitic diseases include early diagnosis and treatment, improved personal hygiene, safer sex practices, community health education, vector control, and improvements in sanitary control of food, water, and waste disposal.

NOSOCOMIAL INFECTIONS

Nosocomial infections are acquired during hospitalization or developed within a hospital setting. They may involve patients, health care workers, visitors, or anyone who has contact with a hospital. Hospitalized patients are more susceptible than healthy persons because of their underlying illnesses, their exposure to virulent infectious agents from other patients, and their exposure to indigenous hospital flora from the hospital staff. Patients have invasive diagnostic and surgical procedures and often are given multiple broad-spectrum antibiotics and immunosuppressive drugs for treatment of neoplastic or chronic diseases. At least 5% of patients admitted to hospitals in the United States develop nosocomial infections, extending the hospital stay by 4 days, directly accounting for 60,000 deaths per year, and adding $10 billion dollars to the national health care expenditure (Mandell, Douglas, and Bennett, 1995). The CDC maintains the National Nosocomial Infection Surveillance (NNIS) system, which is the only source of national data on the epidemiology of nosocomial infections in the United Sates.

Infection control practitioners play a key role in a hospital infection surveillance and control program. Without a qualified and well-trained person in this position, the infection control program is ineffective. Over 95% of infection control practitioners are nurses. Their common job titles are infection control nurse, infection control coordinator and nurse epidemiologist. Nosocomial infections are relevant to the community health nurse in that they are an indicator of the health of one part of the community and as such fall under the surveillance and reportable disease categories.

Universal Precautions

In 1985, in response to concerns regarding the transmission of HIV infection in health care settings, CDC recommended **universal** blood and body fluid precautions. This strategy requires that blood and body fluids from *all* clients be handled as if infected with HIV or other bloodborne pathogens. When in a situation where potential contact with blood or other body fluids exists, health care workers must always wash their hands and wear gloves, masks, protective clothing, and other indicated personal protective barriers. Needles and sharp instruments must be used and disposed of properly. (CDC, 1989). CDC also made recommendations for preventing transmission of HIV and hepatitis B during medical, surgical and dental procedures (CDC, 1991b).

TUBERCULOSIS

Tuberculosis (TB) is a mycobacterial disease caused by *Mycobacterium tuberculosis*. Transmission is usually by exposure to the tubercle bacilli in airborne droplets from persons with pulmonary tuberculosis during talking, coughing, or sneezing. Common symptoms are cough, fever, hemopty-

sis, chest pains, fatigue, and weight loss. The incubation period is 4 to 12 weeks. The most critical period for development of clinical disease is the first 6 to 12 months after infection. About 5% of those initially infected may develop pulmonary tuberculosis or extrapulmonary involvement. The infection in about 95% of those initially infected becomes latent and may be reactivated later in life. Reactivation of latent infections is common in the elderly and the immunocompromised; substance abusers; underweight and undernourished persons; and those with diabetes, silicosis, or gastrectomies (Benenson, 1995).

Resurgence of Tuberculosis

Among adults worldwide, tuberculosis is the leading cause of death from a single infectious agent. It is estimated that if global control of tuberculosis remains at the 1990 level during the next ten years, 30 million people will die from this disease by the year 2000 (Raviglione, Snider, Kochi, 1994). The incidence of tuberculosis in the United States showed a steady decline during the 1970s and early 1980s but began to increase again in 1989. This increase is believed to have been due to the growing incidence of tuberculosis among people with AIDS, the homeless, substance abusers, the elderly, immigrants, people in nursing homes and correctional facilities, and the development of multidrug resistance. During outbreaks due to multidrug-resistant *Mycobacterium tuberculosis*, clients have exhibited mortality rates from 43% to as high as 89% (CDC, 1994i). Since the peak of the resurgence in 1992, total reported tu-

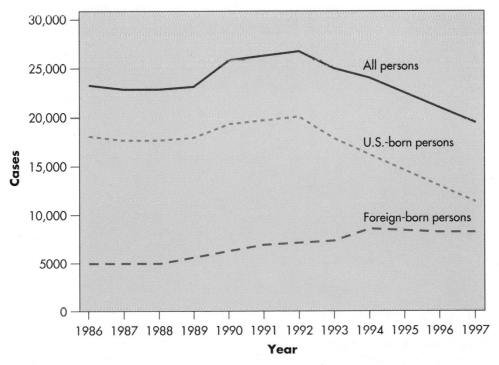

FIG. 38-3 Number of persons with reported cases of tuberculosis, by country of birth—United States, 1986-1997. (From Centers for Disease Control and Prevention: Tuberculosis morbidity—United States, 1997, *MMWR* 47(13):254, 1998.)

berculosis cases in the United States have been falling, although cases in foreign-born persons have continued to increase, as seen in Fig. 38-3. This overall decline has been attributed to improved prevention and control programs at the state and local level as a result of increased federal funding to states beginning in the early 1990s (CDC, 1997g). A national goal has been established for elimination of tuberculosis (less than 1 case per 1 million population) by the year 2010. The key to meeting this goal will be continued funding for prevention and control; the problems that caused the resurgence of cases at the beginning of the decade have not gone away.

Diagnosis and Treatment

TB screening tests used are skin testing with Purified Protein Derivative (sometimes referred to as "putting on a PPD") and chest radiographs for positive skin reactors with pulmonary symptoms. False negative skin test reactions due to anergy may occur in persons who are immunosuppressed by drugs or who have diseases such as advanced tuberculosis, AIDS, and measles. Confirmatory tests include stained sputum smears and other body fluids with demonstration of the acid-fast bacilli (for presumptive diagnosis) and culture of the tubercle bacilli for definitive diagnosis. How to apply and read a PPD test is described below.

HOW TO *Apply and Read a PPD test*

Since nurses usually "put on" the PPD, they need to know the correct procedure for administering this tuberculin skin test and how to interpret the test results.
Applying the PPD test
- *Use intradermal Mantoux test with 0.1 ml of 5 TU PPD tuberculin*
- *Read reaction 48 to 72 hours after injection*
- *Measure only induration*
- *Record results in millimeters*

Reading the PPD test
  Test is positive if greater than or equal to 5 mm in:
- *Persons known or suspected to have HIV infection*
- *Persons who have a chest radiograph suggestive of previous TB*
- *Close contacts of a person with infectious TB*
  Test is positive if greater than or equal to 10 mm in:
- *Persons with certain medical conditions, excluding HIV*
- *Persons who inject drugs (if HIV negative)*
- *Foreign-born persons from areas where TB is common*
- *Medically underserved, low-income populations*
- *Residents of long-term care facilities*
- *Children younger than 4 years of age*
  Test is positive if greater than or equal to 15 mm in:
- *All persons with no risk factors for TB*

From Centers for Disease Control and Prevention: *Screening for TB disease and infection, core curriculum on tuberculosis,* ed 3, Atlanta, 1994, CDC.

Clients with tuberculosis should be treated promptly with the appropriate multiple combination of antimicrobial drugs. Effective drug regimens currently used in the United States include isoniazid (INH) combined with rifampin (RIF), with or without pyrazinamide (PZA) for at least six months. Treatment failure is largely due to poor compliance to long term treatment with resulting development of drug resistance (Benenson, 1995). Community health nurses usually perform tuberculin skin tests and provide client education on the importance of compliance to long-term therapy. They may also be involved in directly observed therapy (DOT), urine testing to check compliance, and contact investigation of cases in the community.

VIRAL HEPATITIS

Viral hepatitis refers to a group of infections that primarily affect the liver. These infections have similar clinical presentations but different causes and characteristics. Brief profiles of these infections are presented in Table 38-6. Hepatitis B is discussed more fully in Chapter 39.

Hepatitis A

The clinical course of hepatitis A ranges from mild to severe and often requires prolonged convalescence. Onset is usually acute with fever, nausea, lack of appetite, malaise and abdominal discomfort followed in several days by jaundice. Hepatitis A is transmitted from person to person via the fecal-oral route. The virus level in the feces appears to peak one to two weeks before symptoms appear, making individuals highly contagious before they realize they are ill.

Hepatitis A is found worldwide. In developing countries where sanitation is inadequate, epidemics are not common because most adults are immune from childhood infection. In countries with improved sanitation, outbreaks are common in daycare centers that enroll children in diapers, among household and sexual contacts of infected individuals and among travelers to countries where hepatitis A is endemic. In the United States cases are most common among school children and young adults. In many outbreaks an individual is the source of an infection that may become community-wide. In other cases, hepatitis A is spread through food contaminated by an infected food-handler, contaminated produce or contaminated water. The source of infection may never be identified in as many as 25% of outbreaks.

Appropriate sanitation and personal hygiene remain the best means of preventing infection. A vaccine for hepatitis A is available and is recommended for those who travel frequently or for long periods to countries where the disease is endemic. In cases of exposure through close contact with an infected individual or contaminated food or water, an injection of prophylactic immune globulin (IG) is indicated. IG should be given as soon as possible, but within 2 weeks of exposure. (Benenson, 1995).

TABLE 38-6 Viral Hepatitis Profiles

	HEPATITIS A	HEPATITIS B	HEPATITIS C	HEPATITIS D	HEPATITIS E	HEPATITIS G
Incubation period	Average 30 days, range 15-50 days	Average 75 days, range 40-120 days	Average 45 days, range 14-175 days	Average 28 days, range 14-43 days.	Average 40 days, range 15-60 days	Unknown
Mode of transmission	Fecal-oral, waterborne, sexual	Bloodborne, sexual, perinatal	Primarily bloodborne; also sexual and perinatal	Superinfection or co-infection of Hepatitis B case	Fecal-oral	Bloodborne; may facilitate other strains of viral hepatitis to progress more rapidly
Incidence	125,00-200,000 cases/yr in the U.S.	140,000-320,000 cases/yr in the U.S.	28,000-180,000 cases/yr in the U.S.	7500 cases/yr in the U.S.	Low in the U.S., epidemic outbreaks worldwide	0.3% of all acute viral hepatitis
Chronic carrier state?	No	Yes, 0.1%-15% of cases	Yes, 85% or more of cases	Yes, 70%-80% of cases	No	Yes, 90%-100% of cases
Diagnosis	Serological tests (anti-HAV), viral isolation	Serological tests (HBsAg), viral isolation	Serological tests (anti-HCV)	Serological tests (anti-HDV), liver biopsy	Serological tests (anti-HEV)	None currently
Sequelae	No chronic infection	Chronic liver disease; liver cancer	Chronic liver disease; liver cancer	Chronic liver disease; liver cancer.	No chronic infection	Rare or may not occur
Vaccine availability	Yes, vaccination of preschool children recommended; travelers to endemic regions	Yes, vaccination of infants recommended; Individuals with expo sure risks	No	No	No	No
Control and prevention	Personal hygiene; proper sanitation	Preexposure vaccination; reduce exposure risk behaviors	Screening of blood/organ donors; reduce exposure risk behaviors	Preexposure or postexposure prophylaxis for HBV	Protection of water systems from fecal contamination	Unknown

clinical application

One of the biggest problems with tuberculosis prevention and control programs is the required lengthy therapy using multiple drug combinations. Failure to comply with therapy over the entire treatment period may result in treatment failure and the development of drug resistance. The South Carolina Department of Health and Environmental Control, Tuberculosis Control Division developed an innovative program in collaboration with the American Lung Association, South Carolina Chapter to provide incentives to clients to adhere to their treatment regimens (Pozsik, 1995). Incentives are monetary or nonmonetary, but are tailored to the wishes of the individual client. Examples of incentives include food, clothing, fish bait, and books.

Tuberculosis control nurses personally administer each dose of treatment drugs to the client, and upon completion of an agreed upon number of treatments, present the client with an incentive item. Each nurse has a regular caseload of clients with whom she meets as the treatment schedule demands. Meetings may be at home or at designated meeting places, such as parking lots, fishing holes, or fast-food restaurants. The incentive program has been so successful in increasing treatment compliance that several other states have replicated this innovative approach. In addition to direct observation of drug therapy, these nurses also aggressively conduct contact investigation of their clients. This investigation may actually involve observing the

Continued

clinical application—cont'd

client's daily activities to identify possible contacts. The vigorous efforts of these community health nurses assigned to the tuberculosis control unit have paid off in the steady decline of tuberculosis cases in South Carolina over the past 10 years.

A. Which of the following would be the first step in developing a directly observed theory (DOT) program?
   1. Develop a proposal to present to potential funding organizations.
   2. Interview clients to determine the best time and place for DOT.
   3. Survey clients for incentive preferences.
   4. Determine whether a DOT program is needed.
B. When developing a proposal to start a DOT program with incentives, what sourt of communicable disease information, aside from need, might be useful to include?
C. When purchasing incentives, the best plan would be to:
   1. Select several items and buy in bulk to cut down on cost.
   2. Ask successful programs in other areas what incentives have worked best for them.
   3. Personally interview clients to determine potential incentives.
   4. Let the funding agency choose the incentives.
D. Why would onsite contact investigation be an important part of a tuberculosis control program?

Answers are in back of book.

KEY POINTS

- The burden of infectious diseases is high in both human and economic terms. Preventing these diseases must be given high priority in our present health care system.
- The successful interaction of the infectious agent, host and environment is necessary for disease transmission. Knowledge of the characteristics of each of these three factors is important in understanding the transmission, prevention, and control of these diseases.
- Effective intervention measures at the individual and community levels must be aimed at breaking the chain linking the agent, host, and environment. An integrated approach attacking all three factors simultaneously is an ideal goal to strive for but may not be feasible for all diseases.
- Health care professionals must constantly be aware of vulnerability to threats posed by emerging infectious diseases. Most of the factors causing the emergence of these diseases are influenced by human activities and behavior.
- Communicable diseases are preventable. Preventing infection through primary prevention activities is the most cost-effective public health strategy.
- Health care professionals must always apply infection control principles and procedures in the work environment. They should strictly practice the universal blood and body fluid precautions strategy to prevent transmission of HIV and other bloodborne pathogens.

- Effective control of communicable diseases requires the use of a multisystem approach focusing on improving host resistance, improving safety of the environment, improving public health systems, and facilitating social and political changes to ensure health for all people.
- Communicable disease prevention and control programs must move beyond providing drug treatment and vaccines. Health promotion and education aimed at changing human behavior must be emphasized.
- Nurses play a key role in all aspects of prevention and control of communicable diseases. Close cooperation with other members of the interdisciplinary health care team must be maintained. Mobilizing community participation is essential to successful implementation of programs.
- The successful global eradication of smallpox proved the feasibility of eradication of communicable diseases. As professionals and concerned citizens of the global village, health care workers must support the current global eradication campaigns against poliomyelitis and dracunculiasis.

critical thinking activities

1. Ride with a nurse who makes home visits. Discuss living situations and other risk factors that may contribute to the development of infectious diseases, as well as possible points where the nurse may intervene to help prevent these diseases, such as checking the immunization status of all individuals in the household.
2. Spend time with the persons who are responsible for reporting communicable disease for your county or city. To become familiar with the reportable diseases that are a problem in the area, look at how many cases have been reported during the past month, 6 months, and year. Contrast these numbers with national statistics. Discuss outbreak procedures that may accompany the reporting of some of these diseases. If possible, go on an outbreak investigation.
3. Accompany a TB outreach nurse to observe case investigation, contact tracing, and directly observed therapy.
4. Visit a clinic that serves a refugee, immigrant, or migrant labor population to observe the infectious diseases commonly seen in these groups. Compare and contrast this visit with a visit to a clinic that serves an inner-city population and a visit to a clinic that serves a rural population.
5. Sit in a clinic waiting room for immunization services and talk with parents about the concerns they may have and the barriers they may perceive in obtaining immunizations for their children.
6. Spend time with a school nurse to see what infectious diseases are routinely encountered in the educational setting. Discuss risk factors for disease in school-age youth and the strategies employed to prevent infectious diseases in this age group.
7. Visit a day care center. Observe potential situations for the communication of infectious diseases and discuss with the director the steps taken to prevent and control infection, including immunization requirements and procedures for hand washing and food preparation.

Bibliography

Bates AS et al: Risk factors for underimmunization in poor urban infants, *JAMA* 272(4):1105, 1994.

Benenson AS, editor: Control of communicable diseases manual, ed 16, Washington DC, 1995, American Public Health Association.

Centers for Disease Control and Prevention: Guidelines for prevention of transmission of HIV and Hepatitis B virus to health care and public safety workers, *MMWR* 38 (S-6):1, 1989.

Centers for Disease Control and Prevention: Rabies prevention-United States: Recommendations of the Immunization Practices Advisory Committee, *MMWR* 40(RR-3), 1991a.

Centers for Disease Control and Prevention: Recommendations for preventing transmission of HIV and Hepatitis B virus to patients during exposure-prone invasive procedures, *MMWR* 40 (RR-8):1, 1991b.

Centers for Disease Control and Prevention: Update: International Task Force for Disease Eradication 1990 and 1991, *MMWR* 41(3):40, 1992a.

Centers for Disease Control and Prevention: Eradication of paralytic poliomyelitis in the Americas, *MMWR* 41(36):681, 1992b.

Centers for Disease Control and Prevention: Public health focus: surveillance, prevention and control of nosocomial infections, *MMWR* 41(42):783, 1992c.

Centers for Disease Control and Prevention: Tuberculosis control laws, 1993: Recommendations of the Advisory Council for the Elimination of Tuberculosis, *MMWR* 42 (RR-15):1, 1993a.

Centers for Disease Control and Prevention: Recommendations of the International Task Force for Disease Eradication, *MMWR* 42 (RR-16):1, 1993b.

Centers for Disease Control and Prevention: Addressing emerging infectious disease threats: a prevention strategy for the U.S., Atlanta, 1994a, CDC.

Centers for Disease Control and Prevention: National notifiable disease reporting, 1994, *MMWR* 43(43):800, 1994b.

Centers for Disease Control and Prevention: Laboratory management of agent associated with hantavirus pulmonary syndrome: interim biosafety guidelines, *MMWR* 43 (RR-7):1, 1994c.

Centers for Disease Control and Prevention: Certification of poliomyelitis eradication—the Americas, 1994, *MMWR* 43(39):720, 1994d.

Centers for Disease Control and Prevention: Rubella and congenital rubella syndrome—United States, January 1, 1991-May 7, 1994, *MMWR* 43(21):391, 1994e.

Centers for Disease Control and Prevention: *Escherichia coli* 0157:H7 outbreak linked to home-cooked hamburger—California, July 1993, *MMWR* 43(12):214, 1994f.

Centers for Disease Control and Prevention: Expanded tuberculosis surveillance and tuberculosis morbidity - U.S., 1993, MMWR 43(20):361, 1994g.

Centers for Disease Control and Prevention: Guidelines for preventing the transmission of *Mycobacterium tuberculosis* in health care facilities, 1994, *MMWR* 43(RR-13):1, 1994h.

Centers for Disease Control and Prevention: *Screening for TB disease and infection: core curriculum on tuberculosis,* ed 3, Atlanta, 1994I, CDC.

Centers for Disease Control and Prevention: Pertussis-United States, 1992-1995, *MMWR* 44(28):525, 1995a.

Centers for Disease Control and Prevention: Outbreaks of *Cyclospora cayenensis* infection-United States, 1996, *MMWR* 54(25):549, 1996a.

Centers for Disease Control and Prevention: Notifiable disease surveillance and notifiable disease statistics-United States, June 1946 and June 1996, *MMWR* 45(25):530, 1996b.

Centers for Disease Control and Prevention: Status report on the Childhood Immunization Initiative: national, state, and urban area vaccination coverage levels among children aged 19-35 months-United States, 1996, *MMWR* 46(29):657, 1997a.

Centers for Disease Control and Prevention: Progress toward global measles control and elimination, 1990-1996, *MMWR* 46(38):893, 1997b.

Centers for Disease Control and Prevention: Measles-United States, 1996 and the interruption of indigenous transmission, *MMWR* 46(11):242, 1997c

Centers for Disease Control and Prevention: Rubella and congenital rubella syndrome-United States, 1994-1997, *MMWR* 46(16):350, 1997d.

Centers for Disease Control and Prevention: Pertussis outbreak-Vermont, 1996, *MMWR* 46(35):822, 1997e.

Centers for Disease Control and Prevention: Lyme disease-United States, 1996, *MMWR* 46(23):531, 1997f.

Centers for Disease Control and Prevention: Tuberculosis morbidity-United States, 1996, *MMWR* 46(30):695, 1997g.

Centers for Disease Control and Prevention: Measles-United States, 1997, *MMWR* 47(14):273, 1998a.

Centers for Disease Control and Prevention: Provisional cases of selected notifiable diseases, United States, weeks ending January 3, 1998, and December 28, 1996 (53rd Week), *MMWR* 46(52 and53):1269, 1998b.

Centers for Disease Control and Prevention: Update: isolation of avian influenza A(H5N1) viruses from humans-Hong Kong, 1997-1998, *MMWR* 46(52 and53):1245, 1998c.

Centers for Disease Control and Prevention: Availability of new rabies vaccine for human use, *MMWR* 47(1):12, 1998d.

Dennis DT, Fikrig E, Schaffner W: Now you can prevent Lyme disease, *Patient Care for the Nurse Practitioner* 2(6):20, 1999.

DeVita VT, Hellman S, Rosenberg SA, editors: *AIDS: etiology, diagnosis, treatment and prevention,* ed 4, Philadelphia, 1997, Lippincott-Raven.

Evans AS: The Eradication of communicable diseases: myth or reality? *Am J Epidemiol* 122 (2):199, 1985.

Fishbein DB, Bernard KW: Rabies virus. In Mandell GL, Bennett JE, Douglas R, editors: *Principles and practice of infectious diseases,* ed 4, New York, 1995, Churchill Livingstone.

Hopkins DR et al: Dracunculiasis eradication: March 1994 Update, *Am J Trop Med Hyg* 52(1):14, 1995.

Kappus KD et al: Intestinal parasitism in the U.S.: update on a continuing problem, *Am J Trop Med Hyg* 50(6):705, 1994.

Krogstad DJ: Malaria. In Mandell GL, Bennett JE, Douglas R, editors: *Principles and practice of infectious diseases,* ed 4, New York, 1995, Churchill Livingstone.

Last JM, editor: *A dictionary of epidemiology,* New York, 1983, Oxford University Press.

Mandell GL, Bennett JE, Douglas R, editors: *Principles and practice of infectious diseases,* ed 4, New York, 1995, Churchill Livingstone.

Martinez A, Suffredini AF, Masur H: *Pneumocystis carinii* disease in HIV-infected persons. In Wormser GP, editor: *AIDS and other manifestations of HIV infection,* ed 2, New York, 1992, Raven Press.

Marwick C: Acellular pertussis vaccine is licensed for infants, *JAMA* 276(7):516, 1996.

McGinnis JM, Foege WH: Actual causes of death in the U.S., *JAMA* 270(18):2207, 1993.

National Center for Health Statistics: Births and deaths: United States, 1995. *Monthly Vital Statistics Report* 45(3)supp 2:21, 1996.

Pozsik C: Personal communication, 1995.

Raviglione MC, Snider DE Jr, Kochi A: Global epidemiology of tuberculosis: morbidity and mortality of a worldwide epidemic, *JAMA* 273(3):220, 1994.

Continued

Bibliography—cont'd

Steere AC: *Borrelia burdorferi.* In Mandell GL, Bennett JE, Douglas R, editors: *Principles and practice of infectious diseases,* ed 4, New York, 1995, Churchill Livingstone.

Stephenson J: Public health experts take aim at a moving target: foodborne infections, *JAMA* 277 (2):97, 1997

Walker, DH, Raoult, D: *Rickettsia rickettsii* and other spotted fever group rickettsiae. In Mandell GL, Bennett JE, Douglas R, editors: *Principles and practice of infectious diseases,* ed 4, New York, 1995, Churchill Livingstone.

Wenzel RP: Control of communicable diseases: overview. In Last JM, Wallace RB, editors: *Public health and preventive medicine,* ed 13, Norwalk, 1992, Appleton & Lange.

Wood D: Reducing missed opportunities to vaccinate during child health visits: how effective are parent education and case management, *Arch Pediatr Adolesc Med* 152(3):238, 1998.

Human Immunodeficiency Virus, Hepatitis B Virus, and Sexually Transmitted Diseases

PATTY J. HALE

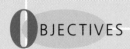

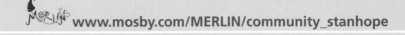

OBJECTIVES

After reading this chapter, the student should be able to do the following:

- Describe the natural history of human immunodeficiency virus (HIV) infection and appropriate client education at each stage.
- Explain the clinical signs of the major sexually transmitted diseases.
- Evaluate the trends in incidence of the major sexually transmitted diseases and groups that are at greatest risk.

- Analyze behaviors that place people at risk of contracting sexually transmitted diseases (STDs).
- Evaluate nursing activities to prevent and control STDs.
- Explain the various roles of nurses in providing care for those with chronic STDs.

KEY TERMS

acquired
  immunodeficiency
  syndrome (AIDS)
chancroid
chlamydia
genital herpes
genital warts
gonorrhea

hepatitis B virus (HBV)
HIV antibody test
HIV infection
human immunodeficiency
  virus (HIV)
human papillomavirus
  (HPV)
incubation period

injection drug use
nongonococcal urethritis
  (NGU)
nonoxynol-9
partner notification
pelvic inflammatory
  disease (PID)

sexually transmitted
  diseases (STDs)
syphilis
trichomoniasis

See Glossary for definitions

CHAPTER OUTLINE

Human Immunodeficiency Virus
Infection
  Pathogenesis
  Natural History of HIV
  Transmission
  Distribution and Trends
  HIV Testing
  Perinatal/Pediatric HIV
    Infection
  AIDS in the Community

Resources
Other Sexually Transmitted
  Diseases
    Trichomoniasis
    Gonorrhea
    Syphilis
    Chlamydia
    Chancroid
    Hepatitis B Virus

Herpes Simplex Virus 2 (Genital
  Herpes)
  Human Papillomavirus
  Infection
Nurse's Role in Preventing STDs
  and Providing Related Services
    Primary Prevention
    Secondary Prevention
    Tertiary Prevention

The study of **sexually transmitted diseases (STDs)** has changed dramatically in recent years. For several decades following the development of antibiotics in the 1940s, STDs were considered to be a problem of the past. Recently, the emergence of new viral STDs and antibiotic-resistant strains of bacterial STDs have posed new challenges. Left unchecked, STDs can cause poor pregnancy outcomes, infertility, and cervical cancers. There is also the problem of coinfection with one STD increasing the susceptibility to other STDs, such as human immunodeficiency virus (HIV).

This concern about STDs has prompted the development of standards for STDs and HIV in *Healthy People 2000–Midcourse Review* (USDHHS, 1996). Box 39-1 gives some of the goals used to evaluate progress toward diminishing STDs as a health threat and providing related services by the year 2000.

Nearly all STDs are acquired through behaviors that can be avoided or changed, and thus intervention efforts by nurses have focused on disease prevention. This is challenging because the population at risk for acquiring STDs has grown, as has the number of people who are living with chronic STD infection and are able to transmit it to others (CDC, 1997a). Thus there is an urgency to develop effective methods to prevent and control STDs, such as through counseling clients on how to make their behavior more healthy.

This chapter describes several STDs and their nursing management. It concludes with implications for community health nursing care for primary, secondary, and tertiary prevention.

HUMAN IMMUNODEFICIENCY VIRUS INFECTION

Human immunodeficiency virus (HIV) infection and **acquired immunodeficiency syndrome (AIDS)** have had an enormous political and social impact on society. Numerous controversies have arisen over many aspects of HIV. The public's fears about HIV have affected many issues and are magnified by the fact that this disease has commonly afflicted two groups that have been largely scorned by society: homosexuals and injection drug users. Debates have arisen over how to control disease transmission and how to pay for related health services. An ongoing debate involves whether clean needles should be distributed to prevent the spread of HIV.

Economic costs are growing since HIV causes premature disability and death. The fact that 88% of afflicted persons are between the ages of 20 and 49 years results in disrupted families and lost creative and economic productivity at a period of life when vitality is the norm. The health care delivery costs of this group are supported largely by Medicaid rather than private insurance or Medicare (Schur and Berk, 1994). This is because many people with HIV are either indigent or fall into poverty when paying for health care over the course of the illness. It is estimated that the total lifetime health care costs for an individual with HIV infection are $119,274 (Hellinger, 1993). HIV/AIDS costs in the United States are estimated to be 5 billion dollars (IOM, 1997).

The Ryan White Comprehensive AIDS Resource Emergency (CARE) Act was passed to provide services for persons with HIV infection in 1990 (CDC, 1997e). This program continues to provide funds for health care in

---

BOX 39-1 Selected *Healthy People 2000* Midcourse Review Objectives Pertaining to Sexually Transmitted Diseases

INFECTION RATES

1. Reduce gonorrhea to an incidence of no more than 100 cases per 100,000 people. (201.6 per 100,000 population in 1992)
2. Reduce *Chlamydia trachomatis* infections among young women under 25 years to no more than 5%. (8.5% in women 20 to 24 and 12.2% in females 19 and younger in 1988)
3. Reduce primary and secondary syphilis to an incidence of no more than 4 cases per 100,000 people. (13.7 per 100,000 population in 1992)
4. Reduce congenital syphilis to an incidence of no more than 40 cases per 100,000 live births. (94.7 per 100,000 population in 1992)
5. Reduce sexually transmitted hepatitis B infection to no more than 30,500 cases. (47,593 cases in 1987)

RISK REDUCTION OBJECTIVES

1. Reduce the proportion of adolescents who have engaged in sexual intercourse to no more than 15% by 15 years of age and no more than 40% by 17 years of age. (Baseline: 27% of females and 33% of males by age 15; 50% of females and 60% of males by age 17 in 1988)
2. Increase to at least 50% the proportion of sexually active, unmarried people who used a condom at last sexual intercourse. (Baseline: 19% unmarried women aged 15 to 44 in 1988)

SERVICE OBJECTIVES

1. Increase to at least 95% schools that provide appropriate instruction in STD transmission prevention in the curricula of all middle and secondary schools, preferably as part of quality school health education. (Interestingly, 95% reported offering at least one class on STD as part of their curricula in 1988)
2. Increase to at least 90% the proportion of primary care providers treating clients with STDs who correctly manage cases, as measured by their use of appropriate types and amounts of therapy. (70% in 1988)

From USDHHS: *Healthy people 2000: midcourse review and 1995 revisions*, Washington, DC, 1996, USDHHS, Public Health Service.

geographical areas with the largest number of AIDS cases. Health services that are covered include emergency services, services for early intervention and care (sometimes including coverage of health insurance), and drug reimbursement programs for HIV-infected individuals.

Pathogenesis

HIV infection is caused by a retrovirus, the human immunodeficiency virus, which was discovered in 1983. Retroviruses produce an enzyme called reverse transcriptase that transcribes the viral genome onto the DNA of the host cell. This results in viral replication by the infected cell. HIV results in immunological deficiencies that leave the host susceptible to opportunistic infections and cancers.

HIV infects mostly lymphoid cells and may remain clinically latent for several months or years, so the person is seemingly well and symptom free. During this symptom-free period the virus continues to replicate in lymphoid tissue.

HIV infects many cells, including the dendritic cells, endothelial cells, Langerhans' cells, lymphocytes, monocytes, and macrophages. The greatest damage is from the infection of the CD4+ T-lymphocyte, the cell that induces nearly every immune response. The progressive decline in numbers of CD4+ T-lymphocytes causes disruptions in immune functioning. Thus HIV adversely affects antibody production and decreases intracellular killing of pathogens following phagocytosis.

Two tests used to track the progress of the infection are the viral load and the CD4+ T-lymphocyte counts (Vlahov et al, 1998). The viral load reflects the level of HIV particles circulating in the blood; as the amount of the virus increases, the number of protective CD4+ T-lymphocytes cells declines. This is depicted in Figure 39-1. The greater the viral load, the more able the person is to transmit the virus and the shorter is the survival time. Antiviral therapy is begun when the CD4 count falls to 500/ml. Therapy may include the common AIDS drugs AZT and 3TC, as well as protease inhibitors, like indinavir, which blocks viral reproduction.

Natural History of HIV

The natural history of HIV is described in Figure 39-1. It includes three stages: the primary infection around 1 month after contracting the virus, a period of time where the body shows no symptoms, called clinical latency, and a final stage of symptomatic disease (Panteleo et al, 1997).

On entering the body, HIV may cause a flu-like syndrome referred to as a primary infection or acute retroviral syndrome. This may go unrecognized. As depicted in Figure 39-1, the body's CD4+ white blood cell count drops for a brief time when the virus is most plentiful in the body. The immune system increases antibody production in response to this initial infection, which is a self-limiting illness. The symptoms are lymphadenopathy, myalgias, sore throat, lethargy, rash, and fever (Pantaleo et al, 1997). Even if the client seeks medical care, at this time the antibody test is usually negative, so it is often not recognized as HIV.

After a variable period of time, commonly from 6 weeks to 3 months, HIV antibodies appear in the blood. Although most antibodies serve a protective role, HIV antibodies do not. However, their presence helps in the detection of HIV infection because tests show their presence in the bloodstream.

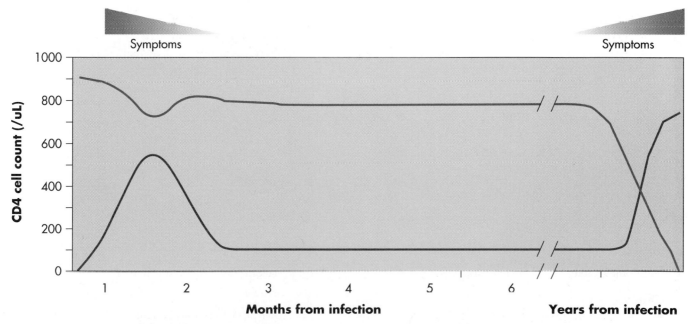

FIG. 39-1 Natural history of HIV disease demonstrating high viral load with low CD4+ levels and symptomatic illness. (From American College of Physicians. Medical Knowledge Self-Assessment Program 10 [MKSAP 10]. Part A, Book 1, HIV Diseases, p. 6, 1994.)

For 80% to 90% of HIV-infected persons, the median survival time is 10 years (Panteleo et al, 1997). During this prolonged **incubation period,** clients have a gradual deterioration of the immune system and can transmit the virus to others.

AIDS is the last stage on the long continuum of HIV infection and may result from damage caused by HIV, secondary cancers, or opportunistic organisms. AIDS is defined as a disabling or life-threatening illness caused by HIV or a CD4+ T-lymphocyte count of less than 200/ml with documented HIV infection.

Many of the AIDS-related opportunistic infections are caused by microorganisms that are commonly present in healthy individuals but do not cause disease in persons with an intact immune system. These microorganisms proliferate in persons with HIV infection because of a weakened immune system.

Opportunistic infections may be caused by bacteria, fungi, viruses, or protozoa. The most common opportunistic diseases are *Pneumocystis carinii* pneumonia and oral candidiasis. On January 1, 1993, an expanded case definition for AIDS was implemented to include pulmonary tuberculosis, invasive cervical cancer, or recurrent pneumonia (CDC, 1992c). Table 39-1 describes diseases commonly associated with AIDS and their clinical symptoms.

Tuberculosis, an infection that is becoming more prevalent because of HIV infection, can spread rapidly among immunosuppressed individuals. Thus HIV-infected individuals who reside in close proximity to one another such as in long-term care facilities, prisons, drug treatment facilities, or other settings must be carefully screened and deemed noninfectious before admission to such settings. For more in-depth coverage of tuberculosis, see Chapter 38.

Transmission

HIV transmission occurs through exposure to blood, semen, vaginal secretions, and breast milk (Levy, 1998). HIV is not transmitted through casual contact; thus it is safe to touch or hug someone or shake hands with someone who has HIV infection. HIV is also not transmitted by insects, coughing, sneezing, office equipment, or sitting next to or eating with someone who has HIV infection. Except for

TABLE 39-1 Clinical Manifestations of AIDS

DISEASE	CLINICAL SIGNS
INFECTIONS	
Varicella zoster (shingles)	Rash, pain
Isosporiasis, chronic interstitial (1 mo)	Diarrhea
Coccidiodomycosis	Fever, fatigue, shortness of breath
Histoplasmosis	Fever, chest pain, dyspnea
Recurrent salmonella septicemia	Fever, vasogenic shock
Candidiasis (respiratory or esophageal)	White patches on tongue, difficulty eating
Cryptococcal meningitis	Fever, headache, stiff neck
Pneumocystis carinii pneumonia or recurrent bacterial pneumonia	Shortness of breath, dry cough, fever, fatigue
Toxoplasmosis of brain	Hemiparesis, seizures, aphasia
Cryptosporidium enteritis infection (1 mo)	Diarrhea, weakness
Mycobacterium tuberculosis infection (pulmonary or extrapulmonary)	Productive, purulent cough; fatigue, weight loss
Mycobacterium avium complex or other mycobacterium	Septicemia, diarrhea
Cytomegalovirus retinitis or CMV disease	Visual blurring
Herpes simplex virus infection	Chronic vesicles (1 mo), bronchitis
Pulmonary tuberculosis	Hemoptysis, night sweats
CANCERS	
Invasive cervical cancer	Cervical dysplasia
Kaposi's sarcoma	Purple skin lesions, localized edema
Lymphoma (Burkitt's or primary of brain)	Weight loss, fever, night sweats
SYNDROMES	
Wasting syndrome caused by HIV	Diarrhea, decreased appetite
HIV-related encephalopathy	Decline in cognition, behavior, or coordination
Progressive multifocal leukoencephalopathy	

those persons who had blood or other body fluid exposure or sexual or needle-sharing contact with an infected person, no one has developed infection (CDC, 1994c). The modes of transmission are listed in Box 39-2. The exposure categories of AIDS are shown in Fig. 39-2.

Potential donors of blood and tissues are screened through interviews and the HIV antibody test to assess for a history of high-risk activities. Blood or tissue is not used from individuals who have a history of high-risk behavior or who are HIV seropositive (antibodies to HIV present in the serum). In addition to screening, coagulation factors used to treat hemophilia and other blood disorders are made safe through heat treatments to inactivate the virus. Such screening has significantly reduced the risk of transmission of HIV by blood products and organ donations. It is estimated that the odds of contracting HIV infection through receiving a blood transfusion are 1 in 450,000 units of blood transfused (Levy, 1998).

When a client is infected with STDs like chlamydia or gonorrhea, the risk of HIV infection increases, and HIV may also increase risk for other STDs. This may result from any of the following: open lesions providing entry of pathogens, such as with syphilis; STDs decreasing host immune status and hastening the progression of HIV infection; and HIV changing the natural history of STDs or the effectiveness of medications used in treating STDs (IOM, 1997).

The nurse serves as an educator about the modes of transmission, as well as a role model for how to behave toward and provide supportive care for those with HIV in-

---

BOX 39-2 Modes of HIV Transmission

HIV can be transmitted in the following ways:
1. Sexual contact, involving the exchange of body fluids, with an infected person.
2. Sharing or reusing needles, syringes, or other equipment used to prepare injectable drugs.
3. Perinatal transmission from an infected mother to her fetus during pregnancy or delivery, or to an infant when breast-feeding.
4. Transfusions or other exposure to HIV-contaminated blood or blood products, organs, or semen.

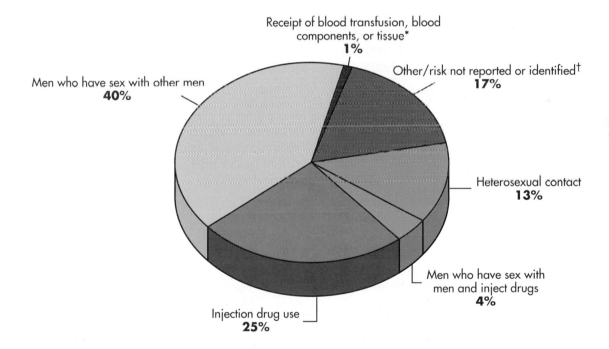

Receipt of blood transfusion, blood components, or tissue*
1%

Other/risk not reported or identified†
17%

Men who have sex with other men
40%

Heterosexual contact
13%

Men who have sex with men and inject drugs
4%

Injection drug use
25%

*Thirty-six adults/adolescents and three children developed AIDS after receiving blood screened negative for HIV antibody. Twelve additional adults developed AIDS after receiving tissue, organs, or artificial insemination from HIV-infected donors. Four of the 12 received tissue, organs, or artificial insemination from a donor who was negative for HIV antibody at the time of donation.

†"Other" includes 49 persons who acquired HIV infection but were diagnosed with AIDS after age 13. These 49 persons are tabulated under the adult/adolescent, not pediatric, exposure category. Incomplete investigation (died, lost to follow-up, or declined interview), transmission mode not identified or still under investigation.

FIG. 39-2 Adult/adolescent AIDS cases by exposure category; 1996, United States. (Data from Centers for Disease Control and Prevention: *HIV/AIDS Surveillance Report* 8(2):10, 1996.)

fection. An understanding of how transmission does and does not occur will help family and community members feel more comfortable in relating to and caring for persons with HIV (see Box 39-2).

Distribution and Trends

Nurses must identify the trends of HIV infection in the populations they serve, so they can screen clients who may be at risk and so they can adequately plan prevention programs and illness care resources. For example, knowing that AIDS disproportionately affects minorities assists the nurse in setting priorities and planning services to these groups. Factors such as geographical location, age, and racial distribution are tracked to more effectively target programs and are discussed below.

The first reported cases of what was later to be known as AIDS occurred in five homosexual men in Los Angeles in 1981. As of June 1997, the total number of cases in the United States is 591,775 (CDC, 1997e). Initially the groups with the highest incidence of HIV infection were homosexual and bisexual males, injection drug users and their sexual partners, and hemophiliacs (CDC, 1989). Although homosexual men still make up the largest group infected with HIV in the United States, the number of women contracting HIV through heterosexual transmission is increasing at a faster rate.

It is estimated that between 600,000 and 900,000 people are infected with HIV in the United States and 13 million people are infected worldwide (CDC, 1997d; World Health Organization, 1993). HIV infection is the third leading cause of death among women 25 to 44 years old in the United States (CDC, 1997c). As of June 1997, 62% of all persons reported to have AIDS in the United States had died (CDC, 1997d). Table 39-2 shows how AIDS was distributed among persons in the United States in 1996.

Gender

In 1996, AIDS incidence decreased by 8% in men, but increased by 2% in women in the United States (CDC, 1997a), the occurrence of new cases is highest in women ages 15 to 24 (Wortley and Fleming, 1997). The rate is much higher in Hispanic and black women than in white women. Since 1992, heterosexual transmission has surpassed injection drug use as the primary mode of HIV transmission in women (Wortley and Fleming, 1997). See the Research Brief.

Pediatric AIDS reflects the infection rate in women, making the disease a family disease. However, the number of perinatally acquired AIDS cases has decreased by 27% between the 1992 and 1995. This drop is a result of the effectiveness of the drug zidovudine when given to HIV-infected pregnant women (CDC, 1996a).

DID YOU KNOW? *There are no protective methods that prevent disease while also preserving a woman's ability to have a baby. Current research is focused on developing products that prevent infection without killing or blocking sperm.*

Age

The largest number of reported AIDS cases (45.3%) is in the age group from 30 to 39 years, and nearly 90% of those with AIDS are between the ages of 20 and 49 years of age (CDC, 1997d). Because the incubation period is so long, the time when the actual transmission took place is likely to have occurred during adolescence and young adulthood. This period of life is characterized by experimentation with various roles and behaviors that may include injectable drug use, sexual experimentation, and other activities that place adolescents and young adults at risk.

TABLE 39-2 **AIDS Cases and Annual Rates per 100,000 Population, by Race/Ethnicity, Age Group, and Sex, Reported in 1998, United States**

| | ADULTS/ADOLESCENTS | | | | | | CHILDREN <13 YEARS OLD | | TOTAL | |
| | MALES | | FEMALES | | TOTAL ADULTS | | | | | |
RACE/ETHNICITY	NUMBER	RATE	NUMBER	RATE	NUMBER	RATE	NUMBER	RATE	NUMBER	RATE
White, non-Hispanic	23,341	29.9	2888	3.5	26,229	16.2	98	0.3	26,327	13.5
Black, non-Hispanic	20,199	177.6	8147	61.7	28,346	115.3	429	5.7	28,775	89.7
Hispanic	10,337	88.9	2629	22.7	12,966	55.8	145	1.7	13,111	41.3
Asian/Pacific Islander	480	13.6	81	2.1	561	7.5	1	0.0	562	5.9
American Indian/ Alaskan Native	166	23.2	41	5.4	207	14.1	3	0.6	210	10.7
TOTAL*	54,653	51.9	13,820	12.3	68,473	31.4	678	1.3	69,151	25.6

*Totals include 166 persons whose race/ethnicity is unknown.
From Centers for Disease Control and Prevention: *HIV/AIDS Surveillance Report* 8(2):17, 1997.

The percentage of all AIDS cases in persons over 50 years of age has remained stable since 1991. However, relative to other categories of age, the group over 50 years has had a greater proportion of persons who present for the first time with an opportunistic disease. Thus many persons over 50 years old with AIDS are not diagnosed as infected with HIV first but are only recognized once they have an AIDS-defining illness (CDC, 1998a).

Race and ethnicity

AIDS has disproportionately affected minority groups. African-Americans made up 12.1% of the total United States population according to the 1990 census, but they represented 43% of those reported to have AIDS (CDC, 1997d). This overrepresentation is associated with economically poor, marginalized populations composed of persons who are likely to be urban residents, may use injection drugs, and use prostitution to obtain illicit drugs (Aral, 1996).

Geographical distribution

The geographical distribution of AIDS is clustered in urban areas, but increasingly it is moving into rural areas. Regionally, the Northeast and Southeast sections of the United States and the U.S. territories of Puerto Rico and the Virgin Islands reflect the highest rates (CDC, 1997d).

States with an incidence greater than 25 per 100,000 population between July 1996 and June 1997 were Florida, New York, Nevada, South Carolina, Maryland, Georgia, Delaware, Connecticut, New Jersey, California, the District of Columbia, Louisiana, and Texas (CDC, 1997d).

HIV surveillance

AIDS is a reportable condition by name of client within the United States. However, the reporting of HIV infection varies among states as shown in Table 39-3. As of January 1998, 31 states had begun name-based HIV reporting in addition to the existing name-based AIDS surveillance systems (CDC, 1998c). Study of already diagnosed cases of AIDS does not reveal current HIV infection patterns because of the long interval between infection with HIV and the onset of clinically-apparent dis-

RESEARCH *Brief*

The purpose of this study was to assess the HIV-related behaviors and mental health of persons who are the closest sources of social support for inner-city women of color. Women who were facing multiple life crises and the person they were closest to were asked about their sexual and drug use history and their psychological well being, then assessed for depression. The most common HIV risk behaviors among the participants were having sex for money, having sex without a condom, and having multiple sex partners. The women scored higher on a depression scale than did their supportive others. When comparing the homeless women with the drug-dependent women, the women in the drug recovery program were significantly more depressed. Thus, although peer support and social support is often assumed to be associated with health benefits, supportive others may also have a negative impact on health. Several other studies have identified that drug use occurs in social networks where needles and drugs are shared and opposition to drug treatment may occur. The researchers conclude that there is a need to provide mental health referral for homeless and drug-addicted women and their supportive others. Future research needs to identify how supportive networks might be used to promote risk reduction.

Nyamathi A, Flaskerud J, Leake B: HIV-risk behaviors and mental health characteristics among homeless or drug-recovering women and their close sources of social support, *Nurs Res* 46(3):1333, 1997.

TABLE 39-3 Reporting Requirements for Human Immunodeficiency Virus (HIV) Infection

By name of infected person	Anonymous	Not required
Alabama	Georgia	Alaska
Arizona	Iowa	California
Arkansas	Kansas	Delaware
Colorado	Kentucky	Florida
Connecticut*	Maine	Hawaii
Idaho	Montana	Louisiana
Indiana	New Hampshire	Maryland
Michigan	Oregon	Massachusetts
Minnesota	Rhode Island	New Mexico
Mississippi		New York
Missouri		Pennsylvania
Nebraska		Vermont
Nevada		Washington
New Jersey		District of Columbia
North Carolina		
North Dakota		
Ohio		
Oklahoma		
Oregon*		
South Carolina		
South Dakota		
Tennessee		
Texas*		
Utah		
Virginia		
West Virginia		
Wisconsin		

*Connecticut and Texas have confidential HIV infection reporting for pediatric cases only; Oregon has reporting for children less than 6 years old.
From Centers for Disease Control and Prevention: *HIV/AIDS Surveillance Report* 9(1):32, 1997.

ease. Moreover, identification of new cases of AIDS does not distinguish between those recently infected and those infected several years ago. The successful use of several new drugs early in the asymptomatic phase of infection also supports determining early identification of illness in this period. Thus several experts, including the CDC, are calling for mandatory reporting of HIV-positive status by name in all 50 states (CDC, 1998a; Gostin, Ward, and Baker, 1997). Opponents express concerns about the government's ability to maintain confidential registries and about potential invasions into personal lives, including housing, employment, and insurance discrimination.

HIV seroprevalence studies involve the anonymous screening of populations for the HIV antibody. Seroprevalence studies can provide information about the number of persons infected with HIV who are carriers and thus how the virus is spreading within populations. This screening has been conducted in emergency rooms, family planning clinics, and military clinics. Based on these studies, estimates of HIV infection have been calculated in several groups. For example, the HIV seroprevalence rate for prisoners was found to range from 2.1% to 14.7% (CDC, 1992b), and 0.9% in a homeless population in Denver (Shlay et al, 1996). Early detection of infected persons enables medical personnel to develop treatment services and decide where to focus prevention efforts.

HIV Testing

The **HIV antibody test** is the most commonly used screening test for determining infection. This test does just as its name implies: it does not reveal whether an individual has AIDS, nor does it isolate the virus. It does indicate the presence of the antibody to HIV. The most commonly used form of this test is the enzyme-linked immunosorbent assay (EIA). The EIA effectively screens blood and other donor products. In cases of false-positive results, a confirmatory test, the Western blot, is used to verify the results. False-negative results may also occur after infection before antibodies are produced. This is sometimes referred to as the window period and can last from 6 weeks to 3 months.

Testing for HIV infection is offered at health department STD clinics and family planning clinics, primary care offices, and freestanding HIV-counseling and HIV-testing sites. Voluntary screening programs for HIV may be either confidential or anonymous: the process for each is unique. With confidential testing the person's name and address is obtained, and this information is considered privileged. With anonymous testing the client is given an identification number that is attached to all records of the test results. Demographic data such as the person's sex, age, and race may be collected, but there is no record of the client's name and address. An advantage of anonymous testing may be that it increases the number of people who are willing to be tested, because many of those at risk are engaged in illegal activities. The anonymity eliminates their concern about the possibility of arrest or discrimination.

Perinatal/Pediatric HIV Infection

Perinatally acquired AIDS accounts for nearly all HIV infection in children. Women who are HIV infected must consider the risk of perinatal infection and the risk to their own health. They should be counseled to prevent pregnancy. The effectiveness of zidovudine therapy in pregnant women toward preventing transmission from mother to fetus or infant has made pediatric HIV rates decline sharply (CDC, 1996a). Based on the effectiveness of zidovudine treatment, recommendations include mandatory prenatal counseling and voluntary testing to identify HIV status early in pregnancy. Zidovudine therapy is not universally effective; estimates of vertical transmission (from mother to fetus or infant) range from 11% to 60% (Levy, 1998). Thus prevention in women must remain the primary focus of efforts to reduce pediatric HIV infection.

Studies are inconclusive about whether pregnancy increases the likelihood of progression to AIDS. Alterations in cell-mediated immunity during pregnancy make the progression to AIDS possible, however with antiviral medication this progression may be halted. Women who become pregnant must consider who will care for their children if they become ill, the effectiveness of current antiviral therapy, and the available health care and financial resources when deciding whether to continue the pregnancy.

The clinical picture of pediatric HIV infection differs greatly from that of adults. The incubation period in infants is shorter as they usually experience symptoms within the first year of life. Children also develop different physical signs and symptoms from adults. These include failure to thrive, diarrhea, developmental delays, and bacterial infections such as otitis media and pneumonia. Children typically have a shorter survival period. Because 89% of children with AIDS contract the disease through maternal transmission, many die within the first 3 years of life (CDC, 1994b).

DID YOU KNOW? *Because of impaired immunity, children with HIV infection are more likely to get childhood diseases and suffer serious sequelae. Therefore DPT (diphtheria-pertussis-tetanus), IPV (inactivated polio virus), and MMR (measles-mumps-rubella) vaccines should be given at regularly scheduled times for children infected with HIV. HIb (Haemophilus influenza type B), hepatitis B, pneumonoccal, and influenza vaccines may be recommended after medical evaluation.*

Detection of HIV infection in infants of seropositive mothers is through different tests from those used in children over 18 months of age. The EIA test is not valid because it tests for antibodies that reflect maternal antibodies, and thus even a seronegative infant may show a positive test result. Thus testing is done by HIV culture, HIV antigen, or polymerase chain reaction (PCR) (CDC, 1994e).

Despite having an infected mother, many children will not acquire AIDS. However, there remains the potential for loss of one or both parents from HIV infection. Many children with AIDS come from impoverished families with limited financial, emotional, social and health care resources. The added strain of this illness makes many families unable to provide for the emotional, physical, and developmental needs of affected children.

AIDS in the Community

Because AIDS is a chronic disease, afflicted individuals live and function in the community. Much of their care is provided in the home. The nurse teaches families and significant others about personal care and hygiene, medication administration, universal precautions to ensure infection control, and healthy lifestyle behaviors such as adequate rest, balanced nutrition, and exercise.

Persons with AIDS have bouts of illness interspersed with periods of wellness when they are able to return to school or work. Policies regarding school and work-site attendance have been developed by most communities and some businesses. These policies provide direction for the community's response when an individual develops HIV infection. Among the roles of the nurse are identifying resources such as social and financial support services and interpreting school and work policies.

Businesses are often unprepared and uninformed about how to deal with situations involving HIV infection (Hale, 1990). The 1974 Vocational Rehabilitation Act protects employees from termination of employment or other discriminatory action based solely on the presence of the disease.

Nurses can assist employers by identifying the importance of sponsoring educational programs on HIV. Educating managers on how to deal with sick or infected workers is vital to reduce the risk of breaching confidentiality or wrongful actions such as termination. Revealing a worker's infection to other workers, terminating employment, and isolating an infected worker are examples of situations that have resulted in litigation between employees and employers. The CDC supports workplace issues through programs offered by its Business and Labor Resource Service. Contact information for this service is included in Box 39-3.

Children who are HIV infected should attend school because the benefit of attendance far outweighs the risk of transmitting or acquiring infections. None of the cases of HIV infection in the United States have been transmitted in a school setting. Decisions regarding educational and care needs should be based on an interdisciplinary team that includes the child's physician, public health personnel, and the child's parent or guardian (CDC, 1996c; CDC, 1988).

Individual decisions about risk to the infected child or others should be based on the behavior, neurological development, and physical condition of the child. Attendance may be inadvisable in the presence of cases of childhood infections, such as chickenpox or measles, within the school, because the immunosuppressed child is at greater risk of suffering complications. Alternative arrangements,

---

BOX 39-3 STD Resources

American Social Health Association (800-227-8922)
Hepatitis Hotline (800-223-0179)
National AIDS Hotline (800-342-2437)
National AIDS Clearinghouse (800-458-5231)
CDC Business Responds to AIDS Resource (800-458-5231)
AIDS Clinical Trials Information Service (800-874-2572)
Hemophilia and AIDS/HIV Network for Dessemination of Information (HANDI) (800-424-2634)
Teens Teaching AIDS Prevention Program (800-234-8336)
AIDS Treatment News (800-873-2812)

See this book's website at www.mosby.com/MERLIN for more information about resources.

---

such as homebound instruction, might be instituted if a child is unable to control body secretions or displays biting behavior.

Resources

As the number of individuals with AIDS has increased, many needs have evolved. Voluntary service organizations, such as community-based organizations or AIDS support organizations, have developed to address these needs. Services commonly provided by these groups include client and family counseling, support groups, legal aid, personal care services, housing programs, and community education programs. Nurses collaborate with workers from community-based organizations in the client's home and may serve to advise these groups in their supportive work.

Each state has established an AIDS hotline. In addition, the federal government and organizations have established toll-free numbers to meet a variety of needs. Box 39-3 presents contact numbers for several different organizations.

OTHER SEXUALLY TRANSMITTED DISEASES

The number of new cases (the incidence) of some STDs, such as syphilis, has been declining recently, while others such as herpes simplex and chlamydia, continue to increase. It is estimated that actual rates of STDs are twice the reported rate. Due to the impact of STDs on long-term health and the emergence of eight new STDs since 1980, continued attention to their prevention and treatment is vital (IOM, 1997).

The common STDs listed in Table 39-4 are categorized by their biological origin: those caused by protozoa, bacteria, or viruses. Trichomonas is a protozoan infection. The bacterial infections include gonorrhea, syphilis, chlamydia, and chancroid. Most of these are curable with antibiotics with the exception of the newly emerging antibiotic-resistant strains of gonorrhea.

STDs caused by viruses cannot be cured. These are chronic diseases resulting in years of symptom management and infection control. The viral infections include

TABLE 39-4 Summary of Sexually Transmitted Diseases

DISEASE/PATHOGENS	INCUBATION	SIGNS AND SYMPTOMS
PROTOZOAN		
Trichomoniasis: *Trichomonas vaginalis*	5-28 days	Frequently asymptomatic; copious, loose yellow or green vaginal discharge; vulvovaginal soreness/irritation; dysuria—internal or external; painful intercourse
BACTERIAL		
Chlamydia: *Chlamydia*	3-21 days	*Male:* nongonococcal urethritis (NGU); painful urination and urethral discharge; epididymitis
		Female: none or mucopurulent cervicitis (MPC), vaginal discharge; if untreated, progresses to symptoms of pelvic inflammatory disease (PID) diffuse abdominal pain, fever, chills
Gonorrhea: *Neisseria gonorrhoeae*	3-21 days	*Male:* urethritis, purulent discharge, painful urination, urinary frequency; epididymitis
		Female: none or symptoms of PID
Syphilis: *Treponema pallidum*	10-90 days	Primary: usually single, painless chancre; if untreated, heals in a few weeks
	6 weeks-6 months	Secondary: low-grade fever, malaise, sore throat, headache, adenopathy, and rash
	With 1 year of infection	Early latency: Asymptomatic, infectious lesions may recur
	After 1 year from date of infection	Late latency: Asymptomatic; noninfectious except to fetus of pregnant women
	Late active: 2-40 years 20-30 years 10-30 years	• Gummas of skin, bone, and mucous membranes, heart, liver • CNS involvement: paresis, optic atrophy • Cardiovascular involvement: aortic aneurysm, aortic value insufficiency
Chancroid: *Haemophilus ducreyi*	3-7 days	Small irregular papule progressing to deep ulcer that is painful and drains pus or blood on the penis, labia, or vaginal opening; inguinal tenderness, dysuria

*FTA-ABS indicates fluorescent treponemal antibody absorption test.
†MHA-TP indicates microhemagglutination—*Treponema pallidum.*
‡VDRL indicates Venereal Disease Research Laboratory test for syphilis.
From Centers for Disease Control and Prevention: Summary of notifable diseases, *MMWR* 45:53, 1996.

DIAGNOSIS	TREATMENT	NURSING IMPLICATIONS
(+) Whiff test; wet mount-visualization of organism and ≥1 PMN per epithelial cell	Metronidazole 2 g PO once; *or* 500 mg PO bid×7 days *or* 250 mg TID×7 days.	Almost always sexually acquired, so treat partners simultaneously; avoid sex until symptoms gone in both client and partners; return for evaluation if symptoms persist; screen for other STDs (gonorrhea, chlamydia, and HIV); medication teaching.
Tissue culture; gram stain of endocervical or urethral discharge: presence of PMNs without gram-negative intracellular diplococci suggests NGU	One of the following treatments: • Doxycycline 100 mg PO bid × 7 days • Azithromycin 1 g PO × 1 • Erythromycin 500 mg qid × 7 days • Ofloxacin 300 mg PO bid × 7 days • Doxycycline—effective/ cheap • Azithyromycin—good because 1-time dose	Refer partners of past 60 days; counsel client to use condoms and to avoid sex until therapy is complete and symptoms are gone in both client and partners; medication teaching
Culture of discharge; Gram stain of urethral discharge, endocervical, or rectal smear	One of the following treatments: • Ceftriaxone 125 mg IM • Ciprofloxacin 500 mg PO × 1 • Ofloxacin 400 mg PO × 1 • Cefixime 400 mg PO × 1 • Azithromycin 1 g PO × 1	Refer partners of past 60 days; return for evaluation if symptoms persist; counsel client to use condoms and to avoid sex until therapy is complete and symptoms are gone in both client and partners; medication teaching
Visualization of pathogen on dark field microscopic examination; single painless ulcer (chancre) FTA-ADS* or MHA-TP† VDRL‡ (reactive 14 days after appearance of chancre)	Benzathine penicillin G 2.4 million U IM once. If penicillin allergy: • Doxycycline 100 mg PO bid × 2 weeks or • Tetracycline 500 mg qid × 14 days • Tetracycline hydrochloride should not be administered to pregnant women or those with neurosyphilis or congenital syphilis	Counsel to be tested for HIV; screen all partners of past 3 months; reexamine client at 3 and 6 months
Clinical signs of secondary syphilis	Benzathine penicillin G 2.4 million U IM once	
VDRL: FTA-ABS or MHA-TP	Benzathine penicillin G	
Lumbar puncture, cerebrospinal fluid (CSF) cell count, protein level determination and VDRL	Penicillin G Benzathine 2.4 million U IM weekly × 3 weeks Penicillins: varying doses depending on diagnosis	
Visual inspection of lesion	Azithromycin 1 g PO ×1 or Ceftriaxone 250 mg IM ×1	Return for exam 3-7 days after treatment begins; partners who had sex within 10 days before client's onset of symptoms should be evaluated; condom use

Continued

TABLE 39-4 Summary of Sexually Transmitted Diseases—cont'd

DISEASE/PATHOGENS	INCUBATION	SIGNS AND SYMPTOMS
VIRAL		
Human Immunodeficiency Virus (HIV)	4 to 6 weeks	Possible: acute mononucleosis-like illness (lymphadenopathy, fever, rash, joint and muscle pain, sore throat)
	Seroconversion: 6 weeks to 3 months	Appearance of HIV antibody
	AIDS: months to years (average 11 years)	Opportunistic diseases: most commonly *Pneumocystis pneumonia*, oral candidiasis, Kaposi's sarcoma
Hepatitis B virus (HBV)	6 weeks to 6 months	Varies greatly from subclinical infection to flu-like symptoms to cirrhosis, fulminant hepatitis; hepatocellular carcinonoma
Genital warts: Human papillomavirus (HPV)	4-6 weeks most common; up to 9 months	Often subclinical infection; painless lesions near vaginal openings, anus, shaft of penis, vagina, cervix; lesions are textured, cauliflower appearance; may remain unchanged over time
Genital herpes: Herpes simplex virus 2 (HSV-2)	2-20 days; average 6 days	Vesicles, painful ulcerations of penis, vagina, labia, perineum, or anus; lesions last 5-6 weeks and recurrence is common; may be asymptomatic

*FTA-ABS indicates fluorescent treponemal antibody absorption test.
†MHA-TP indicates microhemagglutination—*Treponema pallidum*.
‡VDRL indicates Venereal Disease Research Laboratory test for syphilis.
From Centers for Disease Control and Prevention: Summary of notifable diseases, *MMWR* 45:53, 1996.

herpes simplex virus, hepatitis B virus, and human papillomavirus (HPV), also referred to as genital warts. Hepatitis A virus, which may also be transmitted via sexual activity, is discussed in Chapter 38.

Trichomoniasis

Trichomoniasis is a common sexually transmitted disease caused by a unicellular protozoan flagellate, trichomonas vaginalis, that infects the female vulva and vagina, but commonly does not cause symptoms in males (Krieger, 1995). It is transmitted through sexual contact and is easily diagnosed through microscopic identification of the organism. The symptoms vary but include frothy off-white to green vaginal discharge and pruritis. Trichomonas is not

a reportable condition in most states. Although considered a benign STD in comparison with other STDs , it is very common, and recently has been linked with pelvic inflammatory disease, which is a serious condition discussed below (Paisarntantiwong et al, 1995).

Gonorrhea

Neisseria gonorrhoeae is a gram-negative intracellular diplococcus bacterium that infects the mucous membranes of the genitourinary tract, rectum, and pharynx. It is transmitted through genital-genital contact, oral-genital contact, and anal-genital contact.

Gonorrhea is identified as either uncomplicated or complicated. Uncomplicated gonorrhea refers to limited

Diagnosis	Treatment	Nursing Implications
	Prophylactic administration of zidovudine (ZDV) immediately after exposure may prevent seroconversion	HIV education and counseling
HIV antibody test: the enzyme-linked immunosorbent assay (ELISA), or the Western blot test. New test: OraSure made by SmithKline Beechum-an oral HIV-1antibody testing system-test results in about 3 days.	Asymptomatic infection with HIV-1 and CD4 counts ≤500/mm³; treat with ZDV 500-600 mg/day; treatment can be held in those with asymptomatic infection and CD4 counts between 500-200/mm³ until symptoms or CD4 counts	HIV education and counseling; partner referral for evaluation; medication education; assessment and referral
CD4 T-lymphocyte count of less than 200/μL with documented HIV infection, or diagnosis with clinical manifestations of AIDS as defined by the CDC.	Symptomatic infection: start ZDV 20 mg q8h; alternatives to ZDV: didanosine (ddI), stavudine (d4t), zalcitabine (ddC), and the combination of ZDV and ddI; additional treatments necessary for opportunistic infections	
Serum IgM alpha-HBc.	Hepatitis B Immune Globulin within 14 days of last exposure; followed by regular three-dose immunization series	Partners should receive HBIG prophylaxis within 14 days postexposure followed by 3-dose immunization series
Visual inspection for lesions; papanicolaou smear; colposcopy	No cure; one third of lesions will disappear without treatment. Patient-applied: Topical podofilox 0.5% or imiquimod 5% cream. Provider administered: Podophyllin resin 10-25% trichloracetic acid 80%-90% cryotherapy with liquid nitrogen, laser, or surgical removal	Warts and surrounding tissues contain HPV so removal of warts does not completely eradicate virus; examination of partners not necessary since treatment is only symptomatic; condom use may reduce transmission; medication application
Presence of vesicles; viral culture (obtained only when lesions present and before they have scabbed over)	No cure; Acyclovir 400 mg PO tid × 7-10 days or Acyclovir 200 mg five times a day × 7-10 days or Valacyclovir 1 g PO bid × 7-10 days.	Refer partners for evaluation; teach client about likelihood of recurrent episodes and ability to transmit to others even if asymptomatic; condom use; annual Pap smear

cervical or urethral infection. Complicated gonorrhea includes salpingitis, epididymitis, systemic gonococcal infection, and gonococcal meningitis. The signs and symptoms of infection in males are purulent and copious urethral discharge and dysuria, although it is estimated that 10% to 20% of males are asymptomatic.

More females than males tend to be asymptomatic; there may be minimal vaginal discharge or dysuria (Hook and Handsfield, 1990). The asymptomatic state is dangerous because individuals who are unaware of their infection may continue to infect others, whereas those who are symptomatic usually cease sexual activity and seek treatment.

Up to 40% of those infected with gonorrhea are coinfected with *Chlamydia trachomatis* (CDC, 1998b). There-

fore selection of a treatment that is effective against both organisms, such as doxycycline or azithromycin, is recommended (CDC, 1998b).

Gonorrhea rates have declined over time due to the testing of asymptomatic women and follow-up with their partners to prevent reinfection. Although the reported number of cases in the United States in 1996 was just under 300,000, the CDC estimates the actual number of annual cases to be 600,000 (CDC, 1998b). The difference between the actual cases and reported cases occurs because gonorrhea may be unreported by health care providers or clients who are asymptomatic do not seek treatment and are therefore not identified. Groups with the highest incidence of gonorrhea are African-Americans, persons living in the southern United States, and persons 15 to 24 years of age (Division of STD Prevention, 1997).

The number of antibiotic-resistant cases of gonorrhea in the United States has risen at an alarming rate. Penicillin-resistant gonorrhea was first identified in 1976 when 15 cases were reported (Phillips, 1976). By 1990, 64,972 cases were reported (Blount, 1991). Although the number of new cases of drug-resistant gonorrhea is not reported, studies to document antibiotic resistance continue. After resistance to penicillin was identified, a strain of tetracycline-resistant *N. gonorrhoeae* developed. Between 1992 and 1994, another strain was isolated in the United States that is resistant to ciprofloxacin, an antibiotic currently effective against both penicillin- and tetracycline-resistant gonorrhea (CDC, 1994a; Deguchi et al, 1997). The increase in antibiotic-resistant infections is partially attributed to the indiscriminate or illicit use of antibiotics as a prophylactic measure by persons with multiple sexual partners (Zenilman et al, 1988). To ensure proper treatment and cure, those diagnosed with gonorrheal infection should return for health care if symptoms persist, have their partner evaluated for infection, and remain sexually abstinent until antibiotic therapy is completed (CDC, 1998b).

The development of **pelvic inflammatory disease (PID)** is a risk for women who remain asymptomatic and do not seek treatment. PID is a serious infection involving the fallopian tubes (salpingitis) and is the most common complication of gonorrhea but may also result from chlamydia infection. Symptoms of PID include fever, abnormal menses, and lower abdominal pain, however PID may not be recognized because the symptoms vary among women. PID can result in ectopic pregnancy and infertility as a result of fallopian-tube scarring and occlusion. It may also cause stillbirths and premature labor. It has been estimated that the cost of the complications resulting from PID is more than $3.5 billion annually (IOM, 1997).

Syphilis

Syphilis is caused by a member of the *Treponeme* genus of spirochetes called *Treponema pallidum*. It infects moist mucosal or cutaneous lesions and is spread through direct contact, usually by sexual contact or from mother to fetus. In sexual transmission, microscopic breaks in the skin and mucous membranes during sexual contact create a point of entry for the bacteria.

The number of reported cases of syphilis decreased from 26,352 in 1993 to 11,336 in 1996 (Division of STD Prevention, 1997). The number of cases peaked at a 40-year high in 1988 and has since been declining. The highest incidence is in African-Americans and persons age 20 through 39 years (Division of STD Prevention, 1997).

Syphilis is divided into early and late stages. Latency, a period where an individual is free of symptoms, may occur during the early and late stages. As defined by the United States Public Health Service, the early stage is the first full year after infection and includes the primary, secondary, and early latent stages. The late stage is the time after this first year and includes late latency and tertiary syphilis. During latency there are no clinical signs of infection, but the person has historical or serological evidence of infection. The possibility of relapse remains.

Primary syphilis

When syphilis is acquired sexually, the bacteria produce infection in the form of a chancre at the site of entry (Fig. 39-3). The lesion begins as a macula, progresses to a papule, and later ulcerates. If left untreated, this chancre persists for 3 to 6 weeks and then heals spontaneously.

Secondary syphilis

Secondary syphilis occurs when the organism enters the lymph system and spreads throughout the body. Signs include rash, lymphadenopathy, and mucosal ulceration. Symptoms of secondary syphilis include sore throat, malaise, headaches, weight loss, variable fever, and muscle and joint pain.

Tertiary syphilis

Tertiary syphilis may involve the complications of blindness, congenital damage, cardiovascular damage, or syphilitic psychoses. Another potential outcome of tertiary syphilis is the development of lesions of the bones, skin, and mucous membranes, known as gummas. Tertiary syphilis usually occurs several years after initial infection and is rare in the United States because the disease is usually cured in its early stages with antibiotics. Tertiary

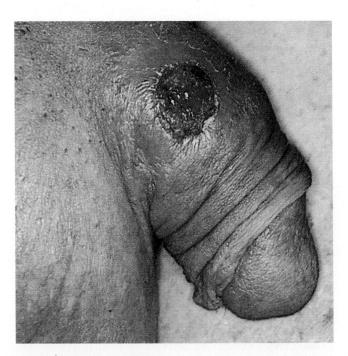

FIG. 39-3 Primary, syphilitic chancre on penile shaft. (Photograph used with permission of Lewis Kaminester, MD. Reproduced with permission of Glaxo-Wellcome Inc.)

syphilis does, however, remain a major problem in developing countries.

Congenital syphilis

Syphilis is transmitted transplacentally and if untreated can cause premature stillbirth, blindness, deafness, facial abnormalities, crippling, or death. Signs include jaundice, skin rash, hepatosplenomegaly, or pseudoparalysis of an extremity. Treatment is penicillin given intravenously or intramuscularly (CDC, 1998b).

Chlamydia

Chlamydia infection results from the bacterium *Chlamydia trachomatis*. It infects the genitourinary tract and rectum of adults and causes conjunctivitis and pneumonia in neonates. Transmission occurs when mucopurulent discharge from infected sites, such as the cervix or urethra, comes into contact with the mucous membranes of a non-infected person. As with gonorrhea, the infection is commonly asymptomatic in women and, if left untreated, can result in PID. When symptoms of chlamydial infection are present in females, they include dysuria, urinary frequency, and purulent vaginal discharge. In males the urethra is the most common site of infection, resulting in **nongonococcal urethritis (NGU).** The symptoms of NGU are dysuria and urethral discharge. Epididymitis is a possible complication.

Chlamydia is the most common reportable infectious disease in the United States with 4 million infections occurring every year (CDC, 1997b). Because it causes PID, ectopic pregnancy, infertility and neonatal complications, it is a major focus of preventive efforts (CDC, 1997b). Rates of chlamydia have increased in recent years, partly because of improved diagnosis and reporting. Risk factors that positively correlate with chlamydial infection include young age and oral contraception use, multiple sexual partners, and the presence of gonorrhea (CDC, 1993). The high frequency of chlamydial infections in individuals infected with gonorrhea requires that effective treatment for both organisms be given when a gonorrheal infection is identified (CDC, 1998a).

Chancroid

Chancroid is caused by *Haemophilus ducreyi* and is spread from person to person through sexual contact. Chancroid is characterized by a type of ulcerative lesion occurring on the penis, labia, or clitoris or at the vaginal orifice. About 1 week after infection, a small papule develops and soon progresses to a painful, deep ulceration (Fig. 39-4). The infection spreads to the inguinal lymph nodes and causes inflammation and tenderness. Usually one or two lesions occur, but there may be as many as 10. In the United States, chancroid is a less-frequent cause of genital ulcers than herpes simplex virus 2 (HSV-2) or syphilis. The reported cases of chancroid have decreased from a high of 4986 in 1987 to 386 in 1996. There is documented underreporting

of the infection because of inadequate laboratory testing, and unclear definition of what signs confirm diagnosis (CDC, 1992a). Although chancroid is not as commonly reported as other STDs in the United States, it is much more prevalent worldwide than gonorrhea or syphilis.

Hepatitis B Virus

The number of new cases of **hepatitis B virus (HBV)** in the United States increased by 37% between 1979 and 1989 (CDC, 1991). Since the use of the HBV vaccine, the numbers have fallen dramatically—from 10.65 cases per 100,000 persons in 1987 to 4.01 cases per 100,000 in 1996. (CDC, 1997g).

The groups with the highest prevalence are users of injection drugs, persons with STDs or multiple sex partners, immigrants and refugees and their descendants who came from areas where there is a high endemic rate of HBV, health care workers, hemodialysis clients, and inmates of long-term correctional institutions.

The HBV is spread through blood and body fluids and, like HIV, is referred to as a bloodborne pathogen. It has the same transmission properties as HIV, and thus individuals should take the same precautions to prevent both HIV and HBV spread. A major difference is that HBV remains alive outside the body for a longer period of time than does HIV and thus has greater infectivity. The virus can survive for at least 1 week dried at room temperature on environmental surfaces, and thus infection control measures are paramount in preventing transmission from client to client (CDC, 1990a; CDC, 1997f).

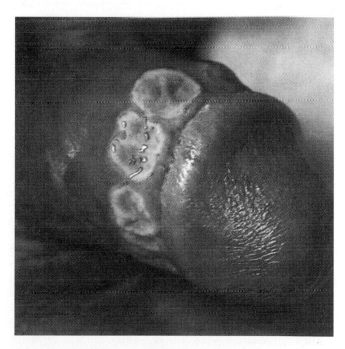

FIG. 39-4 Chancroid: multiple punched-out ulcers on penile shaft. (Photograph used with permission of Lewis Kaminester, MD. Reproduced with permission of Glaxo-Wellcome Inc.)

HIV/AIDS, Hepatitis B, and Sexually Transmitted Diseases

Jo-Ann Ackery, Toronto Public Health

HIV/AIDS

AIDS is a reportable disease in all provinces and territories in Canada. Physicians, hospitals, and laboratories are required under provincial legislation and regulations to report AIDS cases to the local public health department. The local health department transmits case data to the provincial ministry of health, which in turn, provides selected data to the Laboratory Centre for Disease Control (LCDC) at Health Canada in Ottawa.

In Canada the definition for AIDS is "a person who has an illness characterised by the following:

- One or more of the specified indicator diseases." (Canada does not include the definition of "CD4 T-lymphocyte count of less than 200/ml with documented HIV infection") and
- Either a positive test for HIV infection or absence of specified causes of underlying immunodeficiency" (Remis, 1995, p. 1-2).

The first case of AIDS in Canada was reported in 1982. There have been 15,935 AIDS cases reported in Canada from the beginning of the epidemic to June 30, 1998. When adjustments are made for delays in reporting, the total number is estimated to be 20,000 (Health Canada, The AIDS/HIV Files, 1998). There has been a decline in the number of reported AIDS cases each year since 1994 likely due to a combination of improved anti-retroviral treatments and drug prophylaxis regimens. In 1997 there were 54.1% fewer reported AIDS cases than in 1996, while at the same time the proportion of AIDS cases increased among women (14.4% of the annual AIDS diagnoses in 1997) (AIDS/HIV Files, 1998) and injection drug users (IDU) (19.9% of the adult AIDS cases reported in 1997) (Health Canada, 1998b). Injection drug use accounts for 18.3% of all AIDS cases in women compared to 3.7% in adult men, and these percentages are increasing each year (Health Canada, 1998b). Of adult male AIDS diagnoses, 4.8% are due to the combined exposure categories of men who have sex with men/injection drug use (MSM/IDU), while 11,175 cases (71.9%) were attributed to MSM (Health Canada, 1998a; Health Canada, 1998d). Up to December 31, 1997, 78% (133/170) of the reported paediatric AIDS cases were attributed to perinatal transmission (Health Canada, 1998f).

There is a lack of information regarding the HIV/AIDS epidemic among Aboriginal people because of variations in the completeness of reporting ethnic status between provinces. The number of Aboriginal AIDS cases was 255 by the end of 1997 (estimated at 332 when adjusted for reporting delays with a rate of 33.2/100,000 Aboriginal people) (Health Canada, 1998b). The proportion of cases attributed to Aboriginal persons has increased over time from <2% before 1989 to >10% in 1997 (Health Canada, 1998b). Aboriginal people are overrepresented in groups at high risk

for HIV/AIDS (i.e., IDU, inmates in prtison, persons with STDs).

HIV testing is available through confidential, nominal, or coded testing from physicians or clinics. Some provinces have legislated anonymous testing at designated sites. HIV is reportable in the territories and in eight of the ten provinces. British Columbia and Quebec have not yet made HIV reportable. HIV is only collected at the federal level by the reporting of confidential non-nominal laboratory test data, contributed by the provinces and the territories. Through December 1997, it is estimated that 41,681 individuals in Canada have tested positive for HIV, 2598 of which were reported in 1997 (Health Canada, 1998a). There is a significant proportion of persons with risk factors who have never been tested for HIV. The Bureau of HIV/AIDS, STD, and TB has estimated that by the end of 1996 there were between 11,000 and 17,000 HIV-infected Canadians who were not aware of their HIV infection (Division of HIV/AIDS Surveillance et al, 1998). Many provinces have guidelines and/or recommendations for physicians to encourage HIV testing during pregnancy, however the choice remains with the woman.

HEPATITIS B

The number of Hepatitis B (HBV) cases reported in Canada through the National Notifiable Disease Registry System (NNDRS) has decreased from 3001 cases in 1990 (rate 11.3/100,000) to 2385 in 1996 (rate 8.0/100,000) (Division of Disease Surveillance et al, 1998). British Columbia has the highest number of cases, 1309 (rate 33.9/100,000), but it is difficult to compare the provinces due to differences in what is included in the reporting of HBV infection. From a direct contact and mailed survey done in the summer of 1996, information was collected on acute HBV cases that indicates that acute HBV rates in Canada have fallen 29 % between 1992 and 1995 (LCDC, 1997).

Hepatitis B vaccine for high risk groups has been available since 1982 as well as prenatal screening for high risk pregnant women. In addition there are now school-based Hepatitis B vaccination programs (in Grades 3 to 7) in all provinces except Manitoba (Health Canada, 1998g).

CHLAMYDIA TRACHOMATIS

About 84% of reported STDs in Canada are due to genital Chlamydia infections. Although the rate of infection has decreased (169.2/100,000 in 1992 to 114.8/100,000 in 1996) it continues to be disproportionately high in 15- to 19-year-old females (998.1/100,000), in 20- to 24-year-old females (940.6/100,000) (Division of Disease Surveillance et al, 1998), and in street youth.

GONORRHEA

Reported gonorrhea cases in Canada have decreased from a rate of 223/100,000 in 1980 to 16.8/100,000 in 1996. As

HIV/AIDS, Hepatitis B, and Sexually Transmitted Diseases–cont'd

with chlamydia the rates are disproportionately high in young women (86.4/100,000 in 15 to 19 years old and 65/100,000 in 20 to 24 year olds) (Division of Disease Surveillance et al, 1998). Young men 20 to 24 years old also have a high rate (66.6/100,000). Provincial data show the highest rates in the Northwest Territories (187.1), Yukon (31.8), Saskatchewan (39.6), and Manitoba (48.6) (Division of Disease Surveillance et al, 1998).

INFECTIOUS SYPHILIS

The rates for infectious syphilis continue to decline to a national rate in 1996 of 0.3/100,000 (81 cases) (Division of Disease Surveillance et al, 1998). There needs to be a focus on screening and follow-up, especially of women at high risk in their childbearing years to prevent transmission to future children.

Bibliography

Division of Disease Surveillance, Bureau of Infectious Diseases, Laboratory Centre for Disease Control: *Notifiable diseases annual summary 1996*, Ottawa, 1998, Health Canada.

Division of HIV/AIDS Surveillance, Bureau of HIV/AIDS, STDs and TB, Laboratory Centre for Disease Control: *HIV and AIDS in Canada, surveillance report to December 31, 1997*, Ottawa, 1998, Health Canada.

Health Canada, The AIDS/HIV Files: *AIDS*, Ottawa, 1998, Author

Health Canada, HIV/AIDS Epi Update: *AIDS and HIV in Canada 1998*, Ottawa, 1998a, Laboratory Centre for Disease Control.

Health Canada, HIV/AIDS Epi Update: *HIV/AIDS epidemiology among aboriginal people in Canada*, Ottawa, 1998b, Laboratory Centre for Disease Control.

Health Canada, HIV/AIDS Epi Update: *HIV /AIDS among injection drug users*, Ottawa, 1998c, Laboratory Centre for Disease Control.

Health Canada, HIV/AIDS Epi Update: *HIV /AIDS among men who have sex with men*, Ottawa, 1998d, Laboratory Centre for Disease Control.

Health Canada, HIV/AIDS Epi Update: *HIV testing among Canadians*, Ottawa, 1998e, Laboratory Centre for Disease Control.

Health Canada, HIV/AIDS Epi Update: *Perinatally Acquired HIV Infection*, Ottawa, 1998f, Laboratory Centre for Disease Control.

Health Canada, Paediatrics and Child Health Volume 3 Supp B. *Current immunization programs in Canadian provinces and territories*, Ottawa, 1998g, Laboratory Centre for Disease Control.

Laboratory Centre for Disease Control, Health Protection Branch: *Acute Hepatitis B incidence in Canada*, Canada Communicable Disease Report, vol 23-7, Ottawa, 1997, Health Canada.

Remis R: *Laboratory Centre for Disease Control, Health Protection Branch*, Ottawa, 1995, Health Canada.

Canadian spelling is used.

Infection with HBV results in either acute or chronic HBV infection. The acute infection is self-limited, and individuals develop an antibody to the virus and successfully eliminate the virus from the body. They subsequently have lifelong immunity against the virus. Symptoms range from mild symptoms that resemble flu to a more severe response that includes jaundice, extreme lethargy, nausea, fever, and joint pain. Any of these more severe symptoms may result in hospitalization. A second possible outcome from infection is chronic HBV infection, which occurs in 1% to 6% of infected adults (CDC, 1998b). These individuals are unable to rid their bodies of the virus and remain lifelong carriers of the hepatitis B surface antigen (HbsAg). As carriers, they are able to transmit the HBV to others. They may develop hepatic carcinoma or chronic active hepatitis. The signs and symptoms of chronic hepatitis B include anorexia, fatigue, abdominal discomfort, hepatomegaly, and jaundice.

Strategies for preventing HBV infection include immunization, prevention of nosocomial and occupational exposure, and prevention of sexual and injection drug use exposure. Vaccination is recommended for persons with occupational risk, such as health care workers, and for children. The series of vaccines required for protection from HBV consists of three intramuscular injections, with the second and third doses administered 1 and 6 months after the first (Centers for Disease Control, 1991). All pregnant women should be tested for hepatitis B surface antigen (HbsAg), which indicates whether they carry and are able to transmit HBV (Immunization Action Coalition, 1996). If the mother is positive, newborns require hepatitis B immune globulin in addition to the hepatitis B vaccine at birth, then at 1 and 6 months thereafter (CDC, 1996b). Hepatitis B immune globulin is given after exposure to provide passive immunity and thus prevent infection.

OSHA regulations

In 1992 the Occupational Safety and Health Administration (OSHA) released the standard "Occupational Exposure to Bloodborne Pathogens," (OSHA 1992), which mandates specific activities to protect workers from HBV and other bloodborne pathogens. Potential exposures for health care workers are needle-stick injuries and mucous membrane splashes. The OSHA standard requires employers to identify the risk of blood exposure to various employees. If employees do work that involves a potential exposure to others' body fluids, employers are mandated to offer the HBV vaccine to the employee at the employer's expense and annual educational programs on preventing HBV and HIV exposure in the workplace. Employees have the right to refuse the vaccine.

Herpes Simplex Virus 2 (Genital Herpes)

Herpes virus infects genital and nongenital sites. Herpes simplex virus 1 (HSV-1) primarily causes nongenital lesions such as cold sores that may appear on the lip or mouth. Herpes simplex virus 2 (HSV-2) is the primary cause of **genital herpes.**

Because there is no cure for HSV-2 infection, it is considered a chronic disease. The virus is transmitted through direct exposure and infects the genitalia and surrounding skin. After the initial infection, the virus remains latent in the sacral nerve of the central nervous system and may reactivate periodically with or without visible vesicles.

Signs and symptoms of HSV-2 infection include the presence of painful lesions that begin as vesicles and ulcerate and crust within 1 to 4 days (Fig. 39-5). Lesions may occur on the vulva, vagina, upper thighs, buttocks, and penis and have an average duration of 11 days. The vesicles can cause itching and pain and may be accompanied by dysuria or rectal pain. Although infectivity is higher with

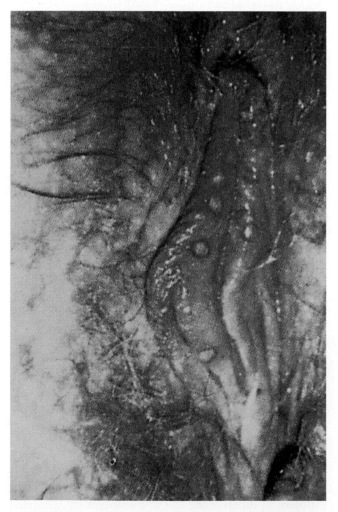

FIG. 39-5 Pustular herpes simplex virus vulvar lesions. (Photograph used with permission of Philip Mead, MD. Reproduced with permission of Glaxo-Wellcome Inc.)

active lesions, some individuals can spread the virus even when they are asymptomatic. Approximately 50% of people experience a prodromal phase. This may include a mild, tingling sensation up to 48 hours before eruption or shooting pains in the buttocks, legs, or hips up to 5 days before eruption (Corey, 1990).

A national survey has identified that one in five Americans is infected with genital herpes, and that it has increased 20% in the last 30 years (Fleming et al, 1997) . The number of people who become infected annually is estimated to be 724,000, and because it is incurable, the prevalence has increased (Fleming et al, 1997). The prevalence is likely to be under-rated because HSV-2 is difficult to identify due to the large proportion of subclinical cases.

The consequences of HSV-2 are of particular concern for women and their children. HSV-2 infection is linked with the development of cervical cancer. There is also an increased risk of spontaneous abortion and risk of transmission to the newborn during vaginal delivery (Brown, et al, 1997). A pregnant woman who has active lesions at the time of birth should have a cesarean delivery before the rupture of amniotic membranes to avoid fetal contact with the herpetic lesions. Mortality for infected neonates is estimated to be as high as 80%, and neurological damage is a major complication (Martens, 1994). The possibility of intrauterine transmission has not been eliminated because some infected neonates are born to women who are asymptomatic at delivery or have had no history of genital HSV (Stone et al, 1989).

Human Papillomavirus Infection

Human papillomavirus (HPV), also called genital warts, can infect the genitals, anus, and mouth. Transmission of HPV occurs through direct contact with warts that result from HPV. However, HPV has been detected in semen, and exposure to the virus through body fluids is also possible. **Genital warts** are most commonly found on the penis and scrotum in men and the vulva, labia, vagina, and cervix in women. Fig. 39-6 shows the textured surface of the lesions, sometimes described as a cauliflower appearance. The warts are usually multiple and vary between 1 and 5 mm in diameter. They may be difficult to visualize, so careful examination is required.

The number of new cases annually of genital HPV infection is estimated to be 500,000 to 1,000,000 (IOM, 1997). Between 10% and 20% of American women of childbearing age and between 5% and 19% of women visiting family planning and university student health clinics (Aral and Holmes, 1990) are infected with genital HPV. As with genital herpes, the actual prevalence is difficult to ascertain because it is not a reported disease, and many infections are subclinical.

Complications of HPV infection are especially serious for women. The link between HPV infection and cervical cancer has been established and is associated with specific types of the virus. It is estimated that 15% of untreated high-grade lesions resulting from HPV develop into cervical cancer (Crum and Nuovo, 1991). HPV infection is exacerbated in both pregnancy and old age as a result of a decrease in cell-mediated immune functioning. HPV may infect the fetus during pregnancy and can result in laryngeal papilloma that can obstruct the infant's airway. Genital warts may enlarge and become friable during pregnancy, and therefore surgical removal may be recommended.

> **DID YOU KNOW?** *The challenge of HPV prevention is that condoms don't necessarily prevent infection. Warts may grow where barriers, such as condoms, do not cover and skin-to-skin contact may occur.*

Because there is no cure for HPV, the goal of therapy is to eliminate the lesions. Genital warts spontaneously disappear over time, as do skin warts. However, because the condition is worrisome for the client and HPV may lead to the development of cervical neoplasia, treatment of the lesions through surgical removal, cytotoxic agents, or immunotherapies is often used.

NURSE'S ROLE IN PREVENTING STDS AND PROVIDING RELATED SERVICES

From prevention to treatment the nurse functions as a counselor, educator, advocate, case manager, and primary care provider. Appropriate interventions for primary, secondary, and tertiary prevention are reviewed. The following discussion of primary prevention applies the nursing

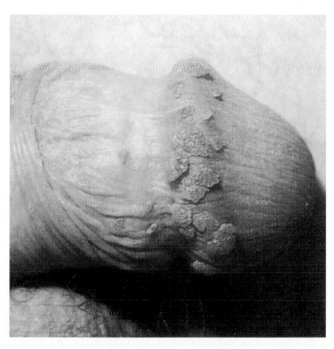

FIG. 39-6 Genital warts. (Photograph used with permission of Lewis Kaminester, MD. Reproduced with permission of Glaxo-Wellcome Inc.)

process to the care of clients with STDs. Nurses are in ideal roles to affect the outcomes often associated with STDs, and their influence begins with primary prevention.

Primary Prevention

Primary prevention consists mainly of activities to keep people healthy before the onset of disease. This begins with assessing for risk behavior and providing relevant intervention through education on how to change risky behaviors.

> **NURSING TIP**
>
> *Assessing a client's risk of acquiring an STD should be done with all sexually active individuals. Such risk assessment should be included as baseline assessment data of those attending all clinics and those who receive school health, occupational health, public health, and home nursing services.*

Assessment

To assess the risk of acquiring STDs, the nurse obtains a sexual and injection drug use history for clients and their partners. The sexual history provides information about the need for specific diagnostic tests, treatment modalities, and partner notification. It also facilitates evaluation of risk factors and is necessary for the nurse to be able to provide relevant education for the client's lifestyle.

A thorough sexual history should include information about the types of relationships, the number of sexual partners and encounters, and types of sexual behaviors practiced. The confidential nature of the information and how it will be used should be shared with the client to establish open communication and goal directed interaction.

Most clients feel uneasy disclosing such personal information. The nurse can ease this discomfort by remaining supportive and open during the interview to facilitate honesty about intimate activities. The nurse serves as a model for discussing sensitive information in a candid manner. When discussing precautions, direct and simple language should be used to describe specific behaviors. This encourages the client to openly discuss sexuality during this interaction and with future partners.

Nurses who are uncomfortable discussing topics such as sexual behavior or sexual orientation are likely to avoid assessing risk behaviors with the client. They will, consequently, be ineffective in identifying risks and in assisting the client in modifying them. It is important that nurses become adept at these skills to prevent and control STDs. Nurses can gain confidence in conducting sexual risk assessments by understanding their own values and feelings about sexuality and realizing that the purpose of the interaction is to improve the client's health. The nurse's comfort in discussing sexual behavior can be improved through practicing role-plays of assessments of sexual and injection drug-using behavior and contracting with clients to make behavior changes.

HOW TO *Improve Taking a Sexual History*

1. *Remain supportive and open to facilitate honesty.*
2. *Use terms client will understand (may need to suggest multiple terms).*
3. *Speak candidly so the client will feel comfortable talking.*
4. *Ask questions in a nonthreatening and nonjudgmental manner.*
5. *Acknowledge that many people are uneasy disclosing personal information.*

Identifying the total number of sexual and injection drug using partners and the number of contacts with these partners provides information about the client's risk. The chance of exposure decreases as the number of partners decreases, so people in mutually monogamous relationships are at low risk for acquiring STDs. This information can be obtained by asking, "How many sex (or drug) partners have you had over the past 6 months?" It is important to avoid assumptions about the sexual partner or partners based on the client's gender, age, race, or any other factor. Stereotypes and assumptions about who people are and what they do are common problems that keep interviewers from asking the right questions that lead to obtaining useful information. For example, it should not be taken for granted that if a male is homosexual he always has more than one partner. Be aware also that the long incubation of HIV and the subclinical phase of many STDs lead some monogamous individuals to assume erroneously that they are not at risk.

It is important to identify whether the person has sexual contact with men, women, or both. This information can be obtained by simply asking, "Do you have sex with men, women, or both?" This lets the client know that the nurse is open to hearing about these behaviors, and thus the nurse is more likely to obtain information that is relevant to sexual practices and risk. Women who are exclusively lesbian are at low risk for acquiring STDs, but bisexual women may transmit STDs between male and female partners. In addition, it is possible for men to have sexual contact with other men and not label themselves as homosexual. Therefore education to reduce risk that is aimed at homosexual males will not be heeded by men who do not see themselves as homosexual. In such situations the nurse can ask, "When was the last time you had sex with another male?"

Certain sexual practices are more likely to result in exposure to and transmission of STDs. Dangerous sexual activities include unprotected anal or vaginal intercourse, oral-anal contact, and insertion of finger or fist into the rectum. These practices introduce a high risk of transmission of enteric organisms or result in physical trauma during sexual encounters. The nurse can obtain information about sexual encounters by asking, "Can you tell me the kinds of sexual practices in which you engage? This will help determine what risks you may have and the type of

---

BOX 39-4 Condoms and Chemical Barriers

Most agency protocols recommend the use of latex condoms. Some may be lubricated with **nonoxynol-9**, a spermicide that is believed to have virucidal properties. The effectiveness of chemical barriers such as nonoxynol-9 has not yet been determined. There is greater emphasis being placed on researching potential chemical barriers as a method of preventing STDs because women control their use. However, for some women, chemical barriers may result in extravasation of the vaginal lining and cervix and therefore may provide breaks in tissue to facilitate transmission of some STDs (Berer, 1992).

---

tests we should do." Clients who engage in genital-anal, oral-anal, or oral-genital contact will need throat and rectal cultures for some STDs as well as cervical and urethral cultures.

Drug use is linked to STD transmission in several ways. Sexual enhancers, such as alcohol or other drugs, put people at risk because they can impair judgment about engaging in risky behaviors. Drugs such as crack cocaine or amyl nitrate (also referred to as poppers) can cause the ability to have multiple orgasms. This increases both the frequency of sexual contacts and the chances of contracting STDs. Addiction to a drug may lead to intense craving of the drug and to trading sex for the drug. Thus the nurse should obtain information on the type and frequency of drug use and the presence of risk behaviors.

The use of oral contraception or Norplant is also important to ascertain, because many clients will believe they are safe and do not have to use barrier precautions such as condoms. Use of contraceptives has been found to decrease condom use (Frank et al, 1993).

Intervention

Based on the information obtained in the sexual history and risk assessment, the nurse is able to identify specific education and counseling needs of the client. Nursing interventions focus on contracting with clients to change behavior and achieving less risky outcomes in regard to sexual practice.

Safer sex. Sexual abstinence is the best way to prevent STDs. However, for many people, sexual abstinence is undesirable; thus information about making sexual behavior safer must be taught. Safer sexual activities include masturbation on intact skin, dry kissing, touching, fantasy, and vaginal and oral sex with a condom. Box 39-4 provides information about condoms.

The use of condoms can prevent the exchange of body fluids during sexual activity. If used correctly and consistently, condoms can prevent both pregnancy and STDs. Although the failure rate of condoms has been estimated to be 3.1%, this is believed to be related to incorrect use rather than condom failure (Novello et al, 1993). Thus information about their proper use and how to communicate about them with a partner is also necessary. The nurse has many opportunities to counsel individuals about this information. Instruction about how to use condoms is presented below. Box 39-4 discusses the pros and cons of using condoms that have chemical lubricants.

HOW TO *Use a Condom*

Correct use of a latex condom requires the following:
1. *Using a new condom with each act of intercourse*
2. *Carefully handling the condom to avoid damaging it with fingernails, teeth, or other sharp objects*
3. *Putting on the condom after the penis is erect and before any genital contact with the partner*
4. *Ensuring no air is trapped in the tip of the condom*
5. *Ensuring adequate lubrication during intercourse, possibly requiring use of exogenous lubricants*
6. *Using only water-based lubricants (e.g., K-Y Jelly or glycerin) with latex condoms; oil-based lubricants (e.g., petroleum jelly, shortening, mineral oil, massage oils, body lotions, or cooking oil) that can weaken latex should never be used*
7. *Holding the condom firmly against the base of the penis during withdrawal and withdrawing while the penis is still erect to prevent slippage.*
8. *Condoms should be stored in a cool, dry place out of direct sunlight and should not be used after the expiration date. Condoms in damaged packages or condoms that show obvious signs of deterioration (e.g., brittleness, stickiness, or discoloration) should not be used regardless of their expiration date.*

Modified from Centers for Disease Control and Prevention: *MMWR* 42(30):520, 1993.

Condom use may be viewed as inconvenient, messy, or decreasing sensation. Moreover, alcohol use may accompany sexual activity, which also may decrease condom use (Hale, 1996). The nurse can encourage clients to become more skilled in discussing safer sex through role modeling and can suggest that condom application be incorporated as part of foreplay. Table 39-5 describes common reasons for refusing to use condoms and ways clients can encourage partners to use them.

Female condoms can also be a barrier to body fluid contact and therefore protect against pregnancy and STDs. The main advantage of the female condom is that its use is controlled by the woman. Made of polyurethane, it may be used if a latex sensitivity develops to regular male condoms. Symptoms of latex allergy include penile, vaginal or rectal itching or swelling after use of a male condom or diaphragm. The female condom consists of a sheath over two rings, with one closed end that fits over the cervix (Fig. 39-7). The cost is about $3 per condom. Figure 39-8 provides instructions on its insertion.

Clients should understand that it is important to know the risk behavior of their sexual partners, including a history of injection drug use and STDs, bisexuality, and any current symptoms. This is because each sexual partner is potentially exposed to all the STDs of all the persons with whom the other partner has been sexually active.

Drug use. **Injection drug use** is risky because the potential for injecting pathogens exists when needles and syringes are shared. During injection drug use, small quantities of drugs are repeatedly injected. Blood is withdrawn into the syringe and is then injected back into the user's vein. Individuals should be advised against using injectable drugs and sharing needles, syringes, or other drug paraphernalia. If equipment is shared, it should be in contact with full-strength bleach for 30 seconds, and then rinsed with water several times to prevent injecting bleach (CDC, 1994d).

People who inject drugs are difficult to reach for health care services. Effective outreach programs include using community peers, increasing accessibility of drug treatment programs combined with HIV testing and counseling, and long-term repeat contacts after completion of the program (CDC, 1990b).

Community outreach. Because of the illegal nature of injectable drugs and the poverty associated with HIV, many people at risk do not have the inclination or resources to seek health care. Nurses may work to establish programs within communities, because the opportunities for counseling on the prevention of HIV and other STDs are increased by bringing services into the neighborhoods of those at risk. Workers go into communities to disseminate information on safer sex, drug treatment programs, and discontinuation of drug use or safer drug use practices (e.g. using new needles and syringes with each injection). Some programs provide sterile needles and syringes, condoms, and literature on anonymous test sites.

WHAT DO YOU THINK? *Several healthcare experts have recommended that sterile needles be given out to injection drug users as a way to prevent HIV. Others have said it supports drug use.*

Community education. Providing accurate health information to large numbers of people is vital for preventing the spread of STDs. Nurses provide educational sessions to community groups about HIV and other STDs. Such educational sessions are most effective in settings where groups normally meet and may include schools, businesses, or churches. When addressing groups about HIV infection, it is important to discuss the number of people who are diagnosed with AIDS, the number infected, modes of transmission of the virus, how to prevent infection, common symptoms of illness, the need for a compassionate response to those afflicted, and available community resources. Teaching about other STDs can be incorporated into these presentations because the mode of transmission (sexual contact) is the same. Other information on these diseases can include the distribution, incidence, and consequences of the infection for individuals and society.

Evaluation

Evaluation is based on whether risky behavior is changed to safe behavior and, ultimately, whether illness is prevented. Condom use is evaluated for consistency of use if the client is sexually active. Other behaviors can be evaluated for their implementation, such as abstinence or monogamy. At the community level, behavioral surveys can be done to measure reported condom use and condom sales, and measures of STD incidence and prevalence can be calculated to evaluate the effectiveness of intervention (APHA, 1991).

Secondary Prevention

Secondary prevention includes screening for STDs to insure their early identification and treatment and follow-up with sex and drug-using partners to prevent further spread.

TABLE 39-5 Discussing Condoms with Resistant, Defensive, or Manipulative Partners

PARTNER RESPONSE	REJOINDER
YOU DON'T NEED IT	
"I'm on the pill. You don't need a condom."	"I'd like to use it anyway. It protects us both from infections we may not realize we have."
"I know I'm clean (disease free); I haven't had sex with anyone in X months."	"Thanks for telling me. As far as I know, I'm disease free too. But I'd still like to use a condom because either of us could have an infection and not know it."
"I'm a virgin."	"I'm not. This protects us both and the relationship."
IT'S A TURNOFF	
"I can't feel a thing when I wear a condom; it's like wearing a raincoat in the shower."	"I know there is some loss of sensation, but there's still plenty left."
"I'll lose my erection by the time I stop and put it on."	"Maybe I can help you put it on—that might give you extra sensations, too."
"By the time you put it on, I'm out of the mood."	"I know it's distracting, but what we feel for each other is strong enough to help us stay in the mood."
"It destroys the romantic atmosphere."	"It doesn't have to be that way. It may be a little awkward the first time or two, but that will pass."
"It's so messy and smells funny."	"Well, sex is that way, but this way, we'll be safe."
"Condoms are unnatural, fake, and a total turnoff."	"There's nothing great about genital infections either. Please let's try to work this out—either give the condom a try or let's look for alternatives."
ALTERNATIVES	
"What alternative do you have in mind?"	"Just petting and maybe some manual stimulation. Or we could postpone orgasm, even though I know we both want it."
MANIPULATIVE PLOYS	
"This is an insult! You seem to think I'm some sort of disease-ridden slut or gigolo."	"I didn't say or imply that. I care about us both and about our relationship. In my opinion, it's best to use a condom."
"None of my other boyfriends use a condom. A real man is not afraid."	"Please don't compare me to them. A real man cares about the women he dates, himself, and their relationship."
"You didn't make Jerry use a condom when you went out with him."	"It bothers me that you and Jerry talk about me that way. If you believe everything Jerry says, I won't argue with you."
"I love you! Would I give you an infection?"	"Not intentionally, of course not. But many people don't know they're infected. I feel this is best for both of us at this time."
"Just this once."	"Once is all it takes."
"I don't have a condom with me."	"I do" or "This time, we can satisfy each other without intercourse."
"You carry a condom around with you?! You were planning to seduce me!"	"I always carry one with me because I care about myself. I made sure I had one with me tonight because I care about us both."
"I won't have sex with you if you're going to use a condom."	"Let's put it off then, until we have a chance to work out our differences" or "OK. But can we try some other things besides intercourse?"

From Greico A: *Medical Aspects Hum Sex* 21:78, 1987. Copyright ©1987 by QUADRANT HEALTHCOM, Inc.

In general, client teaching and counseling should include preventing reinfection with a curable STD, managing symptoms, and preventing the infection of others with chronic STDs. Testing and counseling for HIV are discussed below.

Testing for HIV

The nurse should recommend that persons who have engaged in high-risk behavior be tested. The following people are considered at risk and should be offered the HIV antibody test: those with a history of STDs (which are transmitted through the same behavior and may decrease immune functioning), multiple sex partners, or injection drug use; those who have intercourse without using a condom; those who have intercourse with someone who has another partner and those who have had sex with a prostitute; males with a history of homosexual or bisexual activity; those who have been a sexual partner to anyone in one of these groups; and those who underwent blood transfusion between January 1978 and March 1985.

If HIV infection is discovered before the onset of symptoms, the disease process can be monitored for changes, such as a decrease in the CD4 lymphocyte count or viral load. Prophylactic therapy with antibiotics or protease inhibitors may be started early in the infection to delay the onset of symptomatic illness. Thus, testing enables clients to benefit from early detection and treatment, as well as risk-reduction education.

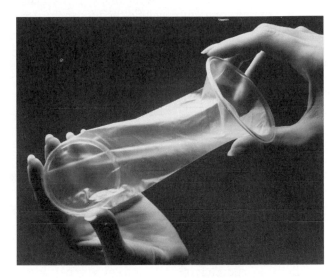

FIG. 39-7 Female condom. (Photograph courtesy of The Female Health Company, Chicago, Ill.)

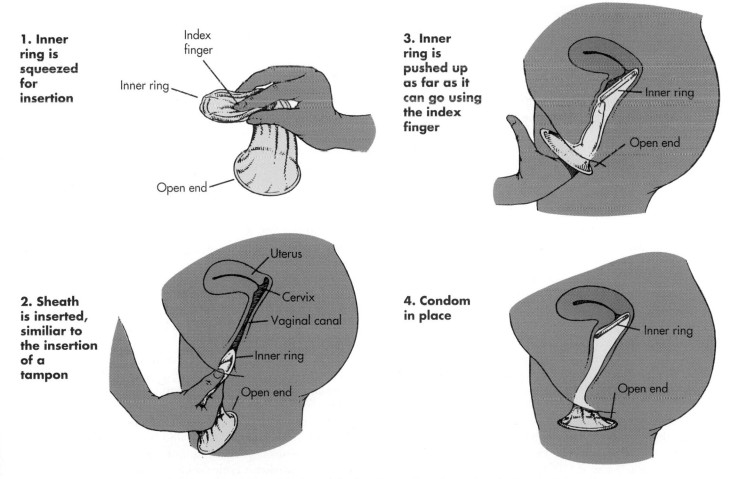

1. Inner ring is squeezed for insertion

Index finger

Inner ring

Open end

2. Sheath is inserted, similiar to the insertion of a tampon

Uterus

Cervix

Vaginal canal

Inner ring

Open end

3. Inner ring is pushed up as far as it can go using the index finger

Inner ring

Open end

4. Condom in place

Inner ring

Open end

FIG. 39-8 Insertion and positioning of the female condom. (Reproduced with permission of The Female Health Company, Chicago, Ill.)

HIV test counseling

An important facet of care is counseling regarding the HIV antibody test. It is essential that the client understand that the antibody test is not diagnostic for AIDS but is indicative of HIV infection. The key activities performed by the nurse during counseling include the following: assessing risk, discussing risk behaviors and how to overcome barriers to change, contracting between the client and the nurse to implement a risk reduction plan, and establishing the follow-up appointment to receive test results and posttest counseling.

Pretest counseling. During pretest counseling the nurse conducts the actual risk assessment, along with relevant teaching as described in the primary prevention section earlier in this chapter. Other activities include exploring how clients will cope with a positive test and assessing support systems. Asking clients to review how they have handled difficult situations in the past can determine how they might cope with learning they are HIV-positive.

Also, during this time, the client is told who will have access to the test results. Although AIDS is reported nationally, the reporting of HIV infection varies among states. States that mandate the reporting of HIV infection are shown in Table 39-3 earlier in the chapter.

Because there is no cure or vaccine available, preventing the transmission of HIV requires a risk assessment of the client's behavior and counseling on how to reduce identified risks. Sexually active individuals who have multiple partners must be encouraged to abstain, to enter a mutually monogamous relationship, or to use condoms. Injection drug users should be advised to enter a treatment program or discontinue drug use. If they continue to use drugs, they should be warned not to share needles, syringes, or any other drug paraphernalia.

Posttest counseling. Persons who have a negative test result are HIV negative, and they should be counseled about risk reduction activities to prevent any future transmission. It is important that the client understand that the test may not be truly negative, because it does not identify infections that may have been acquired several weeks before the test. As noted earlier, seroconversion takes from 6 to 12 weeks. The client must be aware of the means of viral transmission and how to avoid infection.

If pretest counseling was adequate, clients ideally have contemplated the meaning of a positive test result. All clients who are antibody positive should be counseled about the need for reducing their risks and notifying partners. If the client is unwilling or hesitant to notify past partners, partner notification or contact tracing, as described below, is often done by the nurse. The client should visit a primary health care provider so physical evaluation can be performed and, if indicated, antiviral or other therapies begun. Box 39-5 describes responsibilities of an individual who is HIV-positive.

Psychosocial counseling is indicated when positive HIV test results precipitate acute anxiety, depression, or suicidal

---

BOX 39-5 Responsibilities of Persons Who Are HIV Infected

- Have regular medical evaluations and follow-ups.
- Do not donate blood, plasma, body organs, other tissues, or sperm.
- Take precautions against exchanging body fluids during sexual activity.
- Inform sexual or injection drug–using partners of their potential exposure to HIV or arrange for notification through the health department.
- Inform health care providers of their HIV infection.
- Consider the risk of perinatal transmission and follow up with contraceptive use.

---

ideation. Follow-up counseling sessions and telephone calls are important to monitor the client's status. The client should be informed about available counseling services. The person should be cautioned to consider carefully who should be informed of the test results. Many individuals have told others about their HIV-positive test, only to experience isolation and discrimination. Plans for the future should be explored, and clients should be advised to avoid stress, drugs, and infections to maintain optimal health.

Partner notification

Partner notification, also known as contact tracing, is a public health intervention aimed at controlling STDs. It is done by confidentially identifying and notifying exposed sexual and injection drug-using partners of those found to have reportable STDs. Partner notification programs usually occur in conjunction with reportable disease requirements and are carried out by most health departments.

Individuals diagnosed with a reportable STD are asked to provide the names and locations of their partners so that they can be informed of their exposure and obtain the necessary treatment. Clients may be encouraged to notify their partners and to encourage them to seek treatment. If the client agrees to do so, suggestions on how to tell partners and how to deal with possible reactions may be explored. In some instances, clients may feel more comfortable if the nurse notifies those who are exposed. If clients contact their partners about possible infection, the nurse contacts health care providers or clinics to verify examination of exposed partners.

If the client prefers not to participate in notifying partners, the nurse contacts them—often by a home visit—and counsels them to seek evaluation and treatment. The client is offered literature regarding treatment, risk reduction, and the test site's location and hours of operation. The identity of the infected client who names sexual and injection drug-using partners cannot be revealed. Maintaining confidentiality is critical with all STDs but particularly with HIV, because antidiscrimination laws may not be in place or may be inadequate.

Tertiary Prevention

Tertiary prevention can apply to many of the chronic STDs, such as HSV, HIV, and untreated syphilis. For viral STDs, much of this effort focuses on managing symptoms and psychosocial support regarding future interpersonal relations. Many clients report feeling contaminated, and support groups may be available to help clients cope with chronic STDs.

Much of the effort in tertiary prevention focuses on clients with AIDS who return home and are unable to provide care for themselves because of progressing illness. The nurse conducts physical assessments and makes recommendations to the family about obtaining additional care services or maintaining the client in the home. Case management is important in all phases of HIV infection but is a particularly important activity in this stage to ensure that clients have adequate services to meet their needs. This may include ensuring that medication can be obtained through identifying funding resources, maintaining infection control standards, reducing risk behaviors, identifying sources of respite care for caretakers, or referring clients for home or hospice care.

Nursing interventions include teaching families about managing symptomatic illness by preventing deteriorating conditions such as diarrhea, skin breakdown, and inadequate nutrition.

Universal precautions/body substance isolation

The importance of teaching caregivers about infection control in home care is vital. Concerns about the transmission of HIV may be expressed by clients, families, friends, and other groups. Whereas fear may be expressed by some, others who are caring for loved ones with HIV may not take adequate precautions such as glove wearing because of concern about appearing as though they do not want to touch a loved one. Others may believe myths that suggest they cannot be infected by someone they love. Inadequate protection of home-based caregivers has become a concern as a result of eight cases of documented transmission of HIV by individuals living with and caring for an HIV-infected person (CDC, 1994c).

Universal precautions must be taught to caregivers in the home setting. All blood and articles soiled with body fluids must be handled as if they were infectious or contaminated by blood-borne pathogens. Gloves should be worn whenever hands will be expected to touch nonintact skin, mucous membranes, blood, or other fluids. A mask, goggles, and gown should also be worn if there is potential for splashing or spraying of infectious material during any care.

All protective equipment should be worn only once and then disposed. If the skin or mucous membranes of the caregiver come in contact with body fluids, the skin should be washed with soap and water, and the mucous membranes should be flushed with water as soon as possible after the exposure. Thorough hand washing with soap and water—a major infection control measure—should be conducted whenever hands become contaminated and whenever gloves or other protective equipment (mask, gown) is removed. Soiled clothing or linen should be washed in a washing machine filled with hot water using bleach as an additive and dried on a hot air cycle of a dryer.

clinical application

Yvonne Jackson is a 20-year-old woman who visits the Hopetown City Health Department's maternity clinic. Examination reveals she is at 14 weeks' gestation. She is single but has been in a steady relationship for the past 6 months with Phil. She states that she has no other children. The results of the HIV test done as part of the routine prenatal workup is positive.

Yvonne reacts with an expression of disbelief about the positive test results. Understanding that this is a common reaction and that Yvonne will not be able to concentrate on all of the questions and information that need to be covered, the nurse prioritizes essential information to obtain and provide during this visit.

A. What questions does the nurse need to ask regarding controlling the spread of HIV to others?

B. What information should the nurse give to Yvonne?

Answers are in the back of the book.

KEY POINTS

- Nearly all STDs are preventable because they are transmitted through specific, known behaviors.
- STDs are some of the most serious public health problems in the United States. HIV infection has been identified as the most urgent public health problem of this century, and there is an increased incidence of drug-resistant gonococcal infection.
- STDs affect certain groups in greater numbers. Factors associated with risk include being under 25 years of age, being a member of a minority group, residing in an urban setting, being impoverished, and using crack cocaine.
- The increasing incidence, morbidity, and mortality of STDs document the need for nurses to educate clients about STD prevention.
- Many STDs do not produce symptoms in clients. Other STDs, such as HPV (genital warts), HIV, and HSV (genital herpes), are associated with cancer.
- Aside from death, the most serious complications caused by STDs are pelvic inflammatory disease, infertility, ectopic pregnancy, neonatal morbidity and mortality, and neoplasia.
- AIDS is the most extreme stage of HIV infection. As more is learned about methods to prevent disease progression, such as effective medications, stress reduction, and proper nutrition, greater emphasis is being placed on early detection and management of HIV infection.
- HIV testing plays an important role in early detection and treatment and provides opportunities for risk and assessment and preventive counseling.

Continued

KEY POINTS—cont'd

- Partner notification, also known as contact tracing, may be done by the infected client or by the health professional. It is done by identifying, contacting, and encouraging evaluation and treatment of sexual and injectable drug–using partners.
- HIV infection has created an entirely new group of people needing health care. This rapidly growing population is straining a health care system that is already unable to meet the needs of many.
- Most of the care that is provided, both home and outpatient care, is done within the community setting, which reduces direct health care costs but increases the need for financial support of home and community health services.

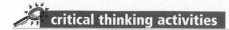 critical thinking activities

1. Identify the number of reported cases of AIDS and the number or reported cases of HIV infection within your state and locale (if reportable in your state). How are the case distributed by age, sex, geographical location, and race?
2. Identify the location or locations of HIV testing services in your community. Are the test results anonymous or confidential? Describe how and to whom the results are reported.
3. Identify counseling and home care services that are available for the person with HIV infection within your community. Are they adequate to meet the needs of those infected? How much do these services cost?
4. Form small groups and role-play a nurse-client interaction involving a risk assessment and counseling regarding safer sex and injection drug-using practices.

Bibliography

American Public Health Association: *Healthy communities 2000 model standards,* ed 3, Washington, DC, 1991, The Association.

Aral SO: The social context of syphilis persistence in the southeastern United States, *Sex Transm Dis* 23(1):9, 1996.

Aral SO, Holmes KK: Epidemiology of sexual behavior and sexually transmitted diseases. In Holmes KK et al, editors: *Sexually transmitted diseases,* New York, 1990, McGraw-Hill.

Berer M: Adverse effects of nonoxynol-9, *Lancet* 340:615, 1992.

Blount J:Personal communication, January 18, 1991.

Brown ZA et al: The acquisition of herpes simplex virus during pregnancy, *N Engl J Med* 337(8):509, 1997.

Centers for Disease Control and Prevention: Guidelines for effective school health education to prevent the spread of AIDS, *MMWR* 37(S-2):1, 1988.

Centers for Disease Control and Prevention: First 100,000 cases of acquired immunodeficiency syndrome: United States, *MMWR* 38:561, 1989.

Centers for Disease Control and Prevention: Nosocomial transmission of hepatitis B virus associated with a spring-loaded fingerstick device-California, *MMWR* 39(35):610, 1990a.

Centers for Disease Control and Prevention: Update: reducing HIV transmission in intravenous-drug users not in drug treatment—United States, *MMWR* 39(31):529, 1990b.

Centers for Disease Control and Prevention: Hepatitis B virus: a comprehensive strategy for eliminating transmission in the United States through universal childhood vaccination-ACIP, *MMWR* 40(RR-13):1, 1991.

Centers for Disease Control and Prevention: Chancroid-United States, 1981-1990: evidence for underreporting of cases, *MMWR* 41(SS-3):57, 1992a.

Centers for Disease Control and Prevention: HIV prevention in the correctional system, 1991, *MMWR* 41(22):389, 1992b.

Centers for Disease Control and Prevention: 1993 revised classification system for HIV infection and expanded surveillance case definition for AIDS among adolescents and adults, *MMWR* 41(RR-17), 1992c.

Centers for Disease Control and Prevention: Recommendations for the prevention and management of chlamydia trachomatis infections, 1993, *MMWR* 42(RR-12), 1993.

Centers for Disease Control and Prevention: Decreased susceptibility of Neisseria gonorrhoeae to fluoroquinolones–Ohio and Hawaii, 1992-1994, *MMWR* 43(18):325, 1994a.

Centers for Disease Control and Prevention: HIV/AIDS surveillance report, *MMWR* 5(4):3, 1994b.

Centers for Disease Control and Prevention: Human immunodeficiency virus transmission in household settings-United States, *MMWR* 43(347):353, 1994c.

Centers for Disease Control and Prevention: Knowledge and practices among injecting-drug users of bleach use for equipment disinfection-New York City, 1993, *MMWR* 43(24):439, 1994d.

Centers for Disease Control and Prevention: 1994 Revised classification system for human immunodeficiency virus infection in children less than 13 years of age, *MMWR* 43(RR-12):1, 1994e.

Centers for Disease Control and Prevention: AIDS among children-United States, *MMWR* 45(46):1006, 1996a.

Centers for Disease Control and Prevention: Prevention of perinantal hepatitis B through enhanced case management–Connecticut, 1994-1995 and United States, 1994, *MMWR* 45(27):584, 1996b.

Centers for Disease Control and Prevention: School-based HIV prevention education–United States, 1994, *MMWR* 45(35):760, 1996c.

Centers for Disease Control and Prevention: CDC reports first-even decline in AIDS diagnoses–treatment and prevention advances spur new trend HIV/AIDS Prevention, December, Atlanta, 1997a, CDC.

Centers for Disease Control and Prevention: Chlamydia trachomatis genital infections–United States, 1995 *MMWR* 46(9):193, 1997b.

Centers for Disease Control and Prevention: Focus on women and HIV, *HIV/AIDS Prevention,* March, Atlanta, 1997c, CDC.

Centers for Disease Control and Prevention: *HIV/AIDS Surveillance Report* 9(1):3,1997d.

Centers for Disease Control and Prevention: CDC, HRSA work to implement CARE act provision, *HIV/AIDS Prevention,* March, Atlanta, 1997e, CDC.

Centers for Disease Control and Prevention: Nosocomial Hepatitis B virus infection associated with resuable fingerstick blood sampling devices–Ohio and New York City, *MMWR* 46(10):217, 1997f.

Centers for Disease Control and Prevention: Summary of notifiable diseases, 1996, *MMWR* 46(53), 1997g.

Centers for Disease Control: AIDS among persons aged >50 years–United States, 1991-1996, *MMWR* 47(2):21, 1998a.

Centers for Disease Control: 1998 guidelines for treatment of sexually transmitted diseases, *MMWR* 47(RR-1), 1998b.

Centers for Disease Control and Prevention: *The role of HIV surveillance as United States enters new era in the epidemic,* http://www.cdc.gov/nchstp/od/surveillances.htm, January, 1998c.

Corey L: Genital herpes. In Holmes KK et al, editors: *Sexually transmitted diseases,* New York, 1990, McGraw-Hill.

Crum CP, Nuovo GJ: *Genital papillomaviruses and related neoplasms,* New York, 1991, Raven Press.

Deguchi T et al: Fluoroquinolone treatment failure in gonorrhea, *Sex Transm Dis* 24(5):247, 1997.

Division of STD Prevention: *Sexually transmitted disease surveillance,* Atlanta, 1996, CDC.

Fleming DT et al: Herpes simplex virus type 2 in the United States, 1976-1984, *N Engl J Med* 337(16):1105, 1997.

Frank ML, Bateman L, Poindexter AN: Planned condom use by women with norplant implants, *Adv Contraception* 9:227, 1993.

Hale PJ: Employer response to AIDS in a low prevalence area, *Fam Community Health* 13(2):38, 1990.

Hale PJ: Women's self-efficacy for the prevention of sexual risk behavior, *Res Nurs Health* 19:101, 1996.

Hellinger F: The lifetime costs of treating a person with HIV, *JAMA* 270:474, 1993.

Hook E, Handsfield H: Gonococcal infections in the adult. In Holmes KK et al, editors: *Sexually transmitted diseases,* New York, 1990, McGraw-Hill.

Immunization Action Coalition Hepatitis B Coalition: *Needle Tips* 6:1, 1996.

Institute of Medicine: *The hidden epidemic: confronting sexually transmitted diseases,* Washington, DC, 1997, National Academy Press.

Krieger JN: Trichomoniasis in men: old issues and new data, *Sex Transm Dis* 22(2):83, 1995.

Levy JA: *HIV and the pathogenesis of AIDS,* Washington, DC, 1998, ASM Press.

Martens KA: Sexually transmitted genital tract infection during pregnancy, *Emerg Med Clin North Am* 12(1):91, 1994.

Novello AC et al: Condom use for the prevention of sexual transmission of HIV infection, *JAMA* 269(22):2840, 1993.

Occupational Health and Safety Administration: *Occupational exposure to bloodborne pathogens,* Richmond, Virginia, 1992, Department of Labor and Industry.

Paisarntantiwong R et al: The relationship of vaginal trichomoniasis pelvic inflammatory disease among women colonized with chlamydia trachomatis, *Sex Transm Dis* 22(6):344, 1995.

Pantaleo G, Grazioso C, Fauci AS: The immunopathogenesis of human immunodeficiency virus infection, *N Engl J Med* 328(5):327, 1993.

Phillips I: Beta-lactamase producing, penicillin-resistant gonococcus, *Lancet* 2:656, 1976.

Schur CL, Berk ML: Health insurance coverage of persons with HIV-related illness: data from the ACSUS screener. In Agency for Health Care Policy Research: *AIDS cost and services utilization survey (ACSUS) Report No 2,* Rockville, Md, 1994, AHCPR.

Shlay JC et al: Human Immunoeficiency virus seroprevalence and risk assessment of a homeless population in Denver, *Sex Transm Dis* 23(4):304, 1996.

Stone K et al: National surveillance for neonatal herpes simplex virus infections, *Sex Transm Dis* 16(3):152, 1989.

US Department of Health and Human Services: *Healthy people 2000: midcourse review and 1995 revisions,* Washington DC, 1996, USDHHS, Public Health Service.

Vlahov D et al: Prognostic indicators for AIDS and infectious disease death in HIV-infected injection drug users: plasma viral load and CD4+ cell count, *JAMA* 279(1):35, 1998.

World Health Organization: *The HIV/AIDS pandemic: 1993 overview.* WHO Global Programme on AIDS, Pub No WHO/GPA/CNP/ EVA/93-1, Geneva, 1993, WHO.

Wortley PM, Fleming PL: AIDS in women in the United States: recent trends, *JAMA* 278:911, 1997.

Zenilman J et al: Penicillinase-producing *Neisseria gonorrhoea* in Dade County, Florida: evidence of core-group transmitters and the impact of illicit antibiotics, *Sex Transm Dis* 15(1):45, 1988.

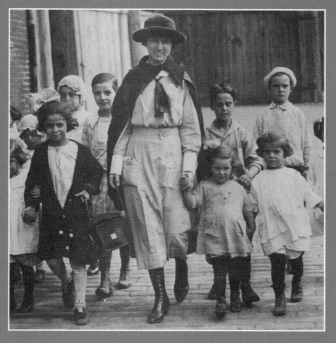

PART Seven

Community and Public Health Nurses: Roles and Functions

At one time the role of the public health nurse primarily included visiting clients at home and identifying cases of communicable disease. Over the decades the role has become multifaceted and now involves community oriented practice. The community health nurse's role is focused on improving the health of individuals and families through the delivery of personal health services with emphasis on primary prevention, health promotion, and health protection. Public health nursing practice emphasizes the delivery of services and interventions aimed at protecting entire populations from illness, disease, and injury. As the health care system has changed, the need for a comprehensive, population-focused public health system has become more evident. Nurses are able to provide care to individuals, families, and communities in a variety of settings and roles.

With increasing emphasis being placed on the community as the client, community health nurses recognize that in order to address community health issues, the nurse must be able to meet the needs of the individuals, families, and groups who are the nucleus of the community. Unlike in the past, when the primary practice setting for the nurse was the hospital, nurses are finding a renewed emphasis on finding their clients in many settings. Regardless of type of client, practice setting, specialty area of practice, or the functional role of the nurse, the community health and public health nurse acts as advocate for clients in meeting their needs through the health care system.

This section discusses the roles of manager, consultant, case manager, clinical nurse specialist, and nurse practitioner with specific emphasis on the development of the advocacy role in community health practice. Throughout the text, content is applicable to a variety of practice settings, including the more traditional public health practice arena, such as the health department. In addition to official agencies, a few other practice settings with close association to community health nursing have been chosen for presentation (e.g., school health, occupational health, home health, and congregational settings).

Community Health Nurse in Home Health and Hospice

LINDA M. SAWYER

OBJECTIVES

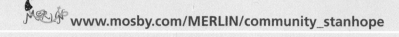

www.mosby.com/MERLIN/community_stanhope

After reading this chapter, the student should be able to do the following:

- Define home health and hospice care.
- Analyze the similarities and differences in the types of home health agencies.
- Discuss the educational requirements and competencies for a home health nurse.
- Relate the nursing process and standards of community health nursing practice to the home health setting.

- Identify the roles and functions of the interdisciplinary health care team.
- Examine the regulatory impact on home health care and nursing practice.
- Analyze the reimbursement mechanisms, issues, and trends relative to home health care.

KEY TERMS

accreditation
benchmarking
care coordination
care planning
certification
charge
client outcomes

cost
distributive care
episodic care
family caregiving
fiscal intermediaries
hospice

interdisciplinary
  collaboration
intermittent care
Outcomes and
  Assessment Information
  Set (OASIS)
palliative care

recertification
regulation
reimbursement system
skilled care
telehealth

See Glossary for definitions

CHAPTER OUTLINE

This chapter presents an important nursing specialty within community health nursing: home health care and the related subspecialty of hospice nursing. Home health differs from other areas of health care in that health care providers practice in the client's environment. Home is a place where nurses have provided care for more than a century in the United States. Nurses provide family care within the context of the community environment.

When working in a client's home, the nurse is a guest and, to be effective, must earn the trust of the family. In this setting nurses have the opportunity to observe family life, a privilege usually reserved for family and friends. Family dynamics; lifestyle choices; communication patterns; coping strategies; responses to health and illness; and social, cultural, spiritual, and economic issues are but a few of the factors nurses assess when visiting in a family's home (Doherty and Hurley, 1994).

Portnoy and Dumas (1994) suggested that when working with an individual client or family in the home the real work is not only within the boundaries of that household. To provide effective, comprehensive care, nurses will want to analyze the strength that clients gain from their neighborhoods, the social network that can be used to support clients in times when they are vulnerable and in crisis. Therefore nurses working in the home will also want to gain the trust of communities by providing for the needs of the clients they serve in that community with caring, honesty, competence, and ethical and cultural sensitivity (Doherty and Hurley, 1994).

The use of home health care continues to expand in response to increased demands for cost-effectiveness, decreased hospital stays, consumer preferences, technologic advancement and simplification, and proven quality of service.

DEFINITION OF HOME HEALTH CARE

Home health care in today's society cannot simply be defined as "care at home." It includes an arrangement of disease prevention, health promotion and episodic illness–related services provided to people in their places of residence. A more comprehensive definition of home health care was prepared by a Department of Health and Human Services interdepartmental work group (Warhola, 1980):

Home health care is that component of a continuum of comprehensive health care whereby health services are provided to individuals and families in their places of residence for the purpose of promoting, maintaining or restoring health, or of maximizing the level of independence while minimizing the effects of disability and illness, including terminal illness. Services appropriate to the needs of the individual client and family are planned, coordinated, and made available by providers organized for the delivery of home care. The agency employed staff, contractual arrangements, or a combination of the two patterns may be used to deliver service.

Home health nursing, according to the American Nurses Association, "refers to the practice of nursing applied to a client with a health condition in the client's place of residence. . . . Home health nursing is a specialized area of nursing practice with its roots firmly placed in community health nursing" (ANA, 1999, p. 3). It involves the same primary preventive focus of care of aggregates of the community health nurses and the secondary and tertiary prevention focuses of the care of individuals in collaboration with the family and other caregivers.

Finally, a third definition, by the National Association of Home Care (NAHC), defines home health care as a broad spectrum of health and social services offered in the home environment to recovering, disabled or chronically ill persons (1994).

These definitions integrate the components of home health care: the individual and family client, caregivers, multidisciplinary health care professionals, and goals to assist the client to return to an optimum level of health and independence. Differences in interpretation and actual delivery of home health care vary according to client needs and the provider and payer of these services.

It is essential to work with the family in the provision of care to an individual client. Family is defined by the individual and includes any caregiver or significant person who assists the client in need of care at home. **Family caregiving** includes assisting clients to meet their basic needs and providing direct care such as personal hygiene, meal preparation, medication administration, and treatments. Care provided in the home today by caregivers was historically only done in the hospital by a health care provider. The caregiver is essential in providing the needed maintenance care between the skilled visits of the professional provider.

A client's place of residence has its own uniqueness in terms of the location for providing care, depending on what the person calls home. Home may be a house, apartment, trailer, boarding and care home, shelter, car, or a makeshift shelter under a bridge or a cardboard box.

Client goals are always related to the principles of health promotion, maintenance, and restoration. By maximizing the level of independence, home health nurses help clients function at the best possible level and prevent dependence. This assistance includes providing a combination of direct care and health education to enhance self-care and through linking the client with community services that provide limited assistance to enable the client to stay at home. In addition, nurses contribute to the prevention of complications in chronically ill persons and help to minimize the effects of disability and illness.

The development of hospice home care programs has improved the care of terminally ill persons. If the client and family accept the hospice concept, most of their care can be handled comfortably at home instead of in the hospital. Reducing of pain and suffering is possible through the use of medications and other measures that are closely supervised by nurses in the home.

In both home health and hospice, nurses continually assess the client's response to treatment modalities, report their findings to the client's physician, and collaborate to modify the treatment plan as needed. Services can be tailored to any client need or problem. When the client's level of independence increases, the need for service decreases. Services are coordinated through an agency obligated to maintain quality care and provide for continuity. Thus the range of services provided in home health care is extensive. The strong connections of home health care to community health nursing practice can be seen by briefly tracing the history of this nursing role.

HISTORY OF HOME HEALTH CARE

Home health care began in the United States in the early 1800s. In these early years, nuns and religious sisters cared for the sick in the home. The Sisters of Charity of St. Joseph was established in Maryland in 1809. The first organized visiting nurse work was done by the Ladies Benevolent Society of Charleston, South Carolina, founded in 1813. At first this society had a visiting committee of 16 ladies who were assigned to a certain portion of the city in which to visit the sick. Later, nurses were hired by the visitors to provide nursing care to the sick at home. This society lasted well over 50 years, until the beginning of the Civil War, and was revived in 1902.

The precursor of modern home care, organized visiting nursing, was established in March 1877 when the women's branch of the New York City Mission sent trained nurses into the homes of the poor and the sick. The first home health nurse, Frances Root, was a member of the Bellevue Hospital Training School's first class. The establishment of the first visiting nurses association (VNA) in the United States occurred in 1885 when Elizabeth Marshall founded the Buffalo District Nursing Association. In 1886 Boston formed the Instructive Visiting Nursing Association. During this same period, Philadelphia's VNA established a pay service.

By 1890, some 13 years after the first nurse was sent out by the New York City Mission, 21 VNAs existed in the United States, most employing only one nurse each. These associations preceded the development, in 1893, of the Henry Street Settlement, founded in New York by Lillian Wald. After 1894, the use of visiting nurses grew rapidly with the country's growing social consciousness (see Chapter 2).

As the demands on nurses visiting in the home increased, nurses began to question whether hospital training was sufficient for public health nurses. The demand for nurses experienced in providing care in the home greatly exceeded the supply of trained nurses. Community after community began nursing associations with untrained nurses. A few undergraduate programs affiliated with a VNA allowed students to leave the hospital for short periods of training in the community. The first postgraduate course in public health nursing was offered in 1906 by the Instructive District Nursing Association of Boston. Following these very simple training programs, Columbia University, in 1910, offered the first university course in public health nursing. This set a precedent for public health nursing education to be provided in universities.

In 1909 the Metropolitan Life Insurance Company began offering home nursing services to its millions of industrial policy holders in the United States and Canada. Initially, arrangements were made with Lillian Wald and the Henry Street Settlement to provide these nursing services. By 1912 Metropolitan was offering home nursing services from 589 nursing centers. These centers provided an opportunity to develop payment mechanisms based on the exact cost of visits to clients and to engage in a number of valuable health studies. Nurses collected data to project future health care needs of policyholders. Sixteen years later, John Hancock Mutual Life Insurance Company established a similar service for its policy holders.

Following the example of the Visiting Nurse Society of Philadelphia (the first to establish a pay service) and of the insurance companies, other nursing organizations began to charge for services. Charges were assessed either on an hourly basis, per visit, or by capitation to meet the needs of those who could pay for these services. The introduction of payment for services marked a change in the philosophy of home nursing services—from providing services only to the "worthy" poor to providing services to people who could afford to pay for the services.

The number of visiting nurses in the United States increased from 136 in 1902 to 3000 in 1912. With funding from both private and public sources, visiting nurses were employed by some 810 agencies, including VNAs, city and state boards of health and education, private clubs and societies, the tuberculosis leagues, hospitals and dispensaries, business concerns, settlements and day nurseries, churches, and charitable organizations.

Public health nursing continued to expand during the 1920s. Then came the dramatic crash of the stock market in October 1929 and the beginning of the financial depression in America. Public health nursing was greatly affected as the budgets of private agencies dwindled and reserve funds disappeared. At the same time, the socioeconomic problems experienced by clients and their families created more need for nursing service. When the country most needed accessible and comprehensive services the quality could not be assured because of reducing staff size, eliminating educational programs, and limited supervision.

At this point, the federal government provided aid to the country and a new relationship among local communities and the state and federal governments developed. The Federal Emergency Relief Administration allocated federal funds to states so that nursing care could be given to the sick receiving federal relief. The Civil Works Administration provided funds for the use of nurses who were unemployed. These nurses worked primarily for official agencies and institutions. A large number of nurses found themselves working in public health without preparation or experience.

In the 1940s, hospitals began to take a more serious interest in home care because of the increased number of chronically ill clients being hospitalized. The Montefiore Hospital Home Care Program in New York began in 1947 and offered comprehensive nursing and social services. Before the enactment of Medicare in 1966, most agencies relied on public contributions and charity for their survival.

Home care reached a turning point with the passage of Medicare, which introduced regulations for home care practice as well as for reimbursement mechanisms. In 1967, one year after Medicare was enacted, there were 1753 Medicare-participating home health agencies in the United States. The majority of agencies were either VNAs or programs in public health departments. By 1980 there were 2924 home health agencies, an increase of about 48%. The Health Care Financing Administration (HCFA) reported 10,027 Medicare-certified home health agencies in 1996, as well as 8034 non–Medicare-certified home health agencies for a total of 18,061. The growth in certified agencies alone represents a 572% growth in 30 years (NAHC, 1998).

WHAT DO YOU THINK? *Throughout its history, home health nurses have epitomized Florence Nightingale's philosophy that nurses are "messengers of health as well as ministers of disease" (Woodham-Smith, 1951).*

The community health nurses working in the home were social reformers, living in immigrant communities and providing nursing clinics, health education, and care for the sick. They provided for the nutritional needs of their communities as well as clothing, hygiene, and adequate shelter. They were responsible for developing needed programs and providing necessary services in communities, including prenatal care, postpartum visits to new mothers and babies, hot lunch school programs, preschool clinics, transportation services, summer camp programs, tuberculosis screening, blood typing, immunization for polio, and "sick room" equipment programs.

This combination of preventive services and illness care continued until the introduction of Medicare in 1966. The Medicare program emphasized an acute disease–care payment program that influenced the services offered through home health and deleted all emphasis on illness prevention and health promotion. Some home health agencies continued to develop programs to benefit their communities, paying for them through their profits or through contributions. Today, a number of agencies are once again offering a combination of preventive and illness care services as a mechanism to decease the long-term costs of health care.

TYPES OF HOME HEALTH CARE AGENCIES

Since the beginning of organized home care, many organizations have established programs to meet the home care needs of people. Home health agencies are divided into the following five general types based on administrative and organizational structures:

- Official
- Private and voluntary
- Combination
- Hospital-based
- Proprietary

These types differ in organization and administration but are similar in terms of the standards they must meet for licensure, certification, and accreditation. Figure 40-1 shows the types of home health agencies. Table 40-1 lists the numbers and kinds of home health agencies, and Box 40-1 presents facts concerning home health agencies.

Official Agencies

Official or public agencies include those agencies operated by the state, county, city, or other local government units, such as health departments. Most official agencies, in addition to having a home care component, also provide health education and disease prevention programs to people in the community.

Community health nurses employed in this setting also provide well-child clinics, immunizations, health education programs, and home visits for preventive health care. Official agencies are funded primarily by tax funds and are nonprofit entities. The home care services provided are reimbursed through Medicare, Medicaid, and private insurance companies. Official agencies offer more comprehensive services for two reasons: their primary objective is health promotion and disease prevention for the community, and they have additional public funding available.

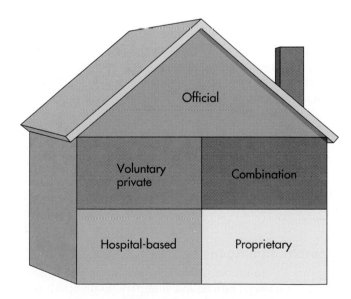

FIG. 40-1 Types of home health agencies.

TABLE 40-1 Number and Kinds of Home Health Agencies

	HOSPITAL	REHABILITATION HOSPITAL	SKILLED NURSING FACILITY	VISITING NURSE ASSOCIATION (VNA)	COMBINATION AGENCY	PUBLIC	PROPRIETARY (NONPROFIT)	PRIVATE	OTHER	TOTAL
1967	133	0	0	549	93	939	0	0	30	1753
1980	359	8	9	515	63	1260	186	484	40	2924
1990	1486	8	101	474	47	985	1884	710	0	5695
1996	2634	4	191	576	34	1177	4658	695	58	10,027

From Health Care Financing Administration, Center for Information Systems, Health Standards and Quality Bureau, Washington DC, 1997, Department of Health and Human Services.

BOX 40-1 Home Health and Hospice Facts

- Medicare-certified agencies in 1996 totaled 20,215 (10,027 home health agencies, 2154 hospice agencies, 8034 other)
- Average cost per home visit: $77 in 1997
- Medicare: $20.5 billion in 1997 for 306,116,000 visits to 3,910,000 clients
- Medicaid: $9.4 billion in 1995 for 1,639,000 clients

From Health Care Financing Administration, Center for Information Systems, Health Standards and Quality Bureau, Washington DC, 1997, Department of Health and Human Services.

Voluntary and Private Nonprofit Agencies

Voluntary and private agencies are grouped together as nonprofit home health agencies. Voluntary agencies are supported by charities such as United Way, as well as by Medicare, Medicaid, other third-party payers, and client payments. The amount of financial assistance the voluntary agency receives depends on the community it serves. Traditionally, VNAs were the principal voluntary type of home health agency. With Medicare in 1966, the private nonprofit agency emerged as an alternative agency to the public-supported program. These agencies included rehabilitation agencies, based in either rehabilitation facilities or in skilled facilities.

Boards of directors that represent the communities they serve govern voluntary and private nonprofit agencies. These agencies are nongovernmental organizations and are exempt from federal income tax. Historically, voluntary agencies were responsible for the initial development of nursing in the home, based on the client's need for service rather than the ability to pay.

Combination Agencies

In some communities, to decrease cost and prevent duplicating of services, official and voluntary home health agencies have merged into combination agencies to provide home health care. The services remain the same, and the board members come from either one of the two existing agencies or a new board is formed. The nurse may serve in several community health nursing roles, as does the nurse in the official type of agency.

Hospital-Based Agencies

Hospitals are frequently a primary site for health care services. In the 1970s, hospital-based agencies emerged in response to the recognized need for continuity of care from the acute care setting and also because of the high cost of institutionalization.

In 1983 implementation of the prospective payment system and diagnosis related groups (DRGs) by the federal government caused a fundamental change in the attitudes of hospital personnel toward home care. Cost of care dictated earlier discharge of sicker clients to control profits. Increased liability risks, the desire for better client care, and the potential for several products and services increased the number of hospital-based home care agencies (Cassak, 1984).

Hospital-based agencies differ from other home health care agencies in that the already-established hospital board of directors is responsible for governing the agency. Moreover, clients of hospital-based home health care have access to existing inpatient services. Whether the agencies are official, voluntary, private nonprofit, or proprietary depends on the hospital structure. Regardless of the form they take, in most cases these agencies are a source of revenue for the hospital and may compete with community-based agencies. Hospital-based agencies outnumber all other types of Medicare-certified agencies except for proprietary agencies (NAHC, 1997).

Proprietary Agencies

Agencies that are not eligible for income tax exemption are called proprietary (profit-making) agencies. Proprietary agencies can be licensed and certified for Medicare by the state licensing agency. The owner of the agency is responsible for governing. Reimbursement is primarily from third-party payers and individual clients if agencies do not accept Medicare. In recent years the number of Medicare-certified proprietary agencies increased significantly as hospitals began implementing quicker discharge of sicker patients (NAHC, 1997).

Managed care and the development of alliances and networks are changing the structure of the health care delivery system. As discussed in Chapter 5, these changes have introduced managed competition into the health care environment. Agencies are reacting to managed competition with a couple of strategies. The first is the creation of a provider network that becomes contracting partners and low-cost providers. A second response to managed competition is the acquisition of or merger with other agencies to gain strength, lower costs, or increase power to compete (McClure, 1994).

Although in 1995 home health care represented only 4% of all health care expenses (Levit et al, 1996), it is the fastest growing market in 1999. Home care and community-based services are projected to increase with continued decreases in institutional services, such as hospitals. Thus home care agencies are expected to move in one of two directions. An agency may either become a contracted partner in a network to provide home care services for a hospital, an HMO, a group of physicians and others, or it may be purchased by other agencies and become the sole provider of home care for that agency. Both of these arrangements are opportunities for nurses to highlight primary prevention and health promotion in their practice. This can reduce the likelihood that clients will need more costly services such as hospital care offered through their network. As a result, home health agencies and nurses need to participate in case management while understanding the cost of care of each client (Dee-Kelly et al, 1994).

Regardless of the type of home health agency existing in a community, the primary goal should be to provide quality home health care based on the community's health needs. Traditionally, most agencies have remained noncompetitive because of their humanitarian mission. Today competition in home health care is on the rise as a result of the federal government's move to deregulate and deinstitutionalize health care. Competition can potentially be a positive force in developing and maintaining quality home health programs. But home health care is a business and can be profit producing, which requires strong utilization review and quality improvement mechanisms (see Chapter 22).

The changing environment in home health care has several implications for the community health nurse. Clients are discharged from acute care at earlier stages of treatment, thereby needing a highly skilled level of care at home. Also, to survive in the competitive arena, agencies must continue to provide quality care and be cost-effective without compromising accountability. These home care changes require that home health nurses, as both clinicians and managers, have highly developed administrative and case management skills (see Chapter 19).

SCOPE OF PRACTICE

A common misconception of home health care is that it is a "custodial" type of nursing. It is important to remember that home health care nursing is part of community health nursing. Thus health promotion and disease prevention activities are a fundamental component of practice. Since home health care is often intermittent, a primary objective for the nurse is to facilitate self-care.

According to Orem (1995, p 104), "Self-care is the practice of activities that individuals initiate and perform on their own behalf in maintaining life, health, and well-being." Home health nurses use this concept for all clients, regardless of the clients' abilities. For example, a client may be recuperating at home after suffering a cerebrovascular accident (CVA, stroke) and be unable to perform activities of daily living (ADL) without assistance. Such clients can be instructed to perform these activities in a modified form. In this way they have some control over their life and self-care activities and they can be taught to prevent possible losses in other self-care areas.

Family caregiving has become an area of concern for home care nursing research over the last 15 years. Although self-care is considered the ideal outcome of home health interventions, in reality many clients require assistance. Schumacher (1995) identified "family caregiving" as a negotiated and shifting combination of self-care and caregiving. Archbold, Stewart and colleagues have developed and tested a research-based intervention, the PREP System of Nursing Interventions, to increase the preparedness and competence of caregivers, identify strategies to enhance caregiving, and increase the ability to predict and control the situation (Archbold et al, 1995). Innovative and cost-effective models of care and interventions are urgently needed in home health care for the next century (see the Research Brief).

A primary goal of home health care is to help prevent the occurrence of illness and to promote the client's well-being. In the home care setting, clients possess more control and determine their own health care needs. The effectiveness of service depends on the client's active involvement and understanding of plans established jointly by the client and nurse. The nurse facilitates the development of positive health behaviors for the individual who has had an episode of illness.

Contracting

Contracting is a vital component of all nurse/client relationships. Constantly evolving legislative guidelines, third-party payer requirements, the high risk of liability, and the level of nurse autonomy require that contracting be used in the home care environment (see Chapter 25).

The process of contracting in home care involves the client, their family, and the nurse. Contracting refers to any working agreement that is continuously renegotiable. The process of contracting is reflected in the client's care plan and clinical notes. Contracting allows the client, family, and nurse to set mutual goals and facilitates the effec-

RESEARCH *Brief*

The authors developed a system of nursing interventions, named PREP, and pilot tested the interventions with 22 families. A quasiexperimental design was used, with 11 families randomly assigned to the control group and 11 to the experimental group. The PREP experimental group received care from one of three nurses over a 3- to 6-month period. The control group received standard home health care over the same time period. Effectiveness and acceptability of the intervention were evaluated through interviews at 2, 7, and 12 weeks after admission to PREP or standard home health and by a mailed survey at 8 to 12 months after completion of the study. Six dependent variables were measured: caregiver role strain, rewards of caregiving, caregiver depression, care effectiveness, hospital utilization, and cost for the care receiver.

The PREP System includes 10 key elements identified through previous research: systematic assessment, family focus, local knowledge of the family, cosmopolitan knowledge brought by nurses, blending of both local and cosmopolitan knowledge, family-nurse collaboration, individualized interventions, multiple strategies, therapeutic relationship, and early detection and intervention during difficult transitions. PREP has three goals:

1. Increasing the preparedness and competence of caregivers through highly individualized interventions
2. Enriching caregiving through engaging in or modifying pleasurable and meaningful activities
3. Increasing the predictability in caregiving situations and the family's control over the environment

The PREP system was delivered through expanded home services, a PREP advice line answered by nurses who knew the family, a "keep-in-touch" system of assessment contacts by telephone after home health discharge, and completion of PREP with a written summary of the family's strengths and progress, as well as a discussion with the family about their learning while on PREP.

There were no significant differences on the nine role strain measures, rewards of caregiving, or the two depression scales between the experimental and control groups. The experimental group rated the PREP nurse as significantly more useful than the nurse or physical therapist in the control group. Caregivers in the experimental group perceived greater changes in preparedness for caregiving, enrichment, and predictability. Mean hospital costs were lower in the PREP group, although not significantly, but the number of hospitalizations in each group were equal. Additionally, the PREP system was acceptable to families. This pilot study supports the need for a larger evaluation of the PREP system.

Home health nurses can use this study as a model to develop effective interventions and assess outcomes of interventions. Family-centered interventions may be the most effective in providing for long-term care in the future.

Archbold PG et al: The PREP system of nursing interventions: a pilot test with families caring for older members, *Res Nurs Health* 18:3, 1995.

---

tiveness of nursing care and the promotion of self-care. Contracting is directly related to use of the nursing process (Fig. 40-2). As an example, during an initial home visit, the nurse gathers data and determines the plan for actions by establishing the contract with the client and family. Contracts can be formal (written) or informal (verbal), depending on the client's needs. In either case, the process is recorded in the client's chart. The most important aspect of contracting is the client's active participation in developing, implementing, and evaluating the process.

DID YOU KNOW? *To avoid what is often referred to as the "home visit ritual," visits that have no predetermined goal or outcome, the home health nurse must establish both short- and long-term goals with clients and families. The goals provide for continuity of care and state the criteria for evaluating the client's condition and progress toward an opotimum level of self-care.*

Practice Functions of the Home Health Nurse

Home health nursing involves both direct and indirect functions. In performing these functions, the home health nurse assumes a variety of roles.

Direct care

Direct care refers to the actual physical aspects of nursing care, anything requiring physical contact and face-to-face interactions. In home health care, direct care activities include performing a physical assessment on the client, changing a dressing on a wound, giving medication by injection, inserting an indwelling catheter, or providing intravenous therapy. Direct care also involves teaching clients and family caregivers how to perform a certain procedure or task. By serving as a role model, the nurse helps the client and family to develop positive health behaviors. Technical skill competency must be demonstrated by the nurse to receive reimbursement by Medicare and Medicaid. Nursing care is covered by Medicare and other third-party payers as long as the care being delivered is **skilled care.** To determine whether a service performed by the nurse is skilled care, several factors are evaluated and must be adequately documented as shown on p. 841.

To adequately answer these questions, the home health nurse must be knowledgeable regarding regulations and be a competent and experienced clinician. Some examples of skilled nursing services include the following:

- Observing and evaluating a client's health status and condition.

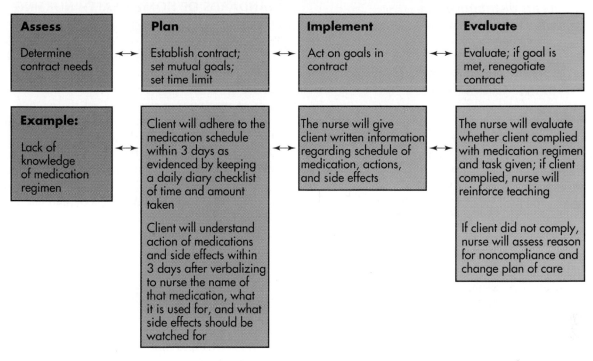

Assess	Plan	Implement	Evaluate
Determine contract needs	Establish contract; set mutual goals; set time limit	Act on goals in contract	Evaluate; if goal is met, renegotiate contract
Example: Lack of knowledge of medication regimen	Client will adhere to the medication schedule within 3 days as evidenced by keeping a daily diary checklist of time and amount taken Client will understand action of medications and side effects within 3 days after verbalizing to nurse the name of that medication, what it is used for, and what side effects should be watched for	The nurse will give client written information regarding schedule of medication, actions, and side effects	The nurse will evaluate whether client complied with medication regimen and task given; if client complied, nurse will reinforce teaching If client did not comply, nurse will assess reason for noncompliance and change plan of care

FIG. 40-2 Contracting in relation to the nursing process.

- Providing direct care in administering treatments, rehabilitative exercises, medications, catheter insertion, colostomy irrigation, and wound care.
- Helping the client and family develop positive coping behaviors.
- Teaching the client and family to give treatments and medications when indicated.
- Teaching the client and family to carry out physician's orders such as treatments, therapeutic diets, or medication administration.
- Reporting to physician changes in the client's condition and arranging for medical follow-up as indicated.
- Helping client and family identify resources that will help client attain a state of optimal functioning.

HOW TO *Determine if the Service Is "Skilled"*

1. *Is the service complex, thereby requiring the knowledge and skill of a registered nurse?*
2. *Does the client's condition warrant skilled intervention?*
3. *Can this service be performed by a nonmedical person?*
4. *Does the instruction of a service to a client involve knowledge, instructions, and demonstrations by a registered nurse?*

Indirect care

Indirect care activities are those that a nurse does on behalf of clients to improve or coordinate care. These activities include consulting with other nurses and health providers, organizing and participating in client care conferences, advocating for clients with the health care system and insurers, obtaining results of diagnostic tests, and documenting care.

Home health care is multidisciplinary care. **Care coordination** of the multidisciplinary team is an essential function of the home health nurse. Team conferences are an ideal time for increasing coordination and continuity of services for optimal client care and use of resources and services. For example, clients with complex conditions or those with inadequate support in the home are presented to the team, and joint **care planning** and problem solving can be done. Supervision of home health aides is both a direct and an indirect function. The home health nurse may evaluate the home health aide's care either by direct observation in the home or by interviewing clients, caregivers, and the aide. If nursing aide services are provided, then regular supervision of the aide by the nurse at least every 2 weeks is mandated. Regular communication with the client's physician is key. There is much indirect care in the home health care setting. It may not be directly visible to the client, but it is necessary to provide quality home care.

Although Medicare places an emphasis on episodic, or acute, care because of its limitations on benefits and requirements for skilled care, the home health nurse cannot entirely separate primary, secondary, and tertiary prevention because of their interrelationship. These levels of prevention have been categorized into two levels of care: episodic and distributive.

DID YOU KNOW? *Home health agencies must provide nursing care as their primary service under Medicare.*

Episodic versus distributive care

Episodic care refers to the curative and restorative aspect of practice, or secondary and tertiary prevention, and **distributive care** refers to health maintenance and disease prevention, or primary prevention. A clinical example can best illustrate the application of these two aspects in home health care.

Mr. Jones, a 70-year-old man discharged from the hospital the previous day, is admitted to home health services for skilled nursing to assess his cardiovascular status after heart surgery for coronary artery disease. Episodic care involves teaching Mr. and Mrs. Jones about medications, exercise, and the signs and symptoms of possible cardiac problems postoperatively. In addition, the home health nurse will provide direct care in assessing Mr. Jones' cardiovascular status, the healing of his incisions, and helping him return to his optimum state of functioning. The Jones family's psychosocial adaptation and needs will also be addressed, in addition to assessing the client's level of self-care and adjustment relative to postcardiac surgery status.

In regard to the distributive aspect, the home health nurse will do additional teaching about ways Mr. Jones can prevent an exacerbation of his condition by maintaining medical follow-up and adapting his lifestyle to increase his compliance with the programs set up for him.

Nursing roles in home health care

The roles of clinician, educator, researcher, administrator, and consultant are seen in home health care. The experienced home health nurse, the nurse manager, or the administrator can fulfill these roles.

Home health nurses in a staff position are clinicians who provide direct nursing care to clients and families. They are also educators because they teach clients and families the "how to" and "why" of self-care. Nurses also participate in the ongoing education of their colleagues as mentors, both formally, providing in-service education, and informally as team members. Additionally, they may teach classes to community groups regarding health education topics. The researcher role in home health care is increasing in importance as the efficacy, or quality, and cost-effectiveness of care becomes mandated by Medicare and other payers. Home health nurses often provide the data required for clinical or administrative changes to occur within their agency of employment. The home health care setting is filled with potential research areas. Research must be a priority in the future if quality and cost effectiveness are to be maintained. A home health administrator can be a nurse who has had advanced education with public health experience; requirements are stipulated by both federal and state rules and regulations. Finally, consultants may provide advice and counsel to staff and clients.

■ WHAT DO YOU THINK? *Disease prevention and health promotion are integral to quality home health care.*

STANDARDS OF HOME HEALTH NURSING PRACTICE

The home health nurse practices in accordance with the Standards of Home Health Nursing Practice developed by the American Nurses Association (ANA, 1999). Periodically, the profession revises the scope of practice and standards of specialty practice to reflect the ongoing changes in the health care system and their effect on nursing care. The Standards of Home Health Nursing Practice were most recently revised in 1999. These latest Standards have two parts: Standards of Care, which follow the six steps of the Nursing Process, and Standards of Professional Performance. Box 40-2 presents both sets of Standards, and they are discussed in detail in this section.

Standards of Care

I. Assessment

The home health nurse is responsible for assessing the client and family during the initial home visit, as well as during all subsequent visits. This process establishes database information for the client and family, consisting of both subjective and objective data. Examples of subjective data include information that the client, family, and physicians relate to the nurse by means of verbal communication. This information is obtained from direct questioning. Information necessary to obtain a thorough database for making accurate nursing diagnoses include the following:

- Primary and secondary diagnoses and past medical history
- Present health status and potential health risks
- Family history and support system
- Socioeconomic status (amount and source of income, educational level, number of dependents, occupation)
- Cultural, spiritual, and religious beliefs
- Daily patterns, functional status, and environmental safety
- Preferred learning style

■ HOW TO *Assess Preferred Learning Style*

How does the client decide how to buy a new piece of equipment for an interest or hobby?
- *Reads a book or magazine—use written materials*
- *Watches a television program—use videos*
- *Talks to expert—verbal teaching*
- *Goes to store and looks at merchandise—use hands-on demonstrations and practice*
- *Belongs to a club and talks with others—group teaching*

Objective data are obtained using a review-of-systems approach to physical examination, physical assessment skills, and direct observation. Assessment findings should be shared with clients, meanings explored, and a plan of care developed in partnership with clients and caregivers.

BOX 40-2 Home Health Nursing Standards of Practice

STANDARDS OF CARE

I. **Assessment:** The home health nurse collects client health data.

II. **Diagnosis:** The home health nurse analyzes the assessment data in determining diagnoses.

III. **Outcome Identification:** The home health nurse identifies expected outcomes customized to the client and client's environment.

IV. **Planning:** The home health nurse develops a plan of care that prescribes interventions to attain expected outcomes.

V. **Implementation:** The home health nurse implements the interventions identified in the plan of care.

VI. **Evaluation:** The home health nurse evaluates the client's progress toward attainment of outcomes.

STANDARDS OF PROFESSIONAL PERFORMANCE

I. **Quality of Care:** The home health nurse systematically evaluates the quality and effectiveness of nursing practice.

II. **Performance Appraisal:** The home health nurse evaluates his or her own nursing practice in relation to professional practice standards, scientific evidence, and relevant statues and regulations.

III. **Education:** The home health nurse acquires and maintains current knowledge and competency in nursing practice.

IV. **Collegiality:** The home health nurse interacts with and contributes to the professional development of peers and other health care practitioners as colleagues.

V. **Ethics:** The home health nurse's decisions and actions on behalf of clients are determined in an ethical manner.

VI. **Collaboration:** The home health nurse collaborates with the client, family, and other health care practitioners in providing client care.

VII. **Research:** The home health nurse uses research finding in practice.

VIII. **Resource Utilization:** The home health nurse assists the client or family in becoming informed consumers about the risks, benefits, and cost in planning and delivering client care.

From American Nurses Association: *The scope and standards of practice for home health nursing*, Washington, DC, 1999, the Association.

Data are recorded in the client's clinical home care record in the form of a flow sheet or assessment chart. It is during the assessment phase that the home health nurse determines that other resources are needed, such as physical therapy, occupational therapy, speech therapy, home health aide, medical social services, Meals on Wheels, transportation assistance, or nutritional counseling. The family is included throughout the entire nursing process because they will assist in the implementation and evaluation of the plan of care.

II. Diagnosis

From the baseline data obtained during the assessment phase the home health nurse develops nursing diagnoses for the problems identified. The Omaha System of Classification of Nursing Diagnosis is one of the best approaches to nursing diagnosis in home health (see Chapter 10). Diagnoses are validated with all who are involved: client, family, physician, and other providers. It is also well-documented so that the plan of care and expected outcomes can be determined

III. Outcome Identification

Identifying appropriate client care and health outcomes is an important part of care. Outcomes that can be expected are to be specific to the client and the client's environment and are derived from the assessment and diagnosis. Outcomes are based on scientific evidence; are culturally sensitive; are mutually agreed upon by all involved, including the client; can be measured; and are attainable. Outcomes are to be documented and provide direction for continuity of care.

IV. Planning

Nursing diagnoses give the home health nurse the necessary information to develop short- and long-term goals with the client and family in addition to formulating an individualized plan for interventions. This plan of care indicates expected **client outcomes** for each identified problem or nursing diagnosis. Goals focus on health promotion, maintenance, restoration, and the prevention of complications. The information is documented on the developed client care plan, which serves as a continuous resource for nurse accountability and as a means to promote continuity of care.

V. Implementation

Implementation of the plan occurs in three phases: before, during, and after the home visit, depending on plan requirements. It is the home health nurse's responsibility to work with the client to facilitate return to an optimal level of functioning and health and to make certain that the client and family are active participants in the care. Instruction and supervision of medications and diet and evaluation of diabetic management are examples of such actions.

VI. Evaluation

Together the client, family, and home health nurse evaluate the client's status and progress toward achieving goals on an ongoing basis. During follow-up visits, previous goals may be replaced with new ones, based on the client's changing health status. The home health nurse prepares the client and family for discharge as early as the initial visit. The short-term nature of the services is explained to the client and family. The frequency of visits and the duration of the service are decreased when the client is able to assume self-care or the family has learned how to care for the client. The nurse provides appropriate referral to other community resources if further assistance is needed upon termination of home care. If the nurse determines that the client or family will not be able to provide the needed care, the nurse must assist the client to make alternative plans for care. Plans may include the potential of moving toward long-term care within a facility or arranging for the employment of a caregiver in the home.

Standards of Professional Performance

I. Quality of care

Quality improvement activities are an important part of nursing care delivery. Nurses willingly participate in such activities as monitoring of care, seeing and analyzing opportunities for improving care, developing guidelines to improve care, collecting data, making recommendations, and implementing activities to enhance quality and to make changes in nursing practice. Results of these activities are used to make changes in health care delivery.

II. Performance appraisal

Community health nurses, as described in Chapter 22, actively participate in quality management activities, including peer review, evaluation of oneself and the entire health team. Professional development is increasing in importance since home health care is changing rapidly to meet society's health care needs.

III. Education

Both the nurse and the employing agency are encouraged to endorse nursing participation in professional development, which includes continuing education and competence in home health nursing.

IV. Collegiality

The nurse shares expertise with others as appropriate and participates in the education and evaluation of students and other colleagues.

V. Ethics

The Code for Nurses (ANA, 1985) provides a guide for nurses facing ethical dilemmas. The home health nurse acts as a client advocate, maintaining client confidentiality, promoting informed consent, and making contacts to see that community resources are available to clients. Ethical conflicts and dilemmas are identified and resolved through formal agency mechanisms designed to address such issues. The nurse is responsible for building a trusting relationship with the family, determining whether the home is a safe and appropriate place to provide care for the particular client, and keeping current on ethical issues related to home care.

VI. Collaboration

The nurse collaborates with the client, family, and health care team to formulate plans of care and goals and to identify and obtain needed services. The nurse initiates referrals and coordinates resources needed by clients.

VII. Research

Home health nurses have a variety of opportunities to participate in research. All nurses should use appropriate research to improve practice. Although the home health nurse may not have formal research training, the nurse may participate in research at some level if agency support and adequate resources are available.

VIII. Resource utilization

The nurse uses appropriate agency and community resources, including delegating tasks to other caregivers, to provide good benefits and resonable cost to the client. The nurse helps the client become an informed consumer.

INTERDISCIPLINARY APPROACH TO HOME HEALTH AND HOSPICE CARE

Interdisciplinary collaboration is required in the home health and hospice settings. Its use is mandated for Medicare-certified home care agencies, and it is also inherent in the definitions of home health care. Without effective collaboration there would be no continuity of care, and the client's home care program would be fragmented.

The collaborative process for home care directed toward secondary and tertiary prevention activities should begin in the hospital with the discharge planner and hospital nurse, who identify a client's need for home care and then review their observations and plans with the physician for approval and orders. The discharge planner then contacts the referral intake coordinator of the home care agency, specifying the services requested by the physician. If persons from several disciplines will be involved, the intake coordinator notifies the appropriate staff and monitors the interdisciplinary collaboration. Either the registered nurse or the physical therapist usually functions as the case manager to ensure that care is coordinated.

In home care, as in other health care settings, professionals may experience stress associated with changing roles and overlapping responsibilities. In collaborating, each home health care provider should carefully analyze the roles of all to determine whether overlapping occurs, and then the team should adjust the plan of care accordingly. Professionals in home care are in a unique setting in which they can truly work together to accomplish the client's care goals.

> **NURSING TIP**
>
> *Convene a client care conference to discuss issues with a family, develop a consistent team approach, and clarify roles.*

In terms of legal accountability and compliance with federal regulations through a Medicare-approved home health agency, it is the physician who must certify the plan of treatment for the client. However, in most instances, it is other health care professionals who evaluate the client's status, report the findings to the physician, and then, in collaboration with the physician, modify the plan of treatment for the client.

Medicare requires that interdisciplinary services be documented. Each professional must document the care provided to demonstrate accountability and provide continuity of care. Interdisciplinary collaboration and coordination through case conferences and contracts made between the caregivers must be documented in the clinical record. Quality improvement mechanisms such as chart audits and peer review verify the appropriate and effective use of collaboration.

Successful interdisciplinary functioning depends on numerous factors, including the knowledge, skills, and attitudes of each team member. Factors necessary for successful interdisciplinary team functioning are shown in Box 40-3. The plan of care should be implemented and reinforced by all involved disciplines. For example, nurses must reinforce the teaching by the physical therapist of the exercise regimen and gait training.

Responsibilities of the Disciplines

The responsibilities and functions of the disciplines in home health care are dictated by Medicare regulations, professional organizations, and state licensing boards. The roles of providers in home health discussed in the following sections may be different from provider roles in other settings. Other specialized services can be provided in home health such as enterostomal therapy, podiatry, pharmaceutical therapy, nutrition counseling, intravenous therapy, respiratory therapy, and psychiatric or mental health nursing. Many of these services can be provided on a consultant basis, either in the form of staff education or through direct care.

Physician

Each client in the Medicare home care programs must be under the current care of a doctor of medicine, podiatry, or osteopathy to *certify* that the client has a medical problem. A nurse can make an assessment visit without physician approval but must have the physician's certification if a plan of care with follow-up is developed. The physician must certify a plan of treatment for the home health agency before care is provided to the client.

A plan of care includes diagnosis, mental status, types of services and equipment required, frequency of visits, prognosis, rehabilitation potential, functional limitations, activities permitted, nutritional requirements, medications and treatments, safety measures, and instructions for timely discharge or referral (NAHC, 1994).

Additionally, the plan of treatment needs to be reviewed by the physician in collaboration with home care professionals at least every 62 days, but more often if the client's condition warrants more frequent assessment and changes in care. This process is called **recertification.**

Physicians in the community also serve in an advisory capacity to the home health agency by assisting in the development of home care policies and procedures relative to client care. Physician involvement in and acceptance of home health care is necessary if the benefits of home health care are to be recognized and appropriately used. The American Medical Association in the early 1960s urged physicians to participate in home health programs, refer clients who would benefit from the services, and promote such programs in their communities. The Physician

---

BOX 40-3 Factors for Interdisciplinary Functioning

KNOWLEDGE
1. Understand how the group process can be used to achieve group goals.
2. Understand problem solving.
3. Understand role theory.
4. Understand what other professionals do and how they see their roles.
5. Understand the conceptual differences between home care and practice versus institutional care and practices.

SKILL
1. Use principles of group process effectively.
2. Communicate clearly and accurately.
3. Communicate without using profession's jargon.
4. Express self clearly and concisely in writing.

ATTITUDE
1. Feel confident in role as a professional.
2. Trust and respect other professionals.
3. Share tasks with other professionals.
4. Work effectively toward conflict resolution.
5. Be flexible.
6. Be "research-minded."
7. Be timely.

Guide to Home Health Care (AMA, 1979) explained the role and benefit of home health care for clients. Today, some physicians are making home visits to provide medical care.

Physical therapist

The physical therapist (PT) provides maintenance, preventive, and restorative treatment for clients in the home. PTs must be licensed by the state in which they practice and are graduates of a baccalaureate or master's-level physical therapy program. Like home health nurses, a PT provides direct and indirect care. Direct care activities include strengthening muscles, restoring mobility, controlling spasticity, gait training, and teaching active-passive resistive exercises. The treatment modalities used include therapeutic exercise, massage, transcutaneous electrical nerve stimulation, heat, water, ultraviolet light, ultrasound, postural drainage, and pulmonary exercises. The therapist is also responsible for teaching the client and family the treatment regimen to promote self-care and responsibility.

Indirect care activities of the PT include consulting with the staff and contributing to client care conferences by sharing skills and expertise. Physical therapy assistants may provide some therapy under the direction of a registered physical therapist. Assistants are high school graduates who have completed an approved assistants' program and have been licensed.

Occupational therapist

The occupational therapist (OT) helps clients achieve their optimal level of functioning by teaching them to develop and maintain the abilities to perform activities of daily living in their home. Occupational therapists focus most of their treatment on the client's upper extremities by helping to restore muscle strength and mobility for functional skills. Occupational therapists earn baccalaureate degrees. When OTs becomes registered by the National Occupational Therapy Association, they are subsequently referred to as OTRs.

Direct functions of the OT include evaluating the client's level of function and ability by testing muscles and joints. The OT teaches self-care activities, assesses the client's home for safety and the need to modify the home to remove barriers, and provides adaptive equipment when needed, such as special spoons and other eating utensils for arthritic clients. Indirect care includes serving as consultants for special client needs regarding self-care activities and adapting the home for the client. Many health care providers have not adequately used OT services because they lack knowledge of OT skills. This discipline is a valuable resource in assisting the client to become independent in self-care, the goal of all home health care professionals.

Certified occupational therapy assistants (COTAs) are high school graduates with an approved continuing education certificate from an occupational therapy program. The COTA works under the supervision of the OTR.

Speech pathologist

The speech pathologist or therapist (ST) is certified by the American Speech, Language, and Hearing Association and is educated at the master's degree level. Speech pathologists work to assist people with communication problems related to speech, language, or hearing. Most clients receive direct care services, such as evaluation of speech and language ability, with specific plans being taught to the client and family for follow-up. The goal of speech therapy is to assist individuals to develop and maintain optimum speech and language ability. Speech pathologists also work with eating and swallowing problems. By serving as a consultant, the speech pathologist can teach other providers of care and families how to encourage development of the best method of communication for clients.

Social worker

The social worker in home health holds a master's degree in social work (MSW) and has at least 1 year of social work experience. The social worker helps clients and families deal with social, emotional, and environmental factors that affect their well-being. Social workers assist directly by identifying and referring clients to appropriate community resources. Often, after an episode in the hospital, clients return home unable to cope with their present state of functioning and need assistance in getting their lives reorganized. The social worker may provide counseling to enhance the client and family's ability to cope with the illness and make difficult decisions about future care. Many indirect care duties are performed by the social worker since consulting and referring constitute the major

focus of their practice. Other functions include identifying resources and filling out applications for them, crisis intervention, and finding equipment when payment is a problem.

Social work assistants are prepared at the baccalaureate level and function similarly to the social worker, who directly supervises the activities of the assistant.

Homemaker/home health aide

With the beginning of Medicare, the home health aide (HHA) became an important member of the home health care team. The home health nurse or physical therapist directly supervises the HHA. The role of the HHA is to help clients reach their level of independence by temporarily helping with personal hygiene and activities of daily living. Additional duties include light housekeeping, laundry, and meal preparation and shopping. The HHA must be experienced as an aide, be trained, and complete a certification program or a competency evaluation to provide home care services. The HHA implements the plan of care developed by the nurse or other professionals to reinforce teaching.

The role of the homemaker, as different from the HHA, helps with housekeeping chores. The homemaker service is one provided by some home health agencies. Although this service is not reimbursed by Medicare, it is a much-needed program and may be provided by some third-party payers or be paid for by clients on a sliding scale.

Aide supervision is required every 2 weeks except in the absence of skilled care; then a visit is required every 60 days. A therapist may make the visit only when therapy and personal care services are being given.

Hospice Care

Historically, the word **hospice** referred to a place of refuge for travelers. The contemporary meaning refers to palliative care of the very ill and dying, offering both respite and comfort (Gurfolino and Dumas, 1994). Originating in nineteenth-century England, the earliest hospices first provided palliative care to terminally ill patients in hospitals and later extended the services into the homes. In 1970 the hospice movement in the United States gained momentum in response to awakened public interest generated by Dr. Elisabeth Kubler-Ross' book *Death with Dignity*. Public-sponsored hospices, successful in meeting the special needs of the dying patient, attracted the attention of Congress. After evaluating a limited hospice benefit as a pilot, Congress enacted legislation in 1985 that provided coverage for hospice services under Medicare. Stringent controls and criteria for quality hospice care are imposed both by the HCFA and the Joint Commission for Accreditation of Healthcare Organizations (JCAHO).

As a result of the hospice movement, persons with terminal diseases now have the option of dying at home with support services available. A variety of hospice care models in the United States use institutional services, home care service, or both. Those that use an existing hospital in conjunction with an established home health

Home Health Care in Canada

Barbara Mildon, Community Health Nurses Association of Canada

HOME CARE AND THE HEALTH CARE SYSTEM

As noted in Chapter 3, the responsibility for funding and administering health care in Canada belongs to the provincial and territorial governments. Nonetheless, the federal government provides provinces with some health care funding as long as the province adheres to the principles and service provisions prescribed in the Canada Health Act (CHA). Home health care was not included in the CHA; however, every province and territory has established a home care program, although the eligibility criteria for the program and the type and extent of services vary considerably. One departure from the provincial responsibility for home care services is that the federal government funds and operates a home care program for Canadian Armed Forces veterans.

SERVICES AVAILABLE FROM HOME CARE PROGRAMS

A scan of home care programs across Canada reveals a wide range of available services, although not all home care programs offer the full range. Services may include nursing care (including complex care such as intravenous therapy, chemotherapy administration, total parenteral nutrition administration, and so on), palliative care, mental health services, respiratory therapy, homemaking, personal care, physiotherapy, occupational therapy, speech therapy, respite care, oxygen therapy, laboratory services including blood and specimen collection, portable x-rays and electrocardiograms, transportation, nutrition counselling, and social work. In addition, many home care programs provide a case management function for clients and serve as the access point for long-term care placement. Home care programs may also offer information on and referral to community services such as meals-on-wheels, friendly visitor programs, and so on. The province of Quebec offers a province-wide 24-hour health information telephone service staffed by nurses that have access to the files of home care clients. The province of New Brunswick also offers to all residents a 24-hour telephone triage service that is staffed by registered nurses.

ADMINISTRATION AND FUNDING OF HOME CARE PROGRAMS

In Canada, home care programs are usually administered by provincial health or social service departments or by local community/regional health boards. The department or board may employ staff to deliver the home care services or may contract out service delivery to external agencies.

In Ontario, home care programs are administered by 43 locally situated Community Care Access Centres (CCACs). CCACs are not-for-profit, independent corporations accountable to the Ministry of Health through a board of directors. They receive funding from the provincial government intended to cover both the case management function performed by CCAC staff and the actual home care services.

The CCACs have adopted a "managed competition" structure in which the services are provided by a variety of contractors selected through a "Request for Proposal" (RFP) process. Criteria for the successful RFP is based on the concept of "best quality and best price."

COST TO THE CLIENT

A review of home care programs across Canada by the Canadian Home Care Association revealed that professional services such as nursing, social work, and physiologic, occupational, or nutrition therapy are usually provided at no cost to the client. Some provinces charge a user fee for support services such as homemaking, personal care, and transportation. The user fee may be a set flat rate or established via a sliding scale based on income. In addition, since the number of hours of support service available is usually limited, clients may choose to purchase extra services. Some programs cover the full cost of supplies, equipment, and medications, whereas clients pay some or all of such costs in others. Some programs offer clients a "self-managed care" option in which the client is given a sum of money that he or she then uses to independently purchase services.

TRENDS INFLUENCING HOME CARE

In Canada, six main trends have been identified as influencing home care. They are:

1. An aging population, with a preference to remain at home in the community, even in the face of physical or cognitive disabilities
2. The expansion of technology such as dialysis equipment and ambulatory pumps that facilitate home care but require more highly skilled staff and longer home visits
3. The need to develop and implement information systems to enable workload measurement, client outcome measurement, service utilisation, and client satisfaction.
4. Increasing demands on the home care programs as a consequence of rising outpatient surgery procedures, earlier discharges, and a reduction in long-term and acute care hospital beds.
5. Consumer demand for a wider range of services and programs.
6. The increasing reliance on informal caregivers such as family members and volunteers due to limitations on service availability.

It is clear that these issues will need to be addressed to ensure that home care programs remain able to identify and meet the needs of the communities they serve.

Bibliography

Canadian Home Care Association: *Portrait of Canada: an overview of public home care programs. Background information prepared for the national conference on home care*, Ottawa, 1998, The Association.

Canadian spelling is used.

The author wishes to acknowledge the assistance of the Canadian Home Care Association, Ottawa, Ontario, for the content in this box.

agency (hospital-based or contracted services) are probably the most cost efficient. Each organization contributes a portion of its resources to this concept of care. In addition to prescribed home care services, core services unique to hospice include volunteers, chaplain support, respite care, financial help with medicines and equipment, and bereavement support of the family after the client's death.

It should be noted that choosing hospice does not mean a client has chosen to die. It is the goal of hospice to increase the quality of remaining life. The hospice team is usually medically directed and nurse coordinated. Pain management, symptom control, and emotional support are primary areas of expertise they offer. One criterion for hospice care is that death is expected within 6 months. Medicare covers this period, and the hospice usually covers the period after 6 months. Clients who improve during care may be discharged and readmitted when their condition changes. In hospice an on-call nurse is available 24 hours a day to monitor changes in the client's condition. After the death of the client, hospice provides bereavement benefits and attends to family needs for up to 1 year. Although a home care agency may provide hospice services, most hospice agencies are freestanding agencies (Gurfolino and Dumas, 1994).

Hospice care requires a multidisciplinary staff with experience in caring for the terminally ill. The primary goal is to help maintain the client's integrity and comfort. *Palliative* (providing comfort) rather than curative care is the objective. Nursing actions such as alleviating symptoms and meeting the special needs of the dying clients and families contribute to **palliative care.**

Health care providers who work with the dying often experience unique stress. Staff stress must be identified and appropriately addressed to help in the delivery of quality care and to maintain the care provider's integrity. Some examples of stress experienced by hospice staff include the following: frustration resulting from clients and caregivers not following the plan of care, difficulty deciding how or when to set limits on involvement with clients and families, and difficulty establishing realistic limitations as to what can be provided by hospice.

The hospice nurse needs a firm foundation in home care skills, knowledge of community resources, the ability to function constructively as a team member, comfort with death and dying, and the mature ability to meet personal emotional needs as well as the emotional needs of the hospice client and family.

Not all terminal clients choose hospice care, and of those who do, not all are eligible for Medicare or covered by private insurance. If reimbursement becomes the primary admission criterion for hospice care, it will no longer be a real option for all terminal clients. The community health nurse choosing hospice as a specialty area must be prepared to deal with this and other ethical issues. End-of-life care is of great concern to nursing, and many issues are hotly debated by the public (e.g., client choice, available hospice services, reimbursement status, admission criteria, and assisted suicide). The Code for Nurses (ANA, 1985) should guide nurses in resolving these dilemmas.

EDUCATIONAL REQUIREMENTS FOR HOME HEALTH PRACTICE

Nurses come to home health from a variety of educational and practice settings. Differences in both experience and educational preparation influence the contributions that nurses make to home health care. Home health nurses should be educated to function at a high level of competency so that they can be relied on not only by their professional colleagues but also by the community. A baccalaureate degree in nursing should be the minimum requirement for entry into professional practice in any community health setting. Nursing education has the responsibility to produce competent, skillful clinicians. A baccalaureate degree does not automatically mean a qualified, mature professional nurse. However, a quality education does lay the foundation for the development of such important characteristics, and the public deserves no less. Life experience, compassion, and awareness of self are factors that are necessary for the delivery of quality client care and professionalism.

In home health care, the nurse with a baccalaureate degree functions in the role of a generalist providing skilled nursing and coordinating care for a variety of home health clients. The nurse with a master's degree is prepared for the advanced practice role as clinical specialist, nurse practitioner, researcher, administrator, or educator. As home care continues to develop its larger role in community health nursing, the need for specialized nurse clinicians will also increase to meet the highly technologic and complex care that has been moved from the hospital into the home setting. In managed care more clinical specialists will be needed to provide case management and to develop programs to meet the needs of the population served by the managed care network. Nurse practitioners can be used to provide primary care to frail elderly and other homebound clients. Educational programs are increasing to prepare nurses for advanced practice roles in home health.

Certification

Home health nurses can seek certification as either a generalist home health nurse or a home health clinical nurse specialist through the American Nurses Credentialing Center. Hospice nurses can be certified by the National Hospice Organization. **Certification** is one means that the profession uses to assure the public of an individual nurse's competence to practice in an area of specialty or in advanced practice. Certification indicates that nurses have met standards set by their peers in the area of practice. Educational and practice requirements, as well as the passing of an examination in the area of specialty, must be met. A baccalaureate degree in nursing is required for the generalist examination and a master's degree for the clinical specialist in home health nursing. Nurses must also demonstrate current practice. Certification is valid for 5 years, and requirements must be met to maintain certification. National certification is required by some states for advanced practice. In a highly competitive health care environment, certification is expected to become more necessary to assure the public of competence and quality.

ACCOUNTABILITY AND QUALITY MANAGEMENT
Quality Control Mechanisms

Since the beginning of Medicare, home health agencies have monitored the quality of care to their clients as a mandatory requirement for certification as a home health agency. All agencies are accountable to their clients, to their reimbursement sources, to themselves as health care providers, and to professional standards. Quality is demonstrated through evaluations reflecting that appropriate and needed care has been given to clients in a professional manner.

Clinical records are of great importance in assessing quality care. The care and services the client receives and any communication between the physicians and other home health providers must be documented. It is in the clinical record that nurses demonstrate that they are delivering quality care and are also identifying means to improve the quality of care. It is the legal method by which quality care can be assessed. This documentation also demonstrates the client's ongoing need for services and shows how the multiple disciplines arrange for continuity and comprehensive care.

Evaluation of the agency is required to monitor the cost and quality of care. Standards serve as requirements for the evaluation in accordance with Medicare certification (HCFA, 1994).

Because individuals from outside the agency participate in the evaluation, the evaluation is viewed as an external means of monitoring the agency's performance. Evaluation requirements are listed in Box 40-4. Representatives from appropriate professional disciplines such as nursing, physical therapy, occupational therapy, speech therapy, and medicine, as well as consumers, objectively report the findings of the review. It is the responsibility of the agency to plan and implement goals for the revision, modification, and correction of problems noted. The evaluation process is valuable to the home health agency. From these reviews the agency can maintain and improve care for the consumers in the community. It is the responsibility of the individual agency to devise the method of implementing the process of clinical review.

Documentation of nursing care is central to home care. The amount of documentation affects the home health nurse more than the nurse in any other setting. As an example, during the initial evaluation visit, the home health nurse assesses the client and family's status. This information becomes a permanent part of the clinical record. Subsequent integrating of health services must be noted. Besides clinical notes of all home visits, progress notes must be sent to the client's physician, including the assessment of the client to verify the application of the plan of care.

Accreditation

Another means of evaluating quality in home health care is **accreditation**. In 1975 the National League for Nursing and the American Public Health Association developed criteria to evaluate community health services. All personnel who deliver community and home health services were represented on the committee. Since then, the criteria were revised and standards to measure quality were added. The purpose of the accreditation process is to evaluate the functioning of the agency in relation to predetermined standards. Components of an accreditation evaluation are:
- Community assessment
- Organization and administration
- Programs
- Personnel
- Performance improvement
- Future plans

Each agency conducts a self-study with the entire staff, including board of directors, executive director, and community advisory committee, participating in the ongoing process of evaluation.

Accreditation is a voluntary process; an agency chooses to participate. The accreditation decision is based on the data in the self-study, the report of the site visit team, and any other relevant information. In the future accreditation may become a requirement for licensure of all home health agencies. Today, home health agencies may be accredited through JCAHO or the Community Health Accreditation Program (CHAP). Both organizations look at the organizational structure through which care is delivered, the process of care through home visits, and the out-

---

BOX 40-4 Requirements for Evaluation

1. The agency must have written policies requiring an overall evaluation of the agency's total program at least once a year by a group of professional personnel, agency staff, and consumers, or by professional people outside the agency working in conjunction with consumers.
2. The evaluation must consist of both an annual policy and an administrative review, and clinical record reviews must be done at least quarterly.
3. The evaluation will assess the extent to which the agency's program is appropriate, adequate, effective, and efficient in promoting client care.
4. Results are reported to and acted upon by those responsible for the agency.
5. A written administrative record of the evaluation is maintained.

comes of client care focusing on improved health status. Performance improvement must be ongoing in the agency.

Regulatory Mechanisms

Home health care is highly regulated. **Regulation** addresses the key aspects of home health care and is an important concern to the home health nurse. The home health nurse is responsible on a daily basis to practice within the guidelines set up by the regulatory agencies. The nurse interprets regulations to colleagues, clients, families, and the community.

The HCFA is accountable for overseeing the Medicare program, federal participation in the Medicaid program, and other health care quality improvement programs. HCFA writes regulations that govern two components of health care: financing and quality improvement (Box 40-5).

Home health regulation is mostly carried out at the state level. State health departments license and certify home health agencies according to state licensing regulations and the HCFA *Conditions of Participation for Home Health Agencies* (1994). These conditions of participation serve as the basis to evaluate each aspect of home health agencies.

Under Medicare regulations, a home health agency is defined as one that meets the following criteria:
- Primarily engages in providing skilled nursing and other therapeutic services.
- Has policies established by a group of professional personnel, including both physicians and nurses, to govern the services that it provides.
- Provides for supervision of services by a physician or registered nurse.
- Maintains clinical records on all clients.

BOX 40-5 Medicare Conditions of Participation

1. Definitions of home health agency terminology
2. Compliance with federal, state, and local laws
3. Organization, services, and administration
4. Group of professional personnel with advisory and evaluation function
5. Acceptance of clients, plan of treatment, and medical supervision
6. Services—skilled nursing, therapies, medical and social work, home health aide
7. Establishment and maintenance of clinical records
8. Evaluation of the agency's total program and behavior
9. Provision of oral and written Clients' Bill of Rights (see Box 40-6)
10. Confidentiality of medical records
11. Disclosure of ownership and management information
12. Compliance with accepted professional standards and principles
13. Qualification to provide outpatient physical or speech pathology services

---

- Is licensed by state or local laws.
- Meets the conditions of participation.

Clients are accepted for treatment on the basis of a reasonable expectation that the client's medical, nursing, rehabilitation, and social needs can be met adequately by the agency in the client's place of residence.

Agencies must provide skilled nursing and at least one other service: physical, speech, or occupational therapy; medical, social, or home health aide services. One service must be provided in its entirety by agency employees. The other services may be contracted. Clients are confined to home and require skilled nursing care on an intermittent basis or speech therapy, physical therapy, or a continual need for occupational therapy.

Intermittent care is defined as follows:
- Up to and including 28 hours per week of skilled nursing and home health aide services provided on a less-than-daily basis.
- Up to 35 hours per week of the above services provided on a less-than-daily basis, subject to review on a case-by-case basis.
- Up to and including full-time service (8 hours per day) needed 7 days per week for temporary periods of up to 21 days.

The state agencies responsible for licensure and certification of home health agencies use these criteria in evaluating whether agencies are conforming to federal regulations. Each criterion has minimum standards to which the program must adhere. Failure to meet these conditions can result in loss of licensure and the closing of the agency. Refer to Chapter 22 for further discussion of quality management and regulatory control.

FINANCIAL ASPECTS OF HOME HEALTH AND HOSPICE CARE

Reimbursement Mechanisms

The **reimbursement system** for home health care is complicated and standard. Before the federal government became involved, home health care was reimbursed either by clients who could pay for the service or by donations that subsidized care for those who could pay only a portion or not at all. Now Medicare and Medicaid are the principal funding sources for home health care, with third-party health insurance providing another major source.

Medicare

Medicare has the most standard payment system of all third-party payers and has traditionally set the criteria followed by other types of reimbursement. Reimbursement of home health services is handled through insurance companies under contract to the Social Security Administration. These **fiscal intermediaries** pay home care agencies for Medicare-covered services rendered to beneficiaries. A beneficiary client must be over 65 years of age or permanently disabled and:
1. Under the care of a physician
2. Confined to the home (homebound)

3. In need of skilled nursing services or physical, occupational, or speech therapy on an intermittent basis
4. Services are medically necessary

Skilled care services are those required by an individual that are reasonable and necessary for treatment of an illness or injury. The following factors are evaluated in determining the degree of skill: complexity of service and condition of client, performing services or supervising of services by a registered nurse or registered physical therapist, teaching of service by skilled professionals, and whether the service can be accomplished by a nonmedical person.

Medicare does not cover services directed toward the prevention of illness or injury. This does not mean, however, that these activities cannot be performed. They must be done in conjunction with a "skilled" service. The following are examples of services that are reimbursable and covered under Medicare because they require the skill, knowledge, and judgment on the part of the provider: observation and evaluation of physical status; teaching and training activities to client, family, or caregiver; therapeutic exercises (for restoration of or loss of function); insertion and irrigation of a catheter or tube; administration of intravenous and intramuscular medications and teaching of medication regimen; and complex wound care.

Medicare beneficiaries usually suffer from chronic conditions with multiple disease processes. Medicare beneficiaries rely on federal reimbursement criteria that definitely influence the providing of care. Medicare places an emphasis on episodic care because of its limitations in benefits and requirements for skilled care. One of the shortcomings of Medicare is its limited protection. Medicare usually reimburses 80% of "usual, customary, and reasonable charges." The remaining 20% is either paid by the client or through supplemental insurance (coinsurance). The nurse should encourage the elderly client to acquire supplemental health insurance to cover the cost of charges that Medicare does not pay. The use of home health services under Medicare has increased significantly since the passage of the 1972 amendments and the implementation of the prospective payment system for hospitals in 1983. New rules and regulations are written for Medicare and intermediaries as needed. These changes are published in bulletins sent to agencies.

Medicaid

Authorized by Title XIX of the Social Security Act, Medicaid provides health services to low-income persons. It is a medical assistance program for eligible people under Title XVI (Aid to Families with Dependent Children) or title XVI (Supplemental Security Income) of the Social Security Act. It is also available for those individuals whose income is not adequate to cover medical services and for disability coverage. Medicaid is administered by the states but is both state and federally funded. Providers are directly reimbursed by the state, which is also responsible for monitoring the operations and enforcing the regulations. Medicaid covers home health services, including skilled and unskilled services such as personal care. Needy children and some low-income elderly are eligible under Medicaid.

Table 40-2 compares Medicare with Medicaid. If a client has both Medicare and Medicaid or a private insurance plan, Medicare is used as the primary payment source provided the services being delivered to the client are "skilled." When the client is no longer eligible for home care under Medicare, the Medicaid benefits can be used.

Private insurance

Third-party payers are represented by private insurance companies in which the person subscribes either individually or with a group such as an employer. Some states (e.g., Connecticut) have laws requiring that home health care be provided in health insurance coverage. Individuals under 65 years of age who need home care after surgery or a prolonged hospitalization use this benefit the most. This ben-

---

TABLE 40-2 Comparison of the Two Major Federally Supported Programs for Home Health Care

MEDICARE (TITLE XVIII)	MEDICAID (TITLE XIX)
Federal insurance program administered by Social Security Administration	Federal and state assistance program administered by the state
Age 65 and over or disabled	Income-based eligibility
Conditions of participation	Conditions of participation
Homebound status	Not necessarily homebound status
Intermittent service	Intermittent service
Skilled service	Not necessarily skilled service
Restorative program	Custodial and maintenance program
Physician certification	Physician certification
Therapies, medical, or social service	State option—therapist, medical, or social service
Pays rental and purchase	Pays purchase
Reimbursement—"reasonable cost"	Reimbursement—maximum allowed at state level

efit can decrease a client's length of stay in the hospital and assist in a faster return to the client's former level of functioning. Managed care organizations authorize a home health agency to provide a limited number of visits. In this environment nurses must advocate for clients and provide good data to justify the need for care.

Payment by individual

Some individuals may pay the home health agency directly. Individuals who do not meet their insurance coverage requirements and still want services pay either the agency charge or on a sliding scale, based on their financial status. For example, clients may not need skilled nursing service for assessment of their condition but may need the help of a home health aide to assist with personal hygiene needs. Some persons may pay for home health services that are needed or desired above and beyond the home health services the Medicare program offers.

Nursing visit changes

Home health care is growing because it is assumed to be more cost-effective than hospital care. It is likely that financial payers will continue to closely monitor home health services, and adjustments and restrictions will occur to maintain cost. Several factors influence the cost and charge data: type of service provided, geographic location of the agency, and current community staffing patterns. The term **cost** refers to the dollar amount agencies spend to provide the service. The term **charge** is the dollar amount billed to the client for the service provided.

The Health Care Financing Administration continuously gathers data regarding use of home care services by analyzing factors such as cost, frequency, duration of services, and number of visits. The federal government is interested in both cost containment and quality of care.

Cost Effectiveness

Refer to Chapter 5 for an in-depth discussion of the economics of health care and its impact on community health nursing. Although public attention has focused on home health care as a cost-effective alternative to institutionalization in the last 15 years, the expansion of services and growth have resulted in greater scrutiny by HCFA and other payers. The federal government has charged fraud and abuse in some home health agencies, and agencies have been closed or have lost reimbursement from Medicare. This close scrutiny is expected to continue. The federal government plans to institute a prospective payment system to pay for home health services.

Nurses in many settings are not directly exposed to the financial aspects of health care. In home health, nurses must be "cost-conscious" and interpret to clients what Medicare will or will not pay for. It is often difficult for an elderly client to understand why Medicare will not pay for the nurse to make home visits to take their blood pressure if the client's condition remains stable. Medicare pays for services only if the client's condition remains unstable. The key words to remember for Medicare home health

coverage are *skilled, homebound, intermittent* or part-time, and *unstable.*

Physician's case management frequently conflicts with Medicare guidelines. It should be noted that services or the frequency of services certified by a physician as being necessary for a particular Medicare client may not meet Medicare's guidelines of "reasonable and necessary" and therefore are not covered by Medicare. For example, a physician might order physical therapy for strengthening exercises for a postsurgical debilitated client. This is not a Medicare-approved physical therapy diagnosis, and therapy would not be provided. However, if skilled nursing is ordered for this same client and is "reasonable and necessary," during the skilled visit the nurse can instruct the family and client regarding a plan of rehabilitation that is developed by collaborating with the therapist.

Hospice Reimbursement

One of the major issues confronting hospice care is the reimbursement structure in the health care delivery system. Initially, many hospices provided free services as a mission of ministering to the dying. Others accepted available payment from third-party payers for billable services. In November 1983, the federal government legislated a Medicare hospice benefit for reimbursement to Medicare hospice-certified agencies (Federal Register, 1983). Originally, the regulation was to be in effect through September 30, 1986, but additional legislation changed the hospice benefit to a permanent status in April 1986 (PL 99-272, 1986).

The hospice reimbursement benefit is optional for the Medicare-eligible client. Hospices may bill for skilled home care services under regular Medicare Part A benefits if the client does not want to use the hospice benefit. Responding to the perceived cost benefit potential of hospice care and the public demand for caring services during end of life, third-party payers are following Medicare's lead in providing hospice service options.

EFFECTS OF LEGISLATION ON HOME HEALTH CARE SERVICES

The federal government plays a significant role in the delivery of home health care services. The information in this section is organized to present an overview of the historical development of the laws affecting home health. Congressional action can change federal legislation regarding home health care. After a law is enacted, the appropriate federal agency develops regulations to implement the law. For updated information concerning amendments, bills presented in Congress, or regulations consult the Federal Register at your local library.

The Social Security Act of 1935 signaled the major entrance of the federal government into the area of social insurance. The Medicare program was enacted on July 30, 1965, as Title XVIII of the Social Security Act and became effective July 1, 1966. The program offers two coordinated insurance coverages: hospital insurance, referred to as Part

A, and supplemental medical insurance, referred to as Part B. Each provides reimbursement for home health services. This legislation established requirements for client eligibility, reimbursement costs, and rules for physician and agency participation.

The Social Security Amendments of 1972 made the following changes in home health coverage to provide incentives for greater use of the benefit:

- In the supplementary insurance section (Part B) the 20% co-insurance requirement was eliminated for services furnished on or after January 1, 1973.
- The Secretary of the Department of Health and Human Services (DHHS) was authorized to establish by diagnoses the permissible periods of coverage of home health care under Part A for clients with specified conditions.
- The numbers of covered services were increased.
- Medicare coverage was extended to individuals receiving Social Security benefits based on disability or end-stage renal disease. This coverage began in July 1973.

The early 1980s brought substantial changes to home health services. In 1980 Congress enacted legislation that modified the existing programs—the Medicare and Medicaid Amendments of 1980, Title IX of the Omnibus Reconciliation Act of 1980 (PL 96-499). This act broadened Medicare coverage for home health services by instituting changes such as eliminating the mandatory 3-day hospital stay as a prerequisite to reimbursement and allowing un-limited visits by home health providers, reimbursement for occupational therapy, and involvement of proprietary agencies. Other important features of the act included the establishment of regional intermediaries for home health agencies by the DHHS and the achievement of more effective administration of the home health benefits (Law, Paragraph 924,097; Committee reports, Paragraph 24,347).

The Medicaid Community Care Act, Section 2176 of the Omnibus Reconciliation Act, recognized and supported the concept of community care as a viable alternative for clients requiring long-term care. States and providers of home health services were afforded the opportunity to develop their own plan and implement their own ideas without the burden of excessive federal regulations. There is a concern that the decrease in federal involvement will result in an increase in fraud and abuse in Medicare home care by some not-so-honest entrepreneurs.

The Patient Self-Determination Act (U.S. Code, 1990), part of the Omnibus Reconciliation Act of 1990 (Box 40-6), requires all health care agencies to provide written information to their clients about their rights and their options to refuse treatment, and to sign advance directives in compliance with state's laws. The clinical record must include whether the client has signed an advance directive and either a copy of the directive or the contents of the directive. These documents communicate the client's wishes and take the form of either a living will or durable power of attorney for health care. The goal of advance directives

---

BOX 40-6 Client's Bill of Rights

1. Client has the right to be informed of his or her rights. The home health agency must protect and promote the exercise of these rights.
2. The Home Health Agency must provide the client with a written notice of the client's rights before furnishing care to the client or during the initial evaluation visit and before the initiation of treatment.
3. The Home Health Agency must maintain documentation showing that it has complied.
4. The client has the right to exercise his or her rights as a client of the agency.
5. The clients' family or guardian may exercise the client's rights when the client has been judged incompetent.
6. The client has the right to have his or her property treated with respect.
7. The client has the right to voice grievances regarding treatment or care that is (or fails to be) furnished or regarding the lack of respect for property by anyone who is furnishing services on behalf of the agency, and must not be subjected to discrimination or reprisal for doing so.
8. The agency must investigate complaints made by a client or the client's family or guardian regarding treatment or care that is (or fails to be) furnished or regarding the lack of respect for the client's property by anyone furnishing services on behalf of the agency, and must document both the existence of the complaint and the resolution of the complaint.
9. The agency must inform and distribute information to the client, in advance, concerning the policies on advance directives, including a description of applicable state law.
10. The client has the right to confidentiality of clinical records.
11. The agency must advise the client of the agency's policies and procedures regarding disclosure of clinical records.
12. The client has the right to be advised, before care is initiated, of the extent to which payment for services may be expected from Medicare or other sources and the extent to which payment may be required from the client.
13. The client has the right to be advised of the availability of the toll-free home health agency hotline in the state, the purpose of the hotline, and the hours of operation.

From US Congress: *Omnibus reconciliation act of 1990*, Washington, DC, 1990, US Government Printing Office; USDHHS: *Federal Register*, Washington, DC, 1990, US Government Printing Office.

Living Will Directive

My wishes regarding life-prolonging treatment and artificially provided nutrition and hydration to be provided to me if I no longer have decisional capacity, have a terminal condition, or become permanently unconscious have been indicated by checking and initialing the appropriate lines below. By checking and initialing the appropriate lines, I specifically:

Designate _____ as my health care surrogate(s) to make health care decisions for me in accordance with this directive when I no longer have decisional capacity. If _____ refuses or is not able to act for me, I designate _____ as my health care surrogate(s).

Any prior designation is revoked.

If I do not designate a surrogate, the following are my directions to my attending physician. If I have designated a surrogate, my surrogate shall comply with my wishes as indicated below:

_____ Direct that treatment be withheld or withdrawn, and that I be permitted to die naturally with only the administration of medication or the performance of any medical treatment deemed necessary to alleviate pain.

_____ DO NOT authorize that life-prolonging treatment be withheld or withdrawn

_____ Authorize the withholding or withdrawal of artificially provided food, water, or other artificially provided nourishment or fluids.

_____ DO NOT authorize the withholding or withdrawal of artificially provided food, water, or other artificially provided nourishment or fluids.

_____ Authorize my surrogate, designated above, to withhold or withdraw artificially provided nourishment or fluids, or other treatment if the surrogate determines that withholding or withdrawing is in my best interest; but I do not mandate that withholding or withdrawing.

In the absence of my ability to give directions regarding the use of life-prolonging treatment and artificially provided nutrition and hydration, it is my intention that this directive shall be honored by my attending physician, my family, and any surrogate designated pursuant to this directive as the final expression of my legal right to refuse medical or surgical treatment and I accept the consequences of the refusal.

If I have been diagnosed as pregnant and that diagnosis is known to my attending physician, this directive shall have no force or effect during the course of my pregnancy.

I understand the full import of this directive and I am emotionally and mentally competent to make this directive.

Signed this _____ day of _____, 19____.

_____

Signature and address of the grantor.

If our joint presence, the grantor, who is of sound mind and eighteen years of age, or older, voluntarily dated and signed this writing or directed it to be dated and signed for the grantor.

_____

Signature and address of witness.

_____

Signature and address of witness.

OR

STATE OF KENTUCKY

_____ County

Before me, the undersigned authority, came the grantor who is of sound mind and eighteen (18) years of age, or older, and acknowledged that he voluntarily dated and signed this writing or directed it to be signed and dated as above.

Done this _____ day of _____, 19____.

_____

Signature of Notary Public or other officers.

_____

Date commission expires.

Execution of this document restricts withholding and withdrawing of some medical procedures. Consult Kentucky Revised Statutes or your attorney.

FIG. 40-3 Example of a living will directive.

KENTUCKY EMERGENCY MEDICAL SERVICES
PREHOSPITAL DO NOT RESUSCITATE
(DNR) ORDER

Patient's Full Legal Name _____

I, the undersigned patient or surrogate who has been designated to make health care decisions in accordance with Kentucky Revised Statutes, hereby direct that in the event of my cardiac or respiratory arrest that this DO NOT RESUSCITATE (DNR) ORDER be honored and that I understand that DNR means that if my heart stops beating or if I stop breathing, no medical procedure to restart breathing or heart function will be instituted by emergency medical services (EMS) personnel.

I understand this decision will NOT prevent emergency medical services personnel from administering other emergency medical care.

I understand that I may revoke this DNR order at any time by physical cancellation, destruction of this form, removal of DNR bracelet, or by expressing a desire to be resuscitated by the EMS personnel. Any attempt to alter or change the content, names, or signatures on the DNR form shall make the DNR form invalid.

I understand that it is my obligation to see that this form, or a standard DNR bracelet, is readily and immediately available to EMS personnel upon their arrival. In the event of my death, the EMS agency which responds shall obtain this form, or the standard DNR bracelet, and it shall become a part of the EMS medical record.

I hereby state that this "Do Not Resuscitate" (DNR) is my authentic wish not to be resuscitated.

_____   _____
Patient/legal surrogate signature   Date

_____
Legal surrogate's relationship to patient

_____   _____
Witness name (print)   Witness signature

This Do Not Resuscitate form has been approved by the Kentucky Board of Medical Licensure. DNR form number (serially numbered).

FIG. 40-4 Example of a "do not resuscitate" order.

is to provide a mechanism for clients to make health care decisions while they are able. The directives can be changed at any time. The durable power of attorney names a person who will make health care decisions when the client is unable, whereas the living will indicates the client's decision to decline or stop treatment. States differ in the implementation of advanced directives. Examples of a living will and a do-not-resuscitate order from the state of Kentucky are presented in Figures 40-3 and 40-4, respectively.

The Omnibus Budget Reconciliation Act of 1993 reduced payments for home health and hospice services and extended Alzheimer Demonstration projects and the ban on physician referral to self-owned agencies. In 1997 Congress passed the Balanced Budget Act of 1997, PL 105-33, which provided for an interim prospective payment system for home health. This system included an annual per-beneficiary limit based on 98% of the 1994 costs through the year 1999. Additionally, agencies are required to post surety bonds of $50,000 or 15% of their Medicare revenues, whichever is greater. Agencies maintain that these regulations will result in clients not receiving needed care and could put home health providers out of business. Strong lobbying and a legal suit brought by the home health industry caused some modifications of these regulations in 1998. Issues related to controlling costs in home care are expected to continue to be high on the federal agenda for some time.

LEGAL AND ETHICAL ISSUES

In any health care system there is the potential for illegal and unethical actions. Much publicity has been given to Medicare fraud and abuse in the last decade. Exploiting the system has been partially caused by the increase in available federal money and the fee-for-service payment system. Examples of such practices include overuse of home health services when the client does not need them, inaccurate billing for services, excessive administrative staff, "kickbacks" for referrals, and billing of noncovered medical supplies. In 1977, the Medicare-Medicaid Anti-Fraud and Abuse Amendments (PL 95-142) were passed to deter such practices. During the late 1990s HCFA stepped up the enforcement of this act.

Home health nurses are confronted with multiple issues in everyday practice. Fiscal intermediaries, insurance companies, have interpreted the definition of skilled care inconsistently over the years. The home health nurse must abide by established federal regulations when delivering care to clients, even when the needs are greater than what is paid for. Frequency of visits poses another issue. Only intermittent visits are reimbursed. If the frequency increases, then full-time skilled services may be required. Continual reassessment of client and family needs is imperative to avoid inappropriate use and overuse of services. Home health nurses must be knowledgeable about which medical supplies are covered. This information is readily available and nurses, as professionals, must work within regulatory guidelines and educate the community as to what is actually covered and what should be.

Several stressors in home health care affect nurses. Documentation is often overwhelming but is an essential part of client care. The home health nurse must justify that care meets reimbursement and legal requirements and is necessary and appropriate. This accountability can be stressful. The role of the home health nurse is complex and continuously expanding, requiring ongoing education and excellent judgement. Home health care may be underused if the hospital orientation or physicians view home care as a burden because of the excess paperwork it entails.

Cost-effectiveness, which is not linked to quality, may raise ethical dilemmas for health care professionals. To exist in the competitive health care arena of today, home health care must be competitive. By properly organizing and using decision-making principles, home health nurses do not have to sacrifice quality for cost-effectiveness. In this environment evidence-based nursing practice is essential.

TRENDS AND ISSUES IN HOME HEALTH CARE

The 1970s began an era of regulation as the government assumed an important role in the financing of health care. Regulations have now been accused of jeopardizing the quality of care. In the 1980s, a different trend emerged—that of deregulation. In the 1990s a more comprehensive restructuring of the health care system with more emphasis on home health care has occurred, with more controls on the services allowed.

Health care providers and consumers are concerned about quality and cost-effective alternatives to institutional care. Home health nurses can play a vital role in providing leadership to see that this realistic dream comes true. Quality care is provided in the home setting. The benefit of home health care is measurable in terms of evaluating client outcomes, as described in the quality management section of this chapter.

The per diem cost of home health care is less than the per diem cost of hospital care. It is assumed that greater self-care is a means to further cut health care costs. Home health care encourages the promotion of self-care. For home health care to thrive nurses must continue to provide quality care while clarifying through research the contributions of home health care as a cost-effective part of the health care delivery system. Home health care should be seen as a primary site to deliver health care, not only as an alternative to institutionalization.

Competition in home health care is on the rise, based primarily on the actions by federal programs to deinstitutionalize and deregulate health care. Clients are being discharged in a more acute condition than previously. The increased level of acuity requires highly skilled clinicians in community health nursing. Administrators of home health agencies are being faced with "marketing" home health care to both consumers and payers. This task, although seemingly difficult, can be easy if accountability and quality are ensured in the agency.

National Health Objectives

In 1991 *Healthy People 2000* presented the nation's health objectives for the year 2000. This document challenged the nation to increase the span of healthy life and reduce health disparities among Americans and to achieve access to preventive services for all. Health promotion, protection, and disease prevention activities are key to meeting these objectives.

Because home health nurses are working with clients and families in the home and community, they are in a position to promote the achievement of some of the key objectives. The nurse can assess the client's status related to key objectives, identify available resources and gaps to meet client needs, and coordinate care with other providers and community agencies. Box 40-7 highlights the objectives the home health nurse can assist the nation in meeting through their client case management activities. Obviously, these objectives relate to lifestyle issues. With appropriate health education and referral to community resources for assistance, numerous lives can be saved or prolonged and chronic disabilities reduced. In this way the nurse can contribute to meeting the national health objectives on a one-to-one client-provider level.

BOX 40-7 National Health Objectives for the Year 2000: Services and Protection Objectives for Home Health Nurse Interventions

2.18	Increase to at least 80% the receipt of home food services by people aged 65 years and older who have difficulty in preparing their own meals or are otherwise in need of home delivered meals.	11.15	Establish programs for recyclable materials and household hazardous waste in 75% of counties.
3.8	Reduce to no more than 20% the proportion of children aged 6 years and younger who are regularly exposed to tobacco smoke at home.	12.3	Increase to at least 75% the proportion of households that routinely refrain from leaving perishable food out of refrigerator for over 2 hours and wash cabinet counters, cutting boards, and utensils after contact with raw meat and poultry.
3.16	Increase to at least 75% the proportion of primary care providers who routinely advise cessation and provide assistance and follow-up for all of their tobacco-using clients.	12.6	Increase to at least 75% the proportion of primary care providers who routinely review with clients aged 65 years and older all prescribed and over-the-counter medicines taken by clients each time a new medication is prescribed.
4.19	Increase to at least 75% the proportion of primary care providers who screen for alcohol and other drug use problems and provide counseling and referral as needed.	13.14	Increase to 70% the proportion of people over aged 35 years using the oral health care system during each year.
6.3	Increase to at least 75% the portion of primary care providers who include assessment of cognitive, emotional, and behavioral functioning with appropriate counseling, referral, and follow-up.	15.13/15.14	Increase to 75% and 90% the proportion of adults who have their cholesterol and blood screened within every 2 to 5 years, respectively.
9.17	Increase the presence of functional smoke detectors to at least one on each habitable floor of all residential dwellings.	16.11/16.12	Increase the number of women receiving clinical breast examinations, Pap smears, and mammograms.
9.21	Increase to at least 50% the proportion of primary care providers who routinely provide age-appropriate counseling on safety precautions to prevent unintentional injury.	17.17	Increase to at least 60% the proportion of providers of care for older adults who routinely evaluate for urinary incontinence and impairments of visual, hearing, cognition, and functional status.
11.6	Increase to at least 40% the proportion of homes in which home occupants have tested for radon and made modification to reduce health risks.	20.14	Increase to at least 90% the proportion of providers who provide information and counseling about immunization and offer age-appropriate immunizations to their clients.
11.11	Perform lead-based paint tests in at least 50% of homes built before 1950.		

From USDHHS: *Healthy People 2000: national health promotion and disease prevention objectives*, Washington, DC, 1991, USDHHS, Public Health Service.

The home health nurse can be instrumental in assisting communities to set and meet these objectives by participating in both community planning activities and in the home health agency to identify which of the objectives the agency can work toward to meet their population needs. The home health nurse can use the protocols developed by the U.S. Preventive Services Task Force in the late 1980s for assessing clients, care planning, and health education (see Appendix A.2).

Healthy People 2000 was evaluated in 1995 and found that the United States was moving toward the set targets for two thirds of the objectives (*Healthy People 2000: Midcourse Review*, 1995). Significant challenges remained for Americans with disabilities, those with low incomes, and minorities who continue to experience disproportionately poorer health outcomes. Several areas that have not been on target include increasing the years of healthy life for persons with chronic conditions, the ability of the elderly to perform self-care activities, and the number of persons experiencing hip fractures, which were 119% below target. These areas are positively affected by home health nursing practice and need to be highlighted to policy makers and payers of health care. Currently, *Healthy People 2010* objectives are in development.

ISSUES FOR THE TWENTY-FIRST CENTURY
Access to Health Care

There is no legal right to health care in the United States, and no recognized constitutional basis exists to solicit this right. The President's Commission for the Study of Ethical Problems in Medicine showed 34 million people were uninsured during some period of 1983 and determined that clients' inability to pay was a major detriment to obtaining health care services (President's Commission, 1983). The number of uninsured rose to 43.4 million by 1997 (US Census Bureau, 1997), and many millions are estimated to be underinsured. Inadequate health care funding, limited resources for private charitable care, and absence of legal recourse to obtain health care as a basic human right adversely affects the medically indigent and limits their access to home care. Additionally, welfare reform implemented in 1998 increased the numbers of persons who work in low-paying jobs and for small businesses, and the increasing costs of both health care and insurance have also contributed to the increased numbers of persons who lack access to health care.

Will health care reform and managed care systems improve access to care for the population? Many home health agencies currently use endowment monies, have United Way funds, or have other charitable funds to provide indigent home health care. Some states have programs in which home health agencies agree to contribute a certain percentage of their time to provide indigent care. By the year 2000 it is projected that 80% of Americans will receive health care through managed care companies (Peters and McKeon, 1998). Nursing is challenged to address access issues through clinical research, public advocacy, and by devising cost-reducing strategies and models of care delivery.

Technology and Telehealth

The Federal Bureau of Labor Statistics (1998) projects that employment in home health care will grow faster in the next decade than in any other health care sector. The main reason for this fast growth is related to technology. The incentives and pressures for early hospital discharge have created a transfer of technology from the hospital to the home care setting (Sheldon, 1994). At the same time, some technologies have been simplified and their reliability increased, allowing their safe use in the home. This trend is expected to continue. Parenteral nutrition, chemotherapy, intravenous therapy for hydration and antibiotics, intrathecal pain management, ventilators, apnea monitors, chest tubes, and skeletal traction are examples of current home care technologies. The home care nurse must be prepared to evaluate the cost and safety of technology for the home. Clients must be screened and meet specific admission criteria. All clients are not suited for home care, and it is up to the nurse to advocate for clients when home care is appropriate and when it is not appropriate. When appropriate, the nurse will become competent to use these technology skills in the home to maximize their performance, to reduce inherent liability risk, to increase client rehabilitation, and to use research to show that nursing is a vital member of this rapidly developing component of health care.

Telehealth is emerging as a viable and acceptable way to provide health care. **Telehealth** is defined as health information sent from one site to another by electronic communication (Thobaben, 1998). Examples of the uses of telehealth include telephone triage and advice and telemonitoring equipment to measure vital signs, cardiac function, and point-of-care diagnostics.

Pediatric and Maternal-Child Home Care

Pediatric home care has changed tremendously over the past years as children are being treated outside the institutional environment. The family is the key to the successful managing of a child at home. A supportive and stable home environment for children can contribute to healing and maintenance of health. Policymakers in the United States are beginning to appreciate the relationship between home care and pediatrics. Legislation has been proposed to require that private insurance companies cover home care in employee benefit packages. New programs, resources, and options for funding are beginning to become available for care of children at home.

Specialized programs for the pediatric population are mandatory. Although infants have been treated in the home for years, the focus on high technology care requires evaluating key issues such as reimbursement, staff competence, and quality improvement. Pediatric needs range from an infant who needs observation and treatment with home phototherapy or a sleep monitor to a child needing ventilator assistance and enteral feeding. Approximately 10 million children are disabled and institutionalized today because of terminal or chronic conditions. Pediatric home care in the future will continue to help parents to care for their children at home if resources and interventions continue to be available.

Although maternal-child home care is not a new concept, there is a revitalized interest in expanding these home care services to reduce maternal and infant mortality and morbidity. The reemerging home care services target high-risk pregnant mothers and provide health education, short-term skilled nursing care, and anticipatory guidance. Recent research has demonstrated long-term positive health outcomes of prenatal and infant home visiting programs by nurses managing pregnancy-induced hypertension, childhood injuries, and subsequent pregnancies among low-income women (Kitzman et al, 1997). Nursing interventions have reduced the use of welfare, child abuse and neglect, and criminal behavior for low-income, unmarried mothers for up to 15 years after the birth of the first child (Olds et al, 1997).

Home care of infants focuses on parent education about infant needs, parenting skills, instructions to improve growth and development outcomes, and skilled medical care. These programs are being shown to be cost-effective. Programs to provide skilled home care to addicted mothers and infants include such services as family counseling, medical treatment, emotional support, methods to improve nutritional state and reduce infant irritability, and training in improving maternal-infant interaction (Struk, 1994). Some hospitals are developing programs that allow a nurse to provide continuity of care from hospital to home. A nurse who provides obstetric inpatient care may follow the mother and baby to the home to provide postpartum care. This trend requires that hospital nurses be well-grounded in community health nursing concepts.

Family Responsibility, Roles, and Functions

The family plays an important role in the delivery of home health care. The term *family*, as discussed previously, refers to a caregiver responsible for the client's well-being. Women have been the traditional caregivers for children and the elderly in the United States. Yet women are less available to provide this care without assistance because they are working outside of the home. At issue is whether home health care services should be used as a respite, or relief, type of care. Sometimes a family member is debilitated and unable to help the client without assistance. Should supportive services be paid by the federal government? On the other hand, some family members are capable of providing the needed care but are unwilling to do so. Who should pay for the service and who should provide the needed care? Family responsibility is an issue that is difficult to resolve in this country. Assistance from social support systems helps in coping with the stress of caring for an ill family member. The goal is to maintain the client at home for as long as possible and to provide high-quality care. To do this, resources must be used appropriately and effectively. However, developing a public consensus to resolve these issues has been a problem.

Measuring the Outcomes of Home Health Care

As a method to ensure quality in health care, regulators are mandating that home health agencies measure and report *client outcome* data. Medicare has funded a multistate research study to develop a standardized patient assessment, the **Outcomes and Assessment Information Set (OASIS)** to measure quality and client satisfaction with care (Federal Register, 1997). OASIS data will be measured and reported to HCFA on admission to home health care, after an episode of hospitalization, at the time of recertification, and on discharge from care. Data will be submitted by each agency to a national databank, and agencies will receive both results and comparisons with similar agencies to determine areas needing improvement. See Appendix C.5 for one part of this assessment.

Accrediting organizations are also mandating the reporting of outcomes as a performance standard. JCAHO (1997) has revised the standards for home health to focus more on performance improvement based on measurable data, including **benchmarking,** or comparing oneself with national standards and guidelines and with other agencies. Clinical guidelines, pathways, and clinical maps are other methods that agencies are using to standardize care and control costs.

These trends will have a great effect on the provision of home health care, the viability of agencies, and the role of the home health nurses in the future. Nursing research will be critical to demonstrate the cost-effectiveness, as well as the quality, of the care provided by professional nurses. The future of home health nursing holds excitement, diversity, and opportunity.

clinical application

The home visit is the hallmark of home health nursing. When a nurse enters a client's home, she or he is a guest and must recognize that the services offered can be accepted or rejected. The first visit sets the stage for success or failure. The initial assessment of the client, their support system, and the environment is critical.

A. What strategies would the nurse consider to develop a trusting relationship during the first visit?
B. What would be the most important elements to assess in the home environment?
C. What is necessary for the nurse to include in the client contract?
D. How can the nurse assess preferred learning style?

Answers are in the back of the book.

KEY POINTS

- Home health care differs from other areas of health care in that the health care providers practice in the client's environment. This unique characteristic affects several components of nursing practice in the home care setting.
- Family is an integral part of home health care, which includes any caregiver or significant persons who takes the responsibility to assist the client in need of care at home.
- Home care reached a turning point with the arrival of Medicare, which provided regulations for home care practice and reimbursement mechanisms.
- Home health agencies are divided into the following five general types based on the administrative and organizational structures: official, private and voluntary, combination, hospital-based, and proprietary.
- Regardless of the type of home health agency existing in a community, the primary goal should be to provide quality home health care to the community based on the health needs of people.
- Demonstration of professional competency is the foremost requirement for home health care nurses.
- Home health care nursing is a division of community health nursing. Thus health promotion activities are a fundamental component of practice.
- There are three accepted components of the concept of self-care: client education, client compliance, and self-help.

KEY POINTS—cont'd

- Contracting is a vital component of all nurse-client relationships. Contracting refers to any working agreement, continuously renegotiable, between the nurse, client, and family.
- The home health care nurse practices in accordance with the Standards of Home Health Nursing Practice developed by the American Nurses Association, Council of Community Health Nurses.
- Interdisciplinary collaboration is a required process in the home health care setting. Its use is mandated for Medicare-certified home care agencies, and it is also inherent in the definition of home health care.
- In home care, as in other care settings, professionals experience stress associated with changing roles and overlapping responsibilities. In collaborating, home health care providers should carefully analyze each others' roles to determine whether overlapping occurs and adjust the plan of care as needed.
- Since the advent of Medicare, home health agencies have monitored the quality of care to their clients as a mandatory requirement for certification as a home health agency. All agencies are accountable to clients and families, to their reimbursement sources, to themselves as a health care provider, and to professional standards.
- The home care nurse today faces many challenges. Ethical issues (reimbursement criteria and indigent care), role development (high technology and hospice nursing), and opportunities for research (quality of care and cost-effectiveness) affect nursing practice in the home.
- The concept of home health care began in the 1800s with an emphasis on health promotion and disease prevention. With the advent of Medicare, the goal became episodic illness care. Today home health is moving back to more of an emphasis on disease prevention and health promotion.
- With the development of managed care networks, home health agencies will be contracting with a group of

health care organizations to provide care or will be purchased by a larger network and provide care only to the network's clients.
- Home care agencies may be accredited through JCAHO or CHAP.
- The Omnibus Reconciliation Act of 1990 introduced the home care clients' bill of rights and advance directives to empower clients with control over their own health care.

critical thinking activities

1. Make a joint home visit with an experienced home health nurse to do the following:
   a. Evaluate the process and content of the nurse-client interaction to determine whether the visit was merely ritual or therapeutic and describe the process of the visit.
   b. Compare actual roles and functions with the Standards of Home Health Nursing Practice.
   c. Assess level of skilled care the clients receive and determine whether the care is needed and appropriate. (Is it within the four criteria described in the section on roles and functions? Answer the four questions in relation to the home visit made.)
2. Make a joint home visit with another home health care professional and assess, as in the preceding activity. Also, attend a client care conference meeting and write a summary of the process of the group.
3. Review a client record and determine what client outcomes were met through home health care.
4. Review your state's laws governing advance directives. Consider the legal and ethical advantages and disadvantages of having such directives.
5. Interview a nurse and determine how the client's bill of rights has affected practice.

Bibliography

American Medical Association: *Physician guide to home health care*, Monroe, Wis, 1979, the Association.

American Nurses Association: *A statement on the scope of home health nursing practice*, Washington, DC, 1992, the Association.

American Nurses Association: *The scope and standards of practice for home health nursing*, Washington, DC, 1999, the Association.

American Nurses Association: *Code for nurses and interpretive statements*, Kansas City, Mo, 1985, the Association.

American Nurses Association: Division of Community Health Nursing: *A conceptual model of community health nursing*, Pub No CH-102M, Kansas City, Mo, 1980, the Association.

American Public Health Association: *Healthy Communities 2000: model standards*, ed 3, Washington, DC, 1991, the Association.

Archbold PG et al: The PREP system of nursing interventions: a pilot test with families caring for older members, *Res Nurs Health* 18:3, 1995.

Cassak D: Hospitals in home health care—an industry in transition, *Health Industry Today* 16:75, 1984.

Community Home Health Accreditation Program (CHAP): *Standards of excellence for home care organizations*, New York, 1993, NLN.

Dee-Kelly P, Heller S, Sibley M: Managed care, *Nurs Clin North Am* 29(3):471, 1994.

Doherty M, Hurley S: Suburban home care, *Nurs Clin North Am* 29(3):483, 1994.

Dolon J: *Goodnow's history of nursing*, Philadelphia, 1958, W.B. Saunders.

Gurfolino V, Dumas V: Hospice nursing, *Nurs Clin North Am* 29(3):533, 1994.

Harvey C: New systems: the restructuring of cancer care delivery and economics, *Oncol Nurs Foundation* 21(1):72, 1994.

Health Care Financing Administration: *Conditions of participation for home health agencies*, Subpart 1, Section 405.1229, Evaluation, Washington, DC, 1994, USDHHS.

Joint Commission for Accreditation of Healthcare Organizations: *1997-98 comprehensive accreditation manual for home care*, Oakbrook Terrace, Ill, 1996, JCAHO.

Kitzman H et al: Effects of prenatal and infancy home visitation by nurses on pregnancy outcomes, childhood injuries, and repeated childbearing: a randomized, controlled trial, *JAMA* 278(8):644, 1997.

Levit KR et al: National health expenditures, 1995, *Health Care Financing Review* 175, 1996.

McClure G: Home care networks, alliances and acquisitions, *Caring* 13:48, 1994.

Medicare Program: Hospice care, *Federal Register* 48:560008-560036, Washington, DC, 1984, US Government Printing Office.

National Association of Home Care: *A providers guide to a Medicare home health certification process,* ed 3, Washington, DC, 1994, the Association.

National Association of Home Care: *1997 national homecare and hospice directory,* ed 9, Washington, DC, 1997, the Association.

National Association of Home Care: *1998 legislative blueprint for action,* Washington, DC, 1998, the Association.

Olds DL et al: Long-term effects of home visitation on maternal life course and child abuse and neglect: fifteen year follow-up of randomized trial, *JAMA* 278(8):637, 1997.

Orem DE: *Nursing: concepts of practice,* ed 3, St Louis, 1995, Mosby.

Peters DA, McKeon T: *Transforming home care: quality, cost and data management,* Gaithersburg, Md, 1998, Aspen.

Portnoy F, Dumas C: Nursing for the public good, *Nurs Clin North Am* 29(3):371, 1994.

President's Commission: *Securing access to health care,* Washington, DC, 1983, US Government President's Office.

Public Health Law 99-272: Omnibus Budget Reconciliation Act of 1985, Medicare and Medicaid Budget Reconciliation Amendments of 1985, CIS-NO: Title IX, December, 1986.

Sheldon P: High technology in home care, *Nurs Clin North Am* 29(3):507, 1994.

Schumacher KL: Family caregiver role acquisition: role-making through situated interaction, *Schol Inq Nurs Pract* 9(3):211, 1995.

Struk C: Women and children, *Nurs Clin North Am* 29(3):395, 1994.

Thobaben M: Health care technology issues in home care, *Home Care Provider* 3(5):244, 1998.

US Census Bureau: *Population profile of the United States, 1997,* Washington, DC, 1998, US Government Printing Office.

US Congress: *Omnibus reconciliation act of 1990,* Washington, DC, 1990, US Government Printing Office.

US Department of Health and Human Services: *Healthy People 2000: national health promotion and disease prevention objectives,* Washington, DC, 1991, USDHHS, Public Health Service.

US Department of Health and Human Services: *Healthy People 2000: Midcourse review and 1995 revisions,* Washington, DC, 1995, USDHHS, Public Health Service.

US Medicare and Medicaid Programs; Revision of Conditions of participation for home health agencies and use of Outcome Assessment Information Set (OASIS); Proposed rules, *Federal Register* 62(46):11003-11064, March 10, 1997.

US Preventive Services Task Force: *Guide to clinical preventive services.* Baltimore, Md, 1989, Williams & Wilkins.

Warhola C: *Planning for home health services: a resource handbook,* Pub No (HRA) 80-14017, Washington, DC, 1980, USDHHS, Public Health Service.

Woodham-Smith C: *Lonely crusader,* New York, 1951, McGraw-Hill.

CHAPTER 41

The Advanced Practice Nurse in the Community

MOLLY A. ROSE

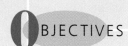

BJECTIVES

MERLIN www.mosby.com/MERLIN/community_stanhope

After reading this chapter, the student should be able to do the following:

- Briefly discuss the historical development of the roles of the clinical nurse specialist and nurse practitioner.
- Describe the educational requirements for community and public health advanced practice nurses.
- Discuss credentialing mechanisms in nursing as they relate to the role of the community health advanced practice nurse.

- Compare and contrast the various role functions of community-oriented advanced practice nurses.
- Identify potential arenas of practice for community-oriented advanced practice nurses.
- Explore current issues and concerns relative to the practice of community-oriented advanced practice nurses.
- Identify five stressors that may affect nurses in expanded roles.

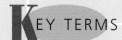

EY TERMS

administrator
block nursing
certification
clinical nurse specialist (CNS)
clinician
collaborative practice

consultant
educator
health maintenance organizations (HMOs)
Healthy People 2000
independent practice
institutional privileges

joint practice
liability
nurse practitioner (NP)
nursing centers
parish nursing
portfolios
prescriptive authority

primary health care
professional isolation
protocols
researcher
third-party reimbursement
See Glossary for definitions

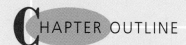

HAPTER OUTLINE

Historical Perspective
Educational Preparation
Credentialing
Advanced Practice Roles
 Clinician
 Educator
 Administrator
 Consultant
 Researcher
Arenas for Practice

Private/Joint Practice
Independent Practice
Institutional Settings
Government
Other Arenas
Issues and Concerns
 Legal Status
 Reimbursement
 Institutional Privileges

Employment and Role
 Negotiation
Role Stress
 Professional Isolation
 Liability
 Collaborative Practice
 Conflicting Expectations
 Professional Responsibilities
Trends in Advanced Practice
 Nursing

The author acknowledges the work of Cynthia S. Selleck, Ann T. Sirles, and Rebecca H. Sloan for the chapters in previous editions, from which this chapter was revised.

This chapter explores roles of the advanced practice nurse in community health. The advanced practice community-oriented nurse is either a licensed professional nurse prepared at the master's level to take leadership roles in applying the nursing process and public health sciences to achieve specific health outcomes for the community, often referred to as a public health or community health **clinical nurse specialist (CNS)**, or a **nurse practitioner (NP)** (ACHNE, 1995). A nurse practitioner is generally a master's prepared nurse who applies advanced practice nursing knowledge with physical, psychosocial, and environmental assessment skills to respond to common health and illness problems (AACN, 1996). The CNS and NP often work in similar settings. However, their client focus differs. The NP's client is an individual and/or family, usually in a fixed setting. The CNS's client may be individuals, families, groups at risk, or communities, with the ultimate goal of health of the community as a whole (APHA 1996). Debate on the similarities and differences in the two roles of CNS and NP has taken place over the past decade. The overlapping of functions of CNSs and NPs are becoming more evident, and future programs may prepare a blended "advance practice nurse" (AACN, 1996; Dunn, 1997; Furlow, 1997; Lindeke, Canedy, and Day, 1997; Pinelli, 1997; Wright, 1997). Table 41-1 lists similarities and differences between a CNS and an NP.

This chapter provides a history on the educational preparation of the advanced practice nurse. Functions in advanced practice and arenas for practice are discussed. Issues and concerns, role negotiation, and areas of role stress relative to the CNS and the NP in the community are also discussed.

HISTORICAL PERSPECTIVE

Changes in the health care system and nursing have occurred in the past few decades because of a shift in society demands and needs. Trends that have influenced the roles of the CNS and NP include a shift from institution-based health care to community-oriented health care, improvements in technology, self-care, cost-containment measures, accountability to the client, third-party reimbursement, and demands for making technology-related care more responsive to the client.

The CNS role began in the early 1960s and grew out of a need to improve client care. CNSs educate clients, communities, populations, families, and individuals; provide social and psychologic support to clients; serve as role models to other nursing staff; consult with communities, nurses and staff in other disciplines; and conduct clinical nursing research (Cukr, 1996).

In the United States during the 1960s, a shortage of physicians occurred, and there was an increasing tendency among physicians to specialize. The number of physicians who might have provided medical care to communities and families across the nation was reduced. As this trend continued, a serious gap in primary health care services developed. **Primary health care** includes both public health and primary care services.

The NP movement was begun in 1965 at the University of Colorado by Dr. Loretta Ford and Dr. Henry Silver. They determined that the morbidity among medically deprived children could be decreased by educating community health nurses to provide well-child care to children of all ages. Nursing practice for these pediatric nurse practitioners included the identification, assessment, and management of common acute and chronic health problems, with appropriate referral of more complex problems to physicians (Silver, Ford, and Stearly, 1967). As a profession, nursing's priorities have traditionally been to care for and support the well, the worried well, and the ill, offering physical care services previously provided only by physicians. Preparing nurses as primary health care providers was not only consistent with traditional nursing but also was responsive to society's critical need for primary health care services, including health promotion and illness prevention (Kozlowski, 1990).

In 1965, as with the NP role, the physician assistant (PA) role was initiated at Duke University. This program was intended to attract former military corpsmen for training as medical extenders (Fisher and Horowitz, 1977). Nurse practitioners are often combined into a single category with other nonphysician providers and are mistak-

---

TABLE 41-1 Similarities and Differences Between Educational Programs for CNS and NP

PREPARATION	TYPE OF ROLE
Comprehensive assessment	Always in NP programs; often in CNS programs
Physiology and pharmacology	Almost always in NP programs; often in CNS programs
Diagnosis and management	Always in NP programs; often in CNS programs
Systems	Individual/family focus in NP programs; CNS programs more systems focused
Leadership	Usually in both types of programs
Program planning and evaluation	More often seen in CNS programs; always in community and public health CNS
Research	Generally in both types of programs

enly portrayed as physician extenders. This misinterpretation of the intended role is addressed by one of the founders, Dr. Loretta Ford (1986).

As conceptualized, the nurse practitioner was always intended to be a nursing model focused on the promotion of health in daily living, growth and development for children in families as well as the prevention of disease and disability. It evolved from such societal needs and opportunities as nursing's development as a discipline and a profession, not because there was a shortage of physicians. Nor did our early plans include preparing nurses to assume medical functions. Our interests were in health and disease prevention for aggregate populations in community settings including underserved groups. These were the hallmarks of community health nursing.

A report issued by the Department of Health, Education, and Welfare, *Extending the Scope of Nursing Practice* (1971), helped convince Congress of the value of NPs as primary health care providers. The Nurse Training Act of 1971 (PL 92-150) and the comprehensive Health Manpower Act of 1971 (PL 92-157) provided education monies for many NP and PA programs through the 1970s and into the 1980s. Similarly, in the 1970s, the concept of an expanded practice role for nurses was garnering interest in Canada. Canadian nurses saw the NP role as an opportunity to expand their scope of practice and perform the role in various settings largely outside tertiary care (Bajnok and Wright, 1993). The United Kingdom has a few advanced practice nurse programs but is continuing to explore the concept in relation to practice and curriculum development issues (Woods, 1997).

EDUCATIONAL PREPARATION

Educational preparation for the public health and community health CNSs includes a master's degree and is based on a synthesis of current knowledge and research in nursing, public health, and other scientific disciplines. In addition to performing the functions of the generalists in community health nursing, specialists possess clinical experience in interdisciplinary planning, organizing, community empowerment, delivering and evaluating service, political and legislative activities, and ability to assume a leadership role in interventions that have a positive effect on the health of the community. The public health and community health CNS's skills are based on knowledge of epidemiology, demography, biometry, community structure and organization, community development, management, program evaluation, and policy development (ACHNE, 1995).

In contrast to the CNS, educational preparation of the NP has not always been at the graduate level. Early NP programs were continuing education certificate programs, and the baccalaureate degree was not always a requirement. The recent trend, however, has been toward graduate education for NPs. The curriculum prepares NPs to perform a wide range of professional nursing functions including assessing and diagnosing, conducting physical ex-

aminations, ordering laboratory and other diagnostic tests, developing and implementing treatment plans for some acute and chronic illnesses, prescribing medications, monitoring client status, educating and counseling clients, and consulting and collaborating with and referring to other providers (AACN, 1996).

WHAT DO YOU THINK? *CNS and NP preparation and functions are continuing to overlap, and future programs may begin to prepare advanced practice nurses who blend the skills of the clinical nurse specialist and the nurse practitioner.*

CREDENTIALING

Certification examinations for advanced practice nurses are offered by the American Nurses Credentialing Center (ANCC). The purpose of professional **certification** is to confirm knowledge and expertise and provide recognition of professional achievement in a defined area of nursing. Certification is a means of assuring the public that nurses who claim to be competent at an advanced level have had their credentials verified through examination (ANCC, 1997). Although certification itself is not mandatory, several state boards of nursing require that nurses in advanced practice, particularly those in an NP role, be nationally certified in order to practice.

The ANA began its certification program in 1973 and has offered NP certification examinations since 1976. The American Nurses Credentialing Center was opened in 1991 and offers certification in six NP and six CNS specialty areas. A nurse can also be certified as a generalist or a BSN-prepared specialist in community health and 11 different specialty areas. Since 1985 the basic qualifications for certification as an NP have been a baccalaureate degree in nursing and successful completion of a formal NP program. As of 1992, a master's or higher degree in nursing is required for NP certification through ANCC.

Examination topics for the NP certification examination include evaluating and promoting client wellness, assessing and managing client illness, nurse/client relationships, professionalism, and health policy and organizational issues (ANCC, 1997). The American Academy of Nurse practitioners also has a national competency-based certification examinations in two areas: family and adult nurse practitioners (AANP, 1998).

The certification examination for CNSs in community health nursing was first offered in October 1990. Qualifications for this examination include a master's or higher degree in nursing with a specialization in community/public health nursing practice. Effective in 1998, eligibility requirements include holding a master's or higher degree in nursing with a specialization in community/public health nursing or holding a baccalaureate or higher degree in nursing and a master's degree in Public Health with a specialization in community/public health nursing. Examination topics for the community health CNS include public health sciences, community assessment process, program administration, trends and issues, theory, research, and the health care delivery system. For the community health CNS certification, the applicant must also meet a practice requirement of an average of 12 hours per week and a minimum of 800 hours in the specialty within the past 24 months (ANCC, 1997).

Certification for the community health CNS and NP is for 5 years. To maintain certification, the nurse must submit documentation of current RN licensure and meet a practice and continuing education requirement within the specialty area.

> **DID YOU KNOW?** *Two certification examinations are available for adult and family nurse practitioners (ANCC and Academy of Nurse Practitioners), and one certification examination is available for community health clinical nurse specialists (ANCC).*

ADVANCED PRACTICE ROLES

Advanced practice nurses holding a master's degree in nursing specializing in public health nursing, community health nursing, or as a family nurse practitioner have many roles, some of which are described below.

Clinician

Most differences between the roles of the CNS and NP are seen in clinical practice. Although the CNS's practice includes nursing directed at individuals, families, and groups, the primary responsibility is to take a leadership role in the overall assessment, planning, development, coordination, and evaluation of innovative programs to meet identified community health needs. The CNS provides the direction for community health care by identifying and documenting health needs and resources in a particular community and in collaborating with community health nurse generalists, other health professionals, and consumers (ACHNE, 1995). Practicing within the role of **clinician,** the CNS is involved in conducting community assessments; identifying needs of populations at risk; and planning, implementing, and evaluating population-focused programs to achieve health goals, including health promotion and disease prevention activities.

> **NURSING TIP**
>
> *Public and community health clinical nurse specialists generally view the community as their client even when caring for individuals, families, and groups.*

The NP applies advanced practice nursing knowledge and physical, psychosocial, and environmental assessment skills to manage common health and illness problems of clients of all ages and both sexes. The NP's primary "client" is the individual and family. In the direct role of clinician, the NP assesses health risks and health and illness status, as well as the response to illness of individuals

and families. The NP also diagnoses actual or potential health problems; decides on treatment plans jointly with clients; intervenes to promote health, protect against disease, treat illness, manage chronic disease, and limit disability; and evaluates with the client and other primary care team members how effective and comprehensive the nursing intervention may be in providing continuity of care (AACN, 1996).

The ability of NPs to diagnose and treat has increased the provision of health care, teaching, and client compliance with treatment plans. The amount of physician involvement in the NP's practice is generally directed through state legislation (Pearson, 1998). Frequently, the NP will use **protocols** or algorithms that have been previously agreed on by the physician and the NP. These documents, required by some states, serve as standing orders for the management of certain illnesses. Over the past few years, 48 state legislatures have broadened the authority of NPs to receive direct payment and write prescriptions (Pearson, 1998).

An important area for both CNSs and NPs to include in their advanced practice is health promotion/disease prevention. Within the past several decades there has been a growing belief that the most effective way of dealing with major health problems is through prevention. This requires refocusing the health care system, identifying aggregates (populations) at risk, introducing risk reduction interventions, teaching people that they control their own health, and encouraging health promotion and disease prevention behaviors. It has been predicted that there will be an even greater emphasis on community-focused care and that nursing will increasingly be viewed as the way to address many of the health care problems that plague society in the 1990s (Mundinger, 1994). The use of *Healthy People 2000* National Health Promotion and Disease Prevention objectives (USDHHS, 1991) and the *Healthy Communities 2000 Model Standards* (APHA, 1991) are essential for CNSs and NPs in working toward the goal of a healthier nation (Gebbie, 1997). It is important that nurses and advanced practice nurses using the Put Prevention into Practice (PPIP) program to help meet one of the three broad goals of *Healthy People 2000,* which states that preventive services will be available to all Americans (Rains and Erickson, 1997). Box 41-1 lists Healthy People objectives and activities.

Educator

Nurses in advanced practice function in several indirect nursing care roles. The **educator** role of the CNS and NP includes health education within a nursing framework (as opposed to *health educators* who may not have a nursing background) and *professional nurse educator* (faculty) roles.

The CNS identifies groups at risk within a community and implements, for example, health education interventions. The CNS and NP increase wellness and contribute to maintaining and promoting health by teaching the importance of good nutrition, physical exercise, stress man-

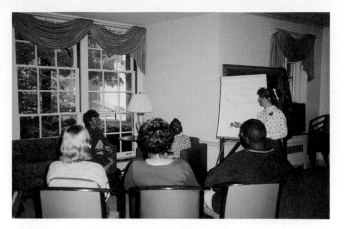

FIG. 41-1 A community health advanced practice nurse leads a training session for a group of congregational nurses.

agement, and a healthy lifestyle. They provide education about disease processes and the importance of following treatment regimens. In addition, they provide anticipatory guidance and educate clients on the use of medications, diet, birth control methods, and other therapeutic procedures (Goodyear, 1995). They also counsel clients, families, groups, and the community on the importance of assuming responsibility for their own health. This education may occur on an individual, family, or group level in an institutional, ambulatory, or home setting, or it may occur in the community with vulnerable at-risk populations.

As professional *nurse educators,* the CNS and NP provide formal and informal teaching of staff nurses and undergraduate and graduate students in nursing and other disciplines (Fig. 41-1). They also serve as role models by instructing/precepting students in advanced practice in the clinical setting.

Administrator

The CNS and NP may function in administrative roles. As a health **administrator,** they may be responsible for all administrative matters within an agency setting. They may be responsible for and have direct or indirect authority and supervision over the organization's staff and client care. In this capacity, nurses in advanced practice serve as decision makers and problem solvers. They may also be involved in other business and management aspects such as supporting and managing personnel; budgeting; establishing quality control mechanisms; and program planning and influencing policies, public relations, and marketing (Lyon, 1996).

Consultant

Consultation is an important part of practice for the CNSs and NPs. Consultation involves problem solving with an individual, family, or community to improve health care

delivery. Steps of the consultation process include assessing the problem, determining the availability and feasibility of resources, proposing solutions, and assisting with implementing solution, if appropriate (AACN, 1996) (see Chapter 42). The CNS and NP may serve as a formal or informal **consultant** to other nurses, providing them with information on improving client care. They may also consult with physicians and other health care providers or with organizations or schools to improve the health care of clients. For example, nurse *consultants* are often used at the district or state level of the public health departments. CNSs and/or NPs work closely with nurse supervisors, other nurse practitioners, and staff public health nurses to develop programs and improve the services provided to clients at clinics and in the home. Nurse consultants in the public health arena may work with all other public health nurses or may work in departments as a member of an interdisciplinary team such as maternal child health, chronic diseases, or family planning.

Researcher

Improvement in nursing practice depends on the commitment of nurses to developing and refining knowledge through research. Practicing CNSs and NPs are in ideal positions to identify research nursing problems related to the communities they serve. They can apply their research findings to the community health practice setting.

All CNSs and most NPs are trained in the research process and, as a **researcher,** can conduct their own investigations and collaborate with doctorally prepared nurses, answering questions related to nursing practice and primary health care. The acts of identifying, defining, and investigating clinical nursing problems and reporting findings encourages peer relationships with other professions and contributes to health care policy and decision making (Pope, 1997). For example, CNSs in administrative, consultant, or practitioner roles daily encounter situations that need further investigating (e.g., noncompliance with cer-

Community Health Clinical Nurse Specialist and Family Nurse Practitioner In Canada

Maureen Cava, Toronto Public Health and University of Toronto

Lianne Jeffs, Registered Nurses Association of Ontario and University of Toronto

Karen Wade, Toronto Public Health and University of Toronto

CLINICAL NURSE SPECIALIST IN CANADA

The Canadian Nurses Association (1993) defines the clinical nurse specialist (CNS) as a registered nurse who holds a master's or doctoral degree in nursing with expertise in a clinical nursing specialty. An expert practitioner, the CNS provides direct care as well as education and consultation to clients and the health care team. The CNS role in Canada was implemented in the 1960s; however, formal educational programs did not develop until the late 1970s (Davies, 1998). The CNS practicing in the community has roles similar to those in the United States—practitioner, educator, consultant, researcher, and leader.

In Canada, the regulation of nursing practice is maintained through a registration/licensure system by examination. There is currently no special certification examinatoin for the CNS. Nursing legislation and standards of practice across Canada rely upon professional responsibility and accountability. All practitioners are thus responsible for their own actions and must not practice beyond their personal level of competence and preparation (Registered Nurses Association of British Columbia, 1997).

The CNS in Canada initially worked in acute care settings, such as hospitals, with a focus on secondary and tertiary prevention. The CNS working in the community brings expertise about disease prevention, health promotion, population health, group process, health education, healthy public policy, community assessment, program planning, and interdisciplinary models of care. The CNS also has knowledge and skills about complex community health issues and practise. The community CNS in Canada works in practice settings similar to those described in this chapter, which include community health centres, public health departments, occupational health settings, visiting nurses agencies, home care agencies, community care access centres, parish nursing services, and community/population health services provided by hospitals (Deane, 1997).

NURSE PRACTITIONER IN CANADA

The nurse practitioner (NP) movement in Canada, particularly in Ontario, is not a new movement. A previous NP movement that occurred in the 1970s and 1980s was undermined by lack of appropriate legislation and materials for compensation (Mitchell et al, 1993). Since that time, in Ontario intense lobbying efforts resulted in legislation (Expanded Nursing Services for Patient Act, 1997) that enables NPs as Extended Class registered nurses (ECs) to independently communicate a diagnosis, prescribe drugs, and order a range of diagnostic tests. NPs who do not have registration in the Extended Class can only perform diagnostic and prescribing activities under the authority of a physician, often by means of a medical directive (College of Nurses of Ontario, 1998).

The NP is a community-based practitioner whose scope of practice includes providing comprehensive health services encompassing health promotion, prevention of diseases and injuries, cure, rehabilitation, and support services to individuals of all developmental stages, and to families and communities (College of Nurses of Ontario, 1998).

Competence areas for the NP in the community health care sector include health assessment and diagnosis; therapeutics (including pharmacological, complementary, and counselling interventions); role and responsibility; health promotion and disease prevention; family health; and community development and planning. Educational preparation for NPs in the community health care sector varies from province to province, from baccalaureate-prepared to postbaccalaureate certificate, to master's-prepared registered nurses.

Variation exists across Canada in the use of NPs in the community health care sector. NPs work in a variety of community health care environments, including community health centres, health services organizations, home care nursing, ambulatory care, sexually transmitted disease clinics, medical services, family practices and solo practices in partnership with physicians, under-serviced areas, fast-track clinics in emergency departments, and other settings offering primary health care.

ADVANCED PRACTICE NURSES IN CANADA

As in the United States, newer nursing roles and titles are emerging in Canada. These nurses are being referred to as *advanced practice nurses*. Although the United States takes the position that education for advanced nursing practice is through a graduate degree program, Canadian nursing organizations have not reached the same consensus. The Canadian Association of University Schools of Nursing believes that preparation for advanced practice nurses should be a graduate or doctoral degree, whereas the Canadian Nurses Association does not specify this requirement. They place emphasis on clinical competencies and education combined. It would appear that while educational requirements will continue to be important indicators of competence, this may not be the only criteria for advanced nursing practice (Registered Nurses Association of British Columbia, 1997).

Bibliography

Canadian Nurses Association: *Policy statement: clinical nurse specialist*, Ottawa, ON, 1993, the Association.

Canadian Nurses Association: Out in front: advanced nursing practice, *Nursing Now: Issues and Trends in Canadian Nursing* 2, 1997.

Community Health Clinical Nurse Specialist and Family Nurse Practitioner In Canada—cont'd

College of Nurses of Ontario: *Standards of practise for registered nurses in the extended class (primary health care nurse practitioners)*, Toronto, 1998, Author.

College of Nurses of Ontario: *A primer on the primary health care nurse practitioner*, Toronto, 1998, Author.

Davies B, Eng B: Implementation of the CNS role in Vancouver, British Columbia, Canada, *Clinical Nurse Specialist* 9(1):23, 1995.

Deane KA: CNS and NP: should the roles be merged? *The Canadian Nurse* 93(6):24, 1997.

Hamilton L et al: Organizational support of the clinical nurse specialist role: a nursing research and professional development directorate, *Can J Nurs Admin* 3(3):9, 1990.

Martin LB: Parish nursing: keeping body and soul together, *The Canadian Nurse* 92(1):20, 1996.

Mitchell A et al: *Utilization of nurse practitioners in Ontario*. A discussion paper requested by the Ontario Ministry of Health, Hamilton, ON, 1993, McMaster University.

Simington J, Olson J, Douglas L: Promoting well-being within a parish, *The Canadian Nurse* 92(1):20, 1996.

Canadian spelling is used.

RESEARCH *Brief*

A descriptive study of the psychologic evaluations, referrals, and follow-up assessments made by nurse practitioners (NP) and a nurse psychotherapist of adolescents (N = 507) in two Southern high schools who experienced Hurricane Hugo was conducted. The NPs' evaluations concluded that 64 adolescents (12%) exhibited symptoms of psychologic distress. The NPs referred 36 of these adolescents to high school counselors for minor distress or school-related problems and 27 for more intensive clinical evaluation by a nurse psychotherapist. Of the 27 adolescents, 10 had symptoms associated with adolescent adjustment reaction, eight showed signs of depression, five revealed symptoms of posttraumatic stress disorder, and four complained of serious family problems. Based on these data, the researchers proposed a model and suggested that adolescent appraisal of stress and crisis is a critical issue to consider when intervening with adolescents who are exposed to major stressors.

Grant SM et al: Psychological evaluations, referrals and follow-up of adolescents after their exposure to Hurricane Hugo, *J Child Adolesc Psychiatr Nurs* 10(1):7, 1997.

tain community/public health regimens or immunization schedules). They may anecdotally identify a trend that, if examined, could be dealt with through community/public health strategies. CNSs and NPs may collaborate with public health nurses at all levels to develop the research design, collect and analyze the data, and determine the implications for further use of community/public health nursing interventions identified. It is important for these studies to be shared through nursing literature.

ARENAS FOR PRACTICE

Positions for NPs and CNSs vary greatly in terms of scope of practice, degree of responsibility, power and authority, work-

ing conditions, creativity, and reward structure (Burgess and Misener, 1997). These factors and their effects on practice are influenced by nurse practice acts and other legislation (e.g., reimbursement and prescriptive privileges) that govern the legal practice in each state (Pearson, 1998). The following areas include traditional as well as alternative practice settings for CNSs and NPs.

Private/Joint Practice

Research indicates that the opportunities for NPs in private practice settings increased throughout the 1980s. This trend is expected to continue (Safriet, 1992). In medical private practice settings, the NP may be the only professional nurse. Negotiating a role is important before entering into an employment contract in this situation. There must be clear communication among NPs and physicians so that there is mutual understanding and respect for each provider's role and contribution each makes to the care of clients (Mundinger, 1994; Steiger, Hagenstad, and Anderson, 1996). Currently, the CNS role in private/**joint practice** is not seen as frequently as that of the NP. This may change as health care continues to shift from primarily acute care settings such as hospitals to innovative models of community-oriented preventive care.

Independent Practice

Nurses form an **independent practice** for several reasons, including personal or professional desire to break new ground for nursing and to meet health care needs within a community. It is important to investigate the state's nurse practice act to determine the limitations and the laws related to this arrangement. For example, NPs may provide a more comprehensive array of health services in states where they have legislative authority to prescribe drugs. Nurses in many states have successfully lobbied for **third-party reimbursement** for all RNs who provide direct care services to individual clients (Pearson, 1998). The independent practice option is more likely to be chosen by NPs and CNSs in states that have established legislation to provide for this nursing practice.

RESEARCH *Brief*

Researchers reported on descriptive data related to encounters, number of visits, and other health variables for participants of a Mobile Health Unit. The Mobile Health Unit was implemented to increase access to nursing services, to improve and/or maintain functional status and health status, and to increase health promotion behaviors of rural elderly residents. The elderly who had difficulty obtaining health care due to illness, transportation problems, or financial factors were targeted for the mobile health care program. Of the 222 elderly project participants, 1773 encounters were completed, with a mean number of visits per individual of 7.9. Elderly participants in the project demonstrated an increased number of breast and cervical cancer screenings; increased immunization rates for influenza, pneumonia, and tetanus; and decreased use of the emergency department.

Alexy BB, Elnitsky C: Rural mobile health unit: outcomes, *Public Health Nurs* 15(1):3, 1998.

Another option for NPs and CNSs interested in independent practice is to contract with physicians or organizations to provide certain services for their clients or staff. Nurses need to define a service package and market it attractively. An example is providing a home visit to new parents after 2 weeks to assess the newborn, respond to parental concerns, and provide counseling and anticipatory guidance about nutrition, development, and immunization needs. This service may be marketed to pediatricians and family practice physicians who would offer or recommend the service to their clients as an option. An NP may negotiate with a local school board to provide preschool children with health examinations or physical assessments before the children participate in sports. Under a contract, CNSs may develop and implement health and safety programs on accident prevention and health promotion activities for small companies.

Nursing centers

Nursing centers or clinics, a type of joint practice developed by advanced practice nurses, provide opportunities for collaborative relationships for CNSs, NPs, baccalaureate-prepared nurses, other health care professionals, and community members (Jenkins and Torrisi, 1997). Primary health services may be provided by NPs, depending upon state legislation. Community health CNSs, along with nurses and nursing students, may identify aggregates at risk and work in a partnership with the community to implement risk reduction activities (Reinhard et al, 1996). Nursing center models are discussed in more detail in Chapter 18.

Block nursing

Block nursing is an innovative nursing model designed to allow the elderly to stay in their homes when they are not totally independent. The beginning of block nursing was seen in the earliest days of professional nursing, when people sought service on a fee basis from nurses who lived in their community. The present model arose from a study by the U.S. General Accounting Office conducted in 1979. The study showed that 20% to 40% of the elderly in nursing homes could have remained in their own homes had they received some support services (Martinson et al, 1985). More recent block nursing models involve NPs and CNSs collaborating with baccalaureate-prepared nurses in the case management of individuals and families in a specific geographic area. These individuals and families receive professional nursing assessment and care from the NP, whereas the CNS mobilizes and coordinates community agencies and volunteers to provide needed supportive services.

An evaluation of a block nursing program in Minnesota revealed that 85% of those persons served would have been institutionalized without the block nursing services and that the total cost of living for families with block nursing was 24% less than it would have been for custodial-care in nursing homes (Jamieson, 1990). Federal agencies and private foundations have granted funds to communities to form block nursing programs. Block nursing may be a future trend that will offer unique opportunities for CNSs and NPs. Block nursing is discussed in more detail in Chapter 45.

Parish nursing

The **parish nursing** concept began in the late 1960s in the United States when increasing numbers of churches employed registered nurses to provide holistic, preventive health care to congregation members. The parish nurse functions as health educator, counselor, group facilitator, client advocate, and liaison to community resources (Magilvy and Brown, 1997). (See nursing tip box.) Since these activities are complimentary to the population-focused practice of public health and community health CNSs, parish nurses either have a strong public health background or work directly with both baccalaureate-prepared public health nurses and CNSs. In a midwestern community, the *Healthy People 2000* (USDHHS, 1991) objectives are being addressed in health ministries through a coalition between public health nurses and parish nurses (King et al, 1993). See Chapter 45 for further discussion about parish nursing.

NURSING TIP

The parish/congregational nurse role is one that has been integrated in some nurses' volunteer activities.

Institutional Settings

Ambulatory/outpatient clinics

NPs and CNSs may be employed in the primary care unit of an institution (e.g., the ambulatory center or outpatient clinic). Ambulatory/outpatient facilities are cost effective and can improve the hospital's image in community service. Hospital clinics generally provide hospital referral, hospital follow-up care, and health maintenance and management for nonemergent problems. The population served is usually more culturally and economically diverse and represents a larger geographic area than that served by private practices. In these outpatient settings, NPs typically practice jointly with physicians to provide acute and chronic primary care. Hospital acute care outpatient services may include clinics for general medicine or family practice, or specialty-oriented clinics, such as pediatric, obstetric-gynecologic, and ENT clinics. Outpatient clinics organized for chronic care may be problem-oriented (e.g., hypertension, diabetes, or AIDS clinics).

Emergency departments

Persons without access to health care, such as the medically uninsured and the homeless, often do not seek health care services until they become ill. Hospital emergency departments are increasingly used for nonemergent primary care. Although this is an inappropriate use of expensive health services, it is a result of the current system, which limits access to routine and preventive health care. Emergency department care is one of the most expensive services offered in health care today.

Emergency services often require long waits for persons who have nonemergency problems. Fast-track/nonemergency sections of ERs have become commonplace to accommodate these situations. NPs in these settings see clients with nonemergent problems and provide the necessary treatment and appropriate counseling. CNSs may also help educate clients on the importance of health care and how to gain access to the preventive health care system. CNSs' knowledge of community health resources helps to see that psychosocial needs are assessed and met. CNSs can act as liaisons or go-betweens for community programs that serve the needs of special populations.

Long-term care facilities

The Census Bureau estimates that between 4% and 5% of Americans over age 75 reside in nursing homes. It is estimated that, by the year 2025, persons 65 and older will make up approximately 22% of the total population of the United States (*Healthy People 2000*, 1991).

Gerontology is an increasingly important field of study, and many courses are available on health needs of the elderly. NPs and CNSs with an interest in geriatrics will need to continue their education in this area to increase their knowledge and skills specific to this at-risk aggregate. Many NPs and CNSs view long-term care facilities as exciting areas for practice and a way of increasing quality of care while containing costs for the elderly and disabled (Safriet, 1992). United States federal legislation provides reimbursement for NPs and CNSs to provide care to clients in Medicare-certified nursing homes and to recertify eligible clients for continued Medicare coverage. In long-term care facilities where clients are not ambulatory, NPs and CNSs may make regular nursing home rounds, assess the health status of clients, and provide care and counseling as appropriate. In long-term care facilities in which the residents are more ambulatory, NPs and CNSs

also may provide health maintenance and other primary health care services to the nursing home clients.

Industry

The *Healthy People 2000* (USDHHS, 1991) objectives include a section on occupational health and safety with goals to reduce work-related injuries and deaths. Thousands of new cases of disease and death occur each year from occupational exposures.

CNSs and NPs are increasingly useful in occupational health programs as business and industry seek ways to control their health care costs and to provide preventive and primary care services on-site. These services help reduce absences from work and increase productibility of workers. The CNS in an industrial setting assesses the health needs of the organization based on claims data, cost/benefit health research, results of employee health screening, and the perceived needs of employee groups. With their advanced administrative and clinical skills, CNSs plan, implement, and evaluate company-wide health programs (Lugo, 1997).

NPs in occupational settings generally practice independently, with physician consultation as needed. The health and welfare of the worker is the major concern. Responsibilities for maintaining employee health include direct nursing care for on-the-job injuries. Often clinical responsibility extends to monitoring work-related illnesses such as diabetes and hypertension. Employees may elect to see the NP for common problems and see a physician for more complicated problems. The role of the occupational health nurse is discussed in Chapter 44.

Government

U.S. Public Health Service

The U.S. Public Health Service operates the National Health Service Corps, which places health providers in federally designated areas with shortages of health workers, and the Indian Health Service, which provides health services to Native Americans.

During the 1970s, both the Corps and the Indian Health Service offered to pay to educate RNs to become nurse practitioners if they would promise to work for a designated period of time with the Public Health Service. These programs were discontinued during the 1980s when more emphasis was placed on physician recruitment. In 1988, Congress reauthorized two loan repayment programs for NPs education—one with the Corps and one with the Indian Health Service. Depending on the needs of the area, an NP employed by the Public Health Service may be the only health care provider in the setting or may practice with a group of providers to serve a rural, urban underserved, or a Native American population.

Armed services

The increased availability of physicians reduced the active recruitment of nurses to advanced degree programs by the armed forces during the 1980s. NPs are used in ambulatory clinics serving active duty and retired personnel and their dependents. *The Civilian Health and Medical Program of the Uniformed Services* (CHAMPUS) provides services to members of the uniformed services and their families when care cannot be obtained from a military hospital. Certified NPs are authorized to provide CHAMPUS services and are directly reimbursed (Mittelstadt, 1993). CNSs use their skills with needs assessment and program planning/evaluation to develop programs aimed at improving the health of the aggregate military population.

Public health departments

Public health departments are increasingly employing advanced practice nurses with master's degrees. These CNSs and NPs have administrative and clinical skills to work collaboratively with physicians and to manage and implement clinical services provided by the health departments. Home care and hospice services are nursing sections in many public health departments and require the services of public and community health nurse clinical specialists.

Health departments also provide primary care services in well-child clinics, family planning clinics, and general adult primary health care clinics. A public health department may use NPs and CNSs, depending on the size of the department, the department's health priorities in the community, and financial constraints.

Schools

School health nursing, discussed in Chapter 43, involves comprehensive assessment and management of care, with particular emphasis on health education, to promote healthy behaviors in children and their families (Adams, Shannon, and Dworkin, 1996; Proctor, 1997). CNSs and NPs may be employed as school health nurses by school boards or county health departments to provide specific services to schools such as confirming that immunization status is current; performing hearing and vision screening; and providing many organizational, community assessment, and political functions. More progressive school systems employ an on-site nurse at each school within their jurisdiction. School-based health services may be staffed by CNSs and/or nurses prepared as school, pediatric, or family nurse practitioners. Services provided by these advanced nurse practitioners include not only basic health screening but also monitoring of children with chronic health problems and finding health care for children with limited access to medical care. These nurses work collaboratively with parents, community leaders, educators, and physicians to ensure that each child within the school community receives needed services. CNSs and NPs may be well suited to manage school health services if they meet specific criteria developed by individual states.

Other Arenas

Health maintenance organizations

Health maintenance organizations (HMOs) emphasize health promotion and disease prevention services to reduce health risks and avoid expensive medical care for the populations they serve. NPs are often employed in HMOs to provide cost-effective basic health care services. Recently HMOs have been contracting with Medicare and Medicaid to provide services to enrollees.

An example of a nursing HMO, the Carondelet Nursing Network HMO in Southern Arizona, provides community care including wellness, home health, and hospice services. All high-risk clients have case managers, most dealing with long-term chronic illness or terminal health problems. The Nursing Network also runs 19 community wellness centers. NPs refer clients when needed to a network of physicians who contract with their HMO. These physicians then often refer their clients to the Nursing Network for case management (Miller, 1994).

Home health agencies

Major legislative changes in Medicare and third-party reimbursement for hospital services have resulted in unprecedented growth in the home health care industry. Home health care is less expensive than extended hospital care and thus is an attractive option for third-party payers (Dick and Burns-Tisdale, 1996). Additionally, equipment and drug companies are developing products for home use, physicians and hospitals are exploring the development of home services, and consumers are demanding more services. CNSs have traditionally been involved in home care in many capacities. Recently NPs have entered the arena of home care nursing (Kelly, 1996).

Because of their knowledge and skills in the following areas, NPs and CNSs are well-qualified to provide home health care that yields positive outcomes for clients and their families:

- Public/community health principles
- Family and individual counseling skills
- Health education and strategies for adult learning
- Increased decision-making.

Correctional institutions

The organizational structure of prisons and jails has long been a barrier to providing or improving health care. Inmates are a population with health needs that can be met by CNSs and NPs.

CNSs are an asset within prison systems, planning and implementing coordinated health programs that include health education as well as health services. Where personnel resources are limited, CNSs provide counseling for inmates and their families to prepare prison clients for going back in to the community upon their release. NPs often practice in health clinics on-site at prisons, providing both primary care services and health education programs (Stevens, 1993).

ISSUES AND CONCERNS
Legal Status

The legal authority of nurses in advanced practice is determined by each state's nurse practice act and, in some states, by additional rules and regulations for practice (Buppert, 1998). In the 1970s, regulations for the direct care role performed by NPs, including diagnosis and treatment, were less defined in state nursing laws than they are today, and the legal statutes of NPs were being questioned. Since 1971, when Idaho revised its nurse practice act to include the practice of NPs, states have amended their nurse practice acts or revised their definitions of nursing to reflect the new nursing roles. CNSs and NPs in 41 states are regulated by their state boards of nursing through specific regulations. In Illinois, Minnesota, and Tennessee, NPs function under a broad nurse practice act but with no specific title protection, meaning that anyone can use the initials NP or CNS after their name. In six states NPs and CNSs are still regulated by both the state board of nursing and the board of medicine (Pearson, 1998).

Legislative authority to prescribe has changed dramatically in the last several years. By 1998, CNSs and NPs in 49 states (including the District of Columbia) had **prescriptive authority,** some with independent authority to prescribe and some dependent on physician collaboration (Pearson, 1998). Although legal problems and unresolved disputes still exist in a few states, tremendous gains have been made because of nurses' active involvement in the political and policy-making arenas.

Reimbursement

The third-party reimbursement system in the United States, both public and private, is complicated. To practice independently or work collaboratively with physicians, NPs and CNSs need to be reimbursed adequately. Because states regulate the insurance industry, available third-party private reimbursement depends in large part on state statute. Advanced practice nurses want direct access to third-party payers. The most common mechanism through which NPs and CNSs get access to direct payment is through benefits-required laws. Laws also include the right to practice without being discriminated against by another provider or a health care agency (Pearson, 1998; Safriet, 1992).

The *Rural Health Clinic Services Act* of 1977 (PL 95-210) was the first breakthrough in third-party reimbursement for nurses in primary care roles. The law authorized Medicare and Medicaid reimbursement to qualified rural clinics for services provided by NPs and PAs, regardless of the presence of a physician (Wasem, 1990). The intent of the act was to improve access to health care in some of the nation's underserved rural areas; however, its use from state to state has varied dramatically. Recent legislative changes to include the coverage of services by certified nurse midwives, clinical psychologists, and social workers, have improved the effective of the Rural Health Clinic Services Act for reimbursement options.

In 1989, Congress mandated reimbursement for services furnished to needy Medicaid clients by a certified family nurse practitioner or certified pediatric nurse practitioner whether or not under the supervision of a physician. Presently, with the 1997 passing of the national reconciliation spending bill, NPs and CNSs can be directly reimbursed, regardless of geographic setting, at 85% of

what a physician would have been paid (if the service is covered under Medicare part B) (Pearson, 1998). NPs and CNSs can now apply to be a Medicare provider. Once an NP/CNS has a provider number, he or she submits bills using the standard government form to the local Medicare insurance carrier agency for each visit or procedure (Buppert, 1998).

DID YOU KNOW? *Landmark U.S. legislation for advanced practice nurses*

1977 Rural Health Clinic Services Act authorized NP and PA services to be directly reimbursed when provided in a rural area.

1989 As part of Omnibus Budget Reconciliation Act (OBRA), Congress recognized NPs as direct providers of services to residents of nursing homes.

1990 Congress established a new Medicare benefit through the Federally Qualified Health Centers where services of NPs are directly reimbursed when provided in these centers.

1997 Passage of the national reconciliation spending bill. NPs and CNSs can now be directly reimbursed, regardless of geographic setting, at 85% of what the physician would have been paid (if the service is covered under Medicare part B).

Institutional Privileges

Because of their direct care role, NPs in the community are more concerned than public and community health CNSs about **institutional privileges.** It is often difficult for NPs to obtain hospital privileges within institutions where their clients are admitted. The traditional hospital nurse is automatically responsible to and governed by the department of nursing as a condition of employment. However, if an NP is employed in a private joint practice with a physician, there is rarely a way for clinical privileges to be granted by the department of nursing because the nurse is not employed by the hospital. There are two reasons for providing a mechanism for community-based NPs to gain access to their hospital clients. First, if people are allowed to choose or purchase direct nursing care, access by NPs to hospital clients is necessary to deliver the care the client is paying for. Second, nursing must be accountable for and regulate the practice of its practitioners. No other group can knowledgeably review or set the standards for nursing practice. Since the nursing department is responsible for writing and upholding nursing care standards within an institution, nurses should have the authority to grant or deny nursing privileges for all nurses within the setting, regardless of whether they are employed by the institution (Burgess and Misener, 1997). However, today when NPs apply for hospital privileges, they are usually received by physicians rather than their nurse peers.

State legislation and the role of the professional organization in encouraging institutional privileges is important.

Legislative action, changes in nurse practice acts, Federal Trade Commission intervention, consumer demands, and pressures by nonphysicians will increase NPs' direct client access (Kelly, 1996; Safriet, 1992).

The changing economy and health care trends are altering the role of the traditional hospital. With competition for clients and nonhospital care increasing, hospitals are more willing to consider alternatives to the medical model. Efforts to obtain third-party reimbursement and institutional privileges for care provided by advanced practice nurses must continue.

Employment and Role Negotiation

For NPs and CNSs to collaboratively provide comprehensive primary health care, they must understand and develop negotiating skills. Positive working relationships with health professionals, organizations, and clients require role negotiation, particularly when few guidelines exist for a role or a role is new and undeveloped. NPs and CNSs need to assess the internal politics of the organization as part of their role negotiation. Networking is another necessary skill. Forums, joint conferences, collaborative practice, and research provide opportunities to expand their functions (Kelly, 1996).

Because NPs and CNSs often seek employment in some locations, as opposed to being sought by employers, assertiveness is needed. Increased financial constraints and new health care legislation have reduced the number of job opportunities. NPs and CNSs should feel comfortable about marketing their skills. Marketing strategies should be designed to project an image that shows a nurse's individual achievement. In assessing and analyzing the needs of target markets, nurses must consider professional, institutional, and the target client groups' goals.

Methods of obtaining positions and negotiating future roles include providing portfolios of credentialed documents and samples of professional accomplishments such as audiovisual materials, program plans and evaluations conducted, client education packets, and history and physical assessment tools developed. **Portfolios** are folders that contain all of these documents to showcase the nurse's abilities. NPs and CNSs should keep these portfolios containing examples of their professional activities. Names, addresses, and telephone numbers of professional and personal references should be furnished in the portfolios only after permission has been obtained for the persons asked to write references.

ROLE STRESS

Factors causing stress for advanced practice nurses include legal issues (as discussed previously), professional isolation, liability, collaborative practice, conflicting expectations, and professional responsibilities. NPs and CNSs should identify self-care strategies to cope with predictable stressors, some of which are discussed below.

Professional Isolation

Professional isolation is a source of conflict for NPs and CNSs. Because they practice across all age groups, NPs and CNSs are likely to be hired in remote practice employment sites. Rural communities unable to support a physician, for instance, may find the NP an affordable and logical alternative for primary care services. The autonomy of practice in these sites attracts many NPs and CNSs, who may fail to consider the disadvantages of isolated practice. Long drives, long hours, lack of social and cultural activities, and lack of opportunity for professional development are often experienced by these rural practitioners. These sources of stress, which could lead to job dissatisfaction, can be reduced or eliminated by negotiating the employment contract to include educational and personal leaves.

Liability

All nurses are liable for their actions. Because more legal action is appearing in the judicial system, specifically concerning NPs and CNSs, the importance of **liability** and/or malpractice insurance cannot be overemphasized. Although malpractice insurance is required to functioning as an NP or CNS, most nurses carry their own liability insurance. It is in the best interest of NPs and CNSs to thoroughly investigate the coverage offered by different companies rather than to assume that the coverage is adequate. Practitioners who function without a physician on site are particularly vulnerable. The scope of the NP's and CNS's authority determines the liability standards applied. The limits of each practitioner's authority are legislated by individual states (Pearson, 1998).

Collaborative Practice

The future of NPs and CNSs depends on whether they make a recognized difference in the health of families and communities and their ability to practice collaboratively with physicians. **Collaborative practice** defines a peer relationship with mutual trust and respect. Working out a collaborative practice takes a considerable amount of time and energy. Until such practice relationships evolve within joint practice situations, the quality health care that nursing and medicine can collaboratively provide will not be achieved. The arrangement demands the professional maturity to work together without territorial disputes, and the structure and philosophy of the organization must support joint practice as a mechanism for health care delivery. The growing pains of establishing such a practice produce stress for all involved; however, the results and benefits to clients and professionals are worth the effort.

Collaborative practice for CNSs and NPs involves more disciplines than just medicine. Advanced practice nurses work with baccalaureate-prepared nurses and other nurses, social workers, public health professionals, nutritionists, occupational and physical therapists, and community leaders and members to meet their goals for the health of individuals, families, groups, and communities. In order to work toward the *Healthy People 2000* objectives, collaboration of multidisciplinary groups is essential. CNSs, NPs, and baccalaureate-prepared nurses can provide leadership in attaining this collaborative effort.

Conflicting Expectations

Services provided by NPs and CNSs in health promotion and maintenance are often more time-consuming and complex than just the management of clients' health problems. NPs and CNSs frequently experience conflict between their practice goals in health promotion and the need to see the number of clients required to maintain the clinic's financial goals. The problem becomes worse when the clinic administrator or physician views NPs or CNSs only as medical extenders and limits reimbursement to the nurse. A practice model that can assist nurses in including health promotion and maintenance activities as well as medical case management into each client visit uses 1) flexible scheduling, 2) health maintenance flow sheets, and 3) problem-oriented recording with nursing goals and plans prominently displayed in the health record. For CNSs, program planning and evaluation based on systematic needs assessments conducted with communities are methods to show the need and benefits of health promotion/disease prevention. Being an educator and role model in carrying out *Healthy People 2000* objectives will also emphasize the importance of health promotion and disease prevention in the health care system.

Professional Responsibilities

Professional responsibilities contribute to role stress. Most states require NPs and CNSs in expanded roles to be nationally certified and to maintain certification. Recertification requires documentation of continuing education hours. Because there may not be many nurse practitioners in an area, continuing education may not be locally available and may require travel and lodging expenses in addition to time away from the practice site. Anticipating professional responsibilities and travel expenses in financial planning decreases these concerns. Negotiating with the employer for educational leave and expenses should be part of any contract.

Quality of client care, however, cannot be measured or ensured by continuing education or the nurse's credentials. Professional responsibility includes monitoring one's own practice according to standards established by the profession and protocols, if used, and a personal feeling of responsibility to the community. Continuous quality improvement is another professional responsibility for NPs and CNSs. This process should evaluate need, cost, and effectiveness of care in relation to client outcomes (Dever, 1997).

TRENDS IN ADVANCED PRACTICE NURSING

Based on a national sample survey of registered nurses in 1996, there were 63,191 NPs, 53,799 CNSs, and 7,802 nurses who were both NPs and CNSs. There has been a rapid increase in NPs between 1992 and 1996, with a slight decrease in CNSs (Division of Nursing, 1997). The need for NPs and CNSs is increasing, especially in light of health care reform, social changes, and complex specialized health problems (Lyon, 1996). More CNSs/NPs are appearing in inpatient settings, as well as in primary health care (Miller, 1998).

Delivery rates for many preventive services are low in the United States, often falling below 50%, for areas such as immunizations, prophylactic measures, and screening (USPHS, 1994). CNSs and NPs in collaboration with nurses, community agencies and members, and other disciplines have the potential to make an impact on health promotion and disease prevention at the individual, family, group, and community levels. Both the roles of community health CNSs and NPs are in excellent positions to use the *Healthy People 2000* National Health Promotion and Disease Prevention objectives (USDHHS, 1991) and the *Healthy Communities 2000* Model Standards (APHA, 1991) in planning their advanced practice nursing interventions. Other suggestions to increase the use of NPs and CNSs include continued reimbursement of services, admitting privileges by hospitals, and more collaborative systems (Miller, 1998).

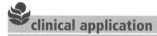 **clinical application**

CASE 1: Clinical Nurse Specialist
Martha Corley is a community health CNS who coordinates the after-care services for a community hospital's early discharge clients. Martha has worked with the nursing staff to develop a nursing history form to identify family and social supports available to clients who are likely to need nursing or supportive care for a limited time after discharge. With this and additional information from head nurses, Martha visits selected clients to begin discharge planning. She consults with each client and family to validate assessed needs. The physician is also consulted about medical therapies to be continued at home. Martha has access to nurses and other resources throughout the community that accept cases on contract. She outlines the initial care plan with nurse case managers assigned to the client and receives regular progress reports. An essential aspect of her practice is to evaluate outcomes of her interventions.

Which of the following is the best example of evaluation of Martha's nursing care?

A. Assessment of client and family satisfaction of her services
B. Reported medical complications of her caseload
C. Review of related literature about home care programs
D. Collected data on hospital readmissions of her clients

CASE 2: Family Nurse Practitioner

Julie Andrews is a master's level NP who practices with two board-certified family practice physicians in an urban office. Julie has her own appointment schedule and sees 12 to 20 adults and children on an average day. Although she sees some acutely ill clients, most of her appointments are for routine health maintenance visits. The two physicians also refer clients to Julie for management of stable chronic health problems such as hypertension and diabetes. She has received a number of referrals from Martha Corley of clients with hypertension and diabetes. Assignment of these clients to Julie by the physicians did not begin until Julie had been with the practice for about a year. During the first months of practice, Julie assessed the numbers and types of client problems seen in a typical week. She found that hypertension was the most frequent chronic problem. Julie reviewed a sample of records of clients with hypertension and found that many had recorded blood pressures indicating uncontrolled hypertension.

Based on this information, what advanced practice nursing intervention could Julie provide?

A. Continue to see the clients referred to her through the physicians and Martha.

B. Conduct an inservice education on the hypertension for the staff in the office.

C. Provide nurse practitioner visits for hypertensive clients and compare the outcomes to hypertension clients seen by the physicians in the office.

D. Provide care for all hypertensive clients in the office.

Answers are in the back of the book.

KEY POINTS

- Changes in the health care system and nursing have occurred in the past few decades because of a shift in society's demands and needs.
- Trends such as a shift of health care from institution-based to the community, an increase in technology, self-care, cost-containment measures, accountability, third-party reimbursement, and demands for humanizing technical care have influenced the new roles of the CNS and NP.
- Educational preparation of the CNS has always been at the graduate level, whereas this has not been true of

NP preparation; however, the trend is for the NP also to be master's prepared.

- Specialty certification began through ANA in 1976 for NPs and ANCC in 1990 for community health CNSs.
- The roles of NP and CNS are merging and many common features exist; however, controversy exists on this blending of roles.
- The major role functions of the NP and CNS in community health are clinician, consultant, administrator, researcher, and educator; typically the NP spends a greater amount of time in direct care clinical activities and less time in indirect activities than the CNS.
- Major arenas for practice for NPs and CNSs in community health include private/joint practice, institutional settings, industry, government, public health agencies, schools, home health, HMOs, correctional health, nursing centers, and health ministry settings.
- Legal status, reimbursement, institutional privileges, and role negotiation are important issues and concerns to nurses who practice in an advanced role in community health nursing.
- Major stressors for NPs and CNSs include professional isolation, liability, collaborative practice, conflicting expectations, and professional responsibilities.
- The use of *Healthy People 2000* objectives is important in emphasizing health promotion and disease prevention in advanced practice nursing and in improving the health of the nation.

critical thinking activities

1. Explore the development of the NP and CNS in community and public health roles locally.
2. Compare and contrast the local, state, and national directors in advanced practice nursing in community and public health.
3. Investigate graduate programs in community health within the state or region to determine the requirements for admission, the type of degree awarded, and whether or not NP and/or CNS preparation is available.
4. Review your state's nurse practice act and any rules and regulations governing advanced practice roles.
5. Negotiate a clinical observation experience with an NP and a CNS in community and public health and compare and contrast their roles.

Bibliography

Adams E, Shannon AR, Dworkin PH: The ready-to-learn program: a school-based model of nurse practitioner participation in evaluating school failure, *J School Health* 66(7):242, 1996.

American Academy of Nurse Practitioners: *National competency-based certification examinations for adult and family nurse practitioner,* Austin, Texas, 1998, The Academy.

American Association of Colleges of Nursing: *The essentials of master's education for advanced practice nursing,* Washington, DC, 1996, the Association.

American Nurses Credentialing Center: *Advanced practice certification catalog,* Washington, DC, 1997, Author.

American Public Health Association: *The definition and role of public health nursing practice in the delivery of health care,* Washington, DC, 1996, APHA, Public Health Nursing Section.

American Public Health Association: *Healthy Communities 2000 model standards: guide-lines for community attainment of the year 2000 national health objectives,* Washington, DC, 1991, the Association.

Association of Community Health Nursing Educators: Community/public health advanced practice nurse position statement, *Newsletter* 13(2):13, 1995.

Bajnok I, Wright J: Revisiting the role of the nurse practitioner in the 1990s: a Canadian perspective, *AACN Clinical Issues in Critical Care Nursing* 4(4):609, 1993.

Continued

Bibliography—cont'd

Buppert C: Reimbursement of nurse practitioner services, *The nurse practitioner* 23(1):67, 1998.

Burgess SE, Misener TR: The professional portfolio: an APN job search marketing tool, *Clin Excellence Nurse Practit* 1(7):468, 1997.

Cukr PL: Viva la difference! The nation needs both types of advanced practice nurses: clinical nurse specialists and nurse practitioners, *Online J Iss Nurs* (Jun 15):1, 1996.

Department of Health, Education, and Welfare: *Extending the scope of nursing practice,* Washington, DC, 1971, US Government Printing Office.

Dever GEA: *Improving outcomes in public health practice,* Gaithersburg, Md, 1997, Sage.

Dick KL, Burns-Tisdale S: Beth Israel home care: a model for practice. In Hickey JC, Ouimette RM, Venegoni SL: *Advanced practice nursing: changing roles and clinical applications,* Philadelphia, 1996. Lippincott-Raven.

Division of Nursing: *Report to American Association of Colleges of Nursing.* Washington, DC, 1997, USDHHS.

Dunn L: A literature review of advanced clinical nursing practice in the USA, *J Adv Nurs* 25(4):814, 1997.

Fisher DW, Horowitz SM: The physician's assistant: profile of a new health profession. In Bliss AA, Cohen ED, editors: *The new health professionals,* Germantown, Md, 1977, Aspen Systems.

Ford LC: Nurses, nurse practitioners: the evolution of primary care (book review), *Image* 18:177, 1986.

Furlow L: Dear editor: . .CNS and NP, an argument for a single title, *Clin Nurse Specialist* 11(1):29, 1997.

Gebbie KM: Using the vision of healthy people to build healthier communities, *Nurs Admin Q* 21(4):83, 1997.

Goodyear R: Concern, continuity, and choice: a health promotion formula for advanced practice nurses, *Adv Pract Nurs Q* 1(3):41, 1995.

Grant SM et al: Psychological evaluations, referrals, and follow-up of adolescents after their exposure to Hurricane Hugo, *J Child Adolesc Psychiatr Nurs* 10(1):7, 1997.

Jamieson MK: Block nursing: practicing autonomous professional nursing in the community, *Nurs Health Care* 11:250, 1990.

Jenkins M, Torrisi D: Community partnership primary care case study: Abbottsford Community Health Center, *Nurse Practit Forum* 8(1):21, 1997.

Kelly M: Primary care across clinical settings, *Nurs Clin North Am,* 31(3):465, 1996.

King JM, Lakin JA, Striepe J: Coalition building between public health nurses and parish nurses, *JONA* 23(2):27, 1993.

Kozlowski D: Nurse practitioners: 25 years of quality health care, *AMA Council Primary Health Care Nurse Practit Newsletter* 13(7):4, 1990.

Lindeke LL, Canedy BH, Day MM: A comparison of practice domains of clinical nurse specialists and nurse practitioners, *J Prof Nurs* 13(5):281, 1997.

Lugo NR: Nurse-managed corporate employee wellness centers, *Nurse Practit Am J Primary Health Care* 22(4):104, 1997.

Lyon BL: Meeting societal needs for CNS competencies: why the CNS and NP roles should not be blended in masters degree programs, *Online J Iss Nurs Adv Pract Nurs* (Jun 15)1, 1996.

Magilvy JK, Brown NJ: Parish nursing: advanced practice nursing model for healthier communities, *Adv Pract Nurs Q* 2(4):67, 1997.

Martinson I et al: The block nurse program, *J Comm Health Nurs* 2(1):21, 1985.

Miller N: An interview with Phyllis Ethridge: challenges for nurse executives, a nursing HMO, chronic patients, and team work, *Nurs Econ* 12(2):65, 1994.

Miller SK: Defining the acute in acute care nurse practitioner, *Clin Excellence Nurse Practit* 2(1):52, 1998.

Mittelstadt PC: Federal reimbursement of advanced practice nurses' services empowers the profession, *Nurse Pract* 18(1):43, 1993.

Mundinger M: Advanced practice nursing: good medicine for physicians? *N Engl J Med* 330:201, 1994.

Pearson LJ: Annual update of how each state stands on legislative issues affecting advanced nursing practice, *Nurs Pract* 23(1):14, 1998.

Pinelli JM: The clinical nurse specialist/nurse practitioner: oxymoron or match made in heaven? *Can J Nurs Admin* 10(1):85, 1997.

Pope RS: The role of nurse practitioners in research, *Nurse Practit Forum* 8(1):2, 1997.

Proctor SE: Nurses and nurse practitioners thinking differently about school nursing, *J School Nurs* 13(4):2, 1997.

Rains JW, Erickson GP: Putting prevention into practice, *J Prof Nurs* 13(2):124, 1997.

Reinhard S et al: Promoting healthy communities through neighborhood nursing, *Nurs Outlook* 44(5):223, 1996.

Safriet BJ: Health care dollars and regulatory sense: the role of advanced practice nursing, *Yale J Regulation* 9:417, 1992.

Silver HK, Ford LC, Stearly SA: A program to increase health care for children: the pediatric nurse practitioner program, *Pediatrics* 39:756, 1967.

Steiger N, Hagenstad R, Anderson A: Budget development and implementation for the APN in independent practice, *Adv Pract Nurs Q* 2(1):41, 1996.

Stevens R: When your clients are in jail, *Nurs Forum* 28(4):5, 1993.

US Department of Health and Human Services: *Healthy People 2000 national health promotion and disease prevention objectives,* Washington, DC, 1991, USDHHS, Public Health Service.

US Department of Health and Human Services, Public Health Service: Put prevention into practice: implementing preventive care, *J Am Acad Nurs Pract* 6:257, 1994.

Wasem C: The Rural Health Clinic Services Act: a sleeping giant of reimbursement, *J Am Acad Nurs Pract* 2(2):85, 1990.

Woods LP: Conceptualizing advanced nursing practice: curriculum issues to consider in the educational preparation of advanced practice nurses in UK, *J Nurs* 25(4):820, 1997.

Wright KB: Advanced practice nursing: merging the clinical nurse specialist and nurse practitioner roles, *Gastroenterol Nurs* 20(2):57, 1997.

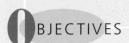

Public and Community Health Nurse Manager and Consultant

JULIANN G. SEBASTIAN & MARCIA STANHOPE

 www.mosby.com/MERLIN/community_stanhope

OBJECTIVES

After reading this chapter, the student should be able to do the following:

- Explain why nurses need effective leadership, management, and consultation skills in today's health care environment.
- Distinguish among nursing leadership, management, and consultation.
- Explain how major trends in the health care environment influence the roles and functions of nurse managers and consultants.
- Explain what is meant by empowerment and how it is related to nursing management and consultation.

- Give examples of ways that micro- and macro-level management theories are used in nursing management.
- Distinguish between content and process theories of consultation and describe their applicability to nursing practice.
- Apply the principles of process consultation in nursing practice.
- Identify consultant and client responsibilities in the various phases of consultation.
- Describe the major skills required to be effective in the nurse manager and consultant roles.
- Understand key fiscal skills required by nurse managers and consultants.

KEY TERMS

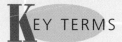

agency report card
alliances
budgets
capitated
coaching
conflict resolution
consultation
consultation contract
contracting

cost-effectiveness analysis
delegation
distribution effects
empowerment
enrollees
external consultant
generative leadership
informal structure
internal consultant

learning organizations
managed care
managed care organizations (MCOs)
negotiation
organically structured agencies
organizational structure
political skills

power dynamics
seamless system of care
service delivery networks
service leadership
supervision
variance analysis
vertical integration

See Glossary for definitions

CHAPTER OUTLINE

Contents of this chapter may reflect contributions of Roberta K. Lee from edition 3 of this text. Excerpts from this chapter were contributed by Rena Alford in edition 3 of this text. The authors gratefully acknowledge the work of both women.

Nurses have an opportunity to provide leadership in creating a new future for healthier communities. Today's changing environment has led more people to ask whether better approaches to health care delivery might be developed. Nurses are relied on more and more to organize clinical services and manage resources and to help others perform these two functions (Stevens, 1995). They perform these functions in a variety of settings, including community-based clinics, schools, health maintenance organizations, and public health departments. The roles of manager and consultant are important to the success of client outcomes that depend heavily on cost-effective, efficient delivery of care. So many aspects of health care are moving from institutional settings to the community. Nurses, therefore, need good managing and consulting skills even if they do not have formal positions as managers or consultants. For these reasons, this chapter examines the roles and functions of nurse managers and consultants in the early twenty-first century, emphasizing nursing leadership in clinical practice, personnel management, and consulting with groups and individuals on a variety of issues affecting clinical nursing services in the community.

MAJOR TRENDS AND ISSUES

The public health system in the United States is undergoing dramatic change, moving from a disorganized state to one that is focusing far more on the core public health functions of assessment, policy, and assurance (Institute of Medicine, 1988; Stevens, 1995). Nurses make up the largest part of the public health workforce and are assuming leadership roles more than ever before. For example, most local programs of maternal-child health case management and direct services are carried out and/or supervised by public health nurses, as are communicable disease programs and clinical preventive services. State directors of public health nursing are usually involved in developing policy, conducting quality assurance, and direct care practice. This means that nurses assume leadership roles at all levels in public health and need the skills necessary to improve the health care system to promote healthier communities.

Six key changes are occurring in health care today (Issel and Anderson, 1996). These are highlighted in Table 42-1.

Health care delivery is focusing on population care, with an emphasis on health rather than illness, cost containment, interdisciplinary care, and information management. Job redesign, the kinds of responsibilities given to individual employees, the ways in which nurses are expected to interact with others, the amount and kind of reimbursement available from payers, new documentation requirements, and, finally, the way the present health system is organized, are all changes designed to make the system better. Management of change is a critical skill for nurses in this environment (McPhail, 1997).

WHAT DO YOU THINK? *Consider the job redesign dilemma that Elizabeth Schaeffer faces in the following case:*

Elizabeth Shaeffer, RN, is the nurse manager of a mobile health clinic for migrant farmworkers. The clinic is owned by the local health department and is housed in a van that travels to migrant camps in a 10-county area providing outreach, casefinding, and primary care services. The clinic employs two nurses, one social worker, one physical therapist, and two lay community health workers. The health department commissioner wants to increase efficiency by instituting cross-training, meaning that the workers can do each other's jobs. The commissioner asked Elizabeth whether it would be possible to train the nurses on the van to do certain physical therapy procedures and train the community health workers to do phlebotomy and run electrocardiograms. Elizabeth is concerned about the effects on quality of care and on employee morale if these jobs are redesigned. She begins her analysis by reading the Standards for Public and Community Health Nursing Practice (ANA; APHA) and the standards for physical therapy services. What do you think Elizabeth should do?

Cost concerns have led to growth of managed care in both the private and public health care sectors. **Managed care** refers to integrating payment for services with delivery of services (Sullivan and Decker, 1997) and emphasizing cost-effective service delivery along a continuum of care (Cohen and DeBack, 1999). In Fig. 42-1, the person at point A may be a low-birth-weight infant requiring multiple costly services. By the time that individual is an adult

---

TABLE 42-1 Six Key Changes in Health Care Delivery

OLD SYSTEM	NEW SYSTEM
Person-as-customer	Population-as-customer
Illness care	Wellness care
Revenue management	Cost management
Autonomy of professionals	Interdependence of professionals
Client as nonconsumer of cost and quality information	Client as consumer of cost and quality information
Continuity of provider	Continuity of information

Modified from Issel LM, Anderson RA: Take charge: managing six transformations in health care delivery, *Nurs Econ* 14(2):78, 1996.

(at point B) the extent and expense of his or her service needs may have declined if the care has been managed well. **Managed care organizations (MCOs)** may both pay for and provide services or they may pay for services and contract with selected health care providers to actually provide services for the enrollees in the MCO. Either way, a close connection exists between service payment and service delivery. In practice, this often means that someone functions as a gatekeeper and approves and monitors the delivery of services for individual enrollees.

Managed care organizations (MCOs) collect payment from **enrollees,** or clients, before services are delivered (usually on a periodic basis, e.g., monthly). Many MCOs are **capitated,** which means that clinical agencies receive a set payment for each MCO enrollee. Any costs over and above this amount are not reimbursed. Therefore MCOs have an incentive to keep their clients healthy, and when it is necessary to provide illness care, they prefer to provide the least expensive, most effective services. As a result more health services are delivered in community settings, where costs are generally assumed to be lower.

⁞ WHAT DO YOU THINK? *Members of vulnerable populations have higher risks of poor health outcomes than others and are likely to require more costly health care. This makes these populations less attractive to managed care organizations. What role should public health agencies play in ensuring that these populations receive high-quality health promotion and illness prevention services? How does this relate to national health goals and priorities?*

Public health nurse managers and consultants are being challenged to develop new, creative health programs focused on health promotion and disease prevention and to obtain payment from MCOs for their clients. Nurse managers and consultants must be able to anticipate the cost of providing nursing services to a certain population over a period of time and to develop a proposal (or bid) for a

contract to provide the services. Because managed care organizations have an incentive to enroll the healthiest people, they may be less likely to actively recruit high-risk, disadvantaged groups. This suggests that the public health sector needs to monitor the health needs of vulnerable populations and ensure that these populations receive the health care services they require (Aiken and Salmon, 1994). In fact, public health nursing is returning to and focusing more attention on the core public health functions of community health assessment, policy making, and assurance of healthy communities.

In many local areas, the health system is being reorganized to provide a full continuum of services within a **seamless system of care.** Large, vertically integrated systems are able to do this. **Vertical integration** means that the system owns all of the services that clients might need, for example, clinics, hospitals, laboratories, and home health agencies. In other cases, free-standing agencies will collaborate and contract with one another to achieve seamlessness. The goal is to reduce fragmentation, which should be helpful for vulnerable populations, such as people who are homeless or abused, and populations with long-term care needs, such as the frail elderly and their caregivers. Nurses traditionally focused on coordinating clients' care across agencies, but this new trend in the health care system places added emphasis on more relationships, such as **alliances,** *agency partnerships, joint programs,* and participation in **service delivery networks.** Nurse managers and consultants actively participate in these groups and need good political and negotiating skills to be effective.

Another important trend is related to the movement toward more partnerships between agencies and between health care providers and community members (Porter O'Grady, 1999). The public has an increasing interest in becoming involved in planning for health services and in being active partners in their own care. It is critical for community members to take a partnership role in identifying community health needs and planning how to meet those needs. Nurse managers and consultants need to be able to listen well and collaborate with lay community members who often have different goals than health care professionals. Related to this is the public's increasing ability to get health information over the Internet and from a wide variety of publications and lay support groups. People need help deciding which information is good and how to best work with their health care providers to adapt information to their own health profiles.

One way of involving community members more actively is through continuous quality improvement programs. Continuous quality improvement includes quality assurance methods as the way to make real improvements in nursing service delivery processes (Sullivan and Decker, 1997). This approach to quality emphasizes combining both formative and summative evaluation methods, actively including clients in the process, and identifying standards upon which an agency's performance can be

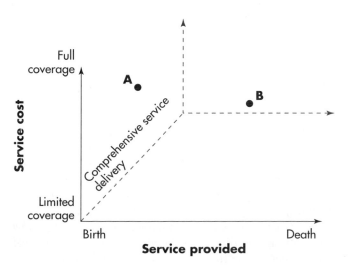

FIG. 42-1 Managed care service pathway.

judged (Simpson, 1994). Continuous quality improvement is a process that focuses on systematically enhancing care delivery to improve outcomes (Sullivan and Decker, 1997). Managed care organizations increasingly use agency report cards in selecting those agencies with which they will contract. An **agency report card** is a written listing of how the agency compares with others in the field on certain key indicators of quality, including morbidity and mortality measures, client satisfaction, and cost of care.

To know whether an agency is performing as expected, nurse managers and consultants must be familiar with their professional standards of care, the standards held by accrediting bodies, such as the Joint Commission on Accreditation of Healthcare Organizations, and guidelines for practice, such as those published by the federal Agency for Health Care Policy and Research. Nurse managers and consultants also need to know the purposes of clinical and management information systems and how to use these systems to link client outcomes with clinical and management processes. They need to be familiar with advances in use of computers in nursing practice and how to use minimum data sets and taxonomies for nursing diagnoses, interventions, and outcomes of nursing actions (Iowa Outcomes Project, 1997; McCloskey and Bulechek, 1996).

DEFINITIONS

Nursing leadership refers to the influence that nurses exert on improving client health, whether clients are individuals, families, groups, or entire communities. *Nursing management,* on the other hand, refers to the ways that nurses manage resources in providing clinical services. These resources might be people, as when a nurse coordinates an interdisciplinary team, or financial resources. An example of managing money resources is when a nurse monitors the budget for an immunization program to make sure that personnel time, supplies, and equipment are being used efficiently. Nurses also manage time. For example, home health nurses must manage their time in order to provide clients with direct and indirect nursing services, such as health education and making referrals (respectively). Nurses must possess strong leadership and management skills to be effective, whether or not they hold management positions.

Consultation has been described as a process in which the helper provides a set of activities that help the client perceive, understand, and act on events occurring in the client's environment. Consultation is similar to learning by experience because consultants help "clients find and learn about new or different ways of behaving in order to overcome some problem or difficulty" (Evans et al, 1992, p 7). Caplan (1970) defined it as a process in which a specialist identifies ways to handle work problems involving the management of clients or the planning and implementing of programs. Consultation is moving away from a focus of only helping another solve a problem to focus-

ing on creating change and developing innovations (McCutcheon and Perkin, 1996).

Management consultation "is any service provided by a qualified person or group of people to increase the effectiveness of a manager or an organization" (Berger et al, 1993, p 65). Nurses have a breadth of knowledge that makes them desirable consultants for colleagues both inside and outside the organizations in which they work. For example, a nurse working in a home health agency might be called on by a school nurse to give suggestions about the most effective way to intervene with a child using a respirator. Another example that occurs frequently is the informal consultation provided by nurses in the community who help nurses working in hospitals make effective community referrals.

Consultation is closely linked with the ideas of empowerment and self-care. When consultants help clients identify and work through problems and learn new skills that clients see as most important, they are enabling clients to solve more of their own problems. This is very similar to the traditional nursing philosophy of helping people to empower themselves, whether they are individuals, families, groups, or communities, to solve their own problems. Empowerment is consistent with Dorothea Orem's nursing theory of self-care (Orem, 1989), in which she states that the nurse's role is to promote clients' self-care abilities.

MANAGEMENT
Goals

The goals of nursing management are as follows:
1. To achieve agency and professional goals for client services and clinical outcomes
2. To help personnel perform their responsibilities effectively and efficiently
3. To develop new services that will enable the agency to respond to emerging community health needs

Theories of Management and Leadership

Leadership and management theories fall into two general categories: *micro-level* theories and *macro-level* theories. Nurses use both micro- and macro-level theories to improve a community's health. Micro-level theories originate in psychology and help explain and predict individual behavior (e.g., motivation theories) and interpersonal issues (e.g., leadership theories, communication theories, and theories of group dynamics). Macro-level theories use a sociology approach and explain issues at a broader, agency level. These theories focus on the best ways to organize work, how to obtain the resources necessary to accomplish agency goals, agency change, and power dynamics (e.g., structural contingency, resource dependence, and institutional theories).

Intrapersonal/interpersonal theories applied to nursing management

Many early management theories tried to predict how to encourage workers to be productive using micro-level approaches. These theories, detailed in Table 42-2, are im-

TABLE 42-2 Micro- and Macro-Level Organizational Theories Relevant to Nurse Managers

AREA	THEORIES	MAJOR EMPHASIS
MICRO-LEVEL THEORIES OF MANAGEMENT AND LEADERSHIP		
Management	Productivity enhancement:	
	Classical management (Taylor, Fayol)	Skill is developed through repetition.
	Neoclassical management (Parker-Follett)	Focus is on workers' human needs and group dynamics.
	Motivation	
	Need theories:	
	Basic human needs (Maslow)	People must fulfill lower level needs before they can move on to higher-level needs.
	ERG theory (Alderfer)	Needs are categorized as existence, relatedness, and growth.
	Job redesign theory (Hackman and Oldham)	Jobs should be organized so they incorporate task identity, task variety, task significance, autonomy, and feedback in order to meet worker growth needs.
	Cognitive theories:	
	Goal-setting theory (Locke)	People are more motivated to meet goals they have helped set
	Expectancy theory (Vroom)	People are more motivated to achieve outcomes they want and can reasonably expect.
	Social reinforcement theories:	
	Reinforcement theory (Skinner)	Behavior is learned based on consequences of actions.
	Social learning theory (Bandura)	People learn from role models with whom they identify. They are most motivated when they feel confident in their ability to achieve a goal.
Leadership	Contingency theory (Fiedler, Blake, and Mouton)	The most effective leadership style depends on characteristics of the task, workers, and situation.
	Path-goal theory (House)	Leaders should facilitate goal achievement through helping to reduce barriers along the path.
	Transformational leadership (Burns)	Leader encourages others to set new goals that are aligned with values.
MACRO-LEVEL ORGANIZATIONAL THEORIES		
Organizational structure	Structural contingency theory (Thompson; Burns, and Stalker)	The optimal organizational structure depends on characteristics of the work to be done, the skills of the workers, and the degree of uncertainty and change in the environment.
	Institutional theory (Meyer and Rowan; Scott)	Organizations are designed more in response to values, beliefs, and norms than as a result of rational planning.
Organizational effectiveness	Resource dependence theory (Pfeffer and Salancik)	Organizational activity is motivated by the need to acquire the resources necessary to survive. Power is a critical issue.
	Systems theory (Von Bertalanffy)	Organizations are interdependent; interorganizational relationships are key to success of individual groups and system-level outcomes.

portant to nurse managers because the cost-containing and job-redesigning trends described earlier encourage productivity. It is unclear about how to measure productivity in health care and many ethical issues relate to decisions about increasing productivity.

WHAT DO YOU THINK? *Sharon Myers is the nurse manager of a home health agency whose case mix is primarily composed of Medicare beneficiaries and enrollees in a large managed care organization (MCO). Changes in Medicare reimbursement and in utilization management policies at the MCO have led the home health agency to increasingly emphasize efficiency and cost containment. Sharon knows one way to do this is to hire fewer staff and ensure that nurses visit as many people as possible each day. She wonders, however, how many people the nurses can be expected to visit. Is an average of five visits per day adequate? What about seven, or eight? She knows of nurses who are paid per visit who make as many as 10 to 12 visits per day. Sharon is not sure how many visits a nurse can make and still provide high-quality care. She also worries about the effects on staff morale if she asks them to increase their visits beyond a certain point. "What is best?" she wonders. What factors enter into the decision? What are the ethical issues? What do you think?*

Classical management theory says that the best way to increase worker productivity is to identify the most efficient way to do the task, usually through time and motion studies and then assign a person to do that task repeatedly (Sullivan and Decker, 1997). If an agency is large enough to organize special teams of nurses, it might be able to increase productivity by doing this. For example, nurses on an intravenous therapy team in a visiting nurse agency are organized according to this theory because they specialize in tasks related to IV therapy. However, one must be aware that repeating the same task bores some individuals, whereas others enjoy the satisfaction of specializing in an area.

Neoclassical management theory, also known as the human relations approach (Sullivan and Decker, 1997), argues that managers should pay attention to workers' human needs and group dynamics and foster cooperation to increase productivity. A nurse manager might consider identifying the types of clinical cases nurses are most interested in and assigning them only these types of clients. However, this could lead to inefficiency because nurses would not always be able to organize their work geographically and may spend more time than necessary in travel. Furthermore, many clients have multiple problems, and nurses work with family groups as well as individuals, so it may be difficult to give assignments based solely on clinical interests.

This emphasis on meeting human needs and encouraging cooperation led to the development of theories of motivation and leadership. *Motivation theories* can be categorized as *need theories, cognitive theories,* and *social/reinforcement theo-*

ries. The most well-known need theory is Maslow's theory of human needs (Maslow, 1970). Clayton Alderfer (1972) modified Maslow's work by proposing that people have only three basic needs: existence, relatedness, and growth needs. His theory became known as *ERG theory,* where people do not constantly strive to meet a higher level need, as Maslow had said, but often remain at a certain level. For example, nurses who are working in an understaffed, high-stress situation may function at the existence level until their situation changes.

Alderfer's theory was adapted by Hackman and Oldham (1976) to predict how to design jobs to increase worker productivity and job satisfaction. According to Hackman and Oldham's *Job Redesign Theory,* persons with high growth needs are most productive and satisfied when their jobs provide the five elements of task variety, task identity, task significance, autonomy, and feedback. A clinic nurse whose primary job responsibility is taking clients' vital signs and assigning them to examination rooms does not have a job that is high in either task variety or task identity. A nurse case manager who works with clients over a long period and helps them manage comprehensive health care needs has much higher task variety and identity.

Most nurses see their roles as high in task significance. Nurses have a great deal of clinical autonomy, which sometimes has challenges related to delegation of authority and supervision. Certain community health functions involve high levels of feedback; for example, working with children, families, and staff in school settings typically gives the nurse many opportunities for feedback from these groups.

If all five job design elements are high this is referred to as *job enrichment.* This differs from *job enlargement,* in which only three elements of task variety, task identity, and/or task significance are enhanced. Workers often do not find job enlargement to be motivating because they view it as simply adding tasks, whereas job enrichment increases individual responsibility, autonomy, and feedback. This is important for nurse managers to know because many workers who are cross-trained or multiskilled may have had their jobs enlarged rather than enriched. Nurses who delegate tasks to others and supervise other workers should know whether these workers are more motivated by existence, relatedness to co-workers, or growth needs and attempt to meet their needs as much as possible. For example, if nursing staff in an adult day care center have high relatedness needs, then these nurses may appreciate opportunities to work together on client retreats and committees.

Cognitive theories explain that motivation results from a person's beliefs and expectations about what will occur as a result of their actions. For example, Locke's *Goal-Setting Theory* (Latham and Locke, 1991) says that people are more motivated to achieve goals they participate in setting, that are challenging, and for which they receive regular feedback. Combining this theory with Victor Vroom's (1964)

Expectancy Theory, the nurse manager should identify each employee's goals and their expectations about which actions will lead to goal achievement and whether they believe themselves to be capable of these actions. In this way, the nurse manager can identify inaccurate perceptions (e.g., the belief that the nurse manager "plays favorites" may be in error) and ways to help workers achieve their own personal goals while achieving agency goals.

Social/reinforcement theories say that human motivation results from learning that occurs following a behavior. Reinforcement theory's basic premise is that behavior is conditioned by reinforcers applied after the behavior occurs. Reinforcers are often very effective ways of increasing productivity and improving worker morale. For example, the nurse manager of a mobile clinic who thanks staff for a job well done with a note or special acknowledgements is more likely to maintain a positive working environment.

A related theory is Albert Bandura's Social Learning Theory (1977). Bandura says that people learn from role models and that confidence in one's ability to reach a goal is a key to motivation and the ability to sustain effort to achieve goals. Nurses should be aware that they serve as role models for other staff and sometimes for lay workers as well. Nurses may wish to consciously use certain behaviors and work with staff to set achievable goals and develop strategies that are realistic to achieve the goal. In this way, they can combine strategies suggested by both cognitive and social/reinforcement motivation theories.

Good leadership skills are essential for nurse managers and consultants. Although many theories of leadership have been proposed, *contingency, path-goal,* and *transformational* leadership theories are especially relevant. *Contingency leadership theory* (Fiedler, 1967) states that the most effective leadership style is contingent (or dependent) on characteristics of the relationships between leaders and followers, the task, and the situation. The most effective leadership style depends on the degree of knowledge and maturity of group members (Hersey and Blanchard, 1996). Contingency theory says that individuals who are less familiar with the task or less self-directed will be more productive when the leader focuses on accomplishing the task through coaching, supervising, and follow-up. On the other hand, individuals who have technical expertise, are highly motivated, and are self-directed primarily need guidance, opportunity, and resources from the leader. In this case, the leader functions more as a facilitator and less as a supervisor. Contingency theory is particularly relevant to community health because so many people work independently in clients' homes or in mobile clinics or other areas where supervision may be difficult. Contingency theory suggests that the nurse manager should know the level of skill, motivation, and maturity of the team members and adjust his or her leadership style accordingly.

Path-goal theory (House, 1971) says that good leaders help others identify their goals and then develop ways to help them achieve those goals. In this way, leaders serve as facilitators who identify a path for achieving the goal and remove barriers along the path. This theory focuses on individual goals and meeting individual needs and is especially compatible with the role of the nurse consultant. A major goal in consultation is helping an individual, program, department, or an entire agency identify its needs and working with it to help it meet those needs.

Finally, *transformational leadership* incorporates both the needs of organizations and individuals. Burns (1978) defined transformational leadership as that form of leadership in which the leader motivates followers to achieve a vision matches their values. Transformational leaders influence others to work toward achieving something new and as yet unimagined—essentially, a new dream. Whereas contingency and path-goal theories focus on identifying the best way to achieve a given goal, transformational leadership addresses the goal itself and the relationship of the goal to values. The transformational leader is able to transform, or change, the situation to one that differs from the status quo. Transformational leaders sometimes are found in **learning organizations** or agencies that not only learn from past experience but also create new visions for their future (Sullivan and Decker, 1997). This form of leadership has been referred to as **generative leadership** (Jaworski and Flowers, 1997) because it results in the generation of new ideas and new ways of working together. The nurse manager or consultant who recognizes opportunities for improving the health of the public and who works with others to design creative nursing programs is just one example of a transformational leader.

Organizational level theories

The macro-level, or organizational-level, theories that are particularly relevant for nurse managers and leaders are *structural contingency theory, institutional theory, resource dependence theory,* and *systems theory* (see Table 42-2). Managers and consultants often ask which form of organizational structure will best promote the efficient achieving of organizational goals. Structural contingency theory predicts that the most effective structure depends on characteristics in the given situation (Thompson, 1967). **Organizational structure** refers to the ways people in an agency organize themselves to accomplish the mission and goals of the agency. A picture is drawn of the organizational chart, which illustrates the formal lines of authority in the agency. Written documents define how the agency will operate and include the mission, goals, philosophy, policies, procedures, and job descriptions. Together, all of these elements show what the agency is trying to accomplish and how employees at all levels will work together to do so. Every agency has an **informal structure,** which is the way people actually work together; it includes informal communication patterns, informal sources of power, and unwritten rules of conduct. Nurse managers and consultants should be familiar with both formal and informal agency structures.

According to the *structural contingency theory,* agencies should have more formal structures 1) when employees perform routine tasks that are not expected to vary a great deal, 2) when employees do not have high levels of special education, and 3) when the industry or environment in which the agency operates is stable and not changing very much (Burns and Stalker, 1961). Typically, as an agency grows larger it becomes more highly structured, or formalized. This is often the case in large health departments, home health agencies, school districts, and ambulatory care clinics. On the other hand, organizations that accomplish their goals through the work of highly skilled professionals, that provide individual services that are expected to vary across clients, and that operate in a turbulent, rapidly changing environment are more likely to be successful if their structures are looser (Burns and Stalker, 1961), allowing employees latitude and autonomy in making decisions. **Organically structured agencies,** or loose organizations, are more likely to be decentralized, with much decision-making authority pushed down to the lowest level in the agency where employees have the information needed for making decisions. In the past, organic structures were most often seen in small agencies. Today, health care organizations of all types are moving toward more organic structures, despite sometimes being very large. Individual units, departments, or programs often operate very autonomously. This places a great deal of authority and responsibility in the hands of nurse managers.

Institutional theory focuses on how formal and informal values and norms affect agency activities. According to this theory, agency members are more likely to respond to widely shared values and norms of behavior than they are to formally written policies and procedures (Meyer and Rowan, 1977). For example, norms for treatment of substance abuse differ greatly from norms for treatment of severe mental illness (D'Aunno et al, 1991). Addiction treatment groups tend to value dependence on a responsible professional and admit powerlessness over the addiction. Mental health professionals, on the other hand, value increasing individual self-reliance and increasing the client's control over their own health. When a community mental health center treats both types of clients, and particularly when treating dually diagnosed clients who are both drug dependent and severely mentally ill, treatment norms may conflict. In such a situation, the written policies and procedures are not good predictors of the actual treatment practices of individual providers (D'Aunno et al, 1991). Nurse managers and consultants must be aware of the powerful influence that values and norms play in agency work and understand the informal norms that exist.

Resource dependence theory (Pfeffer and Salancik, 1978) says that the primary motivator for organizational behavior is the desire to reduce uncertainty about getting the resources necessary to operate. These resources are usually financial but also may include key personnel, seats on influential community boards, or contracts with prestigious organizations. This theory is basically about power—keeping it and maintaining it. To be effective, nurse managers and consultants must be able to accurately analyze power issues both within an agency and within the community. They must be able to predict the resource needs of the agency and how getting and maintaining those resources may affect power issues within the system.

Systems theory emphasizes the interdependence of agency players. Nurses often recognize interdependence of units within an agency but may be less aware of agency interdependence. Economists analyze how distribution affects policies, which players in a system will be influenced by policies, and how they will be influenced. For example, if the federal government reduces money for health and human services, the clients of those services may be negatively affected. Employees of service agencies also are affected because agencies are likely to downsize in order to manage the reduced funding. Consequently, employees may either lose their jobs or have wage cuts. Others likely to be affected include voluntary agencies and religious groups who might be expected to provide more services.

Roy's Adaptation Model of nursing has been extended to include nursing management (Roy and Anway, 1989). Roy argues that agencies are composed of interdependent systems. The role of nurse managers is to help the agency adapt to changing circumstances in the most effective way possible. Roy's Model is particularly helpful for explaining and predicting how nurse managers and consultants can help agencies adapt to change. Nurse managers and consultants should analyze how well interdependent units function to achieve agency goals. Furthermore, nurse managers and consultants function as change agents because they foster agency adaptation.

Nurse Manager Role

First-line nurse managers may be team leaders or program directors (e.g., director of a satellite occupational health clinic or director of a small migrant health clinic), whereas mid-level or executive-level nurse managers may be division directors (including multiple programs or departments), local or state commissioners of health, or directors of large home health agencies with multiple offices. They function as *coaches, facilitators, role models, evaluators, advocates, visionaries,* community health and *program planners,* teachers, and *supervisors.* Nurse managers have ongoing responsibilities for clients', groups', and community's health and for personnel and fiscal resources under their supervision.

CONSULTATION
Goal

The goal of consultation is to help clients to empower themselves to take more responsibility, feel more secure, deal with their feelings and with others in interactions, and use flexible and creative problem-solving skills. The functions of a consultant differ from those of managers because consultation typically is a temporary and voluntary relationship between a professional helper and a client. The similarities between consultants and managers are in their focus on empowerment and helping others develop. Consulting relationships are based on cooperation and respect between consultants and clients, who share equally in problem-solving (Argyris, 1997).

The nurse's job responsibilities may include internal and external consultation. For example, a nurse may be employed to consult with other nurses in the agency about client care problems or, as an employee of the health department, may serve as a consultant to a local community retirement center about the public health care needs of its residents. If the nurse is an **internal consultant,** the nurse is employed on a full-time salaried basis by a community agency in which the consultation takes place. If the nurse is an **external consultant,** the nurse is employed temporarily on a contractual basis by the client. The client of the external nurse consultant may be a colleague, another health provider, or a community group or agency. The nature of the consultation relationship, whether it is internal or external, should not change the goal of consultation.

Theories of Consultation

Several models of consultation have been developed. This chapter focuses on Edgar Schein's models because they are consistent with the nursing process and with nursing values of empowering clients and collaboratively working as partners with clients.

Purchase-of-expertise consultation (Fig. 42-2) is defined as the purchase (hiring) of a professional helper by a client to provide expert information or service (Schein, 1969). Buyers may be individuals, groups, or agencies. In this model the client defines the need for the consultant. The need is defined as information the client seeks or an activity the client wants to implement. The advantage of this popular model is that the client does not have to spend time or energy in solving the identified problem, because that is the responsibility of the "expert consultant." The disadvantage is that the client may question the quality of the consulta-

tion if the client has identified the wrong problem or does not like the consultant's solution.

Although this model often is used, it may be unsatisfactory in effectively and efficiently identifying and solving client problems. Once the consultant has implemented steps to solve the problem, the client must live with the consequences of the changes. This model is likely to be effective by itself only when problems are simple and the client needs specific expert information (Rokwood, 1993).

Another popular consultative model is the *physician-client* **model** (Fig. 42-3), in which the consultant is employed by the client to diagnose the problem and prescribe solutions without assistance from the client (Schein, 1969). Again, the major advantage of this model from the client's viewpoint is the limited time and energy required of the client. This model is often applied in nursing situations requiring consultation services. For example, the director of nursing at the public health department calls in a nurse consultant from the local university. Nurse productivity is poor, according to the director, and the nurse consultant is asked to diagnose what is wrong with the department. If the problem is found to be poor management rather than poor productivity by the staff, the administrator may be reluctant to accept the diagnosis. Since the client does not help diagnose the problem, the goals of consultation may not be met. The purchase-of-expertise and physician-client models are content models of consultation since they deal with the content (or nature) of the problem.

The *process consultation model* focuses on the process of problem solving and collaboration between consultant and the client (Rokwood, 1993). The major goal of the process model, as seen in Fig. 42-4, is to help the client assess both the problem and the kind of help needed to solve the problem (Schein, 1969). Process consultation includes assessing the underlying agency culture that influences the problem and its solution (Schein, 1990). Both consultant and client participate in the problem-solving

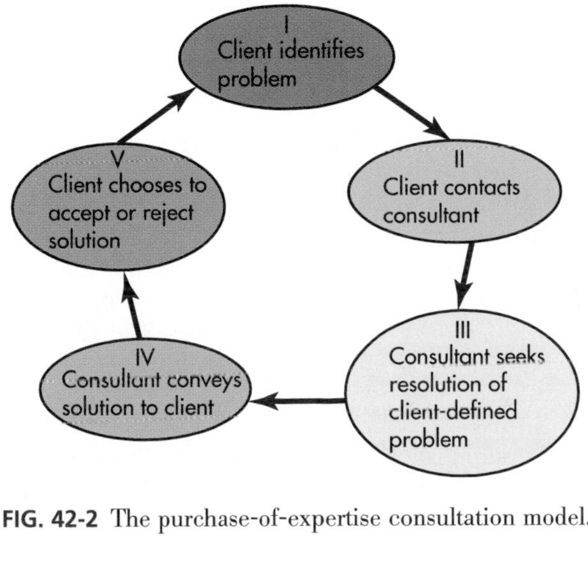

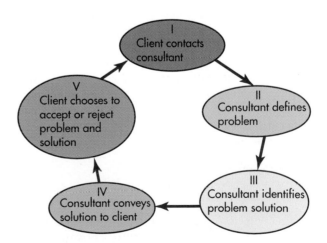

FIG. 42-2 The purchase-of-expertise consultation model.

FIG. 42-3 The physician-client consultation model.

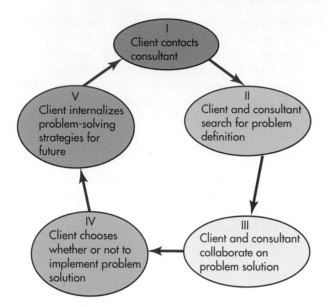

FIG. 42-4 The process consultation model.

steps that lead to changes or to actions for problem solution. The assumptions related to each of the three models are listed in Box 42-1.

Content and process consultation models do not need to be mutually exclusive (Rokwood, 1993; Schein, 1989). Instead, although consultants should emphasize process consultation, they should be willing to share their expert knowledge when appropriate. Because process consultation is collaborative, Schein (1989) recommends that consultants be willing to offer opinions and advice at all stages of the consultation process. Thus, although the major emphasis should be on process consultation, consultants may find it effective to integrate the two models at selected points, using both context and process.

In the process model, the consultant is a resource person whose primary goal is to provide the client with choices for decision making. As shown in Fig. 42-5, the process consultation model includes the same steps as the nursing process, establishing a nurse-client relationship based on trust to assess the problem, plan and implement actions, and evaluate the outcomes of nursing interventions. Nursing interventions may be described as direct client care or as consultation activities, depending on the goal of the intervention. The analysis and synthesis of the process consultation model by Blake and Mouton (1983) serves as the basis for the following discussion and application of this model.

Process Consultation

Process consultation involves a temporary relationship between client and consultant for the purpose of bringing about change. Consultation may be proactive or reactive. *Proactive consultation* is directed toward anticipating a future problem and taking steps to prevent it. *Reactive consultation* is directed toward curing an existing problem through therapeutic intervention. For example, a parent-teacher council developing a school-based family resource center contacts the nurse to assist with options for future nursing and health care for the students and their families. The board wishes to be proactive and plan for the needs of high-risk students and families. The administrator of a minimum-security prison has found that inmates are missing work for minor health problems and that health costs are skyrocketing. The nurse is asked to help explore solutions to the problem. Prison administration is reacting to an existing problem requiring immediate intervention.

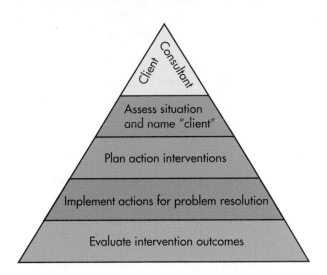

Client

Consultant

Assess situation and name "client"

Plan action interventions

Implement actions for problem resolution

Evaluate intervention outcomes

FIG. 42-5 Integration of the nursing process and the process model of consultation.

: NURSING TIP

One of the most important decisions a nurse makes before accepting or writing a consultation contract is to identify the client in the situation.

The client is identified by determining who in the situation has the problem and needs to change. The following vignette illustrates this point:

Barry Rubin is a school health nurse who receives an inquiry from the school board about ways to get parents to support a school-based clinic. Barry decides that the consultation contract needs to include representatives of the school board and representatives of the parents' group to find effective answers to the question. He realizes that time would be wasted and resistance to change would still be present if the focus were only on one group at a time. If he met separately with the parent group, they may decide such a clinic should be limited to acute illnesses and injuries and should include parental permission for all interventions. At the school board meeting he could find that the board is concerned about teenage pregnancy and sexually transmitted diseases and wishes to provide more comprehensive interventions that ensure confidentiality for the students. After spending much energy meeting with both groups separately, he would find that by being a messenger between the two groups rather than a facilitator for problem solving, the consultant role has been diluted. On the other hand, by meeting with both groups together Barry could serve as a resource for helping the parents and school board explore all viewpoints and alternatives for solving the problem. In this case, both the school board and the parents' group are Barry's clients.

Once the client has been identified, the nurse must decide the best method(s) for intervening in the problem situation. Blake and Mouton (1983) describe five basic intervention modes or techniques that can be applied to the process consultation model: *acceptant, catalytic, confrontation, prescriptive,* and *theory-principles.* These are summarized in the How To table. The *acceptant intervention mode* involves clarifying emotional reactions so that more objective problem solving can begin. This intervention mode benefits the client by improving self-acceptance, emotional health, and the ability to objectively define and deal with problems. Two disadvantages exist with this intervention mode. Expressing emotions may only help the client accept the circumstances leading to the problem rather than taking actions to correct the problem, and this catharsis may be seen by others as hostile and aggressive (Blake and Mouton, 1983).

In the *catalytic intervention mode,* the consultant helps clients broaden their view of the situation by gaining additional information or by considering existing data (Blake and Mouton, 1983). The consultant helps the client clarify understanding of problems by increasing available information, break down barriers to communication by identifying ineffective communication patterns, and raise the awareness of all involved regarding the problem. The consultant is a *facilitator* providing the client with the information needed to solve a problem. Lack of information, however, may be the symptom, not the problem. The disadvantage of having the consultant improve information flow is that the client may rely on the facilitator for data rather than becoming efficient in finding solutions to future problems (Blake and Mouton, 1983; Caplan, 1970).

The *confrontation intervention mode* presents the client with facts that reveal the client's values and assumptions in ways that cannot be denied or disputed (Blake and Mouton, 1983). This intervention mode provides clients with an objective look at how their values and beliefs control their behavior. By looking at present behavior, the consultant and client can examine alternative values to redirect behavior toward improved methods of problem solving. The disadvantage is that the client may not wish to participate in interactions that could be interpreted as criticism (Blake and Mouton, 1983). For example, a consultant may find that the staff nurses in a local public health department are going to resign their positions because they view the director's decisions as autocratic and uncompromising. On the second visit to the agency, the consultant could confront the director with these observations. The director may deny the behavior and point out evidence of having acted democratically. As a result of the confrontation, the director may regard the consultant's observations as personal or be willing to examine and analyze the differences between the perceived and the actual behavior.

The *prescriptive intervention mode* requires less collaboration between consultant and client because the consultant tells the client how to solve the problem (Blake and Mouton, 1983). This mode is best used along with other intervention modes, such as acceptant or catalytic. If clients do not participate in problem solution, they will not be able

HOW TO *Apply Consultation Intervention Modes*

INTERVENTION MODE	DEFINITION	PROBLEM EXAMPLE	CONSULTANT ACTIONS
Acceptance	Consultant urges client to share feelings to move to more objective problem solving	Low morale Feelings of powerlessness to change a situation	Attempt to understand the client's feelings about the situation. Listen actively. Encourage the client to talk. Try to clarify the client's feelings and help the client accept the feelings. Refrain from agreeing or disagreeing with the client's situation. Encourage the client to explore ways of dealing with the problems. Listen for more data to reveal the total scope of the problem.
Catalytic	Consultant broadens client's knowledge of problem by offering new data or clarifying existing data	Standards are violated or changed Inability to meet goals or objectives	Set a nonauthoritarian tone for the interaction by beginning the intervention with social conversation. Ask the client to describe the situation and use the description as a basis for the interaction. Suggest data-gathering techniques that may provide new information of interest to the client. Provide support to the client as the client attempts to accurately perceive the problem. Avoid specific suggestions. Encourage the client to make decisions about problem resolution.
Confrontation	Consultant presents clients with indisputable facts	Additional insight needed Unwillingness to solve problem	Continually question clients about their description of the situation. Present data and logic to test clients' chosen courses of action. Challenge clients' chosen courses of action. Probe for motives and causes of present situation. Provide own thoughts about situation without personally attacking client's values.
Prescriptive	Consultant tells client how to solve problem	Inability to cope Needs immediate answer	Probe for data about the client's situation. Act authoritatively. Control by telling the client how the problem is to be perceived. Tell the client the best solutions. Remind the client if he or she is procrastinating in implementing actions. Offer praise if the client does exactly what the consultant suggests.
Theory-principles	Consultant teaches how to solve problem using theories or principles	Additional insight needed Lack of knowledge to solve problem	Introduce theories for problem-solving to the client. Use techniques to help the client internalize theories. Provide strategies for practical application of the theories, such as problem situations or critiques of application. Offer support when the theory is applied in the actual problem situation.

to solve future problems and may not follow the prescriptions offered. The advantage of the prescriptive intervention mode is its usefulness in situations where clients have lost confidence in their problem-solving ability or have given up in despair (Blake and Mouton, 1983). In the above example, the nurse consultant could decide that the best method of dealing with the problems between the staff and the director is to present a prescription for behavioral conduct to be implemented by the director and the staff. The consultant tells the group when and how follow-up evaluation will be done to look at the progress of both parties in solving their differences.

Use of the *theory-principles intervention mode* requires that the client learn theories, such as behavior theory, and their application to problem solving. This intervention mode introduces the theories after clients have shared their usual methods of problem solving. It also allows the client to apply the theories to problem situations while developing skills in problem diagnosis and solution. The major challenge with this mode is determining how to help clients learn practical ways to apply the theory (Blake and Mouton, 1983). This mode can be combined with another mode because consultation involves facilitating client learning (Evans et al, 1992). Evans and colleagues (1992) explain that theory can be used to help clients better understand what the data are saying, better diagnose the problem, and generate more potentially effective decision alternatives. Before using this mode with the health department staff and director, the consultant may present a conference on leadership theories and principles and a discussion of the responsibilities in administrative decision making. The consultant may be able to show both parties how leadership styles should vary with the types of decisions to be made and with the people involved.

The choice of an intervention mode depends on the client and the problem. Blake and Mouton (1983) identified four categories of problems: *power/authority, morale/cohesion, norms/standards,* and *goals/objectives.* The *power/authority* problem results from questions about who has the right to supervise and who has the right to make decisions. The *morale/cohesion* problem occurs when the client has lost confidence in the ability to solve problems and feels powerless. The *norms/standards* problem occurs when group norms or professional or agency standards are violated or changed. Problems related to *goals/objectives* involve developing new goals, changing goals, or being unable to meet goals.

Several intervention modes may be used with each type of problem. The most common intervention for morale/cohesion or power/authority problems is the acceptant mode because the issue generally causes feelings that block decision making. The catalytic mode is the best choice with norms/standards and goals/objectives problems because it focuses on strengthening the client's perceptions of the most effective decision-making methods. The theory/principles intervention mode may be helpful regardless of

the problem, especially when additional insights are needed. The prescriptive mode may not be helpful unless the client is unable to cope with the situation and needs immediate direction or answers to solve the problem (Blake and Mouton, 1983) or unless the problem is fairly straightforward (Rokwood, 1993).

Consultation Contract

The consultation relationship is based on expectations. The consultant has expectations concerning time, money, resources, and the participation of the client in the process. Clients have expectations about what they will gain from the consultation relationship. Discussing the terms of a **consultation contract** makes expectations explicit, reduces the likelihood of violations of contract terms, and reduces the risk of additional demands being made on either party. Clients will want to know the type of content expertise the consultant has and the consultation processes, communication strategies, and types of feedback the consultant will provide (McCutcheon and Perkin, 1996). Areas to include in the written consultation contract are as follows:
1. Client and consultant goals
2. The identified problem
3. The consultant's resources
4. The time commitment
5. Limitations of the contract
6. Cost
7. Conditions under which the contract may be broken or renegotiated
8. Intervention modes to be used
9. Expected benefits for the client
10. Methods of data collection to be used
11. Client resources
12. Potential interventions
13. Evaluation methods to be used
14. Confidentiality

An example of a consultation contract appears in Fig. 42-6.

Writing a contract for consultation relationships has a number of advantages. The contract terms assist the consultant in determining the number of hours that must be devoted to the interaction and in identifying needed resources and out-of-pocket expenses required to complete the interaction. Negotiation of the contract assists the client in identifying realistic expectations of the consultant and firmly establishes what the consultant will and will not do. The client has the opportunity during the negotiation to place limits on what the consultant can do, and the contract allows for future renegotiation of terms. Pricing methods for consultation services vary with the nature of the services. Consultants may price their services based on the actual number of billable hours required to perform the service, or set a flat fee during the contract negotiation phase. Flat fees are more attractive to clients since they reduce uncertainty over the total cost of the consultation. They create an incentive for consultants to be efficient and

Client Name: J. Hyde, Nurse Manager Address: Residential Complex Phone: 111-2222	Consultant Name: P. Jones, Nursing Student Address: College of Nursing Phone: 333-4444

Estimated costs (external consultant only): $500
(including phone, secretarial assistance, preparation, supplies, travel expenses, and consultant sessions)

Client problem definition: Facility undergoing expansion: residents likely to need more assistance with health promotion & health monitoring. Average resident age is 72.3 yrs. Residents have on avg. 2.5 chronic illnesses each. 10-15 miles from health facilities. Residents are becoming increasingly homebound.

Suggested intervention mode: Catalytic/Prescriptive

Client goals:
A healthy resident population through accessible and ongoing health promotion & monitoring.

Scope of consultation (time & no. of sessions):
3 planning & data gathering sessions in 6 weeks; 3 evaluation sessions at 2 to 3 week intervals during data collection; final evaluation session.

Consultant resources (e.g., computer, secretary, library):
Computer to analyze data; library; assistance from faculty; staff to collect data (3 students).

Contract renegotiation & termination terms:
Renegotiation at 2 to 3 week evaluation conferences. Termination at final evaluation conference.

Client resources (e.g., records, secretary, copy):
Project records available to collect data; secretary type survey questionnaires; conference room for interviews; final report typing; supplies.

Anticipated client benefits:
Residential complex will have a plan for meeting health needs of residents. Residents will have increased access to health promotion & health monitoring services.

Contract limitations (e.g., who, what, when, how data will be shared):
Survey of residents' health needs, and perceptions of staff and administrators by CHN student. Report to nurse manager, facility manager, and college faculty.

Potential interventions (e.g., report shared with administration: meetings held with staff):
Meetings with staff and residents to obtain input on the problem and potential solutions. Review of resources to find the residential complex's ability to manage the problem itself.

Consultant goals:
Collect data as outlined.
Assess and define problem in collaboration with residents, staff, and administration. Identify resources for solving the problem. Develop a realistic method for solving the problem in collaboration with residents, staff, & administration.

Data collection methods:
Interviews: Staff, nurse manager, facility manager, local health care providers
Surveys: Residents
Focus groups: Residents, staff & administrators, faculty
Phone: N/A
Contract evaluation:
                At the end of 12 weeks will look at potential alternatives; choose one that is satisfactory to residents, staff, & administrators.

FIG. 42-6 Example of how to write a consultation contract.

to use an accurate method of estimating their services before the contract negotiation meeting.

Consultation involves seven phases:

1. Initial contact with the client
2. Definition of the relationship
3. Selection of a setting and approach
4. Collection of data and problem diagnosis
5. Intervention
6. Reduction of involvement and evaluation
7. Termination

The initial contact is made when the client or someone in a family, group, agency, or community communicates with the nurse about a potential problem that requires intervention. The communication may be person-to-person during a home visit, may be written, or may occur by telephone. On initial contact, the client and the nurse have an exploratory meeting to define the problem, assess the nurse's ability to help and interest, and formulate future actions. If the nurse has little experience with the type of problem presented, the client may wish to seek assistance elsewhere. Also, if the nurse is quick to make decisions and has a directive approach, the client with a more laissez-faire attitude may have difficulty accepting the nurse's approach. The nurse may also conclude that the situation is not within the nurse's expertise and will want to recommend someone else to work with the client.

Next, the terms of the relationship are discussed. The nurse consultant finds out what the client expects to gain from the relationship and develops terms for the interaction. Finally, in the initial exploratory meeting the setting for the consultation is decided on, the time schedule is set, the goals of the interaction are established, and the mode of intervention is chosen.

When the terms of the contract are agreed upon, the data gathering methods will be part of the agreement. Data gathering methods used by consultants include direct observation, individual and group interviews, use of questionnaires or surveys, and tape recordings. One particularly useful data gathering strategy is the focus group (Krueger, 1994). This is a group of 8 to 10 people who share a common characteristic, such as staff nurses in the same organization or community members living in the same neighborhood. Focus groups are led by one individual, who has prepared five to six open-ended questions to guide the discussion. A recorder takes thorough notes during the session. Focus group sessions are usually 1 hour in length and include refreshments. After the session, the leader and recorder discuss their observations and impressions in order to capture all important data. The outcomes of focus group discussions can guide the development of written surveys (LoBiondo-Wood and Haber, 1998; McDaniel and Bach, 1994). See the Research Brief that il-

RESEARCH *Brief*

This paper reports on the results of focus groups conducted to better understand the causes of underimmunization in children under 2 years of age. Developers of the Consortium for the Immunization of Norfolk's Children designed the study to accomplish three goals: 1) to identify barriers to childhood immunizations from the perspectives of mothers; 2) to supplement data already gathered in structured household interviews about barriers to childhood immunizations; and 3) to enable coalition participants to conduct a component of the community needs assessment. Six focus groups were conducted with mothers of preschool-age children. Study participants represented private, public, and military sectors of the economy, as well as parents who were homeless. The focus groups were conducted by trained moderators. Questions related to mothers' knowledge and attitudes about immunizations, positive and negative experiences in obtaining immunizations, barriers to obtaining immunizations, and suggestions for reducing barriers.

Focus group participants indicated they knew the importance of immunizations but found the process of obtaining both initial and subsequent immunizations to be confusing and complicated. They often did not know where to obtain immunizations, when to return for boosters, or that immunizations were free. They indicated that clinic hours were inconvenient and that public clinics were not "family

friendly" (p. 54). Participants felt these clinics were uncomfortable and that staff were not always sensitive or responsive to them. Transportation and providing care for siblings were difficult, as was scheduling appointments. Suggested strategies to overcome these barriers included implementation of an immunization hotline and mounting a local print media campaign combined with information on billboards, as well as bus and taxi boards. Focus group participants recommended providing immunizations in elementary schools, providing opportunities for walk-in clinic appointments, and considering a community van to transport parents and children to clinic appointments. Consortium members subsequently decided to institute an "Adopt-a-clinic" program (p. 54) to encourage local groups to improve the environments within public clinics (through addition of fresh wallcoverings, furniture, play equipment).

Implications for the nurse: The nurse can more clearly define the health problem and appropriate solutions to the problem that will be used by the clients to be served by having a focus group that includes representatives of all persons affected by the problem and the solution.

Butterfoss FD et al: Use of focus group data for strategic planning by a community-based immunization coalition, *Fam Comm Health* 20(3):49, 1997.

lustrates how focus groups were used for strategic planning related to a community-based immunization program.

While data are being gathered and after the diagnosis has been finalized, the nurse actively engages in the chosen intervention mode. After fulfilling the terms of the contract, the nurse must disengage or reduce the amount of involvement with the client. Decreased contacts allow each side to evaluate the effectiveness of the intervention. During disengagement the nurse reassures the client that future interactions are possible at the client's discretion. When the agreed-upon period of disengagement has passed, the relationship is terminated. The nurse typically provides the client with a written summary of the findings and recommendations resulting from the interactions during the disengagement and termination phases (Ingersoll and Jones, 1992).

The consultation relationship involves responsibilities by both the nurse and the client. Although the contract defines the terms of the relationship, the client can assist in making the consultation process a success. Initially the client must determine whether an internal or external consultant can best assist in solving the problem. An internal nurse consultant knows the agency and the values of the agency and the staff, is a team member, has expertise, and is probably committed to helping solve internal problems. The external nurse consultant brings new ideas and a broader regional or national perspective; has new or proven strategies to offer; can bring objectivity to the problem; and has a short-term, less expensive commitment to the agency. An example of a consultative intervention follows:

Intervention: Prescriptive
Client: Director of Nursing
Consultant: Internal
Problem: Norms/standards

The client telephoned the state nurse consultant and requested a meeting at the local health unit. The purpose of the meeting was to review serious problems the local nursing staff was having in meeting program standards and requirements, as identified in a recent audit. The nurse consultant, Elizabeth, met with the client, Maggie, and reviewed her findings, sharing her analysis of the problems and contributing factors. The central problem was defined as inconsistent supervision of staff with a need for role clarification of supervisory responsibilities. Maggie was immobilized by the situation. Elizabeth directed Maggie to restructure the supervisory job descriptions to clearly reflect supervisory roles and expectations; she also recommended giving supervisors written performance evaluations and guidelines for improving staff performance. Elizabeth maintained contact with Maggie until termination of the consultation occurred and corrective action was completed.

Nurse Consultant Role

An agency that delivers care similar to an official public health service will most likely employ a generalist nurse who provides traditional or nursing consultation for a broad range of community health activities (e.g., a com-

munity or public health nurse clinical specialist). A community health agency that provides a program approach to the delivery of community health services, such as family planning, maternity, child health, handicapped children's services, school health, or home health, will tend to employ specialist consultants. These consultants may have skills and training in specific clinical areas (e.g., a pediatric clinical nurse specialist) in addition to broad community health expertise. Agencies providing primary health care require a consultant with both general knowledge of public health practice and specialized knowledge in a primary care clinical area. This is also a requirement in agencies involved in long-term and home health care.

The nurse consultant employed within an official health agency functions as an internal consultant to the employing agency. As a representative of the agency, the nurse provides nursing and consultation to colleagues, other disciplines, agency administration, and other health and human service agencies and/or community groups. Two primary roles of the internal consultant are resource person and facilitator.

With knowledge of available resources, the nurse consultant can identify gaps in service, identify the critical services provided by the health care delivery system, and promote services for meeting health or social needs of the population. The consultant facilitates staff nurse problem solving about individual client and family needs, health needs of a group of clients, or professional concerns and attitudes. The consultant may assist managers and administrators in solving problems about personnel, program needs, organizational goals, community relationships, and client population needs. The consultant also may facilitate communication across agencies by working with interagency coalitions or alliances.

A generalist nurse in an official community agency is often required to function in a dual supervisor/consultant role. Supervision means decision making and implementing activities in an ongoing relationship, which is the opposite of consultation. Functions of the supervising role could replace the consultation role, and the staff could perceive the supervisor/consultant as being directly aligned with administration. Effective communication is vital.

The internal consultant as a representative of the employing agency has implied authority that may result in conflict between the consultant and the client. The amount of conflict depends on the centralizing or decentralizing of the health agency and the degree of autonomy of the individual units in the organization. One way to decrease potential conflict is to clearly define the role the consultant is to assume. For example, in one state, the state health department has jurisdiction over all the county health departments (centralized). The state has decided to decentralize by making all the county health departments autonomous in their delivery of health services. The state health department will continue to advise the county units about delivery of services but will not supervise the delivery of care. Nurses in the county units will have their own director, and the nurse consultants at the state level will be used as resource persons and facilitators.

Although the state health department was centralized and provided direct supervision to the counties for delivery of health care, the state family planning consultant was also responsible for supervising the county health department staff members who were responsible for delivery of family planning services. In the decentralized system, the supervisory functions are removed from the consultant's responsibilities, and the consultant facilitates the work of other nurses by offering advice and information that will assist them in understanding how to do their work.

The role of external nurse consultant also involves acting as a facilitator or a resource person. The external nurse consultant may represent the employing agency and provide information to the client for planning interagency programs to meet population needs. The external nurse consultant may serve as a resource to health educators, school personnel, psychologists, counselors, dentists, social workers, physicians, legislators, and probation officers, providing data about individual client, group, or community needs. The external consultant may be asked to serve as facilitator to an official agency board to solve problems about community health priorities or to serve as a facilitator or resource person to voluntary agencies, such as the American Red Cross or the American Heart Association.

Consultants from federal agencies often are used as external nurse consultants. The nurse consultant from the federal agency may come to the local or state agency to serve on request as facilitator or resource person helping with program planning, development, and implementation. The primary role function of this consultant is to serve as a resource person, although the consultant may facilitate movement toward identifying actual program objectives.

SKILLS REQUIRED BY MANAGEMENT AND CONSULTANT ROLES

Leadership Skills

Nurse managers and consultants need effective leadership, interpersonal, organizational, and political skills. With today's strong emphasis on teamwork, partnership, and coalitions, management skills are focusing more toward coaching and leading empowered groups (Goodemote, 1995). *Leadership* essential to these roles involves identifying a vision and influencing others to achieve the vision, emphasizing that client needs are the basis for health services, empowering others, balancing attention to people and tasks, delegating tasks and managing time appropriately, and making decisions effectively. Increasingly, leaders must be smart, flexible, able to identify trends, and work comfortably with different types of people and cultures (Lancaster, 1999). Table 42-3 identifies core competencies for nursing leaders in today's health care environment.

The Essential Public Health Services Work Group of the United States Public Health Service (1994) articulated the vision and mission of public health in America, the definition of public health, and essential public health services, which is presented in Box 42-2.

Nurse managers should be involved in developing agency level vision, mission, and goal statements. The American Nurses Association and the American Public Health Association, Public Health Nursing Section, both offer guidance in these areas.

Service leadership

Effective nursing leaders understand the concept of **service leadership.** Greenleaf (1991) points out that customers come first, and the leader's basic function is to serve customers. Expanded to the health care context, nurse managers and consultants need to remember that clients are the reason for their work, whether clients are individual clients in a primary care clinic; families in a home care caseload; aggregates, such as teachers and staff in a school setting; or entire communities. This means that basic organizational assumptions often must change. For example, the assumption of organizational hierarchy as a pyramid with clients at the bottom and administration at the top must be reversed. In a service leadership context, administration is at the bottom of the pyramid and clients are at the top, with staff who work directly with clients located immediately below clients. This alteration in perspective is more than just a picture; it changes the leader's basic assumptions about work rules. For example, in a traditional bureaucracy, organizational efficiency is achieved by developing detailed rules governing how work is done. Often these rules do not match the needs of individual clients. If a single mother brings her three preschool children to a health department clinic for a check-up for her

---

TABLE 42-3 Core Competencies for the Twenty-First Century Leader

COMPETENCIES	KNOWLEDGE AND ABILITIES
Conceptual competencies	Systems thinking Acclimatization to chaos Pattern recognition and synthesis Continuous learning
Participation competencies	Involvement Empowerment Accountability
Interpersonal competencies	Receptivity and similarity Immediacy and equality Facilitation Coaching
Leadership competencies	Technical expertise Transformational style Interactive administering

From Porter-O'Grady T, Wilson CK: *The leadership revolution in health care,* Gaithersburg, Md, 1995, Aspen.

BOX 42-2 Public Health in America

Vision: Healthy People in Healthy Communities
Mission: Promote Health and Prevent Disease

PUBLIC HEALTH

- Prevents epidemics and the spread of disease.
- Protects against environmental hazards.
- Prevents injuries.
- Promotes and encourages healthy behaviors.
- Responds to disasters and assists communities in recovery.
- Ensures the quality and accessibility of health services.

ESSENTIAL PUBLIC HEALTH SERVICES

- Monitor health status to identify community problems.
- Diagnose and investigate health problems and health hazards in the community.
- Inform, educate, and empower people about health issues.
- Mobilize community partnerships and actions to solve health problems.
- Develop policies and plans that support individual and community health efforts.
- Enforce laws and regulations that protect health and ensure safety.
- Link people to needed personal health services and ensure the provision of health care when otherwise unavailable.
- Ensure an expert public health work force.
- Evaluate effectiveness, accessibility, and quality of health services.
- Research for new insights and innovative solutions to health problems.

From Essential Public Health Services Work Group, United States Public Health Service: *The Nation's Health*, p 3, Dec, 1994.

infant and must return at a different time to obtain immunizations for the 4- and 5-year-old children, her needs and the needs of her children have not been met. On the other hand, if the clinic is organized around family needs, as opposed to specializing in the needs of narrow age groups, then all three of her children can be immunized in one visit and the client's needs have been met.

Empowerment

Leaders provide **empowerment** by helping others empower themselves to make organizations more responsive to client needs. This means helping staff acquire the knowledge, skills, and authority to act on behalf of clients (Manthey, 1991). It means removing barriers to decision making and allowing staff nurses the authority to make client decisions in "real time," as needs demand, rather than requiring nurses to obtain numerous approvals. Empowerment is more than simply increasing workers' authority. It includes ensuring that they have the necessary information, knowledge, and skills to effectively make the

decisions for which they are being empowered. For example, nurse managers who are responsible for preparing their own department or program budgets and for approving program spending must be given the opportunity to learn budgetary concepts. The concept of empowerment underpins the consulting process. Consultants assist others in identifying solutions to problems and, more importantly, in developing the ability to manage problems independently in the future.

Balance between people and tasks

A key leadership skill for nurse managers and consultants is the ability to balance attention to people and to tasks (Hersey and Blanchard, 1996). This skill derives from *contingency leadership theory* and means that effective leaders do not focus all of their attention on simply getting the job done; if they do this, they may appear cold and uncaring and reduce staff morale. Similarly, effective leaders do not spend all of their time attending to workers' personal needs and problems. If they did this, the goals of the agency would never be met. Effective leaders must balance their focus, depending on the needs and skills of those with whom they work and on the demands of the situation. In situations in which time is a critical factor, such as in disasters, effective leaders emphasize tasks, such as providing victim triage, meeting basic community needs for safe food and water, and organizing shelter. After the emergency has stabilized somewhat, they should attend to long-term mental health needs, such as shock, grief, and posttraumatic stress syndrome.

Delegation

Effective leaders need to be able to manage time well and to delegate appropriately. For example, nurse consultants must be able to accurately predict the amount of time that will be required for each phase in the consulting process (McCutcheon and Perkin, 1996). The purposes of **delegation** include increasing agency efficiency, developing others' talents, and managing time well (Sullivan and Decker, 1997). Agency efficiency increases when tasks are assigned to the first level in the hierarchy where employees possess the necessary skills and knowledge to complete the task and where the task is related to the goals of those positions. Delegation develops others' talents and can contribute to job satisfaction. Asking a staff nurse in a nursing clinic for the homeless to develop a booklet describing community resources for the homeless helps the staff nurse learn more about community resources, the gaps that exist in local resources, and where opportunities exist for interagency collaboration. The staff nurse also is likely to learn about visual presentation, layout and brochure design issues, and how to present material at the appropriate reading level. Finally, delegation is an important tool in time management. A school nurse may delegate locating resources for a screening clinic to the parent-teacher association and spend the time he or she saves on developing a teaching plan for volunteers who will help with the actual screening. Strategies for effective delegation and time management tips are listed in Box 42-3 and Table 42-4.

Delegation has become an increasingly important skill for nurses, whether they have official roles as a manager or not. As more agencies increase their use of unlicensed assistive personnel and lay community workers, nurses increasingly are delegating selected aspects of practice to others and supervising the completing of those tasks. Two types of delegation occur in clinical practice. *Direct delegation* involves speaking to an individual personally and transferring responsibility for a task to that person (ANA, 1994). *Indirect delegation* results when an agency has policies and procedures in place that stipulate the tasks that may be performed by someone else other than the person who is accountable (ANA, 1994). Sometimes nurses mistakenly think that they are not accountable for tasks that are indirectly delegated through agency policies (e.g., policies for cross-training). However, if nursing care has been delegated, then nurses are accountable for the safe and effective completion of that care.

When planning direct delegation, nurses should first decide when to delegate. The five factors that should be considered when deciding whether to delegate a task are as follows:

1. The potential risk of harming the client
2. The complexity of the nursing task
3. The extent to which the task requires complex problem solving
4. The extent to which the outcome is predictable
5. The degree of interaction involved with the client (Harrell, 1995)

Generally, nurses should not delegate tasks that are high risk, complex, novel, unpredictable, or that will result in nurses having limited contact with clients. Barriers to delegation include inadequate experience or education, lack of confidence, unclear role expectations, and lack of clarity about legal accountability (Harrell, 1995).

BOX 42-3 Time Management Tips

- List goals for 5 years, 1 year, and daily.
- Prioritize the goals.
- Identify the tasks needed to perform to accomplish the goals.
- Identify tasks that can be delegated.
- Group the tasks in a meaningful way (e.g., geographically).
- Plan strategies to minimize time-wasters. For example, plan office hours when people may find you in your office available to respond to questions.
- Plan to work on tasks at times when you are at peak level of efficiency (e.g., plan tasks requiring mental alertness in the morning if you are more alert at that time).
- Plan plenty of time to accomplish tasks with adequate transitional time between tasks.
- Say no to tasks that are not essential to your position or your goals.
- Take adequate breaks from work, including breaks during the day and vacations.
- Maintain personal energy level through good health habits, including proper nutrition and adequate exercise and sleep.

TABLE 42-4 Strategies for Effective Delegation

PROCESS STEPS	PROCESS ACTIVITIES
Assessment	Determine the work that is to be assigned.
	Assess the needs of the clients who will be affected.
	Evaluate the needs of the situation, including professional standards and agency policies.
	Identify relevant laws and regulations and what they say about delegation to various levels and categories of personnel.
Planning	Determine who possesses the knowledge and skills to do the work safely and effectively.
	Develop assignments that allow people to function safely and to grow and develop.
	Identify the components of the tasks to be delegated.
	Develop realistic deadlines for completing the task.
	Determine the best process for delegation—when to ask for feedback, which resources are needed, the amount of supervision required.
Implementation	"Delegate without guilt"
	Communicate expectations clearly and succinctly and provide opportunities to ask questions.
	Explain any procedures or important elements of the task.
	Clarify tasks as necessary, listen to others' points of view, and communicate appreciation for others' efforts to provide quality service.
	Encourage staff to report any observation they feel is important and emphasize the importance of quality and client satisfaction.
Evaluation	Provide feedback at planned intervals.
	Seek out regular progress reports.
	Provide constructive criticism of behaviors, not personalities.
	Provide praise in public, constructive criticism in private.

From Adams D: Teaching the process of delegation, *Sem Nurse Managers* 3(4):171, 1995.

The first source of guidance for delegating tasks to unlicensed individuals is the state nurse practice act. The next source of assistance comes from specialty professional organizations. For example, the National Association of School Nurses, in collaboration with three other national groups (The Joint Task Force for the Management of Children With Special Needs, 1990), issued detailed guidelines about the school nurse's responsibility in delegation. In general, any task involving special knowledge from advanced education cannot be delegated to an unlicensed person. This includes assessment, data analysis, planning, monitoring, and evaluation (National Council on State Boards of Nursing, 1990). For example, a school nurse would assess a child with physical disabilities and develop a plan of care for that child. Selected aspects of that plan of care, such as assisting with feeding or emptying a catheter bag and recording output, could be delegated to an assistant, providing that person had received appropriate training and was competent to perform the task. This means that it is not adequate that the nurse knows the individual has been certified as a nursing assistant; he or she also needs to know that the individual is competent to safely perform the delegated task. The nurse retains the legal accountability for safe client care. This responsibility may be shared with the person to whom one is delegating, but accountability is never transferred. Box 42-4 provides further information on delegation.

Decision making

Finally, a core leadership skill is the ability to make decisions effectively. Along with communication, decision-making skills have been found to be among the most important for nurse managers (Chase, 1994). This is a two-stage process in which nurse managers first must decide how much input they will seek from others and, second, generate alternatives for the decision and choose among the alternatives. Including others in the decision-making process is beneficial in part because others may have information and ideas that would lead to a better decision and because others may support the decision more if they are involved in making it. However, *participatory decision making* is more time-consuming than making decisions alone.

Choosing whether to include others in the decision-making process should be based on the extent to which the manager or consultant needs information and ideas from other people, the extent to which those affected are likely to support a decision they do not participate in making, and the extent to which time pressures are present. A decision tree can be used for selecting a leadership style that varies from a unilateral, independent decision process, to progressively more participative styles, with the most participative style involving delegating authority to a group to be responsible for making the decision. Although many assume that autocratic decision making is not effective, in fact it may be both effective and efficient under certain circumstances, such as emergencies. In other situations, it may be better to seek input from others individually or as a group, to seek suggestions for solutions from the group, or simply to turn a problem over to a group to solve on their own.

The next stage of the decision-making process is to generate alternative solutions and to choose among those solutions. Bernhard and Walsh (1995) developed a useful decision model for nurses. With this model, the nurse determines what characterizes a good decision in the case at hand and then determines what the goal is for that decision. For example, both risk and cost are important dimensions in most situations. The goal is low cost and low risk to clients and staff. Other dimensions might be unique to the situation. Table 42-5 presents the process for deciding whether to develop an in-house wellness program for an occupational setting or to contract with a consulting group for that service. After identifying the key dimensions and goals, the nurse manager ranks each alternative according to how well it is likely to match the goals. For example, if an alternative poses no risk at all, then it completely matches the goal of low risk and receives a ranking of 1. If it poses moderate risk, the nurse might choose to give it a 0.5; if it poses a high level of risk, he or she may give it a 0 because it does not match the goal at all. After rating each alternative along every dimension, the scores are added, and the alternative with the highest score is the one selected for implementation.

In this example, the occupational health nurse manager would choose to develop the wellness program in house rather than using a consultant. The advantages of this model are that it allows for staff participation in identifying key dimensions and goals and brainstorming creative solutions; participants' values are built into the dimensions and goals; and it allows for both creative and logical thinking processes. This is a particularly helpful decision model for nurse consultants.

Critical thinking

Nurse managers and consultants must be adept at critical thinking. *Critical thinking* includes values, makes assumptions explicit, and encourages creativity and innova-

---

> **BOX 42-4 Delegating Responsibility**
>
> Nurse managers share responsibility for any tasks they delegate to others. The nurse manager delegates responsibility for a task but retains final accountability for the safe, effective outcome of the task (ANA, 1994). It is critical, then, that the nurse manager know that the individuals to whom they are delegating responsibility are both prepared and capable of effectively performing the tasks. Nurse managers should plan specific times to obtain progress reports on task completion. This will allow the opportunity to manage problems as they arise and to provide staff with helpful feedback or instruction if needed.

tion (Tappen, 1995). It includes reflection about the connections between sociocultural and biophysiologic aspects of health status and services. Critical thinking may be fostered through the use of guided group discussions, in which group members are assisted to think about the connections just described and about the **distribution effects** that decisions may have on others. It also is fostered through activities to stimulate creativity, such as brainstorming, synectics, and nominal group techniques (Sullivan and Decker, 1997). In the example of the occupational wellness program, the nurse manager would need to critically think about ways to increase program quality.

Interpersonal Skills

Nurse managers and consultants need good interpersonal skills in communicating, motivating, appraisal and coaching, contracting, supervising, team building, and managing diversity.

Communication

Good communication skills, including skills in the use of assertiveness techniques, are essential to being effective in managerial and consultation roles. Nurses have a particular challenge in communicating because many of those with whom they work may be in a different health profession or in a different field altogether. Nurses often communicate with lay workers also. It is especially critical to listen carefully, to make underlying assumptions clear, and to speak in the other's language. This may mean avoiding the use of professional jargon and speaking in more commonly shared language or speaking in the listener's dominant language. For example, a nurse manager working in a migrant clinic with a large Hispanic population would find it helpful to know Spanish.

Communication must be culturally sensitive to be effective. Because communication involves words, tone of voice, posture, eye contact, and space relationships, cultural norms often influence the meanings given to different aspects of body language. For example, whereas most advise direct eye contact when communicating, in some cultures this may be viewed as aggressive, especially when the eye contact is prolonged. Some cultures prefer closer-space relationships that may make others feel they are being crowded. Other aspects of communication are important as well, such as the appropriate place for reprimands. It is never appropriate to reprimand or criticize in public, although public praise is usually an excellent idea. Nurse managers and consultants should be sensitive to the power of written communication and be aware that, although putting a message in writing is a good way to avoid confusion, it also may be seen as aggressive, distrustful, or as a bid for power. On the other hand, managers and consultants must accurately document their assessments and interventions (Ingersoll and Jones, 1992). The key is to make certain that the message that is communicated is the message that was intended. Effective communication skills are listed in Box 42-5.

Motivating others

One of the more difficult skills to master is motivating other people. In fact, one cannot ever really motivate others, since motivation is internal. However, the skillful manager can create a motivating environment, working to make certain that both individual and agency goals are met to the extent possible. Sometimes individual motivation may be low because employees do not believe they have the skills necessary to achieve their goals or they believe that the system will not allow them to do so. The effective nurse manager identifies which perceptions are inaccurate and helps individuals develop plans for improving their personal capacities for achieving goals. Although adequate salaries are clearly important, it is not always possible to in-

TABLE 42-5 Bernhard and Walsh's Decision-Making Model Example Decision: How to Provide Employee Wellness Services

DIMENSION	GOAL	SOLUTION #1 PROVIDE WELLNESS SERVICES USING CURRENT STAFF		SOLUTION #2 CONTRACT FOR WELLNESS SERVICES WITH LOCAL CONSULTANTS		SOLUTION #3 CONTRACT WITH LOCAL CONSULTANTS ONLY FOR EXERCISE PROGRAM	
Feasible	Yes	Probably	0.7	Possibly	0.3	Likely	0.8
Risk	Low	Moderate	0.1	Low	1.0	Moderate	0.2
Cost	Low	Low	1.0	High	0.0	High	0.3
Quality	High	Fair	0.5	Excellent	1.0	Moderate	0.5
Certified instructor	Yes	No	0.0	Yes	1.0	Yes	1.0
Fully utilize staff	Yes	Yes	1.0	No	0.0	Partially	0.5
Consistent with company values	Yes	Yes	1.0	Maybe	0.2	Maybe	0.4
Totals			4.3		3.5		3.7

Modified from Bernhard LA, Walsh M: *Leadership: the key to the professionalization of nursing,* ed 3, St Louis, 1995, Mosby.

BOX 42-5 Effective Communication Skills

- Active listening
- Restating the main points
- Speaking in the listener's language
- Culturally appropriate eye contact and body language
- Appropriate context
- Awareness of the power of written communication
- Simple, direct words
- Use of "I" statements and saying how you feel
- Frequent feedback
- Reflection on the meaning of the message

BOX 42-6 Keys to Motivation

- Identify employee needs and goals.
- Identify beliefs about employees' abilities to meet their goals.
- Discuss with employees their strengths and areas for future development.
- Discuss how the employees' goals and the organization's goals can be aligned.
- Jointly develop job-related goals with employees, including timetables with checkpoints.
- Provide frequent, regular feedback to employees.
- Identify with the employee his or her key reinforcers.
- Provide frequent thanks for a job well done and for progress toward goals.
- Facilitate the development of mentor-protégé relationship and role modeling.
- Provide opportunities for employees to learn new goal-related skills.
- Provide tangible signs of recognition, such as merit pay, employee of the month, special bonuses for achievements.

crease pay in the short run. Nurse managers possess other tools for increasing motivation, even when budgets are tight. One home health aide supervisor is known for the high level of morale among her staff and the unusually low level of turnover, despite low salaries. She makes a point of being available for discussion before the aides leave the agency in the morning and upon their return in the afternoon. Also, she always puts a birthday card and small piece of candy in their mailboxes on their birthdays, and thanks them for a job well done. Other keys to motivation are listed in Box 42-6.

Appraisal and coaching. Employee appraisal and coaching are closely related to motivation and individual development. The purpose of performance evaluation is to assist employees to more effectively meet the objectives of their roles and to help them develop their potential in ways that facilitate achieving agency goals. Performance evaluation should not take place just before an annual appraisal interview is scheduled. It should be a regular part of the job, with the manager providing regular feedback on employee progress toward goals. *Performance appraisal* is particularly challenging for nurse managers because so many community health workers practice independently in the field. For example, nurse managers in home health must plan either to make visits with the nursing staff on a regular basis or to obtain other forms of input on employee performance, such as planning telephone or office conferences with staff.

Coaching involves "directing and closely supervising tasks, and explaining decisions, soliciting suggestions, and supporting progress" (Blanchard et al, 1985, pp 30, 56; cited in Vestal, 1995, p 73). With coaching, managers retain responsibility for decisions but request input and explain decisions. They support progress by helping the employee break the task into manageable parts, providing resources for accomplishing task and for acquiring the necessary skills, and praising task accomplishment. Coaching is most useful with people who may not yet be skillful in a particular area and who are not confident about their skills.

Contracting involves identifying expectations and responsibilities by both parties. Some contracts are informal, verbal agreements between individuals, whereas others (such as the consulting contract) are formal, written agreements.

Supervision

Nurse managers who delegate tasks to others must *supervise* the completion of those tasks and build in mechanisms to make certain that the tasks are completed safely and effectively (ANA, 1994). As stated earlier in the chapter, **supervision** means decision making and implementation of activities in an ongoing relationship. The American Nurses Association defines supervision as "the active process of directing, guiding, and influencing the outcomes of an individual's performance of an activity" (ANA, 1994, p 9). Supervision may occur either on site when the nurse manager is present while the activity is being performed, or off site when the nurse manager "provides direction through various means of written and verbal communication" (ANA 1994, p 9). It is important for nurse managers to build effective means of providing off-site supervision because so many community health activities do not take place within a single agency (e.g., home health care occurs within individual homes, and school health services are provided within individual schools).

Handling criticism is a difficult skill that involves both the give and take of criticism related to job performance. Nurse managers should provide constructive criticism as close as possible to the time they observe a problem with an employee's job performance. Constructive criticism is that which focuses on the behaviors necessary to meet the job expectations and helps identify sources of problems,

TABLE 42-6 Guiding Principles of the Interactive Team

PRINCIPLE	DESCRIPTION	RESULT
Participation and leadership	All team members are viewed as equals, and their participation is encouraged and supported.	Team functions as a cohesive unit.
	Leadership role is assigned in turn to the individual having the greatest expertise.	Promotes equal distribution of leadership responsibilities.
Development of goals	Goals must be developed in a cooperative manner with attention focused on meeting the needs of the client. Secondary focus should be placed on meeting the needs of all team members.	Team functions as a cohesive unit.
Communication	Open communication among team members should be fostered and encouraged, with each member feeling comfortable expressing opinions and thoughts on any and all issues.	Effective team functioning
Decision making	Important decisions should be the joint responsibility of all team members. This should be accomplished through consensus.	Effective team functioning
Conflict resolution	Conflict must be dealt with openly in a productive manner, respectful of all viewpoints. Steps to resolve conflict should be designed when the team is first formed	Effective team functioning

From Coben SS et al: Meeting the challenge of consultation and collaboration: developing interactive teams, *J Learn Disabil* 30(4):430, 1997.

resources for managing problem behavior, and feedback. For example, if an employee is chronically tardy, the nurse manager should speak privately with the employee about the job expectation for promptness, identify why the employee is frequently tardy, establish a behavioral goal with time frames and consequences of achieving or not achieving the goal, and assist the employee to develop a plan for achieving the goal. The employee may simply be unaware of the importance of being punctual and can easily change the behavior. On the other hand, a behavior modification plan based on social learning theory may be useful to help share the desired behavior (Sullivan and Decker, 1997). Behavioral consequences may include both positive reinforcers, such as praise, and disciplinary measures, such as oral and written warnings, limited raises, suspension, and termination. Suspension and termination normally are used only with problems related to safety, inability to perform job duties, breach of confidentiality, and illegal acts and are detailed in agency policies and procedures.

Team building

Finally, team building and managing diversity are group-level skills needed by nurse managers and consultants. Interdisciplinary teams increasingly are used to assess clients, plan client care or services, and manage quality improvement activities. Teams may include members of multiple health disciplines as, for example, with home infusion teams (Sheldon and Bender, 1994). They also may include people from other backgrounds, including lay community health workers, such as Hispanic nurse exten-

ders (Bray and Edwards, 1994). Nurse managers and consultants can facilitate team building by assisting the team to develop goals and ground rules, identifying who will fill various roles and determining how to share leadership, developing strategies for ongoing cooperation and recognition of contributions of each member, and resolving conflict. Key principles of an interactive team are listed in Table 42-6 (Coben, Thomas, Sattler et al, 1997).

Managing diversity

A key challenge to nurse managers is managing diversity in positive, growth-promoting ways that value diversity. Because the demographic profile of the American workforce is changing so rapidly, the nature of the workplace is changing as well. Female and nonwhite groups are increasing the most rapidly in the workforce (AARP, 1993), with projections that 25% of the workforce will be composed of African-Americans, Hispanics, and Asian Americans by the year 2005 (Mancini, 1995). Nurse managers must understand cultural values and norms to communicate effectively and interpret behavior accurately. They must know how to prevent any form of racial, sexual, or ethnic harassment and ensure a positive and welcoming environment in the workplace.

Organizational Skills

Nurse managers and consultants use organizational skills, such as planning, organizing, implementing and coordinating, monitoring and evaluating, improving quality, and managing fiscal resources.

DID YOU KNOW? *Nurse managers and consultants are more likely to be effective when working with people from cultures different from their own if they take the time to learn as much as possible about the culture. This includes learning the language if possible. For example, nurses who are not Native Americans but who work with them should learn about the culture of the tribal groups with whom they are working. Similarly, nurse managers and consultants who work with Vietnamese immigrants (or any other immigrant group) should try to learn about the culture of that group. This helps clarify underlying beliefs, values, and assumptions that may influence managerial or consultative issues and improves communication effectiveness and the effectiveness of change processes. Nurses who are not Hispanic but work with many Spanish-speaking Hispanic persons will find it helpful to learn to speak conversational Spanish or at least hire a translator.*

Planning

Planning includes prioritizing daily activities to achieve goals. It also includes long-range planning, such as working with nurses in a department to plan a new program. Because planning is primarily a cognitive activity, nurse managers and consultants may lessen its importance and allow little time for adequate planning. However, planning is the basis for direct nursing services, so it is important to make adequate time for planning.

Several documents are available to help nurse managers and consultants plan nursing services. *Healthy People 2000* (USDHHS, 1991) defines the national health goals for the United States by the year 2000 and should be the basis for program planning. Progress toward these goals was evaluated in 1995 and is described in the *Mid-Course Review* (USDHHS, 1996). National health goals for the year 2010 are under development and may be reviewed on the USDHHS website (see this book's website at www.mosby.com/MERLIN for a link to this website). The 1998 Presidential Initiative on Racial and Ethnic Health outlines six targets for special efforts to reduce health disparities between racial and ethnic minority groups and the United States population as a whole (Hamburg, 1998). These areas of emphasis should be the special focus of community health programming until goals for reducing health disparities across groups have been met.

Each community has different needs and strengths that should be incorporated into health planning. Model Standards for Community Health Programs (APHA, 1992) provides guidelines for adapting the year 2000 objectives to local conditions and baseline local health indicators. The Assessment Protocol for Excellence in Public Health (APEX-PH) (National Association of County Health Officials, 1991) gives detailed suggestions for maximizing a health department's ability to work with the community in meeting the year 2000 objectives. A Planned Approach to Community Health (PATCH) (Kreuter, 1992) provides guidelines for ways to work in partnership with the community to develop strategies for improving personal and community health.

Collaboration

Nurses and consultants must collaborate with other disciplines to provide coordinated services for target populations requiring multiple services from diverse agencies. For example, high-risk students have problems that are not neatly categorized as health or education problems (Igoe, 1994). Therefore school nurses must work cooperatively with others to plan for comprehensive services. One model for doing this is the Five-Stage Process for Change (Fig. 42-7) (Melaville et al, 1993), which is based on a partnership process built on trust. This model is made up of the following stages:

1. Organizing a group of people interested in the problem
2. Building trust and commitment to solving the problem
3. Developing a strategic plan for managing the problem
4. Taking action
5. Adapting the model to other situations and solidifying the program within the organizational structure

Organizing

Organizing involves determining appropriate sequencing and timelines for the activities necessary to achieve goals and arranging for the appropriate people to carry out the plan. Flow sheets and timetables are helpful tools that allow nurse managers and consultants to visualize how tasks are organized and to identify gaps in the planning. Fig. 42-8 illustrates a timetable for conducting a health fair.

Implementing

Implementing a plan includes not only following the timelines but also making certain that adherence to relevant regulations are followed, appropriate documentation of activities, and coordination of the work of all team members. Nurse managers and consultants should give sufficient attention to the change process by helping those involved identify the need for change, keeping them informed, soliciting their input, and making modifications in the plan as necessary.

Monitoring and evaluating

Monitoring and evaluating are critical to community-oriented nursing services. Nurse managers should monitor nursing services on a regular basis and make improvements as soon as the need for improvements becomes apparent. Professional standards and the standards of various accrediting bodies guide the focus of monitoring and evaluating. The Joint Commission on Accreditation of Healthcare Organizations standards for home health and ambulatory care clinics provides detailed and explicit minimum standards that all such agencies should be expected to meet.

In addition to professional standards of practice available from the American Nurses Association and specialty nursing organizations, the Agency for Health Care Policy and Research has published clinical guidelines for preven-

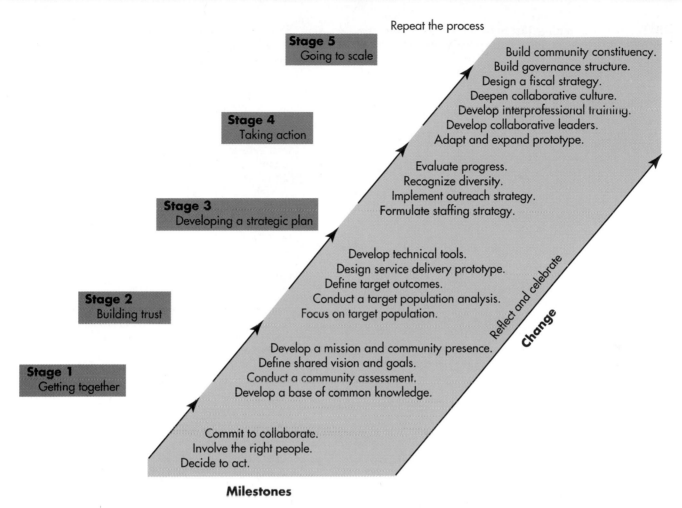

FIG. 42-7 The five-stage process for change. (From Melaville AI, Blank MJ, Asayesh G: *Together we can: a guide for crafting a pro-family system of education and human services,* Washington DC, 1993, US. Government Printing Office.)

Activity	Month 1	Month 2	Month 3	Month 4
Identify planning group	●——→			
Decide which displays to include		●——→		
Reserve location		●——→		
Invite exhibitors		●——→		
Develop referral policies for follow up of screening tests			●————————→	
Arrange for publicity			●————————————→	
Conduct the health fair				●→

FIG. 42-8 Sample timetable for conducting a health fair.

BOX 42-7 Screening Test Sensitivity and Specificity

Sensitivity =

$$\frac{\text{Number of true-positives}}{\text{Number of true-positives} + \text{Number of false-negatives}}$$

$$\times 100$$

Specificity =

$$\frac{\text{Number of true-negatives}}{\text{Number of true-negatives} + \text{Number of false-positives}}$$

$$\times 100$$

CRITERIA FOR A SCREENING PROGRAM

- Test has high sensitivity and specificity.
- Test meets acceptable standards of simplicity, cost, safety, and patient acceptability.
- Disease that is focus of screening should be sufficiently serious in terms of incidence, mortality, disability, discomfort, and financial cost.
- Evidence suggests that the test procedure detects the disease at a significantly earlier stage in its natural history than it would present with symptoms.
- A generally accepted treatment that is easier or more effective than treatment administered at the usual time of symptom presentation must be available.
- The available treatment is acceptable to patients as established by studies on compliance with treatment.
- Prevalence of the target disease should be high in the population to be screened.
- Follow-up diagnostic and treatment service must be available and accompanied by an adequate notification and referral service for those positive on screening.

Modified from Valanis B: *Epidemiology in nursing and health care*, ed 2, Norwalk, Conn, 1992, Appleton & Lange.

BOX 42-8 Components of the Expense Section of an Operating Budget

Salaries
Direct salary costs
   Staff
   Fringe benefits
Expenses
  Direct expenses
    Supplies
    Equipment
    Travel
  Other
Overhead
  Administration
  Depreciation
  Ancillary services
  Marketing
  Other

Modified from Finkler SA, Kovner CT: *Financial management for nurse managers and executives*, Philadelphia, 1993, W.B. Saunders.

---

tion and treatment of selected health problems, such as wound care and pain. Although adhering to the clinical guidelines is voluntary, health professionals may need to justify not following them if client outcomes are poor. Managed care organizations are likely to use guidelines to standardize the process of care and needs for resources. One of the challenges for the nurse manager and consultant is keeping abreast of the numerous standards applicable to his or her practice setting and the changes in those standards.

One example of a guideline that is useful in making programmatic decisions is the concept of screening test sensitivity and specificity. When planning screening clinics, nurse managers must choose tests that are both sensitive and specific. A test is sensitive to a health problem when it is likely to detect all cases of the problem and not give false negatives. On the other hand, to be useful, a test must also be specific to that health problem and not give false positives. These concepts provide a useful decision making tool for the nurse manager. Formulas for determining sensitivity and specificity, and guidelines for screening programs are in Box 42-7.

Fiscal Skills

Forecast costs

Finally, nurse managers must be skilled in the area of fiscal management. Nurse managers and consultants must be able to forecast the cost of nursing services. This is especially important in a managed care environment because the forecast should include risk rating of the likely health and illness experiences of a target population. Combining community health assessment skills, epidemiologic projections, and consultation are key steps in this process. After developing a profile of the anticipated health and illness experiences of a target population, the next step is anticipating the amount and kind of nursing resources needed by the population. These skills are basic to the development of proposals for managed care contracts.

Develop and monitor budgets

Nurse managers have taken on more responsibility for developing and monitoring their own department **budgets** as agencies have decentralized. They must be able to develop a justifiable budget and monitor how actual spending compares with planned spending. Box 42-8 lists the usual expenses to be included in an operating budget. It is helpful to obtain staff input when developing a budget in order to make financial projections as realistic as possible. Combining anticipated volume, revenues, and expenses allows the nurse manager to anticipate a break-even point for new services (i.e., determining when a new program can be expected to be financially self-sufficient).

Table 42-7 shows a portion of a variance report. **Variance analysis** means identifying the variation between ac-

TABLE 42-7 Variance Report

Item	Expected Budget ($)	Actual Budget ($)	Variance ($)
Salaries	40,000	42,000	(2000)
Supplies	750	1000	(250)
Travel	1000	600	(400)
Total	41,750	43,600	(1850)

tual and planned results, determining the cause of the variation, and correcting problems when they exist. Spending more than anticipated is not always negative; it may simply indicate that client or service volume was higher than anticipated. This could, however, be of concern in an agency that is fully capitated since additional services do not bring in additional revenues. Nurses in fully capitated environments have more opportunity than ever before to focus on health promotion and illness prevention services.

Higher expenses than planned are not always under the control of the nurse manager. For example, if the prevailing wage rate increases because of changes in the labor market, an agency may spend more than expected on salaries. On the other hand, spending less than predicted does not always indicate that a program is running efficiently. It may be that client volume is down, or that staff are not providing adequate services.

In the example in Table 42-7, the nurse manager observes that more has been spent on salaries and supplies than originally budgeted and less on travel. Is this desirable or undesirable? To analyze the variance the nurse should ask if the prices for labor and supplies were higher than expected or if the agency has used more nursing time or supplies than planned (Finkler and Kovner, 1993). The answers to these questions will help determine whether the variance resulted from factors under the manager's control, such as inefficiency, or from factors outside of the manager's control, such as higher wage rates or higher prices than expected. The answers also will help determine whether the variance resulted from an increase in client volume or an alteration in case mix, with the agency serving sicker clients. Whether a client volume variance or case mix alteration is seen as desirable will depend partly on whether the agency is paid on a fee-for-service basis or on a capitated basis. In a capitated environment, higher volume will be viewed in a more positive light if the services are primary care health promotion services and more negatively if the services are inpatient acute care services. On the other hand, in the traditional fee-for-service environment, there is a stronger incentive to prefer higher volume in the inpatient acute care areas.

Conduct cost-effectiveness analysis

Regardless of the type of reimbursement system in place, nurses should be able to conduct a **cost-effective-**ness analysis of their interventions. Such analyses are not measurements of the efficiency of a program (see Chapter 21 for a discussion of this distinction) but are comparisons of the money spent for the outcomes across two or more interventions. Cost-effectiveness analyses compare alternative approaches for achieving the same goals. The example in Table 42-8 shows the comparison costs and outcomes of two different approaches to smoking cessation in an occupational health site (Mastroianni and Machles, 1997). The total costs of Intervention A, which includes weekly meetings with a nurse, diaries, and pamphlets, come to $3445. Intervention B does not include planned weekly meetings with the nurse; instead, employees may choose to meet with the nurse as they desire. This intervention also does not include diaries. The total cost of intervention B is $217.

The cost-effectiveness ratio for each intervention is calculated by dividing the total cost by the number of people who quit smoking (the outcome). Another approach is to divide the total cost by the total savings in health costs for clients who quit smoking. Using either approach, the ratio for intervention B is lower, which means that the costs to achieve the outcome were lower than for intervention A. Thus intervention B would be the preferred option.

Political Skills and Power Dynamics

Political skills include negotiation skills, conflict resolution skills, and skills in recognizing and managing power dynamics. *Principled negotiation* (Marriner-Tomey, 1996) involves bargaining based on the characteristics of the issues, rather than focusing on participant personalities. This form of **negotiation** emphasizes collaborative problem solving rather than rigid choice of a single position. It does not imply compromising values or goals, but instead emphasizes development of mutually agreeable ways of achieving goals. **Conflict resolution** strategies can result in win-win, win-lose, or lose-lose outcomes. Strategies most likely to create win-win situations include collaboration, confronting problems directly, and ensuring that all parties have adequate opportunity for input (Sullivan and Decker, 1997).

Nurse managers and consultants must understand **power dynamics.** Because nurses possess altruistic values, they may believe that being powerful is not necessary. However, it is impossible to create health promoting clinical services without some legitimacy in decision-making arenas. Nurse managers need power to ensure that working conditions are conducive to excellent clinical care. Power may originate in information, knowledge, and positioning. Nurse managers who are knowledgeable about health care trends and issues, client needs, and clinical services are more likely to have expert power. Membership on community agency boards and advisory committees puts nurse managers in the position to influence service delivery.

Consultants' advice may be followed because of *perceived expert power.* The client feels that the consultant pos-

TABLE 42-8 Comparing Cost Effectiveness of Two Smoking Cessation Programs for 30 Employees

	INTERVENTION A	INTERVENTION B
DIRECT COSTS		
Development		
Program design implementation (nurse $22/hr)	$176/8 hr	$22/hr
Diary and pamphlet distribution	$44/2 hr	$44/2 hr
Operation		
Program (nurse $22/hr)(30 employees × 15 min/wk × 12 wk)	$1980/90 hr/12 wk	$88/4 hr
Diaries	$150	$0
Pamphlets	$15	$15
INDIRECT COSTS		
Employee time away ($12/hr) (30 employees × 15 min/wk)	$1080/90/12 wk	$48/4 hr
TOTAL COSTS	$3445	$217
3-month quit rate	15.90%	8.90%
Number of employees quit	4	2
Annual health care costs for smoker ($228/yr)	$912	$456
Cost effectiveness ratio for # of employees who quit	861:1	108:1
Cost effectiveness ratio for health care costs of smokers	3.7:1	0.47:1

From Mastroianni K, Machles D: What are consulting services worth? *Am Assoc Occupat Health Nurses J* 45(1):41, 1997.

sesses superior knowledge or skills and is trustworthy and credible. The internal nurse consultant may have *legitimate power* resulting from his or her role in the organization. The external consultant has only *assumed power*, which may result in conflict for the consultant and the client. The client may not feel obligated to implement the recommendations. On the other hand, external consultants may possess *referent power* because of an affiliation with other well-known consultants or a national organization. The consultant's ability to persuade clients by offering reasons, new techniques, or methods of problem solving may establish the consultant's *informational power*.

clinical application

The nurse manager of a nursing clinic in a residential facility for frail elderly approached the local college of nursing for assistance with health promotion and health monitoring activities for the residents. The facility was undergoing renovation and was expected to more than triple its capacity by the time the renovation was completed. The nurse manager thought the health promotion activities that were already in place would be inadequate to serve the growing needs. Most of the residents were over 70 years of age and had several chronic illnesses each. The residential complex was 10 to 15 miles away from health care facilities.

Sheila, the nurse manager, supervised a staff of three nurses and one homemaker aide. She contracted with a local physical therapy firm for services as needed for the residents. Sheila had asked the staff if they thought they could

realistically expand their services and they suggested consultation. The staff commented that residents really needed nurses who could provide health monitoring and skilled nursing services in their apartments, because so many were increasingly homebound. Staff members were hesitant about expanding into home care themselves because they feared it would mean a cutback in the health promotion activities they were currently engaged in. They though the needs and the resources that would be required to meet the needs should be evaluated before making any final decision.

What should the staff do to complete the evaluation of the problem?

A. Call a meeting of persons affected by the problem and decide on using an internal or external consultant to help evaluate the problem.
B. Write a contract and indicate how they want the evaluation to be done.
C. Develop a plan to implement home health services because the plan would include an analysis of needs and resources.
D. Continue with their health promotion activities and decide about home health services when more resources could be identified.

Answer is in the back of the book.

KEY POINTS

• The goals of nursing management are 1) to provide leadership in achieving organization and professional goals for client services and clinical outcomes, 2) to empower personnel to perform their responsibilities effectively and efficiently, 3) to develop new services that will enable the organization to respond to emerging community health needs.

- Nurses use micro-level management theories to help them function in leadership roles, facilitate individual and group motivation, and foster effective group dynamics. Macro-level management theories provide direction for planning and organizing work, obtaining resources necessary to achieve organizational goals, and managing power dynamics.

- Nurse managers may be team leaders or program directors, directors of home health agencies or community-based clinics, or commissioners of health. They function as visionaries, coaches, facilitators, role models, evaluators, advocates, community health and program planners, and teachers. They have ongoing responsibilities for clients, groups, and community health and for personnel and fiscal resources under their direction.

- The goal of consultation is to stimulate clients to take responsibility, feel more secure, deal constructively with their feelings and with others in interaction, and internalize skills of a flexible and creative nature.

- Consultation models can be categorized as content or process models. Both purchase-of-expertise and physician-client models are content models. Purchase-of-expertise model consultation involves hiring an expert to provide information or service. In the physician-client model of consultation, the client hires the consultant to find the problem and offer solutions without background data or assistance from the client. Process model consultation helps the client assess both the problem and the kind of help needed to solve the problem.

- Five basic intervention modes or techniques applied to process consultation are acceptant, catalytic, confrontation, prescriptive, and theory principles. The use of a particular intervention mode is based on the client and the problem. Four categories of problems are power/authority, morale/cohesion, norms/standards, and goals/objectives.

- Consultation involves seven basic phases: initial contact, definition of the relationship, selection of setting and approach, data collection and problem diagnosis, intervention, reduction of involvement and evaluation, and termination.

- Nurse consultants may function as internal consultants within an organization or external consultants outside the client organization.

- Nurse managers and consultants use a wide variety of skills, including leadership, interpersonal, organizational, and political skills. Leadership skills include abilities to influence others to work toward achieving a vision, empower others, balance attention to people and tasks, delegate tasks, manage time, and make decisions effectively.

- Interpersonal skills include communication, motivation, appraisal and coaching, contracting, team building, and diversity management skills.

- Organization skills include planning, organizing, and implementing community health nursing services, monitoring and evaluating services, quality improvement, and managing fiscal resources. Political skills are those used in negotiation and conflict management and managing power dynamics.

- Generally, both nurse managers and consultants must hold a baccalaureate degree in nursing or higher. Organizations employing nurses without this credential should help them obtain additional education in the areas of community and public health nursing, management theories and principles, and theories and principles of consultation.

critical thinking activities

1. Discuss with your class members the implications that managed care has for nurse managers and consultants in community-based organizations and in the public health departments. What other implications can you think of in addition to those described in the text?

2. Draft a vision and mission statement for a nursing clinic with your classmates. Develop goals and objectives that follow the vision and mission you selected. What type of employees would you need to hire? List some of the policies and procedures you would need to have in such a clinic based on your vision, mission goals, and objectives.

3. Have several class members obtain the vision, mission, and philosophy statements from several agencies in which students have community health clinical experiences. Compare these statements in terms of the agencies' target populations, basic values, and essential functions.

4. Interview one or more practicing public health staff nurses. Ask them to describe the activities of their jobs that could be categorized as consultation. During the interview, attempt to determine the following:
   a. How they define consultation
   b. The goals they are attempting to achieve with their consulting activities
   c. The model they seem to be applying in their consulting activities
   d. The intervention modes they use
   e. Whether their activities are of a generalist or a specialist nature and of an internal or external consultative nature
   f. The strengths and limitations they perceive in themselves regarding their consultative functions (e.g., education, experiential, organizational, relational, economic)

5. Interview one or more public health nurse consultants. During the interview, attempt to determine the answers to the preceding questions. Compare the responses of the two groups (consultants and staff nurses). Analyze the factors you think account for the similarities and differences.

Bibliography

Aiken LH, Salmon ME: Health care work-force priorities: what nursing should do now, *Inquiry* 31(3):318, 1994.

Alderfer CP: *Existence, relatedness, and growth: human needs in organizational settings,* New York, 1972, Free Press.

American Association of Retired Persons (AARP): *America's changing workforce,* Washington, DC, 1993, the Association.

American Nurses Association (ANA), Council of Nurses: *Standards of community health nursing practice,* Kansas City, Mo, 1986, the Association.

American Nurses Association (ANA): *Standards for organized nursing services and responsibilities of nurse administrators across all settings,* Kansas City, Mo, 1988, the Association.

American Nurses Association (ANA): *Registered professional nurses and unlicensed assistive personnel,* Washington, DC, 1994, American Nurses Publishing.

American Public Health Association (APHA): *Healthy communities 2000: model standards,* ed 3, Washington, DC, 1992, the Association.

Argyris C: Field theory as a basis for scholarly consulting. *J Soc Iss* 3(4):811, 1997.

Bandura A: *Social learning theory,* Englewood Cliffs, NJ, 1977, Prentice-Hall.

Berger MC, Ray LN, Del Togno-Armanasco V: The effective use of consultants, *J Nurs Adm* 23(7/8):65, 1993.

Bernhard LA, Walsh M: *Leadership: the key to the professionalization of nursing,* ed 3, St Louis, 1995, Mosby.

Blake R, Mouton J: *Consultation,* ed 2, Reading, Mass, 1983, Addison-Wesley.

Bray ML, Edwards LH: A primary health care approach using Hispanic outreach workers as nurse extenders, *Pub Health Nurs* 11(1):7, 1994.

Burns JM: *Leadership,* New York, 1978, Harper & Row.

Burns T, Stalker GM: *The management of innovation,* London, 1961, Tavistock.

Caplan G: *The theory and practice of mental health consultation,* New York, 1970, Basic Books.

Chase, L: Nurse manager competencies, *J Nurs Admin* 24(4S):56, 1994.

Coben SS et al: Meeting the challenge of consultation and collaboration: developing interactive teams, *J Learn Disabil* 30(4):427, 1997.

Cohen EL, DeBack V: *The outcomes mandate: case management in health care today,* St Louis, 1999, Mosby.

D'Aunno T, Sutton RI, Price RH: Isomorphism and external support in conflicting institutional environments: a study of drug abuse treatment units, *Acad Manage J* 34:636, 1991.

Essential Public Health Services Work Group: *Public health in America, the nation's health,* Washington, DC, 1994, US Public Health Service.

Evans B, Reynolds P, Cockman P: Consulting and the process of learning, *J Eur Industr Train* 16(2):7, 1992.

Fiedler FE: *A theory of leadership effectiveness,* New York, 1967, McGraw-Hill.

Final CLIA regulations: Clinical Laboratory Improvement Amendments, *Health Devices* 21:42, 1992.

Finkler SA, Kovner CT: *Financial management for nurse managers and executives,* Philadelphia, 1993, W.B. Saunders.

Goodemote EJ: Managing in the next decade: a new set of skills for nurse managers, *Sem Nurse Managers,* 3(2):84, 1995.

Greenleaf RK: *Servant leadership: a journey into the nature of legitimate power and greatness,* New York, 1991, Paulist Press.

Hackman JR, Oldham GR: Motivation through the design of work, *Organiz Behav Human Perform* 16:250, 1976.

Hamburg M: Eliminating racial and ethnic disparities in health: response to the Presidential initiative on race, *Public Health Rep* 113:372, 1998.

Harrell MS: Practical strategies for delegation and team building in a redesigned environment, *Sem Nurse Managers* 3(4):180, 1995.

Hersey P, Blanchard K: *Management of organizational behavior,* ed 7, Englewood Cliffs, NJ, 1996, Prentice-Hall.

House RJ: A path-goal theory of leader effectiveness, *Adm Sci Q* 16:321, 1971.

Igoe JB: School nursing, *Nurs Clin North Am* 29(3):443, 1994.

Ingersoll GL, Jones LS: The art of consultation, *Clin Nurse Spec* 6(4):218, 1992.

Institute of Medicine. *The future of public health,* Washington, DC, 1988, National Academy Press.

Iowa Outcomes Project (Johnson M, Maas M, editors): *Nursing outcomes classification (NOC),* St Louis, 1997, Mosby.

Issel LM, Anderson RA: Take charge: managing six transformations in health care delivery, *Nursing Economics* 14(2):78, 1996.

Jaworski J, Flowers BS: *Synchronicity: the inner path of leadership,* San Francisco, 1997, Berrett-Koehler.

The Joint Task Force for the Management of Children with Special Health Needs: Guidelines for the delineation of roles and responsibilities for the safe delivery of specialized health care in the educational setting. Unpublished manuscript, Reston, Va, 1990, The Council for Exceptional Children.

Kreuter MW: PATCH: its origins, basic concepts, and links to contemporary public

health policy, *J Health Educ* 23(3):134, 1992.

Krueger RA: *Focus groups: a practical guide for applied research,* ed 2, Thousand Oaks, Calif, 1994, Sage.

Lancaster J: Leading in times of change. In Lancaster J, editor: *Nursing issues in leading and managing change,* St Louis, 1999, Mosby.

Latham GP, Locke E: Self-regulation through goal setting, *Organiz Behav Human Decision Processes* 50:212, 1991.

LoBiondo-Wood G, Haber J: *Nursing research: methods, critical appraisal, and utilization,* ed 4, St Louis, 1998, Mosby.

Mahaffey TL, Kaplan T, Triolo PK: A nursing fellowship: building leadership skills, *Nurs Manage* 29(3):30, 1998.

Mancini M: Managing cultural diversity. In Vestal KW, editor: *Nursing management: concepts and issues,* Philadelphia, 1995, J.B. Lippincott.

Manthey M: Empowering staff nurses: decision on the action level, *Nurs Manage* 22(2):16, 1991.

Marriner-Tomey A: *A guide to nursing management and leadership,* ed 5, St Louis, 1996, Mosby.

Maslow A: *Motivation and personality,* New York, 1970, Harper & Row.

Mastroianni K, Machles D: What are consulting services worth? applying cost analysis techniques to evaluate effectiveness, *AAOHN J* 45(1):35, 1997.

McCloskey JC, Bulechek GM, editors: *Nursing interventions classification,* ed 2, St Louis, 1996, Mosby.

McCutcheon S, Perkin B. Effective consultation in nursing. *Can J Nurs Admin* 9(1):87, 1996.

McDaniel R, Bach C: Focus groups: a data-gathering strategy for nursing research, *Nurs Sci Q* 7(1):4, 1994.

McPhail G: Management of change: an essential skill for nursing in the 1990s, *J Nurs Manag* 5(4):199, 1997.

Melaville AI, Blank MJ, Asayesh G: *Together we can: a guide for crafting a pro-family system of education and human services,* Washington, DC, 1993, US Government Printing Office.

Meyer JW, Rowan B: Institutionalized organizations: formal structure as myth and ceremony, *Am J Sociol* 83:340, 1977.

National Association of County Health Officials: *APEX-PH: assessment protocol for excellence in public health,* Washington, DC, 1991, the Association.

National Council on State Boards of Nursing: Concept paper on delegation. Unpublished manuscript, Chicago, 1990.

Orem D: Nursing administration: a theoretical approach. In Henry B et al, editors:

Dimensions of nursing administration: theory, research, education, and practice, Boston, 1989, Blackwell Scientific Publications.

Pfeffer J, Salancik GR: *The external control of organizations: a resource dependence perspective,* New York, 1978, Harper & Row.

Porter-O'Grady T: Sustainable partnerships: the journey toward health care integration. In Cohen EL, DeBack V, editors: *The outcomes mandate: case management in health care today,* St Louis, 1999, Mosby.

Porter-O'Grady T, Wilson CK: *The leadership revolution in health care,* Gaithersburg, Md, 1995, Aspen.

Rokwood GF: Edgar Schein's process versus content consultation models, *J Counsel Develop* 71:636, 1993.

Roy SC, Anway J: Roy's adaptation model: theories for nursing administration. In Henry B et al, editors: *Dimensions of nursing administration: theory, research, education,*

and practice, Boston, 1989, Blackwell Scientific Publications.

Schein EH: *Process consultation: its role in organizational development,* Reading, Mass, 1969, Addison-Wesley.

Schein EH: Process consultation as a general model of helping, *Consult Psychol Bull* 41:3, 1989.

Schein EH: Organizational culture, *Am Psychol* 45:109, 1990.

Sheldon P, Bender M: High-technology in home care: an overview of intravenous therapy, *Nurs Clin North Am* 6(2):507, 1994.

Simpson RL: Benchmarking MIS performance, *Nurs Manage* 25(1):20, 1994.

Stevens RH: A study of public health nursing directors in state health departments, *Publ Health Nurs* 12(6):432, 1995.

Sullivan EJ, Decker PJ: *Effective leadership and management in nursing,* ed 4, Menlo Park, Calif, 1997, Addison-Wesley.

Tappen RM: *Nursing leadership and manage-*

ment: concepts and practice, ed 3, Philadelphia, 1995, F.A. Davis.

Thompson JD: *Organizations in action,* New York, 1967, McGraw-Hill.

US Department of Health and Human Services: *Healthy People 2000: national health promotion and disease prevention objectives,* Washington, DC, 1991, USDHHS, Public Health Service.

US Department of Health and Human Services, Public Health Service: *Healthy People 2000: midcourse review and 1995 revisions,* Washington, DC, 1995, Government Printing Office.

Valanis B: *Epidemiology in nursing and health care,* ed 2, Norwalk, Conn, 1992, Appleton & Lange.

Vestal KW: *Nursing management: concepts and issues,* Philadelphia, 1995, J.B. Lippincott.

Vroom VH: *Work and motivation,* New York, 1964, Wiley.

Community Health Nurse in the Schools

JULIE C. NOVAK

OBJECTIVES

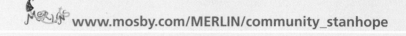

www.mosby.com/MERLIN/community_stanhope

After reading this chapter, the student should be able to do the following:

- Describe the functions of school nurses as generalists and specialists.
- Define the role of the school nurse manager.
- Examine the components of school health.
- Identify health problems of school-age children.
- Plan for school health services.
- Explain the basic requirements for administration of medications in schools.
- Discuss the school health implications of the Individuals with Disabilities Education Act (PL 94:142).
- Cite the goals of health education.
- Describe innovative approaches to the planning, organizing, and delivering of school health programs.

KEY TERMS

absenteeism
area education agencies (AEA)
boards of cooperative education services (BOCES)
case manager
casefinding
Certificates of Immunization Status
Child Find
Child Health Insurance Plan (CHIP)
community health nurse specialist for school-age children
counseling

credentialing
Division of Adolescent and School Health (DASH)
Early Periodic Screening Diagnosis and Treatment Program (EPSDT)
environmental health
exclusion order
family resource/service centers
Growing Healthy
Head Start
health education
Health PACT

International Classification of Diseases (ICD-9)
individualized education plan (IEP)
individualized family service plans (IFSPs)
Individuals with Disabilities Education Act (IDEA)
Know Your Body
neurodevelopmental evaluations
new morbidites
nontraditional health facilities
pivot management

primary health care services
school-based health centers (SBHCs)
school health council
school health managers
school health services
school nurse clinician
school nurse practitioner
screening
Teen Outreach Program (TOP)
Teenage Healthy Teaching Modules (THTM)
vague, nonspecific health complaints
See Glossary for definitions

CHAPTER OUTLINE

Health Problems of School-Age Children
 Most Common Health Problems
 Nutritional Issues
 Vision and Hearing Problems
 Use of Alcohol, Tobacco, and Other Drugs

Teenage Sexual Activity and Pregnancy
Children with HIV/AIDS
Absenteeism
Children Living in Poverty
Children with Disabilities and Chronic Health Conditions

Addressing Children's Health Problems
History of School Nursing
 1900-1940
 World War II to the Present
Components of the School Health Program
 Health Services

The author acknowledges the work of Judith B. Igoe and Sudie Speer for this chapter in previous editions of this book.

Nurses who care for children and adolescents in the school setting cover a variety of developmental groups from preschool to college-age adolescents. In 1996, 83,000,000 children through the age of 21 years made up 31.5% of the total population (U.S. Census Bureau, 1996). Although this number has increased 9.8% since 1990, it is projected that through the year 2000 the numbers will be about the same. Although the absolute numbers are increasing, trends suggest that the school-age population will decline while other age groups increase (e.g., seniors).

The majority of children under 6 (61%) and children age 6 to 17 (76%) have mothers in the workforce. The majority of poor families with children work outside the home (CDF, 1997), composing the fastest-growing segment among poor children–children of the working poor (Annie Casey Foundation, 1996). Although the majority of children living in poverty are white, a disproportionately high percentage of African-American and Hispanic children also live in poverty. These children and adolescents attend 125,000 public and private schools (Digest of Educational Statistics, 1995). Although most of these children can be described as mostly healthy individuals, the stresses of rapid growth and development and society's pressures create health problems.

"Children as children are constantly growing and developing. This basic dynamic characteristic accounts for both their increased vitality and vulnerability and requires specific health approaches in relation to the child's changing needs" (Maternal and Child Health Bureau, 1997).

Nurses who care for children in school settings face many challenges and opportunities as they work with this population. It is unclear how cutting health care and welfare costs will affect health outcomes of school-age children (CDF, 1997). It is clear, however, that innovative partnerships among the schools, university health science centers, managed care agencies, community coalitions, and traditional public health agencies must develop effective, collaborative strategies for meeting the needs of children and youth (Brownson, Kreuter, 1997; SREB, 1998).

HEALTH PROBLEMS OF SCHOOL-AGE CHILDREN

Nurses who work with the school-age population face a variety of psychosocial, physical, developmental, cultural, and environmental problems, issues, and concerns. School nurses are in a unique position to teach children to manage health problems; to care for those needing assistance; and to provide health education for children, their families and school faculty and staff.

Most Common Health Problems

The most significant health problems for elementary through high-school students, reported by grade level, are presented in Table 43-1. It is interesting to note that for school-age children, these problems vary between younger children (5 to 12) and adolescents (13 to 19). The National Health Interview Survey (1997) reveals four major categories of acute conditions of children age 5 through 17 years: respiratory conditions, injuries, infective and parasitic diseases, and digestive system conditions. Pneumonia, the effects of homicide on the victims and the community, upper respiratory infections, malnutrition, dental disease, and chronic illness are the major problems that interfere with school attendance. Since 1977, acute respiratory diseases consistently account for more than 60% of school absences due to illness. Otitis media costs exceed $3 billion due to treatment and lost productivity of parents. If untreated, otitis media may result in chronic ear infection, language delay, and hearing loss. Asthma and chronic bronchitis are the leading chronic conditions limiting children's activity (USDHHS, 1995). There has been a dramatic increase in the prevalence of asthma over the last decade. Attention deficit disorder (ADD) and attention deficit–hyperactivity disorder (ADHD) affects 2% to 9.8% of children worldwide, with as many as two thirds of cases lasting into adulthood. Genetic causes of ADD/ADHD include abnormalities in the basal ganglia of the brain and variations in the dopamine transporter receptor gene D4. Nongenetic factors include premature birth, maternal alcohol and tobacco use, exposure to high levels of lead in early childhood, and brain injuries, particularly those involving the prefrontal cortex (Barkley, 1998).

The leading causes of death for preschool-age children ages 1 to 4 in order of frequency are injuries, congenital anomalies, malignant neoplasms, homicide, heart disease, and HIV/AIDS (Fig. 43-1). For children ages 5 to 14 years, suicide enters the top seven causes of death, ranked at number 4. For leading causes of death among adolescents, refer to Figure 43-2.

Nutritional Issues

The nutritional problems seen in schools have changed over the past two decades. Today fewer children are un-

TABLE 43-1 Most Important Significant Health Problem Reported by Districts at Grade Level (%)

PROBLEM	ELEMENTARY SCHOOL	MIDDLE SCHOOL	HIGH SCHOOL
Accident/injury prevention	6.4	3.1	0.8
Chronic health problem	11.2	5.2	2.9
Communicable disease	5.6	1.9	1.0
Dental problems	1.2	0.6	0.0
Drug/substance abuse	0.6	2.7	6.8
Environmental concerns	0.6	0.0	0.0
High-risk social behaviors	18.9	33.8	45.6
Inadequate immunizations	1.9	0.6	0.2
Infectious disease	3.3	0.8	1.0
Lack of access to health care	9.5	4.1	2.9
Mental illness/emotional problems	4.8	6.4	5.0
Poor school attendance	2.3	2.3	2.9
Poverty	5.8	2.1	2.1
Self-esteem problems	8.7	19.9	7.7
Special health needs	9.1	2.9	1.9
Suicide	0.6	1.0	0.2
Teen pregnancy	0.0	1.7	6.6
Unhealthy lifestyle habits	6.4	8.1	8.5
Violence	0.0	1.2	2.3
Vision problems	0.6	0.2	0.4

From Fryer G, Igoe J: Functions of school nurses and health assistants in US school health programs, *J School Health* 66:55, 1996.

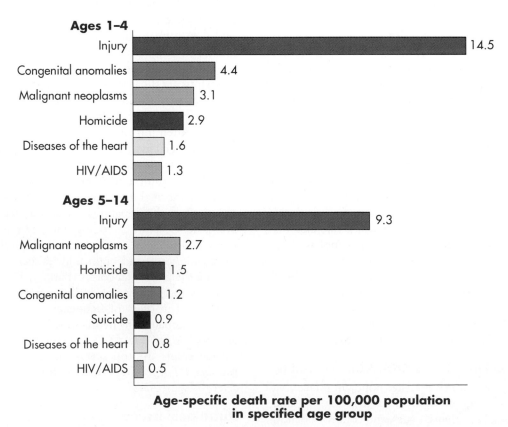

FIG. 43-1 Leading causes of death in children ages 1 to 14: 1995. (From Maternal and Child Health Bureau: *Child health USA 96-97*, DHHS Pub No HRSA-M-DSEA-97-48, Washington, DC, 1997, USDHHS.)

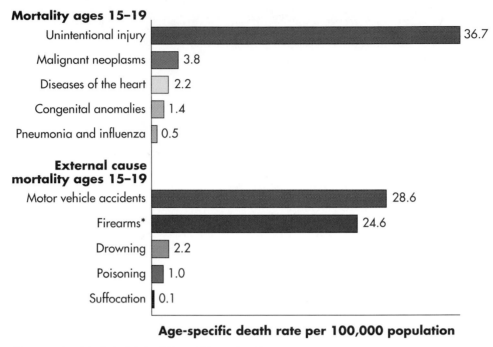

Firearms-related deaths include homicides, suicides, and accidents.

FIG. 43-2 Leading causes of death in adolescents ages 15 to 19: 1995. (From Maternal and Child Health Bureau: *Child health USA 96-97*, DHHS Pub No HRSA-M-DSEA-97-48, Washington, DC, 1997, USDHHS.)

dernourished; modern problems are related to overconsumption, imbalances in the types and amounts of food, and inactivity. In the NHANES III (National Health and Nutrition Examination Survey) study, 26% of children reported watching television for more than 4 hours per day. These children had greater body fat and body mass index (Andersen et al, 1998). Childhood obesity is a serious problem for children ages 2 to 9 years, particularly for females and Hispanic children (Maternal and Child Health Bureau, 1997). Many children consume foods high in sugar, fat, and salt and thus increase their risk of becoming obese and developing diabetes, heart disease, hypertension, and other chronic degenerative diseases later in life (Guide to Clinical Preventive Services, 1995). Eating disorders such as anorexia and bulimia are also increasing in the school-age population, which is strongly influenced by the media emphasis on thinness (Gaesser, 1996).

Vision and Hearing Problems

Many children and adolescents have vision and hearing problems. Sensory motor deficits have increased over the past decade as premature babies weighing less than 1 pound are surviving. The prevalence rate for myopia ranges from 6% to 20%, with the higher rates occurring in children and youth who are neonatal intensive care unit graduates or those 10 to 14 years of age. The National Society for the Prevention of Blindness (NSPB) estimates that 1 in 500 school children in the United States is partially sighted. The Third National Health and Nutrition

Examination Survey (NHANES III) obtained interview data on hearing loss and audiometric screening outcomes in a national sample of 6166 children ages 6 to 19 years. Results indicate a prevalence of 14.9% of either low-frequency hearing loss (lfhl) or high-frequency hearing loss (hfhl) in more than 7 million U.S. children (Niskar et al, 1998). Conductive hearing loss due to otitis media affects 20% to 30% of the preschool and early school-age population. Sensory neural hearing loss results from exposure to ototoxic drugs, hyperbilirubinemia, and serious infections such as meningitis (Donowitz, 1998).

Use of Alcohol, Tobacco, and Other Drugs

Tobacco use among teens has risen steadily in the 1990s (Fig. 43-3) and is being directly related to the introduction of the Joe Camel media campaign. As a result, the federal government has tightened restrictions related to tobacco advertising. Tobacco is considered a "gateway drug" to other substances and high-risk behaviors (American Cancer Society, 1996). Increased smoking rates will have severe lifelong effects for this generation because many of those who become addicted during adolescence will continue to smoke for the rest of their lives. If teens remain smoke-free throughout adolescence it is unlikely that they will use tobacco as an adult.

Alcohol is still the most widely abused substance among teenagers, and drug abuse continues. Recent studies, however, show that alcohol and drug use has declined for this age group. Alcohol use among 12- to 17-year-olds

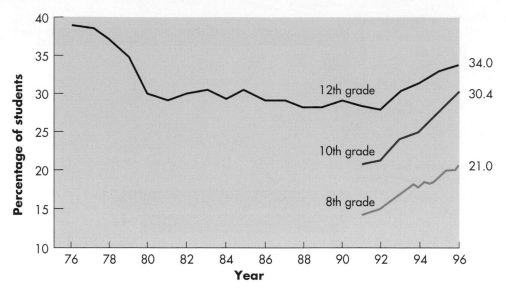

FIG. 43-3 Long-term trends in 30-day prevalence of cigarette smoking for eighth-, tenth-, and twelfth-graders: 1976-1996. (From Maternal and Child Health Bureau: *Child health USA 96-97,* DHHS Pub No HRSA-M-DSEA-97-48, Washington, DC, 1997, USDHHS.)

declined significantly from 21.1% 1995 to 18.8% in 1996. Alcohol use and binge drinking on college campuses, however, remains a serious problem, with 18% to 57% of male students reporting three or more episodes of binge drinking within the 2 weeks before the survey (Harvard School of Public Health, 1997).

Use of marijuana and cocaine decreased from 1988 to 1996. The National Center for Health Statistics reported that marijuana use dropped from 18% in 1977 to 15.5% in 1993 to 7.1% in 1996. Cocaine use by adolescents also was reported to be less, declining from 3.4% in 1988 to 1.3% in 1993 to 0.6% in 1996 (USDHHS, 1994; Maternal and Child Health Bureau, 1997). Not only is the use of alcohol and drugs among those 12 to 17 years of age reported to be down, the awareness of the risks involved in these behaviors also has generally increased. Unfortunately, this profile of declining drug and alcohol use does not hold true for eighth-grade and younger students. Between 1991 and 1996, the proportion using any illegal drug in the previous 12 months more than doubled from 11% to 24% (Johnston, O'Malley, Bachman, 1996). Thus education programs must also target the young school-age population.

Teenage Sexual Activity and Pregnancy

Researchers consistently find four factors that predict sexual intercourse at an early age, adolescent pregnancy, and nonmarital childbearing among teenagers: school failure, early behavior problems, poverty, and family problems/family dysfunction. For teenagers 15 to 19 years of age, one American in 10 becomes pregnant each year, as compared with fewer than one in 20 in Canada, England, and France (Maternal and Child Health Bureau, 1997), making U.S. rates the highest in the industrialized world (Moore,

Snyder, and Glei, 1995). In 1995 there were 65,039 live births among African-American females under the age of 18 years, which represented 10.8% of all births to African-American women. There were 133,019 births to Caucasian females under 18, which represented 4.3% of all births to Caucasian women. In 1997 979,814 teens became pregnant.

Children with HIV/AIDS

Almost 12 million cases of sexually transmitted disease occur annually, 66% in individuals under 25 years of age. As of 1997, 6029 cases of Acquired Immunodeficiency Syndrome (AIDS) were reported in children under 18 years of age (NIH, 1997). Children under the age of 13 years are primarily exposed to HIV through perinatal transmission before or during birth. The transmission rate is 25% in untreated HIV-positive mothers. This rate drops to 7% when these women are treated during pregnancy. Adolescents are primarily exposed to HIV through the receipt of blood products and high-risk behaviors. The American School Health Association (ASHA) suggests a broad-based health education approach, addressing the subject of sexually transmitted diseases (STD) in all grades. Financial resources to provide education regarding AIDS prevention have been substantial. See the Research Brief about the HIV/AIDS educational program.

Absenteeism

Children do not benefit from school when they are not feeling well or are frequently absent from school. For adolescents, pregnancy, alcohol and drug abuse, injuries, suicide, homicide, and sexually transmitted diseases are the most common conditions that lead to school failure and drop out. Students who miss more than 10 days in a 90-

RESEARCH *Brief*

This research study sought to determine the effectiveness of a 1-hour on-site educational program concerning HIV/AIDS, universal precautions, and glove use in the classroom setting by teachers, staff and volunteers. This study was planned in collaboration with the school administrators and PTAs to address the problem identified by the World Health Organization of increased susceptibility of persons in schools to risk for potential transmission of the HIV/AIDS virus. Exposure to nose bleeds, cuts, loss of teeth, and injuries from fights make school personnel vulnerable unless proper precautions are used. The study used a pretest, presentation, and posttest design. The study results showed that although school persons were knowledgeable about HIV/AIDS, they had little knowledge of universal precautions and glove use. The 1-hour presentation resulted in increased glove use in risk situations. This study shows that health education programs to address a health problem or risk can make a difference in the school environment. Involving appropriate administrators, teachers, and parents can help to make programs to address a problem at the aggregate level a success.

Grier E, Hodges H: HIV/AIDS: a challenge in the classroom, *Public Health Nurs* 15(4):257, 1998.

day semester (11% of school days) have difficulty keeping up with their grade level. In 1986, the National Health Interview Survey (NHIS) estimated that students ranging in age from 5 to 17 years lost 226.4 million days of school, or 5 days per child. A missed class day is an absence only when it occurs as the result of an acute or chronic health condition. The absentee rate for girls is slightly higher than for boys, and the rate for Caucasians is somewhat higher than for African-Americans. Children who miss school have a higher rate of visits to the school nurse than other students. Excessive school absence, school failure, and drop-out rates in middle school and high school are often the result of factors such as chaotic family environments, low self-esteem, lack of achievement and motivation, understaffed and uninviting schools, and other societal problems. Poor children and adolescents are at highest risk for **absenteeism.**

Children Living in Poverty

Students from poor families are most likely to miss school and therefore need and deserve special attention from the school nurse. These children often have chronic ear infections that will cause conductive hearing loss, language delay in young children, and possibly sensory neural hearing loss if left untreated. Others have repeated upper respiratory infections, allergies, dental decay, skin disorders, and other clinical disorders that will result in extended periods

of absenteeism if diagnostic and treatment services are not readily available. These students are four times as likely to miss school because of their ailments. They are also two to three times more likely to have a health condition that limits their school activity and are twice as likely to have mental health problems. They frequently go without health care because they are uninsured or their parents cannot leave work to take them to a health care provider without risking job loss. They may fail academically due to a lack of parental involvement and adult supervision. Some are homeless and do not attend school regularly. Others live in homes in which English is a second language, and the children do not speak enough English to understand class discussions. Therefore they soon lose interest in attending school.

Today, 26% of school children in the United States are poor; minority youth are often members of this group (USDHHS, 1997). In 1996, the poverty rate for Hispanics was 2.4 times that for Caucasians but less than the poverty rate for African-Americans (USDHHS, 1996). Because poor children often are enrolled in the federally sponsored free breakfast and lunch programs offered at schools, school nurses can discreetly use enrollment rosters for these programs to identify those students who are in special need of school health care and need access to other community health services.

Measures should be taken to reduce physical and emotional health problems and poor health habits among these children and youth. Offering diagnosis and treatment services at school is a cost- and time-effective way to provide access to quality health care. Identifying and intervening in health-related risk factors prevents a cycle of absenteeism and school failure. The **Child Health Insurance Plan (CHIP),** which was passed by Congress in 1997, will provide school nurses with another option in finding services for children of the working poor who were previously uninsured and not eligible for Medicaid.

Children with Disabilities and Chronic Health Conditions

The number of students who have disabilities and chronic health conditions and are enrolled in regular school has increased since the enactment of the Education for All Handicapped Children legislation (PL 94-142) in 1975. Over a million more children now have access to a free and appropriate education. From 1977 to 1978, about 8.6% of students received special education because of their disabilities; 11.1% received these services in 1987 to 1988. Most of this increase is related to children identified as learning disabled, which rose from 2% of all children in 1977-1978 to 5% of all children in 1987-1988 to 7% to 25% in 1996 (to as high as 41% in some schools) (Digest of Educational Statistics, 1995).

Scientific advances and improved technology make it possible for low-birth-weight babies weighing less than 1 pound to survive, for students with chronic and terminal illnesses to enter remission and live with their diseases, and for severely physically disabled youth to communicate in the school setting. Students in the largest category of those eligible for services under PL94-142 have specific learning disabilities and are usually in otherwise good health. However, the health problems experienced by those who need nursing care at school have become increasingly complex. The proportion of school-age children limited in activity by special health increased from 4% in 1975 to a range of 8% to 30% in 1998. Among the treatments and procedures some students require at school are medications; bladder catheterization; endotrachael suctioning; colostomy, ileostomy, and ureterostomy care; and nasogastric tube feedings.

At the time of the reauthorization of PL 94-142 in 1991, this legislation was retitled the **Individuals with Disabilities Education Act (IDEA).** This federal law guarantees a free public education and related services for every disabled child from 5 to 21 years of age. The IDEA bill PL 101-476 identifies a number of related services, including health care, physical therapy, occupational therapy, speech therapy, and psychologic services. In addition, each state has its own plan for implementing this legislation, which can be more specific. In a growing number of states, school nursing services are designated as a type of health services that must be available for these students.

Addressing Children's Health Problems

Children and adolescents want and need to address their own problems. Several surveys of school-age youth reveal that they are interested in learning about health and that health topics are most often at the top of their priority lists. In surveys of high school students to determine the health needs with which they wanted help, the top five identified were acne, sex education, depression, obesity, and parental disagreements. See the Research Brief about a similar survey of elementary school children.

The health problems of school-age children involve social, emotional, behavioral, and technologic issues that require a complex range of services delivered by individuals and health care systems in a flexible, coordinated, and collaborative manner. Many practitioners, educators, and policymakers have concluded that the school nurse is a key figure in meeting many of the health care needs of students, especially those who are at high risk.

HISTORY OF SCHOOL NURSING
1900-1940

Table 43-2 presents a review of the health, education, and social events that have contributed to the development of school nursing and the school health movement.

In 1902, Lillian Wald, the founder of the Henry Street Settlement House in New York City, discovered a 12-year-old boy excluded from school because of eczema:

In the early 1900s, I had been downtown only a short time when I met Louis. An open door in a rear tenement revealed a

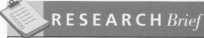

RESEARCH *Brief*

A survey was conducted of 375 inner-city school children to determine their perception of their neighborhood and to solicit suggestions from the children for improving their city. A qualitative word association format was used to determine the children's perceptions of safety, cleanliness, noise, beauty, friendliness, level of happiness, and helpfulness of the neighborhoods in which they lived. Two survey instruments were used; the Kids Place Survey developed in 1984 was used for older children, and a modified version called the Little Kids Survey was used for kindergarten to second grade.

Using a content analysis process it was determined that the children's response often depended on circumstances such as inner-city residence and the values and meaning they brought to the above words. Most of the children studied found family, home, and school safe environments. Although they find fun and happiness in the neighborhood, they often described them as noisy, dirty, and dangerous. The authors found that these children dealt with violence and potential danger daily. The youth suggested projects to clean up their neighborhoods and remove trash while cutting down the noise.

School health nurses through health education programs can assist students in coping with their environments and in finding ways to improve their environments like block parties for neighborhood clean up, family fun at local parks, and identifying safe places to go in the neighborhood in the event of trouble.

Polivka B, Lovell M, Smith B: A qualitative assessment of inner city elementary school children's perceptions of their neighborhood *Public Health Nurs* 15(3):171, 1998.

woman standing over a washtub, a fretting baby on her left arm, while with her right hand she rubbed at the butcher's aprons which she washed for a living. Louis, she explained, was "bad." He did not "cure his head," and what would become of him, for they would not take him into the school because of it? Louis, hanging the offending head, said he had been to the dispensary a good many times, but "every time I go to school Teacher tells me to go home." It needed only intelligent application for the dispensary ointments to the affected area, and in September I had the joy of securing the boy's admittance to school for the first time in his life (Woodfill and Beyrer, 1991).

Public health efforts in the early 1900s concentrated on the control of communicable disease. Thousands of immigrants were crowding into the tenement areas of large cities such as New York and Boston. With the tenements came the diseases that resulted from poverty and overcrowding. Having identified this child and many more like him, Lillian Wald and her staff carefully compiled a data-based report that convinced city officials to introduce

Text continued on p. 920

TABLE 43-2 Chronology: Events Significant in the History of School Health Services

Year	Developments in School Health Services	Developments in Education
1800	First school physicians and nurses hired in Europe (1834-1892)	Child labor reform and emergence of a public education system
1890		Responsibility for school health assigned to local school boards because health departments not in existence in every town Minimal school health instruction
1894	First medical inspections began in Boston schools to identify and exclude students with communicable disease; no follow-up	

COMMUNICABLE DISEASE CONTROL

Year	Developments in School Health Services	Developments in Education
1900	Classroom inspections expand to include screening for ringworm, scabies, impetigo, malnutrition Proper hygiene practices demonstrated in school and home Minor cases of contagion treated at school (e.g., dressing changes)	
1901	Home visits for sanitary inspection, follow-up on excluded students, truancy, social problems; as a result, school attendance escalates	
1910	Emergency services now available in schools School inspections expand to individualized medical examinations to identify and correct defects	School health instruction is combined with medical inspection; teachers rarely participate and health professionals do the health teaching
1920	Red Cross provides school nursing services to rural America	
1924	Employee health services incorporated into school health; Rogers' report recommends teachers have health exams and tuberculin tests	
1930	Mass screenings for early casefinding (e.g., vision, hearing, dental caries, orthopedic defects) increasingly widespread Counseling, health education, and consultation offered in conjunction with health services	Federal school lunch program starts (Department of Agriculture)
1934	School nurses/physicians services are overextended and quality of services deteriorates (National Organization of Public Health Nursing [NOPHN] Study)	

HEALTH GUIDANCE AND CONSULTATION

Year	Developments in School Health Services	Developments in Education
1940	Nonstatutory ban on school-based diagnosis and treatment widely enforced First aid/emergency services closely identified with school nurses despite their "no more bandaides" campaign to delegate more responsibilities for nonnursing tasks to other school personnel Service more public health oriented (e.g., coordinating community services for students)	First coordinated integrated health education curriculum developed
1945	School health councils advocated as a means for organizing school health programs	
1950	School health services under review by American Public Health Association (APHA), American Nurses Association (ANA), American School Health Association (ASHA)	

Developed by J. Igoe and S. Spier for edition 4 of this text.

Continued

TABLE 43-2 Chronology: Events Significant in the History of School Health Services—cont'd

YEAR	DEVELOPMENTS IN SCHOOL HEALTH SERVICES	DEVELOPMENTS IN EDUCATION
PRIMARY CARE		
1960	Comprehensive health histories recommended in lieu of cursory school examinations; record-keeping excessive and not effective for planning purposes	Title I—Elementary and secondary education act authorized provisions for health and nutition services OED
1969	Introduction of the first pilot for school-based primary health care using school nurse practitioners (Denver Public Schools)	
1970		Child Find Screenings begin to identify students eligible for special services under PL 94-142 Handicapped Children's Act White House Conference on Children and Youth recommends for early childhood education and day care Immigration of Vietnamese/Indo-Chinese refugees with third-world health problems; complex cultural and language barriers must be overcome
1974	Special services available for students with disablities, handicaps, chronic illness (e.g., medication administration, catheterization) New school health personnel (clerks, occupational therapist, physical therapist, psychologist, speech pathologist, substance abuse counselors)	
1978		School Health Education Study procedures comprehensive curriculum models for health education (grades K-12)
1979	Private agencies (including hospitals) assume the management of some school health programs on an experimental basis in New York	Growing Healthy curriculum adopted nationwide; well- validated program reported to produce health behavior changes in elementary school students Teenage Health Modules will develop later and also will be disseminated nationally
HEALTH PROMOTION/SPECIAL NEEDS		
1980	National School Health Services Program, Robert Wood Johnson Foundation (1980- 1985); demonstrates the effectiveness of school-based diagnosis and treatment by school nurse practitioners; emphasis on elementary schools	School Reform movement underway; parent participation increases Carnegie Foundation Report *Turning Points* recommends numerous changes in middle school including the establishment of family resource centers and a new role for a health coordinator Student assistance programs to prevent drug and alcohol abuse proliferate under the leadership of guidance counselors
1986	The School Based Adolescent Health Care Program (SBAHC), Robert Wood Johnson Foundation; increased the number of school-based health centers with diagnostic and treatment services (1986-1992); school-based clinics now concentrate on adolescent services Main obstacles: Conservative public opinion, financing, integration with the rest of school health program Disease prevention, health promotion services flourish: health hazard appraisals; fitness/endurance/cardiovascular risk screening; student health fairs	

Developed by J. Igoe and S. Spier for edition 4 of this text.

TABLE 43-2 Chronology: Events Significant in the History of School Health Services—cont'd

YEAR	DEVELOPMENTS IN SCHOOL HEALTH SERVICES	DEVELOPMENTS IN EDUCATION
HEALTH PROMOTION/SPECIAL NEEDS—CONT'D		
1987		Youth 2000 campaign launched by the business community to combat the school dropout problem Division of Adolescent and School Health, Center for Chronic Disease Prevention and Health Promotion, Centers for Disease Control and Prevention established
1990	Clinical services, health education, health promotion, environmental measures increasingly overlap; growing emphasis on environmental health	Numerous initiatives begin to support integrated services between health, education, and social services
1995	Institute of Medicine Study of School Health; proceedings encompass extensive literature review of the field School Health Resource Services program opens at the University of Colorado Office of School Health; first National Resource Center, 1-800-669-9954	

YEAR	DEVELOPMENTS IN PEDIATRICS, NURSING, PUBLIC HEALTH	SOCIAL AND LEGISLATIVE DEVELOPMENTS
1800	Fundamental discoveries in bacteriology	
1897		First appropriation by states for care of handicapped children, Minnesota
1904		Child labor legislation
1908	First Bureau of Child Hygiene established in New York City	
1909	School nursing services provided from visiting nurse associations First White House Conference recommends Federal Children's Bureau	
1912	Discovery of numerous serious health defects among army recruits	Act of 1912, Children's Bureau established
1913	School Nursing Committee created within the National Organization for Public Health Nursing (NOPHN); Lina Rogers Struthers, chairman	
1915		Rockefeller Foundation well-child clinics and clean-milk stations
1918	School of Public Health open	
1919	All cities with population of 100,000+ have maternal and child health services in most state health departments Second White House Conference advocates standards of MCH; consumer education is stressed School nurse established as faculty member in New York State and referred to as School Nurse-Teacher	
1921		Maternity and Infancy Act (Sheppard-Towner) federal grant-in-aid to the states
1924		An alliance develops between the National Education Association and the American Medical Association "Health education, not health services is the proper role for the schools."
1926	National Organization for Public Health Nursing published its first statement on the objectives, scope of work, and methods in school nursing	
1927	American School Health Association (ASHA) is formed	

Continued

TABLE 43-2 Chronology: Events Significant in the History of School Health Services—cont'd

YEAR	DEVELOPMENTS IN PEDIATRICS, NURSING, PUBLIC HEALTH	SOCIAL AND LEGISLATIVE DEVELOPMENTS
1930	American Academy of Pediatrics is formed	
1935		Title V: Social Security Act enacted; Maternal and Child Health Care Services authorized
1937	School nurses became a section of the new Department of School health and Physical Education of the National Education Association; eventually this section evolved into the National Association of School Nurses	
1939	Crippled Children's Services from State Health Department expanded	
1940	Delegation of school nurse tasks to teachers, health clerks, volunteers 50% of all public health nurses are employed in school health	
1941	First edition of *The Nurse in the School* published by the Joint Committee of the National Education Association and the American Medical Association (second edition released in 1955)	
1944	Selective service reports Army recruits have numerous health defects Committee on School Nursing Policies and Practices of the American School Health Association established (Name changed in 1958 to School Nursing Committee and since the late 1960s referred to as the Study Committee on School Nursing)	
1949	Significant increases in number of school nurses employed by health departments	
1950	White House Conference demands a ban on racial public school segregation Concept of school health team develops	
1954		*Brown v. Board of Education;* a civil rights case that overturned the "separate but equal" doctrine in public schools
1960	White House Conference on Children and Youth has youth participation for the first time; profound concern about drug abuse, increases in the incidence of venereal diseases, illegitimate births, inadequate opportunities for youth employment, and concern for the environment	"New Frontier," "Great Society," "War on Poverty" Partnership for Health act—comprehensive neighborhood health centers
1961	National Institute of Child Health and Human Development established, a national center for basic research in child development	
1962	Two-thirds of school nurses are employed by Boards of Education; number of nurses swell to 30,000	
1963		MCH funds authorized for children and youth projects
1965		Headstart Title V; Social Security Act; provides preschool health, education Medicaid, medical services for low-income families (Title XIX) National Health Promotion/Disease Prevention Campaign underway with release of the Surgeon General's report on smoking
1969	School Nurse Practitioner program developed at the University of Colorado in conjunction with Denver Public Schools	

Developed by J. Igoe and S. Spier for edition 4 of this text.

TABLE 43-2 Chronology: Events Significant in the History of School Health Services—cont'd

Year	Developments in pediatrics, nursing, public health	Social and legislative developments
1970	Position statement "Role of the School Nurse Practitioner" developed by various public health, school health and medical associations	Family Planning Services and Population Research Act (PL 94:142); Education of the Handicapped legislation rehabilitation Act of 1973 Early Periodic Screening, Diagnosis and Treatment (EPSDT); (Title XIX, Social Security Act); comprehensive and preventive health services for diagnosis and treatment of physical and mental defects
1973		Child Abuse Act (PL 934-247)
1974		The Education of All Handicapped Children Act (PL 94:142) helps states provide a free and appropriate public education
1975	National Association of State School Nurse Consultants organized	School-based initiative developed, states improve on child-abuse–reporting laws and include school personnel
1976	23 of 50 states have mandatory school nurse certification requirements; 10 states have permissive legislation	
1980	AIDS epidemic fully recognized	Refugee Education Assistance Act
1981		Select Panel for the Promotion of Child Health
1983	*Standards for School Nursing Practice*, a set of guidelines for nursing practice in the schools and developed jointly by five professional health and nursing organizations, published by the American Nurses Association	
1986		Education of the Handicapped Act Amendments (PL 99- 457) (Part H); program for infants and toddlers with handicaps
1989	Position statement *Role of the School Nurse in Disease Prevention, Health Promotion and Health Protection* receives American School Health Association endorsement	
1990	Bureau of Maternal and Child Health reestablished National Health Agenda and Objectives for the Year 2000 launched	
1991	National School Health/Education Coalition established	
1992	National Health Objectives for the Year 2000 related to school health established	
1993	Numerous coordinating councils for school health established by Bureau of Maternal and Child Health; Division of Adolescent and School Health (CDC)	
1994	National Nurses Coalition for School Health formed; representatives include the National Association of School Nurses, National State School Nurses Consultants Association, American School Health Association, American Public Health Association, American Nurses Association	
1995	Child and adolescent health standards established and published by *Bright Futures*	
1997	New options for providing school children previously uninsured with services.	Child Health Insurance Plan Act passed by Congress in 1997.

physicians into schools to examine students and exclude those with contagious diseases. As an isolated event, these daily inspections created more problems than they solved. Follow-up of treatment and counseling was definitely needed because students and their families were frequently unable to understand the instructions on the exclusion card:

In many cases the excluded children, not fully understanding the instructions, played on the street with their companions as they came out of school and lost or destroyed the cards. In other instances the cards were taken home, but the parents, often ignorant of the English language, did not understand what the child tried to explain and the Latin names were uncomprehended. In many instances the cards were never looked at but remained in their sealed envelopes while the child played on the street (Rogers, 1908).

After 5 years of medical inspections in schools, thousands of children were excluded because of trachoma, and classrooms were empty. "In a single school three hundred children were out at one time" (Rogers, 1905). Lillian Wald proposed to the boards of health and education that a nurse be sent into the schools. As a 1-month demonstration project, Lina L. Rogers visited four schools daily, spending an hour in each:

Here she dresses or cleanses all such cases as the physician directs, mild cases of conjunctivitis, minor skin infections, such as ringworm, etc., and the children need not then miss their classwork, as otherwise they would have to do as a matter of protection to the rest. She then visits those who have been sent home, and keeps records of them (Dock, 1902).

Between 1903 and 1904, as a result of the successful demonstration project, 39 nurses were recruited by the New York City Health Department, and they were remarkably successful. According to health department records, 98% of students previously excluded from school were retained in classrooms. Improvised *dispensaries* (clinics) were set up to treat students on-site. Nurses provided the counseling and instruction necessary to overcome parents' fear and indifference.

During home visits, nurses found that many students were out of school for social reasons rather than because of disease, and many were "victims of the temptations of the streets" (Struthers, 1917). Others needed clothing and food before they could come to school, and some were caring for younger children while their mothers worked. In a few instances, these children were providing nursing care to family members who were ill. Steps were taken by the nurses to relieve a number of these social problems, and the children returned to school.

By 1909, municipalities throughout the United States were employing school nurses. Initially, the Visiting Nurses Association provided the nursing service on a demonstration basis. If the project was effective, the tax-supported boards of education or health would take administrative control of the program (Waters, 1909). In 1912, the American Red Cross created a nursing service to meet the school health needs in rural areas (Woodfill and Beyrer, 1991).

The need for school nurses to provide treatment in schools and to focus their efforts almost exclusively on the control of communicable diseases began to diminish around 1916. Different priorities arose with the onset of World War I. In a time when able-bodied men were needed to defend their country, thousands of recruits were found to be physically unfit to serve because of poor eyesight, hearing loss, advanced dental disease, orthopedic problems, and sexually transmitted diseases. Consequently, the importance of early casefinding and corrective follow-up during childhood became clear to public health officials. School nurses soon shifted their attention from communicable disease control to primary prevention efforts, such as vision and hearing screening. It was the first organized large-scale attempt to proactively improve the long-term health status of American children.

By the 1920s, the role of the school nurse had expanded to include the functions of health educator and counselor. The dual role of school nurse-teacher evolved by 1937. A school nurse-teacher group became a section of the newly formed Department of School Health and Physical Education of the National Education Association (NEA). Later a separate department of school nurses was formed, which eventually evolved into the National Association of School Nurses (NASN). Currently, this organization is separate from the NEA, but a close alliance still exists.

World War II to the Present

Over the past 50 years, school nurses have been recognized for their humanitarian, preventive, and educational contributions to child and adolescent health. However, the role of school nurse-teacher has been the subject of continuing debate, and expanded clinical roles for school nurses are emerging. Fortunately, the duties and functions of school nurses are less ambiguous today, largely because of numerous attempts at standardizing the role, as well as state and national certification for the role.

During World War II, the nursing shortage became acute, and the school health program became the responsibility of school personnel other than the school nurse and the few physicians who still worked in the field. Consequently, most school nurses gave up their more labor-intensive roles as health teachers and counselors to take on the role of health consultant/ coordinator/liaison between school, home, and community. Ironically, their school assignments doubled and tripled under this arrangement with no extra personnel to help them (e.g., health assistants carry out the screening programs, simple health instructions, and follow-up activities). Consequently, the quality of school health programs deteriorated.

By the end of the 1960s, many working mothers and worried school administrators recognized the educational and economic advantages of offering services at school. Thus the clinical role of the school nurse practitioner appeared. Over the last 25 years, the importance of the health consultant role and school-teacher roles has diminished, and the **school nurse practitioner** role has become more important. In turn, all school nurses have become more clinically competent while providing more case management services.

Success with the school nurse clinician role requires administrative support, clerical and paraprofessional assistance, available medical consultation, and a collaborative approach for the planning, coordination, operation, and management the school health program. In the past, the only dollars available for school health were salaries for school nurses. The strategy today for finding the resources necessary to develop a comprehensive school health program, in which the **school nurse clinician** is a member of an interdisciplinary team, requires reorganization of schools and community health agencies to include child and adolescent health efforts. Therefore, to be truly effective, school health programs need to include, in addition to the nurse, health, social service, and education personnel who are prepared to deal with the health-related problems of students. These new developments in school health also present new opportunities for nurses to become **school health managers** or health coordinators.

With one foot in the door nursing and the other in education, school nurses often have had to try to balance their talents in both fields. Unfortunately, there has been little power or recognition in either field. However, major changes are underway as the public and policymakers recognize the importance of improving health programs in schools. Here it is possible to increase the health status of all boys and girls and to provide special attention to those who have no other regular source of health care or whose health condition requires special nursing care for them to attend school. The history of school nursing clearly reflects the evolving nature of this role.

COMPONENTS OF THE SCHOOL HEALTH PROGRAM

The components of a comprehensive school health program include an integrated, interdisciplinary approach to school health promotion; coordination of activities between the district and state; effective communication among faculty, staff, parents, and the community; the provision of health services and health education; and the promotion and maintenance of a healthy school community environment. Figure 43-4 presents a model of a school health program based on Bryan's (1973) three perspectives

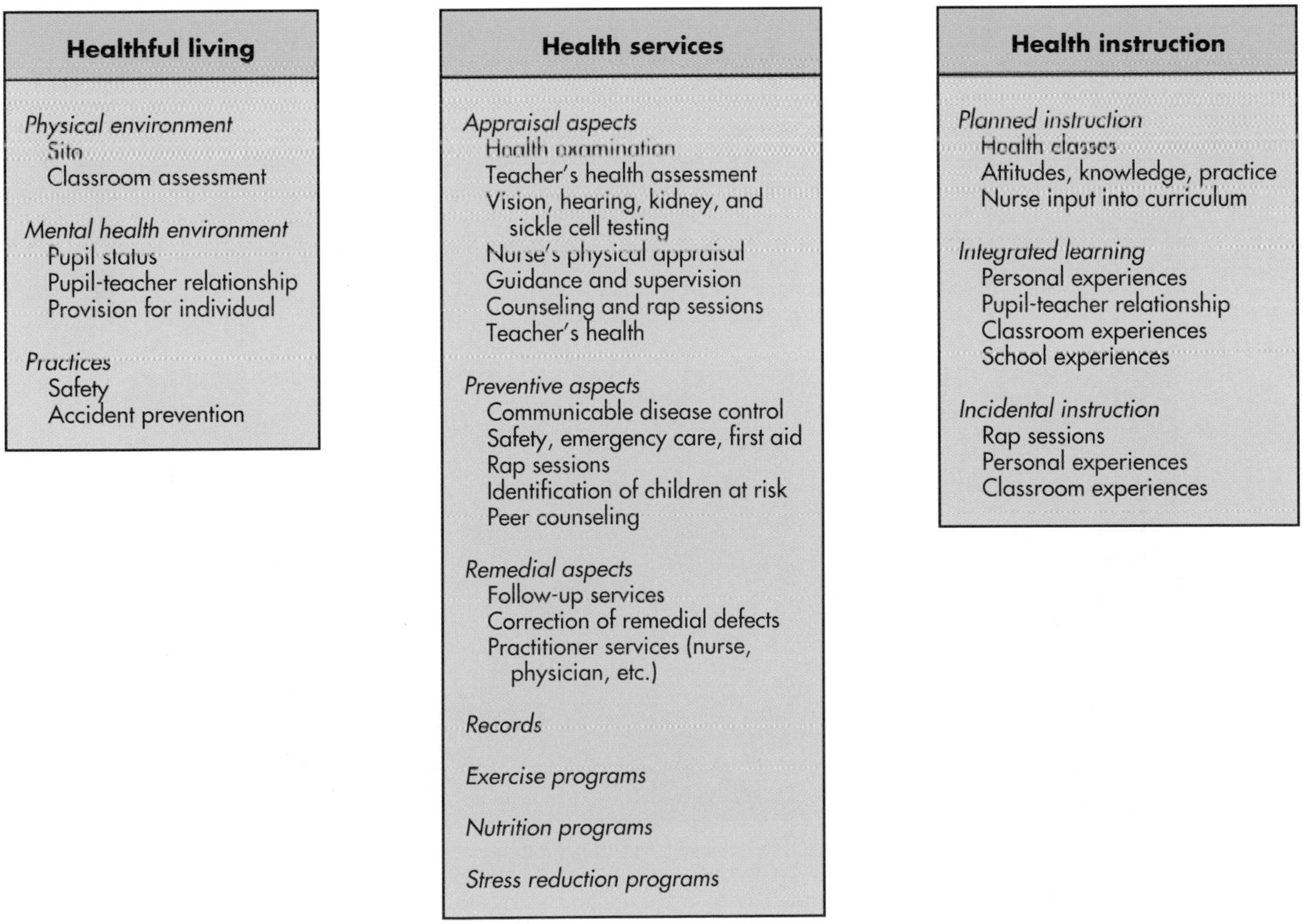

Healthful living	**Health services**	**Health instruction**
Physical environment Site Classroom assessment *Mental health environment* Pupil status Pupil-teacher relationship Provision for individual *Practices* Safety Accident prevention	*Appraisal aspects* Health examination Teacher's health assessment Vision, hearing, kidney, and sickle cell testing Nurse's physical appraisal Guidance and supervision Counseling and rap sessions Teacher's health *Preventive aspects* Communicable disease control Safety, emergency care, first aid Rap sessions Identification of children at risk Peer counseling *Remedial aspects* Follow-up services Correction of remedial defects Practitioner services (nurse, physician, etc.) *Records* *Exercise programs* *Nutrition programs* *Stress reduction programs*	*Planned instruction* Health classes Attitudes, knowledge, practice Nurse input into curriculum *Integrated learning* Personal experiences Pupil-teacher relationship Classroom experiences School experiences *Incidental instruction* Rap sessions Personal experiences Classroom experiences

FIG. 43-4 School health program based on Bryan's three perspectives.

of healthful living, health services, and health instruction. Figure 43-5 depicts a model based on Leavell and Clark's three levels of prevention. Figure 43-6 illustrates an integrated, comprehensive school health program. There is tremendous variety from one state to another regarding school health requirements, nurse:student ratios, scope of practice, and cost, all of which affect the implementation of any model at the local level.

The Centers for Disease Control and Prevention, **Division of Adolescent and School Health (DASH)** defines school health according to an eight-component model:
1. Health services
2. Health education
3. Healthful school environment
4. Physical education
5. Guidance and psychologic services

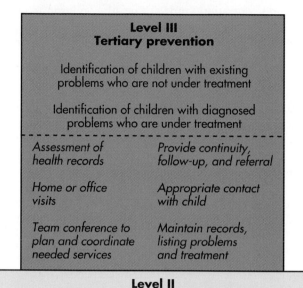

Level III
Tertiary prevention

Identification of children with existing problems who are not under treatment

Identification of children with diagnosed problems who are under treatment

Assessment of health records	*Provide continuity, follow-up, and referral*
Home or office visits	*Appropriate contact with child*
Team conference to plan and coordinate needed services	*Maintain records, listing problems and treatment*

Level II
Secondary prevention

Early identification of children with learning, emotional, physical, communication disorders; substance abuse problems; more than 14 abscences during the school year; or disorganized family life.

Observation and assessment	*Screening*	*Follow-up*
Home vists, telephone calls, and agency referral.	*Assistance with adaptive behaviors*	*Coordination of services*

Level I
Primary prevention

Health promotion	Identification of children and youths at risk	Improvement in the physical environment of the school	Continuous assessment of the emotional climate of the school	Control of communicable diseases
Assistance with developmental crises				

Student counseling	*Teacher workshops in growth and development of children, first aid, CPR, mental health concepts, values clarification, etc.*	*Health education*
Promotion of parental involvement		*Teacher's health appraisal of children*
Exercise programs	*Anticipatory guidance*	*Use of all teachable moments*
Stress reduction programs	*Immunizations*	

Methods selected to achieve levels of prevention are in italics.

FIG. 43-5 School health program based on Leavell and Clark's three levels of prevention. Methods selected to achieve levels of prevention are in italics.

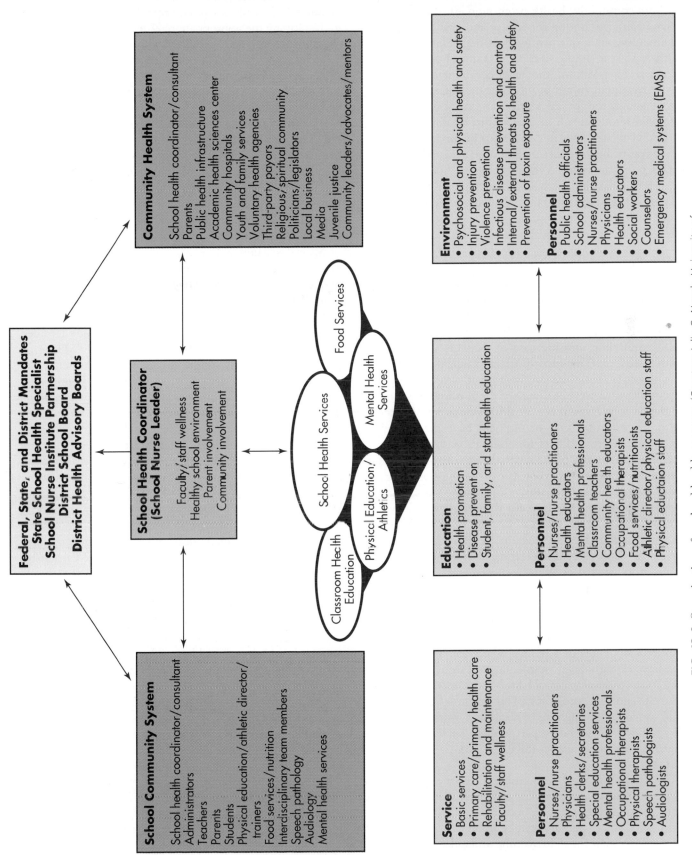

FIG. 43-6 Organization of a school health program. (Courtesy Julie C. Novak, University of Virginia, 1998.)

6. Food services
7. School community health promotion efforts
8. Site health promotion for faculty and staff

Difficulties in implementing this definition of school health suggest a simpler way to explain school health is necessary. In addition, the eight-component model is heavily weighted toward health education. Currently, the rising demand for clinical services at school suggests that additional resources will be required in the future. Hence the DASH model does not appear to be an accurate representation of how resources should be assigned. The important point, however, is the principle of "local control" and the fact that local school districts prefer to develop and define their own programs. Models and definitions of school health should be considered by local policy makers when developing school health programs.

Health Services

School health services generally include health screenings, basic care for minor health problems, administering medications, assessing immunization status, casefinding for the early identification of problems, case management, health counseling, nursing care of students with special health needs, and, in some districts, primary care. All of these activities should be family-centered and should promote health and prevent disease. School nurses are generally the persons responsible for this component of school health. These nurses may or may not have medical and psychologic referral sources for children who need them, depending on the size of the school health program and its level of development.

Recent advances in nursing research have substantially increased the knowledge base for the design and delivery of school health services of high quality. The University of Colorado School Health Program in Denver, Colorado, manages a resource center, clearing house, reference collection, and newsletter. School nurses and others interested in school health have access to this information. The system also provides referrals to nurses working in model school health programs throughout the country. The Southern Region Educational Board (SREB) and its six-member school health advisory board and grant-writing team have recently been awarded a grant from the Helene Fuld Trust to develop school health curriculum for baccalaureate nursing programs. This information will be made available through six educational workshops that will promote collaborative partnerships between nursing programs and school nurses (SREB, 1998).

Screening

The school nurse's responsibility in the **screening** process is to work with families and other team members to do the following:

1. Establish what screening will be done
2. Develop a plan for the screening and a data management system
3. Teach paraprofessionals and others (including students and volunteers) how to conduct the screenings
4. Determine the appropriate resources for additional diagnostic work-up for children with signs and symptoms
5. Refer students in need of further evaluation to other school and community resources
6. Collaborate with others in implementing and evaluating treatment plans

Health promotion and secondary prevention screenings may include vision, hearing, pediculosis, scoliosis, dental, cardiovascular risk factor analysis, and more comprehensive surveys of personal health habits known as behavioral risk surveys. These screenings usually take place as close to the beginning of the school year as possible to reveal problems that may interfere with learning. Table 43-3 lists recommended screenings for school-age youth.

Special screening packages for preschool children are also available in school. One such program is the **Early and Periodic Screening Diagnosis and Treatment Program (EPSDT).** This program is funded through Medicaid (Title XIX of the Social Security Act), a means-tested entitlement program for medical assistance to needy families with dependent children. All states have an EPSDT program that offers early screening, diagnosis, treatment, and periodic follow-up services to children and youth who meet the financial eligibility requirements and who are under 21 years of age.

Two other preschool programs include a number of health screening activities. **Head Start** is an early childhood education program for children who are at risk for academic problems because of poverty and lack of sufficient social stimulation. **Child Find,** funded through the IDEA legislation (PL 104-476), provides early identification of preschool children who are at risk for school failure because of mental retardation, other disabilities, chronic health conditions, or special health needs. Currently, school administrators, including school health personnel, face the challenge of combining all of these preschool programs into a more consolidated screening package to control costs and avoid unnecessary duplication. Although the EPSDT, Head Start, and Child Find programs offer services only to selected children, a national trend is underway to offer early childhood education and health screenings to all students.

Controversy surrounds some screenings. What should be provided, who should do the screening, and who will finance the service are questions that are raised frequently. Epidemiologists from health departments or university health science centers need to work with schools and school nurses to determine which screenings are valid, reliable, cost-effective, simple, and safe. Many states require certain screenings through either laws or regulations. Currently there are questions regarding the safety, quality, and cost-effectiveness of a variety of screening programs, including scoliosis.

TABLE 43-3 Screening and Counseling for School-Age Youth

ISSUE	AGES 7-12	AGES 13-18
Leading Causes of Death	Motor vehicle accidents Injuries (non–motor vehicle) Congenital anomalies	Motor vehicle accidents Homicide Suicide Injuries (non–motor vehicle) Heart disease Malignant neoplasms
Recommended Screening	Height and weight Blood pressure High-risk groups Tuberculin skin test (PPD)	*History* Dietary intake Physical activity Tobacco/alcohol/drug use Sexual practices *Physical Examination* Height and weight Blood pressure High-risk groups Complete skin examination Clinical testicular examination *Laboratory/Diagnostic Procedures* High-risk groups Rubella antibodies VDRL/RPR Chlamydial testing Gonorrhea culture Counseling and testing for HIV PPD Hearing Papanicolaou (Pap) smear
Client and Parent Counseling	*Diet and Exercise* Fat (especially saturated fat), cholesterol, sweets and between-meal snacks, sodium Caloric balance Selection of exercise program *Injury Prevention* Safety belts Smoke detector Storage of firearms, drugs, toxic chemicals, matches Bicycle safety helmets *Dental Health* Regular tooth brushing and dental visits *Other Primary Preventive Measures* High-risk groups Skin protection from ultraviolet light	*Diet and Exercise* Fat (especially saturated fat), cholesterol, sodium, iron, calcium Caloric balance Selection of exercise program *Substance Use* Tobacco: cessation/primary prevention Alcohol and other drugs: cessation/primary prevention Driving/other dangerous activities while under the influence Treatment for abuse High-risk groups Sharing/using unsterilized needles and syringes *Sexual Practices* Sexual development and behavior Sexually transmitted diseases: partner selection, condoms Unintended pregnancy and contraceptive options

From U.S. Preventive Services Task Force: *Guide to clinical preventice services*, ed 2, Baltimore, 1992 and 1996, Williams & Wilkins.

Continued

TABLE 43-3 Screening and Counseling for School-Age Youth—cont'd

Issue	Ages 7-12	Ages 13-18
		Injury Prevention Safety belts Safety helmets Violent behavior Firearms Smoke detectors *Dental Health* Regular tooth brushing, flossing, and dental visits *Other Primary Preventive Measures* High-risk groups Discussion of hemoglobin testing Skin protection from ultraviolet light
Remain Alert For	Vision disorders Diminished hearing Dental decay, malalignment, mouth breathing Signs of child abuse or neglect Abnormal bereavement	Depressive symptoms Suicide risk factors Abnormal bereavement Tooth decay, malalignment, gingivitis Signs of child abuse or neglect

In addition to the traditional school health screenings, the complexity of the school population makes it necessary to deliver more complex clinical services at school. Consequently, selective screening has become available for pregnancy, emotional disorders, and sexually transmitted diseases. In conjunction with this type of screening, students need psychosocial and behavioral counseling and other health promotion and disease prevention services, as well as standard medical treatments.

Casefinding

Casefinding is a form of selective screening that involves a search for certain students whose behavior, family circumstances, or health status place them at particular risk for ill health, absenteeism, and poor school performance. Instead of mass screening, in which all students in variety of grades are involved, casefinding efforts begin by identifying risk factors and then locating students whose behavior suggests they are at risk for certain problems and in need of further assessment and possible referral. Therefore casefinding techniques are more intensive efforts and usually require the clinical judgment of school nurses to determine whether further assessment and diagnosis is necessary.

Casefinding is carried out by practicing careful, systematic observation of all children with whom nurses come in contact, looking for anomalies or suspected symptoms. Casefinding efforts should concentrate on identifying students who have risk factors.

HOW TO *Identify Students Who Are at Risk for Ill Health, Poor School Performance, and Absenteeism*

1. Students who are absent more than 10% of school days.
2. Students frequently sent to the principal's office for illness.
3. Students frequently sent to the principal's office for "acting out" in the classroom.
4. Students who appear chronically ill to the teacher.
5. Students with subtle, as well as obvious, physical defects who are experiencing problems functioning at school.
6. Students with subtle, as well as obvious, emotional problems.
7. Students who frequently seek out the nurse with vague, nonspecific complaints.
8. Students who have been seriously injured or who have a history of repeated injuries.
9. Students who are genetically predisposed to certain conditions, such as sickle cell disease.

Because the frequency rates for absenteeism, visits to the school nurse's office, injuries, referrals to the principal's office, and the practice of various personal health habits vary a great deal from school to school, the first step in casefinding is to establish rates for each school building and for the district as a whole. This is done by keeping track of the students seen by the nurse, reviewing screening results and absenteeism records, collecting information from teachers and school administrators, and having students complete personal lifestyle inventories. Once the overall frequency rates for student behavior in these instances have been established, it becomes possible to determine whether the behaviors of certain students are the same or different from the rest of their classmates. Within most schools there are school administrators with experience in setting up surveillance systems who can help the school nurse in gathering this type of information and learning how to interpret it if a school health supervisor is not available. In 29 states *school nurse consultants* are located in the state departments of health and education who are also available to help.

The most likely place to begin casefinding efforts is with assessment of children who have physical or mental disabilities; recent psychosocial trauma such as parents separating or divorcing; or a move from a rural, mountain, urban, or suburban setting into a totally different social environment. School nurses are especially concerned with detecting children who are victims of maltreatment (e.g., neglect or physical or sexual abuse). The nurse's responsibility in working with children suspected of being abused is to provide a nonthreatening environment—a comfortable, compassionate, safe haven where the child is supported, encouraged, and protected. It is also the nurse's responsibility to report the problem to appropriate authorities, such as to the Child Protective Services (CPS) usually located in the local welfare offices.

Assessment of immunization status

Legally, entry into school requires that students have current, completed immunizations unless exempted for religious or medical reasons. Consequently, up-to-date **Certificates of Immunization Status** must be presented to school personnel for admission. This usually applies to preschool students as well as to boys and girls who are older. Each of the following vaccines are required: polio, measles, mumps, rubella, and diphtheria/tetanus, and for preschoolers the addition of pertussis, *Haemophilus influenzae*, and hepatitis B. Hepatitis A and varicella are also recommended but not required. Because of the measles epidemic of 1989-1991, an MMR booster is required at school entry.

The school should have a procedure for assessment and documentation of immunization status. First, a secretary, health aide or parent volunteer who has received necessary instructions from the school nurse conducts a primary review of the child's health record to determine the immunization status. Next, the information collected from the school is shared with the local county health department. Those children not in compliance with the immunization law are cited with an **exclusion order** by the health department. This information is then routed back to the school, where administrators refuse to admit the unimmunized students. If students do not return to school in a rea-

sonable length of time (i.e., 3 to 4 days), follow-up measures are taken to investigate the truancy. Often families have no access to immunization services because of poverty. Consequently, some schools have reintroduced school-based immunization clinics to alleviate the problem. This alternative is both efficient and economical.

Managing minor complaints

Each school building should have first-aid supplies and equipment in accordance with accepted first-aid guidelines. Local district policies, as well as state and federal occupational health (OSHA) regulations, need to be followed. A clinic area should be available for the delivery of first aid and emergency care, as well as daily care for common complaints including abdominal pain, headaches, earaches, fatigue, nonspecific complaints, and dermatologic problems such as pediculosis and scabies.

Increasingly nurses have begun to involve teachers and students in the responsibilities associated with first aid. Often first-aid kits are located in the classrooms, and nurses work with school personnel and students to enable them to deal directly with minor injuries. American Red Cross classes are an excellent means of preparing persons to do first aid. This approach is especially important if the nurse is not in the building on a full-time basis.

All school nurses need physical assessment skills and equipment to diagnose, treat, or refer students with common health complaints. This type of information needs to be recorded on the student's health record at school and, to provide continuity of care, on written referrals prepared and sent with the student if another health care provider, such as at the private physician, is to see the student. It is also important for the nurse to receive feedback from the other community health care provider; a system of communication must be developed for collaborating. Although this is more complicated in larger communities, the place to begin is to identify the students' health care providers. This is handled by having parents complete emergency cards that not only specify where the parent may be located during the day but also the name of their health care provider and the health facility or managed care system they use.

Innovative school nurses develop partnerships with university health science centers and other community agencies to enhance care delivery through collaborative projects and consultation to foster community support. These community and university leaders may serve on school health advisory boards and may sponsor educational programs, newsletters, and events such as health fairs.

Administration of medications

The administration of medications has rapidly become the number one reason why students visit the school health office. In a 6-month period, over 18,000 visits were made to the school health offices in five middle schools in Albemarle County, Virginia. Fifty percent, or 9,000 visits, were for the purpose of receiving a medication (Albemarle

County Schools, 1997). States vary in their interpretation of the school nurse role, relationship, and responsibility to unlicensed personnel who may be handing out medications. The respective state board of nursing, state department of health, and school board are the agencies responsible for writing medication administration policies. In many schools, nonnursing personnel have this responsibility. In these cases instruction is needed, and manuals do exist for teaching purposes (Virginia Department of Health, 1997).

Medication policies are essential in schools today. However, these policies should not serve as a barrier to gaining access to the classroom and to learning. Some students with chronic disease such as asthma are in special self-management programs to help them learn how to function independently. School nurses need to support this approach by individualizing overall medication policies as appropriate.

HOW TO   *Develop a School-Based Medication Administration Policy: Five Basic Requirements*

1. *Medications are given only with parents' written permission.*
2. *Medications requiring a prescription are given only on the written authorization of a physician or nurse practitioner.*
3. *For medications requiring a prescription there must be an individual, pharmacy-labeled bottle for each student.*
4. *Medications must be recorded by the school personnel who administer them. This record states the student's name, medication, dosage, time, and the person administering the medication.*
5. *Medications must be stored in a secure, locked, clean container or cabinet.*

Improper use of medication is also a problem in the school population. The National Council on Patient Information and Education (1995) found that, in any 2-week period, about 15 million people in the United States under the age of 18 take medicines prescribed or recommended by a physician. Of those, 50% either stop treatment too soon, do not take enough medication, take too much, or refuse to take any at all. When children use medicines improperly, acute illnesses needlessly continue or recur, treatable chronic diseases remain uncontrolled, and lives may be lost. Many of these medications are administered in the school setting; thus school nurses play a vital role in prevention of improper medication use.

Counseling

Counselors must recognize the importance of all children having a stable relationship with at least one adult, a safe environment, adequate health care, and quality life skills (Abu-Nasr, 1997). The ability to counsel students or others skillfully is an art. The counselor's responsibility is to provide information; to listen objectively; and to be supportive, caring, and trustworthy. Effective counselors do not make decisions for their clients; rather they help clients arrive at the decisions that best suit them. Counseling therefore differs from teaching and interviewing. For example, teaching is giving information; interviewing is obtaining information from someone; **counseling** is helping people arrive at workable solutions to their problems or conflicts. See Table 43-3 for recommended counseling topics for school-age youth.

Students usually require counseling when they are unable to make decisions about personal concerns that affect their lives, for example, taking medication and changing lifestyle habits.

WHAT DO YOU THINK?   *Counseling of students with high-risk social behaviors that may result in unintended pregnancy, sexually transmitted diseases, and HIV infection in school districts is considered highly controversial. The health professionals attempting to cope with these issues are viewed negatively and accused of encouraging the very problems they are attempting to resolve.*

If the nurse lacks the ability to counsel or to recognize that counseling is needed, the student may be unable to fully realize the extent of the problem or to find alternatives to solve the problem. Students' peers can be used as counselors. However, students who act as peer counselors must be trained for the role. After providing students who are acting as peer counselors with technical advice, school nurses also should encourage them to use their personal experiences, to role-play, and to be available and accessible to other students.

Students with **vague, nonspecific health complaints** who visit the health room frequently should be of special concern to school nurses. This may be the first warning sign of a student who is not doing well in school and who is at risk for eventually dropping out. Children at risk of becoming school dropouts develop a type of maladaptive response to stress (vague health complaints) during the early school years. This behavior continues into adulthood, thereby affecting work and school performance. These students can be helped to manage their problems more effectively with the right assistance and counseling from the school nurse. This involves making sure the child is not physically ill and developing plans to increase the student's self-esteem, improve their problem-solving skills, and reduce stress levels.

Case management

As a **case manager,** the school nurse performs a number of general activities. Parents need to be contacted to seek permission to discuss their child's health problem with the family physician or nurse practitioner. The nurse also will need to inform teachers and administrators accurately about the nature and prognosis of the health problem and the specific treatments required during the school day. Situations occurring at school that either interfere with the treatment plan or exacerbate the health condition need to be identified, communicated to the parties involved, and managed. Problems that arise from the student's health condition that influence learning also need to be recognized and handled. This usually involves obtaining and conveying information between health and school personnel. The school nurse is usually the person who bridges this gap through the process of case management (see Chapter 19).

Primary health care

School-wide campaigns to improve diet and exercise, individual and small-group counseling to reduce stress and improve self-image, social skills training and cognitive therapies to prevent substance abuse and delay the onset of sexual activity, and contraceptive education are just a few examples of the type of **primary health care services** and health promotion activities now available in most schools. The American School Health Association also recommends fitness screening, school breakfast and lunch programs, physical education, and mental health programs (*Healthy People 2000*, 1991). Detailed handbooks are available to assist school nurses and other school health personnel in developing these programs. If school or pediatric nurse practitioners are available, students will have the opportunity for comprehensive health assessments in the school setting.

An increasing number of boys and girls today need to obtain additional primary care services in their schools. This type of care includes a comprehensive health history, a physical examination, simple laboratory tests, and diagnosis and treatment of minor health problems. A 24-hour-a day, 7 day a week, year-round referral system also must be in place in case students' problems require additional medical attention, or they become ill when school is closed. The National Health Interview Survey found that 4.5 million (14%) students 10 to 18 years of age are from poor and minority households. These students are the ones who are least likely to have health insurance and access to primary care.

Increasingly, school nurse practitioners are becoming involved in more specialized forms of primary care. For example, some nurses serve as sports trainers, offering evaluations and special interventions to reduce the number of sports injuries. Other nurses who are primary care providers work with students experiencing emotional disorders or with students who are medically fragile and technology-dependent, such as a ventilator-dependent child. Still other school nurse practitioners delivery primary care in special settings, such as the diagnostic center for a school system.

Health services for students with special needs

According to the IDEA bill (PL 101-476), students eligible for service must have a comprehensive interdisciplinary evaluation followed by the preparation of an **individualized education plan (IEP)**. This plan is reviewed and modified at regular intervals during the school year and throughout the student's school experience. Parent conferences always occur in conjunction with the evaluation and preparation of the IEP. Students frequently join their parents and school staff for these meetings. For students whose health status significantly interferes with their ability to learn, a health care plan is a component of the IEP.

The health component of the IEP includes the following types of information: specific notes of any special preparations and supervision that may be required in caring for the student; health counseling that is necessary for the student to function in the class; and any changes in the school environment that are necessary, such as the removal of architectural barriers. Also included in the health component of the IEP would be safety measures, measures required to relieve pain and discomfort (e.g., suctioning, skin care), special diet, medications, and special assistance with activities of daily living. Finally, any special adaptations of school health activities (e.g., screenings, health education, casefinding) are described so that the student is able to have full access to this program.

School staff members often need education and supervision by the school nurse to competently manage health care plans and the special health needs of students. Fortunately, the professional organizations for teachers and school nurses have developed policies to define their roles and responsibilities. Unfortunately, it is difficult to enforce policies and guidelines that are issued from professional organizations because they have no legal authority over local school systems.

In 1986, PL94-142 was amended by PL99-457, which changed the limit for required health and education services to include disabled children 3 to 5 years of age. In addition, section H of the amendment, which refers to infants and toddlers, provided the option to extend early intervention services to children from birth to 3 years of age. This included infants and toddlers who are disabled or who have special health needs that could eventually interfere with their ability to learn. In these instances, **individualized family service plans (IFSPs)** are developed by an interdisciplinary team in partnership with parents, developing an early intervention program to prepare the infant/toddler/preschooler for school. Those states involved in section H also designate one community agency to coordinate these efforts. The school has been the designated agency in some states; however, other agencies also have been selected, including departments of health and social services.

Health Education

During the past decade, **health education** has been closely identified with the health promotion movement. Basically, health promotion is a social concept or campaign, as well as a set of health education activities intended to develop healthy lifestyles among Americans. Although not all health educators agree, many believe that the two areas are the same; that health promotion is the more encompassing activity and health education is a technique for its achievement. Health education efforts must therefore relate to the values and beliefs of students and their families. Because the potential exists for health education to infringe on the constitutional rights of individuals, health education at school is best developed locally, by committee, and should be open for public inspection and parents' approval.

The health education component should include instructional efforts that foster wellness, such as health classes and courses to prevent the spread of infectious diseases such as AIDS. Health education also includes education for students with chronic health problems who need to learn more about their diseases, self-care, and how to effectively use the health care system. Three goals for the health education component of school health are as follows:

1. To teach all children about their bodies and how to keep them healthy
2. To instill lifelong healthy habits and the knowledge to make responsible decisions concerning health, the health of their families, and the health of their communities
3. To teach students how to use the health care system wisely and effectively.

DID YOU KNOW? *A number of quality health education curricula are available today. Five programs are particularly well known. The **Growing Healthy** curriculum for elementary grades is a generalized program aimed at improving students' personal lifestyles. At the high-school level, the **Teen Outreach Program (TOP)**, which focuses on building self esteem through volunteering, has been effective in reducing teen pregnancy and drop-out in the experimental groups (Allen, 1998). **Teenage Healthy Teaching Modules (THTM)** have also been widely used. A more targeted type of health instruction is the **Know Your Body** course, which focuses on making students aware of their own cardiovascular risk factors through screening activities followed by special instruction related to risk reduction. The **Health PACT** course is a type of health instruction that is designed as consumer health affairs lessons. It is intended to prepare children to communicate effectively with health professionals during visits for health care.*

The Health PACT program may be used as a supplement to an established health education curriculum, or it may be taught to children in a wide range of locations, including school classrooms, clinics, youth organizations, and at home. It has been implemented in varying degrees and at various times by school nurses, general health educators, dentists, teachers, physicians, clinic and hospital staff, parents, nurses, and physicians' assistants. A variety of program evaluations have been done over the years, with successful outcomes.

Health PACT teaches children to communicate effectively by using five basic communication skills:

1. Talk with the health care provider
2. Listen and learn

3. Ask questions
4. Decide what to do, with help from the provider
5. Do follow through

The letters TLADD are used as an acronym to help children learn and remember their health consumer responsibilities.

The implications from the Health PACT program and its evaluation are threefold: 1) the role of the client/consumer is changing; 2) the concept of the client as partner even during childhood is acceptable; and 3) children can learn consumer behaviors for use in health settings if they have support. The Health PACT program also demonstrates that a new kind of health education is needed and is acceptable. Starting with instruction about active participation in a health facility, children and youth and their parents also need to learn self-help measures (e.g., how to do their own vision screening and how to use an otoscope). They also need to know more about the overall health care system and how it operates so that they can successfully negotiate their way around this system and can change its nature and operation if, as citizens, they see the need for change (Igoe, 1990). Drug abuse prevention curricula and contact information is presented in Table 43-4.

Environmental Health

The third component of the school health program is **environmental health,** which involves physical and psychosocial factors, such as infectious agent control and the physical and psychosocial environment of children. Evaluating the need to improve the psychosocial environment in schools today is complex. Instilling a sense of pride in students; assessing stressors of teachers, parents, and students; and evaluating the attitudes of the rest of the school team for signs of apathy, powerlessness, and hostility is essential (Comer, 1992). With the increase of violent acts in the school setting over the past decade, it is important for all school personnel and families to realize that 40% of American households with children ages 3 to 17 have guns; 7% have handguns, 17% have rifles and shotguns, and 18% have both (Center to Prevent Handgun Violence, 1998). Children who have access to guns are six times more likely to commit violent acts and six times more likely to commit suicide.

The physical environment in schools also needs to be evaluated. School nurses should work closely with local public health officials so that this area of school health is not overlooked. Safety programs are most important. Often nurses actively involve students in identifying areas in the school in which injuries are most frequent and in planning intervention strategies to reduce the risks. Incident reports need to be completed by school personnel when injuries occur, and school health personnel should review this information regularly to improve conditions. Asbestos, lead poisoning, and toxic substances in the chemistry and art classrooms are areas of concern to school administrators. Nurses must be well informed and have a

TABLE 43-4 Drug Abuse Prevention Curricula: Contact Information

CURRICULUM NAME	CONTACT
Alcohol Misuse Prevention Project	University of Michigan Institute for Social Research Room 2349 Ann Arbor, MI 48106-1248 313-647-0587
DARE	DARE America P.O. Box 2090 Los Angeles, CA 90051-0090 800-223-DARE
Growing Healthy	National Center for Health Education 72 Spring Street, Suite 208 New York, NY 10012-4019 800-551-3488
Know Your Body	American Health Foundation 675 Third Avenue, 11th Floor New York, NY 10017 212-551-2509
Life Skills Training	Institute for Prevention Research Cornell University Medical Center 411 East 69th Street New York, NY 10021 212-746-1270
Project Alert	Best Foundation 725 South Figueroa Street, Suite 1615 Los Angeles, CA 90017 800-ALERT10
Project Northland	University of Minnesota Division of Epidemiology School of Public Health 1300 South Second Street, Suite 300 Minneapolis, MN 55445-1015 612-624-0057
Social Competence Promotion Program	Dept of Psychology (M/C 285) University of Illinois at Chicago 1007 West Harrison Street Chicago, IL 60607-7137 312-413-1012
STAR	Institute for Prevention Research 1540 Alcazar Street, CHP 207 Los Angeles, CA 90033 213-457-4000
Teenage Health Teaching Modules	Educational Development Center 55 Chapel Street Newton, MA 02158-1060 800-225-4276

For further information about these and other programs, refer to the WebLinks portion of this book's website at www.mosby.com/MERLIN.

close working relationship with the environmental health personnel at the local health department and nearby universities, so they can be a useful resource to the school community. Often the nurse will be involved in surveying areas for risks, collecting information from students and parents, and providing school administrators, parents, and students with current solutions to complex problems. Web-based educational materials and CDROM environmental health programs are excellent resources for the entire school community.

ROLES, FUNCTIONS, AND CREDENTIALS FOR SCHOOL NURSES

Generalists

The majority of the 30,000 registered professional nurses now employed in school health are generalists prepared at the baccalaureate level who function in the consultant/co-ordinator role. The newer role for school nurses is as *school health manager* or *coordinator.* The functions associated with this role include the following: 1) policy-making activities to ensure a more comprehensive and integrated school health program; 2) case management functions to help families find the help they need; 3) program management duties so that a system of formal school health activities and protocols develops as an integral part of both the private and public community health system; and 4) health promotion and health protection responsibilities, including health education in the curriculum; health screening, follow-up, and referral for potential child health problems; and participation in activities that will make the school environment safe for children (e.g., adequate lunch programs, asbestos monitoring, violence prevention). Because children's health problems are becoming more complex, knowledge of nursing, pediatrics, adolescent health, and public health is essential. These nurses must be prepared to identify health-related situations that place the student at risk and that other school personnel might fail to recognize. In addition, school nurses must be very familiar with community resources and how to gain access to them. Effective communication skills are necessary because this nurse serves as a vital link between the school and community health agencies.

A number of school nurses have dual degrees. Although health education has been a popular second degree, school nurses often attain the guidance and counseling degree. Efforts are underway now to inform school nurses that this content can be found in graduate nursing programs, which should encourage the school nurses to seek degrees in nursing.

Specialists

For nurses who plan to *specialize* in school nursing, a graduate degree in nursing is recommended. Several tracks are available which focus on primary care, case/care management, and health services delivery. When there is a need to reduce costs, there is a tendency to combine clinical and management roles so that the nurse can provide direct care and supervise the school health program.

The most common clinical roles in the schools include: the school nurse practitioner (SNP), pediatric nurse practitioner (PNP) or clinical specialist in community health, mental health, rehabilitation, and/or developmental disabilities. Only 500 certified SNPs are available and employed in schools, whereas approximately 1000 certified PNPs care for children in the school setting. With school health legislation developing in most states, more school health nurse specialists are needed.

School nurse practitioners are registered professional nurses whose advanced practice area is primary care. They can serve as primary care providers for students who have no access to health care or whose parents choose the school setting for primary care. In addition to working with this group of students, SNPs also evaluate students who present in the health office with complaints of illness and injuries. Earlier studies have demonstrated that 1) SNPs send home from school 50% fewer students than regular school nurses, 2) parents are more likely to act on the advice of SNPs, 3) SNPs handle 87% of the health complaints referred to them, and 4) SNPs resolve 96% of the health problems they see. In addition, the difference in cost in relation to other community health facilities is substantial (Igoe, 1990).

In addition to working in a clinical setting, evaluating students in need of primary care and those who are sick and injured, SNPs are also part of the interdisciplinary team involved in screening students with special health needs who may be eligible for services under the IDEA legislation PL 101-476. One of their functions is the performing of **neurodevelopmental evaluations.** These evaluations contribute greatly to the overall assessment of a child by helping primary care providers identify the student's strengths and disabilities in processing information.

The **community health nurse specialist for school-age children** is a role that includes the functions of the school health manager previously described. These nurses function in **nontraditional health facilities** (alternative health care delivery systems), using various community settings, such as schools, juvenile corrections facilities, group homes for the disabled and chronically ill, day care centers, and shelters for the homeless. Special organizational skills and management expertise are needed to provide more accessible public/community health programs in these settings. These settings frequently lack the necessary policies and procedures, data management systems, coordinated networks with other community health systems, and effective financing mechanisms to function effectively. Nurses functioning in this role have the organizational and political skills to design and implement health programs in these settings that cut across systems and produce results (Igoe, 1991).

Credentials

In addition to their nurses' license, school nurses often elect to become certified as a school nurse, school or pediatric nurse practitioner, community health nurse, or other type of clinical nurse specialist through professional nursing associations and certifying bodies. In some states, the State Department of Education offers an additional state certification or **credentialing** program for school nurses. School nurse certification may be obtained through testing offered by the National Association of School Nurses (NASN) or the American Nurses Credentialing Center (ANCC). In some states it may not be possible to be employed in a school system or to receive federal reimbursement for school nursing care for students with disabilities without being certified. Currently, school nurses are promoting credentialing as a way to upgrade the overall quality of school nursing.

MANAGEMENT OF THE SCHOOL HEALTH PROGRAM

A school health program requires good management to operate smoothly and effectively. Essential steps toward reaching this goal include the following: planning, organizing, directing, and controlling the quality of the program through outcome evaluation. Planning for school health should be a joint project involving members of a **school health council.** To ensure broad-based representation, this council should be composed of teachers, school nurses, parents, students, administrators, and community leaders. Members of this team need to set the direction for the program and make certain that the mission of the school health program is consistent with the goals of the school district and the rest of the community health system. The council plans and sets goals for the school health program and develops and then implements strategies to meet these goals. The council also evaluates the program in view of these goals and makes changes as necessary. A school health council is a valuable support mechanism for the proper development, revision, implementation, and evaluation of the school health program. Although traditionally school health councils have been merely advisory bodies, currently these groups strongly influence policy. This has occurred with increased community participation, partnerships, and increased parental involvement.

Education Reform and School Health

In 1990 the National Governor's Association established the following goals for education by the year 2000:
1. All children will start school ready to learn.
2. The high school graduation rate will increase to at least 90% for all groups.
3. All students will leave grades 4, 8, and 12 having demonstrated competency over challenging subject matter in English, mathematics, science, history, and geography.
4. U.S. students will be first in the world in mathematics and science achievement.
5. Every adult will be literate and possess the knowledge and skills necessary to compete in a global economy and to exercise the rights and responsibilities of citizenship.
6. Every school in America will be free of drugs and violence and will offer a disciplined environment conducive to learning (U.S. Department of Education, 1990).

The reason for this action and the need for major reform within education are due to many concerns. Concerns include declining academic achievement scores of American youth; rising dropout rates, particularly in minority communities (Fig. 43-7); increased violence and drug abuse threatening the integrity of school communities; and minority, disabled, or special needs children who do not have equal opportunities for learning. All of these factors threaten the ability of students to become productive adults.

The educational goals for the year 2000, along with *Healthy People 2000: National Health Promotion and Disease Prevention Objectives* (USDHHS, 1991), are the guidelines that have set the course for school health planning. In June 1990 the National Commission on the Role of the School and Community in Improving Adolescent Health issued a planning document for school health in secondary schools, *Code Blue: Uniting for Healthier Youth* (Code Blue, 1990). The commission that authored this report was composed of community leaders from health, education, religious organizations, business, and government. The Commission was co-sponsored by the National Association of State Boards of Education (NASBE) and the American Medical Association (AMA), with funding from the U.S. Centers for Disease Control and Prevention.

Guidelines for Adolescent Preventive Services (GAPS) was developed and used in many settings, including school-based student health centers (Department of Adolescent Health, 1997). In 1991, National Health Objectives Related to School Health were identified (Box 43-1). These objectives provide specific direction, especially in the area of school health education.

Planning

Many school nurses are the managers or coordinators of school health programs. School health requires a unique type of management known as **pivot management.** Under this plan, nurses organize a school health team using the personnel already in the school system or closely associated with it: teachers, students, parents, administrators, psychologists, health educators, social workers, speech pathologists, audiologists, counselors, secretarial staff, and maintenance personnel. With the help of a school health council, this team develops a comprehensive school health plan, and a budget is developed and proposed to school administrators. Program goals, strategies, and activities are designed and organized so that health services, health education, and environmental components of the program are coordinated with one another. If the health program for students with disabilities is separated from the general school health program, special care must be taken to link these efforts to avoid unnecessary duplication and fragmentation.

A needs assessment is the starting point for program development. It is used to determine the problems requiring attention and the way to best meet these needs. Box 43-2 provides an outline of specific areas covered in a needs assessments for school health.

All three areas of school health must be considered when planning is done, and decisions must reflect innovative and economical ways of combining health services with health education and environmental health. Unfor-

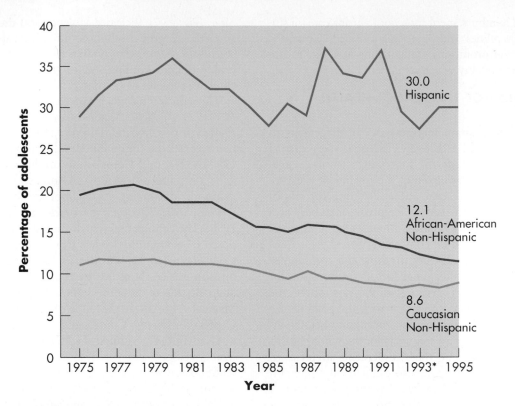

*Because of changes in data collection procedures beginning in 1992, data may not be comparable with figures for earlier years.

Note: Status rates measure the proportion of the population who have not completed high school and are not enrolled at one point in time, regardless of when they dropped out.

FIG. 43-7 Status school dropout rates for young persons ages 16 to 24 by race/ethnicity: 1975-1995. (From Maternal and Child Health Bureau: *Child health USA 96-97*, DHHS Pub No HRSA-M-DSEA-97-48, Washington, DC, 1997, USDHHS.)

tunately, school health programs may be fragmented, with decisions about the health education curriculum made in one department, health services planned and implemented from another office, and the environmental health component attended to in yet another department.

Traditionally, health services have been limited to screening and first aid. However, the beginning of school-based health centers (SBHCs), the increased numbers of uninsured students, and the admission of students with complex health care needs have affected the development of much more complex school health services. In fact, care now being delivered in schools closely resembles the activities of traditional primary care facilities, including on-site diagnostic and treatment services and sophisticated nursing care for students with complex health problems. Rehabilitative services also may be available. Consequently, public health codes governing primary care facilities often apply to SBHCs. By maintaining a close working relationship with the local public health authorities, the school nurse is aware of local health regulations.

Health education requirements are especially important today because the public health agenda increasingly high-

lights health promotion and disease prevention. By obtaining an aggregated (population) lifestyle profile for individual schools and for the total school district, school health planners will be more aware of the level of need for health education in their district. This kind of information can be provided through health appraisal questionnaires that ask students about their knowledge, attitudes, and lifestyle behaviors in relation to diet, nutrition, exercise, dental health, human sexuality, infectious disease, and substance abuse. An audit of student health and school records to determine injury rates and illness-related absences provides administrators and the community with data about the overall health status of the student body. This approach often is effective in gaining school board support for a health education curriculum.

Next, school health planners must decide who will provide the health instruction. Ideally, sufficient numbers of school-employed health educators will teach the classes. More realistically, these same health educators, who are in very short supply, develop the health education curriculum and work with school nurses, teachers, and other community health professionals to implement the program.

BOX 43-1 National Health Objectives Related to School Health By the Year 2000

1. Increase to at least 50% the proportion of children in grades 1 to 12 who participate in daily physical education activities at school.
2. Increase to at least 90% the proportion of school lunch and breakfast programs with menus consistent with nutritional principles contained in Dietary Guidelines for Americans.
3. Increase to at least 75% the proportion of the nation's schools that provide nutrition education from preschool through twelfth grade.
4. Include tobacco-use prevention in the curricula of all elementary, middle, and secondary schools.
5. Provide children in all primary and secondary schools with educational programs on alcohol and other drugs.
6. Increase to at least 85% the proportion of people 10 to 18 years of age who have discussed human sexuality with their parents or received information from parentally endorsed sources, such as schools.
7. Increase to at least 50% the proportion of elementary and secondary schools that teach nonviolent conflict-resolution skills.
8. Provide academic instruction on injury prevention and control in at least 50% of public school systems.
9. Increase to at least 95% the proportion of schools that have age-appropriate HIV education curricula for children in grades 4 to 12.
10. Include in all middle and secondary schools instruction on preventing sexually transmitted diseases.

From USDHHS: *Healthy People 2000: national health promotion and disease prevention objectives*, Washington, DC, 1991, USDHHS, Public Health Service.

BOX 43-2 School Health Needs Assessment

STUDENT HEALTH

Absenteeism: frequency and nature
Health problems presented at school (e.g., illness and the nature, frequency, and location of injuries)
Resolution of health problems: frequency
Chronic health conditions, handicapping conditions
Health status of students
    Immunization level
    Dental
    Vision
    Hearing
    Emotional disorders
    Physical/sexual abuse
    Prevalence of positive health behavior (e.g., nutrition, exercise, safety, and avoidance of substance abuse)
Change in health status of students

RESOURCES

Community resources available
Use of community resources (overuse as well as underuse)
Health care/education available in regular curriculum (e.g., physical education, home economics, special education, science, and health education)
Health services available through current school health programs

EMPLOYEE HEALTH

Health state of school personnel: absenteeism and nature of disability claims

Well-organized school health programs must have clear, relevant written policies and procedures. To be effective, these regulations must address the problems of students living in poverty, students with chronic illnesses or disabilities, and other children with special needs. The **"new morbidities"** affecting school-age children cannot be managed completely by the health care system alone because many problems have psychosocial, political, and physical features. External environmental and sociopolitical forces that lead to these problems must be considered to have an effective school health program. Tools for planning, implementing, and evaluating the school health program should describe a general plan and provide regulations for emergencies, such as anaphylaxis, severe asthma, drug overdose, and head and spinal injuries. Policies and procedures should address these areas and others, including disaster plans, communicable diseases, reportable diseases required by the state, child abuse, and the warning signs and incidence of suicide. If state school nurse consultants are available, they should be consulted during the planning stage (This is a good example of how to plan a program. See Chapter 21 for more details).

Organizing

There are approximately 15,000 to 16,000 public school systems in this country, which are considerably less than the 100,000 districts that existed in 1945 at the end of World War II. School nurses are unevenly distributed from one district to the next and from state to state. Although professional organizations recommend a ratio of 1 nurse for every 750 students, a ratio of 1 nurse to 1000 students is more realistic in terms of the supply of prepared nurses that are available and the costs involved. For students with special health needs, the requirements for care are much different; thus, ratios must be adjusted accordingly. Insufficient data are available about numbers of nurses required to provide good care. Workforce and school health problems data, however, are currently being compiled in most states and at the federal level for better program planning.

A more urgent problem than the number of students per nurse is the number of school buildings the nurse must visit to come in contact with students. For example, 47% of school districts have a total school enrollment of 2500 students (Digest of Educational Statistics, 1995). This means that one or two school nurses often make up the total school health team in these districts, with an assignment of 3 to 5 schools each. This dilemma adds to the credibility of a recommendation that came from a President's Commission on School Health in the early 1970s, which advised that health assistants be placed in schools to handle basic care (first aid, minor complaints), with nurses assuming managerial positions (Igoe, 1991).

The intermediate education district is another network for organizing school health. Known as **area education agencies (AEAs)** or **boards of cooperative education services (BOCES),** these systems frequently provide related services for special education students in school districts of limited size. School nursing, speech pathology, audiology, occupational and physical therapy, and mental health services are some of the services often provided regionally. Nurses working in regional agencies often help local school district personnel develop and implement health care plans for certain students, such as those who are disabled or at high risk for academic difficulty. These specialized school nurses work with the school nurse coordinator in the local district who is responsible for the overall school health program.

School nurses face a tremendous challenge daily in managing their time. Therefore it is important to have a written plan that sets the direction, priorities, and schedule for the school health program. The nurse must organize the day in such a way that low priorities do not keep her from getting to the high-priority problems. For example, many school nurses have discovered that an open-door policy fosters continual interruptions throughout the day. Consequently, school nurses in many school systems now have an appointment system for seeing students and for parent-teacher conferences. Sick-call times are often established as another way of cutting down on the number of unnecessary interruptions.

It is important for school nurses to organize an epidemiologic database that profiles the health status of the student body both individually and as an aggregate. This is accomplished by using a systematic recording system for the problems that nurses see and the care they provide. Well-organized school health programs have policy and procedure manuals that explain the recording system to be used in a particular school system. Software packages for computerized school health records are used, and school nurses include personal computers in their budget requests. School and community health data systems used by school health personnel frequently use the **International Classification of Disease (ICD-9)** codes in recording student health problems.

School health programs may be organized in a single department, office, or division so that needs are met, services do not overlap, and costs are contained. The ideal organizing process would involve and consolidate all health personnel responsible for the care of students in general, for students with special health needs, and for other students at high risk for school failure. Such personnel would include school nurses, speech pathologists, audiologists, occupational therapists, physical therapists, social workers, clinical psychologists, counselors, and student assistant personnel. Although most of these related health service personnel are employed by school districts to carry out the provisions of the IDEA bill, school administrators can integrate these professionals with other school employees, such as school nurses, to achieve a more comprehensive approach to school health.

There are three barriers to reorganizing and consolidating of school health. First, many of the related service personnel do not identify themselves with school health. Second, interdisciplinary interdependent teams may be an unfamiliar or threatening concept. Third, bureaucratic turf battles often interfere with interdisciplinary efforts in which the students' needs are first identified and then the team decides who is the person best suited to provide the care.

One way of overcoming the natural resistance to change would be to organize related service personnel, including the school nurse, into interdisciplinary teams that provide service to a cluster of schools. This organizational arrangement allows various persons with backgrounds in fields other than education to become members of a team and to gain a sense of identity. Interdependent team development work is needed to build trust and a sense of how to operate in this kind of an interdisciplinary environment.

Once the health services component of school health has been unified, the next step in restructuring school health is to strengthen the link between the health service, health education, and environmental health divisions. Regular meetings of the persons responsible for these programs is essential as is the need to develop a comprehensive, coordinated, strategic management plan for school health. The school health advisory board or school health council is the advisory body who drives policy development.

Although schools traditionally have employed their own school health personnel or contracted with the public health agency for these services, new partnerships and organizational arrangements are emerging. School nurses in California and New York are forming their own school health companies and contracting directly with schools. University health sciences centers and community hospitals have also begun to contract with schools to develop partnerships and to administer school health programs.

Directing

Leadership for school health programs needs strengthening at all levels. States currently have school nurse consultants, with approximately 50% of them employed by state health departments and the rest responsible to the state department of education. These individuals frequently provide technical help to local school districts, known as local education agencies (LEA), in the form of in-service education and on-site evaluation of a program, while performing statewide planning for school health.

At the local level, a school nurse supervisor/coordinator usually oversees the health services program and provides supervision for other school nurses. As the health needs of students become increasingly complex and the level of care delivered in school becomes more sophisticated, the school health program needs to be managed by a health professional who knows the clinical aspects of care.

School health managers/coordinators require certain skills to be effective. Among the most frequently cited skills of effective managers are verbal communication and listening skills, managing time and stress, managing individual decisions, recognizing, defining, and solving problems, motivating and influencing others, delegating, setting goals and articulating a vision, self-awareness, team building, and conflict management.

The school nurse's role is expanding rapidly in the area of supervision of school health assistants or unlicensed personnel. As the number of children and the complexity of their health needs continues to rise, the need for assessments and care in the school setting increases. This makes it essential that school nurses have available to them a way to train and credential school health assistants to support the school health program and to work with children with special needs.

Quality Control

Outcome evaluation is a critical component of school health programs. Fortunately, practice standards for the school nurse and school nurse practitioner exist, and these serve as useful guides in determining effectiveness (Guidelines, 1990). Program evaluation is important to determine effectiveness. School nurses are beginning to use outcome measures as well as process evaluations. For example, the number of referred students who now wear glasses should be noted in an evaluation (outcome measures) as should the number of students screened (process variables). Outcome measures of the effectiveness of a particular school health activity also must reflect what impact the activity had on the child's academic performance (see Chapter 21). Another way to improve the quality of school health is to mandate or require that certain services, health education, and environmental measures be provided for students. A regulated approach, however, is not always the best way to proceed. This can turn out to be a highly political process and, once a program is required, it is often difficult to change even if there is evidence that a practice is no longer necessary. Finally, the area of school health that is probably most in need of quality control is the environment. Generally, environmental health standards are not always relevant, available, or enforced. A congressional report issued in 1995 provided evidence of the deterioration of school buildings and called for the need for immediate improvements to safeguard student health.

INNOVATIONS IN SCHOOL HEALTH

School-Based Health Centers

School-based health centers (SBHCs) were established as a result of several demonstration projects conducted during the past two decades. These projects demonstrated that the school can be an effective site for primary care services because most children and youth attend school and have access to this facility. The projects also demonstrated that nurse practitioners with appropriate physician consultation and collaboration provide excellent health care, reduce unnecessary referrals, and cut down on the time away from school. This is particularly true if a student's only other access to care is a public clinic where the waiting time is extensive. Presently, an estimated 350 SBHCs centers in the United States are located in secondary schools. The clinics established in elementary schools, preschools, and school-based after-school day care centers are growing rapidly.

Schools encounter financial problems with even the most basic school health program. Therefore if a community's school-age population is to benefit from the advantages of using the school setting as the student health center, the responsibility for organizing, financing, and delivery of school health services in these sites must be shared with other community health systems, including state and local health departments. SBHCs are cost effective in comparison to other community health facilities, with estimates ranging from $90/student/year to $150/ student/year. Consequently, financing mechanisms must be found to support SBHCs such as third-party reimbursement for services rendered to students who have Medicaid benefits, the *Child Health Insurance Plan* (CHIP), established in 1997, or other state-funded and private health insurance plans.

SBHCs change the school nurse responsibilities in several ways. In some instances the school nurse takes on the responsibility for providing the care as a school nurse practitioner or pediatric nurse practitioner. In other settings the school nurse acts as the manager for the center and designs the programs and activities necessary for its operation. In other settings, nurses serve as team members for the center and their responsibility is triage and case management. However, it should be pointed out that the delivery of individual personal health services is but one aspect of the total school health program.

Family Resource/Service Centers

In Florida, Kentucky, New Jersey, Minnesota, and numerous other states the idea of **family resource/service centers** is attracting attention. Within this organizational structure, a number of school and community resources for families are consolidated into one agency for the sake of efficiency and reducing costs. Various public agencies, including the school, pool their child and adolescent health and child care resources and reduce their overhead and management expenses by offering a one-stop shopping arrangement. An extension of the school health program logically belongs within these centers.

Family resource centers may be either geographically located in the school or linked to the school in some other way. In addition to student services, education and employment opportunities for parents also are offered.

Employee Health

Another key aspect of some school health programs is that the program should meet some of the health needs of the teaching staff and other employees of the school system. Currently a number of school districts have wellness programs for employees, as well as medical services (e.g., physical examinations, smoking cessation programs, counseling for drug and alcohol abuse) and in-house evaluations for workmen's compensation claims. These services are often highly valued by the school board and school administrators because of the potential for health care cost containment and reduction in absences. School nurses have offered a variety of consumer health education programs, such as an adult version of the Health PACT course, in an effort to enhance teacher satisfaction with the health care system and to improve their use of their health care benefits.

clinical application

The school board and the school-based council of ANY county, Virginia has agreed to develop a school health program. Such a program was necessary because an assessment of the school environment found an unhealthy environment with a high rate of absenteeism.

A. A school health program involves which of the following?
 1. Health services
 2. Health education
 3. Environmental health
B. How could the school health nurse best address the problem of absenteeism?
 1. Keep track of the students seen by the nurse in the school clinic
 2. Collect information from teachers and administrators
 3. Set up a surveillance system for casefinding

Answers are in the back of the book.

KEY POINTS

- The health problems of school-age youth vary substantially between the younger years and the adolescent years.
- Health problems are major risk factors for absenteeism and academic failure.
- Children and adolescents who are poor are at high risk for absenteeism and school failure.
- The three core components of school health are health services, health education, and promotion of a healthy environment.
- School health services generally include health screenings, basic care for minor complaints, administration of medications, surveillance of immunization status, casefinding for the early identification of problems, and nursing care of students with special needs.
- Historically, reducing absenteeism has been the single most important reason for school nursing services. With the current emphasis on education reform and acade-

mic performance, reducing absenteeism continues to be a top priority for school nurses.
- The role of the school nurse includes the functions of health education and counseling, as well as the delivery of clinical care to students with disabilities. Coordination of the overall school health program and case management of individual student health problems are other responsibilities of the nurse.
- School health activities are family centered and are intended to promote health and reduce the incidence of disease.
- Although health screenings are an integral component of school health services, nurses must prepare other school personnel, students, and volunteers for this work.
- Administration of medications and clinical care of students with disabilities in school is increasing in frequency. Nevertheless the risks associated with these practices can be managed successfully provided there are well-developed policies and procedures.
- School health education involves health promotion instruction for all students to develop their positive personal health habits; self-help classes for students with special health needs; and consumer education for all so that the next generation will be prepared to use the health care system effectively.
- The school environment requires attention, and certain measures are necessary if the climate at school is to be both physically and psychologically healthy.
- Schools are nontraditional health care settings. Consequently, it is important to establish health policies, procedures, and plans to provide direction for the school health program.
- Planning and operation of the school health program involves parents and community health professionals, as well as school personnel.

critical thinking activities

1. Visit a school. Observe the activities and interactions of students as a group both inside and outside the classroom. What are the advantages and disadvantages of learning collectively as opposed to being tutored? What are the implications for health teaching and counseling?
2. Interview a school nurse, school nurse practitioner, or community health nurse clinical specialist for school-age youth working in schools. How do they explain their roles in the school? What are the rewards? What are the frustrations?
3. Visit a school with a school nurse. Observe how the nurse works with individual children with disabilities and with boys and girls who are at high risk for academic failure because of chronic illness, poverty, and family problems. Inquire about any special procedures and precautions they observe in caring for these students. Look at the record-keeping system. Ask to review an individual education plan (IEP) and an individualized family service plan (IFSP). Find out whether the school nurse is involved with the school district's preschool program. Does the school also have a program for those infants and toddlers 0 to 3 years of age who have disabilities? How is the nurse involved with this effort?

4. Find a journal or textbook for school teachers. Review the table of contents to determine the areas of interest and importance to them. Select and read one of these articles/chapters. Compare and contrast the school teacher's approach to problem solving with the way nurses solve problems. What benefits and constraints could these differences present when nurses and teachers try to work together?

5. Attend a school board meeting. In preparation for this activity find out whether the board members are appointed or elected. Also find out something about the board members: their names, occupations, special concerns about education. At the time of the meeting, review the agenda, notice the amount of preparatory work the board members must do before meetings, and observe the interactions between the board, school administrators, and members of the audience. What are the chief concerns expressed at this meeting? How will this affect the school health program and school nurses?

6. Find a group of children or adolescents. Ask them to draw you a picture of (or explain) the nature of the health program at their school. What services are provided? What health classes are taught? What activities go on at school to keep it a safe and healthy environment for students? Ask the students to identify one change in the school health program that they would like to make.

7. Contact a parent who is a member of the Parent-Teachers Organization (PTO). Discover the purpose and functions of this organization. Find out whether the PTO is involved in school health locally or nationally. Also discover whether the PTO represents all parents. Are parents who are poor or from minority groups involved?

8. Is there a state school nurse consultant in your state? Find out by contacting the state Department of Health and the state Department of Education/Instruction. If a nurse consultant is available, find out the answers to these questions:
   a. How many school nurses are in your state?
   b. Is a current statewide policy/procedure manual for school health available to guide the practice of all school health personnel, especially those people working in districts too small to develop their own? How is this manual developed?
   c. What is the major school health concern right now in your state and the nurse consultant's strategy for addressing this issue?
   d. Where are the school health programs in your state that work well? What are the ingredients in these school systems that make these programs successful?

9. Review the Chronology of School Health Events in Table 43-2 and predict what type of school health program will be needed in the year 2015.

Bibliography

Abu-Nasr D: Volunteer vision turns into reality, *The Ann Arbor News*, April 27, 1997, pp A-1, A-11.

Albemarle County School Health Advisory Board: *Visits to the middle school health office: a data analysis,* Charlottesville, Virginia, 1997, The School Board.

American Cancer Society (ACS). *Research progress report, cancer facts and figures,* Atlanta, 1996, ACS.

American School Health Association: School Health Nursing Services Progress Review, *J School Health* 68(1):1, 1998.

Andersen RE et al: Relationship of physical activity and television watching with body weight and level of fatness among children, *JAMA* 279(12):938, 1998.

Annie Casey Foundation: *Kids count data book: 1996,* Baltimore, 1996, Author.

Barkley RA: Attention-deficit hyperactivity disorder, *Scientific American,* www.sciam.com/1998/0998issue/0998barkley.html.

Barkley RA: *Nature of self-control,* New York, 1997, Guilford Press.

Barkley RA: *ADHD: a handbook for diagnosis and treatment,* New York, 1998, Guilford Press.

Bradley BJ: The school nurse as health educator, *J School Health* 67:3,1997.

Brownson RC, Kreuter MW: Future trends affecting public health, *JPH Management Pract* 3(2):49,1997.

Bryan DS: *School nursing in transition,* St Louis, 1973, Mosby.

Center to Prevent Handgun Violence: *Guns in American schools 1998,* www.handgun-control.org/protecting/D1/dlgunsch.htm

Centers for Disease Control and Prevention: AIDS among children—US, 1998, *MMWR* 45:1005, 1996.

Centers for Disease Control and Prevention: *School health programs: an investment in our future,* Atlanta, 1995, CDC.

Children's Defense Fund: *The state of America's children yearbook 1997,* Washington, DC, 1997, CDF.

Code blue: uniting for healthier youth: a call to action, The National Commission on the Role of the School and Community in Improving Adolescents Health, Alexandria, Va, 1990, NASBE.

Comer JP: Environmental health: the psychosocial climate In Wallace et al: *Principles and practices of student health,* Oakland, 1992, Third Party Publishing.

Committee on Vision: *Myopia: prevalence and progression,* Commission on Behavioral and Social Sciences and Education, National Research Council, Washington, DC, 1995, National Academy Press.

Department of Adolescent Health, American Medical Association: *Guidelines for adolescent preventive services (GAPS),* Chicago, Ill, 1997, American Medical Association.

Digest of Educational Statistics, NCES86 643, Washington, DC, 1995, US Department of Education Office of Educational Research and Improvement.

Dock LL: School-nurse experiment in New York, *Am J Nurs* 3:108, 1902.

Donowitz L: *Infection control in the child care center and preschool,* ed 3, Baltimore, 1996, Williams & Wilkins.

Dusenbury L, Falco M, Lake A: A review of 47 drug abuse prevention curricula available nationally, *J School Health* 67:127, 1997.

Fryer G, Igoe J: Functions of school nurses and health assistants in US school health programs, *J School Health* 66:55, 1996.

Gaesser GA: *Big fat lies: the truth about your weight and your health,* New York, 1996, Fawcett Columbine.

Green M, editor: *Bright futures: guidelines for health supervision on infants, children and adolescents,* Arlington, Va, 1997, National Center for Education in Maternal and Child Health.

Guide to Clinical Preventive Services: *Report of the US preventive services task force,* Baltimore, 1995, Williams & Wilkins.

Guidelines for the delineation of roles and responsibilities for the safe delivery of specialized health care in the educational setting, Developed by the joint task force for the management of children with spe

Continued

Bibliography—cont'd

cial health needs of the American Federation of Teachers (AFT), The Council for Exceptional Children (CEC), National Association of School Nurses (NASN), National Education Association (NEA), Scarborough, Maine, 1990, National Association of School Nurses.

Igoe J: School nursing and school health. In Natapoff J, Wieczarek R, editors: *Maternal child health policy: a nursing perspective,* New York, 1990, Springer.

Igoe J: Is health a school issue? School-based health services. In Aiken L, Fagin C, editors: *Nursing and health policy: issues of the 1990s,* Philadelphia, 1991, J.B. Lippincott.

Igoe J, Campos EL: Report of a national survey of school nurse supervisors, *Sch Nurs* 6:8, 1991.

Igoe J, Giordano B: *Expanding school health services to serve families in the 21st century,* Washington, DC, 1992, American Nurses Publishing.

Johnston L, O'Malley P, Bachman J: *News release, the rise in drug use among American teens continues,* Ann Arbor, 1996, University of Michigan Institute for Social Research.

Kids count data book: state profiles of child wellbeing, Washington, DC, 1996, The Center for the Study of Social Policy.

Marx E, Wooley S: *Health is academic,* Kent, Ohio, 1998, American School Health Association.

Maternal and Child Health Bureau: *Child health USA 96-97,* USDHHS Pub No HRSA-M-DSEA-97-48, Washington, DC, 1997, USDHHS.

Moore K, Snyder N, Glei D: *Facts at a glance,* Flint, Mich, February, 1995, Charles Mott Foundation.

Nader P: *School health policy and practice,* Evanston, Ill, 1993, AAP.

National Association of School Nurses: *Guidelines for a model school nursing services program,* Scarborough, Maine, 1990, the Association.

National Center for Health Statistics: *Current estimates from the National Health Interview Survey: vital and health statistics,* Series 10, Washington, DC, 1997, NCHS.

Niskar AS et al: Prevalence of hearing loss 6-19 years of age, *JAMA* 279(14):1071, 1998.

Redican K, Olsen L, Baffi C: *Organization of school health programs,* ed 2, Dubuque, Ia, 1993, Brown & Benchmark.

Resnicow K, Allensworth D: Conducting a comprehensive school health program, *J School Health* 66:59, 1996.

Rogers L: The nurse in the public school, *Am J Nurs* 5:763, 1905.

Rogers L: Some phases of school nursing, *Am J Nurs* 8:966, 1908.

Schneider M, Friedman S, Fisher M: Stated and unstated reasons for visiting a high school nurse's office, *J Adolesc Health* 16:35, 1995.

School health in America, Kent, Ohio, 1996, American School Health Association.

Schwab N, Hass M: Delegation and supervision in school settings: standards, issues and guidelines for practice (Part 1), *J Sch Nurs* 11(1):26, 1995.

Shi L, Singh D: *Delivering health care in America: a systems approach,* Gaithersburg, Md, 1998, Aspen.

Southern Region Educational Board (SREB): *Developing a school health nursing curriculum,* Fuld trust grant, 1998.

Stoto M, Behrens R, Rosemont C, editors: *Healthy People 2000: citizens chart the course,* Institute of Medicine, Washington, DC, 1990, National Academy Press.

Struthers LR: *The school nurse,* New York, 1917, GP Putnam's Sons.

Sultz H, Young K: *Health care USA: understanding its organization and delivery,* Gaithersburg, Md, 1997, Aspen.

US Department of Education Teachers and Goals 2000: *Leading the journey toward high standards for all students,* June 1995. www.ed.gov/GsK/teachers

US Census Bureau: *Current population reports,* Series P-60, No 161, US Department of Commerce, Washington, DC, 1996, Author.

US Department of Education: *National goals for education,* Washington, DC, 1990, Author.

US Department of Health and Human Services: *Health: United States, 1993,* USDHHS Pub No (PHS) 73-1232, Washington, DC, 1994, USDHHS.

US Department of Health and Human Services: *Health: United States.* USDHHS Pub. No. (PHS) 76-1232, Washington, DC, 1997, USDHHS.

US Department of Health and Human Services: *Healthy People 2000 midcourse review 1995,* Washington, 1995, USDHHS.

US Department of Health and Human Services: *Healthy People 2000: national health promotion and disease prevention objectives,* Washington, DC, 1991, USDHHS, Public Health Service.

Virginia Department of Health: *School Health Data,* Richmond, Virginia, 1997, Author.

Waters Y: *Visiting nursing in the United States,* New York, 1909, Charities Publications Committee.

Wechsler H et al: Binge drinking among college students, *J Am Coll Health* 45:273, 1997.

Woodfill M, Beyrer M: *The role of the nurse in the school setting: an historical view as reflected in the literature,* Kent, Ohio, 1991, American School Health Association.

Community Health Nurse in Occupational Health

BONNIE ROGERS

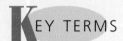

OBJECTIVES

 www.mosby.com/MERLIN/community_stanhope

After reading this chapter, the student should be able to do the following:

- Describe the nursing role in occupational health.
- Describe current trends in the American workforce.
- Describe examples of work-related illness and injuries.
- Use the epidemiologic model to explain work-health interactions.

- Cite at least three host factors associated with increased risk from an adverse response to hazardous workplace exposure.
- Explain one example each of biologic, chemical, environmental/mechanical, physical, and psychosocial workplace hazards.
- Complete an occupational health history.
- Describe functions of OSHA and NIOSH.
- Describe an effective disaster plan.

KEY TERMS

agents
environment
Hazard Communication
    Standard
host

National Institute for
    Occupational Research
    Agenda (NORA)
National Institute for
    Occupational Safety and
    Health (NIOSH)

occupational health
    hazards
occupational health
    history
work-health interactions

worker's compensation
worksite walk-through

See Glossary for definitions

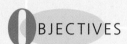

CHAPTER OUTLINE

In America, work is viewed as important to one's life experiences, and most adults spend about one third of their time at work (Rogers, 1994). Work—when fulfilling, fairly compensated, healthy, and safe—can help build long and contented lives and strengthen families and communities. Such work can reduce health care costs and improve agency effectiveness and profits. Although some workers may never face more than minor adverse health effects from exposures at work, such as occasional eye strain resulting from poor office lighting, every single industry grapples with serious hazards (USDHHS, NIOSH, 1996). No work is completely risk-free, and all health care professionals should have some basic knowledge about workforce populations, work and related hazards, and methods to control hazards and improve health.

There have been many and substantial changes in the nature of work and workplace risks, the work environment, workforce composition and demographics, and health care delivery mechanisms. An analysis of these trends suggests that work-health interactions will continue to grow in importance affecting how work is done, how hazards are controlled or minimized, and how health care is managed and integrated into workplace health delivery strategies. As a result, significant developments are occurring in occupational health and safety programs designed to prevent and control work-related illness and injury and to create environments that foster and support health-promoting activities. Occupational health nurses have performed critical roles in planning and delivering worksite health and safety services, which must continue to grow as comprehensive and cost-effective services. In addition, the continuing increase of health care costs and the concern about health care quality have prompted the including of primary care and management of nonwork-related health problems in the health services programs. In some settings, family services are also provided.

Health at work is an important issue for most individuals for whom the nurse provides care. As many individuals spend much time at work, the workplace has significant influence on health and can be a primary site for the delivery of health promotion and illness prevention. As a result of the influence of health care reform and the movement toward managed care, a shift in the delivery of health care will become more focused. The home, the clinic, the nursing home, and other community sites such as the workplace will become the dominant areas where health and illness care will be sought (Adams, 1995; Burgel, 1993).

This chapter describes the nurse's role with the working population. It introduces work-related health and safety and the principles for prevention and control of adverse work-health interactions. The focus is on the knowledge and skills needed to promote the health and safety of workers through occupational health programs. The prevalence and significance of the interactions between health and work underscore the importance of including principles of occupational health and safety in nursing practice. The types of interactions and the frequent use of the general health care system for identifying, treating, and preventing occupational illnesses and injuries require nurses to use this knowledge in all practice settings. The epidemiologic triad is used as the model for understanding these interactions, as well as risk factors, and effective nursing care for promoting health and safety among employed populations. The assessment, management, and prevention of occupational health problems are skills that can be applied in all types of nursing care settings.

DEFINITION AND SCOPE OF OCCUPATIONAL HEALTH NURSING

Adapted from the American Association of Occupational Health Nurses (AAOHN, 1999), occupational health nursing is defined as:

The specialty practice that focuses on the promotion, prevention, and restoration of health within the context of a safe and healthy environment. It involves the prevention of adverse health effects from occupational and environmental hazards. It provides for and delivers occupational and environmental health and safety services to workers, worker populations, and community groups. It is an autonomous specialty, and nurses make independent nursing judgments in providing health care.

Occupational health nurses work in traditional manufacturing, industry, service, healthcare facilities, construction sites, consulting, and government settings. Their scope of practice is broad and includes worker/workplace assessment and surveillance, primary care, case management, counseling, health promotion/protection, administration and management, research, legal-ethical monitoring, and a community orientation. The knowledge in occupational health and safety is applied to the workforce aggregate.

HISTORY AND EVOLUTION OF OCCUPATIONAL HEALTH NURSING

Nursing care for workers began in 1888 and was called industrial nursing. A group of coal miners hired Betty Moulder, a graduate of the Blockley Hospital School of Nursing in Philadelphia (now Philadelphia General Hospital) to take care of their ailing co-workers and families (AAOHN, 1976). Ada Mayo Stewart, hired in 1885 by the Vermont Marble Company in Rutland, Vermont, is often considered the first industrial nurse. Riding a bicycle, Miss Stewart visited sick employees in their homes, provided emergency care, taught mothers how to care for their children, and taught healthy living habits (Felton, 1985). In the early days of occupational health nursing, the nurse's work was family centered and holistic.

Employee health services grew rapidly during the early 1900s as companies recognized that the provision of worksite health services led to a more productive workforce. At that time, workplace accidents were seen as an inevitable part of having a job. However, the public did not support this attitude, and a system for **worker's compensation** arose that remains today (McGrath, 1995).

Industrial nursing grew rapidly during the first half of the twentieth century. Educational courses were established, as were professional societies. By World War II there were approximately 4000 industrial nurses (Brown, 1981). The American Association of Industrial Nursing (AAIN) (now called the American Association of Occupational Health Nurses), was established as the first national nursing organization in 1942. The aim of the AAIN was to improve industrial nursing education and practice and to promote interdisciplinary collaborative efforts (Rogers, 1994).

Passage of several laws in the 1960s and 1970s to protect workers' safety and health led to an increased need for occupational health nurses. In particular, the passing of the landmark *Occupational Safety and Health Act* in 1970, which created the Occupational Safety and Health Administration (OSHA) and the *National Institute for Occupational Safety and Health* (NIOSH), discussed later in this chapter, created a large need for nurses at the worksite to meet the demands of the many standards being implemented. The Act focused primarily on education and research. In 1988, the first occupational health nurse was hired by OSHA to provide technical assistance in standards development, field consultation, and occupational health nursing expertise. In 1993 the Office of Occupational Health Nursing was established within the agency.

PROFESSIONAL ROLES AND PROFESSIONALISM IN OCCUPATIONAL HEALTH NURSING

As American industry has shifted from agrarian (agriculture) to industrial to highly technologic processes, the role of the occupational health nurse has continued to change. The focus on work-related health problems now includes the spectrum of human responses to multiple, complex interactions of biopsychosocial factors that occur in community, home, and work environments. The customary role of the occupational health nurse has extended beyond emergency treatment and prevention of illness and injury to include the promotion and maintenance of health, overall risk management, and efforts to reduce health-related costs in businesses. The interdisciplinary nature of occupational health nursing has become more critical as occupational health and safety problems require more complex solutions. The occupational health nurse frequently collaborates closely with multiple disciplines and industry management, as well as representatives of labor.

Occupational health nurses constitute the largest group of occupational health professionals. The most recent national survey of registered nurses indicates that there are approximately 23,000 licensed occupational health nurses (USDHHS, 1996). Occupational health nurses hold positions as *nurse practitioners, clinical nurse specialists, managers, supervisors, consultants, educators,* and *researchers.* Data also show that approximately 65% of occupational health nurses report that they are employed to single-managed occupational health nurse units in a variety of businesses. The occupational health nursing role is unique in that the nurse adapts to an agency's needs as well as to the needs of specific groups of workers.

The professional organization for occupational health nurses is the American Association of Occupational Health Nurses (AAOHN). The AAOHN's mission is comprehensive. It supports the work of the occupational health nurse and advances the specialty. The AAOHN also does the following:

- Promotes the health and safety of workers
- Defines the scope of practice and sets the standards of occupational health nursing practice
- Develops the Code of Ethics for occupational health nurses with interpretive statements
- Promotes and provides continuing education in the specialty
- Advances the profession through supporting research
- Responds to and influences public policy issues related to occupational health and safety

The AAOHN describes 10 job roles for occupational health nurses: *clinician, case manager, coordinator, manager, nurse practitioner, corporate director, health promotion specialist, educator, consultant,* and *researcher* (AAOHN, 1997). The majority of occupational health nurses work as solo clinicians, but increasingly, additional roles are being included the specialty practice. In many companies, the occupational health nurse has assumed expanded responsibilities in job analysis, safety, and benefits management. Many occupational health nurses also work as independent contractors or have their own businesses providing occupational health and safety services to industry, as well as consultation. With the current changes in health care delivery and the movement toward managed care, occupational health nurses will need increased skills in primary care, health promotion, and disease prevention. The aim of the occupational health nurse will be to devote much attention to keeping workers and, in some cases, their families healthy and free from illness and worksite injuries. Specializing in the field is often a requirement.

Academic education in occupational health and safety is generally at the graduate level (Morris, 1994). Training grants from NIOSH support master's and doctoral education with emphases in occupational health nursing, industrial hygiene, occupational medicine, and safety. These programs are offered through Occupational Safety and Health Education and Research Centers throughout the country. A listing of these programs can be found in Box 44-1. Certification in occupational health nursing is provided by the American Board for Occupational Health Nurses (ABOHN) and is met through experience, continuing education, professional activities, and examination.

WORKERS AS A POPULATION AGGREGATE

The population of the United States is expected to increase from approximately 272 million people in 1999 to an estimated 297 million people by the year 2010 (US Census Bureau, 1999). By 2010 the U.S. population will be older, with a median age of more than 37 years, compared

BOX 44-1 National Institutes for Occupational Safety and Health Education and Research Centers*

ALABAMA EDUCATION & RESEARCH CENTER
University of Alabama at Birmingham
School of Public Health
Birmingham, AL 32594-0008
205-934-7032

CALIFORNIA EDUCATION & RESEARCH CENTER NORTHERN
University of California, Berkeley
School of Public Health
322 Warren
Berkeley, CA 94720
510-642-0761

CALIFORNIA EDUCATION & RESEARCH CENTER SOUTHERN
University of Southern California
Inst. of Safety and Systems Management
University Park
Los Angeles, CA 90089-0021
213-740-4038

CINCINNATI EDUCATION & RESEARCH CENTER
University of Cincinnati
Department of Environmental Health
3223 Eden Avenue
Cincinnati, OH 45267-0056
513-558-5701

HARVARD EDUCATION & RESEARCH CENTER
Harvard School of Public Health
Department of Environmental Health
665 Huntington Avenue
Boston, MA 02115
617-432-3325

ILLINOIS EDUCATION & RESEARCH CENTER
University of Illinois at Chicago
School of Public Health
PO Box 6998, M/C 922
Chicago, IL 60680
312-996-7887

JOHNS HOPKINS EDUCATION & RESEARCH CENTER
Johns Hopkins University
School of Hygiene and Public Health
615 North Wolfe Street
Baltimore, MD 21205
301-955-3602

MICHIGAN EDUCATION & RESEARCH CENTER
University of Michigan
School of Public Health
Dept. of Environmental and Industrial Health
Ann Arbor, MI 48109
313-936-0735

MINNESOTA EDUCATION & RESEARCH CENTER
University of Minnesota
School of Public Health
1158 Mayo Memorial Building
420 Delaware Street, SE
Minneapolis, MN 55455
612-626-0900

NEW YORK/NEW JERSEY EDUCATION & RESEARCH CENTER
Department of Community Medicine
Mt. Sinai School of Medicine
PO Box 1057
10 E 102nd Street
New York, NY 10029
212-966-5001

NORTH CAROLINA EDUCATION & RESEARCH CENTER
University of North Carolina
School of Public Health
Rosenau Hall, CB #7400
Chapel Hill, NC 27599-7410
919-966-5001

TEXAS EDUCATION & RESEARCH CENTER
The University of Texas Health Science Center at Houston
School of Public Health
PO Box 20186
Houston, TX 77225
713-792-4638

UTAH EDUCATION & RESEARCH CENTER
University of Utah
Rocky Mountain Center for Occupational and Environmental Health, Building 512
Salt Lake City, UT 84112
801-581-8719

WASHINGTON EDUCATION & RESEARCH CENTER
University of Washington
Department of Environmental Health, SC-34
Seattle, WA 98195
206-543-6991

*Occupational Health Nursing Programs are located in the centers. For futher information on these centers, see this book's website at www.mosby.com/MERLIN.

to 29 years in 1975. The greatest growth will be among people over age of 65, representing 14% of the population, with a reduction of the under 25-year-olds. This will be reflected in the workforce with a decrease in the number of young job seekers. It is estimated that by the year 2010 28% of the workforce will be between the ages of 35 and 54. The number of elderly (65 years of age and older) will more than double between now and the year 2050, to 80 million. By that year, 1 in 5 Americans will be elderly.

There are more than 138 million civilian wage and salary workers over 16 years of age in the United States, employed in about 6.3 million different work sites (Bureau of Labor Statistics, March, 1999). More than 91% of those who are able to work outside of the home do so for some

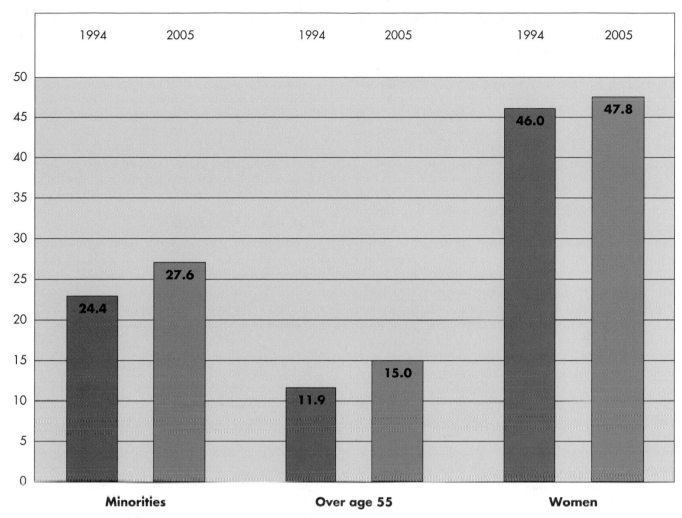

FIG. 44-1 Projected changes in civilian labor force 1994 to 2005. (From Fullerton H: The 2005 labor force: growing, but slowly, *Monthly Labor Review* 118(11):29, 1995.)

portion of their lives (Bureau of Labor Statistics, 1999). Neither of these statistics indicates the full number of individuals who have potentially been exposed to work-related health hazards. Although some individuals may currently be unemployed or retired, they continue to bear the health risks of past occupational exposures. The number of affected individuals may be even larger as work-related illnesses are found among spouses, children, and neighbors of exposed workers.

Americans are employed in diverse industries that range in size from one to tens of thousands of employees. Types of industries include traditional manufacturing (e.g., automotive and appliances), service industries (e.g., banking, health care, and restaurants), agriculture, construction, and the newer high-technology firms, such as computer chip manufacturers. Approximately 95% of business organizations are considered small, employing fewer than 500 people (Bureau of Labor Statistics, 1995). Although some industries are noted for the high degree of hazards associated with their work (e.g., manufacturing, mines, construction, and agriculture), no worksite is free of occupational health

and safety hazards. The larger the company, the more likely it is that there will be health and safety programs for employees. Smaller companies are more apt to rely on the external community to meet their needs for health and safety services.

Characteristics of the Workforce

The U.S. workplace is rapidly changing (USDHHS, NIOSH, 1996). Jobs in the economy continue to shift from manufacturing to service. Longer hours, compressed workweeks, shift work, reduced job security, and part-time and temporary work are realities of the modern workplace. New chemicals, materials, processes, and equipment are developed and marketed at an ever-increasing pace.

The workforce is also changing. As the U.S. workforce grows to approximately 147 million by the 2005, it will become older and more racially diverse. By the year 2005, minorities will represent 28% of the workforce, and women will represent approximately 48% of the workforce (Fig. 44-1). These changes will present new challenges to protecting worker safety and health.

The demographic trends in the American workforce describe a changing population aggregate that has implications for the prevention services targeted to that group. Major changes in the working population are reflected in the increasing numbers of women, older individuals, and those with chronic illnesses who are part of the workforce. Because of changes in the economy, extension of life span, legislation, and society's acceptance of working women, the proportion of the employed population that these three groups represent will probably continue to grow.

In an era in which the demand for workers is expected to outstrip the available supply, businesses must be concerned about strategies to increase health status, employment longevity, and satisfaction of workers. For example, although nearly 60% of all women are employed (representing 48% of the workforce), it is predicted that women will account for 67% of the increase in the labor force over the next decade (Bureau of Labor Statistics, 1997; Rix, 1990). These workers tend to be married, with children and aging parents for whom they are responsible. This aggregate of workers presents new issues for individual and family health promotion, such as child care and elder care, that can be addressed in the work environment. In 1990, more than half of the female labor force was concentrated in three areas: administrative support/clerical (26%), service (14%), and professional specialty (14%). Twelve percent were employed in fields such as labor, transportation and moving, machine operation, precision products, crafts, farming, forestry, or fishing. In the male labor force nearly 20% worked in precision production, crafts, or repair occupations, 13% in executive positions, 11% in professional specialty occupations, and 10% in sales. Other trends shaping the profile of the workforce include more education and mobility, as well as increasing mismatches in the 1990s between skills of workers and types of employment.

Characteristics of Work

There has been a dramatic shift in the types of jobs held by workers. Following the evolution from an agrarian (agriculture) economy to a manufacturing society and then to a highly technologic workplace, the greatest proportion of paid employment is now in the occupations of service (e.g., health care, information processing, banking, and insurance), professional and technical positions (e.g., managers and computer specialists), and clerical work (e.g., word processors and secretaries). Of the new jobs created from 1984 to 1994, 73% were in the categories of professional administrative, sales and technical, and precision crafts (Bureau of Labor Statistics, 1995). During the 1996 to 2000 period, service-providing industries accounted for virtually all of the job growth. Only construction added jobs in the goods-producing business sector, offsetting declines in manufacturing and mining. Health services, business services, social services, and engineering, management, and related services are expected to account for

almost one in every two worker jobs. The 10 fastest-growing occupations include six health-related and four computer-related occupations (Bureau of Labor Statistics, 1998) (Box 44-2).

This change in the nature of work has been accompanied by many new occupational hazards such as complex chemicals, nonergonomic workstation design (the adaptation of the workplace or work equipment to meet the employee's health and safety needs), and job stress. In addition, the emerging of a global economy with free trade and multinational corporations presents new challenges for health and safety programs that are culturally relevant.

Work-Health Interactions

The influence of work on health, or **work-health interactions,** is shown by statistics on illnesses, injuries, and deaths associated with employment. Each day, an average of 137 individuals die from work-related diseases, and an additional 16 die from injuries on the job. Every 5 seconds a worker is injured, and every 10 seconds a worker is temporarily or permanently disabled (BLS, 1998). In 1997 2.9 million reported work-related illnesses and injuries resulted in lost time from work. Of these, approximately 82,000 were severe enough to result in temporary or permanent disabilities that prevented the workers from returning to their usual jobs (BLS, 1998). Over the past few years, the incidence and severity of work-related injuries have increased (BLS, 1995). Employers reported 5.7 million work injuries and 430,000 newly reported cases of occupational illnesses in 1997. That same year, occupational injuries alone cost $132 billion in lost wages and lost productivity, administrative expenses, health care, and other costs (BLS, 1998). This figure does not include the cost of occupational diseases. These figures are often described as the "tip of the iceberg" because many work-related health problems go unreported. But even the recorded statistics are significant in describing the amount of human suffering, financial loss, and decreased productivity associated

---

BOX 44-2 The 10 Occupations with the Fastest Employment Growth

1. Database administrators, computer support specialists, and all other computer scientists
2. Computer engineers
3. Systems analysts
4. Personal and home care aides
5. Physical and corrective therapy assistants and aides
6. Home health aides
7. Medical assistants
8. Desktop publishing specialists
9. Physical therapists
10. Occupational therapy assistants and aides

From Bureau of Labor Statistics: *Employment projections, 1998,* Washington, DC, 1998, US Government Printing Office.

with workplace hazards. The high number of work injuries and illnesses can be drastically reduced. In fact, significant progress has been made in improving worker protection since Congress passed the 1970 Occupational Safety and Health Act. This progress has been largely based on actions—sometimes voluntary, sometimes regulatory—directed by the science and knowledge generated from occupational safety and health research (Klinger, 1994). For example, vinyl chloride-induced liver cancers and brown lung disease (byssinosis) from cotton dust exposure have been almost eliminated. Reproductive disorders associated with certain glycol ethers have been recognized and controlled (Katz, 1994). Fatal work injuries have declined substantially through the years (Occupational Health and Safety, 1993). Notably, since 1970, fatal injury rates in coal miners have been reduced by more than 75%, and there has been a general downward trend in the prevalence of coal miner's pneumoconiosis.

The U.S. workplace is rapidly changing and becoming more diverse. Major changes are also occurring in the way work is organized, with increased shiftwork, reduced job security, and part-time and temporary work as realities of the modern workplace. In addition, new chemicals, materials, processes, and equipment (such as latex gloves in health care, or fermentation processes in biotechnology)

continue to be developed and marketed at an ever-accelerating pace.

APPLICATION OF THE EPIDEMIOLOGIC MODEL

The epidemiologic triad can be used to understand the relationship between work and health (Fig. 44-2) (Campos-Outcalt, 1994). With a focus on the health and safety of the employed population, the **host** is described as any susceptible human being. Because of the nature of work-related hazards, nurses must assume that all employed individuals and groups are at risk of being exposed to occupational hazards. The **agents,** factors associated with illness and injury, are occupational exposures that are classified as *biologic, chemical, ergonomic, physical,* or *psychosocial* (Box 44-3). The third element, the **environment,** includes all external conditions that influence the interaction of the host and agents. These may be workplace conditions such as temperature extremes, crowding, shiftwork, and inflexible management styles (Callahan, 1994). The basic principle of epidemiology is that health status interventions for restoring and promoting health are the result of complex interactions among these three elements. To understand these interactions and to design effective nursing strategies for dealing with them in a proactive manner, nurses must look at how each element influences the others.

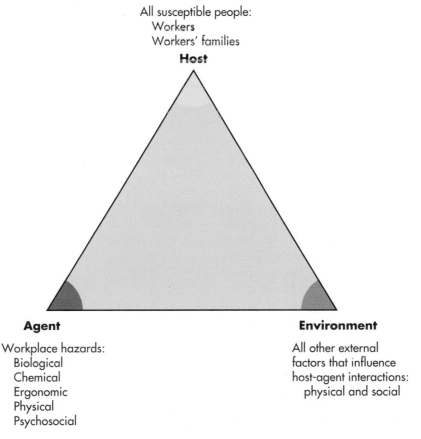

FIG. 44-2 The epidemiologic triad.

BOX 44-3 Categories of Work-Related Hazards

Biologic and infectious hazards. Infectious/biologic agents, such as bacteria, viruses, fungi, or parasites, that may be transmitted via contact with infected patients or contaminated body secretions/fluids to other individuals.

Chemical hazards. Various forms of chemicals, including medications, solutions, gases, vapors, aerosols, and particulate matter, that are potentially toxic or irritating to the body system.

Environmental and mechanical hazards. Factors encountered in the work environment that cause or potentiate accidents, injuries, strain, or discomfort (e.g., unsafe/inadequate equipment or lifting devices, slippery floors, work station deficiencies).

Physical hazards. Agents within the work environment, such as radiation, electricity, extreme temperatures, and noise, that can cause tissue trauma.

Psychosocial hazards. Factors and situations encountered or associated with one's job or work environment that create or potentiate stress, emotional strain, and/or interpersonal problems.

From Rogers B: *Occupational health nursing: concepts and practice,* Philadelphia, 1994, W.B. Saunders.

Host

Each worker represents a host within the worker population group. Certain host factors are associated with increased risk of adverse response to the hazards of the workplace. These include age, gender, health status, work practices, ethnicity, and lifestyle factors (Barratt, 1994; Girgis, 1994; Jeffry, 1993). For example, the population group at greatest risk for experiencing work-related accidents with subsequent injuries are men (18 to 30 years old) with less than 6 months experience on the current job. The host factors of age, gender, and work experience combine to increase this group's risk of injury because of characteristics such as risk taking, lack of knowledge, and lack of familiarity with the new job. Older workers may be at increased risk in the workplace because of diminished sensory abilities, the effects of chronic illnesses, and delayed reaction times (Stine and Brown, 1996). A third population group that may be very susceptible to workplace exposure is women in their child-bearing years (Bellows and Rudolph, 1993; Stellman, 1994). The hormonal changes during these years, along with the increased stress of new roles and additional responsibilities, as well as transplacental exposures, are host factors that may influence this group's response to potential toxins.

In addition to these host factors, there may be other, less well-understood individual differences in responses to occupational hazard exposures. Even if employers maintain exposure levels below the level recommended by occupational health and safety standards, 15% to 20% of the population may have health reactions to the "safe" low-level exposures (Levy and Wegman, 1995). This group has been termed *hy-persusceptible.* A number of host factors appear to be associated with this hypersusceptibility: light skin, malnutrition, compromised immune system, glucose 6-phosphate dehydrogenase deficiency, serum alpha 1-antitrypsin deficiency, chronic obstructive pulmonary disease, sickle cell trait, and hypertension. Individuals who have known hypersusceptibility to chemicals that are respiratory irritants, hemolytic chemicals, organic isocyanates, and carbon disulfide may also be hypersusceptible to other agents in the work environment (Levy and Wegman, 1995). Although this has prompted some industries to consider preplacement screening for such risk factors, the associations between these individual health markers and hypersusceptible response are speculative and require further research.

Agent

Work-related hazards, or agents (see Box 44-3), present potential and actual risks to the health and safety of workers in the millions of business establishments in the United States. Any worksite commonly presents multiple and interacting exposures form all five categories of agents. Table 44-1 lists some of the more common workplace exposures, their known health effects, and the types of jobs associated with these hazards.

Biologic agents

Biologic agents are living organisms whose excretions or parts are capable of causing human disease, usually by an infectious process. Biologic hazards are common in workplaces such as health care facilities and clinical laboratories where employees are potentially exposed to a variety of infectious agents, including viruses, fungi, and bacteria. Of particular concern in occupational health are infectious diseases transmitted by humans (e.g., from client to worker or from worker to worker) in a variety of work settings (USDHHS, NIOSH, 1996). Bloodborne and airborne pathogens represent a significant class of exposures for the 6 million U.S. health care workers. Occupational transmission of bloodborne pathogens (including the hepatitis B and C viruses and the human immunodeficiency virus [HIV]), occurs primarily by means of needlestick injuries but also through exposures to the eyes or mucous membranes (Jagger, 1994). The risk of hepatitis B virus infection following a single needlestick injury with a contaminated needle varies from 2% to greater than 40%, depending on the antigen status of the source person and nature of exposure. Similarly, the risk of hepatitis C virus transmission also depends on the same factors and ranges from 3.3% to 10%.

Transmission of tuberculosis (TB) within health care settings (especially multidrug-resistant TB) has reemerged as a major public health problem (USDHHS, NIOSH, 1996; Sepkowitz, 1994; Wenger, 1995). Since 1989, outbreaks of this type of TB have been reported in hospitals and some workers have developed active drug-resistant TB. In addition, among workers in health care, social service, and corrections facilities who work with populations at in-

TABLE 44-1 Selected Job Categories, Exposures, and Associated Work-Related Diseases and Conditions

JOB CATEGORIES	EXPOSURES	WORK-RELATED DISEASES AND CONDITIONS
All workers	Workplace stress	Hypertension, mood disorders, cardiovascular disease
Agricultural workers	Pesticides, infectious agents, gases, sunlight	Pesticide poisoning, "farmer's lung," skin cancer
Anesthetists	Anesthetic gases	Reproductive effects, cancer
Automobile workers	Asbestos, plastics, lead, solvents	Asbestosis dermatitis
Butchers	Vinyl plastic fumes	"Meat wrappers' asthma'
Caisson workers	Pressurized work environments	"Caisson disease," "the bends"
Carpenters	Wood dust, wood preservatives, adhesives	Nasopharyngeal cancer, dermatitis
Cement workers	Cement dust, metals	Dermatitis, bronchitis
Ceramic workers	Talc, clays	Pneumoconiosis
Demolition workers	Asbestos, wood dust	Asbestosis
Drug manufacturers	Hormones, nitroglycerin, etc.	Reproductive effects
Dry cleaners	Solvents	Liver disease, dermatitis
Dye workers	Dyestuffs, metals, solvents	Bladder cancer, dermatitis
Embalmers	Formaldehyde, infectious agents	Dermatitis
Felt makers	Mercury, polycyclic hydrocarbons	Mercuralism
Foundry workers	Silica, molten metals	Silicosis
Glass workers	Heat, solvents, metal powders	Cataracts
Hospital workers	Infectious agents, cleansers, radiation	Infections, latex allergies, unintentional injuries
Insulators	Asbestos, fibrous glass	Asbestosis, lung cancer, mesothelioma
Jack hammer operators	Vibration	Raynaud's phenomenon
Lathe operators	Metal dusts, cutting oils	Lung disease, cancer
Office computer workers	Repetitive wrist motion on computers and eye strain	Tendonitis, carpal tunnel syndrome, tenosynovitis

creased risk of TB, hundreds have experienced tuberculin skin test conversions. Reliable data are lacking on the extent of possible work-related TB transmission among other groups of workers at risk for exposure. Many workers in these settings are employed as maintenance workers, security guards, aides, or cleaning people, who tend not to be well-protected from inadvertent exposures which include contaminated bed linen in the laundry, soiled equipment, and trash containing contaminated dressing or specimens (CDC, 1996).

Chemical agents

Over 300 billion pounds of chemical agents are produced annually in the United States. Of the approximately 2 million known chemicals in existence, less than 0.1% have been adequately studied for their effects on humans. Of those chemicals that have been linked to carcinogens, approximately half test positive as animal carcinogens. Most chemicals have not been studied epidemiologically to determine the effects of exposure on humans (Levy and Wegman, 1995). As a consequence of general environmental contamination with chemicals from work, home, and community activities, a variety of chemicals are found

in the body tissues of the general population (Stine and Brown, 1996). These tissue loads may result in part from the accidental release of chemicals into the environment, such as that which occurred in Love Canal when chemicals leached out from buried industrial wastes.

DID YOU KNOW? *Only 0.1% of the nearly 2 million known chemicals produced have been tested for their effect on humans.*

In many workplaces, significant exposure to a daily, low-level dose of workplace chemicals may be below the exposure standards but may still carry a potentially chronic and perhaps cumulative assault on workers' health. Predicting human responses to such exposures is further complicated because several chemicals are often combined to create a new chemical agent. Human effects may be associated with the interaction of these agents rather than with a single chemical. Another concern about occupational exposure to chemicals is reproductive health effects. Workplace reproductive hazards have become important legal and scientific issues. Toxicity to male and female reproductive systems has been demonstrated from exposure to common agents such as lead, mercury, cadmium, nickel, and zinc, as well as in antineoplastic drugs. Since data for predicting human responses to many chemical agents are inadequate, workers should be assessed for all potential exposures and cautioned to work preventively with these agents. High-risk or vulnerable workers should be carefully screened and monitored for optimal health protection, such as those workers with latex allergy, which is a widely recognized health hazard (McCormick, 1995; NIOSH, 1997a). It is essential that the nurse have a good understanding of the basic principles of toxicology, including routes of exposure, dose-response relationships, and differences in effects (i.e., acute vs. chronic toxicity) in order to be able to accurately assess and evaluate the exposure and recommend changes for abatement.

Environmental/mechanical agents

Environmental/mechanical agents are those that can potentially cause injury or illness and are related to the work process, or cause postural or other strains that can produce adverse health effects when certain tasks are performed repeatedly. Examples are repetitive motions, poor workstation-worker fit, and lifting heavy loads. Carpal tunnel syndrome, tendonitis, and tenosynovitis are the most frequently seen occupational diseases observed in workers who are chronically exposed to repetitive motion. In 1995 705,800 musculoskeletal disorders due to repeated trauma were reported in the U.S. workplace. This figure represents nearly 62% of all illness cases reported to the Bureau of Labor Statistics (NIOSH, 1997b). The most frequently reported upper-extremity musculoskeletal disorders affect the hand/wrist region. In 1993, carpal tunnel syndrome, the most widely recognized condition, occurred at a rate of 5.2 per 10,000 full-time workers. This syndrome required the longest recuperation period of all conditions resulting in lost workdays, with a median 30 days away from work.

Back pain and injury is one of the most common and significant musculoskeletal problems in the world (NIOSH, 1997b; Jorgensen, 1994; Larese, 1994). In 1995, back injuries and disorders accounted for 38% of all nonfatal occupational injuries and illnesses involving days away from work in the United States. While the exact costs of back disorders is unknown, the estimates are staggering. In a recent study, the average cost of a workers' compensation claim for a low back disorder was $8300, which was more than twice the average cost of $4075 for all other paid claims combined. A conservative estimate of back injury costs is $13 billion per year (USDHHS-NIOSH, 1996). Others estimate the cost as $20 billion annually (AFL-CIO, 1997). Regardless of the estimates used, the problem is large both in health and economic terms. Of these costs, about $11 billion are paid by the workers' compensation system. Moreover, as many as 30% of American workers are employed in jobs that routinely require them to perform activities that may increase risk of developing low back disorders. The research on these hazards, related human responses, and prevention is evolving. Injuries and illnesses related to this category of agents have been termed cumulative trauma, which composes the largest category of work-related illness and disability claims in the United States. The most productive strategy in preventing these exposures appears to be redesigning the workplace and the work machinery or processes.

Physical agents

Physical agents are those that produce adverse health effects through the transfer of physical energy. Commonly encountered physical agents in the workplace include temperature extremes, vibration, noise, radiation, and lighting (Payling, 1994; Platt, 1993). For example, vibration, which accompanies the use of power tools and vehicles such as trucks, affects internal organs, supportive ligaments, the upper torso, and the shoulder-girdle structure. Localized effects are seen with handheld power tools; the most common is Raynaud's phenomenon. The control of worker exposure to these agents is usually accomplished through engineering strategies such as eliminating or containing the offending agent. In addition, workers must use preventive actions, such as practicing safe work habits and wearing personal protective equipment when needed. Examples of safe work habits include taking appropriate breaks from environments with temperature extremes and not eating or smoking in radiation-contaminated areas. Personal protective equipment includes hearing protection, eye guards, protective clothing, and devices for monitoring exposures to agents such as radiation. This class of agents is considered one of the most easily controlled.

Psychosocial agents

Psychosocial agents are conditions that create a threat to the psychologic and/or social well-being of individuals and groups (Rogers, 1994a). A psychosocial response to the work environment occurs as an employee acts selectively toward his environment in an attempt to achieve a harmonious relationship. When such a human attempt at adaptation to the environment fails, an adverse psychosocial response may occur. Work-related stress or burn-out is fast becoming a significant problem for many individuals (Fielding, 1994). Responses to negative interpersonal relationships, particularly those with authority figures in the workplace, are often the cause of vague health symptoms and increased absenteeism. Epidemiologic work in mental health has pointed to environmental variables such as these in the incidence of mental illness and emotional disorder (see the Research Brief).

The psychosocial environment includes characteristics of the work itself, as well as the interpersonal relationships required in the work setting and shiftwork. An estimated 11.5 million Americans do some form of shiftwork that has the potential to lead to a variety of psychologic and physical problems including exhaustion, depression, anxiety, and gastrointestinal disturbance. Strategies to minimize the

RESEARCH *Brief*

The authors of this study were interested in how organizations and the psychosocial environment of work affect morbidity and mortality, especially related to heart disease. The authors investigated previously established risk factors for heart disease in a sample of 2682 men from Kuopio, Finland.

Baseline assessments were completed of biologic, behavioral, and psychosocial factors related to each participant, as well as an assessment of the prevalence of current illnesses and an evaluation of each person's work environment, income, and education.

The study concluded that there were risks of mortality from a number of causes for men in low-income jobs that were high in demand but had few resources to complete the job. Mortality also increased in all-low income jobs that had also lots of resources regardless of the job demands. However, men in high-demand, low-income jobs with few resources were at greater risk for heart disease than other workers.

It is thought by the authors that, considering all factors related to the individual and the workplace, the results over time of the effects of poor working conditions and low income lead to feelings of hopelessness, depression, poor behavior, psychologic risk profiles, higher levels of morbidity, and increased mortality risk.

Because the low-income worker is at greater risk for mortality, occupational nurses can be aware of the organization of the workplace, the job demands, and the work environment on the population of low-income workers. Increasing the skills of the workers, creating a democratic work environment, and focusing on job satisfaction and economic rewards for enhancing worker skills are a few recommended interventions. Health education and counseling directed to the population, spending quality family time, and encouraging hobbies and recreational events can help.

Lynch J et al: Workplace conditions, socioeconomic status and the risk of mortality and acute myocardial infarction: the Kuopio ischemic heart disease risk factor study, *Am J Public Health* 87(4):617, 1997.

adverse effects of shiftwork such as rotating shifts clockwise will be beneficial. Job characteristics such as low autonomy, poor job satisfaction, and limited control over the pace of work have been associated with an increased risk of heart disease among clerical and blue-collar workers.

Interpersonal relationships among employees and coworkers or bosses and managers are often sources of conflict and stress. Another aspect is *organizational culture*. This refers to the norms and patterns of behavior that are sanctioned within a particular organization. Such norms and patterns set guidelines for the types of work behaviors that will enable employees to succeed within a particular firm.

Examples include following organizational norms for working overtime, expressing constructive dissatisfaction with management, and making work a top priority. These factors and the employee's response to them must be assessed if strategies for influencing the health and safety of workers are to be effective.

Nonfatal violence in the health care worker's workplace is a serious problem that seems to be underreported. Much of the study of health care worker violence has been in psychiatric settings; however, reports in other areas such as the emergency department have been reported. Risk factors associated with this type of violence must be identified and strategies implemented to reduce the risk (Poster, 1994).

Environment

Environmental factors influence the occurrence of host-agent interactions and may direct the course and outcome of those interactions. The physical environment involves the geologic and atmospheric structure of an area and the source of such elements as water, temperature, and radiation, which may serve as positive or negative stressors. Although aspects of the physical environment (e.g., heat, odor, or ventilation) may influence the host-agent interaction, the social and psychologic environment can be of equal importance (Hodgson, 1994).

New environmental problems continue to arise, such as an increase in industrial wastes and toxins and indoor and outdoor environmental pollution, which present opportunities for significant health threats to the working and general population. The social aspects of the environment encompass the economic and political forces affecting society and its health. This includes factors such as sanitation/hygiene practices, housing conditions, level and delivery of health care services, development and enforcement of health-related codes (e.g., occupational health and safety, pollution), employment conditions, population crowding, literacy, ethnic customs, extent of support for health-related research, and equal access to health care. In addition, addictive behaviors such as alcohol and substance abuse and various forms of psychosocial stress may be an outgrowth of negative social environments. Consider an employee who is working with a potentially toxic liquid. Providing education about safe work practices and fitting the employee with protective clothing may not be adequate if the work must occur in a very hot and humid environment. As the worker becomes uncomfortable in the hot clothing, his or her protection may be compromised by rolling up a sleeve, taking off a glove, or wiping his face with a contaminated piece of clothing. If the psychosocial norms in the workplace condone such work practices (e.g., "Everyone does it when it's too hot"), the interventions that address only the host and agent will be ineffective. The epidemiologic triad can be used as the basis for planning interventions to restore and promote the health of workers. These efforts are influenced by society and organization activities related to occupational health and safety (Rabinowitz, 1994; Snyder, 1994).

The occupational environment, within the context of the social environment, is represented by the workplace and work setting and the interactive effects of this environment on the worker. One must consider the hazards and threats posed by this environment and the commitment of the employer to providing a safe and healthful workplace through use of preventive strategies and controls (e.g., engineering, substitution) (Rogers, 1994a).

ORGANIZATIONAL AND PUBLIC EFFORTS TO PROMOTE WORKER HEALTH AND SAFETY

Promotion of worker health and safety is the goal of occupational health and safety programs (Porro, 1993). These programs are offered primarily by the employer at the workplace, but the range of services and the models for delivering them have bee changing dramatically over the past few years. In addition to specific services, legislation at the federal and state levels has had a significant effect on efforts to provide a healthy and safe environment for all workers. Under the Occupational Safety and Health Act and increased public concern about worker health and safety, there have recently been citations of companies that do not meet minimal occupational health and safety standards. Criminal charges have been filed against business owners when preventable work-related deaths occurred. These events have redirected an emphasis on preventive occupational health and safety programming.

Unless a company has OSHA-regulated exposures, business firms are not required to provide occupational health and safety services that meet any specified standards. With few exceptions, there is no legal request for specific services or level of personnel provided by employers to protect worker health and safety. Therefore the range of services offered and the qualifications of the providers of occupational health and safety vary widely across industries. An important stimulus for health and safety programs is avoiding cost that can be attributed to the effectiveness of prevention services, as well as the need to support occupational health and safety and health promotion at the worksite.

On-Site Occupational Health and Safety Programs

Optimally, on-site occupational health and safety services are provided by a team of occupational health and safety professionals. The core members of this team are the occupational health nurse, occupational physician, industrial hygienist, and safety professional. The largest group of health care professionals in business settings are occupational health nurses; therefore the most frequently seen model is that of the one-nurse unit. This nurse collaborates with a community physician or occupational medicine physician who provides consultation and accepts referrals where medical intervention is needed. The collaboration may occur primarily through telephone contact, or the physician may be under contract with the company to spend a certain amount of time on-site each week. As companies become larger, they are likely to hire additional nurses, safety professionals, industrial hygienists, and physicians, the latter usually on a part-time or consultant basis. An increasingly popular option is to contract some health, safety, and industrial hygiene work to external providers. The largest firms often have corporate occupational health and safety professionals who set policy and participate in company decision making at the corporate level. These professionals work with the nurses employed at the individual sites within the company. Depending on the needs of the company and the workers, additional professionals may be on the occupational health and safety team, including employee assistance counselors or social workers, health educators, physical fitness specialists, toxicologists, and ergonomists.

The services provided by on-site occupational health programs range from those focused only on work-related health and safety problems to a wide scope of services that includes primary health care (Box 44-4). In industries that have exposures regulated by law, certain programs are required, such as respiratory protection or hearing conservation. The ability of a company to offer additional programs depends on employee needs, management's attitudes and understanding about health and safety, acceptance by the workers, and the economic status of the firm. A significant increase in the number of health promotion and employee assistance programs offered in industry has occurred over the past few years. Health promotion programs focus on lifestyle choices that cause risks to health (e.g., job stress, obesity, smoking, stress responses, or lack of exercise) (Paskett, 1994; Rigotti, 1994). Employee assistance programs are designed to address personal problems (e.g., marital/family issues, substance abuse, or financial difficulties) that affect the employee's productivity. Since such efforts are cost-effective for businesses, they should continue to increase.

Similar types of occupational health and safety programs are available on a contractual basis from community-based providers. These may be offered by free-standing industrial clinics, health maintenance organizations, hospitals, emergency clinics, and other health care organizations. In addition, consultants in each discipline work in the private sector (self-employed, in group practice, or in insurance companies) and in the public sector (in local and state health departments or departments of labor and industry). These services may be provided on site, delivered elsewhere in the community, or offered through a mobile van that visits companies. These multiple resources have increased the options for companies that need occupational health and safety services and have also broadened the employment opportunities for health and safety professionals.

NURSING CARE OF WORKING POPULATIONS

The nurse is often the first health care provider seen by an individual with a work-related health problem. Consequently, nurses are in key positions to intervene with working populations at all levels of prevention.

Worker Assessment

The initial step of assessment involves the traditional history and physical assessment, emphasizing exposure to occupational hazards and individual characteristics that may predispose the client to increased health risk of certain jobs. The **occupational health history** is an indispensable component of the health assessment of individuals (Rogers, 1994a). Since work is a part of life for most people, including an occupational health history into all routine nursing assessments is essential. Many workers in the United States do not have access to health care services in their workplaces. Yet it is not unusual to find health care providers in the community who have little or no knowledge about workplaces or expertise in occupationally-related illnesses and injuries. Because of the large number of small businesses that do no have the resources for maintaining on-site health care, injured and ill workers are first seen in the public and private health care sector (e.g., in clinics, emergency rooms, physicians' offices, hospitals, HMOs, and ambulatory care centers). Nurses are often the first-line assessors of these individuals and perhaps the only contact for education about self-protection from workplace hazards. The identifying of workplace exposures as sources of health problems may influence the client's course of illness and rehabilitation and also prevent similar illnesses among others with potential for exposure.

Including occupational health data into client assessments begins with recognizing the possible relationship between health and occupational factors (Rabinowitz, 1994). The next step is to integrate into the history-taking procedure some routine assessment questions that will provide the data necessary to confirm or rule out occupationally induced symptoms. Symptoms of hazardous workplace exposures may be indicated by vague complaints involving any body system. These complaints are often similar to common medical problems. Three points that occupational health histories should include are a list of current and past jobs the client has held; questions about exposures to specific agents and relationships between the symptoms and activities at work, their job titles, or history of exposures; and other factors that may enhance the client's susceptibility to occupational agents (e.g., smoking history, underlying illness, previous injury, or handicapping condition).

Questions about the employee's occupational history can be included in existing assessment tools. The more complete the data collected, the more likely the nurse is to notice the influence of work-health interactions. All employees should be questioned about their employment history. To describe only a current status of "retired" or "housewife" may lead to the omission of needed data. The nurse should be aware that not all workers are well-informed about the materials with which they work or about potential hazards. For this reason the nurse must develop basic knowledge about the types of jobs held by clients and the possible hazards associated with them. Since there is an increased likelihood of multiple exposures from other environments, like home and yard, that may interact with workplace exposures, the nurse should extend the questioning to include this information.

Identifying work-related health problems does not require an extensive knowledge of occupational agents and their effects. A systematic approach for evaluating the potential for workplace exposures is the most effective intervention for detecting and preventing occupational health risks. Fig. 44-3 shows one short assessment tool that can be incorporated into routine history taking. Similar questions can be included in the assessment of workers' spouses and dependents, who may receive second-hand or indirect exposure to occupational hazards.

During these health assessments, the nurse has the opportunity to teach about workplace hazards and preventing measures the worker can use. At the same time, the nurse is obtaining information that will be valuable in optimizing work-job fit. Such assessments may be done as preplacement examinations before the client begins a job, on a periodic basis during employment, or with the onset of a

I. Present Job

A.   What is your job title? _____

B.   What do you do for a living? _____

C.   How long have you had this job? _____

D.   Describe the specific tasks of this job: _____
_____

E.   What product or service is produced by the company where you work:? _____
_____

F.   Are you exposed to any of the following on your present job?
Metals   Radiation   Stress
Vapors, gases   Vibration   Others: _____
Dusts   Loud noise
Solvents   Extreme heat or cold

G.   Do you feel you have any health problems that may be associated with your work?
If yes, describe: _____
_____

H.   How would you describe your satisfaction with your job? _____
_____

I.   Have any of your co-workers complained of illness or injuries that they associate with their jobs?
If yes, describe: _____
_____

II. All Past Work

Starting with your first job, please provide the following information:

Job title	Years held	Description of work	Exposures	Injuries/Illnesses	Personal protection equipment used

III. Other Exposures

A.   Do you have any hobbies which involve exposure to chemicals, metals or any of the other agents mentioned before? If yes, describe: _____

B.   Are any other members of your household exposed to any of the substances listed above? If yes, describe:
_____

C.   Do you live near any factories, dump sites, or other sources of pollution? If yes, describe: _____
_____

FIG. 44-3 Occupational health history form.

work-related health problem or exposure. Work-related health assessments can also be conducted when an employee is being transferred to another job with different requirements and exposures, at termination, and at retirement. The goal of these assessments is to identify agent and host factors that could place the employee at risk and to determine prevention steps that can be taken to eliminate or minimize the exposure and potential health problem.

WHAT DO YOU THINK? *There is an acceptable level of risk in any job.*

When the health data from such assessments are considered collectively, the nurse may determine some patterns in risk factors associated with the occurrence of work-related injuries and illnesses in a total population of workers. For example, a nurse practitioner in a clinic noted a dramatic increase in the number of bladder cancer cases among her clients. When she looked at factors in common among these individuals, she determined that they all worked at a company that used benzidine dyes, which are known bladder carcinogens. She worked with the union and the company to assess the environmental exposure to the employees. This nursing intervention led to a safer work environment and a decrease in bladder cancer among this population group. Such an approach can be used at the company, industry, and community levels. The initial collection of data and the questioning about workplace exposures are vital steps for any intervention.

Workplace Assessment

The nurse may conduct a similar assessment of the workplace itself. The purpose of this assessment, known as a **worksite walk-through** or survey, is to become knowledgeable about the work processes and the materials, the requirements of various jobs, the presence of actual or potential hazards, and the work practices of employees (AAOHN, 1994). Figure 44-4 shows a brief outline that can be used to guide a worksite assessment. More complex surveys are performed by industrial hygienists and safety professionals when the purpose of the walk-through is environmental monitoring or a safety audit. However, most occupational health nurses have developed expertise in these areas and include such tasks as part of their functions. For any health care provider who assesses workers, this information makes up an important database. For the on-site health care provider, worksite walk-throughs assist the professional in developing rapport with and being seen as a credible worker among the employees.

A worksite survey begins with an understanding of the type of work that occurs in the workplace. All business organizations are classified by the U.S. Department of Commerce with a numerical code, the Standard Industrial Classification (SIC) Code. This code, usually a two- to four-digit number, indicates a company's product and, therefore, the possible types of **occupational health hazards** that may be associated with the processes and materials used by its employees. SIC codes are used to collect and report data on businesses. For example, illness and injury rates of one company are compared to the rates of other companies of similar size with the same SIC code to determine whether the company is having an excess of illness or injury.

HOW TO *Assess a Worker and the Workplace*

Assessing the worker for a work-related problem is a critical practice element. You need to do the following:
- *Complete general and occupational health history taking with emphasis on workplace exposure assessment, job hazard analysis, and list of previous jobs.*
- *Conduct a health assessment to identify agent and host factors that interact to place workers at risk.*
- *Identify patterns of risk associated with illness/injury.*

Assessing the work environment is necessary to determine workplace exposures that create worker health risk. You need to do the following:
- *Understand the work being done*
- *Evaluate the work-related hazards*
- *Understand the work process*
- *Gather data about incidence/prevalence of work-related illness/injuries and related hazards*
- *Examine control strategies in place for eliminating exposures*

All OSHA and workers' compensation data are reported by the SIC code. In addition, by knowing the SIC code of a company, a health care professional can access reference books that describe the usual processes, materials, and by-products of that kind of company. A simple drawing of the work processes and work areas shows information by jobs or locations in the workplace. These preliminary data provide clues about what hazards may be present and an understanding of the types of jobs and health requirements that may be involved in a particular industry. A description of the work environment is next and provides an overall picture of general appearances, physical layout, and safety of the environment. Are safety signs posted and readable where needed? Is there clutter or dampness on the floor that could cause slips or falls?

A description of the employee group is necessary information to know the demographics and the work distribution in the company. Knowing about shiftwork and productivity can be helpful in pinpointing potential stressors. Human resources management and corporate commitment to health and safety, is necessary to develop a support culture for effective and efficient programming. Assessing the status of policies and procedures, as well as opportunities for input into improving service, are important to establish the organization's strength in occupational health and safety management. Gathering data about the incidence and prevalence of work-related illnesses and injuries, and the cost patterns for these condi-

Name of company: _____ Date: _____

Address: _____

Telephone: _____

Parent company (if any): _____

Location of corporate offices: _____

SIC code: _____

The Work:

Major products: _____

Major processes and operations, raw materials, by products: _____

_____

Type of jobs: _____

_____

Potential exposures: _____

_____

Work Environment

General conditions: _____

Safety signs: _____

Physical environment: _____

Worker Population

Employees

Total number: _____ Number in production: _____ Others: _____

% Fulltime: _____ % Men: _____ % Women: _____

% First shift: _____ % Second shift: _____ % Third shift: _____

Age distribution: _____

% Unionized: _____ Names of Unions: _____

Human Resources Management

Corporate commitment to health

Personnel

Policies/procedures

Input/surveys/committees

Recordkeeping

Health Data

Work related illnesses, injuries, deaths per annum: _____

OSHA recordable: _____ Workers' Compensation: _____

Other: _____ Most frequent complaints: _____

Average number of monthly calls to the health unit: _____

Absenteeism rate: _____

Occupation Health and Safety Services

Examinations

Employee assistance

Treatment of illness/injury

Health Education

Physical fitness, health promotion activities

Mandatory programs

Safety audits

Environmental monitoring

Health risk appraisal

Screenings

Health promotion

Control Strategies

Engineering

Work practice

Administrative

Personal protective equipment

FIG. 44-4 Worksite assessment guide.

tions, provides useful epidemiologic trend data. It also targets high-cost areas. The types of occupational safety and health services and programs are important to know. This will show whether required programs are being offered and include health promotion and disease prevention strategies.

Finally, examining control strategies that are effective in eliminating or reducing exposure is important in determining risk reduction. Engineering controls can reduce worker exposure by modifying the exposure source, such as putting needles in a puncture-proof container.

Work practice controls include good hygiene, waste disposal, and housekeeping. Administrative controls reduce exposure through job rotation, workplace monitoring, and employee training and education. Personal protective control is the last resort and requires the worker to actively engage in strategies for protection such as use of gloves, masks, and gowns to prevent blood/body fluid exposure (Rogers, 1994a).

> **NURSING TIP**
>
> *Both corporate culture and cost-effective programs are key factors in influencing the development of occupational health services.*

The more information that can be collected before the walk-through, the more efficient will be the process of the survey. After the survey is conducted, the nurse can use the information with the aggregate health data to evaluate the effectiveness of the occupational health and safety program and to plan future programs.

HEALTHY PEOPLE 2000 AND 2010 RELATED TO OCCUPATIONAL HEALTH

In an attempt to meet the goal of increasing the span of healthy life for Americans, health protection strategies are proposed to address the needs of large population groups such as the American Workforce. The *Healthy People 2000* and the draft *Healthy People 2010* documents identify the national occupational safety and health strategy: that is, the promotion of good health and well-being among workers, including the elimination of factors in occupational environments that cause death, injury, disease, or disability. In addition, this document promotes the minimizing of personal damage from existing occupationally related illness.

LEGISLATION RELATED TO OCCUPATIONAL HEALTH

The occupational health and safety services provided by an employer are influenced by specific legislation at federal and state levels. Although the relationship between work and health has been known since the second century (Ramazzini, 1713), public policy that effectively controlled occupational hazards was not enacted until the

1960s. The Mine Safety and Health Act of 1968 was the first legislation that specifically required certain prevention programs for workers. This was followed by the Occupational Safety and Health Act of 1970, which established two agencies to carry out the Act's purpose of ensuring "safe and healthful working conditions for working men and women" (PL 91-596, 1970).

Within the context of the OSH Act, the Occupational Safety and Health Administration (OSHA), a federal agency within the U.S. Department of Labor, was created to develop and enforce workplace safety and health regulations. OSHA sets the standards that regulate workers' exposure to potentially toxic substances, enforcing these at the federal, regional, and state levels. Specific standards and information about compliance can be obtained from federal, regional, and state OSHA offices.

The **National Institute for Occupational Safety and Health (NIOSH)** was established by the Occupational Safety and Health Act of 1970 and is part of the Centers for Disease Control and Prevention (CDC). In 1996, NIOSH and its partner agencies (the National Institute of Arthritis and Musculoskeletal and Skin Diseases, the National Institute of Environmental Health Sciences, and the National Heart, Lung, and Blood Institute) unveiled the **National Institute for Occupational Research Agenda (NORA),** a framework to guide occupational safety and health research into the next decade. The NIOSH agency identifies, monitors, and educates about the incidence, prevalence, and prevention of work-related illnesses and injuries and examines potential hazards of new work technologies and practices (USDHHS-NIOSH, 1999). NORA, with its research-priority agenda (Box 44-5), is responsible for providing targeted research in areas with the highest likelihood of reducing the still-significant toll of workplace illness and injury.

Although NIOSH and OSHA were both created by the same act of Congress, they have discrete functions (Box 44-6).

> **NURSING TIP**
>
> *NIOSH publications, many of which are free, are available by writing or faxing a request to: NIOSH Publications, Mail Stop C-13, 4676 Columbia Parkway, Cincinnati, OH 45226-1998. See this book's website at www.mosby.com/MERLIN for additional contact information.*

One of the most far-reaching OSHA standards is the **Hazard Communication Standard.** Also known as the federal "right-to-know" law, this standard is based on the premise that working environments cannot eliminate all potentially toxic agents; therefore an important line of defense is an educated workforce. The Hazard Communication Standard, which took effect in 1983, required that all manufacturing firms inventory their toxic agents, label them, and develop information sheets, called Material

BOX 44-5 National Occupational Research Agenda (NORA) Priority Research Areas

DISEASE AND INJURY
- Allergy and irritant dermatitis
- Asthma and chronic obstructive pulmonary disease
- Fertility and pregnancy abnormalities
- Hearing loss
- Infectious diseases
- Low back disorders
- Musculoskeletal disorders of the upper extremities
- Traumatic injuries

WORK ENVIRONMENT AND WORKFORCE
- Emerging technologies
- Indoor environment
- Mixed exposures
- Organization of work
- Special populations at risk

RESEARCH TOOLS AND APPROACHES
- Cancer research methods
- Control technology and personal protective equipment
- Exposure assessment methods
- Health services research
- Intervention effectiveness research
- Risk assessment methods
- Social and economic consequences of workplace illness and injury
- Surveillance research methods

From Centers for Disease Control and Prevention, USDHHS-National Institute for Occupational Safety and Health, National Occupational Research Agenda, Publication Number 99-108, 1999.

BOX 44-6 Functions of Federal Agencies Involved in Occupational Health and Safety

OSHA
Determine and set standards for hazardous exposures in the workplace.
Enforce the occupational health standards (including the right of entry for inspection).
Educate employers about occupational health and safety.
Develop and maintain a database of work-related injuries, illnesses, and deaths.
Monitor compliance with occupational health and safety standards.

NIOSH
Conduct research and review of research findings to recommend permissible exposure levels for occupational hazards to OSHA.
Identify and research occupational health and safety hazards.
Educate occupational health and safety professionals.
Distribute research findings relevant to occupational health and safety.

From Centers for Disease Control and Prevention, USDHHS-National Institute for Occupational Safety and Health, National Occupational Research Agenda, Publication Number 99-108, 1999.

Safety Data Sheets (MSDSs), for each agent. In addition, the employer must have in place a Hazard Communication Program that provides workers with education about these agents. This education must include agent identification, toxic effects, and protective measures. In 1988, this standard was extended to all employers covered by the Occupational Safety and Health Act. Similar right-to-know legislation exists at many state and local levels. The next legislative approach will focus on the right-to-act standards and guidelines that protect workers' rights to use the information from right-to-know efforts to change unsafe or unhealthy working conditions.

Workers' compensation acts are important state laws that govern financial compensation of employees who suffer work-related health problems. These acts vary by state; each state sets rules for the reimbursement of employees with occupational health problems for medical expenses and lost work time associated with the illness or injury. Workers' compensation claims and the experience-based insurance premiums paid by industry have been important motivators for increasing the health and safety of the workplace.

DISASTER PLANNING AND MANAGEMENT

Although disaster planning and management have been functions of occupational health and safety programs, this is an area of new legislation that affects businesses and health professionals. The legislation of the *Superfund Amendment and Reauthorization Act* (SARA) requires that written disaster plans be shared with key resources in the community, such as fire departments and emergency rooms. Public concern about disasters, such as the methyl isocyanate leak in Bhopal, India, or the community exposure to chemicals at Times Beach, Missouri, has mandated more attention to disaster planning.

The goals of a disaster plan are to prevent or minimize injuries and deaths of workers and residents, minimize property damage, provide effective triage, and facilitate necessary business activities. A disaster plan requires the cooperation of different personnel within the company and community. The nurse is often a key person on the disaster planning team, along with safety professionals, physicians, industrial hygienists, the fire chief, and company management. The potential for disaster (e.g., explosions, fires, and leaks) must be identified; this is best achieved by completing an exhaustive chemical and hazard inventory of the workplace. The Material Safety Data Sheets and plant blueprints are critical for correctly identifying substances and work areas that may be hazardous. Work site surveys are the first step to completing this inventory.

Effective disaster plans are designed by those with knowledge of the work processes and materials, the workers and workplace, and the resources in the community. Specific steps must be detailed for actions to be put in place by specific individuals in the event of a disaster. The written plan must be shared with all who will be involved. Employees should be prepared in first aid, CPR, and fire brigade procedures. Plans must be clear, specific, and comprehensive (i.e., covering all shifts and all work areas) and must include activities to be conducted within the worksite and those that require community resources. Transportation plans, fire response, and emergency response services should be coordinated with the agencies that would be involved in actual disaster. The disaster plan, emergency and safety equipment, and the first response team's abilities should be tested at least annually with a drill. Practice results should be carefully evaluated, with changes made as needed.

Hospitals and other emergency services, such as fire departments, should be involved in developing the disaster plan and should receive a copy of the plan and a current hazard inventory. It is imperative that the plan and hazard inventory be periodically updated. The occupational health nurse or another company representative should provide emergency health care providers with updated clinical information on exposures and appropriate treatment. It should never be assumed that local services will have current information on substances used in industry. Representatives of these agencies should visit the work site and accompany the nurse on a work site walk-through so that they are familiar with the operations.

In disaster planning, the nurse is often assigned or assumes the responsibility for coordinating the planning and implementing efforts, working with appropriate key people within the company and in the community to develop a workable, comprehensive plan. Other tasks include providing ongoing communication to keep the plan current; planning the drills; educating the employees, management, and community providers; and assessing the equipment and services that may be used in a disaster.

In the event of a disaster, the nurse should play a key role in coordinating the response. Principles of triage may be used as the response team determines the extent of the disaster and the ability of the company and community to respond. Postdisaster nursing interventions are also critical. Examples include identifying of ongoing disaster-related health needs of workers and community residents, collecting epidemiologic data, and assessing the cause and the necessary steps to prevent a recurrence.

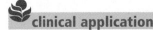

clinical application

An insurance company recently renovated its claims processing office area. All typewriters were replaced with video display terminals (VDTs) and associated hardware for handling all future work by computer. The company's occupational health nurse noticed an increase in visits to the health unit for complaints of headaches, stiff neck muscles, and visual disturbances. These health problems have been associated with VDT operation.

To conduct a complete investigation of this problem, the nurse assessed the workers, the new agent (the VDTs), previously existing potential agents, and the work environment. Interventions focused on designing the health hazard out of the work process, if possible. In the present example, the first level of intervention was design of the workstation, the component used by the VDT operations in doing their work. Minimizing the possible hazards of the agent involved recommendations for desks, chairs, and lighting designs that would accommodate the individual worker and allow shielding of the VDT. The nursing interventions included strengthening the resistance of the host by prescribing appropriate rest breaks, eye exercises, and relaxation strategies. Recognizing that previous cervical neck injury or impaired vision may increase the risk of adverse effects from VDT work, the nurse would include assessment for these factors in employees' preplacement and periodic health examinations.

For the environmental concerns, the nurse educated the manager about the health risks of paced, externally controlled work expectations and recommended alternatives.

This case is an example of which of the following:

A. The application of the occupational health history.
B. A work site assessment or walk-through.
C. A work-health interaction
D. The use of the epidemiologic triad in exploring occupational health problems.

Answer is in the back of the book.

KEY POINTS

- Occupational health nursing is an autonomous practice specialty.
- The scope of occupational health nursing practice is broad, including worker/workplace assessment and surveillance, case management, health promotion, primary care, management/administration, business and finance skills, and research.
- The workforce and workplace are changing dramatically requiring new knowledge and new occupational health services.
- The type of work has shifted from primarily manufacturing to service and technologic jobs.

Continued

KEY POINTS

- Workplace hazards include exposure to biologic, chemical, environmental/mechanical, physical, and psychosocial agents.
- Each day an average of 137 people die from work-related disease and an additional 16 die from on-the-job injuries.
- In 1994, occupational injuries alone cost an estimated $121 billion.
- The Occupational Safety and Health Act of 1970 states that workers must have a safe and healthful work environment.
- The interdisciplinary occupational health team usually consists of the occupational health nurse, occupational medicine physician, industrial hygienist, and safety specialist.
- Work-related health problems must be investigated and control strategies implemented to reduce exposure.
- Control strategies include engineering, work practice, administration, and personal protective equipment.
- The Occupational Safety and Health Administration enforces workplace safety and health standards.
- The National Institute for Occupational Safety and Health is the research agency that provides grants to investigate the causes of workplace illness and injuries.
- Worker's Compensation Acts are important laws that govern financial compensation of employees who suffer work-related health problems.
- The occupational health nurse should play a key role in disaster planning and coordination.
- Academic education in occupational health nursing is generally at the graduate level.

critical thinking activities

1. Arrange to visit a local industry to observe work processes and discuss working conditions. See if you can identify the work-related hazards and make recommendations for eliminating them.
2. Interview the occupational health nurse in an industry setting and ask questions about scope of practice, job functions, and contributions to the business.
3. Contact the American Association of Occupational Health Nurses and ask what the most pressing trends are in the specialty.
4. Obtain a proposed standard for the Occupational Safety and Health Administration, critique it, and submit your comments.
5. Attend a worker's compensation hearing, analyze the problem, and critique the outcome.

Bibliography

Adams J: Primary care at the worksite: the use of health risk appraisal in a nursing center, *AAOHN J* 43(1):17, 1995.

American Association of Occupational Health Nurses: *Guidelines for developing job descriptions in occupational and environmental health nursing:* Atlanta, 1997, the Association.

American Association of Occupational Health Nurses: *Standards for occupational health nursing practice,* Atlanta, 1999, the Association.

American Association of Occupational Health Nurses: *The nurse in industry,* New York, 1976, the Association.

Barratt A: Worksite-cholesterol screening and dietary intervention: the Staff Healthy Heart Project, Steering Committee, *Am J Publ Health* 84(5):779, 1994.

Bellow J, Rudolph L: The initial impact of a workplace lead-poisoning project, *Am J Publ Health* 83(3):406, 1993.

Brown M: *Occupational health nursing,* New York, 1981, MacMillan.

Bureau of Labor Statistics: *Handbook of labor statistics,* Washington, DC, 1995, US Department of Labor.

Bureau of Labor Statistics: *Employment projections: 1997,* Washington, DC, 1997, US Department of Labor.

Bureau of Labor Statistics: *Employment projections: 1998,* Washington, DC, 1998, US Department of Labor.

Bureau of Labor Statistics: *Employment projections: 1999,* Washington, DC, 1999, US Department of Labor.

Burgel B: *Innovations at the worksite: delivery of nurse-managed primary care services,* Washington, DC, 1993, American Nurses Association.

Callahan E: Quality in occupational health care: management's view, *J Occupat Med* 36(4):410, 1994.

Campos-Outcalt D: Occupational health epidemiology and objectives for the year 2000: primary care, *Clin Office Pract* 21(20):213, 1994.

Centers for Disease Control and Prevention: Prevalence of work disability, United States, 1990, *MMWR* 42(39):757, 1993.

Centers for Disease Control and Prevention: Tuberculosis morbidity–United States, 1995, *MMWR* 45(18):365, 1996.

Concerning occupational illness, *Emerg Med* 15:22, 1990.

Felton J: The genesis of American occupational health nursing, Part 1, *Occupat Health Nurs* 33:615, 1985.

Fielding J, Weaver SM: A comparison of hospital- and community-based mental health nurses: perceptions of their work environment and psychological health, *J Adv Nurs* 19:1196, 1994.

Girgis A: A workplace intervention for increasing outdoor workers' use of solar protection, *Am J Public Health* 84(1):77, 1994.

Hodgson M, Storey E: Patients and the sick building syndrome, *J Allergy Clin Immunol* 94(2 Pt 2):335, 1994.

Jagger J: Report on blood drawing: risky procedures, risky devices, risky job, *Adv Exposure Prevent* 1(1):4, 1994.

Jeffrey RW et al: The Healthy Worker Project: a work-site intervention for weight control and smoking cessation, *Am J Public Health* 83(3):395, 1993.

Jorgensen S, Hein HO, Gyntelberg F: Heavy lifting at work and risk of genital prolapse and herniated lumbar disc in assistant nurses, *Occupat Med* 44(1):47, 1994.

Katz E et al: Exposure assessment in epidemiologic studies of birth defects by industrial hygienic review of maternal interviews, *Am J Indust Med* 26(1):1, 1994.

Klinger C, Jones M: The OSHA standard setting process...role of the occupational health nurse, *AAOHN J* 42(8):374, 1994.

Larese F, Fiorit A: Musculoskeletal disorders in hospital nurses: a comparison between two hospitals, *Ergonomics* 37:1205, 1994.

Levy BS, Wegman DH: *Occupational health: recognizing and preventing occupational disease,* Boston, 1995, Little, Brown.

McGrath B: Fifty years of industrial nursing, *Public Health Nurse* 37:119, 1995.

Morris S: Academic occupational safety and health training programs, *Occupat Med* 9(2):189, 1994.

National Institute for Occupational Safety and Health: *Latex allergy,* Pub No 97-135, Washington, DC, 1997a, US Government

Printing Office [on-line: www.cdc.gov/noish/latexfs.html].

National Institute for Occupational Safety and Health: *Musculoskeletal disorders (MSDs) and workplace factors,* Washington, DC, 1997b, US Government Printing Office [on-line: www.cdc.gov/noish/ergtx1l.html].

National Institute for Occupational Safety and Health: *National occupational research agenda,* Washington, DC, 1999, USDHHS, Publication Number 99-108.

Paskett ED et al: Breast cancer screening education in the workplace, *J Cancer Educ* 9(2):101, 1994.

Payling K: A hazard we can no longer ignore: effects of excessive noise on wellbeing, *Prof Nurse* 9(6):418, 1994.

Platt J: Radon: its impact on the community and the role of the nurse, *AAOHN J* 41(11):547, 1993.

Porro S et al: The utility of health education among lead workers: the experience of one program, *Am J Indust Med* 23(3):473, 1993.

Poster E, Ryan J: A multiregional study of nurses' beliefs and attitudes about work safety and patient assault, *H & CP* 45(11):1104, 1994.

Rabinowitz S et al: Teaching interpersonal skills to occupational and environmental health professionals, *Psycho Rep* 74(3 Pt 2):1299, 1994.

Ramazzini B: *De Morbis Artificum* [Diseases of Workers], 1713. Translated by W.C. Wright, Chicago, 1940, University of Chicago Press.

Rigotti N et al: Do businesses comply with a no-smoking law? Assessing the self-enforcement approach, *Prevent Med* 23(2):223, 1994.

Rix S: *The American woman, 1990-1999,* New York, 1990, Norton.

Rogers B: *Occupational health nursing: concepts and practice,* Philadelphia, 1994a, W.B. Saunders.

Rogers B: The role of the occupational health nurse. In McCunnery RM, Brandt-Rauf PW, editors: *A practical approach to occupational and environmental medicine,* Boston, 1994b, Little, Brown.

Sepkowitz K: Tuberculosis and the health care worker: a historical perspective, *Ann Intern Med* 120(1):71, 1994.

Snyder M et al: Environmental and occupational health education: a survey of community health nurses' need for educational programs, *AAOHN J* 42(7):325, 1994.

Stellman J: Where women work and the hazards they may face on the job, *J Occupat Med* 36(8):814, 1994.

Stine D, Brown T: *Principles of toxicology,* Boca Raton, 1996, Lewis.

US Census Bureau: *Resident population of the United States: middle series projections, 2006-2010, by age and sex,* Washington, DC, 1996, US Government Printing Office [on-line: www.census.gov/population/projections/nation/nas/npas0610.txt].

US Department of Health and Human Services: *Data from the national sample survey of registered nurses,* Rockville, Md, 1996, Bureau of Health Professions.

US Department of Health and Human Services: *Healthy People 2000: national health promotion and disease prevention objectives,* Washington, DC, 1991, USDHHS, Public Health Service.

US Department of Health and Human Services, National Institute for Occupational Safety and Health: *National Occupational Research Agenda,* Cincinnati, 1996, Author.

US Department of Health and Human Services, National Institute for Occupational Safety and Health: *NORA fact sheet,* Pub No 99-108, Washington, DC, 1999, US Government Printing Office [on-line: www.cdc.gov/niosh/99-108.html].

Wenger PN et al: Control of nosocomial transmission of multidrug-resistant *Mycobacterium tuberculosis* among health care workers and HIV-infected patients, *Lancet* 345:235, 1995.

Workplace injury/illness rates for 1991 show a 10-year record drop in incidence, *Occupat Health Safety* 62(1):8, 1993.

Community Health Nurse as Parish Nurse and Block Nurse

RUTH D. BERRY

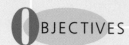BJECTIVES

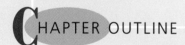 www.mosby.com/MERLIN/community_stanhope

After reading this chapter, the student should be able to do the following:

- Describe the heritage of health and healing in faith communities
- Describe models of the parish nurse and block nurse
- Develop awareness of the community health nurse's role as parish nurse in faith communities for health promotion and disease prevention
- Identify characteristics of the philosophy of parish nursing

- Help communities of faith include *Healthy People 2000* and *2010* guidelines in program planning
- Collaborate with key partners to implement congregational health ministries relevant for the faith community
- Use models of parish nursing with the nursing process in a faith community
- Evaluate programs for healthy congregations throughout the life span
- Examine the legal, ethical, and financial issues related to parish nursing

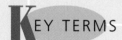EY TERMS

block nursing	healing	neighborhood nursing	pastoral care staff
circle of care	health ministries	parish nurse coordinator	polity
congregants	holistic care	parish nurses	wellness committee
congregational model	Holistic Health Centers	parish nursing	
faith communities	institutional model	partnerships	*See Glossary for definitions*

CHAPTER OUTLINE

Definitions in Parish Nursing
Heritage and Horizons
  Faith Communities
  Nursing Community
  Health Care Delivery
Parish Nursing Practice
  Characteristics of the Practice

Scope and Standards of Parish
  Nursing Practice
Educational Preparation for a
  Parish Nurse
Issues in Parish Nurse Practice
  Professional Issues
  Ethical Issues

Legal Issues
Financial Issues
National Health Objectives and
  Faith Communities
Functions of the Parish Nurse
Block Nursing

arish nursing has long established roots in the healing and health professions. Throughout historical accounts of nursing, caring for members of communities has been important. The earliest accounts of concern for others stem from communities of faith. Wholeness in health and being in "right" relationships with one's creator have sustained individuals and groups during times of illness, brokenness, stress, and when cure was not possible (Dossey, 1993; Rydholm, 1997; Solari-Twadell, 1990). Today parish nurses help individuals, families and congregations become more aware of the relationship of wholeness in body, mind, and spirit (McDermott et al, 1998; Schacht, 1992; Schank, Weis, and Matheus, 1996; Solari-Twadell et al, 1994).

Parish nurses address universal health problems of individuals, families, and groups of all ages. The members of congregation populations experience birth, death, acute and chronic illness, stress, dependency concerns, challenges of life transitions, growth, and development, and also face decisions regarding healthy lifestyle choices. Congregational members live in communities that make decisions regarding policies for financing and managing health care and for keeping environments safe and communities healthy for present and future generations.

Parish nursing is gaining prominence as nurses reclaim their traditions of healing, acknowledge gaps in service delivery, and, along with the rise of nursing centers, affirm the independent functions of nursing. In 1998 the American Nurses Association (ANA) accepted *parish nursing* as the most recognized term for the practice of nurses working with congregations or faith communities. With the Health Ministries Association, the ANA published the *Scope and Standards of Parish Nursing* (HMA/ANA, 1998). Although most parish nurses are in Protestant congregations, the concept is evident in most faith communities, including communities that serve diverse cultures. Parish nurses are also serving faith communities in countries such as Korea, Australia, Russia, and Canada (Bondine, 1997; Culp, 1997; Granberg-Michaelson, 1997; McDermott, 1998; Van Loon, 1996).

DEFINITIONS IN PARISH NURSING

Faith communities are congregational communities that gather in churches, cathedrals, synagogues, or mosques and acknowledge common faith traditions. **Parish nursing** is the most commonly used term that denotes the professional advanced nurse practice role in this context. **Parish nurses** respond to health and wellness needs within the context of populations of faith communities and are partners with the church in fulfilling the mission of health ministry. A parish nurse in the church may be referred to as a *congregational health minister, emergency church nurse,* or *health ministries nurse.*

The faith community includes persons throughout the life span. This includes active and less active members, as well as those confined to homes or in nursing homes. Often the church's mission also includes individuals and groups in the geographic community who are not designated church members. The services may be extended to those beyond the congregation. **Health ministries** are those activities and programs in faith communities organized around health and healing foci to promote wholeness in health across the life span. The services may be specifically planned or may be more informal. A professional or a lay person may provide them. These services include visiting the homebound, providing meals for families in crisis or when returning home after hospitalization, prayer circles, volunteering in community AIDS care groups, serving "healthy heart" church suppers, or holding regular grief support groups. The parish nurse emphasizes the nursing discipline's spiritual dimension while incorporating physical, emotional, and social aspects of nursing with individuals, families, and congregational communities.

Parish nurse models that have been widely implemented include congregational-based and institutional-based models. In the **congregational model,** the nurse is usually autonomous. The development of a parish nurse/health ministry program arises from the individual community of faith. The nurse is accountable to the congregation and its governing body. The **institutional model** includes greater collaboration and partnerships; the nurse may be in a contractual relationship with hospitals, medical centers, long-term care establishments, or educational institutions. Within either model, nurses work closely with professional health care members, **pastoral care staff,** and lay volunteers who represent various aspects of the life of the congregational community. To promote **healing,** the nurse builds on strengths to promote the connecting and integrating of inner spiritual knowing and healthy lifestyle choices for optimal wellness in life's many circumstances faced by individuals and families. Intentional and compassionate presence of a spiritually mature professional nurse in individual or group situations is vital. In this role, providing such **holistic care** with congregation populations is important. Holistic care is concerned with the body, mind, and spirit relationship in a constantly changing environment (Dossey, 1995). The nurse and members of the congregation assess, plan, implement and evaluate programs. The process of providing holistic care is enhanced by an active **wellness committee** or health cabinet. These committees are most effective when members represent the broad spectrum of the life of the church. The parish nurse uses all the knowledge and skills of this specialty to give effective services. The outcome is a truly caring congregation that supports healthy, spiritually fulfilling lives. Box 45-1 lists resources for parish nursing.

DID YOU KNOW? *Parish nurses are employed by senior living complexes and nursing homes to offer a spiritual focus to the nursing practice within various levels of living arrangements for elders, as well as serving one or more congregations in the community.*

BOX 45-1   Resources for Parish Nursing

International Parish Nurse Resource Center
205 W. Touhy Avenue, Suite 104
Park Ridge, IL 60068-1174
1-800-556-5368
(Publication: *Perspectives in Parish Nursing Practice*)

Health Ministries Association
601 Riverview Avenue
Dayton, OH 45406
1-800-280-9919
(Publication: *Connections*)

Interfaith Health Program of the Carter Center
453 Freedom Parkway
Atlanta, GA 30307
(Publication: *Faith & Health)*

See the WebLinks on this book's website at ʃₑₐᵣₚ www.mosby.com/
MERLIN for further information about resources.

HERITAGE AND HORIZONS
Faith Communities

In the roots of many faith communities are concerns for justice, mercy, and the need for spiritual and physical healing. The appeal for caring, the healing of diseases, and acknowledging periods of illness and wellness is universal. Throughout a major portion of the twentieth century religion has continued to play an important role in the lives of many in this country. More than half of the population prays daily. Eighty-five percent of clients state that they would like to have their health care provider pray with them, and at least 60% to 85% of the U.S. population indicates that they have some religious affiliation or an attachment to a house of worship (Princeton, 1994). Researchers in the last decade have become intrigued with relationships between spirituality and religion (Dossey, 1993; Koenig et al, 1997; Matthews et al, 1998; Oman and Reid, 1998; Oxman et al, 1995) (see the Research Brief about religious commitment and health status). An important aspect of living out one's spirituality and religion is being a part of a community of faith from birth to death, throughout wellness and illness. Participating as individuals or as families, all benefit from the associations with the supportive faith community or congregation.

The biblical account of Phoebe (Romans 16:1-2) exemplifies the tradition of health and healing within a congregation. Additionally, many Old Testament accounts and healing stories in the New Testament provide additional faith foundations (Psalms 106, 107, 113, Mark, Luke, Acts). So, too, nuns, deacons, deaconesses, the *Gemeindeschwester* or *Fuersorgerin* in Europe, and "emergency nurses" in African-American congregations are all examples of the healing professions serving in communities as they encounter more caring congregations. Support from mem-

RESEARCH *Brief*

The authors reviewed epidemiologic and clinical studies dealing with the relationship among selected religious factors such as frequency of religious attendance, private religious practices, reliance on religious beliefs, and the physical and mental health status in the areas of prevention, coping, and recovery. Studies characteristic of primary, secondary, and tertiary levels of prevention examined involvement in the prevention of illness, coping with current illnesses, and factors to facilitate recovery. A large proportion of the information gathered suggests that religious commitment plays a beneficial role in preventing mental and physical illness, enhances coping with these illnesses, and aids in the recovery from the illness. The authors contend that although increased studies with special attention directed to religious involvement and health status are needed, the implication for all health care clinicians is that interventions that recognize and involve clients' religious commitments may enhance health care outcomes. Beneficial interventions included incorporating religious orientation in preparing the care plan; praying with clients; encouraging clients to pray alone and with others, to continue attendance to meditations, faith rituals, worship services, and to seek and ask for forgiveness from others in their lives; reading holy writings; and offering referrals to clergy or chaplains. The implications for the parish nurse are to implement the appropriate interventions following assessment of the importance of religious commitment in one's life and supporting other health care professionals in their practice with the individual or family.

Matthews DA et al: Religious commitment and health status: a
review of the research and implications for family medicine,
Arch Fam Med 7:118, 1998.

bers of groups that are meaningful to a person's total well-being aids in recovery and healing (Matthews et al, 1998; Oman et al, 1998; Oxman et al, 1995). Asking for help and using strengths from earliest faith, traditions, family support, and teachings assist individuals, groups, and communities in interpreting brokenness, disasters, joys, births, deaths, illness, and recovery

The origins of wholeness and salvation are derived from similar concepts of *Sodzo* (Greek) and shalom or wholeness. These terms and harmony in health are common to most faith communities and have a biblical base. Writings in Christian and Jewish sources address the individual and community relationship with God as the source for a wise use of resources of self, environment, and one's community. Hygiene, health, and healing were a part of the Holiness Code of Leviticus. Throughout history, health existed at the center of the interaction between one's creator and

RESEARCH *Brief*

The authors administered several scales including an intrinsic and extrinsic religiosity index and a spiritual well-being scale to 100 elderly persons diagnosed with cancer. The mean age was 73 years old. Relationships among spiritual well-being, religiosity, hope, depression, and other mood states were examined to determine whether differences existed in those with high and low intrinsic religiosity and spiritual well-being. Outcomes found that there were consistent positive correlations among intrinsic religiosity, spiritual well-being, hope, and other positive mood states and negative correlations among intrinsic religiosity, depression, and other negative mood states. There were higher levels of hope and positive moods in those elderly who had high levels of intrinsic religiosity. The challenge for professional nursing is to assess and support intrinsic religiosity and promote spiritual well-being in elderly people coping with terminal illnesses.

Fehring RJ, Miller JF, Shaw C: Spiritual well-being, religiosity, hope, depression and other mood states in elderly people coping with cancer, *Oncol Nurs Forum* 24:663, 1997.

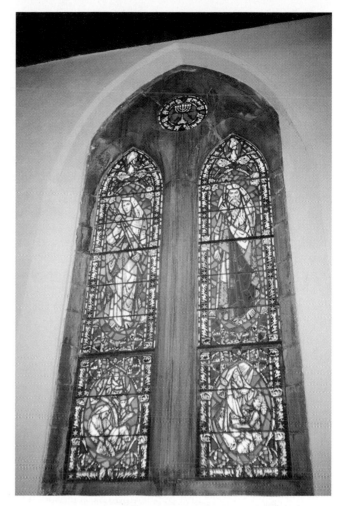

Religious symbols and rituals are a significant part of a faith lifestyle and practice for many people.

mankind. The integration of faith and health within the caring community results in beneficial outcomes. Persons who encounter assaults with physical and emotional illness and brokenness and who are able to call upon their faith beliefs and religious traditions are able to increase coping skills and realize spiritual growth (see the Research Brief about elderly clients with cancer). These coping skills and spiritual strengths extend beyond the current situation and help with future life challenges and total well being. Foege (1996) identifies three conditions needed for persons to be responsive to life in the future. These are equity, kinship, and continuity. These faith beliefs include equality in the eyes of one's Creator; global connectedness; and traditions that are inherited and handed down to future generations. Woodward and Underwood (1997) describe the consolation of sacred liturgies, religious rituals, and communal events in order for grieving to become a healing process and to affirm transcendent life.

Some of the major Protestant faith communities in the late nineteenth and early twentieth centuries used missionaries to develop multipurpose activities in communities, which included education and health activities along with religious messages. Hospitals were built in the United States and abroad, and underserved populations were targeted. As political and economic forces have changed through the years, so health ministry strategies of the churches have altered their approaches. Some churches have identified with community development efforts in helping people empower themselves to meet their needs for food, education, clean environments, social support, and primary health care. Some churches have also recognized and increased their emphasis on individual responsibility, the escalating cost of health care, the need for cost containment, the increasing numbers of uninsured and underserved, and the ever-increasing dilemma of interpreting the many changes in the health care delivery system. These efforts have been translated into a variety of positions endorsed by the governing bodies of the faith communities.

The **Holistic Health Centers** of the 1970s emphasized a comprehensive team approach to total health care. The teams in these Centers included family and clergy, who emphasized personal responsibility for health and encouraged preventive health practices. The formulation of parish nursing in the early 1980s built on the strengths of the Holistic Health Centers and focused on the team of nurses and clergy, working with individuals with their families. Nurses used their abilities to listen to the spoken and unspoken concerns of individuals and made assessments and judgments based on their knowledge of the health sciences and humanities. The attributes of the nurses were recognized by clergy and acute care institutions in the upper Midwest. By the mid-1980s Lutheran General Hospital and the Reverend Granger Westberg embarked on a pilot project with six Chicago congregations that included four Protestant and two Roman Catholic communities (Solari-Twadell et al, 1994). Loyola University and Swedish Covenant Hospital were among the forerunners in the revitalizing of the nurse's role in the healing traditions, acknowledging the importance of body, mind, and spirit connections, by incorporating education and providing health promotion services within congregations.

As with the early history of the development of public health nursing in this country, parish nurses found that health promotion services were needed in underserved and rural areas. Nurses identified gaps in the delivery of service. Nurses acknowledged strength within persons to increase healing, the vital role of families on healthy outcomes, and the community support needed and individuals and families. In 1986, the Northwest Aging Association began with 12 nurses and within 6 years had expanded to 90 parish nurses (Solari-Twadell et al, 1990). In 1989, W.K. Kellogg Foundation funded a collaborative study of rural communities in northwest Iowa where the average county population was 15,000 persons (Striepe, 1990). Partnerships with medical centers, mental health centers, health care providers, and parish nurses were formed. As a part of this study, coalitions of parish nurses and networks were formed and found to be important as the congregations developed into centers of support and caring. Nurses considered their environment and population characteristics and addressed the identified needs for health promotion, disease prevention, and an understanding of the importance of the body, mind, and spirit.

DID YOU KNOW? *The International Parish Nurse Resource Center/Advocate Health Care resources the outgrowth of the early visions of the Rev. Granger Westberg. As a Lutheran clergyman who was involved with the W.K. Kellogg Wholistic Health Centers, Westberg recognized that nurses were central to the endeavors and that they enhanced minister/doctor communication to promote a "whole person" approach. Westberg suggested placing nurses on the staff of churches and proposed the church as another "health agency" in the community in the mid-1980s (Solari-Twadell et al, 1990).*

Parish nurses affiliate with coalitions of inner city churches, hospitals, and health departments or they may work closely with a network of rural churches of one or more faiths. In addition to activities in the Lutheran and Roman Catholic faith communities in the rural and urban Midwest, other denominations also show interest in health ministries and parish nursing.

The Presbyterian Church (USA) is cited as an example of a long-standing tradition if encouraging members to be good stewards or responsible managers of body, mind, the

environment, and total resources. Studies in the late 1980s, the publication of essays titled *Health Care and Its Costs,* and the meetings of the Task Force on Health Costs and Policies resulted in a 1988 Policy Statement, *Life Abundant: Values, Choices and Health Care* (OGA, 1988). Congregations were asked to take responsibility to model holistic and compassionate concern for health and the providing of care. Further, the Policy Statement endorsed employing parish nurses or other health professionals as agents of the congregation's mission to encourage the role of "communities of health and healing" (PC, USA, p. 20).

The Presbyterian Health Network was formed in 1989. Nurses joined the efforts in 1991 and within 1 year held the first Parish Nurse Seminar. The seminar's purpose was to further implement the 1988 policy statement, increase awareness of the parish nurse concept, provide a forum for networking and support, provide nurturing for the nurse healers, encourage adequate education and skill preparation, and encourage implementation of parish nurse services in congregations or groups of congregations throughout the country.

Nursing Community

The beginnings of the parish nurse movement coincided with the recognition of more independent functions of the nurse, the articulation and proliferation of advanced practice nursing roles, the growth of nursing centers, and technologic advances. Hospitals discharged clients earlier and clients returned to their homes sicker with few, if any, caregivers available. Caregivers were faced with multiple tasks of coordinating employment, finances, learning new caregiving tasks, and maintaining former and ongoing family responsibilities. Consumer demand for involvement in health care decisions was also increasing, and society was emphasizing individual responsibility for health because many diseases were indeed preventable and health care costs needed to be cut. These numerous interacting and overlapping forces were burdensome for the population. Fragmented care and inadequate caregiver training and availability were problems for the disenfranchised, underserved, and uninsured, as well as for the economically well situated and better-educated persons. Suburban and rural families were challenged to seek ways to best meet the multiple demands of young children, teens and aging parents. Parish nurse services were one of the responses to assist with coordination of care and to foster continuity of care. The parish nurse services emphasized health promotion and disease prevention and provided the benefits of holistic care through the supportive faith community. The spiritual dimension of health was and is optimized by complementing the nursing role with pastoral care.

The International Parish Nurse Resource Center has as its mission the promotion and development of quality parish nurse programs through research, education, and consultation (International Parish Nurse Resource Center, 1998). To this end, the Center offers resources, catalogs, regular newsletters, and consultation and reference packets with information about the parish nurse concept and services offered by the Center. Information about accessing the Center appears in Box 45-1. The Center has also endorsed curricula for the parish nurse and **parish nurse coordinator** (McDermott et al, 1998).

Parish nurse interventions augment services of faith community populations in a variety of practice arrangements. Community health nurses functioning as parish nurses need to have leadership skills and astute, articulate nonverbal and verbal communication, negotiation, and collaboration skills. As with other population groups, the parish nurse attempts to include those persons who are less vocal or visible in the community of faith. If the vision of the congregation extends beyond its immediate membership, then those outside of the immediate faith community who would benefit from the services are also potential recipients. This may be accomplished by including the concept of block nursing or nursing in the neighborhood surrounding the church. Block and neighborhood nursing are discussed later in the chapter. As both advanced practice nurses and parish nursing practices increase in numbers and varieties of arrangements, evaluation of practice trends within the health care delivery system environment and the needs of society are necessary. Nursing must be accountable and responsive to those being served, as well as to those who provide opportunities to serve.

Health Care Delivery

Early chapters in Parts One and Two of this text familiarize the reader with the historical, economic, social, political, environmental, and ethical trends in the past years. The health care delivery system is challenged to work within parameters of tighter financial constraints while also welcoming advanced technology and addressing new health concerns. Consumers have increased interest in their own well-being and have expressed needs for more current health information to be available in a wider variety of formats.

In addition to consumer interest and a heightened awareness of responsibility for one's own health, health care providers and managed care systems have found it a financial advantage for their participants to be healthy and remain out of the system. Thus with rising costs of care, scarce resources for populations, and the complex system demands on individuals and families to seek health, the challenge for the consumer now is how to cope with these forces. Information and guidance is available in schools, workplaces, via the media, and through faith communities.

Community health nursing professionals are aware of the necessity of collaborative practices and formation of **partnerships** to care for groups and individuals throughout the age span. Parish nurses share these and other functions as they serve populations through faith communities. These nurses also advocate for healthy lifestyle choices in exercise, nutrition, substance use, and stress management. Nurses recognize the need for health promotion and disease prevention at all levels and regularly assess the need for interpreting care plans given to clients by health care providers. A primary position of the community health nurse is to coordinate care and to link health care providers, groups, and community resources as the client tries to understand the health plan. Negotiating with individuals, agencies, and community partnerships within the complex maze of the broader health care environment demands a knowledgeable and seasoned professional. At the close of the twentieth century consumers and health care providers are still muddling through the complexity and fragmentation of the delivery system as it affects young, old, and very old; poor, middle income, and well-to-do; and those of all ethnic origins.

PARISH NURSING PRACTICE
Characteristics of the Practice

Parish nursing's goal is to develop and sustain health ministries within faith communities. Health ministry promotes wholeness in health, emphasizes health promotion and disease prevention, and does this within the context of linking healing with the person's faith belief and level of spiritual maturity. The author participated in a 1994 invitational conference that included 26 professionals consisting of nurse educators, practicing parish nurses, and staff of the Parish Nurse Resource Center to discuss and design a document outlining educational guidelines for the rapidly growing new nursing specialty. The final product included five characteristics identified as central to the philosophy of parish nursing (Solari-Twadell et al, 1994).

The *spiritual dimension* is central to the practice of parish nursing. Nursing embodies the physical, psychologic, social, and spiritual dimensions of clients into professional practice, and whereas parish nursing includes all four, it focuses on intentional and compassionate care, which stems from the spiritual dimension of all humankind. Secondly, the *roots of the role balance both knowledge and skills* of nursing, using nursing sciences, the humanities, and theology. The nurse combines nursing functions with *pastoral care* functions. Visits in the office, home, hospital, or nursing home often involve prayer, and may include a reference to scripture, symbols, sacraments, and liturgy of the faith community represented by the nurse. The values and beliefs of the faith community are integral to the supportive care given. Nurses also assist with worship services as appropriate within the faith community.

The third characteristic is that the *focus of the specialty is the faith community and its ministry.* The faith community is the source of health and healing partnerships, which result in creative responses to health and health-related concerns. Partnerships may be among individuals, groups, and health care professionals within the congregation. Partnerships may also be among various congregations or community agencies, institutions, or individuals. Partnerships also evolve as the congregation visualizes its health-related

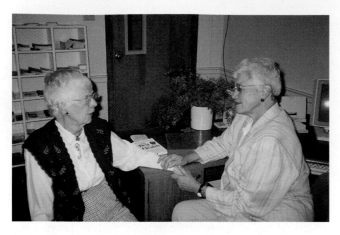

A parish nurse provides support for spiritual and emotional needs as well as physical needs.

mission beyond the walls, stones, and steeples of its own place of worship.

As within other areas of community health nursing, parish nurse services *emphasize strengths* of individuals, families, and communities. Parish nurses endorse this fourth characteristic in their practice. As congregations realize the need for and care for one another, their individual and corporate relationship with their Creator often is enhanced. This provides additional coping strength for future crisis situations within the family and community. Finally, *health, spiritual health, and healing* are considered an ongoing, dynamic process. Since spiritual health is central to well-being, influences are evident in the total individual and noted in a healthy congregation. Well-being and illness may occur simultaneously; spiritual healing or well-being *can* exist in the absence of cure. Faith communities that value individual and congregational health can move beyond their "congregational" boundaries to address health-related concerns in the geopolitical communities locally, nationally, and globally. Studying health care reform issues, domestic and youth violence, and safe environmental conditions in light of faith beliefs prepares members to participate in policy-making activities to promote the ethical principle of justice (see Chapter 6).

Scope and Standards of Parish Nursing Practice

Based on the minimum level of professional nursing practice delineated in *Standards of Clinical Nursing Practice (HMA/ANA, 1998),* nurses well-versed in the parish nursing practice field developed a document for the new specialty's scope and standards to be submitted to the American Nurses Association. The Practice and Education Committee of Health Ministries Association consulted with many colleagues to review and submit recommendations for the document. Health Ministries Association members are professional and lay persons from various health and faith disciplines. Professional nurse members who specialized in the practice of parish nursing prepared the document. Some of these same nurses were also present at the initial conference called by the Parish Nurse Resource Center. The document addressing the scope and standards was approved by the American Nurses Association in February, 1998, published in June, 1998, and is known as *Scope and Standards of Parish Nursing Practice.*

The *unique* practice of parish nursing and the *minimum* scope and standards of care for the independent practice of the profession related to activities of "health promotion within the context of the client's values, beliefs and faith practices." The parish nurse *"client focus . . . is the faith community, including its family and individual members and the community it serves"* (ANA, 1998, p. 3). Nurses encourage individuals, families and entire faith communities to promote health and healing within the context of the faith community to arrive at wellness outcomes. As in other arenas of nursing, the client level is multidimensional. "The clients of a parish nurse represent the total life span of three client levels: the faith community and its families and individuals" (p. 17). Using the nursing process for assessment, program planning, and evaluation, the parish nurses target specified age groups or health-related concerns.

The *Scope and Standards* delineate examples of the parish nurse's independent functions. These functions are in compliance with and reflect current nursing practice, client health promotion needs, professional standards, and the legal scope of professional nursing practice. Nurses function within the nurse practice act of their jurisdiction (state). If dependent functions are practiced, parish nurses must be in compliance with the legal criteria of the jurisdiction's nurse practice act (ANA, 1998). For example, when influenza vaccine or immunization clinics are offered, appropriate arrangements are made to use nurses from the cooperating agency (health department), or the parish nurse must have a contractual policy agreement with the cooperating agency to provide the immunizations. In addition to a narrative description and glossary of terms, the 1998 document outlines standards of care and standards of professional performance. In keeping with wise use of persons and materials, standards of professional performance elaborate on collaboration and resource use. The parish nurse collaborates with those who "share a commitment to promoting health" and "facilitates a health ministry that maximizes resources to achieve the desired health outcomes for all clients" (ANA, 1998, pp 20, 22).

> **NURSING TIP**
>
> *The parish nurse benefits from several years of practice experience following the basic undergraduate preparation since the nature of the position demands a seasoned professional.*

Educational Preparation for a Parish Nurse

Adoption of the *Scope and Standards of Parish Nursing Practice* has paralleled the International Parish Nurse Resource

Center's efforts on standardization of, first, a basic curriculum for preparation of parish nurses and, second, a curriculum for *coordinators of parish nurses.* A third curriculum is intended for faculty who plan to implement teaching programs of the basic curriculum in parish nursing. Following successful completion of the courses, parish nurses adapt to individual local community needs to gain outcomes congruent with goals established by the congregation and communities they serve.

Before the standard basic course recommendations, the practice generally requires that parish nurses have a baccalaureate degree in nursing and hold a valid license in the state of practice. A basic understanding or introduction to the parish nurse concept, 3 to 5 years experience in professional nursing, and evidence of a mature faith are also required. Varying routes of preparation are evident. The International Parish Nurse Resource Center offered the earliest orientation courses beginning in 1984. A graduate program in "parish health nurse" preparation at Georgetown University, diverse continuing education offerings, and some undergraduate courses are available. Several seminars have offered opportunities to raise awareness of the practice and have provided networking and nurturing support for nurses. An intensive continuing education program through Marquette University in Milwaukee has been offered in locations throughout the nation. The annual Westberg Symposium held in Chicago each September offers comprehensive sessions and a forum for nurses to network, gain new knowledge, and stay abreast of current resources and trends in the practice. Although these efforts have been valuable to the parish nurse specialty in its beginning stages, and the need for continuing education networking opportunities are ongoing, the standardization of basic programs provides similar learning modules and a common knowledge base.

Specialty areas within professional nursing achieve a major milestone in the evolving practice when the standards and scope common to that practice are recognized. Advanced practice opportunities then enrich the specialty. Master's-prepared nurses with specialization in community health nursing, holistic nursing, or mental health nursing and nurse practitioners have found niches in parish nursing. A 1500-member congregation in Florida employs a full-time master's-prepared nurse who is certified in holistic nursing by the American Holistic Nurses' Association. A Kentucky congregation has a collaborative faculty practice agreement with the University of Kentucky College of Nursing. The University of Colorado School of Nursing also has a faculty member who practices in parish nursing. These two arrangements provide clinical experiences for doctorate and master's-level community health nursing students (Magilvy, 1997). A consortium of rural churches pool resources for a parish nurse to facilitate health ministries programs. A Charlotte, North Carolina hospital system employs a parish nurse coordinator who

facilitates differing arrangements with several faith communities of varying backgrounds.

Many parish nurses function in a part-time capacity. Some nurses are responsible for service with several congregations, whereas others engage in parish nursing as part of a full-time commitment in other capacities. Working in several arenas adds distinctive perspectives to a parish nurse service. Depending on the practice model, the nurse has a narrowly defined or a wider realm of responsibility. Parish nurse practices may be integrated into a health care facility or into practices that collaborate with related professional practice areas such as health departments or Colleges of Nursing. Practices in which several parish nurses are supervised by a coordinator have built-in opportunities for sharing, partnering, and mentoring. Parish nurses may also have regional responsibilities that correspond to intermediate governing areas of the faith community. These regions may be clusters of churches or areas such as districts, synods, presbyteries, or jurisdictions.

Preparation and continuing education must continue to include the basics and enrichment courses in the nursing profession and the theologic/pastoral care field. Additionally, the nurse needs updates in areas of public health, medicine, sociology, cultural diversity, and human growth and development throughout the life span. Improving collaboration, negotiation, and coordination skills, as well as consultation, leadership, management, and research skills, is essential. Parish nurses accept responsibility for ongoing professional education within nursing and pastoral care arenas.

The challenge for the evolving practice is to document trends, maintain and enhance quality of preparation and services offered, use increased numbers of advanced practice nurses, network within professional organizations, and become involved in outcomes-oriented research. It is anticipated that the specialty will be considered for professional certification. Certification recognizes competency among practitioners in a specialty. Both the profession and consumers will increasingly consider credentialing and attention to keeping it current as a mark of excellence.

ISSUES IN PARISH NURSING PRACTICE

Every new discipline or care area must be alert to issues of accountability to populations served, as well as to those who entrust the nurse with the responsibility to serve a designated population. Discussions of health promotion plans include the individual, the family, and the faith community. Additionally, negotiations with the pastoral staff, congregations, institutions, and the wider community may be involved in job description preparation or program planning. Issues such as privacy, confidentiality, group concerns, access, and record management must be discussed with the pastoral staff or the contracting agency at the outset of any parish nurse agreement. This facilitates positive outcomes and avoids conflicts with individual/group rights and state regulations.

Professional Issues

Annual and periodic evaluations of parish nurse practices, as well as assessments and evaluations of services needed, are certainly indicated. These evaluations include self, peer, congregational, and/or institutional evaluations. Professional appraisal is standard in nursing practice. The appraisals guide professional development as well as program development and planning. Since the scope of parish nursing practice is broad and focuses on the independent practice of the discipline, the nurse must consider a wide variety of issues such as position descriptions, professional liability, professional educational, experiential preparation, collaborative agreements, and working with lay volunteers as well as retired professionals. Abiding by the professional nursing code is understood; however, the nurse must also know the **polity,** expectations and mission of the particular faith community. The nurse also continually interprets the profession for the faith community.

The nurse must be knowledgeable about lines of authority and channels of communication in the congregation as well as in the collaborative institutions. Nurses need to become well acquainted with the personnel committees of the congregation. Personnel committees provide guidance and contribute to the evaluation. They also advocate for parish nurse services and raise awareness with the congregational staff members and programs.

> **NURSING TIP**
>
> *Developing a keen sense of the value of the congregation within the geopolitical community and appreciating its associations within the local and wider community is beneficial.*

Nurses in parishes advocate for well-being and thus are in unique positions to highlight justice issues in local and national legislation. As the faith community reflects on the implications of legislation for their congregation and national faith community, the nurse contributes information to policy makers about the implications for health and well-being for the parish, the local community, and globally. Active participation in political activities contributes to spiritual growth and healthy functioning.

Ethical Issues

Issues evolve from client, faith community, and professional arenas. The nurse's interventions are guided by professional responsibilities that include the Code for Nurses (ANA, 1985), individual and group rights, Statements of Faith, and polity of the faith community served. Professional and therapeutic relationships are maintained at all times; consulting and counseling with minors and individual members of the opposite sex are conducted using professional ethical principles. Policies about these issues are established at the outset of the practice in conjunction with the pastoral team, the wellness committee, the parish nurse, and the local congregation's governing body.

As in other community health situations, the parish nurse, along with the client, identifies parameters of ethical concerns, plans ahead with clients to consider healthy options in making ethical decisions, and supports clients in their journey to choose alternatives that will strengthen coping skills and allow them to grow stronger in faith and health. "In addition, parish nurses ought to consider the virtue ethics, such as caring, forgiveness, and compassion, in their decision making" (ANA, 1998, p 19).

Communities of faith strive to be caring communities and value the fellowship among its members. However, confidentiality is of utmost importance in parish nursing practice. The parish nurse values client confidentiality while at the same time delicately assisting the client and client family to "share" concerns with pastoral staff and fellow **congregants.** This sharing gains valuable support to promote optimal healing. The nurse is often the staff member who helps the family to the stage of acceptance of a health concern. How much to share and when to share a concern is indeed a private affair and a part of the important journey of healing. A joyous event for one family may be a devastating event or even a depressing reminder of a past event for another family. The celebrations and joys of a healthy new infant one week may raise guilt and ambivalence for congregational members when, within a brief time, another family's long-awaited child dies at birth.

> **WHAT DO YOU THINK?** *The young couple who has contributed their time, enthusiasm, and skills assisting as church youth group leaders are expecting a first child. What a valuable learning experience for the teens, the parish nurse contends. Having a couple experience healthy life events is indeed beneficial for youth. Upon birth, the infant is diagnosed with Down syndrome. Now there are not the normal celebrations and visions for the future. Instead of parties, what information is to be shared, and with whom, and when? How much privacy is granted? The manner in which the family, other youth leaders, and the nurse work with the team, use the strengths of the congregation, and reflect on the spiritual needs of all concerned is most important for healthy outcomes. The learning opportunities are valuable growth experiences for the young teens as well as for the new parents. Having opportunities to describe one's feelings and dealing with them in supportive groups reaps benefits in the healing process.*

Legal Issues

As an advocate of client and group rights, the nurse identifies and reports neglect, abuse, and illegal behaviors to the appropriate legal sources. The nurse appropriately refers members to pastoral or community resources if the scope of the problem is beyond the realm of the professional nurse. Referral is also indicated if conflict between nurse and client is such that no further progress is possible. The parish nurse who has a positive relationship that values open dialogue with the pastoral team will be supported in efforts to select the most appropriate community resource for clients.

The nurse must personally and professionally abide by the parameters of the nurse practice act of the jurisdiction and maintain an active license of that state. Additional legal concerns are those of institutional contractual agreements, records management, release of information, and volunteer liability. Resources would include the faith community's legal consultant, the faith community's national position statements, and Parish Nurse Resource Center guides (Solari-Twadell et al, 1994).

Financial Issues

Innovative arrangements for variations of the basic models mentioned earlier call for sustained financial support. The nurse is called on to partner in finding funds and partnering with potential supporters. The nurse is accountable for money spent and for fundraising whether the position is salaried or volunteer. Educational and promotional materials, equipment, travel time, continuing education, and malpractice insurance are selected areas that need to be included in the budget of the parish nurse. If these materials are not budget items, services may be limited and this needs to be interpreted to the faith community.

NATIONAL HEALTH OBJECTIVES AND FAITH COMMUNITIES

The 1990 health objectives, most recently *Healthy People 2000*, and the currently developing *Healthy People 2010* encourage communities to cooperatively lend support to individuals and families to attain an improved health status that can be passed on to future generations. One of the oldest and strongest partnerships is that established between communities and religious or faith communities. The Carter Center in Atlanta and the Park Ridge Center in Chicago collaborated with health care professionals and leaders of faith traditions to identify roles of faith communities to address national health objectives and approaches to improving overall public health. The faith communities recognized the strengths of the attainment of almost half of the 1990 objectives and affirmed the development of the goals and objectives of *Healthy People 2000* (Marty, 1990).

Since faith communities are rooted in healing traditions and also have justice issues as a priority agenda, the goals to reduce health disparities among Americans and provide improved access to health care can be readily addressed. Examples of congregational models addressing the specific objectives encouraging *Healthy People 2000* guidelines are increasingly being documented (Berry, 1994; Carter Center, 1990; Magilvy and Brown, 1997; Weiss et al, 1997). Additionally, the National Heart, Lung and Blood Institute urges partnerships with faith communities and offers suggestions for program planning (USDHHS, 1992).

A third national level effort to strengthen the potential partnerships between faith communities and health care

professionals is the Caucus on Public Health and the Faith Community of the American Public Health Association (APHA). The caucus' first gathering at the 1995 American Public Health Association annual meeting was addressed by then-APHA President Dr. Caswell Evans. Health care professionals of many faiths welcomed the opportunity to voice their interest in holistically supporting their communities and clients.

Specific national objectives dealing with nutrition; physical activity; use of tobacco, alcohol, and other drugs; improved maternal and infant health; immunization status; environmental health; and prevention of unintentional injuries are within the realm of the health education role of the parish nurse. Parish nurse activities are helping the attainment of nine *Year 2000* objectives as described by Weiss (Box 45-2). Additionally, alerting entire congregation communities to the benefits of health promotion to prevent onset of chronic disease helps to minimize sickness visits to health care professionals, improve quality of life, and increase savings of scarce individual, government, and private insurance health care dollars. The nurse as well as the supportive faith community plays a major role in caring for those families who are experiencing alterations of functional and emotional health because of chronic illness. Monitoring disabling physical functioning, encouraging adherence to treatment plans, interpreting rehabilitation programs, noting specific progress, and offering support from the entire faith community are approaches to address health status objectives dealing with chronic illness.

Wellness committees and parish nurses with the faith community's input may regularly review the various health status objectives, make comparisons between national and specific state objectives, and then assess to what extent the specific congregation or groups of congregations are in need of risk reduction. Health promotion activities such as regular blood pressure screening and monitoring activities address Objective 15, which focuses on heart disease and stroke prevention and disability. Age appropriate discus-

---

BOX 45-2 *Healthy People (HP) 2000* Objectives Identified by Parish Nurses for 1 Year

Blood pressure knowledge and control (HP15.4/.5/.13)
Overweight prevalence and weight loss practices (HP1.2/.7 2.3/.7)
Vigorous physical activity (HP 1.4)
BSE and mammogram (HP 16.11)
Home fire safety (HP 9.6/.17)
Stress management (HP 6.5)
Reduce heart disease and stroke (HP 15.1/.2)
Reduce child abuse (HP 7.4)
Maintain ADLs 65+ (HP 1.13)

From Weis D, Mathews R, Schank MJ: Health care delivery in faith communities: the parish nurse model, *Public Health Nurs* 14(2):370, 1997.

sion of preventive activities can be held with various groups. Signs and symptoms of heart attack and stroke can be noted and described in newsletters and posted in strategic areas. The nurse can coordinate healthy low-fat church suppers and encourage "moms and tots" groups to choose healthy fruit and vegetables as snacks following their faith discussion meetings. The nurse can coordinate a series of classes for families of adolescents on stress management as well as sessions on the use and misuse of alcohol, tobacco, and other drugs. Additionally, the nurse can encourage regular exercise for individuals as a part of ongoing church activities. Examples of interventions related to selected portions of Objective 15 listed below.

HOW TO *Provide Interventions for Selected Healthy People 2000 Risk Reduction Objectives within Faith Communities*

- *15.4 Increase to at least 50% the proportion of people with high blood pressure whose BP is under control.*
  Intervention: *Schedule regular BP screening for elevated blood pressure; monitor blood pressure regularly.*
- *15.5 Increase to at least 90% the proportion of people with high blood pressure who are taking action to help control their blood pressure.*
  Intervention: *Facilitate and encourage activities related to healthy nutrition, healthful and regular exercise, stress management, and avoidance of tobacco, alcohol, and other drug activity*
- *15.9 Reduce dietary fat intake to an average of 30% calories or less.*
  Intervention: *Work with committees planning dinners, festive events; individual counseling with all BP screening, incorporate information in youth activities; discuss nutrition during visits to families with new infants*
- *15.10 Reduce overweight to a prevalence of no more than 20% among people ages 20 and older and no more than 15% among adolescents ages 12 to 19.*
  Intervention: *Encourage involvement in regular exercise, facilitate groups when possible; encourage wellness committee to have activities available throughout the age span*

The congregation's health and wellness committee can similarly address the remaining objectives to identify activities in which to engage individuals, groups or the congregation as a whole. To promote healthy families, faith communities can address objectives with a maternal and infant health focus (see the How To below). Most advantageous for the faith community would be to engage in partnership activities with other community efforts such as health fairs. Health fairs are effective strategies for health promotion efforts guided by the *Healthy People 2000* framework. Dillon and Sternas (1997) describe steps to successfully plan, implement, and evaluate health fairs that sup-

port health promotion and disease prevention efforts. These and similar activities promote increased health of the entire community and include persons of all ages, encourage enthusiastic fellowship and leisure, and reduce duplication of effort.

HOW TO *Intervene in Maternal and Infant Health*

- *Visit family immediately following the birth of a new infant to further assess parenting skills and parent/infant bonding, reinforce holistic reflection of life transition, and plan for faith community support as indicated in those areas not addressed by family or other community agencies.*
- *Augment community prenatal classes or facilitate classes in faith community stressing growth and development of prenatal and postnatal period, family transitions, adequate health monitoring needed by parents, children, and new family members.*
- *Facilitate expectant parent support group to reinforce positive health during pregnancy, interpret plans negotiated with health care provider, promote spiritual reflection of family life transition to encourage connectedness with Creator and beliefs of faith community; provide emotional, social, community support to family.*

As *Healthy People 2010* goals are being identified, congregational committees are encouraged to revisit their activities so that they may focus their programs. Since spring of 1997, work groups have met to develop the new objectives. Currently, all interested persons in the country are invited to comment or to join the effort on the Internet by suggesting areas of need. The *Healthy People 2010* Web site requests "public" input. (This Web site can be accessed through the WebLinks portion of the book's Web site at www.mosby.com/MERLIN.) This is a valiant effort to involve persons in responsibility for their own health and that of their community. Following a period designated for public comment on the draft objectives, the release of the final objectives is slated for January of 2000.

The proposed *Healthy People 2010* categories will incorporate leading health indicators. The 2010 authors hope that use of "leading health indicators" will result in a more precise and accurate way to reflect the intent of *Healthy People 2010*. Hopefully, the current process will also improve communication among the general public and new health and social service partners within the community. Communities of faith will be among the new health-related partners, which includes members such as managed care organizations and business partners. The indicators will strive to do the following:

- Increase years of healthy life
- Promote healthy behaviors
- Protect health
- Ensure access to quality health care
- Strengthen community prevention efforts

Selected areas for emphases in the last months of 1998 include reducing the increasing prevalence of obesity by exploring new and effective ways to influence girls and women to engage in physical activity in and out of schools and to continue regular physical activity throughout life. Parish nurses working with these population groups are pivotal as supportive links to implementing healthy behaviors. The recognition that persons are at greater risk of HIV infection when other sexually transmitted diseases are present is another cue for faith communities to encourage community-based programs to prevent sexually transmitted diseases, especially among adolescents and minorities. As young persons develop values and make lifestyle choices, their growth in character in a faith community can provide direction, support, and coping skills to select healthy options.

As faith communities continue to address the three major goals of *Healthy People 2000,* they will be assured that the authors of the new *Healthy People 2010* aim for continued periodic surveillance of these goals. However, the authors are also keenly aware that a major challenge for the next decade is to focus on the prominence of health disparities (USDHHS, March 1998). The disparities in the national health objectives are identified among groups differing in racial-ethnic background, age, gender, income, disabilities, and geographic location. Nurses working in collaboration with faith community wellness committees can be key members of efforts to address these justice and social righteousness issues, since faith communities draw members from varied groups.

FUNCTIONS OF THE PARISH NURSE

Examples of parish nursing interventions have been cited throughout this chapter. This section summarizes and expands some of the usual functions and describes activities. A primary independent function is that of *personal health counseling.* Parish nurses discuss health risk appraisals, spiritual assessments, plan for healthier lifestyles, and provide support and guidance related to numerous acute and chronic actual and potential health problems. Parish nurses carry out their practice in groups or individually; they make visits to homes, hospitals, and nursing homes and see persons in the faith community's house of worship. Some nurses have designated offices, whereas others use space that is most conducive to the particular activity or client need.

A second function is that of *health education.* Parish nurses publish information in congregation news bulletins, distribute information, and have available a variety of resources for the physical, mental, and spiritual health of the congregation. Classes are held to address identified needs, individual teaching is done as needed, and discussions are held for targeted groups or meetings. Parish nurses strive to promote wholeness in health and create a fuller understanding of total physical, mental, and spiritual well-being.

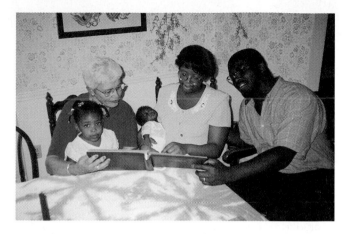

A parish nurse visits with a family of the congregation in their home.

As a *liaison* between resources in the faith community and the local community, the parish nurse again creates awareness of the resources, helps individuals and families create the appropriate resource match, and links them with the services. The parish nurse is also a *facilitator.* The nurse links congregational needs to the establishment of and referral to support groups and facilitates changes in the congregation to increase disability access or to extend meals and services to those who are homebound. If needed, the nurse would also work with the volunteer coordinator to train volunteers or ensure that interested persons acquire training to function as lay caregivers to meet congregational needs. Box 45-3 is an example of how the parish works with other providers and community resources to meet the health needs of a client.

An important function underlying all of the previously mentioned functions is that of *pastoral care.* The nurse stresses the spiritual dimension of nursing and lends support during times of joy and sorrow; the nurse guides the person through health and illness throughout life and helps to identify the spiritual strengths that assist in coping with particular events. The nurse may use hymns, favorite scripture verses, psalms, pictures, church windows, stories, or other images that are important for the individual or group to hold to the connectedness between faith, health, and well-being.

Healthy activities to be encouraged in congregations are numerous and the nurse often works with the congregation to stretch beyond its immediate borders to augment services in the community that promote health and wellness. Congregations are keenly aware that more than half of the members of mainline churches are part of the growing aging population of our country. Increased numbers of persons who are either uninsured or underinsured are in their communities. Thus food pantries, day care for seniors, congregate meals, preschool and latch-key arrangements, tutoring, meals on wheels, visiting less-mobile members, and outreach for vulnerable populations are not

BOX 45-3 Parish Nursing as Healing Ministry . . .
An Adult Daughter's Reflection

What a pleasure to be able to commend (parish nurse's) personal friendship and professional help! Without her support it would have been difficult, if not impossible, for my father to live at home during his last 6 years. But she had, along with his doctor, the sure feeling that it was the right thing for him and that it could be done. When the time came that he needed caregivers around the clock, she skillfully conveyed suggestions in such a way that the caregivers' cultural differences were not a barrier. She helped them grow as caregivers, appreciating their accomplishments, even to having a blackberry-picking "outing" at her home.

My father in his earlier years had been a deacon and had loved visiting shut-ins. It brought him so much happiness that he in turn received his church's caring, healing ministry through his parish nurse. He attended church on Sundays beyond what one would expect of one in his 90s, and almost his last Sunday was the day he celebrated turning 96.

Thank you, (parish nurse), for our "Mission Accomplished"!

With permission, A.F.H.

BOX 45-4 A Sampling of Parish Nurse
Interventions and Activities

- *Sharing the joys* of a new member in the family; *sharing sorrows* of losses
- *Anticipating changes* in health status or in growth and development
- *Being present* for questions that seem difficult or unacceptable to ask the health care provider
- *Explaining and assisting in considering choices* when new living and care arrangements must be made
- *Listening* to the concerns of a youngster anticipating diagnostic procedures
- *Praying* with the spouse of a dying parishioner
- *Helping individuals and families make decisions* regarding advance directives in light of faith beliefs
- *Helping teens* consider options when overwhelmed with serious life issues
- *Providing information, support, and prayer* regarding advance directives
- *Seeking community resources/opportunities* for fitness and nutrition classes
- *Working with the wellness committee* to ensure that fellowship meals meet nutritional and spiritual needs of the elderly
- *Offering educational opportunities* about health care legislation changes and its influence on the congregation and community
- *Accompanying* a faith community member to 12-step meeting
- *Participating in worship leadership* with pastoral staff

From Berry R: A parish nurse. In Office of Resourcing Committees on Preparation for Ministry: *A day in the life of. . . . A kaleidoscope of specialized ministries*, Louisville, Ky, 1994, Presbyterian Church (USA): Distribution Management Service.

only services offered, but also provide volunteers with opportunities to gain a feeling of worth.

Box 45-4 lists several selected activities of parish nurses (Berry, 1994). However the creative implementing of the parish nurse concept by each individual nurse with a unique faith community will result in a wealth of possibilities that most certainly can be inexhaustible.

BLOCK NURSING

Parish nursing grew out of the public health nursing specialty. Neighborhood or **block nursing** was one of the first approaches used in public health nursing both in England and in the United States. The term reappeared in the early 1980s, growing out of a need to address concerns arising in communities experiencing the social and political environmental changes of the decade. The health care delivery system has undergone many changes as a result of health advances and new technologies while at the same time being asked to reduce costs. This has resulted in growing personal responsibility for acquiring health information; unequal availability of care; and a lack of information about the outcomes of high-tech care. The health care delivery system changes have created lack of care for some segments of the population with much confusion about getting care.

Lillian Wald's introduction to the many problems on New York City's lower east side in the nineteenth century and the example she set of going into the community to intimately sense the needs, gather a mix of partners from the community, attempt to address the gaps of care, and to reach out to the most vulnerable would be replicated once more through block nursing. Parallel to the parish nursing movement, other innovative examples reminiscent of Wald's population-focused attempts of almost a century earlier were projects such as block nursing, neighborhood nursing, and circles of care (Jamieson, 1983, 1990; Magilvy et al, 1994; Reinhard et al, 1996). In these examples, professional nurses considered the needs of the community and collaborated with formal and informal partners in the community to address the needs.

Using nurses who live in close proximity to individuals and families needing care, block nurse arrangements were found to be capable of decreasing costs to families and society, encourage community involvement, address needs of a dying child at home, and provide quality care for frail elderly living alone with meager resources. The block nurse program provides direct nursing care coupled with supportive services such as social services. Professional nurses and well-prepared volunteers coordinate the various levels of services needed. Public health nursing services in a St. Paul, Minnesota/Ramsey County Health Department developed block nurse services; more than a decade later the program continues as a nonprofit company. The Living at Home/Block Nurse program is a Health Care Financing Administration (HCFA) Community Nursing Center demonstration site and "works with communities to plan and implement community programs that enable senior citizens to remain in their homes and communities" (Jamieson, 1998, p. 161).

A second trend responding to needs of communities while using a population-focused approach is **neighborhood nursing.** This approach, implemented in communities affiliated with the Visiting Nurse Association of Central Jersey (Reinhard, 1996), focuses on continuity of care and linking individual, family, and community. The agency provides education, process, and structural changes to support the shift in scope of services. The nurse is envisioned as the key community designee to enhance accessibility to care and to reduce fragmentation. Wellness and illness phases of the community are addressed; the entire age span is included; home, school, and workplace are considered. While they collaborate with the community, unlike block nurses, the neighborhood nurses do not live in the community nor do they focus on a narrow dimension of the community. Sustaining the momentum of the renewed population-focused philosophy in public health requires committed staff at all levels. A major barrier faced within the broad neighborhood nursing approach is health care financing. Nursing and other health and health related professionals must subscribe to public private community partnerships if the core public health function of assurance of services to the unserved is to be realized. The nurse and the community partners must communicate regularly and creatively engage in seeking adequate financial support.

In Colorado, nurses identified some essential components of a workable system that could result in population focused care for aggregates at risk (Magilvy, 1994). The **circle of care** developed from ethnographic studies of frail elderly in two rural, culturally different communities. Careful networking, collaboration, and formal as well as informal use of health professionals, lay persons, and community groups supported this vulnerable population and provided quality care with meager resources. Nurses lived in close proximity and were indeed part of the fabric of the community. Nurses shopped at the same stores and were members of the same churches; their families worked together, they attended school together, and together nurses and community members experienced the joys and hardships of rural life. Neighbors "keep a watchful eye on people" in rural communities (Maglivy, 1994, p 29). Although a population focus was not the intention of nor integral to the Colorado example, the networking and strong sense of community support are major strengths on which this advanced public health nursing practice will build. The for-

mal and informal parts of this service within a rural community can lay the groundwork for transcending effective community-based practices into population-focused practices. Nurses actively involved in policy development for effective health care delivery can advocate for consumers within these communities.

The strength of all of the foregoing programs is that they have demonstrated strong, collaborative, community partnerships. Community health nurses as parish nurses or block nurses can envision comprehensive population-focused practices or implement programs at beginning levels as community-based practices to ensure seamless care for individuals and families. The challenge for nurses, other health care providers, and the communities will continue to be how to garner government, foundation, and private funding and combine it with support from volunteer activities, family involvement, and community groups to create the unique mix needed for the distinctiveness of each community. Nurses are asked to partner with community members where they live, work, attend school, and gather for worship; to closely partner with these same members to advocate for those who are powerless; to keenly identify health and health-related needs; to detect and address those needs to prevent costly use of the health care system; and to be closely aligned with those who can implement visionary policy that improves health care for community members through the life span.

 clinical application

The nursing process is a method that can be used to begin program planning and evaluation with faith communities. Such an approach can involve congregational members and parish nurses in a dynamic endeavor to jointly learn about the members' individual health status, as well as that of the faith community and the local and broader geographic community. Parish nurse programs are derived in various ways. Initially, the impetus for parish nursing may stem from an unmet health need within the congregation; from visions of a lay or health professions member concerned about caring within the congregation; or from discussions of a committee dealing with health and wellness issues.

Which of the following activities is most likely to increase the interest and involvement of the congregation's members?

A. Writing a contract for parish nurses services
B. Surveying the faith communities' environment
C. Gathering information on leaders and valued activities in the congregation through focus groups of pastoral staff
D. Assessing the needs of the congregational members through a survey
E. Holding a health fair

Answer is in the back of the book.

KEY POINTS

- Parish nurse services respond to health, healing, and wholeness within the context of the church. Although the emphasis is on health promotion and disease prevention throughout the life span, the spiritual dimension of nursing is central to the practice.
- The parish nurse partners with the wellness committee and volunteers to plan programs and consider health-related concerns within faith communities.
- To promote a caring faith community, usual functions of the parish nurse include personal health counseling, health teaching, facilitating linkages and referrals to congregation and community resources, advocating and encouraging support resources, and providing pastoral care.
- Parish nurses collaborate to plan, implement, and evaluate health promotion activities considering the faith community's beliefs, rituals, and polity. *Healthy People 2000/ Healthy People 2010* guidelines are basic to the partnering for programs.
- Nurses in congregational or institutional models enhance the health ministry programs of the faith communities if carefully chosen partnerships are formed within the congregation, with other congregations, and also with local health and social community agencies.
- Nurses working in the parish nursing specialty must seek to attain adequate educational and skill preparation for the accountability to those served and to those who have entrusted the nurse to serve.

- Nurses are encouraged to consider innovative approaches to creating caring communities. These may be in congregations as parish nurses, among several faith communities in a single locale, or regionally; or in partnership with other community agencies or models such as block nursing.
- To sustain oneself as a parish nurse healer, the nurse takes heed to heal and nurture self while supporting individuals, families and congregation communities in their healing process.

critical thinking activities

1. Contact the local council of churches to see if there is a parish nurse in your community. If so, contact the nurse and arrange to spend a day with the nurse.
   a. Interview the nurse regarding the parish nurse role functions.
   b. Ask how the parish nurse standards of practice are integrated into the practice.
2. Discuss with classmates the similarities and differences between block nursing and parish nursing. Review the content in this chapter and compare your answers.
3. Choose a *Healthy People 2010* objective to implement in a block nursing or parish nursing setting. Discuss plans for implementing the objective and evaluating the outcomes. What data did you use to develop a plan for implementing? How did you choose your population?

Bibliography

Abbott B: Parish nursing, *Home Healthcare Nurse* 16(4):265, 1998.

American Nurses Association: *Standards of clinical nursing practice*, Washington, DC, 1998, the Association.

American Nurses Association: *Code for nurses with interpretive statements*, Washington, DC, 1985, the Association.

Berry R: A parish nurse. In Office of Resourcing Committees on Preparation for Ministry: *A day in the life of . . . A kaleidoscope of specialized ministries*, Louisville, Ky, 1994, Presbyterian Church (USA): Distribution Management Service.

Bondine D: Parish nursing, *Perspectives* 21(2):8, 1997.

Bunkers SS, Michaels C, Ethridge P: Advanced practice nursing in community: nursing's opportunity, *Adv Pract Nurs Q* 2(4):79, 1997.

Bunkers S: A nursing theory-guided model of health ministry: human becoming in parish nursing, *Nurs Sci Q* 11(1):7, 1998.

Can spirituality uplift your health? *Consum Rep Health* 10(6):7, 1998.

Chandler E: Theology and ethics. In Weist WE, editor: *Healthcare and its costs: a challenge for the church*, Lanham, Md, 1988, University Press of America.

Christopher MA et al: Neighborhood nursing: the community as partner, *Caring Mag* 12(1):44, 1993.

Culp L: Health ministries: caring for body and soul, *Reg Nurse J* 9(3):8, 1997.

Dillon DL, Sternas K: Designing a successful health fair to promote individual, family, and community health, *J Comm Health Nurs* 14(1):1, 1997.

Djupe AM, Olson H, Ryan JA: *Reaching out: parish nursing services*, ed 2, Chicago, 1994, Lutheran General Healthsystem.

Djupe AM, Solari-Twadell A: The community: the parish nurse, *Home Health Focus* 2(7):53, 1995.

Dossey BM et al: *Holistic nursing: a handbook for practice*, ed 2, Gaithersburg, Md, 1995, Aspen.

Dossey L: *Healing words: the power of prayer and the practice of medicine*, New York, 1993, Harper Collins.

Dossey L: *Prayer is good medicine*, San Francisco, 1996, Harper.

Fehring RJ, Miller JR, Shaw C: Spiritual well-being, religiosity, hope, depression, and other mood states in elderly people coping with cancer, *Oncol Nurs Forum* 24(4):663, 1997.

Foege W: A strategy for change, *Faith Health* Summer:2, 1996.

Granberg-Michaelson K: Staying healthy: the spiritual dimension, *Contact* 155:3, 1997.

Health Ministries Association/American Nurses Association: *Scope and standards of parish nursing practice*, Washington, DC, 1998, American Nurses Publishing.

Huggins D: Parish nursing: a community-based outreach program of care, *Orthopaed Nurs* March/April:26, 1998.

International Parish Nurse Resource Center: *Role of parish nurse, mission and resources* (brochure), Park Ridge, IL, 1998, Author.

Jamieson MK, Martinson I: Block nursing: neighbors caring for neighbors, *Nurs Outlook* 31(5):270, 1983.

Jamieson MK: Block nursing: practicing autonomous professional nursing in the community, *Nurs Health Care* 11(5):250, 1990.

Jamieson MK: Expanding the associate degree curriculum without adding time, *Nurs Health Perspect* 19:161, 1998.

Koenig HG et al: Religious coping in the nursing home: a biopsychosocial model, *Internat J Psychiatr Med* 27(4):365, 1997.

Kucey M: Professional practice and parish nurses, *Can Nurse* Jan:51, 1999.

Lenehan G: Free clinics and parish nursing offer unique rewards, *J Emerg Nurs* 24:3, 1998.

Magilvy JK, Congdon JG, Martinez R: Circles of care: home care and community support for rural older adults, *Adv Nurs Sci* 16(3):22, 1994.

Magilvy JK, Brown NJ: Parish nursing: advanced practice nursing model for healthier communities, *Adv Pract Nurs Q* 2:67, 1997.

Martinson IM et al: The block nurse program, *J Comm Health Nurs* 2(1):21, 1985.

Marty M, editor: *Healthy people 2000: a role for America's religious communities,* Chicago, 1990, Park Ridge Center.

Matthews DA et al: Religious commitment and health status, *Arch Fam Med* 7(2):118, 1998.

McDermott MA, Solari-Twadell PA, Mathews R: Promoting quality education for the parish nurse and parish nurse coordinate, *Nurs Health Care Perspect* 19(1):4, 1998.

Miller L: Can you go back? *Wall Street J* pp. W1, W10, April 10, 1998.

Miskelly S: A parish nursing model: applying the community health nursing process in a church community, *J Comm Health Nurs* 12(1):1, 1995.

Mustoe K: The unbroken circle, *Health Progress* May-June:47, 1998.

Nouwen HJ: *The wounded healer,* New York, 1979, Image Books.

Office of the General Assembly: *Life abundant: values, choices, and health care,* Louisville, Ky, 1988, Presbyterian Distribution Services.

Olson J, Simington J, Clark M: Educating parish nurses, *Can Nurse* Sept:40, 1988.

Oman D, Reed D: Religion and mortality among the community-dwelling elderly, *Am J Public Health* 88(10):1469, 1998.

Oxman TE, Freeman DH, Manheimer ED: Lack of social participation or religious strength and comfort as risk factors for death after cardiac surgery in the elderly, *Psychosom Med* 57(1):5, 1995.

Parish nurses offer support, *Case Manage Advis* 9(3):41, 1998.

Princeton Religion Research Center: *Religion in America, 1993-1994,* Princeton, NJ, 1994, Princeton Religion Research Center.

Reinhard SC et al: Promoting healthy communities through neighborhood nursing, *Nurs Outlook* 44(5):223, 1996.

Rydholm L: Patient-focused care in parish nursing, *Holist Nurs Pract* 11(3):47, 1997.

Schacht AR: The parish nurse, *Horizons* 5:16, 1992.

Schank MJ, Weis D, Matheus R: Parish nursing: ministry of healing, *Geriatr Nurs* 17(1):11, 1996.

Sibbald B: Hospital brings parish nursing to the community, *Can Nurse* 92(7):22, 1997.

Silverman HD: Creating a spirituality curriculum for family practice residents, *Altern Therap* 3(6):54, 1997.

Solari-Twadell A, McDermott MA, editors: *Parish nursing: promoting whole person health within faith communities,* Thousand Oaks, 1999, Sage .

Solari-Twadell A et al: *Assuring viability for the future: guideline development for parish nurse education programs,* Park Ridge, Ill, 1994, Lutheran General HealthSystem.

Solari-Twadell PA, Djupe AM, McDermott MA, editors: *Parish nursing: the developing practice,* Park Ridge, Ill, 1990, International Parish Nurse Resource Center.

Striepe J: The developing practice of the parish nurse: a rural experience. In Solari-Twadell PA, Djupe AM, McDermott MA, editors: *Parish nursing: the developing practice,* Park Ridge, Ill, 1990, International Parish Nurse Resource Center.

Tolley M: Experiencing the neighborhood: the parish as clinical site, *Oklahoma Nurse* 43(3):31, 1998.

US Department of Health and Human Services: *Leading indicators for HP 2010: a report from health and human services working group on sentinel objectives.* Section One: Healthy People 2000 and Leading Health Indicators, Washington, DC, 1998, Author.

Van Loon A: International: Faith community nursing. *Internat J Nurs Pract* 2(3):168, 1996.

Van Loon A: The Development of Faith community nursing programs as a response to changing Australian health policy, *Health Educ Behav* 25(6):790, 1998.

Weis D, Mathews R, Schank MJ: Health care delivery in faith communities: the parish nurse model, *Public Health Nurs* 14(6):368, 1997.

Weist WE, ed: *Health care and its cost: a challenge for the church,* Lanham, Md, 1988, University Press of America.

Woodward KL, Underwood A: The ritual solution, *Newsweek* 130(12):62, 1997.

Public Health Nursing in the Local Health Department

MARY EURE FISHER

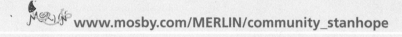

www.mosby.com/MERLIN/community_stanhope

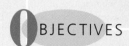

OBJECTIVES

After reading this chapter, the student should be able to do the following:

- Define public health, public health nursing, and local roles
- Describe the similarities and differences in local health department roles
- Identify trends in public health nursing
- Describe examples of public health nursing roles
- Discuss changes in the current health care environment that affect public health nursing
- Describe collaborative partnerships of public health nursing

- Identify educational preparation of nurses and skills essential to practice at different levels
- Explain effect of health maintenance organizations on local public health nurses/nursing
- Examine the effect of changes in payment sources on the at-risk populations served by public health nurses
- Discuss lessons learned from the past that may affect the future of public health nursing
- Describe the role of the public health nurse in a disaster
- Explore team concepts in public health settings

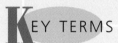

KEY TERMS

local public health departments	**public health**	**public health nursing**	**public health programs** *See Glossary for definitions*

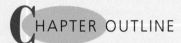

CHAPTER OUTLINE

Definitions in Public Health Nursing
History and Trends of Public Health
Scope, Standards, and Roles of Public Health Nursing

Issues and Trends in Public Health Nursing
Education and Knowledge Requirements for Public Health Nurses

Certification for Public Health Nursing
National Health Objectives
Functions of Public Health Nurses

"Just as all politics is local, all health is local" (Bunker, 1994, p 87). To understand public health nursing at the local level it is important to understand the different responsibilities and characteristics of the local public health department. **Local public health departments** have responsibilities that vary depending on the locality, but they are the agencies that are responsible for implementing and enforcing local, state, and federal public health codes and ordinances and providing essential public health programs to a community. The health department's authority is delegated by the state for specific functions (Box 46-1). Because of this delegation of specific duties, local public health agencies vary greatly from state to state, as well as within states, depending on the expectations of local governments.

The goal of the local public health department is to safeguard the public's health and to improve the community's health status. Public health nurses work with a wide range of staff within the health department to meet, this goal including physicians, nutritionists, environmental health professionals, paraprofessional home visitors, and other public health workers.

Changes in local, state, and federal governments affect public health services, and public health nursing has to develop strategies for dealing with these changes. To meet the changing needs of a community, public health nurses must identify new public health concerns and help develop programs to provide needed services.

DEFINITIONS IN PUBLIC HEALTH NURSING

Public health nursing focuses on the individuals, families, communities, and populations where public health nurses live, work, and play. The American Public Health Association Public Health Nursing Section (1996) defines **public health nursing** as "the practice of promoting and protecting the health of populations using knowledge from nursing, social and public health sciences." The Institute of Medicine defined **public health** in its 1988 Report as "fulfilling society's interest in assuring conditions in which people can be healthy (p. 7)."

In 1920, C.E.A. Winslow defined public health as "the science and art of preventing disease, prolonging life and promoting health and efficiency through organized community effort" (Turnock, 1997, p 9). This definition is still recognized by public health textbooks because it focuses on the relationship between social conditions and health across all levels of society.

Additional knowledge, efforts, and skills are necessary for a nurse to go beyond focusing on the health needs of the individual to focusing on the health needs of populations (see Chapters 1 and 15). This additional effort distinguishes the public health nurse from the nurse who is simply practicing in the community setting.

Public health nursing practices arise from knowledge gained from the physical and social sciences, psychologic and spiritual fields, environmental areas, political arena, economics, community organization, and life experience. Jan Wallinder's (1997, p 77) explanation that "public health nurses define and redefine their roles as they live them" describes the essence of the spirit of commitment most practicing public health nurses experience or they would not still be practicing in this complex area.

Public health programs are often designed with the goal of improving a population's health status. Public health programs go beyond the administration of health care to include public education, outreach, record keeping, professional education for providers, surveillance, compliance to regulations for some institutions/agencies and school systems, and follow-up of noncompliant populations, such as persons with active, untreated tuberculosis. Public health programs are frequently implemented by the development of partnerships or coalitions with other providers, agencies, and groups in the location being served.

The duties of local health departments vary depending on the state and local public health codes and ordinances and the responsibilities assigned by the state and local governments. Usually the local public health department provides for the administration, regulatory oversight, public health, and environmental services for a geographic area. The majority of local public health agencies will be involved in the following:
- Collecting and analyzing vital statistics (Chapter 11)
- Providing health education and information to the population served (Chapter 14)
- Receiving reports, investigating and controlling communicable diseases (Chapters 38 and 39)
- Protecting the environment to reduce the risk to health (Chapter 8)
- Providing some health services to particular populations at risk or with limited access to care (Chapters 24 to 30, 32 to 40, 43 to 45)
- Identifying public health problems for at-risk and high-risk populations

Public health nurses will be involved in most of these activities in various ways depending on the local public health agency and the local needs.

Public health is not a branch of medicine; it is an organized community approach designed to prevent disease, promote health, and protect populations. It works across many disciplines and is based on the scientific core of epi-

---

BOX 46-1 Public Health Agency Functions

Generally, local public health agencies perform the following functions:
- Provide and disseminate health information
- Provide leadership in health planning
- Provide essential public health and environmental services
- Collect statistics on births
- File a certificate for every birth or death in that area

demiology (IOM, 1988). Public health nurses work with multidisciplinary teams of people both within the public health areas and in other human services agencies.

HISTORY AND TRENDS OF PUBLIC HEALTH

A person born today can expect to live 30 years longer than the person born in 1900. Medical care accounts for 5 years of that increase, but public health is responsible for the additional 25 years through prevention efforts brought about by changes in social policies, community actions, and individual and group behavior changes (Milbank, 1994, p 225). Historically, public health nurses were valued by and important to society and functioned in an autonomous setting. They worked with populations and in settings that were not of interest to other health care disciplines or groups. Much of the public health services were delivered to the poor and to women and children, who did not have political power or voice.

In 1996 nearly 900,000 fewer cases of measles were reported than in 1941 (Turnock, 1997, p 1). Public health nurses were a major factor in accomplishing the immunizations that accounted for this dramatic decrease in measles. The general public was not informed about how this immunization activity was accomplished and the resulting effect on improving health and lowering health care cost. Today most of the public does not understand what public health nurses do, because these nurses have been busy "doing" and not providing education to the public about their public health activities. For public health services to receive adequate funding it is necessary for the public and government to be aware of the benefits provided to a community by public health nurses. Public health nurses must be at the table when issues are being discussed and decisions are being made to make certain that public health programs are provided for the populations at risk and that funds are available to cover those services.

> **WHAT DO YOU THINK?** *In this era of managed care a critical question is whether public health will take a position as an advocate for the community or as a part of the medicine market place and become just another commodity. Once medicine was seen as a "mission-driven, value-laden" profession, but now it is seen as a partner with managed care bargaining for roles and resources and not as a profession serving society for the common good (Citrin, 1998, p 351). What will be the role of public health nurses in the twenty-first century?*

SCOPE, STANDARDS, AND ROLES OF PUBLIC HEALTH NURSING

Public health nurses integrate community involvement and knowledge about the entire population with personal, clinical understandings of the health and illness experiences of individuals and families within the population. They translate and articulate the health and illness experiences of diverse, often vulnerable individuals and families in the population to health

planners, and policy makers, and assist members of the community to voice their problems and aspirations. Public health nurses are knowledgeable about multiple strategies for intervention, from those applicable to the entire population, to those for the family, and the individual. Public health nurses translate knowledge from the health and social sciences to individuals and population groups through targeted interventions, programs, and advocacy . . . Public health nurses are directly engaged in the interdisciplinary activities of the core public health functions of assessment, assurance and policy development. . . . In any setting, the role of public health nurses focuses on the prevention of illness, injury or disability, the promotion of health, and maintenance of the health of populations. (APHA PHN Definition and Role of Public Health Nursing, 1996)

In Virginia, a statewide committee looked at the role of public health nursing in light of the changes in health care. The committee developed a document that was intended to identify roles within the context of the core public health functions (see Chapter 1) and to identify the educational program needs of staff that would prepare them to function effectively in the changing public health care area. Essential elements of the role were identified, which are presented below.

> **HOW TO** *Implement the Core Public Health Functions in a Community: Essential Elements of the Public Health Role*
>
> - *Conduct community assessments*
> - *Prevent and control epidemics*
> - *Provide a safe and healthy environment*
> - *Measure performance, effectiveness, and outcomes of health services*
> - *Promote healthy lifestyles*
> - *Provide laboratory testing*
> - *Provide targeted outreach to vulnerable populations and form partnerships*
> - *Provide personal health care services*
> - *Conduct research and create innovations (in programs)*
> - *Mobilize the community for action*
>
> From National Association of City and County Health Officials: *Blueprint for a healthy community: a guide for local health departments,* Washington, DC, 1994, the Association.

These essential elements will be implemented through multidisciplinary public health teams. A matrix was developed to show the relationship of the public health functions defined by the essential elements to the public health nursing roles at the local level as well as the role of the state in this responsibility (see Appendix K.1).

Local public health nurses make a significant difference in improving the health of a community by monitoring critical health status indicators, such as immunization levels, infant mortality rates, and communicable diseases. Local public health nurses provide the "linkage between epidemiological data and clinical understanding of health and illness as it is experienced in peoples' lives" (APHA, 1996).

In the effort to contain costs and develop leaner, more efficient workforces at all levels of government, public agencies such as local public health departments have had major changes over the last decade, and more changes will come in the new millennium. These changes may be seen as an opportunity to return to the core values of public health, allowing public health to focus on the prevention of disease, promotion of health, and protection of populations and the environment. In the past several decades public health has moved away from its intended mission of implementing the core functions and has provided primary care services.

A driving force behind these changes is the economy and the increase in managed care providers. To meet local public health needs there has been a shift from the local health department being the primary care clinical provider to the development of partnerships with a variety of existing individuals, groups, institutions, and hospitals to meet the needs of the populations in a community for health promotion and disease prevention activities. There are many concerns about the available health care for the uninsured and underinsured in these new arrangements. The public health nurses' role in this latest shift in health care delivery is still being developed for many agencies. Case management at the community level is a renewed effort in public health nursing rather than having case management done at the institution (see Chapter 19) (see the Research Brief).

In 1998 about 43 million American citizens lacked health insurance. These uninsured individuals seek services on a sliding payment scale from such sources as university or public hospital clinics or from a variety of free clinics. Public health nurses can serve as a bridge between these populations and the resource needs for this at-risk group by approaching health care providers on behalf of individuals seeking medical/health services and keeping the needs of this population on the political agenda.

Frequently the indigent and low-income populations lack the knowledge and skills to negotiate the complex medical system made up of physicians and hospitals. This population needs education and training in identifying their problems, approaches to self-care, and illness prevention strategies and lifestyle choices that will have an effect on their health. Public health nurses are skilled in working with this population, which is often defined by other health providers as noncompliant since this population often faces barriers, like transportation, in keeping appointments and lacks knowledge to understand and follow medical instructions.

Although indigent and low-income populations have always benefited from public health nursing services, the populations that are most acutely in need of public health nursing services have changed dramatically over the last couple of decades. Of particular concern are the number of young women and their partners who are substance abusers and have risky behaviors, such as hostility and ag-

RESEARCH *Brief*

This descriptive study looked at a health department parenting project to see whether teen mothers' self-esteem, social support, and parenting competence improved while receiving case management services from public health nurses during the first 18 months of motherhood. A sample of 56 first-time teen mothers participated in the study; 45% were Hispanic. Public health nurses received special training in assessment of and intervention with teen mothers. The nurses provided assessments, interventions, referrals for medical care, vocational training and finances, and education in prenatal and postnatal care, diet, family planning, child care and child health, and safe-baby environment. The nurses also provided for transportation for mothers to keep appointments and encouraged the teens to stay in school. The nurses used home visits and phone calls to maintain contact with the mothers.

Data were collected at 6, 12, and 18 months using the Rosenberg Self-Esteem Scale, the Inventory of Socially Supportive Behaviors by Barrera, and Parental Sense of Competency Scale by Gibard et al. The study results indicated that mothers need special attention during the first months of parenting to enhance that self-esteem and to encourage better parenting. Social support was found to decrease as the child moved toward 18 months and the parents' competence in caring for the baby slightly increased.

Teen pregnancy is a national concern because it usually results in less education and less future earning power for the teen mother. Early intervention to promote self-esteem and to encourage social support from family, friends, and agencies and competent parenting skills for the mother may make a difference for the health of the baby and the mother's ability to become a happy, healthy, productive adult.

Parenting, competence, social support, and self-esteem in teen mothers case managed by public health nurses, *Public Health Nurs* 15(6):432, 1998.

gression, that put their pregnancy or children at high risk of injury or abuse. Public health nurses and local public health departments have had to provide innovative, collaborative approaches to prepare their staff to work effectively with this population. As with any profession, ongoing educational resources are essential for public health nursing staff to develop new skills to meet ever-changing public health challenges.

At the 1998 annual meeting of the Association of State and Territorial Directors of Nursing, Kristine Gebbie, a leader in public health nursing and former national AIDS czar in the Clinton administration, presented the curriculum plan that was developed with help from the Centers for Disease Control and Prevention (CDC), Health Resources and Services Administration (HRSA) the Division of Nursing, and the Preventive Health and Health Promotion Office (PHHPO) to use a satellite link teleconference approach to retraining and updating public health nurses for their future job responsibilities.

HOW TO *Educate Nurses for Roles in Public Health: Curriculum Objectives for Public Health Nursing*

The nurse should be able to do the following:
* *Articulate similarities and differences between individual and population-focused nursing practice*
* *Describe the history and current perspectives of public health nursing practice*
* *Demonstrate skills in applying key nursing contributions to public health practice (core functions and essential services) in a community*
* *Apply principles and skills of population health to his or her practice in the public health agency*
* *Use current information and communication technology in all public health agencies*
* *Communicate the benefits of public health and public health nursing practice*

The functioning of the local public health nurse varies significantly depending on the education and practice skills of the staff. However, all nursing staff should be able to function at the same level. Public health nurses focus on health rather than disease in working with populations. There is a tremendous difference in public health nursing practice from nursing practiced in other settings where the emphasis is usually on illness care and cure. Although public health nurses perform direct hands-on care in many instances, they also perform tasks that one may not be able to see or touch. Knowledge is imparted in many complex and subtle ways that result in changes in health status and behavior at the population level.

NURSING TIP

Many of the epidemics of the future will be defined by social problems such as substance abuse and teen pregnancy.

ISSUES AND TRENDS IN PUBLIC HEALTH NURSING

Some of the current issues facing public health nursing services today are violence in society, substance abuse, welfare reform effects on families and children, multicultural and biracial integration into society, lack of health and medical resources for the uninsured and underinsured, and managed care. Public health nurses must keep abreast of the issues that are affecting all of society. Assessments need to be changed to include these factors that affect the populations that they serve. When child care is an issue for the welfare mother returning to work, consideration must be given to

effects on the individual, family, community, and population. Public health nurses cannot say "that's a shame," and go on about other business, but must look at the problem and determine what is wrong with the system that wants parents to go to work so they can be removed from welfare but does not provide services such as child care so parents can be successful? "What will it take to change the system?" Is the question to be answered by a nurse? Partnerships and collaboration among groups are much more powerful in making change than the individual client and public health nurse working alone. These types of problems have not developed in a day and will not be solved overnight. As another example, the depressed, nonfunctional mother in need of counseling is of significant public health concern because the mother's, children's, and family's needs are not being met. Frequently the presenting problem may not be obvious to the health professional seeing this woman for the first time. Public health nurses have special preparation to help them identify both the individual client's problem and then to look at the effect on the broader community. Some of the problems that may result are children who grow to be adults may have mental health problems of their own. The community mental health services will need to be able to handle the growing population. Children may become violent adults, resulting in need for more corrections facilities. Mothers may need additional mental health services or children may be absent from school often and may not be able to contribute to society and be as productive in the workplace because of lack of skills learned when absent from school. Mothers may not be able to provide financially, and the monies from welfare are needed. Often one problem of the single individual places great burdens on the community.

Some macro-level trends affecting public health today are as follows (Brownson and Kreuter, 1997):
* Changes in health care delivery systems
* Changing patterns in the racial and ethnic composition in the U.S. population
* The aging of the population
* Rapid development of information technologies
* Development of numerous and diverse health-related partnerships
* Educational needs and changes within the public health work force
* The antigovernment sentiment and polarization of some factions of the population

---

WHAT DO YOU THINK? *Changes have occurred in public health nursing (Frank, 1959, p. vii). Changes are occurring in public health nursing. Change will continue to occur in public health nursing. Public health nurses have to learn to function in an organization that must deal with many changes, as changes occur continually, due to the many internal and external factors from people, programs, politics, and the unknown, as well as known local, state, and federal actions. Which skills help the public health nurse to adapt to changes?*

EDUCATION AND KNOWLEDGE REQUIREMENTS FOR PUBLIC HEALTH NURSES

The American Public Health Association's Public Health Nursing Section (1996) states the educational preparation of public health nurses should be at least a baccalaureate degree, because "All public health nurses should have a background in the social and behavioral sciences, epidemiology, environmental health, current treatment modalities, and health care delivery options in order to fully understand health policy, research, and treatment choices and to translate this knowledge into the promotion of healthy populations" The reality is that about two thirds of the practicing public health nurses do not have baccalaureate degrees but are providing public health services based on skills acquired through experience (APHA, PHN Section, 1996).

The Core Public Health Functions Steering Committee (1994) identified 10 activities that need to be implemented in a community to meet the public health core functions of assessment, assurance, and policy development:

1. Health status monitoring and surveillance
2. Investigation and control of disease and injuries
3. Protection of environment, workplace, housing, food, and water
4. Laboratory services to support disease control and environmental protection
5. Health education and information
6. Community mobilization for health-related issues
7. Targeted outreach and linkage to personal services
8. Health services quality assurance and accountability
9. Training and education of public health professionals
10. Leadership, policy, planning and administration

Many of these core public health functions are provided by public health nurses who have learned these skills in the workplace while gaining knowledge slowly through years of practice. Rapid changes in public health are providing a challenge to public health nurses in that there is neither the time nor staff to provide as much on-the-job training as is needed to learn and upgrade skills and knowledge of staff. Therefore nurses with baccalaureate or master's preparation will be needed to provide a strong public health system (see Chapter 1).

CERTIFICATION FOR PUBLIC HEALTH NURSING

At this point two levels of certification are available for nurses in community health and public health nursing. Both are offered through the American Nurses Credentialing Center. Although certification is voluntary, being recognized as competent in a specialty area says to clients and employers that the nurse has knowledge and skills that are essential to nursing practice. The nurse who is certified focuses on a holistic approach to care of the total population including the promotion and maintenance of health, health education, case management, coordination, and the provision of continuity of care. To be eligible to write the certification examination at the generalist level, one must be a registered nurse and licensed in the United States or its territories, have a baccalaureate or higher degree in nursing or related field, have at least 30 contact hours of continuing education applicable to the field in the past 3 years, and have practiced in the community health field a minimum of 1500 hours in the last 3 years. Nurses are examined on such topics as public health science, individual, family and community as client, areas of practice, public health issues/problems, and professional issues. The clinical specialist in community and public health is discussed in Chapter 41.

NATIONAL HEALTH OBJECTIVES

State health departments play a key role in implementing the *Healthy People 2000* objectives. In Virginia, as an example, the State Health Department (1997) helps set local goals using the *Healthy People 2000* objectives as a framework. Knowing that the public health departments do not have the resources to accomplish these goals independently, collaboration is essential to quality nursing practice and is encouraged at the local level with existing groups. New partnerships are developed and related to specific goals. For example, to improve pregnancy outcomes, the Year 2000 objectives are to decrease infant mortality (with each local health department using local data to set goals), to decrease low weight births, to improve the percentage of entry into prenatal care in the first trimester, to decrease pregnancies of 15- to 17-year-old females, to decrease smoking during pregnancy, and to decrease nonmarital births. Since the addition of the objective to decrease nonmarital births, several communities developed new coalitions to address the objectives to include all of the local community players such as social services, mental health, education, justice and courts, recreation, government, and businesses. Membership varies from community to community depending on that community's formal and informal structure. The groups join the coalition for a variety of reasons. For example, businesses see the value of developing a productive work force that will be of importance to them and the community in the future.

The Year 2000 objectives focus on decreasing deaths from coronary heart diseases, strokes, cancers, and diabetes. Public health nurses help clients identify unhealthy behaviors and then help them develop strategies to improve their health. Some of the behaviors addressed by public health nurses are tobacco use, physical activity, and obesity, all of which affect these chronic diseases.

Some Year 2000 communicable disease areas of focus are immunizations, STD, HIV, and AIDS. Public health nurses provide clients with instructions on the use of barrier methods of contraception and information on the hazards of multiple sexual partners and street drug use in order to help clients reduce their risk of acquiring a communicable disease. Getting a complete sexual history on all clients coming to the health department for services takes special skills but is essential to determine the behaviors that have brought the client to the local health de-

Community Health Nursing in the Traditional Setting in Canada

Karen Wade, Toronto Public Health and University of Toronto
Maureen Cava, Toronto Public Health and University of Toronto

ORGANIZATION OF PUBLIC HEALTH SERVICES IN CANADA

A recent survey that assessed the status of provincially and territorially-mandated public health authorities and administrations in Canada revealed that the organization of public health and its linkages with other health and nonhealth sectors varies considerably across the country (Canadian Public Health Association, 1997). In all provinces and territories, with the exception of British Columbia, public health is the responsibility of the Ministry of Health or its equivalent. In British Columbia public health functions are the shared responsibility of the Ministries of Health, Seniors, Children, and Families. Funding for public health services also varies. Programs and services that are integrated into comprehensive health organizations are usually funded through a health board. The legislative mandate for public health focuses primarily on health protection and control of communicable diseases. Other secondary acts and regulations include legislation regarding second-hand smoke, environmental contaminants, and health standards in public places.

SCOPE OF PUBLIC HEALTH NURSING IN CANADA

In some areas of Canada the terms *community health nurse* and *public health nurse* are used interchangeably. In others, the term *community health nurse* encompasses the speciality of public health nursing. In Canada, the focus of community/public health nursing practice is primarily health promotion, illness and injury prevention, health protection, and health maintenance (Canadian Public Health Association, 1990). The Canadian Public Health Association (CPHA) (1990) has taken the position that a baccalaureate degree in nursing is essential for community/public health nursing practice. Currently community/public health nurses in Canada do not write certification examinations.

The Canadian Public Health Association (1990) defines community/public health nursing as "an art and a science that synthesizes knowledge from the public health sciences and professional nursing theories. Its goal is to promote and preserve the health of populations and is directed to communities, groups, families, and individuals across their life span, in a continuous rather than episodic process . . . (They) work in collaboration with, among others, communities, families, individuals, other professionals, voluntary organizations, self-help groups, informal health care providers, governments, and the private sector" (p 3). Community/public health nurses are proactive regarding social and health care trends, changing needs of communities, policies, and legislation that affect on the health of communities, families, and individuals and/or the health care system (CPHA, 1990). Public health nurses provide education, counselling, support, referral, and coordination services for underserviced communities, whether underserviced for reasons of geography or social structure (Hayward et al, 1993). One of the unique features of public health nursing in Canada has been its direct accessibility to the population through self-referral.

The CPHA (1990) identified eleven key activities of community/public health nurses in Canada, which are similar to the roles and functions of public health nurses in the United States. These are listed below.

KEY ACTIVITIES OF COMMUNITY/PUBLIC HEALTH NURSES IN CANADA

Care/Service Provider: Assesses client's health status and plans and implements and evaluates care, in partnership with the client, using health promotion, illness, and injury prevention strategies.

Communicator: Uses effective communication skills a) with individual clients, b) to represent the views of individuals, groups, and communities, c) to facilitate interagency and intersectoral cooperation, and d) to strive for sufficient community resource allocation.

Community Developer: Applies knowledge of community assessment and community development models to facilitate public participation in identifying and decision making regarding health issues.

Consultant: Provides expertise/information to clients, lay helpers, professionals, social and community agencies, professional associations, and all levels of government.

Educator: Provides formal/informal presentations/teaching and educational programs to individuals, groups, families, aggregates, and communities.

Facilitator: Acts as a *Leader* in developing a proactive approach to health issues and/or encouraging individuals or communities to take action on issues; acts as an *Enabler* in supporting the community to participate in identifying and taking ownership of health issues; acts as an *Advocate* for the disadvantaged.

Policy Formulator: Identifies the need for and participates in the development of and evaluation of policy conducive to health.

Researcher/Evaluator: Identifies and investigates key issues and approaches to community health; uses research/program evaluation findings to inform programming and to allocate resources.

Resource Manager/Planner/Coordinator: Involves communities in health services planning, priority setting, and allocation.

Social Marketer: Uses marketing techniques and skills to promote healthy living as well as health promotion programs.

Team Member/Collaborator: Fosters team building as well as interdisciplinary, interagency, and intersectoral cooperation and collaboration.

continued

Community Health Nursing in the Traditional Setting in Canada—cont'd

Bibliography

Canadian Public Health Association: *Community health–public health nursing in Canada–preparation and practice*, Ottawa, 1990, the Association.

Canadian Public Health Association: *Public health infrastructure in Canada*, Ottawa, 1997, the Association.

Hayward S et al: *Public health nursing and health promotion: a background paper for the systematic overviews of the effectiveness of public health nursing interventions*, Hamilton, ON, 1993, Quality of Nursing Worklife Research Unit Working Paper Series, 93-2.

Canadian spelling is used.

partment. Abstinence as a birth control method can be addressed with all populations. Education of young persons before they become sexually active has helped reduce the incidence of some sexually transmitted diseases in this population.

Each local health department or district reviews the data and can develop specific goals based on the *Healthy Communities 2000 Model Standards* format. A 3- or 5-year average is used to compare data to see if trends are changing in health behaviors and health status, because the numbers are often extremely small. It is essential to have data that is comparable with other similar populations in other communities or states to know if public health strategies are working.

FUNCTIONS OF PUBLIC HEALTH NURSES

Public health nurses play many roles depending on the needs and resources of an area. *Advocate* is one of the many roles of the public health nurse. As an advocate, the public health nurse collects data and discusses with the client which services are needed, whether an individual, family, community, or population. The public health nurse and the client then develop the most effective plan and approach to take, and the nurse helps the client implement the plan so that the client can become more independent in making decisions and getting the services they need. At the community and population levels public health nurses promote safe water, air, and sanitation. They advocate for healthy policies that will develop healthy communities (see Chapter 17).

Case manager is a major role for public health nurses. Public health nurses use the nursing or scientific process of assessing, planning, implementing and evaluating outcomes to meet clients' needs. Clear and complex communications are frequently an important component of case management. Other health and social agency participants may not be familiar with the home and community living conditions that are known to the public health nurse. It is the nurse who has been there and seen the living conditions and who can tell the story for the client or assist the individual or family with the telling of their story. Case managers assist clients in identifying the services they need the most at the least cost. They also assist communities and populations in identifying services that will increase the overall community health status.

Public health nurses are a major *referral resource.* Because of necessity they have had to keep up to date on the services that are available to their populations. They know what resources will be acceptable to the client within the social and cultural norms for that group. The nurse educates the client to enable them to use the resources and to learn self-care. Nurses refer to other services in the area, and other services refer to the public health nurse for care or follow-up. For example, the mother and new baby may be referred to the public health nurse for postnatal with postpartum home visit follow-up to hospital care.

Assessment of literacy is a large part of public health nursing. Many individuals are limited in their ability to read, write, and communicate clearly. The public health nurse has to be culturally sensitive and aware of the specific areas of unique problems of clients, such as financial limitations that may in turn limit educational opportunities. Frequently, when a person goes to a physician's office, clinic, or hospital, they are clean and neatly dressed. The assumption is made that when they nod at the health care provider it means that they understand what has been said. This is frequently not the case, but the client is embarrassed to admit that he or she does not understand what has been said. Being illiterate does not mean a person is mentally slow. It is important for the public health nurse to follow up on the many contacts the individual or family has with medical, social, and legal services to clarify what is understood and to find an answer to the questions that have not been asked by the client or answered by the services.

The public health nurse is a strong *role model* for many of the clients they serve. These clients may not have had a positive, mature individual to interact with in their family of origin. The public health nurse becomes an example for the children and family and may encourage them to seek education or employment so they can improve their social and financial status (see Chapter 24). The nurse is also an educator, teaching to the level of the client so that information received is information that can be used. Patience and repetitions over time are necessary to develop the trust and to enable the client to use the relationship with the nurse for more information.

Counselor is another important public health nursing role. The client frequently cannot define or identify the problem that needs to be handled, much less develop solutions. At-risk populations frequently lack problem-solving skills. For example, a sexually active teenage female is unaware that she has made a decision to be sexually active. Frequently she thinks "things" just happen. Knowing this is a beginning step in problem identification, which can lead to safe contraception. This is an active decision the girl can control. The nurse can help her to set goals and to accomplish these goals.

Public health nurses are direct *primary caregivers* in many situations both in the clinic and in the community. As primary caregiver the public health nurse assesses the clients' health and social status. The nurse then helps to define the problems and to marshal the resources available to solve the problems. In visiting a mother and a newborn baby, the public health nurse's assessment can identify physical and other problems that might have been seen in the hospital in the past, when hospital stays were more than 24 to 48 hours. Teaching before discharge is limited because of the short hospital stays, and many mothers need reinforcement of that teaching after they return to the community. Regardless of the educational, social, or economic level of the family, the public health nursing assessment is essential for the majority of families. Frequently it may be to reassure the family that everything is normal. When nurses are not providing direct care they are working to ensure that direct care services are available in the community for at-risk populations by developing programs that will meet the needs of those populations.

Currently no system of *outreach* service in the medical models of care addresses the multiple needs of high-risk populations. High-risk populations frequently do not understand the medical, social, educational, or judicial system and the professional languages, codes of behavior, or expected outcomes of these services. Clients need a case manager, health educator, advocate, and role model to enable them to benefit from these services and to teach them how to avoid complex and expensive problems in the future. The above roles and many more are filled by the local public health nurse for this population.

An essential and unique role for public health nurses exist in the area of communicable disease control. Public health nursing skills are necessary for education and prevention, *surveillance* and outbreak investigation. Public health nurses can find infected individuals, notify contacts, refer, administer treatments, educate the individual, family, community, professionals and populations, act as an advocate, and in general be a state-of-the-art resource needed to reduce the individual of communicable disease in the community (see Chapters 38 and 39).

These are examples of the difficult clinical issues that public health nurses have to face in making ethical and professional decisions. They work for the greater good and must have great patience to work with diverse players in some very complex situations, knowing that not everyone will be satisfied with the outcome.

The public health nurse's role is unique and essential in many situations because through his or her access to homes the nurse has information that usually cannot be gathered in the hospital or clinic setting. The public health nurse learns to ask intimate questions creatively and to seek information that will facilitate case management and provide the clinical and social care needed, including other community resources. Careful attention must be paid to privacy and confidentiality in delivering public health nursing services. The credibility of the nurse and the agency is dependent on the professional handling of the public health information of each and every staff member.

When a *disaster* (see Chapter 20) occurs public health nurses have multiple roles in assessment, planning, implementing, and evaluating needs and resources for the different populations being served. Whether the disaster is local or national, small or large, natural or manmade, public health nurses are skilled professionals essential to the team. As a health care facility, the local public health department has a disaster plan, as well as a role in the local, regional, and state disaster plans. Local public health nurses' roles vary from providing education, such as CPR or first aid instruction, to preparing individuals and communities to cope with disasters to providing professional triage for local shelters. Their presence may be required in other regions of the state or country to provide official public health nursing duties in a time of crises, such as a hurricane, that requires a lengthy period of recovery. Each local government unit has a local emergency plan, and the public health department is expected to provide planning and staffing for the local area. These local emergency preparedness plans may be multigovernmental, which requires coordination between communities.

In Virginia an electrical company has a nuclear plant that requires disaster drills that are multijurisdictional. They are routinely planned and practiced with all the agencies assigned specific roles and responsibilities. These disaster planning and practice sessions are an opportunity for local public health nurses to get to know other agencies' representatives and to let them know what public health nursing can offer. Because public health nurses are out in the communities and have assessment skills, they are essential in evaluating how the disaster was handled and making suggestions about how future events might be managed. Public health nurses have to be a part of the team before an emergency to be most effective as a *disaster responder.* Knowing what type of disaster is likely to occur in a community is essential for planning. Types of disasters will vary from place to place, but there is a history of past events and how they were handled, as well as resources and training from regional, state, and federal agencies. Public health nurses can help educate the public regarding the individual responsibilities and preparations that can be in place both for the person and the community.

DID YOU KNOW? *It is important for public health nurses to practice confidentiality when they have knowledge about an individual, family, communicable disease outbreak, community-level problem, or any special knowledge obtained in the public health work setting.*

clinical application

A retirement community in a small town reported to the local health department 24 cases of severe gastrointestinal illness that had occurred among residents and staff of the facility during the past 24 to 36 hours. It was determined that the ill clients became sick within a short, well-defined period, and most recovered within 24 hours without treatment. The communicable disease outbreak team composed of public health nurses, public health physicians, and an environmental health specialist was called to respond to this possible epidemic.

How should they respond to this situation? (Refer to Chapter 11 for help in answering this question).

A. Call the Centers for Disease Control and Prevention and ask for help with surveillance
B. Send all of the retirement community ill persons to the hospital
C. Evaluate the agent, host, and environment relationships to determine the cause of the problem
D. Close the dining room and find another source to provide food to the residents

Answer is in the back of the book.

KEY POINTS

- Local public health departments are responsible for implementing and enforcing local, state, and federal public health codes and ordinances while providing essential public health services.

- The goal of the local health department is to safeguard the public's health and improve the community's health status.
- Public health nursing is the practice of promoting and protecting the health of populations using knowledge from nursing and social and public health sciences.
- Public health is based on the scientific core of epidemiology.
- Marketing of public health nursing is essential to inform both professionals and the public about the opportunities and challenges of populations in public health care.
- A driving force behind public health nursing changes is the economy and the increase in managed care.
- Public health nurses need ongoing education and training as public health changes.
- Some of the roles public health nurses function in are advocate, case manager, referral source, counselor, primary care provider, educator, outreach worker, disaster responder, and many more.
- Public health nurses have an important role in helping with local disasters, including planning, staffing, and evaluating events.

critical thinking activities

1. What are some of the various roles of the public health nurse in the local health department?
2. How can public health nurses prepare themselves for change?
3. What can today's public health nurses learn from the past practice of public health nurses?
4. Describe collaborative partnerships that public health nurses have developed.
5. What are some external factors that have an affect on public health nursing?
6. If you were a public health nurse for a day, what would you like to accomplish? Why?
7. How would you determine the most pressing public health issue in your community?
8. Give an example of policy change or effect from the work of public health nurses.

Bibliography

American Public Health Association: *Definition and role of public health nursing,* Washington, DC, 1996, APHA Public Health Nursing Section.
American Public Health Association: *Healthy Communities 2000: model standards,* ed 3, Washington, DC, 1991, the Association.
Badovinac K: Policy advocacy for public health practitioners: workshops on policy change, *Public Health Nurs* 14(5):280, 1997.
Brownson R, Kreuter M: Future trends affecting public health: challenges and opportunities, *J Public Health Manage Pract* 2(3):49, 1997.
Bunker JP et al: Improving health: measuring effects of medical care, *Milbank Q* 72:225, 1994.

Citrin T: Topics for our times: public health–community or commodity? reflections on healthy communities, *Am J Public Health* 88(3):351, 1998.
Coughlin S, Beauchamp T: *Ethics and Epidemiology,* New York, 1996, Oxford University Press.
Detels R et al: *Oxford textbook of public health,* ed 2, New York, 1997, Oxford University Press.
Downing D: Reframing the quest: health for all, *Public Health Nurs* 15(2):65, 1998.
Frank CM Sr: *Foundations of nursing,* ed 2, Philadelphia, 1959, W.B. Saunders.
Grason H, Guyer B: *Public MCH program functions framework,* Health Services and

Resources Administration, Washington, DC, 1995, NMCHC, USDHHS.
Harkness G: *Epidemiology in nursing practice,* St Louis, 1995, Mosby.
Hickey T et al: *Public health and aging,* Baltimore, 1997, The Johns Hopkins University Press.
Huston C, Fox S: The changing health care market: implications for nursing education in the coming decade, *Nurs Outlook* 46(3):109, 1998.
Institute of Medicine: *Healthy communities,* Washington, DC, 1996, National Academy Press.
Institute of Medicine: *The future of public health,* Washington, DC, 1988, National Academy Press.

988 PART *Seven* Community and Public Health Nurses: Roles and Functions

Bibliography—cont'd

Kuss T et al: A public health nursing model, *Public Health Nurs* 14(2):81, 1997.

Mechanic D: Topics for our times, managed care and public health opportunities, *Am J Public Health* 88(6):874, 1998.

Milio N: *Engines of empowerment,* Chicago, 1996, Health Administration Press.

National Association of City and County Health Officials: *Blueprint for a healthy community: a guide for local health departments,* Washington, DC, 1994, the Association.

Richards, T: Maternal and child health essential public health services, *J Public Health Manage Pract* 3(5):11, 1997.

Savage A, Pratt A: Case study. In Helvie C, editor: *Advanced practice nursing in the community,* Thousand Oaks, Calif, 1998, Sage.

Scutchfield E, Keck CW: *Principles of public health practice,* Albany, 1997, Delmar.

Stanhope M, Knollmueller R: *Public and community nurse's consultant,* St Louis, 1997, Mosby.

Turnock BJ: Public health: what it is and how it works, Gaithersburg, Md, 1997, Aspen.

US Department of Health and Human Services: *Healthy People 2000: national health promotion and disease prevention objectives,* Washington, DC, 1991, USDHHS, Public Health Services.

Virginia Department of Health: *Healthy Virginia communities,* Richmond, Virginia, 1997, Author.

Wallinder J: Supporting one another: the definition of PHN, *Public Health Nurs* 14(2):77, 1997.

Appendixes

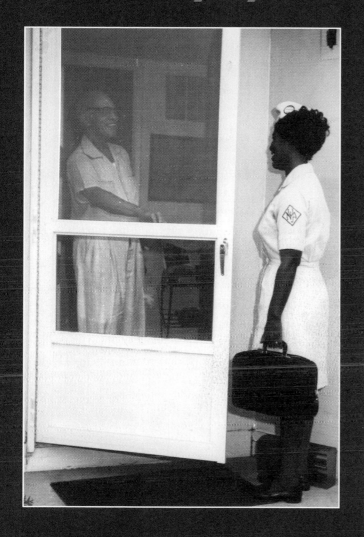

Contents

International/National Agendas for Health Care Delivery

A.1 Year 2000: National Health Objectives

(1995 Midcourse Additions have been included)

1. PHYSICAL ACTIVITY AND FITNESS
Health Status Objectives

1.1 Reduce coronary heart disease deaths to no more than 100 per 100,000 people.

1.2 Reduce overweight to a prevalence of no more than 20% among people aged 20 and older and no more than 15% among adolescents 12 through 19.

Risk Reduction Objectives

1.3 Increase to at least 30% the proportion of people aged 6 and older who engage regularly, preferably daily, in light to moderate physical activity or at least 30 minutes per day.

1.4 Increase to at least 20% the proportion of people aged 18 and older and to at least 75% the proportion of children and adolescents aged 6 through 17 who engage in vigorous physical activity that promotes the development and maintenance of cardiorespiratory fitness 3 or more days per week for 20 or more minutes per occasion.

1.5 Reduce to no more than 15% the proportion of people aged 6 and older who engage in no leisure-time physical activity.

1.6 Increase to at least 40% the proportion of people aged 6 and older who regularly perform physical activities that enhance and maintain muscular strength, muscular endurance, and flexibility.

1.7 Increase to at least 50% the proportion of overweight people aged 12 and older who have adopted sound dietary practices combined with regular physical activity to attain appropriate body weight.

Services and Protection Objectives

1.8 Increase to at least 50% the proportion of children and adolescents in first through twelfth grade who participate in daily school physical education.

1.9 Increase to at least 50% the portion of school physical education class time that students spend being physically active, preferably in lifetime physical activities.

+ 1.10 **Increase the proportion of work sites offering employer-sponsored activity and fitness programs.**

1.11 Increase community availability and accessibility of physical activity and fitness facilities.

1.12 Increase to at least 50% the proportion of primary care providers who routinely assess and counsel their patients regarding the frequency, duration, type, and intensity of each patient's physical activity practices.

1995 MIDCOURSE ADDITION
Health Status Objective

1.13 **Reduce to no more than 90 per 1000 people the proportion of all people aged 65 and older who have difficulty in performing two or more personal care activities, thereby preserving independence.**

2. NUTRITION
Health Status Objectives

2.1 Reduce coronary heart disease deaths to no more than 100 per 100,000 people.

2.2 Reverse the rise in cancer deaths to achieve a rate of no more than 130 per 100,000 people.

2.3 Reduce overweight to a prevalence of no more than 20% among people aged 20 and older and no more than 15% among adolescents aged 12 through 19.

+ 2.4 **Reduce growth retardation among low-income children aged 5 and younger to less than 10%.**

Risk Reduction Objectives

2.5 Reduce dietary fat intake to an average of 30% of calories or less and average saturated fat intake to less than 10% of calories among people aged 2 and older.

2.6 Increase complex carbohydrate and fiber-containing foods in the diets of adults to five or more daily servings for vegetables (including legumes) and fruits, and to six or more daily servings for grain products.

2.7 Increase to at least 50% the proportion of overweight people aged 12 and older who have adopted sound dietary practices combined with regular physical activity to attain appropriate body weight.

2.8 Increase calcium intake so at least 50% of youth aged 12 through 24 and 50% of pregnant and lactating women consume 3 or more servings daily of foods rich in calcium, and at least 50% of people aged 25 and older consume two or more servings daily.

2.9 Decrease salt and sodium intake so at least 65% of home meal preparers prepare foods without adding salt, at least 80% of people avoid using salt at the table, and at least 40% of adults regularly purchase foods modified or lower in sodium.

2.10 Reduce iron deficiency to less than 3% among children aged 1 through 4 and among women of childbearing age.

2.11 Increase to at least 75% the proportion of mothers who breastfeed their babies in the early postpartum period and to at least 50% the proportion who continue breastfeeding until their babies are 5 to 6 months old.

2.12 Increase to at least 75% the proportion of parents and caregivers who use feeding practices that prevent baby tooth decay.

2.13 Increase to at least 85% the proportion of people aged 18 and older who use food labels to make nutritious food selections.

Services and Protection Objectives

2.14 Achieve useful and informative nutrition labeling for virtually all processed foods and at least 40% of fresh meats, poultry, fish, fruits, vegetables, baked goods, and ready-to-eat carry-away foods.

+ **2.15 Increase to at least 5000 brand items the availability of processed food products that are reduced in fat and saturated fat.**

2.16 Increase to at least 90% the proportion of restaurants and institutional food service operations that offer identifiable low-fat, low-calorie food choices, consistent with the Dietary Guidelines for Americans.

2.17 Increase to at least 90% the proportion of school lunch and breakfast services and child care food services with menus that are consistent with the nutrition principles in the Dietary Guidelines for Americans.

2.18 Increase to at least 80% the receipt of home food services by people aged 65 and older who have difficulty in preparing their own meals or are otherwise in need of home-delivered meals.

2.19 Increase to at least 75% the proportion of the nation's schools that provide nutrition education from preschool through twelfth grade, preferably as part of quality school health education.

2.20 Increase to at least 50% the proportion of work sites with 50 or more employees that offer nutrition education and/or weight management programs for employees.

2.21 Increase to at least 75% the proportion of primary care providers who provide nutrition assessment and counseling and/or referral to qualified nutritionists or dietitians.

1995 MIDCOURSE ADDITIONS
Health Status Objectives

2.22 **Reduce stroke deaths to no more than 20 per 100,000 people.**

2.23 **Reduce colorectal cancer deaths to no more than 13.2 per 100,000 people.**

2.24 **Reduce diabetes to an incidence of no more than 2.5 per 1000 people and a prevalence of 25 per 1000 people.**

Risk Reduction Objectives

2.25 Reduce the prevalence of blood cholesterol levels of 240 mg/dl or greater to no more than 20% of adults.

2.26 Increase to at least 50% the proportion of people with high blood pressure whose blood pressure is under control.

2.27 Reduce the mean serum cholesterol level among adults to no more than 200 mg/dl.

3. TOBACCO
Health Status Objectives

3.1 Reduce coronary heart disease deaths to no more than 100 per 100,000 people.

3.2 Slow the rise in lung cancer deaths to achieve a rate of no more than 42 per 100,000 people.

3.3 Slow the rise in deaths from chronic obstructive pulmonary disease to achieve a rate of no more than 25 per 100,000 people.

Risk Reduction Objectives

3.4 Reduce cigarette smoking to a prevalence of no more than 15% among people aged 20 and older.

3.5 Reduce the initiation of cigarette smoking by children and youth so that no more than 15% have become regular smokers by age 20.

3.6 Increase to at least 50% the proportion of cigarette smokers aged 18 and older who stopped smoking cigarettes for at least one day during the preceding year.

3.7 Increase smoking cessation during pregnancy so that at least 60% of women who are cigarette smokers at the time they become pregnant quit smoking early in pregnancy and maintain abstinence for the remainder of their pregnancy.

3.8 Reduce to no more than 20% the proportion of children aged 6 and younger who are regularly exposed to tobacco smoke at home.

3.9 Reduce smokeless tobacco use by males aged 12 through 24 to a prevalence of no more than 4%.

Services and Protection Objectives

3.10 Establish tobacco-free environments and include tobacco-use prevention in the curricula of all elementary, middle, and secondary schools, preferably as part of quality school health education.

3.11 Increase to at least 75% the proportion of worksites with a formal smoking policy that prohibits or severely restricts smoking in the workplace.

3.12 Enact in all 50 states comprehensive laws on clean indoor air that prohibit or strictly limit smoking in the workplace and enclosed public places (including health care facilities, schools, and public transportation).

+ 3.13 Enact and enforce in all 50 states laws prohibiting the sale and distribution of tobacco products to youths under age 19.

3.14 Increase to 50 the number of states with plans to reduce tobacco use, especially among youth.

3.15 Eliminate or severely restrict all forms of tobacco product advertising and promotion to which youths under age 18 are likely to be exposed.

3.16 Increase to at least 75% the proportion of primary care and oral health care providers who routinely advise cessation and provide assistance and follow-up for all of their tobacco-using patients.

1995 MIDCOURSE ADDITIONS
Health Status Objectives

3.17 Reduce deaths due to cancer of the oral cavity and pharynx to no more than 10.5 per 100,000 men aged 45 to 74 and 4.1 per 100,000 women aged 45 to 74.

3.18 Reduce stroke deaths to no more than 20 per 100,000 people.

Risk Reduction Objectives

3.19 Increase by at least 1 year the average age of first use of cigarettes, alcohol, and marijuana by adolescents aged 12 to 17.

3.20 Reduce the proportion of young people who have used alcohol, marijuana, cocaine, or cigarettes in the past month. (Target percentages vary with age and substance.)

3.21 Increase the proportion of high school seniors who perceive social disapproval of heavy use of alcohol (70%), occasional use of marijuana (85%), and experimentation with cocaine (95%), or regular use of cigarettes (95%).

3.22 Increase the proportion of high school seniors who associate physical or psychologic harm with heavy use of alcohol (70%), occasional use of marijuana (90%), and experimentation with cocaine (80%), or regular use of tobacco (95%).

Service and Protection Objectives

3.23 Increase the average (state and federal combined) tobacco excise tax to at least 50% of the average retail price of all cigarettes and smokeless tobacco.

3.24 Increase to 100% the proportion of health plans that offer treatment of nicotine addiction (e.g., tobacco use cessation counseling by health care providers, tobacco use cessation classes, prescriptions for nicotine replacement therapies, and/or other cessation services.)

3.25 Reduce to zero the number of states that have clean indoor air laws preempting stronger clean indoor air laws on the local level.

3.26 Enact in 50 states and the District of Columbia laws banning cigarette vending machines except in places inaccessible to minors.

+ **4. ALCOHOL AND OTHER DRUGS**
Health Status Objectives

4.1 Reduce deaths caused by alcohol-related motor vehicle crashes to no more than 8.5 per 100,000 people.

4.2 Reduce cirrhosis deaths to no more than 6 per 100,000 people.

4.3 Reduce drug-related deaths to no more than 3 per 100,000 people.

4.4 Reduce hospital emergency department visits related to drug abuse by at least 20%.

Risk Reduction Objectives

+ 4.5 Increase by at least 1 year the average age of first use of cigarettes, alcohol, and marijuana by adolescents aged 12 through 17.

4.6 Reduce the proportion of young people who have used alcohol, marijuana, and cocaine in the past month (met for ages 12 to 25 years).

4.7 Reduce the proportion of high school seniors and college students engaging in recent occasions of heavy drinking of alcoholic beverages to no more than 28% of high school seniors and 32% of college students.

4.8 Reduce alcohol consumption by people aged 14 and older to an annual average of no more than 2 gallons of ethanol per person.

4.9 Increase the proportion of high school seniors who perceive social disapproval associated with heavy use of alcohol, occasional use of marijuana, and experimentation with cocaine.

4.10 Increase the proportion of high school seniors who associate risk of physical and psychologic harm with the heavy use of alcohol, regular use of marijuana, and experimentation with cocaine.

4.11 Reduce to no more than 3% the proportion of male high school seniors who use anabolic steroids.

Services and Protection Objectives

4.12 Establish and monitor in all 50 states comprehensive plans to ensure access to alcohol and drug treatment programs for traditionally underserved people.

4.13 Provide to children in all school districts and private schools primary and secondary school educational programs on alcohol and other drugs, preferably as a part of quality school health education.

4.14 Extend adoption of alcohol and drug policies for the work environment to at least 60% of worksites with 50 or more employees.

4.15 Extend to all 50 states administrative driver's license suspension/revocation laws or programs of equal effectiveness for people determined to have been driving under the influence of intoxicants.

4.16 Increase to 50 the number of states that have enacted and enforce policies to reduce access to alcoholic beverages by minors.

4.17 Increase to at least 20 the number of states that have enacted statutes to restrict promotion of alcoholic beverages that is focused principally on young audiences.

4.18 Extend to all 50 states legal blood alcohol concentration tolerance levels of .04% for motor vehicle drivers aged 21 and older and .00% for those younger than age 21.

4.19 Increase to at least 75% the proportion of primary care providers who screen for alcohol and other drug use problems and provide counseling and referral as needed.

1995 MIDCOURSE ADDITION
Services and Protection Objective

4.20 Increase to 30 the number of states with hospitality resource panels (including representatives from state regulatory, public health, and highway safety agencies; law enforcement; insurance associations; and alcohol retail and licensed beverage associations) to ensure a process of management and server training and define standards of responsible hospitality.

5. FAMILY PLANNING
Health Status Objectives

5.1 Reduce pregnancies among girls aged 17 and younger to no more than 50 per 1000 adolescents.

5.2 Reduce to no more than 30% the proportion of all pregnancies that are unintended.

5.3 Reduce the prevalence of infertility to no more than 6.5%.

Risk Reduction Objectives

5.4 Reduce the proportion of adolescents who have engaged in sexual intercourse by age 15 to no more than 15% and by age 17 to no more than 40%.

5.5 Increase to at least 40% the proportion of adolescents aged 17 and younger who have ever been sexually active that have abstained from sexual activity for the previous 3 months.

5.6 Increase to at least 90% the proportion of sexually active unmarried people aged 19 and younger who use contraception, especially combined-method contraception that both effectively prevents pregnancy and provides barrier protection against disease.

5.7 Increase the effectiveness with which family planning methods are used, as measured by a decrease to no more than 5% in the proportion of couples experiencing pregnancy despite use of a contraceptive method.

Services and Protection Objectives

5.8 Increase to at least 85% the proportion of people aged 10 through 18 who have discussed human sexuality, including values surrounding sexuality, with their parents and/or have received information through other parentally endorsed sources, such as school, religious, or youth programs.

5.9 Increase to at least 90% the proportion of pregnancy counselors who offer positive, accurate information about adoption to their unmarried patients with unintended pregnancies.

5.10 Increase to at least 60% the proportion of primary care providers who provide age-appropriate preconception care and counseling.

5.11 Increase to at least 50% the proportion of the following kinds of clinics that screen, diagnose, treat, counsel, and provide (or refer for) partner notification services for HIV infection and bacterial sexually transmitted diseases (gonorrhea, syphilis, and chlamydia): family planning clinics, maternal and child health clinics, sexually transmitted disease clinics, tuberculosis clinics, drug treatment centers, and primary care clinics.

1995 MIDCOURSE ADDITION
Risk Reduction Objectives

5.12 Increase to at lest 95% the proportion of all females aged 15 to 44 at risk of unintended pregnancy who use contraception.

6. MENTAL HEALTH AND MENTAL DISORDERS
Health Status Objectives

6.1 Reduce suicides to no more than 10.5 per 100,000 people.

6.2 Reduce by 15% the incidence of injurious suicide attempts among adolescents aged 14 through 19.

6.3 Reduce to less than 10% the prevalence of mental disorders among children and adolescents.

6.4 Reduce the prevalence of mental disorders (exclusive of substance abuse) among adults living in the community to less than 10.7%.

6.5 Reduce to less than 35% the proportion of people aged 18 and older who within the past year have experienced adverse health effects from stress.

Risk Reduction Objectives

6.6 Increase to at least 30% the proportion of people aged 18 and older with severe, persistent mental disorders who use community support programs.

6.7 Increase to at least 45% the proportion of people with major depressive disorders who obtain treatment.

6.8 Increase to at least 20% the proportion of people aged 18 and older who seek help in coping with personal and emotional problems.

6.9 Decrease to no more than 5% the proportion of people aged 18 and older who report experiencing significant levels of stress who do not take steps to reduce or control their stress.

Services and Protection Objectives

6.10 In order to facilitate identification and appropriate intervention to prevent suicide by jail inmates, increase to 50 the number of states with officially established protocols that engage mental health, alcohol, drug, and public health authorities with corrections authorities.

6.11 Increase to at least 40% the proportion of work sites employing 50 or more people that provide programs to reduce employee stress.

+ **6.12 Establish mutual-help clearinghouses in at least 25 states.**

6.13 Increase to at least 50% the proportion of primary care providers who routinely review with patients their patients' cognitive, emotional, and behavioral functioning and the resources available to deal with any problems that are identified.

6.14 Increase to at least 75% the proportion of providers of primary care for children who include assessment of cognitive, emotional, and parent-child functioning, with appropriate counseling, referral, and follow-up, in their clinical practices.

1995 MIDCOURSE ADDITION
Health Status Objective

6.15 Reduce the prevalence of depressive (affective) disorders among adults living in the community to less than 4.3%.

7. VIOLENT AND ABUSIVE BEHAVIOR
Health Status Objectives

7.1 Reduce homicides to no more than 7.2 per 100,000 people.

7.2 Reduce suicides to no more than 10.5 per 100,000 people.

7.3 Reduce weapon-related violent deaths to no more than 12.6 per 100,000 people.

7.4 Reverse to less than 25.2 per 1000 children the rising incidence of maltreatment of children younger than age 18.

7.5 Reduce physical abuse directed at women by male partners to no more than 27 per 1000 couples.

7.6 Reduce assault injuries among people aged 12 and older to no more than 10 per 1000 people.

+ **7.7 Reduce rape and attempted rape of women aged 12 and older to no more than 107 per 100,000 women.**

7.8 Reduce by 15% the incidence of injurious suicide attempts among adolescents aged 14 to 19.

Risk Reduction Objectives

7.9 Reduce by 20% the incidence of physical fighting among adolescents aged 14 through 17.

7.10 Reduce by 20% the incidence of weapon-carrying by adolescents aged 14 through 17.

7.11 Reduce by 20% the proportion of weapons that are inappropriately stored and therefore available and dangerous.

Services and Protection Objectives

7.12 Extend protocols to at least 90% of hospital emergency departments for routinely identifying, treating, and properly referring victims of sexual assault; victims of spouse, elder, and child abuse; and those who have attempted suicide.

7.13 Extend to at least 45 states implementation of unexplained child death review systems.

7.14 Increase to at least 30 the number of states in which at least 50% of children identified as physically or sexually abused receive physical and mental evaluation with appropriate follow-up as a means of breaking the intergenerational cycle of abuse.

7.15 Reduce to less than 10% the proportion of battered women and their children turned away from emergency housing because of lack of space.

7.16 Increase to at least 50% the proportion of elementary and secondary schools that teach nonviolent conflict resolution skills, preferably as part of quality school health education.

7.17 Extend coordinated, comprehensive violence prevention programs to at least 80% of local jurisdictions with populations over 100,000.

7.18 In order to facilitate identification and appropriate intervention to prevent suicide by jail inmates, increase to 50 the number of states with officially established protocols that engage mental health, alcohol, drug, and public health authorities with corrections authorities.

1995 MIDCOURSE ADDITION
Services and Protection Objective

7.19 Enact in 50 states and the District of Columbia laws requiring that firearms be properly stored to minimize access and the likelihood of discharge by minors.

8. EDUCATIONAL AND COMMUNITY-BASED PROGRAMS
Health Status Objective

8.1 Increase years of healthy life to at least 65 years.

Risk Reduction Objective

8.2 Increase the high school graduation rate to at least 90%, thereby reducing risks for multiple problem behaviors and poor mental and physical health.

Services and Protection Objectives

8.3 Achieve for all disadvantaged children and children with disabilities access to high-quality and developmentally appropriate preschool programs that help prepare children for school, thereby improving their prospects with regard to school performance, behavior, and mental and physical health.

8.4 Increase to at least 75% the proportion of the nation's elementary and secondary schools that provide planned and sequential quality school health education from kindergarten through twelfth grade.

8.5 Increase to at least 50% the proportion of postsecondary institutions with institution-wide health promotion programs for students, faculty, and staff.

8.6 Increase to at least 85% the proportion of workplaces with 50 or more employees that offer health promotion activities for their employees, preferably as part of a comprehensive employee health promotion program.

8.7 Increase to at least 20% the proportion of hourly workers who participate regularly in employer-sponsored health promotion activities.

8.8 Increase to at least 90% the proportion of people aged 65 and older who during the preceding year had the opportunity to participate in at least one organized health promotion program through a senior center, lifecare facility, or other community-based setting serving older adults.

8.9 Increase to at least 75% the proportion of people aged 10 and older who have discussed issues related to nutrition, physical activity, sexual behavior, tobacco, alcohol, other drugs, or safety with family members on at least one occasion during the preceding month.

8.10 Establish community health promotion programs that separately or together address at least three of the Healthy People 2000 priorities and reach at least 40% of each state's population.

8.11 Increase to at least 50% the proportion of counties that have established culturally and linguistically appropriate community health promotion programs for racial and ethnic minority populations.

8.12 Increase to at least 90% the proportion of hospitals, health maintenance organizations, and large group practices that provide patient education programs, and to at least 90% the proportion of community hospitals that offer community health programs addressing the priority health needs of their communities.

8.13 Increase to at least 75% the proportion of local television network affiliates in the top 20 television markets that have been become partners with one or more community organizations in working toward one of the health problems addressed by the Healthy People 2000 objectives.

8.14 Increase to at least 90% the proportion of people who are served by a local health department that is effectively carrying out the core functions of public health.

9. UNINTENTIONAL INJURIES

Health Status Objectives

+ 9.1 **Reduce deaths caused by unintentional injuries to no more than 29.3 per 100,000 people.**

+ 9.2 **Reduce nonfatal unintentional injuries so that hospitalizations for this condition are no more than 754 per 100,000 people.**

+ 9.3 **Reduce deaths caused by motor vehicle crashes to no more than 1.9 per 100 million vehicle miles traveled and 17 per 100,000 people.**

9.4 Reduce deaths from falls and from fall-related injuries to no more than 2.3 per 100,000.

9.5 Reduce deaths by drowning to no more than 1.3 per 100,000 people.

9.6 Reduce deaths resulting from residential fire to no more than 1.2 per 100,000 people.

9.7 Reduce hip fractures among people aged 65 and older so that hospitalizations for this condition are no more than 620 per 100,000 people.

+ 9.8 **Reduce nonfatal poisoning to no more than 88 emergency department treatments per 100,000 people.**

+ 9.9 **Reduce nonfatal head injuries so that hospitalizations for this condition are no more than 106 per 100,000 people.**

+ 9.10 **Reduce nonfatal spinal cord injuries so that hospitalizations for this condition are no more than 4.5 per 100,000 people.**

9.11 Reduce the incidence of secondary disabilities associated with head injuries to no more than 16 per 100,000 people and the incidence of secondary disabilities associated with spinal cord injuries to no more than 2.6 per 100,000 people.

Risk Reduction Objectives

9.12 Increase use of occupant protection systems, such as safety belts, inflatable safety restraints, and child safety seats, to at least 85% of motor vehicle occupants.

9.13 Increase use of helmets to at least 80% of motorcyclists and at least 50% of bicyclists.

Services and Protection Objectives

9.14 Extend to all 50 states laws requiring safety belt and motorcycle helmet use for all ages.

9.15 Enact in all 50 states laws requiring that new handguns be designed to minimize the likelihood of discharge by children.

9.16 Extend to 2000 the number of jurisdictions whose codes address the installation of fire-suppression sprinkler systems in those residences at highest risk for fires.

9.17 Increase the presence of functional smoke detectors to at least one on each habitable floor of all inhabited residential dwellings.

9.18 Provide academic instruction on injury prevention and control, preferably as part of quality school health education, in at least 50% of public school systems (grades K through 12).

+ **9.19 Extend requirement of the use of effective head, face, eye, and mouth protection to all organizations, agencies, and institutions sponsoring sporting and recreation events that pose risks of injury.**

9.20 Increase to at least 30 the number of states that have design standards for signs, signals, markings, lighting, and other characteristics of the roadway environment to improve the visual stimuli and protect the safety of older drivers and pedestrians.

9.21 Increase to at least 50% the proportion of primary care providers who routinely provide age-appropriate counseling on safety precautions to prevent unintentional injury.

9.22 Increase to 50 the number of states having emergency medical services and trauma systems that link prehospital, hospital, and rehabilitation services in order to prevent trauma deaths and long-term disability.

1995 MIDCOURSE ADDITIONS

Health Status Objective

9.23 Reduce deaths caused by alcohol-related motor vehicle crashes to no more than 5.5 per 100,000 people.

Services and Protection Objectives

9.24 Extend to 40 states laws requiring helmets for bicycle riders.

9.25 Enact in 50 states laws requiring that firearms be properly stored to minimize access and the likelihood of discharge by minors.

9.26 Increase to 35 the number of states having a graduated driver licensing system for novice drivers and riders under the age of 18.

10. OCCUPATIONAL SAFETY AND HEALTH

Health Status Objectives

10.1 Reduce deaths from work-related injuries to no more than 4 per 100,000 full-time workers.

10.2 Reduce work-related injuries resulting in medical treatment, lost time from work, or restricted work activity to no more than 6 cases per 100 full-time workers.

10.3 Reduce cumulative trauma disorders to an incidence of no more than 60 cases per 100,000 full-time workers.

10.4 Reduce occupational skin disorders or diseases to an incidence of no more than 55 per 100,000 full-time workers.

+ **10.5 Reduce hepatitis B infections among occupationally exposed workers to an incidence of no more than 1250 cases.**

Risk Reduction Objectives

10.6 Increase to at least 75% the proportion of work sites with 50 or more employees that mandate employee use of occupant protection systems, such as seat belts, during all work-related motor vehicle travel.

10.7 Reduce to no more than 15% the proportion of workers exposed to average daily noise levels that exceed 85 decibels.

10.8 Eliminate exposures that result in workers having blood lead concentrations greater than 25 mg/dl of whole blood.

10.9 Increase hepatitis B immunization levels to 90% among occupationally exposed workers.

Services and Protection Objectives

10.10 Implement occupational safety and health plans in all 50 states for the identification, management, and prevention of leading work-related diseases and injuries within each state.

+ **10.11 Establish in all 50 states exposure standards adequate to prevent the major occupational lung diseases to which their worker populations are exposed (byssinosis, asbestosis, coal workers' pneumoconiosis, and silicosis).**

10.12 Increase to at least 70% the proportion of work sites with 50 or more employees that have implemented programs on worker health and safety.

10.13 Increase to at least 50% the proportion of work sites with 50 or more employees that offer back injury prevention and rehabilitation programs.

10.14 Establish in all 50 states either public health or labor department programs that provide consultation and assistance to small businesses to implement safety and health programs for their employees.

10.15 Increase to 75% the proportion of primary care providers who routinely elicit occupational health exposures as part of patient history and provide relevant counseling.

1995 MIDCOURSE ADDITIONS

Health Status Objectives

10.16 Reduce deaths from work-related homicides to no more than 0.5 per 100,000 full-time workers.

10.17 Reduce the overall age-adjusted mortality rate for four major preventable occupational lung diseases (byssinosis, asbestosis, coal workers' pneumoconiosis, and silicosis).

Services and Protection Objectives

10.18 Increase to 100% the proportion of worksites with a formal smoking policy that prohibits or severely restricts smoking at the workplace.

10.19 Enact in 50 states and the District of Columbia comprehensive laws on clean indoor air that prohibit smoking or limit it to separately ventilated areas in the workplace and enclosed public places.

10.20 Reduce to zero the number of states that have clean indoor air laws preempting stronger clean indoor air laws on the local level.

11. ENVIRONMENTAL HEALTH
Health Status Objectives

11.1 Reduce asthma morbidity, as measured by a reduction in asthma hospitalizations to no more than 160 per 100,000 people.

11.2 Reduce the prevalence of serious mental retardation among school-aged children to no more than 2 per 1000 children.

11.3 Reduce outbreaks of waterborne disease from infectious agents and chemical poisoning to no more than 11 per year.

+ **11.4** **Reduce among children aged 6 months through 5 years the prevalence of blood lead levels exceeding 15 mg/dl and 25 mg/dl to no more than 500,000 and zero, respectively.**

Risk Reduction Objectives

11.5 Reduce human exposure to criteria air pollutants, as measured by an increase to at least 85% in the proportion of people who live in counties that have not exceeded any Environmental Protection Agency standard for air quality in the previous 12 months.

11.6 Increase to at least 40% the proportion of homes in which homeowners/occupants have tested for radon concentrations and that have either been found to pose minimal risk or have been modified to reduce risk to health.

11.7 Reduce human exposure to toxic agents by confining total pounds of toxic agents released into the air, water, and soil each year to no more than:
- 0.24 billion pounds of those toxic agents included on the Department of Health and Human Services list of carcinogens.
- 2.6 billion pounds of those toxic agents included on the Agency for Toxic Substances and Disease Registry list of the most toxic chemicals.

11.8 Reduce human exposure to solid waste–related water, air, and soil contamination, as measured by a reduction in the average amount of municipal solid waste produced per person each day to no more than 3.6 pounds.

11.9 Increase to at least 85% the proportion of people who receive a supply of drinking water that meets the safe drinking water standards established by the Environmental Protection Agency.

11.10 Reduce potential risks to human health from surface water, as measured by a decrease to no more than 15% in the proportion of assessed rivers, lakes, and estuaries that do not support beneficial uses, such as fishing and swimming.

Services and Protection Objectives

11.11 Perform testing for lead-based paint in at least 50% of homes built before 1950.

11.12 Expand to at least 35 the number of states in which at least 75% of local jurisdictions have adopted construction standards and techniques that minimize elevated indoor radon levels in those new building areas locally determined to have elevated radon levels.

11.13 Increase to at least 30 the number of states requiring that prospective buyers be informed of the presence of lead-based paint and radon concentrations in all buildings offered for sale.

11.14 Eliminate significant health risks from National Priority List hazardous waste sites, as measured by performance of clean-up at these sites sufficient to eliminate immediate and significant health threats as specified in health assessments completed at all sites.

11.15 Establish programs for recyclable materials and household hazardous waste in at least 75% of counties.

11.16 Establish and monitor in at least 35 states plans to define and track sentinel environmental diseases.

1995 MIDCOURSE ADDITION
Risk Reduction Objective

11.17 **Reduce to no more than 20% the proportion of children aged 6 and younger who are regularly exposed to tobacco smoke at home.**

12. FOOD AND DRUG SAFETY
Health Status Objectives

+ **12.1** **Reduce infections caused by key foodborne pathogens (e.g., *Salmonella*, *Campylobacter jejuni*, *Escherichia coli* 0157:H7, and *Listeria monocytogenes*).**

12.2 Reduce outbreaks of infections due to *Salmonella enteritidis* to fewer than 25 outbreaks yearly.

Risk Reduction Objective

12.3 Increase to at least 75% the proportion of households in which principal food preparers routinely refrain from leaving perishable food out of the refrigerator for over 2 hours and wash cutting boards and utensils with soap after contact with raw meat and poultry.

Services and Protection Objectives

12.4 Extend to at least 70% the proportion of states and territories that have implemented model food codes for institutional food operations and to at least 70% the proportion that have adopted the new uniform food protection code ("Unicode") that sets recommended standards for regulation of all food operations.

12.5 Increase to at least 75% the proportion of pharmacies and other dispensers of prescription medications that use linked systems to provide alerts to potential adverse drug reactions among medications dispensed by different sources to individual patients.

12.6   Increase to at least 75% the proportion of primary care providers who routinely review with their patients aged 65 and older all prescribed and over-the-counter medicines taken by their patients each time a new medication is prescribed.

1995 MIDCOURSE ADDITION
Services and Protection Objectives

12.7   **Increase to at least 75% the proportion of the total number of adverse event reports voluntarily sent directly to the FDA that are regarded as serious.**

12.8   **Increase to at least 75% the proportion of people who receive useful information verbally and in writing for new prescriptions from prescribers or dispensers.**

13. ORAL HEALTH
Health Status Objectives

13.1   Reduce dental caries (cavities) so that the proportion of children with one or more caries in permanent or primary teeth is no more than 35% among children aged 6 through 8 and no more than 60% among adolescents aged 15.

13.2   Reduce untreated dental caries so that the proportion of children with untreated caries in permanent or primary teeth is no more than 20% among children aged 6 through 8 and no more than 15% among adolescents aged 15.

13.3   Increase to at least 45% the proportion of people aged 35 through 44 who have never lost a permanent tooth due to dental caries or periodontal disease.

13.4   Reduce to no more than 20% the proportion of people aged 65 and older who have lost all of their natural teeth.

13.5   Reduce the prevalence of gingivitis among people aged 35 through 44 to no more than 30%.

13.6   Reduce destructive periodontal diseases to a prevalence of no more than 15% among people aged 35 through 44.

13.7   Reduce deaths due to cancer of the oral cavity and pharynx to no more than 10.5 per 100,000 men aged 45 through 74 and to 4.1 per 100,000 women aged 45 through 74.

Risk Reduction Objectives

13.8   Increase to at least 50% the proportion of children who have received protective sealants on the occlusal (chewing) surfaces of permanent molar teeth.

13.9   Increase to at least 75% the proportion of people served by community water systems providing optimal levels of fluoride.

13.10   Increase use of professionally or self-administered topical or systemic (dietary) fluorides to at least 85% of people not receiving optimally fluoridated public water.

13.11   Increase to at least 75% the proportion of parents and caregivers who use feeding practices that prevent baby bottle tooth decay.

Services and Protection Objectives

13.12   Increase to at least 90% the proportion of all children entering school programs for the first time who have received an oral health screening, referral, and follow-up for necessary diagnostic, preventive, and treatment services.

13.13   Extend to all long-term institutional facilities the requirement that oral examinations and services be provided no later than 90 days after entry into these facilities.

13.14   Increase to at least 70% the proportion of people aged 35 and older using the oral health care system during each year.

13.15   Increase to at least 40 the number of states that have an effective system for recording and referring infants with cleft lips and/or palates to craniofacial anomaly teams.

13.16   Extend requirement of the use of effective head, face, eye, and mouth protection to all organizations, agencies, and institutions sponsoring sporting and recreation events that pose risks of injury.

1995 MIDCOURSE ADDITION
Risk Reduction Objectives

13.17   **Reduce smokeless tobacco use by males aged 12 to 24 to a prevalence of no more than 4%.**

14. MATERNAL AND INFANT HEALTH
Health Status Objectives

14.1   Reduce the infant mortality rate to no more than 7 per 1000 live births.

14.2   Reduce the fetal death rate (20 or more weeks of gestation) to no more than 5 per 1000 cases of live births and fetal deaths combined.

14.3   Reduce the maternal mortality rate to no more than 3.3 per 100,000 live births.

14.4   Reduce the incidence of fetal alcohol syndrome to no more than 0.12 per 1000 live births.

Risk Reduction Objectives

14.5   Reduce low birth weight to an incidence of no more than 5% of live births and very low birth weight to no more than 1% of live births.

14.6   Increase to at least 85% the proportion of mothers who achieve the minimum recommended weight gain during their pregnancies.

14.7   Reduce severe complications of pregnancy to no more than 15 per 100 deliveries.

14.8 Reduce the caesarean delivery rate to no more than 15 per 100 deliveries.

14.9 Increase to at least 75% the proportion of mothers who breastfeed their babies in the early postpartum period and to at least 50% the proportion who continue breastfeeding until their babies are 5 to 6 months old.

14.10 Increase abstinence from tobacco use by pregnant women to at least 90% and increase abstinence from alcohol, cocaine, and marijuana by pregnant women by at least 20%.

Services and Protection Objectives

14.11 Increase to at least 90% the proportion of all pregnant women who receive prenatal care in the first trimester of pregnancy.

14.12 Increase to at least 60% the proportion of primary care providers who provide age-appropriate preconception care and counseling.

14.13 Increase to at least 90% the proportion of women enrolled in prenatal care who are offered screening and counseling on prenatal detection of fetal abnormalities.

14.14 Increase to at least 90% the proportion of pregnant women and infants who receive risk-appropriate care.

+ **14.15 Increase to at least 95% the proportion of newborns screened by state-sponsored programs for genetic disorders and other disabling conditions and to 90% the proportion of newborns testing positive for disease who receive appropriate treatment. (for galactosemia only)**

14.16 Increase to at least 90% the proportion of babies aged 18 months and younger who receive recommended primary care services at the appropriate intervals.

1995 MIDCOURSE ADDITION
Health Status Objective

14.17 Reduce the incidence of spina bifida and other neural tube defects to 3 per 10,000 live births.

15. HEART DISEASE AND STROKE
Health Status Objectives

15.1 Reduce coronary heart disease deaths to no more than 100 per 100,000 people.

15.2 Reduce stroke deaths to no more than 20 per 100,000 people.

15.3 Reverse the increase in end-stage renal disease (requiring maintenance dialysis or transplantation) to attain an incidence of no more than 13 per 100,000.

Risk Reduction Objectives

15.4 Increase to at least 50% the proportion of people with high blood pressure whose blood pressure is under control.

15.5 Increase to at least 90% the proportion of people with high blood pressure who are taking action to help control their blood pressure.

15.6 Reduce the mean serum cholesterol level among adults to no more than 200 mg/dl.

+ **15.7 Reduce the prevalence of blood cholesterol levels of 240 mg/dl or greater to no more than 20% of the adult population.**

15.8 Increase to at least 60% the proportion of adults with high blood cholesterol who are aware of their condition and are taking action to reduce their blood cholesterol to recommended levels.

15.9 Reduce dietary fat intake to an average of 30% of calories or less and average saturated fat intake to less than 10% of calories among people aged 2 and older.

15.10 Reduce overweight to a prevalence of no more than 20% among people aged 20 and older and no more than 15% among adolescents aged 12 through 19.

15.11 Increase to at least 30% the proportion of people aged 6 and older who engage regularly, preferably daily, in light to moderate physical activity for at least 30 minutes per day.

15.12 Reduce cigarette smoking to a prevalence of no more than 15% among people aged 20 and older.

Services and Protection Objectives

15.13 Increase to at least 90% the proportion of adults who have had their blood pressure measured within the preceding 2 years and can state whether their blood pressure was normal, high, or low.

15.14 Increase to at least 75% the proportion of adults who have had their blood cholesterol checked within the preceding 5 years.

15.15 Increase to at least 75% the proportion of primary care providers who initiate diet for patients with high blood cholesterol and, if necessary, drug therapy at levels of blood cholesterol consistent with current management guidelines.

15.16 Increase to at least 50% the proportion of work sites with 50 or more employees that offer high blood pressure and/or cholesterol education and control activities to their employees.

15.17 Increase to at least 90% the proportion of clinical laboratories that meet the recommended accuracy standard for cholesterol measurement.

16. CANCER
Health Status Objectives

16.1 Reverse the rise in cancer deaths to achieve a rate of no more than 130 per 100,000 people.

16.2 Slow the rise in lung cancer deaths to achieve a rate of no more than 42 per 100,000 people.

16.3 Reduce breast cancer deaths to no more than 20.6 per 100,000 women.

16.4 Reduce deaths from cancer of the uterine cervix to no more than 1.3 per 100,000 women.

+16.5 Reduce colorectal cancer deaths to no more than 13.2 per 100,000 people.

Risk Reduction Objectives

16.6 Reduce cigarette smoking to a prevalence of no more than 15% among people aged 20 and older.

16.7 Reduce dietary fat intake to an average of 30% of calories or less and average saturated fat intake to less than 10% of calories among people aged 2 and older.

16.8 Increase complex carbohydrate and fiber-containing foods in the diets of adults to five or more daily servings for vegetables (including legumes) and fruits, and to six or more daily servings for grain products.

16.9 Increase to at least 60% the proportion of people of all ages who limit sun exposure, use sunscreens and protective clothing when exposed to sunlight, and avoid artificial sources of ultraviolet light (e.g., sun lamps, tanning booths).

Services and Protection Objectives

+16.10 Increase to at least 75% the proportion of primary care providers who routinely counsel patients about tobacco use cessation, diet modification, and cancer screening recommendations.

16.11 Increase to at least 80% the proportion of women aged 40 and older who have ever received a clinical breast examination and a mammogram, and to at least 60% those aged 50 and older who have received them within the preceding 1 to 2 years.

+16.12 Increase to at least 95% the proportion of women aged 18 and older with uterine cervix who have ever received a Pap test, and to at least 85% those who received a Pap test within the preceding 1 to 3 years.

16.13 Increase to at least 50% the proportion of people aged 50 and older who have received fecal occult blood testing within the preceding 1 to 2 years, and to at least 40% those who have ever received proctosigmoidoscopy.

16.14 Increase to at least 40% the proportion of people aged 50 and older visiting a primary care provider who have received oral, skin, and digital rectal examinations during a visit within the preceding year.

16.15 Ensure that Pap tests meet quality standards by monitoring and certifying all cytology laboratories.

16.16 Ensure that mammograms meet quality standards by monitoring and certifying at least 80% of mammography facilities.

1995 MIDCOURSE ADDITION
Health Status Objective

16.17 Reduce deaths due to cancer of the oral cavity and pharynx to no more than 10.5 per 100,000 men aged 45 to 74 and 4.1 per 100,000 women aged 45 to 74.

17. DIABETES AND CHRONIC DISABLING CONDITIONS
Health Status Objectives (Chronic Disabling Conditions)

17.1 Increase years of healthy life to at least 65 years.

17.2 Reduce to no more than 8% the proportion of people who experience a limitation in major activity due to chronic conditions.

17.3 Reduce to no more than 90 per 1000 people the proportion of all people aged 65 and older who have difficulty in performing two or more personal activities, thereby preserving independence.

17.4 Reduce to no more than 10% the proportion of people with asthma who experience activity limitation.

17.5 Reduce activity limitation due to chronic back conditions to a prevalence of no more than 19 per 1000 people.

17.6 Reduce significant hearing impairment to a prevalence of no more than 82 per 1000 people.

17.7 Reduce significant visual impairment to a prevalence of no more than 30 per 1000 people.

17.8 Reduce the prevalence of serious mental retardation in school-aged children to no more than 2 per 1000 children.

Diabetes

17.9 Reduce diabetes-related deaths to no more than 34 per 100,000.

17.10 Reduce the most severe complications of diabetes (i.e., end-stage renal disease, blindness, lower extremity amputation, perinatal mortality, and major congenital malformations).

17.11 Reduce diabetes to an incidence of no more than 2.5 per 1000 people and a prevalence of no more than 25 per 1000 people.

Risk Reduction Objectives

17.12 Reduce overweight to a prevalence of no more than 20% among people aged 20 and older and no more than 15% among adolescents aged 12 through 19.

17.13 Increase to at least 30% the proportion of people aged 6 and older who engage regularly, preferably daily, in light to moderate physical activity for at least 30 minutes per day.

Services and Protection Objectives

17.14 Increase to at least 40% the proportion of people with chronic and disabling conditions who receive formal patient education including information about community and self-help resources as an integral part of the management of their conditions.

17.15 Increase to at least 80% the proportion of providers of primary care for children who routinely refer or screen infants and children for impairments of vision, hearing, speech, and language, and assess other developmental milestones as part of well-child care.

17.16 Reduce the average age at which children with significant hearing impairment are identified to no more than 12 months.

17.17 Increase to at least 60% the proportion of providers of primary care for older adults who routinely evaluate people aged 65 and older for urinary incontinence and impairments of vision, hearing, cognition, and functional status.

17.18 Increase to at least 90% the proportion of perimenopausal women who have been counseled about the benefits and risks of estrogen replacement therapy (combined with progestin, when appropriate) for prevention of osteoporosis.

+17.19 **Increase to at least 75% the proportion of work sites with 50 or more employees that have a voluntarily established policy or program for hiring people with disabilities.**

17.20 Increase to 50 the number of states that have service systems for children at risk of or having chronic and disabling conditions, as required by Public Law 101-239.

1995 MIDCOURSE ADDITIONS
Health Status Objectives

17.21 **Reduce the prevalence of peptic ulcer disease to no more than 18 per 1000 people aged 18 and older by preventing its recurrence.**

17.22 **Develop and implement a national process to identify significant gaps in the nation's disease-prevention and health-promotion data, including data for racial and ethnic minorities, people with low incomes, and people with disabilities, and establish mechanisms to meet these needs.**

Services and Protection Objective

17.23 **Increase to 75% the proportion of people with diabetes who have an annual dilated eye examination.**

18. HIV INFECTION
Health Status Objectives

18.1 Confine annual incidence of diagnosed AIDS cases to no more than 98,000 cases.

18.2 Confine the prevalence of HIV infection to no more than 800 per 100,000.

Risk Reduction Objectives

18.3 Reduce the proportion of adolescents who have engaged in sexual intercourse by age 15 to no more than 15% and by age 17 to no more than 40%.

18.4 Increase to at least 50% the proportion of sexually active unmarried people who used a condom during last sexual intercourse.

18.5 Increase to at least 50% the estimated proportion of all intravenous drug users who are in drug abuse treatment programs.

+18.6 **Increase to at least 50% the estimated proportion of intravenous drug users not in treatment who use only uncontaminated drug paraphernalia ("works").**

18.7 Reduce to no more than 1 per 250,000 units of blood and blood components the risk of transfusion-transmitted HIV infection.

Services and Protection Objectives

18.8 Increase to at least 80% the proportion of HIV-infected people who have been tested for HIV infection.

18.9 Increase to at least 75% the proportion of primary care and mental health care providers who provide age-appropriate counseling on the prevention of HIV and other sexually transmitted diseases.

18.10 Increase to at least 95% the proportion of schools that have age-appropriate HIV education curricula for students in fourth through twelfth grade, preferably as part of quality school health education.

18.11 Provide HIV education for students and staff in at least 90% of colleges and universities.

18.12 Increase to at least 90% the proportion of cities with populations over 100,000 that have outreach programs to contact drug users (particularly intravenous drug users) to deliver HIV risk reduction messages.

18.13 Increase to at least 50% the proportion of the following kinds of clinics that screen, diagnose, treat, counsel, and provide (or refer for) partner notification services for HIV infection and bacterial sexually transmitted diseases (gonorrhea, syphilis, and chlamydia): family planning clinics, maternal and child health clinics, sexually transmitted disease clinics, tuberculosis clinics, drug treatment centers, and primary care clinics.

+18.14 Extend to all facilities where workers are at risk for occupational transmission of HIV regulations to protect workers from exposure to bloodborne infections, including HIV infection.

1995 MIDCOURSE ADDITIONS
Risk Reduction Objectives

18.15 **Increase to at least 40% the proportion of ever sexually active adolescents aged 17 and younger who have not had sexual intercourse for the previous 3 months.**

18.16 **Increase to at least 50% the proportion of large businesses and to 10% the proportion of small businesses that implemented a comprehensive HIV/ AIDS workplace program.**

18.17 **Increase to at least 40% the number of federally funded primary care clinics that have formal established linkages with substance abuse treatment programs that have formal established linkages with primary care clinics.**

19. SEXUALLY TRANSMITTED DISEASES
Health Status Objectives

+ **19.1** **Reduce gonorrhea to an incidence of no more than 225 cases per 100,000 people.**

19.2 Reduce *Chlamydia trachomatis* infections, as measured by a decrease in the incidence of nongonococcal urethritis, to no more than 170 cases per 100,000 people.

19.3 Reduce primary and secondary syphilis to an incidence of no more than 10 cases per 100,000 people.

19.4 Reduce congenital syphilis to an incidence of no more than 50 cases per 100,000 live births.

+ **19.5** **Reduce genital herpes and genital warts, as measured by reductions to 142,000 and 385,000, respectively, in the annual number of first-time consultations with a physician for the conditions (for genital warts only).**

+ **19.6** **Reduce the incidence of pelvic inflammatory disease, as measured by a reduction in hospitalizations for the condition, to no more than 250 per 100,000 women aged 15 through 44.**

19.7 Reduce sexually transmitted hepatitis B infection to no more than 30,500 cases.

19.8 Reduce the rate of repeat gonorrhea infection to no more than 15% within the previous year.

Risk Reduction Objectives

19.9 Reduce the proportion of adolescents who have engaged in sexual intercourse by age 15 to no more than 15% and by age 17 to no more than 40%.

19.10 Increase to at least 50% the proportion of sexually active unmarried people who used a condom during last sexual intercourse.

Services and Protection Objectives

19.11 Increase to at least 50% the proportion of the following kinds of clinics that screen, diagnose, treat, counsel, and provide (or refer for) partner notification services for HIV infection and bacterial sexually transmitted disease (gonorrhea, syphilis, and chlamydia): family planning clinics, maternal and child health clinics, sexually transmitted disease clinics, tuberculosis clinics, drug treatment centers, and primary care clinics.

19.12 Include instruction in preventing transmission of sexually transmitted diseases in the curricula of all middle and secondary schools, preferably as part of quality school health education.

19.13 Increase to at least 90% the proportion of primary care providers treating patients with sexually transmitted diseases who correctly manage cases, as measured by their use of appropriate types and amounts of therapy.

19.14 Increase to at least 75% the proportion of primary care and mental health care providers who provide age-appropriate counseling on the prevention of HIV and other sexually transmitted diseases.

19.15 Increase to at least 50% the proportion of all patients with bacterial sexually transmitted diseases (gonorrhea, syphilis, and chlamydia) who are offered provider referral services.

1995 MIDCOURSE ADDITION
Risk Reduction Objective

19.16 **Increase to at least 40% the proportion of ever sexually active adolescents aged 17 and younger who have not had sexual intercourse for the previous 3 months.**

20. IMMUNIZATION AND INFECTIOUS DISEASES
Health Status Objectives

+ **20.1** **Reduce indigenous cases of vaccine-preventable diseases (i.e., diphtheria, tetanus, polio [wild-type virus], measles, rubella, congenital rubella syndrome, mumps, and pertussis).**

20.2 Reduce epidemic-related pneumonia and influenza deaths among people aged 65 and older to no more than 7.3 per 100,000 people.

+ **20.3** **Reduce viral hepatitis (for hepatitis B and C only).**

20.4 Reduce tuberculosis to an incidence of no more than 3.5 cases per 100,000 people.

20.5 Reduce by at least 10% the incidence of surgical wound infections and nosocomial infections in intensive care patients.

20.6 Reduce incidence among international travelers of typhoid fever, hepatitis A, and malaria.

20.7 Reduce bacterial meningitis to no more than 4.7 cases per 100,000 people.

20.8 Reduce infectious diarrhea by at least 25% among children in licensed child care centers and children in programs that provide an Individualized Education Program (IEP) or Individualized Health Plan (IHP).

20.9 Reduce acute middle ear infections among children aged 4 and younger, as measured by days of restricted activity or school absenteeism, to no more than 105 days per 100 children.

+ **20.10** **Reduce pneumonia-related days of restricted activity (met for ages 0 to 4 only).**

Risk Reduction Objectives

20.11 Increase immunization levels as follows:
- Basic immunization series among children under age 2: at least 90%.
- Basic immunization series among children in licensed child care facilities and kindergarten through postsecondary education institutions: at least 95%.
- Pneumococcal pneumonia and influenza immunization among institutionalized chronically ill or older people: at least 80%.
- Pneumococcal pneumonia and influenza immunization among noninstitutionalized, high-risk populations, as defined by the Immunization Practices Advisory Committee: at least 60%.

- Hepatitis B immunization among high-risk populations, including infants of surface antigen-positive mothers, to at least 90%; occupationally exposed workers to at least 90%; IV drug users in drug treatment programs to at least 50%; and homosexual men to at least 50%.

20.12 Reduce postexposure rabies treatments to no more than 9000 per year.

Services and Protection Objectives

20.13 Expand immunization laws for schools, preschools, and day care settings to all states for all antigens.

20.14 Increase to at least 90% the proportion of primary care providers who provide information and counseling about immunizations and offer immunizations as appropriate for their patients.

20.15 Improve the financing and delivery of immunizations for children and adults so that virtually no American has a financial barrier to receiving recommended immunizations.

20.16 Increase to at least 90% the proportion of public health departments that provide adult immunization for influenza, pneumococcal disease, hepatitis B, tetanus, and diphtheria.

20.17 Increase to at least 90% the proportion of local health departments that have ongoing programs for actively identifying cases of tuberculosis and latent infection in populations at high risk for tuberculosis.

20.18 Increase to at least 85% the proportion of people found to have tuberculosis infection who completed courses of preventive therapy.

20.19 Increase to at least 85% the proportion of tertiary care hospital laboratories and to at least 50% the proportion of secondary care hospital and health maintenance organization laboratories possessing technologies for rapid viral diagnosis of influenza.

21. CLINICAL PREVENTIVE SERVICES
Health Status Objective

21.1 Increase years of healthy life to at least 65 years.

Risk Reduction Objective

21.2 Increase to at least 50% the proportion of people who have received, as a minimum within the appropriate interval, all of the screening and immunization services and at least one of the counseling services appropriate for their age and sex as recommended by the U.S. Preventive Services Task Force.

Services and Protection Objectives

21.3 Increase to at least 95% the proportion of people who have a specific source of ongoing primary care for coordination of their preventive and episodic health care.

21.4 Improve financing and delivery of clinical preventive services so that virtually no American has a financial barrier to receiving, at a minimum, the screening, counseling, and immunization services recommended by the U.S. Preventive Services Task Force.

21.5 Assure that at least 90% of people for whom primary care services are provided directly by publicly funded programs are offered, at a minimum, the screening, counseling, and immunization services recommended by the U.S. Preventive Services Task Force.

21.6 Increase to at least 50% the proportion of primary care providers who provide their patients with the screening, counseling, and immunization services recommended by the U.S. Preventive Services Task Force.

21.7 Increase to at least 90% the proportion of people who are served by a local health department that assesses and assures access to essential clinical preventive services.

21.8 Increase the proportion of all degrees in the health professions and allied/associated health profession fields awarded to members of underrepresented racial/ethnic minority groups.

22. SURVEILLANCE AND DATA SYSTEMS
Objectives

+22.1 **Develop a set of health status indicators appropriate for federal, state, and local health agencies and establish use of the set in at least 40 states.**

22.2 Identify, and create where necessary, national data sources to measure progress toward each of the Year 2000: National Health Objectives.

22.3 Develop and disseminate among federal, state, and local agencies procedures for collecting comparable data for each of the Year 2000: National Health Objectives and incorporate these into Public Health Service data collection systems.

22.4 Develop and implement a national process to identify significant gaps in the nation's disease prevention and health promotion data, including data for racial and ethnic minorities, people with low incomes, and people with disabilities, and establish mechanisms to meet these needs.

+22.5 **Implement in all states periodic analysis and publication of data needed to measure progress toward objectives for at least 10 of the priority areas of the National Health Objectives.**

+22.6 **Expand in all states systems for the transfer of health information related to the National Health Objectives among federal, state, and local agencies.**

22.7 Achieve timely release of national surveillance and survey data needed by health professionals and agencies to measure progress toward the National Health Objectives.

From US Department of Health and Human Services: *Healthy People 2000: national health promotion and disease prevention objectives,* Washington, DC, 1991, USDHHS, Public Health Service; and US Department of Health and Human Services: *Healthy People 2000: midcourse review and 1995 revisions,* Washington, DC, 1996, USDHHS, Public Health Service.

+, *Objectives known to be met or exceeded by 1995 midcourse review. Data for some objectives were not available.*

A.2 Schedule of Clinical Preventive Services

1.   Birth to 10 years

Interventions considered and recommended for the periodic health examination

LEADING CAUSES OF DEATH

Conditions originating in perinatal period
Congenital anomalies
Sudden infant death syndrome (SIDS)
Unintentional injuries (non–motor vehicle)
Motor vehicle injuries

INTERVENTIONS FOR THE GENERAL POPULATION

Screening
Height and weight
Blood pressure
Vision screen
Hemoglobinopathy screen (birth)[1]
Phenylalanine level (birth)[2]
T_4 and/or TSH (birth)[3]

Counseling

Injury prevention

Child safety car seats (age <5yr)
Lap-shoulder belts (age ≥5 yr)
Bicycle helmet; avoid bicycling near traffic
Smoke detector, flame retardant sleepwear
Hot water heater temperature <120° to 130° F
Window/stair guards, pool fence
Safe storage of drugs, toxic substances, firearms, and matches
Syrup of ipecac, poison control phone number
CPR training for parents/caretakers

Diet and exercise

Breastfeeding, iron-enriched formula and foods (infants and toddlers)
Limit fat and cholesterol; maintain caloric balance; emphasize grains, fruits, vegetables (age ≥2 yr)
Regular physical activity*

Substance use

Effects of passive smoking*
Anti-tobacco message*

Dental health

Regular visits to dental care provider*
Floss, brush with fluoride toothpaste daily*
Advice about baby bottle tooth decay*

Immunizations

Diphtheria-tetanus-pertussis (DTP)[4]
Oral poliovirus (OPV)[5]
Measles-mumps-rubella (MMR)[6]
H. influenzae type b (Hib) conjugate[7]
Hepatitis B[8]
Varicella[9]

Chemoprophylaxis

Ocular prophylaxis (birth)

---

*The ability of clinician counseling to influence this behavior is unproven.
[4]2, 4, 6, and 12 to 18 mo; once between ages 4 to 6 yr (DtaP may be used at 15 mo and older).
[5]2, 4, 6 to 18 months; once between ages 4 to 6 yr.
[6]12 to 15 mo and 4 to 6 yr.
[7]2, 4, 6 and 12 to 15 mo; no dose needed at 6 mo if PRP-OMP vaccine is used for first 2 doses.
[8]Birth, 1 mo, 6 mo; or 0 to 2 mo., 1 to 2 mo later, and 6 to 18 mo. If not done in infancy: current visit, and 1 and 6 mo later.
[9]12 to 18 mo; or any child without hx of chickenpox or previous immunization. Include information on risk in adulthood, duration of immunity, and potential need for booster doses.

---

[1]Whether screening should be universal or targeted to high-risk groups will depend on the proportion of high-risk individuals in the screening area and other considerations (see Chapter 43).
[2]If done during first 24 hr of life, repeat by age 2 wk.
[3]Optimally between day 2 and 6, but in all cases before newborn nursery discharge.

INTERVENTIONS FOR HIGH-RISK POPULATIONS

POPULATION	POTENTIAL INTERVENTIONS
Preterm or low birth weight	Hemoglobin/ hematocrit (HR1)
Infants of mothers at risk for HIV	HIV testing (HR2)
Low income; immigrants	Hemoglobin/hematocrit (HR1); PPD (HR3)
TB contacts	PPD (HR3)
Native American/Alaska Native	Hemoglobin/hematocrit (HR1); PPD (HR3); hepatitis A vaccine (HR4); pneumococcal vaccine (HR5)
Travelers to developing countries	Hepatitis A vaccine (HR4)
Residents of long-term care facilities	PPD (HR3); hepatitis A vaccine (HR4); influenza vaccine (HR6)
Certain chronic medical conditions	PPD (HR3); pneumococcal vaccine (HR5); influenza vaccine (HR6)
Increased individual or community lead exposure	Blood lead level (HR7)
Inadequate water fluoridation	Daily fluoride supplement (HR8)
Family history of skin cancer; nevi; fair skin, eyes, hair	Avoid excess/midday sun, use protective clothing* (HR9)

*The ability of clinician counseling to influence this behavior is unproven.

From U.S. Preventive Services Task Force: *Guide to clinical preventive services*, ed 2, Baltimore, 1996, Williams & Wilkins.

HIGH-RISK DEFINITIONS

HR1 = Infants age 6 to 12 months who are: living in poverty, black, Native American or Alaska Native, immigrants from developing countries, preterm and low birth weight infants, infants whose principal dietary intake is unfortified cow's milk.

HR2 = Infants born to high-risk mothers whose HIV status is unknown. Women at high risk include: past or present injection drug use; persons who exchange sex for money or drugs, and their sex partners; injection drug-using, bisexual, or HIV-positive sex partners currently or in past; persons seeking treatment for STDs; blood transfusion during 1978 to 1985.

HR3 = Persons infected with HIV, close contacts of persons with known or suspected TB, persons with medical risk factors associated with TB, immigrants from countries with high TB prevalence, medically underserved low-income populations (including homeless), residents of long-term care facilities.

HR4 = Persons ≥2 yr living in or traveling to areas where the disease is endemic and where periodic outbreaks occur (e.g., countries with high or intermediate endemicity; certain Alaska Native, Pacific Island, Native American, and religious communities). Consider for institutionalized children aged ≥2 yr. Clinicians should also consider local epidemiology.

HR5 = Immunocompetent persons ≥2 yr with certain medical conditions, including chronic cardiac or pulmonary disease, diabetes mellitus, and anatomic asplenia. Immunocompetent persons ≥2 yr living in high-risk environments or social settings (e.g., certain Native American and Alaska Native populations).

HR6 = Annual vaccination of children >6 mo who are residents of chronic care facilities or who have chronic cardiopulmonary disorders, metabolic diseases (including diabetes mellitus), hemoglobinopathies, immunosuppression, or renal dysfunction.

HR7 = Children about age 12 mo who: (1) live in communities in which the prevalence of lead levels requiring individual intervention, including residential lead hazard control or chelation, is high or undefined; (2) live in or frequently visit a home built before 1950 with dilapidated paint or with recent or ongoing renovation or remodeling; (3) have close contract with a person who has an elevated lead level; (4) live near lead industry or heavy traffic; (5) live with someone whose job or hobby involves lead exposure; (6) use lead-based pottery; or (7) take traditional ethnic remedies that contain lead.

HR8 = Children living in areas with inadequate water fluoridation (<0.6 ppm)

HR9 = Persons with a family history of skin cancer, a large number of moles, atypical moles, poor tanning ability, or light skin, hair, and eye color.

2. Ages 11 to 24 years

Interventions considered and recommended for the periodic health examination

LEADING CAUSES OF DEATH

Motor vehicle/other unintentional injuries
Homicide
Suicide
Malignant neoplasms
Heart diseases

INTERVENTIONS FOR THE GENERAL POPULATION

Screening
Height and weight
Blood pressure[1]
Papanicolaou (Pap) test[2] (females)
Chlamydia screen[3] (females <20 yr)
Rubella serology or vaccination hx[4] (females >12 yr)
Assess for problem drinking

Counseling

Injury prevention
Lap/shoulder belts
Bicycle/motorcycle/ATV helmets*
Smoke detector*
Safe storage/removal of firearms*

[1]Periodic BP for persons aged ≥21 yr.
[2]If sexually active at present or in the past: q ≤3 yr. If sexual history is unreliable, begin Pap tests at age 18 yr.
[3]If sexually active.
[4]Serologic testing documented vaccination history, and routine vaccination against rubella (preferably with MMR) are equally acceptable alternatives.

Substance use
Avoid tobacco use
Avoid underage drinking and illicit drug use*
Avoid alcohol/drug use while driving, swimming, boating, etc.*

Sexual behavior
STD prevention: abstinence; avoid high-risk behavior*; condoms/female barrier with spermicide*
Unintended pregnancy: contraception

Diet and exercise
Limit fat and cholesterol; maintain caloric balance; emphasize grains, fruits, vegetables
Adequate calcium intake (females)
Regular physical activity*

Dental health
Regular visits to dental care provider*
Floss, brush with fluoride toothpaste daily*

Immunizations

Tetanus-diphtheria (Td) boosters (11 to 16 yr)
Hepatitis B[5]
MMR (11 to 12 yr)[6]
Varicella (11 to 12 yr)
Rubella[4] (females >12 yr)

Chemoprophylaxis

Multivitamin with folic acid (females planning/capable of pregnancy)

[5]If not previously immunized: current visit, 1 and 6 mo later.
[6]If susceptible to chickenpox.
*The ability of clinician counseling to influence this behavior is unproven.

INTERVENTIONS FOR HIGH-RISK POPULATIONS

POPULATION	POTENTIAL INTERVENTIONS
High-risk sexual behavior	RPR/VDRL (HR1); screen for gonorrhea (female) (HR2), HIV (HR3), chlamydia (female) (HR4); hepatitis A vaccine (HR5)
Injection or street drug use	RPR/VDRL (HR1); HIV screen (HR3); hepatitis A vaccine (HR5); PPD (HR6); advice to reduce infection risk (HR7)
TB contacts; immigrants; low income	PPD (HR6)
Native Americans/Alaska Natives	Hepatitis A vaccine (HR5); PPD (HR6); pneumococcal vaccine (HR8)
Travelers to developing countries	Hepatitis A vaccine (HR5)
Certain chronic medical conditions	PPD (HR6); pneumococcal vaccine (HR8); influenza vaccine (HR9)
Settings where adolescents and young adults congregate	Second MMR (HR10)
Susceptible to varicella, measles, mumps	Varicella vaccine (HR11); MMR (HR12)
Blood transfusion between 1975 and 1985	HIV screen (HR3)
Institutionalized persons; health care/lab workers	Hepatitis A vaccine (HR5); PPD (HR6); influenza vaccine (HR9)
Family history of skin cancer; nevi; fair skin, eyes, hair	Avoid excess/midday sun, use protective clothing* (HR13)
Prior pregnancy with neural tube defect	Folic acid 4.0 mg (HR14)
Inadequate water fluoridation	Daily fluoride supplement (HR15)

*The ability of clinician counseling to influence this behavior is unproven.
From U.S. Prevention Services Task Force: *Guide to clinical preventive services*, ed 2, Baltimore, 1996, Williams & Wilkins

HIGH-RISK DEFINITIONS

HR1 = Persons who exchange sex for money or drugs, and their sex partners; persons with other STDs (including HIV); and sexual contacts of persons with active syphilis. Clinicians should also consider local epidemiology.

HR2 = Females who have: two or more sex partners in the last year; a sex partner with multiple sexual contacts; exchanged sex for money or drugs; or a history of repeated episodes of gonorrhea. Clinicians should also consider local epidemiology.

HR3 = Males who had sex with males after 1975; past or present injection drug use; persons who exchange sex for money or drugs, and their sex partners; injection drug-using, bisexual, or HIV-positive sex partner currently or in the past; blood transfusion during 1978 to 1985; persons seeking treatment for STDs. Clinicians should also consider local epidemiology.

HR4 = Sexually active females with multiple risk factors including: history of prior STD; new or multiple sex partners; age under 25; nonuse or inconsistent use of barrier contraceptives; cervical ectopy. Clinicians should consider local epidemiology of the disease in identifying other high-risk groups.

HR5 = Persons living in, traveling to, or working in areas where the disease is endemic and where periodic outbreaks occur (e.g., countries with high or intermediate endemicity; certain Alaska Native, Pacific Island, Native American, and religious communities); men who have sex with men; injection or street drug users. Vaccine may be considered for institutionalized persons and workers in these institutions, military personnel, and day-care, hospital, and laboratory workers. Clinicians should also consider local epidemiology.

HR6 = HIV positive, close contacts of persons with known or suspected TB, health care workers, persons with medical risk factors associated with TB, immigrants from countries with high TB prevalence, medically underserved low-income populations (including homeless), alcoholics, injection drug users, and residents of long-term facilities

HR7 = Persons who continue to inject drugs

HR8 = Immunocompetent persons with certain medical conditions, including chronic cardiac or pulmonary disease, diabetes mellitus, and anatomic asplenia. Immunocompetent persons who live in high-risk environments or social settings (e.g., certain Native American and Alaska Native populations).

HR9 = Annual vaccination of: residents of chronic care facilities; persons with chronic cardiopulmonary disorders, metabolic diseases (including diabetes mellitus), hemoglobinopathies, immunosuppression, or renal dysfunction; and health care providers for high-risk patients.

HR10 = Adolescents and young adults in settings where such individuals congregate (e.g., high schools and colleges), if they have not previously received a second dose.

HR11 = Healthy persons aged ≥13 yr without a history of chickenpox or previous immunization. Consider serologic testing for presumed susceptible persons aged ≥13 yr.

HR12 = Persons born after 1956 who lack evidence of immunity to measles or mumps (e.g., documented receipt of live vaccine on or after the first birthday, laboratory evidence of immunity, or a history of physician-diagnosed measles or mumps).

HR13 = Persons with a family or personal history of skin cancer, a large number of moles, atypical moles, poor tanning ability, or light skin, hair, and eye color.

HR14 = Women with prior pregnancy affected by neural tube defect who are planning pregnancy.

HR15 = Persons aged <17 yr living in areas with inadequate water fluoridation (<0.6 ppm)

3. Ages 25 to 64 years

Interventions considered and recommended for the periodic health examination

LEADING CAUSES OF DEATH

Malignant neoplasms
Heart diseases
Motor vehicle and other unintentional injuries
Human immunodeficiency virus (HIV) infection
Suicide and homicide

INTERVENTIONS FOR THE GENERAL POPULATION

Screening

Blood pressure
Height and weight
Total blood cholesterol (men age 35 to 64, women age 45 to 64)
Papanicolaou (Pap) test (women)[1]
Fecal occult blood test[2] and/or sigmoidoscopy (≥50 yr)
Mammogram clinical breast examination[3] (women 50 to 69 yr)
Assess for problem drinking
Rubella serology or vaccination hx[4] (women of childbearing age)

---

[1]Women who are or have been sexually active and who have a cervix: q ≤3 yr.

[2]Annually

[3]Mammogram q1-2 yr, or mammogram q1-2 yr with annual clinical breast examination.

[4]Serologic testing, documented vaccination history, and routine vaccination (preferably with MMR) are equally acceptable.

Counseling

Substance use

Tobacco cessation

Avoid alcohol/drug use while driving, swimming, boating, etc.*

Diet and exercise

Limit fat and cholesterol; maintain caloric balance; emphasize grains, fruits, vegetables

Adequate calcium intake (women)

Regular physical activity*

Injury prevention

Lap/shoulder belts

Motorcycle/bicycle/ATV helmets*

Smoke detector

Safe storage/removal of firearms*

Sexual behavior

STD prevention: avoid high-risk behavior*
 condoms/female barrier with spermicide

Unintended pregnancy: contraception

---

*The ability of clinician counseling to influence this behavior is unproven.

Dental health

Regular visits to dental care provider*

Floss, brush with fluoride toothpaste daily*

Immunizations

Tetanus-diphtheria (Td) boosters

Rubella[4] (women of childbearing age)

Chemoprophylaxis

Multivitamin with folic acid (women planning or capable of pregnancy)

Discuss hormone prophylaxis (perimenopausal and postmenopausal women)

---

[4]Serologic testing, documented vaccination history, and routine vaccination (preferably with MMR) are equally acceptable.

*The ability of clinician counseling to influence this behavior is unproven.

INTERVENTIONS FOR HIGH-RISK POPULATIONS

POPULATION	POTENTIAL INTERVENTIONS
High-risk sexual behavior	RPR/VDRL (HR1); screen for gonorrhea (female) HR2, HIV (HR3), chlamydia (female) (HR4); hepatitis B vaccine (HR5); hepatitis A vaccine (HR6)
Injection or street drug use	RPR/VDRL (HR1); HIV screen (HR3); hepatitis B vaccine (HR5); hepatitis A vaccine (HR6); PPD (HR7); advice to reduce infection risk (HR8)
Low income; TB contacts; immigrants; alcoholics	PPD (HR7)
Native Americans/Alaska Natives	Hepatitis A vaccine (HR6); PPD (HR7); pneumococcal vaccine (HR9)
Travelers to developing countries	Hepatitis B vaccine (HR5); hepatitis A vaccine (HR6)
Certain chronic medical conditions	PPD (HR7); pneumococcal vaccine (HR9); influenza vaccine (HR10)
Blood product recipients	HIV screen (HR3); hepatitis B vaccine (HR5)
Susceptible to measles, mumps, or varicella	MMR (HR11); varicella vaccine (HR12)
Institutionalized persons	Hepatitis A vaccine (HR6); PPD (HR7); pneumococcal vaccine (HR9); influenza vaccine (HR10)
Health care/lab workers	Hepatitis B vaccine (HR5); hepatitis A vaccine (HR6); PPD (HR7); influenza vaccine (HR10)
Family history of skin cancer: fair skin, eyes, hair	Avoid excess/midday sun, use protective clothing* (HR13)
Previous pregnancy with neural tube defect	Folic acid 4.0 mg (HR14)

*The ability of clinician counseling to influence this behavior is unproven.

From U.S. Preventive Services Task Force: *Guide to clinical preventive services*, ed 2, Baltimore, 1996, Williams and Wilkins

HIGH-RISK DEFINITIONS

HR1 = Persons who exchange sex for money or drugs, and their sex partners; persons with other STDs (including HIV); and sexual contacts of persons with active syphilis. Clinicians should also consider local epidemiology.

HR2 = Women who exchange sex for money or drugs, or who have had repeated episodes of gonorrhea. Clinicians should also consider local epidemiology.

HR3 = Men who had sex with men after 1975; past or present injection drug use; persons who exchange sex for money or drugs, and their sex partners; injection drug-using, bisexual, or HIV-positive sex partner currently or in the past; blood transfusion during 1978 to 1985; persons seeking treatment for STDs. Clinicians should also consider local epidemiology.

HR4 = Sexually active women with multiple risk factors including: history of STD; new or multiple sex partners; nonuse or inconsistent use of barrier contraceptives; cervical ectopy. Clinicians should also consider local epidemiology.

HR5 = Blood product recipients (including hemodialysis patients), persons with frequent occupational exposure to blood or blood products, men who have sex with men, injection drug users and their sex partners, persons with multiple recent sex partners, persons with other STDs (including HIV), travelers to countries with endemic hepatitis B.

HR6 = Persons living in, traveling to, or working in areas where the disease is endemic and where periodic outbreaks occur (e.g., countries with high or intermediate endemicity; certain Alaska Native, Pacific Island, Native American, and religious communities); men who have sex with men; injection or street drug users. Consider for institutionalized persons and workers in these institutions, military personnel, and day care, hospital, and laboratory workers. Clinicians should also consider local epidemiology.

HR7 = HIV positive, close contacts of persons with known or suspected TB, health care workers, persons with medical risk factors associated with TB, immigrants from countries with high TB prevalence, medically underserved low-income populations (including homeless), alcoholics, injection drug users, and residents of long-term care facilities.

HR8 = Persons who continue to inject drugs.

HR9 = Immunocompetent institutionalized persons aged ≥50 yr and Immunocompetent persons with certain medical conditions, including chronic cardiac or pulmonary disease, diabetes mellitus, and anatomic asplenia. Immunocompetent persons who live in high-risk environments or social settings (e.g., certain Native American and Alaska Native populations).

HR10 = Annual vaccination of residents of chronic care facilities; persons with chronic cardiopulmonary disorders, metabolic diseases (including diabetes mellitus), hemoglobinopathies, immunosuppression or renal dysfunction; and health care providers for high-risk patients.

HR11 = Persons born after 1956 who lack evidence of immunity to measles or mumps (e.g., documented receipts of live vaccine on or after the first birthday, laboratory evidence of immunity, or a history of physician-diagnosed measles or mumps).

HR12 = Healthy adults without a history of chickenpox or previous immunization. Consider serologic testing for presumed susceptible adults.

HR13 = Persons with a family or personal history of skin cancer, a large number of moles, atypical moles, poor tanning ability, or light skin, hair, and eye color.

HR14 = Women with previous pregnancy affected by neural tube defect who are planning pregnancy.

4. Age 65 and older

Interventions considered and recommended for the periodic health examination

LEADING CAUSES OF DEATH

Heart diseases
Malignant neoplasms (lung, colorectal, breast)
Cerebrovascular disease
Chronic obstructive pulmonary disease
Pneumonia and influenza

INTERVENTIONS FOR THE GENERAL POPULATION

Screening

Blood pressure
Height and weight
Fecal occult blood test[1] and/or sigmoidoscopy
Mammogram ±clinical breast examination[2] (women ≤69 yr)
Papanicolaou (Pap) test (women)[3]
Vision screening
Assess for hearing impairment
Assess for problem drinking

Counseling

Substance use

Tobacco cessation
Avoid alcohol/drug use while driving swimming, boating, etc.*

Diet and exercise

Limit fat and cholesterol; maintain caloric balance; emphasize grains, fruits, vegetables
Adequate calcium intake (women)
Regular physical activity*

Injury prevention

Lap/shoulder belts
Motorcycle and bicycle helmets*

---

[1]Annually.

[2]Mammogram q1-2 yr. or mammogram q1-2 yr with annual clinical breast examination.

---

[3]All women who are or have been sexually active and who have a cervix. Consider discontinuation of testing after age 65 yr if previous regular screening with consistently normal results.

*The ability of clinician counseling to influence this behavior is unproven.

Fall prevention*
Safe storage/removal of firearms*
Smoke detector*
Set hot water heater to <120° to 130°F
CPR training for household members
Dental health
Regular visits to dental care provider*
Floss, brush with fluoride toothpaste daily*
Sexual behavior
STD prevention: avoid high-risk sexual behavior*; use
 condoms

Immunizations
Pneumococcal vaccine
Influenza[1]
Tetanus-diphtheria (Td) boosters
Chemoprophylaxis
Discuss hormone prophylaxis (perimenopausal and
 postmenopausal women)

---

*The ability of clinician counseling to influence this behavior is un-
proven.

[1]Annually.

INTERVENTIONS FOR HIGH-RISK POPULATIONS

POPULATION	POTENTIAL INTERVENTIONS
Institutionalized persons	PPD (HR1); hepatitis A vaccine (HR2); amantadine/rimantadine (HR4)
Chronic medical conditions; TB contacts; low income; immigrants; alcoholics	PPD (HR1)
Persons ≥75 yr; or ≥70 yr with risk factors for falls	Fall prevention intervention (HR5)
Cardiovascular disease risk factors	Consider cholesterol screening (HR6)
Family history of skin cancer; nevi; fair skin, eyes, hair	Avoid excess/midday sun, use protective clothing * (HR7)
Native Americans/Alaska Natives	PPD (HR1); hepatitis A vaccine (HR2)
Travelers to developing countries	Hepatitis A vaccine (HR2); hepatitis B vaccine (HR8)
Blood product recipients	HIV screen (HR3); hepatitis B vaccine (HR8)
High-risk sexual behavior	Hepatitis A vaccine (HR2); HIV screen (HR3); hepatitis B vaccine (HR8); RPR/VDRL (HR9)
Injection or street drug use	PPD (HR1); hepatitis A vaccine (HR2); HIV screen (HR3); hepatitis B vaccine (HR8); RPR/VDRL (HR9); advice or reduce infection risk (HR10)
Health care/lab workers	PPD (HR1); hepatitis A vaccine (HR2); amantadine/rimantadine (HR4); hepatitis B vaccine (HR8)
Persons susceptible to varicella	Varicella vaccine (HR11)

*The ability of clinician counseling to influence this behavior is unproven.
From U.S. Preventive Services Task Force: *Guide to clinical preventive services*, ed 2, Baltimore, 1996, Williams and Wilkins

HIGH-RISK DEFINITIONS

HR1 = HIV positive, close contacts of persons with known or suspected TB, health care workers, persons with medical risk factors associated with TB, immigrants from countries with high TB prevalence, medically underserved low-income populations (including homeless), alcoholics, injection drug users, and residents of long-term care facilities.

HR2 = Persons living in, traveling to, or working in areas where the disease is endemic and where periodic outbreaks occur (e.g., countries with high or intermediate endemicity; certain Alaska Native, Pacific Island, Native American, and religious communities); men who have sex with men; injection or street drug users. Consider for institutionalized persons and workers in these institutions, and day-care, hospital, and laboratory workers. Clinicians should also consider local epidemiology.

HR3 = Men who had sex with men after 1975; past or present injection drug use; persons who exchange sex for money or drugs, and their sex partners; injection drug-using, bisexual, or HIV-positive sex partner currently or in the past; blood transfusion during 1978 to 1985; persons seeking treatment for STDs. Clinicians should also consider local epidemiology.

HR4 = Consider for persons who have not received influenza vaccine or are vaccinated late; when the vaccine may be ineffective due to major antigenic changes in the virus; for unvaccinated persons who provide home care for high-risk persons; to supplement protection provided by vaccine in persons who are expected to have a poor antibody response; and for high-risk persons in whom the vaccine is contraindicated.

HR5 = Persons aged 75 years and older; or aged 70 to 74 with one or more additional risk factors including: use of certain psychoactive and cardiac medications (e.g., benzodiazepines, antihypertensives); use of ≥4 prescription medications; impaired cognition, strength, balance, or gait. Intensive individualized home-based multifactorial fall prevention intervention is recommended in settings where adequate resources are available to deliver such services.

HR6 = Although evidence is insufficient to recommend routine screening in elderly persons, clinicians should consider cholesterol screening on a case-by-case basis for persons aged 65 to 75 with additional risk factors (e.g., smoking, diabetes, or hypertension).

HR7 = Persons with a family or personal history of skin cancer, a large number of moles, atypical moles, poor tanning ability, or light skin, hair, and eye color.

HR8 = Blood product recipients (including hemodialysis patients), persons with frequent occupational exposure to blood or blood products, men who have sex with men, injection drug users and their sex partners, persons with multiple recent sex partners, persons with other STDs (including HIV), travelers to countries with endemic hepatitis B.

HR9 = Persons who exchange sex for money or drugs and their sex partners; persons with other STDs (including HIV); and sexual contacts of persons with active syphilis. Clinicians should also consider local epidemiology.

HR10 = Persons who continue to inject drugs.

HR11 = Healthy adults without a history of chickenpox or previous immunization. Consider serologic testing for presumed susceptible adults.

5. Pregnant Women*

Interventions considered and recommended for the periodic health examination

INTERVENTIONS FOR THE GENERAL POPULATION
Screening
First visit
Blood pressure
Hemoglobin/hematocrit
Hepatitis B surface antigen (HbsAg)
RPR/VDRL
Chlamydia screen (<25 yr)
Rubella serology or vaccination history
D(Rh) typing, antibody screen
Offer CVS (<13 wk)[1] or amniocentesis (15 to 18 wk)[1] (age ≥35 yr)
Offer hemoglobinopathy screening
Assess for problem or risk drinking
Offer HIV screening[2]

Follow-up visits
Blood pressure
Urine culture (12 to 16 wk)
Offer amniocentesis (15 to 18 wk)[1] (age ≥35 yr)
Offer multiple marker testing[1] (15 to 18 wk)
Offer serum α-fetoprotein[1] (16 to 18 wk)
Counseling
Tobacco cessation; effects of passive smoking
Alcohol/other drug use
Nutrition, including adequate calcium intake
Encourage breastfeeding
Lap/shoulder belts
Infant safety car seats
STD prevention: avoid high-risk sexual behavior; use condoms

Chemoprophylaxis
Multivitamin with folic acid[3]

---

[1]Women with access to counseling and follow-up services, reliable standardized laboratories, skilled high-resolution ultrasound, and, for those receiving serum marker testing, amniocentesis capabilities.

[2]Universal screening is recommended for areas (states, counties, or cities) with an increased prevalence of HIV infection among pregnant women. In low-prevalence areas, the choice between universal and targeted screening may depend on other considerations.

*See A.2-2 and A.2-3 for other preventive services recommended for women of this age group.

---

[1]Women with access to counseling and follow-up services, reliable standardized laboratories, skilled high-resolution ultrasound, and, for those receiving serum marker testing, amniocentesis capabilities.

[3]Beginning at least 1 mo before conception and continuing through the first trimester.

INTERVENTIONS FOR HIGH-RISK POPULATIONS

POPULATION	POTENTIAL INTERVENTIONS
High-risk sexual behavior	Screen for chlamydia (1st visit) (HR1), gonorrhea (1st visit) (HR2), HIV (1st visit) (HR3); HbsAg (3rd trimester) (HR4); RPR/VDRL (3rd trimester) (HR5)
Blood transfusion 1978 to 1985	HIV screen (First visit) (HR3)
Injection drug use	HIV screen (HR3); HbsAg (3rd trimester) (HR4); advice to reduce infection risk (HR6)
Unsensitized D-negative women	D(Rh) antibody testing (24-28 wk) (HR7)
Risk factors for Down syndrome	Offer CVS[1] (1st trimester), amniocentesis[1] (15-18 wk) (HR8)
Prior pregnancy with neural tube defect	Offer amniocentesis[1] (15-18 wk), folic acid 4.0 mg3 (HR9)

[1]Women with access to counseling and follow-up services, reliable standardized laboratories, skilled high-resolution ultrasound, and, for those receiving serum marker testing, amniocentesis capabilities.
From U.S. Preventive Services Task Force: *Guide to clinical preventive services*, ed 2, Baltimore, 1996, Williams and Wilkins

HIGH-RISK DEFINITIONS

HR1 = Women with history of STD or new or multiple sex partners. Clinicians should also consider local epidemiology. Chlamydia screen should be repeated in third trimester if at continued risk.

HR2 = Women under age 25 with two or more sex partners in the last year, or whose sex partner has multiple sexual contacts; women who exchange sex for money or drugs; and women with a history of repeated episodes of gonorrhea. Clinicians should also consider local epidemiology. Gonorrhea screen should be repeated in the third trimester if at continued risk.

HR3 = In areas where universal screening is not performed due to low prevalence of HIV infection, pregnant women with the following individual risk factors should be screened: past or present injection drug use; women who exchange sex for money or drugs; injection drug-using, bisexual, or HIV-positive sex partner currently or in the past; blood transfusion during 1978 to 1985; persons seeking treatment for STDs.

HR4 = Women who are initially HbsAg negative who are at high risk due to injection drug use, suspected exposure to hepatitis B during pregnancy, multiple sex partners.

HR5 = Women who exchange sex for money or drugs, women with other STDs (including HIV), and sexual contacts of persons with active syphilis. Clinicians should also consider local epidemiology.

HR6 = Women who continue to inject drugs.

HR7 = Unsensitized D-negative women

HR8 = Prior pregnancy affected by Down syndrome, advanced maternal age (≥35 yr), known carriage of chromosome rearrangement.

HR9 = Women with previous pregnancy affected by neural tube defect.

6. Conditions for which clinicians should remain alert

CONDITION	POPULATION
Symptoms of peripheral arterial disease	Older persons, smokers, diabetic persons
Skin lesions with malignant features	General population, particularly those with established risk factors
Symptoms and signs of oral cancer and premalignancy	Persons who use tobacco, older persons who drink alcohol regularly
Subtle or nonspecific symptoms and signs of thyroid dysfunction	Older persons, postpartum women, persons with Down syndrome
Signs of ocular misalignment	Infants and children
Symptoms and signs of hearing impairment	Infants and young children (<3 yr)
Large spinal curvatures	Adolescents
Changes in functional performance	Older persons
Depressive symptoms	Adolescents, young adults, persons at increased risk for depression
Evidence of suicidal ideation	Persons with established risk factors for suicide
Various presentations of family violence	General population
Symptoms and signs of drug abuse	General population
Obvious signs of untreated tooth decay or mottling, inflamed or cyanotic gingiva, loose teeth, and severe halitosis	General population
Evidence of early childhood caries, mismatching of upper and lower dental arches, dental crowding or malalignment, premature loss of primary posterior teeth (baby molars) and obvious mouth breathing	Children

From U.S. Preventive Services Task Force: *Guide to clinical preventive services*, ed 2, Baltimore, 1996, Williams & Wilkins.

A.3 Select Major Historical Events Depicting Financial Involvement of Federal Government in Health Care Delivery

1798 Marine Hospital Service Act was passed to provide medical care to Merchant Marines.

1878 Port Quarantine Act was passed to prevent epidemic diseases from entering the country through seaports.

1879 National Health Department was established by Congress with a budget of $500,000.

1887 Laboratory of Hygiene at Staten Island Marine Hospital marked the beginning of Public Health Service research activities. This bacteriologic research laboratory later evolved into the National Institutes of Health.

1890 Marine Hospital Service was given authority to inspect all immigrants to bar "lunatics and others unable to care for self" from entering the country.

1902 National Health Department was renamed the Public Health and Marine Hospital Service.

1912 National Institute of Health functions were expanded to study and investigate diseases of persons and the conditions influencing the origin and spread of disease.

1912 The Public Health and Marine Hospital Service was renamed the United States Public Health Service.

1912 The Child Health Bureau was established within the USPHS.

1917 National leprosarium was established at Carville, Louisiana under the aegis of the USPHS.

1917 USPHS became responsible for the physical and mental examination of all aliens.

1917 Congress appropriated $25,000 to USPHS to study and provide demonstration projects sharing state and federal cooperative rural health services.

1918 Because of increased venereal disease incidence during World War I, the Division of Venereal Disease was established in USPHS, providing for cooperative federal and state control and prevention programs.

1921 Shepherd-Towner Maternity Infancy Act was passed to provide for the establishment of state maternal and infant programs. The Act provided for mother-child health conferences, home delivery supplies, improved prenatal care, improved infant and child care, more public health nurses, and health education.

1929 USPHS Narcotics Division was developed to provide facilities for the confinement and treatment of drug addicts (renamed Division of Mental Hygiene in 1939).

1935 Congress passed the Social Security Act. Title VI of the Act was written for the purpose of assisting states, counties, health districts, and other political subdivisions in establishing and maintaining adequate public health service, including the training of personnel for state and local health work.

1935 The Social Security Act provided for grants-in-aid to states to finance the public's health. Grants-in-aid resulted in increased numbers of new health departments and the strengthening and expansion of existing health departments.

1937 National Cancer Act called for the establishment of the National Cancer Institute for research into the causes, diagnosis, and treatment of cancer; for assistance to public and private agencies; and for the promotion of the most effective prevention and treatment.

1938 The second Federal Venereal Disease Control Act was passed to promote investigation and control and to provide funds for the development and maintenance of state and local programs.

1939 The Federal Security Agency was established to bring health, welfare, and education services of the federal government together.

1940 Communicable Disease Center (National Center for Disease Control) was established in Atlanta for the purpose of conducting epidemiologic studies, providing health personnel training, and establishing methods of communication and education.

1940 National Office of Vital Statistics (National Center for Health Statistics) was authorized to provide data about health, illness, injuries, and death.

1941 Nurse training appropriations provided monies to nursing programs to increase enrollment and improve programs.

1943 Nurse Training Act established the U.S. Nurse Cadet Corps in USPHS to support nurse training.

1946 National Mental Health Act was passed for constructing and equipping hospitals and laboratories to stimulate research and training in mental health.

1946 Hill-Burton Act provided for hospital services and construction.

1947 National Institute of Health Division of Research Grants were established to administer and award grants for research projects and training.

1947 A permanent Nursing Corps in the Army and Navy was established.

1948 National Heart Institute was established (renamed Heart, Lung, and Blood Institute in 1976).

1948 Microbiological, Experimental Biology, and Medicine Institutes were established (renamed National Institute of Allergy and Infectious Diseases in 1955).

1948 National Institute of Dental Research was authorized.

1948 National Institute of Health became National Institutes of Health (NIH).

1949 National Institute of Mental Health was established (renamed Alcoholism, Drug Abuse, and Mental Health Administration in 1974).

1950 National Institute of Neurological Diseases and Blindness was established (renamed National Eye Institute in 1968 and the National Institute of Neurological and Communicative Disorders and Strokes in 1975).

1950 Health Manpower Training Acts evolved to provide for training of health personnel.

1953 National Clinical Center was founded to accelerate research and to confirm and apply research findings. A 600-bed research hospital evolved.

1954 Congress extended Hill-Burton Act to allow monies for construction of other types of health facilities, such as general, mental, tuberculosis, and chronic disease hospitals; public health centers; diagnostic and treatment centers; rehabilitation facilities; nursing homes; state health laboratories; and nurse training facilities.

1954 Taft Sanitary Engineering Center was founded in Cincinnati for research and training in environmental health.

1955 National Institutes of Health Division of Biological Standards was established to oversee the growth of the pharmaceutical industry and market.

1955 Polio Vaccination Assistance Act was passed to aid state vaccination programs.

1956 U.S. Army Medical Library was transferred to USPHS, which became the Library of Medicine at the National Institutes of Health. The library provides MEDLARS, the Medical Literature Analysis and Retrieval System.

1956 CHAMPUS program was established for dependents of military personnel.

1956 National Health Survey was established for continuous monitoring of sickness and disability in the United States.

1959 National Institute of Arthritis and Metabolic Diseases was established (renamed National Institute of Arthritis, Metabolic, and Digestive Diseases in 1981).

1960 Social Security Amendments provided grants to states for medical assistance to the aged.

1962 National Institute of Child Health and Human Development was founded.

1962 Program for state assistance in preschool vaccination programs was authorized.

1963 Aid program was established for the construction of mental retardation and community mental health facilities and the development of programs to combat health problems (e.g., maternal health, crippled children, and the mentally retarded).

1965 Heart disease, cancer, and stroke legislation was provided for the establishment of Regional Medical Programs to coordinate existing services for these three health problems.

1965 Appalachian Regional Development Act was passed to provide for construction of health services facilities in economically depressed area.

1965 Social Security Act was amended to provide for Medicare and Medicaid programs.

1966 Division of Environmental Health Services was established in Public Health Service.

1966 Partnership for health legislation consolidated preexisting projects and formula grants to states through a new system of grants for comprehensive health planning. The legislation allowed health planning but did not give authority to control program development, spending, or construction of health facilities.

1968 Fogarty International Center for Advanced Study in Health Sciences was founded at NIH for international collaboration, study, and research by world scholars.

1970 Occupational Health and Safety Act was passed to ensure safe and healthy working conditions.

1971 Environmental Protection Agency was founded to establish an umbrella agency for all environmental programs.

1971 National Center for Toxicological Research was established at Pine Bluff, Arkansas under the aegis of the Food and Drug Administration of USPHS.

1972 National programs were established for research, screening, counseling, and treatment of sickle cell anemia and Cooley's anemia.

1972 Social Security Act amended to encourage Professional Standards Review Organizations (PSRO). PSROs were designed to review hospital services ordered by physicians to determine overuse and underuse of services for patient care.

1972 National commission was established to study and investigate causes, cures, and treatment of multiple sclerosis.

1973 Social Security Act was amended to provide for the development of health maintenance organizations (HMOs)—prepaid comprehensive health care delivery systems designed to introduce competition into the health care arena.

1973 Program of grants (contracts for establishing and operating emergency medical services systems) was authorized.

1974 National Health Planning and Resources Development Act was passed to provide a triad health planning system. The system was designed as a comprehensive planning structure to review health services and facilities and to control and limit the expenditure of federal monies by discouraging the development and continuation of unnecessary new and existing programs.

1974 National Diabetes Mellitus Research and Education Act was passed to authorize NIH to establish a National Commission on Diabetes to formulate long-range plans to combat the disease.

1974 Sudden Infant Death Syndrome Act was passed to provide a program of dissemination of research and information to the public.

1976 National Swine Flu Immunization Program was established and implemented.

1976 Toxic Substances Control Act was passed to require testing of certain chemical substances to protect human health and environment.

1977 Rural Health Clinics Services Act was passed to provide for the establishment of health clinics in rural underserved communities. The clinics were to be staffed by nurse practitioners or physician assistants. The bill marked the first national legislation passed for reimbursement of nurse practitioner and physician assistant services under Medicare and Medicaid.

1980 Civil Rights of Institutionalized Persons Act was passed to protect mentally ill, disabled, retarded, chronically ill, or handicapped persons from flagrant conditions in state-affiliated institutions.

1980 Infant Formula Act was passed to require that such formulas meet certain standards of nutrition, quality, and safety in manufacturing.

1980 Department of Health, Education, and Welfare reorganized. Department of Health and Human Services oversees the regulation of health programs.

1981 Omnibus Budget Reconciliation Act (OBRA) provided for maternal and child health block grants to states under Title V of the Social Security Act to assist the states in advancing the health of mothers and children. Legislation allows states to make decisions on how to spend monies for nine maternal-child health programs.

1981 Omnibus Budget Reconciliation Act provided preventive health services block grants to allow states to make decisions about monies spent for 10 preventive health programs like hypertensive screening, rape crisis centers, etc.

1981 Omnibus Budget Reconciliation Act provided alcohol, drug abuse, and mental health block grants for states to provide direct service through community health centers and alcohol and drug abuse programs.

1981 Omnibus Budget Reconciliation Act provided primary care block grants to states for community health center funding.

1982 Defense appropriations amendments allowed for direct, independent nurse practitioner reimbursement under CHAMPUS.

1982 The Tax Equity and Fiscal Responsibility Act established reductions in Medicare and Medicaid spending, called for the development of a prospective reimbursement system, authorized Medicare payments for hospice service, and replaced PSRO with a new utilization and quality control peer review program.

1983 Public Health Emergency Act provided for a permanent revolving fund for use by the Secretary of DHHS in responding to public health emergencies.

1983 Social Security Amendments of 1983 contained provisions providing for the establishment of a prospective payment system under Medicare.

1983 Amendments to the Public Health Act authorized grants, contracts, and loans for the development of home health agencies and training of home health personnel.

1985 Health Research Extension Act establishes a new National Center for Nursing Research.

1986 Supplemental appropriations bill passed to allow hospitals to include capital building costs in payment requests under PPS beginning in 1987.

1987 Omnibus Budget Reconciliation Act provided increased quality control measures for the nursing home industry, and required nurse aid training for nursing home and home health.

1989 Medicare/Medicaid regulations established a PPS for ambulatory surgery; provided Medicaid coverage for children 6 years of age and under and pregnant women with incomes of 133% of poverty level; provided reimbursement of certified pediatric nurse practitioners and family nurse practitioners for Medicaid services; and provided for nurse practitioners and clinical nurse specialists to certify patients needs for nursing home care.

1990 Americans with Disabilities Act prohibits discrimination against disabled individuals in employment, public transportation, accommodations, and services.

1992 The Older Americans Act Amendments were established to revise and extend assistance programs for the elderly. Authorizes grants to states and localities for services to the elderly, including food assistance and nutrition services, in-home services for the frail elderly, disease prevention, and health promotion programs.

1992 The Preventive Health Amendments to the Public Health Service Act revise and extend the program of block grants for preventive health and health services.

1993 Family and Medical Leave Act grants eligible employees of up to 12 weeks unpaid medical leave for a serious health condition, childbirth, adoption, care of infants or seriously ill children, spouses, or parents.

1993 National Institute of Health Revitalization Act amends the Public Health Service Act to revise and extend the programs of the National Institutes of Health, including the formation of the National Institute of Nursing Research.

1996 Health Insurance Portability and Accountability Act enacted to protect health insurance coverage for laid off or displaced workers.

1998 Third Party Reimbursement for Medicare, Part B, services under Public Law 105-33 for clinical nurse specialists and nurse practitioners.

1998 Child Health Insurance Plan to cover uninsured children in poverty

*Sources for this listing were Hanlon J, Pickett G: *Public health administration and practice*, ed 2, St Louis, 1984, Mosby; Congressional Research Service: *Summary of health legislation, 1959-1981*, Library of Congress, Pub No 82-127 EPW, Washington, DC, May 7, 1981, US Government Printing Office; Congressional Research Service: *Major legislation of the 97th Congress*, Library of Congress, Pub No 9, Washington, DC, Oct 6, 1982, US Government Printing Office; Congressional Research Service: *Major legislation of the 98th Congress*, Library of Congress, Pub No 9, Washington, DC, Oct, 1986, US Government Printing Office; Congressional Information Service Index, 1990, 1992, 1993, 1996, and 1998 editions of the *Legislative histories of US public laws.*

A.4 Delaration of Alma Ata

The International conference on primary health care, meeting in Alma-Ata this twelfth day of September in the year nineteen hundred and seventy-eight, expressing the need for urgent action of all governments, all health and development workers, and the world community to protect and promote the health of all the people of the world, hereby makes the following Declaration:

I

The Conference strongly reaffirms that health, which is a state of complete physical, mental, and social well-being, and not merely the absence of disease or infirmity, is a fundamental human right and that the attainment of the highest possible level of health is a most important worldwide social goal, whose realization requires the action of many other social and economic sectors in addition to the health sector.

II

The existing gross inequality in the health status of the people, particularly between developed and developing countries and within countries, is politically, socially, and economically unacceptable and is therefore of common concern to all countries.

III

Economic and social development, based on a new international economic order, is of basic importance to the fullest attainment of health for all and to the reduction of the gap between the health status of developing and developed countries. The promotion and protection of the health of the people are essential to sustained economic and social development and contribute to a better quality of life and to world peace.

IV

The people have the right and duty to participate individually and collectively in the planning and implementation of their health care.

V

Governments have a responsibility for the health of their people, which can be fulfilled only by the provision of adequate health and social measures. In the coming decades a main social target of governments, international organizations, and the whole world community should be the attainment by all peoples of the world by the year 2000 of a level of health that will permit them to lead a socially and economically productive life. Primary health care is the key to attaining this target as part of development in the spirit of social justice.

VI

Primary health care is essential health care based on practical, scientifically sound, and socially acceptable methods and technology made universally accessible to individuals and families in the community through their full participation and at a cost that the community and country can afford to maintain at every stage of their development in the spirit of self-reliance and self-determination. It forms an integral part both of the country's health system, of which primary health care is the central function and main focus, and of the overall social and economic development of the community. It is the first level of contact for individuals, the family, and the community with the national health system bringing health care as close as possible to where people live and work, and it constitutes the first element of a continuing health care process.

VII

Primary health care

1. Reflects and evolves from the economic conditions and sociocultural and political characteristics of the country and its communities and is based on the application of the relevant results of social, biomedical, and health services research and public health experience;
2. Addresses the main health problems in the community, providing promotive, preventive, curative, and rehabilitative services accordingly;
3. Includes at least education concerning prevailing health problems and the methods of preventing and controlling them; promotion of food supply and proper nutrition; an adequate supply of safe water and basic sanitation; maternal and child health care, including family planning; immunization against the major infectious diseases; prevention and control of locally endemic diseases; appropriate treatment of common diseases and injuries; and provision of essential drugs;
4 Involves, in addition to health sector, all related sectors and aspects of national and community development, in particular agriculture, animal husbandry, food indus-

try, education, housing, public works, communication, and other sectors; and demands the coordinated efforts of all those sectors;
5. Requires and promotes maximum community and individual self-reliance and participation in the planning, organization, operation, and control of primary health care making fullest use of local, national and other available resources; and to this end, develops through appropriate education the ability of communities to participate;
6. Should be sustained by integrated, functional, and mutually supportive referral levels, on health workers, including physicians, nurses, midwives, auxiliaries, and community workers, as applicable, as well as on traditional practitioners as needed, suitably trained socially and technically to work as a health team and to respond to the expressed health needs of the community; and
7. Relies, at local and referral levels, on health workers, including physicians, nurses, midwives, auxiliaries, and community workers, as applicable, as well as on traditional practitioners as needed, suitably trained socially and technically to work as a health team and to respond to the expressed health needs of the community.

VIII

All governments should formulate national policies, strategies, and plans of action to launch and sustain primary health care as part of a comprehensive national health system and in coordination with other sectors. To this end, it will be necessary to exercise political will, to mobilize the country's resources, and to use available external resources rationally.

IX

All countries should cooperate in a spirit of partnership and service to ensure primary health care for all people because the attainment of health by people in any one country directly concerns and benefits every other country. In this context the joint WHO-UNICEF report* on primary health care constitutes a solid basis for the further development and operation of Primary Health Care through the world.

X

An acceptable level of health for all the people of the world by the year 2000 can be attained through a fuller and better use of the world's resources, a considerable part of which is now spent on armaments and military conflicts. A genuine policy of independence, peace, détente, and disarmament could and should release additional resources that could well be devoted to peaceful aims and in particular to the acceleration of social and economic development of which primary health care, as an essential part, should be allotted its proper share.

---

*World Health Organization: *Primary health care: report of the International Conference on Primary Health Care, Alma-Ata, USSR, Sept 6-12, 1978*, Geneva, 1978, WHO.

Community Resources

Please refer to this book's website at www.mosby.com/MERLIN/community_stanhope for detailed information about the community resources listed below.

HEALTH-RELATED ORGANIZATIONS

This list contains a description of and detailed contact information for 100 major health-related organizations, such as Alcoholics Anonymous, American Diabetes Association, Children's Foundation, and National Kidney Foundation.

AAPCC-CERTIFIED REGIONAL POISON CONTROL CENTERS

This list presents, state by state, the poison control centers certified by the American Association of Poison Control Centers (AAPCC).

COMPUTERIZED INFORMATION SYSTEMS FOR ENVIRONMENTAL AND OCCUPATIONAL HEALTH

This list provides a description of the major electronic databases related to environmental and occupational health.

ENVIRONMENTAL AND OCCUPATIONAL HEALTH HOTLINES

This is a list of the hotlines associated with environmental and occupational health.

SELECTED RESOURCES FOR WORKING WITH DISABLED CLIENTS

This is a list of certain organizations and programs for disabled clients.

END-OF-LIFE HOTLINES

This is a list of websites for organizations associated with end-of-life issues.

Contracts and Forms: Samples

C.1 Community-Oriented Health Record (COHR)

COMMUNITY HEALTH ASSESSMENT MODEL

Definition of community: A locality-based entity—composed of systems of formal organizations reflecting societal institutions, informal groups, and aggregates, which are interdependent—whose function (expressed intent) is to meet a wide range of collective needs.

Definition of community health: The meeting of collective needs through identifying problems and managing interactions within the community and between the community and the larger society. This requires commitment, self-other awareness and clarity of situational definitions, articulateness, effective communication, conflict containment and accommodation, participation, management of relations with the larger society, and machinery for facilitating participant interaction and decision making.

COMMUNITY HEALTH ASSESSMENT GUIDE CATEGORIES

A. Community
  1. Place
     a. Geopolitical boundaries of community
     b. Local or folk name for community
     c. Size in square miles/areas/blocks/census tracts
     d. Transportation avenues
     e. Physical environment
  2. People
     a. Number and density of population
     b. Demographic structure of populations
     c. Informal groups
     d. Formal groups
     e. Linking structures
  3. Function
     a. Production—distribution—consumption of goods and services
     b. Socialization of new members
     c. Maintenance of social control
     d. Adapting to ongoing and unexpected change
     e. Provision of mutual aid
B. Community health
  1. Status
     a. Vital statistics
     b. Disease incidence and prevalence for leading causes of mortality and morbidity
     c. Health risk profiles
     d. Functional ability levels
  2. Structure
     a. Health facilities
     b. Health-related planning groups
     c. Health manpower
     d. Health resource utilization patterns
  3. Process
     a. Commitment
     b. Self-other awareness and clarity of situational definitions
     c. Articulateness
     d. Effective communication
     e. Conflict containment and accommodation
     f. Participation
     g. Management of relations with larger society
     h. Machinery for facilitating participant interaction and decision making

DATABASE

This form provides a structured method for recording data. The name of the community and the assessment category and/or subcategory are noted at the top of the page. These categories correspond to those of the assessment guide. The data are collected and the source of the information and the data are recorded. Data are often entered using the SOAP format. An example of the COHR Database form is depicted on the next page.

COMMUNITY HEALTH NURSING DIAGNOSIS OF THE PROBLEM

Headings of columns for the Community Health Diagnosis List are Date, Number, Diagnosis/Concern, and Supportive Data (title of appropriate section of database and capsule summary of relevant data).

COMMUNITY CAPABILITY LIST

Heading of columns for this list are Date, Number, Capability, Supportive Data (title of appropriate section of database and capsule summary of relevant data).

PROBLEM ANALYSIS

Problems come from the Community Health Nursing Diagnosis. A line labeled Problem/Statement is included at the top of the form below Name of Community. Heading of columns are Problem Correlates, Relationship of Correlates of Problem, and Data Supportive to Relationships (refer to appropriate sections of database and relevant research findings in current literature). An example of a completed Problem Analysis is depicted on p. 319.

PROBLEM PRIORITIZATION

Headings of columns are Criteria, Criteria Weights (1-10), Problem, Problem Rating (1-10), Rationale for Rating, Problem Ranking/(Weight × Rate).

DATABASE

Name of community _____

Assessment category _____ Subcategory _____

Date	Data Source	Data*

*Note with an asterisk the themes identified and meanings given.

Goals and Objectives
This form includes a line labeled Problem/Concern as well as lines for Goal Statement at the top under Name of Community. Column headings are Date, Objectives (number and statement) depicted on p. 321.

Plan
A line labeled Objective Number and Statement is included under Name of Community. Column headings are Date, Intervener Activities/Means, Value (1-10), and Activity/Means Selected for Implementation. Sample plan sheets from the interventions to infant malnutrition are presented on p. 322.

Progress Notes
A line labeled Goal is included under Name of Community. Column headings are Date, Narrative, Assessment. Plan (NAP), and Budget and Time. A footnote to the second column explains the NAP procedure: Record both objective and subjective data. Interpret these data in terms of (1) whether the objectives were achieved and (2) whether the intervener activities utilized were effective. The plan is dependent on the assessment and may include both new (or revised) objectives and activities. Progress Notes reflecting evaluation of interventions aimed at the Nursing Diagnosis: Risk of infant malnutrition are presented in the chapter.

C.2 Windshield Survey Components

ELEMENT	DESCRIPTION
Housing and zoning	What is the age of the houses, architecture? Of what materials are they constructed? Are all neighborhood houses similar in age, architecture? How would you characterize their differences? Are they detached or connected to others? Do they have space in front or behind? What is their general condition? Are there signs of disrepair—broken doors, windows, leaks, locks missing? Is there central heating, modern plumbing, air conditioning?
Open space	How much open space is there? What is the quality of the space—green parks or rubble-filled lots? What is the lot size of the houses? Lawns? Flower boxes? Do you see trees on the pavements, a green island in the center of the streets? Is the open space public or private? Used by whom?
Boundaries	What signs are there of where this neighborhood begins and ends? Are the boundaries natural—a river, a different terrain; physical—a highway, railroad; economic—difference in real estate or presence of industrial or commercial units along with residential? Does the neighborhood have an identity, a name? Do you see it displayed? Are there unofficial names?
"Commons"	What are the neighborhood hangouts? For what groups, at what hours (e.g., schoolyard, candy store, bar, restaurant, park, 24-hour drugstore)? Does the "commons" area have a sense of "territoriality," or is it open to the stranger?
Transportation	How do people get in and out of the neighborhood—car, bus, bike, walk, etc.? Are the streets and roads conducive to good transportation and also to community life? Is there a major highway near the neighborhood? Whom does it serve? How frequently is public transportation available?
Service centers	Do you see social agencies, clients, recreation centers, signs of activity at the schools? Are there offices of doctors, dentists; palmists, spiritualists, etc.? Are there parks? Are they in use?
Stores	Where do residents shop—shopping centers, neighborhood stores? How do they travel to shop?
Street people	If you are traveling during the day, whom do you see on the street—an occasional housewife, mother with a baby? Do you see anyone you would not expect—teenagers, unemployed males? Can you spot a welfare worker, an insurance collector, a door-to-door salesman? Is the dress of those you see representative or unexpected? Along with people, what animals do you see—stray cats, pedigreed pets, "watchdogs"?
Signs of decay	Is this neighborhood on the way up or down? Is it "alive"? How would you decide? Trash, abandoned cars, political posters, neighborhood-meeting posters, real estate signs, abandoned houses, mixed zoning usage?
Race	Are the residents Caucasian, African-American, or of another minority, or is the area integrated?
Ethnicity	Are there indices of ethnicity—food stores, churches, private schools, information in a language other than English?
Religion	Of what religion are the residents? Do you see evidence of heterogeneity or homogeneity? What denominations are the churches? Do you see evidence of their use other than on Sunday mornings?
Health and morbidity	Do you see evidence of acute or of chronic diseases or conditions? Of accidents, communicable diseases, alcoholism, drug addiction, mental illness, etc.? How far it is to the nearest hospital? Clinic?
Politics	Do you see any political campaign posters? Is there a headquarters present? Do you see an evidence of a predominant party affiliation?
Media	Do you see outdoor television antennas? What magazines, newspapers do residents read? Do you see *Forward Times, Hampton Post, Enquirer, Readers' Digest* in the stores? What media seem most important to the residents—radio, television, print?

From Anderson ET, McFarlane J: *Community as partner: theory and practice in nursing,* Philadelphia, 1996, J.B. Lippincott.

C.3 The Living Will Directive

The Living Will Directive

My wishes regarding life-prolonging treatment and artificially provided nutrition and hydration to be provided to me if I no longer have decisional capacity, have a terminal condition, or become permanently unconscious have been indicated by checking and initialing the appropriate lines below. By checking and initialing the appropriate lines, I specifically:

_____ Designate _____ as my health care surrogate(s) to make health care decisions for me in accordance with this directive when I no longer have decisional capacity. If _____ refuses or is not able to act for me, I designate _____ as my health care surrogate(s).

Any prior designation is revoked.

If I do not designate a surrogate, the following are my directions to my attending physician. If I have designated a surrogate, my surrogate shall comply with my wishes as indicated below:

_____ Direct that treatment be withheld or withdrawn, and that I be permitted to die naturally with only the administration of medication of the performance or any medical treatment deemed necessary to alleviate pain.

_____ DO NOT authorize that life-prolonging treatment be withheld or withdrawn.

_____ Authorize the withholding or withdrawal of artificially provided food, water, or other artificially provided nourishment or fluids.

_____ DO NOT authorize the withholding or withdrawal of artificially provided food, water, or other artificially provided nourishment or fluids.

_____ Authorize my surrogate, designated above, to withhold or withdraw artificially provided nourishment or fluids, or other treatment if the surrogate determines that withholding or withdrawing is in my best interest; but I no not mandate the withholding or withdrawing.

In the absence of my ability to give directions regarding the use of life-prolonging treatment and artificially provided nutrition and hydration, it is my intention that this directive shall be honored by my attending physician, my family, and any surrogate designated pursuant to this directive as the final expression of my legal right to refuse medical or surgical treatment and I accept the consequences of the refusal.

If I have been diagnosed as pregnant and that diagnosis is known to my attending physician, this directive shall have no force or effect during the course of my pregnancy.

I understand the full import of this directive and I am emotionally and mentally competent to make this directive.

Signed this _____ day of _____ 19 _____ .

_____
Signature and Address of the Grantor

In our joint presence, the grantor, who is of sound mind and eighteen years of age, or older, voluntarily dated and signed this writing or directed it to be dated and signed for the grantor.

_____   _____
Signature and Address of Witness   Signature and Address of Witness

or

STATE OF _____)
COUNTY OF _____)

Before me, the undersigned authority, came the grantor who is of sound mind and eighteeen (18) years of age, or older, and acknowledged that he voluntarily date and signed this writing or directed it to be signed and dated as above.

Done this _____ day of _____ 19 _____ .

_____
Signature or Notary Public or Other Officer

Date Commission Expires _____

Execution of this document restricts withholding of some medical procedures. Consult Revised Statutes or your attorney.

C.4 Audit Form (SIMP-H)

	Best care		Average care		Worst care	Not applicable	Not observed
	5	4	3	2	1	0	0

I. Assessing

Objective: To measure the quality of nursing care observed for the *intervention* component of the nursing process.

	5	4	3	2	1	0	0
1. The nurse collects data about the client's response to his/her medical illness.	5	4	3	2	1	0	0
2. The nurse collects data about the client's ability to care for self in the home.	5	4	3	2	1	0	0
3. The nurse collects data about client and/or family strengths that maintain or promote health.	5	4	3	2	1	0	0
4. During the visit, the nurse obtains pertinent data by questioning the client and/or family.	5	4	3	2	1	0	0
5. During the visit, the nurse's objective examination (auditory visual, palpable) of the client if either indicated* and made or *not* indicated and *not* made.	5	4	3	2	1	0	0
6. During the visit, the client is given an opportunity (time and encouragement) to initiate discussion or questions.	5	4	3	2	1	0	0
7. The nurse inquires about financial conditions of the client that affect his/her health.	5	4	3	2	1	0	0
8. Environmental data is collected (home, neighborhood, community).	5	4	3	2	1	0	0
9. The nurse collects data about cultural beliefs that affect his/her health.	5	4	3	2	1	0	0
10. The nursing diagnoses are validated with the client and/or family during the visit.	5	4	3	2	1	0	0
11. The nurse collects data about client use and/or ability to use community health care resources.	5	4	3	2	1	0	0
12. The nurse asks questions about health history.	5	4	3	2	1	0	0
13. The data gathered supports the nursing diagnosis, which is noted in the record.	5	4	3	2	1	0	0
14. Nursing diagnoses are prioritized with the client during the visit.	5	4	3	2	1	0	0
15. The nursing diagnosis can be treated by nursing interventions.	5	4	3	2	1	0	0

II. Planning

Objective: To measure the quality of nursing care observed for the *planning* component of the nursing process.

	5	4	3	2	1	0	0
16. The client and family participate in goal setting.	5	4	3	2	1	0	0
17. A long-term goal (hoped for outcome) is established.	5	4	3	2	1	0	0
18. Short-term goals (steps to meet long-term goal) are established.	5	4	3	2	1	0	0
19. Action plans (steps to achieve goals) are established.	5	4	3	2	1	0	0
20. The client participates in action planning.	5	4	3	2	1	0	0
21. The nurse and client discuss the resources (community, agency, family, personal, etc.) needed to fulfill the plan.	5	4	3	2	1	0	0
22. The nurse and client mutually decide upon an expected date of goal accomplishment.	5	4	3	2	1	0	0
23. The nurse discusses costs and benefits of the nursing plan.	5	4	3	2	1	0	0
24. The plan includes community resources.	5	4	3	2	1	0	0
25. The plan is revised as goals are achieved or changed.	5	4	3	2	1	0	0
26. Goals are measurable.	5	4	3	2	1	0	0
27. Goals are achievable.	5	4	3	2	1	0	0
28. Goals are based on the nursing diagnosis.	5	4	3	2	1	0	0
29. The nursing plan indicates what the nurse will do.	5	4	3	2	1	0	0
30. The nursing plan indicates what the client will do.	5	4	3	2	1	0	0

*"Indicated" means that there was evidence of a problem requiring assistance of someone other than the nurse.

Continued

	Best care		Average care		Worst care	Not applicable	Not observed
	5	4	3	2	1	0	0

III. Intervention

Objective: To measure the quality of nursing care observed for the *intervention* component of the nursing process.

	Best care		Average care		Worst care	Not applicable	Not observed
31. The nurse periodically reinforces client and family strengths.	5	4	3	2	1	0	0
32. Nursing actions provide for client participation in health promotion, maintenance, or restoration.	5	4	3	2	1	0	0
33. During the visit, one of the following takes place regarding a referral to another agency or discipline: referral indicated* and made or referral *not* indicated and *not* made.	5	4	3	2	1	0	0
34. The communication pattern that illustrates the decision-making process during this visit is:							

Nurse ⟶⟵ Client
⟶
⟵

	Best care		Average care		Worst care	Not applicable	Not observed
35. Teaching regarding the client's problems or need is done during the visit.	5	4	3	2	1	0	0
36. The client participates in the intervention(s) if capable.	5	4	3	2	1	0	0
37. The intervention is performed to reach the nursing care goal.	5	4	3	2	1	0	0
38. The nurse explains the rationale for the intervention.	5	4	3	2	1	0	0
39. The nursing action reflects currently accepted standards of practice.	5	4	3	2	1	0	0
40. The nurse coordinates health care services when more than one discipline is involved.	5	4	3	2	1	0	0
41. The nurse advocates for the client.	5	4	3	2	1	0	0
42. The nurse informs the client about nursing interventions being carried out.	5	4	3	2	1	0	0
43. The nurse assists the client to modify the environment according to need.	5	4	3	2	1	0	0
44. The nurse explores the use of health care resources with the client and/or family.	5	4	3	2	1	0	0
45. The nurse adapts or uses alternative interventions based on the client's response.	5	4	3	2	1	0	0

IV. Evaluating

Objective: To measure the quality of nursing care observed for the *evaluation* component of the nursing process.

	Best care		Average care		Worst care	Not applicable	Not observed
46. The nurse refers to the nursing care goal set at the previous visit.	5	4	3	2	1	0	0
47. The communication pattern used to illustrate the evaluation of the client's progress to goal achievement is:							

Nurse ⟶⟵ Client
⟶
⟵

	Best care		Average care		Worst care	Not applicable	Not observed
48. The family and nurse discuss the accomplishment of the nursing care goal(s).	5	4	3	2	1	0	0
49. The nurse informs the client about his/her health status.	5	4	3	2	1	0	0
50. There is mutual consideration of the short-term goals.	5	4	3	2	1	0	0
51. There is mutual consideration of the long-term goals.	5	4	3	2	1	0	0
52. New data is validated with the client and family.	5	4	3	2	1	0	0
53. The nurse and the client discuss how actions will be evaluated.	5	4	3	2	1	0	0
54. Changes in the care plan are discussed with the client and family.	5	4	3	2	1	0	0
55. During the visit, there is evidence of ongoing assessment.	5	4	3	2	1	0	0
56. During the visit, there is consideration of priorities.	5	4	3	2	1	0	0
57. Revision of the nursing care plan is based on progress toward the goal.	5	4	3	2	1	0	0
58. The nurse and the client and/or family discuss progress toward goal achievement.	5	4	3	2	1	0	0
59. The client's ongoing response to the medical illness is discussed.	5	4	3	2	1	0	0
60. The client and/or family demonstrates the ability to follow the nursing care plan.	5	4	3	2	1	0	0

*"Indicated" means that there was evidence of a problem requiring assistance of someone other than the nurse.

Continued

C.5 OASIS–Start of Care Assessment

START OF CARE ASSESSMENT FOR_____

(Patient's Name)

DEMOGRAPHICS AND PATIENT HISTORY

1. (M0080) Discipline of Person Completing Assessment:

① RN
② PT
③ SLP/ST
④ OT

> **USE BLUE OR BLACK PEN**
> **FILL-IN EACH OVAL COMPLETELY**
> ☑Wrong! ☒Wrong! ●Right!!!

2. (M0100) This Assessment is Currently Being Completed for the Following Reason:

Start/Resumption of Care

① **Start of care--further visits planned**
② **Start of care–no further visits planned**
③ **Resumption of care (after inpatient stay)**

Follow-Up
   Recertification (follow-up) reassessment [Go to *M0150*]
   Other follow-up [Go to *M0150*]
Transfer to an Inpatient Facility
   Transferred to an inpatient facility–patient not discharged from agency [Go to M0830]
   Transferred to an inpatient facility–patient discharged from agency [Go to M0830]
Discharge from Agency–Not to an Inpatient Facility
   Death at home [Go to *M0906*]
   Discharge from agency [Go to *M0150*]
   Discharge from agency–no visits completed after start/resumption of care assessment [Go to *M0830*]

3. (M0140) Race/Ethnicity (as identified by patient):

① American Indian or Alaska Native
② Asian
③ Black or African-American
④ Hispanic or Latino
⑤ Native Hawaiian or Pacific Islander
⑥ White
⑦ UK-Unknown

4. (M0150) Current Payment Sources for Home Care: (Mark all that apply.)

○ 0 - None; no charge for current services
○ 1 - Medicare (traditional fee-for-service)
○ 2 - Medicare (HMO/managed care)
○ 3 - Medicaid (traditional fee-for-service)
○ 4 - Medicaid (HMO/managed care)
○ 5 - Workers' compensation
○ 6 - Title programs (e.g., Title III, V, or XX)
○ 7 - Other government (e.g., CHAMPUS, VA, etc.)
○ 8 - Private insurance
○ 9 - Private HMO/managed care
○ 10 - Self-pay
○ 11 - Other (specify)_____
○ UK - Unknown

5. (M0160) Financial Factors limiting the ability of the patient/family to meet basic health needs: **(Mark all that apply.)**

⓪ None
① Unable to afford medicine or medical supplies
② Unable to afford medical expenses that are not covered by insurance/Medicare (e.g., copayments)
③ Unable to afford rent/utility bills
④ Unable to afford food
⑤ Other (specify)_____

6. (M0170) From which of the following **Inpatient Facilities** was the patient discharged <u>during the past 14 days</u>?
(Mark all that apply.)

① Hospital
② Rehabilitation facility
③ Nursing home
④ Other (specify)_____
Ⓝ NA-Patient was not discharged from an inpatient facility
   ↓ **[If NA, go to *M0200* (Question 9)]**

7. (M0180) Inpatient Discharge Date

    ⓤ UK-Unknown

Month	Day	Year
○ Jan		
○ Feb		
○ Mar	⓪ ⓪	⓪ ⓪ ⓪ ⓪
○ Apr	① ①	① ① ① ①
○ May	② ②	② ② ② ②
○ Jun	③ ③	③ ③ ③ ③
○ Jul	④ ④	④ ④ ④ ④
○ Aug	⑤ ⑤	⑤ ⑤ ⑤ ⑤
○ Sep	⑥ ⑥	⑥ ⑥ ⑥ ⑥
○ Oct	⑦ ⑦	⑦ ⑦ ⑦ ⑦
○ Nov	⑧ ⑧	⑧ ⑧ ⑧ ⑧
○ Dec	⑨ ⑨	⑨ ⑨ ⑨ ⑨

8. (M0190) Inpatient Diagnoses and ICD code categories (three digits required; five digits optional) <u>for only those conditions treated during an inpatient facility stay within the last 14 days</u> (no surgical or V-codes):

    <u>Inpatient Facility Diagnosis</u>

a. _____

b. _____

a. **ICD-9 Code**　　b. **ICD-9 Code**

9. (M0200) Medical or Treatment Regimen Change Within Past 14 Days: Has this patient experienced a change in medical or treatment regimen (e.g., medication, treatment, or service change due to new or additional diagnosis, etc.) within the last 14 days?

    ⓪ No
    ↓ [If No, go to *M0220* (Question 11)]
    ① Yes

10. (M0210) List the patient's Medical Diagnoses and ICD code categories (three digits required; five digits optional) <u>for those conditions requiring changed medical or treatment regimen</u> (no surgical or V-codes):

    <u>Changed Medical Regimen Diagnosis</u>

a. _____

b. _____

c. _____

d. _____

a. **ICD-9 Code**　　b. **ICD-9 Code**　　c. **ICD-9 Code**　　d. **ICD-9 Code**

11. **(M0220) Conditions Prior to Medical or Treatment Regimen Change or Inpatient Stay Within Past 14 Days:** If this patient experienced an inpatient facility discharge or change in medical or treatment regimen within the past 14 days, indicate any conditions which existed prior to the inpatient stay or change in medical or treatment regimen. **(Mark all that apply.)**

  ① Urinary incontinence
  ② Indwelling/suprapubic catheter
  ③ Intractable pain
  ④ Impaired decision-making
  ⑤ Disruptive or socially inappropriate behavior
  ⑥ Memory loss to the extent that supervision required
  ⑦ None of the above
  Ⓝ NA-No inpatient facility discharge and no change in medical or treatment regimen in past 14 days
  Ⓤ UK-Unknown

12. **(M0230/M0240) Diagnoses and Severity Index:** List each medical diagnosis or problem for which the patient is receiving home care and ICD code category (three digits required; five digits optional - no surgical or V-codes) and rate them using the following severity index. (Choose one value that represents the most severe rating appropriate for each diagnosis.)

Severity Rating Index

0 = Asymptomatic, no treatment needed at this time
1 = Symptoms well controlled with current therapy
2 = Symptoms controlled with difficulty, affecting daily functioning; patient needs ongoing monitoring
3 = Symptoms poorly controlled, patient needs frequent adjustment in treatment and dose monitoring
4 = Symptoms poorly controlled, history of rehospitalizations

(M0230) Primary Diagnosis   **Severity Rating**

_____   ⓪ ① ② ③ ④

(M0240) Other Diagnoses

a. _____   ⓪ ① ② ③ ④

b. _____   ⓪ ① ② ③ ④

c. _____   ⓪ ① ② ③ ④

d. _____   Ⓤ ① ② ③ ④

e. _____   ⓪ ① ② ③ ④

Primary   **Other**

ICD-9 Code	a. ICD-9 Code	b. ICD-9 Code	c. ICD-9 Code	d. ICD-9 Code	e. ICD-9 Code

(Scannable bubble grids for ICD-9 Codes, digits 0–9 for each position)

13. **(M0250) Therapies** the patient receives at home: **(Mark all that apply.)**

  ① Intravenous or infusion therapy (excludes TPN)
  ② Parenteral nutrition (TPN or lipids)
  ③ Enteral nutrition (nasogastric, gastrostomy, jejunostomy, or any other artificial entry into the alimentary canal)
  ④ None of the above

14. **(M0260) Overall Prognosis:** BEST description of patient's overall prognosis for recovery from this episode of illness.

  ⓪ Poor: little or no recovery is expected and/or further decline is imminent
  ① Good/Fair: partial to full recovery is expected
  Ⓤ UK-Unknown

15. **(M0270) Rehabilitative Prognosis:** BEST description of patient's prognosis for <u>functional status</u>.

⓪ Guarded: minimal improvement in functional status is expected; decline is possible
① Good: marked improvement in functional status is expected
ⓤ UK-Unknown

16. **(M0280) Life Expectancy:** (Physician documentation is not required.)

⓪ Life expectancy is greater than 6 months
① Life expectancy is 6 months or fewer

17. **(M0290) High Risk Factors** characterizing this patient: **(Mark all that apply.)**

① Heavy smoking
② Obesity
③ Alcohol dependency
④ Drug dependency
⑤ None of the above
ⓤ UK-Unknown

LIVING ARRANGEMENTS

18. **(M0300) Current Residence:**

① Patient's owned or rented residence (house, apartment, or mobile home owned or rented by patient/couple/ significant other)
② Family member's residence
③ Boarding home or rented room
④ Board and care or assisted living facility
⑤ Other (specify)_____

19. **(M0340) Patient Lives With: (Mark all that apply.)**

① Lives alone
② With spouse or significant other
③ With other family member
④ With a friend
⑤ With paid help (other than home care agency staff)
⑥ With other than above

20. **(M0310) Structural Barriers** in the patient's environment limiting independent mobility: **(Mark all that apply.)**

⓪ None
① Stairs inside home which <u>must</u> be used by the patient (e.g., to get to toileting, sleeping, eating areas)
② Stairs inside home which are used optionally (e.g., to get to laundry facilities)
③ Stairs leading from inside house to outside
④ Narrow or obstructed doorways

21. **(M0320) Safety Hazards** found in the patient's current place of residence: **(Mark all that apply.)**

○ 0 - None
○ 1 - Inadequate floor, roof, or windows
○ 2 - Inadequate lighting
○ 3 - Unsafe gas/electric appliance
○ 4 - Inadequate heating
○ 5 - Inadequate cooling
○ 6 - Lack of fire safety devices
○ 7 - Unsafe floor coverings
○ 8 - Inadequate stair railings
○ 9 - Improperly stored hazardous materials
○ 10 - Lead-based paint
○ 11 - Other (specify) _____

22. **(M0330) Sanitation Hazards** found in the patient's current place of residence: **(Mark all that apply.)**

○ 0 - None
○ 1 - No running water
○ 2 - Contaminated water
○ 3 - No toileting facilities
○ 4 - Outdoor toileting facilities only
○ 5 - Inadequate sewage disposal
○ 6 - Inadequate/improper food storage
○ 7 - No food refrigeration
○ 8 - No cooking facilities
○ 9 - Insects/rodents present
○ 10 - No scheduled trash pickup
○ 11 - Cluttered/soiled living area
○ 12 - Other (specify) _____

SUPPORTIVE ASSISTANCE

23. **(M0350) Assisting Person(s) Other than Home Care Agency Staff: (Mark all that apply.)**

① Relatives, friends, or neighbors living outside the home
② Person residing in the home (EXCLUDING paid help)
③ Paid help
④ None of the above
   ↓ **[If None of the above, go to *M0390* (Question 27)]**
ⓤ UK-Unknown
   ↓ **[If Unknown, go to *M0390* (Question 27)]**

24. **(M0360) Primary Caregiver** taking <u>lead</u> responsibility for providing or managing the patient's care, providing the most frequent assistance, etc. (other than home care agency staff):

⓪ No one person
   ↓ **[If No one person, go to *M0390* (Question 27)]**
① Spouse or significant other
② Daughter or son
③ Other family member
④ Friend or neighbor or community or church member
⑤ Paid help
ⓤ UK-Unknown
   ↓ **[If Unknown, go to *M0390* (Question 27)]**

25. **(M0370) How Often** does the patient receive assistance from the primary caregiver?

① Several times during day and night
② Several times during day
③ Once daily
④ Three or more times per week
⑤ One to two times per week
⑥ Less often than weekly
⑦ UK-Unknown

26. **(M0380) Type of Primary Caregiver Assistance: (Mark all that apply.)**

① ADL assistance (e.g., bathing, dressing, toileting, bowel/bladder, eating/feeding)
② IADL assistance (e.g., meds, meals, housekeeping, laundry, telephone, shopping, finances)
③ Environmental support (housing, home maintenance)
④ Psychosocial support (socialization, companionship, recreation)
⑤ Advocates or facilitates patient's participation in appropriate medical care
⑥ Financial agent, power of attorney, or conservator of finance
⑦ Health care agent, conservator of person, or medical power of attorney
⓪ UK-Unknown

SENSORY STATUS

27. **(M0390) Vision** with corrective lenses if the patient usually wears them:

⓪ Normal vision: sees adequately in most situations; can see medication labels, newsprint.
① Partially impaired: cannot see medication labels or newsprint, but <u>can</u> see obstacles in path, and the surrounding layout; can count fingers at arm's length.
② Severely impaired: cannot locate objects without hearing or touching them <u>or</u> patient non-responsive.

28. **(M0400) Hearing and Ability to Understand Spoken Language** in patient's own language (with hearing aids if the patient usually uses them):

⓪ No observable impairment. Able to hear and understand complex or detailed instructions and extended or abstract conversation.
① With minimal difficulty, able to hear and understand most multi-step instructions and ordinary conversation. May need occasional repetition, extra time, or louder voice.
② Has moderate difficulty hearing and understanding simple, one-step instructions and brief conversation; needs frequent prompting or assistance.
③ Has severe difficulty hearing and understanding simple greetings and short comments. Requires multiple repetitions, restatements, demonstrations, additional time.
④ <u>Unable</u> to hear and understand familiar words or common expressions consistently, <u>or</u> patient nonresponsive.

29. **(M0410) Speech and Oral (Verbal) Expression of Language** (in patient's own language):

⓪ Expresses complex ideas, feelings, and needs clearly, completely, and easily in all situations with no observable impairment.
① Minimal difficulty in expressing ideas and needs (may take extra time; makes occasional errors in word choice, grammar or speech intelligibility; needs minimal prompting or assistance).
② Expresses simple ideas or needs with moderate difficulty (needs prompting or assistance, errors in word choice, organization or speech intelligibility). Speaks in phrases or short sentences.
③ Has severe difficulty expressing basic ideas or needs and requires maximal assistance or guessing by listener. Speech limited to single words or short phrases.
④ <u>Unable</u> to express basic needs even with maximal prompting or assistance but is not comatose or unresponsive (e.g., speech is nonsensical or unintelligible).
⑤ Patient nonresponsive or unable to speak.

30. **(M0420) Frequency of Pain** interfering with patient's activity or movement:

⓪ Patient has no pain or pain does not interfere with activity or movement
① Less often than daily
② Daily, but not constantly
③ All of the time

31. **(M0430) Intractable Pain:** Is the patient experiencing pain that is <u>not easily relieved</u>, occurs at least daily, and affects the patient's sleep, appetite, physical or emotional energy, concentration, personal relationships, emotions, or ability or desire to perform physical activity?

⓪ No
① Yes

INTEGUMENTARY STATUS

32. **(M0440)** Does this patient have a **Skin Lesion** or an **Open Wound?** This excludes "OSTOMIES."

⓪ No
↓ [If No, go to *M0490* (Question 45)]
① Yes

33. **(M0445)** Does this patient have a **Pressure Ulcer?**

⓪ No
↓ [If No, go to *M0468* (Question 37)]
① Yes

34. **(M0450) Current Number of Pressure Ulcers at Each Stage:** (one response for each stage.)

Pressure Ulcer Stages

Number of Pressure Ulcers

a) Stage 1: Nonblanchable erythema of intact skin; the heralding of skin ulceration. In darker-pigmented skin, warmth, edema, hardness, or discolored skin may be indicators.

⓪ ① ② ③ ④ or more

b) Stage 2: Partial thickness skin loss involving epidermis and/or dermis. The ulcer is superficial and presents clinically as an abrasion, blister, or shallow crater.

⓪ ① ② ③ ④ or more

c) Stage 3: Full-thickness skin loss involving damage or necrosis of subcutaneous tissue which may extend down to, but not through, underlying fascia. The ulcer presents clinically as a deep crater with or without undermining of adjacent tissue.

⓪ ① ② ③ ④ or more

d) Stage 4: Full-thickness skin loss with extensive destruction, tissue necrosis, or damage to muscle, bone, or supporting structures (e.g., tendon, joint capsule, etc.)

⓪ ① ② ③ ④ or more

e) In addition to the above, is there at least one pressure ulcer that cannot be observed due to the presence of eschar or a nonremovable dressing, including casts?

⓪ No   ① Yes

35. **(M0460) Stage of Most Problematic (Observable) Pressure Ulcer:**

① Stage 1
② Stage 2
③ Stage 3
④ Stage 4
Ⓝ NA-No observable pressure ulcer

36. **(M0464) Status of Most Problematic (Observable) Pressure Ulcer:**

① Fully granulating
② Early/partial granulation
③ Not healing
Ⓝ NA-No observable pressure ulcer

37. **(M0468)** Does this patient have a **Stasis Ulcer?**

⓪ No
↓ [If No, go to *M0482* (Question 41)]
① Yes

38. **(M0470) Current Number of Observable Stasis Ulcer(s):**

⓪ Zero
① One
② Two
③ Three
④ Four or more

39. **(M0474)** Does this patient have at least one **Stasis Ulcer that Cannot be Observed** due to the presence of a nonremovable dressing?

⓪ No
① Yes

40. **(M0476) Status of Most Problematic (Observable) Stasis Ulcer:**

① Fully granulating
② Early/partial granulation
③ Not healing
Ⓝ NA-No observable stasis ulcer

41. **(M0482) Does this patient have a Surgical Wound?**

⓪ No
↓ [If No, go to *M0490* (Question 45)]
① Yes

42. **(M0484) Current Number of (Observable) Surgical Wounds:** (If a wound is partially closed but has <u>more</u> than one opening, consider each opening as a separate wound.)

  ⓪ Zero
  ① One
  ② Two
  ③ Three
  ④ Four or more

43. **(M0486)** Does this patient have at least one **Surgical Wound that Cannot be Observed** due to the presence of a nonremovable dressing?

  ⓪ No
  ① Yes

44. **(M0488) Status of Most Problematic (Observable) Surgical Wound:**

  ① Fully granulating
  ② Early/partial granulation
  ③ Not healing
  Ⓝ NA-No observable surgical wound

RESPIRATORY STATUS

45. **(M0490)** When is the patient dyspneic or noticeably **Short of Breath?**

  ⓪ Never, patient is not short of breath
  ① When walking more than 20 feet, climbing stairs
  ② With moderate exertion (e.g., while dressing, using commode or bedpan, walking distances less than 20 feet)
  ③ With minimal exertion (e.g., while eating, talking, or performing other ADLs) or with agitation
  ④ At rest (during day or night)

46. **(M0500) Respiratory Treatments** utilized at home: **(Mark all that apply.)**

  ① Oxygen (intermittent or continuous)
  ② Ventilator (continually or at night)
  ③ Continuous positive airway pressure
  ④ None of the above

ELIMINATION STATUS

47. **(M0510)** Has this patient been treated for a **Urinary Tract Infection** in the past 14 days?

  ⓪ No
  ① Yes
  Ⓝ NA-Patient on prophylactic treatment
  ⓤ UK-Unknown

48. **(M0520) Urinary Incontinence or Urinary Catheter Presence:**

  ⓪ No incontinence or catheter (includes anuria or ostomy for urinary drainage)
    ⬇ **[If No, go to *M0540* (Question 50)]**
  ① Patient is incontinent
  ② Patient requires a urinary catheter (i.e., external, indwelling, intermittent, suprapubic)
    ⬇ **[Go to *M0540* (Question 50)]**

49. **(M0530) When** does **Urinary Incontinence** occur?

  ⓪ Timed-voiding defers incontinence
  ① During the night only
  ② During the day and night

50. **(M0540) Bowel Incontinence Frequency:**

  ⓪ Very rarely or never has bowel incontinence
  ① Less than once weekly
  ② One to three times weekly
  ③ Four to six times weekly
  ④ On a daily basis
  ⑤ More often than once daily
  Ⓝ NA-Patient has ostomy for bowel elimination
  ⓤ UK-Unknown

51. **(M0550) Ostomy for Bowel Elimination:** Does this patient have an ostomy for bowel elimination that (within the last 14 days): a) was related to an inpatient facility stay, <u>or</u> b) necessitated a change in medical or treatment regimen?

  ⓪ Patient does <u>not</u> have an ostomy for bowel elimination.
  ① Patient's ostomy was <u>not</u> related to an inpatient stay and did <u>not</u> necessitate change in medical or treatment regimen.
  ② The ostomy <u>was</u> related to an inpatient stay or <u>did</u> necessitate change in medical or treatment regimen.

NEURO/EMOTIONAL/BEHAVIORAL STATUS

52. **(M0560) Cognitive Functioning:** (Patient's current level of alertness, orientation, comprehension, concentration, and immediate memory for simple commands.)

   ⓪ Alert/oriented, able to focus and shift attention, comprehends and recalls task directions independently.
   ① Requires prompting (cueing, repetition, reminders) only under stressful or unfamiliar conditions.
   ② Requires assistance and some direction in specific situations (e.g., on all tasks involving shifting of attention), or consistently requires low stimulus environment due to distractibility.
   ③ Requires considerable assistance in routine situations. Is not alert and oriented or is unable to shift attention and recall directions more than half the time.
   ④ Totally dependent due to disturbances such as constant disorientation, coma, persistent vegetative state, or delirium.

53. **(M0570) When Confused (Reported or Observed):**

   ⓪ Never
   ① In new or complex situations only
   ② On awakening or at night only
   ③ During the day and evening, but not constantly
   ④ Constantly
   Ⓝ NA-Patient nonresponsive

54. **(M0580) When Anxious (Reported or Observed):**

   ⓪ None of the time
   ① Less often than daily
   ② Daily, but not constantly
   ③ All of the time
   Ⓝ NA-Patient nonresponsive

55. **(M0590) Depressive Feelings Reported or Observed in Patient: (Mark all that apply.)**

   ① Depressed mood (e.g., feeling sad, tearful)
   ② Sense of failure or self reproach
   ③ Hopelessness
   ④ Recurrent thoughts of death
   ⑤ Thoughts of suicide
   ⑥ None of the above feelings observed or reported

56. **(M0600) Patient Behaviors (Reported or Observed): (Mark all that apply.)**

   ① Indecisiveness, lack of concentration
   ② Diminished interest in most activities
   ③ Sleep disturbances
   ④ Recent change in appetite or weight
   ⑤ Agitation
   ⑥ A suicide attempt
   ⑦ None of the above behaviors observed or reported

57. **(M0610) Behaviors Demonstrated <u>at Least Once a Week</u> (Reported or Observed): (Mark all that apply.)**

   ① Memory deficit: failure to recognize familiar persons/places, inability to recall events of past 24 hours, significant memory loss so that supervision is required
   ② Impaired decision-making: failure to perform usual ADLs or IADLs, inability to appropriately stop activities, jeopardizes safety through actions
   ③ Verbal disruption: yelling, threatening, excessive profanity, sexual references, etc.
   ④ Physical aggression: aggressive or combative to self and others (e.g., hits self, throws objects, punches, dangerous maneuvers with wheelchair or other objects)
   ⑤ Disruptive, infantile, or socially inappropriate behavior (**excludes** verbal actions)
   ⑥ Delusional, hallucinatory, or paranoid behavior
   ⑦ None of the above behaviors demonstrated

58. **(M0620) Frequency of Behavior Problems (Reported or Observed)** (e.g., wandering episodes, self abuse, verbal disruption, physical aggression, etc.):

   ⓪ Never
   ① Less than once a month
   ② Once a month
   ③ Several times each month
   ④ Several times a week
   ⑤ At least daily

59. **(M0630)** Is this patient receiving **Psychiatric Nursing Services** at home provided by a qualified psychiatric nurse?

   ⓪ No
   ① Yes

ADL/IADLs

For M0640-M0800, complete the "Current" column for all patients. For these same items, complete the "Prior" column only at start of care and at resumption of care; mark the level that corresponds to the patient's condition 14 days prior to start of care date (M0030) or resumption of care date (M0032). In all cases, record what the patient is able to do.

60. **(M0640) Grooming:** Ability to tend to personal hygiene needs (i.e., washing face and hands, hair care, shaving or make up, teeth or denture care, fingernail care).

Prior Current

- ⓪ ⓪ Able to groom self unaided, with or without the use of assistive devices or adapted methods.
- ① ① Grooming utensils must be placed within reach before able to complete grooming activities.
- ② ② Someone must assist the patient to groom self.
- ③ ③ Patient depends entirely upon someone else for grooming needs.
- ⓤ UK-Unknown

61. **(M0650) Ability to Dress <u>Upper</u> Body** (with or without dressing aids) including undergarments, pullovers, front-opening shirts and blouses, managing zippers, buttons, and snaps:

Prior Current

- ⓪ ⓪ Able to get clothes out of closets and drawers, put them on and remove them from the upper body without assistance.
- ① ① Able to dress upper body without assistance if clothing is laid out or handed to the patient.
- ② ② Someone must help the patient put on upper body clothing.
- ③ ③ Patient depends entirely upon another person to dress the upper body.
- ⓤ UK-Unknown

62. **(M0660) Ability to Dress <u>Lower</u> Body** (with or without dressing aids) including undergarments, slacks, socks or nylons, shoes:

Prior Current

- ⓪ ⓪ Able to obtain, put on, and remove clothing and shoes without assistance.
- ① ① Able to dress lower body without assistance if clothing and shoes are laid out or handed to the patient.
- ② ② Someone must help the patient put on undergarments, slacks, socks or nylons, and shoes.
- ③ ③ Patient depends entirely upon another person to dress lower body.
- ⓤ UK-Unknown

63. **(M0670) Bathing:** Ability to wash entire body. **<u>Excludes</u> grooming (washing face and hands only).**

Prior Current

- ⓪ ⓪ Able to bathe self in <u>shower or tub</u> independently.
- ① ① With the use of devices, is able to bathe self in shower or tub independently.
- ② ② Able to bathe in shower or tub with the assistance of another person:
  - (a) for intermittent supervision or encouragement or reminders, <u>OR</u>
  - (b) to get in and out of the shower or tub, <u>OR</u>
  - (c) for washing difficult to reach areas.
- ③ ③ Participates in bathing self in shower or tub, <u>but</u> requires presence of another person throughout the bath for assistance or supervision.
- ④ ④ <u>Unable</u> to use the shower or tub and is bathed in <u>bed or bedside chair</u>.
- ⑤ ⑤ Unable to effectively participate in bathing and is totally bathed by another person.
- ⓤ UK-Unknown

64. **(M0680) Toileting:** Ability to get to and from the toilet or bedside commode.

Prior Current

- ⓪ ⓪ Able to get to and from the toilet independently with or without a device.
- ① ① When reminded, assisted, or supervised by another person, able to get to and from the toilet.
- ② ② <u>Unable</u> to get to and from the toilet but is able to use a bedside commode (with or without assistance).
- ③ ③ <u>Unable</u> to get to and from the toilet or bedside commode but is able to use a bedpan/urinal independently.
- ④ ④ Is totally dependent in toileting.
- ⓤ UK-Unknown

65. **(M0690) Transferring:** Ability to move from bed to chair, on and off toilet or commode, into and out of tub or shower, and ability to turn and position self in bed if patient is bedfast.

Prior Current

- ⓪ ⓪ Able to independently transfer.
- ① ① Transfers with minimal human assistance or with use of an assistive device.
- ② ② <u>Unable</u> to transfer self but is able to bear weight and pivot during the transfer process.
- ③ ③ Unable to transfer self and is <u>unable</u> to bear weight or pivot when transferred by another person.
- ④ ④ Bedfast, unable to transfer but is able to turn and position self in bed.
- ⑤ ⑤ Bedfast, unable to transfer and is <u>unable</u> to turn and position self.
- ⓤ UK-Unknown

66. **(M0700) Ambulation/Locomotion:** Ability to <u>SAFELY</u> walk, once in a standing position, or use a wheelchair, once in a seated position, on a variety of surfaces.

<u>Prior</u> <u>Current</u>

⓪ ⓪ Able to independently walk on even and uneven surfaces and climb stairs with or without railings (i.e., needs no human assistance or assistive device).

① ① Requires use of a device (e.g., cane, walker) to walk alone <u>or</u> requires human supervision or assistance to negotiate stairs or steps or uneven surfaces.

② ② Able to walk only with the supervision or assistance of another person at all times.

③ ③ Chairfast, <u>unable</u> to ambulate but is able to wheel self independently.

④ ④ Chairfast, unable to ambulate and is <u>unable</u> to wheel self.

⑤ ⑤ Bedfast, unable to ambulate or be up in a chair.

① UK-Unknown

67. **(M0710) Feeding or Eating:** Ability to feed self meals and snacks. **Note: This refers only to the process of <u>eating</u>, <u>chewing</u>, and <u>swallowing</u>, <u>not preparing</u> the food to be eaten.**

<u>Prior</u> <u>Current</u>

⓪ ⓪ Able to independently feed self.

① ① Able to feed self independently but requires:
    (a) meal set-up; <u>OR</u>
    (b) intermittent assistance or supervision from another person; <u>OR</u>
    (c) a liquid, pureed or ground meat diet.

② ② <u>Unable</u> to feed self and must be assisted or supervised throughout the meal/snack.

③ ③ Able to take in nutrients orally <u>and</u> receives supplemental nutrients through a nasogastric tube or gastrostomy.

④ ④ <u>Unable</u> to take in nutrients orally and is fed nutrients through a nasogastric tube or gastrostomy.

⑤ ⑤ Unable to take in nutrients orally or by tube feeding.

① UK-Unknown

68. **(M0720) Planning and Preparing Light Meals** (e.g., cereal, sandwich) or reheat delivered meals:

<u>Prior</u> <u>Current</u>

⓪ ⓪ (a) Able to independently plan and prepare all light meals for self or reheat delivered meals; <u>OR</u>
    (b) Is physically, cognitively, and mentally able to prepare light meals on a regular basis but has not routinely performed light meal preparation in the past (i.e., prior to this home care admission).

① ① <u>Unable</u> to prepare light meals on a regular basis due to physical, cognitive, or mental limitations.

② ② Unable to prepare any light meals or reheat any delivered meals.

① UK-Unknown

69. **(M0730) Transportation:** Physical and mental ability to <u>safely</u> use a car, taxi, or public transportation (bus, train, subway).

<u>Prior</u> <u>Current</u>

⓪ ⓪ Able to independently drive a regular or adapted car; <u>OR</u> uses a regular or handicap-accessible public bus.

① ① Able to ride in a car only when driven by another person; <u>OR</u> able to use a bus or handicap van only when assisted or accompanied by another person.

② ② <u>Unable</u> to ride in a car, taxi, bus, or van, and requires transportation by ambulance.

① UK-Unknown

70. **(M0740) Laundry:** Ability to do own laundry -- to carry laundry to and from washing machine, to use washer and dryer, to wash small items by hand.

<u>Prior</u> <u>Current</u>

⓪ ⓪ (a) Able to independently take care of all laundry tasks; <u>OR</u>
    (b) Physically, cognitively, and mentally able to do laundry and access facilities, <u>but</u> has not routinely performed laundry tasks in the past (i.e., prior to this home care admission).

① ① Able to do only light laundry, such as minor hand wash or light washer loads. Due to physical, cognitive, or mental limitations, needs assistance with heavy laundry such as carrying large loads of laundry.

② ② <u>Unable</u> to do any laundry due to physical limitation or needs continual supervision and assistance due to cognitive or mental limitation.

① UK-Unknown

71. **(M0750) Housekeeping:** Ability to safely and effectively perform light housekeeping and heavier cleaning tasks.

<u>Prior</u> <u>Current</u>

⓪ ⓪ (a) Able to independently perform all housekeeping tasks; <u>OR</u>
    (b) Physically, cognitively, and mentally able to perform <u>all</u> housekeeping tasks but has not routinely participated in housekeeping tasks in the past (i.e., prior to this home care admission).

① ① Able to perform only <u>light</u> housekeeping (e.g., dusting, wiping kitchen counters) tasks independently.

② ② Able to perform housekeeping tasks with intermittent assistance or supervision from another person.

③ ③ <u>Unable</u> to consistently perform any housekeeping tasks unless assisted by another person throughout the process.

④ ④ Unable to effectively participate in any housekeeping tasks.

① UK-Unknown

72. **(M0760) Shopping:** Ability to plan for, select, and purchase items in a store and to carry them home or arrange delivery.

Prior Current

- ⓪   ⓪   (a) Able to plan for shopping needs and independently perform shopping tasks, including carrying packages; OR
       (b) Physically, cognitively, and mentally able to take care of shopping, but has not done shopping in the past (i.e., prior to this home care admission).
- ①   ①   Able to go shopping, but needs some assistance:
       (a) By self is able to do only light shopping and carry small packages, but needs someone to do occasional major shopping; OR
       (b) Unable to go shopping alone, but can go with someone to assist.
- ②   ②   Unable to go shopping, but is able to identify items needed, place orders, and arrange home delivery.
- ③   ③   Needs someone to do all shopping and errands.
- ⓤ   ⓤ   UK-Unknown

73. **(M0770) Ability to Use Telephone:** Ability to answer the phone, dial numbers, and effectively use the telephone to communicate.

Prior Current

- ⓪   ⓪   Able to dial numbers and answer calls appropriately and as desired.
- ①   ①   Able to use a specially adapted telephone (i.e., large numbers on the dial, teletype phone for the deaf) and call essential numbers.
- ②   ②   Able to answer the telephone and carry on a normal conversation but has difficulty with placing calls.
- ③   ③   Able to answer the telephone only some of the time or is able to carry on only a limited conversation.
- ④   ④   Unable to answer the telephone at all but can listen if assisted with equipment.
- ⑤   ⑤   Totally unable to use the telephone.
- ⓝ   ⓝ   NA-Patient does not have a telephone.
- ⓤ   ⓤ   UK-Unknown

MEDICATIONS

74. **(M0780) Management of Oral Medications:** Patient's ability to prepare and take all prescribed oral medications reliably and safely, including administration of the correct dosage at the appropriate times/intervals. **Excludes injectable and IV medications. (NOTE: This refers to ability, not compliance or willingness.)**

Prior Current

- ⓪   ⓪   Able to independently take the correct oral medication(s) and proper dosage(s) at the correct times.
- ①   ①   Able to take medication(s) at the correct times if:
       (a) individual dosages are prepared in advance by another person; OR
       (b) given daily reminders; OR
       (c) someone develops a drug diary or chart.
- ②   ②   Unable to take medication unless administered by someone else.
- ⓝ   ⓝ   NA-No oral medications prescribed.
- ⓤ   ⓤ   UK Unknown

75. **(M0790) Management of Inhalant/Mist Medications:** Patient's ability to prepare and take all prescribed inhalant/mist medications (nebulizers, metered dose devices) reliably and safely, including administration of the correct dosage at the appropriate times/intervals. **Excludes all other forms of medication (oral tablets, injectable and IV medications).**

Prior Current

- ⓪   ⓪   Able to independently take the correct medication and proper dosage at the correct times.
- ①   ①   Able to take medication at the correct times if:
       (a) individual dosages are prepared in advance by another person, OR
       (b) given daily reminders.
- ②   ②   Unable to take medication unless administered by someone else.
- ⓝ   ⓝ   NA-No inhalant/mist medications prescribed.
- ⓤ   ⓤ   UK-Unknown

76. **(M0800) Management of Injectable Medications:** Patient's ability to prepare and take all prescribed injectable medications reliably and safely, including administration of correct dosage at the appropriate times/intervals. **Excludes IV medications.**

Prior Current

- ⓪   ⓪   Able to independently take the correct medication and proper dosage at the correct times.
- ①   ①   Able to take injectable medication at correct times if:
       (a) individual syringes are prepared in advance by another person, OR
       (b) given daily reminders.
- ②   ②   Unable to take injectable medications unless administered by someone else.
- ⓝ   ⓝ   NA-No injectable medications prescribed.
- ⓤ   ⓤ   UK-Unknown

Patient's Name _____

If no bar code label present, please fill in this section.

Patient's Gender _____ Patient's Birth Date _____

Patient's Medicare Number _____

Patient's Medicaid Number _____

Patient's Zip Code _____ State _____

Primary Referring Physician ID _____

Agency ID Number _____

Place Bar Code Here

(M0030)
Start of Care Date

Month	Day	Year
○ Jan		
○ Feb		
○ Mar	⓪⓪	⓪⓪⓪⓪
○ Apr	①①	①①①①
○ May	②②	②②②②
○ Jun	③③	③③③③
○ Jul	④④	④④④④
○ Aug	⑤⑤	⑤⑤⑤⑤
○ Sep	⑥⑥	⑥⑥⑥⑥
○ Oct	⑦⑦	⑦⑦⑦⑦
○ Nov	⑧⑧	⑧⑧⑧⑧
○ Dec	⑨⑨	⑨⑨⑨⑨

(M0090)
Date Assessment Completed

Month	Day	Year
○ Jan		
○ Feb		
○ Mar	⓪⓪	⓪⓪⓪⓪
○ Apr	①①	①①①①
○ May	②②	②②②②
○ Jun	③③	③③③③
○ Jul	④④	④④④④
○ Aug	⑤⑤	⑤⑤⑤⑤
○ Sep	⑥⑥	⑥⑥⑥⑥
○ Oct	⑦⑦	⑦⑦⑦⑦
○ Nov	⑧⑧	⑧⑧⑧⑧
○ Dec	⑨⑨	⑨⑨⑨⑨

(M0032)
Resumption of Care Date
○ Not Applicable

Month	Day	Year
○ Jan		
○ Feb		
○ Mar	⓪⓪	⓪⓪⓪⓪
○ Apr	①①	①①①①
○ May	②②	②②②②
○ Jun	③③	③③③③
○ Jul	④④	④④④④
○ Aug	⑤⑤	⑤⑤⑤⑤
○ Sep	⑥⑥	⑥⑥⑥⑥
○ Oct	⑦⑦	⑦⑦⑦⑦
○ Nov	⑧⑧	⑧⑧⑧⑧
○ Dec	⑨⑨	⑨⑨⑨⑨

Caregiver ID Number

⓪⓪⓪⓪⓪⓪⓪⓪⓪⓪
①①①①①①①①①①
②②②②②②②②②②
③③③③③③③③③③
④④④④④④④④④④
⑤⑤⑤⑤⑤⑤⑤⑤⑤⑤
⑥⑥⑥⑥⑥⑥⑥⑥⑥⑥
⑦⑦⑦⑦⑦⑦⑦⑦⑦⑦
⑧⑧⑧⑧⑧⑧⑧⑧⑧⑧
⑨⑨⑨⑨⑨⑨⑨⑨⑨⑨

(M0064)
Patient's SSN

⓪⓪⓪⓪⓪⓪⓪⓪⓪⓪
①①①①①①①①①①
②②②②②②②②②②
③③③③③③③③③③
④④④④④④④④④④
⑤⑤⑤⑤⑤⑤⑤⑤⑤⑤
⑥⑥⑥⑥⑥⑥⑥⑥⑥⑥
⑦⑦⑦⑦⑦⑦⑦⑦⑦⑦
⑧⑧⑧⑧⑧⑧⑧⑧⑧⑧
⑨⑨⑨⑨⑨⑨⑨⑨⑨⑨

Mark Reflex® by NCS MM222237-1   654321   Printed in U.S.A.

FEED THIS DIRECTION

SCAN THIS SIDE UP

EQUIPMENT MANAGEMENT

77. **(M0810) Patient Management of Equipment (includes <u>ONLY</u> oxygen, IV/infusion therapy, enteral/parenteral nutrition equipment or supplies):** <u>Patient's ability</u> to set up, monitor and change equipment reliably and safely, add appropriate fluids or medication, clean/store/dispose of equipment or supplies using proper technique. **(NOTE: This refers to ability, not compliance or willingness.)**

⓪ Patient manages all tasks related to equipment completely independently.
① If someone else sets up equipment (i.e., fills portable oxygen tank, provides patient with prepared solutions), patient is able to manage all other aspects of equipment.
② Patient requires considerable assistance from another person to manage equipment, but independently completes portions of the task.
③ Patient is only able to monitor equipment (e.g., liter flow, fluid in bag) and must call someone else to manage the equipment.
④ Patient is completely dependent on someone else to manage all equipment.
Ⓝ NA-No equipment of this type used in care
↓ [If NA, skip M0820 (skip question 78)]

78. **(M0820) Caregiver Management of Equipment (includes <u>ONLY</u> oxygen, IV/infusion equipment, enteral/parenteral nutrition, ventilator therapy equipment or supplies):** <u>Caregiver's ability</u> to set up, monitor, and change equipment reliably and safely, add appropriate fluids or medication, clean/store/dispose of equipment or supplies using proper technique. **(NOTE: This refers to ability, not compliance or willingness.)**

⓪ Caregiver manages all tasks related to equipment completely independently.
① If someone else sets up equipment, caregiver is able to manage all other aspects.
② Caregiver requires considerable assistance from another person to manage equipment, but independently completes significant portions of task.
③ Caregiver is only able to complete small portions of task (e.g., administer nebulizer treatment, clean/store/dispose of equipment or supplies).
④ Caregiver is completely dependent on someone else to manage all equipment.
Ⓝ NA-No caregiver
Ⓤ UK-Unknown

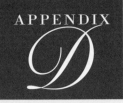
Drug and Immunization Information

D.1 Recommendations for Prophylaxis of Hepatitis A

1. **Close personal contact.** Immune globulin (IG) is recommended for all household and sexual contacts of persons with hepatitis A.

2. **Day care centers.** Day care facilities with children in diapers can be important settings for HAV transmission. IG should be administered to all staff and attendees of day care centers or homes if (1) one or more hepatitis A cases are recognized among children or employees, or (2) cases are recognized in two or more households of center attendees. When an outbreak (hepatitis cases in three or more families) occurs, IG should also be considered for members of households whose diapered children attend. In centers not enrolling children in diapers, IG need only be given to classroom contacts of an index case.

3. **Schools.** Contact at elementary and secondary schools is usually not an important means of transmitting hepatitis A. Routine administration of IG is not indicated for pupils and teachers in contact with a patient. However, when epidemiologic study clearly shows the existence of a school- or classroom-centered outbreak, IG may be given to those who have close personal contact with patients.

4. **Institutions for custodial care.** Living conditions in some institutions, such as prisons and facilities for the developmentally disabled, favor transmission of hepatitis A. When outbreaks occur, giving IG to residents and staff who have close contact with patients with hepatitis A may reduce spread of disease. Depending on the epidemiologic circumstances, prophylaxis can be limited or can involve the entire institution.

5. **Hospitals.** Routine IG administration is not indicated. Rather, sound hygienic practices should be emphasized. Staff education should point out the risk of exposure to hepatitis A and emphasize precautions regarding direct contact with potentially infective materials. Outbreaks of hepatitis A among hospital staff occur occasionally, usually in association with an unsuspected index patient who is fecally incontinent. Large outbreaks have occurred among staff and family contacts of infected infants in neonatal intensive care units. In outbreaks, prophylaxis of persons exposed to feces of infected patients may be indicated.

6. **Offices and factories.** Routine IG administration is not indicated under the usual office or factory conditions for persons exposed to a fellow worker with hepatitis A. Experience shows that casual contact in the work setting does not result in virus transmission.

7. **Common-source exposure.** IG might be effective in preventing foodborne or waterborne hepatitis A if exposure is recognized in time. However, IG is not recommended for persons exposed to a common source of hepatitis infection after cases have begun to occur in those exposed, because the 2-week period during which IG is effective will have been exceeded.

   If a food handler is diagnosed as having hepatitis A, common-source transmission is possible but uncommon. IG should be administered to other food handlers but is usually not recommended for patrons. However, IG administration to patrons may be considered if (1) the infected person is directly involved in handling, without gloves, foods that will not be cooked before they are eaten; (2) the hygienic practices of the food handler are deficient; and (3) patrons can be identified and treated within 2 weeks of exposure. Situations in which repeated exposures may have occurred, such as in institutional cafeterias, may warrant stronger consideration of IG use.

   For postexposure IG prophylaxis, a single intramuscular dose of 0.02 ml/kg is recommended.

D.2 Summary Description of Hepatitis A-G

Type	Definition/Incubation	Risk	Symptoms	Precautions	Prevention of spread
A	Liver disease caused by picornavirus, commonly called "infectious hepatitis" 30 days incubation	• Live in house with infected person • Inject drugs • Travel internationally to areas with high prevalence of hepatitis A • Eat infected shell fish • Consume contaminated food and water • Anal sex	• Skin, eye yellowing • Loss of appetite • Nausea • Vomiting • Fever • Fatigue • Diarrhea • Stomach/joint pain • Unable to work for extended periods • Usually no symptoms in children	• Stricter handwashing by food handler • Improved sanitary conditions • Improved personal hygiene	• Immune gamma globulin injections 2 to 3 weeks before or 2 weeks after exposure • Hepatitis A vaccine • Infection leads to immunity
B	A major cause of acute and chronic liver disease that can lead to cirrhosis and hepatocellular cancer; "serum hepatitis" 7 days incubation	• Exposure to human blood • Live with someone who is a carrier • Inject drugs • Have a sex partner infected with B • Have sex with more than one partner • A child born in Asia, Africa, Amazon, South America, Pacific Islands, or the Middle East	• Skin, eye yellowing • Loss of appetite • Nausea • Vomiting • Diarrhea • Stomach/joint pain • No symptoms—carrier • Itching • Skin eruptions	Vaccinate: • Babies at birth • Adolescents and others who have sex or inject drugs • Persons whose job places them at risk	• Hepatitis B vaccine within 14 days of exposure • Interferon alpha-2B and Lamivudine
C	Virus causing chronic liver disease, found in blood caused by non-A and non-B hepatitis virus. May develop cirrhosis and liver failure 7-9 weeks incubation; may be 28 weeks	• Drug injection • Exposure to human blood/contaminated objects • Hemodialysis patients • Receipt of blood transfusion • Multiple sex partners • Live with person with C • Snorting cocaine	• Same as hepatitis B • Symptoms usually occur after liver damage	• Do not take blood, organs, tissue, or sperm from C-infected person • Do not share toothbrushes, razors, or other items possibly contaminated with blood (including needles) • Cover open sores or other skin breaks	• Practice safe sex • Have only one sex partner • Routine screening of blood/other donors • Interferon

Type	Definition	Risk	Symptoms	Precautions	Prevention of spread
D	An incomplete virus requiring hepatitis B to be present to cause infection. This results in a more severe acute liver disease, leading to chronic liver disease with cirrhosis	• Injection drug users • Hemophilia clients • Developmentally disabled persons who are hospitalized • Sexual contact with hepatitis B	Same as hepatitis B	• Avoid sexual contact with injection drug users • Do not use needle used by others • Proper sterilization technique in institutions	• Individual screening for hepatitis B • Blood screening for B and D • Early vaccination for hepatitis B • Interferon alpha
E	• Enterically transmitted non-A and non-B hepatitis virus. Usually acute and does not usually cause chronic disease • 2-9 weeks	• Ingestion of fecally contaminated water • Pregnant women • International travelers • Persons in Asia and Indian countries	Same as hepatitis B	• Avoid contaminated waters	None at this time
F	A few cases described. Scientists not certain that this is a separate hepatitis virus.				
G	Non-A-E hepatitis virus described as a flavivirus. Present in 1% to 2% of blood donors in USA. Causes acute liver disease	• Any IV therapy • Injected drugs and end-stage renal disease • Pregnancy • Hemophilia	• Same as B/C • Liver inflammation • Liver failure	• Avoid multiple transfusions • Avoid IV drug use • Check new babies for perinatal transmission • Avoid all unnecessary IVs • Monitor persons for hemodialysis	• Individual screening for HGV • See precautions • No treatment at this time

Data compiled from multiple sources provided by the Centers for Disease Control and Prevention, Atlanta, 1995; *Science News* 149(15):238, 1996; National Institutes of Health, HCV International Symposium, June 1999.

D.3 Immunization Information

1. Recommended childhood immunization schedule, United States, January–December 1999

Vaccines[1] are listed under routinely recommended ages. Bars indicate range of recommended ages for immunization. Any dose not given at the recommended age should be given as a "catch-up" immunization at any subsequent visit when indicated and feasible. Ovals indicate vaccines to be given if previously recommended doses were missed or given earlier than the recommended minimum age.

Age ▶ / Vaccine ▼	Birth	1 mo	2 mo	4 mo	6 mo	12 mo	15 mo	18 mo	4-6 yr	11-12 yr	14-16 yr
Hepatitis B[2]	Hep B	Hep B			Hep B					Hep B	
Diphtheria, Tetanus, Pertussis[3]			DTaP	DTaP	DTaP		DTaP[3]		DTaP	Td	
H. influenzae type b[4]			Hib	Hib	Hib	Hib					
Polio[5]			IPV	IPV	Polio[5]				Polio		
Rotavirus[6]			Rv[6]	Rv[6]	Rv[6]						
Measles, Mumps, Rubella[7]						MMR			MMR[7]	MMR[7]	
Varicella[8]						Var				Var[8]	

Approved by the Advisory Committee on Immunization Practices (ACIP), the American Academy of Pediatrics (AAP), and the American Academy of Family Physicians (AAFP).

1 This schedule indicates the recommended ages for routine administration of currently licensed childhood vaccines. Combination vaccines may be used whenever any components of the combination are indicated and its other components are not contraindicated. Providers should consult the manufacturers' package inserts for detailed recommendations.

2 **Infants born to HBsAg-negative mothers** should receive the 2nd dose of hepatitis B vaccine at least 1 month after the 1st dose. The 3rd dose should be administered at least 4 months after the 1st dose and at least 2 months after the 2nd dose, but not before 6 months of age for infants.

Infants born to HBsAg-positive mothers should receive hepatitis B vaccine and 0.5 mL hepatitis B immune globulin (HBIG) within 12 hours of birth at separate sites. The 2nd dose is recommended at 1-2 months of age and the 3rd dose at 6 months of age.

Infants born to mothers whose HBsAg status is unknown should receive hepatitis B vaccine within 12 hours of birth. Maternal blood should be drawn at the time of delivery to determine the mother's HBsAg status; if the HBsAg test is positive, the infant should receive HBIG as soon as possible (no later than 1 week of age).
All children and adolescents (through 18 years of age) who have not been immunized against hepatitis B may begin the series during any visit. Special efforts should be made to immunize children who were born in or whose parents were born in areas of the world with moderate or high endemicity of HBV infection.

3 DTaP (diphtheria and tetanus toxoids and acellular pertussis vaccine) is the preferred vaccine for all doses in the immunization series, including completion of the series in children who have received 1 or more doses of whole-cell DTP vaccine. Whole-cell DTP is an acceptable alternative to DTaP. The 4th dose (DTP or DTaP) may be administered as early as 12 months of age, provided 6 months have elapsed since the 3rd dose and if the child is unlikely to return at age 15-18 months. Td (tetanus and diphtheria toxoids) is recommended at 11-12 years of age if at least 5 years have elapsed since the last dose of DTP, DTaP, or DT. Subsequent routine Td boosters are recommended every 10 years.

4 Three H. influenzae type b (Hib) conjugate vaccines are licensed for infant use. If PRP-OMP (PedvaxHIB and COMVAX [Merck]) is administered at 2 and 4 months of age, a dose at 6 months is not required. Because clinical studies in infants have demonstrated that using some combination products may induce a lower immune response to the Hib vaccine component, DTaP/Hib combination products should not be used for primary immunization in infants at 2, 4, or 6 months of age, unless FDA-approved for these ages.

5 Two poliovirus vaccines currently are licensed in the United States: inactivated poliovirus vaccine (IPV) and oral poliovirus vaccine (OPV).
The ACIP, AAP, and AAFP now recommend that the first two doses of poliovirus vaccine should be IPV. The ACIP continues to recommend a sequential schedule of two doses of IPV administered at ages 2 and 4 months, followed by two doses of OPV at 12-18 months and 4-6 years. Use of IPV for all doses also is acceptable and is recommended for immunocompromised persons and their household contacts.
OPV is no longer recommended for the first two doses of the schedule and is acceptable only for special circumstances such as: children of parents who do not accept the recommended number of injections, late initiation of immunization which would require an unacceptable number of injections, and imminent travel to polio-endemic areas. OPV remains the vaccine of choice for mass immunization campaigns to control outbreaks due to wild poliovirus.

6 Rotavirus (Rv) vaccine is shaded and italicized to indicate: 1) health care providers may require time and resources to incorporate this new vaccine into practice; and 2) the AAFP feels that the decision to use rotavirus vaccine should be made by the parent or guardian in consultation with their physician or other health care provider. The first dose of Rv vaccine should not be administered before 6 weeks of age, and the minimum interval between doses is 3 weeks. The Rv vaccine series should not be initiated at 7 months of age or older, and all doses should be completed by the first birthday.

7 The 2nd dose of measles, mumps, and rubella vaccine (MMR) is recommended routinely at 4-6 years of age but may be administered during any visit, provided at least 4 weeks have elapsed since receipt of the 1st dose and that both doses are administered beginning at or after 12 months of age. Those who have not previously received the second dose should complete the schedule by the 11- to 12-year-old visit.

8 Varicella vaccine is recommended at any visit on or after the first birthday for susceptible children, ie, those who lack a reliable history of chickenpox (as judged by a health care provider) and who have not been immunized. Susceptible persons 13 years of age or older should receive 2 doses, given at least 4 weeks apart.

Immunization Protects Children
Regular checkups at your pediatrician's office or local health clinic are an important way to keep children healthy.
By making sure that your child gets immunized on time, you can provide the best available defense against many dangerous childhood diseases. Immunizations protect children against: hepatitis B, polio, measles, mumps, rubella (German measles), pertussis (whooping cough), diphtheria, tetanus (lockjaw), *Haemophilius influenzae* type b, chickenpox, and rotavirus. All of these immunizations need to be given before children are 2 years old in order for them to be protected during their most vulnerable period. Are your child's immunizations up-to-date?

The chart on the other side of this fact sheet includes immunization recommendations from the American Academy of Pediatrics. Remember to keep track of your child's immunizations—it's the only way you can be sure your child is up-to-date. Also, check with your pediatrician or health clinic at each visit to find out if your child needs any booster shots or if any new vaccines have been recommended since this schedule was prepared.
If you don't have a pediatrician, call your local health department. Public health clinics usually have supplies of vaccine and may give shots free.

The information contained in this publication should not be used as a substitute for the medical care and advice of your pediatrician. There may be variations in treatment that your pediatrician may recommend based on individual facts and circumstances.

2. Recommended schedule of vaccinations for adolescents ages 11 to 12 years

IMMUNOBIOLOGIC	INDICATIONS	NAME	DOSE	FREQUENCY	ROUTE
Hepatitis A vaccine	Adolescents who are at increased risk of hepatitis A infection or its complications	HAVRIX (R)* VAQTA (R)*	720 EL.U.+/ 0.5 ml‡ 25 U/0.5 ml	A total of two doses at 0,§ 6-12 mo A total of two doses at 0, 6-18 mo	IM‖ IM
Hepatitis B vaccine	Adolescents not vaccinated previously for hepatitis B	Recombivax HB (R)* Engerix-B (R)*	5 μg/0.5 ml 10 μg/0.5 ml	A total of three doses at 0, 1-2, 4-6 mo A total of three doses at 0, 1-2, 4-6 mo	IM IM
Influenza vaccine	Adolescents who are at increased risk for complication caused by influenza or who have contact with persons at increased risk for these complications	Influenza virus vaccine¶	0.5 ml	Annually (September-December)	IM
Measles, mumps, and rubella vaccine (MMR)	Adolescents not vaccinated previously with two doses of measles vaccine at ≥12 mo of age	MMR II (R)*	0.5 ml	One dose	SC#
Pneumococcal polysaccharide vaccine	Adolescents who are at increased risk for pneumococcal disease or its complications	Pneumococcal vaccine polyvalent¶	0.5 ml	One dose	IM or SC
Tetanus and diphtheria toxoids (Td)	Adolescents not vaccinated within the previous 5 yr	Tetanus and diphtheria toxoids, absorbed (for adult use)¶	0.5 ml	Every 10 yr	IM
Varicella virus vaccine	Adolescents not vaccinated previously and who have no reliable history of chickenpox	VARIVAX (R)*	0.5 ml	One dose**	SC

* Manufacturer's product name.
† Enzyme-limned immunosorbent assay (ELISA) unit.
‡ Alternative dosage and schedule of 360 EL.U./0.5 ml and a total of three doses administered at 0, 1, and 6-12 months.
§ 0 months represents timing of the initial dose, and subsequent numbers represent months after the initial dose.
‖ Intramuscular injection.
¶ Generic name.
# Subcutaneous injection.
** Adolescents ≥13 years of age should be administered a total of two doses (0.5 ml/dose) subcutaneously at 0 and 4-8 weeks.

3. Recommended postexposure prophylaxis for percutaneous or permucosal exposure to hepatitis B virus, United States

VACCINATION AND ANTIBODY RESPONSE STATUS OF EXPOSED PERSON	TREATMENT WHEN SOURCE IS		
	HBsAG* POSITIVE	HBsAg NEGATIVE	SOURCE NOT TESTED OR STATUS UNKNOWN
UNVACCINATED	HBIG† × 1; initiate HB vaccine series‡	Initiate HB vaccine series	Initiate HB vaccine series
PREVIOUSLY VACCINATED			
Known responder§	No treatment	No treatment	No treatment
Known nonresponder	HBIG × 2 or HBIG × 1 and initiate revaccination	No treatment	If known high-risk source, treat as if source were HBsAg positive
Antibody response unknown	Test exposed person for anti-HBs‖ 1. If adequate§, no treatment 2. If inadequate§, HBIG × 1 and vaccine booster	No treatment	Test exposed person for anti-HBs 1. If adequate§, no treatment 2. If inadequate§, initiate revaccination

* Hepatitis B surface antigen.
† Hepatitis B immune globulin; dose 0.06 ml/kg intramuscularly.
‡ Hepatitis B vaccine.
§ Responder is defined as a person with adequate levels of serum antibody to hepatitis B surface antigen (i.e., anti-HBs ≥10mIU/ml); inadequate response to vaccination defined as serum anti-HBs
‖ Antibody to hepatitis B surface

4. Recommended poliovirus vaccination schedules for children

VACCINATION SCHEDULE	CHILD'S AGE			
	2 MO	4 MO	12-18 MO	4-6 YR
Sequential IPV*/OPV†	IPV	IPV	OPV	OPV
OPV*	OPV	OPV	OPV‡	OPV
IPV†	IPV	IPV	IPV	IPV

* Inactivated poliovirus vaccine.
† Live, oral poliovirus vaccine.
‡ For children who receive only OPV, the third dose of OPV may be administered as early as 6 months of age.
IPV, Inactivated poliovirus vaccine; *OPV*, oral poliovirus vaccine.

5. Suggested intervals between administration of immune globulin preparations for various indications and vaccines containing live measles virus*

INDICATION	DOSE	TIME INTERVAL (MONTHS) BEFORE MEASLES VACCINATION
Tetanus (TIG) prophylaxis	250 units (10 mg IgG/kg) IM	3
Hepatitis A (IG) prophylaxis		
Contact prophylaxis	0.02 ml/kg (3.3 mg IgG/kg) IM	3
International travel	0.06 ml/kg (10 mg IgG/kg) IM	3
Hepatitis B prophylaxis (HBIG)	0.06 ml/kg (10 mg IgG/kg) IM	3
Rabies immune globulin (HRIG)	20 IU/kg (22 mg IgG/kg) IM	4
Varicella prophylaxis (VZIG)	125 units/10 kg (20 to 40 mg IgG/kg) IM (maximum 625 units)	5
Measles prophylaxis (IG)		
Standard (i.e., nonimmuno-compromised contact)	0.25 ml/kg (40 mg IgG/kg) IM	5
Immunocompromised contact	0.50 ml/kg (80 mg IgG/kg) IM	6
Blood transfusion		
Red blood cells (RBCs), washed	10 ml/kg (negligible IgG/kg) IV	0
RBCs, adenine-saline added	10 ml/kg (10 mg IgG/kg) IV	3
Packed RBCs (Hct 65%)†	10 ml/kg (60 mg IgG/kg) IV	6
Whole blood cells (Hct 35% to 50%)	10 ml/kg (80-100 mg IgG/kg) IV	6
Plasma/platelet products	10 ml/kg (160 mg IgG/kg) IV	7
Replacement therapy for immune deficiencies	300 to 400 mg/kg IV‡ (as IGIV)	8
Treatment of:		
Immune thrombocytopenic purpura§	400 mg/kg IV (as IGIV)	8
Immune thrombocytopenic purpura§	1000 mg/kg IV (as IGIV)	10
Kawasaki disease	2 g/kg IV (as IGIV)	11

*This table is not intended for determining the correct indications and dosage for the use of immune globulin preparations. Unvaccinated persons may not be fully protected against measles during the entire suggested time interval, and additional doses of immune globulin and/or measles vaccine may be indicated after measles exposure. The concentration of measles antibody in a particular immune globulin preparation can vary by lot. The rate of antibody clearance after receipt of an immune globulin preparation can also vary. The recommended time intervals are extrapolated from an estimated half-life of 30 days for passively acquired antibody and an observed interference with the immune response to measles vaccine for 5 months after a dose of 80 mg (g/kg).

†Assumes a serum IgG concentration of 16 mg/ml.

‡ Measles vaccination is recommended for most HIV-infected children who do not have evidence of severe immunosuppression, but it is contraindicated for patients who have congenital disorders of the immune system.

§ Formerly referred to as idiopathic thrombocytopenic purpura.

6. Immunizing agents and immunization schedules for health care workers*

Generic name	Primary schedule and boosters (s)	Indications	Major precautions and contraindications	Special considerations
IMMUNIZING AGENTS STRONGLY RECOMMENDED FOR HEALTH CARE WORKERS				
Hepatitis B (HB) recombinant vaccine	Two doses IM 4 weeks apart; third dose 5 months after second; booster doses not necessary.	Preexposure: HCWs at risk for exposure to blood or body fluids. Postexposure: See Appendix D.3.2.	On the basis of limited data, no risk of adverse effects to developing fetuses is apparent. Pregnancy should not be considered a contraindication to vaccination.	The vaccine produces neither therapeutic nor adverse effects on HBV-infected persons. Prevaccination serologic screening is not indicated for persons being vaccinated because of occupational risk. HCWs who have contact with patients or blood should be tested 1 to 2 months after vaccination to determine serologic response.
Hepatitis B immune globulin (HBIG)	0.06 ml/kg IM as soon as possible after exposure. A second dose of HBIG should be administered 1 month later if the HB vaccine series has not been started.	Postexposure prophylaxis (see Appendix D.3.3): For persons exposed to blood or body fluids containing HbsAg and who are not immune to HBV infection—0.06 ml/kg IM as soon as possible (but no later than 7 days after exposure).		
Influenza vaccine (inactivated whole-virus and split-virus vaccines)	Annual vaccination with current vaccine. Administered IM.	HCWs who have contact with patients at high risk for influenza or its complications; HCWs who work in chronic care facilities; HCWs with high-risk medical conditions or who are aged ≥65 years.	History of anaphylactic hypersensitivity to egg ingestion.	No evidence exists of risk to mother or fetus when the vaccine is administered to a pregnant woman with an underlying high-risk condition. Influenza vaccination is recommended during second and third trimesters of pregnancy because of increased risk for hospitalization.

*Persons who provide health care to patients or work in institutions that provide patient care, e.g., physicians, nurses, emergency medical personnel, dental professionals and students, medical and nursing students, laboratory technicians, hospital volunteers, and administrative and support staff in health-care institutions

HAV, Hepatitis A virus; *HBV*, hepatitis B virus; *HbsAg*, hepatitis B surface antigen; *HCW*, health-care worker; *HIV*, human immunodeficiency virus; *IgA*, immune globulin A; *ID*, intradermal; *IM*, intramuscular; *MMR*, measles, mumps, rubella vaccine; *SC*, subcutaneous; *TB*, tuberculosis.

GENERIC NAME	PRIMARY SCHEDULE AND BOOSTERS (S)	INDICATIONS	MAJOR PRECAUTIONS AND CONTRAINDICATIONS	SPECIAL CONSIDERATIONS
IMMUNIZING AGENTS STRONGLY RECOMMENDED FOR HEALTH CARE WORKERS—cont'd				
Measles live-virus vaccine	One dose SC; second dose at least 1 month later.	HCWs† born during or after 1957 who do not have documentation of having received 2 doses of live vaccine on or after the first birthday or a history of physician-diagnosed measles or serologic evidence of immunity. Vaccination should be considered for all HCWs who lack proof of immunity, including those born before 1957.	Pregnancy; immuno-compromised persons‡ including HIV-infected persons who have evidence of severe immunosuppression; anaphylaxis after gelatin ingestion or administration of neomycin; recent administration of immune globulin.	MMR is the vaccine of choice if recipients are likely to be susceptible to rubella and/or mumps as well as to measles. Persons vaccinated during 1963 to 1967 with a killed measles vaccine alone, killed vaccine followed by live vaccine, or with a vaccine of unknown type should be revaccinated with 2 doses of live measles virus vaccine.
Mumps live-virus vaccine	One dose SC; no booster.	HCWs† believed to be susceptible can be vaccinated. Adults born before 1957 can be considered immune.	Pregnancy; immuno-compromised persons‡; history of anaphylactic reaction after gelatin ingestion or administration of neomycin.	MMR is the vaccine of choice if recipients are likely to be susceptible to measles and rubella as well as to mumps.
Rubella live-virus vaccine	One dose SC; no booster.	Indicated for HCWs†, both men and women, who do not have documentation of having received live vaccine on or after their first birthday or laboratory evidence of immunity. Adults born before 1957, except women who can become pregnant, can be considered immune.	Pregnancy; immuno-compromised persons‡; history of anaphylactic reaction after administration of neomycin.	The risk for rubella vaccine–associated malformations in the offspring of women pregnant when vaccinated or who become pregnant within 3 months after vaccination is negligible. Such women should be counseled regarding the theoretical basis of concern for the fetus. MMR is the vaccine of choice if recipients are likely to be susceptible to measles or mumps as well as to rubella.
Varicella zoster live-virus vaccine	Two 0.5-mL doses SC 4 to 8 weeks apart if ≥13 years of age.	Indicated for HCWs† who do not have either a reliable history of varicella or serologic evidence of immunity.	Pregnancy, immuno-compromised persons‡, history of anaphylactic reaction following receipt of neomycin or gelatin. Avoid salicylate use for 6 weeks after vaccination.	Vaccine is available from the manufacturer for certain patients with acute lymphocytic leukemia (ALL) in remission. Because 71% to 93% of persons without a history of varicella are immune, serologic testing before vaccination is likely to be cost-effective.

†All HCWs (medical or nonmedical, paid or volunteer, full-time or part-time, student or nonstudent, with or without patient-care responsibilities) who work in health care institutions (e.g., inpatient and outpatient, public and private) should be immune to measles, rubella, and varicella.

‡ Persons immunocompromised because of immune deficiency disease, HIV infection (who should primarily not receive BCG, OPV, and yellow fever vaccines), leukemia, lymphoma or generalized malignancy, or immunosuppressed as a result of therapy with corticosteroids, alkylating drugs, antimetabolites, or radiation.

Generic name	Primary schedule and boosters (s)	Indications	Major precautions and contraindications	Special considerations
IMMUNIZING AGENTS STRONGLY RECOMMENDED FOR HEALTH CARE WORKERS—cont'd				
Varicella-zoster (VZIG)	Persons <50 kg: 125 U/10 kg IM, persons ≥50 kg: 625 U§	Persons known or likely to be susceptible (particularly assessing whether to those at high risk for complications, e.g., pregnant women) who have close and prolonged exposure to a contact case or to an infectious hospital staff worker or patient.	Serologic testing may help in immune globulin, administer VZIG. If use of VZIG prevents varicella disease, patient should be vaccinated subsequently.	
Bacille Calmette-Guérin (BCG) vaccine (tuberculosis)	One percutaneous dose of 0.3 ml; no booster dose recommended.	Should be considered only for HCWs in areas where multidrug tuberculosis is prevalent, a strong likelihood of infection exists, and where comprehensive infection control precautions have failed to prevent TB transmission to HCWs.	Should not be administered to immunocompromised persons‡ and pregnant women.	In the United States tuberculosis-control efforts are directed towards early identification, treatment of cases, and preventive therapy with isoniazid.
OTHER IMMUNOBIOLOGICS THAT ARE OR MAY BE INDICATED FOR HEALTH CARE WORKERS				
Immune globulin (Hepatitis A)	Postexposure—One IM dose of 0.02 ml/kg administered ≥2 weeks.	Indicated for HCWs exposed to feces of infectious patients.	Contraindicated in persons with IgA deficiency; do not administer within 2 weeks after exposure, after MMR vaccine, or 3 weeks after varicella vaccine. Delay administration of MMR vaccine for ≥3 months and varicella vaccine ≥5 months after administration of IG.	Administer in large muscle mass (deltoid, gluteal).
Hepatitis A vaccine	Two doses of vaccine either 6 to 12 months apart (HAVRIX [R]), or 6 months apart (VAQTA [R]).	Not routinely indicated for HCWs in the United States. Persons who work with HAV-infected primates or with HAV in a research laboratory setting should be vaccinated.	History of anaphylactic hypersensitivity to alum or, for HAVRIX (R), the preservative 2-phenoxyethanol. The safety of the vaccine in pregnant women has not been determined; the risk associated with vaccination should be weighed against the risk for hepatitis A in women who may be at high risk for exposure to HAV.	

‡ Persons immunocompromised because of immune deficiency disease, HIV infection (who should primarily not receive BCG, OPV, and yellow fever vaccines), leukemia, lymphoma or generalized malignancy, or immunosuppressed as a result of therapy with corticosteroids, alkylating drugs, antimetabolites, or radiation.

§ Some experts recommend 125 U/10 kg regardless of total body weight.

Generic name	Primary schedule and boosters (s)	Indications	Major precautions and contraindications	Special considerations
OTHER IMMUNOBIOLOGICS THAT ARE OR MAY BE INDICATED FOR HEALTH CARE WORKERS—cont'd				
Meningococcal polysaccharide vaccine (tetravalent A, C, W135, and Y)	One dose in volume and by route specified by manufacturer; need for boosters unknown.	Not routinely indicated for HCWs in the United States.	The safety of the vaccine in pregnant women has not been evaluated; it should not be administered during pregnancy unless the risk for infection is high.	
Typhoid vaccine, IM, SC, and oral	IM vaccine: One 0.5 ml dose, booster 0.5 ml every 2 years. SC vaccine: two 0.5 ml doses, ≥4 weeks apart, booster 0.5 ml SC or 0.1 ID every 3 years if exposure continues. Oral vaccine: Four doses on alternate days. The manufacturer recommends revaccination with the entire four-dose series every 5 years.	Workers in microbiology laboratories who frequently work with *Salmonella typhi*	Severe local or systemic reaction to a previous dose. Ty21a (oral) vaccine should not be administered to immunocompromised persons‡ or to persons receiving antimicrobial agents.	Vaccination should not be considered an alternative to the use of proper procedures when handling specimens and cultures in the laboratory.
Vaccinia vaccine (smallpox)	One dose administered with a bifurcated needle; boosters administered every 10 years.	Laboratory workers who directly handle cultures with vaccinia, recombinant vaccinia viruses, or orthopox viruses that infect humans.	The vaccine is contraindicated in pregnancy, in persons with eczema or a history of eczema, and in immunocompromised persons‡ and their household contacts.	Vaccination may be considered for HCWs who have direct contact with contaminated dressings or other infectious material from volunteers in clinical studies involving recombinant vaccinia virus.
OTHER VACCINE-PREVENTABLE DISEASES				
Tetanus and diphtheria (toxoids [Td])	Two IM doses 4 weeks apart, third dose 6 to 12 months after second dose; booster every 10 years.	All adults.	Except in the first trimester, pregnancy is not a precaution. History of a neurologic reaction or immediate hypersensitivity reaction after a previous dose. History of severe local (Arthus-type) reaction after a previous dose. Such persons should not receive further routine or emergency doses of Td for 10 years.	Tetanus prophylaxis in wound management‖.

‖ See (15) Centers for Disease Control and Prevention: Update on adult immunization: recommendations of the Advisory Committee on Immunization Practices (ACIP), *MMWR* 1991;40(No. RR-12):1-94.

Generic name	Primary schedule and boosters (s)	Indications	Major precautions and contraindications	Special considerations
OTHER VACCINE-PREVENTABLE DISEASES				
Pneumococcal polysaccharide vaccine (23 valent)	One dose, 0.5 ml, IM or SC; revaccination recommended for those at highest risk >5 years after the first dose.	Adults who are at increased risk of pneumococcal disease and its complications because of underlying health conditions; older adults, especially those age ≥65 who are healthy.	The safety of vaccine in pregnant women has not been evaluated; it should not be administered during pregnancy unless the risk for infection is high. Previous recipients of any type of pneumococcal polysaccharide vaccine who are at highest risk for fatal infection or antibody loss may be revaccinated ≥5 years after the first dose.	

Guidelines for Practice

E.1 Infection Control Guidelines for Home Care

The practice of universal precautions means that all blood and body fluids are treated as potentially infectious. Universal precautions are implemented to prevent exposure and infection of caregivers. It is an important practice because many infections are subclinical.

- Use extreme care when handling needles, scalpels, and razors to prevent injuries. Do not recap, bend, break, or remove the needle from a syringe before disposal. Discard needles and syringes in puncture-resistant containers made of plastic or metal and dispose of them in a local landfill.
- Barrier precautions, such as gloves, masks, eye covering, and gowns, should be worn when contact with blood and body fluids is expected. Gloves must be worn when in contact with body fluids, mucous membranes, nonintact skin, and when drawing blood. Masks and eye cover are recommended when droplets or splashes of blood or other body fluids is expected. Wear gowns, aprons, or smocks to protect regular clothing from splashes of blood or body fluids.
- Handwashing is the single most important practice in preventing infections. Handwashing should be done before and after providing client care and before and after preparing food, eating, feeding, or using the bathroom.
- Soiled dressings and perineal pads should be placed inside polyethylene garbage bags by using two bags and double lining them.
- HIV is easily decontaminated by common disinfectants such as Lysol and is rapidly killed by household bleach. Surfaces can be disinfected with a solution of 1 part bleach to 10 parts water. This solution must be mixed daily to retain its disinfectant properties. Bathrooms and kitchens can be safely shared with persons infected with HIV, but towels, razors, and toothbrushes should not be shared. Household cleaning can be done in a regular manner unless there are spills of blood or body fluids. If a spill occurs, wear gloves and decontaminate the area by flooding the spill with a disinfectant, then use paper towels to remove visible debris and reapply disinfectant.
- Kitchen counters, dishes, and laundry should be cleaned in warm water and detergent after use. Bathrooms may be cleaned with a household disinfectant.

E.2 Safer Sex Guidelines

The following information is intended to be given to clients during risk-reduction counseling: Discuss injectable drug use, sexual history, and safer sex practices with potential partners before sexual activity. If you are infected with any sexually transmitted disease, such as genital herpes, HIV, or genital warts, let sexual partners know. Drugs and alcohol may impair judgment and reduce your ability to make wise decisions.

RECOMMENDATIONS FOR USE OF CONDOMS

Use latex condoms to prevent exchange of body fluids because they offer greater protection against STD than natural-membrane condoms. The use of condoms that contain spermicides, such as nonoxynol-9, can be effective in rendering HIV inactive. Nonoxynal-9 can also be put in the condom before putting it on. Oil-based lubricants, such as petroleum jelly (Vaseline), are unsafe because they weaken condoms and diminish protection. Only water-based lubricants, such as K-Y jelly, should be used. Condoms should be put on before any genital contact. Hold the tip of the condom and unroll it onto the erect penis. Leave a space at the tip for collection of semen but make sure that no air is trapped in the tip of the condom. Withdrawal should occur before loss of erection. The base of the condom should be held throughout withdrawal, and the condom should be removed slowly to avoid tearing it or spilling body fluids. If the penis relaxes before withdrawal, the condom may fall off and body fluids may spill, thus causing potential exposure. Avoid mouth contact with the penis, vagina, or anus. Wear condoms during oral sex. Condoms should never be reused and should be stored in a cool, dry place.

E.3 Guide for Evaluation of Group Effectiveness

The following questions focus evaluation on group task accomplishment, member satisfaction, conflict management, and group purpose. Answer each question for the group, then write a descriptive summary of group effectiveness.

1. Describe the group's task goal. List the steps proposed or acted on by members relative to the goal. How well do members achieve these steps?
2. Describe leadership behavior for the group. How well do members carry out other group roles?
3. Describe comfort level for group members. Do members support each other? Is the level of tension conducive to productive behavior?
4. Is disagreement expressed clearly and openly? How do members manage and resolve conflict?
5. By what bonds are members attracted to each other and to the group?
6. Are there implicit goals for the group, and do these goals interfere with the group's work toward the explicit goal?

E.4 Normal Variations and Minor Abnormalities in Newborn Physical Characteristics

VARIANT	CAUSE	COURSE	NURSING ANTICIPATORY GUIDANCE
HEAD			
Cephalhematoma	Usually caused by trauma of birth.	Soft, fluctuant, well-outlined mass of blood trapped beneath the pericranium and confined to one bone. This is a subperiosteal hematoma with no extension across suture lines.	Observe for any changes in the size or shape of the hematoma. Reassure parents. May not resolve for weeks to months.
Caput succedaneum	Caused by head pressing on the pelvic outlet in the last period of labor.	Clear fluid trapped between the scalp and bone. It is ill-defined, pits on pressure, not fluctuant. Fluid usually disappears in 1 to 2 weeks.	Explain the cause to parents and reassure them it will disappear.
Facial asymmetry	Overriding of the cranial sutures at birth caused by intrauterine molding or molding from delivery. Bones are soft and pliable.	Flattening of part of head or face. Generally disappears a few days after birth.	If the occipital area is flat because of labor and delivery, reassure parents about its disappearance in a few days. If it is caused by the "same" positioning of the child in the crib, instruct the parents to alternate the positioning of the child in the crib daily.
Asymmetry of the scalp	Usually occurs from molding during delivery or the use of forceps during delivery. Also can be caused by positioning the infant repeatedly on the same side without rotating.	Flattening of part of head.	Same as facial asymmetry.
Craniotabes	Unknown.	Softening of localized areas in the cranial bone. Sometimes found in the parietal bones at the vertex near the sagittal suture. The areas are spongelike and can be indented by the pressure of a fingertip. They resume their shape when the pressure is removed.	Usually inconsequential, but if they persist, could be indicative of a pathologic cause. There is no specific treatment. It is normal for these craniotabes to persist for months. They should eventually disappear.

Compiled by Nancy Dickenson-Hazard, RN, CPNP, MSN, for the third edition of this text.

VARIANT	CAUSE	COURSE	NURSING ANTICIPATORY GUIDANCE
HEAD—cont'd			
Fontanelle	An irregular area enclosed by a membrane that occurs where the sutures of the bone of the skull meet. These areas are called anterior fontanelle, posterior fontanelle, and temporal fontanelles.	The anterior fontanelle should be open; the posterior fontanelle may be closed.	Explain to the parents that the open fontanelle helped to protect the baby's head during the birth process. The fontanelle allows the brain to grow and will continue to do so for the next 18 months. Reassure parents that fontanelle can be touched and scalp scrubbed without ill effect.
MOUTH			
Bednar's aphthae (ulcers)	Unknown. May be caused by vigorous sucking.	Usually located on hard palate posteriorly; generally bilateral.	Reassure and support parents. Explain to the parents that there is no specific treatment, and condition will disappear without any treatment.
Epstein's epithelial pearls	Small epithelial cysts.	Located along both sides of the middle of the hard palate or along the alveolar ridge.	Reassure parents that cysts will disappear. There is no specific treatment.
Bohn's pearls (nodules)	Small white papules.	Located on each side of the midline of the hard palate. They disappear spontaneously in several weeks.	Reassure and support parents. Parents sometimes think that these lesions look like thrush. Reassure that these lesions are not thrush and will go away without treatment.
High palatal arch		Of no significance if there are no other findings present.	Reassure, support, and explain the lack of significance.
EYES			
Chemical conjunctivitis	Irritation from silver nitrate solution instilled after birth.	Eyes red with purulent exudate. Lids swollen. Onset occurs within first 24 hours and lasts about 2 to 4 days.	Cleanse eyelids with cotton balls soaked in warm saline solution. Wipe the eyes from the inner canthus out toward the outer canthus. Reassure parents that the infant's eyesight will not be affected.
Subconjunctival hemorrhage	Caused from pressure in the birth process.	Occurs at the limbus. It may be crescent shaped or may form a red halo around the iris. The hemorrhage resolves itself without any specific treatment in a few days.	Reassure parents that no residual defects occur from the hemorrhage. The blood will reabsorb itself in a few days.
Pseudostrabismus	Poor muscle coordination of the eye.	Movements of the newborn's eyes are poorly coordinated. The eyes do not necessarily move together. Very common and usually disappears spontaneously.	Reassure parents that this generally disappears spontaneously as the eye muscles strengthen and the infant's eyes continue to develop and grow.
SKIN			
Vernix caseosa	Cheeselike material that sticks to the skin. Protective covering for infant in utero.	Skin of newborn covered with varying amounts of this substance.	Will dry and disappear within a few days. Discourage mother from trying to vigorously rub it off. Encourage good skin care.
Lanugo	Fine, downy type of hair.	Usually found on the back, shoulders, and ear lobes.	Usually disappears in time as a result of the friction of the skin rubbing on the bassinet linens. Reassure parents.

VARIANT	CAUSE	COURSE	NURSING ANTICIPATORY GUIDANCE
SKIN—cont'd			
Desquamation	Skin in the newborn is very tender and soft. Following birth, the skin reacts to the changed environment by becoming very red. When the redness subsides, desquamation of the skin tends to occur.	Shedding, flaking, or peeling of the skin. Usually occurs during the first week of life. Can vary from extensive to so slight it almost goes unnoticed.	Reassure, support, and explain the cause to parents. Encourage good skin care, which avoids use of lotions, oils, and powders.
Ecchymosis	Blood under the skin caused by superficial trauma to the skin.	Bruise—disappears as the blood is reabsorbed.	Provide reassurance.
Acrocyanosis	Venous stasis.	Blue hands and feet.	No specific treatment. Make sure the baby is warm and that the cause of the acrocyanosis is not being cold.
Erythema toxicum	Unknown.	A rash consisting of small red, flat, or raised lesions. Looks splotchy and sometimes resembles chickenpox or flea bites. Usually occurs during the first 2 weeks.	No specific treatment. Reassure, support, and explain.
Nevi, pigmented	Increased pigmentation.	Range from smooth, flat, hairless pigmented areas to those with hair; some can look like warts.	No treatment unless for cosmetic reasons. Provide reassurance.
Nevus flammeus (telangiectatic) or "storkbite"	Widening of surface capillaries.	Small red areas attributable to widening of surface capillaries; disappear momentarily with blanching of skin, but usually do not disappear completely. Dull pink spots at the nape of the neck, eyelids, globella, or nasolabial folds. Gradually fade; usually disappear by 2 years (nape of the neck patches may persist).	Provide reassurance and support. No specific treatment.
Mongolian spots	Large aggregations of melanin-rich dark cells, which give the affected area a purple or blue/black color. Occur most frequently in black children but may occur in white children.	Generally found over the sacrum and coccygeal area of a large percentage of infants of black, Hispanic, Mediterranean, and Asiatic Indian origin. They do not have any significance and most disappear with time.	Explain cause and reassure parents. The spots usually disappear within the first year of life.
Mottling (Cutis marmorata)	Vasoconstriction— general circulatory instability.	Overall red and white coloration of the skin. Generally occurs in fair children who become chilled. Disappears when child becomes warm.	Explain causes and reassure parents; use a blanket to warm the infant.
Milia	Retained sebum in the skin.	Yellow-white, pinpoint-size lesions located on the bridge of the nose, the chin, or the cheeks. Disappear after first few weeks of life.	No specific treatment necessary. Explain to parents that lesions will disappear.
Café au lait spot	Variations in pigment.	Light to dark brown pigmented spots. One or two patches considered normal. If infant has several patches, may indicate fibromas or neurofibromatosis.	Assess nature of spots. If number of spots exceeds five to six, refer to physician or neurologist. Reassurance and support.
Accessory nipples (supernumerary nipples)	Not adequately explained (sometimes referred to as developmental cutaneous defect).	Occurs in a unilateral or bilateral distribution along the "mammary lines" from midaxilla to the inguinal area.	Reassure parents that the nipples may be excised for cosmetic reasons.

Compiled by Nancy Dickenson-Hazard, RN, CPNP, MSN, for the third edition of this text.

Variant	Cause	Course	Nursing anticipatory guidance
SKIN—cont'd			
Harlequin coloring	Thought to be caused by poorly developed vasomotor reflexes.	Half of the infant's body appears red/white, the other half is pale. Transitory condition, which usually occurs when the infant cries forcefully.	Explain to parents that this is not significant. It is apparently harmless and the cause is not adequately explained.
Cyanosis (localized)	Inadequate oxygen-attain of tissues; localized cyanosis because of immature peripheral circulation and venous stasis.	Usually involves lips, hands and feet, or cyanosis of the presenting parts. Usually present at birth and for variable number or days afterwards.	Keep child warm; cyanosis will decrease as peripheral circulation improves. Reassure and support parents. Explain cause.
Cyanosis (general)	Numerous causes of general cyanosis (e.g., atelectasis, congenital heart disease, central nervous system damage, obstructed airway).	Depends on the cause.	Reassurance and support. Try to determine the relationship of cyanosis to crying, (e.g., if cyanosis is relieved or improved when the child cries, then the cause may be atelectasis). Crying tends to make infants with cardiac malformations worse. Refer to physician.
ABDOMEN			
Umbilical cord variations	Natural process for sloughing tissues.	Blue/white at birth. Dull and yellow/brown within 24 hours, then black/brown and dry. Usually drops off at the end of the second week.	Keep cord area clean and dry. Reassure parents. Instruct parents in cord care.
Umbilical hernia	Occurs at the defect in the musculature of the abdominal wall near the umbilicus.	Skin-covered protuberance at the umbilicus. Very common in black infants and some Italian infants. Usually disappears spontaneously at the end of 1 to 3 years.	Reassure parents that it will probably disappear spontaneously. If it does not, it can be treated surgically when the child is older. Discourage home remedies (e.g., coin taped to hernia, binding, etc.)
OTHER			
Vaginal discharge	Physiologic manifestation of increased maternal hormonal influences.	Milky white discharge, sometimes blood-tinged or whole blood. Usually disappears in 2 weeks.	Reassure mother that this is nothing to worry about. It occurs quite frequently and is considered normal. Explain that it will disappear in a few weeks.
Brachial palsy	Sometimes caused when lateral traction is exerted on the head and neck during delivery of the shoulder in a vertex presentation, in a breech presentation when the arms are extended over the head, or when there is excessive traction on the shoulders.	Should be suspected when there is asymmetric response of the upper extremities during a Moro response. The asymmetric response occurs because there is paralysis of the muscles of the upper arm or paralysis of the entire arm. Prognosis depends on the extent of damage to the nerves.	Treatment usually consists of partial immobilization, range of motion, and appropriate positioning. Problem needs to be evaluated and the appropriate treatment initiated. Depending on the severity of damage, there could be complete return of function within a few months or there may be permanent damage. Teach parents the importance of carrying out the immobilization-positioning treatment on a daily basis. Reassure and support parents. Observe for any changes in the movement of the upper extremities.

E.5 Common Concerns and Problems of First Year (Neonate and Infant)

Problem or concern	Assessment	Nursing intervention
Burping	Swallowed air bubbles trapped in stomach; occurs more frequently in bottle-fed infants who cry during feeding.	Burp frequently during feeding (i.e., before, during, and after, after every 1 ounce of formula, or after every 4 to 5 minutes at breast). Use upright position to burp (gently rub infant's back while baby sits on parent's knee and rests forward against parent's arm). Sit upright in infant seat for 30 to 45 minutes after feeding if awake or position with head elevated and on right side if sleeping.
Colic	Unexplained bouts of crying frequently occurring at same time of day (usually busiest) and often accompanied by abdominal distention, spasms, drawing up legs to stomach, and/or passing gas. May be caused by feeding problems, maternal anxiety, or allergy, and is aggravated by tension in household. Can last 3 months. Also see Crying.	Review basic infant needs with parents (i.e., is infant hungry or wet, have air bubble, in uncomfortable position)? Review feeding method, technique, and burping; review maternal diet for offending foods if breastfed. Record time when colic episodes occur. Soothe and comfort before "attack." Walk, rock, and hold infant over shoulder. Try a monotonous soothing noise (music, ticking clock) or activity (ride in a car). Change infant position from stomach to side to back to sitting position. Rest infant on abdomen on warm, hard surface (e.g., parent's knee, warmed crib surface). Change household routine if indicated; create a quiet environment. Try pacifier or sugar water; if bottlefed, try soy formula. Reassure parents that infant is not ill, that they are providing good care, and that colic will definitely go away. Provide support to parents, giving opportunity to discuss feelings. Explain theories about origin and cycle of colic.
Crying	Periodic crying for unexplained reason; ascertain if a pattern exists for crying spells; may be related to colic; obtain a detailed history of time and length of spell; feeding frequency, method, technique, and burping; stool patterns; meeting contact and sucking needs; parental handling of crying and feelings about crying; other household factors (i.e., siblings, relative advice, parental support of each other, presence of other symptoms and/or allergies).	See previous section on colic. Reinforce that babies cry for a reason. Best to respond to crying versus letting baby cry it out. Try to identify different types of cry (hungry, wet, sleepy, pain, boredom). Crying is a release and/or exercise for infant. One or two periods a day of 5 to 10 minutes is normal for most infants. Assist parents to develop positive, relaxed approach. Reassure and support parents in this time of stress. Suggest parents alternate infant care and alternate meeting infant demands.
Constipation	Consistency of stool that is hard, pebbly, rock-like. Not related to frequency, straining, grunting, or number of days between stools. Ascertain color, consistency, and frequency, as well as presence of blood or mucus. Review infant diet and verify parent perception of constipation and expectation of normal stool patterns.	Discuss normal elimination/stool patterns for type of feeding method (i.e., breastfed stools versus bottlefed stools). Reassure that straining, grunting, infrequent number are normal. Reinforce that each infant has individual stool pattern and educate parents about what constipation actually is (i.e., consistency). Discuss parents' attitude regarding toilet habits and expectations about stool patterns. If constipated, increase liquids in diet; may offer water between meals.

Compiled by Nancy Dickenson-Hazard, RN, CPNP, MSN, for the third edition of this text.

PROBLEM OR CONCERN	ASSESSMENT	NURSING INTERVENTION
Constipation —cont'd		If introduced to solids too early or in too large a quantity, discontinue use until constipation clears, then begin again with smaller amounts. If appropriate for feeding stage, add prunes (up to 3 tbsp) or prune juice to diet.
Flatus	Air in stomach or intestines causing abdominal distress, distention, and discomfort, frequently expelled through anus. May be caused by excess swallowing of air, overfeeding, underfeeding, or allergy. Ascertain details about feeding (e.g., frequency and size of nipple, type of bottle used, breastfeeding technique, maternal diet, use of pacifier, propping of bottle, burping).	Burp frequently during and after feedings. See first section. Calm infant when crying and burp after crying. Place on left side to ease expulsion of gas. If suspect allergies, try soy formula or elimination diet. Reassure parents. May offer water between feeding—5 to 10 ml may increase gastric mobility.
Hiccoughs	Sudden sharp involuntary spasms of diaphragm; usually occur following a meal.	Reassure client that infant will cry if truly distressed. Offer infant something to suck (pacifier, breast, bottle with warm water).
Pacifier	Infants demonstrate a need for nonnutritive sucking.	Assist parents to understand aspects of positive and negative use of pacifier. Positive use: indicated immediately after birth before newborn can manipulate thumb into mouth; assists in developing sucking function; contributes to establishment of breastfeeding; good means of satisfying sucking need, especially for bottlefed infants who need extra sucking time; does not usually become a habit unless child sucks beyond infancy; most infants substitute thumb for pacifier around 3 to 4 months. Parents should look for clues to eliminate pacifier use at this time and provide stimulation suitable for the age. Negative use: pacifiers do not replace holding, stimulation, or needs satisfaction; pacifiers should not be used constantly, especially before tending to infant's needs; parents should be encouraged to discontinue use by 5 months since continued use may become a hard habit to overcome. If thumb is substituted, generally it is used less frequently than pacifier.
Spoiling	Ascertain parent definition of spoiling. Generally it is the result of basic needs not being met in early infancy, leading to a demanding, undisciplined child because need for gratification continues beyond normal time. Overgratification usually occurs then. Generally it is believed that infants cannot be spoiled under 6 months of age.	Parents require counseling and education that reinforces the following: Early infant needs must be gratified. A child cannot handle frustrations well until 8 to 9 months and is unable to delay gratification of needs until this age. A gradual and gentle approach to limits and delaying gratification is best. A relaxed, positive approach is helpful. Parents often find support groups helpful in dealing with this problem.
Biting	In first year, frequently related to teething. Particularly a problem for breastfeeding mothers. In toddlerhood related to normal aggressive impulses.	If related to teething, see later section on teething for alleviation of discomfort. Breastfeeding mothers should remove infant from breast at every occurrence and may accompany with a "no"; should also allow time to lapse before finishing feeding. If related to impulsivity of toddlerhood, see first section of Appendix A.6 on p. A-74.

PROBLEM OR CONCERN	ASSESSMENT	NURSING INTERVENTION
Separation anxiety	Occurs at 9 to10 months as infant is learning to differentiate self from mother. Can occur again in toddlerhood as child is learning to distance and separate self from mother in attempt to establish autonomy.	Reassure mother that this is normal developmental process. Advise parents, especially mother, to do the following: Play "peek-a-boo" games. Allow sufficient time (30 to 45 minutes) for child to acquaint him/herself with new person (e.g., visitor, babysitter). Avoid "sneaking out." Tell child firmly that "mommy leaves, mommy comes back." Reinforce this with "peek-a-boo" or "hide and seek" games. Avoid making major changes in child's or household routines during this period (e.g., mother returning to work; changing child's room; changing regular babysitter or day care situation).
Stranger anxiety	Begins at 6 to 8 months, gradually diminishing by 18 months. Process of child development.	See preceding section on separation anxiety. Advise parents, particularly mother, to hold infant in presence of strangers. If infant is to be left, mother should spend a short time with stranger.
Infant sleep patterns	Some infants have difficulty releasing into sleep or awaken easily. Separation anxiety, teething, illness are among the common causes. Ascertain history of problem to include how long infant sleeps, what feeding schedule is, bedtime and household routines, presence of illness or teething, and how problem is handled.	Counseling should be directed toward education of parents; infants need gratification and normal sleep patterns, emphasizing the following: Differences in temperament and incidence of sleep problems can be related. Infants generally sleep through the night by 6 months. Infant may need help transitioning to sleep by rocking, holding, pacifier, walking, etc., but should be put to bed drowsy, but awake. Environment and atmosphere conducive to sleep, (e.g., quiet, dim) should be provided. If sleep problem is related to a physical problem, measures to remedy should be implemented.
Teething	Eruption of primary or deciduous teeth starting at about 6 months, usually with lower incisors. Will continue every 2 months for first 2 years. Signs may include, but are not always present: red, swollen gums; irritable; crying and rubbing gums. Since other events in infant development are occurring simultaneously, nursing must assist parents to distinguish between these and teething as follows: • Drooling, which normally occurs at 3 to 4 months and has little to do with teething, although it may persist throughout teething. • Fevers do not usually accompany teething. Must be assessed separately because maternal antibody protection is diminishing and presence of fever is suspect for infectious process. • Separation anxiety, sleep disturbances, or fussiness from other causes are all common developmental symptoms associated with infant age group, as is reaching for and mouthing objects.	Recommend to parents hard, clean objects for baby to chew on, such as rubber teething rings, or beads, hard rubber toys, cool spoon, teething biscuits or pretzels, etc. Parents should avoid use of teething toys or rings filled with liquid because plastic covers are easily broken and liquid can be ingested.

Compiled by Nancy Dickenson-Hazard, RN, CPNP, MSN, for the third edition of this text.

PROBLEM OR CONCERN	ASSESSMENT	NURSING INTERVENTION
Diaper rashes	Rashes of varying types occurring in diaper area. Persistent rashes that do not respond to home management or continue to occur in spite of preventive measures should be referred for medical evaluation.	Preventive measures to keep area clean, dry, and aerated: Frequent diaper changing. Cleansing with water (and mild cleaner after bowel movement) at each changing, dry area well. Thick diapers and/or absorbent pads are recommended; plastic or rubber pants are not suggested. A *thin* film of protection may be used, such as A and D ointment, petroleum jelly, zinc oxide. Remove diapers for short periods every day. Wash diapers well as follows: 1. Soak soiled diapers in Borateen or borax solution (½ cup to 1 gallon of water). 2. Prerinse before washing. 3. Wash in full cycle with mild soap such as Ivory, Dreft, or Lux. 4. Avoid softeners and strong detergents. 5. Rinse diapers 2 to 3 times; may add ¼ to ½ cup vinegar to final rinse. 6. Dry in sun if possible.
	Home management of diaper rash:	Follow preventive measures with emphasis on leaving diaper off more frequently, changing when wet, and cleaning area thoroughly during changes. Zinc oxide ointment often is helpful in checking early nonfungal rashes. Cornstarch is never recommended for rashes or their prevention. Seek medical help if rash worsens or does not improve.
Cradle cap	Form of seborrheic dermatitis in neonate characterized by scalping, flaking of scalp skin, especially over anterior fontanelle. May persist beyond neonate into infancy period.	Preventive measures: Teach parents how to shampoo infant head and recommend shampooing every other day. Reassure that vigorous scrubbing will not injure fontanelle or skull. Home management for mild cases: Shampoo head daily with warm water and soap, using firm pressure on scalp. Loosen cap by applying mineral or baby oil to scalp 15 to 20 minutes before shampooing. Remove with shampoo. Comb scalp with fine comb to loosen and dislodge scaly cap. Severe cases will require medical attention and are generally managed with nonsalicylate antiseborrheic shampoos.

PROBLEMS RELATED TO FEEDING

Parental concerns about over-feeding or under-feeding	Some parents find it difficult to determine appropriate amount of milk and/or solid food to give infant. Ascertain parent understanding, knowledge, and perceptions through the following: • Diet history. • Height and weight measurement and charting on growth curve. • Elimination habits and description.	Assist parents to construct a workable feeding schedule. Discuss normal feeding patterns for breastfed and bottlefed infants. Discuss infant need for nonnutritive sucking. Convey that infants will eat more than they need or require if food is offered at each cry. Offer water between feedings to postpone next feeding to reasonable time. Suggest schedule of solid food introduction (Appendix E.9). Reassure parents that if infant is gaining weight he is not underfed. Explain growth and appetite spurts.

PROBLEM OR CONCERN	ASSESSMENT	NURSING INTERVENTION
Refusal of solids	Infant may refuse new foods for a number of reasons, e.g., temperature, texture, manner presented by person feeding, or too-early introduction. Ascertain through diet history which foods accepted, likes and dislikes, and parental feelings and perception regarding solid foods.	Discuss normal feeding patterns for age. Review indications for starting or not starting solid foods: No need before 4 to 6 months. Digestion begins with salivation around 4 months. Feeding of solid foods is not necessarily related to sleeping through the night. Tongue thrusting of solid food is normal and not a refusal. Discuss ways to encourage solid food acceptance: Allow infant to feed self. Avoid forcing infant to eat since this will only increase resistance. Solids may be stopped for a while, offering only ones that infant likes. Offer solid foods before milk when infant is hungriest. Offer food in calm, positive manner.
Refusal of food and variations in appetite	Once solid foods have been introduced and established, infants and especially toddlers will go through periods of refusal, pickiness, and preference. Obtain diet history as reviewed in preceding section (Refusal of solids).	See preceding section (Refusal of solids). Discuss following with parents: Refusal may be due to loss of interest in food when more active or due to form of negativism and means to control. Avoid use of food as substitute for attention or stimulation. Some degree of refusal and variation in appetite is normal for age. Try following approaches: Offer small amounts food frequently. Emphasize favorite foods as much as possible. Use as few nonnutritive foods as possible. Allow child to feed self if child desires to, and provide finger foods. Be patient as child tries to master use of utensils. Eating should be an enjoyable and sociable time. If hunger does not permit infant to wait until family dinner time, feed before and offer nibbles during family meal. Give older infant and toddler place, chair, utensils, plate at the table.
Spitting up	Regurgitation commonly following a feeding. Usually related to air swallowed with food, inability to relax esophageal sphincter, possible overfeeding, allergy to milk, gastroesophageal reflux. Ascertain nature of regurgitation (frequency, amount, color, consistency), as well as diet history and data regarding weight gain. Frequently outgrown by time infant is sitting well in upright position.	Reinforce the following with parents: Correct preparation of formula. Use of appropriate size nipple and nipple hole. Regular and frequent burping is needed. Place infant in an upright position for 30 minutes after feeding. Correct position of infant during feeding. Determine need to change method of feeding or formula.

Compiled by Nancy Dickenson-Hazard, RN, CPNP, MSN, for the third edition of this text.

PROBLEM OR CONCERN	ASSESSMENT	NURSING INTERVENTION
Weaning	A transition of feeding methods. May be from bottle to cup or from breast to bottle and/or cup. Weaning from breast is difficult if parents (especially mother) have ambivalent feelings or if infant refuses alternative methods. Ascertain who wants baby weaned and why, as well as schedule of feedings. Weaning from bottle should be attempted gradually, when child is ready, usually around 1 year. Ascertain who wants child weaned, what has been tried, feeding schedule and number of bottles, and ability to use cup. Babies often begin to lose interest in one or two bottles between 9 and 12 months. Offering a cup at that time may ease weaning.	Assist parents to make decision to wean: Should be discussed and decided by both parents. Positive attitude toward weaning is essential, especially for breastfeeding mothers. Weaning at times of separation anxiety is not advised, especially in breastfed infants. If possible, an infant should be weaned from breast to cup. This avoids having to wean from bottle later on. Active weaning for breastfeeding mothers: Start by substituting bottle or cup for breast at one feeding and allow 5 to 6 days before substituting for second breast feeding. If resistance is encountered, try giving water or juice in bottle or cup before weaning starts, using nipple similar to breast or pacifier if one is used, heating milk before offering, and having someone other than mother offer bottle or cup. Keep to a schedule and be firm, positive, and patient. Active weaning to cup: continue preceding steps with following additions: Reinforce idea of accomplishment in using a cup to child. May give one bottle a day but should contain only water to avoid incidence of dental caries. Avoid forcing child to wean; forcing use of cup may increase need to suck. Calm, relaxed, positive approach is essential.

E.6 Common Concerns and Problems of Toddler and Preschool Years

PROBLEM AND ASSESSMENT	NURSING INTERVENTION

AGGRESSIVE AND NEGATIVE BEHAVIORS

Biting and Hitting

Temporary behaviors occurring as a result of normal aggressive impulses and most frequently happening in new or difficult situations, when tired, hungry, or frustrated; or when expectations are too high in terms of social behaviors (ability to play with peers); used as a means of asserting control or power.

Reassure parents that behaviors are normal; discuss development and tasks child is trying to accomplish.
Advise parents to:
Avoid retaliation by hitting or biting back.
Cup chin or hold hand, giving reminder that biting and/or hitting is unacceptable.
Anticipate circumstances in which behaviors occur and circumvent them.
Use limits, such as isolation, if helpful.
Limit playmates and playtime to what is reasonable for child and age.
Allow child and playmate to work out difficulties as much as possible, redirecting their play when necessary.

Verbal Negativism

Use of the word "no" as means of control in striving for independence; often used indiscriminately and inappropriately.

Advise parents to:
Offer child a choice when possible, making alternatives simple.
Avoid bargaining and arguments.
If no choice is available, do not offer one—approach with a matter-of-fact attitude.
Develop strategy for times when child will choose and then change his mind.

Temper Tantrums

Developmental behavior directed at gaining control; Frequently triggered by unmet needs (tired, hungry), frustration. and/or overgratification and need for limits; ascertain when tantrums occur and how they are handled.

Management by parents should be directed at finding cause and prevention; counseling is directed toward approaches to discipline and limit setting (see section on discipline) and the following:
Discussion of child's needs for limits at this age.
Diary can be kept to identify pattern when tantrums occur.
Intervention is made before tantrum begins.
Should tantrum occur, possible approaches include the following:
Calm, matter-of-fact approach by parents.
Isolation of child by removal to neutral place until control is achieved (time-out).
Hold child until control is achieved, possibly offering substitute for desired object or activity that triggered tantrum.
Discourage use of corporal punishment (spanking) to achieve control.

DISCIPLINE

Discipline is guidance offered by parents to assist child in demonstrating correct, acceptable, safe behaviors; discipline is based on the parent's concepts, feelings, and attitudes regarding desirable behaviors and rules of conduct for them; mechanisms of discipline will set limits and control undesirable behaviors.

Advise parents regarding different approaches to discipline:
Permissiveness
Overpermissiveness
Authoritarianism.
Advise parents that setting limits should permit self-respect and protection of parent and child integrity; parents should be aware that discipline is essential to healthy growth.
Parent techniques include the following:
Set examples of desirable behaviors (honesty, unselfishness, good manners).

Compiled by Nancy Dickenson-Hazard, RN, CPNP, MSN, for the third edition of this text.

Problem and assessment	Nursing intervention

DISCIPLINE—cont'd

Be fair, clear, and consistent.
Agree on methods of discipline.
Give simple clear directions; bend a little by giving warnings.
Allow child to express feelings.
Respect your child; be sure to praise, show approval, and encourage.
Be realistic in behaviors expected.
Avoid arguing, threatening, promising, sermonizing, over-permissiveness, and an overly authoritarian manner.
Discipline (punishing the act).

PUNISHMENT

A method of controlling behaviors when limits are exceeded and based on child being made to feel responsible for misdeed; child will eventually learn to inhibit impulse to commit act; punishment may be verbal, restrictive, or physical and should always be appropriate to the act; punishment should not be the result of parental loss of temper.

Advise parents to:
Allow a cooling-off period.
Direct anger at situation or act, not child.
Avoid retaliation by hitting, belittling, sarcasm, ridicule, humiliation, or shame.
Avoid sending to bed or going without food.
Avoid depriving child of love.
Review points discussed in discipline section.

BREATH HOLDING

Characterized by child holding breath and turning blue. May occur with episode of anger or crying. It has a high familial incidence.
Ascertain circumstances that trigger episodes and how handled by parents.

Counseling directed toward guidance and education regarding parent-child relationship; parents will need reassurance and support as they attempt to ignore breath holding in an attempt to prevent child satisfaction in gaining control.
See section on discipline.

ROCKING, HEAD BANGING, BED SHAKING

Forms of self-stimulation frequently occurs at bedtime; ascertain how child's needs are met.

Counseling directed toward advising parents regarding:
Gratification of needs.
Provision of comfort and extra stimulation time.
Provision of relaxed, calm atmosphere through holding, singing, music.

MASTURBATION

A normal reaction, which is an exploration of body that results in stimulation of pleasurable sexual feelings; generally occurs at bedtime and starts accidentally, becoming more purposeful and frequent around 4 years.
Ascertain frequency, how parents handle, and their attitude and feelings.

Advise parents that masturbation is normal and that censoring of open masturbation is appropriate; otherwise parents should convey to child that they are aware of and understand the behavior.
Avoidance of placing excessive importance on masturbation, which may only encourage it; it is best to ignore it and/or set limits as appropriate to situation.
A punitive attitude should be avoided.

PERSISTENT THUMB SUCKING

A form of self-comfort occurring in times of stress or as a habit and persisting beyond 3 to 4 years; generally sporadic sucking is harmless and regular sucking until 2 or 3 is considered normal.

Assist parents to identify source of stress and ways to alleviate it.
Reassure and support parents when thumb sucking is within normal range.
Suggest parents remove fingers or thumb from mouth after asleep.
Suggest parents avoid constant nagging and reminding; pulling thumb from mouth; and use of restraints.
Contracting with child, rewarding alternate behaviors, and bad-tasting nail treatments may be useful to diminish thumb sucking.

PROBLEM AND ASSESSMENT	NURSING INTERVENTION

FEEDING-RELATED PROBLEMS

Loss or Variations of Appetite; Refusal of Food

Common problems related to: "too busy to eat"; development of food preferences; a normal decrease in amount of food required; and/or an attempt to control and assert independence.

See Chapter 26 for anticipatory guidance.

SLEEP-RELATED PROBLEMS

Nightmares

Problems may follow a tiring, busy day, be associated with illness, or be the result of working things out in dreams. Nightmares are frightening dreams that awaken child who feels fear and helplessness; they generally occur as a result of increased aggressive urges.

Review normal sleep patterns with parents (see Chapter 26).
Reassure parents that dreams and terrors are normal and tend to disappear spontaneously.
Parents should comfort child when awakened by dream—may attempt to explain why they are not "real."
Parents should avoid making a fuss over these sleep problems.

Night Terrors

These are dreams, generally frightening in nature, from which a child does not awaken; after acting out dream and/or a period of disorientation, child returns to sleep.

TOILET TRAINING

Achievement of control over bodily elimination; development of habits that make child self-sufficient in toileting; parents need to understand child's development and readiness before instituting a toilet training regimen (see following); parent must ascertain attitude and expectations regarding toilet training, as well as measures previously used.

Direct counseling toward parental understanding of realistic expectations, readiness of child, types of toilet training, and frequent problems encountered.
Types of toilet training:
A. Early training from ages 10 to 15 months; points to emphasize:
1. Child is not physiologically able to use toilet at this age.
2. Parents may be ready to train child, but they will be the ones who will have to pick up signals, put child on toilet, undress and dress, etc.; therefore, they should be highly motivated.
3. Bowel training may be accomplished but accidents will happen and will be due to trainer (parent), not trainee (child).
4. Training should not be stressful for parent or child.
B. Training at 18 to 30 months; points to emphasize:
1. Review readiness signs and check off which ones child has accomplished. If the majority has been achieved, probably appropriate to start training.
2. Select a good time, such as:
When there are no major changes in household and child has shown some interest after observing others.
When nursery school friends are trained.
When child is aware of wet and dirty versus dry and clean.

Indicators of readiness to toilet train	Approximate age (yr)
1. Manipulates sphincter muscles	1½ to 2
2. Manual dexterity needed to manipulate clothing	2 to 2½
3. Can hold urine for up to 4 to 5 hours	2 to 2½
4. Can understand simple directions	1½ to 2
5. Can communicate needs using words or gestures	1½ to 2
6. Developed a sense of self	1 to 2
7. Demonstrates trust in mother and desire to please	1½ to 2
8. Demonstrates sense of independence and a desire to do for self	2 to 2½
9. Is proud of own accomplishments	2 to 2½
10. Demonstrates behavioral control	2 to 2½

Compiled by Nancy Dickenson-Hazard, RN, CPNP, MSN, for the third edition of this text.

PROBLEM AND ASSESSMENT	NURSING INTERVENTION

TOILET TRAINING—cont'd

3. Select a method and stick to it.
4. Training should not be stressful; if child resists it is best to forget for awhile, then try again.
5. Accomplishment of training is variable; it may be a few days or several weeks or months.
6. Parents need to develop a relaxed, positive attitude.
7. Alternative methods include:
   Placing child on own potty chair at given intervals during the day.
   Placing child on potty before elimination is expected.
   Placing child on potty when parent goes.
   Always positively reinforce a successful attempt.

C. "Natural" toilet training (children training themselves), points to emphasize:
1. Toileting is brought to child's attention when readiness is indicated.
2. Child handles situation by himself.
3. Child needs to know parents are willing to help.
4. Although enjoying a sense of independence and accomplishment, child also needs limits set at this age.
   Problems are frequently encountered; reassure parents about naturalness, normalcy, and transient nature of these problems:
1. Problem with sitting or standing for boys; suggest starting training with sitting progressing to standing.
2. Problem using large toilet; suggest potty chair with portable seat, which can be taken on excursions.
3. Regression; suggest reinforcing as little as possible; depending on severity, may require going back to diapers for a while.
4. Need help with wiping; suggest allowing child to try if wants to clean self.
5. Being able to communicate toilet needs to others; suggest parents make sure other caretakers are aware of child's progress in training, how he communicates need, what words and what degree of independence have been achieved.
6. Child does not wish to flush bowel movements; suggest this point not be emphasized; flush toilet later.
7. Playing with feces; suggest play with clay or fingerpaints; parent should matter-of-factly state displeasure when this occurs.

E.7 Common Behaviors of School-Age Child and Adolescent

BEHAVIOR	DEVELOPMENT	GUIDANCE
SCHOOL-AGE		
Cheating	Testing right and wrong; generally follow parents' rules and authority but may succumb to peer pressure to break rules; becoming more aware of their parents' "cheating" in different ways.	Assist parents to: Reinforce positive, "good" behaviors. Maintain limits and discipline standards. Recognize that most children confess or are caught and that disciplinary action must be immediate. Identify what prompted cheating.
Lying	Differentiating between fantasies and realities; use of untruth to avoid the unpleasant; becoming more aware of parents not always telling the truth.	Confront and assess problem with assistance from teacher and involvement of child Reassure child that a real world of absolute truthfulness does not exist. Point out to child untruths that are fantasies, emphasizing the real component. Use discipline for act and discuss meaning of untruths. Reinforce honest behaviors positively.
Stealing	Curiosity about other possessions; continue to learn and internalize concept of "mine" versus "yours"; not easy to resist temptations; limited idea of property.	Act as role model; respect child's property and spouse's property; ask before use. Reinforce concept of property and ownership verbally as well as behaviorally. Discipline for petty acts (e.g., have child return or pay back item; use verbal disapproval). Assess, help, and seek referral if problem is persistent.
Fighting	More boys than girls fight; siblings usually fight; an attempt to establish position for self; may be result of frustration.	Act as role model; parents who verbally and physically fight indicate behavior is acceptable. Establish behaviors that are acceptable vents for frustration and anger. Emphasize the need to share, exchange, and interact in positive manner. Separate siblings when fighting; then allow them to work out differences once composure is regained. Avoid condoning physical assault as a means of retaliation with peers; assist child to find other solutions. Discover reason for fighting if it is continual.
Scatology	Uses dirty words as means of attention and testing parents; frequently has no understanding of meaning.	Set an example; do not use dirty words in front of child. Indicate unacceptability of dirty words; remind when child uses. Avoid a struggle, argument, or excessive discipline unless profound problem exists. Seek help if persistent.
Fears	Often learned from parents; indicative of struggle to cope with unknown or unpleasant experience; may be result of learning right from wrong.	Deal with each fear separately. Avoid overemphasis of own fear. Identify what specifically about situation evokes fear. Reassure child; reinforce that some fears are healthy and protective in nature. Seek help if fears interfere with daily life.

Compiled by Nancy Dickenson-Hazard, RN, CPNP, MSN, for the third edition of this text.

Behavior	Development	Guidance
ADOLESCENT		
Moodiness/ noncommunication	Result of emotional conflicts of establishing an identity, developing sexually, and worries over body image and social relationships.	Assist adolescent and parents to: Feel reassured about normalcy of wanting to be alone, mood swings, and fears. Recognize and discuss family conflicts and possible solutions. Recognize and discuss importance of communication and need to validate feelings.
Preoccupation with body image and sexuality	Physical changes are dramatic; need to be the same as peers; sexual fantasies and erotic urges and behaviors are heightened with physiologic changes.	Recognize normalcy of feelings and preoccupation. Understand normal physical growth, physiologic changes, and individual patterns. Accept self; develop constructive coping behaviors (e.g., sublimate into activity; need to verbalize feelings). Identify other resources of information: courses at school, books, etc. Encourage physical activity as tension release.
Rebellion	Need to establish own value and belief system.	Alleviate conflicts through open communication and validation of feelings. Role-play and offer reflective feedback to each other. Focus on individual needs and place value and pressure from others in perspective.
Conformity	Need for allegiance and belonging; assists in challenge of authority and developing of self; serves as validation mechanism.	Reinforce positive aspects of peer group and what is taught by them. Recognize normalcy of need. Find solutions when conformity interferes with adolescent's and family's goals.
Inferiority feelings	Result of feelings of loneliness and being different when unable to conform to peer group.	Relate importance of social involvement to individual goals. Explore interest and participation in after-school activities. Recognize feelings about self (what he or she likes and dislikes and what are desired changes). Identify solutions to problem behaviors identified.
Poor study habits	May result from disinterest, preoccupation, excessive parent expectations.	Identify cause of poor habits; may need remedial help or assistance in developing constructive habits. Avoid nagging or conflict over issue. Identify constructive solutions. Identify feelings and attitudes. Discuss individual goals, methods of meeting goals as related to ability and consequences.
Ambivalence	An attempt to identify dependent versus independent needs; reflects conflict between parental rules and own wishes.	Identify conflict and possible solutions. Maintain a system of accountability for behavior and compliance with rules of system. Deal with feelings constructively (e.g., verbally, physical exercise). Recognize importance and normalcy of behavior.

E.8 Health Problems of School-Age Child and Adolescent

HEALTH PROBLEM	ETIOLOGY	INCIDENCE
Acne	Sebaceous glands overproduce sebum, which occludes skin pores.	70% of adolescents experience acne.
Impetigo	Superficial skin lesion invaded by staphylococci or streptococci, spread by direct contact, with incubation of 2 to 10 days.	
Cellulitis	Bacterial invasion of skin (both dermis and subcutaneous tissue) caused by *Staphylococcus aureus,* group A beta-hemolytic *streptococcus,* or *Haemophilus influenzae.* Less communicable than impetigo but suspect throughout infection; more apt to lead to septicemia.	Frequently a secondary infection to impetigo or other skin lesions. 70% of adolescents experience acne.
Reye's syndrome	Acute encephalopathy may be sequelae of influenzae or varicella and is linked to aspirin and possibly ibuprofen use with viral illnesses.	Typical age of onset is 6 to 8 years of age. Incidence has declined in the past 10 to 15 years.
Streptococcal pharyngitis	Group A-beta hemolytic *streptococcus.*	Increased incidence in winter and spring. 30% to 50% of cases appear in school-age children. At risk for complications of cervical adenitis, otitis media, peritonsillar abscess, sinusitis, acute glomerulonephritis, acute rheumatic fever.
Toxic shock syndrome	*Staphylococcus aureus* is causative agent, with use of super-absorbant tampons a significant contributing factor.	42% of cases are adolescents.

Compiled by Nancy Dickenson-Hazard, RN, CPNP, MSN, for the third edition of this text.

ASSESSMENT	MANAGEMENT	PREVENTION
Noninflamed comedones or inflamed papules, pustules, and nodulocystic lesions on face, neck, upper chest, back, and shoulders; hair and skin are often oily.	Use of benzoyl peroxide agent; more severe cases may require retinoic acid and/or antibiotics; thorough cleansing of the skin two or three times a day using warm water and a mild soap; drying and peeling lotions may be used overnight; avoid exposure to sun and wind; frequent shampooing of the scalp; proper diet with added liquids; no diet restrictions are indicated, but should the adolescent feel a certain food aggravates the acne, it should be avoided; avoid greasy make-up, powder is better.	No known prevention, but severity of symptoms can be reduced with appropriate management.
Appearance of discolored spots that form vesicles or bullae; these vesicles break and form yellow, honey-colored, seropurulent lesions. Most frequently on hands, face, or perineum and accompanied by regional lymphadenopathy. Culture fluid from lesion or at base of lesion.	Topical treatment with Bacitracin or neomycin ointment after soaking with warm compresses. Systemic antibiotic if numerous lesions are present. Follow-up if not improved within 3 days.	Teach child not to pick or scratch insect bites, healing lesions, etc. Keep nails short and clean. Frequent handwashing. Isolate child's washing and bed linen, drinking glass, and clothes. Inspect other family members. Adequate rest and nutrition.
Warm, tender, erythematous, swollen, and indurated area on skin. Lymphangitis seen on extremities. Fever, malaise, lymphadenopathy often present.	Warm compresses. Immobilization of affected part. Rest and symptomatic measures. Systemic antibiotic therapy.	Prevention as for impetigo. All family members should be cultured and those with positive cultures treated.
Characterized by encephalopathy, severe brain edema, increased intracranial pressure, hypoglycemia, and fatty infiltration of liver.	Immediate hospitalization and medical treatment of neurologic symptoms.	Educate parents and particularly school-age and adolescent children to eliminate use of aspirin for self-treatment of viral illnesses; develop school and/or community program about Reye's syndrome, its prevention and early recognition.
Must differentiate from viral pharyngitis. Obtain throat culture.	10-day course of appropriate antibiotic when strep confirmed by culture. Symptomatic treatment for fever reduction; normal saline gargles, hard sour candy for sore throat; hot or cold compresses for tender cervical nodes.	Culture all symptomatic exposed family contacts. Avoid contact with infected child and his eating/drinking utensils. Education regarding illness and necessity of full treatment course of medication.
Sudden onset of fever, headache, sore throat, nausea, vomiting, and diarrhea, abdominal pain, hypotension, rash, arthralgia, and desquamation of soles and palms.	Immediate hospitalization, antibiotics, and monitoring and treatment of shock.	Counseling to avoid use of tampons; if must use tampons, use regular, not superabsorbant, and change every 3 to 4 hours; use sanitary pads at night; employ general genitourinary hygiene measures.

HEALTH PROBLEM	ETIOLOGY	INCIDENCE
Tuberculosis	Communicated through sputum and cough spray of infected person. Causative organism are *Mycobacterium tuberculosis* and *M. bovis.* Incubation range is 2 to 10 weeks.	Most at risk in first 3 years and the second year preceding puberty. For children of all ages, an average of 4000 new cases are reported annually. Predisposing factors include state of health and nutrition; age; environmental and socioeconomic circumstances (crowding, poor sanitation); virulence and number of bacilli.
Urinary tract infections	Bacteria enter urinary tract through urethra.	5% to 10% of girls and 1% of boys experience a UTI before 18 years.
	Predisposing factors include: Short female urethra. Obstruction. Foreign body. Poor hygiene and/or fecal contamination. Incomplete bladder emptying resulting in urine stasis. Chemical irritants. Pinworms. Indwelling catheter or catheterization. Sexual intercourse. Pregnancy. Causative organisms: *Escherichia coli* accounts for 80% to 85% of cases. Gram-positive organisms *(Staphylococcus aureus),* *Klebsiella, enterobacteria, Pseudomonas,* and *Proteus* species.	More frequent in girls than boys.
Osteomyelitis	Causative organisms are *Staphylococcus aureus* in older children and *Haemophilus* in younger children; organisms may enter directly to bone or through a preexisting infection.	Occurs most frequently between the ages of 5 and 14 years and more commonly in boys than girls.

PARASITIC INFECTIONS

Scabies	Caused by parasite, female mite that burrows into stratum corneum of skin and lays eggs in the tunnel. Transmitted by direct contact with infected person; can be contracted from infected bedding and clothing.	Pandemic in United States since 1974.

Compiled by Nancy Dickenson-Hazard, RN, CPNP, MSN, for the third edition of this text.

ASSESSMENT	MANAGEMENT	PREVENTION
Development of overt symptoms occurs in small percentage. Demonstrated systemic hypersensitivity as evidenced by positive skin test. Chest x-ray examination to determine presence and extent of active lesions. Sputum smears.	Rest, adequate diet, and gradual return to normal activity; prevention of other infection. Drug therapy. Counseling and support.	Screening tests, particularly for at-risk population. Identify, screen, and treat contacts. Hygiene and sputum precautions/measures.
History of signs and symptoms: urgency, frequency, burning, dribbling, foul-smelling urine, fever, irritability, GI symptoms; *may be asymptomatic.*	Medication course based on causative organism, age, weight of child, sensitivity of organism to drug, and previous occurrences.	
Laboratory signs: bacteria on clean-catch urine culture of greater than 100,000 colonies of a single bacteria per ml of urine confirms infection in symptomatic child.	Medications frequently used: Sulfonamides Penicillins Cephalosporins Nitrofurantoin	Hygiene education: Wipe front to back. Frequent voiding (3 to 4 hours) with complete bladder emptying. Avoid bubble baths and harsh detergents. Use cotton versus nylon panties. Avoid tight clothing. Adequate fluid intake. Prompt attention for recurrent symptoms.

	Increased fluid and rest.
	Symptomatic measures for generalized signs.
	Follow-up is essential:
	  Urine culture 48 to 72 hours after medication is instituted.
	  Urine culture on completion of medication.
	  Further follow-up includes radiographic studies and regular urine cultures.	

Frequently a history of trauma usually localized tenderness, warmth, and redness with pain on movement. Laboratory signs: marked leukocytes, elevated erythrocyte sedimentation rate, and positive blood culture.	Antibiotic therapy for 3 to 4 weeks; complete bedrest and immobilization.	Prompt attention to penetrating injuries or suspect skin lesions. Proper treatment and hygiene of injuries and skin lesions.
Vesicular or papulovesicular rash occurring typically on genitals, buttocks, between fingers and in folds of wrist, elbows, armpits, and at beltline. Appear as fine wavy line; gray to pink in color. Pruritus. Skin scrapings from over lesion reveal mite presence under microscope.	Scabicide applied to affected areas; one application is generally sufficient. Clothing and bedding should be washed.	Avoid contact with infected person's bedding and clothing. Family members should do self-skin inspection.

HEALTH PROBLEM	ETIOLOGY	INCIDENCE
PARASITIC INFECTIONS—cont'd		
Tinea capitis (scalp), corporis (body), pedis (foot)	Fungal infection easily transmitted among children. Most frequently caused by *Trichophyton tonsurans.*	Permanent baldness may occur with severe capitis.
Pinworms	Ova are swallowed after scratching anal area and transfers fingers to mouth or inhaled from contaminated clothing or linens.	Most common of helminthic parasites in humans.
Pediculosis capitis (head lice)	Causative agent is parasite, and lice infestations are communicable.	Very common among school children.
Insect bites	A variety of stinging and biting insects.	Very common in children of all ages.
Lyme disease	Causative agent is a spirochete, *Borrelia burdorferi.* Transmitted by tick bite.	High in Northeastern, coastal, Great Lakes, and western states.
DENTAL		
Caries	Progressive lesions of calcified dental tissue characterized by tooth structure loss. Bacteria, carbohydrates, and plaque are definite factors producing tooth decay.	50% to 97% of children have 1 or more cavities by 6 years of age. Greatest incidence occurs between 4 to 8 years and 12 to 18 years.

Compiled by Nancy Dickenson-Hazard, RN, CPNP, MSN, for the third edition of this text.

ASSESSMENT	MANAGEMENT	PREVENTION
Capitis: bald patches with erythema, gray scaling, and crusting.	Capitis: griseofulvis—follow-up cultures should be done.	Capitis: avoid exchange of head gear; avoid/treat infected animal; wash scalp after haircuts; avoid use of infected person's personal care articles.
Corporis: macule that enlarges peripherally, healing in center to present as scaly, circular lesions found on face, upper extremities, and trunk; may have mild pruritus.	Corporis: tolnaftate (Tinactin) 1% solution or cream.	Corporis: preceding plus avoiding exchange of clothing and community showers or bathing places.
Pedis: vesicular eruptions with skin maceration between toes.	Pedis: tolnaftate (Tinactin) solution or cream and Desenex or Tinactin powder prophylactically.	Pedis: preceding plus thoroughly dry between toes; use cotton socks and change frequently; wear well-ventilated shoes; air feet; wear rubber sandals in community showers.
Laboratory procedures: (1) microscopic examination with KOH; (2) ultraviolet light fluoresces *Microsporum* infections; (3) microscopic culture.		
Nocturnal perianal or vaginal pruritus without systemic symptoms. Worm is seen as a whitish-yellow thread 8 to 13 mm long. Scotch tape test to confirm diagnosis.	Antihelmintic such as Piperzine citrate, Mebendazole, or Pyrantel pamoate. Clothing and linen should be washed.	Personal hygiene: Handwashing and trimming nails Education regarding transmission.
Itching of occipital area, behind ears and nape of neck; diagnosis made by observation of eggs attached to hair shafts, which fluoresce white under wood light.	Application of pediculocidal shampoo, with manual removal of nits.	Wash clothing and bed linen of infected person in hot water; vacuum furniture; wash hair care items with louse shampoo; advise child against sharing hair care items or head coverings.
Localized erythema, itching, and a local wheal are common.	Cool compresses, antipruritic agents, and antihistamines are recommended; removal of stinger.	Wear shoes outside, avoid wooded, overgrown areas; use insect repellants; avoid scratching to prevent secondary infections.
Maculopapular rash at tick bite site progressing to an expanded area of erythema; progresses to neurologic and cardiac symptoms if not treated.	Careful removal of tick, pulling out with tweezers close to its mouth. Antibiotic therapy. Monitoring of progressive symptoms.	Avoid wooded, grassy areas; wear light-colored clothing for easier visualization of ticks; wear hats, long-sleeved shirts tucked inside pants, and white socks; check thoroughly for ticks if in woods; inspect children everyday if playing outside especially checking head, neck, ears, axilla, navel, buttocks, and groin; use DEET-containing insect repellants approved for children.
Characterized as discolored areas or actual lesion in fissures of chewing surfaces of teeth. May be visible on inspection. Dental equipment and x-rays most reliable in detecting caries.	Dental referral. Prevention.	Preventive measures: Early institution of dental care and visits. Brushing and flossing after every meal. Water fluoridation; oral supplemental fluoride if indicated; fluoride rinses. Topical fluoride application and use of toothpaste containing fluoride. Limit carbohydrate content of diet.

Health problem	Etiology	Incidence
DENTAL—cont'd		
Malocclusion	Irregularities of tooth alignment and improper fitting of teeth. Causative factors: abnormal jaw alignment; abnormal muscle function; incompatibility of tooth and jaw size, creating abnormal spacing, crowding, or teeth irregularities; delayed permanent teeth eruption; prolonged retention of primary teeth; neglected teeth; prolonged occurrence of lip biting, mouth breathing, tongue twisting, teeth grinding, thumb sucking.	Most frequently recognized in early school-age years. Not common in deciduous teeth.
PSYCHOGENIC		
Enuresis	Exact cause is not known but potential factors include: delayed development of neuromuscular control, organic causes, deep sleep, and high threshold for nocturnal arousal; psychologic/emotional factors.	Up to 15% of 6- to 7-year olds and 3% of 13- to 14-year olds. Males affected more than females.

Compiled by Nancy Dickenson-Hazard, RN, CPNP, MSN, for the third edition of this text.

ASSESSMENT	MANAGEMENT	PREVENTION
Variation of normal occlusion of top molars meeting firmly on opposing bottom posterior teeth with upper incisors barely overlapping and touching bottom anterior incisors.	Dental referral. Prevention.	Preventive measures: Meeting early sucking needs. Avoidance of prolonged use of bottle over 2 years. Weaning to cup at 1 year to promote jaw and mouth development after sucking. Gentle reminder about finger/thumb sucking, lip biting, etc. Remove finger, thumb from mouth when child is sleeping.
Primary: In children who have never achieved bladder control. *Secondary:* In children who have achieved bladder control for 3 to 6 months, then lose it. Complete history to include: Amount and times of fluid intake. Number of enuretic episodes per week/month. Sleeping patterns. Voiding patterns. Any recent stressful events. Occurrence at home and/or away from home or both. Child's response to enuresis. Emotional atmosphere of home. Details of toilet training. Family history of enuresis. Past medical history. Laboratory tests. Routine urinalysis.	INITIAL MEASURES Fluids are restricted after supper. Child voids before bedtime. Before retiring for night, parents should wake child to void. A night light is provided. CONDITIONING Moisture-sensitive device that sounds an alarm upon initiation of wetting, can be used. PHARMACOLOGIC Imipramine (Tofranil), which exerts an anticholinergic effect on bladder muscle and/or an antidepressant effect on central nervous system, can be used. DDAVD (desmopressin acetate) a nasal spray that is a synthetic analogue of ADH (antidiuretic hormone) to achieve night dryness). BLADDER TRAINING (A BEHAVIOR MODIFICATION PROCEDURE) Child drinks large fluid amount during day and retains urine as long as possible. When child must void, urine is measured and recorded in a daily log. Dry nights are recorded. Wall charts are maintained. Positive reinforcers, such as stars or points, are maintained for advances (e.g., two dry nights, dry all day, breaking record of previous voiding volume). COUNSELING Family and child should be encouraged to express feelings about enuresis. Parents and child should be informed that enuresis is not intentional and is no one's fault. Punitive or shaming techniques should be avoided. Explanation of the many variables involved in enuresis is essential for parents and child.	Preventive measures: Avoid too-early toilet training. Avoid negative reinforcement if accidents happen. Empty bladder before bedtime. Get up at night to void. Decrease fluid intake from dinner time on. Be supportive if accidents happen. Identify stresses child may have and help resolve.

HEALTH PROBLEM	ETIOLOGY	INCIDENCE
DENTAL—cont'd Enuresis—cont'd		
Encopresis	Commonly caused by chronic constipation or psychogenic problems. Fecal incontinence with constipated movements; frequently impactions occur.	Occurs in children over 5 years. Boys affected more frequently than girls.
EATING DISORDERS Anorexia	Psychosomatic disorder that frequently begins with weight reduction diet even though weight is within normal range.	Primarily affects adolescent girls.
Bulimia	Psychosomatic disorder of recurrent episodes of binge eating followed by self-induced vomiting.	Primarily affects adolescent girls.

Compiled by Nancy Dickenson-Hazard, RN, CPNP, MSN, for the third edition of this text.

ASSESSMENT	MANAGEMENT	PREVENTION
	COUNSELING—cont'd Nurse should assist parents and child to accept problem. Nurse should help provide support for child. Nurse should maintain a positive attitude and assist parents and child to do the same.	
Primary: children have never been toilet trained. *Secondary:* children had established bowel control. Children state they are unaware of having bowel movement. Complete history focusing on patterns of occurrence, bowel habits, and toilet training. Explore psychosocial development for significant factors (i.e., illness, loss, stress).	Removal of fecal impactions by use of enemas. Use of stool softeners. High-residue diet. Counseling and support to child and parents. Establishment of regular bowel routine. Assist parents to help child deal with anxiety. Identify practical solutions (e.g., wear extra underwear) Skin care measures.	Preventive measures: Avoid too-early toilet training. Avoid punitive techniques in toilet training. Avoid negative feedback when incontinent. Increase fluid intake. High-residue diet.
Weight loss and refusal of food accompanied by denial of hunger. Definitive diagnostic criteria include (1) loss of at least 25% of original body weight; (2) delay or cessation of menstruation for at least 3 months; and (3) distorted body image.	Frequently requires hospitalization for both anorexic and/or bulimic adolescent.	Promote healthy eating habits and attitudes; early recognition of behavioral indicators, such as: obsessive-compulsive traits; setting of perfectionistic standards for self; neat, clean, well-behaved manner; a general immaturity; and difficulty with peer and social relationships. Other nursing activities include (1) liaison contracts with the client, family, and tertiary care management team; (2) provision of support and reassurance; and (3) facilitation of home management and follow-up care by assisting the discharged client and family to maintain normal eating patterns through use of a food journal and education about balancing caloric intake requirements and exercise. See measures under anorexia.
Rapid consumption of large amounts of high-calorie, easily digested food in a short time period, sudden weight loss or dramatic weight fluctuations are common, dental erosion, electrolyte imbalance, and menstrual irregularities.		

HEALTH PROBLEM	ETIOLOGY	INCIDENCE
EATING DISORDERS—cont'd		
Obesity	Causes are related to organic problem and imbalance between caloric intake and energy expenditure. Influencing factors: Genetic. Activity patterns. Metabolic rate. Number and size of fat cells. Nutritional habits. Attitude about feeding. Quantity of food ingested.	Approximately 10% to 30% of American children are considered obese.
DEVELOPMENTAL		
Stuttering	Child's advancing mental ability and level of comprehension exceeds vocabulary ability.	Common until 6 years, reversal difficult after 7 years.
PSYCHOSOCIAL		
Latch-key children	Increased number of single-, working-parent families and inadequacy of child-care options.	As many as 10 million children lack adequate adult supervision after school.

Compiled by Nancy Dickenson-Hazard, RN, CPNP, MSN, for the third edition of this text.

ASSESSMENT	MANAGEMENT	PREVENTION
Clinically, children with weight 20% above the mean for their age and height are obese, with those 10% to 20% over mean defined as overweight. Organic problems must be ruled out. Nutritional status and diet history.	Referral, if organic problem indicated. Weight control or reduction plan that modifies eating habits, reduces caloric intake, increases energy expenditure, and promotes sense of well-being and self-esteem. Early prevention.	Preventive measures: Encourage breastfeeding. Avoid overfeeding in infancy/early childhood, including milk. Teach nutritional needs to parents. Encourage healthful eating habits. Avoid extra-caloric foods (sweetened water, candy as reward). Delay early introduction of solids. Encourage home-prepared baby foods and meals for older children. Avoid commercially prepared baby dinners and meals for older children. Encourage physical activity.
Hesitancy or dysfluency in speech pattern.	Avoid helping child to speak; speak clearly to child, avoid rushing child, look at child when speaking, praise fluent speech.	Understand normalcy of dysfluency to age 6, avoid situations where stuttering increases.
Inadequacy of care leaves children vulnerable to injury, delinquent behavior, feeling lonely, isolated, and fearful.	Teach self-help skills to children; develop programs that focus on safety, how to handle telephone calls, answering door, calling parent when arrives at home; explore alternative after-school activities; discuss feelings of loneliness, isolation, and fear with child and explore ways to reduce these feelings; promote employer-based day care and after-school care; assist parent and child to plan time alone with activities.	

E.9 Feeding and Nutrition Guidelines for Infants

AGE	TYPE OF FEEDING	SPECIFIC RECOMMENDATIONS
Birth to 6 months	Breastfeeding	Most desirable complete diet for first half year of life. Requires supplement of iron by 6 months of age (may be accomplished with solid foods). Average number of daily feedings: 6 to 8 in first 2 weeks, decreasing to 4 to 5 by 6 months.
	Formula	Iron-fortified commercial formula is a complete food for the first half year of life. Requires fluoride supplements (0.25 mg) when the concentration of fluoride in the drinking water is below 0.3 parts per million (ppm). Average total of 22 oz at 2 weeks; 28 to 30 oz at 2 months; 32 to 34-oz at 3 months; 32 to 38-oz at 6 months. Frequency and amount ranges from 2 to 3 oz 6 to 8 times a day at 2 weeks to 5 oz 5 to 6 times a day at 2 months to 7 to 8 oz 4 to 5 times a day at 5 months
6 to 12 months	Solid foods	May begin to add solids by 4 to 6 months of age; earlier introduction tends to contribute to overfeeding, choking, and allergies. Cereals are offered first. First foods are strained, pureed, or finely mashed. "Finger foods" such as teething crackers, raw fruit, or vegetables can be introduced by 6 to 7 months. Chopped table food or commercially prepared junior foods can be started by 9 to 12 months. With the exception of cereal, the order of introducing foods is variable; a recommended sequence is weekly introduction of other foods, beginning with fruit or vegetables and then meat. As the quantity of solids increases, the amount of formula may be limited to 28 to 30 oz daily. Solids should be given with a spoon, not in a bottle or "feeder."
	Cereal	Introduce commercially prepared iron-fortified infant cereals and offer daily until 12 to 18 months of age. Rice cereal is usually introduced first because of its low allergenic potential.
	Fruits and vegetables	Applesauce, bananas, and pears are usually well tolerated. Avoid canned fruits and vegetables that are not specifically designed for infants because of variable and sometimes high lead content and addition of salt, sugar, or preservatives.
	Meat, fish, and poultry	Avoid fatty meats. Prepare by baking, broiling, steaming, or poaching. Include organ meats such as liver, which has a high content of iron, vitamin A, and vitamin B complex. If soup is given, be sure all ingredients are familiar in child's diet.
	Eggs and cheese	Serve egg yolk hard-boiled and mashed, soft cooked, or poached. Introduce egg white in small quantities (1 tsp) toward end of first year to detect any allergic manifestation. Use cheese as a substitute for meat and as "finger food."

Modified from Wong D: *Whaley and Wong's nursing care of infants and children*, ed 6, St Louis, 1999, Mosby.

AGE	TYPE OF FEEDING	SPECIFIC RECOMMENDATIONS
6 to 12 months— cont'd	Suggested progression of starting solids	Start enriched baby cereal 2 to 2½ tb at breakfast and supper at 4 to 6 months; progress to 3 tb at breakfast and supper by 6 to 7 months. Continue to progress not to exceed ½ cup by 9 months.
		Add 1½ to 3 tb strained fruits for breakfast and supper at 6 months; progress to 3 tb at breakfast and supper. Continue to progress, not to exceed 2 to 3 tb 2 to 3 times a day at 8 months.
		Add 1 to 2 tb strained vegetables at lunch at 6 to 7 months; progress to 2 to 3 tb. Continue to progress, not to exceed 3 tb 2 to 3 times a day by 8 to 9 months.
		Add strained meats, 1 to 2 tb at lunch at 7 to 9 months; progress to 1 to 2 tb at lunch and supper. Continue to progress to 2 to 2½ tb 2 to 3 times a day at 9 to 10 months.
		Add egg yolk, 1 yolk or 2 tb at 7 months.
		Add bread and starch at 8 to 9 months.
		Progress to mashed table food at 8 to 9 months and finger foods at approximately same time.
	Food texture	Liquids, birth to 4 months.
		Baby-soft, 4 to 6 months.
		Thickened soft, 6 to 7 months.
		Mashed table food, 8 to 9 months.
		Finger foods, 9 months.
		Finely cut, 11 to 12 months.

E.10 Infant Stimulation

BIRTH TO 1 MONTH
Babies like to
    Suck
    Listen to repeated soft sounds
    Stare at movement and light
    Be held and rocked
Give your baby
    Your talking and singing
    Lamps throwing light patterns
    Your arms
    Rocking

1 MONTH
Babies like to
    Listen to your voice
    Look up and to the side
    Hold things placed in their hands
Give your baby
    A lullaby record
    A mobile overhead
    Pictures on the walls
    Your face near his or hers
    A change in scenery and position

2 MONTHS
Babies like to
    Listen to musical sounds
    Focus, especially on their hands
    Reach and bat nearby objects
    Smile
Give your baby
    A music box or a soft musical toy
    A soft security cuddle toy tied to crib
    Your smile
    Play time with you

3 MONTHS
Babies like to
    Reach and feel with open hands
    Grasp crudely with two hands
    Wave their fists and watch them
Give your baby
    Musical records
    Rattles
    Dangling toys
    Textured toys

4 MONTHS
Babies like to
Grasp things and let go
Kick
Laugh at unexpected sights and sounds
Make consonant sounds
Give your baby
Bells
A crib gym
More dangling toys
Space to kick and move

5 MONTHS
Babies like to
Shake, feel, and bang things
Sit with support
Play peek-a-boo
Roll over
Give your baby
A high chair with a rubber suction toy
A play pen
A kicking toy
Toys that make noise

6 MONTHS
Babies like to
Shake, bang and throw things down
Gum objects
Recognize familiar faces
Give your baby
Many household objects
Tin cups, spoons, and pot lids
Wire whisks
A clutch ball and squeaky toys
A teether and gumming toys
Bouncing, swinging seat

7 MONTHS
Babies like to
Sit alone
Use their fingers and thumb
Notice cause and effect
Bite on their first tooth
Give your baby
Bath tub toys
More "things"
String
More squeaky toys
Finger foods

8 MONTHS
Babies like to
Pivot on their stomachs
Throw, wave, and bang toys together
Look for toys they have
Make vowel sounds
Give your baby
Space to pivot and creep
2 toys at once to bang together
Big soft blocks
A jack-in-the-box
Nested plastic cups
Your conversation

9 MONTHS
Babies like to
Pull themselves up
Creep
Place things generally where they're wanted
Say "da-da"
Play pat-a-cake
Give your baby
A safe corner of the room to explore
Toys tied to the high chair
A metal mirror
Jack-in-the-box

10 MONTHS
Babies like to
Poke and prod with their forefingers
Put things in other things
Imitate sounds
Give your baby
A big pegboard (small pegs could be dangerous at this age)
Some cloth books
Motion toys
Textured toys

11 MONTHS TO 1 YEAR
Babies like to
Use their fingers
Lower themselves from standing
Drink from a cup
Mark on paper
Give your baby
Pyramid disks
A large crayon
A baking tin with clothespins
Personal drinking cup
More picture books

E.11 Accident Prevention in Children

Age	Development	Major accidents	Anticipatory guidance
Neonate to 1 month	Is unable to protect self; when on abdomen can lift and turn head; dependent, requires protection; little control over body and movements.	Motor vehicles	Use approved car seat. Do not hold infant in lap. Never leave infant in car unattended.
		Strangulation	Spacing between crib bars should be no more than 2⅜ inches apart. Avoid tying anything, including pacifiers, around neck. Fasten mobiles securely.
		Suffocation and injuries	Crib mattress should fit firmly to sides. Do not use pillows; use bumper pads. Support infant's head when lifting, holding, or bathing.
		Burns, including sunburn	Avoid bathing near hot water faucets. Test water temperature before bath. Set home water temperature less than 120° to 130° F. Avoid handling hot liquids, and do not smoke while handling infant. Keep out of direct sunlight and use sunscreen. Use flame-resistant clothing and furniture. Have smoke detectors and fire extinguishers in the home. Develop a fire plan for the home.
2 to 3 months	Begins gross motor movements of wiggling, squirming, thrashing, rolling.	Falls	Never leave infant unattended (at any age) for any reason. Keep one hand on infant while giving care. Keep crib sides up. Use infant seat on floor or playpen.
4 to 5 months	Mouths objects; brings hands to mouth.	Aspiration and choking	Do not prop bottles (at any age). Burp well before putting infant in crib. Toys should be too large for infant to swallow, nonbreakable, and free of sharp edges, strings, and detachable parts. Keep diaper pins closed during changing. Keep small objects (e.g., buttons, coins) out of reach. Use only one-piece pacifiers with a large shield.
		Suffocation	Keep all plastic bags out of reach. Keep stuffed animals out of crib.
		Lead poisoning	Check toys and other objects for lead-free paint.
6 to 7 months	Sits without support; has a firm grasp; rolls and creeps.	Falls and falling objects	Use safety strap in stroller or high chair. Use sturdy high chair or feeding table. Keep doors to stairs and outside locked; use safety gates. Avoid use of hanging tablecloths. Remove knickknacks and breakables.

Compiled by Nancy Dickenson-Hazard, RN, CPNP, MSN, for the third edition of this text.

Age	Development	Major accidents	Anticipatory guidance
6 to 7 months—cont'd		Ingestion	Keep small objects, medicine, and plants out of reach.
			Keep ipecac on hand and understand use.
			Have poison control number posted.
			Lock up medicine, cleaning agents, insecticides, etc.
			Keep trashcans out of reach or use locklids.
		Injuries and electric shock	Cover wall outlets.
			Place furniture so cords are inaccessible.
			Check furniture for sharp corners—pad or remove.
			Inspect toys for breakage.
			Keep sharp objects out of reach.
8 to 12 months	Pulls to stand; crawls, grabs; beginning to walk; enjoys exploring.	Burns	Crawl around on floor and investigate what child could reach or get into.
			Keep all hot food and drinks away from table edge; turn pot handles inward on stove.
			Keep matches and lighters out of reach.
			Keep kitchen closed up or gated.
			Never leave child unattended near fireplace or stove.
			Place guards around open hearths, registers, stoves, and fans.
			Do not iron when child is crawling nearby.
		Choking	Do not give child small hard foods, such as peanuts, raw vegetables, popcorn.
			Inspect toys for broken parts.
			Keep floors, counters, tables free of small objects.
		Motor vehicle accidents	Continue use of car seat.
			Keep doors locked.
		Poisoning	See previous discussion.
1 to 2 years	Walks up and down stairs; stoops and recovers; climbs; likes to take things apart.	Falls and injuries	Supervise children in most activities, especially up and down stairs, out of doors, and at playgrounds.
			Lock all windows; when opening, do so from top only.
			Remove any objects or furniture in front of window that child could use as a ladder.
			Permit climbing within child's capabilities.
			Remove bumper pads or toys in crib which child could use to climb on.
			Check toys, especially riding ones, for damage.
			Keep small, pointed, or sharp objects out of reach.
			Keep out of way of swings.
		Burns	Teach child meaning of hot.
			Avoid use of flowing clothing.

Compiled by Nancy Dickenson-Hazard, RN, CPNP, MSN, for the third edition of this text.

AGE	DEVELOPMENT	MAJOR ACCIDENTS	ANTICIPATORY GUIDANCE
1 to 2 years— cont'd		Drowning	Continue to supervise bath/toilet use.
			Supervise all water sport activity (e.g., wading pools, swimming, boating); use floats and/or life jackets.
			Teach child to respect water and seek swimming lessons.
		Automobile-related accidents	Continue to use appropriate car seat.
			Keep doors and windows locked.
			Do not permit child to hang out of windows.
			Hold onto child when crossing street or in parking lots.
			Do not permit child to ride toys near street.
		Poisoning and ingestion	Have ipecac in any household child frequents (babysitter, grandparents).
			Use childproof caps on medications.
			Do not regard medicine as candy.
			Do not give one child another's prescription.
2 to 4 years	More adventuresome and curious; explores body orifices; more independent, with limited cognition, imitates.	Falls and injuries	Teach child to be cautious around strange animals.
			Supervise play at playground.
			Keep out of reach small objects and foods (peanuts, beans) that can be inserted into orifices; check buttons on clothes and toys.
			Discontinue use of crib when height of crib rail is ¾ of toddler's height.
			Keep stairs well-lighted and free of clutter.
			Give toys a safety check.
			Discourage running in house and limit outdoor running to safe places.
			Teach child to respect street and cars.
			Teach child to stay away from and out of old appliances.
		Drowning	Continue to teach water safety.
			Supervise all water activities.
			Continue with swimming lessons.
		Automobile-related accidents	See previous discussion.
	Play increases to include rougher games and bike riding.	Burns	Teach child what to do if fire breaks out; hold household drills.
	Cognition improving and can identify good and bad.		Teach child to roll and smother clothes if they catch on fire.
		Drowning	Continue swimming lessons.
			Use floats or lifejacket if child cannot swim.
			Swim only where supervision is available (parent or lifeguard).
		Automobile-related accidents	Teach pedestrian safety, providing example for child.
			Do not permit playing in street.
			Use adult seat belt, if child is over 40 pounds.
			If over 55 inches tall, use shoulder restraints.
			If under 55 inches tall, only lap belt is used.

AGE	DEVELOPMENT	MAJOR ACCIDENTS	ANTICIPATORY GUIDANCE
2 to 4 years— cont'd		Falls, injuries	Make periodic checks on playground or play area used frequently. Check on child when out playing. Instruct child in safe use of toys; keep in good condition. Keep away from driveways and streets. If possible, provide fenced-in play area. Set a good example by using seat belt, looking before crossing street, etc.
		Burns	Teach child about danger of matches, lighters, stove. Recheck radiators, space heaters, fireplaces, and protective guards.
		Poisoning and ingestions	Do not become lax about keeping medication, etc., locked up. Teach child to respect harmful objects and use a symbol to indicate "danger or harmful" to child. Routinely check house, basement, and garage for harmful substances within reach.
4 to 6 years	Continues to be curious, daring, and imitative; frequently plays out of sight.		Involve child in safety discussions. Continue previously described activities when using household tools and equipment.
School age	Increased motor coordination and cognitive ability; increased peer and group activity and involvement in sports; assumes more responsibility for self and well-being.	Motor vehicle and bicycle accidents	Involve child in safety discussion and planning. Assign safety responsibilities, such as checking bike. Teach child not to ride with strangers. Teach child how to contact police and fire department and physician. Be certain child knows address and phone number. Discuss bicycle and pedestrian safety. Discuss bicycle riding rules: Always wear an approved bike helmet. Do not hitch ride on moving vehicles. Do not ride on dark street. Use headlight or reflector light at night; wear bright clothes. Do not dart from behind parked cars. Do not carry passengers on bicycle. Keep bike in good repair. Do not use street as a playground. Use seat belts.
		Injuries	Teach child to participate in sports safely using appropriate gear. Permit only supervised sport activities. Teach child proper use of household gadgets and equipment; supervise as necessary.
		Drowning	Teach the following swimming rules: Swim only where a lifeguard is present. Use buddy system. Know water depth before diving. Wear life jacket while boating or skiing or if nonswimmer. No horseplay or calling for help jokingly.

Compiled by Nancy Dickenson-Hazard, RN, CPNP, MSN, for the third edition of this text.

Age	Development	Major accidents	Anticipatory guidance
School age—cont'd		Falls	See bicycle rules. Discuss climbing trees: Avoid slippery shoes. Avoid weak or dead branches. Keep a secure handhold.
		Burns	Continue household drills. Camp with supervision. Teach proper campfire and barbecue care. Use safe camping gear, including flame-retardant clothes.
Adolescence	Seeking identity and establishment of independence; subject to strong peer pressure; rejects unsought advice; has a need for physical activity; spends most of free time away from home.	Drowning	Most important to have cooperation of adolescent when discussing and implementing safety measures. See previous sections. Never too late to learn to swim. Enroll in lifesaving classes.
		Firearms accidents	Avoid having loaded guns in household. Learn safety handling if involved in sport hunting. Keep guns in locked closet and ammunition in separate locked area. Never assume gun is not loaded. Never point gun at another.
		Automobile-related accidents	Take drivers' education. Use seat belts for self and passengers. Practice pedestrian safety. Do not drive under influence of drugs or alcohol. Do not hitchhike or pick up hitchhikers.
		Alcohol, drugs, and tobacco	Discuss effects of substance use and abuse. Assist teen to identify other ways to achieve self-esteem, independence, and peer acceptance.

E.12 Nursing Intervention for Child Abuse Prevention

OBSERVATIONS OF PARENTS-TO-BE

1. Are the parents overconcerned with the baby's sex?
2. Are they overconcerned with the baby's performance? Do they worry that he or she will not meet the standard?
3. Is there an attempt to deny that there is a pregnancy (mother not willing to gain weight, no plans whatsoever, refusal to talk about the situation)?
4. Is this child going to be one child too many? Could he or she be the "last straw"?
5. Is there great depression over this pregnancy?
6. Is the mother alone and frightened, especially by the physical changes caused by the pregnancy? Do careful explanations fail to dissipate these fears?
7. Is support lacking from husband and/or family?
8. Where is the family living? Do they have a listed telephone number? Are there relatives and friends nearby?
9. Did the mother and/or father formerly want an abortion but not go through with it or wait until it was too late?
10. Have the parents considered relinquishing of their child? Why did they change their minds?

Modified from Kempe CH: Approaches to preventing child abuse, *Am J Dis Child* 130:941, 1976.

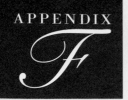

Screening Tools

F.1 Infant Reflexes

Reflex	How to elicit	Response of infant	Clinical implications
Acoustic blink	Produce a sharp, loud noise (a clap of the hands) about 30 cm from the head.	By second or third day of life infant blinks both eyes. Disappearance of reflex is variable.	Absence may indicate decreased hearing.
Ankle clonus	Flex the leg at the hip and knee, sharply dorsiflex the foot, and maintain pressure.	Rhythmic flexions and extensions of the foot at the ankle.	Abnormal if more than 10 beats during the first 3 months or more than 3 beats after 3 months. Sustained clonus indicates upper motor neuron disease.
Babinski	Stroke lateral aspect of the plantar surface of foot from heel to toes. Use a blunt object.	Hyperextension or fanning of toes occurs. As myelinization is completed, the normal response becomes flexion (downward curling) of all toes; the positive (pathologic) sign is hyperextension (dorsiflexion) of the great toe with or without fanning of the remaining toes.	After 2 years of age, a positive sign is the most significant clinical symptom of the presence of an upper motor neuron (pyramidal tract) lesion.
Blinking	Shine a light suddenly at the infant's open eyes.	Eyelids close in response to light. Disappears after first year.	Absence may indicate poor light perception or blindness.
Landau	Suspend infant carefully in prone position by supporting infant's abdomen with examiner's hand.	By 3 months of age the expected response consists of extension of head, trunk, and hips. Head is slightly above horizontal plane. Disappears by 2 years of age.	If newborn collapses into a limp, concave position, response is abnormal.
Moro	With infant in supine position, gently support head and lift it a few centimeters off the surface. As soon as neck relaxes, suddenly release the head and let it drop back to the surface. *or* Produce sudden loud noise, or jar the table or crib suddenly.	Normal response is present at birth and is one in which the arms extend outward, the hands open, and then are brought together in midline. The legs flex slightly. Usually disappears by 3 to 4 months. Infant may cry.	Asymmetry indicates possible paralysis. Absence suggests severe neurologic problem. Persistence beyond 4 months may indicate neurologic disease. If it lasts longer than 6 months, definitely abnormal.
Neck righting	With infant in supine position, turn head to one side.	Infant's trunk rotates in direction in which head is turned. Appears at 4 to 6 months. Disappears at 24 months.	Absent or decreased reflex may indicate spasticity.
Palmar grasp	With infant's head positioned in midline, place examiner's index fingers from ulnar side into infant's palm and press against palm.	Normal response is flexion of all fingers around examiner's fingers. Present at birth and disappears by 4 months when infant is ready to reach.	Note symmetry and strength. Persistence of grasp beyond 4 months suggests cerebral dysfunction.

REFLEX	HOW TO ELICIT	RESPONSE OF INFANT	CLINICAL IMPLICATIONS
Parachute	Infant is held in a prone position and is quickly lowered toward the surface of the examining table or floor.	Normal response is extension of arms, hands, and fingers, as if to break a fall. Appears by 9 months and persists.	Asymmetry or absence of response is abnormal.
Perez	Infant is held in a suspended prone position in one of the examiner's hands. The thumb of the other hand is moved firmly from sacrum along entire spine.	Normal response is extension of head and spine, flexion of knees on the chest, a cry, and emptying of the bladder. Present at birth and disappears by 3 months.	Absence indicates severe neurologic disease.
Placing	Infant is held erect and the dorsum of one foot touches the undersurface of the examining table top.	Infant flexes hip and knee and places stimulated foot on top of the table. Present at birth and disappears at 6 weeks or variable.	Absent in paralysis or in infants born by breech delivery.
Plantar grasp	Examiner's finger is placed firmly across base of infant's toes.	Toes curl downward. Present at birth and disappears by 10 to 12 months.	Absent in defects of lower spinal column. Infant cannot walk until this reflex disappears.
Rooting	Infant is held in supine position with head in midline and hands against chest. Examiner strokes perioral skin at corner of mouth or cheek.	Infant opens mouth and turns head toward stimulated side. Present at birth and disappears by 3 to 4 months (awake); by 7 months (asleep).	Absence indicates severe central nervous system disease or depressed infant.
Rotation test	Infant is held upright facing examiner and rotated in one direction and then the other.	Infant's head turns in the direction in which the body is being turned. If head is restrained, the eyes will turn in the direction in which the infant is turned.	If head and eyes do not move, it indicates a vestibular problem.
Spontaneous crawling (Bauer's response)	Infant is lying prone and examiner presses soles of feet.	Infant makes crawling movements. Present at birth.	Crawling is absent in weak or depressed infants.
Stepping	Infant is held upright and soles of feet are put in touch with solid surface.	Infant "walks" along surface. Present at birth and disappears at 6 weeks.	Absence indicates depressed infant, breech delivery, or paralysis.
Sucking	With infant in supine position, place nipple or finger 3 to 4 cm into mouth.	Vigorous sucking of finger or nipple. Present at birth and disappears by 3 to 4 months (awake) and 7 months (asleep). Tongue action should push finger up and back. Note rate of suck, amount of suction, and patterns or groupings of sucks.	Absence in term infants indicates central nervous system depression. Weak reflex may lead to feeding problems.
Tonic neck	With infant in supine position, passively rotate head to one side.	Arm and leg on side to which head is turned extend, and opposite arm and leg flex (fencer's position). Sometimes present at birth but usually by 2 to 3 months. Disappears by 6 months.	Obligatory response is always abnormal. Persistence beyond 6 months is abnormal and indicates central motor lesions (e.g., cerebral palsy).
Trunk incurvation (Galant)	Infant is held prone in examiner's hand. With the other hand the examiner moves a finger down the paravertebral portion of the spine, first on one side, then on the other.	Infant's trunk should curve to the side being stimulated. Present at birth and disappears by 2 months.	Presence of spinal cord lesions interrupts this reflex.
Vertical suspension positioning	Infant is held upright; head is maintained in midline.	Legs are flexed at the hips and knees. Present at birth and disappears after 4 months.	Scissoring or fixed extension indicates spasticity.

F.2 Vision and Hearing Screening Procedures

Method	Age	Procedure	Normal response
VISION			
Following	Infancy	Shine light or hold bright object directly in front of infant's line of vision; move slowly from side to side.	Follow light or bright object up to 180 degrees.
Turn to light response	Infancy	Hold back of head to bright light source.	Eyes turn toward source of light.
Optokinetic drum	Infancy	Twirl drum with stripes slowly in front of infant's eyes.	Nystagmus occurs.
Herschberg reflex (corneal light reflex)	Infancy through adolescence	Shine penlight into child's eyes; note where light reflex falls. For older children: have child focus and stare at point 14 inches and then 20 inches away before shining light into eyes.	Light reflex falls in same position in eye.
Cover test	Toddler through adolescence	Have child focus on specified spot first 14 inches, then 20 inches away. While child is focusing, one eye is completely covered for 5 to 10 seconds. Cover is then removed and eye observed for movement. Procedure repeated for other eye.	No wandering or sharp, jerky movement of eyes noted, indicating ability to focus.
Snellen E	Preschool	Child is instructed to point finger in direction that the E or table legs are pointing from a distance of 20 feet. Test each eye separately, then together. Test as far down on chart as child can go.	Visual acuity of 20/30 to 20/40.
Snellen alphabet	School age through adolescence	Child stands 20 feet from chart and reads letters. Each eye is tested separately and then together. Testing usually started at 20/30 or 20/40 line and child allowed to test as far down chart as possible. Passing score consists of reading majority of letters (or Es) on each line.	Visual acuity of 20/20.
HEARING			
Startle reflex	Newborn	Loud noise or bang made near infant's ears.	Jumps at noise, blinks, cries, or widens eyes.
Tracks sound	3 to 6 months	Make noise, call name, or sing.	Eyes shift toward sound; responds to mother's voice; coos to verbalization.
Recognizes sound	6 to 8 months	As preceding, from out of line of vision.	Turns head toward sound; responds to name, babbles to verbalization.
Localization of sound	8 to 12 months	Call name or use tuning fork or say words.	Localizes source of sound; turns head (and body at times) toward sound, repeats words.
Pure tone screening—play	Toddler to preschool	Demonstrate to child by putting headphones on and making believe you hear sound. As you say "I hear it," put a block in box or ring on holder. Put headphones on child and give block or ring to use. Sound a 50 dB tone at 1000 Hz and guide child's hand with block to box. When child can do this alone, begin screening. Set at 25 dB at 1000 Hz. If child responds, go to 200, 4000, and 6000 Hz. Praise child and place new block in hand. Switch to other ear and test.	Should respond at 25 dB at any frequency.

METHOD	AGE	PROCEDURE	NORMAL RESPONSE
HEARING—cont'd			
Pure-tone audiometry	School age through adolescence	Explain procedure to child. Place headphones on ears. Test one ear at a time in sequence as preceding (i.e., 25 dB at 1000, 2000, 4000, and 6000 Hz). Have child raise hand to indicate sound is heard.	Should respond at 25 dB at any frequency.
Tuning fork test	Some preschoolers; school age through adolescence		
A. Weber test		Strike tuning fork to make it vibrate and place the stem in midline of scalp. Ask child if sound is same in both ears or louder in either ear.	Sound heard equally well in both ears.
B. Rinne test		Strike tuning fork until it vibrates, place stem on child's mastoid until he or she no longer hears it. Then place vibrating fingers of fork 1 to 2 inches in front of concha. Ask child if he or she can still hear sound.	Sound from fingers of fork vibrating in air should be heard when child can no longer hear sound with stem against mastoid (i.e., air conduction is greater than bone conduction).

F.3   Screening for Common Orthopedic Problems

DEFORMITY	SCREENING
CONGENITAL HIP DISLOCATION (CHD)	
Complete or partial displacement of femoral head out of the acetabulum	Barlow's maneuver (for dislocation of femoral head): Flex hip to 90 degrees; grasp symphysis in front and sacrum in back with one hand; with other hand, apply lateral pressure to medial thigh with thumb and longitudinal pressure to knee with palm; abduct flexed hip. A positive sign is sensation of abnormal movement. Reverse hands for examining other hip (Fig. F-1). Ortolani's maneuver (for reduction of femur): Abduct hip to 80 degrees, lifting proximal femur anteriorly with fingers placed on lateral thigh. A positive sign is sensation of a jerk or snap with reduction into socket (Fig. F-2). Limited full abduction of hips: With child flat on back, abduct hips one at a time, then together. See Figure F-3 for degrees of hip abduction.

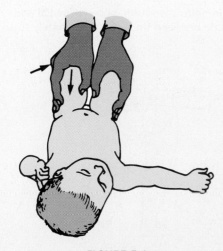

FIGURE F-1

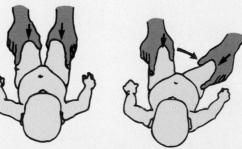 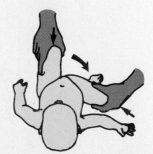

FIGURE F-2

DEFORMITY	SCREENING

METATARSUS ADDUCTUS (VARUS)

Adduction or turning in of forefoot with high longitudinal arch and wide space between first and second toes. Commonly associated with tibial torsion.

Apparent shortening of femur:
1. Allis sign: With child lying on back, pelvis flat, knees flexed, and feet planted firmly, observe knees. If the knee projects further anteriorly, femur is longer; if one knee is higher, the tibia is longer.
2. With child on back, both legs are extended out with pressure on knees. Heels are matched and observed for equal or unequal length.
3. Trendelenburg's sign: With child standing on one leg, observe pelvis. When child stands on abnormal leg, the pelvis drops on normal side. (Fig. F-4).

PES PLANUS (FLAT FEET)

When child is weight bearing, longitudinal arch of foot appears flat on floor.
1. Pseudo flat feet: Very common until ages 2 to 3; created by plantar fat pad. Feet are flexible, exhibit hypermobility of joint, and have a low arch.
2. Rigid flat feet: Uncommon; created by tightness of heel cord or tarsal coalition (a cartilaginous fibrous or bony connection between bones)

Test foot for flexibility and elicit tonic foot reflexes. Rigidity is indicated by eversion or inversion when foot does not move beyond neutral position or does not respond to toe grasping or by dorsiflexing. Signs of metatarsus adductus are illustrated in Figure F-5.
1. Observe feet in weighted and unweighted position
2. Stand child on toes. Arch disappears with weight bearing in flexible flat foot and reappears when on toes (Fig. F-6).
3. Elicit dorsal and plantar flexion to rule out tight heel cord.
4. Elicit eversion and inversion flexion to rule out tarsal coalition.

GENU VALGUM (KNOCK KNEES)

A deviant axis of thighs and calves of more than 10 to 15 degrees (normal from ages 2 to 6).

Same as for preceding No. 1 (pseudo flat feet)

GENU VARUM (BOWLEGS)

Deviant axis of thighs and calves, which is:
1. Physiologic: Normal until ages 2 to 3; occurs with internal tibial torsion and genu valgum.
2. Pathologic.

1. Observe axis of thighs and calves with child standing. Normally axes are parallel with 10 to 15 degrees deviance (Fig. F-7).
2. Observe space between the knees from front to back. Normal spacing is 1½ inches.
3. Observe space between ankles from front and back. Normal spacing between medial malleoli at heel is 2 inches.

INTERNAL TIBIAL TORSION

Twisting or torsion of tibia usually accompanied by metatarsus adductus.

Same as for genu valgum.

SCOLIOSIS

S-shaped lateral curvature of spine with rotation of vertical bodies.

1. Examine legs for range of motion and flexibility of ankle and elicit tonic foot reflexes.
2. Holding knee firmly with foot in neutral position, observe medial and lateral malleoli. The normal angle between them is approximately 15 to 20 degrees (Fig. F-8).

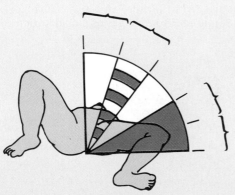

FIGURE F-3

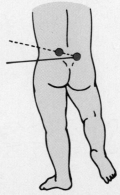

FIGURE F-4

Deformity   Screening

SCOLIOSIS—cont'd

3. Have child sit on examining table and draw a circle over patellar and external malleoli. With patella facing forward, only anterior edge of malleolar circle should be seen (Fig. F-9).

Screening is implemented as follows:

1. Ask the child to bend forward in a 50% flexing position with shoulders drooping forward and arms and head dangling. Observe the spine from above the head and inspect for any lateral curvature or prominent projection of the rib cage on one side (Fig. F-10).
2. While the child is standing erect with weight equal on both feet, observe for the following:
    a. Difference in levels of shoulders, scapula, and hips
    b. Differences in the size of the spaces between the arms and the trunk
    c. Prominence of either scapula or hip
    d. A curve in the vertebral spinous process alignment
3. Ask the child to walk and make observations discussed in No. 2 and observe for the presence of a waddle, limp, or tilt.

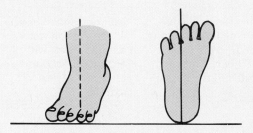

FIGURE F-5

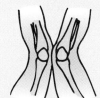

FIGURE F-6

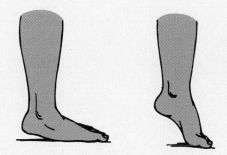

FIGURE F-7

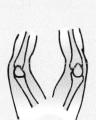

FIGURE F-8

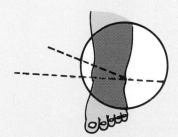

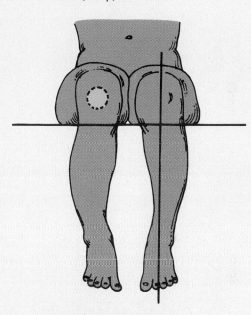

FIGURE F-9

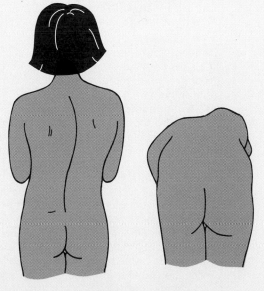

FIGURE F-10

F.4 Development Characteristics: Summary for Children

AGE	PHYSICAL AND MOTOR DEVELOPMENT	INTELLECTUAL DEVELOPMENT	SOCIALIZATION AND VOCALIZATION	EMOTIONAL DEVELOPMENT
1 month	Physiologically more stable than in newborn period. Waves hands as clenched fists. Objects placed in hands are dropped immediately. Momentary visual fixation on objects and human face. Tonic neck reflex position frequent and Moro reflex brisk. Able to turn head when prone, but unable to support head. Responds to sounds of bell, rattle, etc. Makes crawling motions when prone. Sucking and rooting reflex present. Coordinates sucking, swallowing, and breathing.	Reflexive. No attempt to interact with environment. External stimuli do not have meaning.	Cries, mews, and makes throaty noises. Responds in terms of internal need states. Interested in the human face.	Response limited generally to tension states. Panic reactions, with arching of back and extension and flexion of extremities. Derives satisfaction from the feeding situation when held and pleasure from rocking, cuddling, and tactile stimulation. Maximum need for sucking pleasures. Quiets when picked up.
2 months	Moro reflex still brisk. Posture still toward tonic neck reflex position. Has visual response to patterns. Eye coordination to light and objects. Follows objects vertically and horizontally. Responds to objects placed on face. Listens actively to sounds. Able to lift head momentarily from prone position. Turns from side to back. Able to swallow pureed foods.	Recognition of familiar face. Indicates inspection of the environment. Begins to show anticipation before feeding.	Begins to vocalize; coos. Beginning of social smile. Actively follows movement of familiar person or object with eyes. Crying becomes differentiated. Vocalizes to mother's voice. Visually searches to locate sounds of mother's voice.	Maximum need for sucking pleasures. Indicates more active satisfaction when fed, held, rocked.
3 months	Frequency of tonic neck reflex position and vigor of Moro response rapidly diminishing. Uses arms and legs simultaneously but not separately. Able to raise head from prone position; may get chest off bed. Holds head in fairly good control. Begins differentiation of motor responses. Hands are beginning to open, and objects placed in hands are retained for brief inspection; able to carry objects to mouth.	Shows active interest in environment. Can recognize familiar faces and objects such as bottle; however, objects do not have permanence. Recognition is indicative of recording of memory traces. Begins playing with parts of body. Follows objects visually. Begins to be able to coordinate stimuli from various sense organs. Shows awareness of a strange situation.	More ready and responsive smile. Facial and generalized body response to faces. Preferential response to adult voices. Has longer periods of wakefulness without crying. Begins to use prelanguage vocalizations, babbling, and cooing. Laughs aloud and shows pleasure in vocalization. Shows anticipatory preparation to being lifted.	Maximum need for sucking pleasure. Wishes to avoid unpleasant situations. Not yet able to act independently to evoke response in others.

From Waechter EH, Blake FG: *Nursing care of children*, ed 9, Philadelphia, 1976, JB Lippincott.

Age	Physical and motor development	Intellectual development	Socialization and vocalization	Emotional development
3 months —cont'd	Indicates preference for prone or supine position. "Stepping" reflex disappears. Landau reflex appears. Eyes converge as objects approach face. Has necessary muscular control to accept cereal and fruit.		Turns head to follow familiar person. Ceases crying when mother enters the room.	
4 months	Ability to carry objects to mouth. Inspects and plays with hands. Grasps objects with both hands. Turns head to sound of bell or bottle. Reaches for offered objects. Eyes focus on small objects. Begins to demonstrate eye-hand coordination. Ability to pick up objects. Rooting reflex disappears; tonic neck reflex disappearing. Sits with minimum support with stable head and back. Turns from back to side. Breathing and mouth activity coordination in relation to vocal cords. Holds head up when pulled to sitting position. Begins to drool.	Recognizes bottle on sight. Becomes bored when left alone for long periods of time. Actively interested in environment. Indicates beginnings of intentionality and interest in affecting the environment. Indicates beginning anticipation of consequences of action.	Vocalizes frequently and vocalizations change according to mood. Begins to respond to "no, no." Enjoys being propped in a sitting position. Turns head to familiar noise. Chuckles socially. Demands attention by fussing; enjoys attention.	Interest in mother heightens. Is affable and lovable. Shows signs of increasing trust and security.
5 months	Ability to recover near objects. Reaches persistently. Grasps with whole hand. Ability to lift objects. Begins to use thumb and finger in "pincer" movement. Able to sustain visual inspection. Able to sit for longer periods of time when well supported. Begins to show signs of tooth eruption. Ability to sleep through night without feeding. Moro reflex and tonic neck reflex finally disappear.	Able to discriminate strangers from family. Turns head after fallen object. Shows active interest in novelty. Attempts to regain interesting action in environment. Ability to coordinate visual impressions of an object. Begins differentiation of self from environment.	Enjoys play with people and objects. Smiles at mirror image. More exuberantly playful but also more touchy and discriminating.	Other members of the family become important as the baby's emotional world expands. Begins to be able to postpone gratification. Awaits anticipated routines with happy expectation. Begins to explore mother's body.

continued

Age	Physical and motor development	Intellectual development	Socialization and vocalization	Emotional development
6 months	Ability to pick up small objects directly and deftly. Ability to lift cup by handle. Grasps, holds, and manipulates objects. Ability to pull self to sitting position. Begins to "hitch" in locomotion. Momentary sitting and hand support. When lying in prone position, supports weight with hands. Weight gain begins to decline. Ability to turn completely over.	Increasing awareness of self. Responds with attentiveness to novel stimuli. Begins to be able to recognize mother when she is dressed differently. Objects begin to acquire permanence; searches for lost object for brief period.	Very interested in sound production. Playful response to mirror. Laughs aloud when stimulated. Great interest in babbling, which is self-reinforcing. Begins to recognize strangers.	Begins to have sense of "self." Increased growth of ego
7 months	Ability to transfer objects from one hand to another. Holds object in one hand. Gums or mouths solid foods; exploratory behavior with food. Ability to bang objects together. Palmar grasp disappears. Bears weight when held in standing position. Sits alone for brief periods. Rolls over adeptly.	Ability to secure objects by pulling on string. Repeats activities that are enjoyed. Discovers and plays with own feet. Drops and picks up objects in exploration. Searches for lost objects outside perceptual field. Has consciousness of desires. Growing differentiation of self from environment. Rudimentary sense of depth and space.	Vocalizes four different syllables. Produces vowel sounds and chained syllables. Makes "talking sounds" in response to the talking of others. Crows and squeals.	Begins to show signs of fretfulness when mother leaves or in presence of strangers. Shows beginning fear of strangers. Orally aggressive in biting and mouthing.
8 months	Ability to ring bell purposively. Ability to feed self with finger foods. Begins to experience tooth eruption. Sits well alone. Ability to release objects at will.	Uncovers hidden toy. Increased interest in feeding self. Differentiation of means from end in intentionality. Has lively curiosity about the world.	Listens selectively to familiar words. Says "da da" or equivalent. Babbles to produce consonant sounds. Vocalizes to toys. Stretches out arms to be picked up.	Plays for sheer pleasure of the activity. Anxiety when confronted by strangers indicates recognition and need of mother; attachment behavior begins to be obvious and strong.
9 months	Rises to sitting position. Creeps and/or crawls, maybe backward at first. Tries out newly developing motor capacities. Ability to hold own bottle. Drinks from cup or glass with assistance. Begins to show regular patterns in bladder and bowel elimination. Good ability to use thumb and finger in pincer grasp. Pulls self to feet with help.	Ability to put objects in container. Examines object held in hand; explores objects by sucking, chewing, and biting.	Responds to simple verbal requests. Plays interactive games, such as peek-a-boo and patty cake.	Mother is increasingly important for her own sake; reacts violently to threat of her loss. Begins to show fears of going to bed and being left alone. Increasing interest in pleasing mother. Active search in play for solutions to separation anxiety.

From Waechter EH, Blake FG: *Nursing care of children*, ed 9, Philadelphia, 1976, JB Lippincott.

AGE	PHYSICAL AND MOTOR DEVELOPMENT	INTELLECTUAL DEVELOPMENT	SOCIALIZATION AND VOCALIZATION	EMOTIONAL DEVELOPMENT
10 months	Ability to unwrap objects. Pulls to standing position. Uses index finger to poke and finger and thumb to hold objects. Finger feeds self; controls lips around cup. Plantar reflex disappears. Neck-righting reflex disappears. Sits without support; recovers balance easily. Pulls self upright with use of furniture.	Begins to imitate. Looks at and follows pictures in book.	Extends toy to another person without releasing. Responds to own name. Inhibits behavior to "no, no" or own name. Begins to test reactions to parental responses during feeding and at bedtime. Imitates facial expressions and sounds.	Has powerful urge toward independence in locomotion, feeding; beginning to help in dressing. Experiences joy when achieving a goal and mastering fear.
11 months	Ability to hold crayon adaptively. Ability to push toys. Ability to put several objects in container; releases objects at will. Stands with assistance; may be beginning attempts to walk with assistance. Begins to be able to hold spoon. "Cruises" around furniture.	Works to get toy out of reach. Growing interest in novelty. Heightened curiosity and drive to explore environment.	Repeats performance laughed at by others. Imitates definite speech sounds. Uses jargon. Communicates by pointing to objects wanted.	Reacts to restrictions with frustration, but has ability to master new situations with mother's help (weaning).
12 months	Turns pages in book; can make marks on paper. Babinski sign disappears. Begins standing alone and toddling. "Cruises" around furniture. Lumbar curve develops. Hand dominance becomes evident. Ability to use spoon in feeding.	Dogged determination to remove barriers to action. Further separation of means from ends. Experiments to reach goals not attained previously. Concepts of space, time, and causality begin to have more objectivity.	Jabbers expressively. Has words that are specific to parents. Few, simple words. Experimentation with "pseudo-words" of great interest and pleasure.	Ability to show emotions of fear, anger, affection, jealousy, anxiety. Is in love with the world.
15 to 18 months	Uses spoon and cup with little spilling; builds 2-cube tower; can undress; has refined pincer grasp.	Stoops and recovers; walks well; pushes furniture to climb; walks up stairs one at a time with assistance.	Rolls ball back and forth with one other person; imitates household chores; indicates desires without crying; drinks from a cup.	Vocabulary of 10 to 20 words; understands simple questions; forms 2-word phrases; beginning to name pictures.
2 years	Builds a 6-cube tower; turns pages of a book one at a time; begins to dress self; washes and dries hands.	Runs; walks up and down stairs alone; walks backwards; jumps in place; throws ball overhand.	Removes clothes; awareness of ownership; helps out; eats with family but cannot sit through entire meal.	Points to body parts; has 300 to 400 word vocabulary; uses "my" pronouns and prepositions; forms 3- to 4-word phrases.
3 years	Opens and closes doors using knob by self; uses fingers to hold pencil; builds 8- to 10-block tower; zips zippers; does simple buttoning.	Walks up and down stairs alternating feet; rides tricycle; broad jumps; dresses with assistance.	May have imaginary playmates; can put on simple garment; washes and dries hands; likes to have a choice.	Uses plurals; forms 3- to 4-word sentences, using correct grammatical structures.

continued

Age	Physical and motor development	Intellectual development	Socialization and vocalization	Emotional development
4 years	Draws a 3-part man; buttons easily; can cut out pictures.	Catches ball with hands; broad jumps; climbs up and down stairs, alternating feet; balances on one foot momentarily.	Separates easily from mother; can button clothing; plays interactive and associative games, demonstrating some control; able to share.	Comprehends and uses opposites; has increased vocabulary and about 90% comprehensibility; speaks in full sentences, using prepositions, pronouns, adverbs, and adjectives.
5 years	Copies a square accurately; draws a 5-part man; begins to tie shoelaces.	Runs with speed and agility; dresses without supervision; skips crudely.	Developing attachment outside of family; engages in cooperative play; strives for independence.	Vocabulary expanding to 3-syllable words; composition increasing to spoken paragraphs.

From Waechter EH, Blake FG: *Nursing care of children*, ed 9, Philadelphia, 1976, JB Lippincott.

F.5 Developmental Behaviors: School-Age Children

Age (yr)	Physical competency	Intellectual competency	Emotional-social competency	Play	Safety
6 to 12 (General)	Gains an average of 2.5 to 3.2 kg/year (5½ to 7 lb/yr). Overall height gains of 5.5 cm (2 in) per year; growth occurs in spurts and is mainly in trunk and extremities. Loses deciduous teeth; most of permanent teeth erupt. Progressively more coordinated in both gross and fine motor skills. Caloric needs increase with growth spurts.	Masters concrete operations. Moves from egocentrism; learns he or she is not always right. Learns grammar and expression of emotions and thoughts. Vocabulary increases to 3000 words or more; handles complex sentences.	Central crisis: industry vs. inferiority; wants to do and make things. Progressive sex education needed. Wants to be like friends; competition important. Fears body mutilation, alterations in body image; earlier phobias may recur, nightmares; fears death. Nervous habits common.	Plays in groups, mostly of same sex; "gang" activities predominate. Books for all ages. Bicycles a must. Sports equipment. Cards, board, and table games. Most of play is active games requiring little or no equipment.	Enforce continued use of safety belts during car travel. Bicycle safety must be taught and enforced. Teach safety related to hobbies, handicrafts, mechanical equipment.

Age (yr)	Physical competency	Intellectual competency	Emotional-social competency	Play	Safety
6 to 7	Depth perception developed. Vision reaches adult level of 20/20. Gross motor skill exceeds fine motor coordination. Balance and rhythm are good—runs, skips, jumps, climbs, gallops. Throws and catches ball. Dresses self with little or no help.	Vocabulary of 2500 words. Learning to read and print; beginning concrete concepts of numbers, general classification of items. Knows concepts of right and left; morning, afternoon, and evening; coinage. Intuitive thought process. Verbally aggressive, bossy, opinionated, argumentative. Likes simple games with basic rules.	Boisterous, outgoing, and know-it-all, whiny; parents should sidestep power struggles, offer choices. Becomes quiet and reflective during seventh year; very sensitive. Can use telephone. Likes to make things: starts many, finishes few. Give some responsibility for household duties.	Still enjoys dolls, cars, and trucks. Plays well alone but enjoys small groups of both sexes; begins to prefer same-sex peer during seventh year. Ready to learn how to ride a bicycle. Prefers imaginary, dramatic play with real costumes. Begins collecting for quantity, not quality. Enjoys active games such as hide-and-seek, tag, jump rope, roller skating, kickball. Ready for lessons in dancing, gymnastics, music. Restrict TV time to 1 to 2 hours/day.	Teach and reinforce traffic safety. Still needs adult supervision of play. Teach to avoid strangers, never take anything from strangers. Teach cold prevention and reinforce continued practice of other health habits. Restrict bicycle use to home ground; no traffic areas; teach bicycle safety. Teach and set examples regarding harmful use of drugs, alcohol, smoking.
8 to 10	Myopia may appear. Secondary sex characteristics begin in girls. Hand eye coordination and fine motor skills well established. Movements are graceful, coordinated. Cares for own physical needs completely. Constantly on move; plays and works hard; enforce balance in rest and activity. Vision and hearing fully developed.	Learning correct grammar and to express feelings in words. Likes books can read by self; will read funny papers, scan newspaper. Enjoys making detailed drawings. Mastering classification, seriation, spatial and temporal, numerical concepts. Uses language as a tool; likes riddles, jokes, chants, word games. Rules guiding force in life now. Very interested in how things work, what and how weather, seasons, etc., are made.	Strong preference for same-sex peers; antagonizes opposite-sex peers. Self-assured and pragmatic at home; questions parental values and ideas. Has a strong sense of humor. Enjoys clubs, group projects, outings, large groups, camp. Modesty about own body increases over time; sex conscious. Works diligently to perfect skills he or she does best. Happy, cooperative, relaxed and casual in relationships. Increasingly courteous and well-mannered with adults. Gang stage at a peak; secret codes and rituals prevail. Responds better to suggestion than dictatorial approach.	Likes hiking, sports. Enjoys cooking, woodworking, crafts. Enjoys cards and table games. Likes radio and records. Begins qualitative collecting now. Continue restriction on TV time.	Stress safety with firearms. Keep them out of reach and allow use only with adult supervision. Know who the child's friends are; parents should still have some control over friend selection. Teach water safety; swimming should be supervised by an adult.

continued

Age (yr)	Physical competency	Intellectual competency	Emotional-social competency	Play	Safety
11 to 12	Vital signs approximate adult norms. Growth spurt for girls; inequalities between sexes increasingly noticeable; boys attain greater physical strength. Eruption of permanent teeth complete except for third molars. Secondary sex characteristics begin in boys. Menstruation may begin.	Able to think about social problems and prejudices; sees others' points of view. Enjoys reading mysteries, love stories. Begins playing with abstract ideas. Interested in whys of health measures and understands human reproduction. Very moralistic; religious commitment often made during this time.	Intense team loyalty; boys begin teasing girls and girls flirt with boys for attention; best-friend period. Wants unreasonable independence. Rebellious about routines; wide mood swings; needs some times daily for privacy. Very critical of own work. Hero worship prevails. "Facts of life" chats with friends prevail; masturbation increases. Appears under constant tension.	Enjoys projects and working with hands. Likes to do errands and jobs to earn money. Very involved in sports, dancing, talking on phone. Enjoys all aspects of acting and drama.	Continue monitoring friends; stress bicycle safety on streets and in traffic.

F.6   Tanner Stages of Puberty

Both sexes	Pubic hair
Stage 1	Prepubescent: no pubic hair
Stage 2	Sparse growth along labia or at base of penis; long, slightly pigmented, downy
Stage 3	Darker, coarser, curly hair spreading sparsely over junction of the pubes
Stage 4	Dark, coarse, adult-like in texture but smaller area of distribution
Stage 5	Adult-like in quantity and distribution; spread to medial surface of thighs
Stage 6	Spread up linea alba

Boys	Genitalia Development
Stage 1	Prepubescent: no change from childhood
Stage 2	Scrotum and testes enlarge; scrotal skin reddened and thicker in texture
Stage 3	Penis elongates; further enlargement of scrotum and testes
Stage 4	Penis enlarges with increased size of glans; scrotal skin continues to darken
Stage 5	Genitalia adult-like in size, shape, and pigmentation

Girls	Breast Development
Stage 1	Prepubescent: elevation of papilla only
Stage 2	Development of breast bud; diameter of areola increases; papilla and breast form small mound
Stage 3	Enlargement of breast and areola with no separation of contours
Stage 4	Areola and papilla form secondary mound above the level of the breast
Stage 5	Mature stage: Projection of papilla only, due to recession of the areola to the general contour of the breast

F.7 Sources of Screening and Assessment Tools

Denver Articulation Screening Examination (DASE) by AF Drumwright
Source: LADOCA Project and Publishing Foundation
East 51st Avenue and Lincoln Street
Denver, CO 80216

Denver Developmental Screening Test (Denver II) by WK Frankenberg, JB Dodds, A Fandal, E Kazuk, and M Cohrs
Source: LADOCA Project and Publishing Foundation
East 51st Avenue and Lincoln Street
Denver, CO 80216

Developmental Profile II by GD Alpern. TJ Boll, and MS Shearer
Source: Western Psychological Services
12031 Wilshire Blvd
Los Angeles, CA 90025

Early Language Milestone Scale
Source: Modern Educational Corp
PO Box 721
Tulsa, OK 74101

Neonatal Behavioral Assessment Scale by TB Brazelton
Source: Spastic International Medical Publications
Lippincott Publications
Philadelphia, PA

Temperament Scales
Source: William Carey, MD
Division of General Pediatrics
Childrens Hospital of Philadelphia
Philadelphia, PA 19104

For more information about these and other screening and assessment tools, see the Community Resources section on this book's website at www.mosby.com/MERLIN/community_stanhope.

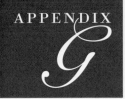
Health Risk Appraisal

G.1 Lifestyle Assessment Questionnaire

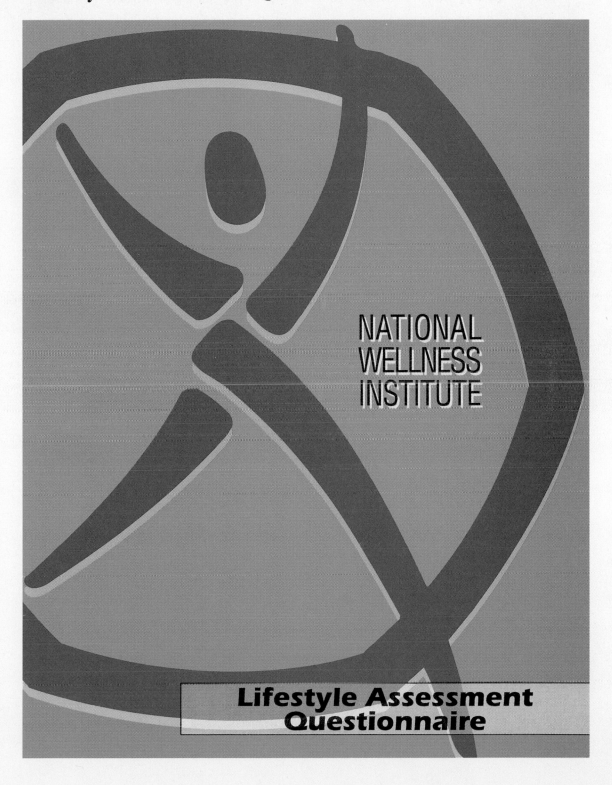

NATIONAL
WELLNESS
INSTITUTE

**Lifestyle Assessment
Questionnaire**

Purpose

This assessment tool and the analysis it provides are designed to help you discover how the choices you make each day affect your overall health.

By participating in this assessment process, you will also learn how you can make positive changes in your lifestyle, enabling you to reach a higher level of wellness.

Some of the questions are personal. While you may leave them blank, the more information you provide about your current lifestyle, the more accurately the LAQ can assess your current level of wellness and risk areas.

Confidentiality

The National Wellness Institute, Inc. subscribes to the guidelines established by the Society of Prospective Medicine concerning confidentiality in the use of health risk appraisals and risk reduction systems. These guidelines specifically state that only the participant and health professionals authorized by the participant should receive copies of his/her own health risk appraisal results.

The National Wellness Institute, Inc. strongly encourages all users of the LAQ to strictly follow these guidelines and maintain the confidentiality of all answers.

What is Wellness?

Wellness is an active process of becoming aware of and making choices toward a higher level of well-being. **Remember,** leading a wellness lifestyle requires your **active involvement.** As you gain more knowledge about what enhances your well-being, you are encouraged to use this information to make informed choices which lead to a healthier life.

General Instructions

The enclosed answer sheet is for you to record your answers to the Lifestyle Assessment Questionnaire. Please make certain that you complete all of the information at the top of the answer sheet including your zip code, group code, and social security number. If a group code has not been provided for you, leave this item blank.

Your questionnaire will be scored by an optical mark reading instrument; therefore, please use only a No. 2 (soft) pencil for marking your responses. To assure the most accurate results, follow the instructions shown on the answer sheet. Only your answer sheet needs to be returned for scoring. You may keep this questionnaire.

The Lifestyle Assessment Questionnaire was written by the National Wellness Institute, Inc.'s Cofounders; Dennis Elsenrath, Ed.D., Bill Hettler, M.D., and Fred Leafgren, Ph.D.

LIFESTYLE ASSESSMENT QUESTIONNAIRE ANSWER SHEET

Please Do Not Mark In This Box

129920

NAME

INSTRUCTIONS

SAMPLE

LAST FIRST

RETURN ADDRESS

- USE #2 PENCIL ONLY
- MARK BUBBLE COMPLETELY
- DO NOT MAKE ANY STRAY MARKS
- ERASE ONLY MARKS YOU WISH TO CHANGE

ZIP CODE

GROUP CODE

SOCIAL SECURITY #

Printed in U.S.A. NCS Trans-Optic® MP30-78818- 161514 ED08

SECTION 1-PERSONAL DATA

1. Ⓐ Ⓑ
2. Ⓐ Ⓑ Ⓒ Ⓓ Ⓔ Ⓕ
3.
4.
5.
6. Ⓐ Ⓑ Ⓒ
7. Ⓐ Ⓑ Ⓒ Ⓓ Ⓔ Ⓕ
8. Ⓐ Ⓑ Ⓒ Ⓓ Ⓔ Ⓕ Ⓖ
9. Ⓐ Ⓑ Ⓒ Ⓓ Ⓔ Ⓕ
10. Ⓐ Ⓑ Ⓒ Ⓓ
11. Ⓐ Ⓑ Ⓒ Ⓓ
12. Ⓐ Ⓑ Ⓒ Ⓓ Ⓔ

SECTION 2-LIFESTYLE

A. Physical Exercise

1. Ⓐ Ⓑ Ⓒ Ⓓ Ⓔ
2. Ⓐ Ⓑ Ⓒ Ⓓ Ⓔ
3. Ⓐ Ⓑ Ⓒ Ⓓ Ⓔ
4. Ⓐ Ⓑ Ⓒ Ⓓ Ⓔ
5. Ⓐ Ⓑ Ⓒ Ⓓ Ⓔ
6. Ⓐ Ⓑ Ⓒ Ⓓ Ⓔ
7. Ⓐ Ⓑ Ⓒ Ⓓ Ⓔ
8. Ⓐ Ⓑ Ⓒ Ⓓ Ⓔ
9. Ⓐ Ⓑ Ⓒ Ⓓ Ⓔ
10. Ⓐ Ⓑ Ⓒ Ⓓ Ⓔ

B. Nutrition

11. Ⓐ Ⓑ Ⓒ Ⓓ Ⓔ
12. Ⓐ Ⓑ Ⓒ Ⓓ Ⓔ
13. Ⓐ Ⓑ Ⓒ Ⓓ Ⓔ

14. Ⓐ Ⓑ Ⓒ Ⓓ Ⓔ
15. Ⓐ Ⓑ Ⓒ Ⓓ Ⓔ
16. Ⓐ Ⓑ Ⓒ Ⓓ Ⓔ
17. Ⓐ Ⓑ Ⓒ Ⓓ Ⓔ
18. Ⓐ Ⓑ Ⓒ Ⓓ Ⓔ
19. Ⓐ Ⓑ Ⓒ Ⓓ Ⓔ
20. Ⓐ Ⓑ Ⓒ Ⓓ Ⓔ
21. Ⓐ Ⓑ Ⓒ Ⓓ Ⓔ
22. Ⓐ Ⓑ Ⓒ Ⓓ Ⓔ
23. Ⓐ Ⓑ Ⓒ Ⓓ Ⓔ

C. Self-Care

24. Ⓐ Ⓑ Ⓒ Ⓓ Ⓔ
25. Ⓐ Ⓑ Ⓒ Ⓓ Ⓔ
26. Ⓐ Ⓑ Ⓒ Ⓓ Ⓔ
27. Ⓐ Ⓑ Ⓒ Ⓓ Ⓔ
28. Ⓐ Ⓑ Ⓒ Ⓓ Ⓔ
29. Ⓐ Ⓑ Ⓒ Ⓓ Ⓔ
30. Ⓐ Ⓑ Ⓒ Ⓓ Ⓔ
31. Ⓐ Ⓑ Ⓒ Ⓓ Ⓔ
32. Ⓐ Ⓑ Ⓒ Ⓓ Ⓔ
33. Ⓐ Ⓑ Ⓒ Ⓓ Ⓔ
34. Ⓐ Ⓑ Ⓒ Ⓓ Ⓔ
35. Ⓐ Ⓑ Ⓒ Ⓓ Ⓔ
36. Ⓐ Ⓑ Ⓒ Ⓓ Ⓔ
37. Ⓐ Ⓑ Ⓒ Ⓓ Ⓔ

D. Vehicle Safety

38. Ⓐ Ⓑ Ⓒ Ⓓ Ⓔ
39. Ⓐ Ⓑ Ⓒ Ⓓ Ⓔ
40. Ⓐ Ⓑ Ⓒ Ⓓ Ⓔ
41. Ⓐ Ⓑ Ⓒ Ⓓ Ⓔ
42. Ⓐ Ⓑ Ⓒ Ⓓ Ⓔ

43. Ⓐ Ⓑ Ⓒ Ⓓ Ⓔ
44. Ⓐ Ⓑ Ⓒ Ⓓ Ⓔ
45. Ⓐ Ⓑ Ⓒ Ⓓ Ⓔ
46. Ⓐ Ⓑ Ⓒ Ⓓ Ⓔ
47. Ⓐ Ⓑ Ⓒ Ⓓ Ⓔ
48. Ⓐ Ⓑ Ⓒ Ⓓ Ⓔ

E. Drug Usage Awareness

49. Ⓐ Ⓑ Ⓒ Ⓓ Ⓔ
50. Ⓐ Ⓑ Ⓒ Ⓓ Ⓔ
51. Ⓐ Ⓑ Ⓒ Ⓓ Ⓔ
52. Ⓐ Ⓑ Ⓒ Ⓓ Ⓔ
53. Ⓐ Ⓑ Ⓒ Ⓓ Ⓔ
54. Ⓐ Ⓑ Ⓒ Ⓓ Ⓔ
55. Ⓐ Ⓑ Ⓒ Ⓓ Ⓔ
56. Ⓐ Ⓑ Ⓒ Ⓓ Ⓔ
57. Ⓐ Ⓑ Ⓒ Ⓓ Ⓔ
58. Ⓐ Ⓑ Ⓒ Ⓓ Ⓔ
59. Ⓐ Ⓑ Ⓒ Ⓓ Ⓔ
60. Ⓐ Ⓑ Ⓒ Ⓓ Ⓔ
61. Ⓐ Ⓑ Ⓒ Ⓓ Ⓔ
62. Ⓐ Ⓑ Ⓒ Ⓓ Ⓔ
63. Ⓐ Ⓑ Ⓒ Ⓓ Ⓔ

F. Social/ Environmental

64. Ⓐ Ⓑ Ⓒ Ⓓ Ⓔ
65. Ⓐ Ⓑ Ⓒ Ⓓ Ⓔ
66. Ⓐ Ⓑ Ⓒ Ⓓ Ⓔ
67. Ⓐ Ⓑ Ⓒ Ⓓ Ⓔ
68. Ⓐ Ⓑ Ⓒ Ⓓ Ⓔ
69. Ⓐ Ⓑ Ⓒ Ⓓ Ⓔ
70. Ⓐ Ⓑ Ⓒ Ⓓ Ⓔ
71. Ⓐ Ⓑ Ⓒ Ⓓ Ⓔ

72. Ⓐ Ⓑ Ⓒ Ⓓ Ⓔ
73. Ⓐ Ⓑ Ⓒ Ⓓ Ⓔ
74. Ⓐ Ⓑ Ⓒ Ⓓ Ⓔ
75. Ⓐ Ⓑ Ⓒ Ⓓ Ⓔ
76. Ⓐ Ⓑ Ⓒ Ⓓ Ⓔ
77. Ⓐ Ⓑ Ⓒ Ⓓ Ⓔ
78. Ⓐ Ⓑ Ⓒ Ⓓ Ⓔ
79. Ⓐ Ⓑ Ⓒ Ⓓ Ⓔ
80. Ⓐ Ⓑ Ⓒ Ⓓ Ⓔ
81. Ⓐ Ⓑ Ⓒ Ⓓ Ⓔ
82. Ⓐ Ⓑ Ⓒ Ⓓ Ⓔ
83. Ⓐ Ⓑ Ⓒ Ⓓ Ⓔ
84. Ⓐ Ⓑ Ⓒ Ⓓ Ⓔ

G. Emotional Awareness & Acceptance

85. Ⓐ Ⓑ Ⓒ Ⓓ Ⓔ
86. Ⓐ Ⓑ Ⓒ Ⓓ Ⓔ

H. Emotional Management

87. Ⓐ Ⓑ Ⓒ Ⓓ Ⓔ
88. Ⓐ Ⓑ Ⓒ Ⓓ Ⓔ
89. Ⓐ Ⓑ Ⓒ Ⓓ Ⓔ
90. Ⓐ Ⓑ Ⓒ Ⓓ Ⓔ
91. Ⓐ Ⓑ Ⓒ Ⓓ Ⓔ
92. Ⓐ Ⓑ Ⓒ Ⓓ Ⓔ
93. Ⓐ Ⓑ Ⓒ Ⓓ Ⓔ
94. Ⓐ Ⓑ Ⓒ Ⓓ Ⓔ
95. Ⓐ Ⓑ Ⓒ Ⓓ Ⓔ
96. Ⓐ Ⓑ Ⓒ Ⓓ Ⓔ
97. Ⓐ Ⓑ Ⓒ Ⓓ Ⓔ
98. Ⓐ Ⓑ Ⓒ Ⓓ Ⓔ
99. Ⓐ Ⓑ Ⓒ Ⓓ Ⓔ
100. Ⓐ Ⓑ Ⓒ Ⓓ Ⓔ
101. Ⓐ Ⓑ Ⓒ Ⓓ Ⓔ

102. Ⓐ Ⓑ Ⓒ Ⓓ Ⓔ
103. Ⓐ Ⓑ Ⓒ Ⓓ Ⓔ
104. Ⓐ Ⓑ Ⓒ Ⓓ Ⓔ
105. Ⓐ Ⓑ Ⓒ Ⓓ Ⓔ
106. Ⓐ Ⓑ Ⓒ Ⓓ Ⓔ
107. Ⓐ Ⓑ Ⓒ Ⓓ Ⓔ
108. Ⓐ Ⓑ Ⓒ Ⓓ Ⓔ
109. Ⓐ Ⓑ Ⓒ Ⓓ Ⓔ
110. Ⓐ Ⓑ Ⓒ Ⓓ Ⓔ
111. Ⓐ Ⓑ Ⓒ Ⓓ Ⓔ
112. Ⓐ Ⓑ Ⓒ Ⓓ Ⓔ
113. Ⓐ Ⓑ Ⓒ Ⓓ Ⓔ
114. Ⓐ Ⓑ Ⓒ Ⓓ Ⓔ
115. Ⓐ Ⓑ Ⓒ Ⓓ Ⓔ
116. Ⓐ Ⓑ Ⓒ Ⓓ Ⓔ
117. Ⓐ Ⓑ Ⓒ Ⓓ Ⓔ
118. Ⓐ Ⓑ Ⓒ Ⓓ Ⓔ
119. Ⓐ Ⓑ Ⓒ Ⓓ Ⓔ
120. Ⓐ Ⓑ Ⓒ Ⓓ Ⓔ
121. Ⓐ Ⓑ Ⓒ Ⓓ Ⓔ
122. Ⓐ Ⓑ Ⓒ Ⓓ Ⓔ
123. Ⓐ Ⓑ Ⓒ Ⓓ Ⓔ
124. Ⓐ Ⓑ Ⓒ Ⓓ Ⓔ
125. Ⓐ Ⓑ Ⓒ Ⓓ Ⓔ
126. Ⓐ Ⓑ Ⓒ Ⓓ Ⓔ
127. Ⓐ Ⓑ Ⓒ Ⓓ Ⓔ
128. Ⓐ Ⓑ Ⓒ Ⓓ Ⓔ
129. Ⓐ Ⓑ Ⓒ Ⓓ Ⓔ
130. Ⓐ Ⓑ Ⓒ Ⓓ Ⓔ
131. Ⓐ Ⓑ Ⓒ Ⓓ Ⓔ

132. Ⓐ Ⓑ Ⓒ Ⓓ Ⓔ
133. Ⓐ Ⓑ Ⓒ Ⓓ Ⓔ
134. Ⓐ Ⓑ Ⓒ Ⓓ Ⓔ
135. Ⓐ Ⓑ Ⓒ Ⓓ Ⓔ
136. Ⓐ Ⓑ Ⓒ Ⓓ Ⓔ
137. Ⓐ Ⓑ Ⓒ Ⓓ Ⓔ
138. Ⓐ Ⓑ Ⓒ Ⓓ Ⓔ
139. Ⓐ Ⓑ Ⓒ Ⓓ Ⓔ
140. Ⓐ Ⓑ Ⓒ Ⓓ Ⓔ

I. Intellectual

141. Ⓐ Ⓑ Ⓒ Ⓓ Ⓔ
142. Ⓐ Ⓑ Ⓒ Ⓓ Ⓔ
143. Ⓐ Ⓑ Ⓒ Ⓓ Ⓔ
144. Ⓐ Ⓑ Ⓒ Ⓓ Ⓔ
145. Ⓐ Ⓑ Ⓒ Ⓓ Ⓔ
146. Ⓐ Ⓑ Ⓒ Ⓓ Ⓔ
147. Ⓐ Ⓑ Ⓒ Ⓓ Ⓔ
148. Ⓐ Ⓑ Ⓒ Ⓓ Ⓔ
149. Ⓐ Ⓑ Ⓒ Ⓓ Ⓔ
150. Ⓐ Ⓑ Ⓒ Ⓓ Ⓔ
151. Ⓐ Ⓑ Ⓒ Ⓓ Ⓔ
152. Ⓐ Ⓑ Ⓒ Ⓓ Ⓔ
153. Ⓐ Ⓑ Ⓒ Ⓓ Ⓔ
154. Ⓐ Ⓑ Ⓒ Ⓓ Ⓔ
155. Ⓐ Ⓑ Ⓒ Ⓓ Ⓔ

J. Occupational

156. Ⓐ Ⓑ Ⓒ Ⓓ Ⓔ
157. Ⓐ Ⓑ Ⓒ Ⓓ Ⓔ
158. Ⓐ Ⓑ Ⓒ Ⓓ Ⓔ
159. Ⓐ Ⓑ Ⓒ Ⓓ Ⓔ
160. Ⓐ Ⓑ Ⓒ Ⓓ Ⓔ

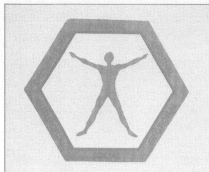

Lifestyle Assessment Questionnaire ™

Answer Sheet

SIDE 2

J. Occupational (Cont.)

SECTION 3-HEALTH RISK APPRAISAL

161 Ⓐ Ⓑ Ⓒ Ⓓ Ⓔ   1 Ⓐ Ⓑ
162 Ⓐ Ⓑ Ⓒ Ⓓ Ⓔ   2 Ⓐ Ⓑ Ⓒ
163 Ⓐ Ⓑ Ⓒ Ⓓ Ⓔ   3 Ⓐ Ⓑ Ⓒ Ⓓ
164 Ⓐ Ⓑ Ⓒ Ⓓ Ⓔ   4 Ⓐ Ⓑ
165 Ⓐ Ⓑ Ⓒ Ⓓ Ⓔ   5a
166 Ⓐ Ⓑ Ⓒ Ⓓ Ⓔ
167 Ⓐ Ⓑ Ⓒ Ⓓ Ⓔ
168 Ⓐ Ⓑ Ⓒ Ⓓ Ⓔ   5b
169 Ⓐ Ⓑ Ⓒ Ⓓ Ⓔ
170 Ⓐ Ⓑ Ⓒ Ⓓ Ⓔ
171 Ⓐ Ⓑ Ⓒ Ⓓ Ⓔ   6 Ⓐ Ⓑ Ⓒ

K. Spiritual   7
172 Ⓐ Ⓑ Ⓒ Ⓓ Ⓔ
173 Ⓐ Ⓑ Ⓒ Ⓓ Ⓔ
174 Ⓐ Ⓑ Ⓒ Ⓓ Ⓔ   8
175 Ⓐ Ⓑ Ⓒ Ⓓ Ⓔ
176 Ⓐ Ⓑ Ⓒ Ⓓ Ⓔ
177 Ⓐ Ⓑ Ⓒ Ⓓ Ⓔ   9
178 Ⓐ Ⓑ Ⓒ Ⓓ Ⓔ
179 Ⓐ Ⓑ Ⓒ Ⓓ Ⓔ   10
180 Ⓐ Ⓑ Ⓒ Ⓓ Ⓔ
181 Ⓐ Ⓑ Ⓒ Ⓓ Ⓔ   11
182 Ⓐ Ⓑ Ⓒ Ⓓ Ⓔ
183 Ⓐ Ⓑ Ⓒ Ⓓ Ⓔ   12 Ⓐ Ⓑ Ⓒ
184 Ⓐ Ⓑ Ⓒ Ⓓ Ⓔ   13
185 Ⓐ Ⓑ Ⓒ Ⓓ Ⓔ
14a
14b

15a
15b
16 Ⓐ Ⓑ Ⓒ Ⓓ Ⓔ Ⓕ Ⓖ Ⓗ
17
18 Ⓐ Ⓑ Ⓒ Ⓓ
19
20
21
22
23
24 Ⓐ Ⓑ Ⓒ Ⓓ Ⓔ
25
26 Ⓐ Ⓑ Ⓒ
27 Ⓐ Ⓑ Ⓒ Ⓓ Ⓔ
28 Ⓐ Ⓑ Ⓒ
29 Ⓐ Ⓑ Ⓒ Ⓓ Ⓔ
30 Ⓐ Ⓑ Ⓒ Ⓓ Ⓔ
31 Ⓐ Ⓑ Ⓒ Ⓓ Ⓔ
32 Ⓐ Ⓑ Ⓒ

33 Ⓐ Ⓑ Ⓒ
34 Ⓐ Ⓑ Ⓒ Ⓓ Ⓔ
35 Ⓐ Ⓑ Ⓒ Ⓓ
36 Ⓐ Ⓑ Ⓒ Ⓓ
37 Ⓐ Ⓑ Ⓒ
38 Ⓐ Ⓑ Ⓒ Ⓓ

39 Ⓐ Ⓑ
40 Ⓐ Ⓑ
41 Ⓐ Ⓑ Ⓒ
42 Ⓐ Ⓑ Ⓒ

SECTION 4-TOPICS FOR PERSONAL GROWTH

1 ◯   23 ◯
2 ◯   24 ◯
3 ◯   25 ◯
4 ◯   26 ◯
5 ◯   27 ◯
6 ◯   28 ◯
7 ◯   29 ◯
8 ◯   30 ◯
9 ◯   31 ◯
10 ◯   32 ◯
11 ◯   33 ◯
12 ◯   34 ◯
13 ◯   35 ◯
14 ◯   36 ◯
15 ◯   37 ◯
16 ◯   38 ◯
17 ◯   39 ◯
18 ◯   40 ◯
19 ◯   41 ◯
20 ◯   42 ◯
21 ◯   43 ◯
22 ◯

Section 1: PERSONAL DATA

INSTRUCTIONS:

Please complete the following general information about yourself by marking your answers in the appropriate places on the LAQ answer sheet. Please take your time and read each question carefully.

1. Sex
   a) male
   b) female
2. Race
   a) White
   b) Black
   c) Hispanic
   d) Asian
   e) American Indian
   f) other
3. Age
4. Height (feet and inches)
5. Weight (pounds)
6. Body frame size
   a) small
   b) medium
   c) large
7. Marital Status
   a) married
   b) widowed
   c) separated
   d) divorced
   e) single
   f) cohabiting
8. What was the total gross income of your household last year?
   a) under $12,000
   b) $12,000-$20,000
   c) $20,001-$30,000
   d) $30,001-$40,000
   e) $40,001-$50,000
   f) $50,001-$60,000
   g) over $60,000
9. What is the highest level of education you have completed?
   a) grade school or less
   b) some high school
   c) high school graduate
   d) some college or technical school
   e) college graduate
   f) postgraduate or professional degree
10. On the average day, how many hours do you watch television?
    a) 0 hours
    b) 1-3 hours
    c) 4-7 hours
    d) more than 8 hours
11. Where do you live?
    a) in the country
    b) in a city
    c) suburb
    d) small town
12. If you live in a city, suburb, or small town, what is the population?
    a) under 20,000
    b) 20,000-50,000
    c) 50,001-100,000
    d) 100,001-500,000
    e) over 500,000

Section 2: LIFESTYLE

INSTRUCTIONS:

This section will help determine your level of wellness. It will also give you ideas for areas in which you might improve. Some questions touch on very personal subjects. Therefore, if you prefer to skip certain questions, you may. However, the more questions you answer, the more you will learn about your health and how to improve it.

Please respond to these statements using the following responses. If an item does not apply to you, do not mark it.

A Almost always (90% or more of the time)
B Very often (approximately 75% of the time)
C Often (approximately 50% of the time)
D Occasionally (approximately 25% of the time)
E Almost never (less than 10% of the time)

PHYSICAL EXERCISE

Measures one's commitment to maintaining physical fitness.

1. I exercise vigorously for at least 20 minutes three or more times per week.
2. I determine my activity level by monitoring my heart rate.
3. I stop exercising before I feel exhausted.
4. I exercise in a relaxed, calm, and joyful manner.
5. I stretch before exercising.
6. I stretch after exercising.
7. I walk or bike whenever possible.
8. I participate in a strenuous activity (tennis, running, brisk walking, water exercise, swimming, handball, basketball, etc.).
9. If I am not in shape, I avoid sporadic (once a week or less often), strenuous exercise.
10. After vigorous exercise, I "cool down" (very light exercise such as walking) for at least five minutes before sitting or lying down.

NUTRITION

Measures the degree to which one chooses foods that are consistent with the dietary goals of the United States as published by the Senate Select Committee on Nutrition and Human Needs.

11. When choosing non-vegetable protein, I select lean cuts of meat, poultry, fish, and low-fat dairy products.
12. I maintain an appropriate weight for my height and frame.
13. I minimize salt intake.
14. I eat fruits and vegetables, fresh and uncooked.
15. I eat breakfast.
16. I intentionally include fiber in my diet on a daily basis.
17. I drink enough fluid to keep my urine light yellow.
18. I plan my diet to insure an adequate amount of vitamins and minerals.
19. I minimize foods in my diet that contain large amounts of refined flour (bleached white flour, typical store bread, cakes, etc.).
20. I minimize my intake of fats and oils including margarine and animal fats.

1

21. I include items from all four basic food groups in my diet each day (fruits and vegetables; milk group; breads and cereals; meat, fowl, fish or vegetable proteins).

22. To avoid unnecessary calories, I choose water as one of the beverages I drink.

23. I avoid adding sugar to my foods. I minimize my intake of pre-sweetened foods (sugarcoated cereals, syrups, chocolate milk, and most processed and fast foods).

SELF-CARE

Measures the behaviors which help one prevent or detect early illnesses.

24. I use footgear of good quality designed for the activity or the job in which I participate.

25. I record immunizations to maintain up-to-date immunization records.

26. I examine my breasts or testes on a monthly basis.

27. I have my breasts or testes examined yearly by a physician.

28. I balance the type and amount of food I eat with exercise to maintain a healthy percent body fat.

29. I take action to minimize my exposure to tobacco smoke.

30. When I experience illness or injury, I take necessary steps to correct the problem.

31. I engage in activities which keep my blood pressure in a range which minimizes my chances of disease (e.g., stroke, heart attack, and kidney disease).

32. I brush my teeth after eating.

33. I floss my teeth after eating.

34. My resting pulse is 60 or less.

35. I get an adequate amount of sleep.

36. If I were to have sex, I would take action to prevent unplanned pregnancy.

37. If I were to have sex, I would take action to prevent giving and/or getting sexually transmitted disease.

VEHICLE SAFETY

Measures one's ability to minimize chances of injury or death in a vehicle accident.

38. I do not operate vehicles while I am under the influence of alcohol or other drugs.

39. I do not ride with drivers who are under the influence of alcohol or other drugs.

40. I stay within the speed limit.

41. I practice defensive driving techniques.

42. When traffic lights change from green to yellow, I prepare to stop.

43. I maintain a safe driving distance between cars based on speed and road conditions.

44. Vehicles which I drive are maintained to assure safety.

45. Because they are safer, I use radial tires on cars that I drive.

46. When I ride a bicycle or motorcycle, I wear a helmet and have adequate lights/reflectors.

47. Children riding in my car are secured in an approved car seat or seat belt.

48. I use my seat belt while driving or riding in a vehicle.

DRUG USAGE AND AWARENESS

Measures the degree to which one functions without the unnecessary use of chemicals.

49. I use prescription drugs and over-the-counter medications only when necessary.

50. If I consume alcohol, I limit my consumption to not more than one drink per hour and no more than two drinks per day.

51. I avoid the use of tobacco.

52. Because of the potentially harmful effects of caffeine (e.g., coffee, tea, cola, etc.), I limit my consumption.

53. I avoid the use of marijuana.

54. I avoid the use of hallucinogens (LSD, PCP, MDA, etc.).

55. I avoid the use of stimulants ("uppers"—e.g., cocaine, amphetamines, "pep pills," etc.).

56. I avoid the use of nonmedically prescribed depressants ("downers"—e.g., barbituates, quaaludes, minor tranquilizers, etc.).

57. I avoid using a combination of drugs unless under medical supervision.

58. I follow the instructions provided with any drug I take.

59. I avoid using drugs obtained from illegal sources.

60. I understand the expected effect of drugs I take.

61. I consider alternatives to drugs.

62. If I experience discomfort from stress or tension, I use relaxation techniques, exercise, and meditation instead of taking drugs.

63. I get clear directions for taking my medicine from my doctor or pharmacist.

SOCIAL/ENVIRONMENTAL

Measures the degree to which one contributes to the common welfare of the community. This emphasizes interdependence with others and nature.

64. I conserve energy at home.

65. I consider energy conservation when choosing a mode of transportation.

66. My social ties with family are strong.

67. I contribute to the feeling of acceptance within my family.

68. I develop and maintain strong friendships.

69. I do my part to promote a clean environment (i.e., air, water, noise, etc.).

70. When I see a safety hazard, I take action (warn others or correct the problem).

71. I avoid unnecessary radiation.

72. I report criminal acts I observe.

73. I contribute time and/or money to community projects.

74. I actively seek to become acquainted with individuals in my community.

75. I use my creativity in constructive ways.

76. My behavior reflects fairness and justice.

77. When possible, I choose an environment which is free of **noise** pollution.

78. When possible, I choose an environment which is free of **air** pollution.

79. I participate in volunteer activities benefiting others.

80. I help others in need.

81. I beautify those parts of my environment under my control.

2

82. Because of limited resources, I do my part to conserve.

83. I recycle aluminum, glass, and paper products.

84. I involve myself with people who support a positive lifestyle.

EMOTIONAL AWARENESS AND ACCEPTANCE

Measures the degree to which one has an awareness and acceptance of one's feelings. This includes the degree to which one feels positive and enthusiastic about oneself and life.

85. I have a good sense of humor.

86. I feel positive about myself.

87. I feel there is a satisfying amount of excitement in my life.

88. My emotional life is stable.

89. I am aware of my needs.

90. I trust and value my own judgment.

91. When I make mistakes, I learn from them.

92. I feel comfortable when complimented for jobs well done.

93. It is okay for me to cry.

94. I have feelings of sensitivity for others.

95. I feel enthusiastic about life.

96. I find it easy to laugh.

97. I am able to give love.

98. I am able to receive love.

99. I enjoy my life.

100. I have plenty of energy.

101. My sleep is restful.

102. I trust others.

103. I feel others trust me.

104. I accept my sexual desires.

105. I understand how I create my feelings.

106. At times, I can be both strong and sensitive.

107. I am aware when I feel angry.

108. I accept my anger.

109. I am aware when I feel sad.

110. I accept my sadness.

111. I am aware when I feel happy.

112. I accept my happiness.

113. I am aware when I feel frightened.

114. I accept my feelings of fear.

115. I am aware of my feelings about death.

116. I accept my feelings about death.

EMOTIONAL MANAGEMENT

Measures the degree to which one controls and expresses feelings, and engages in effective, related behaviors.

117. I share my feelings with those with whom I am close.

118. I express my feelings of anger in appropriate ways.

119. I express my feelings of sadness in healthy ways.

120. I express my feelings of happiness in desirable ways.

121. I express my feelings of fear in appropriate ways.

122. I compliment myself for a job well done.

123. I accept constructive criticism without reacting defensively.

124. I set appropriate limits for myself.

125. I stay within the limits that I have set.

126. I recognize that I can have wide variations of feelings about the same person (such as loving someone even though you are angry with her/him at the moment).

127. I am able to develop close, intimate relationships.

128. I say "no" without feeling guilty.

129. I would feel comfortable seeking professional help to better understand and cope with my feelings.

130. I reduce feelings of failure by setting achievable goals.

131. I relax my body and mind without using drugs.

132. I can be alone without feeling lonely.

133. I am able to be spontaneous in expressing my feelings.

134. I accept responsibility for my actions.

135. I am willing to take the risks that come with making change.

136. I manage my feelings to avoid unnecessary suffering.

137. I make decisions with a minimum of stress and worry.

138. I accept the responsibility for creating my own feelings.

139. I can express my feelings about death.

140. I recognize grieving as a healthy response to loss.

INTELLECTUAL

Measures the degree to which one engages her/his mind in creative, stimulating mental activities, expanding knowledge, and improving skills.

141. I read a newspaper daily.

142. I read twelve or more books yearly.

143. On the average, I read one or more national magazines per week.

144. When I watch TV, I choose programs with informational/educational value.

145. I visit a museum or art show at least three times yearly.

146. I attend lectures, workshops, and demonstrations at least three times yearly.

147. I regularly use some of my time participating in hobbies such as photography, gardening, woodworking, sewing, painting, baking, art, music, writing, pottery, etc.

148. I read about local, state, national, and international political/public issues.

149. I learn the meaning of new words.

150. I engage in some type of writing activity such as a regular journal, letter writing, preparation of papers or manuscripts, etc.

151. I am interested in understanding the views of others.

152. I share ideas, concepts, thoughts, or procedures with others.

153. I gather information to enable me to make decisions.

154. I listen to radio and/or TV news.

155. I think about ideas different than my own.

OCCUPATIONAL

Measures the satisfaction gained from one's work and the degree to which one is enriched by that work. Please answer these items from your primary frame of reference, (e.g., your job, student, homemaker, etc.).

156. I enjoy my work.

157. My work contributes to my personal needs.
158. I feel that my job in some way contributes to my well-being.
159. I cooperate with others in my work.
160. I take advantage of opportunities to learn new work-related skills.
161. My work is challenging.
162. I feel my job responsibilities are consistent with my values.
163. I find satisfaction from the work I do.
164. I find healthy ways of reducing excessive job-related stress.
165. I use recommended health and safety precautions.
166. I make recommendations for improving worksite health and safety.
167. I am satisfied with the degree of freedom I have in my job to exercise independent judgments.
168. I am satisfied with the amount of variety in my work.
169. I believe I am competent in my job.
170. My co-workers and supervisors respect me as a competent individual.
171. My communication with others in my work place is enriching for me.

SPIRITUAL

Measures one's ongoing involvement in seeking meaning and purpose in human existence. It includes an appreciation for the depth and expanse of life and natural forces that exist in the universe.

172. I feel good about my spiritual life.
173. Prayer, meditation, and/or quiet personal reflection is/are important part(s) of my life.
174. I contemplate my purpose in life.
175. I reflect on the meaning of events in my life.
176. My values guide my daily life.
177. My values and beliefs help me to meet daily challenges.
178. I recognize that my spiritual growth is a lifelong process.
179. I am concerned about humanitarian issues.
180. I enjoy participating in discussions about spiritual values.
181. I feel a sense of compassion for others in need.
182. I seek spiritual knowledge.
183. My spiritual awareness occurs other than at times of crisis.
184. I believe in something greater or that I am part of something greater than myself.
185. I share my spiritual values.

Section 3: HEALTH RISK APPRAISAL

INSTRUCTIONS:

This section is intended to help you identify the problems most likely to interfere with the quality of your life. It will also show you choices you can make to stay healthy and avoid the most common causes of death for a person your age and sex.

This Health Risk Appraisal is not a substitute for a checkup or physical exam that you get from a doctor or nurse. It only gives you some ideas for lowering your risk of getting sick or injured in the future. It is NOT designed for people who already have HEART DISEASE, CANCER, KIDNEY DISEASE, OR OTHER SERIOUS CONDITIONS. If you have any of these problems and you want a Health Risk Appraisal anyway, ask your doctor or nurse to read this section of the printout with you.

If you don't know or are unsure of an answer, please leave that item blank.

1. Have you ever been told that you have diabetes (or sugar diabetes)?
   a. yes
   b. no
2. Does your natural mother, father, sister or brother have diabetes?
   a. yes
   b. no
   c. not sure
3. Did either of your natural parents die of a heart attack before age 60? (If your parents are younger than 60, mark no).
   a. yes, one of them
   b. yes, both of them
   c. no
   d. not sure
4. Are you now taking medicine for high blood pressure?
   a. yes
   b. no
5. What is your blood pressure now?
   a. _____ systolic (high number)
   b. _____ diastolic (low number)
6. If you *do not* know the number, select the answer that describes your blood pressure.
   a. high
   b. normal or low
   c. don't know
7. What is your TOTAL cholesterol level (based on a blood test)?
   _____ (mg/dl)
8. What is your High Density Lipoprotein (HDL) cholesterol level (based on a blood test)?
   _____ (mg/dl)
9. How many cigars do you usually smoke per day?
   _____
10. How many pipes of tobacco do you usually smoke per day? _____
11. How many times per day do you usually use smokeless tobacco (chewing tobacco, snuff, pouches, etc.)? _____
12. How would you describe your cigarette smoking habits?
    a. never smoked **Go to 15**
    b. used to smoke **Go to 14**
    c. still smoke **Go to 13**

13. How many cigarettes a day do you smoke?
    _____ cigarettes per day **Go to 15**

14. a. How many years has it been since you smoked cigarettes regularly?
    _____ years
    b. What was the average number of cigarettes per day that you smoked in the 2 years before you quit?
    _____ cigarettes per day

15. In the next 12 months, how many thousands of miles will you probably travel by each of the following? (NOTE: U.S. average = 10,000 miles)
    a. car, truck, or van: _____,000 miles
    b. motorcycle: _____,000 miles

16. On a typical day how do you USUALLY travel? (Check one only)
    a. walk
    b. bicycle
    c. motorcycle
    d. sub-compact or compact car
    e. mid-size or full-size car
    f. truck or van
    g. bus, subway, or train
    h. mostly stay home

17. What percent of the time do you usually buckle your safety belt when driving or riding?
    _____%

18. On the average, how close to the speed limit do you usually drive?
    a. within 5 mph of limit
    b. 6-10 mph over limit
    c. 11-15 mph over limit
    d. more than 15 mph over limit

19. How many times in the last month did you drive or ride when the driver had perhaps too much alcohol to drink?
    _____ times last month

20. When you drink alcoholic beverages, how many drinks do you consume in an average day? (If you *never* drink alcoholic beverages, write 0.)
    _____ alcoholic beverages/average day

21. On the average, how many days per week do you consume alcohol?
    _____ days/week

(MEN GO TO QUESTION 31)

WOMEN ONLY (QUESTIONS 22-30)

22. At what age did you have your first menstrual period?
    _____ years old

23. How old were you when your first child was born (if no children, write 0)?
    _____ years old

24. How long has it been since your last breast x-ray (mammogram)?
    a. less than 1 year ago
    b. 1 year ago
    c. 2 years ago
    d. 3 or more years ago
    e. never

25. How many women in your natural family (mother and sisters only) have had breast cancer?
    _____ women

26. Have you had a hysterectomy?
    a. yes
    b. no
    c. not sure

27. How long has it been since you had a pap smear test?
    a. less than 1 year ago
    b. 1 year ago
    c. 2 years ago
    d. 3 or more years ago
    e. never

28. How often do you examine your breasts for lumps?
    a. monthly
    b. once every few months
    c. rarely or never

29. About how long has it been since you had your breasts examined by a physician or nurse?
    a. less than 1 year ago
    b. 1 year ago
    c. 2 years ago
    d. 3 or more years ago
    e. never

30. About how long has it been since you had a rectal exam?
    a. less than 1 year ago
    b. 1 year ago
    c. 2 years ago
    d. 3 or more years ago
    e. never

WOMEN GO TO QUESTION 35

MEN ONLY (QUESTIONS 31-34)

31. About how long has it been since you had a rectal or prostate exam?
    a. less than 1 year ago
    b. 1 year ago
    c. 2 years ago
    d. 3 or more years ago
    e. never

32. Do you know how to properly examine your testes for lumps?
    a. yes
    b. no
    c. not sure

33. How often do you examine your testes for lumps?
    a. monthly
    b. once every few months
    c. rarely or never

34. About how long has it been since you had your testes examined by a physician or nurse?
    a. less than one year ago
    b. 1 year ago
    c. 2 years ago
    d. 3 or more years ago
    e. never

35. How many times in the last year did you witness or become involved in a violent fight or attack where there was a good chance of a serious injury to someone?
    a. 4 or more times
    b. 2 or 3 times
    c. 1 time or never
    d. not sure

36. Considering your age, how would you describe your overall physical health?
    a. excellent
    b. good
    c. fair
    d. poor

37. In an average week, how many times do you engage in physical activity (exercise or work which lasts at least 20 minutes without stopping and which is hard enough to make you breathe heavier and your heart beat faster)?
    a. less than 1 time per week
    b. 1 or 2 times per week
    c. at least 3 times per week

38. If you ride a motorcycle or all-terrain vehicle (ATV), what percent of the time do you wear a helmet?
    a. 75% to 100%
    b. 25% to 74%
    c. less than 25%
    d. does not apply to me

39. Do you eat some food every day that is high in fiber, such as whole grain bread, cereal, fresh fruits, or vegetables?
    a. yes
    b. no

40. Do you eat foods every day that are high in cholesterol or fat, such as fatty meat, cheese, fried foods, or eggs?
    a. yes
    b. no

41. In general, how satisfied are you with your life?
    a. mostly satisfied
    b. partly satisfied
    c. not satisfied

42. Have you suffered a personal loss or misfortune in the past year that had a serious impact on your life? (For example, a job loss, disability, separation, jail term, or the death of someone close to you.)
    a. yes, 1 serious loss or misfortune
    b. yes, 2 or more
    c. no

Section 4: TOPICS FOR PERSONAL GROWTH

This section will help you identify areas in which you would like more information. In response to your selection from the following topics, we will provide you with resources or services to meet your requests.

Select topics on which you would like information. (Maximum of 4 topics.)

1. Responsible alcohol use
2. Stop-smoking programs
3. Sexuality
4. Gay issues
5. Depression
6. Loneliness
7. Exercise programs
8. Weight reduction
9. Self-breast exam
10. Medical emergencies
11. Nutrition
12. Relaxation
13. Stress reduction
14. Parenting skills
15. Marital or couples problems
16. Assertiveness training (how to say "no" without feeling guilty)
17. Biofeedback for tension headache and pain
18. Overcoming fears (i.e., high places, crowded rooms, etc.)
19. Educational career goal setting/planning
20. Spiritual or philosophical values
21. Communication skills
22. Automobile safety
23. Suicide thoughts or attempts
24. Substance abuse
25. Anxiety associated with public speaking, tests, writing, etc.
26. Enhancing relationships
27. Time-management skills
28. Death and dying
29. Learning skills (i.e., speed-reading, comprehension, etc.)
30. Financial management
31. Divorce
32. Alcoholism
33. Men's issues
34. Women's issues
35. Medical self-care
36. Dental self-care
37. Self-testes exam
38. Aging
39. Self-esteem
40. Premenstrual syndrome (PMS)
41. Osteoporosis
42. Recreation and leisure
43. Environmental issues

> **IMPORTANT**— **If you have finished completing all sections of the LAQ, please make sure you have answered the questions in Section 1 requesting your sex, race, age, height and weight. Results cannot be generated for the Health Risk Appraisal section without this information.**

You and Your Lifestyle Are the Major Determinants for Joyful Living

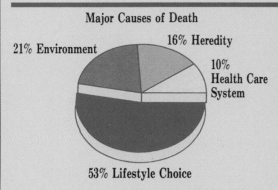

Major Causes of Death

21% Environment

16% Heredity

10% Health Care System

53% Lifestyle Choice

The circle graph to the left indicates the factors which contribute to your enjoyment and quality of life. While medical professionals contribute to the quality of your life, this graph clearly shows that the majority of those factors which contribute to your well-being are controlled by you. As you make responsible, informed choices, your chances of improving your health and well-being increase.

The LAQ's Role . . .

We believe this instrument is useful in helping individuals identify the most likely causes of death and disability. More importantly, it identifies those areas of self-improvement which will lead to higher levels of health and well-being.

The areas assessed in the LAQ emphasize the importance of creating a balance among the many different aspects of your lifestyle. Each of these areas affects one another and determines your overall wellness status. Also, each provides an opportunity for learning, making responsible decisions, and personal growth.

We invite you to use the information provided by the LAQ to your best advantage to increase your level of wellness.

Words from the Past

Wellness is a term that has enjoyed growing popularity during the past several decades. Although the term was introduced relatively recently, the concept of prevention has been present for centuries. The following passages provide a brief glimpse of the wellness philosophy through the years. Wellness is a movement which has become a major part of modern culture and is the most important weapon available to combat lifestyle illnesses.

"For many years, while engaged in the practice of medicine, the author of this volume has been more and more impressed with the idea that the causes of suffering, diseases, and premature deaths, which we witness around us on every hand, lie near our own doors . . . and that the men and women of today, are, at least, equally as responsible for existing suffering, as those who have gone before them, and often much more so. In fact, he feels satisfied that by far the greatest portion of all the suffering, disease, deformity, and premature deaths which occur are the direct result of either the violation of, or the want of compliance with the laws of our being; calamities, which, were the requisite knowledge possessed by the community, can and should be avoided."

— JOHN ELLIS, M.D., 1859

"It is universally admitted at the present time that preventive medicine is of far greater importance than curative medication, and many of the most eminent members of the profession are devoting themselves exclusively to this branch."

— J. H. KELLOGG, M.D., 1902

"To ward off disease or recover health, men as a rule find it easier to depend on the healers than to attempt the more difficult task of living wisely."

— RENE DUBOS, Ph.D., 1959

"It's what you do hour by hour, day by day, that largely determines the state of your health; whether you get sick, what you get sick with, and perhaps when you die."

— LESTER BRESLOW, M.D., 1969

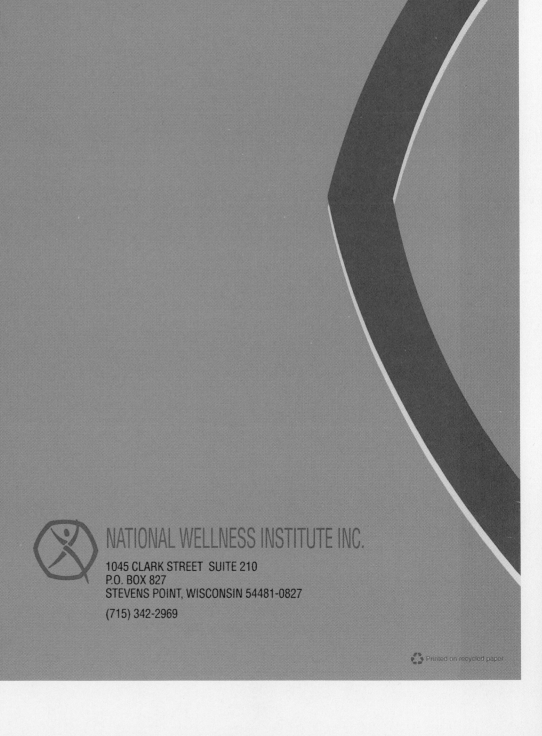

NATIONAL WELLNESS INSTITUTE INC.

1045 CLARK STREET SUITE 210
P.O. BOX 827
STEVENS POINT, WISCONSIN 54481-0827

(715) 342-2969

Printed on recycled paper

G.2 Healthier People Health Risk Appraisal

Form C

The HEALTHIER PEOPLE NETWORK, Inc.

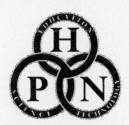

. . . linking science, technology, & education to serve the public interest . . .

IDENTIFICATION NUMBER

☐☐☐☐☐☐☐☐☐

The health risk appraisal is an educational tool, showing you choices you can make to keep good health and avoid the most common causes of death (for a person of your age and sex). This health risk appraisal is **not** a substitute for a check-up or physical exam that you get from a doctor or nurse; however, it does provide some ideas for lowering your risk of getting sick or injured in the future. It is NOT designed for people who already have HEART DISEASE, CANCER, KIDNEY DISEASE, OR OTHER SERIOUS CONDITIONS; if you have any of these problems, please ask your health care provider to interpret the report for you.

DIRECTIONS:
To get the most accurate results, **answer as many questions as you can**. If you do not know the answer leave it blank.

The following questions __must__ be completed or the computer program cannot process your questionnaire:

1. SEX   2. AGE   3. HEIGHT   4. WEIGHT   15. CIGARETTE SMOKING

Please write your answers in the boxes provided. ✏	**(Examples:** ☒ or ☐ 98 **)**

1.	**SEX**	1 ☐ Male 2 ☐ Female
2.	**AGE**	☐ Years
3.	**HEIGHT** (Without shoes) (No fractions)	☐ Feet ☐ Inches
4.	**WEIGHT** (Without shoes) (No fractions)	☐ Pounds
5.	Body frame size	1 ☐ Small 2 ☐ Medium 3 ☐ Large
6.	Have you ever been told that you have diabetes (or sugar diabetes)?	1 ☐ Yes 2 ☐ No
7.	Are you now taking medicine for high blood pressure?	1 ☐ Yes 2 ☐ No
8.	What is your blood pressure now?	☐ / ☐ Systolic (High Number)/Diastolic (Low Number)
9.	If you do **not** know the numbers, check the box that describes your blood pressure.	1 ☐ High 2 ☐ Normal or Low 3 ☐ Don't Know

10. What is your TOTAL cholesterol level (based on a blood test)?	☐ mg/dl
11. What is your HDL cholesterol (based on a blood test)?	☐ mg/dl
12. How many cigars do you usually smoke per day?	☐ cigars per day
13. How many pipes of tobacco do you usually smoke per day?	☐ pipes per day
14. How many times per day do you usually use smokeless tobacco? (Chewing tobacco, snuff, pouches, etc.)	☐ times per day
15. **CIGARETTE SMOKING** How would you describe your cigarette smoking habits?	1 ☐ Never smoked ☛ **Go to 18** 2 ☐ Used to smoke ☛ **Go to 17** 3 ☐ Still smoke ☛ **Go to 16**
16. **STILL SMOKE** How many cigarettes a day do you smoke? ☛ **GO TO QUESTION 18**	☐ cigarettes per day ☛ **Go to 18**
17. **USED TO SMOKE** a. How many years has it been since you smoked cigarettes fairly regularly? b. What was the average number of cigarettes per day that you smoked in the 2 years before you quit?	☐ years ☐ cigarettes per day
18. In the next 12 months, how many thousands of miles will you probably travel by each of the following? (NOTE: U.S. average = 10,000 miles) a. Car, truck, or van: b. Motorcycle:	☐ ,000 miles ☐ ,000 miles
19. On a typical day, how do you USUALLY travel? (Check one only)	1 ☐ Walk 2 ☐ Bicycle 3 ☐ Motorcycle 4 ☐ Sub-compact or compact car 5 ☐ Mid-size or full-size car 6 ☐ Truck or van 7 ☐ Bus, subway, or train 8 ☐ Mostly stay home
20. What percent of time do you usually buckle your safety belt when driving or riding?	☐ %
21. On the average, how close to the speed limit do you usually drive?	1 ☐ Within 5 mph of limit 2 ☐ 6-10 mph over limit 3 ☐ 11-15 mph over limit 4 ☐ More than 15 mph over limit
22. How many times in the last month did you drive or ride when the driver had perhaps too much alcohol to drink?	☐ times last month
23. How many drinks of an alcoholic beverage do you have in a typical week? ☛ *MEN GO TO QUESTION 33*	(Write the number of each type of drink) ☐ Bottles or cans of beer ☐ Glasses of wine ☐ Wine coolers ☐ Mixed drinks or shots of liquor

Form C

WOMEN ONLY

24. At what age did you have your first menstrual period?	[ ] years old
25. How old were you when your first child was born?	[ ] years old (If no children, write 0)
26. How long has it been since your last breast x-ray (mammogram)?	1 ☐ Less than 1 year ago 2 ☐ 1 year ago 3 ☐ 2 years ago 4 ☐ 3 or more years ago 5 ☐ Never
27. How many women in your natural family (mother and sisters only) have had breast cancer?	[ ] Women
28. Have you had a hysterectomy operation?	1 ☐ Yes 2 ☐ No 3 ☐ Not sure
29. How long has it been since you had a pap smear test?	1 ☐ Less than 1 year ago 2 ☐ 1 year ago 3 ☐ 2 years ago 4 ☐ 3 or more years ago 5 ☐ Never
★30. How often do you examine your breasts for lumps?	1 ☐ Monthly 2 ☐ Once every few months 3 ☐ Rarely or never
★31. About how long has it been since you had your breasts examined by a physician or nurse?	1 ☐ Less than 1 year ago 2 ☐ 1 year ago 3 ☐ 2 years ago 4 ☐ 3 or more years ago 5 ☐ Never
★32. About how long has it been since you had a rectal exam? ☞ *WOMEN GO TO QUESTION 34*	1 ☐ Less than 1 year ago 2 ☐ 1 year ago 3 ☐ 2 years ago 4 ☐ 3 or more years ago 5 ☐ Never

MEN ONLY

★33. About how long has it been since you had a rectal or prostate exam? ☞ *MEN CONTINUE ON QUES. 34*	1 ☐ Less than 1 year ago 2 ☐ 1 year ago 3 ☐ 2 years ago 4 ☐ 3 or more years ago 5 ☐ Never
★34. How many times in the last year did you witness or become involved in a violent fight or attack where there was a good chance of a serious injury to someone?	1 ☐ 4 or more times 2 ☐ 2 or 3 times 3 ☐ 1 time or never 4 ☐ Not sure
★35. Considering your age, how would you describe your overall physical health?	1 ☐ Excellent 2 ☐ Good 3 ☐ Fair 4 ☐ Poor

★ Questions with a star symbol are not used by the computer to calculate your risks; however, answering these questions may help you plan a more healthy lifestyle.

Form C

★36. In an average week, how many times do you engage in physical activity (exercise or work which lasts at least 20 minutes without stopping and which is hard enough to make you breathe heavier and your heart beat faster)?	1 ☐ Less than 1 time per week 2 ☐ 1 or 2 times per week 3 ☐ At least 3 times per week
★37. If you ride a motorcycle or all-terrain vehicle (ATV), what percent of the time do you wear a helmet?	1 ☐ 75% to 100% 2 ☐ 25% to 74 % 3 ☐ Less than 25% 4 ☐ Does not apply to me
★38. Do you eat some food every day that is high in fiber, such as whole grain bread, cereal, fresh fruits or vegetables?	1 ☐ Yes 2 ☐ No
★39. Do you eat foods every day that are high in cholesterol or fat, such as fatty meat, cheese, fried foods, or eggs?	1 ☐ Yes 2 ☐ No
★40. In general, how satisfied are you with your life?	1 ☐ Mostly satisfied 2 ☐ Partly satisfied 3 ☐ Not satisfied
★41. Have you suffered a personal loss or misfortune in the past year that had a serious impact on your life? (For example, a job loss, disability, separation, jail term, or the death of someone close to you.)	1 ☐ Yes, 1 serious loss or misfortune 2 ☐ Yes, 2 or more 3 ☐ No
★42a. Race	1 ☐ Aleutian, Alaska native, Eskimo or American Indian 2 ☐ Asian 3 ☐ Black 4 ☐ Pacific Islander 5 ☐ White 6 ☐ Other 7 ☐ Don't know
★42b. Are you of Hispanic origin, such as Mexican-American, Puerto Rican, or Cuban?	1 ☐ Yes 2 ☐ No
★43. What is the highest grade you completed in school?	1 ☐ Grade school or less 2 ☐ Some high school 3 ☐ High school graduate 4 ☐ Some college 5 ☐ College graduate 6 ☐ Post graduate or professional degree

Name _____

Address_____

City _____State ___ ___   Zip ___ ___ ___ ___ ___

(Note: Name and address are optional, depending on how your report will be returned to you. If you wish to remain anonymous, copy your Identification Number onto a receipt form. You can then use this receipt to claim your computerized report.)

The
HEALTHIER PEOPLE NETWORK, Inc.

Participant's Guide to Interpreting the
HEALTH RISK APPRAISAL REPORT

Unhealthy habits lead to early death or chronic illness. Every year, 1.3 million people in the United States die prematurely from conditions which could be prevented or delayed. This Health Risk Appraisal may help you avoid becoming one of these statistics by giving you a picture of how your health risks relate to your particular characteristics and habits.

WHAT IS A HEALTH RISK APPRAISAL?

The Health Risk Appraisal is an estimation of your risk of dying in the next ten years from each of 42 causes of death. The twelve most important of these are printed individually on your report. The others are grouped together and printed as "All Other". These risks are calculated by a computer program which compares your characteristics to national mortality statistics using equations developed by epidemiologists. This Health Risk Appraisal does not tell you how long you will live, nor does it diagnose or treat disease.

RISK FACTORS

Most chronic diseases develop slowly in the presence of certain risk factors. Risk factors are either controllable or uncontrollable. Controllable risk factors include lifestyle habits that you can change such as smoking, exercise, diet, stress and weight. Uncontrollable risk factors include items such as your age and sex, and the health history of your family.

The Health Risk Appraisal uses both controllable and uncontrollable risk factors in calculating health risks. Your focus, however, should be on controllable risk factors.

To help you decide which controllable risk factors to concentrate on, the Health Risk Appraisal identifies your controllable risk factors for each cause of death. Your report gives you an idea of their relative importance by indicating the number of risk years you could gain by controlling these factors.

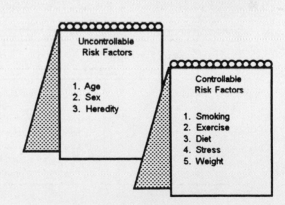

To identify your personal risks, to see what the numbers on your report mean, and to learn which risk factors you need to control, turn the page.

Participant's Guide to Interpreting the Health Risk Appraisal Report Form

An example using a 48 year old woman: 5'7", 250 mg/dl cholesterol, 160/95 BP, 30 cigarettes/day, 9 drinks/week, seat belt use 15%, drives 4,000 mi/yr, menarche 13 yrs, 1st child at 32

1 | YOUR | NOW | TARGET | ← Risks are elevated due to
| RISK AGE | 68.91 | 60.82 | diabetes and family breast cancer

Mrs. Lopez **6**
Female Age 48

THIS REPORT CONTAINS ESTIMATES DUE TO MISSING ITEMS, INCLUDING THE FOLLOWING **7**
Cigars per day. Pipes smoked per day. Smokeless tobacco.

Many serious injuries and health problems can be prevented. Your Health Risk Appraisal lists factors you can change to lower your risk. For causes of death that are not directly computable, the report uses the average risk for a person of your age and sex.

MOST COMMON CAUSES OF DEATH	NUMBER OF DEATHS IN NEXT 10 YEARS FOR 1000 WOMEN AGE 48			MODIFIABLE RISK FACTORS
	2 YOUR GROUP	**3** TARGET	**4** POPULATION AVERAGE	
Heart Attack	104	22	5	Avoid Tobacco Use, Blood Pressure, Cholesterol Level, **8** HDL Level, Weight
Breast Cancer	42	42	5	A Low-Fat Diet and Regular Exercise Might Reduce Risk
Diabetes Mellitus	21	21	1	Control Your Weight and Follow Your Doctor's Advice
Stroke	19	5	2	Avoid Tobacco Use, Blood Pressure
Lung Cancer	13	7	5	Avoid Tobacco Use
Emphysema/Bronchitis	2	<1	1	Avoid Tobacco Use
Kidney Failure	2	2	<1	"
Colon Cancer	1*	1*	1	A High-Fiber and Low-Fat Diet Might Reduce Risk
Ovary Cancer	1*	1*	1	Get Regular Exams
Pancreas Cancer	1	1	1	Avoid Tobacco Use
Cirrhosis of Liver	1	1	1	Continue to Avoid Heavy Drinking
All Other	21	19	20	* = Average Value Used
TOTAL:	228	122	46	Deaths in Next 10 Years Per 1,000 Women, age 48

For Height 5'7" and Large Frame, 175 pounds is about 20% Overweight. Desirable Weight Range: 139-153 **9**

GOOD HABITS **5**	TO IMPROVE YOUR RISK PROFILE:	RISK YEARS GAINED **10**
+ Regular pap tests	- Quit smoking <estimate>	3.57
+ Safe driving speed	- Lower your blood pressure	1.88
	- Lower your cholesterol	1.56
	- Improve your HDL level	.92
	- Bring your weight to desirable range	.13
	- Always wear your seat belts	.03

Total Risk Years you could gain = 8.09 **11**

❶ Your **RISK AGE** compares your total risk from all causes of death to the total risk of those who are your age and sex. It gives you an idea of your risks compared with the population average in terms of an age. Your **TARGET** risk age indicates what your risk age would be if you made the changes recommended below.

❷ The numbers in the **YOUR GROUP** column refer to the number of predicted deaths for each cause of death in the next 10 years from among 1,000 people who have habits and characteristics just like you.

❸ The numbers in the **TARGET** column refer to those predicted to die in the next 10 years from among 1,000 people who have characteristics just like you, but who have adopted the habits recommended below in the **TO IMPROVE YOUR RISK PROFILE** box.

❹ The numbers in the **POPULATION AVERAGE** column refer to the national average of deaths in 10 years for people of your same sex and age.

❺ This box lists your **GOOD HABITS**. Congratulations!

❻ Your I.D., sex and actual age is here.

❼ If you did not answer items on the questionnaire which are used for calculations, these missing items will be listed here. The computer substitutes national average values for the items you left blank and calculates your risks with these numbers.

❽ Beside each cause of death are listed the modifiable risk factors which your questionnaire responses indicate you need to work on. The list is specific for you unless you have none of the risk factors or if there are no known risk factors for a cause of death. In this case, a short statement of general advice related to risk reduction is printed.

❾ Your **DESIRABLE WEIGHT RANGE** is based on your height and frame size.

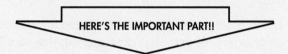

HERE'S THE IMPORTANT PART!!

❿ In this box is our prescription to lengthen your life and a prediction of how many **RISK YEARS** you can expect to gain by adopting these health habits.

⓫ The **TOTAL RISK YEARS** you could gain by making these habit changes are printed here. This is also the difference between your **Risk Age Now** and your **Target Age**. Also important are the recommendations on page 2.

Page 2 of your report lists some **ROUTINE PREVENTIVE SERVICES** that are specific for people of your age and sex. The report also lists some **GENERAL RECOMMENDATIONS FOR EVERYONE.** For the 48 year old woman used in this example, the following messages were printed:

ROUTINE PREVENTIVE SERVICES FOR WOMEN YOUR AGE	GENERAL RECOMMENDATIONS FOR EVERYONE
Blood Pressure and Cholesterol test	* Exercise briskly for 15-30 minutes at least three times a week.
Pap Smear test	
Breast cancer screening (check with your doctor or clinic)	* Use good eating habits by choosing a variety of foods that are low in fat and high in fiber.
Rectal exam (or Sigmoidoscopy)	
Eye exam for glaucoma	* Learn to recognize and handle stress - get help if you need it.
Dental Exam	
Tetanus-Diphtheria booster shot (every 10 years)	

The standard report can also print health education messages.

HEALTH RISK APPRAISAL LIMITS

Health Risk Appraisal is an educational tool. It does not take into consideration whether or not you already have a medical condition and it does not consider rare diseases and other health problems which are not fatal but can limit your enjoyment of life, such as arthritis.

Health Risk Appraisal does not predict when you will die or specifically what diseases you might get. It does tell you, however, your chances of getting a disease relative to a large group of people your age and sex, who answered the questionnaire just as you did.

Health Risk Appraisal does take into consideration lifestyle factors which account for a large number of premature deaths. When you become familiar with your particular risks, you can then do something about them!

CHOOSING A HABIT TO WORK ON

Health Risk Appraisal is intended to encourage you to work on habits you can change by showing you which behaviors should have top priority. If you can't change the behavior that is at the top of your list (the one that would give the largest number of **RISK YEARS GAINED**), try to concentrate on changing the next highest one. You don't have to change your entire lifestyle overnight. In fact, trying to change too many habits at once is probably the quickest way to become discouraged and fail.

MAKE A PLAN FOR CHANGING HABITS

Make a plan for changing the habit you choose as your first priority, write it down and keep it in sight. Be prepared for temptation! Observe the time, situation, or place that most often triggers your unhealthy habit and be ready to combat it when it appears. Let family and friends know of your goals and ask for their encouragement.

REWARD YOURSELF

Rewards are an important part of changing behavior. Give yourself a reasonable reward when you accomplish your goal. Don't eat half a gallon of ice cream after losing 10 pounds! Choose a healthy and enjoyable reward and you'll be on the road to good health!

G.3 1999 Youth Risk Behavior Survey*

This survey is about health behavior. It has been developed so you can tell us what you do that may affect your health. The information you give will be used to develop better health education for young people like yourself.

DO NOT write your name on this survey. The answers you give will be kept private. No one will know what you write. Answer the questions based on what you really do.

Completing the survey is voluntary. Whether or not you answer the questions will not affect your grade in this class. If you are not comfortable answering a question, just leave it blank.

The questions that ask about your background will be used only to describe the types of students completing this survey. The information will not be used to find out your name. No names will ever be reported.

Make sure to read every question. Fill in the ovals completely. When you are finished, follow the instructions of the person giving you the survey.

Thank you very much for your help.

DIRECTIONS
• Use a #2 pencil only.
• Make dark marks.
• Fill in a response like this: A B C D.
• To change your answer, erase completely.

1. How old are you?
   A. 12 years old or younger
   B. 13 years old
   C. 14 years old
   D. 15 years old
   E. 16 years old
   F. 17 years old
   G. 18 years old or older

2. What is your sex?
   A. Female
   B. Male

3. In what grade are you?
   A. 9th grade
   B. 10th grade
   C. 11th grade
   D. 12th grade
   E. Ungraded or other grade

4. How do you describe yourself? **(Select one or more responses.)**
   A. American Indian or Alaska Native
   B. Asian
   C. Black or African American
   D. Hispanic or Latino
   E. Native Hawaiian or Other Pacific Islander
   F. White

5. How tall are you without your shoes on?

DIRECTIONS
Write your height in the shaded blank boxes. Fill in the matching oval below each number.

EXAMPLE

HEIGHT		HEIGHT	
FEET	INCHES	FEET	INCHES
5	7		
③	⓪	③	⓪
④	①	④	①
⑤	②	⑤	②
⑥	③	⑥	③
⑦	④	⑦	④
	⑤		⑤
	⑥		⑥
	⑦		⑦
	⑧		⑧
	⑨		⑨
	⑩		⑩
	⑪		⑪

6. How much do you weigh without your shoes on?

Directions: Write your weight in the shaded blank boxes. Fill in the matching oval below each number.

EXAMPLE

WEIGHT (LB)			WEIGHT (LB)		
1	5	2			
⓪	⓪	⓪	⓪	⓪	⓪
①	①	①	①	①	①
②	②	②	②	②	②
③	③	③	③	③	③
	④	④		④	④
	⑤	⑤		⑤	⑤
	⑥	⑥		⑥	⑥
	⑦	⑦		⑦	⑦
	⑧	⑧		⑧	⑧
	⑨	⑨		⑨	⑨

*From Centers for Disease Control and Prevention: [www.cdc.gov/mccdphp/dash/yrbs/survey99.htm] August, 1999.

The next five questions ask about personal safety.

7. **When you rode a motorcycle** during the past 12 months, how often did you wear a helmet?
   A. I did not ride a motorcycle during the past 12 months
   B. Never wore a helmet
   C. Rarely wore a helmet
   D. Sometimes wore a helmet
   E. Most of the time wore a helmet
   F. Always wore a helmet

8. **When you rode a bicycle** during the past 12 months, how often did you wear a helmet?
   A. I did not ride a bicycle during the past 12 months
   B. Never wore a helmet
   C. Rarely wore a helmet
   D. Sometimes wore a helmet
   E. Most of the time wore a helmet
   F. Always wore a helmet

9. How often do you wear a seat belt when **riding** in a car driven by someone else?
   A. Never
   B. Rarely
   C. Sometimes
   D. Most of the time
   E. Always

10. During the past 30 days, how many times did you **ride** in a car or other vehicle **driven by someone who had been drinking alcohol?**
   A. 0 times
   B. 1 time
   C. 2 or 3 times
   D. 4 or 5 times
   E. 6 or more times

11. During the past 30 days, how many times did you **drive** a car or other vehicle **when you had been drinking alcohol?**
   A. 0 times
   B. 1 time
   C. 2 or 3 times
   D. 4 or 5 times
   E. 6 or more times

The next 10 questions ask about violence-related behaviors.

12. During the past 30 days, on how many days did you carry **a weapon** such as a gun, knife, or club?
   A. 0 days
   B. 1 day
   C. 2 or 3 days
   D. 4 or 5 days
   E. 6 or more days

13. During the past 30 days, on how many days did you carry **a gun?**
   A. 0 days
   B. 1 day
   C. 2 or 3 days
   D. 4 or 5 days
   E. 6 or more days

14. During the past 30 days, on how many days did you carry a weapon such as a gun, knife, or club **on school property?**
   A. 0 days
   B. 1 day
   C. 2 or 3 days
   D. 4 or 5 days
   E. 6 or more days

15. During the past 30 days, on how many days did you **not** go to school because you felt you would be unsafe at school or on your way to or from school?
   A. 0 days
   B. 1 day
   C. 2 or 3 days
   D. 4 or 5 days
   E. 6 or more days

16. During the past 12 months, how many times has someone threatened or injured you with a weapon such as a gun, knife, or club **on school property?**
   A. 0 times
   B. 1 time
   C. 2 or 3 times
   D. 4 or 5 times
   E. 6 or 7 times
   F. 8 or 9 times
   G. 10 or 11 times
   H. 12 or more times

17. During the past 12 months, how many times were you in a physical fight?
   A. 0 times
   B. 1 time
   C. 2 or 3 times
   D. 4 or 5 times
   E. 6 or 7 times
   F. 8 or 9 times
   G. 10 or 11 times
   H. 12 or more times

18. During the past 12 months, how many times were you in a physical fight in which you were injured and had to be treated by a doctor or nurse?
   A. 0 times
   B. 1 time
   C. 2 or 3 times
   D. 4 or 5 times
   E. 6 or more times

19. During the past 12 months, how many times were you in a physical fight **on school property?**
    A. 0 times
    B. 1 time
    C. 2 or 3 times
    D. 4 or 5 times
    E. 6 or 7 times
    F. 8 or 9 times
    G. 10 or 11 times
    H. 12 or more times

20. During the past 12 months, did your boyfriend or girl-friend ever hit, slap, or physically hurt you on purpose?
    A. Yes
    B. No

21. Have you ever been forced to have sexual intercourse when you did not want to?
    A. Yes
    B. No

The next five questions ask about sad feelings and attempted suicide. Sometimes people feel so depressed about the future that they may consider attempting suicide, that is, taking some action to end their own life.

22. During the past 12 months, did you ever feel so sad or hopeless almost every day for **two weeks or more in a row** that you stopped doing some usual activities.
    A. Yes
    B. No

23. During the past 12 months, did you ever **seriously** consider attempting suicide?
    A. Yes
    B. No

24. During the past 12 months, did you make a plan about how you would attempt suicide?
    A. Yes
    B. No

25. During the past 12 months, how many times did you actually attempt suicide?
    A. 0 times
    B. 1 time
    C. 2 or 3 times
    D. 4 or 5 times
    E. 6 or more times

26. **If you attempted suicide** during the past 12 months, did any attempt result in an injury, poisoning, or overdose that had to be treated by a doctor or nurse?
    A. **I did not attempt suicide** during the past 12 months
    B. Yes
    C. No

The next 12 questions ask about tobacco use.

27. Have you ever tried cigarette smoking, even one or two puffs?
    A. Yes
    B. No

28. How old were you when you smoked a whole cigarette for the first time?
    A. I have never smoked a whole cigarette
    B. 8 years old or younger
    C. 9 or 10 years old
    D. 11 or 12 years old
    E. 13 or 14 years old
    F. 5 or 16 years old
    G. 17 years old or older

29. During the past 30 days, on how many days did you smoke cigarettes?
    A. 0 days
    B. 1 or 2 days
    C. 3 to 5 days
    D. 6 to 9 days
    E. 10 to 19 days
    F. 20 to 29 days
    G. All 30 days

30. During the past 30 days, on the days you smoked, how many cigarettes did you smoke **per day?**
    A. I did not smoke cigarettes during the past 30 days
    B. Less than 1 cigarette per day
    C. 1 cigarette per day
    D. 2 to 5 cigarettes per day
    E. 6 to 10 cigarettes per day
    F. 11 to 20 cigarettes per day
    G. More than 20 cigarettes per day

31. During the past 30 days, how did you **usually** get your own cigarettes? (Select only **one** response.)
    A. I did not smoke cigarettes during the past 30 days
    B. I bought them in a store such as a convenience store, supermarket, or gas station
    C. I bought them from a vending machine
    D. I gave someone else money to buy them for me
    E. I borrowed them from someone else
    F. I stole them
    G. I got them some other way

32. **When you bought cigarettes** in a store during the past 30 days, were you ever asked to show proof of age?
    A. I did not buy cigarettes in a store during the past 30 days
    B. Yes
    C. No

33. During the past 30 days, on how many days did you smoke cigarettes **on school property**?
    A. 0 days
    B. 1 or 2 days
    C. 3 to 5 days
    D. 6 to 9 days
    E. 10 to 19 days
    F. 20 to 29 days
    G. All 30 days

34. Have you ever smoked cigarettes regularly, that is, at least one cigarette every day for 30 days?
    A. Yes
    B. No

35. Have you ever tried **to quit** smoking cigarettes?
    A. Yes
    B. No

36. During the past 30 days, on how many days did you use **chewing tobacco or snuff,** such as Redman, Levi Garrett, Beechnut, Skoal, Skoal Bandits, or Copenhagen?
    A. 0 days
    B. 1 or 2 days
    C. 3 to 5 days
    D. 6 to 9 days
    E. 10 to 19 days
    F. 20 to 29 days
    G. All 30 days

37. During the past 30 days, on how many days did you use **chewing tobacco or snuff on school property**?
    A. 0 days
    B. 1 or 2 days
    C. 3 to 5 days
    D. 6 to 9 days
    E. 10 to 19 days
    F. 20 to 29 days
    G. All 30 days

38. During the past 30 days, on how many days did you smoke **cigars, cigarillos, or little cigars**?
    A. 0 days
    B. 1 or 2 days
    C. 3 to 5 days
    D. 6 to 9 days
    E. 10 to 19 days
    F. 20 to 29 days
    G. All 30 days

The next five questions ask about drinking alcohol. This includes drinking beer, wine, wine coolers, and liquor such as rum, gin, vodka, or whiskey. For these questions, drinking alcohol does not include drinking a few sips of wine for religious purposes.

39. During your life, on how many days have you had at least one drink of alcohol?
    A. 0 days
    B. 1 or 2 days
    C. 3 to 9 days
    D. 10 to 19 days
    E. 20 to 39 days
    F. 40 to 99 days
    G. 100 or more days

40. How old were you when you had your first drink of alcohol other than a few sips?
    A. I have never had a drink of alcohol other than a few sips
    B. 8 years old or younger
    C. 9 or 10 years old
    D. 11 or 12 years old
    E. 13 or 14 years old
    F. 15 or 16 years old
    G. 17 years old or older

41. During the past 30 days, on how many days did you have at least one drink of alcohol?
    A. 0 days
    B. 1 or 2 days
    C. 3 to 5 days
    D. 6 to 9 days
    E. 10 to 19 days
    F. 20 to 29 days
    G. All 30 days

42. During the past 30 days, on how many days did you have five or more drinks of alcohol in a row, that is, within a couple of hours?
    A. 0 days
    B. 1 day
    C. 2 days
    D. 3 to 5 days
    E. 6 to 9 days
    F. 10 to 19 days
    G. 20 or more days

43. During the past 30 days, on how many days did you have at least one drink of alcohol **on school property**?
    A. 0 days
    B. 1 or 2 days
    C. 3 to 5 days
    D. 6 to 9 days
    E. 10 to 19 days
    F. 20 to 29 days
    G. All 30 days

APPENDIX Health Risk Appraisal   A-139

The next four questions ask about marijuana use. Marijuana also is called grass or pot.

44. During your life, how many times have you used marijuana?
    A. 0 times
    B. 1 or 2 times
    C. 3 to 9 times
    D. 10 to 19 times
    E. 20 to 39 times
    F. 40 to 99 times
    G. 100 or more times

45. How old were you when you tried marijuana for the first time?
    A. I have never tried marijuana
    B. 8 years old or younger
    C. 9 or 10 years old
    D. 11 or 12 years old
    E. 13 or 14 years old
    F. 15 or 16 years old
    G. 17 years old or older

46. During the past 30 days, how many times did you use marijuana?
    A. 0 times
    B. 1 or 2 times
    C. 3 to 9 times
    D. 10 to 19 times
    E. 20 to 39 times
    F. 40 or more times

47. During the past 30 days, how many times did you use marijuana **on school property**?
    A. 0 times
    B. 1 or 2 times
    C. 3 to 9 times
    D. 10 to 19 times
    E. 20 to 39 times
    F. 40 or more times

The next nine questions ask about cocaine and other drugs.

48. During your life, how many times have you used **any** form of cocaine, including powder, crack, or freebase?
    A. 0 times
    B. 1 or 2 times
    C. 3 to 9 times
    D. 10 to 19 times
    E. 20 to 39 times
    F. 40 or more times

49. During the past 30 days, how many times did you use **any** form of cocaine, including powder, crack, or freebase?
    A. 0 times
    B. 1 or 2 times
    C. 3 to 9 times
    D. 10 to 19 times
    E. 20 to 39 times
    F. 40 or more times

50. During your life, how many times have you sniffed glue, breathed the contents of aerosol spray cans, or inhaled any paints or sprays to get high?
    A. 0 times
    B. 1 or 2 times
    C. 3 to 9 times
    D. 10 to 19 times
    E. 20 to 39 times
    F. 40 or more times

51. During the past 30 days, how many times have you sniffed glue, breathed the contents of aerosol spray cans, or inhaled any paints or sprays to get high?
    A. 0 times
    B. 1 or 2 times
    C. 3 to 9 times
    D. 10 to 19 times
    E. 20 to 39 times
    F. 40 or more times

52. During your life, how many times have you used **heroin** (also called smack, junk, or China White)?
    A. 0 times
    B. 1 or 2 times
    C. 3 to 9 times
    D. 10 to 19 times
    E. 20 to 39 times
    F. 40 or more times

53. During your life, how many times have you used **methamphetamines** (also called speed, crystal, crank, or ice)?
    A. 0 times
    B. 1 or 2 times
    C. 3 to 9 times
    D. 10 to 19 times
    E. 20 to 39 times
    F. 40 or more times

54. During your life, how many times have you taken **steroid pills or shots** without a doctor's prescription?
    A. 0 times
    B. 1 or 2 times
    C. 3 to 9 times
    D. 10 to 19 times
    E. 20 to 39 times
    F. 40 or more times

55. During your life, how many times have you used a needle to inject any **illegal** drug into your body?
    A. 0 times
    B. 1 time
    C. 2 or more times

56. During the past 12 months, has anyone offered, sold, or given you an illegal drug **on school property**?
    A. Yes
    B. No

The next eight questions ask about sexual behavior.

57. Have you ever had sexual intercourse?
    A. Yes
    B. No

58. How old were you when you had sexual intercourse for the first time?
    A. I have never had sexual intercourse
    B. 11 years old or younger
    C. 12 years old
    D. 13 years old
    E. 14 years old
    F. 15 years old
    G. 16 years old
    H. 17 years old or older

59. During your life, with how many people have you had sexual intercourse?
    A. I have never had sexual intercourse
    B. 1 person
    C. 2 people
    D. 3 people
    E. 4 people
    F. 5 people
    G. 6 or more people

60. During the past 3 months, with how many people did you have sexual intercourse?
    A. I have never had sexual intercourse
    B. I have had sexual intercourse, but not during the past 3 months
    C. 1 person
    D. 2 people
    E. 3 people
    F. 4 people
    G. 5 people
    H. 6 or more people

61. Did you drink alcohol or use drugs before you had sexual intercourse the **last time**?
    A. I have never had sexual intercourse
    B. Yes
    C. No

62. The **last time** you had sexual intercourse, did you or your partner use a condom?
    A. I have never had sexual intercourse
    B. Yes
    C. No

63. The **last time** you had sexual intercourse, what **one** method did you or your partner use to **prevent pregnancy**? (Select only **one** response.)
    A. I have never had sexual intercourse
    B. No method was used to prevent pregnancy
    C. Birth control pills
    D. Condoms
    E. Depo-Provera (injectable birth control)
    F. Withdrawal
    G. Some other method
    H. Not sure

64. How many times have you been pregnant or gotten someone pregnant?
    A. 0 times
    B. 1 time
    C. 2 or more times
    D. Not sure

The next seven questions ask about body weight.

65. How do **you** describe your weight?
    A. Very underweight
    B. Slightly underweight
    C. About the right weight
    D. Slightly overweight
    E. Very overweight

66. Which of the following are you trying to do about your weight?
    A. **Lose** weight
    B. **Gain** weight
    C. **Stay** the same weight
    D. I am **not trying to do anything** about my weight

67. During the past 30 days, did you **exercise** to lose weight or to keep from gaining weight?
    A. Yes
    B. No

68. During the past 30 days, did you **eat less food, fewer calories, or foods low in fat** to lose weight or to keep from gaining weight?
    A. Yes
    B. No

69. During the past 30 days, did you **go without eating for 24 hours or more** (also called fasting) to lose weight or to keep from gaining weight?
    A. Yes
    B. No

70. During the past 30 days, did you **take any diet pills, powders, or liquids** without a doctor's advice to lose weight or to keep from gaining weight? (Do **not** include meal replacement products such as Slim Fast.)
    A. Yes
    B. No

71. During the past 30 days, did you **vomit or take laxatives** to lose weight or to keep from gaining weight?
    A. Yes
    B. No

The next seven questions ask about food you ate or drank during the past 7 days. Think about all the meals and snacks you had from the time you got up until you went to bed. Be sure to include food you ate at home, at school, at restaurants, or anywhere else.

72. During the past 7 days, how many times did you drink **100% fruit juices** such as orange juice, apple juice, or grape juice? (Do **not** count punch, Kool-Aid, sports drinks, or other fruit-flavored drinks.)
    A. I did not drink 100% fruit juice during the past 7 days
    B. 1 to 3 times during the past 7 days
    C. 4 to 6 times during the past 7 days
    D. 1 time per day
    E. 2 times per day
    F. 3 times per day
    G. 4 or more times per day

73. During the past 7 days, how many times did you eat **fruit**? (Do **not** count fruit juice.)
    A. I did not eat fruit during the past 7 days
    B. 1 to 3 times during the past 7 days
    C. 4 to 6 times during the past 7 days
    D. 1 time per day
    E. 2 times per day
    F. 3 times per day
    G. 4 or more times per day

74. During the past 7 days, how many times did you eat **green salad**?
    A. I did not eat green salad during the past 7 days
    B. 1 to 3 times during the past 7 days
    C. 4 to 6 times during the past 7 days
    D. 1 time per day
    E. 2 times per day
    F. 3 times per day
    G. 4 or more times per day

75. During the past 7 days, how many times did you eat **potatoes**? (Do **not** count french fries, fried potatoes, or potato chips.)
    A. I did not eat potatoes during the past 7 days
    B. 1 to 3 times during the past 7 days
    C. 4 to 6 times during the past 7 days
    D. 1 time per day
    E. 2 times per day
    F. 3 times per day
    G. 4 or more times per day

76. During the past 7 days, how many times did you eat **carrots**?
    A. I did not eat carrots during the past 7 days
    B. 1 to 3 times during the past 7 days
    C. 4 to 6 times during the past 7 days
    D. 1 time per day
    E. 2 times per day
    F. 3 times per day
    G. 4 or more times per day

77. During the past 7 days, how many times did you eat **other vegetables**? (Do **not** count green salad, potatoes, or carrots.)
    A. I did not eat other vegetables during the past 7 days
    B. 1 to 3 times during the past 7 days
    C. 4 to 6 times during the past 7 days
    D. 1 time per day
    E. 2 times per day
    F. 3 times per day
    G. 4 or more times per day

78. During the past 7 days, how many **glasses of milk** did you drink? (Include the milk you drank in a glass or cup, from a carton, or with cereal. Count the half pint of milk served at school as equal to one glass.)
    A. I did not drink milk during the past 7 days
    B. 1 to 3 glasses during the past 7 days
    C. 4 to 6 glasses during the past 7 days
    D. 1 glass per day
    E. 2 glasses per day
    F. 3 glasses per day
    G. 4 or more glasses per day

The next eight questions ask about physical activity.

79. On how many of the past 7 days did you exercise or participate in physical activity for **at least 20** minutes **that made you sweat and breathe hard,** such as basketball, soccer, running, swimming laps, fast bicycling, fast dancing, or similar aerobic activities?
    A. 0 days
    B. 1 day
    C. 2 days
    D. 3 days
    E. 4 days
    F. 5 days
    G. 6 days
    H. 7 days

80. On how many of the past 7 days did you participate in physical activity for **at least 30** minutes that did **not** make you sweat or breathe hard, such as fast walking, slow bicycling, skating, pushing a lawn mower, or mopping floors?
    A. 0 days
    B. 1 day
    C. 2 days
    D. 3 days
    E. 4 days
    F. 5 days
    G. 6 days
    H. 7 days

81. On how many of the past 7 days did you do exercises to **strengthen or tone your muscles,** such as push-ups, sit-ups, or weight lifting?
    A. 0 days
    B. 1 day
    C. 2 days
    D. 3 days
    E. 4 days
    F. 5 days
    G. 6 days
    H. 7 days

82. On an average school day, how many hours do you watch TV?
    A. I do not watch TV on an average school day
    B. Less than 1 hour per day
    C. 1 hour per day
    D. 2 hours per day
    E. 3 hours per day
    F. 4 hours per day
    G. 5 or more hours per day

83. In an average week when you are in school, on how many days do you go to physical education (PE) classes?
    A. 0 days
    B. 1 day
    C. 2 days
    D. 3 days
    E. 4 days
    F. 5 days

84. During an average physical education (PE) class, how many minutes do you spend actually exercising or playing sports?
    A. I do not take PE
    B. Less than 10 minutes
    C. 10 to 20 minutes
    D. 21 to 30 minutes
    E. More than 30 minutes

85. During the past 12 months, on how many sports teams did you play? (Include any teams run by your school or community groups.)
    A. 0 teams
    B. 1 team
    C. 2 teams
    D. 3 or more teams

86. During the past 12 months, how many times were you injured while exercising, playing sports, or being physically active and had to be treated by a doctor or nurse?
    A. 0 times
    B. 1 time
    C. 2 times
    D. 3 times
    E. 4 times
    F. 5 or more times

The next question asks about AIDS education.

87. Have you ever been taught about AIDS or HIV infection in school?
    A. Yes
    B. No
    C. Not sure

This is the end of the survey.
Thank you very much for your help.

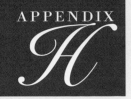

Community Assessment Tools

H.1 Community-As-Partner Model

The community-as-partner model was developed to illustrate public health nursing as a synthesis of public health and nursing. The model, originally titled community-as-client, has evolved to incorporate the philosophy that nurses work with communities as partners. This is congruent with what was learned about how communities (and people, for that matter) change and grow best, that is, by full involvement and self-empowerment, not by imposed programs and structures.

The model's "heart" is the assessment wheel (Fig. H-1), which depicts that the people actually are the community—the core elements. Without people there is no community, and it is the people (their demographics, values, beliefs, history) that is of interest to the public health nurse. Surrounding the people, and integral with them, are the identified eight subsystems of a community. These subsystems (physical environment, education, safety and transportation, politics and government, health and social services, communication, economics, and recreation) both affect and are affected by the people. To understand this interaction, one must understand each subsystem; therefore incorporate its assessment into assessment of the people.

The "wheel" (actually the entire community, including the people and subsystems) is shown with broken lines between each subsystem to show that these are not discrete, but that all subsystems affect each other. Within the community are lines of resistance, those "strengths" that defend against stressors (e.g., a school-based program to prevent teen violence); identifying strengths in the community is as important as identifying "problems." Surrounding the community are lines of defense, depicted in the model as "flexible" and "normal" to indicate that there are two types of defense: one is the usual (normal) "health" of a community and the other is more dynamic (flexible) and changes more rapidly. Two illustrations may assist in clarifying these lines. The flexible line of defense may be a temporary response to a stressor. For instance, an environmental stressor like flash flooding or a major fire may call into play resources from within the community and from surrounding areas; these resources are considered the flexible lines of defense. The normal line of defense is the usual level of health a community has reached over time. Examples of normal lines of defense include the immunization rate, adequate housing, or access to Meals On Wheels for shut-ins; all of these contribute to the health of the community.

Stressors affect the community and may be of the community or from outside the community. Either way, the community's response to stressors is mitigated by its overall health state, that is, by the strength of its lines of resistance and defense. Knowing these strengths is one purpose of the community assessment. In the analysis phase of the nursing process, the nurse will weigh the stressor and the degree of reaction it causes in order to describe a community nursing diagnosis that, in turn, will give direction to goals and interventions. One method for stating the community nursing diagnosis is to state the "problem" as the degree of reaction (from which the goal is derived) and the "as related to" as stressors ("causes" that help define needed interventions). Using this method, an example of a community nursing diagnosis might be as follows: High rate of tuberculosis (the problem, the degree of reaction) related to poor hygiene and sanitation, crowded living conditions, poverty, and consumption of raw milk (stressors) as manifested by open garbage, and poor ventilation; an average of 5.6 persons per household; and sale of raw milk for income (the "data" collected in your assessment).

Think for a moment how each subsystem contributes to the health of the community. The nurse can see how an inadequate infrastructure, such as modern sewage treatment or unemployment, can affect the health of all of the citizens.

Many models exist to provide a framework for assessing a community. This systems model gives one other way to describe a community. Working with the community is a vital and challenging task for nurses. Using a model wherein the community is viewed as a partner will help formulate community-focused interventions and promote the health of the entire community.

Elizabeth T. Anderson, RN, FAAN, DrPH
Professor and Chair, Department of Community Health and Gerontology
University of Texas School of Nursing at Galveston
University of Texas Medical Branch
Galveston, Texas

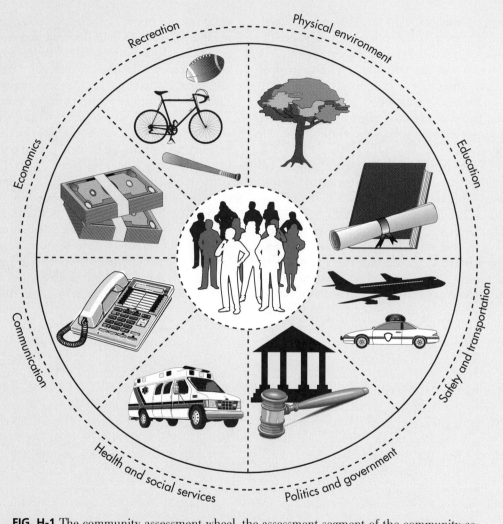

FIG. H-1 The community assessment wheel, the assessment segment of the community-as-partner model. (From Anderson ET, McFarlane J: *Community-as-partner: theory and practice in nursing,* Philadelphia, 1996, J.B. Lippincott.)

H.2 Communities with Physically Compromised Members: Assessment Tools

ASSESSMENT TOOL	PURPOSE	REFERENCES
Adequacy of Prenatal Care Utilization Index	Assesses the adequacy of prenatal care utilization and its association with low birth weight in the United States	Kotelchuck M: An evaluation of the Kessner Adequacy of Prenatal Care Index and a proposed adequacy of prenatal care utilization index, *Am J Public Health* 84(9):1414. Kotelchuck M: The adequacy of prenatal care utilization index: its U.S. distribution and association with low birth-weight, *Am J Public Health* 84(9):1486.
Attitude Towards Disabled People (ATDP)	Measures attitudes of people in community towards those who are disabled	Yuker HE, Block JR, Campbell WJ: *A scale to measure attitudes towards disabled persons,* Albertson, NY, 1960, Human Resources Foundation.
Community Integration Questionnaire (CIQ)	Assesses three components of community integration: home integration, social integration, and productive activities	Corrigan JK, Deming R: Psychometric characteristics of the Community Integration Questionnaire: replication and extension, *J Head Trauma Rehabil* 10(4):41, 1995.
Environmental Status Scale (ESS)	Assesses area of handicap status	Steward G, Kidd D, Thompson AJ: The assessment of handicap: an evaluation of the Environmental Status Scale, *Disabil Rehabil* 17(6):312, 1995.
Health Related Quality of Life	Evaluates efforts in the prevention of disabling chronic diseases	Hennessey CH, Moriarty DG, Zack MM, et al: Measuring health-related quality of life for public health surveillance, *Public Health Rep* 109(5):655, 1994.
Readily Available Checklist	Determines the frequency of architectural barriers to persons with disabilities	Ahn HC, McGovern EE, Walk EE, Edlich RF: Architectural barriers to persons with disabilities in businesses in an urban community, *J Burn Care Rehabil* 15(2):176, 1994
Revised Screening Survey	Measures the extent that populations are served by local health departments carrying out core function of public health	Miller CA, Moore, KS, Richards TB, McKaig C: A screening survey to assess local public health performance, *Public Health Rep* 109(5):659, 1994.
Wheelchair Accessibility Checklist	Assesses the accessibility of buildings to those who use wheelchairs	McClain L et al: Restaurant wheelchair accessibility, *Am J Occup Ther* 47(7):619, 1993. McClain L, Todd D: Food store accessibility, *Am J Occup Ther* 44(6):487, 1990.

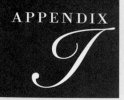

Family Assessment Tools

I.1 List of Family Assessment Tools

ASSESSMENT TOOL	PURPOSE	REFERENCES
Calgary Family Assessment Model (CFAM)	Assessment based on strengths critical to healthy family functioning. Addresses family structure, development, and function.	Wright LM, Leahey M: *Nurses and families–a guide to family assessment and intervention,* Philadelphia, 1984, FA Davis.
Chronicity Impact and Coping Instrument: Parent Questionnaire (CICI:PQ)	Assessment of parent perception of the effect of chronic childhood disorder on family and how families cope with the problems associated with the child's condition.	Hymovich D: The chronicity impact and coping instrument: parent questionnaire, *Nurs Res* 32, 1983.
Family Assessment for School Nurses and Other Professions (FAT)	Assessment of home and environment; family interaction styles; child's growth, development, and health history; and family health and social history.	Holt S, Robinson T: The school nurse's family assessment tool, *Am J Nurs* 79(5), 1979.
Family Health Protective Behavior Assessment Tool	Assessment of specific health behaviors for each family developmental stage.	Dandzari JK, Howard JR: *The well family: a developmental approach to assessment,* Boston, 1981, Little, Brown.
Feetham Family Functioning Survey (FFFS)	Assessment of accomplishment of family tasks and functioning of families with normal or impaired child. Identifies specific areas of dysfunction during a period of stress.	Feetham S, Humenick S: The Feetham family functioning survey. In Humenick S, editor: *Analysis of current assessment strategies in the health care of young children and childbearing families,* New York, 1982, Appleton-Century-Crofts.
Friedman's Guidelines for Function Assessment of the Family	Assessment of variables (communication, role, power, values, and coping) and the effect on affective, socialization, and health care functions.	Friedman M: *Family nursing: theory and assessment,* ed 2, New York, 1986, Appleton-Century-Crofts
Home Observation for Measurement of the Environment (HOME)	Assessment of family influence through the child's environment. Assesses animate and inanimate aspects of the environment that support development. Identifies family strengths and weaknesses.	Caldwell BM: *Home observation for measurement of the environment,* Little Rock, 1979, University of Arkansas

I.2   Family Systems Stressor-Strength Inventory (FS³I)

Karen B. Mischke, RN, OGNP/WHCNP, PhD, CFLE
Hillsboro Women's Clinic
620 SE Oak Street
Hillsboro, OR 97123

Shirley M. H. Hanson, RN, PMHNP, PhD, FAAN, CFLE, LMFT*
Professor, School of Nursing
Department of Family Nursing
Oregon Health Sciences University
Portland, OR 97201
Telephone: (503) 494-3869
Fax: (503) 494-3878
E-Mail: hanson@ohsu.edu

INSTRUCTIONS FOR ADMINISTRATION

The Family Systems Stressor-Strength Inventory (FS³I) is an assessment/measurement instrument intended for use with families. It focuses on identifying stressful situations occurring in families and the strengths families use to maintain healthy family functioning. Each family member is asked to complete the instrument on an individual form before an interview with the clinician. Questions can be read to members unable to read.

Following completion of the instrument the clinician evaluates the family on each of the stressful situations (general and specific) and the available strengths they possess. This evaluation is recorded on the family member form.

The clinician records the individual family member's score and the clinician perception score on the Quantitative Summary. A different color code is used for each family member. The clinician also completes the Qualitative Summary synthesizing the information gleaned from all participants. Clinicians can use the Family Care Plan to prioritize diagnoses, set goals, develop prevention/intervention activities, and evaluate outcomes.

*Respondent to inquiries.

From Mischke-Berkey K, Hanson SMH: *Pocket guide to family assessment and intervention,* St Louis, 1991, Mosby.

FAMILY SYSTEMS STRESSOR-STRENGTH INVENTORY (FS³I)

Family Name _____   Date _____

Family Member(s) Completing Assessment _____

Ethnic Background(s) _____

Religious Background(s) _____

Referral Source _____

Interviewer _____

Family members	Relationship in family	Age	Marital status	Education (highest degree)	Occupation
1.					
2.					
3.					
4.					
5.					
6.					

Families current reasons for seeking assistance?

_____

_____

_____

Part I: Family Systems Stressors (General)

DIRECTIONS: Each of the 25 situations/stressors listed here deals with some aspect of normal family life. They have the potential for creating stress within families or between families and the world in which they live. We are interested in your overall impression of how these situations affect your family life. Please circle a number (0 through 5) that best describes the amount of stress or tension they create for you.

Stressors:	Not applicable	Little stress	Medium stress		High stress	Clinician perception Score
1. Family member(s) feel unappreciated 0		1	2	3	4 5	_____
2. Guilt for not accomplishing more 0		1	2	3	4 5	_____
3. Insufficient "me" time 0		1	2	3	4 5	_____
4. Self-image/self-esteem/feelings of unattractiveness 0		1	2	3	4 5	_____
5. Perfectionism 0		1	2	3	4 5	_____
6. Dieting 0		1	2	3	4 5	_____
7. Health/Illness 0		1	2	3	4 5	_____
8. Communication with children 0		1	2	3	4 5	_____
9. Housekeeping standards 0		1	2	3	4 5	_____
10. Insufficient couple time 0		1	2	3	4 5	_____
11. Insufficient family playtime 0		1	2	3	4 5	_____
12. Children's behavior/discipline/sibling fighting 0		1	2	3	4 5	_____
13. Television 0		1	2	3	4 5	_____
14. Over-scheduled family calendar 0		1	2	3	4 5	_____
15. Lack of shared responsibility in the family 0		1	2	3	4 5	_____
16. Moving 0		1	2	3	4 5	_____
17. Spousal relationship (communication, friendship, sex) 0		1	2	3	4 5	_____
18. Holidays 0		1	2	3	4 5	_____
19. In-laws 0		1	2	3	4 5	_____
20. Teen behaviors (communication, music, friends, school) 0		1	2	3	4 5	_____
21. New baby 0		1	2	3	4 5	_____
22. Economics/finances/budgets 0		1	2	3	4 5	_____
23. Unhappiness with work situation 0		1	2	3	4 5	_____
24. Overvolunteerism 0		1	2	3	4 5	_____
25. Neighbors 0		1	2	3	4 5	_____

Additional stressors: _____

Family remarks: _____

Clinician: Clarification of stressful situations/concerns with family members.
Prioritize in order of importance to family members: _____

Part II: Family Systems Stressors (Specific)

DIRECTIONS: The following 12 questions are designed to provide information about your specific stress producing situation, problem, or area of concern influencing your family's health. Please circle a number (1 through 5) that best describes the influence this situation has on your family's life and how well you perceive your family's overall functioning.

The specific stress producing situation/problem or area of concern at this time is _____

_____

Stressors:	Family perception score			Clinician perception
	Little	Medium	High	Score

1. To what extent is your family bothered by this problem or stressful situation? 1   2   3   4   5
(e.g., effects on family interactions, communication among members, emotional, and social relationships)

    Family remarks: _____

    Clinician remarks: _____

    Score: _____

2. How much of an effect does this stressful situation have on your family's usual pattern of living? 1   2   3   4   5
(e.g., effects on life-style patterns and family developmental tasks)

    Family remarks: _____

    Clinician remarks: _____

    Score: _____

3. How much has this situation affected your family's ability to work together as a family unit? 1   2   3   4   5
(e.g., alteration in family roles, completion of family tasks, following through with responsibilities)

    Family remarks: _____

    Clinician remarks: _____

    Score: _____

Has your family ever experienced a similar concern in the past?
    1. YES   If YES, complete question 4.
    2. NO   If NO, complete question 5.

4. How successful was your family in dealing with this situation/problem/concern in the past? .1   2   3   4   5
(e.g., workable coping strategies developed, adaptive measures useful, situation improved)

    Family remarks: _____

    Clinician remarks: _____

    Score: _____

5. How strongly do you feel this current situation/problem/concern will affect your family's future? 1   2   3   4   5
(e.g., anticipated consequences)

    Family remarks: _____

    Clinician remarks: _____

    Score: _____

6. To what extent are family members able to help themselves in this present situation/problem/concern? 1   2   3   4   5
(e.g., self-assistive efforts, family expectations, spiritual influence, and family resources)

    Family remarks: _____

    Clinician remarks: _____

    Score: _____

Stressors:	Family perception score				Clinician perception
	Little	Medium		High	Score
7. To what extent do you expect others to help your family with this situation/problem/concern? . . . . 1 (e.g., What roles would helpers play? How available are extra-family resources?) Family remarks: _____ _____ Clinician remarks: _____ _____	2	3	4	5	____

Stressors:	Family perception score				Clinician perception
	Poor	Satisfactory		Excellent	Score
8. How would you rate the way your family functions overall? . . . . 1 (e.g., how your family members relate to each other and to larger family and community) Family remarks: _____ _____ Clinician remarks: _____ _____	2	3	4	5	____
9. How would you rate the overall physical health status of each family member by name? (Include yourself as a family member; record additional names on back.)					
a. _____ 1	2	3	4	5	____
b. _____ 1	2	3	4	5	____
c. _____ 1	2	3	4	5	____
d. _____ 1	2	3	4	5	____
e. _____ 1	2	3	4	5	____
10. How would you rate the overall physical health status of your family as a whole? . . . . 1 Family remarks: _____ _____ Clinician perceptions: _____ _____	2	3	4	5	____
11. How would you rate the overall mental health status of each family member by name? (Include yourself as a family member; record additional names on back.)					
a. _____ 1	2	3	4	5	____
b. _____ 1	2	3	4	5	____
c. _____ 1	2	3	4	5	____
d. _____ 1	2	3	4	5	____
e. _____ 1	2	3	4	5	____
12. How would you rate the overall mental health status of your family as a whole? . . . . 1 Family remarks: _____ _____ Clinician perceptions: _____ _____	2	3	4	5	____

Part III: Family Systems Strengths

Directions: Each of the 16 traits/attributes listed below deals with some aspect of family life and its overall functioning. Each one contributes to the health and well-being of family members as individuals and to the family as a whole. Please circle a number (0 through 5) that best describes the extent that the trait applies to your family.

My family:	Not applicable	Seldom		Usually		Always	Clinician perception Score
			Family perception score				
1. Communicates and listens to one another 0		1	2	3	4	5	____
Family remarks:							
Clinician remarks:							
2. Affirms and supports one another 0		1	2	3	4	5	____
Family remarks:							
Clinician remarks:							
3. Teaches respect for others 0		1	2	3	4	5	____
Family remarks:							
Clinician remarks:							
4. Develops a sense of trust in members 0		1	2	3	4	5	____
Family remarks:							
Clinician remarks:							
5. Displays a sense of play and humor 0		1	2	3	4	5	____
Family remarks:							
Clinician remarks:							
6. Exhibits a sense of shared responsibility 0		1	2	3	4	5	____
Family remarks:							
Clinician remarks:							
7. Teaches a sense of right and wrong 0		1	2	3	4	5	____
Family remarks:							
Clinician remarks:							
8. Has a strong sense of family in which rituals and traditions abound 0		1	2	3	4	5	____
Family remarks:							
Clinician remarks:							
9. Has a balance of interaction among members 0		1	2	3	4	5	____
Family remarks:							
Clinician remarks:							
10. Has a shared religious core .0		1	2	3	4	5	____
Family remarks:							
Clinician remarks:							

My family:	Family perception score						Clinician perception
	Not applicable	Seldom		Usually		Always	Score
11. Respects the privacy of one another 0		1	2	3	4	5	_____
Family remarks: _____							
Clinician remarks: _____							
12. Values service to others 0		1	2	3	4	5	_____
Family remarks: _____							
Clinician remarks: _____							
13. Fosters family table time and conversation 0		1	2	3	4	5	_____
Family remarks: _____							
Clinician remarks: _____							
14. Shares leisure time 0		1	2	3	4	5	_____
Family remarks: _____							
Clinician remarks: _____							
15. Admits to and seeks help with problems 0		1	2	3	4	5	_____
Family remarks: _____							
Clinician remarks: _____							
16a. How would you rate the overall strengths that exist in your family? 0		1	2	3	4	5	_____
Family remarks: _____							
Clinician remarks: _____							

16b. Additional Family Strengths: _____

_____

_____

16c. Clinician: Clarification of family strengths with individual members: _____

_____

_____

_____

_____

SCORING SUMMARY

The Family Systems Stressor-Strength Inventory (FS³I) Scoring Summary is divided into two sections: Section 1, Family Perception Scores and Section 2, Clinician Perception Scores. These two sections are further divided into three parts: Part I, Family Systems Stressors: General; Part II, Family Systems Stressors: Specific; and Part III, Family Systems Strengths. Each part contains a Quantitative Summary and a Qualitative Summary.

Quantifiable family and clinician perception scores are both graphed on the Quantitative Summary. Each family member has a designated color code. Family and clinician remarks are both recorded on the Qualitative Summary. Quantitative summary scores, when graphed, suggest a level for initiation of prevention/intervention modes: primary, secondary and tertiary. Qualitative summary information, when synthesized, contributes to the development and channeling of the Family Care Plan.

Section 1: Family Perception Scores

Part I   **Family Systems Stressors (General)**

Add scores from questions 1 to 25 and calculate an overall numerical score for Family System Stressors (General). Ratings are from 1 (most positive) to 5 (most negative). The Not Applicable (0) responses are omitted from the calculations. Total scores range from 25 to 125.

Family Systems Stressor Score: General

$$\frac{(\ \ )}{25} \times 1 = \underline{\hspace{2cm}}$$

Graph score on Quantitative Summary, Family Systems Stressors: General, Family Member Perception. Color code to differentiate family members.

Record additional stressors and family remarks in Part I, Qualitative Summary: Family and Clinician Remarks.

Part II   **Family Systems Stressors: Specific**

Add scores from questions 1-8, 10, and 12 and calculate a numerical score for Family Systems Stressors: Specific. Ratings are from 1 (most positive) to 5 (most negative). Questions 4, 6, 7, 8, 10, and 12 are reverse scored.* Total scores range from 10-50.

Family Systems Stressor Score: Specific

$$\frac{(\ \ )}{10} \times 1 = \underline{\hspace{2cm}}$$

Graph score on Quantitative Summary: Family Systems Stressor: Specific. (Family Member Perceptions). Color code to differentiate family members.

Summarize data from questions 9 and 11 (reverse scored) and record family remarks in Part II, Qualitative Summary: Family and Clinician Remarks

Part III   **Family Systems Strengths**

Add scores from questions 1 to 16 and calculate a numerical score for Family Systems Strengths. Ratings are from 1 (seldom) to 5 (always). The Not Applicable (0) responses are omitted from the calculations. Total scores range from 16 to 80.

Family Systems Strength Score

$$\frac{(\ \ )}{16} \times 1 = \underline{\hspace{2cm}}$$

Graph score on Quantitative Summary: Family Systems Strengths (Family Member Perception).

Record additional family strengths and family remarks in Part III, Qualitative Summary: Family and Clinician Remarks.

*Reverse Scoring:
   Question answered as (1) is scored 5 points
   Question answered as (2) is scored 4 points
   Question answered as (3) is scored 3 points
   Question answered as (4) is scored 2 points
   Question answered as (5) is scored 1 point

Section 2: Clinician Perception Scores

Part I   **Family Systems Stressors (General)**

Add scores from questions 1 to 25 and calculate an overall numerical score for Family System Stressors (General). Ratings are from 1 (most positive) to 5 (most negative). The Not Applicable (0) responses are omitted from the calculations. Total scores range from 25 to 125.

Family Systems Stressor Score: General

$$\frac{(\ \ )}{25} \times 1 = \underline{\hspace{2cm}}$$

Graph score on Quantitative Summary, Family Systems Stressors: General (Clinician Perception).

Record Clinicians' clarification of general stressors in Part I, Qualitative Summary: Family and Clinician Remarks

Part II   **Family Systems Stressors: Specific**

Add scores from questions 1-8, 10 and 12 and calculate a numerical score for Family Systems Stressors: Specific. Ratings are from 1 (most positive) to 5 (most negative). Questions 4, 6, 7, 8, 10, and 12 are reverse scored.* Total scores range from 10-50.

Family Systems Stressor Score: Specific

$$\frac{(\ \ )}{10} \times 1 = \underline{\hspace{2cm}}$$

Graph score on Quantitative Summary: Family Systems Stressor: Specific. (Clinician Perception).

Summarize data from questions 9 and 11 (reverse order) and record clinician remarks in Part II, Qualitative Summary: Family and Clinician Remarks

Part III   **Family Systems Strengths**

Add scores from questions 1 to 16 and calculate a numerical score for Family Systems Strengths. Ratings are from 1 (seldom) to 5 (always). The Not Applicable (0) responses are omitted from the calculations. Total scores range from 16 to 80.

Family Systems Strength Score

$$\frac{(\ \ )}{16} \times 1 = \underline{\hspace{2cm}}$$

Graph score on Quantitative Summary: Family Systems Strengths (Clinician Perception).

Record clinicians' clarification of family strengths in Part III, Qualitative Summary: Family and Clinician Remarks.

*Reverse Scoring:
   Question answered as (1) is scored 5 points
   Question answered as (2) is scored 4 points
   Question answered as (3) is scored 3 points
   Question answered as (4) is scored 2 points
   Question answered as (5) is scored 1 point

Scores for Wellness and Stability			Scores for Wellness and Stability		
5.0			5.0		
4.8			4.8		
4.6			4.6		
4.4			4.4		
4.2			4.2		
4.0			4.0		
3.8			3.8		
3.6			3.6		
3.4			3.4		
3.2			3.2		
3.0			3.0		
2.8			2.8		
2.6			2.6		
2.4			2.4		
2.2			2.2		
2.0			2.0		
1.8			1.8		
1.6			1.6		
1.4			1.4		
1.2			1.2		
1.0			1.0		

Sum of strengths
available for
prevention/
intervention
mode

5.0
4.8
4.6
4.4
4.2
4.0
3.8
3.6

3.4
3.2
3.0
2.8
2.6
2.4
2.2

2.0
1.8
1.6
1.4
1.2
1.0

Qualitative Summary Family and Clinician Remarks

Part I: Family Systems Stressors: General

Summarize general stressors and remarks of family and clinician. Prioritize stressors according to importance to family members.

_____

_____

_____

Part II: Family Systems Stressors: Specific

A. Summarize specific stressor and remarks of family and clinician.

_____

_____

_____

B. Summarize differences (if discrepancies exist) between how family members and clinician view effects of stressful situation on family.

_____

_____

_____

C. Summarize overall family functioning.

_____

_____

_____

D. Summarize overall significant physical health status for family members.

_____

_____

_____

E. Summarize overall significant mental health status for family members.

_____

_____

_____

Part III: Family Systems Strengths

Summarize family systems strengths and family and clinician remarks that facilitate family health and stability.

_____

_____

_____

Family Care Plan*					
Diagnosis general and specific family system stressors	Family systems strengths supporting family care plan	Goals family and clinician	Prevention/Intervention mode		Outcomes evaluation and replanning
			Primary, secondary or tertiary	Prevention/intervention activities	

*Prioritize the three most significant diagnoses.

I.3 Friedman Family Assessment Model (Short Form)

Before using the following guidelines in completing family assessments, two words of caution. First, not all areas included below will be germane for each of the families visited. The guidelines are comprehensive and allow depth when probing is necessary. The student should not feel that every subarea needs to be covered when the broad area of inquiry poses no problems to the family or concern to the health worker. Second, by virtue of the interdependence of the family system, one will find unavoidable redundancy. For the sake of efficiency, the assessor should try not to repeat data, but to refer the reader back to sections where this information has already been described.

IDENTIFYING DATA

1. Family Name
2. Address and Phone
3. Family Composition (see table)
4. Type of Family Form
5. Cultural (Ethnic) Background
6. Religious Identification
7. Social Class Status
8. Family's Recreational or Leisure-time Activities

DEVELOPMENTAL STAGE AND HISTORY OF FAMILY

9. Family's Present Developmental Stage
10. Extent of Developmental Tasks Fulfillment
11. Nuclear Family History
12. History of Family of Origin of Both Parents

ENVIRONMENTAL DATA

13. Characteristics of Home
14. Characteristics of Neighborhood and Larger Community
15. Family's Geographic Mobility
16. Family's Associations and Transactions with Community
17. Family's Social Support Network (ecomap)

FAMILY STRUCTURE

18. Communication Patterns
    Extent of Functional and Dysfunctional Communication (types of recurring patterns)
    Extent of Emotional (Affective) Messages and How Expressed
    Characteristics of Communication within Family Subsystems
    Extent of Congruent and Incongruent Messages
    Types of Dysfunctional Communication Processes Seen in Family
    Areas of Open and Closed Communication
    Familial and External Variables Affecting Communication

19. Power Structure
    Power Outcomes
    Decision-making Process
    Power Bases
    Variables Affecting Family Power
    Overall Family System and Subsystem Power
20. Role Structure
    Formal Role Structure
    Informal Role Structure
    Analysis of Role Models (optional)
    Variables Affecting Role Structure
21. Family Values
    Compare the family to American or family's reference group values and/or identify important family values and their importance (priority) in family.
    Congruence Between the Family's Values and the Family's Reference Group or Wider Community
    Congruence Between the Family's Values and Family Member's Values
    Variables Influencing Family Values
    Values Consciously or Unconsciously Held
    Presence of Value Conflicts in Family.
    Effect of the Above Values and Value Conflicts on Health Status of Family.

FAMILY FUNCTIONS

22. Affective Function
    Family's Need-Response Patterns
    Mutual Nurturance, Closeness, and Identification
    Separateness and Connectedness
23. Socialization Function
    Family Child-rearing Practices
    Adaptability of Child-rearing Practices for Family Form and Family's Situation
    Who Is (Are) Socializing Agent(s) for Child(ren)?
    Value of Children in Family
    Cultural Beliefs That Influence Family's Child-rearing Patterns
    Social Class Influence on Child-Rearing Patterns
    Estimation About Whether Family Is at Risk for Child-rearing Problems and, if so, Indication of High-Risk Factors
    Adequacy of Home Environment for Children's Needs to Play
24. Health Care Function
    Family's Health Beliefs, Values, and Behavior
    Family's Definitions of Health-Illness and Their Level of Knowledge
    Family's Perceived Health Status and Illness Susceptibility
    Family's Dietary Practices
    Adequacy of family diet (recommended 24-hour food history record).

Function of mealtimes and attitudes toward food and mealtimes.

Shopping (and its planning) practices.

Person(s) responsible for planning, shopping, and preparation of meals.

Sleep and Rest Habits

Physical Activity and Recreation Practices (not covered earlier)

Family's Drug Habits

Family's Role in Self-care Practices

Medically Based Preventive Measures (physicals, eye and hearing tests, and immunizations)

Dental Health Practices

Family Health History (both general and specific diseases—environmentally and genetically related)

Health Care Services Received

Feelings and Perceptions Regarding Health Services

Emergency Health Services

Source of Payments for Health and Other Services

Logistics of Receiving Care

FAMILY STRESS AND COPING

25. Short- and Long-term Familial Stressors and Strengths

26. Extent of Family's Ability to Respond, Based on Objective Appraisal of Stress-producing Situations

27. Coping Strategies Utilized (present/past)
    Differences in family members' ways of coping
    Family's inner coping strategies
    Family's external coping strategies

28. Dysfunctional Adaptive Strategies Utilized (present/past; extent of usage)

FAMILY COMPOSITION FORM

NAME (LAST, FIRST)	GENDER	RELATIONSHIP	DATE AND PLACE OF BIRTH	OCCUPATION	EDUCATION
1. (Father)					
2. (Mother)					
3. (Oldest child)					
4.					
5.					
6.					
7.					
8.					

From Friedman MM: *Family nursing research, theory, and practice,* Stamford, Conn, 1998, Appleton & Lange.

I.4   Case Example of Family Assessment

The Jeddi family is a real family in a real situation. They came to the attention of the nurse when the family was referred to the county home health agency for a baseline family assessment with their impending adoption of a 4-year-old boy from Russia. This upper middle class Caucasian family consists of Ben (age 51), Mare (age 43), and the son they will adopt, Alex (age 4). See Figure I-1 for the Jeddi family genogram and Figure I-2 for the Jeddi family ecomap.

Ben and Mare have been married for 8 years. Ben has a PhD in chemical engineering and does consulting work. His business is located in the caretaker apartment located in the basement of their home. Mare has a PhD, is a pediatric nurse, and teaches at a private university. They are adopting a 4-year-old boy from Russia. Mare has a diagnosis of infertility after 2 years of trying to have a biologic child and extensive testing. The infertility issue was a significant loss for both Ben and Mare. The couple considered in vitro fertilization. Mare decided against this approach because she felt the risks of failure of pregnancy

and miscarriage were too great. Ben felt that this was Mare's decision to make as it more directly involved her physical and mental health. He supported Mare's decision to not pursue in vitro fertilization.

Mare initiated the discussions about adoption. The decision to adopt a child was reached in May of this year after a year and a half of discussion and investigation. Initially, Ben was not equally committed to the concept of adoption and had a longer grieving process over their inability to have a child together than Mare. The issue of biologic heritage and the loss of blood lineage were more significant to Ben. The significant issue for Mare was the loss of being parent and raising a child.

The couple investigated several adoption agencies and attended potential adoptive parent classes a year and a half ago. At that time, Ben was not ready to make a commitment to adoption. The topic of adoption repeatedly was discussed by the couple over the course of the next year. In January 1994, the couple again seriously considered adoption. Mare investigated several adoption agencies

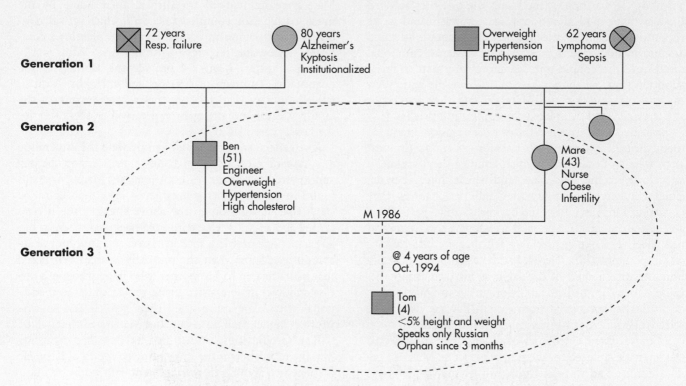

FIG. I.1

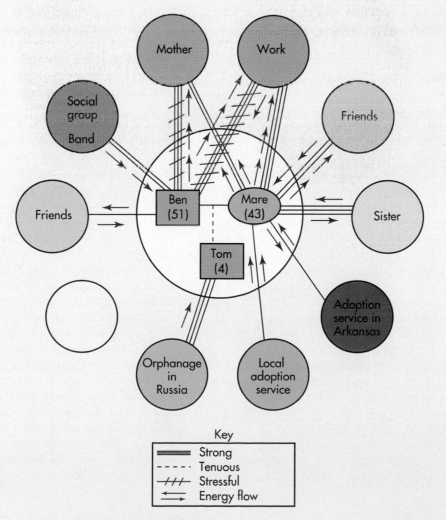

Key

═══════	Strong
- - - - -	Tenuous
⫽⫽⫽	Stressful
←——→	Energy flow

FIG. I.2

again, as she was not satisfied with the one they selected the last time. A local adoption agency was found to be supportive and informative for them. The couple attended an information meeting. After much intense emotional discussion, the couple pursued more information about adoption with the support personnel from the agency. At the end of May, Ben and Mare decided they wanted to adopt a child and completed the application process.

Both Ben and Mare feel this was an emotional time for them. After they made their decision to adopt, the next steps were to decide from which country they wanted to adopt a child, the child's age, and which child. They decided that, given their lifestyles and personalities, they wanted to adopt an older child between 3 and 5 years of age and not an infant. Ben wanted to adopt a son. Mare was not selective of the gender. Ben felt that the issue of race was important to him. He felt that he might have difficulty bonding with a child of dark skin as his own family. Because of Ben's immediate family origins from Finland, they decided to adopt a child from eastern Europe. Russia was selected because of its historical ties with Finland.

Mare reviewed videotapes of 40 children and selected the top male children for them to select from. Mare is a pediatric nurse and was determined to be the one to make the decisions about health. After viewing the films numerous times and reviewing a medical examination, Alex was the young child of choice. Ben and Mare made a formal petition to adopt Alex.

The process has taken 6 months. They are currently waiting for the final paperwork to arrive from the Russia government, which is expected in the next few days. They are in the midst of preparing their home for the arrival of Alex. They will both travel to Russia in 2 weeks to pick him up, complete the formal adoption process in Russia, and travel home together as a new family.

They are nervous and excited about the adoption. They are concerned about how Alex will adjust to them and the move to America. They are concerned about how adopting a 4-year-old will change their lifestyle. The preparation of their home for the arrival of Alex has been time consuming. The arrangements for travel to Russia are being finalized. Ben has taken 2 years of Russian 20 years ago; both are currently taking individual language tutoring in Russian. Ben and Mare are currently working full time. Mare plans to continue working full time after they adopt Alex, but she does have a reduced workload for the next 4 months. They plan to have Alex attend full-time preschool.

The initial assessment of the Jeddi family involved the use of two assessment approaches with their respective instruments, guidelines, a genogram, and an ecomap. A summary of the findings from this assessment follows.

FAMILY SYSTEMS STRESSOR STRENGTH INVENTORY

The FS³I is presented, which focused on the Jeddi family stressors and strengths to create a plan of action. Ben and

Mare were interviewed together in their home by the nurse. Each person completed the FS³I, which provided individual and composite scores. Figure I-1 presents a completed genogram. Figure I-2 shows the Jeddi family ecomap. Figure I-3 and I-4 provide the scoring for the quantitative summary of stressors and strengths. A qualitative summary (Fig. I-5) presents a brief picture of the family stresses and strengths and served as the guide for the family care plan (Fig. I-6).

The general stressors of the family were the impending adoption of Alex, issues of family nutrition and dieting, and lowered self-image for both Ben and Mare. Mare was found to have a higher general stress level than Ben. She states that in addition to the above stressors she is concerned about: stress relative to housekeeping issues, an ongoing physical problem with her knee, and guilt for not accomplishing more than she presently is able. Ben noted that issues related to his mother, who has Alzheimer's disease and lives in an assisted living center, causes him additional stress. The nurse rated their general and specific stressors higher than both Ben and Mare rated themselves.

The specific stressor identified by Ben that is causing him the most stress is the impending adoption of Alex. He is concerned about time management with work and a new family member. The additional stress of his mother's care is requiring a lot of his time. She is well taken care of in an assisted living center, but he is concerned about her advancing dementia. At present he is actively involved in renting out his mother's home. The specific stressor identified by Mare was how she is going to manage food preparations and meal times after they adopt Alex. She stated that cooking and meal preparation are currently a big problem for her. Mare stated that Ben does not help with food preparation or clean up now. They both eat on different schedules. She is concerned about family dinners and feels this is an important time for them with Alex. Food preparation is not a new issue for them. She stated that she feels pressured and "like a failure" because she does not manage this aspect of their family life well now, before the addition of Alex. In the past the family has hired a cook which was a "excellent solution" for them. The have been without a cook for 2 years now after their previous cook moved out of state.

The strengths of this family are many. They scored their individual strengths inventory almost identically, which demonstrates a similar perception of their family unit. Both Ben and Mare viewed their family and each other as experienced problem solvers. They have good, open communication between them and feel that the adoption of Alex has even brought them closer together. They recognized that much of their current stress is related to the unknown about Alex. They feel that once they meet Alex that they will be able to work together to solve their problems.

The nurse concluded that this family has the strengths they need to adapt to their new family life cycle of a family with a preschooler. In looking at the ecomap, the fam-

Text continued on p. A-167

Family Systems Stressor—Strength Inventory (FS^3I)
Quantitative Summary
Family Systems Stressors: General and Specific
Family and Clinician Perception Scores

Directions: Graph the scores from each family member inventory by placing an **"X"** at the appropriate location. (Use first name initial for each different entry and different color code for each family member.)

Scores for Wellness and Stability	Family Systems Stressors: General — Family Member Perception Score	Family Systems Stressors: General — Clinician Perception Score	Scores for Wellness and Stability	Family Systems Stressors: Specific — Family Member Perception Score	Family Systems Stressors: Specific — Clinician Perception Score
5.0			5.0		
4.8			4.8		
4.6			4.6		
4.4			4.4		
4.2			4.2		
4.0			4.0		
3.8			3.8		
3.6			3.6		
3.4			3.4		M O
3.2			3.2	B X	B X
3.0			3.0		
				M O	
2.8			2.8		
2.6			2.6		
2.4			2.4		
		M O			
2.2	M O		2.2		
2.0			2.0		
1.8		B X	1.8		
	B X				
1.6			1.6		
1.4			1.4		
1.2			1.2		
1.0			1.0		

• **PRIMARY**	Prevention/Intervention Mode: Flexible Line	1.0 - 2.3
• **SECONDARY**	Prevention/Intervention Mode: Normal Line	2.4 - 3.6
• **TERTIARY**	Prevention/Intervention Mode: Resistance Lines	3.7 - 5.0

• Breakdown of numerical scores for stressor penetration are suggested values

FIG. I.3

Family Systems Stressor—Strength Inventory (FS³I)
Quantitative Summary
Family Systems Strengths
Family and Clinician Perception Scores

Directions: Graph the scores from the inventory by placing an **"X"** at the appropriate location and connect with a line. (Use first name initial for each different entry and different color code for each family member.)

Sum of strengths available for prevention/ intervention mode	Family Systems Strengths	
	Family Member Perception Score	Clinician Perception Score
5.0		
4.8		
4.6		
4.4		
4.2		
4.0		
3.8		
3.6	MO B X	MO B X
3.4		
3.2		
3.0		
2.8		
2.6		
2.4		
2.2		
2.0		
1.8		
1.6		
1.4		
1.2		
1.0		

- **PRIMARY**   Prevention/Intervention Mode: Flexible Line   1.0 - 2.1
- **SECONDARY**   Prevention/Intervention Mode: Normal Line   2.2 - 3.6
- **TERTIARY**   Prevention/Intervention Mode: Resistance Lines   3.7 - 5.0

- Breakdown of numerical scores for stressor penetration are suggested values

FIG. I.4

Family Systems Stressor—Strength Inventory (FS³I)
Qualitative Summary
Family and Clinician Remarks

Part I: Family Systems Stressors: General

Summarize general stressors and remarks of family and clinician. Prioritize stressors according to importance to family members.

Ben: General stressors are: Lower self image, dieting, and adopting new child.

Mare: General stressors are: Guilt for not doing more; adopting new child;

lower self image; dieting; housekeeping; lack of shared responsibility; knee problem

Part II: Family Systems Stressors: Specific

A. Summarize specific stressor and remarks of family and clinician.

Both Ben & Mare feel the adoption of new child is the most important stessor specifically,

Ben is concerned about time management and Mare about time management relative to

cooking healthy meals for the family. Nurse sees these stressors higher than Ben & Mare.

B. Summarize differences (if discrepancies exist) between how family members and clinician view effects of stressful situation on family.

Both Ben & Mare see this stressor similarly, but Mare also sees several other related

family stressors particularly lack of shared responsibilities.

C. Summarize overall family functioning.

Family overall is functioning well with this stressor, but as adoption gets closer the stress

level will continue to rise; both are perfectionists and first time parents; they communicate

well and are now open to help from the outside.

D. Summarize overall significant physical health status for family members.

Ben - OK, but stressed

Mare - Stressed and concerned about knee problem which increases her emotional lability

Alex - Healthy, small for age both height and weight; mild developmental delay

E. Summarize overall significant mental health status for family members.

The family members are stressed but not in a crisis mode. They openly talk about concerns

and help each other emotionally.

Part III: Family Systems Strengths

Summarize family systems strengths and family and clinician remarks that facilitate family health and stability.

The major strengths are the open honest communication between Ben & Mare and their

experience with solving problems together and independently. They recently have opened

their closed family boundary to help from extended family, friends and professionals.

FIG. I.5

Family Systems and Stressor—Strength Inventory (FS³I)
Family Care Plan*

Diagnosis General and Specific Family System Stressors	Prognosis Goals Family and Clinician	Family Systems Strengths Supporting Family Care Plan	Prevention/Intervention Mode		Outcomes Evaluation and Replanning
			Primary, Secondary or Tertiary	Prevention/Intervention Activities	
1. Family life cycle transition: stress related to adoption of 4yr old boy from Russia	1. Excellent prognosis with anticipatory guidance, information and history of problem solving	Family communication Family commitment to adoption	Primary	1.a. Offer educational material on families with preschool child 1.b. Introduce family to adoption support groups and networks	1.a. Discuss normal family stressors 1.b. Attend support group
2. Family nutrition management: Stressed related to adoption, ongoing eating patterns and family health problems	2. Good prognosis as had faced this problem before- Investigate prior problems family had with last cook. Poor self images will take time to affect	Family communication Family known problem solvers	Secondary	2.a. Provide sources to contact where family can hire a cook 2.b. Investigate why they did not follow through with their last cook 2.c. Education on nutrition for 4yr old	2.a+b. Contact and hire a cook 2.c. Design healthy family meal plan for 1 month

*Prioritize the three most significant diagnoses

FIG. I.6

ily is found to be well supported by resources. They are responsive to information provided to them and ideas suggested by others for them to consider in their problem solving.

FRIEDMAN'S FAMILY ASSESSMENT FORM

Identifying Data

Ben and Mare Jeddi
Portland, Maine
Type of family: Nuclear
Ethnic background: Ben comes from a Finnish background. Mare has no particular ethnic identity
Religious: No affiliation
Social Class: Upper middle class
Leisure activities: Travel, gardening, music
Occupations: Ben, consulting chemical engineer. Mare, pediatric nurse and university faculty

Developmental Stage and History of Family

The family's present developmental stage cannot be defined in the conventional family life cycle. Ben and Mare have been married for 8 years, so they do not fit the categories for beginning families or families with children. However, they are in transition and, with the adoption of a 4-year old boy, the family will fit into the classical family life cycle stage of family with preschooler.

Ben comes from a nuclear family of origin; however, his parents were divorced after 30 years of marriage. Mare comes from a nuclear family of origin.

Environmental Data

The family live in an upper middle class urban neighborhood that is ethnically diverse. They are within close distance of schools, hospitals, fire department, and shopping areas. The neighborhood is clean and relatively safe, as there have been a few burglaries in the neighborhood. Both attend the neighborhood community meetings. The family is centrally located only 8 blocks from freeways around town, 2 miles from downtown, and 5 blocks from a bus route. Ben works in the home, where the basement caretaker apartment has been converted into his office and laboratories. Mare works at the university, which is 4 miles away. She often rides her bike to work.

Their home is a 75-year-old brick home that has four levels. It is situated on the edge of a hollow. The home is well kept but old. Both Ben and Mare enjoy their home and spend a lot of time there. They are slowing remodeling. The house is safe, but with the adoption of a 4-year-old boy, several safety factors need to be addressed. There is no medicine cabinet in the bathroom and medicines are easily within reach of a 4-year-old. The cleaning solutions are kept under the sinks in the kitchen and the bathroom. The patio above the garage does have a railing, but a 4-year-old may be tempted to walk on it. A fire plan needs to be made for the family because all of the bedrooms are on the top floor, which is three levels above the ground.

Family Structure

Communication is a strength of this family. There is an open relationship and communication pattern between Ben and Mare. Both are very verbal and expressive about their feelings, opinions, and needs. Because of this openness, they state that there is often conflict and arguing between them. However, they feel that they are good at conflict resolution. At times, however, the argument does get out of control and takes a personal attack format. When they realize this, usually Mare suggests that they take up the conversation at later time when they can both approach the topic more calmly. They are not worried about arguing in front of their son. They feel that their open, honest communication will be helpful in raising their son.

The decision making of the family is by consensus for important issues that affect the lives of both members. Otherwise, the decision making style is accommodation. The power and decision making is more situational in that whoever has more experience with certain issues will influence the decisions. For example, Mare is a nurse and has the referent power in health-related issues. Ben is a chemical engineer. He has referent power for concerns about fixing things in the house or with cars. Both state that a strength of their family is that they are both known problem solvers.

The role structure is typical relative to gender. Mare does the cooking, laundry, house cleaning, shopping, and kinship roles. Ben does the lawn mowing, carries out the garbage, and services the cars. Mare feels that she has more roles and expected behaviors of her than Ben does. They both work full-time outside the home. Both state they are concerned about role overload and time management issues with the adoption of their 4-year-old. Mare knows that she will be the primary caregiver but is not sure how much or in what way Ben will assist with these new role requirements. Ben is concerned about how much time the new child will demand and his ability to juggle all of these work responsibilities and family responsibilities.

The family values are clear and shared by both Ben and Mare. The family values: education, open, honest communication, family, health, diversity, caring and compassion for others.

Family Functions

Affective function

Ben and Mare have a close, caring relationship and demonstrate a reciprocal emotional relationship. They are a close, cohesive family. They are excited about expanding their family with the adoption of Alex. They each state that the other is a major support person in their lives. The family has closed boundaries but does look to extended family members for needed support. They express concern about their son's adjustment to them as parents, since he has lived in an orphanage in Russia since the age of 3 months. They have investigated as much as possible about how other children adapt to their new situations. They plan to go to Russia to pick up their son, which will give them access to information about rules and rituals he is familiar with in the orphanage, and plan to institute them in their home.

Socialization function

Ben and Mare talk about the importance of parenting their son. They have openly discussed discipline to be used, which will be time out. They plan to be involved in the child-rearing practices of their son. Their son will be in full-time preschool. They plan to be active in the education process of their son.

Health care function

The family has a primary care physician for Ben and Mare, but they have not selected a pediatrician for their son. Ben sees the physician regularly for management of hypertension and high cholesterol. Mare rarely sees the doctor. The have a medical report for their son. He appears to be in good health, except that he is below the fifth percentile for height and weight. He is current on immunizations except hepatitis. They both have dental cleaning and examinations every 6 months. They value health, yet both are overweight. Mare is obese. A major concern for Mare is regular meal preparation for their son. At present, Ben and Mare do not eat together for dinner on a regular basis. In the past they have hired a cook to ensure that healthful meals were available, especially with Mare working full time.

Family Coping

The short-term stressors for this family are the imminent adoption of their 4-year-son from Russia in 3 weeks. They are concerned about his adaptation to his new environment, his ability to learn English, and how there lives will change with this adoption. Long-term stressors are not an issue at this time.

The family has a large repertoire of successful coping strategies. They have a pattern of problem-solving issues to the best of their ability. They are seeking out information and garnering support from people and resources acceptable to them. They are a well-adjusted family unit. The family is open to education and information.

Summary of Assessments

In summary, both assessment approaches provided important information for the nurse and family to create a plan of action. There was some overlap of information, but the whole picture of the family was enhanced by merging data from both assessment tools.

I.5 Families with Physically Compromised Members: Assessment Tools

ASSESSMENT TOOL	PURPOSE	REFERENCES
The Caregiver Reaction Assessment (CRA)	Assess the reaction of family members caring for elderly persons with physical impairments.	Given CS et al: The Caregiver Reaction Assessment (CRA) for caregivers to persons with chronic physical and mental impairments, *Res Nurs Health* 15(4):271, 1992.
Coping Health Inventory for Parents (CHIP)	Assess parents' appraisal of their coping responses to management of family life when a child is seriously or chronically ill.	McCubbin HI, Thompson AI, McCubbin MA: *Family assessment: resiliency, coping, and adaptation,* Madison, Wis, 1996, University of Wisconsin Publishers.
Demands-of-Illness Scale	Can be used with individuals or families to assess impact of disease on entire family's health, coping, and functioning.	Haberman MR, Woods NF, Packard NJ: Demands of chronic illness: reliability and validity assessment of a Demands-of-Illness inventory, *Holistic Nurs Practice* 5(1):25, 1990.
Family Hardiness Index (FHI)	Measures the characteristic of hardiness as a stress resistance and adaptation resource in families. Available in English and Spanish.	McCubbin HI, Thompson AI, McCubbin MA: *Family assessment: resiliency, coping, and adaptation,* Madison, Wis, 1996, University of Wisconsin Publishers.
Family Needs Assessment Tool	Assesses needs of families of chronically ill children.	Rawlins PS, Rawlins RD, Horner M: Development of the Family Needs Assessment Tool, *Western J Nurs Res* 12(2):201, 1990.
Family Pressures Scale—Ethnic (FPRES-E)	Assesses pressure related to life experiences of families of color; provides index of severity of these pressures on the family system.	McCubbin HI, Thompson AI, McCubbin MA: *Family assessment: resiliency, coping, and adaptation,* Madison, Wis, 1996, University of Wisconsin Publishers.
Impact-on-Family Scale	Measures stressors related to childhood illness.	Stein R, Riessman C: The development of an Impact-on-Family Scale: preliminary findings, *Med Care* 18(2):324, 1980.
Parent/Caretaker Involvement Scale (P/CIS)	Assesses dyadic family interactions.	Comfort M, Farran DC: Parent-child interaction assessment in family-centered intervention, *Infants Young Children* 6(4):33, 1994.
Parents of Children with Disabilities Inventory (PCDI)	Measures perceived disability-related stress, to be used with mothers of children with physical disabilities.	Noojin AB, Wallander JL: Development and evaluation of a measure of concerns related to raising a child with a physical disability, *J Pediatric Psychology* 21(4):483, 1996.

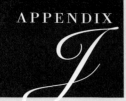

APPENDIX J Individual Assessment Tools

J.1 Discharge Patient Questionnaire

VNA of Eastern Montgomery County/Department of Abington Memorial Hospital Discharge Patient Questionnaire

---

DISCHARGE PATIENT QUESTIONNAIRE # _____

1. What services were provided?

Nursing	—	Occupational Therapy —
Home Health Aide (personal care)	—	Speech Therapy —
Social Worker	—	Physical Therapy —

2. Was the service what you expected it to be? _____

_____

3. VNA personnel considered my family's special needs.

Poor	Fair	Satisfactory	Very Good	Excellent
1	2	3	4	5

4. I was satisfied with the personnel.

Poor	Fair	Satisfactory	Very Good	Excellent
1	2	3	4	5

5. Were there other services you would have liked us to provide? _____

_____

6. Instructions provided by VNA personnel related to my health care needs were clear.

Poor	Fair	Satisfactory	Very Good	Excellent
1	2	3	4	5

7. Questions were answered adequately.

Poor	Fair	Satisfactory	Very Good	Excellent
1	2	3	4	5

8. This service helped me achieve my health care goals.

Poor	Fair	Satisfactory	Very Good	Excellent
1	2	3	4	5

9. Would you use this service again? _____

_____

10. Would you recommend this service to others? _____

_____

11. What suggestions would you make to improve the services? _____

_____

Reprinted with permission of the Visiting Nurse Association of Eastern Montgomery County/Dept of Abington Memorial Hospital, Willow Grove, Penn.

VNA of Eastern Montgomery County/Department of Abington Memorial Hospital Discharge Patient Questionnaire—cont'd

12. Additional Comments: _____
_____
_____

Signature: _____   Date: _____

Please complete for those services received:

1. The nurse understood what my main health problem was.

Poor	Fair	Satisfactory	Very Good	Excellent
1		3	4	5

2. The nurse appeared skillful in carrying out procedures.

Poor	Fair	Satisfactory	Very Good	Excellent
1		3	4	5

3. The home health aide considered my individual needs.

Poor	Fair	Satisfactory	Very Good	Excellent
1		3	4	5

4. The home health aide provided personal care to my satisfaction.

Poor	Fair	Satisfactory	Very Good	Excellent
1		3	4	5

5. The physical therapist explained things in language that I could understand.

Poor	Fair	Satisfactory	Very Good	Excellent
1		3	4	5

6. The exercise program that the physical therapist gave me helped me achieve my goals.

Poor	Fair	Satisfactory	Very Good	Excellent
1		3	4	5

7. The social worker acted in a supportive manner.

Poor	Fair	Satisfactory	Very Good	Excellent
1		3	4	5

8. The social worker gave me information about available resources.

Poor	Fair	Satisfactory	Very Good	Excellent
1		3	4	5

9. The speech therapist visited according to the plan.

Poor	Fair	Satisfactory	Very Good	Excellent
1		3	4	5

10. The speech therapist helped me communicate.

Poor	Fair	Satisfactory	Very Good	Excellent
1		3	4	5

11. The occupational therapist enabled me to improve in my activities of daily living.

Poor	Fair	Satisfactory	Very Good	Excellent
1		3	4	5

12. The occupational therapy visit schedule met my needs.

Poor	Fair	Satisfactory	Very Good	Excellent
1		3	4	5

J.2   Instrumental Activities of Daily Living (IADL) Scale

Name _____ Rated by _____ Date _____

1. **Can you use the telephone**
   without help,   3
   with some help, or   2
   are you completely unable to use the telephone?   1

2. **Can you get to places beyond walking distance**
   without help,   3
   with some help, or   2
   are you completely unable to travel unless special
   arrangements are made?   1

3. **Can you go shopping for groceries**
   without help,   3
   with some help, or   2
   are you completely unable to do any shopping?   1

4. **Can you prepare your own meals**
   without help,   3
   with some help, or   2
   are you completely unable to prepare any meals?   1

5. **Can you do your own housework**
   without help,   3
   with some help, or   2
   are you completely unable to do any housework?   1

6. **Can you do your own handyman work**
   without help,   3
   with some help, or   2
   are you completely unable to do any handyman
   work?   1

7. **Can you do your own laundry**
   without help,   3
   with some help, or   2
   are you completely unable to do any laundry
   at all?   1

8a. **Do you take medicines or use any medications?**
    Yes (If yes, answer Question 8b.)   1
    No (If no, answer Question 8c.)   2

8b. **Do you take your own medicine**
    without help (in the right doses at the right time),   3
    with some help (if someone prepares it for
    you and/or reminds you to take it), or   2
    are you completely unable to take your own
    medicine?   1

8c. **If you had to take medicine, could you do it**
    without help (in the right doses at the right time),   3
    with some help (if someone prepared it for
    you and/or reminded you to take it), or   2
    would you be completely unable to take your own
    medicine?   1

9. **Can you manage your own money**
   without help,   3
   with some help, or   2
   are you completely unable to manage money?   1

From Philadelphia Geriatric Center, Philadelphia, Penn. Used with permission.

J.3   Comprehensive Older Persons' Evaluation

Name (print): _____ Date of Visit: _____

Chief complaint: _____

Today, I will ask you about your overall health and function and will be using a questionnaire to help me obtain this information. The first few questions are to check your memory.

Preliminary Cognition Questionnaire: Record if answer is correct with (+); if answer is incorrect with (−).

1. What is the date today?   _____
2. What day of the week is it?   _____
3. What is the name of this place?   _____
4. What is your telephone number or room number?
   record answer: _____
   If subject does not have phone, ask:
   What is your street address?   _____
5. How old are you? record answer: _____   _____
6. When were you born? Record answer from records if
   patient cannot answer: _____
7. Who is the president of the United States now? _____

8. Who was the president just before him?   _____
9. What was your mother's maiden name?   _____
10. Subtract 3 from 20 and keep subtracting from each new
    number until you get all the way down   _____
    Total errors: _____

If more than 4 errors, ask 11. If more than 6 errors, complete questionnaire for informant.

11. Do you think you would benefit from a legal guardian, someone who would be responsible for your legal and financial matters? Do you have a living will? Would you like one?
    a. no
    b. has functioning legal guardian for sole purpose of managing money-describe:
    c. has legal guardian
    d. yes

From Pearlman R: Development of a functional assessment questionnaire for geriatric patients: the comprehensive older persons evaluation, *J Chronic Disease* 40(56):85S, 1987.

J.3   Comprehensive Older Persons' Evaluation—cont'd

Demographic Section:
1. Patient's race or ethnic background—record: _____
2. Patient's gender (circle)   male   female
3. How far did you go in school?
   a. post-graduate education
   b. four-year degree
   c. college or technical school
   d. high school complete
   e. high school incomplete
   f. 0-8 years

Social Support Section: Now there are a few questions about your family and friends.
4. Are you married, widowed, separated, divorced, or have you never been married?
   a. now married
   b. widowed
   c. separated
   d. divorced
   e. never married
5. Who lives with you? (circle all responses)
   a. spouse
   b. other relative or friend—specify: _____
   c. group living situation (non-health)
   d. lives alone
   e. nursing home, number of years: _____
6. Have you talked to any friends or relatives by phone during the last week?
   a. yes
   b. no
7. Are you satisfied by seeing your relatives and friends as often as you want to, or are you somewhat dissatisfied about how little you see them?
   a. satisfied—skip to #8
   b. dissatisfied—ask A
      A. Do you feel you would like to be involved in a Senior Citizens Center for social events, or perhaps meals?
         1. no
         2. is involved—describe: _____
         3. yes
8. Is there someone who would take care of you for as long as you needed if you were sick or disabled?
   a. yes—skip to C
   b. no—ask A
      A. Is there someone who would take care of you for a short time?
         1. yes—skip to C
         2. no—ask B
      B. Is there someone who could help you now and then?
         1. yes—ask C
         2. no—ask C
      C. Who would we call in case of an emergency? Record name and telephone: _____
      _____

Financial Section: The next few questions are about your finances and any problems you might have.
9. Do you own, or are you buying, your own home?
   a. yes—skip to #10
   b. no—ask A
      A. Do you feel you need assistance with housing?
         1. no
         2. has subsidized or other housing assistance
         3. yes—describe: _____
      B. What type of housing did you have prior to coming here?
10. Are you covered by private medical insurance, Medicare, Medicaid, or some disability plan? (Circle all that apply)
    a. private insurance—specify and skip to #11:
    _____
    b. medicare
    c. medicaid
    d. disability—specify and ask A:
    _____
    e. none
    f. other—specify: _____
       A. Do you feel you need additional assistance with your medical bills?
          1. no
          2. yes
11. Which of these statements best describes your financial situation?
    a. my bills are no problem to me—skip to #12
    b. my expenses make it difficult to meet my bills—ask A
    c. my expenses are so heavy that I cannot meet my bills—ask A
       A. Do you feel you need financial assistance such as: (circle all that apply)
          1. food stamps
          2. social security or disability payments
          3. assistance in paying your heating or electrical bills
          4. other financial assistance? describe: _____

Psychological Health Section: The next few questions are about how you feel about your life in general. There are no right or wrong answers, only what best applies to you. Please answer yes or no to each question.
12. Is your daily life full of things that keep you interested?   _____
13. Have you, at times, very much wanted to leave home?   _____
14. Does it seem that no one understands you?   _____
15. Are you happy most of the time?   _____
16. Do you feel weak all over much of the time?   _____
17. Is your sleep fitful and disturbed?   _____

Continued.

J.3   Comprehensive Older Persons' Evaluation—cont'd

18. Taking everything into consideration, how would you describe your satisfaction with your life in general at the present time?
    a. good
    b. fair
    c. poor

19. Do you feel you now need help with your mental health; for example, a counselor or psychiatrist?
    a. no
    b. has—specify: _____
    c. yes

Physical Health Section: The next few questions are about your health.

20. During the past month (30 days), how many days were you so sick that you couldn't do your usual activities, such as working around the house or visiting with friends? _____

21. Relative to other people your age, how would you rate your overall health at the present time?
    a. excellent—skip to #22
    b. very good—skip to #22
    c. good—ask A
    d. fair—ask A
    e. poor—ask A
        A. Do you feel you need additional medical services such as a doctor, nurse, visiting nurse or physical therapy?
            1. doctor
            2. nurse
            3. visiting nurse
            4. physical therapy
            5. none

22. Do you use an aid for walking, such as a wheelchair, walker, cane or anything else? (circle aid usually used)
    a. wheelchair
    b. other—specify _____
    c. visiting nurse
    d. walker
    e. none

23. How much do your health troubles stand in the way of your doing things you want to do?
    a. not at all—skip to #24
    b. a little—ask A
    c. a great deal—ask A
        A. Do you think you need assistance to do your daily activities; for example, do you need a live-in aide or choreworker?
            1. live-in aide
            2. choreworker
            3. has aide, choreworker or other assistance describe _____
            4. none needed

24. Have **you had**, or do you currently have, any of the following **health** problems? (if yes, place an "X" in appropriate **box** and describe; medical record information may **be used** to help complete this section.)

	HX	Current	Describe
a. **Arthritis** or **rheuma**tism?			
b. **Lung or** breathing problem?			
c. **Hypertension?**			
d. **Heart trouble?**			
e. **Phlebitis** or poor circulation problems in arms **or legs?**			
f. **Diabetes** or low blood sugar?			
g. **Digestive ulcers?**			
h. **Other digestive problem?**			
i. **Cancer?**			
j. **Anemia?**			
k. **Effects of stroke?**			
l. **Other neurological problem?** specify: _____			
m. **Thyroid or other glandular problem?** specify: _____			
n. **Skin disorders** such as pressure sores, leg ulcers, burns?			
o. **Speech problem?**			
p. **Hearing problem?**			
q. **Vision or eye problem?**			
r. **Kidney or bladder problems, or incontinence?**			
s. **A problem of falls?**			
t. **Problem with eating or your weight?** specify: _____			
u. **Problem with depression?** specify: _____			
v. **Problem with your behavior?** specify: _____			
w. **Problem with your sexual activity?**			
x. **Problem with alcohol?**			
y. **Problem with pain?**			
z. **Other health problems?** specify: _____			

J.3   Comprehensive Older Persons' Evaluation—cont'd

Immunizations: _____

_____

_____

25. What medications are you currently taking, or have been taking, in the last month? (May I see your medication bottles?) (If patient cannot list, ask categories a-r and note dosage and schedule, or obtain information from medical or pharmacy records and verify accuracy with the patient.)

Allergies: _____

		Rx (dosage and Schedule)
a.	Arthritis medication	_____
b.	Pain medication	_____
c.	Blood pressure medication?	_____
d.	Water pills or pills for fluid?	_____
e.	Medication for your heat	_____
f.	Medication for your lungs	_____
g.	Blood thinners	_____
h.	Medication for your circulation	_____
i.	Insulin or diabetes medication	_____
j.	Seizure medication	_____
k.	Thyroid pills	_____
l.	Steroids	_____
m.	Hormones	_____
n.	Antibiotics	_____
o.	Medicine for nerves or depression	_____
p.	Prescription sleeping pills	_____
q.	Other prescription drugs	_____
r.	Other nonprescription drugs	_____

26. Many people have problems remembering to take their medications, especially ones they need to take on a regular basis. How often do you forget to take your medications? Would you say you forget often, sometimes, rarely or never?
    a. never
    b. rarely
    c. sometimes
    d. often

Activities of Daily Living: The next set of questions asks whether you need help with any of the following activities of daily living.

27. I would like to know whether you can do these activities without any help at all, or if you need assistance to do them. Do you need help to: (If yes, describe, including patient needs.)

		Yes	No	Describe (include needs)
a.	Use the telephone?			
b.	Get to places out of walking distance? (using transportation)			
c.	Shop for clothes and food?			
d.	Do your housework?			
e.	Handle your money?			
f.	Feed yourself?			
g.	Dress and undress yourself?			
h.	Take care of your appearance?			
i.	Get in and out of bed?			
j.	Take a bath or shower?			
k.	Prepare your meals?			
l.	Do you have any problem getting to the bathroom on time?			

28. During the past six months, have you had any help with such things as shopping, housework, bathing, dressing and getting around?
    a. yes—specify: _____
    b. no

Signature of person completing the form:

_____

J.4 The Geriatric Depression Scale

Choose the best answer for how you felt the past week.

1. Are you basically satisfied with your life?	YES	NO*
2. Have you dropped many of your activities and interests?	YES*	NO
3. Do you feel that your life is empty?	YES*	NO
4. Do you often get bored?	YES*	NO
5. Are you hopeful about the future?	YES	NO*
6. Are you bothered by thoughts you can't get out of your head?	YES*	NO
7. Are you in good spirits most of the time?	YES	NO*
8. Are you afraid that something bad is going to happen to you?	YES*	NO
9. Do you feel happy most of the time?	YES	NO*
10. Do you often feel helpless?	YES*	NO
11. Do you often get restless and fidgety?	YES*	NO
12. Do you prefer to stay at home, rather than going out and doing new things?	YES*	NO
13. Do you frequently worry about the future?	YES*	NO
14. Do you feel you have more problems with memory than most?	YES*	NO
15. Do you think it is wonderful to be alive now?	YES	NO*
16. Do you often feel downhearted and blue?	YES*	NO
17. Do you feel pretty worthless the way you are now?	YES*	NO
18. Do you worry a lot about the past?	YES*	NO
19. Do you find life very exciting?	YES	NO*
20. Is it hard for you to get started on new projects?	YES*	NO
21. Do you feel full of energy?	YES	NO*
22. Do you feel that your situation is hopeless?	YES*	NO
23. Do you think that most people are better off then you are?	YES*	NO
24. Do you frequently get upset over little things?	YES*	NO
25. Do you frequently feel like crying?	YES*	NO
26. Do you have trouble concentrating?	YES*	NO
27. Do you enjoy getting up in the morning?	YES	NO*
28. Do you prefer to avoid social gatherings?	YES*	NO
29. Is it easy for you to make decisions?	YES	NO*
30. Is your mind as clear as it used to be?	YES	NO*

From Yesavage HA et al: Development and validation of a geriatric depression scale: a preliminary report, *J Psychiatric Res* 17:37, 1983. Elsevier Science Ltd, Pergamon Imprint, Oxford, England. Reprinted with permission.

*Each answer indicated by an asterisk counts 1 point. Scores between 15 and 22 suggest mild depression; scores above 22 suggest severe depression. Fifteen-item short form includes questions 1-4, 7-10, 12, 14, 17, 21-23. On the short form, scores between 5 and 9 suggest depression, scores above 9 generally indicate depression.

J.5 Mini-Mental State Examination

	Points
I. Orientation (Maximum score: 10) Ask "What is today's date?" Then ask specifically for parts omitted, such as "Can you also tell me what season it is?"	Date (e.g., January 21) . . . 1 ____ Year . . . . .2 ____ Month . . . .,3 ____ Day (e.g., Monday) . . . . . . 4 ____
Ask "Can you tell me the name of this hospital?" "What floor are we on?" "What town (or city) are we in?" "What county are we in?" "What state are we in?"	Season . . . . .5 ____ Hospital . . . . 6 ____ Floor . . . . 7 ____ Town/City . . . . 8 ____ County . . . . 9 ____ State . . . . .10 ____

II. Registration (Maximum score: 3)
Ask the patient if you may test his memory. Then say "ball", "flag", "tree" clearly and slowly, allowing about one second for each. After you have said all three words, ask the patient to repeat them. This first repetition determines the score (0-3), but continue to say them (up to six trials) until the patient can repeat all three words. If he does not eventually learn all three, recall cannot be meaningfully tested.

"ball" . . . . .11 ____
"flag" . . . . .12 ____
"tree" . . . . .13 ____

Number of trials: _____

III. Attention and calculation (Maximum score: 5)
Ask the patient to begin at 100 and count backward by 7. Stop after five subtractions (93, 86, 79, 72, 65). Score one point for each correct number.

If the subject cannot or will not perform this task, ask him to spell the word "world" backward (D, L, R, O, W). Score one point for each correctly placed letter, e.g., DLROW=5, DLORW=3.
Record how the patient spelled "world" backward: _____

"93" . . . . .14 ____
"86" . . . . .15 ____
"79" . . . . .16 ____
"72" . . . . .17 ____
"65" . . . . .18 ____
or
Number of correctly placed letters . . . . .19 ____

IV. Recall (Maximum score: 3)
Ask the patient to recall the three words you previously asked him to remember (learned in Registation).

"ball" . . . . .20 ____
"flag" . . . . .21 ____
"tree" . . . . .22 ____

V. Language (Maximum score: 9)
Naming: Show the patient a wristwatch and ask "What is this?"
Repeat for a pencil. Score one point for each item named correctly.

Watch . . . . .23 ____
Pencil . . . . .24 ____

Repetition: Ask the patient to repeat "No if's, and's or but's." Score one point for correct repetition.

Repetition . . . . .25 ____

Three-stage command: Give the patient a piece of blank paper and say "Take the paper in your right hand, fold it in half and put it on the floor." Score one point for each action performed correctly.

Takes in right hand . . . .26 ____
Folds in half . . . . .27 ____
Puts on the floor . . . . . .28 ____

Reading: On a blank piece of paper, print the sentence "Close your eyes" in letters large enough for the patient to see clearly. Ask the patient to read it and do what it says. Score correct only if he actually closes his eyes.

Closes eyes . . . . .29 ____

Writing: Give the patient a blank piece of paper and ask him to write a sentence. It is to be written spontaneously. It must contain a subject and verb and make sense. Correct grammar and punctuation are not necessary.

Writes sentence . . . . . . .30 ____

Copying: On a clean piece of paper, draw intersecting pentagons as illustrated, each side measuring about 1 inch, and ask the patient to copy it exactly as it is. All 10 angles must be present and two must intersect to score 1 point. Tremor and rotation are ignored.

Draws pentagons . . . . . .31 ____

Score: Add number of correct responses. In Section III, include items 14 through 18 or item 19, not both. (Maximum total score: 30).

Level of consciousness: ____ coma ____ stupor ____ drowsy ____ alert   **Total Score:** _____

From Folstein MS, Folstein SE, McHugh PR: Mini-mental examination, *J Psychiatric Res* 12:189, 1995. Elsevier Science Ltd, Pergamon Imprint, Oxford, England. Reprinted with permission.

J.6 Assessment Tools for Physically Compromised Individuals

ASSESSMENT TOOL	PURPOSE	REFERENCES
Abilities Index	Provides a profile of child's individual characteristics; cross-cultural applicability	Simeonsson RJ, Chen J, Hu Y: Functional assessment of Chinese children with the ABILITIES index, *Disabil Rehabil* 17(7):400, 1995.
Activities Scales for Kids	Assesses children's perceptions of their own physical performances	Young NL et al: The role of children in reporting their physical disability, *Arch Phys Med Rehabil* 76(10):913, 1995.
Alcohol Consumption Questionnaire	Administered after the Semi-Quantitative Food Frequency Questionnaire as a way to enhance self-report of alcohol use.	King AC: Enhancing the self-report of alcohol consumption in the community: two questionnaire formats, *Am J Public Health* 84(2):294, 1994.
Assessment of older drivers: History and initial tests	Assesses older drivers' capacity to operate a motor vehicle safely.	Reuben DB: Assessment of older drivers, *Clin Geriatr Med* 9(2):449, 1993.
Available Motions Inventory (AMI)	Assesses the abilities of a specific individual in performing a specific task	Malzhan DE, Fernandez JE, Kattel BP: Design-oriented functional capacity evaluation: The Available Motions Inventory–a review, *Disabil Rehabil* 18(8):382, 1996.
Barriers to Health-Promoting Activities for Disabled Persons Scale	Measures perceived barriers to health promotion behaviors of adults with disabilities.	Stuifberger AK, Becker H, Sands D: Barriers to health promotion for individuals with disabilities, *Fam Community Health* 13(1):11, 1990.
Coping Health Inventory for Children (CHIC)	Designed to provide systematic assessment of coping behaviors of chronically ill school-age children.	Austin JK, Patterson JM, Huberty TJ: Development of the Coping Health Inventory for Children, *J Pediatr Nurs* 6(3)166, 1991.
Denver II	Screen for developmental problems in children 1 month to 6 years of age.	Frankenburg WK: Preventing developmental delays: is developmental screening sufficient? *Pediatrics* 93(4)586, 1994.
Dietary Behavior Questionnaire	Measures dietary practices related to fat intake.	Beerman KA, Dittus K: Assessment of a Dietary Behavior Questionnaire, *Health Values* 18(2):3, 1994.
Epilepsy Self-Efficacy Scale (ESES)	Assesses a person's confidence in managing epilepsy; explores epilepsy self-management.	Dilorio C, Faherty B, Manteuffel B: The development and testing of an instrument to measure self-efficacy in individuals with epilepsy, *J Neuroscience Nurs* 24(1):9, 1992.
Functional Disability Inventory	Measures functional limitations of children.	Walker LS, Greene JW: The Functional Disability Inventory: measuring a neglected dimension of child health status, *J Pediatr Psychol* 16(1):39, 1991.
Functional Independence Measure (FIM)	Assesses client functional status to determine rehabilitation need, set goals, and evaluate outcomes.	Stineman MG et al: The Functional Independence Measure: Tests of scaling assumptions, structure and reliability across 20 diverse impairment categories, *Arch Phys Med Rehabil* 77(1):1101, 1996.
Groningen Activity Restriction Scale (GARS)	Measures disability severity of several chronic conditions and changes over time in adults.	Suurmeijer TP et al: The Groningen Activity Restriction Scale for measuring disability: its utility in international comparison, *Am J Public Health* 84(8):1270, 1994.
Health Assessment Questionnaire	Self-administered questionnaire. Disability score is specifically for function with arthritis.	Goeppinger T et al: A nursing perspective on the assessment of function in persons with arthritis, *Res Nurs Health* 11(5):321, 1998.

ASSESSMENT TOOL	PURPOSE	REFERENCES
The Hearing Handicap Inventory for Adults	Questionnaire for adults <64 years of age to help describe a person's reaction to his hearing loss.	Newman CW, Weinstein BE, Jacobson GP, Huy GA: The Hearing Handicap Inventory for Adults Psychometric adequacy and audiometric correlates, *Ear and Hearing* 11(6):430, 1990.
Metro-Manila Developmental Screening Test (MMDST)	A Philippine version of the Denver Developmental Screening Test.	Williams PD: The Metro-Manila Developmental Screening Test: a normative study, *Nurs Res* 33:204, 1984.
Neurobehavioral Assessment Scale (NAS)	Tests the modifiability of the infant's performance in response to changes of environmental inputs.	Bottos M et al: The Neurobehavioral Assessment Scale as an instrument for early long-term prognosis and intervention in major disability in high-risk infants, *J Pediatr Psychol* 21(6):755, 1996.
Pain Thermometer	Assesses chronic pain in elderly women.	Benesh LB et al: Tools for assessing chronic pain in rural elderly women, *Home Healthcare Nurse* 15(3):207, 1997.
Pediatric Evaluation of Disability Inventory (PEDI)	Assessment of children with physical disabilites.	Reid DT, Boschen K, Wright V: Critique of the Pediatric Evaluation of Disability Inventory (PEDI), *Phys Occup Ther Pedatr* 13(4):434, 1990.
Pediatric Functional Independence Measure (WeeFIM)	Assesses and tracks functional abilities of children from 6 months to 7 years.	McCabe MA: Pediatric Functional Independence Measure: Clinical trials with disabled and nondisabled children, *Applied Nurs Res* 9(3):136, 1997. Sperle PA et al: Equivalence reliability of the Functional Independence Measure for children (WeeFIM) administration methods, *Am J Occupat Ther* 51(1):35, 1997.
Physical Performance Test (PPT)	Determines the effects on the functional capacity of several common chronic conditions in elderly people.	Rozzini R et al: The effect of chronic diseases on physical function, *Age Aging* 26(4):281, 1997.
"PRESTON Profile"	Assesses the quality of life in clients with malignant glioma; a disease-specific tool for this condition.	Lyons GJ: The 'PRESTON Profile'–the first disease-specific tool for assessing quality of life in patients with malignant glioma, *Disabil Rehabil* 18(9):460, 1996.
RECursive Partition and AMalgamation (RECPAM)	Defines risk profiles that can easily be applied to allow an estimation of the risk of permanent work disability.	Mau W et al: Prediction of permanent work disability in a follow-up study of early rheumatoid arthritis: results of a tree structured analysis using RECPAM, *Br J Rheumatol* 35(7):652, 1996.
Tinnitus Handicap Questionnaire	Compares a person's tinnitus handicap with the norm, identifies specific areas of handicaps, and monitors progress with particular treatment programs.	Kuk FK et al: The psychometric properties of a Tinnitus Handicap Questionnaire, *Ear Hearing* 11(6):434, 1990.
Torabi Cancer Prevention Behavior Scale	Measures behavior of college students with regard to cancer prevention.	Torabi MR: A cancer prevention behavior scale, *Health Values* 15(3):12, 1991.
Development	Children	Fewell RR: Trends in the assessment of infants and children with disabilities. *Exceptional Children* 58(2):166, 1991. Glascoe FP, Martin ED, Humphrey S: A comparative review of developmental screening tests, *Pediatrics* 86(4):547, 1990.

continued

ASSESSMENT TOOL	PURPOSE	REFERENCES
Disability	Adults	Kinney WB, Coyle CP: Predicting life satisfaction among adults with physical disabilities, *Arch Phys Med Rehab* 73(9):863, 1992. Delitto A: Are measures of function and disability important in low-back care? *Phys Ther* 74(5):452, 1994. Duncan PW: Stroke disability, *Phys Ther* 74(5):452, 1994. Haley SM, Coster WI, Binda-Simdbert K: Measuring physical disablement: the contextual challenge, *Phys Ther* 74(5):443, 1994.
	Children	Goffin R, Adler B: A seven item scale for the assessment of disabilities after child and adolescent injuries, *Injury Prevention* 3(2):120, 1997.

J.7 Comprehensive Occupational and Environmental Health History

WORK HISTORY

1. List your current and past longest held jobs, including the military:

COMPANY	DATES EMPLOYED	JOB TITLE	KNOWN EXPOSURES

2. Do you work full-time? NO ___   YES ___ How many hours per week? ___

3. Do you work part-time? NO ___   YES ___ How many hours per week? ___

4. Please describe any health problems or injuries that you have experienced in connection with your present or past jobs:

5. Have you ever had to change jobs due to health problems or injuries? YES ___   NO ___
   If yes, describe:

   Did any of your coworkers experience similar problems?

6. In what type of business do you currently work?

7. Describe your work (what you actually do):

8. Have you had any current or past exposure (through breathing or touching) to any of the following?

__acids	__alkalis	__arsenic	__benzene	__cadmium
__chlorinated	__chloroprene	__coal dust	__dichlorobenzene	__ethylene dichloride
naphthalenes	__isocyanates	__lead	__mercury	__nickel
__halothane	__perchloroethylene	__phenol	__radiation	__silica powder
__PBBs	__TDI or MDI	__trichloroethylene	__vibration	__welding fumes
__styrene	__ammonia	__asbestos	__beryllium	__carbon tetrachloride
__alcohols	__chromates	__cold (severe)	__ethylene dibromide	__fiberglass
__chloroform	__ketones	__manganese	__methylene chloride	__noise (loud)
__heat (severe)	__pesticides	__phosgene	__rock dust	__solvents
__PCBs	__toluene	__trinitrotoluene	__vinyl chloride	__x-rays
__talc				

9. Did you receive any safety training about these agents? YES __ NO __
   Explain:

10. Are you involved in any work processes such as grinding, welding, soldering, or polishing that create dust, mists, or fumes? YES __ NO __ (If yes, describe):

11. Did you use any of the following personal protective equipment when exposed?

__boots	__respirator	__safety shoes
__gloves	__sleeves	__welding mask
__shield	__earplugs/muffs	__glasses/goggles
__coveralls		

12. Is your work environment generally clean? YES __ NO __ If no, describe:

13. What ventilation systems are used in your workplace?

14. Do they seem to work? Are you aware of any chemical odors in your environment (if so, explain)?

15. Where do you eat, smoke, and take your breaks when you are on the job?

continued

16. Do you use a uniform or have clothing that you wear only to work? YES __ NO __

17. How is your work clothing laundered (at home, by employer, etc.)?

18. How often do you wash your hands at work and how do you wash them? (running water, special soaps, etc.)

19. Do you shower before leaving the worksite? YES __ NO __

20. Do you have any physical symptoms associated with work? YES __ NO __
    If yes, describe:

21. Are other workers similarly affected? YES __ NO __

HOME EXPOSURES

1. Which of the following do you have in your home?

__air conditioner   __fireplace   __electric stove
__central heating (gas or oil?)   __air purifier   __woodstove

2. In approximately what year was your home built?_____

3. Have there been any recent renovations? YES __ NO __
   If yes, describe:

4. Have you recently installed new carpet, bought new furniture, or refinished existing furniture? YES __ NO __
   If yes, explain:

5. Do you use pesticides around your home or garden? YES __ NO __
   If yes, describe:

6. What household cleaners do you use? (List most common and any new products you use.)

7. List all hobbies done at your home:

8. Are any of the agents listed earlier for work exposures encountered in hobbies or recreational activities?
   YES __ NO __

9. Is any special protective equipment or ventilation used during hobbies? YES __ NO __
   Explain:

10. What are the occupations of other household members?

11. Do other household members have contact with any form of chemicals at work or during leisure activities?
    YES __ NO __ If yes, explain:

12. Is anyone else in your home environment having symptoms similar to yours? YES __ NO __
    If yes, explain briefly:

COMMUNITY EXPOSURES

1. Are any of the following located in your community?

__industrial plant   __major source of air pollution   __waste site
__landfill   __toxic spill   __other_____

2. What is your source of drinking water?

__private well   __public water source   __other

3. Are neighbors experiencing any health problems similar to yours? YES __ NO __
   If yes, explain:

KEY OCCUPATIONAL AND ENVIRONMENTAL HEALTH QUESTIONS TO BE ASKED WITH ALL HISTORIES

1. What are your current and past longest held jobs?

2. Have you been exposed to any radiation or chemical liquids, dusts, mists, or fumes? YES __ NO __

3. Is there any relationship between current symptoms and activities at work or at home? YES __ NO __

From Pope AM, Snyder MA, Mood LH, editors: *Nursing, health, and environment: strengthening the relationship to improve the public's health,* Washington, DC, 1995, National Academy Press.

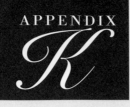

Essential Elements of Public Health Nursing

K.1 Examples of Public Health Nursing Roles and Implementing Public Health Functions

This document is intended to clearly present the role of public health nurses in Virginia as members of the multidisciplinary public health team in a changing health care environment. The following matrices present the role of public health nursing in Virginia. The following definitions were used to develop these matrices.

Essential Element is taken from the National Association of City and County Health Officials' (NACCHO) Document "Blueprint for a Healthy Community." The following public health essential elements are used as a framework to present the role of public health nursing in Virginia:

- Conducting Community Assessments
- Preventing and Controlling Epidemics
- Providing a Safe and Healthy Environment
- Measuring Performance, Effectiveness, and Outcomes of Health Services
- Promoting Healthy Lifestyles
- Providing Targeted Outreach and Forming Partnerships
- Providing Personal Health Care Services

- Conducting Research and Innovation
- Mobilizing the Community for Action

Public Health Function is defined as a broad public health activity needed to ensure a strong, flexible, accountable public health structure. It may require a multidisciplinary team to carry out.

Public Health Nurse Role is the activity the public health nurse is responsible for, either alone or as a member of a team, to accomplish the stated public health function. This can be the public health nurse at the local level or at the state level.

State Role is what public health nurses need from the state level to do their jobs (e.g., policy, aggregate data, training). This refers to any Central Office program or staff, not just nurses.

A process was implemented that would involve all public health nurses in Virginia. Although this lengthened the timeline to completion, it will ensure that the final document represents a consensus developed through creative open dialogue.

From National Association of City and County Health Officials: *Blueprint for a healthy community: a guide for local health departments*, Washington, DC, 1994, the Association.

ESSENTIAL ELEMENT 1: Conduct Community Assessment: Systematically collect, assemble, analyze, and make available health-related data for the purpose of identifying and responding to community and state level public health concerns and conducting epidemiologic and other population-based studies.

PUBLIC HEALTH FUNCTION	PHN ROLES	STATE ROLES
Develop frameworks, methodologies, and tools for standardizing data collection and analysis and reporting across all jurisdictions and providers.	• Provide, review, and comment on proposed methodologies and tools for data collection • Field test tools and methods	• Collaborate with professional organizations and academic and governmental institutions to develop and test tools and methods. • Provide educational opportunities in areas of and use of tools. • Work with local level agencies to standardize definitions, data collected, etc. across jurisdictions and amongst all stakeholders (schools, community-based organizations, and private providers).
Collect and analyze data.	• Collaborate with the community to identify population-based needs and gaps in service. • Analyze data and needs, knowledge, attitudes, and practices of specific populations. • Identify patterns of diseases; illness and injury and develop or stimulate development of programs to respond to identified trends.	• Provide aggregated data to the local level in a timely and accurate manner. • Provide census tract–level aggregated data to the local level. • Provide national and state comparisons to be used with local data to obtain trends and assist localities in documenting need, progress, etc. to attain standard outcomes.

ESSENTIAL ELEMENT 2: Preventing and Controlling Epidemics: Monitoring disease trends and investigating and containing diseases and injuries.

Develop programs that prevent, contain, and control the transmission of diseases and danger of injuries (including violence).	• Provide community-wide preventive measures in the form of health education and mobilization of community resources • Ensure isolation/containment measures when necessary. • Ensure adequate preventive immunizations. • Implement programs that control the transmission of diseases and danger of injuries during disasters	• Work with local jurisdictions to develop tools such as videos, PSAs, and/or posters that local jurisdictions can use. • Work with local jurisdictions to develop disaster plans for the control of the transmission of diseases and danger of injuries during disasters. • Facilitate state level partnerships that promote health, healthy lifestyles, and wellness (individual and family).
Develop regulatory guidelines for the prevention of targeted diseases.	• Implement regulatory measures. • Implement OSHA Guidelines for Blood Borne Pathogens and the Prevention of the Transmission of TB in Health Care Settings.	• In partnership with localities, develop regulatory guidelines. • Serve as clearinghouse or source of information.

continued

ESSENTIAL ELEMENT 3: Providing a Safe and Healthy Environment: Maintaining clean and safe air, water, food, and facilities both in the community and the home environment.

Public health function	PHN roles	State roles
Develop methods/tools for collection and analysis of health-related data (occurrence of mortality and morbidity relating to both communicable and chronic diseases, injury registries, sentinel event establishment, environmental quality, etc.).	• Provide reporting guidelines and consultation regarding disease prevention, diagnosis, treatment, and follow-up of cases/contacts to physicians and institutions (emergency department, university and secondary school student health, prisons, industries, etc.) • Conduct/participate in community needs assessments to determine customer/provider knowledge deficits and perceptions of need. • Provide education to individuals, providers, targeted populations, etc., in response to knowledge deficits, disease outbreaks, toxic waste emissions, etc. • Provide individual follow-up/case management of communicable diseases that are transmitted by air, water, food and fomites (TB, hepatitis A, salmonella, and staphylococcus, etc.).	• Develop standard methodology and tools for collection and analysis of health-related data. • Provide training in area of data collection and analysis. • Evaluates activities and outcomes of interactions. • Work in partnership with localities to develop program based on data analysis needs.
Develop programs that promote a safe environment in the home,	• Provide childhood lead poisoning screenings and follow-up • Teach clients to inspect homes for safety violations and toxic substances and to practice safe behaviors; assist families to access/use available resources/safety devises. • Assess/teach regarding safe food selection, preparation, and storage. • Train/supervise volunteers/auxiliary personnel in performance of the above tasks • Teach families that all men, women, and children have a right to a safe environment free of physical or mental abuse.	• Provides consultation and technical assistance to state/local organizations regarding laws and regulations that protect health and ensure safety. • In partnership with localities, develops and evaluates educational programs.
Develop programs that promote a safe environment in the workplace.	• Provide consultation in implementation of OSHA regulations relating to occupational exposure to diseases. • Provide educational program related to healthy lifestyles (smoking cessation, back protection, etc). • Ensure provision of screenings for individuals to determine baselines and occurrence of infectious diseases and preventable deterioration of health and function: hearing, back soundness, lung capacity, RMS indicators, PPDs, etc. • Assist in policy/practice development to address prevention of the above. • Provide immunizations.	• Monitor and assist localities to implement prevention activities. • Assist localities in developing and evaluating educational programs. • Monitor outcomes of screening activities and evaluate interventions.

Public health function	PHN roles	State roles
Develop programs that promote a safe environment in the school setting.	• Provide consultation on implementation of OSHA regulations relating to occupational exposure to diseases. • Provide educational programs related to healthy lifestyles (smoking cessation, etc.) • Ensure provision of screenings for students to determine baselines and occurrence of infectious disease and preventable deterioration of health and function. • Assist in policy/practice development to address prevention of the above. • Provide immunizations.	• Develop guidelines that ensure accountability in meeting standards set forth. • Ensure that policy is developed to protect children in the school environment. • Monitor immunization status of children and provide immunizations during outbreaks and evaluate activities.
Develop programs that promote a safe environment in the community.	• Identify population clusters exhibiting an unhealthy environment; provide consultation/group education regarding preventive measures • Participate in development of local disaster plans to ensure provision of safe water, food, air, and facilities. • Respond in time of natural disasters such as floods, tornadoes, hurricanes. • Participate in developing plans for shelter management during disasters, especially "Special Needs" shelters that may require nursing staff.	• In times of disaster, facilitate availability of resources across jurisdictions. • Have a statewide plan. • Ensure that localities have developed plans to protect the public in time of national and/or other disasters. • Coordinate efforts statewide. • Assist localities in responding. • Evaluate efforts.
Develop and issue standards that guide regulations, mandate, policy, and program development. Develop protocols to ensure accountability of all health care providers, public and private. Provide inservice to all providers of health care services.	• Survey worksites, schools, institutions, etc. for compliance to regulations that protect health and ensure safety. • Provide technical assistance, i.e., interpretation, implementation and evaluation processes. • Share and implement knowledge gained in inservices.	• Develop a systematic evaluation tool for collection of data to measure trends. • Assist localities in developing standards to mandate accountability. • Provide consultation/technical assistance to localities.

ESSENTIAL ELEMENT 4: Measuring Performance, Effectiveness, and Outcomes of Health Services: Monitoring health care providers and the health care system to identify gaps in service, deteriorating health status indicators, effectiveness of interventions, and accessibility and quality of personal and population-wide health services.

Promote competency in public health issues throughout the health delivery system.	• Provide educational and technical assistance in areas such as case management and appropriate treatment and control of communicable diseases to be community.	• Develop appropriate regulatory, educational and technical assistance programs. • Provide technical assistance and training to local health department for local forecasting and interpretation of data.

continued

ESSENTIAL ELEMENT 4: Measuring Performance, Effectiveness, and Outcomes of Health Services—cont'd

PUBLIC HEALTH FUNCTION	PHN ROLES	STATE ROLES
Collect data.	• Participate in data collection with a target population. • Ensure that the data collection system supports the objectives of programs serving the community by participating in the design and operation of data collection systems. • Collect data via surveys, polls, interviews, focus groups that will enable assessment of the community's perception of health status and understanding how the system works and how to obtain needs service.	• Work with localities (health districts, private providers, other state and local agencies) to develop standard data elements and definitions across jurisdictions and among all stakeholders, especially for consistency in coding of population-based data. • Identify data collection and analytic issues related to monitoring the impact of health system changes such as costs and benefits of record linkage, strategies for ensuring confidentiality, and strategies for analyzing trends in health within a broader social and economic context. • Advocate for uniform data collection from all managed care plans so that outcomes and health trends can be analyzed and tracked and sentinel events reported.
Analyze data to ensure accurate diagnosis of health status, identification of threats to health, and assessment of health service needs.	• Participate in a systematic approach to convert data into information that will identify gaps in service at the local and state level and will lead to action. • Monitor health status indicators to identify emerging problems and facilitate community-wide response to identified problems. • Facilitate data analysis as part of a local collaborative effort.	• Develop a systematic, integrated statewide approach to converting data into information that directs action. • Ensure that resources, such as hardware and software, to analyze data are available at the local level. • Work with localities (health districts, private providers, other state and local agencies) to address issues related to variable access to technology, confidentiality issues. • Educate and train currently employed public health nurses in areas of epidemiology and population-based services.
Monitor health status indicators for the entire population and for specific population groups and/or geographic areas.	• Identify target populations that may be at risk for public health problems such as communicable diseases, unidentified and untreated chronic diseases. • Conduct surveys or observe targeted populations such as preschools, child care centers, high-risk census tracks to identify health status. • Monitor health care utilization of vulnerable populations at the local and regional level.	• Develop methodology for identification, measurement, and analysis of key indicators of health care utilization of vulnerable populations

PUBLIC HEALTH FUNCTION	PHN ROLES	STATE ROLES
Monitor and assess availability, cost-effectiveness, and outcomes of personal and population-based health services	• Identify gaps in services (e.g., a neighborhood with deteriorating immunization rates may indicate lack of available primary care services). • Ensure that all receive the same quality of care, including comprehensive preventive services. • Monitor the impact of health system reforms on vulnerable populations. • Evaluate the effectiveness and outcomes of care. • Plan interventions based on the health of the overall population, not just for those in the health care system. • Identify interventions that are effective and replicable.	• Develop analyses that demonstrate the cost effectiveness of investment in public health services. • Develop protocols and technical assistance for ensuring accountability of Medicaid managed care plans and other government-funded plans for service delivery and overall health status of their covered populations. • Identify standard theoretical, methodological, and measurement issues that are specific to population subgroups for monitoring the impact of health system changes on vulnerable populations.
Disseminate information	• Disseminate information to the public on community health status, including how to access and use services appropriately. • Disseminate information to other health care providers regarding gaps in services or deteriorating health status indicators.	• Ensure a mechanism for public accountability of performance and outcomes through public dissemination of information and in particular ensure that underservice, a risk inherent in capitated plans, is measurable through available data. • Ensure that information is provided to communities, local health departments, managed care plans, and other appropriate state agencies.

ESSENTIAL ELEMENT 5: Promoting Healthy Lifestyles: Providing health education to individuals, families, and communities.

Promote informed decision making of residents about things that influence their health on a daily basis.	• Exert influence through contact with individuals and community groups • Accept and issue challenge of healthy lifestyles to all contacts. • Reinforce and reward positive informed decisions made for healthy lifestyles.	• Develop and monitor standards or the changes to determine changes in behavior.
Promote effectiveness use of media to encourage both personal and community responsibility for informed decision making.	• Be a resource for the community • Gather data and address findings as appropriate. • Work with community groups to promote accurate information for healthy lifestyle through the media. • Utilize current information and other agencies' resources to maximize information accessible to public.	• Assist localities to provide current information to community organizations and other state organizations. • Serve as a resource for localities and work with media.
Develop a public awareness/marketing campaign to demonstrate the importance of public health to overall health improvement and its proper place in the health delivery system.	• Provide education to special groups, e.g., local politicians, school boards, PTAs, churches, civic groups, news media, regarding the benefits of preventive health.	• Develop training activities to assist localities in marketing

continued

ESSENTIAL ELEMENT 5: Promoting Healthy Lifestyles—cont'd

PUBLIC HEALTH FUNCTION	PHN ROLES	STATE ROLES
Develop public information and education systems/programs through partnerships	• Provide educational sessions/programs to public regarding components of healthy lifestyles. • Access grants/other funding sources to promote healthy lifestyle decisions; (e.g., cervical and breast cancer prevention; bike helmets, hypertension). • Provide/promote teaching for individual and families at every opportunity (home, clinic, community settings).	• Assist localities in developing and evaluating educational programs. • Assist localities in funding. • Hold regional/state training sessions. • Evaluate outcomes and plan ongoing educational systems/program.

ESSENTIAL ELEMENT 6: Providing Targeted Outreach and Forming Partnerships: Ensuring access to services, including those that lead to self-sufficiency, for all vulnerable populations and ensuring the development of culturally appropriate care.

Ensure accessibility to health services that will improve morbidity, decrease mortality, and improve health status outcomes.	• Provide family-centered case management services for high-risk and hard-to-reach populations that focus on linking families with needed services. • Improve access to care by forming partnerships with appropriate community individuals and entities. • Increase influence of cultural diversity on system design and on access to care, as well as on individual services rendered. • Ensure that translation services are available for the non–English speaking population. • Participate in ongoing community assessment to identify areas of concern and above needs for rules. • Provide outreach services that focus on preventing epidemics and the spread of disease, such as tuberculosis and sexually transmitted diseases.	• Provide funds in cooperation with locality. • Ensure policy development that includes case management and is culturally sensitive. • Provide adequate ongoing continuing education for staff (especially in areas common to all localities). • Participate in state-level contract development to ensure that contracts with health plans require and include incentives for health plans to offer and deliver preventive health services in the minimum benefits package. • Educate financing officials about the roles of public health both in performing core public health services and in ensuring access to personal health services.

ESSENTIAL ELEMENT 7: Providing Personal Health Care Services: Provide targeted direct services to high-risk populations.

Provide direct services for specific diseases that threaten the health of the community and develop programs that prevent, contain, and control the transmission of infectious diseases	• Plan, develop, implement, and evaluate: • Sexually transmitted disease services • Communicable disease services • HIV/AIDS services • Tuberculosis control services • Develop and implement guidelines for the prevention of the above targeted disease.	• Establish standards/criteria for personal health care • Work with local health departments to assist in developing infrastructure and management techniques to facilitate record-keeping and appropriate financial monitoring and tracking systems, which enable local health departments to enter into contractual arrangements for preventive health and primary care services.
Provide health services, including preventive health services, to high-risk and vulnerable populations (e.g., the uninsured working poor), and in geographic areas where primary health care services are not readily accessible or available in a privatized setting.	• Provide coordination, follow-up, referral, and case management as indicated. • Integrate supportive services, such as counseling, social work, nutrition, into primary care services. • Assess existing community medical capacity for referral and follow-up.	• Continue to work at the state and local level to build primary and preventive health services capacity, particularly in traditionally underserved areas, to ensure availability to providers and primary care sites essential to primary care access.

ESSENTIAL ELEMENT 8: Conducting Research and Innovation: Discovering and applying improved health care delivery mechanisms and clinical interventions.

PUBLIC HEALTH FUNCTION	PHN ROLES	STATE ROLES
Ensure ongoing prevention research relating to biomedical and behavioral aspects of health promotion and prevention of disease and injury.	• Develop outcome measures. • Identify research priorities for target communities and develop and conduct scientific and operations research for health promotion and disease/injury prevention.	• Provide training in area of measuring program effectiveness
Implement pilot or demonstration projects	• Develop and implement linkages with academic centers, ensuring that clients and populations who participate in research projects benefit as a result of the research	• Support evaluations and research that demonstrate the benefits of public health, as well as the consequences of failure to support public health interventions.

ESSENTIAL ELEMENT 9: Mobilizing the Community for Action: Providing leadership and initiating collaboration.

Provide leadership to stimulate development of networks or partnerships that will ensure the availability of comprehensive primary health care services to all regardless of ability to pay. Initiate collaboration with other community organizations to ensure the leadership role in resolving a public health issue.	• Advocate for improved health. • Disseminate of health information. • Build coalitions. • Make recommendations for policy implementation or revision. • Facilitate resources that manage environmental risk and maintain and improve community health. • Provide information for a community group working on impacting policy at the local, state, or federal level. • Use results of community health assessments to stimulate the community to develop a plan to respond to identified gaps in service.	• Facilitate the establishment and enhancement of statewide high-quality, needed health services • Administer quality improvement programs. • Uses information-gathering techniques of assessment to assist policy/legislature activities to develop needed health services and functions that require statewide action or standards. • Recommend programs to carry out policies

K.2 Public Health Guidelines for Practice

AMERICAN PUBLIC HEALTH ASSOCIATION DEFINITION OF PUBLIC HEALTH NURSING

Public health nursing is a systematic process by which:

1. The health and health care needs of a population are assessed in order to identify subpopulations, families, and individuals who would benefit from health promotion or who are at risk of illness, injury, disability, or premature death.
2. A plan for intervention is developed with the community to meet identified needs that takes into account available resources, the range of activities that contribute to health, and the prevention of illness, injury, disability, and premature death.
3. The plan is implemented effectively, efficiently, and equitably.
4. Evaluations are conducted to determine the extent to which the interventions have an impact on the health status of individuals and the population.
5. The results of the process are used to influence and direct the current delivery of care, deployment of health resources, and the development of local, regional, state, and national health policy and research to promote health and prevent disease.

This systematic process for public health nursing practice is based on and is consistent with 1) community strengths, needs, and expectations; 2) current scientific knowledge; 3) available resources, 4) accepted criteria and standards of nursing practice, 5) agency purpose, philosophy, and objectives, and 6) the participation, cooperation, and understanding of the population. Other services and organizations in the community are considered and planning is coordinated to maximize the effective use of resources and enhance outcomes.

The title "public health nurse" designates a nursing professional with educational preparation in public health

From American Public Health Association: *The definition and role of public health nursing: a statement of APHA Public Health Nursing Section,* Washington, DC, 1996, the Association.

and nursing science with a primary focus on population-level outcomes.

Examples of Activities of Public Health Nurses

The activities of public health nurses include the following:

1. They provide essential input to interdisciplinary programs that monitor, anticipate, and respond to public health problems in population groups, regardless of which disease or public health threat is identified.
2. They evaluate health trends and risk factors of population groups and help determine priorities for targeted interventions.
3. They work with communities or specific population groups within the community to develop public policy and targeted health promotion and disease prevention activities.
4. They participate in assessing and evaluating health care services to ensure that people are informed of programs and services available and are assisted in the use of available services.
5. They provide health education, care management, and primary care to individuals and families who are members of vulnerable populations and high-risk groups.

AMERICAN NURSES ASSOCIATION STANDARDS OF PUBLIC HEALTH NURSING PRACTICE*

Standards of Care

Standard I. Assessment: The public health nurse assesses the health status of populations using data, community resources identification, input from the population, and professional judgment.

Standard II. Diagnosis: The public health nurse analyzes collected assessment data and partners with the people to attach meaning to that data and determine opportunities and needs.

Standard III. Outcome Identification: The public health nurse participates with other community partners to identify expected outcomes in the populations and their health status.

Standard IV. Planning: The public health nurse promotes and supports the development of programs, policies, and services that provide interventions that improve the health status of populations.

Standard V. Assurance: Action Component of the Nursing Process for Public Health Nursing: The public health nurse ensures access and availability of programs, policies, resources, and services to the population.

Standard VI. Evaluation: The public health nurse evaluates the health status of the population.

Standards of Professional Performance

Standard I. Quality of Care: The public health nurse systematically evaluates the availability, accessibility, acceptability, quality, and effectiveness of nursing practice for the population.

Standard II. Performance Appraisal: The public health nurse evaluates his or her own nursing practice in relation to professional practice standards and relevant statutes and regulations.

Standard III: Education: The public health nurse acquires and maintains current knowledge and competency in public health nursing practice.

Standard IV: Collegiality: The public health nurse establishes collegial partnerships while interacting with health care practitioners and others and contributes to the professional development of peers, colleagues, and others.

Standard V. Ethics: The public health nurse applies ethical standards in advocating for health and social policy and delivery of public health programs to promote and preserve the health of the population.

Standard VI. Collaboration: The public health nurse collaborates with the representatives of the population and other health and human service professionals and organizations in providing for and promoting the health of the population.

Standard VII. Research: The public health nurse uses research findings in practice.

Standard VIII. Resource Utilization: The public health nurse considers safety, effectiveness, and cost in the planning and delivery of public health services when using available resources to ensure the maximum possible health benefit to the population.

---

*Because the ANA's publication of the 1999 scope and standards had not yet published when this book went to press, this list is reproduced from a draft of the ANA publication.

From American Nurses Association: *Scope and standards of public health nursing practice*, Washington DC, 1999, American Nurses Publishing.

Answers to Clinical Applications

CHAPTER 1

C and G are population-focused, looking at the needs of their subpopulation and planning programs to meet their needs. A, B, D, and F are likely to be practicing community health nursing if their focus is health protection, health promotion, and disease prevention of the individuals/families in their subpopulations. B and D are more likely to be practicing community-based nursing, caring for clients who are ill.

CHAPTER 2

A. It is easier to use a population-focused approach to solving these problems. If you can show through a community needs assessment that these are problems for a large number of people in the community and are putting the community at risk for increased health problems, more costly health care, and less social and economic growth, then one can convince policy makers to establish programs directed at these problems. With limited health care dollars the emphasis is on the greatest good for the greatest number.

B. A historical approach will build understanding of the public policy elements limiting care of various populations, in exploring what attempts have been made in the past to innovate or reform services for these populations; determining what has limited these attempts; and identifying examples of programs or policies that have been successful.

CHAPTER 3

The correct answer is D. The nurse's responsibility is to educate clients about appropriate health care resources in their community and to allow families to choose care based on their own unique needs and preferences.

CHAPTER 4

A. Identify what experiences each nurse has had in dealing with similar public health problems. Find out what the other nurses see as important to do first. Avoid forcing the "Western view" on local people who may be comfortable with a non-Western approach.

B. Find out if the water is safe. Is there sufficient, safe food? Is there shelter? Do people need (have) clothes?

C. Deal first with injuries and illnesses, then move to teaching first aid and safe eating and drinking water practices. Also set up groups or other arenas for people to deal emotionally with the stress of the traumas experienced.

CHAPTER 5

A. Agencies are reimbursed for visits either by private insurance or Medicare or by clients through self-pay.

B. The payment for the visit is determined by using a cost basis or a charge basis. Cost basis reflects the actual cost to the agency to deliver the service. Charge basis reflects the cost plus additional monies charged for the visit, which may include indigent care visits or profit to be paid to stockholders if the agency is a for-profit agency.

C. Nursing care costs, while they may be known, are usually not used alone to determine the costs of a visit. The visit cost includes money for lights, water, supplies, secretarial and administrative salaries and benefits, as well as nurse salaries and benefits.

D. There is rationing in all of health care. Home health visits are rationed by the criteria set by the federal government for Medicare clients, such as a limited number of visits per year, and by private insurance, which also limits the number of visits per year. The individual client who must pay out of pocket sets his or her own limits and self-rations the amount he or she may be willing to pay for home health visits.

CHAPTER 6

A. First, Sharon might consider calling the case manager and persuading her that more nursing home visits are necessary. However, without more evidence that Mrs. Callahan's health is failing, this is unlikely.

Second, Sharon can advise the Callahans that if Mrs. Callahan exhibits signs of infection, they should call an ambulance and go to the hospital. If this occurs, the client will likely be admitted to the hospital and then more home visits will be authorized. This option, however, is not a very good one. It places the client at risk, uses more health care resources, and is more costly.

Third, Sharon could call Mrs. Callahan's physician, describe the client's home situation and the need for more home visits, and ask him to order more care for the client. With the physician's support and help, it is likely that the HMO will authorize more visits. Sharon can then continue to visit Mrs. Callahan and provide care for her.

B. Sharon might be tempted to say that this situation is out of her control and she has done all that is reasonable for her to do. It will take time for Sharon to call the physician and to wait for the HMO to respond to Mrs. Callahan's need for more visits. The Callahans will just have to cope. It is not her responsibility to plead for more home visits; it is the responsibility of the health care system to change so that clients receive the care they need. Given the number of clients in Sharon's case load, she might not want to spend this time to deal with the need for more home visits, preferring to go ahead with other clients' needs. If Sharon does this, however, she is essentially leaving Mrs. Callahan at risk to develop infection and not progress toward health. Sharon would not be fulfilling her nursing obligation to reduce harm and promote good.

C. First, nurses need to develop good relationships with case managers of HMOs. Many nurses find that when they develop good relationships with case managers, they are more likely to accept the judgments of nurses about the need for more home visits. The case manager is one more person in the health care system who the nurse needs to collaborate with in order to obtain quality care for clients.

    Second, nurses need to participate in their professional organizations to promote the needs of clients for quality care. They might also need to speak out about the risks that clients experience under HMO-sponsored care systems and help clients to decide which type of health care plan is best for their needs.

    Last, nurses need to use their clinical judgment skills to identify unsafe client care situations and to use their communication skills to bring these situations to the attention of supervisors, professional organizations, and the public.

CHAPTER 7

The correct answer is A. The nurse should first find out from the client what he heard the doctor say. This is important because what the client heard would have a significant effect on his perception of health and what decisions he makes about treatment modalities.

CHAPTER 8

A. You would include in your assessment a Denver II on Billy to determine the neurologic effects of the lead on his growth and development; an assessment of the population to find the total child population under 6 years of age who may benefit from screening; and a community assessment to find the number of older homes in the community that may have lead-based paint.

B. Prevention strategies would include assisting the parents in enrolling Billy in Head Start to stimulate his development, because of his altered growth and development state; a blood level screening program for children under 6 years of age in the community to determine other children who may need to be referred for treatment; and a community-wide lead poisoning prevention program that includes educational materials about where lead is found in home environments and how to test for it. The nurse can target parent group leaders, local newspapers, and the school system to distribute educational materials.

CHAPTER 9

A plan of action to influence the health department about its decision to close the prenatal clinic would include the following:

A. In the law library, the state register was reviewed to see if regulations for the block grants had been finalized.

B. State health statistics were checked, which included vital statistics providing the current infant and maternity mortality rates in the state, and compared to national statistics.

C. The literature was reviewed for research that would show the relationships between prenatal care, normal deliveries, and complications of pregnancy and delivery.

D. After discussion, the group met with the state nurses association to create answers. Together the groups contacted their local senators and representatives and asked for a meeting to discuss the issue.

E. The legal aid society was contacted to find a lawyer interested in consulting with them in preparing written and oral testimony.

F. The testimony was presented to the state health department during the process of preparing the regulations for the block grants.

CHAPTER 10

The correct answer is D. It is becoming increasingly important for nurses to collect standardized assessment data, document care using standardized intervention terms, and generate standardized outcomes of care. However, it is also essential that nurses use their critical thinking skills and judgment and an individualized approach as they apply all the steps of the nursing process.

CHAPTER 11

The correct answer is D. There is controversy about prostate cancer screening, and the experts disagree. The revised American Cancer Society recommends that prostate cancer screening be offered only after men are informed of their risk and benefits. Age recommendations for screening are 45 years and older in African-American men and 50 years and older in Caucasian men. Prostate cancer screening should be offered to men who have 10 years or more of life expectancy left.

    Population risks include incontinence and impotence for some but not all forms of treatment for prostate cancer. Individual risks for Tom are increased due to his family history of prostate cancer, as well as personal lifestyle habits of smoking and consumption of a high-fat diet. It is believed that hereditary cancer is more aggressive than regular cancer.

Population benefits include increased survival rate when prostate cancer is detected in the early stages rather than the advanced stages, 100% vs. 31%. Personal benefits may include decreased psychologic stress from fear of dying from prostate cancer, especially with family history of father dying from prostate cancer.

Two loci have been identified for hereditary prostate cancer: one on chromosome 1 and one on chromosome x. However, additional research is needed before the gene is available for cancer susceptibility testing in high-risk men. High risk for cancer susceptibility testing is usually defined as having several family members with cancer and/or earlier age of onset than normal for the cancer. Cancer susceptibility testing is not appropriate for all persons with cancer, only persons in the high-risk group. Genetic testing is new and there are many misconceptions. Community health nurses are often some of the first health professionals who come into contact with at-risk persons and/or who are asked questions by the public. Therefore it is critical that community health nurses know and understand the basic concepts of cancer susceptibility testing. In addition, community health nurses need to know referral sources for additional genetic information that include genetic counselors.

CHAPTER 12

The correct answer is B. Although all of the answers relate to the students' overall goal, number two is directly related to their plan for collecting data for purposes of research. The plan for collection of the data would first need to be approved by the Institutional Review Board of the university.

CHAPTER 13

A. The population of interest is elementary school children and their parents, a community group. The problem, that a large percentage of elementary school children are not receiving standard immunizations for communicable childhood diseases, is a public health problem. The nurse educator needs to have a solid foundation in community and public health nursing to meet the community needs and to prevent serious public health threats, such as communicable diseases.

B. If the nurse had used behavioral theory to understand how individuals learn, the target behavior—immunizing children against communicable childhood diseases—would have been identified. Then, either a reinforcer (such as receipt of money or a health plaque) or a punishment (such as a fine or removing children who have not had their immunizations from school) would be identified and instituted to change the target behavior.

C. The nurse might distribute a brief survey at the end of the "town meeting" that asks satisfaction and knowledge questions about immunizations as well as whether parents feel that they enjoyed and benefited from the program. The nurse may then compile and tabulate the answers to these questions to determine the community's response to the educational program.

D. No. Long-term evaluation to determine the number of children who receive immunizations and the number of children who do not receive immunizations is needed to evaluate whether the identified community problem has been resolved.

CHAPTER 14

A. One useful approach is to organize evaluation efforts according to the client systems and the focuses of care. In the outreach program the targeted client systems are specific aggregates (indigent or vulnerable groups) and the community (rural county), and the focuses of care are health promotion and illness prevention. This strategy involves examining existing data for the client systems (e.g., population demographics and health statistics; data related to the foci of care, such as clinic utilization patterns; and the amount and type of health education materials disseminated at different locations). In addition, focus groups can be organized, targeting neighborhood or clinic related populations, to assess perceived needs, utilization, and self-reported behavior change.

B. Departments of health at the local and state levels are an excellent resource for vital statistics and health data. Extensive information is accessible on the Internet from national, state, and local government agencies: census data and demographics, morbidity, mortality, and age-specific death rates. These community health indicators are available from the government documents section of many university libraries, the Centers for Disease Control and Prevention (CDC), and the National Centers for Health Statistics (NCHS). In addition, many local communities and community health systems publish health-related report cards with updated information about use of existing health services.

C. Successful community health promotion and illness prevention interventions are based on theories of health behavior change and social learning. Health programs must be individualized and culturally relevant to meet the needs of a specific population. It is essential to assess the clients' values, prior health-related behaviors, and health care utilization patterns to design effective interventions.

D. It is important to identify key informants in this rural community who are involved with the target population in a variety of institutional and community settings. These informants include nurses, physicians, social workers, mental health personnel, community and religious leaders, and health program consumers.

E. The local media (e.g., local radio, television, and newspapers) can be used to communicate important targeted messages about the health outreach program to concerned citizens and to build the informational foundation for partnerships. Nurses can solicit concerned citizens, community leaders, and health professionals to participate in a community coalition to seek funding and support for future program activities.

CHAPTER *15*

The correct answer is B. A high level of community motivation is critical for any community-focused intervention and will help to ensure active community involvement in the planning process and commitment to the intervention itself.

CHAPTER *16*

A. Liz might coordinate getting nutritious food for Ethyl by arranging for Meals-On-Wheels to deliver a hot meal daily and extra meals for the weekend to be delivered on Friday.

B. Because Ethyl is alone a lot, the Meals-On-Wheels driver can be taught to observe any unusual or out-of-the-ordinary behaviors. Should anything be noticed, the driver should call the Coordinating Assessment and Monitoring (CAM) Agency in the hospital emergency department.

C. Liz might also arrange through the Senior Center for their van to take Ethyl into town weekly to shop and/or visit the physician.

D. After the episode where Ethyl was found in her yard, Liz coordinated with her neighbor to organize a rotating system among other neighbors so that one person went by to see Ethyl daily.

E. A remote monitoring system was put into Ethyl's home so she can call the CAM whenever she feels not "up to par."

F. Liz can also arrange for Ethyl's sister, Suzanna, to call Ethyl each day to check on her.

G. The most significant outcome achieved by Liz's case management would be to arrange sufficient basic services to allow Ethyl to remain at home. These include the following:
- Coordination of food (both Meals-On-Wheels and grocery shopping).
- Organizing a team of people to regularly check on Ethyl both to determine her health status and also for stimulation and socialization.
- Arranging transportation to get regular health care.

CHAPTER *17*

The true statements are A, B, C, and D. These examples pertain to local communities and rely on participation, cooperation, equity, and the use of technology.

CHAPTER *18*

LSNNC pursued option A. During the summer of 1998, the nurse practitioner coordinator and the Director of the Neighborhood Nursing Center, with the support of the Advisory Board, submitted the CHIPLINK proposal to a private foundation. This one-year, $50,000 grant-funded program enables LSNNC to provide primary health care for uninsured children from birth through 18 years of age while linking them with available health insurance programs. The programs are CHIP and medical assistance. Outreach, health coverage registration, case management, and primary health care services are components of the program. The first 300 income-eligible children will be accepted into CHIPLINK from November 1 to October 30 of the following year. Select quantitative and qualitative data regarding CHIPLINK services, as well as family experiences with medical assistance or CHIP enrollment, are collected and analyzed. Lessons learned and future initiatives are shared with the funder.

CHAPTER *19*

The correct sequence is C, B, A, D. The first piece of information (C) is essential to understanding the level, amount, and nature of services the client is eligible to receive. The client must be informed, her needs assessed, and her options discussed (B). Family care options must be understood to formulate resource possibilities for the client (A). Arrangement for a facility site visit may or may not be essential but may be preferred (D).

CHAPTER *20*

The correct answer is A. Sharing her feelings with a trained professional who is familiar with the devastating circumstances in which Paula is involved will be most helpful. Although calling home might be comforting, family members with no experience in disaster work would not be able to fully appreciate the stress that Paula is experiencing.

CHAPTER *21*

Eva would include all the steps in planning her project.

She contacted the pastor of the church who was planning to open the soup kitchen to discuss the issue (formulation and assessment). She found him most receptive to the idea of developing a solution to the health care needs of the homeless. In her assessment, Eva found that no other health services were available to the homeless in the community. She looked at national data to estimate needs and size of the population. She talked with the community health nursing faculty to discuss potential solutions to the problem. She talked to members of the homeless population to get their perceptions of their needs.

On completing her assessment, Eva conceptualized the solutions. Several solutions were possible: work with the health department, attempt to provide better care through the local medical center, or open a clinic on site at the soup kitchen where most of the people gathered so that transportation would not be a problem.

After considering the solutions, Eva detailed the plan looking at the resources needed for opening a clinic at the soup kitchen. She considered supplies, equipment, facilities, and acceptability to the clients. She also considered the time involved, the activities required to implement a program, and funding sources.

In evaluating the possibilities, Eva considered the cost, the client and community benefits, and acceptability to clients, self, faculty, and the church. Although it would have been easier for her to choose to work with the health department or the medical center, she knew that the solution most acceptable to the clients would be to have a clinic located at the soup kitchen. The clinic would be more accessible, transportation would not be needed, and health services through the clinic could possibly prevent more costly hospital and emergency care (value).

Eva presented her plan to the faculty and the church. She convinced them that it would not be a costly endeavor. She had nurses in the community who volunteered to help, she had a carpenter who would donate his time to build an examining room in the back of the soup kitchen, and she had equipment promised to her by community physicians. The client assessment indicated that a first-aid and health assessment clinic was what was needed most. With approval from all (implementation), Eva began the clinic in 1981, seeing 25 to 35 clients a week, 1 hour per day for 5 days per week.

Eva evaluated the relevance of the program via the needs assessment process. She tracked the progress of the program by keeping records of her activities. She kept track of the resources in relation to the number of persons served (efficiency) and used these data to convince the church and the college of nursing to fund the ongoing clinic operation after she graduated. A summative evaluation of the clinic was completed by the faculty at the end of 4 years. The program's impact was outstanding. The clinic had grown. The client demand was high; most of the health problems could be handled at the clinic, which eliminated the cost burden to the community for more expensive health care; and it was highly acceptable to the clients (effectiveness). This clinic began as a service to 25 people for 1 hour per day. Today this clinic is open all day, 5 days per week, has more than 900 clients per year, and provides for more than 5000 client visits per year. The success of this clinic shows the effect that one community health nursing student can have on a community.

CHAPTER 22

Both of these questions would be important in determining outcome elements. After answering these questions with the committee, Margaret decides she would like to perform a self-evaluation or, preferably, have a peer review by fellow students to determine the quality of care she has given through the semester. She uses the client satisfaction survey in Appendix J.1 to determine how the clients feel about the services she has delivered. She applies the SIMP audit instrument (see Appendix C.4) to review and evaluate several records of clients she has cared for. She interprets the data, makes adjustments in her care, and shares findings with her faculty advisor. Margaret feels good about the process and outcomes of her clients' care. She has functioned under the agency policies and knows that she has contributed to the overall quality of care as defined by the agency structure.

CHAPTER 23

A. Several contributing factors should be considered, including each of the following:
- The group was unwilling to confront conflict when three members failed to carry out their expected parts.
- Member responsibilities may have been incompletely described when the agreement to work together was specified.
- Students showed a lack of commitment to the project purpose.

B. Lifestyle behavior changes are best sustained through continuing support from family and friends. As individuals develop healthier attitudes and behavior, a variety of family, school or work, and neighborhood supports is needed. Nurses, in partnership with important others in the community, must initiate, participate in, facilitate, and encourage formal and informal groupings within that community that advocate positive practices and contest norms that promoted or ignored risk taking activities.

CHAPTER 24

A. No. The idealized version never existed. There have always been stressors, which presented challenges for families. While not as prominent, there have always been differing family structures within U.S. society.

B. According to a report from the National Commission on Children, people are both discouraged and encouraged about the status of America's families. The contradictions in this report indicate a disparity between people's perceptions of their own families (healthy) and the perception of families outside their own (unhealthy or dysfunctional).

C. There are liberal people in our society who believe the definition of family should be and is expanding and should include two-parent, single-parent, remarried, gay, adoptive, foster, and many other alternative family forms. That is, families are what people define them to be and the government with its health and economic sanctions should be supportive of all family groups. However, there are conservative people who believe that the definition of families should remain limited to the blood, legal, and adoptive guidelines.

D. How we ourselves define family will influence how we live, how we provide nursing care to families, and what health and welfare programs we are willing to support in the society.

CHAPTER 25

A. A home visit would allow for a more extensive assessment of the family within the four models of health: clinical, role-performance, adaptive, and eudaimonistic. The community health nurse phoned the home to make an appointment for a home visit. Amy's mother answered the phone and indicated that Amy was at school during the day. The nurse introduced herself and explained that the counselor at the high school had talked with Amy about the possibility of having a community health nurse from the health department help her to learn more about her pregnancy, labor and delivery, and caring for a new infant. Amy's mother sounded both relieved and enthusiastic about having the nurse visit. Although Amy was in school during the day, she could arrange to be at home so the nurse could meet her at the end of the agency working day. An appointment was made for later in the week to meet with Amy and her mother. At this point, the initiation and previsit phases of the home visit process were completed by the nurse.

B. At the first home visit, it became apparent that Amy and her mother were interested in continuing community health nursing service. During her visit with Amy and her mother, the nurse added to her assessment by exploring with them what they saw as problems and concerns. This is consistent with an approach focused on empowerment. Amy and her mother identified a number of questions and concerns. How could Amy finish her education and care for a child? What would labor and delivery be like? How could Amy and her boyfriend avoid unplanned pregnancies in the future? How could the family members be supportive and yet have their own needs met?

C. A second visit was scheduled to include Amy's boyfriend and father. During the second visit, additional areas related to clinical health of the family, in terms of acute or chronic conditions, were assessed using a family genogram. Because it was apparent that there was a potential conflict between individual and family development needs that had implications for the adaptive processes of the family, time was spent identifying both family needs and individual needs and how best to meet these needs.

D. A contract was negotiated to continue visiting with Amy, but the visits would occur at school during a study period. The focus would be on prenatal teaching on the nurse's part, with Amy agreeing to attend a group for pregnant students offered at the school.

Visits also were arranged with Amy's mother to discuss her concerns. These approaches reflected acknowledgment of the family's abilities to be actively and competently involved in resolving problems they had identified. Over time, the contract was modified and expanded to include well-child supervision during the year following the birth of a healthy baby boy.

CHAPTER 26

A. The correct answer is 3. John is dealing with issues of industry verses inferiority. Encouraging him to be a part of his plan is a strategy to give him control. Choosing a reward system and using concrete activities acknowledge his level of cognitive development.

B. The correct answer is 2. Parents set examples by adhering to healthy lifestyles. It would be appropriate for the nurse to also offer Mrs. D. information to help her stop smoking.

C. Peer involvement is very important to John. School-age children compare themselves to others to determine their own adequacy. He compares himself to his friends at school. He may be reluctant to use his inhalers at school because he sees himself as different than others.

D. He needs MMR#2. If he has not had chickenpox, he needs the varicella vaccine. He should also begin the hepatitis B series, although it is acceptable to wait until he is 11 or 12. If it is fall, he is an excellent candidate for the influenza vaccine (see Chapter 38)

CHAPTER 27

A. The nurse should determine Mrs. Johnson's understanding of the heart and hypertension, the significance of her medication, and the risk associated with her dietary and smoking habits. A health risk appraisal would provide additional information and serve as an educational tool to teach Mrs. Johnson her specific risk factors.

B. A major nursing diagnosis is "Alteration in health maintenance due to limited financial resources and access problems." Another diagnosis might be "Income deficit as evidenced by difficulty buying prescribed medications."

C. The nurse should include Mrs. Johnson in the planning process. Client input is essential to the success of any plan of care. A plan of care should include nursing diagnoses based on a thorough assessment, measurable objectives, nursing interventions, and evaluation.

D. In addition to heart disease, Mrs. Johnson is at risk for lung cancer and caregiver burden. Mrs. Johnson and her family are also at risk for violence.

E. Two of the most significant issues creating stress in Mrs. Johnson's life are a lack of money and her caregiving responsibilities.

F. Many communities have a local resource directory that is useful to community health nurses. Resource directories provide a listing of services provided by community agencies. For example, the Council on Aging is a social service agency that can provide transportation assistance, meals, and emergency financial assistance.

CHAPTER 28

A. Lab test: CBC with differential, CD4+ T-cell count/percentage and CD4+/CD8+ ratio, HIV RNA viral load test, multichannel chemistry panel, urinalysis, TB test, and chest x-ray. Conduct a history and physical assessment: assess general appearance including weight changes and muscle wasting; eye examination; skin assessment and breakdown, including swollen, tender lymph nodes, mouth lesions, painful swollen gums, skin rashes, and lesions; neurologic and genitourinary examination; and nutrition screen.

B. Hyperthermia, social isolation, risk for infection, fluid volume deficit, ineffective coping, body image disturbance, altered nutrition, altered health maintenance, and altered family processes.

C. Ensure adequate hydration and nutrition; control fever and replace fluid loss; facilitate the restoration of usual bowel patterns; and prevent skin breakdown.

D. There is no cure at this time; however, goals should focus on the quality of life. Antiviral therapy suppresses the replication of HIV infection in the body. Retrovir is an antiviral agent most frequently used to treat AIDS. Monitor and treat opportunistic infections such as *Pneumocystis carinii* pneumonia as they occur. Develop an achievable plan that integrates psychosocial and health care goals. Link John to the needed services and continue to monitor/track the services for achievements.

E. Begin with the dietitian, social worker, and the CNS in HIV management at the local public health department. Community-based and national AIDS organizations that should be consulted and for assistance include Aids for AIDS, Aids Service Center, HIV/AIDS Legal, Homeless Health Care, and Project New Hope.

F. Preservation and efficient use of energy. Enhanced self-esteem. Increased sense of personal control. Maintenance of supportive family structure. Anxiety decreased to manageable levels.

CHAPTER 29

The correct answers are C, D, and E. First, the nurse completed a physical examination and administered the Mini-Mental Status Examination short form (to assess cognitive function) and found that Mrs. Eldridge had eight errors.

The medications, an antihypertensive and a diuretic, were verified with the physician and the pharmacist. One pill bottle did not have a label, and the pharmacist said the unknown medication was probably a sleeping pill because its description fit one that had been prescribed. The pharmacist said that the sleeping pill was an old prescription and had not been refilled in some time.

A meeting was arranged with the son at the health department after a neighbor agreed to stay with Mrs. Eldridge. After revealing what had been observed, the son was both shocked and saddened. He went on to say that he had an uneasy feeling about his mother for the past couple of weeks but that he "just couldn't put a finger on what was going on." Because of Mrs. Eldridge's obvious cognitive impairment, the nurse asked for validation of what information she had been able to obtain. She learned that Mrs. Eldridge had been hypertensive for several years and had always been faithful about taking her medications, keeping appointments, and eating a healthy diet. He went on to say that he had been dreading the day when he would have to look for a nursing home for his mother for an extended stay.

Mrs. Eldridge's son and nurse met again 2 weeks later at Mrs. Eldridge's home. The home and Mrs. Eldridge were clean, and Mrs. Eldridge apologized for not remembering the first meeting. It appeared that the sleeping pill, which she had taken to help with the sad feeling and insomnia that accompanied the anniversary of her husbands death, had caused Mrs. Eldridge's intellectual impairment. Mrs. Eldridge and her son had a frank discussion about her living arrangements, and both agreed she would stay in her apartment. Mrs. Eldridge also wished that should her health deteriorate to a point that all hope for recovery was lost, she be allowed to die a peaceful death. The nurse suggested that both mother and son discuss this issue and come to an agreement on the advance directive measure; both agreed.

CHAPTER 30

The nurse planned to evaluate the safety of the home environment and to begin her assessment of the family's understanding of the situation and their concerns. She found that Joel's mother and grandmother were optimistic about the future and delighted to bring him home after such a long hospitalization. They recognized that he would probably suffer motor and visual impairments, yet they wanted to participate in a program to help him develop to his best potential.

The nurse also assessed knowledge of infant care and availability of infant care items. The nurse recommended the purchase of a cool mist humidifier. Because the family had been so involved in providing Joel's daily care in the nursery, they had become skilled in this area and no knowledge deficits were identified.

In planning for early intervention services, several factors were considered. Joel's family expressed a desire for developmental services. Joel's chronic lung disease made him susceptible to complications of respiratory tract infections, making it unwise to expose him to groups of young children. Lack of financial resources limited access to services. Later the community development center would serve as the main program.

During the week following Joel's discharge from the hospital, he was seen at the health department by the pediatrician and nurse to establish a baseline health appraisal. The DDT Denver II was administered using Joel's corrected age (birth age in weeks minus number of weeks premature). Results showed delays in all areas. Nutritional assessment showed that weight gain was only minimally acceptable but consistent with the growth demonstrated in the hospital.

The nurse planned to continue biweekly home visits with the physical therapist to develop further intervention techniques and establish goals in self-help, social, emotional, cognitive, and language skills. Periodic evaluations were performed by the multidisciplinary staff at the follow-up clinic. In collaboration with the physician and nutritionist, the nurse also planned a schedule of health appraisal, nutritional assessments, and family assessments to identify health problems and to guide well-child care.

CHAPTER 31

A. Check Ms. Green for proteinuria (because of her pitting edema and complaints of a mild headache). Contact the health department and arrange for her to be seen soon by the NP to determine what medication she needs; what dietary restrictions and additions she needs; what are the intervals of work/rest that will help her; and whether she needs any meals brought to her or she needs to get some meals from a local shelter.

B. Ms. Green is likely approaching preeclampsia. She may be on the brink of an emergence of her psychotic illness. Her nutrition may be inadequate with too much salt and fat. Her psychotropic medicine needs to be regulated and taken regularly. What help can she get to be able to afford the medicine? How can she get vitamins? Investigate whether she can really take care of this infant. Is the father a source of support?

CHAPTER 32

The correct answer is C. An assessment may have revealed that Tonya did not have transportation and was also responsible for caring for some of the other children in the household. Advocating for support services to assist Tonya in providing for her children raises her self-esteem and opens the door for the nurse to assist Tonya in finding a way out of her situation.

CHAPTER 33

The correct answer is B. Some states have mandatory reporting in cases of partner violence; if so, this will also be an important step. However, student safety and support from her family are important to establish initially.

CHAPTER 34

A. Collection of a family database via meeting with family at a comfortable time and place. In keeping in mind cultural needs, permission should be obtained from the male head of family.
   - Family composition: extended family, housing, education, work/vocation, financial resources, religious practices, ritual, recreation.
   - Family environment: housing, furnishings, living space; sleeping arrangements; bathroom facilities; food preparation arrangements; eating arrangement; adequate water, sewer, lights, ventilation, etc.; condition of yard; pets, transportation; provisions for emergencies; environmental hazards; family attitudes toward home, neighborhood, and community.
   - Goals for the future: type of home, neighborhood to live in.
   - Neighborhood: sociocultural characteristics; traffic patterns; street lighting; resources such as shopping, transportation, education, health and illness, environmental stressors such as noise, crime, substance abuse, crowding; environmental hazards: air quality, neighbors' attitudes; family involvement in neighborhood.
   - Family structure: organization; roles; socialization processes for roles; division of labor, authority, and power; values, beliefs, stresses related to family structure and roles.
   - Emotional, social coping: conflict, life changes, support systems.
   - Life satisfaction: What is going well in life? how happy are you?
   - Health behavior: present health status; perception of vulnerability to disease; perception of present health problems; potential health problems; belief about cause, cure, treatment; risk behaviors; health beliefs; self-care, health care resources.

B. Public health department, migrant health care centers, free clinics, emergency rooms, client may be eligible for Medicaid, but eligibility and resources vary from state to state. Another issue is legality of their stay (are they legal)? Many states/clinics will want evidence of legal entry.

C. Potential barriers are lack of money for treatment or medication; language; need for male presence, which may inhibit client and provider; transportation to clinics; attitudes of health care workers; clinic times that are during prime work hours; fear of being unable to work; need for follow-up; fear of being reported if illegal; limitation of medical record and health history.

CHAPTER 35

A. Many caregivers receive strong support from other family members, neighbors, and their church or religious group. Former coworkers may also be a source of support.

B. If Jason shows signs of emotional disturbance, information can be gathered from the systems that he is involved with. In the school system, the teacher, counselor, and health nurse are important sources of information. Cub scout leaders or athletic directors are also good sources of information. When collecting information, caregiver approval and confidentiality are essential.

C. Important case management activities for Ann would include observation for functional deficits, ability to meet basic nutrition and shelter needs, and medication monitoring.

D. If Mary's depression is treated with medications, the first nursing care activity is to know the name, type, and nature of the drug. Second, assess to determine if she is taking other prescribed or over-the-counter medications. Third, assess her understanding about the medication and determine if there is resistance to medication management. Fourth, monitor for expected and unexpected outcomes of the medication including those related to pharmacokinetics.

CHAPTER 36

A. Consider Mr. Jones' readiness for change, educational needs regarding health effects of smoking, and risks to family members from sidestream smoke.

B. Consider support groups such as AA for Mr. Jones and Alanon for Anne and how this could be helpful. Is it realistic for Anne to stop her grandfather from drinking if he doesn't want to? What else would be helpful to know about his drinking (e.g., where he drinks, what his behavior is like when he is drinking, health risks related to drinking, effects of his drinking on her children) and how would this affect the interventions?

C. Is there evidence of Anne's concern about her children's health as a place to begin? If Anne is not ready to stop "cold turkey," what steps can she begin to take towards the ultimate goal of stopping? What local resources are available?

D. Consider Anne's knowledge of good parenting skills. Consider counseling needs—what stressors are Anne and her children dealing with in their family and environment? How does age affect the potential interventions? Which child is at greater risk? Consider school resources, day care possibilities, and community resources for recreational activities.

E. Consider what the local neighborhood can do to help as well as what community resources are available. Which community leaders might be helpful? Could Jane facilitate a meeting between the local neighbors and law enforcement to help establish helpful communication and relationships? What prevention and treatment programs are available and at what cost? Are legislators aware of the cost benefits of drug treatment compared with law enforcement?

CHAPTER 37

A. The nurse needs to listen carefully to the pain and anguish the daughter felt about hitting her mother. She can convey a nonjudgmental attitude and help the daughter and mother explore ways in which both of their needs could be more effectively met. She can provide information and resources to allow the daughter some respite from constant caretaking and a way to continue her own activities.

B. 1. Assess the situation: Mrs. Smith felt stiff and seemed to have more joint pain from her arthritis in the mornings. With further assessment it became clear that, by late afternoon, her joints were more flexible and less painful.

2. Discuss options with the family: When nurse, daughter, and client discussed their options, they decided that Mary would wash only her mother's anal area in the morning and put clean pads under her if indicated. Total hygienic care would be done in the late afternoon.

3. Teach alternative approaches: Mrs. Jones demonstrated to Mary alternative ways to move, turn, and wash her mother to minimize the strain on her arthritic joints and to incorporate some effective exercise into the bath.

4. Make appropriate referrals and coordinate services: On two mornings each week, a home health care aide was engaged to stay with Mrs. Smith. Mary could then do family shopping and errands and participate in activities in which she had previously been involved.

C. Mrs. Jones will need to monitor the situation carefully for any further signs of abuse. Any further instance of violence must be discussed with the daughter and immediately reported. In a subsequent visit, the nurse evaluated the effectiveness of her teaching and learned that Mary and her mother were working much more cooperatively on Mrs. Smith's care.

CHAPTER 38

A. The correct answer is 4. Historical and current TB surveillance data should be consulted to see if the number of TB cases has been increasing or not falling as would be expected and if noncompliance with treatment has been a contributing factor.

B. Justification for such a program would include a brief description of the difficulties in TB treatment, the resultant problems with noncompliance, and the implications for development of resistance and the potential for continued infection of the public.

C. The correct answer is 3. The success of the incentive program appears to be linked with identifying an incentive that has a strong personal value to the client. Of course, the incentive must also be acceptable to all parties involved. For example, alcohol and tobacco would probably not be considered appropriate incentives.

D. Identifying contacts for treatment or prophylaxis is an important part of preventing the continued spread of TB infection. Clients may be reluctant for personal reasons to reveal contacts or they may simply not realize who all their contacts are. Observing client daily activity provides an opportunity to investigate all possibilities for transmitting disease.

CHAPTER 39

A. Questions the nurse asks Yvonne seek information about past injection drug use and sexual partners. The nurse evaluates Yvonne's comfort in sharing the information with Phil as she explores what she believes Phil's response might be. The nurse offers to role-play the situation of Yvonne telling Phil about the possibility of his infection, risks, and the importance of testing for the HIV antibody. Rather than contacting other previous sexual and drug-using partners herself, Yvonne requests that health department staff contact them about being tested for possible infection. She gives the nurse the names and addresses of two additional drug-using partners.

B. The most immediate concerns for Yvonne are the need to seek ongoing care to monitor the HIV infection and to decide whether to continue the pregnancy. The nurse asks Yvonne whether she has a primary health care provider. The information given includes providing Yvonne a list of providers and counseling about the importance of establishing an ongoing relationship with a primary health care provider for follow-up of the HIV infection. She tells Yvonne that important information about her health may be identified that will help to determine her ability to carry and deliver the baby if she chooses to continue the pregnancy. Other important information includes the implications of the test results, such as how they may affect the infant's and mother's health.

The nurse explains that transmission to the fetus is possible during the pregnancy and she may have a greater chance of progressing from asymptomatic infection to symptomatic HIV disease but that medications would be given to try to prevent this from happening. The nurse explores possibilities with Yvonne about the decision regarding her ability to physically, emotionally, and financially cope with rearing a child that possibly may be ill. Family members and other potential resources are assessed. The need for Yvonne to tell health care providers or blood handlers about the HIV infection is reviewed. The nurse schedules a second appointment for follow-up counseling 1 week after the initial test results are given. She also gives Yvonne the telephone number of the local AIDS support group and arranges to make a home visit to her in 2 days.

At the follow-up home and clinic visits, specific information is given regarding infection control in the home and safer sexual relations. The nurse ensures that Yvonne is taking steps toward receiving prenatal care and medical care for the HIV infection. The nurse reviews information about how to maintain health and avoid stressors and contracts with Yvonne to initiate home visits to provide reinforcement of adequate prenatal nutrition and teaching and to assess Yvonne's physical health as the pregnancy progresses.

CHAPTER 40

A. 1. Respecting the family's customs and space, as well as sensitivity to the timing of questions, will help develop a trusting relationship.
   2. Flexibility and keeping promises is even more important in the home.
   3. Give the family a time range when making an appointment to allow for delays at other homes and for traffic.
   4. Provide the client and family information about the referral, the purpose of your visit, what services are available, and how to contact the agency.
   5. Deal first with the issue that is uppermost on the client's mind, not what is first on your agenda. This strategy will decrease client anxiety and improve the ability to understand and focus on what you need to tell them.

B. 1. Taking a detailed history.
   2. Doing a physical assessment.
   3. Walking through the important parts of the house (bedroom, bathroom, kitchen, and hallways) provides baseline data for forming the plan of care.
   4. Listening to clients provides the most important clues to health status and effective teaching strategies.
   5. Begin completing necessary forms. Some clients will not be able to complete all the forms and required information on the first visit because of pain or fatigue. Focus on the essentials and complete the rest on a second visit.

C. 1. Set short- and long-term goals with clients.
   2. Have a plan for every visit to progress toward the goals.
   3. Clients and families must be informed that home health services are time limited and that they need to learn to provide their own care.
   4. Nurses need to set limits, model expected behaviors, and write in the behaviors of the client.
   5. Develop principles to facilitate and encourage self-care.
   6. Plan for modifying care to allow as much independence as possible.
   7. Writing plans to teach client rather than do for the client.

D. 1. Understand adult learning principles.
   2. Identify the characteristics that indicate client's preferred learning style by asking.

CHAPTER 41

Case 1: The best method of evaluation would be D. Client outcome data on rehospitalization and/or medical complications are used to evaluate the service. Also evaluating the aftercare service and assessing client and family satisfaction by questionnaire and telephone is a useful evaluation approach.

Case 2: The most correct answer is C. After her assessment, Julie could negotiate with the physicians to randomly assign 30 hypertensive clients to her for follow-up care. Then at a later date (6 to 9 months later), she could compare blood pressure measurements in the two groups.

CHAPTER 42

The correct answer is A. The nurse manager thus used a participative decision-making approach at the meeting, and the group decided to obtain external consultation through the local college of nursing.

The community health faculty member assigned Patricia, a community health student, to assess this community's request for consultation. Patricia met with the nurse manager and the manager of the residential complex to discuss the problem, assess her ability to help, and explore the client's expectations for herself and for the College of Nursing. After careful consideration, Patricia and the nurse manager determined that a survey of residents' needs, community resources, and staff perceptions would assist them in planning the alternatives they could explore for providing additional health promotion and health monitoring to the residents.

With the approval of the community health faculty member, Patricia and her fellow students agreed to implement a health screening survey project and to collect data about the residential program, such as the physical facilities, the available equipment and supplies, and staff available to provide assistance with health screening and promotion activities. They collected data on existing relationships with community referral sources, including local home care programs, money available to support program expansion at the residential facility, and the attitudes of staff and residents toward expansion. Anticipated outcomes to be evaluated for the consultation included recommending to the management of the residential program that home care services be made more accessible for residents using one of several options. The facility might contract for such a program with the college of nursing, develop a service contract with the health department for a satellite home care agency on facility grounds, or provide space for a proprietary home care agency to operate within the facility.

At the evaluation conference, Patricia and her colleagues shared the results of their data collection. After careful consideration of the data, the nurse manager and the manager of the residential facility agreed that residents needed more access to home care and decided to develop a contract with the College of Nursing for provision of home nursing services on site. This would enable the current staff to devote their energies to aggregate health promotion activities.

CHAPTER 43

A. A school health program involves all three: health services, health education, and environmental health. School health services help to screen and identify children who have unmet health problems or need monitoring of chronic illnesses, either of which can affect the child's ability to learn. Health education is important and should begin in kindergarten so children can understand the meaning of and begin practicing health habits early. Heath education throughout the school experience can affect how children learn and can lead to healthy productive adults. Attention to the physical environment of the school–climate, safety, esthetics–all affect the child's ability to pay attention and to want to learn. Reducing stress in the environment for teachers and students and creating a climate of acceptance for all may reduce violent acts and can improve attitudes toward learning.

B. The answer is 3. Creating a surveillance system will assist the nurse in defining the problem at the population level. The surveillance system will provide a system for tracking rates at each school and for the school system as a whole. Tracking students seen by the nurse, reviewing absence records, collecting data from teachers, and assessing students at risk through a personal lifestyle inventory are all a part of the surveillance system.

CHAPTER 44

The correct answer is D. This is an example of how the epidemiologic triad can be used to assess clients and plan nursing care. It illustrates the usefulness of approaching occupational health problems with an epidemiologic perspective.

CHAPTER 45

Regardless of the earliest beginnings, discussions; questions; eliciting statements of healthy and unhealthy events in the lives of the members; and surveying the physical, social, emotional, and spiritual environmental conditions of the faith community will begin to shape the path. Formation of a broadly representative wellness committee will help to plan the formal and informal assessment methods and careful documentation of activities and communication.

Building on strengths of the congregation, gathering information on leaders and valued activities in the congregation, and becoming informed regarding lines of authority and communication help to provide a foundation for the service. The best answer is D, planning a congregational survey. This increases interest and involvement of the members. Results assist in focusing a possible goal. If the majority of the congregation is over the age of 55 years, it would be helpful to assess areas such as needs for retirement planning, current health status and adequacy of health financing options, involvement in caregiving for parents as well as adult children, needs for involvement in meaningful volunteer activities, and ability to holistically engage in activities appropriate for the life stage. Assessment would also include the impact of the over-55 age group on the remainder of the congregation and the surrounding community. Information regarding resources within the church and geopolitical community is helpful.

Organizing and implementing a health fair to address identified needs often is beneficial in creating awareness of health needs, providing information to act on identified health concerns, increasing visibility of the value of health and faith connection, and promoting interest for additional congregational members to become involved in the parish nurse/health ministry program. The greater involvement by the members, the greater the ownership of the program by the total faith community. Evaluation of the activity will yield information regarding which areas or activities should be continued or reinforced, which need to change focus, and which should be omitted.

In addition to the group and population activities, the parish nurse meets regularly with the pastoral staff and coordinates with other committee chairs. Together, they identify individuals requiring further assessment or support; become aware of issues that need to be clarified, supported, or addressed; and determine individuals, groups, or issues that have not yet become a part of the parish nurse or congregational wellness program. Home visits, phone calls, and visits to hospitals or community agencies are also part of the parish nurse's weekly activities. Agendas might include advocacy and interpretation with a health care provider, monitoring dementia progress, supporting a new mother embarking on a "new" career at home, leading a support group, therapeutic touch, prayer, and visualization.

CHAPTER 46

The team organized to develop the case definition, plan the interview questions and sampling, and organize the specimen collection. Interviews were used to determine characteristics of the illness and to attempt to identify the source by dietary recall and living arrangements. The dietary recall was focused on the food consumed during the three meals before illness onset. While the interviews were being conducted, an environmental investigation concentrated on food preparation, service, and storage, along with housekeeping procedures. The administrative staff of the retirement community kept a daily log documenting all interventions implemented to determine what effect the measures undertaken to stop the spread of illness may have actually had on controlling the spread of illness.

It was initially thought that the infectious agent was a "Norwalk-like" virus, classified under the heading of human caliciviruses (HCV). Specimen testing, however, confirmed the presence of a virus strain similar to the Mexican virus, also an HCV, but classified in a different genogroup than the Norwalk virus. Clinically, symptoms are indistinguishable. The outbreak was revealed to have been caused by a virus strain closely related to the Mexican virus. Fecal-oral spread through food contamination, close person-to-person contact, and possible respiratory spread were hypothesized for this highly contagious virus.

There is a great deal to be learned about the transmission from persons who are asymptotic. A majority of the residents of the facility became ill even after the institutional precautions were implemented, such as closing the dining room and limiting contacts between residents, encouraging disinfection of common areas of the retirement community, and placing emphasis on personal hygiene and glove use by staff. Ill staff were told to stay home until at least 2 days after their symptoms subsided. Handwashing by the staff was emphasized using antibacterial soap and drying with paper towels. The use of disposable items was encouraged when possible. Due to the recent increase in gastrointestinal illness in older populations in the state and the fragile state of health of many of the residents, as a result of this investigation, recommendations for control measures during gastroenteritis outbreaks in institutions became incorporated into a checklist for long-term care facilities to increase the level of awareness of the importance of strict adherence to hygienic practices in institutional settings.

Glossary

A

abortion: Termination of a pregnancy by spontaneous expulsion of a human fetus during the first 12 weeks of gestation or by induced abortion.

absenteeism: The lack of attending school.

acceptant intervention mode: Consultative mode of client intervention that is a process of catharsis intended to clear emotional blocks in order to engage in objective problem solving.

accommodation: Ways in which children modify their view of the world as they have new experiences that influence their responses.

accountability: Being answerable legally, morally, ethically, or socially to someone for something one has done.

accreditation: A credentialing process used to recognize health care agencies or educational programs for provision of quality services and programs.

acquired immunity: The resistance acquired by a host due to previous natural exposure to an infectious agent. May be induced by passive or active immunization.

acquired immunodeficiency syndrome (AIDS): The final stages of HIV infection, which follows a protracted and debilitating course, characterized by specific opportunistic diseases that have a poor prognosis.

active immunization: Administration of all or part of a microorganism to stimulate active response by the host's immunological system, resulting in complete protection against a specific disease.

activities of daily living (ADLs): Basic personal care activities that include eating, toileting, dressing, bathing, transferring, walking, and getting outside.

addiction treatment: Focuses on the addiction process by helping clients view addiction as a chronic disease and assisting them to make lifestyle changes to halt the progression of the disease.

administrative law: Branch of law dealing with organs of government power; prescribes the manner of their activity (e.g., state board of nurse examiners).

administrative order: A legal document issued and signed by the U.S. Environmental Protection Agency, EPA, or a state environmental organization requiring an individual, business, or other entity to take corrective actions or refrain from an activity in order to achieve compliance with federal or state pollution laws, regulations, or standards. The order also can include a civil penalty.

administrator: One who manipulates the resources within an organization to meet the organizational goals.

adolescent period: Period from onset of puberty (approximately age 11) to end of puberty (approximately age 21).

adoption: The action of taking by choice into a relationship; to take voluntarily as one's own child.

advance directives: Written or oral statements by which a competent person makes known treatment preferences and/or designates a surrogate decision-maker.

Advanced Practice Nurse: Nurse with advanced education beyond the baccalaureate degree who is prepared to manage and deliver health care services to individuals, families, groups, communities, and populations; includes clinical nurse specialists, nurse practitioners, nurse midwives, nurse anesthetists, and others.

advocacy: Activities for the purpose of protecting the rights of others while supporting the client's responsibility for self-determination; involves informing, supporting, and affirming a client's self-determination in health care decisions.

aeration: The process of being supplied with air. Aeration is used in wastewater treatment to foster biologic and chemical purification.

aerobic: Life or processes that require or are not destroyed by the presence of oxygen.

affective domain: A domain of learning that includes changes in attitudes and the development of values.

affirming: Ratifying, asserting, or giving strength to the declarations of self or others.

ageism: A term for prejudice about older people that is similar to racism or sexism.

Agency for Toxic Substances and Disease Registry (ATSDR): Federal agency mandated to prevent exposure and adverse health effects associated with exposure to hazardous substances from waste sites, unplanned releases, and other sources of environmental pollution.

agency report card: A written listing of how the agency compares with others in the field on certain key indicators of quality, including morbidity and mortality measures, client satisfaction, and cost of care.

agent: Causative factor invading a susceptible host through an environment favorable to produce disease, such as a biologic or chemical agent.

aggregate: Population or defined group.

Aid to Families with Dependent Children: A federal and state program to provide financial assistance to needy children deprived of parental support because of death, disability, absence from the home, or, in some states, unemployment. Now known as Temporary Assistance to Needy Families (TANF).

air quality or emission standard: The maximum amount of air polluting discharge legally allowed from a single source, stationary or mobile, in a specified time.

Al-Anon: Lay, self-help group for family members and/or significant others of alcoholics with a structure similar to Alcoholics Anonymous.

Alcoholics Anonymous: Lay, self-help group that practices a 12-step approach to recovery for persons suffering from alcoholism.

alcoholism: Addiction to alcohol.

alliance: A formal relationship between two agencies in which they agree to cooperate in some way.

allocation: The distribution or designation of something for a specific purpose or to particular persons or things.

ambient air: The outside air that surrounds us. The air we live in and breathe.

ambulatory care centers: Hospital or community-based facilities that offer a wide range of outpatient services to treat mental and physical health problems.

American Nurses Association: The national professional association of registered nurses in the United States, founded in 1896.

American Public Health Association: A national organization founded in 1872 to facilitate interdisciplinary efforts and to promote the health of the public.

American Red Cross: A national organization that seeks to reduce human suffering through various health, safety, and disaster relief programs in affiliation with the International Committee of the Red Cross.

Americans with Disabilities Act (ADA): An act passed in 1990 that mandated that individuals with mental and physical disabilities be brought into the mainstream of American life.

amplification: Expanding a statement or idea; an objective of communication.

anaerobic: A life or process that occurs in, or is not destroyed by, the absence of oxygen.

analytic epidemiology: An epidemiologic study designed to investigate associations between exposures or characteristics and health or disease outcomes, often with a goal of understanding the etiology (or origins and causal factors) of disease.

anorexia: Intense fear of becoming obese and disturbances in body image result in strict dieting and excessive weight loss. Occurs most commonly in females between the ages of 12 and 21 but may occur on older women and men.

anovulatory: The lack of production and discharge of an ovum.

antibody: An organism formed in the body that identifies and destroys initial and subsequent invasions of an identified disease-producing organism.

anticipatory guidance: Providing advice to clients before an event and discussing potential problems or risks so clients will be aware and may be able to prevent the occurrence of the problem.

antiprohibitionists: Persons who are against the government's authority/laws to prohibit what drugs/substances adults may choose to ingest.

antitoxin: Solution of antibodies derived from the serum of animals immunized with specific antigens (e.g., diphtheria, tetanus); used to achieve passive immunity.

APEXH: Acronym for *Assessment Protocol for Excellence in Public Health.* A guideline publication for community intervention to obtain health objectives. APEXH emphasizes local level activity and focuses on improving the public health of communities by increasing the capacity of the location health care agencies to provide core functions, such as assessment and policy development.

appropriate technology: Affordable social, biomedical, and health services that are relevant and acceptable to individuals' health, needs, and concerns.

aquifer: A geologic formation underneath the earth's surface that stores groundwater.

area education agencies (AEAs): Provide services for special education students in school districts of limited size.

artificially acquired immunity: Immune state that results from immunization or vaccination for a specific disease.

assault: A violent physical or verbal attack

assertiveness: The ability to present one's own needs.

assessment: Systematic use of data to assist in identifying needs, questions to be addressed, or abilities and available resources.

assessment of community resources: Procedure similar to the process used on behalf of individual clients. The scope of the investigation is more detailed and includes examination of data from health planning groups, including the number of public health facilities, availability of health personnel, availability of funds, and a multitude of other statistics, such as those on mortality and morbidity.

assessment of need: Verifying and mapping out the extent and location of a problem and the target population.

assimilation: (a) Process of a minority group becoming absorbed into the dominant or majority culture by adopting its behaviors. Also the process of a child's responding to the environment in accordance with his or her cognitive structures so that elements in the environment are incorporated into his or her cognitive structures. (b) The conversion or incorporation of absorbed nutrients into protoplasm. Also refers to the ability of a body of water to purify itself of pollutants.

assisted living: Living arrangements, primarily for elders, that provide services in an environment that resembles a home. Assisted-living facilities have common areas (dining room, game room) that are available but also provide privacy and independence to the residents, fostering an increased sense of self.

assumption: A characteristic of the research situation that is not explored, usually because it has been well demonstrated in previous research.

assurance activities: Monitoring access to health services, determining the effectiveness of the services provided in relation to the needs of the people, and working to improve continually the quality of the health services.

attack rates: A type of incidence rate defined as the proportion of persons exposed to an agent who develop the disease, usually for a limited time in a specific population.

attention deficit disorder: Inappropriate degree of inattention, impulsiveness, and hyperactivity for age and development.

attributable risk: Statistical measure that estimates the reduction in the occurrence of a particular disease that could be affected by elimination of a specific causal agent.

audit process: A six-step process used concurrently or retrospectively for nursing peer review.

autoimmunity: Abnormal condition in which the body reacts against parts of its own tissues.

autonomy: Freedom of action as chosen by an individual.

B

barriers to access: Financial or nonfinancial impediments to obtaining health care. May include lack of funds to pay for health care or inadequate insurance coverage. Also may include cultural obstacles and practical problems, such as lack of transportation or inconvenient clinic hours.

battered child syndrome: Term coined by Kempe to describe the pattern of abuse against children.

behavioral theory: A theory that approaches the study of learning by concentrating on behaviors that can be observed and measured.

benchmarking: Comparing national standards and guidelines to other agencies.

beneficence: Ethical principle stating that one should do good and prevent or avoid doing harm.

benefit cost analysis: A method of comparing the monetary gains and expenses associated with a health care program or service, including start-up and maintenance costs.

bias: A systematic deviation of observed values from the true value.

biodegradable: The ability to break down or decompose under natural conditions or processes.

biodegradation: Alteration of waste product to a less toxic form through chemical intervention.

biologic agent: Disease-producing hazards primarily consisting of bacteria, viruses, and other microorganisms and parasites.

birth control: Control of the number of children born, especially by preventing or lessening the frequency of conception.

block grant: Sum of money given to a state or local government whereby the federal government offers a general purpose for the use of the money but allows the state or local area to spend the money without meeting specific conditions.

block nursing: A contemporary term for district nursing.

blood alcohol concentration—BAC (also called blood alcohol level—BAL): The amount of alcohol in the blood, commonly expressed as grams of alcohol per 100 milliliters of blood. Most state legal limits of intoxication while driving are 0.08% or 0.1%.

boards of cooperative education services (BOCES): Provides services for special education students in school districts of limited size.

boundary: In systems theory, the line or border that defines the elements making up the system.

brainstorming: To generate as many alternatives as possible without critical evaluation.

Breckinridge, Mary: A leader in public health nursing who established the Frontier Nursing Service (FNS) in Kentucky. The FNS nurses were trained in nursing, public health, and midwifery.

brief intervention: An intervention that is sometimes made by health care professionals who are not treatment experts and has been found to be effective in helping ATOD abusers and addicts reduce their consumption or follow through with treatment referrals. It can have six parts: feedback, responsibility, advice, menu of options, empathy, and self-efficacy.

brokering health services: Coordinating services provided by multiple agencies. Case managers often coordinate services to provide comprehensive care for clients.

budget: A plan stated in financial terms that identifies the costs associated with implementing a program.

budget constraint: The amount of money available to an individual or organization to spend on a particular good or service.

bulimia: Persistent concern with body shape and weight. Recurrent episodes of binge eating followed by extreme methods to prevent weight gain such as purging, fasting, or vigorous exercise.

business cycle: A natural, recurring expansion and contraction within business.

business plan: Operational and fiscal plan that enables an organization to meet goals and objectives; includes activities/services, marketing and public relations, staff, administrative and overhead costs of operations, sources of and methods for generating revenue, research and development for the future.

C

capitation: A payment system whereby one fee is charged the client to pay for all services received or needed.

care coordination: Linking clients with services.

caregiver burden: The physical, psychologic, emotional, social, and financial problems that can be experienced by those who provide care for impaired others.

caregivers: Those persons, professional and nonprofessional, who provide for the social and health needs of others.

CareMaps: A tool developed by Zander showing cause and effect and identifying expected client/family and staff behaviors against a time line. It has four components: index of problems with intermediate and outcome criteria, time line, critical path, and variance record.

care management: See *case management*.

care planning: Home health nurse and clients work together to give adequate service at home.

caring: Behavior that is directed toward the protection and maintenance of the health and welfare of clients. Indication of a commitment toward the protection of human dignity and the preservation of human health.

case-control study: An epidemiologic study design in which subjects with a specified disease or condition (cases) and a comparable group without the condition (controls) are enrolled and assessed for the presence or history of an exposure or characteristic.

case finding: Careful, systematic observations of people to identify present or potential problems.

case law: A decision by the courts; a judicial opinion.

case management: Interchangeable term with care management. Used to describe a service given to clients that contains the following activities: screening, assessment, care planning, arranging for service delivery, monitoring, reassessment, evaluation, and discharge. Case management is a process that enhances continuity and appropriateness of care. Most often used with clients whose health problems are actually or potentially chronic and complex.

case manager: A school nurse who performs a number of general activities concerning health problems of the children.

case register: Systematic registration of acute, chronic, and contagious diseases.

case study: A written analysis of program development and implementation throughout the life of the program; a historical depiction of the program.

catalytic intervention mode: A situation whereby a consultant assists a client to broaden his or her view of an existing situation by gaining additional information or by unifying existing data.

causality: The relationship of one factor to another such that the presumed causal factor produces or contributes to the occurrence of some outcome.

census data: Composite data provided by the federal government on the population of states, local and political jurisdictions, and defined geographic tracts in organized areas.

Centers for Disease Control and Prevention: Branch of the U.S. Public Health Service whose primary responsibility is to propose, coordinate, and evaluate changes in the surveillance of disease in the United States.

certificate of need: Determination in any given community of the need for new health care facilities on the basis of currently available resources and anticipated demands for use.

Certificates of Immunization Status: Shows if a child has up-to-date immunizations needed to attend school.

certification: A mechanism, usually by means of written examination, that provides an indication of professional competence in a specialized area of practice.

chancroid: A sexually transmitted disease caused by a bacteria, *Haemophilus ducreyi,* that results in a highly infectious ulcer located on the penis, urethra, vulva, or anus.

change agent: Nursing role that facilitates change in client or agency behavior to more readily achieve goals. This role stresses gathering and analyzing facts and implementing programs

change partner: Nursing role that facilitates change in client or agency behavior to more readily achieve goals. This role includes the activities of serving as an enabler-catalyst, teaching problem-solving skills, and activist advocate.

charge: Dollar amount billed to the client for the service provided.

charter: A mechanism by which a state government agency under state laws grants corporate status to institutions with or without rights to award degrees.

chemical agents: Home, workplace, and community manmade hazards found in the environment that can produce disease.

chemical contamination: Contamination of food, either deliberately or accidentally, by chemical additives.

chemical dependency: Addiction to alcohol or other drugs.

child abuse: Active forms of maltreatment of children.

Child Find: Provides early identification of preschool children at risk for school failure because of disabilities such as mental retardation, chronic health conditions, or other special needs. It is funded through IDEA legislation.

Child Health Insurance Plan: Provides school nurses with option in finding services for children of the working poor who are uninsured and not eligible for Medicaid.

child neglect: Physical or emotional neglect. Physical neglect refers to failure to provide adequate food, clothing, shelter, hygiene, or necessary medical care; emotional neglect refers to the omission of basic nurturing, acceptance, and caring essential for healthy development.

chlamydia: A sexually transmitted disease caused by the organism *Chlamydia trachomatis* that causes infection of the urethra and cervix. Infections may be asymptomatic and, if untreated, result in severe morbidity.

chlorofluorocarbons: A family of chemicals containing chlorine and fluorine that damages the ozone layer in the air; found in furniture and bedding foam, carpet padding, foam egg cartons and coffee cups, and insulation.

chronically homeless: Long-term homelessness.

circle of care: Neighbors who keep watch out for the frail and elderly in rural communities.

CITYNET process: A nine-step community problem-solving process in *Healthy Cities* that provides broad community participation in all steps.

clarification: The process of attempting to make communication or expression clear or easier to understand.

Clean Water Act: A federal law passed in 1972. The act, one of the most comprehensive laws passed by Congress, limits or controls point source discharges into navigable waters, making sure U.S. waters are fishable and swimmable. The act also delegates federal authority to those states with the resources and technical expertise to enforce the regulations.

client outcome: A change in client health status as a result of care or program implementation.

client population: Individuals, groups, families, organizations, or communities that are the targets of the consultant's interventions.

client problem: A current, historic, or potential matter of difficulty or concern that adversely affects any aspect of a client's well-being.

client responsibilities: Those tasks or areas for which the client is accountable. In the case of an individual health care client, responsibilities might be related to self-care or actively participating in a referral. In a consulting relationship, the client may be expected to provide information and engage in active problem solving.

clients' rights: Those services, programs, goods, and provider behaviors to which consumers are entitled in order to maintain or achieve health or to exist.

client system: (a) The variety of systems toward which interventions are directed. (b) The client system in the integrative model is multidimensional and includes various levels of client, individual, family, aggregate, and community toward which community health nursing care is targeted.

clinical nurse specialist: An advanced practice nurse who provides direct care to clients and participates in consultative, health education, and program management.

clinician: A nurse prepared at any level who provides direct care.

coaching: Encouraging another in the acquisition of certain skills, including making suggestions, giving feedback at incremental intervals, and praising as goals are met.

code for nurses: The American Nurses Association professional statement prescribing moral behavior and actions of nurses based on moral principles.

code of ethics: A set of statements encompassing rules that apply to people in professional roles.

codependency: A condition characterized by preoccupation and extreme dependency (emotionally, socially, and sometimes physically) on a person. Eventually this dependence on another person becomes a pathologic condition that affects the person in all of his or her relationships.

codes of regulation: Federal and state legal documents in which finalized regulations are published.

coercive health measures: Health care treatment and services required regardless of the client's wishes, choices, or life plans. Such care is usually regulated by law and is instituted to protect the public's health.

coercive sex: Sexual relations that occur with force, intimidation, or authority.

cognitive development: The progressive process of acquisition of skills for thinking, reasoning, and language use.

cognitive domain: A domain of learning that includes memory, recognition, understanding, and application and is divided into a hierarchic classification of behaviors.

cognitive theory: A theory that maintains that by changing thought patterns and providing information, learners' behavior will change.

cohesion: Attraction of group members to one another and to the group.

cohort: Group of people born during the same era who are influenced by some of the same biologic, psychologic, and social factors.

cohort study: An epidemiologic study design in which subjects without an outcome of interest are classified according to past or present (or future) exposures or characteristics and followed over time to observe and compare the rates of some health outcome in the various exposure groups.

coliform index: A rating of the purity of water based on a count of fecal bacteria.

collaboration: Mutual sharing and working together to achieve common goals in such a way that all persons or groups are recognized and growth is enhanced.

collaborative practice: Professionals working together in a collegial relationship to provide primary health care to a given population.

combination agency: A health care agency that provides home health and hospice services.

common law: Law based on the opinion of the courts; comes from past court decisions or opinions based on fairness, respect for individuals, autonomy, and self-determination.

common vehicle: Transportation of the infectious agent from an infected host to a susceptible host via water, food, milk, blood, serum, or plasma.

communicable disease: A disease of human or animal origin caused by an infectious agent and resulting from transmission of that agent from an infected person, animal, or inanimate source to a susceptible host. Infectious disease may be communicable or noncommunicable (e.g., tetanus is infectious but not communicable).

communicable period: The time or times when an infectious agent may be transferred from an infected source directly or indirectly to a new host.

communication structure: A descriptive framework that identifies message pathways and member participation in sending and receiving messages utilized for a group or groups.

community: People and the relationships that emerge among them as they develop and use in common some agencies and institutions and a physical environment; a locality-based entity composed of systems of formal organizations reflecting society's institutions, information groups, and aggregates.

Community-as-Partner model: An assessment guide model developed by Anderson and McFarlane in 1995 that illustrates how communities change and grow best by full involvement and self-empowerment. It presents an assessment wheel with people in the center and eight subsystems that affect and are affected by people surrounding them (see Appendix H1 for this model).

community assessment: Process of critically thinking about the community and getting to know and understand the community as a client. Assessments help identify community needs, clarify problems, and identify strengths and resources.

community-based care: A process initiated by community members to provide health care to the community.

community-based nursing: Setting-specific practice whereby care is provided for "sick" individuals and families where they live, work, and go to school. The emphasis of practice is acute and chronic care and the provision of comprehensive, coordinated, and continuous services. Nurses who deliver community-based care are generalists or specialists in maternal-infant, pediatric, adult, or psychiatric-mental health nursing.

community client: Target of service (i.e., the population group for whom healthful change is sought).

community collaboration: Health services with an emphasis on health promotion and disease prevention, community involvement, multisectoral cooperation, appropriate technology; includes accessible, acceptable, and affordable public and primary health care services.

community competence: Process whereby the competence of a community—organizations, groups, and advocates—are able to collaborate effectively in identifying the problems and needs of the community, can achieve a working consensus on goals, and can collaborate effectively in the required actions.

community forum: An open meeting for members of a particular community or group to address an issue of interest.

community health: The meeting of collective needs by identifying problems and managing interactions within the community itself and between the community and the larger society; a function of the energy, the individuality, and the relationships of the community as a whole and of all its constituents.

community health nurse consultant: A community health nurse who assists another individual or organization with problem solving regarding provision of community health nursing services.

community health nurse specialist for school-age children: The person who evaluates the children to identify their strengths and weaknesses.

community health nursing: The synthesis of nursing theory and public health theory applied to promoting, preserving, and maintaining the health of populations through the delivery of personal health care services to individuals, families, and groups. The focus of practice is health of individuals, families, and groups and the effect of their health status on the health of the community as a whole.

community health nursing leadership: Refers to the influence that community health nurses exert to improve client health, whether clients are individuals, families, groups, or entire communities.

community health nursing management: Refers to the ways that community health nurses manage resources in the provision of clinical services. Resources include people, time, supplies and equipment, and financial resources.

community health problem: An actual or potential difficulty or need for action within a target population with identifiable causes and consequences in the environment.

community health strength: Resources or abilities available to meet a community health need.

community health workers: Paraprofessionals who staff nursing centers. Typically they have a high school or 2-year college degree and want to work in their community.

community mental health: Orientation toward health care that seeks to provide a program of continuing and comprehensive mental health care to a specific population.

Community Mental Health Centers (CMHCs): Comprehensive centers that implement community mental health model of care.

Community Nursing Center: Community facility that delivers accessible primary care and is managed and staffed by nurses.

community-oriented practice: A clinical approach in which the nurse and community join in partnership and work together for healthful change.

Community-Oriented Primary Care (COPC): A community-responsive model of health care delivery that integrates aspects of both primary care and public health. It combines the care of individuals and families in the community with a focus on the community and its subgroups when services are planned, provided, and evaluated.

community participation: Well-informed and motivated community members who participate in planning, implementing, and evaluating health programs.

community partnership: Collaborative decision-making process participated in by community members and professionals.

community preparedness: A process whereby communities prepare and update a disaster plan and participate in regular mock disaster drills.

community resident survey: A direct assessment of the population of a community to identify the need for a service, the acceptability of the service to the population, and the willingness of the people to use and pay for the service.

community support program: Funded by the National Institute of Mental Health; provides grant monies to states for the purpose of developing comprehensive services for persons discharged from psychiatric institutions.

compliance: Processes for ensuring that permitting requirements are met.

Comprehensive Environmental Response, Compensation and Usability Act (CERCLA): More popularly known as the "Superfund," it is a federal law passed in 1980 that authorized $1.6 billion over 5 years for a comprehensive program to clean up the worst abandoned or inactive waste sites in the nation. CERCLA funds used to establish and administer the cleanup program are derived primarily from taxes on crude oil and 42 commercial chemicals. CERCLA was amended and extended in 1986.

Comprehensive Health Planning and Public Health Services Amendments of 1966 (CHP): Landmark legislation that emphasized regional planning; the first time each person's "right to health care" was acknowledged.

comprehensive primary health care center: A center that provides multiple and complete health care services such as community outreach, physical and mental/behavioral health care, linkages to specialized health care and social support, health education, screening, immunizations, home visiting, child care, and policy development.

comprehensive services: Services that completely meet an individual's or family's needs.

compromise: An agreement between two or more people or groups with goals that cannot be met without modification of the positions of each person or group; implies "give and take" in the negotiating process.

concept: A category or class of objects or phenomena that represents either an abstract version of the real world (e.g., an ideal) or a concrete idea (e.g., a chair or bench).

conceptual framework: A group of concepts and a set of propositions that spells out the relationships between them.

conceptual model: A set of concepts and the assumptions that integrate them into a meaningful configuration.

concurrent audit: A method of evaluating quality of ongoing care through appraisal of the nursing process.

confidentiality: Information kept private, such as between health care provider and client.

conflict: Difference in perception, opinion, or priorities between people; can be spoken or unspoken.

conflict resolution: Methods of handling conflict between individuals or groups. Some methods may lead to desirable outcomes for all parties, for only some parties, or for none of the parties involved.

confounding: A bias that results from the relation of both the outcome and study factor (exposure or characteristic) with some third factor not accounted.

confrontation intervention mode: Consultant intervention mode that provides for presentation of ideas and facts to the client and reveals the client's values and assumptions that cannot be disputed.

congenital disability: A disability that has existed since birth. Do not use the term *birth defect;* the word "defect" is not a synonym of "disability."

congregants: People of the congregation of a church.

congregational model: An individual community of faith where the nurse is accountable to the congregation and its governing body.

constituency: A group or body that patronizes, supports, or offers representation.

constituents: Clients, individuals, families, peers, groups, or communities represented by another person(s).

constitutional law: Branch of law dealing with organization and function of government.

constructs: Conceptual components that are not directly observable; deliberately created ideas or references that cannot be seen but allow for explanation and analysis.

consultant: One who provides professional advice, services, or information.

consultation: Interactional or communication process between two or more persons; one is a consultant, the other is the consultee. The consultant seeks to help the consultee solve a problem or improve or broaden skills.

consultative contract: A working agreement between the consultant and consultee for services provided by the consultant. The contract stipulates the responsibilities held by both the consultant and the consultee.

consultee: Person seeking the help of an outside, usually impartial, person in problem resolution.

consumer: The recipient of health care. Primary clients are the current or former recipients of care; secondary consumers are the client's family or significant others.

consumer advocacy: A group dedicated to the protection of the rights of consumers, particularly those of people with mental illness.

consumerism: Organized movement and commitment to the belief that people have both a right and a responsibility to be knowledgeable about the choices they make for health and illness care.

consumer price index: The basic indicator of inflation—a measurement of inflation by comparison of prices overall and of categories of consumed goods and services purchased by urban wage earners and their families over a certain period of time.

contaminant: Any biologic, chemical, or radiologic substance or matter that has an adverse effect on air, water, or soil.

continuous quality improvement: An approach to managing quality that emphasizes continual improvement in real time, empowering employees to manage quality themselves, including client and family perceptions of quality, and making changes in organizational systems to better enable workers to provide high-quality services.

contract: A promissory agreement between two or more persons that creates, modifies, or destroys a legal relation. It is a legally enforceable promise between two or more persons to do or not to do something.

contracting: Developing any working agreement, continuously renegotiable and agreed upon by nurse and client.

Controlled Substances Act of 1970: A federal law that regulates psychoactive plants and chemicals. It provides for five levels of control, or Schedules, with Schedule I being the most restricted, including such drugs as heroin, mescaline, LSD, and marijuana.

cooperation: Working together or associating with others for common benefit, a common effort.

coordination: Conscious activity of assembling and directing the work efforts of a group of health providers so that they can function harmoniously in the attainment of the objective of client care.

core metropolitan: Densely populated counties with more than 1 million inhabitants.

cost-accounting studies: Studies finding the actual budgetary cost of a program, procedure, or technique.

cost-benefit studies: Studies assessing the desirability of a program, procedure, or technique by placing a specific quantifiable value (a dollar amount) on all costs and benefits of the variable to be evaluated.

cost effectiveness: Cost of resources to produce and allocate interventions/health services that are beneficial and result in desired outcomes.

cost-effectiveness analysis: Compares alternative approaches for achieving the same goals between two or more interventions.

cost-effectiveness studies: Studies measuring the quality of a program, procedure, or technique relative to cost.

cost-efficiency studies: Studies analyzing the actual costs of performing a number of services at different volumes when the same standards are applied.

cost-plus reimbursement: Method of payment whereby an agency receives actual costs of services delivered plus added allowable expenses, such as depreciation of facilities and equipment and administrative costs.

cost shifting: The process of making up for revenue lost when caring for the uninsured by charging more to those who are able to pay.

cottage industry: An industry whose labor force is small or may consist of family units working at home with their own equipment. A single-purpose industry.

counseling: Helping people achieve workable solutions for their problems or conflicts.

credentialing: A mechanism that seeks to produce performance of acceptable quality by individuals and programs of education and service. The four fundamental features of credentialing are quality, identify, protection, and control.

crisis poverty: A situation of hardship and struggle; may be transient or episodic. Can result from lack of employment, lack of education, domestic violence, or similar issues. These issues can lead to persistent poverty.

critical path method (CPM): A planning technique that focuses on activities, best use of time and resources, and estimated time to complete activities. The technique can be used for planning programs or individual client care as it is related to a specific diagnosis.

critical theory: A theory that approaches learning as an ongoing dialogue. The process of discourse ultimately changes thinking and behavior.

cross-sectional study: An epidemiologic study in which health outcomes and exposures or characteristics of interest are simultaneously ascertained and examined for association in a population or sample, providing a picture of existing levels of all factors.

cross-tolerance: Condition in which tolerance to one drug results in a lessened response to another drug in the same general category.

crude rates: Statistical rates in which the events in the numerator and the denominator refer to the entire population.

cultural accommodation: Negotiation with clients to include aspects of their folk practices with the traditional health care system to implement essential treatment plans.

cultural assessment: A systematic identification of the culture care beliefs, meanings, symbols, and practices of individuals or groups within a holistic perspective, including the worldview, life experiences, environmental context, ethnohistory and social structure factors.

cultural attitudes: The beliefs and perspectives that a society values.

cultural awareness: An appreciation of and sensitivity to a client's values, beliefs, practices, life-style and problem-solving strategies.

cultural blindness: When differences between cultures are ignored and persons act as though these differences do not exist.

cultural brokering: Advocating, mediating, negotiating, and intervening on behalf of the client between the health care culture and the client's culture.

cultural competence: An interplay of factors that motivate persons to develop knowledge, skill, and ability to care for others.

cultural conflict: A perceived threat that may arise from a misunderstanding of expectations between clients and nurses when neither is aware of their cultural differences.

cultural differences: Differences that derive from cultural aspects.

cultural encounter: Interactions with clients related to all aspects of their lives.

cultural imposition: The process of imposing one's values on others.

cultural knowledge: The information necessary to provide nurses with an understanding of the organizational elements of cultures and to provide effective nursing care.

cultural preservation: Use by clients of those aspects of their culture that promote healthy behaviors.

cultural relativism: The value of the culture as defined by its meaning to its members.

cultural repatterning: Working with clients to make changes in health practices when the client's cultural behaviors are harmful or decrease their wellbeing.

cultural sensitivity: Appreciation for and receptiveness to another's cultural heritage and values.

cultural skill: The effective integration of cultural knowledge and awareness to meet client needs.

cultural values: The prevailing and persistent guides influencing thinking and actions of people within a culture.

culturally sensitive communication: Communication that recognizes the cultural meanings and values of multiple ways of communicating. Community health nurses that practice culturally sensitive communication are sensitive to diverse interpretations at a minimum and, ideally, develop ways of communicating that the receiver of the communication understands and is comfortable with.

culturally sensitive health education strategies: Strategies that are based on respect for cultural diversity and demonstrate that the culture of the participants is respected.

culture: The learned ways of behaving that are communicated by one group to another in order to provide tested solutions to vital problems.

culture-bound illnesses: Illnesses specific to a particular culture (e.g., mal ojo [evil eye] in the Mexican-American culture).

culture change: The constant process of adding or deleting elements within a culture, such as language, customs, beliefs, attitudes, values, goals, laws, traditions, and moral codes.

culture of poverty: A status not merely of economic deprivation but also entailing personality traits passed from one generation to another.

culture shock: Feelings of helplessness, discomfort, and disorientation experienced by a person attempting to understand or effectively adapt to a different cultural group because of dissimilarities in practices, values, and beliefs.

cumulative risks: The additive effects of multiple risk factors

cycle of vulnerability: The feedback effect of factors that predispose one to vulnerability and lead to negative health outcomes, which then increase the predisposing factors and so on.

D

database: Collection of gathered and generated data.

data collection: The process of acquiring existing information or developing new information.

data gathering: The process of obtaining existing, readily available data.

data generation: The development of data, frequently qualitative rather than numerical, by the data collector.

data interpretation: The process of analyzing and synthesizing data, which culminates in the identification of community health problems and strengths.

data management: A method of collecting, organizing, and prioritizing information to use in resolving client problems.

death rates: A statistical indicator comparing the number of deaths to the total population.

Declaration of Alma Ata: A resolution first adopted by the 30th World Health Organization (WHO) Health Assembly in 1977 that accepted the goal of attaining a level of health that permitted all citizens of the world to live socially and economically productive lives. In 1978 at the international conference in Alma Ata, USSR, it was determined that this goal was to be met through primary health care. This resolution has become known as the slogan "Health for All (HFA) by the Year 2000" and captured the official health target for all of the member nations of the WHO.

deductive approach: The reasoning process of developing specific predictions or ideas from general principles.

deinstitutionalization: Effort to move long-term psychiatric patients out of the hospital and back into their own community.

delayed stress reaction: Stress that occurs after a disaster that is related to the disaster; workers' feelings of exhaustion; frustration and guilt over not having been able to do more; disappointment from family and friends who don't seem as interested in what the worker has been through; and a general inability to adjust to the slower pace of work and home.

delegation: Sharing responsibility for a task with another who is competent to perform the task. The person who delegates the task retains responsibility and ultimate accountability for the effective completion of the task.

demand: Willingness, ability, and desire to purchase a commodity or service.

demand management: A program which provides to consumers, at the point at which they are deciding how to enter the health care system, information and support to access care. A telephone clinical triage system is an activity in which nurses talk to clients about their presenting problem and provide advice and coordination of care.

demographic trends: Population trends related to age at first marriage; fertility patterns; birth rates; numbers of individuals engaging in singlehood, divorce, and remarriage; number of dependent children experiencing divorce, life with a never-married parent; and the number of persons in specific age categories.

denial: A primary symptom of addiction. The person may lie about use, play down use, and blame; also may use anger or humor to avoid acknowledging the problem to self and others.

deontology: Doctrine that moral duty or obligation is binding; also: what makes acts right are nonconsequential characteristics such as fidelity, veracity, justice, and honesty.

depressants: Drugs that reduce the activity of the central nervous system.

dermal absorption: Absorption through the skin.

descriptive epidemiology: An epidemiologic study designed to describe the distribution of health outcomes according to person, place, and time.

determinants: Factors that influence the risk for or distribution of health outcomes.

detoxification: Process of allowing time for the body to metabolize and/or excrete accumulations of a drug. Often called *social* detoxification if the withdrawal symptoms are not life-threatening and do not require medication, or *medical* detoxification if the symptoms require medical management.

developed country: A country with a stable economy and a wide range of industrial and technologic development, such as the United States, Canada, Japan, the United Kingdom, Sweden, and France.

development: Increase in complexity of the function and progression of physical, social, and mental skills throughout life.

developmental disability: Any mental or physical disability manifested before the age of 22 that may continue indefinitely and result in substantial limitation in three or more of the following life activities: self-care, receptive and expressive language, learning mobility, self-direction, independent living, economic sufficiency.

developmental theory: A theory that maintains that learning occurs in concert with developmental stages. Readiness to learn depends on the individual's developmental stage.

diagnosis-related groups (DRGs): A client classification scheme that defines 468 illness categories and the corresponding health care services that are reimbursable under Medicare.

differential vulnerability hypothesis: Vulnerable population groups are those who are not only particularly sensitive to risk factors but also possess multiple, cumulative risk factors.

digital rectal examination: A procedure used to assess the condition of the prostate and rectum; generally used for early detection of cancer.

dilution: The act of making thinner or more liquid or reducing the strength or flavor by mixing with another substance.

disability: A physical or mental impairment that substantially limits a person in some major life activity, such as walking, talking, breathing, or working; has a record of such an impairment; and/or is regarded as being "disabled."

disability-adjusted life years: An economic term that measures the years of loss of healthy life that is a result of disability.

disadvantaged: Lacking in the basic resources or conditions believed to be necessary for an equal position in society.

disaster: Any man-made or natural event that causes destruction and devastation *that* cannot be alleviated without assistance.

disaster action team: A group of specially trained persons who can assist communities in implementing their disaster plans.

disaster medical assistance teams (DMAT): A team consisting of approximately 30 volunteers including physicians, nurses, and other allied health personnel who train as a group to perform specific emergency functions during a disaster. Upon activation of the National Disaster Medical System, each member becomes an automatic and temporary employee of the U.S. Public Health Service.

disaster planning: The process of developing organized actions to prevent or minimize injuries or deaths of workers or residents, and property damage. To effectively triage and facilitate the resumption of normal activities.

discharge planning: The process of activities facilitating the client's movement from one setting to another. Discharge planning is a process that enhances continuity of care.

disease: An indication of a physiological dysfunction or a pathological reaction to an infection.

disease/illness prevention: Behavior directed toward reducing the threat of illness, disease, or complications.

disease management: A proactive treatment approach focused on a specific diagnosis that seeks to manage a chronic health condition and minimize acute episodes in a population.

disease self-management: Self-care practices of individuals with a chronic condition done in an effort to influence their comfort, ability to function, and other illness outcomes.

disenfranchisement: A sense of social isolation; a feeling of separation from mainstream society.

distribution: The pattern of a health outcome in a population; the frequencies of the outcome according to various personal characteristics, geographic regions, and time.

distribution effects: The effects that a policy may have on people other than those for which it was intended.

distributive care: Health care services that emphasize health promotion, maintenance, and disease prevention.

distributive outcomes: An outcome in which one person enlarges their share at another person's expense.

district nursing: Early public health nursing whereby a nurse was assigned to each district in a town to provide home health care to needy people.

Division of Adolescent and School Health (DASH): Part of The Centers for Disease Control and Prevention. They define school health according to eight components.

Division of Nursing: A component of the Public Health Service, part of the Health Resources and Services Administration, which oversees nursing education and special nursing demonstration projects in the United States.

documentation: The process of recording data in client records.

dose: Standard amount.

drug addiction: A pattern of abuse characterized by an overwhelming preoccupation with the use (compulsive use) of a drug, securing its supply, and a high tendency for relapse if the drug is removed.

drug dependence: A state of neuroadaptation (a physiologic change in the central nervous system) caused by the chronic, regular administration of a drug in which continued use of the drug becomes necessary to prevent withdrawal symptoms.

dysfunctional family: A family unit that inhibits clear communication within family relationships and does not provide psychologic support for individual members.

E

early adopters: Individuals and/or groups with cosmopolitan rather than local orientations, with abilities to adopt new ideas from mass media rather than face-to-face information sources, and with specialized rather than global interests.

Early Periodic Screening Diagnosis and Treatment Program (EPSDT): A special screening for preschool children that is funded through Medicaid and gives medical assistance to needy families with dependent children.

ecologic fallacy: A bias that may occur in ecologic studies because associations observed at the group level may not hold true for the individuals that compose the groups, or associations that actually exist may be masked.

ecologic studies: An epidemiologic study in which only aggregate or group data, such as population rates, are used rather than data on individuals.

ecology: The science of the relationship between living and nonliving things; concerned with both structure and function.

economic growth: An increase in the output of a nation.

economics: Social science concerned with the problems of using or administering scarce resources in the most efficient way to attain maximum fulfillment of society's unlimited wants.

ecosystem: All living things and nonliving parts that support a chain of life within a selected area.

educator: A nurse in advanced practice may function in several indirect nursing care roles, such as teaching and faculty.

effectiveness: A measure of an organization's performance as compared to its philosophy, goals, and objectives.

efficiency: The process of meeting goals in a way that minimizes costs and maximizes benefits.

effluent: Wastewater, treated or untreated, that flows out of a treatment plant, sewer, or industrial outfall. Generally refers to waste discharged into surface waters.

egalitarian theory: A theory of justice that holds that the distribution of goods in the community takes the needs of all citizens into account equally.

elder abuse: A form of family violence against older members. May include neglect and failure to provide adequate food, clothing, shelter, and physical and safety needs; can also include roughness in care and actual violent behavior toward the elderly.

elimination: Focuses on removing a disease from a large geographic area such as a country or region of the world.

Elizabethan poor laws: Laws during the reign of Queen Elizabeth I of England that address poverty and assistance measures.

emergency support functions: Activities that must be carried out as part of the Federal Response Plan by each of 26 federal agencies and the American Red Cross.

emerging infectious diseases: Diseases in which the incidence has increased in the past 2 decades or has the potential to increase in the near future.

emotional abuse: Extreme debasement of a person's feelings so that he or she feels inept, uncared for, and worthless.

emotional neglect: The omission of the basic nurturing, acceptance, and caring essential for healthy personal development.

employee assistance programs: The range of services offered in the workplace to assist employees to cope with personal and work-related problems.

empowerment: Helping people acquire the skills and information necessary for informed decision making and ensuring that they have the authority to make decisions that affect them.

enabling: The act of shielding or preventing the addict from experiencing the consequences of the addiction. Also applies to shielding individuals from the consequences of their actions more generally.

enabling legislation: A bill or law passed by Congress to support the development of a specific program or service.

enculturation: The process of acquiring knowledge and internalizing values or learning about a culture.

endemic: The constant presence of an infectious disease within a specific geographic area.

enforcement: The act of obtaining by force.

enrollee: Someone who is in a managed care organization.

entitlement theory: Theory that people have rights to resources as determined by the natural lottery and may increase their possessions in any way possible (by purchase, gift, or legitimate exchange), as long as they do not cheat others or acquire the possessions in an unjust manner.

entropy: A concept stating that elements in a closed environment will proceed toward greater randomness or less order.

environment: All of those factors internal and external to the client that constitute the context in which the client lives and that influence and are influenced by the host and agent-host interactions. The sum of all external conditions affecting the life, development, and survival of an organism.

environmental health: Aspect of community health concerned with those forms of life, substances, forces, and conditions in the surroundings of people that may exert an influence on their health and well-being. The study of environmental conditions in relation to human health.

environmental impact statement: A document required of federal agencies by the National Environmental Policy Act for major projects or legislative proposals significantly affecting the environment. The statement, which is a tool for decision making, describes the positive and negative potential effects of the undertaking and lists other actions.

environmental media: An element of the environment, such as air, water, or soil.

Environmental Protection Agency (EPA): Established in 1970 to be responsible for air, water, and land pollution control; never achieved its full goal.

epidemic: The occurrence of an infectious agent or disease within a specific geographic area in greater numbers than would normally be expected.

epidemiologic triad: Infectious agent, host, and environment.

epidemiology: The study of the distribution of states of health and of the causes of deviations from health in populations and the application of this study to control the health problems.

episodic care: Curative and restorative aspect of nursing practice.

episodically homeless: Frequently being without permanent shelter.

equalitarian theory: Doctrine that takes the needs of all people into account equally.

equity: Providing accessible services to promote the health of populations most at risk to health problems.

eradication: The irreversible termination of all transmission of infection by extermination of the infectious agents worldwide.

ergonomic agent: Agents that cause mechanical strain on the body resulting in illness (e.g., vibrations).

ergonomics: The study of people at work in order to understand the complex relationships associated with work.

established group: An existing group of persons linked by membership and group purpose.

estimation of risk: Assessing the nature of a problem, size of the problem, and need for a program within a community to prevent occurrence of the problem.

estrogen replacement therapy: Single hormone estrogen used for women who have had a hysterectomy.

estuaries: Areas where fresh water meets salt water. Examples include bays, mouths of rivers, salt marshes, and lagoons. Estuaries are delicate ecosystems. They serve as nurseries, spawning and feeding grounds for large groups of marine life, and provide shelter and food for birds and wildlife.

ethical decision making: Making decisions in an orderly process that considers ethical principles, client values, and professional obligations.

ethical principles: Abstract guides that serve as foundations for moral rules.

ethical theories: Collection of principles and rules providing theoretic foundations for deciding what to do when moral principles or rules conflict.

ethics: The science or study of moral values; also, a code of principles and ideals that guide action.

ethnicity: Shared feeling of peoplehood among a group of individuals.

ethnocentrism: Belief that one's own group or culture is superior to others.

eudaimonistic model of health: A model in which health is viewed as maximizing individual and family well-being and potential.

evaluation: Provision of information through formal means, such as criteria, measurement, and statistics, for making rational judgments necessary about outcomes of care.

evaluation of program effectiveness: Examination of the level of client and provider satisfaction with a program.

evaluative research: A method of collecting information according to the rigors of scientific inquiry for the purpose of evaluating the long-term effect of a program.

evaluative studies: Systematic method for collecting information to assess the relevance, progress, effectiveness, efficiency, and impact of a program.

exclusion order: An unimmunized student is given this when he or she is not in compliance with the immunization law.

experimental epidemiology: Third stage of epidemiologic investigation, which uses experimental design for studies to confirm the causal nature of relationships identified through observational studies.

exposure: The intake into the body of a hazardous pollutant. The primary routes of exposure to substances are through the skin, mouth, and lungs.

exposure pathway: The process by which an individual is exposed to contaminants that originate from some source of contamination.

external consultant: A nurse who is employed temporarily on a contractual basis by the client.

F

facilitator: One who provides an environment in which the client is assisted in meeting health care needs and is a participant in decision making.

faith communities: Congregational communities that gather in churches, cathedrals, synagogues, or mosques and acknowledge faith traditions.

familialism: A culture belief that family needs take priority over individual needs.

family: Two or more individuals coming from the same or different kinship groups who are involved in a continuous living arrangement, usually residing in the same household, experiencing common emotional bonds, and sharing certain obligations toward each other and toward others.

family assessment: Systematic collection, classification, and analysis of family data for the purpose of identifying the family's health-related strengths and problems.

family caregiving: Assisting the client to meet his or her basic needs and providing direct care such as personal hygiene, meal preparation, medication administration, and treatments.

family-centered care: A care arrangement enabling families to assume the role of advocates, decision makers, and caregivers.

family crisis: A situation whereby the demands of the situation exceed the resources and coping capacity of the family.

family demography: The study of the structure of families and households and the family-related events, such as marriage and divorce, that alter the structure through the number, timing, and sequence of the events.

family developmental framework: A model that assumes that family development follows orderly, sequential changes throughout the family's lifespan.

family developmental task: A growth responsibility that arises at a certain stage in the life of a family, the successful achievement of which leads to satisfaction, approval, and success with later tasks.

family dynamics: Interactions and relationships within the family that influence the work of the family and its ability to complete its functions and tasks.

family functions: Behaviors or activities performed to maintain the integrity of the family unit and to meet the family's needs, individual members' needs, and society's expectations.

family health: A condition including the promotion and maintenance of physical, mental, spiritual, and social health for the family unit and for individual family members.

family health risks: Those factors that predispose or increase the family's likelihood of ill health.

family life cycle: A developmental theory that divides family life into a series of stages or phases over time. The stages are qualitatively and quantitatively different from the preceding and succeeding stages.

family nurse practitioner/clinician: A registered nurse with additional education through a master's degree program in nursing or a nondegree or certificate continuing education program preparing the nurse to deliver primary health care to individuals, groups, and communities of all ages.

family planning nurse practitioner (obstetric/gynecologic nurse practitioner): A registered nurse with additional education through a master's degree program in nursing or a nondegree or certificate continuing education program preparing the nurse to deliver obstetric and gynecologic primary care to women.

family resource/service centers: School and community resources for families that are consolidated into one agency for the sake of efficiency and reducing costs.

family roles: Behaviors assumed by family members to maintain the organizational structure of the family and to define the division of labor and the family processes.

family self-care: A decision-making process that involves the family in self-observation, symptom perception and labeling, judgment of severity, and choice and assessment of treatment options.

family strengths: Those factors or forces that contribute to family unity and solidarity and foster the development of the potentials inherent within the family.

family structure (configuration): Refers to the characteristics of the individual members (gender, age, number) who constitute the family unit.

farm residency: Residence outside area zoned as "city limits"; usually infers involvement in agriculture industry.

Federal Emergency Management Agency (FEMA): The government agency responsible for directing the federal response to disasters.

Federal Income Poverty Guidelines: A definition of poverty drafted by the Social Security Administration in 1964. The federal government defines poverty in terms of income, family size, the age of the head of household, and the number of children under 18 years of age. The guidelines change annually to be consistent with the consumer price index.

federal poverty level: The income level for a certain family size that the federal government uses to define poverty.

Federal Register: A legal document in which all U.S. government–proposed new regulations are published.

federal response plan: A federal emergency response system that may become activated when a disaster is assumed to overwhelm the capability of state and local governments to carry out the extensive emergency operations necessary to save lives and protect property. Twenty-six federal agencies and the American Red Cross are responsible for coordinating efforts in a particular area with all of its designated support agencies.

feedback: Process in which the output of a system is returned as input to the same system.

fee-for-service: List of health care services with monetary or unit values attached that specifies the amounts third parties must pay for specific services.

fetal alcohol syndrome: A condition that may occur when a woman has consumed alcohol regularly during pregnancy (about six drinks per day). Infants tend to be of low birth weight and mentally retarded and may have behavioral, facial, limb, genital, cardiac, or neurologic impairments.

fiscal intermediaries: Insurance companies under contract to the Social Security Administration to pay home care agencies for Medicare-covered services rendered to beneficiaries.

flexible lines of defense: In the Neuman Systems Model, the outer concentric ring, which characterizes an open system that exchanges energy with the environment.

focus of care: The foci of care in the integrative model include health promotion, illness (disease or disability) prevention, and illness care.

forensic: Pertaining to the law.

formal group: Persons having a defined membership and specified purpose. The group may or may not have an official or public place in the community's organization.

formal structure: The established power and communication relationships within an organization.

formative evaluation: An ongoing evaluation instituted for the purpose of assessing the degree to which objectives are met or activities are being conducted.

fossil fuels: Coal, oil, and natural gas, so-called because they are derived from the remains of ancient plant and animal life.

frontier: Regions having fewer than six persons per square mile.

Frontier Nursing Service: A rural nursing service founded by Mary Breckinridge in Kentucky in the early 1900s. It led to the development of other rural public health programs.

functional family: A family unit that provides autonomy and is responsive to the particular interests and needs of individual family members.

G

general systems theory: As defined by von Bertalantfy, a complex of elements in mutual interaction. The elements are wholeness, organization, and order.

generative leadership: Leadership that results in the generation of new ideas and new ways of working together.

genital herpes: A virus that attacks genitalia and sacral nerves. Infection is characterized by painful lesions that present as vesicles and progress to ulcerations on the male and female genitalia, buttocks, or upper thighs.

genital warts: Lesions caused by the human papillomavirus.

gentrification: Move to upgrade urban housing.

gerontology: A field of study that explores the biopsychosocial issues of aging.

global burden of disease: A world wide mortality indicator (death rate) that combines premature deaths and losses of healthy life that result from disability.

goal: The end or terminal point toward which intervention efforts are directed.

goal attainment: A process for assessing the efficacy of a program by examination or measurement of predetermined goals.

goals/objectives: A consultative problem that involves the inability of a group or individual to accept new goals, change goals, or meet established goals.

gonorrhea: A sexually transmitted disease caused by a bacteria, *Neisseria gonorrhoeae*, usually resulting in inflammation of the urethra and cervix and dysuria, although it may result in no symptoms.

government: The ultimate authority in society, designated to enforce the policy whether it is related to health, education, economics, social welfare, or any other societal issue.

government organizations: Organizations that enter into bilateral agreements with organizations in other countries, most often between less-developed countries and more economically advanced countries.

grant: A source of public funds paid by a central to a local government in aid of a public undertaking.

gross domestic product (GDP): A statistical measure used to compare health care spending between countries.

gross national product (GNP): The total value of all final goods and services produced in the United States in 1 year.

ground water: The supply of fresh water under the surface of the earth that feeds springs, wells, and aquifers.

group: A collection of interacting individuals who have a common purpose or purposes.

group cohesion: Measurement of degree of attraction among members and toward the group.

group culture: A composite of the group norms that comes to dictate perceptions and behaviors.

group member: An individual who comes together with others to comprise a group.

group norms: Unwritten and often unspoken standards for group members that guide their behavior and influence their attitudes and perceptions.

group purpose: The reason two or more people come together; may be subtle or obvious and easily stated by members.

group structure: The particular arrangement of group parts that comprise the whole.

Growing Healthy: A curriculum for elementary grades that is a generalized program aimed at improving students' personal lifestyles.

growth: Increase in size of the whole or parts of an organism.

growth charts: Standardized tools that serve as norms to compare an individual's growth to a population.

gynecological age: Number of years from menarche.

H

half-life: The time it takes certain materials to lose half their strength.

hallucinogens (also known as psychedelics): Drugs that stimulate the nervous system and produce varied changes in perception and mood.

harm reduction (also called harm minimization): A public health approach to substance abuse problems. This approach acknowledges, without judgement, that licit and illicit drug use is a reality, and the focus of interventions is to minimize these drugs' harmful effects rather than to simply ignore or condemn them.

hazard communication standard: Known as the "right-to-know" law. This was developed since the working environments cannot eliminate all potentially toxic agents; therefore an important line of defense is an educated workforce.

Hazardous and Solid Waste Amendments: The federal law, passed in 1984, that amended the Resource Conservation and Recovery Act (RCRA) of 1976. The amendments changed the focus of waste management in many ways. HSWA required the EPA to focus on permitting land disposal facilities and eventually phasing out land disposal of some waste. It expanded the RCRA-regulated community to include businesses that generate small amounts of hazardous waste. HSWA also addressed previously exempted underground storage tanks containing petroleum and some other hazardous substances.

hazardous waste: By-products of society that can pose a substantial or potential hazard to human health or the environment when improperly disposed of or managed. Hazardous waste possesses at least one of four characteristics: it may ignite easily; it may be corrosive, capable of dissolving metals, other materials or burning the skin; it may be reactive or unstable, or may undergo rapid or violent chemical reactions with water or other materials; it may be toxic, capable of causing serious illness or other health problems.

hazardous waste landfill: A land disposal site for hazardous waste, Sites are selected to minimize the chance of release of hazardous waste into the environment. There are about 30 commercial hazardous waste landfills in the United States.

Head Start: An early childhood education program for children at risk for academic problems because of poverty and lack of sufficient social stimulation.

healing: Strengthening the inner spirit and choosing healthy lifestyles so that families and individuals can face life's circumstances.

health: Four models of health ordered from narrow to broad are: (1) clinical health, the absence of disease; (2) role-performance health, the ability to satisfactorily perform one's social roles; (3) adaptive health, flexible adaptation to the environment; and (4) eudaemonistic health, self-actualization and the attainment of one's greatest human potential.

health behavior: Any health-related action undertaken by a person to prevent or detect disease, protect health, or promote a higher level of health.

health belief model: Developed to provide a framework for understanding why some people take specific actions to avoid illness, whereas others fail to protect themselves.

health commodification: The buying and selling of health and health care products.

health economics: Branch of economics concerned with the problems of producing and distributing the health care resources of the nation in a way that provides maximum benefit to the most people.

health education: Any combination of learning experiences designed to facilitate adaptations of behavior conducive to health.

health field concept: A model of health that states that health results from the interactions between individual behavior, biology, the environment, and the health care system. Originally described by LaFramboise (1973) and expanded by Lalonde (1974) (both in Denver, 1988).

Health for All by the Year 2000 (HFA 2000) Agreement developed at Alma Alta conference that states that the major social goal for all World Health Assembly member agencies should be "the attainment by all citizens of the world by the year 2000 a level of health that will permit them to lead a socially and economically productive life" (WHO, 1986a, p. 65).

health hazards: Biologic, physical, chemical, or psychosocial threats to health that arise from the environment.

health index: A summary of the health features of a community that enables the determination of health care delivery needs.

health maintenance: Behavior directed toward keeping a current state of health.

health maintenance behavior: A behavior directed toward keeping a current state of health. Similar to tertiary prevention.

Health Maintenance Organization (HMO): Organized system of health care that provides a fixed fee for all needed health care services with an emphasis on primary care.

health ministries: Activities and programs in faith communities organized around health and healing foci to promote wholeness in health through life.

Health PACT: Health instruction intended to prepare children to communicate with health professionals during visits for health care.

health planning: A continuous social process by which data about a client are collected and evaluated for the purpose of creating a plan to guide change in health care delivery.

health policy: Public policy that affects health and health services. Delineates options from which individuals and organizations make their health-related choices. Made within a political context.

health professional shortage areas (HPSAs): Geographic areas that have insufficient numbers of health professionals according to criteria established by the federal government. Often a rural area where a doctor, nurse practitioner, or community health nurse often provides services to residents who live in several counties.

health program planning: Five-step process of formulation of plan, conceptualization, detailing, evaluation, and implementation.

health promotion: "The process of enabling people to increase control over, and to improve, their health" (Ottawa Charter, 1986, p. 1). Five major aspects of health promotion, in order of priority, are: building health-promoting public policy, creating supportive environments, strengthening community action, developing personal skills, and reorienting health services.

health promotion behavior: Behavior directed toward achieving a greater level of health.

health promotion model: Developed as a complement to other health-protecting models such as the health belief model. This model explains the likelihood that healthy lifestyle patterns or health-promoting behaviors will occur.

health risk appraisal: Process of identifying and analyzing an individual's prognostic characteristics of health and comparing them with those of a standard age group, thereby providing a prediction of a person's likelihood of prematurely developing the health problems that have high morbidity and mortality in this country.

health risk/health risk factor: Disease precursor whose presence is associated with higher-than-average morbidity and/or mortality. Disease precursors include demographic variables, certain individual behaviors, positive individual and/or family history, and some physiologic changes.

health risk reduction: Application of selected interventions to control or reduce risk factors and minimize the incidence of associated disease and premature mortality. Risk reduction is reflected in greater congruity between appraised and achievable ages.

health status: The state or level of health of an individual, family, or community at a given time.

Healthy Cities: An international movement of cities focused on mobilizing local resources and political, professional, and community members to improve the health of the community.

healthy city: A city whose priority is to improve its environment and expand its resources so that community members can support each other in achieving their highest potential.

Healthy People 2000: A government document that outlines the nation's health goals and objectives. The national health objectives were set through collaboration among government, voluntary, and professional organizations, businesses, and individuals as the means of providing access to "health for all" and improving health outcomes for Americans by the year 2000.

Healthy People 2010: The United States' health promotion and disease prevention agenda with outcome objectives to be achieved by the year 2010 and particularly emphasizing healthy communities, elimination of health disparities and increasing years of quality healthy life; represents consensus among government, voluntary and professional organizations, businesses, and individuals.

healthy public policy: Future-oriented health policies that deal with local and global health problems and issues that are based on an ecologic perspective with multisectoral and participatory strategies.

hepatitis: Inflammatory condition of the liver caused by viral or bacterial infection, parasites, alcohol, drugs, toxins, or transfusions of incompatible blood.

hepatitis B virus (HBV): A virus that is transmitted through exposure to body fluids. Infection results in a clinical picture that ranges from a self-limited acute infection to fulminant hepatitis or hepatic carcinoma, possibly leading to death.

herd immunity: Immunity of a group or community.

HFA 2000: The 1977 goal of the World Health Assembly of WHO of the attainment of a level of health for all world citizens that will permit them to lead socially and economically productive lives.

hidden homeless: Individuals who are not usually visible to members of a community because they may have shelter while they are in that community, but not on a permanent basis. Migrant workers are often among the hidden homeless.

Hill-Burton Act: First U.S. legislation to focus on planning as a major area of concern. Its primary purpose was to provide for a more equal distribution of hospitals across the nation by matching federal funds for one third to two thirds of the total cost of a facility.

historical factors: Historical acts, ideas, and events that have shaped current attitudes.

HIV antibody test: Enzyme linked immunosorbent assay (ELISA) is the test commonly used in screening blood for the antibody to HIV; the Western Blot is used as a confirmatory test.

HIV disease: A disease involving a defect in cell-mediated immunity that is caused by HIV and has a spectrum of clinical expressions that includes AIDS and other symptoms not included in the clinical definition of AIDS.

HIV infection: Infection with the human immunodeficiency virus. A phase of this infection is subclinical, but infected individuals remain capable of transmitting the virus through specific behaviors.

HIV seronegative/HIV seropositive: Blood serum showing a positive or negative result to a specific test.

HIV seroprevalence: The number of new and old cases of persons in the United States identified with human immunodeficiency virus in their blood.

HMO Act: Legislation enacted in 1973 to provide a demonstration program for the development of health maintenance organizations.

holistic care: Understanding the changes of the body, mind, and spirit of the congregation as a whole in an environment that is always changing.

holistic health centers: A comprehensive team that includes family and clergy that encourages personal responsibility for health and preventive health practices.

home health agency: An organization that provides skilled nursing and other related skills in the home.

homeless child syndrome: Combination of the effects of homelessness on children resulting in health problems, environmental dangers, and stress.

homeless: The federal government defines a homeless person as one who lacks a fixed, regular, and adequate address or has a primary nighttime residence in a supervised publicly or privately operated shelter for temporary accommodations.

home visits: Provision of community health nursing care where the individual resides.

homicide: A killing of one human being by another.

homophobia: An unfounded fear or hatred of lesbians and gays.

horizontal transmission: Person-to-person spread of infection through one or more of the following routes: direct/indirect contact, common vehicle, airborne, or vectorborne.

hormone replacement therapy (HRT): Hormone combination of estrogen and progesterone used for postmenopausal women who have not had a hysterectomy.

hospice: Palliative system of health care for terminally ill people; takes place in the home with family involvement under the direction and supervision of health professionals, especially the visiting nurse. Hospice care takes place in the hospital when severe complications of terminal illness occur or when there is family exhaustion or loss of commitment.

host: A living organism, human or animal, in which an infectious agent can exist under natural conditions.

household: A single dwelling (apartment or house) occupied by an individual or a group of two or more individuals (related or untreated).

human capital: The combined human potential of the people living in a community.

human immunodeficiency virus (HIV): The virus that causes AIDS and HIV disease.

human papillomavirus infection (HPV): A sexually transmitted disease that results in genital warts (condyloma acuminata) that grow in the vulva, vagina, cervix, urinary meatus, scrotum, or perianal area. A link exists between HPV infections and cancer.

human subject review committees: Groups of representatives of various disciplines or departments brought together to review research proposals. Their major concerns are protecting human research participants from physical or mental harm, as well as protecting the researcher from undue complaints.

humanist theory: A theory that describes the influence that feelings, emotions, and personal relationships have on behavior. If people are given free choice, they will do what is best for themselves.

hypothesis: A supposition or question that is raised to explain an event or guide investigation.

I

ICD-9: International classification of disease that contains codes to help record health problems.

illness prevention: Behavior directed toward reducing the threat of illness or disease.

immune globulin (IG): Sterile solution containing antibodies from human blood. IG is primarily indicated for routine maintenance of certain immunodeficient individuals and for passive immunization.

immunity: Natural or acquired ability to ward off disease.

immunization: A process of protecting an individual from a disease through introduction of a live, killed, or partial component of the invading organism into the individual's system.

impairment: A disturbance in structure or function resulting from anatomic, physiologic, and/or psychologic abnormalities.

implementation: Carrying out a plan that is based on careful assessment of need.

incest: Sexual abuse among family members, typically a parent and a child.

incidence rate: The frequency or rate of new cases of an outcome in a population; provides an estimate of the risk of disease in that population over the period of observation.

incineration: A treatment technology involving destruction of waste by controlled burning at high temperatures.

incubation period: The time between first contact with an infectious agent and the first appearance of clinical signs of the resultant disease.

independent practice: Private practice of a professional who works independently from other professionals.

Individuals with Disabilities Education Act (IDEA): A federal law that guarantees a free public education and related services for every disabled child from 5 to 21 years of age.

individualized education plan (IEP): An evaluation prepared by the school staff for each student that is reviewed and modified at regular intervals during the school year and throughout the student's school experience.

individualized family service plans (IFSP): An early intervention program to prepare the infant/toddler/preschooler for school that is developed by an interdisciplinary team along with the parents.

inductive approach: The reasoning process of developing general rules or ideas from specific observations.

infancy: One month of age through 12 months.

infant stimulation: Activities to encourage development of the infant, such as cognitive, emotional, and social development.

infection: The state produced by the invasion of a host by an infectious agent. Such infection may or may not produce clinical signs.

infectiousness: A measure of the potential ability of an infected host to transmit the infection to other hosts.

inflation: A sustained upward trend in the prices of goods and services.

informal caregiver: A voluntary caregiver who may or may not be related to the client. This caregiver usually does not receive payment for the caregiving services rendered but may actually give care more hours of the day than the formal (professional or ancillary) health care worker.

informal group: A group whose membership and purposes are not articulated but are understood by members.

informal structure: The way people actually work together; it includes informal communication patterns, informal sources of power, and unwritten rules of conduct.

informant interviews: Directed conversation with selected members of a community about community members or groups and events; a direct method of assessment.

information management: The management of the accumulation and distribution of information through electronic means.

informed consent: The client agrees to a treatment plan after receiving sufficient information concerning the proposal, its incumbent risks, and the acceptable alternatives.

informing: A communication process in which the nurse interprets facts and shares knowledge with clients.

ingestion: The act of taking in for or as if for digestion.

inhalants: Category of gases and solvents that are inhaled to produce a psychoactive effect.

inhalation: The act of drawing in by breathing.

injection drug user: Includes intravenous and subcutaneous drug injection, with the latter usually being over the abdominal area and called "popping." The sharing of paraphernalia to prepare or inject the drug can result in transmission of bloodborne pathogens, such as HIV.

institutional licensure: A mechanism for allowing employing agencies to be responsible for the competence of the people they hire.

institutional models: A nurse that is in a larger partnership. His/her contract would be with hospitals, medical centers, long-term care facilities, or educational institutions.

institutional privileges: Rights and responsibilities awarded to a nurse not employed by the agency to practice autonomously in the agency.

instrumental activities of daily living: Those activities of daily living that help individuals manage their lives, such as cooking, shopping, paying bills, cleaning house, and using the telephone.

integrated system: A system of care delivery that provides linkages between a variety of health care providers and agencies.

integrative outcomes: An outcome in which mutual advantages override individual gains.

interacting group: A cluster of individuals who are linked by personal relationships. The links may be either primary, such as in a family, or secondary, such as in a voluntary association.

Interagency Council on the Homeless: A council composed of the heads of 16 federal agencies that have programs or activities for the homeless; created by the Stewart B. McKinney Act to coordinate and direct federal homeless activities.

intercessor: One who acts on behalf of the client when the client could act for self.

interdependent: The involvement between different groups or organizations within the community that are mutually reliant upon each other.

interdisciplinary: Activities involving the collaboration among personnel representing different disciplines (occupational therapists, nurses, physical therapists, physicians, environmental hygienists, and so on).

interdisciplinary collaboration: Each home health care provider carefully analyzes their role in determining the best plan for the client's care.

intergovernmental organizations: Those agencies supported by more than one nation's government, e.g., WHO.

intermediate criteria: Incremental incidents that serve to monitor progress toward outcomes.

intermittent care: Clients who are confined to home and required skilled care for one of the following: speech therapy, physical therapy, or occupational therapy. The amount of time could range from 28 or 35 hrs per week to full-time services.

internal consultant: A nurse who is employed on a full-time salaried basis by a community agency in which the consultation takes place.

international cooperation: Health promotion efforts that transcend national borders to ensure that all individuals have access to accessible, affordable, acceptable health care that incorporates community participation in achieving social, physical, and mental health.

intervention: Means or strategies by which objectives are achieved and change is effected.

iterative assessment process: Obtaining only as much assessment data as necessary at one time, then obtaining additional data as it is needed.

J

joint practice: A nurse practitioner (NP) and physician work together as a team, sharing the responsibility for a client.

judicial law: Law based on court or jury decisions.

justice: Ethical principle that claims that equals should be treated equally and those who are unequal should be treated differently according to their differences.

K

key informants: Professional experts, community leaders, politicians, and entrepreneurs who are in touch with the needs of the community and who are in positions to support new community programs.

Know Your Body: A course that focuses on making students aware of their own cardiovascular risk factors through screening activities followed by special instruction related to risk reduction.

knowledge: That which we know; our range of information.

L

landfilling: Burial of waste in the soil.

land use planning: Authority for planning and zoning of land use to promote livable and sustainable communities and minimize waste.

late adopters: Individuals and/or groups who are the last to embrace change.

law: The sum total of man-made rules and regulations by which society is governed in a formal and legally binding manner.

lay advisors: Individuals who are influential in approving or disapproving new ideas and who seek advice and information from others about these things.

leachate: A liquid that results from water collecting contaminants as it trickles through waste, pesticides, or fertilizers. Leaching may occur in farming areas, feedlots, and landfills and may result in hazardous substances entering ground water, surface water, or soil.

leader: An individual who is given informal power in an organization by followers.

leadership: Influencing others to achieve a goal.

learning disability: A disorder in one or more of the basic psychologic processes involved in understanding or using spoken or written language, which may affect one's ability to listen, think, speak, read, write, spell, or do mathematical calculations. The term includes such conditions as perceptual handicaps, brain injury, minimal brain dysfunction, dyslexia, and developmental aphasia.

learning organization: Refers to organizations in which people not only learn to improve the way they work, but are encouraged to question even the basic assumptions and goals of work in an effort to constantly increase value.

legislation: Bills introduced by Congress for the purpose of establishing laws that direct policy.

legislative process: The process used within governments to make laws.

lesser developed country: A country that is not yet stable with respect to its economy and technologic development, such as Bangladesh, Zaire, Haiti, Guatemala, and Indonesia.

level I disaster: A disaster that requires activation by the local emergency medical system in cooperation with local community organizations.

level II disaster: A disaster that requires activation of the local emergency medical system and local community organizations in cooperation with the regional response system.

level III disaster: A disaster that requires activation of the federal emergency system to work in cooperation with local and regional emergency medical systems.

levels of prevention: A three-level model of interventions based on the stages of disease, designed to prevent, halt, or reverse the process of pathologic change as early as possible, thereby preventing damage.

Lexis: A computerized search tool of the legal literature.

liability: An obligation one has incurred or might incur through any act or failure to act, or responsibility for conduct falling below a certain standard that is the cause of client injury.

licensure: Legal sanction to practice a profession after attaining the minimum degree of competence to ensure protection of public health and safety.

life care planning: A tool used in case management to assess the current and future needs of a client. It is a customized, medically based document that provides assessment of all present and future needs, services, equipment, supplies, and living arrangements for a client.

life events: Occurrences that are normative (generally expected to occur at a particular stage of life) and nonnormative (unanticipated) in a person or family's life.

life expectancy: The average number of years that a man or woman can expect to live from the time of birth.

life review: A universal process that can occur at any point in life where an individual is forced to confront his or her mortality.

lifestyle: A general way of living and individual patterns of behavior, which may be beneficial or detrimental to health

lifestyle risk: Factors that predispose a family to ill health that are caused by the personal health behaviors of the members.

limitations: Uncontrollable elements of the research that limit the certainty of the findings or their applicability to the population in general.

lines of resistance: In the Neuman Systems Model, refers to a series of circles between the normal lines of defense and the basic care that support the defense lines and protect the basic structure.

liposuction: The surgical removal of excess fatty tissue through the insertion of suction tubes in specific areas.

local public health department: The agency that is responsible for implementing and enforcing local, state, and federal public health codes and ordinances and providing essential public health programs to a community.

locus of control: An individual's feeling of whether he or she controls his/her destiny (internal locus of control) or if his/her destiny is controlled by outside forces such as luck (external locus of control).

long-term care: Care that is delivered to individuals who are dependent on others for assistance with basic tasks over a sustained period.

long-term evaluation: Geared toward following and assessing the behavior of an individual, family, or community over time.

low birth weight: Birth weight of less than 5.5 pounds.

low-level radioactive waste (LLRW): Waste less hazardous than most of those generated by a nuclear reactor. Usually generated by hospitals, research laboratories, and certain industries.

M

machismo: The male quality of dominance, defined as courage, strength, honor, virility, pride, and dignity.

macroeconomic theory: Branch of economics that deals with the total or aggregate of all individuals and organizations.

macro-level management theories: Sociologic theories that explain and predict the best ways to organize work, obtaining organizational resources, power dynamics, and organizational change.

mainstream smoke: Smoke inhaled and exhaled by the smoker.

maintenance functions: Behaviors that provide physical and psychologic support and therefore hold the group together.

maintenance norms: Norms that create group pressures to ensure affirming actions for members and are helpful in maintaining comfort.

malpractice: Professional misconduct, improper discharge of professional duties, or a failure to meet the standard of care by a professional that results in harm to another.

malpractice litigation: A lawsuit resulting from client dissatisfaction with the provider and the content or quality of care received; a quality assurance measure.

managed care: Refers to integrating payment for services with delivery of services and emphasizing cost-effective service delivery along a continuum of care.

managed care organizations (MCOs): May both pay for and provide services and contract with selected health care providers to actually provide services for the enrollees in the MCO.

managed competition: A creation of market conditions in which the more efficient providers will survive and the more costly will be put out of business.

mandatory credentialing: Certification requiring statutory law (e.g., state nurse practice acts).

mandatory nurse licensure: A law that requires all who practice nursing for compensation to be licensed.

man-made disaster: An act of individuals that causes devastation and destruction, such as war, terrorist bombings, or riots.

Marijuana Tax Act of 1937: Primarily a federal tax law that marked the beginning of the marijuana prohibition. This was originally supported by the Bureau of Narcotics and Dangerous Drugs (now called the Drug Enforcement Agency) and was not supported by the American Medical Association.

market model: Type of model that assumes that people who have the resources to purchase services are the ones entitled to those services. Also assumes that consumers have the information and opportunity to make free choices about where to purchase services.

mass media: Newspapers, TV, radio, or other modes of communication to large audiences.

maximum theory: Economic theory of distribution of goods and resources to maximize the minimum position in society while at the same time allowing exercise of liberty on the span of all people.

Meals on Wheels: A local nutritional program in which one hot meal and sometimes a cold breakfast and sack lunch are delivered to elderly people in their homes.

media discourse: Communication of thoughts and attitudes through literature, film, art, television, and newspapers.

mediating structures: Institutions standing between the individual in private life and the larger institution of public life, such as one's neighborhood, family, church, or voluntary associations.

mediator: A role in which the nurse acts to assist parties to understand each other's concerns and to determine their conclusion of the issues. The mediator has no authority to decide on behalf of another.

Medicaid: A jointly sponsored state and federal program that pays for medical services for the aged, poor, blind, disabled, and families with dependent children.

medically indigent: A portion of the population that is usually above the recognized poverty level and has money to buy the necessities of life but that cannot afford a catastrophic illness or an acute illness crisis.

medically underserved: Not having an adequate number of health care providers and/or services.

Medicare: A federally funded health insurance program for the elderly, disabled, and persons with end-stage renal disease.

member interaction: The ways that group members behave and relate toward each other.

menopause: Permanent cessation of menstruation resulting from loss of ovarian follicular activity.

men's health care practitioner: A registered nurse who has advanced education and clinical training in the health care of men.

mental health problems: Difficulties related to a person's ability to manage daily life events without experiencing undue social isolation, emotional distress, or behavioral incapacity.

men-to-women death ratio: A statistical comparison of death rates between men and women.

Metropolitan Life Insurance Company: With assistance from Lillian Wald, instituted the first community health program for employees in 1909. It also began a cooperative program with visiting nurse associations to provide care for sick policyholders.

microeconomic theory: The branch of economics that deals with the behaviors of individuals and organizations and the effects of those behaviors on prices, costs, and the allocation and distribution of resources.

micro-level management theories: Psychologic theories that help explain and predict individual behavior in organizations (e.g., work motivation) and interpersonal dynamics (e.g., leadership theories, group dynamics).

migrant farm worker: A laborer whose principal employment involves moving from farm to farm, planting or harvesting agriculture, and attaining temporary housing.

Migrant Health Act: U.S. legislation that funds more than 100 migrant health projects that have 364 actual clinic sites and serve more than 500,000 farm workers and their families in 40 states and Puerto Rico.

migration: To move from one country, place, or locality to another.

minority: A group of people who, because of physical or cultural characteristics, are singled out in society for differential and unequal treatment.

mitigation: Actions designed to either prevent something (e.g., a disaster) from happening or reduce the severity of its effects

model: A representation of reality.

moral accountability: A moral obligation that directs the professional nurse to act in a particular way according to moral norms and requires the nurse to be answerable for what has been done.

moral obligation: Duty to act in a particular way in response to moral norms.

moral virtue: Ideal standard of human behavior or thinking; excellence in response to moral norms, such as goodness.

morbidity: Relative disease rate, usually expressed as incidence or prevalence of a disease.

mortality: Relative death rate; the proportion of deaths at a particular time and place.

multi-level intervention: Strategies for personal, organizational, environmental and policy development to achieve health goals by addressing the array of causative and contributing factors in health and illness.

multiproblem family: A family unit that faces a number of events within and without the family environment and does not have the ability to solve its own problems.

multisectoral cooperation: Coordinated health care action by all parts of a community, from local government officials to grass-roots community members.

multiskilled workers: Refers to persons with a broad range of skills. Such individuals are considered to be more productive in day-to-day situations than more specialized workers because they are able to respond quickly and in a flexible way to needs in the work environment.

N

Narcotics Anonymous: Lay, self-help support group for drug addicts.

National Advisory Council on Migrant Health: Advises, consults with, and makes recommendations concerning the organization, operation, selection, and funding of migrant centers. Meets three times a year.

National Alliance for the Mentally Ill (NAMI): An organization that advocates for better services for people with mental illness.

national disaster: Acts of nature that cause devastation and destruction, such as floods, tornadoes, earthquakes.

National Disaster Medical System (NDMS): A system comprised of approximately 75 local disaster medical assistance teams (DMAT) that can be activated (1) in a presidential declaration of a disaster (2) by request for major medical assistance from a state health official under provisions of the Public Health Service Act, or (3) in a foreign military conflict involving U.S. Armed Forces, where casualty levels are likely to exceed the capacity of the Department of Defense-Veterans' Administration Medical System.

National Emission Standards for Hazardous Air Pollutants (NESHAP): Federal air quality standards for sources of hazardous air pollutants, for example, benzene, lead, and mercury.

national health objectives: Indicate major health concerns for different age groups and provide specific standards that researchers can use to evaluate program progress.

National Health Planning and Resources Development Act of 1974 (P.L. 93-641) Legislation set forth to coordinate and direct national health policy via state and regional regulatory agencies; its major goal was to establish a nationwide network of health system agencies.

National Health Service Corps: Program established in 1970 by the Public Health Service to recruit health providers to areas experiencing shortages in health work forces.

National Institute for Nursing Research: One of the National Institutes of Health charged with promoting the growth and quality of research in nursing.

National Institute for Occupational Research Agenda (NORA): Identifies, monitors, and educates the incidence, prevalence, and prevention of work-related illnesses and injuries and examines potential hazards of new work technologies and practices.

National Institute of Mental Health (NIMH): The federal agency charged with developing and supporting education and research programs for mental health.

National Institute of Occupational Safety and Health (NIOSH): The branch of the USPHS responsible for investigating workplace illnesses, accidents, and hazards.

National Institute on Alcohol Abuse and Alcoholism (NIAAA): The lead federal agency under the National Institutes for Health charged with research on alcohol-related problems.

National Institute on Drug Abuse (NIDA): The lead federal agency under the National Institutes of Health charged with drug abuse research.

National Joint Practice Commission: Organization established by the American Nurses Association and the American Medical Association to promote collaborative efforts between medicine and nursing; disbanded in 1981.

National Labor Relation Act Amendments of 1974 (P.L. 93-8360): Amended the Taft-Hartley Act of 1947 and extended the right to organize collectively for matters concerning wages, hours, and working conditions to all employees of nonpublic health care facilities.

National Labor Relations Act: Passed in 1935 and known as the Wagner Act; it protected employees' rights to organize and join unions and also provided for action against unfair labor practices of employers.

National League for Nursing: A national organization for nurses that is composed of nurses and consumers.

National Organization for Public Health Nursing: An early organization for public health nurses, founded in 1912. It was dissolved in 1952, and many of its functions were distributed primarily to the National League for Nursing.

National Pollution Discharge Elimination System (NPDES): A provision of the federal Clean Water Act that prohibits discharge of pollutants into waters of the United States unless a special permit is issued by the EPA, a state, or a tribal delegation on an Indian reservation.

National Priorities List (NPL): EPA's list of the most serious abandoned hazardous waste sites identified for possible long-term cleanup under Superfund. A site must be on the NPL to receive money from the national Superfund's Trust Fund.

National Response Center (NRC): The federal operations center that receives notification of all releases of oil and hazardous substances into the environment, The center, located in Washington, D.C., is operated by the U.S. Coast Guard, which evaluates all reports and notifies the appropriate agency.

nationally notifiable conditions: Certain communicable diseases defined by the Centers for Disease Control and Prevention as requiring weekly, monthly, and annual reports of occurrence by all states.

natural disaster: Any naturally occurring (without human intervention) event that causes devastation and destruction, such as hurricanes, blizzards, and earthquakes.

natural history of disease: The course of disease process from onset to resolution without intervention by humans.

natural immunity: Species-determined innate resistance to an infectious agent.

natural radiation: Radiation that comes from soil, certain rocks, body potassium, and ultraviolet sun rays.

near poor: People who earn slightly more than the government-defined poverty level, are unable to meet living expenses, and are not eligible for government assistance programs.

needs assessment: Systematic appraisal of type, depth, and scope of problems as perceived by clients, health providers, or both.

negative predictive value: Proportion of persons with a negative test who are disease-free.

negentropy: Energy in a system that propels toward order or can be used for work.

negligence: Failure to act as an ordinary, prudent person; conduct contrary to that of a reasonable person under a specific circumstance.

negotiation: Working with others in a formal way to achieve agreement on areas of conflict, using principles of communication, conflict resolution, and assertiveness. Negotiation may be relatively informal, as when two staff members negotiate which vacation times they will have. It may also be formal, as when labor and management negotiate a contract in a unionized environment.

neighborhood nursing: Also known as block nursing. A person who responds to the needs of the community.

neighborhood poverty: Refers to spatially defined areas of high poverty, characterized by dilapidated housing and high levels of unemployment.

neoclassical management: A theoretical approach to management based on the idea that human needs, group dynamics, and cooperation are important to successful achievement of organizational goals.

neonatal period: Between birth and 1 month of age.

Neuman Systems Model: Model that depicts an open system in which persons and their environments are in dynamic interaction. Client system includes five variables: physiologic, psychologic, sociocultural, developmental, and spiritual.

neurodevelopmental evaluations: Assessment of a child by helping primary care providers identify the student's strengths and disabilities.

neurotransmitter: An endogenous chemical released by one neuron that alters the chemical activity of another neuron involved in the transmission of information by nerves.

new morbidities: Illnesses and conditions that are associated with the problems of students living in poverty, students with chronic illnesses or disabilities, and other children with special needs. Affecting school-age children, these cannot be managed completely by the health care system alone because many of them have psychosocial, political, and physical features. External environmental and sociopolitical forces that lead to these problems must be considered to have an effective school health program.

New Source Performance Standards (NSPS): Federal air quality standards for major industrial sources, including steel mills, paper mills, and refineries.

Nightingale, Florence: Considered to be the founder of nursing. She led a mission to the Crimea while the British were fighting a war there and began developing nursing procedures. She wrote the first texts on nursing and founded a training school for nurses.

Noise Control Act: Legislation passed by Congress in 1972 to identify major sources of noise, establish noise emission standards, and provide a mechanism for people to take civil action on their own behalf when a person or agency violates the Act.

nominal group: A group in which individuals work in the presence of one another but do not interact.

nonfarm residency: Residence within area zoned as "city limits."

nongonococcal urethritis (NGU): Inflammation of the urethra from microorganisms other than *Neisseriae gonorrhea; Chlamydia trachomatis* has been implicated as the cause of 50% of cases.

non-metropolitan statistical area (non-MSA): Counties that do not meet SMSA criteria.

Nonoxynol-9: A spermicidal gel found in some contraceptive foams and jellies, in condoms, and in some sexual lubricants. Nonoxynol-9 has viricidal and bactericidal properties and can be used as a lubricant to protect against HIV.

non-point source: A pollution source that does not have a single point of origin or is not introduced into a receiving stream from a specific outlet. The pollutants are generally carried off the land when it rains. Commonly used categories for non-point sources are agriculture, forestry, urban, mining, construction, dams and channels, land disposal, and saltwater intrusion.

nontraditional family: Alternative family structures composed of two or more individuals coming from the same or different kinship groups who are involved in a continuous living arrangement, usually residing in the same household, experiencing common emotional bonds, and sharing certain obligations toward each other and toward others.

nontraditional health facilities: Alternative health care delivery systems, using various community settings.

normal lines of defense: In the Neuman System's Model, is dynamic and defines the stability and integrity of the system.

norms: Standards that guide, regulate, and control.

nuclear (traditional) family: A unit composed of mother, father, and young children.

nuclear reactor: A device in which a fission chain reaction can be initiated, maintained, and controlled. Its essential component is a core with fissionable fuel. It usually has a moderator, shielding, coolant, and control mechanisms.

nurse midwifery: "The independent nursing management and care of essentially normal newborns and women antepartally, intrapartally, postpartally, and gynecologically, occurring within a health care system that provides for medical consultation, collaborative management, and referral . . ." (Rooks and Haas, 1986, p. 9).

Nurse Practice Act: See *Practice Acts*

nurse practitioner: Nursing role that includes a primary care component that focuses on health maintenance and client counseling.

nursing centers: (a) Health care facilities in which the primary aim is to offer nursing services, including health assessment, promotion, screening, and health teaching. (b) Organizations that give the client direct access to professional nursing services. Using nursing models of care, professional nurses diagnose and treat human responses to actual and potential health problems and promote health and optimal functioning among target populations and communities. These services are holistic, client centered, and reimbursable at a reasonable level. Accountability and responsibility for client care and professional practice remain with the professional nurse. Overall accountability and responsibility remain with the nurse executive. Nursing centers are not limited to any particular organizational configuration; they may be affiliated with universities, community organizations, hospitals, or other service organizations, or may be free standing. The primary characteristic of the organization is responsiveness to the health needs of the population.

nursing diagnosis: A clinical judgment about individual, family, or community responses to actual or potential health problems/life processes.

nursing intervention: Any treatment based on clinical judgement and knowledge that a nurse performs to enhance patient/client outcomes.

nursing practice: Nurse clinical activities and behaviors that are performed on behalf of clients.

O

OASIS: Outcomes and Assessment Information Set—A multistate research study funded by Medicare to develop a standardized patient assessment to measure quality and client satisfaction with care.

objective: A precise behavioral statement of the achievement that will accomplish partial or total realization of a goal. The date by which the achievement is expected is specified.

occupational health: The state in which a worker is able to function at an optimum level of well-being (see HEALTH) at the worksite; reflected by higher employee productivity, an increase in work attendance, a reduction in workers' compensation claims, and an increase in longevity in employment status.

occupational health hazards: Dangerous processes or materials within a work environment that result in harm to an employee.

Occupational Safety and Health Administration (OSHA): Federal agency charged with improving worker health and safety by establishing standards and regulations and by educating workers.

official health agencies: Agencies operated by state or local governments to provide home health care.

Older Americans Act: Legislation enacted in 1965 to mandate and provide funds for services, programs, and activities deemed essential to accomplish certain goals for older Americans meeting specified criteria.

Omaha System: A system of nursing diagnoses, interventions, and evaluations of outcomes of care developed by the Omaha Visiting Nurses Association.

Omaha System Intervention Scheme: A systematic arrangement of nursing actions or activities designed to help nurses and other health care professionals document both plans and interventions. Intended for use with nursing diagnoses.

Omaha System Problem Classification Scheme: A client-focused taxonomy of nursing diagnoses comprised of simple terms.

Omaha System Problem Rating Scale for Outcomes: A five-point Likert-type scale that provides a systematic, recurring way of measuring client progress throughout the time of service.

openness: The extent to which a system exchanges energy with the environment. In an open system, a continuous give-and-take occurs with the environment.

operating budget: An agency's budget that includes all anticipated revenues and projected expenses that are related to the day-to-day costs of achieving the organization's goals.

operational framework: Infrastructure of an organization or project needed to support efforts to carry out its mission; typically includes executive leadership, services, operational administration, and support.

opportunity costs: Dollar value of a good or service not purchased.

organically structured agencies: An organization that is loose in decision-making authority. Decisions are made at the lowest level of the agency, and employees have the information needed to make a decision.

organization: The arrangement of the elements of a system and their relationship to each other.

organization structure: The way people in an agency organize themselves to accomplish the mission and goals of the agency.

organizational structure: The formal and informal relationships that operationalize accomplishment of organizational goals.

osteoporosis: Condition characterized by increased bone brittleness.

other metropolitan: Fringe counties of core metropolitan areas; suburban areas.

Ottawa Charter for Health Promotion (1986): Provides a definition for health promotion and a framework for the Healthy Cities movement. Includes six elements: health promotion, building healthy public policy, creating supportive environments, strengthening community action, developing personal skills, and reorienting health services.

outcome criteria: Measurable ends to be achieved based on the problems presented by the client's condition of health or illness.

outcome evaluation: Assessment of the effects of a program on the ultimate objectives, including changes in health and social benefits or quality of life, in contrast to evaluation of program development efforts or its impact on participant.

outrage factors: Characteristics of risk that contribute to the public's feeling of outrage.

outreach: Making a special, focused effort to find people with a specific health problem for the purpose of increasing their access to health services.

P

palliative care: Alleviating symptoms of, meeting the special needs of, and providing comfort for the dying clients and families by the nurse.

Pan American Health Organization: One of the oldest continuously functioning international health organizations, it focuses its efforts on working to improve health and living standards of the countries of the Americas.

pandemic: A worldwide outbreak of an epidemic disease.

parent organization: An umbrella organization that oversees or manages another organization or separately incorporated units of the organization.

parish nurse: Responds to health and wellness needs within the context of populations of faith communities and is a partner with the church in fulfilling the mission of health ministry.

parish nurse coordinator: A parish nurse who has completed a certificate program designed to develop the nurse as a coordinator of a parish nursing service.

parish nursing: A nursing service provided by a church as a community outreach to its parishioners, usually focused on primary prevention.

participant observation: Conscious and systematic sharing in the life activities and occasionally in the interests and activities of a group of persons; observational methods of assessment; a direct method of data collection.

partner notification: Also known as contact tracing. Identifying and locating sexual and injectable drug-use partners of people who have been diagnosed with a sexually transmitted disease in order to notify them of exposure and encourage them to seek medical treatment.

partnership: A relationship between individuals, groups, or organizations in which the parties are working together to achieve a joint goal. Often used synonymously with coalitions and alliances, although partnerships usually have focused goals, such as jointly providing a specific program. Partnerships generally involve shared power.

passive immunization: Immunization by a transfer of specific antibody from an immunized person to one who is not immunized.

pastoral care staff: Represents various aspects of the life of the congregational community and works closely with the congregational model or the institutional model.

PATCH: Acronym for *Planned Approach To Community Health.* A guideline publication for community intervention to obtain health objectives. PATCH emphasizes the prevention of identified chronic disease and health promotion programs and their planning and implementation processes.

paternity: Fatherhood.

pathogenicity: An agent's relative ability to produce disease.

Patient's Bill of Rights: A document prepared by the American Hospital Association that defines the provider-client relationship within an organization.

peer pressure: Influence that teens (or others) place on each other to engage in certain behaviors. Generally considered in areas of negative influence, including smoking cigarettes, using controlled substances, engaging in sexual activity, and getting pregnant.

pelvic inflammatory disease (PID): Also known as salpingitis. Infection of the female reproductive organs, especially the fallopian tubes and endometrium, resulting in infertility and/or ectopic pregnancy. Acute symptoms and signs include lower abdominal pain, increased vaginal discharge, urinary frequency, vomiting, and fever. PID results from untreated gonorrhea and chlamydia.

performance budget: A financial plan that shows clearly and concisely the services to be provided in return for the funds available or income generated.

perimenopause: The period immediately before menopause when endocrinologic, biologic, and clinical features of approaching menopause commence, continuing for at least the first year after permanent cessation of menstruation.

permit: An authorization, license, or equivalent control document issued to implement the requirements of an environmental regulation; for example, a permit to operate a wastewater treatment plant. A permit sets standards or criteria by which to regulate.

permitting: Process of granting a permit.

persistent poverty: Refers to individuals and families who remain poor for long periods of time.

personal beliefs: Ideas about the world that an individual believes to be true.

personal preparedness: A process whereby the nurse keeps self healthy and plans for family and work responsibilities to continue in an organized manner if the nurse is called to participate in a disaster.

personalismo: The cultural preference to see health care providers with backgrounds, culture, and language similar to one's own.

pesticide exposure: Health risk to farm workers who work in fields that have been treated with pesticides. Residue from pesticides also enter farm worker's homes and their food. Risks include mild psychologic and behavioral deficits, and acute severe poisoning can result in death.

pharmacokinetics: The absorption, distribution, metabolism, and elimination of drugs in the body.

philanthropic organizations: Those agencies that receive funds through private endowments and use those funds to support health-related projects.

physical abuse: One or more episodes of extreme discipline or displaced aggression or frustration, often resulting in serious physical damage to the internal organs, bones, central nervous system, or sense organs.

physical agent: Extremes of temperature, noise, radiation, and lighting that may cause illness.

physical neglect: Failure to provide adequate food, proper clothing, shelter, hygiene, or necessary medical care.

physician assistant: Health practitioner role created in the 1960s to free physician's time by completing tasks such as taking medical histories and conducting physical examinations.

physician-client model of consultation: A consulting mode in which the consultant is employed to diagnose a problem and suggest a remedy.

pivot management: A plan in which the nurse organizes a school health team using the personnel already in the school system or closely associated with it.

planning: Selecting a series of actions designed to achieve stated goals.

plume: A visible or measurable discharge of a contaminant from a given point of origin. A plume can be visible or thermal in water, or visible in the air, for example, a plume of smoke.

point epidemic: A concentration in space and time of a disease event, such that a graph of frequency of cases over time shows a sharp point, usually suggestive of a common exposure.

point source: A stationary location or fixed facility like an industrial plant or factory from which pollutants are discharged or emitted. Also, any single identifiable source of pollution.

police power: States' power to act to protect the health, safety, and welfare of their citizens.

policy: Settled course of action to be followed by a government or institution to obtain a desired end.

political skills: Bargaining and negotiation skills based on an understanding of others' wants and needs and the effects of decisions on others' goals achievement.

politics: The art of influencing others to accept a specific course of action.

polity: The expectations and mission of a particular faith community.

polysubstance abuse: Use of drugs from different categories used together or at different times to regulate how the person feels.

population: Collection of individuals who have one or more personal or environmental characteristic in common.

population-focused: Action directed toward an aggregate or community versus an individual.

population-focused practice: Problems and solutions are implemented for or with a defined population or subpopulation in mind.

portfolio: Folders that contain documents that show the nurses' abilities and competency to practice.

positive predictive value: The proportion of persons with a positive screening or diagnostic test who do have the disease (the proportion of "true positives" among all who test positive).

poverty: Refers to having insufficient financial resources to meet basic living expenses. These expenses include cost of food, shelter, clothing, transportation, and medical care.

poverty threshold guidelines: A definition of poverty drafted by the Social Security Administration in 1964. The federal government defines poverty in terms of income, family size, the age of the head of household, and the number of children under 18 years of age. The guidelines change annually to be consistent with the consumer price index.

power dynamics: Use of power to promote effective health care by influencing decision makers in organizations, in governments, and on community boards.

Practice Acts: State laws that govern the practice of health providers.

practice-based research: Questions and key concepts of primary health care and health promotion, as defined by the World Health Organization, are appropriate to guide research and to develop concepts for community health nursing.

practice setting: Context and/or environment within which nursing care is given.

precedent: An earlier occurrence of something similar. Something said or done, such as a legal decision, that may serve as an example or rule to authorize or justify a subsequent act of the same or a similar kind.

PRECEDE-PROCEED Model: (a) Focuses primarily on planning and evaluating community health education programs. (b) A health education model that is outcome oriented and asks "why" before it asks "how"; it can be used with individuals, families, groups, or the community.

preconceptional counseling: Education, assessment, diagnosis, and intervention to address risk of pregnancy and birth before conception.

Preferred Provider Organization (PPO): An organization of providers who contract on a fee-for-service basis with third-party payers to provide comprehensive medical services to subscribers.

prejudice: The emotional manifestation of deeply held beliefs about other groups; involves negative attitudes.

prematurity: Birth that occurs before 37 weeks' gestation.

prenatal care: Care of a pregnant woman during the entire term of her pregnancy, includes consistent monitoring of fetus, recommending vitamins, ultrasounds, and so on. Half of all teenage girls who are pregnant do not get prenatal care until the second trimester; one quarter of all women wait until the second trimester.

preparedness: The pre-disaster stage in which individuals and communities plan for and coordinate their response efforts.

prepathogenesis: A stage in the natural history of a disease in which the disease has not yet developed, although the groundwork has been laid through the presence of factors that favor its occurrence.

preschool period: Between 3 and 5 years of age.

prescriptive authority: A legal right granted to nurses by states to write prescriptions for clients.

prescriptive intervention mode: An intervention requiring less collaboration between consultant and client because the consultant explicitly tells the client how to solve the problem.

prevalence: The proportion of existing cases of a health outcome in a population at a particular time.

Prevention of Significant Deterioration (PSD): Federal air quality standards designed to protect air quality in pristine areas like national parks and wilderness areas.

price inflation: Increases in costs of all goods and services in the United States.

primary care: Typically the entry point into the health care system; emphasizes management of commonly occurring diseases or chronic disease.

primary care generalist: Primary care providers who possess skills in health promotion and disease prevention, assessment/evaluation of undiagnosed symptoms and physical signs, management of common acute and chronic medical conditions, and identification and appropriate referral for other needed health care services. Includes family physicians, general internists, general pediatricians, nurse practitioners, physician assistants, and nurse midwives.

primary health care: Meeting the basic needs of a community by providing readily accessible primary and public health services through full community participation at an affordable cost.

primary prevention: Actions that reduce the incidence of disease by promoting health and preventing disease processes from developing.

principles: The foundations for rules.

private and commercial organizations: Organizations that provide financial and technical backing for investment, employment, and access to market economies and health care. Includes Nestlé and Johnson and Johnson companies.

private sector: An individual or any part of society that is not part of the government.

private voluntary organizations: Includes both religious and secular groups. They work together to improve efforts with health care, community development, and other needed projects.

probability: Likelihood that an intervention activity can be implemented.

problem analysis: Process of identifying problem correlates and interrelationships and substantiating them with relevant data.

problem correlates: Contributing factors to a problem.

problem prioritization: Evaluation of problems and establishment of priorities according to predetermined criteria.

problem-purpose-expansion method: A way to broaden limited thinking involving restating the problem and expanding the problem statement so that different solutions can be generated.

problem solving: A process of seeking to find solutions to situations that present difficulty or uncertainty.

process: The ongoing activities and behaviors of health providers engaged in conducting client care.

process consultation: A consultation model in which the consultant and client work in the partnership to identify and solve client problems. The consultant works more as a facilitator and coach, encouraging the client to identify the problem and helping the client develop a problem-solving strategy.

professional and technical organizations: Organizations that are focused on specific technical research, like the Institut Pasteur, whose laboratories have developed sera and vaccines for many countries.

professional isolation: The act of practicing in a setting where there are no colleagues.

professional negligence: An unreasonable act or a failure to act when a duty is owed to another, leading to injuries that can be legally compensated.

professional preparedness: A process whereby the nurse becomes aware and understands disaster plans in the workplace and the community.

professional standards review organizations/professional review organizations Organizations established by law to monitor delivery of health care to clients of Medicaid, Medicare, and Maternal/Child health programs and to monitor implementation of prospective reimbursement.

program: A health care service designed to meet identified health care needs of clients.

program budget: A financial plan that shows expenses and income related to a specific service.

program evaluation: Collection of methods, skills, and activities necessary to determine whether a service is needed, likely to be used, conducted as planned, and actually helps people.

Program Planning Model: Proposed by Delbecq and Van de Ven in 1971 as a model to encourage lay people to participate in defining problems. The model shows how to use active community participation in problem definition and program planning, making the most of contributions from groups with diverse interests, skills, and knowledge.

prohibition: Originally referred to the period during 1920 to 1933, during which the sale of alcoholic beverages was prohibited in the United States. Currently, drug prohibition refers to the outlawing of the manufacturing (or growing), sale, and/or use of certain drugs.

promotor: An advocacy role in which the nurse partners with the client and pushes the client's right to make his or her own decision.

proprietary agencies: For-profit organizations.

prospective payment system: The diagnosis-related group payment mechanism for reimbursing hospitals for inpatient health care services through Medicare.

prospective reimbursement: Method of payment to an agency for services to be delivered based on predictions of what an agency's costs will be for the coming year.

protocols (algorithms): Written, standing orders that have been mutually agreed on by the nurse practitioner and the physician. The nurse practitioner uses them as a guide to manage certain illnesses or conditions.

provider service records: A written summary of the provider's work activities on a daily, weekly, or monthly basis.

psychoactive drugs: Drugs that affect mood, perception, and thought.

psychomotor domain: A domain of learning that includes the performance of skills that require some degree of neuromuscular coordination.

psychosocial development: Combination of emotional and social development.

psychosocial agents: Workplace hazards that affect the emotional and social well-being of a worker.

public health: Organized community efforts designed to prevent disease and promote health

public health core functions: The core functions of public health are assessment, policy development, and assurance.

public health ethic: Principle of providing health care services that will offer the greatest good for the greatest number.

public health nursing: The synthesis of nursing theory and public health theory applied to promoting and preserving the health of populations. The focus of practice is the community as a whole and the effect of the community's health status (resources) on the health of individuals, families, and groups. Care is provided within the context of preventing disease and disability and promoting and protecting the health of the community as a whole.

public health program: A program designed with the goal of improving a population's health status.

Public Health Service: An arm of the Department of Health and Human Services that fulfills the function of overseeing health care services within the United States.

public sector: A government entity.

purchase-of-expertise consultation: A model of consultation in which the client hires an expert to provide information or suggest solutions to client-identified problems.

Q

qualitative methods: A tool of science that is characterized by inductive reasoning, subjectivity, discovery, description, and the meaning of an experience or phenomenon to an individual or group.

quality: Continuous striving for excellence and a conformance to specifications or guidelines.

quality assurance: Monitoring of the activities of client care to determine the degree of excellence attained in the implementation of the activities.

quality improvement: See *total quality management/improvement.*

quantitative methods: Traditional scientific inquiry that advocates objectively gathering data that can be verified by another researcher and generalized to other populations. These methods are characterized by deductive reasoning, objectivity, quasi-experiments, statistical techniques, and control.

quasivoluntary: A form of accreditation that is linked to governmental regulations and encourages programs to participate in a voluntary accrediting process.

R

race: A biologic designation whereby group members share distinguishing features (e.g., skin color, bone structure, and genetic traits such as a blood grouping).

racism: A form of prejudice that refers to beliefs that persons who are born into particular groups are inferior in intelligence, morals, beauty, and self-worth.

rape: Natural or unnatural sexual intercourse forced on an unwilling person by threat of bodily injury or loss of life.

rates: Measures of the frequency of a health event in a defined population during a specified period of time.

Rathbone, William: A British philanthropist who founded the first district nursing association, in Liverpool, England. He and Florence Nightingale then spread the concept throughout England.

ratio: Statistical measure in which the numerator is not included in the denominator.

rationing: Limits placed on health care that may not be beneficial to a client's well-being.

reality norms: Group members' perceptions of reality, upon which daily behavior is based. Influences decision-making and action-taking processes.

receptor population: Population that is within the exposure pathway for harm to human health.

recertification: In home health care, the review and certification performed at least every 62 days by the health care team; it demonstrates that the client continues to need a specified plan of care.

recidivism: Readmission to a clinical agency for treatment of a problem for which treatment had been received earlier.

reciprocity: The recognition and acceptance of a professional's licensure between certain states.

recognition: Process whereby one agency accepts the credentialing status of and the credentials conferred by another.

records: Documentation of all aspects of an organization, required by law. They provide complete information about a client, indicate the extent and quality of services rendered, resolve legal issues in malpractice suits, and provide information for education and research.

recovery: The stage of a disaster in which all involved agencies and individuals pull together to restore the economic and civic life.

referral: Guiding clients toward problem resolution and assisting them in using available resources.

regulations: Specific statements of law that relate to and clarify individual pieces of legislation.

reimbursement: Payment for nurses services through direct fees for service, service contracts with organizations or businesses, and third-party payments from private insurers, government, and managed care organizations.

reimbursement systems: The process by which home health care services receives payment, either by the client or by three major funding sources: Medicare, Medicaid, and third-party health insurance.

relapse management: Activities of a case manager designed to foster coping and competency and manage symptoms to prevent a relapse of illness.

relative risk ratio: Statistical measure of how much the risk of acquiring a particular disease increases with exposure to a specific causal agent or risk factor.

relative standard: Defines poverty in terms of the society's median standard of living.

reliability: The consistency of a measure from person to person or over time.

religious organizations: Organizations consisting of several denominations and religious interests, which support many different kinds of health care programs.

remediation: The act or process of remedying or correcting a problem.

repeat pregnancy: A closely spaced second pregnancy. For teen mothers, leads to poorer education and economic outcomes.

report card: A written listing of how an agency or professional group compares with others in the field on certain key indicators of quality, including morbidity and mortality measures, consumer satisfaction, and cost of care.

representative group: Type of community group whose members are elected, appointed, or selected from various community sectors.

research process: A problem-solving method of scientific inquiry that involves assessment, planning, implementation, evaluation, and, preferably, action.

resilience: The ability to withstand stressors and multiple problems without developing health problems.

resistance: The ability of the host to withstand infection.

Resource Conservation and Recovery Act (RCRA): A federal law passed in 1976 to promote "cradle-to-grave" management of hazardous waste from the point of generation to the final disposal location. The law works through requirements for hazardous waste generators, transporters, and treatment, storage, and disposal facilities.

respite care: Relief time provided by others to a caregiver from responsibilities for care of a family member.

respondeat superior: When a nurse is employed and functioning within the scope of that job, the employer is responsible for the nurse's negligent actions. By directing a nurse to carry out a particular function, the employer becomes responsible for negligence, along with the individual nurse.

response: Responsibilities assumed and activities occurring as a result of a specific level of disaster.

retrospective audit: A method of evaluating quality of care through appraisal of the nursing process after the client's discharge from the health care system.

retrospective reimbursement: Method of payment to an agency based on units of service delivered.

right: That to which a person has a just claim; legal claim recognized as valid by a legal system; moral claim recognized as valid by moral principles that in turn may or may not be recognized by legal rules.

right to health: Right to not have one's health affected by others (a negative right).

right to health care: Right to goods, resources, and services to maintain and improve one's state of health (a positive right).

risk: The probability of some event or outcome within a specified period of time.

risk appraisal: Data about health risks experienced by an individual or group are collected and analyzed, and a health risk profile is generated.

risk assessment: (a) Assessing the probability of developing a disease. (b) The qualitative and quantitative evaluation performed in an effort to define the risk posed to human health and the environment by the presence or potential presence and/or use of specific pollutants.

risk communication: Communicating the magnitude and probability of risk.

risk factor: Disease precursor, the presence of which is associated with higher than average mortality. Disease precursors include demographic variables, certain everyday health practices, family history of disease, and some physiologic changes.

risk management: Intervention designed to induce and/or sustain changes in health-compromising behaviors, such as counseling, mass media campaigns, or increased production of low-fat dairy goods.

risk reduction: Helps individuals and groups maximize their self-care activities. The goal is to prevent disease or detect it at its earliest stages.

role: Identifiable social position associated with a set of behavioral expectations.

role ambiguity: Lack of clarity about what is expected.

role behavior: What an actor in a position actually does in response to role expectations.

role conflict: Presence of contradictory and often competing role expectations.

role negotiation: Two or more persons deciding together which tasks, activities, or responsibilities each will accept in a defined situation.

role overload: A situation that occurs when there is insufficient time to carry out all of the expected role functions.

role performance model of health A model in which health is viewed as the individual's ability to effectively perform roles and the family's ability to effectively meet their functions and developmental tasks.

role sequence: Positions within the family and related behaviors that change over time.

role sharing: Arrangement in which both partners have equal claims to the breadwinning role and equal responsibilities for the care of the home and children, including the obligations to contribute equally or equitably to family expenses.

role strain: A situation resulting from conditions requiring complex role demands and the fulfillment of multiple roles.

role structure: Arrangement of group-member positions according to the expected functions of members.

route of exposure: Manner in which exposure occurs. May be through inhalation, ingestion, or skin absorption.

rule of confidentiality: Nondisclosure of personal information about others, such as clients, to those not authorized to have this information; also, a rule grounded in the principle of autonomy.

rule of utility: Rule derived from the principle of beneficence. Includes the moral duty to weigh and balance benefits and reduce the occurrence of harms.

rules: Guidelines, principles, or regulations that govern conduct.

rural: Communities having less than 20,000 residents or fewer than 99 persons per square mile.

Rural Health Clinic Act: Legislation enacted in 1978 to provide for the development of rural health clinics staffed by new health professionals in existing medically underserved areas of the United States.

rural-urban continuum: Residence ranging from living on a remote farm, to a village or small town, to a larger town or city, to a large metropolitan area with a "core inner city."

S

sampling: Selecting a portion of the population to study; can use random or deliberate sampling techniques.

schemes: Actions and mental processes allowing the child to understand the environment.

school-age adolescent period: Between 6 and 20 years of age.

school-based health centers (SBHC): Health care that is provided at school.

school health council: A council composed of teachers, school nurses, parents, students, administrators, and community leaders that plans school health.

school health manager: Coordinator of a health program within a school.

school health services: Includes several activities that should be family-centered, promote health, and prevent disease.

school nurse clinic: Facilities run by nurses that provide physical and/or mental health services to school-age children that are located within or near schools.

school nurse practitioner: Registered nurse with certificate or master's-level advanced education in the areas of health assessment, diagnosis, and treatment who is prepared to deliver primary health care to school-age children.

school phobia: The persistent and abnormal fear of going to school.

scientific management: The earliest theoretic approach to management; the best way to increase work productivity is to help people become expert at their jobs through repeating the same tasks over and over.

scope of practice: The usual and customary practice of a profession taking into account how legislation defines the practice of a profession within a particular jurisdiction (local, state, community, or nationally).

Scorpio: A service provided by the Library of Congress to assist in topic searches in the legal literature.

screening: The application of a test to people who are as yet asymptomatic for the purpose of classifying them with respect to their likelihood of having a particular disease.

seamless system of care: With vertical integration, freestanding agencies that are all owned by one system are able to collaborate and contract with one another to provide clients with smooth, continuous service.

secondary analysis: Analysis using previously gathered data.

secondary care: Actions to treat disease in the early, acute phase.

secondary prevention: Programs, such as screening, designed to detect disease in the early stages (early pathogenesis), before clinically evident signs and symptoms, in order to intervene with early diagnosis and treatment.

second-hand smoke: Smoke in an environment inhaled by someone who is not currently smoking.

secular organizations: Nonreligious organizations that work to improve efforts with health care, community development, and other needed projects around the world.

secular trend: Long-term patterns of morbidity or mortality (i.e., over years or decades).

selected membership group: A group of persons brought together for a specific purpose, such as health assessment or promotion. Some members may be linked to others through previous association, or members may be unacquainted before group formation.

self-care: Any activity that individuals initiate and perform on their own behalf to maintain life, health, and well-being.

self-determination: The right and responsibility of a person to decide and direct his or her own choices.

self-efficacy: A sense of competence and capability.

self-regulation: An essential characteristic of a profession involving activities that have as their goals the overseeing of the rights, obligations, responsibilities, and relationships of a provider to society, to the profession, and to the client. On the individual level, one's ability to exert self-control.

sensitivity: The proportion of persons who actually have a disease who will have a positive screening or diagnostic test; or the probability that a person with a disease will be correctly classified by the test.

seroconversion: The appearance of antibodies in serum.

seroprevalence: The overall occurrence of HIV antibodies within a specific population at any point in time.

service delivery network: A group of organizations that provide health and human services. Generally, the services are complementary, although some overlap is often seen. Clients may receive comprehensive services from the agencies in the network.

service leadership: A form of leadership that emphasizes the leader's role in providing service as a partner with others, as opposed to a more hierarchic approach to leadership.

set: Expectation, including unconscious expectation, as a variable determining a person's reaction to a drug.

setting: The environment—physical, social, and cultural—as a variable determining a person's reaction to a drug.

settlement houses: Early agencies for visiting nurses.

severe mental disorders: Disorders that are persistent and disabling; they are determined by diagnoses and criteria that evaluate degree of functional disability.

sexual abuse: Abuse ranging from fondling to rape; robs children of the feeling of being in control of themselves and emphasizes their vulnerability.

sexual debut: First intercourse.

sexual victimization: Suffering from a destructive or injurious sexual action.

sexually transmitted diseases (STDs): Communicable diseases, such as gonorrhea, chlamydia, and HIV infection, that can be passed on during sexual activity.

Sheppard-Towner Act: Maternity and Infancy Act of 1921, which provided federal matching funds to establish maternal and child health divisions in state health departments. It was ended in 1929 in response to concerns that it gave too much power to the federal government and too closely resembled socialized medicine.

short-term evaluation: Focuses on identifying behavioral effects of health education programs and determining whether or not changes are caused by the educational program.

sibling relationship: The interaction among brothers and sisters.

sidestream smoke: Smoke that comes off a cigarette from the outside rather than being drawn through the cigarette.

simpatia: Some cultures have a goal of polite, respectful, nonconfrontational relationships with others; these tendencies may prevent clients from asking questions of health care providers.

skilled care: Care provided to a client that requires the knowledge and skill of a registered nurse.

social Darwinism: A sense that only those people who are skillful and hardworking deserve to obtain social goods, such as a good income and comfortable lifestyle.

social isolation: Socially withdrawn; separated or removed from society. Not having friends or confidants.

social learning theory: A theory that builds on the principles of behavioral theory; says that behavior is a function of an individual's expectations about the value of an outcome or self-efficacy. If individuals believe that an outcome is desired and attainable, they are more likely to change their behavior to achieve that goal.

social network: Individuals who may or may not include family members with whom others have contact because of proximity or reciprocity.

Social Security Act of 1935: Federal legislation that attempted to overcome the national setbacks of the Depression. Title VI of this act provided funding for expanded opportunities for health protection and promotion through education and employment of public health nurses and provided funds to establish and maintain adequate health services.

source of harm: Agents in the environment that can cause illness or injury to a person: chemical, physical, or psychological.

sovereign immunity: Doctrine by which an agency may be exempt from a lawsuit for particular kinds of actions.

special care nursing centers: Nursing centers that have a particular focus.

special population groups: Groups identified as needing special consideration in *Healthy People 2000*. The special population groups include low-income groups, minority groups, and people with disabilities.

specialist: A nurse who provides services that are specific to an area of concentration of nursing (e.g., pediatric care).

specificity: The proportion of persons who do not have a disease who will have a negative screening or diagnostic test, or the probability that a person without disease will be correctly classified by the test.

spouse abuse: Physical or emotional mistreatment of one's partner.

staff review committees: Committees whose function is to monitor client-specific aspects of care appropriate for certain levels of care.

stakeholders: All those who have an investment, or stake, in the outcomes of a program and therefore have reasons to be interested in the evaluation of a program.

Standard Metropolitan Statistical Area (SMSA): Region with a central city of at least 50,000 residents.

standard of care: Those acts performed or omitted that an ordinarily prudent person in the defendant's position would or would not have done; a measure by which the defendant's conduct is compared to ascertain negligence.

standardized rates (adjusted rates): Artificial rates of disease that are calculated to allow comparison of rates in populations with differing distributions of characteristics, such as age or race.

standards: Criteria for measuring conformity to established practice.

statistical indicators: Measures of incidence, prevalence, mortality, and other data to estimate client problems, magnitudes of problems, and needs for programs to resolve the problems.

statutes: Legislative enactments declaring, commanding, or prohibiting something.

statutory law: Law enacted by a legislative body.

statutory rape: Sexual intercourse with a female who is below the statutory age of consent. Varies by state.

stereotyping: The basis for ascribing certain beliefs and behaviors about a group to an individual without giving adequate attention to individual differences.

Stewart B. McKinney Homelessness Act: Public Law 100-77 passed in 1987 officially involved the federal government with meeting the needs of homeless persons. It was intended to respond to the range of emergency needs facing homeless Americans, such as food, shelter, and health care.

stimulants: Drugs that increase the activity of the CNS, causing wakefulness.

strategic plan: Immediate, intermediate, and long-term goals, objectives, and activities of an organization to carry out its mission; includes anticipated outcomes, programs and services to be provided, and community and organizational infrastructure, training, development, and support needed to carry out activities.

strength of the association: Degree of a relationship between a causal factor and disease occurrence, usually measured by the relative risk ratio.

structure: In groups, the particular arrangement of group parts that helps to describe the group as a whole. An organizational arrangement including mission, goals, services, and work force.

subpopulations: Particular segments of a population.

substance abuse: Use of any substance that threatens a person's health or impairs his or her social or economic functioning.

suburbs: Area adjacent to highly populated city.

suicide: The act or an instance of taking one's own life voluntarily and intentionally.

summative evaluation: A method used to assess program outcomes or as a follow-up of the results of program activities.

Superfund Amendments and Reauthorization Act (SARA): A federal law passed in 1986 amending CERCLA and providing $8.5 billion for the cleanup program and $500 million for cleanup of leaks from underground storage tanks. SARA also strengthened EPA's mandate to focus on permanent cleanup at Superfund sites, involve the public in decision processes at sites, and encourage states to actively participate as partners with EPA to address these sites. SARA expanded EPA's research, development, and training responsibilities and the agency's enforcement authority to get others to clean up hazardous waste problems for which they are responsible.

supervision: The process of directing, coaching, and monitoring the work of others to whom tasks have been delegated.

supply: Quantity or amount of goods or services available.

surveillance: Systematic and ongoing observation and collection of data concerning disease occurrence in order to describe phenomena and detect changes in frequency or distribution.

survey: Method of assessment in which data from a sample of persons are reported to the data collector.

survivors: Family members and friends of victims of violent acts, especially those victims who have died.

susceptibility: The stage before the development of disease at which a person is subject to or at risk of disease.

sustainability: Efforts and resources needed to deliver health programs and services in an effective, consistent, and reliable manner over time so as to achieve desired outcomes.

syphilis: An infectious, chronic sexually transmitted disease caused by a bacteria, *Treponema pallidum*; characterized by the appearance of lesions or chancres that may involve any tissue. Relapses are frequent, and after the initial chancre syphilis may exist without symptoms for years.

systems theory: A useful framework for community mental health practice because it emphasizes the relationship of the elements of a unit to the whole.

T

Taft-Hartley Act: Passed in 1947, a revision of the Wagner Act of 1935. Included in the 1947 law was a provision that professional employees should not be organized in the same bargaining unit with nonprofessionals unless a majority of the professional employees voted for such an inclusion.

target of service: Population group for whom healthful change is sought.

task: Function with work or labor overtones assigned to or demanded of a person.

task functions: Behaviors that focus or direct movement toward the main work of the group.

task norm: Group's commitment to return to the central goals of the groups when it has strayed from its purpose.

taxonomy: A framework that provides order to a set of related terms or concepts.

Teen Outreach Program: Focuses on building self-esteem through volunteering.

Teenager Healthy Teaching Modules: Health education program that has been effective in reducing teen pregnancy and dropout in the experimental groups.

telehealth: Health information sent from one site to another by electronic communication.

Temporary Assistance to Needy Families (TANF): Formerly called Aid to Families with Dependent Children (AFDC), a federal and state program to provide financial assistance to needy children deprived of parental support because of death, disability, absence from the home, or in some states, unemployment.

tertiary care: Actions taken to limit the progression of disease or disability.

tertiary prevention: Programs directed toward persons with clinically apparent disease, with the aim of ameliorating the course of disease, reducing disability, or rehabilitating.

testicular self-examination: A procedure performed by oneself to assess the condition of the testicles and detect abnormalities.

theories of justice: Doctrines that indicate how to distribute goods and resources among the population.

theory: A clearly stated, operationally defined set of concepts, statements, and hypotheses. A collection of principles and rules.

theory principles intervention mode: A consultation mode in which the client learns theories and their application to problem solving.

third-party payments: Reimbursement made to health care providers by an agency other than the client for the care of the client (e.g., insurance companies, governments, or employers).

third-party reimbursement: Reimbursement given to a third person (e.g., someone in an independent practice) who has provided direct care service to an individual client.

timelines: Landmarks of an episode of health or illness care from initial encounter to the transfer of accountability to the client or another health care agency.

toddler period: Between 1 and 3 years of age.

tolerance: In pharmacology, the need for increasing doses of a drug over time to maintain the same effect.

tort: Legal or civil wrong committed by one person against the person or property of another.

total quality management/improvement: An approach to managing quality that emphasizes continual improvement, employee empowerment, client input, and systems change as key principles.

Town and Country Nursing Service: The later name of the American Red Cross's Rural Nursing Service.

toxic wastes: Poisons, inflammables, infectious contaminants, explosives, and radionuclides.

toxicity: Ability of a substance to cause injury to biologic tissues.

tracer method: A method of evaluating programs based on the premise that health status and care can be evaluated by observing the care and outcomes of specific health problems.

treatment, storage, and disposal facility: A site where hazardous waste is treated, stored, or disposed. TSD facilities are regulated by the EPA and states.

trend: An event that occurs over time and shows a series of fluctuations in its patterns.

triage: Deciding which injured or sick individuals need the most immediate attention and by whom.

triangulation: Use of multiple assessment methods. In relationships, the involvement of a third party or object to avoid communication, closeness, or conflict between two individuals.

trichomoniasis: A common STD transmitted by *Trichomonas vaginalis* that results in infection of the female vulva and vagina and may not cause male symptoms. It is curable through effective treatment.

triggers: Specific activities or objects that, when encountered, may lead to (trigger) a relapse in drug use.

typology: The study or classification of communities by types.

U

United Nations Children's Fund (UNICEF): Formed shortly after WWII to assist children in the war-ravaged countries of Europe, its mission has expanded to assist children throughout the world. Supported by the United Nations.

unit of service: An entity—individual, family, aggregate, organization, or community—to whom nursing care is given; the level at which service is delivered.

urban: Geographic areas described as nonrural and having a higher population density; more than 99 persons per square mile; cities with a population of at least 20,000 but less than 50,000.

urban nonmetropolitan: Urban areas having fewer than 50,000 persons.

urinary incontinence (UI): A condition in which involuntary loss of urine is a social or hygienic problem.

U.S. Department of Health and Human Services (USDHHS): A regulatory agency of the executive branch of government charged with overseeing health and welfare needs of U.S. citizens.

utilitarian theory: Economic theory that holds that the best way to distribute resources among people is to decide how expenditures or the use of resources will bring about the greatest net total of good and serve the largest number of people.

utility: Level of satisfaction from consuming a particular product or service.

utilization management: A continual process of evaluating the appropriateness, necessity, and efficiency of health service over a period of time. Includes data obtained during preadmission certification, service delivery, and postdischarge periods to determine the extent to which the service meets established guidelines (May et al, 1997).

utilization review: Review directed toward ensuring that care is actually needed and cost is appropriate for the level of care provided.

V

vaccine: Immunizing agent.

vague, nonspecific health complaints: The first sign of a student who may be having difficulty in school and may drop out.

validity: The accuracy of a test or measurement; how closely it measures what it claims to measure. In a screening test, validity is assessed in terms of the probability of correctly classifying an individual with regard to the disease or outcome of interest, usually in terms of sensitivity and specificity.

values: (a) Idea of life, customs, and ways of behaving that members of a society regard as desirable. (b) Likelihood that an activity will help meet an objective.

variables: Key characteristics of the problem under study.

variance: Difference between what is expected and what is occurring with the client.

variance analysis: Analyzing variations from the expected goals or standards. It can be applied to analyzing variances from budgeted expenditures or to analyzing situations in which client goals on a critical pathway were not met.

vector: A nonhuman organism, often an insect, that either mechanically or biologically plays a role in the transmission of an infectious agent from source to host.

veracity: A duty to tell the truth and not lie or deceive others.

verification: A communication process used by a nurse advocate to establish accuracy and reality of facts.

vertical integration: The system owns all of the services that clients might need, for example, clinics, hospitals, laboratories, and home health agencies.

vertical transmission: Passing the infection from parent to offspring via sperm, placenta, milk, or contact in the vaginal canal at birth.

violence: Nonaccidental acts, interpersonal or intrapersonal, that result in physical or psychologic injury to one or more of the people involved.

virulence: Ability to produce severe disease.

voluntary agency: An agency that relies on staff and volunteers to provide a wide range of services; must seek operating funds from a variety of sources, including gifts, dues, and fees.

voluntary certification: Process of education, experience, or examination in which a professional elects to engage to be recognized as a specialist.

voluntary credentialing: The choice made by an agency or institution to participate in an accreditation process.

vulnerable population group: A subgroup of the population that is more likely to develop health problems as a result of exposure to risk or to have worse outcomes from these problems than the population as a whole.

W

Wald, Lillian: The first public health nurse in the United States and a social reformer. She founded the Henry Street Settlement in New York, the first established public health agency in 1883.

waste minimization: Efforts to reduce waste.

water discharge: Interruption of exposure pathway through disposal in water by treating the water so that the dosage in the water is not great enough to cause harm or alter the waste product to a less toxic form.

web of causality: The complex interrelations of factors interacting with each other to influence the risk for or distribution of health outcomes.

weight gain: Strong predictor of infant birth weight. It is recommended that women gain between 26 and 35 pounds during pregnancy. If less weight is gained, the risk of a low birth weight baby is greater.

wellness: Dynamic state of health in which individuals progress toward a higher level of functioning, thus maximizing their potential in the environment.

wellness centers: Nursing centers that focus on health promotion and disease prevention and serve as linking agents to community resources.

wellness committee: A health cabinet made up of a nurse and members of the congregation that supports healthy, spiritually fulfilling lives.

wholeness: Condition of a system in which a collection of parts responds as an integrated single part.

wife abuse: See *spouse abuse.*

willingness to pay: A consumer's choice to purchase a particular good or service and not other things.

windshield survey: A community assessment, the motorized equivalent of a physical assessment for an individual; *windshield* refers to looking through the car windshield as the community health nurse drives through the community collecting data.

withdrawal: Physical and psychologic symptoms that occur when a drug upon which a person is dependent is removed.

women's health: A relatively new and growing body of knowledge that documents the distinctive nature of women's well-being.

Women's Health Movement: A grassroots movement that began in the 1960s to address women's health issues.

Women, Infants, and Children (WIC): A special supplemental food program administered by the Department of Agriculture through the State Health Departments. Provides nutritious foods that add to the diets of pregnant and nursing women, infants, and children under 5 years of age. Eligibility is based on income and nutritional risk as determined by a health professional.

work-health interactions: Influence of work on health shown by statistics on illnesses, injuries, and deaths associated with employment.

worker's compensation: Compensation given to an employee for an injury that occurred while working.

Worker's Compensation Act: Law requiring employers to assume financial responsibility for wages lost by employees because of occupational injury or illness.

working conditions: Conditions one faces while engaged in work.

worksite walk-through: An assessment of the workplace conducted by the nurse.

World Bank: Facilitates significant interventions to improve the health status of individuals living in areas that lack economical development.

World Health Organization: An arm of the United Nations that provides worldwide services to promote health.

worthiness: A sense that some people are deserving of help from the community as a whole.

Index

A

AA; *see* Alcoholics Anonymous
AAIN; *see* American Association of Industrial Nursing
AAOHN; *see* American Association of Occupational Health Nurses
AAP; *see* American Academy of Pediatrics
Ability in psychomotor learning, 273-274
ABOHN; *see* American Board for Occupational Health Nurses
Abortion, teen pregnancy and, 686-688, 693
Absenteeism, school nursing and, 912-913
Abstinence for drug addiction, 751
Abuse
  in case management, 395
  child, 643, 764-766
  drug; *see* Drug abuse
  elder, 605, 768-769
  family, 763-769
  physically compromised and, 624
Academic education
  in occupational health and safety, 943
  in quality improvement, 442
Acceptant intervention mode, 887, 888
Access to health care
  barriers to, 647
  in home, 857-858
  research and, 259
  resource allocation and, 109
  in rural environments, 335-336
  systems of, 43-44
Accidents
  in agriculture industry, 622*t*
  in children, 543-545, *544*, 544*t*
  in men, 589*t*, 589-590
Accommodation
  in cognitive development, 537
  in conflict management, 393
  cultural, 146
Accountability, 117
  in community-oriented nursing, 134, *135*
  ethics and, 125-126
  in quality management, 439
Accounting in program management, 432
Accreditation
  for home health practice, 849
  in quality improvement, 442
ACIP; *see* Advisory Committee on Immunization Practices
ACOA; *see* Adult Children of Alcoholics
Acquired immunity, 782
Acquired immunodeficiency syndrome; *see also* Human immunodeficiency virus
  in children, 912, 913
  emergence of, 783-784
  historical and current perspectives of, 780-781
  homelessness and, 677
  international health care and, 71-72
  in men, 590-591
  parasitic opportunistic infections in, 798
  vulnerable populations and, 643-644
  in women, 568-569
Action
  in environmental standards, 161*t*
  of quality assurance/quality improvement program, 452-453
  in research, 258
  social
    advocacy and, 171
    in community practice, 351
Action on Smoking and Health, 752

Active immunity, 541
Active immunization, 782
Activities of daily living
  chronic disease and, 618-619
  in elder health, 598, *598*
Activity theory of aging, 599
Acute illness in children and adolescents, 545
ADA; *see* Americans with Disabilities Act
Adaptive model
  of family health, 508, 509*t*
  of nursing, 884
ADD; *see* Attention deficit disorder
Addiction
  biopsychosocial model of, 743
  denial and, 746
  treatment for, 750-752
ADL; *see* Activities of daily living
Administrative controls, in workplace assessment, 957
Administrator
  advanced practice nurse as, 866
  in public health nursing, 13
Adolescents, 685-686, 687
  chronic illness and, 617-618
  drug use and, 747
  growth and development of, 531-534, 535, 536*t*
  homelessness and, 678
  injuries and accidents in, 544
  mental health problems in, 722-723
  migrants and, 703, 705
  nutrition for, 541
  physically compromised, 616-618
    effects on community and, 621
    effects on family and, 619 620
  poverty and, 672
  pregnancy in; *see* Teen pregnancy
  sexual behavior of
    in Canada, 691
    school nursing and, 912
  trends in, pregnancy and, 686-688
  women's health in, 557-558
Adopters, early, 324
Adopters, late, 324
Adoption, teen pregnancy and, 689, 693
Adult Children of Alcoholics, 753
Adult day health, 606-607
Adult Personal Health Guide, 294
Adulthood
  middle
    male psychosocial development in, 582
    women's health in, 558-559
  older
    homeless, 678
    mental health problems in, 723
    poverty and, 673
    women's health in, *559*, 559-560
  young
    male psychosocial development in, 582, *583*
    women's health in, 557-558
Advance directives
  elder health and, 605-606
  ethics and, 119
  home health care and, 853-855, *854*, *855*
Advanced planning methods and evaluation models, *428*, 428-432, 429*t*, *430*
Advanced practice nurse, 48, 862-876
  arenas for practice of, 868-871
  clinical application for, 874-875
  credentialing of, 864-865
  educational preparation for, 863, 863*t*, 864
  historical perspective of, 863-864

Advanced practice nurse—cont'd
  issues and concerns for, 871-873
  nursing centers and, 367-368
  roles of, 865-868, *866*
  stress for, 873-874
  trends in, 874
Advice in brief interventions, 749
Advisory Committee on Immunization Practices, 541, 542*t*, 543*t*
Advocacy
  case management and, 388-392, 391*t*
  environmental health and, 166, 170-172
  ethics and, 124
  men's health and, 594
  mental health and, 715, 719
  physically compromised and, 628-629
  poor or homeless care and, 680
  public health nurse in, 985
  right to health and, 118
AEAs; *see* Area education agencies
AFDC; *see* Aid to Families with Dependent Children
Affective domain, 273, 273*t*
Affirming in case management, 390-391, 391*t*
African Americans
  chronic conditions in, 618*t*
  food preferences of, 154*t*
  health care needs and nursing skills for, 338*t*
Age
  human immunodeficiency virus and, 810-811
  vulnerability and, 653
Age-specific mortality rate, 236*t*
Ageism, 599
Agency for Health Care Policy and Research, 51, 184
Agency report card, 880
Agent
  in communicable diseases, 781, *781*
  in community health, 323
  in epidemiologic triangle, *231*, 231-232, *233*
  in occupational health nursing, 947, *947*, 948-951, 949*t*
  in physically compromised care, 629
Aggregate, 307
  definition of, 9
  in Neuman Systems Model, 213
  in occupational health nursing, 943-947, *945*
Aggressive behavior of toddler and preschooler, 529-530
Aging
  definition of, 599
  multidimensional influences on, 601*t*, 601-603, *602*
  theories of, 599-601, 600*t*
Agriculture
  Department of, 52, 184
  disability and, 62*t*, 621-622
  health risks and, 338
AHCPR; *see* Agency for Health Care Policy and Research
Aid to Families with Dependent Children, 187, 669
AIDS; *see* Acquired immunodeficiency syndrome
Air, human dependence on, 158
Air pollutants, 162
Airborne pathogens, 948-949
Al-Anon, 753
Alabama Education & Research Center, 944
Alameda County Study, 296
Alaskans, 338*t*
Alateen, 753

Alcohol, tobacco, and other drug problems, 732-756
  attitudes and myths of, 733-735
  clinical application for, 753-754
  definitions in, 735-736
  disorders from, 592
  historical overview of, 733, *734*
  paradigm shift in, 735
  predisposing/contributing factors in, 742-743
  prevention of
    primary, 743-745
    secondary, 745-749
    tertiary, 749-753
  psychoactive drugs in, 736*t*, 736-742; *see also* Psychoactive drugs
  in school-age children, 911-912, *912*
  vulnerability and, 642-643
  withdrawal in, 750
Alcohol Misuse Prevention Project, 931*t*
Alcoholics Anonymous, 753
Alcoholism, 736
  Healthy People 2000 and, 433*t*
Alderfer's theory of management, 881*t*, 882
Alliances, 879
Allocation
  nurse advocate and, 392
  resource, 108-110
Alma Ata
  Declaration of, 46
  research and, 254
Alternative healing, 151*t*
Ambivalence in victim blaming, 651
Ambulatory clinics, 869-870
Ambulatory Payment Classes, 105
American Academy of Pediatrics
  guidelines for childhood immunization, 541, 542*t*, 543*t*
American Association of Industrial Nursing, 943
American Association of Occupational Health Nurses, 942, 943
American Board for Occupational Health Nurses, 943
American Cancer Society, 752
American Heart Association, 752
American Lung Association, 752
American Nurses Association, 35
  code of ethics of, 121
  health care delivery and, 111
  primary prevention and, 110, 111
  quality management and, 441
  Steering Committee on Data Bases of, 214, 214*t*
American Nurses Credentialing Center, 864
American Public Health Association, 28
  public health nursing definition of, 205, 979
  quality management guidelines of, 444
American Red Cross, 26
  disaster management and, 403
Americans for Nonsmokers Rights, 752
Americans with Disabilities Act
  men's health and, 581-582
  mental health and, 717*t*, 718-719
  physically compromised and, 624, 629-631
Amphetamines, 740
Amplification in case management, 390
Amyl nitrite inhalation, 742
ANA; *see* American Nurses Association
Analytic economic tools, 84-85
Analytic epidemiology, 241-245, 242*t*, *243*, *244*
  definition of, 227
Analytical stage in research, 257-258

I-1

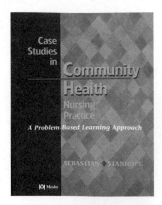

Sebastian & Stanhope
CASE STUDIES IN COMMUNITY HEALTH NURSING: A Problem-Based Learning Approach

This unique text and workbook teaches nursing students to think critically and apply nursing knowledge to solving problems. A case-study approach helps them ask the right questions, gather supporting data, sort through options, and identify optimal solutions.

1999. 224 pp. Soft cover. **#0-323-00260-9.**

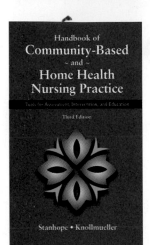

Stanhope & Knollmueller
HANDBOOK OF COMMUNITY-BASED AND HOME HEALTH NURSING PRACTICE: Tools for Assessment, Intervention, and Education, Third Edition

This portable resource offers users quick access to all the information they need to provide care in a community-based setting.
Features. . .
- 295 tool and reference documents
- Many lists, tables, charts, and forms
- Clinical decision-making guides
- Teaching and assessment tools

Oct. 1999. Over 635 pp. Illustrated. **#0-323-00875-5**

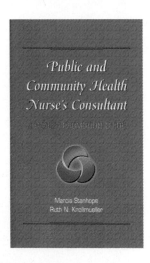

Stanhope & Knollmueller
PUBLIC AND COMMUNITY HEALTH NURSE'S CONSULTANT: A Health Promotion Guide

This comprehensive reference delivers the information that public and community health nurses need when teaching and discussing disease prevention, promoting healthy lifestyles, managing cases, and coordinating care. Comprised primarily of tables, charts, forms, and lists, this book includes a wide range of assessment tools, risk indicators, and client teaching tips.

1997. 800 pp. 90 illustrations. **#0-8151-9003-4**

To purchase or for more information regarding these resources please visit your local health sciences or campus bookstore, call customer service at **1-800-545-2522,** or visit our website at **www.mosby.com**.